GYNECOLOGIC, OBSTETRIC, AND RELATED SURGERY

Visit our website at **www.mosby.com**

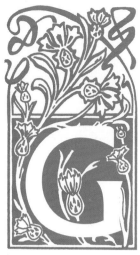

Gynecologic, Obstetric, and Related Surgery

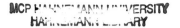

Edited by

DAVID H. NICHOLS, M.D.

Professor of Obstetrics and Gynecology
Brown University School of Medicine;
Senior Consultant in Reconstructive Pelvic Surgery
Women and Infants Hospital
Providence, Rhode Island

DANIEL L. CLARKE-PEARSON, M.D.

J. M. Ingram Professor of Gynecologic Oncology
Director, Division of Gynecologic Oncology
Duke University Medical Center
Durham, North Carolina

SECOND EDITION

with **966** illustrations including **15** Color Plates

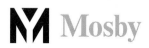

St. Louis Baltimore Boston Carlsbad Chicago Minneapolis New York Philadelphia Portland
London Milan Sydney Tokyo Toronto

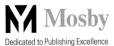

Senior Developmental Editor: Anne Gunter
Project Manager: Patricia Tannian
Production Editor: John Casey
Design Manager: Gail Morey Hudson
Cover Designer: Teresa Breckwoldt

SECOND EDITION

Mosby, Inc.
A Harcourt Health Sciences Company
11830 Westline Industrial Drive
St. Louis, Missouri 63146

Printed in the United States of America
Composition by The Clarinda Co.
Lithography/color film by Coral Graphics
Printing/binding by Maple-Vail Book Mfg Group

Library of Congress Cataloging in Publication Data

Gynecologic, obstetric, and related surgery / edited by David H. Nichols, Daniel L.
    Clarke-Pearson. — 2nd ed.
        p.   cm.
    Rev. ed. of: Gynecologic and obstetric surgery / edited by David H. Nichols.
c1993.
    Includes bibliographical references and index.
    ISBN 0-8151-3670-6
    1. Generative organs, Female—Surgery.   2. Obstetrics—surgery.
I. Gynecologic and obstetric surgery.
    [DNLM: 1. Genital Diseases, Female—surgery.   2. Breast—surgery.
3. Delivery.   4. Genitalia, Female—surgery.   5. Pregnancy Complications—
surgery.   6. Urinary Tract—surgery.   WP 660 G9965 1999]
RG104.G93   1999
618′.0459—dc21
DNLM/DLC
for Library of Congress   99-27194
                                                                                CIP

99 00 01 02 03 / 9 8 7 6 5 4 3 2 1

Contributors

RONY A. ADAM, M.D.
Assistant Professor, Department of Gynecology and Obstetrics
Emory University School of Medicine
Atlanta, Georgia

LEILA V. ADAMYAN, M.D.
Professor and Chief, Department of Operative Gynecology
Scientific Center for Obstetrics, Gynecology,
and Perinatology
Moscow, Russia

MICHAEL S. BAGGISH, M.D.
Professor, Department of Obstetrics and Gynecology
University of Cincinnati School of Medicine;
Chairman
Department of Obstetrics and Gynecology
Good Samaritan Hospital
Cincinnati, Ohio

DAVID L. BARCLAY, M.D.
Professor, Department of Obstetrics and Gynecology
University of Arkansas for Medical Sciences
Little Rock, Arkansas

IVOR BENJAMIN, M.D.
Assistant Professor, Department of Obstetrics and Gynecology
Division of Gynecologic Oncology;
Co-Editor-in-Chief, Oncolink
Associate Director for Clinical Information Systems
University of Pennsylvania Medical Center
Philadelphia, Pennsylvania

DOUGLAS BROWN, Ph.D.
Chief Education and Development Officer
Dayspring Family Health Center
Jellico, Tennessee

MARSHALL W. CARPENTER, M.D.
Director, Division of Maternal-Fetal Medicine
Women and Infants Hospital
Providence, Rhode Island

CHRISTOPHER R. CHAPPLE, M.D.
England

JOEL M. CHILDERS, M.D.
Gynecologic and Laparoscopic Surgery
Arizona Oncology Associates
Tucson, Arizona

DONALD R. COUSTAN, M.D.
Obstetrician and Gynecologist-in-Chief
Department of Obstetrics and Gynecology
Women and Infants Hospital
Providence, Rhode Island

DANIEL F. G. DARGENT, M.D.
Professeur, Gynecologue Accoucheur des Hopitaux
Chef de Service a l'Hopital E. Herriot
Universite Claude Bernard
Lyon, France

RAPHAEL DURGEE, M.D.
Retired Professor of Reproductive Medicine
University of California School of Medicine
San Diego, California

H. ALEXANDER EASLEY III, J.D., M.D.
Clinical Faculty, Department of Obstetrics and Gynecology
East Carolina University School of Medicine
Greenville, North Carolina

†THOMAS E. ELKINS, M.D.
Professor and Chief of Gynecology
Director of Reconstructive Pelvic Surgery
Johns Hopkins School of Medicine
Baltimore, Maryland

SEBASTIAN FARO, M.D., Ph.D.
John M. Simpson Professor and Chairman
Director, Section of Infectious Diseases
Department of Obstetrics and Gynecology
Rush-Presbyterian-St. Luke's Medical Center
Chicago, Illinois

AUGUSTO G. FERRARI, M.D.
Professor
Milano, Italy

---

†Deceased.

v

DONALD G. GALLUP, M.D.
Clinical Professor, Department of Obstetrics and Gynecology
Medical College of Georgia, Augusta, Georgia;
Professor, Department of Obstetrics and Gynecology
Mercer University School of Medicine, Macon, Georgia;
Associate Director, Department of Gynecologic Oncology
Memorial Medical Center
Savannah, Georgia

CELSO-RAMON GARCIA, M.D.
The William Shippen, Jr., Emeritus Professor of Obstetrics and
    Gynecology
University of Pennsylvania Medical Center
Philadelphia, Pennsylvania

E. CATHERINE HAMLIN, M.D.
Medical Director
Addis Ababa Fistula Hospital
Addis Ababa, Ethiopia

CHARLES B. HAMMOND, M.D.
E.C. Hamblen Professor and Chairman
Department of Obstetrics and Gynecology
Duke University Medical Center
Durham, North Carolina

JAROSLAV F. HULKA, M.D.
Professor Emeritus
University of North Carolina
Chapel Hill, North Carolina

ROBERT B. HUNT, M.D.
Clinical Instructor, Obstetrics and Gynecology
Harvard Medical School
Beth Israel Hospital
Boston, Massachusetts

W. GLENN HURT, M.D.
Professor, Department of Obstetrics and Gynecology
Medical College of Virginia
Virginia Commonwealth University
Richmond, Virginia

NEIL D. JACKSON, M.D.
Clinical Professor of Obstetrics and Gynecology
Brown University School of Medicine;
Director of Urogynecology and Reconstructive Pelvic Surgery
Women and Infants Hospital
Providence, Rhode Island

RAYMOND A. LEE, M.D.
Professor, Department of Obstetrics and Gynecology;
Consultant, Departments of Obstetrics and Gynecology and
    Surgery
Mayo Clinic and Mayo Foundation
Rochester, Minnesota

CHARLES M. MARCH, M.D.
Professor, Department of Obstetrics and Gynecology
University of Southern California School of Medicine
Los Angeles, California

DOUGLAS J. MARCHANT, M.D.
Emeritus Director, Breast Health Center
Departments of Obstetrics and Gynecology and Women's
    Oncology
Women and Infants Hospital
Providence, Rhode Island

DAN C. MARTIN, M.D.
Clinical Associate Professor
Department of Obstetrics and Gynecology
University of Tennessee College of Medicine
Memphis, Tennessee

KUNIO MIYAZAWA, M.D.
Colonel (Ret.) Medical Corps, US Army
Professor, Department of Obstetrics and Gynecology
Uniformed Services University of the Health Sciences
Kaneohe, Hawaii;
Professor, Department of Obstetrics and Gynecology
Tripler Army Medical Center
Honolulu, Hawaii

FREDERICK J. MONTZ, M.D.
Professor and Director of Gynecologic Oncology
Department of Obstetrics and Gynecology
Johns Hopkins School of Medicine
Baltimore, Maryland

GEORGE W. MORLEY, M.D.
Department of Obstetrics and Gynecology
University of Michigan Medical School
Ann Arbor, Michigan

BETH E. NELSON, M.D.
Professor and Director of Gynecologic Oncology
Department of Obstetrics and Gynecology
University of Massachusetts Medical Center
Worcester, Massachusetts

JOHN PATRICK O'GRADY, M.D.
Professor, Department of Obstetrics and Gynecology
Tufts University School of Medicine
Boston, Massachusetts;
Director, Obstetrical Services
Baystate Medical Center
Springfield, Massachusetts

JOHN R. OLIVER, M.D.
Pasadena, California

RICHARD H. PAUL, M.D.

SAMANTHA M. PFEIFER, M.D.
Assistant Professor, Department of Obstetrics and Gynecology
University of Pennsylvania Medical Center
Philadelphia, Pennsylvania

GUNTHER REIFFENSTUHL, M.D.
Professor, Department of Obstetrics and Gynecology
Baden, Austria

R. KEVIN REYNOLDS, M.D.
Chief, Division of Gynecologic Oncology
University of Michigan Medical School
Ann Arbor, Michigan

JOHN A. ROCK, M.D.
James Robert McCord Professor and Chairman
Department of Gynecology and Obstetrics
Emory University School of Medicine
Atlanta, Georgia

STEPHEN C. RUBIN, M.D.
Professor and Director
Department of Obstetrics and Gynecology
Chief, Division of Gynecologic Oncology
University of Pennsylvania Medical Center
Philadelphia, Pennsylvania

DEVEREUX N. SALLER, JR., M.D.
Associate Professor of Obstetrics and Gynecology
Division of Maternal-Fetal Medicine
Associate Professor, Division of Pediatric Genetics
University of Rochester Medical Center
Rochester, New York

PETER E. SCHWARTZ, M.D.
The John Slade Ely Professor of Obstetrics and Gynecology
Vice Chairman and Director, Gynecologic Oncology
Yale University School of Medicine
New Haven, Connecticut

EILEEN M. SEGRETI, M.D.
Assistant Professor, Department of Obstetrics and Gynecology
Medical College of Virginia
Virginia Commonwealth University
Richmond, Virginia

SUMNER A. SLAVIN, M.D.
Assistant Clinical Professor
Harvard Medical School;
Associate in Plastic and Reconstructive Surgery
Beth Israel Hospital
Boston, Massachusetts

JOHN T. SOPER
Professor, Department of Obstetrics and Gynecology
Division of Gynecologic Oncology
Duke University Medical Center
Durham, North Carolina

JOHN F. STEEGE, M.D.
Professor and Chief, Department of Obstetrics and Gynecology
Division of Gynecology
University of North Carolina School of Medicine
Chapel Hill, North Carolina

THOMAS G. STOVALL, M.D.
Professor, Department of Obstetrics and Gynecology
University of Tennessee College of Medicine
Memphis, Tennessee

PHILLIP G. STUBBLEFIELD, M.D.
Chairman, Department of Obstetrics and Gynecology
Boston University Medical Center
Boston, Massachusetts

ROBERT L. SUMMITT, Jr., M.D.
Associate Professor and Chief
Department of Obstetrics and Gynecology
Section of Urogynecology
University of Tennessee College of Medicine
Memphis, Tennessee

RICHARD TURNER-WARWICK, M.D.
England

DIONYSIOS K. VERONIKIS, M.D.
Chief of Gynecology
Director, Reconstructive Pelvic Surgery and Urogynecology
St. John's Mercy Medical Center
St. Louis, Missouri

PAUL J. WENDEL, M.D.
Assistant Professor, Department of Obstetrics and Gynecology
Division of Maternal-Fetal Medicine
University of Arkansas for Medical Sciences
Little Rock, Arkansas

ROBERT F. ZACHARIN, M.D.
Consultant Gynecologist
Alfred Hospital
Melbourne, Australia

Dedicated to
my beloved husband—
that whoever reads this book will have a better
understanding of the author and his devotion to his vocation.

What a wondrous man is he; yes *"is,"* because to know him (and as proven
through the words of this book) one cannot think of him any other way than in the
present and as a true visionary.

Many have asked what motivated him to do so much during his lifetime. David
was a prolific reader. His personal medical library was his pride and joy. He
eagerly devoured the latest in scientific research and development and equally had
a passion for searching as far back into medical history as he could reach, all
while embracing as many cultures and languages as possible. He was gifted with
an extraordinary ability to retain what he read and learned, enabling him to use
this knowledge in developing creative ways to move forward. More important,
David was a deeply spiritual man, and I believe that, along with his thirst for
knowledge, his desire to give and to share was his motivation.

This book is but one example of his extraordinary inner drive to share his discoveries and offer his visions to all those willing to absorb them. Most of all he gave
generously of himself every day and in every way of his life. David was never
outwardly too weary, too sick, too tired, or too frustrated or angry to let it slow
him down. He was infinitely patient with his family, friends, colleagues, and patients. Because he was strong, confident in his knowledge and skills, and coura-
geous, he did not hesitate to correct but never as to offend anyone. It would seem
that he was not only gifted as a physician, writer, and teacher, but perfect as a
human being and most certainly as a husband and father. "Together," as he said to
me many, many times, "we can do anything." Together fifty precious and glorious
years, more than half our ages, facing many challenges but also blessed with many
opportunities we *did* do the "anythings" together and then some. For that I am
most grateful.

David continues to live in the hearts of all of us who love him so deeply. His
work lives on in the patients that were healed through him, the doctors he has
trained, the surgical techniques and helpful instruments he has developed, and the
vision contained in this and all his books.

I pray now that the readers of this book will embrace the wealth of knowledge
presented here. With confidence and creativity, think "beyond," as he did. Find
guidance in his words and in the words of so many who generously contributed
here so that David's lifelong mission *to improve the quality of life for women everywhere* will continue. I am sure *"together"* he will help you, his readers, to
succeed in what might seem to be impossible—as he did.

Lorraine L. Nichols

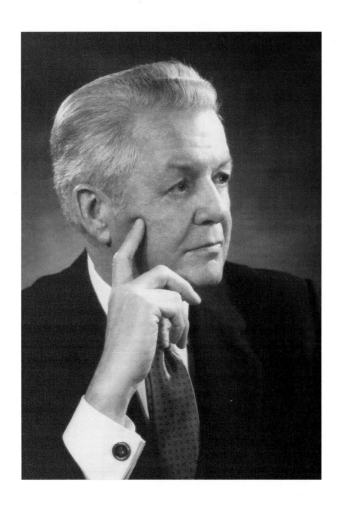

David H. Nichols

1925-1998

Preface

The second edition of *Gynecologic, Obstetric, and Related Surgery* is conceived to address issues relevant to the practicing pelvic surgeon—the traditions of surgical teaching held dearest by David H. Nichols, MD. Dr. Nichols was first and foremost concerned with the expert care of women with surgical problems. He was one of the preeminent surgeons of his generation, and we are indebted to him for his excellence as a teacher. For as many patients as he could help personally, he knew that the message and skills of pelvic surgery must be disseminated to thousands of surgeons worldwide. Those who came to his operating room, who heard his lectures, or who read his books carry on his mission.

It is not our intent to produce a text that reviews the world's literature on a topic, as we feel that it is more important to clearly communicate the skills that we have found effective in our years of collective surgical experience. Our goal therefore is to convey a clear description of our personal surgical philosophy and techniques, which we hope will enhance the expertise of gynecologists, obstetricians, and others who perform pelvic surgery.

Since the first edition of this text, gynecologic surgery has undergone many changes, and even more changes have occurred in how we provide health care. The true effect of managed care, reduced reimbursement for surgery, and the additional administrative paperwork is yet to be fully appreciated by surgeons or the women whom we serve. The diminishing satisfaction of many physicians has been discussed broadly and is reflected in the decreasing numbers of those who will provide obstetric care or who are retiring from practice earlier than they had anticipated. Yet I feel that the pelvic surgeon derives great satisfaction in surgical procedures performed with excellence of technique and outcome. The ultimate reward of the pelvic surgeon is the woman who has been relieved of her symptoms and restored to normal function.

This second edition updates the current practice of gynecologic and obstetric surgery. Many of the chapter topics are the same, yet each has been refined and is based on the author's current experience. I believe that evidence-based medicine is an important part of our continued evaluation of how we practice surgery. Although it would be ideal to base decisions on the outcomes of well-designed clinical trials (and many randomized trials in surgery are under way), we must acknowledge that we will never be able to evaluate all surgical procedures on the basis of a randomized trial. Dr. Nichols continually assessed his surgical techniques and outcomes. For example, those familiar with Dr. Nichols' teachings regarding sacrospinous ligament fixation for the correction of vaginal vault prolapse will recognize that he has continued to update the technique, ever refining it to achieve safer, more effective results. It is therefore our challenge to honestly evaluate our experiences and refine our techniques on the basis of careful, thoughtful analysis of our own work. Surgeons who does not reflect on their personal series and critically review their results is likely to miss the opportunity to improve the surgical outcome of their patients.

In recent years laparoscopic surgery has gained center stage in gynecologic surgery. Many procedures that were previously performed through abdominal incisions may now be performed through the laparoscope. Of the many laparoscopic procedures described in the past decade, we have added to this text those that we believe are true contributions to our specialty and are being performed commonly in our surgical community. Where a surgical procedure is truly advanced we wish to broadly disseminate the technique to other surgeons. Outcomes research will aid in our evaluation of these newer techniques. This must evaluate not only the surgical outcome, but also the economic outcome. For example, what is the additional cost of the laparoscopic procedure given the additional operating room time? Given the cost of the disposable instruments? Given the shorter hospitalization? Given the faster return to normal function and to the workplace? Randomized trials of laparoscopically assisted vaginal hysterectomy offer us an opportunity to critically evaluate this particular technique. Ongoing randomized trials of laparoscopic staging of ovarian cancer and endometrial cancer, being conducted by the Gynecologic Oncology Group, will assist in our understanding of the role of laparoscopy in surgery for gynecologic cancers.

In the second edition of *Gynecologic, Obstetric, and Related Surgery* we have continued to present the breadth of gynecologic and obstetric surgery and have included related operations such as breast and intestinal surgery, which are often relevant to our patients' care. The authors have been selected because they are active surgeons who have a wealth of experience in the procedures they describe. They are also excellent teachers who effectively communicate the nuances of surgery to the reader.

This text is intended to be a resource for residents in training, board-certified obstetricians and gynecologists, and other pelvic surgeons. For the resident, we hope it will explain all of the procedures he or she would need to master. For the practicing surgeon, we hope it may serve as a refresher before performing a case, as well as an update of new procedures that have been added to our surgical armamentarium since completing formal training.

We are aware of the rare surgeon who will perform all the procedures described in this text. As obstetrics and gynecology has become subspecialized, many obstetricians and gynecologists have restricted their surgical practice to the more commonly performed procedures and refer their patients to a subspecialist for treatment of more complex surgical problems. We view this trend as entirely reasonable, and we should continue to draw on the expertise of the subspecialist to deliver the highest quality of care to women with an unusual problem. However, we must guard against the potential of gynecologic and obstetric surgery being restricted to a point at which a generalist can no longer capably and safely perform surgery if the case becomes complex or difficult. We hope therefore that by presenting the details of many surgical techniques to a broad audience of surgeons many will continue to hone their surgical skills. In addition, by presenting subspecialty procedures it is our intent that the general obstetrician and gynecologist may better understand the concepts, techniques, and instruments used in performing subspecialty procedures and that these skills and techniques might be incorporated into his or her general practice. This cross-pollination in our specialty is vitally important.

The contributors to this text have done a wonderful job of presenting their chosen topic clearly and completely. The opportunity to publish a text that is up to date yet broadly comprehensive is a tribute to each author.

Despite modern concepts, improved techniques, subspecialization, and new equipment, we must continually uphold the principles that are the basis of gynecologic and obstetric surgery. Those basic principles, such as the proper selection of the operation for the individual patient, careful anatomic dissection, delicate tissue handling, and attention to the details of preoperative and postoperative care, are reiterated in this edition.

I would like to acknowledge the support and unfailing assistance of Mosby editor Anne Gunter. Her gentle prodding has expedited the completion of this work. Lori Vaskalis has done a fantastic job in rendering many new illustrations for this edition. Pelvic anatomy and surgical techniques are superbly demonstrated through her pen and greatly enhance the entire text.

Finally, I am indebted to David H. Nichols, MD, for the privilege, confidence, and trust of asking me to assist him in editing this text. It is a true honor to have collaborated with such a renowned surgeon, caring physician, gentleman, and teacher.

Daniel L. Clarke-Pearson, M.D.

Contents

1 History of Gynecologic Surgery

RAPHAEL DURFEE

Gynecologic surgery, as well as other surgery, could not have evolved without the development of hemostasis, surgical anesthesia, and asepsis plus antisepsis. These, in turn, would not have been possible without advances in (1) instruments, sutures, ligatures, and bandaging, (2) wound treatment, (3) the art of examination, (4) knowledge of human anatomy, (5) use of drugs, (6) awareness of physiologic principles, and (7) ability to transmit this knowledge through formal instruction. Operations on the human female pelvis involve a highly vascular area, which can lead to extensive blood loss, and an area exquisitely sensitive to pain and especially vulnerable to infection. These factors had to be addressed to allow the successful development of gynecologic surgery.

This chapter explores the origins of current gynecologic surgical procedures. A list of suggested readings is included as a resource for readers who want additional information.

SURGICAL MILESTONES

Initial medical care was heavily influenced by magic, astrology, religion, mythology, and the supernatural. These elements were separated from medicine only after many centuries. Yet the earliest accounts of manipulation of the human body, the most complicated of which we know as surgery, began with and have always included procedures associated with complicated childbirth.

Surgery in the ancient world was characterized by practical responses to the situations found by observation of the patient. Although some medical knowledge was noted in early documents (Fig. 1-1), such as the *Sushruta,* most was transmitted by word of mouth or by tradition.

Seventeenth Century

Improvements in surgery, specifically gynecologic surgery, were stimulated by the Renaissance. The first major developments in procedures and instruments occurred in the seventeenth century. For example, Trautmann, in 1600, performed the first successful cesarean operation, without anesthesia or asepsis. De Castro used a silk or horsehair suture dipped in aqua sublimati to ligate a hypertrophied clitoris; in addition, he excised a prolapsed uterus by daily application of increased tension on a ligature.

Van Roonhuyze, the outstanding gynecologic surgeon of the seventeenth century, wrote the first text on gynecologic surgery, performed cesarean sections, described vaginal atresia and obstruction, reported a case of ruptured uterus, repaired vesicovaginal fistulae, extirpated totally prolapsed uteri, opened an obstructed urethra, and performed plastic surgery on a deformed urethra. He revived the method of wound drainage that was used by Greek surgeons and is considered by some to be the father of surgical gynecology.

Eighteenth Century

Although advances in gynecologic surgical practice in this period were not extensive, some of the following developments are notable:

1. Excision of ovarian cysts found in extensive hernias was proposed.
2. Increased numbers of perineal lacerations were repaired successfully.
3. Abdominal tumefactions that contained abdominal pregnancies were opened and the contents were removed.
4. Intrapelvic abscesses were incised and drained, primarily through the vagina.

Advances were also made in instrumentation.

The identification of specific gynecologic abnormalities was the foremost contribution of the eighteenth century. All kinds of uterine abnormalities, from congenital to positional to prolapses to cancer and benign tumors, were described. Vaginal relaxations, without any terms attached, were considered; variations of ectopic pregnancy were recognized and categorized. Urinary incontinence was differentially diagnosed, which revealed causes other than vesicovaginal fistula.

Nineteenth Century

The 1800s ushered in the explosive growth in the practice of gynecologic surgery. Although advances were not as profound as those made in the twentieth century, much of the basis for modern gynecologic surgery was established at this time. Surgical methods evolved with some carryover from the 1700s, which included solutions to the three obstructions to operative therapy: hemostasis, pain relief, and antisepsis and asepsis.

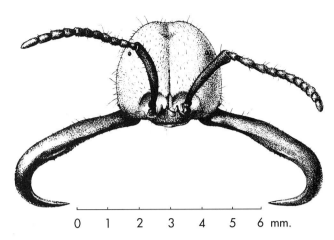

Fig. 1-1 The ant—the first surgical wound clip. (From The *Sushruta*, in Topoff HR: The social behaviour of army ants, *Scientific American*, Nov, 1972, Scientific American, New York.)

Before the nineteenth century, gynecologic surgery was limited to the external genitalia, cervix and vagina, perineal lacerations, vesicovaginal fistula, ovariotomy (occasionally), hysterectomy (although extremely hazardous), laparotomy (rarely), and incision and drainage of pelvic abscess. These were often beyond the ability of many surgeons, and failures were numerous.

The etiology of uterine infection, malposition, and vaginal discharges attracted great interest in the early 1800s. The first text of the era was devoted entirely to gynecologic surgery; it was fairly complete and well illustrated. The terms *anteflexion* and *retroflexion* were proposed.

In the nineteenth century, hemostasis was addressed, and many clamps and methods were devised for individual vessel ligation. Yet it remained for twentieth century surgeons to perfect instruments and procedures for their use.

Twentieth Century

The first 40 to 50 years of the 1900s were dedicated to the surgical treatment of many gynecologic problems and disease. Laparotomy had become just barely reasonable, as had both vaginal and abdominal hysterectomy.

Knowledge of fallopian tube disease, endometriosis, and pelvic pain led to specific operations to treat some of the more common of these. The invention of Bovie cautery in 1928 led to its use in the treatment of endometriosis and pelvic inflammatory disease. Improvements in surgical techniques were universal, with new instruments, improved sutures, self-retaining retractors, better surgeon's gloves, the use of sterile caps, and improved masks with sterile gowns and shoe covers and scrub clothes; all occurred in the early 1900s and greatly decreased wound infection rates.

The establishment of residency programs and a well-developed examination in obstetrics and gynecology improved the capability of the surgeon immensely and created a true specialty. Bolstered by the American Board in the 1930s, gynecology was divorced from general surgery. By

1945, at least 75 to 100 procedures were generally used to treat female pelvic organs.

The antibiotic era enlarged the scope of gynecologic surgery. The availability of blood from established blood banks further increased the amount and kind of gynecologic surgery that was attempted. Methods for sterilization were developed, and in the 1950s a simple, safe, and effective procedure for removal of uterine contents through suction was introduced in England.

Development of many new diagnostic instruments and techniques greatly expanded the possibilities of surgical treatment. Laparoscopy, which followed culdoscopy in the middle 1900s, permitted a wide variety of operations in the pelvis, from new methods of tubal ligation to lysis of adhesions, treatment of pelvic inflammatory disease and endometriosis, excision of benign disease of the ovary, and several other procedures, even myomectomy. Posterior colpotomy and culdoscopy allowed the introduction of simple invasive pelvic operations. All of these were greatly enhanced, if not replaced, by laparoscopically guided surgery. A final contribution was the innovation of laser surgery, which, combined with laparoscopy and hysteroscopy, has revolutionized much of gynecologic surgery.

Microsurgery was introduced into gynecology in the mid-1970s and has developed into a major area of expertise in gynecologic surgery. Residual tubal disease, pelvic adhesions, ectopic pregnancy, endometriosis, and many other pelvic problems are managed by combinations of the new methods.

Microsurgery is used extensively in reanastomosis of the fallopian tube either after partial excision for sterilization or after resection for correction of the tubal tissue associated with ectopic pregnancy. Microsurgical repair of the tube during the removal of an early ectopic pregnancy has been reported. Techniques for fimbriaplasty have been improved in the past 5 years, resulting in improved pregnancy rates. Microsurgery in combination with the laser for lysis of adhesions has proven to be a superior method for the correction of this vexing problem. The operating microscope facilitates more complete removal of endometriotic implants by improving the visual field. It also facilitates closure of the uterine serosa after surgery of the uterine fundus following myoma excision, after the removal of a cornual pregnancy, or after uterine unification operations.

Microsurgical techniques yield improved ovarian suspension after ovarian cyst excision or after the now-rare wedge resection. One of the more interesting uses of the microscope is the direct insertion of viable sperm into a fertilizable ovum. Microsurgical insertion of a fertilizable ovum with or without sperm into the fimbria of the fallopian tube allows for optimal placement of such small tissues. The microscope also is helpful in uterotubal implantation in cases of cornual blockage. Other methods of surgery in the female pelvis seem crude and bulky in comparison to microsurgery.

From 1992 to the present, many changes have occurred in the application of diagnostic and surgical procedures in the management of gynecologic and obstetric diseases and abnormalities. Previous principles and techniques in these areas have been abandoned or almost completely altered. Diagnosis has proceeded from educated guesswork to more exact establishment of objective findings. The full range of gynecologic disease and obstetric complications has been dramatically influenced by the addition and substitution of electronic, optical, and ultrasonographic manipulation.

Basic examinations such as pelvic, rectovaginal, or breast palpation have been practically replaced except when making a preliminary diagnosis in a triage or emergency situation or when conducting a primary general screening during an initial visit or consultation.

Direct, hands-on intrapelvic abdominal surgery involving a large abdominal access incision has been replaced by surgery involving one or more considerably smaller incisions. Access is made with an operating or diagnostic laparoscope combined with specialized devices for organ incision and excision, small biopsy, hemostasis, organ suspension (e.g., suprapubic suspension of the bladder neck without peritoneal invasion) and other suspension operations, tissue removal, and suture placement. Intraabdominal laser surgery for lysis of adhesions and obliteration of diseases such as endometriosis is now common. These procedures are enhanced by laparoscopes fitted with mini-cameras, or in some cases by ultrasound, for viewing images on a color monitor. The hand-eye coordination necessary for direct vision and instrument contact with remote observation on a color monitor involves a difficult integration of skills. Considerable learning time is necessary, as is a great deal of combined manual and mental practice.

The value of a direct, manual, tactile sense is lost, but a different "feel" is established involving visualization of the operative area, which is assisted by the enlargement of images on a color monitor. Ancillary assistance provided by medical observers in the operating suite can be helpful, since several individuals can see the screen and offer suggestions as requested by the operator.

This integrated approach is not for everyone, and for some it is impossible. In general, contemporary gynecologic surgery offers several advantages and causes few complications. Multiple, small (1 to 1.5 cm) incisions are easily closed, heal readily with minimal discomfort as compared with the usual surgical abdominal wounds, and minimize postoperative hospital stay. Even more important is the avoidance of the bowel. It is not necessary to remove the bowel from the pelvic area, since newer instruments distend the abdominal wall and provide unimpeded operative space in the pelvis with full exposure of the pelvic organs. The former practice of "packing the bowel away" frequently led to potentially serious postoperative problems, ranging from ileus to adhesion formation; modern procedures avoid these difficulties.

Laparoscopy and ultrasound have opened up a wide and entirely new vista in both diagnosis and treatment that will not only enhance the future of gynecology, but also ensure less discomfort for the patient, with long-term cure, reduced cost, and shorter hospitalization.

Progress has been made in the treatment of gynecologic cancer by surgical methods, but not at the same pace as other gynecologic surgery, primarily because of the characteristics of the disease. This is especially true in ovarian malignancy.

SPECIFIC AREAS
Diagnosis

Hysterosalpingography. The 1895 discovery of x-rays was quickly followed by discovery of many of their uses. For example, liquid bismuth was injected through the cervical canal to explore possible ectopic pregnancy, and collargol injection was used to diagnose uterine tumors, as well as examine tubal patency. A delayed film was used to verify tubal patency, and this technique combined with peritoneography came to be termed *hysterosalpingography* (HSG). Water-soluble Hypaque is used for hysterosalpingography, but a modified Lipiodol still has value in diagnosing and treating tubal obstruction. The technique has been improved with better cannulas, water-soluble injection media, local anesthesia for the cervix, relaxation premedication, possible use of antiprostaglandins, use of the fluoroscopic monitor together with a magnifier, cinematography, spot and delayed films, and image intensification. When combined with ultrasound, the potential for this medium increases.

Cystoscopy. In 1805, Bozzini tried to visualize the interior of the urethra with a double catheter and candlelight; he was reprimanded by the Medical Society of Vienna, but this proved to be the origin of endoscopy. With improvements, the method was used to identify polyps in the uterine cavity in 1869. Nitze put a light and an endoscope together and made the first truly functional cystoscope that could be used for endoscopy in parts of the body other than the bladder. With the invention of the air cystoscope, gynecologic urology was born.

The Brown-Buerger water cystoscope has been the workhorse for the urologist and gynecologist. The use of CO_2 and placement of the patient in a lithotomy rather than the awkward knee-chest position were added in the 1970s. The visualization of the bladder through the clear, weightless medium was superb, but of even greater importance was the observation of the urethrovesical junction and the action of the bladder neck with passage of urine in normal and abnormal states. Voiding cystograms illustrated the passage of urine with absolute clarity. As a result, various forms of urinary incontinence can be identified and classified, even if the cause remains unknown, as does the act of the release of urine and the maintenence of continence.

In the past 8 years several reports have advocated the value of intraoperative cystoscopy in reconstructive pelvic surgery, including urogynecologic procedures. This was summarized by Harris et al. in 1997. In general, few urinary tract injuries have been discovered by intraoperative cystoscopy, and almost all have been corrected at the time of injury. Several of these were ureteral traumas, and a few indicated the presence of suture material through the bladder wall. It is clear that this simple, noncomplicated addition to the usual techniques for pelvic repair is extremely valuable not only for detecting unwanted trauma but also for guiding proper anatomic replacement in operations for stress incontinence and vaginal resuspension. The ability to maneuver catheters and even microcameras into the ureters for diagnosis and dilation and other treatment requires detailed knowledge of various cystoscopes and their uses. Intraoperative cystoscopy also can be used to facilitate the position of the bladder, vesical neck, and even the urethra by virtue of lighted organ. This especially is true if the anatomy of the area is occluded by scar tissue or disease; more accurate dissection or suture placement is permitted, and traumatic damage to the urinary tract is avoided. In some cases of radical pelvic dissections, a light in the ureter permits accurate anatomic placement and avoids unnecessary injury.

Hysteroscopy. From its first use in 1880 until as recently as 1980, hysteroscopy has been regarded as everything from limited to dangerous. Serious visualization problems occurred, some related to insufficient dilation of the endometrial cavity and some to inadequate lighting. Difficulties with controlling blood loss were also common.

The fiberoptic light introduced in the 1950s was a great improvement, but blood was still problematic. An ingenious balloon hysteroscope unfortunately pressed on the endometrium, causing blood to obstruct the view through the balloon wall and preventing any manipulation through the instrument. In 1968, a glass-fiber hysteroscope allowed visualization of a fetus, the inner surface of the uterine wall in pregnancy, the onset of labor, and the inner surface and lumen of the fallopian tube. Concentrated dextran, which is still in use today, was introduced in 1971, as was a cervical cap and CO_2. A colpohysteroscope, developed in 1979, revolutionized the applications of diagnostic hysteroscopy.

The hysteroscope is no longer a single diagnostic device. Endometrial ablation by several methods including "rollerball" tissue removal, laser tissue vaporization, polyp excision, myoma removal, tissue biopsy, uterine septum excision, and intrauterine correction of some uterine anomalies are all possible with the hysteroscope. It may be even more possible to include some of the more simple intrauterine fetal surgery procedures by combining the necessary instruments with the hysteroscope. As the extent of all ancillary materials and concepts broadens, the future use of this method of diagnosis and treatment will expand.

Culdoscopy. As early as 1898, posterior colpotomy incisions were used to treat intrapelvic diseases. Endoscopic observation of the pelvic cavity originated in 1935, using the principle of negative intraabdominal pressure and the knee-chest position. With a straight endoscope, the negative pressure distended the abdominal cavity for observation through the cul-de-sac attained by a posterior colpotomy incision. Culdocentesis had been used for hundreds of years, and the proximity of the posterior vaginal wall to the pouch of Douglas provided a natural avenue for endoscopy. By 1942, this was pronounced a success, and in 1944 the term *culdoscopy* was established. Photography was accomplished by 1953. However, because of the unwieldy position, difficul-

ties with anesthesia, and somewhat limited observational capability, culdoscopy gave way to peritoneoscopy.

Laparoscopy. *Laparoscopy,* which is a much better term for the process of intraabdominal observation with distention, eventually eliminated culdoscopy. As early as 1900, a cystoscope was inserted through a paracentesis wound. Abdominal endoscopy was performed with the patient in Trendelenburg's position, marking the first time laparoscopy was used to view the female pelvis. Laparoscopy was used successfully to diagnose ectopic pregnancy, coagulate the fallopian tubes, aspirate ovarian and paraovarian cysts, lyse pelvic adhesions, and identify ruptured and unruptured ectopic pregnancies.

Despite its potential diagnostic and therapeutic effect, laparoscopy fell into disfavor for a few years. But Palmer, in 1947, published several cases of laparoscopy. The first atlas on laparoscopy was published in 1968, and the American Association of Gynecologic Laparoscopists was founded in 1972. Public courses of instruction were given, and the procedure regained popularity. The combination of hysteroscopy and laparoscopy has proven invaluable in many cases, but, more important, the extent to which endoscopic surgery has expanded in the past 20 years is amazing. The effect of these procedures on obstetrics and gynecology cannot be estimated, and the future possibilities remain limitless.

As predicted, laparoscopy has completely changed the practice of gynecologic surgery. Aside from simple diagnostic procedures or simple therapeutic advances, the use of various forms and sizes of laparoscopes for performing multiple complex intrapelvic and abdominal surgeries is profound. Laparoscopes are used with gas distention or balloon dissecters retroperitoneally to explore the pelvis, to remove tissue, and to observe and operate on the ureter. Their most effective application is exploration of retroperitoneal lymph nodes as high as the aortic chain.

Gasless laparoscopy has become an alternative approach to the abdominal cavity. It requires an entirely new set of instruments to elevate the abdominal wall from the inside. These "lifters" elevate the anterior abdominal wall to a height sufficient to permit laparoscopic observation and surgery of the pelvis and abdomen. Inflatable balloons and inflatable flat disks positioned at the edge of long retractable metal rods are used to push away the bowel and eliminate any other tissue obstruction.

Open laparoscopy with a Hasoon cannula is still used occasionally and is especially helpful in obese patients. When no distention is created before a trocar is inserted, the potential risk for trauma to internal organs is great; despite this risk, open laparoscopy without distention has been reported.

Inevitably, as laparoscopic use has increased, so has the potential for complications, which include urinary tract injuries to the bladder and ureters, trauma to both large and small bowel (usually after an electric burn or tears or perforation) and to adjacent tissues, and problems with abdominal wall wounds such as hematoma or infection. Related problems include failed hemostasis, suture and ligature failure, inability to remove excised tissue, and failure to perform the operation necessary to achieve the treatment goal. Controversy surrounds the techniques used in laparoscopically assisted hysterectomy.

Ultrasonography. The use of ultrasound as a diagnostic medium developed as a spin-off from the studies of sonar (underwater sound) by the U.S. military in World War II, especially through the investigative committee for antisubmarine detection. It was first applied to the brain, and, in 1961, the first biparietal measurements of the fetal head were made. In the late 1900s ultrasound was used in combination with surgery. Vaginal ultrasound better demonstrates the adnexal areas.

Ultrasound has become almost as useful and applicable for diagnosis and as a guidance system for invasive procedures as laparoscopy. Ultrasound may be more valuable and may have a broader range of application in obstetrics, infertility, and fetal surgery. Color ultrasound is effective in specialized diagnosis and treatment. Ultrasound use in infertility manipulations of all kinds has expanded remarkably in the past 5 years. It is especially useful in harvesting extra, unwanted pregnancies after intrauterine placement of multiple fertilized ova, leaving one or two gestations intact to progress to maturity.

Ultrasound use has brought together the fields of radiology, perinatology, specialized infertility, and fetal surgery. Transvaginal techniques have recently been further developed and applied.

Transvaginal ultrasound has many uses, and modifications continue to be made to improve the quality of specific studies. Among these is hydrosonography for detection of intrauterine abnormalities, especially abnormal uterine blood loss. The injection of sterile saline solution into the uterine cavity before commencing ultrasound imaging was proposed in 1986, and some applications continue to be used today. Recent studies have confirmed the procedure's safety and low complication rate, as well as its accuracy, except in rare instances when hysteroscopy has been necessary. False-positive results usually are caused by endometrial tissue folds or irregular endometrial lining. Hydrosonography is easier to perform than hysteroscopy and is effective in establishing an accurate diagnosis in all cases of abnormal uterine blood loss in the absence of pregnancy. If endometrial malignancy is highly suspected, biopsy is preferred to decrease the possibility of spread.

Transvaginal ultrasound is useful in analyzing the endometrium in patients who have breast cancer and are taking tamoxifen. If ultrasound indicates an endometrial thickness greater than 10 mm, transvaginal pulsed Doppler color flow imaging can be used, but it does not provide enough information to warrant the added expense. Sonohysterography may be the method of choice for examining endometrial thickening or irregularity because it may help to detect space-occupying lesions and to differentiate endometrial polyps from other masses. Positive sonohysterographic findings necessitate hysteroscopy, and biopsy is necessary when tissue thickness is greater than 10 mm. Sonohysterography verifies complete removal of endometrial disease.

Fetal surgery has been performed to correct fetal defects believed to be reversible and those that can be prevented from progressing. Frequently this is a matter of fetal death in utero. Ultrasound makes the initial diagnosis possible. Fetal surgery requires highly specialized knowledge and technical expertise. Not all fetal abnormalities can be corrected, and some are corrected directly by extrauterine procedures. Not all these surgeries are successful; some fetuses do not survive and others are prematurely delivered. The potential risk is great, but the severity of the fetal disease may justify the risk. Continued use of ultrasound for diagnosis and therapy undoubtedly will lead to dramatic corrections of many fetal anomalies. These operations are subject to rigid ethical standards, and patient information and total consent are completely necessary.

Papanicolaou Cervical Smear. In 1943, Papanicolaou and Traut published a procedure that is now one of the most important in gynecology: the diagnosis of uterine cancer by the vaginal smear. This has been the most widespread, reliable, and inexpensive cancer screening device ever conceived. Refinements have been made in the manner of collection of material for the smears and to some extent in differential cytologic stains. The validity of the test is based on research establishing the fundamentals of cytology.

The thin Pap test has been recently introduced. Smears are obtained with a brush and placed immediately in liquid fixative. The liquid is then processed by the TP technique and stained in the usual manner, producing a thin, even smear that decreases the number of hidden cells. The Papnet, a computerized screening process, as well as auto-Pap, has improved the quality of microexaminations. The auto-Pap identifies abnormal cells by a dot placed on the slide, which should increase the value of the test and help to reduce the cost in the long run.

The continued high level of false cervical smears has prompted efforts to improve not only the process of sampling the tissue surface for cells, but also the preparation of cell collection for screening (e.g., the thin Pap test). Others have not yet been accepted. Computerized screening devices are not yet totally dependable, but may prove to be effective in the future. Other methods to improve the value of cytologic screens are discussed under colposcopy.

Colposcopy. Invention of an optical instrument that permitted high magnification of the surface of the uterine cervix made possible a process named *colposcopy*. Earlier descriptions of cervical atypia had motivated production of this magnification instrument. One of the difficulties with colposcopy centers on the confusion in the terminology used to describe the tissues observed.

The colposcope was invented in Europe in the early 1900s but was not used in the United States until 1968 when Coppelson et al. published a fine text and toured the nation with descriptions and photographs of the procedure and its value. The instrument was used mostly in large institutions and medical schools, primarily because of its cost. Information on cervical anatomy and physiology derived from its continued use brought about a new appreciation of the dynamics of the human cervix. Correlation with the Pap smear and integration of colposcopy made it possible to diagnose cervical malignancy earlier and, even more important, to identify cellular changes indicating ongoing pathologic processes that eventually lead to malignancy. Because of some discrepancies and the discovery of the relationship between cervical pathology and human papillomavirus (HPV), seven different tests for virus identification have been developed over a short period, most of which focus on HPV DNA.

To further establish this relationship, Stafl developed a technique in 1981 that used a high-intensity strobe and a macrolens camera to produce fine color photographs of the cervix that could be reproduced and used for studying and monitoring ongoing changes on the cervical surface. This technique is called cervicography. Although this technique has been criticized, lower specificity and higher sensitivity of cervicography have been verified. Although cervicography cannot be used to screen the endocervix, its valuable for evaluating the ectocervical transformation zone.

Speculoscopy is a new process used for studying this area. This technique, introduced by Massad et al. in 1993, uses specialized "blue-white" chemiluminescent light with acetic acid and low-power magnification to screen for abnormalities of the cervical epithelium. A peroxyoxalate chemical is attached to the upper blade of a speculum, and under dim room light the cervix and vagina are studied with low-magnification "loupes." Acetowhitening is considered positive. Because this examination does not include atypical vessels, its use requires further study.

Another approach for studying the cervix originated in Australia and is called Polarprobe (Polartechnics Ltd., Sidney, Australia). Polarprobe is an optoelectronic instrument that detects malignant and premalignant tissues by using voltage decay and various wavelengths of scattered light. Polarprobe depends on tissue transmission and the scattering of light, both of which depend on the density of the tissue examined. By a complicated analysis system, positive findings are almost immediately available. Because the device is portable and can be used in areas where colposcopy and other methods may not be as available, it has a high value for screening in many areas of the world.

Female Genital Tract Biopsy. Methods for cervical biopsy and uterine curettage of the endometrial cavity were not readily used until the 1900s.

Cervical Biopsy. Many methods have been developed for collecting tissue samples from suspected areas of the cervix. Some have used simple Lugol's stain and others have involved acetic acid markers and other stains. The biopsy and cytopathologic study correlations with gross observation have made earlier diagnosis of cervical malignancy possible. Various methods have been devised to obtain untainted tissues. The most important innovation has been selective tissue biopsy with colposcopic guidance. Several articles have examined the value and accuracy of this directed tissue sample method; some have been contentious but not totally negative, and others have been more

positive. New methods have been introduced to increase accuracy and to obtain tissue from the proper areas, especially when the transformation zone is located in the endocervical canal. This condition may require a conization, which is discussed elsewhere. Small, sharp curettes of various shapes have been devised to remove adequate tissue samples from the endocervix, but suction devices are not always quantitative or complete.

Endometrial Biopsy. Biopsy of the internal uterine tissues was developed in the nineteenth century and refined and improved in the first half of the twentieth century. The Novak suction endometrial curette, while not the first, was the easiest to use and caused minimal trauma. Several devices have since been invented, but most have merely altered the size or shape of the curette. More important was the introduction of endometrial dating by Noyes, which offered a more sophisticated approach to tissue sampling because it emphasized hormonal influences on endometrial tissues. The next improvement came with the hysteroscope, which provided directed biopsy capability; this also has been expanded and modified. Ultrasound also has been used with success for biopsy.

Vaginal and Vulvar Biopsy. Biopsy specimens of the vagina and vulva have been obtained directly, and only recently biopsy of these organs has been further directed by the use of materials similar to those used for the cervix. Diethylstilbestrol adenocarcinoma of the vagina led to significant improvement in biopsy of the upper vagina through direct microscopic guidance. The many variable changes in the vulva and introitus, which includes Bartholin's gland, have encouraged multiple biopsy of suspicious tissues. Various stains have been helpful, but the colposcope is more effective for observing the most suspicious areas. Almost all biopsies are now directed.

Cone biopsy of the cervix ultimately resolves some of the problems with single or even directed biopsy. This form of tissue sampling has become an integral part of the diagnosis of early and premalignant change.

Because this can be a bloody procedure, techniques to control blood loss were developed, and sutures were used for hemostasis and for covering the raw area after the cone was used. A new procedure using a high-frequency electrical loop has been devised for obtaining cervical tissue samples.

Other devices have been developed to improve on the conization operation. Laser use for conizations is relatively innovative, and by now most problems related to this method have been solved. Deep conization, which includes most of the endocervix, may well be therapeutic in some well-delineated cases.

Ureteroscopy and Tubaloscopy. Both of these procedures are products of the expertise of the late 1980s and early 1990s. The highly refined visualization instruments of contemporary times have enabled the extensive exploration of the ureter and the fallopian tube lumens. Internal tubal disease can be visualized to an extent that makes decisions regarding therapy possible.

Instruments

Vaginal Speculum. The design of the vaginal speculum has varied dramatically over the centuries. Among the earliest was a complicated speculum that consisted of four blades that tapered inward and were attached to a ring. The blades had four rods attached, which opened inside the vagina by applying external pressure.

Plastic instruments are now commonly used to expose the vaginal tract and the cervix. Plastic speculae have several advantages including increased comfort, avoidance of temperature excesses or changes, reduction of annoying reflections from metals, and unlimited adaptation to suit any purpose, size, or shape, all of which help to facilitate the intended procedure. Black, nonreflective speculae are an example of this, as are plastic speculae used with lasers or electrocautery, which help to prevent injury. Some specialized speculae have been developed to carry attached visual aids to improve available light and to direct small cameras for record production or even transmission to a color monitor, as in laparoscopically assisted pelvic surgery. Adjunctive fixed or movable and removable features can be added to the plastic speculum to support instruments of all types to improve the surgeon's manual capability.

Laser. Development of the laser was based on the quantum theory of Planck (1900) and Bohr's description of the energy system in the hydrogen atom (1913). The gaseous laser had particular application in medicine, with CO_2 and YAG lasers proving the most useful in gynecology. Colposcopy is essential for use of the laser for cervical procedures. Laparoscopy combined with the laser facilitates treatment of various pelvic diseases. It is widely used for vulvar and cervical disease and has been used in the treatment of vaginal intraepithelial neoplasm (VAIN).

Laser photoradiation treatment for various cancers of the genital tract has been used since 1982. The more promising areas of laser surgery are infertility and debilitating pelvic disease (endometriosis). The following operations have benefited greatly from laser application:

1. Midsegment tubal obstruction for anastomosis
2. Proximal and distal tubal occlusion
3. Lysis of adhesions
4. Endometriosis ablation
5. Myomectomy and plastic operations of the uterus
6. Microsurgery
7. Hysteroscopic laser total ablation of the endometrium
8. Resection of Asherman's adhesions
9. Resection of intrauterine septa

These were all introduced in the 1980s. Clearly the future holds incredible possibilities for the application of lasers in gynecology.

Electronically produced specialized light modified through a crystal, such as a ruby, was found to vaporize cells and has been adapted for surgical use. The control of the light beam is absolute and is the key to the success of the instrument. This type of laser has been used to treat cervical disease and to obtain a cone biopsy. When modified for superficial use, it can remove adhesions and leave no residual tissue, which prevents reformation. The laser is very useful in treating endometriosis, because when correctly applied it vaporizes endometrial nodules completely. This decreases the potential for recurrence and prevents adhesions. The superficial surface of the ovary can be cleared of residual tissue after pelvic infection. The ovary has been drilled successfully in cases of polycystic ovarian disease. Laser treatment of vaginal and especially vulvar disease has gained prominence.

The laser also has been adapted for hemostasis. Although laser use is somewhat limited to hemostasis of smaller blood vessels, with selection of its superficial mode, the laser can readily control blood loss from a large dissection area with ooze. The laser can be changed from incision mode to hemostasis almost simultaneously, which permits making incisions while controlling blood loss, such as when accessing the abdominal cavity. The lowest power that will cut prevents the possible production of a local burn.

Hemostasis

The control of blood loss is one of the most important factors in the development of gynecologic surgery because of the extensive vascularity of the female pelvic area. Yet it took many years to produce the simple process of blood vessel ligation, even though ancient people developed remarkable capability with bandages and showed surprising inventiveness with the creation of surgical instruments. The concept of the tourniquet was established but not applied to hemostasis. Manual compression and pressure with tight wrapping with pliable materials defined the hemostasis of early times, but it is probable that other materials were applied to bleeding wounds.

Greco-Roman medicine, which included the Alexandrian school, was advanced for its time and used ligation to accomplish hemostasis (Fig. 1-2). Hot iron cautery and boiling oil also were used to control blood loss.

The origin of the hemostatic forceps may well have been described by Erasistratus, who stated that a lead forceps used for dental purposes was in the temple of the oracle at Delphi. A much finer and smaller forceps was greatly needed. The Roman tenaculum was revived and soon was generally used to pull up a vessel for ligation; it was modified to become a ligature carrier. A dissection forceps was developed out of similar necessity, and a device for holding it closed was added. In about 1829, surgeons began twisting the cut ends of vessels with a square-beaked forceps with two nuts and a bar that moved.

For the remainder of the 1800s, surgeons followed the principle for forci-pressure and clamps. Another contribution to the application of ligature was, of course, the use of sterilized, chromacized catgut by Lister.

Hemostasis in the modern sense began with Pare and his invention of a clamp known as the "bec de corbin" (Fig. 1-3) or "raven's beak." In the years that followed, variations were invented such as a "crane's bill forceps" with long pincers. Many devices were created to manage the stump of the ovarian pedicle after ovariotomy; one example is Cintrat's

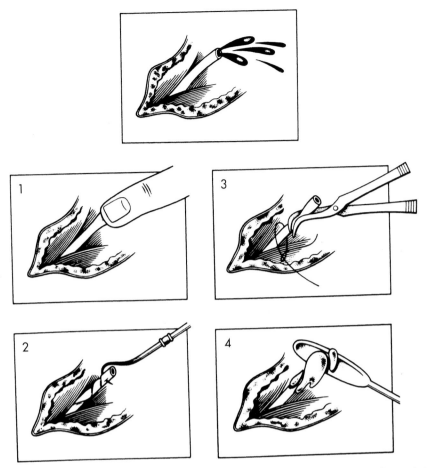

Fig. 1-2   Hemostasis methods by Galen. (From Majno G: *The healing hand,* Cambridge, Mass, 1975, Harvard University Press.)

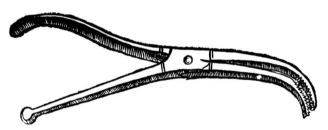

Fig. 1-3   Hemostatic clamp "bec de corbin." (From Pare A: *The collected works of Ambrose Pare,* Pound Ridge, NY, 1968, Milford House [Translated by T Johnson].)

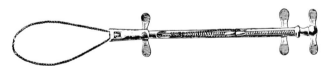

Fig. 1-4   Pedicle constrictor by Cintrat. (From Doyen E: *Surgical therapeutics and operative technique,* vol 1, New York, 1917, William Wood [Translated by H Spencer-Browne].)

constrictor (Fig. 1-4). The further pursuit of a compression forceps brought about crude instruments for constriction of blood vessels, such as the use of two wooden pieces tied with cord.

The development of the hemostatic clamp was enhanced in the United States by Halsted with the introduction of a fine-nosed, small instrument and clear emphasis on the techniques of arterial ligation, both free and within tissue.

Improvement in clips of all kinds and sizes for hemostasis has considerably reduced blood loss. Development of various lasers also has improved hemostasis, especially in controlling blood loss from small vessels and in ooze for-

mation associated with broad denudation. Clips to secure broad tissues such as broad ligaments or the ovarian pedicle help to reduce blood loss and cause less tissue necrosis than ligation. Refined, highly controllable cautery devices, especially bipolar machines, have improved hemostasis and also can be used as tissue cutters.

Materials also have been developed to control blood loss in massive dissection areas (e.g., in oncologic surgery of the pelvis). Hemostatic, nontraumatic clamps to secure the larger vessels that supply the operative area prevent significant blood loss, facilitate dissection, and can be removed at any time without causing demonstrable damage to the blood vessel wall. There is no substitute for knowledge of the blood supply to the area under manipulation.

Cautery

Many kinds of cautery instruments have been used throughout surgical history, and the one thing they all shared was the causing of unimaginable pain.

In the early 1900s, Cushing devised a silver clip for vessel occlusion. Steel eventually replaced silver, and tantalum or tellurium clips are currently used for occlusion. Together with Bovie, Cushing developed the "sparking" device, which used controlled electricity. Since 1928, the Bovie machine, with modifications, has been the instrument of choice for cautery in gynecologic surgery, especially pelvic surgery. Despite the efficiency of the Bovie machine, broad areas of constant discharge of blood have made it necessary to use various substances, including treated cottons and Gel-Foam. More recently, other substances have been created to produce local hemostasis without forming adhesions.

Position

It is essential for patients to be positioned in a comfortable, practical manner to permit examination of or surgery on internal and external genitalia. A basic position for such purposes has been illustrated in ancient Hindu medicine texts. Descriptions and illustrations of a wide lithotomy position for extirpation of a bladder stone have been found in the records of early Greece. Other early illustrations demonstrated a procedure called *succussion* (shaking), in which the body was tied upside down to a ladder to reduce genital prolapse in women and large hernias in men.

The lithotomy position was adapted in numerous ways in the 1800s (Fig. 1-5). One of the problems with lithotomy was the uncomfortable way in which the legs were supported, especially when an assistant was not available. Several ingenious devices that included many variations of stirrups were created to meet this need. These ranged from complicated mechanical apparati to simple bands mounted on a vertical bar. The knee-chest position was popularized in the 1800s and was revived in the 1900s for examinations such as culdoscopy. Prone positions with lateral abduction of the thighs, which rest on a table, permit a better approach to the anterior vaginal wall. Variations of the lateral abduction position are used for combined vaginoabdominal operations. Lateral abduction positions are most adaptable to laparoscopically assisted hysterectomy, both abdominal and vaginal. A lateral position has been recommended to facilitate retroperitoneal diagnosis and surgical procedures such as lymphadenectomy or biopsy. Modified Trendelenburg positions are currently used for laparoscopically guided operations, with abdominal wall elevators used in cases of gasless laparoscopy.

Anesthesia

The ancient recorded instances of the use of anesthetic agents are few. In Greece about 1000 BC, *nepenthe* was used to anesthetize patients for surgery, and Helen of Troy used a form of opium dissolved in wine to produce insensibility.

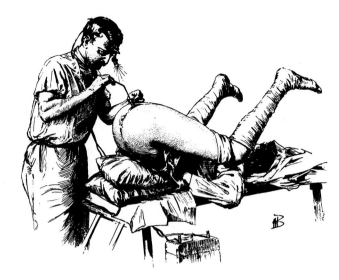

Fig. 1-5 Exaggerated lithotomy for air cystoscopy. (From Kelly H: *Operative gynecology*, vol 1, New York, 1902, D Appleton.)

In India, a drug named *samohini*, presumably a narcotic herb or a combination of herbs, was used to put a patient to sleep; another drug, *samojani*, apparently a stimulant, was used to awaken the patient. Mention has also been made of the use of henbane and hashish for anesthesia and another drug to reverse their action. In China (225 BC), wine loaded with hashish was used for pain relief during surgery.

"Sweet vitriol" (later named *ether*) was apparently discovered in Spain, but it was Paracelsus in 1540 who described the potential for insensibility with the mixture (sulfuric acid and alcohol); it was not named for almost 200 years. Paracelsus also described the value of a mixture of opium and alcohol known as *laudanum.*

Anesthesia in the 1600s was attempted by the use of cold and compression. Mesmer introduced a form of hypnosis to produce lack of sensibility to pain. Oxygen and nitrous oxide were discovered in the late 1700s, and experiments were done with the inhalation of nitrous oxide ("laughing gas"), which produced a loss of cerebral control, a concept that led to the development of inhalation anesthesia.

Morphine was extracted from opium in 1806; ether was inhaled to allay painful stimuli; and chloroform was discovered in 1831. During the mid-eighteenth century in the United States, various uses of ether and nitrous oxide were demonstrated, with a public presentation of surgery using ether anesthesia at Massachusetts General Hospital. Also at this time, ether and chloroform were used to ease the pain of childbirth, which was promoted by Simpson in England. Morphine was introduced as a preanesthetic medication, and cyclopropane was suggested for anesthesia. Corning used cocaine for epidural anesthesia, which led to the use of spinal anesthesia. In 1899, Tuffier developed "twilight sleep" for management of the pain of labor, but this often proved lethal for the child.

Caudal anesthesia was promoted in the early twentieth century. Continuous caudal anesthesia was introduced in

1942, and, with the development of continuous epidural anesthesia, pain control in labor could be extended to cesarean section. The intravenous use of pentothal was further developed in the early 1900s and became almost routine when its safety was ensured by the development of intratracheal intubation. Nitrous oxide and cyclopropane have been made practical, and many newer agents have been used successfully for pain relief.

Asepsis

Based on the improvements in the microscope, the discoveries and theories of Pasteur, the development of the etiology of postpartum sepsis (streptococci), and the support of this theory, Lister in 1869 introduced the concept of sterility needed for all aspects of surgery, which included the patient's skin.

The introduction of sterile gloves by Halsted in the late nineteenth century facilitated the prevention of infection during surgery. This was followed by the use of the surgical mask, which prevents contamination of surgical wounds by personnel in the surgical suite. The evolution of the surgical uniform soon followed, with caps, shoe covers, scrub suits, gowns, and tight-fitting gloves. This completed the improvement in prevention of outside contamination of surgical wounds.

The steam autoclave eliminated another potential cause of bacterial contamination during surgery by employing high temperature sterilization of all materials that come into contact with the patient. Elaborate skin preparation, including removal of body hair the night before surgery, was simplified by the use of iodine preparations, which are highly effective skin cleaners.

The surgeon's scrub techniques, also once long and arduous with soaps and dips with bacteriostatic solutions, have been simplified by modern chemicals; studies have reported a proper, easier method for achieving satisfactory, virtually bacteria-free hands and fingernails. However, none of this compares with the cataclysmic advent of the antibiotic era, which began in the 1920s and 1930s and crystallized in the 1940s with the sulfa drugs, penicillins, mycotics, and others. When properly used, these medications revolutionized all surgery, especially gynecologic surgery. Although the vagina, by its structure and location, has never been bacteria free, antibiotic drugs have greatly reduced the threat of sepsis. Prophylactic antibiotics, although still a controversial subject, have probably reduced morbidity significantly, as demonstrated in many studies of vaginal hysterectomy and suspected uterine or tubal infections. Postoperative antibiotics have been even more effective in the management of wounds and infections.

Disorders

Fallopian Tube Disease

Ectopic Pregnancy. Extrauterine pregnancy was known in ancient times, with accounts of abdominal pregnancy going back at least 1000 years. In addition, spontaneous drainage from abdominal abscesses, usually from near the umbilicus, commonly contained decomposed fetal elements. Almost all ectopic pregnancies were found at the time of anatomic dissection, which was when the first lithopedion was described, or at a postmortem autopsy, which is when tubal ectopic pregnancies were recognized.

In the mid-1800s, laparotomy was suggested for ectopic pregnancy; however, this was disregarded in favor of exotic methods for destruction of the tubal fetus, which ranged from poisons, to hormones, to electricity. In 1883, a successful exploratory laparotomy and adnexectomy was performed. Once the surgery had been established for ruptured ectopic pregnancy, lives were saved by this procedure.

The development of a reliable pregnancy test improved the management of early ectopic pregnancy. Although the early urine test took too long to be of benefit in cases of severe internal hemorrhage, it was helpful in nonemergent situations. With later developments, the rapidity and reliability of early pregnancy tests have saved not only lives, but also fallopian tubal tissues. Contemporary tests are read in minutes and can be performed anywhere.

The etiology and management of extrauterine gestation were reassessed in 1976. Several reports have noted the success of laparoscopic diagnosis and management for early unruptured tubal ectopic pregnancies. Early diagnosis and conservative treatment have reduced mortality from this problem to nearly nothing except in developing countries.

Ultrasound has increased the ability to diagnose ectopic pregnancy. Factors leading to a diagnosis of ectopic pregnancy include a rise in human chorionic gonadotropin (HCG), the absence of ultrasound findings indicating intrauterine gestation, ultrasound findings in the adnexa or elsewhere of probable products of conception, and a general suspicion. In the rare case of heterotopic pregnancy, it is possible to diagnose coexistent intrauterine and extrauterine pregnancies, but this is not always possible. In this case, a rise in HCG does not contribute to the diagnosis.

Treatment should be planned once a diagnosis is made, except in cases of obvious tubal rupture with intraabdominal blood loss. Expectant treatment carries the risk of such an accident, and early management permits preservation of tissues and protection for possible future pregnancy. In recent years, single dose methotrexate with an occasional repeated small dose has become the method of choice in certain cases. Surgery, some of which is laparoscopically guided, and conservative preservation of the tube have increased the chances of normally placed pregnancies, decreased the risk of hemorrhage, and reduced the need for costly hospitalization. If an ectopic pregnancy persists after a single dose of methotrexate, the drug may be repeated and the HCG levels carefully monitored. Occasionally salpingectomy is necessary if the tube is irreparably damaged; in such cases preservation of the contralateral tube is mandatory.

Pelvic Inflammatory Disease. Inflammation and severe pelvic infections have been recognized for several hundred years and were commonly attributed to cellulitis of the uterus. Tubal involvement was always secondary and was rarely diagnosed by pelvic examination. Hunter in 1775 was the first to recognize chronic tubal infections. Other reports were published, but tubal infections were neither recognized nor accepted as involving the pelvis primarily; rather the uterus was always considered the primary infected organ.

Pelvic abscesses that pointed into the vagina had been incised and drained since before the Middle Ages, a practice continuing until the early 1800s (Fig. 1-6). Conservative preservation of the ovaries with tubal excision and salpingostomies to preserve fertility found support.

In the United States, the first laparotomy for salpingitis was done in 1887 with excision of just one tube; a bilateral adnexectomy and hysterectomy were also performed at the same time. This radical procedure gained acceptance among surgeons in both the United States and Europe.

Hot cautery also was used for hemostasis. From 1886 until 1890, several surgeons in the United States and Europe treated pyosalpingitis and hydrosalpingitis with surgery and drainage.

Partial adnexal removal proved ineffective, and severe bilateral disease was treated by supravaginal hysterectomy. Conservative cures were lengthy, and recurrence of the infection frequently resulted in a "pelvic clean-out." The infection was widespread and severely debilitated the patient. Antibiotics revolutionized the treatment of pelvic inflammatory disease and allowed for more conservative surgery. Techniques of tuboplasty improved significantly with the introduction of microtubal surgery.

Severe, irreversible adnexal disease is no longer seen except in developing countries. The role of pelvic and tubal infection in the etiology of tubal ectopic pregnancy became well recognized in the twentieth century, and therapeutic surgery for pelvic inflammatory disease was performed with this in mind.

Pelvic Organ Prolapse. This gynecologic problem is one of the oldest on record, even older than vesicovaginal fistula, which has been demonstrated in an Egyptian mummy. Uterine prolapse, including inversion, was treated in several ways, ranging from pleasant medications to entice the uterus back into the abdominal cavity, to odorous ones to drive it up into place, to one method in which the woman

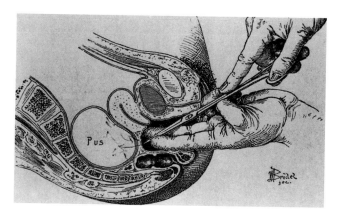

Fig. 1-6 Culdocentesis for both treatment and diagnosis. (From Kelly H: *Operative gynecology,* vol 2, New York, 1902, D Appleton.)

was inverted and shaken severely. Hundreds of combinations of materials have been placed in the vagina and the woman's legs tied together sometimes for long periods. Probably the first pessary was one half of a sun-dried pomegranate. Ancient medical documents are filled with prescriptions of all kinds for treatment of pelvic organ prolapse.

By the time of the Renaissance, diagnoses of genital prolapse were made with greater accuracy, and the specifics of the insertion of pessaries were demonstrated. Very little progress was made until the 1800s, when interest in the subject was high; types of prolapse were differentiated, and congenital prolapse, even in children, was identified.

Surgical procedures were developed in the 1800s; one of the first was a vaginal constriction operation. Later, mucosal denudation and bringing the round ligaments up through the inguinal canal were used. *Elytrorrhaphy* was the term used to describe procedures involving the vaginal mucosa. The vaginal walls were burned with cautery and caustic chemicals and even purposely infected to produce dense scars to cure the prolapse. The vulva and labia were attacked in the 1840s and 1850s. Forms of infibulation and several methods of suture of the labia that included apposition were used. The use of cautery and permanent silver sutures together with all of the above were eventually abandoned, but not until after some women were terribly tortured.

In the middle 1800s, there was a return to cervical amputation and destruction by pressure to produce a heavy cicatrix at the vaginal apex. Perineoplastic surgery was also advocated. Sims in 1866 described a cystocele and inadvertently performed an anterior vaginal repair that resembled the technique used in modern times. In 1877, Le Fort introduced his vaginal occlusion operation, which has survived to contemporary times. Many complicated combined operations were practiced in the late 1800s.

Hadra in 1884 introduced the idea that obstetric injury to the pelvic structures was the probable cause of pelvic organ prolapse. A combined multiple procedure was created involving amputation of the cervix and imbrication of the uterine ligaments into the vaginal apex with silver wires. The operation was modified by Fothergill in 1908 and came to be known as the "Manchester operation"; it was very popular in England but not in the United States. Kelly suggested anterior and posterior repairs; his suburethral Lembert-style stitch tightened the urethrovesical junction and has proved to be the best method for restoring urinary continence in cases of symptomatic cystocele. Almost all vaginal repairs use some form of the Kelly suture.

The first vaginal hysterectomy for the treatment of prolapse was done in 1861, the first suprapubic suspension of the vagina in 1890. Abdominal hysterectomy has been used for prolapse, and the broad and cardinal ligaments have been shortened and imbricated into the cervical stump.

Vaginal prolapse proved to be difficult to correct. Uterine inversion was seriously considered but rejected because of the mortality associated with it. Several methods for both manual and instrument reduction of inversion were suggested, some of which were very strange. Vaginal surgery with reversion to cervical amputation in chronic cases was used, as was an abdominal operation.

Surgery for pelvic organ prolapse increased in the twentieth century. Operations were performed simply because the tissues hung down into or out of the vagina or because the prolapsed tissues produced severe symptoms of pain and pressure. Also, some were associated with urinary incontinence with or without difficult defecation. Much of the surgery was associated with vaginal hysterectomy for prolapse with asymptomatic anterior and posterior vaginal relaxation. In these cases, a token anterior and posterior vaginal repair was recommended without extensive dissection.

Overcorrection of the posterior vagina and perineum resulted in criticism of posterior vaginal repairs. Recent attempts have been made to carefully correct this error. Prophylactic procedures have been performed to prevent recurrence of uterine or vaginal prolapse.

Enterocele and Massive Vaginal Prolapse. Enterocele, which is the true pelvic hernia, was adequately described in the 1800s. As early as 1912, surgery was suggested for the correction of enterocele, as well as other vaginal wall relaxations. An abdominal procedure was developed for elevation of the rectum, which works equally well for obliteration of cul-de-sac hernias in women. Although transvaginal colpopexy was first reported in 1892, it lay forgotten until rediscovered in 1951 by an operation that obliterated the cul-de-sac and repaired the hernia. Before the 1950s, enterocele repairs were usually done vaginally. In general, these followed the basic surgical principles of herniorrhaphy. By the mid-1960s, postoperative vaginal prolapse was sometimes treated by colpocleisis and vaginectomy. The Le Fort operations were used frequently for these problems but had been modified so that more vaginal mucosa could be removed than in the initial procedure. Prophylactic imbrication of the sacrouterine ligaments at the time of hysterectomy was suggested to prevent formation of an enterocele, and fascia lata strips were used to correct enterocele or the prolapsed vagina. Other recent surgeries include an abdominal surgery for vaginal and uterine prolapse; a composite vaginal vault suspension with fascia lata; pulsion enterocele and use of a levator muscle plication with vaginal vault fixation for repair of vaginal prolapse or enterocele; and uterosacral ligament and cardinal ligament suspension of the vagina. A unique, simple vaginal suspension by use of specially placed nonabsorbable suture through the vaginal apex and the sacrospinous ligament has been especially effective. Variations of these techniques have been implemented over the past 15 to 20 years with the addition of Dacron tape supports for relaxed pelvic organs and the continued use of Marlex mesh slings and replacement of destroyed support in the pelvis.

Analysis and follow-up of the long-term results of operations for pelvic organ prolapse and correction of urinary incontinence are necessary. Recent use of multichannel urodynamic evaluation of the results of laparoscopic Burch vaginal suspensions has proven valuable.

Standardized evaluation of the surgical results of pelvic organ prolapse should include description of the population, anatomic changes, objective physiologic function tests, laboratory analysis when relevant, records of the exact operation, morbidity and perhaps mortality related to the operative procedures, patient follow-up, expense of total care, and quality of life. Such studies will lead to improvement in the overall management of these complicated cases and permit extended use of all methods available.

Collagen periurethral injection, which includes the area near the external urethrovesical junction, has been increasingly used in the past 5 years with encouraging short-term results; long-term records are not available. Urethral prolapse after such treatment has recently been reported. Since collagen begins to biodegrade at various times, the persistence of the cure may lapse. Plastic surgeons and dermatologists who have used collagen injection to correct facial wrinkles have noted this degradation.

Sacrospinous ligament fixation for repair of vaginal vault prolapse—the Nichols operation—has become a standard operative procedure in modern gynecology and an integral part of fellow and resident instruction. The operation is used to correct vaginal prolapse, perineal pressure, urination problems including incontinence, difficult defecation, and dyspareunia or impossible intercourse. One essential requirement for a successful operation is adequate exposure, which always requires help with retraction; long, deep-bladed convex retractors are effective. A Deschamps ligature carrier is an excellent instrument for ensuring proper suture placement. Postoperative complications include urinary tract infection, febrile course, hematoma in the operative site, rectovaginal fistula, and some persistent neuralgia. Additional surgery of the anterior vaginal wall prevents or cures vesical incontinence. Posterior vaginal vault repair is indicated in certain cases of complete vaginal prolapse; a herniated peritoneal sac, if present, should be obliterated as well. This operation has begun to take precedence over other surgical methods for treating these problems, especially abdominal sacropexy. Follow-up should be extensive, and the patient should be carefully advised regarding precautions and personal care. All patients should have a preoperative urinary tract evaluation, Pap smear, uterine ultrasound with endometrial biopsy as indicated, and a general physical examination that includes laboratory studies and detailed information concerning the procedure and expectations.

Endometriosis. Endometriosis probably was first described by Rokitansky in 1861 when he referred to a complicated term for an adenomatous cystosarcoma of uterine tissue origin in the ovary. Russell described endometriosis as aberrant portions of the müllerian duct found in an ovary. Sampson in 1921 described endometriosis and its possible etiology in a landmark article. Aside from adhesions and carcinoma in the pelvis, this was a fairly common but unrecognized disease.

The use of hysterectomy for endometriosis has allowed ovarian preservation, but this has been a point of contention for several years. Description of the anatomy of the pelvic autonomic nerves helped to properly identify the tissue to be removed using presacral neurectomy, a procedure designed to relieve pain in the pelvis, including that caused by endometriosis. Several studies of endometriosis have observed the effect of suppressive hormones on the disease (1950 to 1962). Numerous definitive surgical procedures have been proposed for the treatment of pelvic endometriosis. In contemporary times, combined hormone therapy, laser, and microsurgery have continued the therapeutic approach to this increasingly common disease.

Fistula

Vesicovaginal Fistula. This entity has often been difficult to diagnose, is always difficult to treat, and has been one of the worst nonlethal gynecologic problems. Van Roonhuyse was one of the few in the past who successfully used surgery to treat vesicovaginal fistula. In the 1700s, very little could be done; Desault in 1799 provided the prevalent views of the time for management of the fistula: the use of a lint, a wax vaginal pessary, and an inlying bladder catheter.

In 1834, Gosset enunciated the basic principles of the surgical treatment of vesicovaginal fistula. With the patient in the knee-chest position, the fistula edges were freshened, interrupted sutures of gilded wire were twisted closed, a catheter was left in the bladder, and the patient remained in a prone position postoperatively. This combination was forgotten until Sims.

It remained, however, for Sims to provide the procedure of choice for many years. Sims placed his patient in the lateral prone position that carries his name, used silver sutures with lead bars and perforated shot, and was eminently successful. One of his followers, Emmet, had done more than 300 cases of both vesical and rectal vaginal fistulae by 1868 and achieved a very high success rate; Emmet is considered the first great vaginal plastic surgeon in the United States. In the latter third of the nineteenth century, many modifications and additions were made, among them a repair of the fistula from the vesical side by Trendelenburg. Other improvements occurred in the twentieth century.

Rectovaginal Fistula. Rectovaginal fistula was another entity that had been recognized for a long time but unsuccessfully treated. Information gained from the difficulties with repair of a totally ruptured perineum formed the basis for surgical treatment of rectovaginal fistulae. These fistulae were categorized according to cause, including obstetric trauma, syphilis, malignancy, or congenital disorder.

Over most of the eighteenth century, the concept was to consider the area a complete perineal rupture that included the fistula, and treat the entire area. A series of many operations was created for repair of the ruptured perineum. A form of dedoublement was used for this repair; such wide dissection allowed for the excellent apposition of tissues and also encouraged movement of the rectum, which disturbed the continuity of the fistula. When the fistula was high up in the vagina, the tissues were separated and the rectal side was sutured first with some displacement; then the vagina was closed so that the original tract was disrupted. Lembert sutures were placed in the fistulous orifice of the rectal wall, after a transverse incision, and then

the vagina and perineum were closed by dedoublement. An autoplastic movable flap was created, and silver wire was frequently used for these procedures.

About 1880, a flap of vaginal mucosa was created to cover the defect. This was improved in the early 1900s and, in modified form, is still used in modern practice.

Contemporary suture material has eliminated silver wire and encourages the process of repair by reducing local tissue irritation.

Malignancy. In 1595, Schenck reported several rare lesions, including a large tumor that forced the vagina open and was successfully excised; a large ovarian tumor in an amenorrheic young girl; several congenital anomalies, among them a bicornuate uterus; and a tumor of the ovary filled with hair, wax, pus, and fluid. These are the first clear descriptions of ovarian carcinoma and dermoid cyst. Schenck used the term *molea aquea,* which probably was a hydatid mole; a mole described by de Vega in 1564 weighed 12 pounds. Schenck described both fleshy mola and fibroids and the calcified variety.

Surgical treatment of gynecologic carcinoma was not a successful enterprise until the twentieth century. Vulvar and clitoral disease was known to ancient surgeons, and the amputation or excision attempted failed miserably. Innumerable benign measures were attempted to treat carcinoma, also to no avail. Amputation of prolapsed carcinomatous tissue has been practiced from time to time throughout the course of history. Many of these tissues were literally burned away with red iron cautery in a fashion similar to the treatment of breast tumors. Ovarian cancer was relieved by both vaginal and abdominal drainage with obvious failure.

Treatment of cervical malignancy was attempted more than other gynecologic cancers, perhaps partially because of its accessibility and the many variations of observable growth. Clark in 1812 first described an unusual change in the cervix that he called a "cauliflower excrescence" because of its appearance. Clarke introduced the term *carcinoma uteri* in 1821. It was not until Virchow in 1850 that the cellular nature of these cancers was recognized. By 1870, galvanocautery had been used for amputation because its use reduced blood loss immeasurably.

The definition and results of treatment of early cervical malignancy continue to be debated. Creasman et al. reported on the risk factors and prognosis of early invasive cervical carcinoma. In 1985 The International Federation of Obstetrics and Gynecology (FIGO) quantified the histologic definition of cervical cancer as follows: stage 1A(1), the earliest form of invasion, with minimum foci observed only by the microscope; and stage 1A(2), macroscopically measurable microcarcinoma not deeper than 5 mm nor wider than 7 mm. Stage 1A(1) cancers have been redefined as 0 to 3 mm of invasion, and stage 1A(2) as no more than 3 to 5 mm with limited width of 7 mm. Either venous or lymphatic space involvement does not alter the staging.

Patients who had conization of the cervix followed by radical hysterectomy and lymphadenectomy and 3 to 5 mm of invasion measured had no lymph node involvement and no recurrences; the 5-year apparent cure rate was 100%, with no deaths from cancer. The vascular space was involved in one fourth of patients, but obviously did not influence the recovery rate. No cancer was found in the hysterectomy specimens.

Other recent studies have reported that invasive malignancy, defined using the same definition as above, was associated with 2% lymph node involvement. These studies may not have followed the strict criteria used in the Gynecologic Oncology Group study. These and other reports cause some concern about minimal treatment even in early cases. Simple adequate conizations or standard hysterectomy, while desirable, may be insufficient for actual cure.

Vaginal hysterectomy was introduced for removal of a malignant uterus, and abdominal hysterectomy was also tried in an effort to cure the disease. These operations fostered the development of both types of uterine extirpation but did not affect the cancer. By 1888, the use of abdominal hysterectomy for both cervical and endometrial carcinoma had advanced considerably; at that time, Pawlik passed a catheter into the left ureter before a vaginal hysterectomy, providing some protection against ureteral trauma from surgery. Catheterization of the ureters was not used again until 1892. Halsted's radical breast surgery in 1895 encouraged a more radical approach to the surgical treatment of both kinds of uterine cancer. Clark in 1895 performed a wide dissection abdominal hysterectomy and ligated the uterine arteries next to the internal iliac. He then dissected the ureter free and ligated the broad and cardinal ligaments as far lateral as possible; he did not remove the pelvic lymph nodes. Rumpf, however, actually dissected the pelvic nodes in a live patient in 1895.

Kelly had used a straight-tube cystoscope with the patient in the knee-chest position and passed catheters into both ureters before these extensive hysterectomies. Wertheim in 1900 performed a logical and meticulous radical hysterectomy for cervical cancer.

Endometrial carcinoma was recognized and accurately described in 1813, with fundal sarcoma identified in 1845. Virchow described carcinosarcoma of the fundus, and coexistent squamous and adenocarcinoma were identified by Kaumann in 1894. Vaginal hysterectomy had been done for endometrial carcinoma but most surgeons were more comfortable with abdominal hysterectomy, and some preferred to leave the adnexa intact.

Salpingitis isthmica nodosa was diagnosed by Chiari in 1887, who suspected possible malignancy and found an inflammatory lesion instead. In 1896, Cullen identified uterine adenomyosis; at one time this was thought to be carcinoma.

Ovarian disease had been known for many years. Hodgkin in 1829 was the first to describe papillomatous ovarian growths. Virchow in 1848 attempted to classify ovarian disease, but an appropriate and comprehensive system has never been developed. Waldeyer in 1870 and Olshausen in 1877 established the histogenesis of ovarian tumors. Various benign and malignant ovarian tumors were described in the 1800s including papillary cystomata, the germ cell origin tumors, fibromas, hemorrhagic cysts, and corpus luteum cysts to sclerocystic ovaries. The management of these tumors is described in the sections on ovarian surgery.

Vulvar and vaginal carcinomas, although identified and locally treated by excision or cautery much earlier, were more adequately managed in the twentieth century. Wide local excision of the clitoris was popular for malignant and benign disease; in the early 1900s, a true radical vulvectomy was done for carcinoma of the clitoris, which established the possibility of this operation for all kinds of vulvar cancer, including carcinoma of Bartholin's gland. Lymph gland excision with this operation was also introduced.

Gynecologic pathology as divulged by persons such as Novak, who may well be the first gynecologic pathologist, led to specific surgical approaches to all gynecologic malignancy. Diagnosis was enhanced by the screening Pap smear, tissue biopsy, increased cytologic knowledge, and colposcopy.

Myomata Uteri. Uterine tumors have been described under the term *mola* since the establishment of Greek medicine. Galen referred to a solid uterine tumor as a "scleroma." For the next several centuries, solid uterine tumors were confused with all other pelvic masses. Salius in the 1500s called it "uterine stone." It was not until postmortem autopsy became possible that any true knowledge of these tumors was obtained. Hunter in the late 1700s wrote a treatise on fibroids that defined their nature; they were then variously called "fleshy tubercles" or "tubercular tumors." Vogel in 1843 established the characteristic tissues microscopically. Uterine carcinoma was clearly differentiated from myomas in the early 1800s; by 1862, Klob identified malignant changes in a fibroid.

The treatment, as noted in 1868, involved slough, absorption, excision, ecrasement (crushing), enucleation, and "gastrotomy" (laparotomy). Other techniques included morselization, hot iron cautery, incision of the capsule and removal of the fibroid by finger dissection, and electrolysis. In 1861, an extensive removal of a myoma, including morselization, was accomplished per vaginum. Atlee in the United States did a myomectomy in 1843 and classified fibroids as extrauterine, intrauterine, and intramural.

Because laparotomy was so lethal, vaginal myomectomy became popular. By 1901, hundreds of cases were reported. Cervical myomectomy was first done in the late 1800s. Myomectomy in a pregnant woman was done in 1874.

As the techniques for hysterectomy improved in the early 1900s, the indications for the operation for myomata increased. Mayo in 1911 advocated hysterectomy or myomectomy for uterine fibroids; he followed Kelly and Cullen who in 1907 had produced a classic book on myomata uteri. Bonney in England (1948) introduced the use of a flap of tissue to cover any large areas that were left after removal of an extensive amount of tissue; this was known as the Bonney hood.

Since 1976, hysterectomy and myomectomy have been advocated to treat myomas. Meigs delineated the syndrome bearing his name and suggested that in some cases a myoma could stimulate a similar production of fluid. Malignant changes in myomas were noted over the next few years.

Myomectomy in infertility was reported in 1975; this stimulated several other reports of similar conditions and successes. Symptoms of large myomas included stress incontinence. Tomographic studies of these tumors were done in 1981, and the endocrine relationships of these tumors with the pituitary and ovary were postulated. The analogue of GnRh was investigated as a tool to shrink myomas.

Hysteroscopic removal of submucous myomas was introduced in 1983 and has become very popular. The procedure has been combined with the use of a resectoscope or with the adaptation of the laser for tumor ablation. This has made the procedure much easier for the patient with a minimal hospital stay and no painful incisions. The laser has been used with the laparoscope for pedunculated myomas and in some reports of subserosal and intramural tumors as well. An excellent mastery of intraabdominal laser surgery through the laparoscope is required.

Recent methods for the management of large or symptomatic myomas and those associated with abnormal uterine blood loss have included laparoscopic-assisted excision, morselization, and removal, laser destruction, hysteroscopic internal excision, and hormone treatment for tumor regression. A new method was introduced in 1995 and used again in 1998 in which uterine artery embolization is used with polyvinyl alcohol particles. This technique has been employed in interventional radiology for several years for other purposes. Bilateral artery injection appears to be more effective than unilateral application, and larger alcohol molecules also produce fewer postoperative symptoms. The results are very gratifying, and if long-term observation does not reveal a high level of recurrence or growth of additional tumors, the procedure has great potential merit. Extensive necrosis may produce large fluid masses that, if symptomatic and febrile, can lead to hysterectomy and exploratory laparotomy. Arterial embolization should be performed by an interventional radiologist.

PROCEDURES
Surgery of the Vagina

The conditions of the vagina for which primary surgery is indicated include benign tumors, cysts, malignancy, endometriosis, and local abscesses in the vaginal wall. Other surgical conditions that engage the vagina are in association with adjacent organs and pelvic relaxation, congenital anomalies, and posttraumatic residual problems.

Benign tumors of the vagina have been managed by sharp and blunt dissection and excision; many are removed by Bovie cautery or, more recently, the laser. Retention cysts in old vaginal lacerations or incisions are removed by local excision.

Vaginal malignancy has been treated by surgery almost exclusively in the twentieth century and only under very strict protocols. Olshausen in 1895 introduced a procedure for extirpation of the vagina for primary malignancy, and a

few total vaginectomies were performed in the early 1900s. By the middle 1900s, the treatment of choice was irradiation, but it has been suggested that low-placed cancers could be treated much the same as carcinoma of the vulva. Total vaginectomy with pelvic exenteration has been performed since the invention of the Bricker ileal loop bladder. Total vaginectomy for severe adenosis has been suggested since the importance of eradicating this potentially premalignant lesion, particularly in diethylstilbestrol (DES)–exposed young women, was realized. Total vaginectomy with radical hysterectomy has been performed successfully for clear cell adenocarcinoma. Partial vaginectomy for confined carcinoma in situ of the vagina has been recommended in contemporary times.

Metastatic malignant lesions, most commonly from endometrial carcinoma, have been managed by combined vaginectomy and radical hysterectomy with or without lymphadenectomy, but several oncologists favor irradiation for such lesions. Other metastatic lesions such as melanoma, choriocarcinoma, or breast carcinoma usually are managed conservatively unless radical surgery is thought to be the best therapeutic method. Endometriosis of the vagina is probably best treated by wide excision, especially if it is in or near the adjacent bladder or rectum. Use of the laser in the past 15 years has been helpful in the treatment of vaginal endometriosis. Local abscesses are incised and drained with added antibiotic therapy.

Surgery of the Cervix

The cervix is the most abused organ in the female genital tract. From the earliest of times, some form of treatment of cervical disease has been used. Growths of the cervix were removed, and many applications of various medications were common. Leeches were used in the genital tract for treatment of cervical disease. Archigenes treated cervical carcinoma by surgery; there is a question as to the use of hysterectomy for that purpose, but this was probably amputation of the cancerous cervix; blood loss was probably controlled by cautery.

Soranus identified the cervix even more accurately than his predecessors; it may be that many reported prolapsed uteri were primarily the cervix. Polybos, Hippocrates' son, clearly described the cervix in the first written text of gynecology ever recorded. Galen stated that midwives examined the cervix for diagnostic purposes, spoke of cervical "erosion," and quoted Celsus on the use of gold or silver dilators to dilate the cervix and also to hold the vagina open after surgery.

Aetios described cervical stenosis, laceration, ulcer (erosion), and spongy tents to dilate the cervix; ligated polyps with waxed silk thread; and stated that cervical carcinoma was incurable.

Cophon from Salerno described the cervix and its orifice; it was open in intercourse and closed in pregnancy. He identified it as a site for sexual pleasure, and he was the originator of the term "seven-celled uterus." Lanfranchi, the father of French surgery, described the dilation of a hard cervix with sounds made of lead; in some cases, it was necessary to incise as well as dilate. The first accurate delineation of the cervical canal was by Eustachio. Fallopio detailed a description of the cervix and stated that it should never be included as part of the vagina.

In the eighteenth century, interest in anatomy expanded again. Verheyen properly used the term *fundus*, wrote of a fundal-cervical sphincter, and identified the cervical mucosa. Bianchi and Naboth both described the rugae of the cervical canal; the latter identified the occlusion cysts that carry his name.

This was an era of preoccupation with cervical and uterine polyps. Literally hundreds of complicated instruments were created for polyp removal. Polyps were excised, crushed, cauterized, and ligated. No hysterectomies for cervical carcinoma were authenticated, but amputations were done, obviously without a cure. Of interest is that no mention of hemostasis was made in any of these reports.

The instruments used in cervical surgery carried exotic names: *ecraseur, uterotomist, uteroceps, hysterotomist,* and *hysterotome*. Despite a myriad of vaginal speculae invented at this time, cervical amputation was barbaric; the cervix was exposed by use of a speculum, it was grasped with a double-toothed Museaux vulsellum, the speculum was then removed, and by slow and heavy traction the cervix was pulled down external to the vulva! This task commonly took 20 to 30 minutes to complete. Many women died of hemorrhage. Amputation fortunately did not persist and yielded instead to an even more potentially hazardous operation known as vaginal hysterectomy.

The mid-nineteenth century was marked by an explosion in gynecologic surgery. Baker-Brown wrote the first definitive book on gynecologic surgery in 1854; in it, only cervical stenosis, polyps, and cancer were considered. Many new instruments were devised to facilitate removal of the cervix especially for cancer, but these were still bloody and without adequate hemostasis. De L'Isere invented very complicated devices to amputate or crush the cervix.

Cautery amputation began to be used for conditions other than cancer (e.g., prolapse). Sims was the first to cover the cervical stump with mucous membrane. Lisfranc pulled the cervix down to the vulva for amputation by use of Muzeux forceps. The operation lost favor but once more was brought back with the performance of excision of cone-shaped tissue in the late 1800s, probably the precursor of the cone biopsy.

In 1950, a proposal was made for a plastic procedure to treat the incompetent cervix. This involved a surgical reduction of the widespread internal cervical os by local excision and application of sutures. In 1952, a cervical ligation was done with a strip of fascia lata to reinforce a damaged or congenitally abnormal cervix that could not hold a pregnancy past the fifth month. A strip of exocervix was denuded for about 1 cm and closed with catgut.

In 1965, Benson and Durfee introduced the idea of abdominal cervical cerclage in pregnancy when the vaginal procedure was not possible. Several other modifications of cerclage followed the original. One was very simple and ef-

fective, employing a heavy suture in and out of the tissue. One advantage of this was that it could be cut and removed when the patient was ready for labor. Different kinds of foreign material have been used for cerclage: nylon, horsehair, heavy silk (Wurm procedure), and Mersilene. Glass or plastic ring pessaries also have been used to hold the cervix closed, but it is difficult to keep them at the proper level. An inflatable silicone cuff has been applied to the internal cervical os, and Smith-Hodge pessaries also have been used with some success.

Several modifications of cerclage have been introduced in the past 15 to 25 years, none of which is much of an improvement over the original operation.

The use of a vertical position to serve as a method for cervical shortening has been proposed. In patients who had been diagnosed with a shortened cervix by vaginal ultrasound in the supine position, greater shortening was demonstrated in the vertical position. This led to consideration of expectant treatment of either bed rest or cerclage. In other patients with no evidence of a shortened cervix, no difference in cervical length was noted in the vertical position. This is another clue as to the possible progression of early cervical integrity failure accentuated by the pull of gravity.

Interest has increased in transabdominal cervical cerclage in patients who are not candidates for vaginal cervical cerclage and who have repeated failed pregnancies due to early spontaneous cervical dilation with a residual short cervical canal. The tape can be placed during pregnancy or in some cases in the nonpregnant state. Despite its risk, cerlage may be easier to perform during the fourteenth to sixteenth of gestation because then it is easier to delineate the anatomy of the upper cervix and the level of the uterine arteries. The procedure has stood the test of time and is definitely indicated in some cases.

Cervix Conization

The first to suggest a circular excision of the central cervix was Lisfranc in 1815, but not until Emmet in 1874 was this recognized as an important procedure. Hyams in 1928 suggested electroconization; Ayre devised a special knife for the purpose of a cone biopsy (1948); and Sturmdorf in 1961 devised a method for covering the raw surface, which has stood the test of time.

Several attempts have been made to improve the occlusion of the defect in the cervix that remains after conization, but none of them has been entirely successful. A modification of the original Sturmdorf procedure is still widely used.

Recently, cylindrical conization by the laser has been used extensively. Bellina and Baggish have emphasized how important it is that the careful exact technique of laser tissue removal be done to preserve a usable specimen for the pathologist. Those areas that remain apparently epithelialize readily, eliminating the problem of a proper mucosal cover.

Since approximately 1988 Townsend and others have used another method for conization that employs a high-frequency electrical loop for incision of a portion of the external cervix for examination. This method has several advocates, but the skill and agility of the operator are still the most important factors because it is very easy to overheat the tissue sample. LEEP, as it is called, has an excellent therapeutic application in superficial cervical lesions.

Surgery of the Ovaries

The East Indians performed laparotomies and bilateral ovarian extirpation for "control of lust"; this operation is claimed to have been done for the Lydian kings to control "oversexed" women. Other historians have stated that the operation was done for hypersexuality even many years later.

Ovarian excision was apparently practiced in the 1500s, but there are no details. Australian natives also removed ovaries.

Houston (1701) performed a partial ovarian cystectomy and evacuated a great deal of material through a 4-inch incision, which had been enlarged a little at a time. When the cyst had been entirely emptied, the base of it was sutured to the abdominal wall. Hunter advocated removal of an ovarian cyst but did not actually do it. Pott removed an ovary that was in a hernial sac in 1756. Ovarian cysts were tapped through the vagina in 1760 and 1777; a cyst that obstructed the pelvis in a woman in labor was drained through the vagina in 1815; in the same year, a cyst was drained through the rectum.

Theden recorded the first ovariectomy in 1771, but this went largely unnoticed. Theden outlined the use of an inguinal incision, exposure of the cyst, puncture, evacuation, delivery of the sac, and ligation of the pedicle; this was a definitely proper method for the operation. McDowell, who has been called the "father of abdominal surgery," created a landmark in surgery in 1809 by a successful extirpation of an ovarian cyst without anesthesia; he sutured the ovarian pedicle to the abdominal incision for drainage. In 1821, Smith did an ovariotomy, without knowing of McDowell's technique. He sutured the pedicle and dropped it into the abdomen. All bleeding points, as well as the pedicle, were sutured with leather sutures. Clearly he was ahead of his time as to the details of the technique. Eight years later, Rogers ligated the pedicle vessels separately and tied each with animal suture.

Simpson coined the term *ovariotomy* in 1844, and the operation became fairly common in the United States and Europe.

Wells was the great ovariotomist of England. He achieved a high success rate not only because of his meticulous technique but also because of his high regard for cleanliness. He invented a clamp for the ovarian pedicle, then created a forci-pressure clamp for arteries. Tait, another great English gynecologic surgeon, devised many methods for ovarian surgery and performed many gynecologic operations, including the first laparotomy for ectopic pregnancy (1837).

For the remainder of the century, the only additions to the procedure were to leave the ligated ovarian pedicle in the abdominal cavity and eventually use the peritoneum to cover it.

Wedge resection for polycystic ovarian disease was common for about 40 years in the 1900s but has lost favor in view of endocrine management of the problem. Excision of endometriomas expanded with increased knowledge of that disease. Procedures for ovarian suspension have waxed and waned over the years, with very clear indications only in modern times. Ovarian transplantation into the uterine wall in certain cases of infertility was popular in the middle years, but complications have almost eliminated the procedure.

Surgery can be curative for stage Ia grade I ovarian carcinoma, but the diagnosis must be certain. Preservation of the contralateral ovary in these cases has become very controversial; in general, it may be limited to young women who desire to maintain fertility, and even then in only very carefully selected cases with clear recognition of the risks. Many surgeons believe the diagnosis must establish a well-differentiated mucinous malignancy to justify the risk. Bilateral ovarian excision with hysterectomy is the most accepted treatment today.

Omentectomy in the obvious absence of metastases in ovarian carcinoma is also a contentious subject and may be a matter of judgment. Until the latter part of the 1900s, lymph node dissection either for excision or for a diagnostic sample was usually not performed, but with the advent of magnetic resonance imaging (MRI) and computed tomography (CT) scans, positive nodes are more common than formerly believed; therefore, node dissection is now included in surgery for ovarian carcinoma. Peritoneal cell samples are mandatory at the start of any laparatomy for ovarian carcinoma or even suspected disease. Since 1950, the second-look operation has become common but is still controversial; laparoscopy is not as reliable or successful as second-look operation.

Operations to debulk massive amounts of tumor have evolved over the past 50 years and are still a part of the surgical approach.

The application of a special catheter into the peritoneal cavity to implement improved direct dosage of chemotherapeutic agents has been another recent innovation. Bilateral ovarian excision was highly recommended for several years for breast carcinoma, but this is no longer generally performed. It is still generally accepted to remove the ovaries in all but very early cases of endometrial carcinoma.

Placement of the ovary in an accessible location for harvest of ova for IVF or GIFT programs has been common since 1975. Ovarian transplants, both autogenous or donor, have not realized accountability. Microsurgical lysis of adhesions with or without the laser has greatly improved ovarian reclamation.

Despite all surgical efforts to treat ovarian malignancy, success has not improved greatly, but some changes in overall management combined with some laparoscopic techniques, such as retroperitoneal exploration and lymphadenectomy, have improved the outcome of the disease.

One of the most controversial subjects is the prophylactic use of ovariectomy at the time of hysterectomy. Positive indications are a strong family history of ovarian cancer, avoidance of postsurgical pelvic pain and dyspareunia with residual ovaries, abolishing the ovarian cycle syndrome, and the avoidance of potentially benign cystic changes that may become symptomatic or cause concern of possible malignancy. Conversely, women with no history of ovarian cancer who wish to retain their ovaries may not opt for castration. This attitude fails to acknowledge the many problems related to postmenopausal uterine bleeding, which, of course, is not a factor with hysterectomy. Some women may wish to preserve reproductive capacity even when ovariectomy for bilateral endometriosis is indicated; this leaves an intact uterus so that modern methods of artificial insemination with ovarian donors is more and more possible. Some researchers believe the intact ovary, even after menopause, still produces some hormones that otherwise would be lacking. Usually ovarian removal is performed in women older than 45 years of age, except in women who have severe disease, such as pelvic inflammatory disease or endometriosis with ovarian involvement, or those who have a persistent tendency to form benign bilateral ovarian cysts. In the absence of any real indication for ovarian removal, the patient's attitude is an important consideration, since the psychologic effect of castration can be powerful.

Clomiphene and other ovulation-stimulating drugs are preferred in the treatment of polycystic ovarian disease. When these have failed, the next choice was abdominal ovarian wedge resection. Diathermy or several kinds of laser application are now used with variable success. Ovarian drilling can be accomplished by either the laser or diathermy. Some findings indicate that diathermy produces more adhesions, but in general more ovulatory successes are achieved with electrocautery.

Hormonal treatment of small benign endometriotic lesions diagnosed by laparoscopy and laparoscopic laser ablation of abnormal residual tissue constitute the method of choice for treating such lesions. Ovarian suspension is another procedure that lends itself to laparoscopy.

Surgical Treatment of Vulvar Disease

Surgery for diseases of the vulva is derived from ancient medicine. Amputation of a hypertrophied clitoris is found in medical literature over the past 2000 years. Excision of external growth and pedunculated tumors and incision and drainage of abscesses are among the few gynecologic operations performed for over 1000 years.

Specific extensive removal of vulvar tissue was first accomplished by Basset for clitoral carcinoma in 1912. Taussig in 1929 introduced the importance of recognizing lymphatic metastases and lymphadenectomy. Conservative surgery for vulvar disease involved local excision and inguinal gland resection for melanoma unless the disease was extensive and deeply invasive. Pringle was among the first to discuss surgery for melanoma (1908). Conservative excision of superficial, confined, microinvasive carcinoma has been a method of choice.

The "skinning vulvectomy" was used for carcinoma precursors and for extensive symptomatic benign diseases. Simple vulvectomy has been the method of choice for sev-

eral lesions, including carcinoma in situ, for the past 40 years. A modified simple vulvectomy has been used for intractable irritation and itch, as has intraepithelial injection with alcohol.

Extensive radical vulvectomy with inguinal gland resection and deep iliac lymph gland resection has also been used. Exenteration procedures that included the vulva and the vagina have been performed.

Combined irradiation and surgery has had mixed results. In extensive malignant vulvar or Bartholin's gland involvement, wide radical vulvectomy with exenteration has been suggested.

Transsexual surgery with successful conversion of otherwise normal males to females was of interest in the 1960s. In the early 1950s, a team composed of a urologist, a gynecologist, and a plastic surgeon and directed by a psychiatric expert in transsexualism performed these conversion operations. Acceptable, functional external female genitalia and vagina were produced in genetic males with the otherwise unsolvable problem of confused sex identification. The knowledge gained from these procedures has helped immeasurably with plastic operations required because of burns or trauma in contemporary gynecology.

Recent reports of rare basal cell cancer of the vulva have found it is often diagnosed late and also has low mortality. Local excision is the treatment of choice. Cases of local extension probably require lymphadenectomy. Recurrence may be treated with further excision if the patient can tolerate it, otherwise irradiation must be used.

One of the most difficult problems in gynecology is the persistence of symptoms of vestibulitis after previous surgery. Therefore conservative therapy of all kinds should be initially attempted. Inadequate surgery is usually the main reason for most of these failures. It has been more successful to extend the primary incision line halfway down the perineum toward the anus and advance the vagina to facilitate closure of the wound. The remaining scar is thus inside the introitus, so dyspareunia due to an exterior scar also is inside the vagina. The psychologic trauma caused by the irritation of the disease must be kept in mind, as well as the interruption of sexual intercourse, with resultant general abnormal response of the pelvic muscles. Many patients need psychologic assistance.

Plastic Surgery

Uterine Reunification. Plastic surgery of the uterus consists of the correction of intrauterine adhesions or synechiae, especially repair of the cavity that remains after myomectomy and of congenital anomalies. Although Fritsch first described uterine cavity adhesions in 1894, Asherman between 1948 and 1957 established the entire syndrome, which generally carries his name.

Hysteroscopic lysis of intracavitary adhesions is now accepted as the method of choice for management and treatment of this problem.

Excision of a rudimentary uterine horn and surgical correction of similar anomalies were done if indicated; on occasion, abdominal hysterectomy was performed. Rudimentary horns have been fused or unified by excision and suturing. Diagnosis of a true bicornuate uterus may be made, and a classification of the variants together with the septate uterus is very valuable in the selection of treatment. In 1907, a unification operation for a double, as well as a true and partial bicornuate uterus, was introduced and proved very effective; it was later moderately modified and proved to be not as applicable to septate uteri. Wedge excision and plastic repair of various types of septate uteri were also introduced; these operations became the standard for plastic uterine reunification.

Recent operations for correction of congenital defects of the uterus have used both hysteroscopy and laparoscopy, with ultrasound employed for establishing diagnosis. Direct surgery is performed in the uterine cavity with resection of partial and complete uterine septae. The results have been very good. Blood loss can be a problem, but proper use of hemostatic cautery usually controls it. Laparoscopic surgery has been used to correct uterus didelphys and variants thereof, which only requires the placement of an intrauterine device from below to hold the healing uterine cavity open.

Creation of a Neovagina. Preliminary work was done in the 1880s to construct a neovagina. The advent of antibiotics, increased information about the use of skin grafts and intravaginal molds, and the apparent success with bowel transplantation paved the way for the invention of many procedures. Frank in 1940 proposed a method for creation of a neovagina that used dilators of increased size and length to invert the external tissue between the rectum and the urethra into a vaginal "pit." In 1977, Broadbent used a modification of this method, and Ingram in 1981 proposed the ingenious idea of using a bicycle seat with vertical dilators of various sizes placed so that the patient's weight would cause the desired penetration of the tissues of the area.

The surgical methods have frequently been very complicated, especially those using bowel transplantation. Skin flaps from the thighs and labia have been turned into a potential vaginal space. In 1895, Abbe created a procedure using an obturator and a skin graft that was highly successful; it was redescribed by McIndoe in 1938 and is one of the preferred methods in contemporary gynecology. Among the many variations is the stimulation of tissue growth over a mold. A vulvovaginal pouch that functioned externally as a vagina suitable for intercourse was especially useful in exenteration cases.

Hysterectomy

Hysterectomy, which was the proper term for any uterine extirpation, was introduced by Tillaux in 1879 and is the accepted designation.

Vaginal Hysterectomy through the Nineteenth Century. Surgical procedures on the cervix preceded the evolution of vaginal hysterectomy, which was not performed until after a long period of experimentation with various medical therapies and many operations. These included amputations for all possible problems, among them carcinoma.

Vaginal hysterectomy for malignancy was first done in 1813. Recamier in 1829 performed a successful vaginal hys-

terectomy but injured the bladder. He was the first to consider the possibility of injury to the ureter in performance of the operation and to realize the importance of systematic ligation of the vessels and attention to a secure ligation of the ligaments of the uterus; in fact, vaginal hysterectomy has been named "Recamier's operation." Recamier held the severed uterine ligaments with his left hand and passed a curved needle mounted on a handle threaded with a strong suture to secure the tissues.

An improved method that included anesthesia, hemostasis, and antisepsis was developed and probably was the first operation for vaginal extirpation of a myomatous uterus. It also promoted the use of vaginal hysterectomy for benign conditions.

From the late 1890s to the early 1900s there was a division in the approach to pelvic operations. Vaginal and abdominal surgeons almost never used the alternative method, but, with time, most surgeons used both.

Schauta in 1890 performed a radical vaginal hysterectomy for cervical carcinoma and continued the procedure as late as 1909 in direct competition with the abdominal operation of Wertheim. Schauta incorporated the deep perineal incision introduced by Schuchardt in 1894. In that same year, Richelot in Paris published a text on vaginal hysterectomy and outlined nine benign indications for the operation. Benign conditions were now included more and more as indications for vaginal extirpation of the uterus.

The clamp operation was promoted by Hunter in New York in 1889; he left as many as 14 pairs of clamps attached to vessels and ligaments (Fig. 1-7).

Vaginal Hysterectomy in the Twentieth Century. By the turn of the century, vaginal hysterectomy had begun to be an acceptable surgical procedure. Vaginal techniques were extremely varied and included the use of clamps alone, step-by-step ligation of small amounts of tissue and all ves-

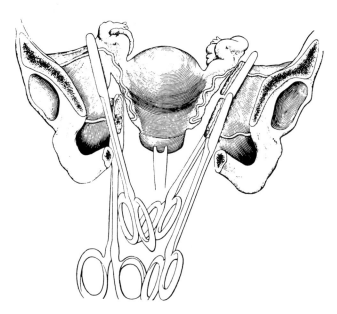

Fig. 1-7 Hysterectomy by clamp method, no ligatures or sutures. (From Pozzi S: *A treatise on gynecology,* vol 2, London, 1893, New Sydenham Society.)

sels, use of braided Chinese silk or catgut, and use of cautery in place of a scalpel. There were as many variations in closure of the operative area as there were in the extirpation of the uterus and adnexa. By 1903, Pryor introduced clamps with detachable handles, which were removed at the completion of the operation and provided more postoperative comfort for the patient. Kennedy and Price reportedly did thousands of vaginal hysterectomies by the clamp method from 1918 to 1927. By 1909, Schauta had perfected his radical vaginal hysterectomy.

Heany in 1934 introduced a technique for vaginal hysterectomy that has endured the passage of time and is the basic technical method for the operations (Fig. 1-8). Lash in 1941 proposed a method for reduction of uterine size that removed the myometrium and left a shell of uterine tissue, which could easily be removed. In 1942, Heaney secured the details of Lash's operation and indicated vaginal repair at the same time. The clear practical aspects of his technique cannot be denied.

Throughout the late 1940s, most of the 1950s, and then through the 1960s, many reports were published by many well-respected gynecologic surgeons in the United States.

In 1952, Ricci and Thom clearly identified the difference between total prolapse of the pelvic organs and a simulated condition of persistent hypertrophy and elongation of the cervix.

In 1953, Tauber presented his "stump stitch." Allen led in the use of vaginal hysterectomy, using preoperative curettage and an immediate posterior colpotomy to explore the

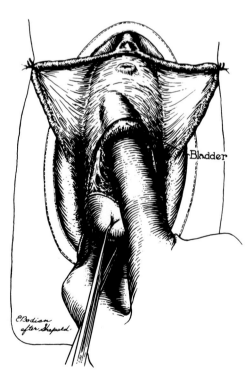

Fig. 1-8 Vaginal hysterectomy—start of dissection. (From Mattingly R, Thompson J: *Operative gynecology,* ed 6, Philadelphia, 1985, JB Lippincott.)

pelvis, both of which prevented many serious mistakes. There were many modifications in the procedure and several reports of complications. The use of drains in the operative area was considered, and the concept of preoperative and postoperative antibiotics, which still has not been resolved, was introduced.

In 1957, McCall popularized the important contribution of imbrication of the sacrouterine ligaments and obliteration of the cul-de-sac after uterine removal, which prevented the development of postoperative enterocele.

In 1958, Werner and Sederl wrote on abdominal surgery by the vaginal route.

In 1959, Mitra presented his radical vaginal hysterectomy for cervical carcinoma combined with an extraperitoneal lymph gland dissection.

In 1962, Hofmeister and Wolfgram extensively studied anatomic variance in the relationship of the ureter in the cardinal ligament to the clamps and sutures of hysterectomy.

In the mid-1970s, recommendation was made for routine placement of a T-tube in the operative area for 24 hours, suggesting that there is some degree of accumulation of bloody fluid under the flaps and tissues that is invariably a source of infection. Suction drainage of the same areas had been suggested 10 years before. There has been considerable opposition to drains after this operation. About the same time, obesity was noted as an indication for the vaginal operation instead of the abdominal approach, because there is a much lower morbidity with the former.

Today, by use of the advances over the past 25 years, detailed techniques of vaginal hysterectomy have been developed by many operators. Injection with saline or hemostatic medications before the initial incisions in the vaginal mucosa have reduced operative blood loss. The newer synthetic suture materials have greatly improved the postoperative recovery, which, when combined with preoperative and postoperative prophylactic antibiotics, have made this almost an outpatient procedure. In the 1990s, vaginal hysterectomy combined with laparoscopic dissection of the uterine ligaments, with the exception of the cardinal ligaments and uterine arteries, has broadened the indications for vaginal hysterectomy.

Abdominal Hysterectomy. Abdominal hysterectomy was derived from laparotomy and, to some degree, from vaginal hysterectomy. It was based on Guterblat's combined vaginal and abdominal operation (1813), which was followed by Delpech in 1830 and by others who used the combined approach.

The early history of this operation is divided by the evolution of its use in benign versus malignant disease.

Abdominal Hysterectomy for Benign Disease. The first abdominal hysterectomies for benign disease (myomata) followed the experience of Lizars (1825), Atlee (1849), and others, all of whom had begun a laparotomy for ovarian cysts and found large, multiple myomata that caused them to abandon the procedure. Clay (1843) and Heath (1845) performed uterine amputation at the level of the internal cervical os for myomas; Clay removed the adnexa bilaterally with the uterus and thus carried out the first so-called panhysterectomy.

Schroder in 1878 introduced intraperitoneal management of the cervical stump (Fig. 1-9). An important step in this procedure was destruction of the mucous portion of the cervical canal using either Paquelin's cautery or strong carbolic acid; the cervical stump was then carefully sutured with silk and catgut sutures to achieve secure closure.

Bardenhauer in 1881 performed a total abdominal hysterectomy and left the ligament ligatures to drain into the vagina. This report included an account of a broad transverse abdominal incision that extended nearly from one anterior superior spine to the other, which preceded all other transverse incisions that transected the rectus muscles.

Although hysterectomy for carcinoma may have been questionably acceptable, total hysterectomy for treatment of benign disease was even more questionable.

In an effort to decrease mortality, Fritsch in 1886 curetted a carcinoma and packed the uterus with iodoform gauze, using a permanganate wash in other situations. Freund in 1888 performed hysterectomy for myomata, used iodoform gauze, placed drains as indicated, and advocated bilateral excision of the ovaries when the operation was not considered possible. Martin in 1889 suggested oil-soaked sponges for protection of the intestines, used a temporary elastic ligature, freed the cervix through the vagina, and removed the uterus abdominally. Clifford used an ecraseur for supravaginal operations in 1889. Chrobak in 1891 shelled the uterus out of the serosa and amputated it very low into the cervix, leaving just a ring of tissue, and sutured the serosa to it. He achieved great success with this operation.

Abdominal Hysterectomy for Malignancy. Apparently, the first total hysterectomy for carcinoma of the cervix was performed by Jones in the United States in 1867. In 1878, Freund reported a total hysterectomy for cervical carcinoma; his outline of the technique was remarkably progressive in that the procedure was highly disciplined with attention to the details of hemostasis and asepsis. Schroeder in 1879 did a total hysterectomy and vaginectomy for carcinoma.

Freund's later operations for uterine fundal carcinoma were done as a combined procedure with the cervix freed vaginally and the uterus and cervix then removed abdominally. In 1880, Rydygier revived the combined operation, freed the cervix through the vagina, placed the patient in Trendelenburg's position, and used a midline incision. In cases where the rectus muscles were rigid, he transected them at the insertion on the pubis (clearly a predecessor to the Cherney incision). Crede excised part of the abdominal wall in such cases; when more space was needed, he packed the intestines and, on occasion, eventrated them onto the abdominal wall and kept them warm and wet. In 1889, Martin did a supravaginal hysterectomy first and then removed the cervix through the vagina. As of 1886, the mortality associated with abdominal hysterectomy for carcinoma was more than 67% from the procedure alone.

Abdominal Hysterectomy in the Twentieth Century. The 1900s were the new era not only for hysterectomy for carcinoma, with the Wertheim procedure, but also for the onset of gynecologic surgery at its finest. Wertheim recorded his technique for radical hysterectomy with pelvic lymph node dissection in 1900. This was a classic example of the kind of perfection of technique that came to distinguish gynecologic surgery toward the middle and end of the century.

Abdominal hysterectomy came to be used more frequently for benign diseases in the early 1900s, with indications in myomata, endometriosis and adenomyosis, persistent uterine blood loss, pelvic inflammatory disease, and several less common problems (Fig. 1-10). Worrall in Aus-

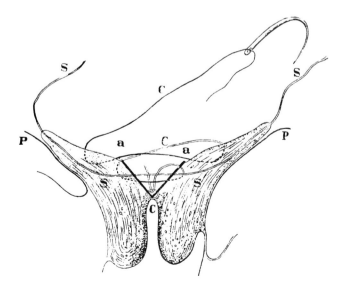

Fig. 1-9 Cervical stump closure at abdominal hysterectomy by Schroeder. (From Pozzi S: *A treatise on gynecology,* vol 1, London, 1896, New Sydenham Society.)

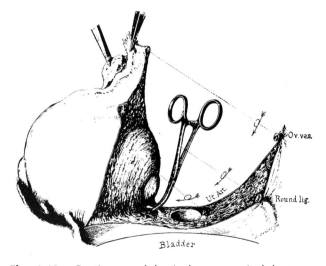

Fig. 1-10 Continuous abdominal supracervical hysterectomy by Kelly. (From Kelly H: *Operative gynecology,* vol 2, New York, 1902, D Appleton.)

tralia devised the first intrafascial abdominal hysterectomy in 1914, and Masson at the Mayo Clinic in 1927 reported on a similar operation. Richardson in 1929 standardized the technique for hysterectomy on which almost all other such operations are based (Fig. 1-11); he further described a form of "intrafascial" dissection technique that employed a T-shaped incision in the pericervical fascia, facilitating its identification. The Mayo operation, patterned somewhat on Richardson, became a popular procedure by 1947 but was an extrafascial operation, as most hysterectomies are now.

In the 1940s, Meigs perfected the radical hysterectomy in the United States. By 1948, Brunschwig published details of his extensive exenteration with radical hysterectomy for cervical cancer; this was involved and consisted of removal of the pelvic organs, which included both bladder and rectum with the vagina and internal genitalia, with extensive lymph node dissection and the creation of abdominal stomas for both urine and fecal streams. His eventration of the intestines is a reminder of the work done in the 1800s.

Hysterectomy remained more or less static, with great improvements in mortality and morbidity primarily as a result of the judicious application of antibiotic medications. The advent of the surgical clip was the newest innovation in hysterectomy in several decades. The use of clips for intestinal anastomosis was introduced by the Russians and used extensively in the United States but saw only limited application in hysterectomy. In 1968, staples were used to close the vagina in abdominal hysterectomy, supposedly isolating

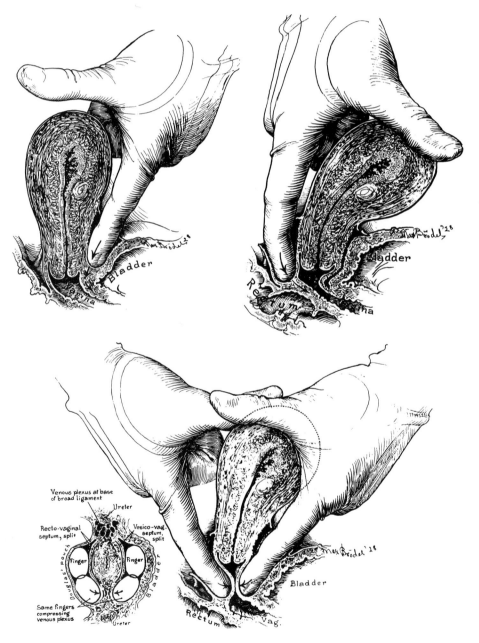

Fig. 1-11 The Richardson abdominal hysterectomy. (From Richardson EH: *A simplified abdominal panhysterectomy,* Chicago, 1929, Surgical Publishers of Chicago.)

the vagina from the surgical field before the uterus and cervix were removed. By 1977, problems were noted with the metal staples in the apex of the vagina, namely, severe dyspareunia. Absorbable ligature clips were introduced and applied to vaginal closure with much greater success.

The first to perform a hysterectomy with cesarean section was Storer in Boston in 1876. He was literally forced to do this operation because of hemorrhage after delivery of the child caused by the presence of myomata. This was a supravaginal operation. Unfortunately, the patient died about 3 days postoperatively.

In the past 6 or 7 years, interest has increased in laparoscopically assisted hysterectomy; this is composed of a dissection of the round, broad, uteroovarian, and sometimes uterosacral ligaments through a laparoscope, in the 1990s with the use of clips. Once this has been accomplished, the cervix is dissected through the vagina, the cardinal ligaments are secured, the uterine vessels are also ligated vaginally, and the total hysterectomy is completed from below. This is an interesting exercise; the overall advantages, if any, are still to be realized.

Confusion has surfaced regarding the terminology used to describe assisted hysterectomy. If one removes the pelvic organs by small abdominal incisions with tissue dissection down to the uterine artery level and then completes the operation through the vagina by a technique similar to vaginal hysterectomy, is such an operation an assisted vaginal hysterectomy or an assisted abdominal hysterectomy? If the cardinal ligaments and the uterine arteries are dissected and ligated abdominally with removal of the cervix vaginally, then this is primarily an abdominal operation. On the other hand, if the adnexal structures and the round and broad ligaments are only excised and ligated abdominally and the base of the broad ligaments and the cardinal ligaments, which include the uterine arteries, are incised and ligated vaginally with ultimate uterine removal by that route, the operation technically is an assisted vaginal hysterectomy.

Although terminology may not be important, some delineation of technique and consistent use of terms make for clarity in recording. Although these procedures have been criticized, a properly selected and performed hysterectomy by the combined method definitely reduces postoperative morbidity, discomfort, and length of hospital stay and allows for a less painful recovery with an improved return to normal life.

Abdominal hysterectomy through a small or minilaparotomy has been performed by Hoffman and Lynch. A small number of selected patients had a total abdominal hysterectomy and bilateral salpingo-oophorectomy performed through 6 cm incision either transverse or low vertical without any obvious difficulty. The fascial incision was extended in some cases beyond the length of the skin incision. Recovery was noted as being better than for standard procedures. For those not inclined to perform laparoscopically assisted hysterectomy, this may prove to be an acceptable abdominal hysterectomy and is certainly an innovative change.

In a recent collaborative study, Hillis et al. found that women who had been sterilized had an increased incidence of hysterectomy (4.6 to 7.9). This apparently was caused by several factors, among which was the type of sterilization. The highest incidence was found in those with partial or complete salpingectomy, and the lowest was in those with a ring. Aside from obvious reasons, it appears that women who have had surgery are inclined to elect hysterectomy for the management of other gynecologic problems.

Careful choice of the type of pelvic operation creates an improved result. This is evidenced by some improvement in the postoperative recovery of patients who undergo radical surgery for malignancy. Recovery is enhanced by judicious management of the bowel, absolute hemostasis with retroperitoneal lymphadenectomy, minimal manipulation of both bladder and the ureters, and minimal peritonization whenever possible.

Surgery for Vesicourinary Incontinence

Identification and classification of various urination situations were correlated with proper terminology before 1980. Enhorning established the urethral closure pressure profile in 1981.

Cystometry, electromyography, and microtransducers were introduced; simultaneous measurement of intravesical and intraurethral pressures was made possible. This work helped establish a postresidency fellowship in gynecologic urology.

Robertson in the 1970s devised a straight urethroscope based, in part, on the previous Kelly air cystoscope, which used CO_2 for bladder distention and provided a direct internal observation of the bladder neck and urethrovesical junction at all phases of the urination process; it also provided direct observation of the urethra throughout its entire length. It serves as a cystoscope as well and is used for urethrocystometrogram studies. The patient is in the lithotomy position, which preserves the normal anatomic relationships.

Diagnostic procedures were evaluated, and three important areas were noted: (1) the value of the Q-tip test, (2) the importance of the history with a description of urination in the patient's own words, and (3) the physical examination designed specifically to identify neurologic, muscular, and anatomic defects in incontinence cases. The Bonney stress test with upward movement of the vaginal wall was used to determine if anatomic replacement would solve the problem of stress urinary loss. Other studies included the use of posterior downward pull on the perineum with a Sims speculum or the posterior blade of Graves, the levator test, cystometry, urethral pressure profiles, electromyelography, uroflowmetry, radiographic studies such as urination video cystograms, and the use of direct cystoscopy.

In 1907, George R. White described transvaginal reattachment of the anterior vaginal fornix to the arcus tendineus as a treatment for cystocele. This concept is not unlike the transabdominal paravaginal fixation operation. Kelly first illustrated his suture in 1911, and it is still the basis for most vaginal repairs of cystocele and urinary incontinence due to stress. Kennedy added an important procedure to these repairs in suggesting reinforcement of the integrity of the posterior length of the urethra. The invention of polyglycolic suture material has improved anterior vaginal repairs if for no other reason than the elimination of much of the scar tissues. In the last 15 years, various authors have reported greater than 90% success with the basic Kelly-Kennedy vaginal repair in the treatment of urinary stress incontinence, but these results are not universal.

Furniss was the first in the 1900s to attempt suprapubic suspension of the vagina and urethra. The Marshal-Marchetti-Krantz (MMK) suprapubic elevation of the anterior vaginal wall, and with it the urethra (after some modification), has been highly successful since 1949. Burch in 1968 attached the suspension sutures to Cooper's ligament, also with success; however, even if popular because it is relatively easier, it is not anatomically correct. Various modifications of these procedures have been developed. Durfee simplified the MMK operation and facilitated suprapubic cystocele obliteration by the placement of vaginal suspension sutures in the undersurface of the cartilaginous central portion of the symphysis as well as one bilaterally to the condensed connective tissue of the obturator orifices.

Suspension of the urethrovesical region by a supportive "strap" of strong permanent tissue was another approach to the problem. Goebell demonstrated a "sling" operation using strips of abdominal rectus muscle fascia, which he brought down under the urethrovesical area and used to elevate the tissues anteriorly in 1910; this was modified later by Stoeckel and Frangenheim. Williams and TeLinde used a narrow synthetic strap for this purpose in 1962 but had to abandon it because of trauma to the undersurface to the bladder and urethra. A high percentage of these operations are unsatisfactory because of obstruction due to excessive scar formation.

Transplantation of other tissues under the relaxed anterior vaginal wall was attempted in 1918 by Taussig, who used tissues from the levator ani muscles. Other muscles used were the gracilis, the pyramidalis, the bulbocavernosis, and the pubococcygeus.

Procedures in which artificial materials have been used include the epiurethral suprapubic vaginal suspension by Sexton, who used both an artificial tape and a tendon from the forearm as a sling to suspend the vagina by inducing the perivaginal tissues to raise the anterior vaginal wall to the conjoined tendon bilaterally. Moir suggested a 1-inch-wide Mersilene gauze hammock for support of this area. A fibrin bean implantation was performed in 1975. The Politano procedure consists of endoscopic injection of Teflon under the mucosa of the bladder neck.

Surgical management of detrusor dysfunction was first approached by Ingelman-Sundberg in 1959 when he transsected the infravesical nerves. The key to success in this treatment lies in identifying those patients who will profit from the operations.

Several other exotic procedures have persisted, and there are many pharmaceutical approaches to these problems. The proper surgical procedure accurately and carefully done in cases where the problem has been definitely diagnosed has provided relief for many women.

TUBAL STERILIZATION AND ALTERNATIVE METHODS

Tubal sterilization and tubal ligation were first suggested by Blundell in 1823. Ovarian castration may have been practiced by ancient peoples for sterilization as well as for nymphomania, but this is unsubstantiated. Lungren in 1880 ligated the tubes for the first time. Porro performed a cesarean hysterectomy with the secondary intention of sterilization in 1876; Thomas in 1885 suggested tubal ligation as opposed to Porro's operation. Several surgeons performed the operation over the next 200 years. Duhrssen used a double ligature and was the first to perform tubal ligation by colpotomy. Fehrer and Buettner divided the tubes between two sutures in 1897, and Fritsch in 1897 suggested that at least 1 cm of tubal tissue be removed. Ruhl in 1898 cut the tube 5 cm from the uterus and sutured the ends to a vaginal incision. The tubes were removed at the cornua by Rose in 1898, and the cornual area was sutured closed. Intrauterine cauterization of the tubes was done with the use of silver nitrate and galvanocautery. Uchida's procedure is the most effective.

Laparoscopy in the 1950s led to unipolar electrocoagulation tubal ligation, the Hulka spring clip, the Yoon plastic Falope ring, and bipolar cautery. Laparoscopy is the most popular method of sterilization in nonpregnant or recently pregnant women, although minilaparotomy immediately postpartum has many advocates. Pomeroy ligation with use of a large plain catgut double tie at cesarean section is very satisfactory.

SUGGESTED READING

Baas J: *Outlines of the history of medicine,* 2 vols, Huntington, New York, 1971, R Krieger (Translated by H Handerson).

Baggish M: *Basic and advanced laser surgery in gynecology,* Norwalk, Conn, 1985, Appleton-Century-Crofts.

Baker-Brown I: *Surgical diseases of women,* ed 2, London, 1861, John W Davies.

Baker VV, Deppe G: *Management of perioperative complications in gynecology,* Philadelphia, 1997, WB Saunders.

Benshushan A, Brzezinski A, Shoshani O, Rojansky N: Periurethral injection for the treatment of urinary incontinence, *Obstet Gynecol Surv* 53:383, 1998.

Benson R: *Current obstetric and gynecologic diagnosis and treatment,* Los Altos, Calif, 1978, Lange Medical Publications.

Bhisgratna K: *Sushruta samhita,* ed 2, Varanasi, India, 1963, Chowkhamba Sanskrit Series Office.

Breasted J: *The Edwin Smith surgical papyrus,* Chicago, 1930, University of Chicago Press.

Bonney V: *Gynecological surgery,* ed 3, London, 1974, Balliere & Tindall.

Bornstein J, Goldik Z, Alter Z: Persistent vulvar vestibulitis: the continuing challenge, *Obstet Gynecol Surv* 53:39, 1998.

Brubaker L, Benson JT, Bent A, et al: Transvaginal electrical stimulation for female urinary incontinence, *Am J Obstet Gynecol* 177:536, 1997.

Buchanan DJ, Schlaerth J, Kurosaki T: Primary vaginal melanoma: thirteen-year disease-free survival after wide local excision and review of recent literature, *Am J Obstet Gynecol* 178:1177, 1998.

Bucknell T, Ellis H: *Wound healing for surgeons,* London, 1984, Balliere & Tindall.

Channing W: *A treatise on etherization in childbirth,* London, 1848, W Ticknor (special edition, Birmingham, Ala, 1990, Gryphon editions).

Cohen I, Beyth Y, Tepper R: The role of ultrasound in the detection of endometrial pathologies in asymptomatic postmenopausal breast cancer patients with tamoxifen treatment, *Obstet Gynecol Surv* 53:429, 1998.

Craig S, Fliegner JR: Treatment of cervical incompetence by transabdominal cervicoisthmic cerclage, *Aust N Z J Obstet Gynaecol* 37:407, 1997.

Creasman WT, Zaino RJ, Major FJ, et al: Early invasive carcinoma of the cervix (3 to 5 mm invasion): risk factors and prognosis. A Gynecologic Oncology Group study, *Am J Obstet Gynecol* 178:62, 1998.

Creinin MD, Vittinghoff E, Schaff E, et al: Medical abortion with oral methotrexate and vaginal misoprostol, *Obstet Gynecol* 90:611, 1997.

Cullen T: *Adenomyomata uteri,* New York, 1890, D Appleton.

Cullen T: *Cancer of the uterus,* New York, 1900, D Appleton.

Cushing H, Bovie W: Electro-surgery as an aid to removal of intracranial tumors, *Surg Gynecol Obstet* 47:751, 1928.

Darzi A, et al: *Retroperitoneoscopy,* Oxford, 1996, Isis Medical Media.

DeLancey J, Starr R: Histology of the connection between the vagina and levator ani muscles, *J Reprod Med* 35:765, 1990.

Dionis P: *Cours d'operations de chirugie,* ed 4, Paris, 1750, Chez D'Houry.

Doderlein ASG, Kronig B: *Operative gynakologie,* ed 5, Leipzig, 1924, Georg Thieme.

Doyen C: *Surgical therapeutics and operative technique,* New York, 1917, William Wood (Translated by H Spencer-Browne).

Durfee R: Anterior vaginal suspension operation, *Am J Obstet Gynecol* 78:628, 1959.

Emge L, Durfee R: Pelvic organ prolapse, 4000 years of treatment, *Clin Obstet Gynecol* 4:997, 1961.

Engelmann G: The early history of vaginal hysterectomy, *Am Gynecol Obstet J* 31:521, 1895.

Evans MI, Johnson MC, Moghissi KS: *Invasive outpatient procedures in reproductive medicine,* Philadelphia, 1997, Lippincott-Raven.

Fisk NM, Moise KA Jr: *Fetal therapy,* Cambridge, 1997, Cambridge University Press.

Fong YF, Lim FK, Arulkumaran S: Prophylactic oophorectomy a continuing controversy, *Obstet Gynecol Surv* 53:493, 1998.

Fylstra DL: Tubal pregnancy: a review of current diagnosis and treatment, *Obstet Gynecol Surv* 53:320, 1998.

Garrison F: *An introduction to the history of medicine,* ed 4, Philadelphia, 1929, WB Saunders.

Gomel V: *Microsurgery in female infertility,* Boston, 1983, Little, Brown.

Gomel V: *Laparoscopy and hysteroscopy in gynecologic practice,* Chicago, 1986, Mosby.

Goodwin SC, Vendentham S, McLucas B, et al: Preliminary experience with uterine artery embolization for uterine fibroids, *J Vasc Intervent Radiol* 8:517, 1997.

Gray L: *Vaginal hysterectomy,* ed 3, Springfield, Ill, 1983, Charles C Thomas.

Gupta GH, Dinas K, Khan KS: To peritonealize or not to peritonealize? A randomized trial of abdominal hysterectomy, *Am J Obstet Gynecol* 178:796, 1998.

Hajenius PJ, Engelsbel S, Mol BWJ, et al: Randomised trial of systemic methotrexate versus laparoscopic salpingostomy in tubal pregnancy, *Lancet* 350:774, 1997.

Halban J, Seitz L: *Biologie und Pathologie des Weibes,* Berlin, 1924, Urban & Schwarzenberg.

Halsted W: *Surgical papers,* Baltimore, 1924, Johns Hopkins Press.

Harris RL, Cundiff W, Coates KW, Addison WA: Urethral prolapse after collagen injection, *Am J Obstet Gynecol* 178:614, 1998.

Harris RL, Cundiff GW, Theofrastus JP, et al: The value of intraoperative cystoscopy in urogynecologic and reconstructive pelvic surgery, *Am J Obstet Gynecol* 177:1367, 1997.

Harvey S: *History of hemostasis,* New York, 1929, Paul Hoeber.

Hillis SD, Marchbanks PA, Tylo LR, Peterson HB: Higher hysterectomy risk for sterilized than nonsterilized women: findings from the U.S. Collaborative Review of Sterilization, *Obstet Gynecol* 91:242, 1998.

Hopman EH, Kenemans P, Helmerhorst TJ: Positive predictive rate of colposcopic examination of the cervix uteri: an overview of the literature, *Obstet Gynecol Surv* 53:97, 1998.

Hughes A: *A history of cytology,* London, 1959, Abelard Schuman.

Hunt R: *Atlas of female infertility surgery,* Chicago, 1985, Mosby.

Hunt R, Seigler A: *Hysterosalpingography: techniques and interpretation,* Chicago, 1988, Mosby.

Jaffe R, Abramowicz JS: *Manual of obstetric and gynecologic ultrasound,* Philadelphia, 1997, Lippincott-Raven.

Jones H, Rock J: *Reparative and constructive surgery of the female generative tract,* Baltimore, 1983, Williams & Wilkins.

Kelly H: *Operative gynecology,* ed 2, New York, 1900, Appleton & Co.

Kelly H, Cullen T: *Myomata of the uterus,* Philadelphia, 1909, WB Saunders.

Kelly H, Noble CP: *Operative gynecology,* ed 3, New York, 1911, Appleton & Co.

Keys T: *The history of surgical anesthesia,* ed 2, Boston, 1950, Milford House.

Kovac SR: Guidelines to determine the role of laparoscopically assisted vaginal hysterectomy, *Am J Obstet Gynecol* 178:1257, 1998.

Leonardo R: *The history of surgery,* New York, 1943, Froben.

Leonardo T: *The history of gynecology,* New York, 1944, Froben.

Li TC, Saravelos H, Chow MS, et al: Factors affecting the outcome of laparoscopic ovarian drilling for polycystic ovarian syndrome in women with anovulatory infertility, *Br J Obstet Gynaecol* 105:338, 1998.

Ling FW, Smith RP, Vontver LA, Laube DW: *Comprehensive gynecology review,* St Louis, 1997, Mosby.

Lipscomb GH, Bran D, McCord ML, et al: Analysis of 315 ectopic pregnancies treated with single dose methotrexate, *Am J Obstet Gynecol* 178:1354, 1998.

Lister J: *Collected papers,* Oxford, 1909, Clarendon Press.

Lower A, Sutton C, Grudzinskas G: *Introduction to gynecological endoscopy,* Oxford, 1996, Isis Medical Media.

Maino G: *The healing hand,* Cambridge, 1975, Harvard University Press.

Malgaigne J: *Surgery and Ambrose Pare,* Norman, Okla, 1965, University of Oklahoma Press (Translated by W Hamby).

Malpas P: *Genital prolapse and allied conditions,* New York, 1955, Grune & Stratton.

Mann M: *American system of gynecology,* Philadelphia, 1888, Lea Brothers.

Marshall V, Marchetti A, Krantz K: Suprapubic urethral vesical suspension, *Surg Gynecol Obstet* 78:628, 1959.

Martius N: *Die Gynekologischen Operationen,* Stuttgart, 1954, Georg Thieme.

Mattingly R, Thompson J: *TeLinde's operative gynecology,* ed 6, Philadelphia, 1985, JB Lippincott.

McDowell E: Three cases of expiration of diseases ovaria, *The Eclectic Repertory and Analytical Review* 7:242, 1817.

McKay W: *The history of ancient gynecology,* New York, 1901, Wiliam Wood.

Meigs J: *Surgical treatment of carcinoma of the cervix,* New York, 1954, Grune & Stratton.

Milne J: *Surgical instruments in Greek and Roman times,* Oxford, 1907, Clarendon Press.

Mishell DK, Herbst AL, Kirschbaum TH: *1997 Year Book of obstetrics, gynecology, and women's health,* St Louis, 1997, Mosby.

Monahan EG: Medical clearance for gynecologic surgery, *Obstet Gynecol Surv* 53:117, 1998.

Mukhopadhyaya G: *The surgical instruments of the Hindus,* Calcutta, 1913, Calcutta University.

Neuwirth R: *Hysteroscopy,* Philadelphia, 1975, WB Saunders.

Nichols DH: Sacrospinous fixation for massive eversion of the vagina, *Am Obstet Gynecol* 4:901, 1982.

Nichols D: *Clinical problems, injuries and complications of gynecologic surgery,* ed 2, Baltimore, 1988, Williams & Wilkins.

Nichols D, Randall C: *Vaginal surgery,* ed 3, Baltimore, 1989, Williams & Wilkins.

Novak E: *Gynecological and obstetrical pathology,* Baltimore, 1945, Williams & Wilkins.

O'Connell, Fries MH, Zeringue E, Brehm W: Triage of abnormal postmenopausal bleeding: a comparison of endometrial biopsy and transvaginal sonohysterography versus fractional curettage with hysteroscopy, *Am J Obstet Gyncol* 178:956, 1998.

Ostrenzenski A, Ostrenzenska KM: Bladder injury during laparoscopic surgery, *Obstet Gynecol Surv* 53:175, 1998.

Paolucci V, Schaeff B, et al: *Gasless laparoscopy in general surgery and gynecology,* Stuttgart, 1996, Thieme.

Pare A: *The collected works of Ambrose Pare,* New York, 1968, Milford House (Translated by T Johnson from the first English edition, 1634).

Parsons L, Ulfelder H: *An atlas of pelvic operations,* New York, 1968, WB Saunders.

Patton G, Kistner R: *Atlas of infertility surgery,* ed 2, Boston, 1985, Little, Brown.

Peham H, Amreich J: *Operative gynecology,* Philadelphia, 1934, JB Lippincott (Translated by L Ferguson).

Penalever M, Mekki Y, Lafferty H, et al: Should sacrospinous ligament fixation for the management of pelvic support defects be part of a residency program procedure? *Am J Obstet Gynecol* 178:325, 1998.

Phillips J: *Endoscopy in gynecology,* Downey, Calif, 1978, AAGL.

Ploss H, Bartels M, Bartels P: In Dingwell E, editor: *Woman,* St Louis, 1938, Mosby.

Possover M, Frause N, Kuhn-Heid R, Schneider A: Value of laparoscopic evaluation of paraaortic and pelvic lymph nodes for treatment of cervical cancer, *Am J Obstet Gynecol* 178:806, 1998.

Pozzi SA: *Treatise on gynecology,* London, 1898, New Sydenham Society.

Preuss J: *Biblical and Talmudic medicine,* New York, 1978, Sanhedrin Press (Translated by F Rosner).

Reich W, Nechtow M: *Pitfalls in gynecologic diagnosis and surgery,* New York, 1962, McGraw-Hill.

Reiffenstuhl G, Platzer W: *Atlas of vaginal surgery,* Philadelphia, 1974, WB Saunders (Translated by E Friedman and J Friedman).

Ricci J: *One hundred years of gynecology,* Philadelphia, 1945, Blakiston.

Ricci J: *The development of gynecological surgery and instruments,* Philadelphia, 1949, Blakiston.

Ricci J: *The cystocele in America,* Philadelphia, 1950, Blakiston.

Ricci J: *The geneology of gynecology,* Philadelphia, 1950, Blakiston.

Richardson E: A simplified technique for abdominal panhysterectomy, *Surg Gynecol Obstet* 48:248, 1929.

Roberts JM, Gurley AM, Thurloe JK, et al: Evaluation of the thin Pap test as an adjunct to the conventional Pap smear, *Med J Aust* 167:466, 1997.

Sammarco MJ, Stovall TG, Steege JF, et al: *Gynecologic endoscopy,* Baltimore, 1996, Williams & Wilkins.

Scultetus J: *Armamentarium surgicum,* 1655, Ulm edition (photocopy by Sautter K, 1919, Editions Medicina Rara Ltd; original by Agathon Presse, Baiersbraun, W Germany).

Sims J: On the treatment of vesico-vaginal fistulas, *Am J Med Sci* 23:59, 1852.

Spitzer M: Cervical screening adjuncts: recent advances, *Am J Obstet Gynecol* 179:544, 1998.

Spitzer M, Chernys AE, Shifrin A, Ryskin M: Indications for cone biopsy: pathologic correlation, *Am J Obstet Gynecol* 178:74, 1998.

Tamussino KF, Lanf PFJ, Breini E: Ureteral complications with operative gynecologic laparoscopy, *Am J Obstet Gynecol* 178:967, 1998.

Thomas T: *A practical treatise on the diseases of women,* ed 4, Philadelphia, 1874, Henry Lea.

Timor-Tritsch IE: Is it safe to use methotrexate for selective injection in heterotopic pregnancy? *Am J Obstet Gynecol* 178:193, 1998.

Timor-Tritsch I, Rottem S: *Transvaginal ultrasound,* New York, 1988, Eleesevier.

Ulin A, Gollub S: *Surgical bleeding,* New York, 1966, McGraw-Hill.

Wertheim E: Zur frage der radikal operation beim uterus krebs, *Arch Gynak* 61:627, 1900.

White GR: An anatomical operation for the cure of cystocele, *JAMA* 53:1707, 1909.

Wind G, Dudai M: *Applied laparoscopic anatomy: abdomen and pelvis,* Baltimore, 1997, Williams & Wilkins.

2 Pelvic Anatomy for the Gynecologic Surgeon

GUNTHER REIFFENSTUHL

PELVIC CONNECTIVE TISSUE PLANES AND SPACES

An exact knowledge of the anatomy of the firm pelvic connective tissue is necessary for the gynecologic surgeon to find the appropriate blood vessels running within these tissues and thereby save the patient's blood during surgery. A precise knowledge of the location of the loose connective tissue also is essential, since this tissue fills both the actual and potential spaces between the pelvic organs and the firm connective tissue ligaments that have to be exposed.

The term *pelvic connective tissue* includes the entire system of connective tissue that surrounds the pelvic organs and extends into the subperitoneal area. This is bounded cranially by the pelvic peritoneum, caudally by the muscular pelvic floor, anteriorly by the symphysis, posteriorly by the sacrum, and laterally by the obturator and piriform muscles.

Operating in the correct layer—one of the most important prerequisites for successful vaginal and pelvic surgery— is possible only if the surgeon has exact knowledge of the anatomy of the connective tissue matrix and of the spaces filled with parenchyma (the *paraspaces*) and enters them correctly.

This chapter uses the nomenclature of Amreich,[77] which is the most practical for gynecologic surgery.

Connective Tissue Matrix (Firm Pelvic Connective Tissue)

The vessels of the female pelvis always course precisely from the pelvic wall through the extraperitoneal tissue to the uterus, vagina, bladder, and rectum and in the opposite direction from the pelvic organs to the pelvic wall. Because of the concentration of the connective tissue surrounding the vessels, the columns extend in different directions. This connective tissue matrix originally was thought to be a fixation device of the pelvic viscera, but after detailed study by Amreich it became evident that the primary functions of the matrix are to convey blood and lymphatic vessels and to cover the organs. The following subsections of the connective tissue matrix are differentiated based on their position and course.

Horizontal Connective Tissue Matrix

The horizontal connective tissue ground bundle, or matrix, extends horizontally from the symphysis—beginning with the pubovesical ligament, mainly on the side of the vagina— sacrally up to the ischial spine and curves in accordance with the angle between the vagina and uterus into a frontal plate (frontal connective tissue matrix). The horizontal connective tissue matrix sends the vaginal and cervical column in a medially and ultimately forms the connective tissue "fascial" sheath for the vagina and cervix. Laterally, the horizontal part of the connective tissue matrix originates in the tendinous arch (arcus tendineus) of the endopelvic fascia. Just ventral to this is a concentration of the levator fascia, described as the arcus tendineus of the levator ani, which is the lateral origin of the levator ani muscle arising from the surface of the obturator internus muscle. The distance between these two arches and their relative strengths vary considerably (Fig. 2-1). According to Baden,[2] these two tendinous arches may fuse at a point about halfway to the ischial spine, becoming the arcus tendineus communis. The horizontal portion of this connective tissue matrix begins as a narrow insertion to the rear surface of the symphysis and broadens gradually in a posterior direction against the frontal connective tissue matrix, so from above it has the shape of a horizontal triangle.

Frontal Connective Tissue Matrix

The frontal connective tissue matrix is a continuation of the horizontal connective tissue matrix as it curves upward at the large ischial foramen and rises to the point of separation of the uterine artery from the internal iliac artery. In sagittal section, the entire connective tissue matrix has the shape of a sled runner, the point of which extends sacrally. The horizontal part of the sled runner rests on the levator fascia; the curved part comes up in a cranial direction to a frontal plate. The frontal connective tissue matrix, also called the *cardinal ligament of Mackenrodt,* slowly decreases in mass in the caudocranial direction, so on sagittal section it assumes the shape of a wedge. It runs almost transversely from the uterus to the pelvic wall and therefore is often called the *lateral parametrium.* Medially, the firm connective tissue of the cardinal, or Mackenrodt's, ligament joins with the uterine vessels into the edge of the uterus, and laterally it continues upward along the pelvic sidewall into the firm connective tissue of the hypogastric vessels.

The frontal section of the connective tissue matrix can be anatomically described easily because all vessels of the urogenital tract are united within it and its lateral end is attached firmly to the pelvic wall. This fixation is especially tight because all the vessels of the pelvic viscera either originate at this section or run through it as they move toward the larger vessels of the pelvic wall.

The pelvic floor is mainly formed anatomically by the le-

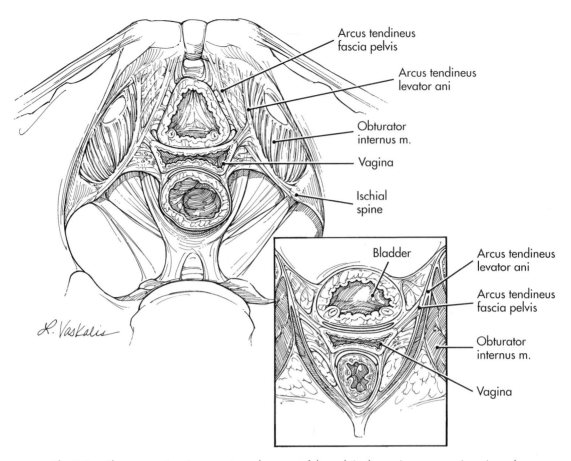

L. Vaskalis

Fig. 2-1 The connective tissue septa and spaces of the pelvis shown in cross-section viewed from above *(left)* and through the pelvis *(insert)*. In the view from above, the dome of the bladder and the uterus has been removed. Notice the bridges of connective tissue that connect the vaginal sulci to the respective arcus tendineus. The paravesical spaces are shown lateral to the bladder. The ischial spine is in the lateral wall of the pararectal space on each side. The prevesical space, vesicovaginal space, rectovaginal space, and retrorectal space are shown in the midline. Note the attachment of the vaginal sulci to the arcus tendineus and ventral surface of the levator ani. The levator ani forms the lateral wall of the pararectal spaces. The ureters are shown. The rectal pillar separating the rectovaginal space from the pararectal space is made up of two layers, although these may be fused, as shown.

vator ani muscle and investing fascia and in front by the urogenital diaphragm. The levator leaves a hiatus that is penetrated by the pelvic hollow organs (urethra, vagina, rectum). In the levator hiatus, the urethra (urinary bladder), vagina, and rectum are located one upon another, but then follow a curve of almost 90 degrees, typical for the genital tract, and are then located one behind another. The connective tissue matrix also follows this curve.

Ascending and Sagittal Bladder Pillars

Three layers separate from the horizontal connective tissue matrix: (1) a connective tissue sheet that ascends to the bladder (ascending bladder pillar), (2) a connective tissue sheet that descends caudally to the rectum (descending rectal pillar), and (3) a connective tissue sheet that extends medially to the vagina (horizontal vaginal column). The frontal connective tissue matrix also passes the same three layers on to the pelvic organs, but these sheets have a different

course because the pelvic organs are located behind one another. The bladder pillar branches off from the ventral surface of Mackenrodt's ligament and extends forward sagittally to the bladder (sagittal bladder pillar). Because of its importance as a vessel-conducting cord, this sagittal section of the bladder pillar also has its own name—*vesicouterine ligament.* (The name is not quite correct because the cord, as one might conclude from the name, does not go from the bladder to the side of the uterus, but instead from the bladder to the anterior surface of the frontal connective tissue matrix.) The second layer originating from Mackenrodt's ligament runs from the posterior surface of this ligament in a sacral direction to the rectum (sagittal rectal pillar). This pillar also is called the *rectouterine ligament,* but, like the vesicouterine ligament, it also is falsely designated because it does not run from the rectum to the side of the uterus, but instead to the posterior surface of the frontal connective tissue matrix. The third layer originating from Mackenrodt's ligament runs as a frontal cervical column to the uterine neck. It contains the uterine vessels and forms the shell for the cervix.

Rectal Pillar

The part of the rectal column that proceeds sacrally (sagittal rectal column, uterosacral ligament) originates at the posterior surface of Mackenrodt's ligament and runs along the pelvic wall to the rectum. At its rear end, near the side wall of the rectum, the rectal pillar splits into an anterior layer that surrounds the rectum as fascia and into a posterior layer that attaches to the lateral mass of the sacrum at the level of S2-S4. The part of the rectal pillar that proceeds caudally from the posterior surface of Mackenrodt's ligament (descending rectal column) is located next to the pelvic wall.

Vaginal Cervical Column

The connective tissue matrix in its entire expansion splits off lamellae in a medial direction to provide the fascial envelope for the pelvic organs (vaginal cervical fascia). To expose the ureter vaginally, knowledge of the connective tissue matrix and the subperitoneal hollow spaces filled with loose connective tissue is an absolute prerequisite.

Loose Connective Tissue

Between the firm columns of the connective tissue matrix on the one hand and the pelvic organs and the pelvic wall on the other, a series of actual or potential spaces is formed that are filled with loose connective tissue. If this loose connective tissue is removed or if it is pushed aside with dissection scissors, the artificial, or potential, spaces form. The formation of the spaces exposes the firm connective tissue columns in which the blood vessels are contained (Fig. 2-2).

Prevesical Space (of Retzius)

Laterally, the prevesical space borders on the lateral umbilical ligament. It can be exposed by bluntly separating the bladder from the rear surface of the symphysis in a downward direction using finger dissection. The space is filled with fat and loose connective tissue. Visualization of this space is important mainly during operations involving restoration of urinary continence.

Paravesical Spaces

The paravesical spaces border laterally on the fascia of the obturator and the levator ani muscles, medially on the bladder and the bladder pillar, and in back the space runs up to Mackenrodt's ligament. A paravesical space can be opened up from above by boring a hole with closed scissors from the lateral parametrium laterally from the lateral umbilical ligament. Because the paravesical space is filled with fragile connective tissue and fat, it can be bluntly exposed easily all the way to the pelvic floor.

Vesicocervical and Vesicovaginal Spaces

Laterally, these spaces border on the ascending and sagittal bladder pillars, frontally on the urinary bladder, and behind on the cervix and vagina, respectively. The roof of these spaces is formed by the peritoneum (plica vesicouterina). These two spaces are separated because the rear flap of the bladder fascia is fixed to the front wall of the vagina and cervix by a small number of stronger connective tissue cords (supravaginal septum).

The vesicocervical and vesicovaginal spaces can be opened from above by transversely splitting the vesicouterine peritoneum in the midline, pushing the urinary bladder off the anterior wall of the cervix, and again in the midline by sharp dissection with scissors, cutting through the supravaginal septum. In this way the vesicocervical space is united with the vesicovaginal space. Then with a dissecting swab in the midline, the bladder can be bluntly pushed from the vagina. Bluntly pushing the urinary bladder away from the midline is not easy; it also is unsafe because this is where vessel-containing ascending and sagittal bladder pillars are located. (In the cranial parts of the bladder pillars, the outlet veins of the vesical plexus run to Mackenrodt's ligament to empty into the uterine veins, or to get directly into the veins of the pelvic wall.) The superior vesical artery also runs between these veins of the vesical plexus; it originates from the uterine artery and uses the bladder pillar (vesicouterine ligament) as passage to the bladder. The ureter runs in the lowest part of the sagittal bladder pillar (the lateral wall of the vesicocervicovaginal space) in a kind of channel. If one works exactly in the midline when exposing the vesicocervical and vesicovaginal spaces, the potential for bleeding or ureteral injury is eliminated and the urinary bladder can be pushed off bluntly.

Rectovaginal Space

The rectovaginal space posteriorly borders on the rectum, anteriorly on the vagina, and laterally on the rectal pillars. (The sagittal rectal pillars are also called *rear parametrium* or *rectouterine ligaments*.) A thin layer of peritoneal fusion fascia (of Denonvilliers) is fused to the undersurface of the posterior vaginal wall and extends from the most caudal portion of the cul-de-sac of Douglas to the most cranial portion of the perineal body. The roof of the rectovaginal space is formed by the peritoneum of the cul-de-sac of Douglas, which may be of varying depths—the deeper, the more infantile.[28] Caudally the vaginal fascia and rectal fascia come closer together just above the pelvic floor. The rectovaginal space, which contains loose connective tissue, can be exposed by transversely cutting the peritoneum at the lowest point of the cul-de-sac of Douglas and then bluntly separating the rectum from the vagina in the midline.

Pararectal Space

The pararectal space medially borders on the rectal pillar and laterally borders on the large blood vessels of the pelvic wall or the levator and piriform muscles. Anteriorly it borders on Mackenrodt's ligament and posteriorly on the lateral parts of the sacrum. The roof is formed by the peritoneum. The caudal part of this space is entered (e.g., during a Wertheim radical hysterectomy) by penetrating with a finger around the curve of the connective tissue matrix. Here it is important to stay close to the sacrospinal ligament to separate the connective tissue matrix from the pelvic floor in the area of its knee. If the finger goes a little higher, in the area of the ischial foramen, it hits the appendage of Mackenrodt's ligament and can injure the genital veins.

After completely opening up the caudal sections of the pararectal space, one's finger arrives in the already exposed paravesical space and can reach into the front surface of Mackenrodt's ligament around the bend of the connective tissue matrix. In this way, the vessel-carrying ligament of Mackenrodt is exposed as a completely isolated condensation, which is important during a radical abdominal operation for carcinoma. After exposing the pararectal and paravesical spaces, the isolated Mackenrodt ligaments with their vessels can be ligated easily.

The pararectal space can be opened if, after separating the infundibulopelvic ligament, one splits the rear sheet of the broad ligament downward to the ureter and pushes the latter with its connective tissue layer aside.

Retrorectal Space

Posteriorly, the retrorectal space borders on the sacrum, anteriorly on the rectal fascia, and laterally at the height of S2-S4 on the rectal pillars, which also represent the separating wall of the pararectal spaces. Cranially, the retrorectal

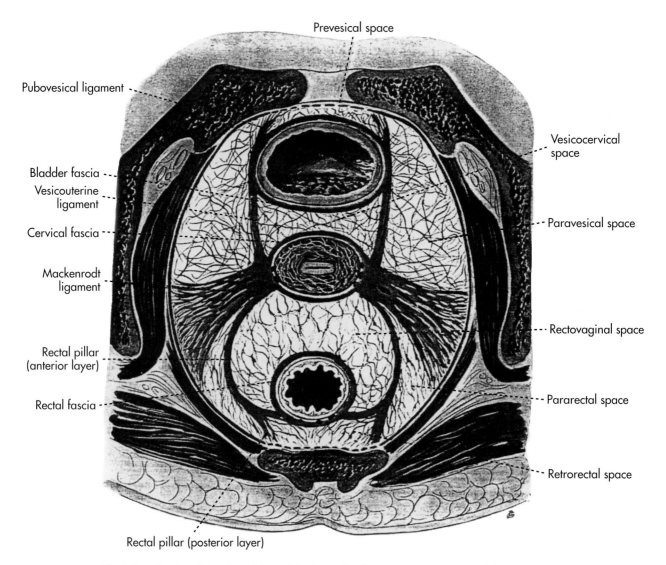

Prevesical space

Pubovesical ligament

Bladder fascia

Vesicouterine ligament

Cervical fascia

Mackenrodt ligament

Rectal pillar (anterior layer)

Rectal fascia

Vesicocervical space

Paravesical space

Rectovaginal space

Pararectal space

Retrorectal space

Rectal pillar (posterior layer)

Fig. 2-2 Sectional drawing of the pelvis shows the firm connective tissue and the paraspaces (Amreich). The bladder, cervix, and rectum are surrounded by a connective tissue covering. Mackenrodt's ligament extends from the lateral cervix to the lateral abdominal pelvic wall. The vesicouterine ligament originating from the anterior edge of Mackenrodt's ligament leads to the covering of the bladder on the posterior side. The sagittal rectum column spreads both to the connective tissue of the rectum and the sacral vertebrae, closely nestled against the back of Mackenrodt's ligament and the lateral pelvic wall. Loose connective tissue (paraspaces) is between the firm connective tissue bundles. (From Von Peham H, Amreich JA: *Gynäkologische Operationslehre,* Berlin, 1930, S Karger.)

space becomes the retroperitoneal space, whereas caudally, the space ends at the levator. The retrorectal space can be exposed by bluntly separating the rectum from the sacrum.

ARTERIES, VEINS, AND NERVES OF THE INTERNAL GENITALIA
Arteries of the Internal Genitalia (Fig. 2-3)

The main nutritional artery of the uterus is the uterine artery. In almost every patient it branches together with the residual umbilical artery from the internal iliac artery; rarely, it may originate directly from the hypogastric artery about 1 to 1.5 cm below the linea terminalis. The uterine artery has to be exposed when joining the so-called ovarian fascia at the lateral pelvic wall. The uterine artery then makes a medial turn and follows Mackenrodt's ligament on its upper edge further medially. Inside this lateral parametrium, the uterine artery crosses the ureter. The crossing is located near the cervix about 1.5 to 2 cm lateral to the uterus. At the ureteral crossing, a small ramus uretericus branches from the uterine artery, crossing cranially and caudally along the ureter. The uterine artery sends off the vaginal artery either before or after crossing the ureter. The uterine artery turns upward approximately 0.5 cm lateral to the uterus, crossing onto the lateral margin of the uterus, and sending off the rami uterini to the front and back of the uterus, anastomosing to the opposite side.

At the angle of the fallopian tube, the uterine artery finally branches into its four terminal arteries. The *fundus ramus,* penetrating into the muscle tissue of the uterine fundus, and the *round ligament ramus* are the weakest of the four branches leading underneath the fallopian tube to the round ligament, accompanying the round ligament to the inguinal canal and finally anastomosing to a branch of the inferior epigastric artery. The *tubal ramus* leads into the mesosalpinx and sends small branches to the fallopian tube until it reaches the infundibulopelvic ligament, where it anastomoses with the ovarian artery. The *ovarian ramus,* originating from the uterine artery below the ovarian proprium ligament, sends numerous branches to the ovary and continues into the ovarian artery, which originally had perfused the ovary alone. Branching almost immediately after the crossing of the uterine artery and the ureter, the cervical vaginal artery feeds the uterine cervix and the vagina.

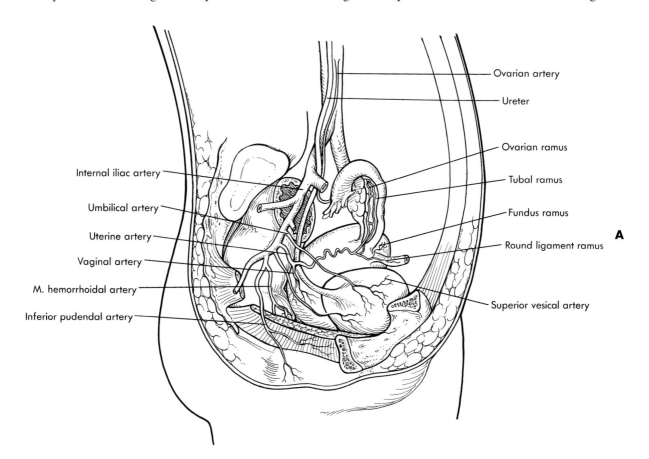

Fig. 2-3 Arteries of the internal female genitalia. **A,** Sagittal view of the right side of the pelvic arteries. Notice the origin of the right ovarian artery from the aorta, which divides into an ovarian ramus and tubal ramus, and at the sides of the uterus anastomoses with the uterine artery, with ramus to the fundus and round ligament. The right ureter is shown coursing over the common iliac artery en route to the bladder. The common iliac artery divides into internal and external branches. The significant branches of the internal iliac are the umbilical, uterine, vaginal, middle hemorrhoidal, and inferior pudendal.

Continued

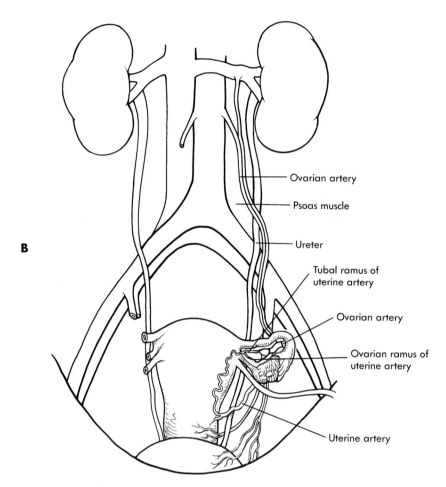

B

- Ovarian artery
- Psoas muscle
- Ureter
- Tubal ramus of uterine artery
- Ovarian artery
- Ovarian ramus of uterine artery
- Uterine artery

Fig. 2-3, cont'd **B,** Frontal view. Note the ovarian artery and ureter coursing over the surface of the psoas muscle.

The second largest artery in the internal genital area is the ovarian artery. Originating from the aorta below the renal arteries, it runs on the psoas muscle downward and crosses the ureter at the entrance of the small pelvis, reaching the ovary inside the infundibulopelvic ligament. A strong collateral branch connects the ovarian artery to the ovarian ramus and the tubal ramus of the uterine artery. The third artery involved with perfusion of the internal genitals is the medial hemorrhoidal artery, which usually originates from the pudendal artery. It divides within Mackenrodt's ligament into a smaller branch, reaching the rectum through the descending rectal pillar, and a stronger anterior branch, extending into the horizontal connective tissue and the vaginal pillar to the vagina.

In the most caudal part of the vesicouterine ligament, the inferior vesical artery is surrounded by the draining veins of the vaginal plexus. This artery is a direct branch of the internal iliac artery in the area of Mackenrodt's ligament. It uses the vesicouterine ligament to approach the bladder and vagina. Only the proximal part of the umbilical artery, being the main branch of the internal iliac in fetal life, is preserved. The distal part became the lateral umbilical ligament. The proximal part of the umbilical arteries and the superior vesical artery often consist of two branches parting on the upper edge of the sagittal pillar of the bladder (vesico-uterine ligament). Similar to the inferior vesical artery, these two branches provide the bladder and the neighboring ureter with blood. The gynecologic surgeon must have detailed knowledge of the ureteral segments near the bladder because damaging any artery in the operative field can cause insufficient blood supply and perfusion followed by necrosis.

Veins of the Internal Genitalia (Fig. 2-4)

The veins of the internal genitalia include the superior and inferior gluteal veins and the iliolumbar, laterosacral, and obturator veins. The visceral branches of the veins are the internal pudendal vein (corresponding to the internal pudendal artery), which drains the deep vein of the clitoris; the posterior labial veins; and the inferior rectal veins. Entering the pelvis, the internal pudendal veins join the inferior gluteal veins. The vein plexus of the bladder, which drains the caudal segments of the bladder, flows into the internal iliac vein. The rectal vein branches surrounding the caudal segments of the rectum can drain either into the superior hemorrhoidal vein, which leads to the caudal vein, or into the medial hemorrhoidal vein, which flows into the internal iliac vein. The uterine and vaginal venous plexuses are located between the posterior rectal vein plexus and the ante-

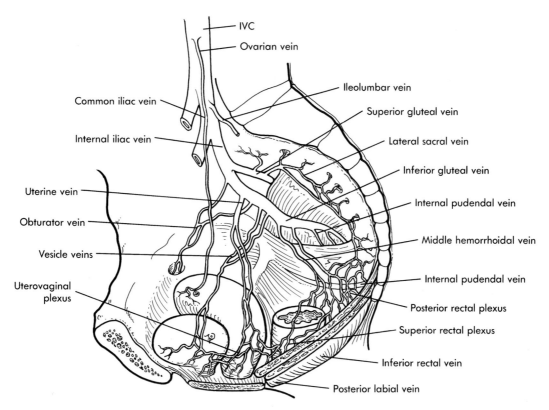

Fig. 2-4 The pelvic veins. Sagittal section shows the principal veins of the right side. Notice the uterovaginal plexuses, the superior and inferior plexuses, the middle hemorrhoidal veins, and internal pudendal vein and inferior gluteal vein. Together with the vesical veins, obturator veins, and uterine vein, they join the lateral and superior gluteal veins to form the internal iliac vein. The latter, in company with the external iliac vein, become the common iliac vein, which proceeds directly to the vena cava. The right ovarian vein is shown.

rior vesical vein plexus. Combined, these are called the *uterovaginal plexus.* The uterovaginal plexus lies lateral to the vagina and the uterus, and it flows into the internal iliac veins. The vein draining the fundus of the uterus mainly uses the ovarian veins leading to the inferior vena cava. The venous drainage of the vagina is performed by the uterovaginal plexus situated in the walls of the paraspaces and flows into the internal iliac veins. All these vein plexuses communicate with each other. The internal iliac vein combines with the external iliac vein, coming from the side to form the common iliac vein. The two common iliac veins join the inferior vena cava on the right side of the aorta.

The uterine and vaginal veins pass directly from Mackenrodt's ligament to the veins of the pelvic wall, creating the extraordinarily firm attachment of Mackenrodt's ligament to the pelvic wall. Occasionally, the right obturator vein flows directly into the external iliac vein, and, in that case, the uterine, vaginal, and vesical veins are drained by the obturator vein. This newly created, strong vein is called the *medial iliac vein.*[30]

A perfect collated circulation of the venous backflow from the genitals is generally present because of the numerous venous connections and drainage into various drainage systems. Even if the hypogastric vein has been ligated, there is still enough drainage of the bladder coming from the genital into the caudal vein and the medial and superior hemorrhoidal veins. In addition, because the obturator iliac ramus is a communicating vessel between internal and external genitals, blood may flow into the external iliac vein. If the hypogastric vein is being ligated, only the drainage of the uterine, vaginal, vesical, and internal pudendal veins into the hypogastric vein is closed.

Special Innervation of the Internal Genitalia

The celiac ganglion situated near the celiac artery is supposed to be the origin for the genital nerves. This ganglion receives parasympathetic branches from the pneumogastric (phrenic) and vagus nerves and sympathetic branches from the splanchnic nerves. The celiac ganglion is the origin for a number of nerve fibers covering the aorta (aortic plexus). The aortic plexus also receives fibers from the renal and the upper mesenteric ganglion. A bit below the renal arteries are the generally bilateral genital ganglia and the lower mesenteric ganglia (Fig. 2-5). The plexus of the prevertebral sympathetic nervous system reaches about 1 cm in front of the fifth lumbar vertebra in the branch of the aorta and can be seen, at least in thin persons, through the peritoneum

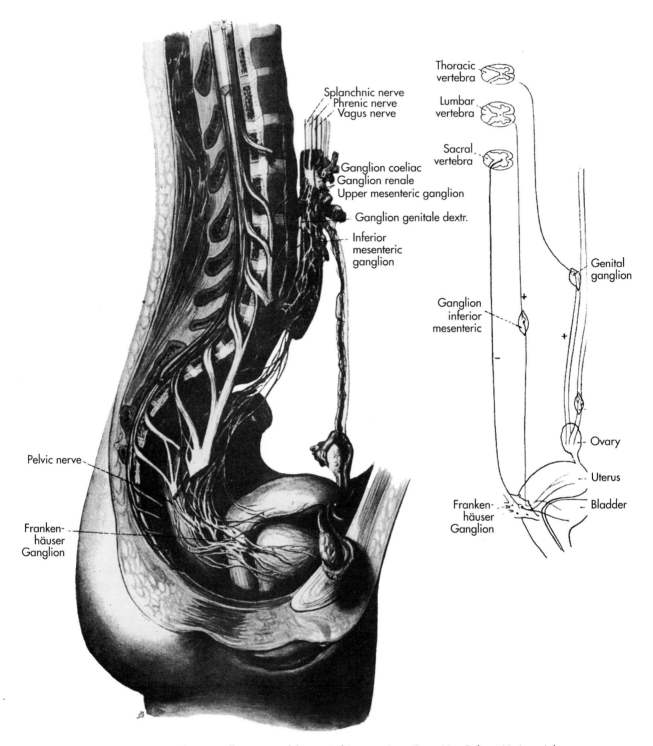

Fig. 2-5   Semischematic illustration of the genital innervation. (From Von Peham H, Amreich JA: *Gynäkologische Operationslehre,* Berlin, 1930, S Karger.)

of the posterior abdominal wall. In front of the sacral promontory, the plexus branches into the bilateral hypogastric plexus. This plexus borders the rectum very closely on both lateral faces and follows inside the rectal column to the posterior face of Mackenrodt's ligament. The largest ganglion located in that area is called *Frankenhäuser's ganglion* (Fig. 2-6). This ganglion receives parasympa-

thetic branches from S2 to S4 (pelvic nerves), where the sensitive branches of the uterus also can be found. Frankenhäuser's ganglion is the origin of the nerve fibers of the uterus and vagina.

The fallopian tubes and ovaries are innervated by the "spermatic" plexus. The origin of this plexus is the superior part of the aortic plexus. It accompanies the ovarian artery

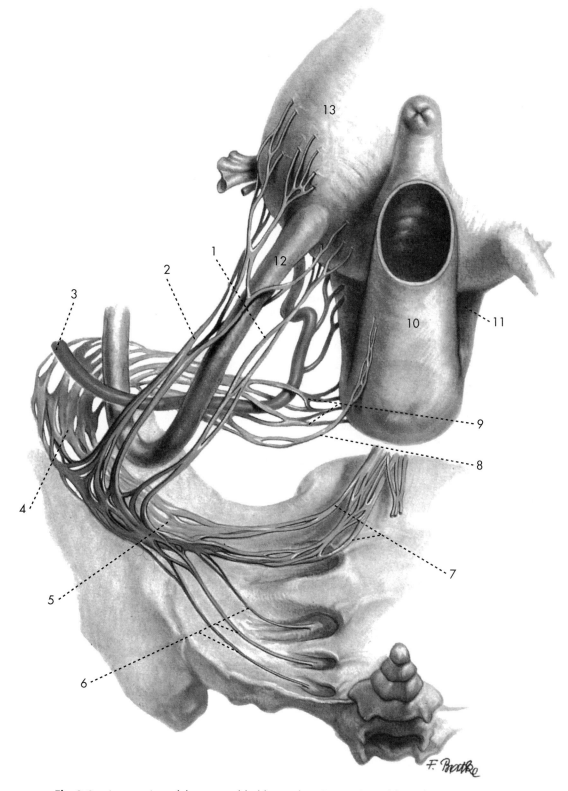

Fig. 2-6 Innervation of the uterus, bladder, and vagina as viewed from the perineum. *1,* Inferior vesical nerves; *2,* superior vesical nerves; *3,* uterine artery; *4,* uterine plexus (uterovaginal); *5,* plexus pelvinus (pelvic ganglion, inferior hypogastric plexus); *6,* pelvic nerves (parasympathetic); *7,* superior hypogastric plexus (sympathetic); *8,* vaginal ramus; *9,* uterine nerves; *10,* vagina; *11,* uterus; *12,* ureter; *13,* urinary bladder. (From Reiffenstuhl G, Platzer W: *Die Vaginalen Operationen: Chirurgie, Anatomie und Operationslehre,* Berlin, 1974, Urban-Schwarzenberg.)

downward and reaches the adnexa inside the infundibulopelvic ligament. In summary, nerves innervating the uterus, vagina, bladder, and rectum come from the lumbosacral bundle (sympathetic) and the sacral plexus (parasympathetic).

ARTERIES, VEINS, AND NERVES OF THE EXTERNAL GENITALIA
Urogenital and Anal Region

The internal pudendal artery and vein and the pudendal nerve, after passing the minor ischiatic fossa, are located in the pudendal (Alcock) canal inside the internal obturator fascia (Fig. 2-7). The inferior rectal vein and artery (hemorhoidal or anal vein and artery) branch here, and the inferior rectal nerves reach the anus through the fat tissues of the ischiorectal fossa.

Arteries. The internal pudendal artery branches into the perineal and clitoral artery at the posterior edge of the urogenital diaphragm. The perineal artery passes the perineum in the superficial perineal space of the urogenital region and finally forms the posterior labial rami, which supply the major and minor labia with blood. The clitoral artery, which is a continuation of the internal pudendal artery, sends out the vestibular artery at the region of the posterior edge of the urogenital diaphragm penetrating into the bulbus vestibuli. The clitoral artery is embedded in the urogenital diaphragm tissue. The two terminal branches of the clitoral artery are the profundus and dorsal clitoral artery. The profundus artery penetrates into the crural of the clitoris coming from the diaphragm. The dorsal clitoral artery leads to the dorsum of the clitoris, leaving the diaphragm closely underneath the symphysis. Clitoral erection is caused by the terminal branches of the internal pudendal artery (dorsal clitoral artery and vestibular artery); in amputations of the clitoris, both dorsal and clitoral arteries need to be ligated for hemostasis. Although bleeding coming from the corpora cavernosa can easily be stopped by compression, it is more exact to suture the corpora.

Veins. The main vein is the internal pudendal vein, which does not drain the whole volume of the area. Another pond flows underneath the symphysis toward the vesicopudendal plexus. The dorsal superficial clitoral vein drains the corpus of the clitoris and the glands. The internal pudendal vein receives blood coming from the bulbus vestibuli in the bulbovestibular vein, where the profundus clitoral vein also contributes. In addition, the internal pudendal vein drains the dorsal part of the labia through the posterior labial veins. The internal pudendal vein crosses along the posterior edge of the urogenital triangle and goes into the pudendal canal to the minor ischiadic foramen. Passing the infrapiriform foramen, it enters the small pelvis and flows into the internal iliac vein. The perineal veins do not have venous valves; therefore, if the tension of the pelvic floor muscles decreases, venous blood flow will be obstructed. Chronic venous stasis causes varices, including the area of the draining hemorrhoidal veins. Reconstruction of the pelvic floor

muscles causes increasing tension in the pelvic floor and stops chronic venous stasis. The blood congestion of the erectile phases (clitoris and bulbocavernosus body) probably is a secondary phenomenon.[39] Most of this blood comes from the arterial side.

Nerves. The pudendal nerve is thought to be the main nerve of the urogenital region. It passes the pudendal canal, sending inferior rectal nerves (anal nerves) to innervate the external sphincter muscle of the anus and the anal skin area. At the posterior edge of the urogenital diaphragm, the pudendal nerve finally branches into the perineal and clitoral nerves. The perineal nerves terminate in the urogenital diaphragm into the posterior labial nerves, which innervate the dorsal part of the labia. Some of its fibers innervate the transverse superficial perineal muscle and the muscles of the swelling body. The clitoral nerve supplies the dorsum of the clitoris, the muscle of the urethra, and the deep transverse perineal muscle. These nerves are all branches of the pudendal nerve. The anococcygeal nerves also participate in the innervation of the urogenital and anal skin, originating from the coccygeal nerve and penetrating the pelvic diaphragm near the coccyx. They innervate the area around the coccyx toward the anus. The skin around the ischial tuberosity is innervated by perineal rami that originate from the posterior femoral nerve.

Perineal Region

Arteries. The main vessel is the internal pudendal artery. The lateral and anterior segments of the labia are perfused by the anterior labial rami, which originate from the external pudendal and, therefore, from the femoral artery.

Veins. The deep veins have been discussed previously. A superficial vein is located on the dorsum of the clitoris. This subcutaneous dorsal vein of the clitoris connects to the deep vessels of the clitoris but also to the subcutaneous veins of the pubic mons. More important are the anterior labial veins, which flow into the external pudendal veins and finally are drained by the femoral veins.

Nerves. The pudendal nerve is the most important nerve for this region. Its posterior labial nerves innervate the dorsal segment of the labia, and the dorsal clitoral nerve covers the area of the clitoris. The anterior labial nerves, which are branches of the ilioinguinal nerve, reach the pubic mons, the ventral part of the major labia, and the clitoral prepuce.

The genital rami of the genital femoral nerves participate in the neural supply of the major labia reaching the area accompanying the teres uteri ligament.

LYMPHATIC SYSTEM OF THE FEMALE GENITALS
Pelvic Lymph Nodes

The pelvic lymph nodes are concentrated mostly around the large arteries and veins, resulting in the blood vessels of the pelvis being entwined by lymphatic nerves and vessels. It is more useful to base the discussion of lymphatics on their lo-

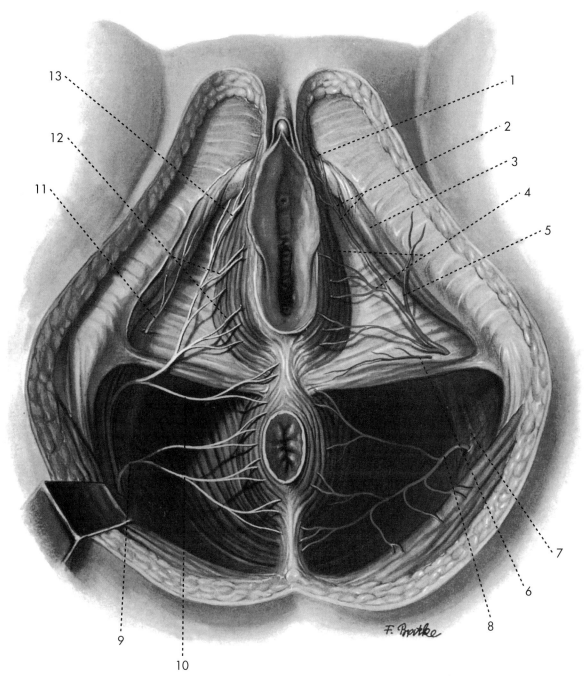

Fig. 2-7   The arteries and nerves of the pelvic floor as seen from below, demonstrating the branching of the internal pudendal artery and the pudendal nerve. *1,* Dorsal clitoral artery; *2,* deep clitoral artery; *3,* ischiocavernosus muscle; *4,* bulbocavernosus muscle and the artery of the vestibular bulb; *5,* posterior labial artery; *6,* perineal artery; *7,* internal pudendal artery in Alcock's canal; *8,* inferior rectal artery; *9,* anal nerve; *10,* perineal nerve; *11,* branch innervating the ischiocavernosus muscle; *12,* posterior labial nerves; *13,* dorsal clitoral nerve. (From Reiffenstuhl G, Platzer W: *Die Vaginalen Operationen: Chirurgie, Anatomie und Operationslehre,* Berlin, 1974, Urban-Schwarzenberg.)

cation near the arteries, although no other system in the body is as well connected and transitional as the lymphatic system of the pelvis (Fig. 2-8).

Aortic Lymph Nodes. These nodes are located anteriorly, laterally, and superiorly to the aorta (see Fig. 2-8, *A*).

Lateral Common Iliac Lymph Nodes. These nodes are located on the lateral face of the common iliac artery. The superficial lymph nodes can be seen easily at the lateral phase of the common iliac artery (see Fig. 2-8, *B*). The deep lymph nodes of this group are attached to the posterior face

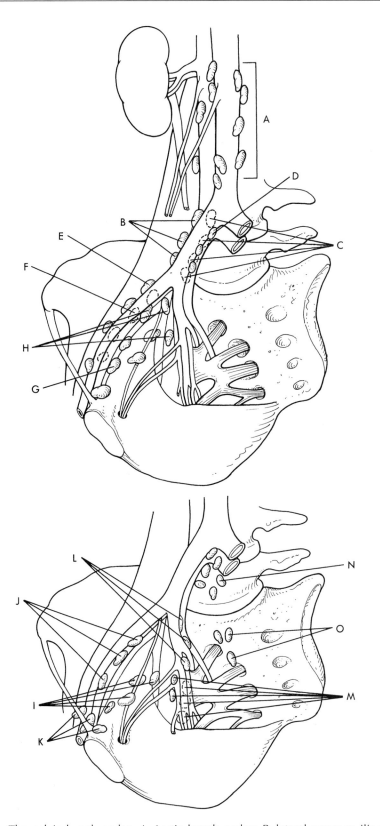

Fig. 2-8 The pelvic lymph nodes. *A,* Aortic lymph nodes; *B,* lateral common iliac lymph nodes (superficial); *C,* lateral common iliac lymph nodes (deep); *D,* medial common iliac lymph nodes; *E,* lateral external iliac lymph nodes (superficial); *F,* lateral external iliac lymph nodes (deep); *G,* interiliac lymph nodes; *H,* hypogastric lymph nodes; *I,* obturator lymph nodes; *J,* medial external iliac lymph nodes; *K,* femoral ring lymph nodes; *L,* superior gluteal lymph nodes, *M,* inferior gluteal lymph nodes; *N,* subaortic (promontorial) lymph nodes; *O,* sacral lymph nodes. (See also Fig. 2-20.) (Adapted and redrawn from Reiffenstuhl G: *Das Lymphsystem des weiblichen Genitale,* Vienna, 1957, Urban-Schwarzenberg.)

of the common iliac vessels and therefore are hidden (see Fig. 2-8, *C*). They can be exposed by following the lateral margins of the common iliac artery into the depths lying between the posterior face of the vessels and the psoas muscle.

Medial Common Iliac Lymph Nodes. These nodes are located on the medial face of the common iliac artery (see Fig. 2-8, *D*).

Lateral External Iliac Lymph Nodes. These nodes are located on the lateral edges of the external iliac artery. The superficial (see Fig. 2-8, *E*) and deep lymph nodes (see Fig. 2-8, *F*) are found caudal to the common iliac lymph nodes. These lymph nodes are not often exposed but can be found on the posterior surface of the external iliac vessels between the vessels and the psoas muscle.

Interiliac Lymph Nodes. All lymph nodes are located on the pelvic wall in the obturator fossa, which is limited by the medial face of the external iliac artery, by the lateral face of the internal iliac artery, and by the superior face of the obturator artery (see Fig. 2-8, *G*). They can be divided into three groups: hypogastric lymph nodes located in the hypogastric angle (see Fig. 2-8, *H*), obturator lymph nodes located along the obturator vessels and the obturator nerve (see Fig. 2-8, *I*), and medial external iliac lymph nodes located on the medial face of the external iliac artery (see Fig. 2-8, *J*). Usually the interiliac lymph nodes form a bunch that is surrounded by plenty of fat tissue. Starting distally at the femoral annulus extending cranially to the hypogastric angle, the lymph node packet caudally borders the obturator artery. The group of lymph nodes surrounding the femoral annulus where the external iliac vessels meet the pelvic vessels consist primarily of three lymph nodes called *annuli femoralis* lymph nodes (see Fig. 2-8, *K*). In this group, the lateral lymph node corresponds to the most distal lateral external iliac lymph node. The middle one is located on the external iliac vessels, and the medial one corresponds to the most distal obturator lymph node, known as *Rosenmüller's node.*

Superior Gluteal Lymph Nodes. These are located at the branch of the internal iliac artery and the cranial gluteal artery situated on the medial phase of the cranial gluteal artery (see Fig. 2-8, *L*).

Inferior Gluteal Lymph Nodes. These are located on the branch of and along the inferior gluteal and internal pudendal artery, caudal to the obturator artery (see Fig. 2-8, *M*). At the lateral insertion of Mackenrodt's ligament, they lie on the internal obturator muscle and the piriform muscle, on the sacral pelvis plexus. These lymph nodes can be found along the pelvic wall down to the lateral part of the infrapiriform foramen where the pudendal artery exits the pelvis. This area corresponds to the region around the spine of the ischiatic bone. These lymph nodes are found on the pelvic wall partly anterior and partly posterior to the blood vessels.

Subaortic Lymph Nodes (Promontoric). These are located in the aortic bifurcation on the fifth lumbar vertebra and the promontory (see Fig. 2-8, *N*).

Sacral Lymph Nodes. These are located on the anterior face of the sacral bone in the basin of the medial and lateral sacral arteries (see Fig. 2-8, *O*).

Cranial Rectal Lymph Nodes. These are located at the posterior wall of the rectum in the basin of the cranial rectal artery.

The lymphatic drainage of the uterus and vagina can be traced by following the blood vessels of these organs to the lymphatic nodes on the pelvic wall.

Draining Lymphatics of the Cervix Uteri. Fig. 2-9 shows schematically the lymphatics leaving the cervix uteri. All groups of lymph nodes from numbers 1 to 10 are the station of the drainage of the cervix uteri. The actual extension of the lymphatics connecting the cervix uteri and the pelvic lymph nodes is shown in Figs. 2-10 to 2-14.

Draining Lymphatics of the Corpus Uteri and the Vagina. Figs. 2-15 and 2-16 show schematics of the lymphatics originating at the corpus uteri and the vagina. Numbers 1, 5, 6, 8, and 9 are marked more prominently because they belong to the lymph node stages mainly frequented by the lymphatics of the corpus uteri and vagina.

Lymphatic Cord of Poirier-Seelig. At the lateral edge of the uterus resides a lymphatic cord first described by Poirier and confirmed by Seelig (Fig. 2-17). This lymphatic cord connects the uterine lymph vessels to the vaginal lymph vessels and even the ovarian and fallopian tube lymph vessels. This anatomic situation allows carcinoma of the portio, above all cervical carcinoma, to metastasize cranially into the myometrium of the corpus uteri. The carcinoma cells can then use the meridionally running anastomosis. For that reason, cervical carcinoma cells can infiltrate the muscles of the corpus uteri with numerous cords of carcinoma and isolated fields or clusters right up to the uterine fundus. Because of the spread of metastases from the meridional to the radial lymph vessels and by retrograde cell transport, cervical cancer might produce isolated islands of tumor inside the mucous membrane of the corpus uteri. Even the more cranially situated internal genitals, the fallopian tubes and ovaries, can be invaded by cervical carcinoma cells. This is more likely with corpus uteri carcinoma than with uterine cervical carcinoma.

Cervical cancer usually spreads into the vagina by continuous growth and local infiltration of a superficial cancer cell population that destroys the vaginal epithelium. In rare cases, metastatic disease carries carcinoma cells of the cervix in the lymph vessels of the cord of Poirier downward to the vagina by reversing the direction of lymphatic flow. Small carcinoma cell aggregations may infiltrate the rectal or vaginal septum, inside the paravaginal connective tissue.

Draining Lymph Vessels of Bladder and Urethra. The course of the lymphatics between the bladder and the lymph nodes of the pelvic wall is illustrated in Fig. 2-16, *A*. The lymphatics of the extrapelvic segment of the urethra are shown in Fig. 2-16, *B* and *C*.

Draining Lymph Vessels of Labia and Clitoris. The courses of the lymph vessels from the labia and clitoris to the inguinal lymph nodes, and also to the pelvic lymph nodes, are illustrated in Figs. 2-18 and 2-19.

Text continued on p. 47

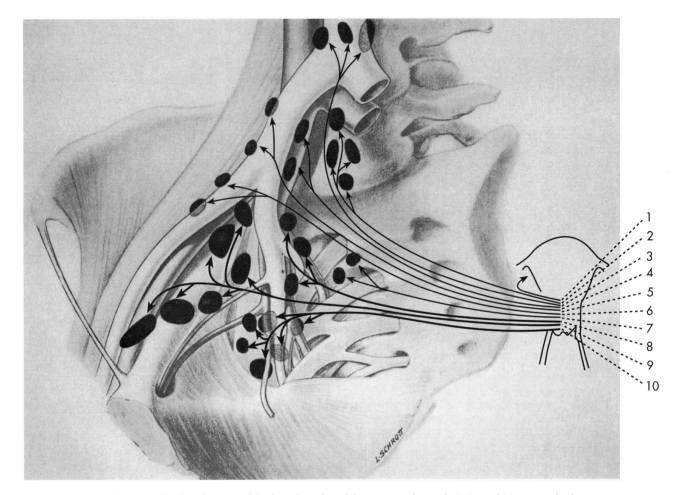

1
2
3
4
5
6
7
8
9
10

Fig. 2-9 Regional stages of the lymph nodes of the cervix. Channels 8, 9, and 10 are marked in bold because they feed main lymphatics of the cervix. Nevertheless, it must be remembered that, in cases of carcinoma of the cervix, tumor cells easily could be spread directly to the pelvic lymph nodes by lymphatic numbers 1 to 7. Remember that the inferior gluteal lymph nodes, being near the ischiatic spine, can be totally or partly hidden because of their location behind the bigger vessels. Therefore in Wertheim's radical procedure and modified procedures, it is technically very difficult if not relatively impossible to remove these lymph nodes (except for Brunschwig's exenteration, discussed later on). These facts explain the occurrence of so-called *ischial spinous recurrence* in cancer of the cervix, which is not a real recurrence but a primary infiltration of carcinoma cells to the gluteal inferior lymph nodes, including the rectal *(1)*, subaortic (promontorial) *(2)*, aortic *(3)*, medial common iliac *(4)*, lateral common iliac *(5)*, lateral external iliac *(6)*, sacral *(7)*, superior gluteal *(8)*, interiliac *(9)*, and inferior gluteal *(10)*. (From Reiffenstuhl G: *Das Lymphsystem des weiblichen Genitale,* Vienna, 1957, Urban-Schwarzenberg.)

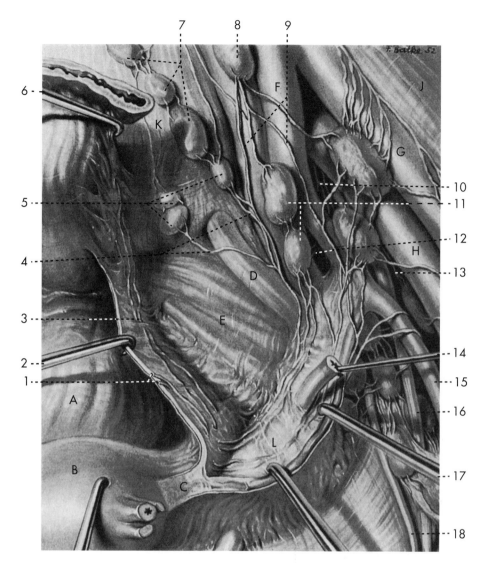

Fig. 2-10 Lymphatic drainage of the cervix to the pelvic wall and rectum. The rectouterine ligaments (sagittal/rectal pillar or column) are drawn medially by a small retractor *(2).* The lymphatics of the cervix *(3)* inside the sagittal/rectal pillar reach the posterior face of the rectum flowing into the superior rectal lymph nodes (not seen). The lymphatics marked with *(1)* extend cranially to the ureter sheet. Originating from the superior gluteal lymph nodes *(11),* efferent vessels lead to the medial common iliac lymph nodes *(8).* Notice that cervical lymphatics *(4)* reach the sacral lymph nodes *(5)* located on the anterior sacrum without any interruption. These lymph nodes are likewise regional lymph node stage of the cervix. *A,* Rectum; *B,* uterus (intestinal surface); *C,* Mackenrodt's ligament (medial portion); *D,* first sacral nerve, *E,* piriform muscle; *F,* internal, and *G,* external iliac arteries; *H,* external iliac vein; *J,* psoas muscle; *K,* promontory; *L,* Mackenrodt's ligament (posterior surface); *1,* cervical lymph vessels; *2,* rectouterine ligament; *3* and *4,* cervical lymph vessels; *5,* sacral lymph nodes; *6,* rectum; *7,* subaortic (promontorial), and *8,* medial common iliac lymph nodes; *9,* cervical lymph vessels; *10,* efferent vessels; *11,* superior gluteal lymph nodes; *12* and *13,* efferent vessels; *14,* ureter; *15,* lateral umbilical ligament; *16,* obturator nerve; *17,* uterine, and *18,* obturator arteries. (From Reiffenstuhl G: *Das Lymphsystem des weiblichen Genitale,* Vienna, 1957, Urban-Schwarzenberg.)

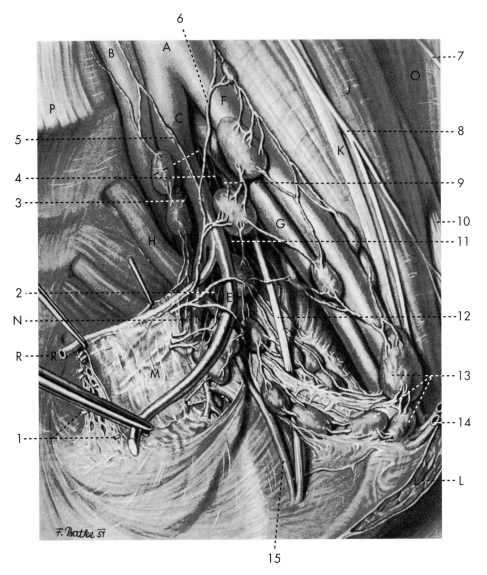

Fig. 2-11   Lymphatic drainage of the cervix. Mackenrodt's ligament was divided from the ureter. The superior border of the ligament is the uterine artery followed by several lymphatics flowing into the hypogastric and obturator lymph nodes. Efferent vessels of the cervix *(6)* pass the hypogastric lymph nodes and reach (without any interruption) the nodes of the lateral face of the external iliac artery. Further lymphatic vessels of the cervix pulled out by a small retractor follow at first the uterine artery and then join the superior gluteal lymph nodes surrounding the artery of the same name *(D)*. Other lymphatic drainages of the cervix flow into the inferior gluteal and the hypogastric lymph nodes located caudally to the obturator artery and partly covered by the lateral umbilical ligament. Notice the deep draining vessels *(2, 11, and 4)* coming from the inferior gluteal and the hypogastric lymph nodes, crossing underneath the big vessels of the pelvic wall to empty into the profound common iliac lymph nodes situated at the posterior face of the common iliac vessels *(A, B)* (see also Fig. 2-13). *A,* Common iliac artery; *B,* common iliac vein; *C,* internal iliac artery; *D,* superior gluteal artery; *E,* lateral umbilical ligament; *F,* external iliac artery; *G,* external iliac vein; *H,* first sacral nerve; *J,* psoas major and *K,* psoas minor muscles (tendon); *L,* internal oblique and transverse abdominal muscles; *M,* Mackenrodt's ligament; *N,* inferior gluteal–internal pudendal artery; *O,* iliac muscle; *P,* promontory; *R,* uterine artery; *1,* cervical lymph vessels; *2 to 4,* efferent vessels; *5 and 6,* cervical lymph vessel; *7,* lateral femoral cutaneous nerve; *8,* genitofemoral nerve; *9,* deep lateral external lymph node; *10,* femoral nerve; *11,* efferent vessel; *12,* obturator nerve; *13,* femoral ring lymph nodes; *14,* inferior epigastric vessel; *15,* obturator artery. (From Reiffenstuhl G: *Das Lymphsystem des weiblichen Genitale,* Vienna, 1957, Urban-Schwarzenberg.)

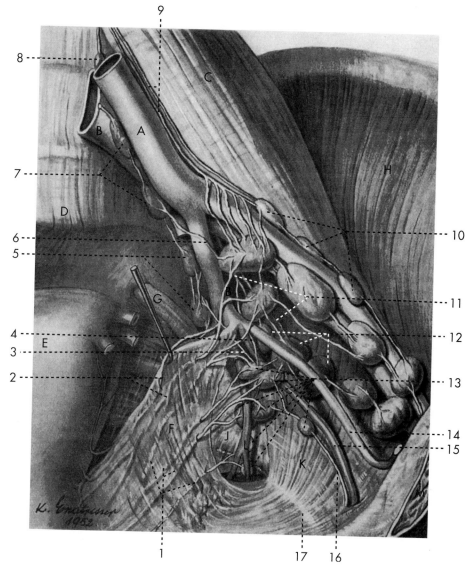

Fig. 2-12 Lymphatic vessels of the cervix *(1)* to the inferior gluteal lymph nodes. They go mainly to the pelvic wall in the basal segments of the lateral parametrium and then empty into the inferior gluteal lymph nodes *(13)* predominately. These nodes extend along the inferior gluteal–internal pudendal artery down as far as the infrapiriform foramen and, in part, lie behind the parietal blood vessels and are hidden by them. *A,* Common iliac artery; *B,* common iliac vein; *C,* psoas muscle; *D,* promontory; *E,* uterus; *F,* Mackenrodt's ligament; *G,* first sacral nerve; *H,* iliac muscle; *J,* sacral plexus; *K,* internal obturator muscle; *L,* internal pudendal–inferior gluteal artery; *M,* internal oblique and transverse abdominal muscles; *1* and *2,* cervical lymph vessels; *3* and *4,* efferent vessels; *5,* superior gluteal lymph nodes; *6,* efferent vessel; *7,* medial common iliac, and *8,* deep lateral common iliac lymph nodes; *9,* lymphatic vessels; *10,* lateral external iliac lymph nodes; *11,* efferent vessels; *12,* interiliac (obturator) and *13,* inferior gluteal lymph nodes; *14,* lateral umbilical ligament; *15,* obturator artery; *16,* lymphatic vessel; *17,* tendinous arch of the levator ani muscle. (From Reiffenstuhl G: *Das Lymphsystem des weiblichen Genitale,* Vienna, 1957, Urban-Schwarzenberg.)

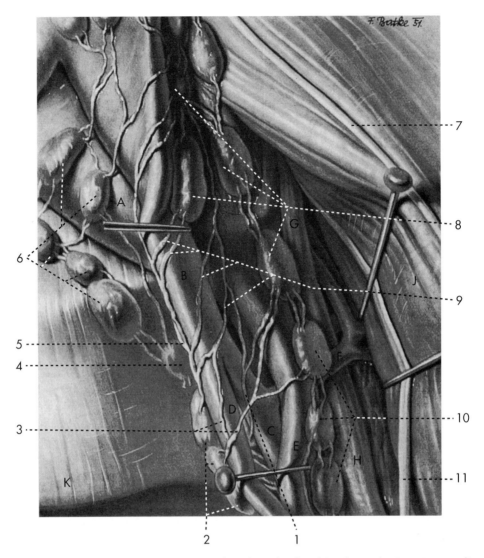

Fig. 2-13 Deep, or profound, iliac lymph nodes. The iliac blood vessels *(B to E)* were divided from the psoas muscle and pulled medially. The obturator nerve *(11)* and the psoas muscle *(J)* are forced laterally by two needles. In the deep recess of the fourth lumbar nerve *(G)*, the lumbosacral trunk *(H)* and the iliolumbar artery *(F)* are exposed. They are accompanied by the deep lateral common iliac lymph nodes *(8)* and the deep lateral external iliac lymph nodes *(10)*. These lymph nodes are located behind the parietal blood vessels and are normally hidden by those vessels. During extirpation of the deep external and common iliac lymph nodes, the iliolumbar artery *(F)* has to be exposed carefully to avoid damage. *A,* Left common iliac vein; *B,* left common iliac artery (posterior aspect); *C,* internal iliac artery (posterior aspect); *D,* external iliac artery (posterior aspect); *E,* external iliac vein (posterior aspect); *F,* iliolumbar artery; *G,* half of fourth lumbar nerve; *H,* lumbosacral trunk; *J,* psoas muscle; *K,* promontory; *1,* efferent vessels; *2,* lateral external iliac lymph nodes; *3,* efferent vessels; *4,* medial common iliac lymph node; *5,* lymph vessels; *6,* subaortic (promontorial) lymph nodes; *7,* genitofemoral nerve; *8,* deep lateral common iliac lymph nodes; *9,* efferent vessels; *10,* deep lateral external iliac lymph nodes; *11,* obturator nerve. (From Reiffenstuhl G: *Das Lymphsystem des weiblichen Genitale,* Vienna, 1957, Urban-Schwarzenberg.)

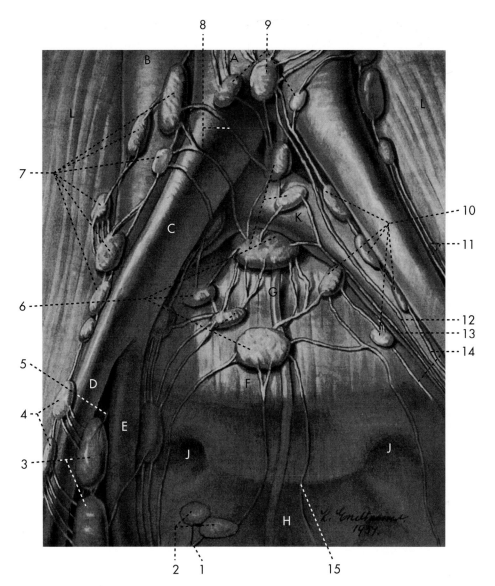

Fig. 2-14   Inflow and outflow of the subaortic (promontory) lymph nodes *(6)* that lie on the promontory *(F)* and in the aortic bifurcation angle and are interconnected by numerous lymph vessels, creating a picture of a lymphatic plexus on the promontory. They are also regional lymph nodes of the cervix and the uterus because they are supplied by lymph vessels *(13)* coming from the cervix and being intermitted for the first time here. Other lymphatics of the cervix *(12)* pass the subaortic lymph nodes without emptying into them and first being interrupted by the aortic lymph nodes *(9)*. Even the aortic lymph nodes are a regional lymph node station of the lymphatic drainage of the cervix. Notice the deep lymphatic vessels *(5)* starting from the hypogastric lymph nodes, undercrossing the internal iliac artery, running upward, and making a connection to the deep common iliac lymph nodes. These are located behind the blood vessels of the same names and are not visible here. (Compare with Figs. 2-10, 2-11, and 2-13.) *A,* Aorta; *B,* inferior vena cava; *C,* right common iliac artery; *D,* external iliac artery; *E,* internal iliac artery; *F,* promontory; *G,* medial sacral artery; *H,* sacrum; *J,* first sacral foramen; *K,* left common iliac vein; *L,* psoas muscle; *1,* cervical lymph vessels; *2,* sacral, *3,* interiliac, and *4,* lateral external iliac lymph nodes; *5,* efferent vessels; *6,* subaortic (promontorial) and *7,* lateral common iliac lymph nodes; *8,* efferent vessels; *9,* aortic, and *10,* medial common iliac lymph nodes; *11,* lymph vessels; *12* to *15,* cervical lymph vessels. (From Reiffenstuhl G: *Das Lymphsystem des weiblichen Genitale,* Vienna, 1957, Urban-Schwarzenberg.)

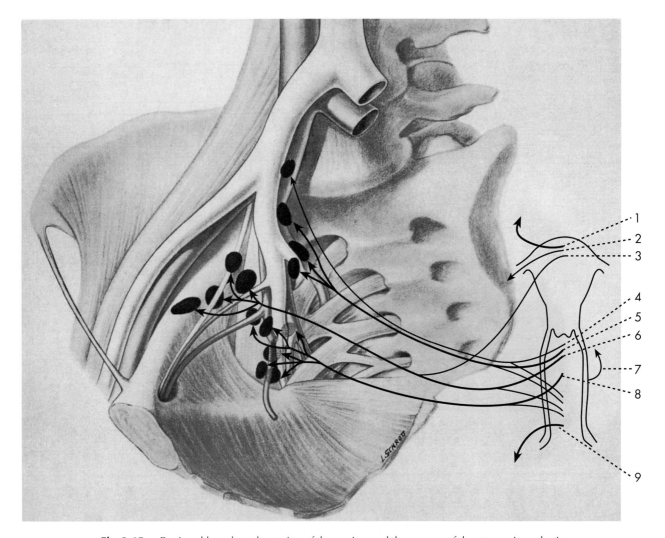

Fig. 2-15   Regional lymph node staging of the vagina and the corpus of the uterus. Lymphatic vessels numbers *1, 5, 6, 8,* and *9* are marked in bold because they are emptying into the regional lymph node groups, mostly draining from the uterus, fundus, and vagina. Notice in comparison to Fig. 2-9 the partly hidden location of the inferior gluteal lymph node *(gray)* reached by vessel number 8. To *(1)* aortic, *(2)* inguinal, *(3)* interiliac, *(4)* medial common iliac, *(5)* superior gluteal, *(6)* interiliac, *(7)* rectal, *(8)* inferior gluteal, and *(9)* inguinal lymph nodes. (From Reiffenstuhl G: *Das Lymphsystem des weiblichen Genitale,* Vienna, 1957, Urban-Schwarzenberg.)

LYMPHADENECTOMY

Every operation on a carcinoma should fulfill the following three demands:

1. If possible, the cancerous organ must be totally removed.
2. As much as possible of the surrounding tissue must be resected.
3. The regional lymph nodes must be extirpated or resected.

It is probably impossible to remove all the lymph nodes of the cervix uteri in a surgical procedure. The usual methods of lymph node resection will always be incomplete because in procedures modeled after Wertheim-Meigs, Latzko, or Okabayashi, the inferior gluteal lymph nodes are not removed. Radical extirpation of these lymph nodes would be complete only with resection of the gluteal pudendal vessels, which technically is not possible. Resection of these vessels of the pelvic wall fails because the veins accompanying the gluteal pudendal artery are very wide, have thin walls, and are transformed into a cavernous system, having numerous anastomoses and buried in the fascia of the pelvic wall. Many people have tried to modify and extend the Wertheim procedure, but most procedures have failed to remove the gluteal lymph nodes. However, Brunschwig's radical method of pelvic exenteration has been successful even in very advanced cases. To remove the inferior gluteal lymph nodes, the hypogastric artery must be ligated near its branch from the common iliac artery. Then the gluteal pudendal arteries are exposed and ligated. The hypogastric vein that lies underneath needs to be ligated with all its branches and then removed together with the surrounding lymphatic and fatty tissue. After that, the sciatic nerve and its roots are exposed totally on each side. It is commonly felt that Brunschwig's procedure is too extended and dangerous to perform as a palliative operation for uterine or cervical carcinoma.

Inguinal Lymph Nodes

The inguinal lymph nodes are divided into superficial and deep. The superficial lymph nodes can be divided into a horizontal tract (parallel to the groin and vertical tract) along the great saphenous vein. The deep inguinal lymph nodes lie directly on the iliopsoas muscle and are covered by the superficial layer of the fascia lata. The fascia lata of the thigh is divided into two layers: the superficial one has a very small, oval opening—lamina cribriformis fossae ovalis—and goes medially into the ductus muscles fascia. The deep layer covers the psoas and pectinate muscles on the medial side and also the ductus muscle group. The superficial and deep inguinal lymph nodes are connected by anastomoses. The draining vessels of the vertical tract mainly go through the lateral group of the horizontal tract of the inguinal lymph nodes. The draining vessels of the horizontal tract of the inguinal lymph nodes can be divided into the following three groups:

1. Numerous efferent vessels of the lateral inguinal lymph nodes pass the lateral side of the femoral artery and reach the pelvis by passing the lacuna of vessels (Fig. 2-20). On the lateral and dorsal side of the external iliac artery, they turn upward and reach the lateral external iliac lymph nodes. From there, the lymph fluid flows through the common iliac and aortic lymph nodes. Interesting variations in the direction taken by the lymph vessels have been noted. Lymphatics move from the lateral inguinal lymph nodes through the most lateral part of the lacuna of vessels along the intralacunal ligament into the pelvic cavity, which empty either into the distal external iliac lymph nodes and turn upward or turn without any intermission by the distal external iliac lymph nodes directly to the iliac or psoas muscle inside the iliac fossae and then flow cranially to the common iliac lymph nodes. In this way, there are lymphatic anastomoses of the lateral inguinal or distal external iliac lymph nodes into the common iliac lymph nodes.

2. Numerous efferent vessels of the inguinal lymph nodes pass centrally with the femoral vein (and also femoral artery). They flow into the lymph nodes of the femoral ring (see Fig. 2-8, *K*) and mainly reach the medial external iliac nodes (see Fig. 2-8, *J*). The most medially situated lymph node of the group around the femoral ring is called *Rosenmüller's lymph node*. Its anterior part touches the femoral vein medially inside the lacuna of vessels and extends, depending on its size, over the horizontal ramus of the pubic bone. If Rosenmüller's lymph node has not developed, a bunch of narrow lymph vessels is found in its place. These vessels flow from the lateral pelvic wall toward and into the external medial iliac lymph node. Starting from the external medial iliac lymph nodes, lymph vessels may lead to the obturator (Fig. 2-8, *I*), hypogastric (Fig. 2-8, *H*), and external iliac lymph nodes at the external iliac artery (Fig. 2-8, *J*).

3. After injection of contrast into the medial superficial inguinal lymph nodes, many efferent vessels exiting these lymph nodes and turning medially to the femoral vein on the iliopsoas and pectineal muscles fascia, later on the lacunar ligament upward, enter the pelvis through the most medial part of the vessel. Later they turn around the horizontal ramus of the pubic bone, crossing underneath the pubic branches of the inferior epigastric artery and vein. They do not flow into the femoral ring lymph nodes, as expected, but pass Rosenmüller's lymph node medially and empty into the obturator and the inferior gluteal lymph nodes. The most caudal vessel of those lymphatics perform anastomosis with the lymph vessel entering the pelvis by the obturator foramen. The lymphatic fluid flows farther from the obturator lymph nodes and the inferior gluteal lymph nodes to the hypogastric, the superior gluteal, and sacral lymph nodes. The inferior gluteal lymph nodes also receive fluid from the gluteal region by lymphatics that enter the pelvis through the infrapiriform foramen.

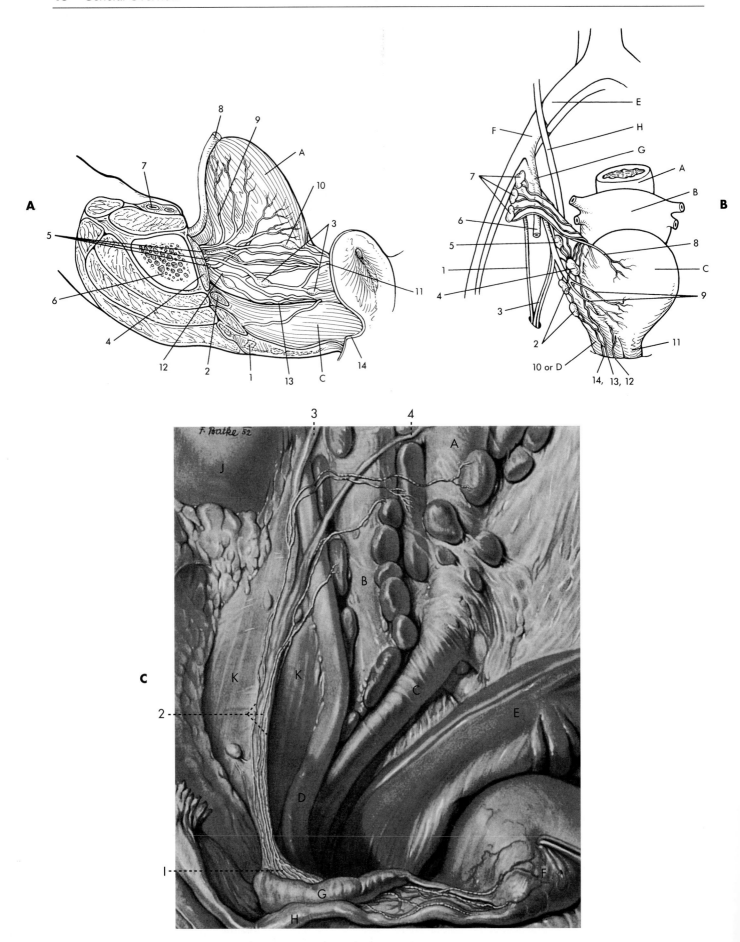

Fig. 2-16   For legend see opposite page.

Fig. 2-16 **A,** Lymphatic drainage of vagina, urethra, and bladder. Vaginal lymph vessels *(13)* follow the vaginal artery upward to the lymph nodes of the pelvic wall. The course is interrupted by small paravaginal or juxtavaginal lymph nodes *(3)*. Other vaginal lymphatics *(15)* extend to the posterior face of the rectum *(C)* flowing into the rectal (anorectal) lymph nodes (therefore lymph node metastasis on the back side of the rectum from carcinoma of the vagina is possible). The draining lymph vessels of the intrapelvic segment of the urethra *(11)* sometimes are interrupted by an anterior vesical lymph node *(10)* and later proceed to the pelvic wall and are accompanied by the efferent lymphatic vessels of the bladder *(A)*. A, Urinary bladder; B, vagina; C, rectum; D, labium pudendi; *1,* sacral os; *2,* ischiatic nerve; *3,* juxtavaginal lymph nodes; *4,* internal obturator muscle; *5,* obturator nerve, artery, and vein; *6,* os; *7,* femoral artery and vein; *8,* lateral umbilical ligament; *9,* lymph vessels of the urinary bladder; *10,* anterior vesical lymph node; *11,* urethral lymph vessels; *12,* vaginal artery; *13,* vaginal lymph vessel; *14,* anus. **B,** Lymphatic drainage of the superior half of the vagina. The fatty lymphoidal tissue of the obturator fossa was taken down the pelvic wall and clipped in a medial direction. Several vaginal lymph vessels *(12)* go upward to the draining lymph vessels of the cervix and turn along the superior vesical artery *(8)*; all empty into the hypogastric lymph nodes *(7)*. Other vaginal lymph vessels *(13)* flow into an obturator node *(4)*, which has been medially exposed. From there, lymphatic connections go to a superior gluteal lymph node *(5)*. Notice further the course of the draining vaginal lymph vessels *(14)* flowing into an inferior gluteal lymph node *(2)*. A, Rectum; B, uterus (vesical surface); C, urinary bladder; D, vagina; E, common iliac artery; F, external iliac artery; G, internal iliac artery; H, ureter; *1,* obturator nerve; *2,* inferior gluteal lymph nodes; *3,* obturator artery; *4,* interiliac (obturator) lymph node; *5,* superior gluteal lymph node; *6,* lateral umbilical ligament; *7,* hypogastric lymph nodes; *8,* superior vesical artery; *9,* inferior vesical veins; *10,* vagina; *11,* urethra; *12 to 14,* vaginal lymph vessels. **C,** Lymphatic drainage of the fallopian tube, ovary, and fundus of the uterus. Lymphatic vessels originating at the tube go either directly to the subovarian lymphatic plexus *(1)* or flow first into the lymph vessels draining the uterine fundus *(F)*. The lymphatics of the fundus follow the ovarian proprium ligament and mesosalpinx until reaching the subovarian plexus, which mainly drains the ovary area. From there the lymphatic vessels *(2)* extend along the ovarian blood vessels cranially, leave the blood vessels near the lower kidney edge *(J)*, turn medially across the ureter *(D)*, and flow into the upper aortic lymph nodes. A, Aorta; B, inferior vena cava; C, right common iliac artery; D, ureter; E, sigmoid; F, uterine fundus; G, right ovary; H, right fallopian tube; J, right kidney; K, psoas muscle; *1,* subovarian plexus; *2,* lymph vessels; *3,* ovarian vein; *4,* ovarian artery. (Adapted and redrawn from Reiffenstuhl G: *Das Lymphsystem des weiblichen Genitale,* Vienna, 1957, Urban-Schwarzenberg.)

Fig. 2-17 Lymphatic cord of Poirier. Possible metastasis of cervical carcinoma into the uterine corpus. Advanced cases of cancer in both the portio vaginalis and primarily the cervix can metastasize upward into the myometrium of the uterine corpus. For such dissemination, it needs anastomoses of the mucosal and myometrial lymphatics of Seelig, which radiate to the meridionally coursing Poirier lymphatics, located along the border of the uterus. In this way they can intersperse the musculature of the uterine corpus with cancerous areas and also lead to development of metastatic colonies in the mucosa of the uterine corpus. (From Amreich IA: *Biologie und Pathologie des Weibes: Handbuch der Frauenheilkunde und Geburtshilfe,* Bd IV, Berlin, 1955, Urban & Schwarzenberg.)

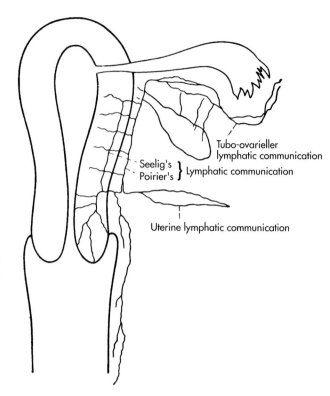

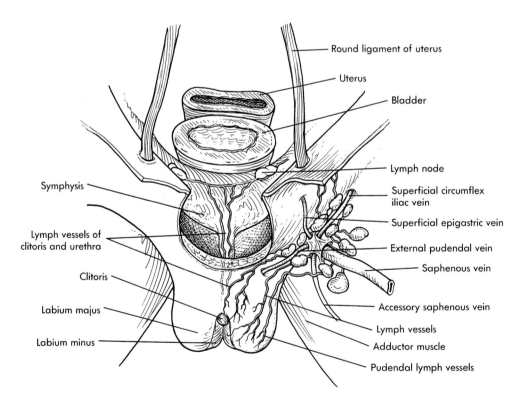

Fig. 2-18 Lymph drainage. (Adapted and redrawn from Reiffenstuhl G: *Das Lymphsystem des weiblichen Genitale,* Vienna, 1957, Urban-Schwarzenberg.)

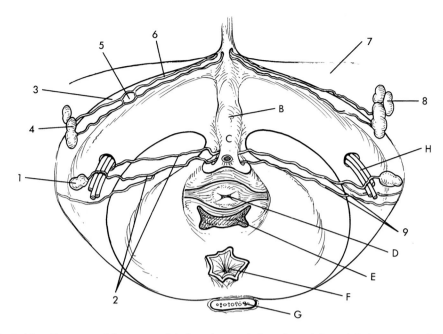

Fig. 2-19   Entrance of the extrapelvic lymph vessels into the pelvis and their course to the intrapelvic lymph nodes. View into the small pelvis from above. On the upper edge of the symphysis several lymph vessels *(6)* enter the pelvic cavity medially between the insertion of the rectus abdominal muscle *(A)*. Then following the superior ramus of the pubic bone *(3)*, they may reach on both sides the femoral ring lymph nodes *(4, 8)*. Other lymph vessels *(2)* reach the pelvis together with the dorsal vein of the clitoris *(C)*, following the inferior surface of the symphysis, then turn laterally and reach an obturator lymph node *(1)* on the left side, whereas on the right side they *(9)* empty finally into the hypogastric lymph nodes. In this manner, efferent lymphatic channels of the external genitals have reached lymph nodes of the pelvic wall as their regional stations. *A,* Rectus abdominis muscle; *B,* symphysis (posterior aspect); *C,* dorsal clitoridic vein; *D,* urethra; *E,* vagina; *F,* rectum; *G,* sacrum; *H,* obturator nerve, artery and vein; *1,* obturator lymph node; *2,* lymph vessels; *3,* superior ramus of the pubic bone; *4,* femoral ring lymph nodes; *5,* lymph node; *6,* lymph vessels; *7,* inguinal ligament; *8,* femoral ring lymph nodes; *9,* lymph vessels. (Adapted and redrawn from Reiffenstuhl G: *Das Lymphsystem des weiblichen Genitale,* Vienna, 1957, Urban-Schwarzenberg.)

URETER

The ureter plays an important part in gynecologic operations. Its topographic relation to the organs and structures within the pelvis and on the pelvic wall is especially important. Finding it and sometimes exposing it are absolute prerequisites for its protection.

The ureter enters the small pelvis in front of or slightly medial to the sacral iliac junction; both sides are the same distance from the midline. To the outside convex arc, both ureters run along the small pelvic wall caudally to the back side of Mackenrodt's ligament; at this point, they are farther from each other than when entering the pelvis. The relation to the big vessels is not always constant. The ureter crosses either the common iliac artery or the external iliac artery. This is not caused by the location of the ureter but rather by the length of the common iliac artery.

After crossing the blood vessel, the right ureter lies either medially or medially and in front of the internal iliac artery and reaches the ovarian fossa. The ovarian fossa is a depression of the peritoneum between the internal and external iliac arteries. On the left side, the ureter generally proceeds along the common iliac artery, crosses at a sharp angle at the beginning of the internal iliac artery, and reaches the ovarian fossa in front of the internal iliac artery. The ureter is covered by the parietal peritoneum, to which it also is fixed by the connective tissue surrounding itself. In some women the ureter produces a fold that can be followed from the entrance of the pelvis onto Mackenrodt's ligament. Laterally from the ureter are branches of the internal iliac vessels, the obturator artery, and the obturator vein, as well as the beginning of the lateral umbilical ligament. Above the pelvic floor, the ureter turns medially and ventrally into Mackenrodt's ligament. It remains on the back side of the ligament, then penetrates the parametrial connective tissue. It passes the uterine cervix laterally for a short distance while coursing medially and ventrally. Of course, the proximity of the ureter to the cervix varies with the position of the uterus, which generally is not strictly median nor strictly in the midline. The distance between the right and left ureter and the cervix can vary, so it is important during surgery to stay close to the uterus to avoid damaging the ureter. Inside the parametrium, the ureter is located very close to the vessels. The uterine artery

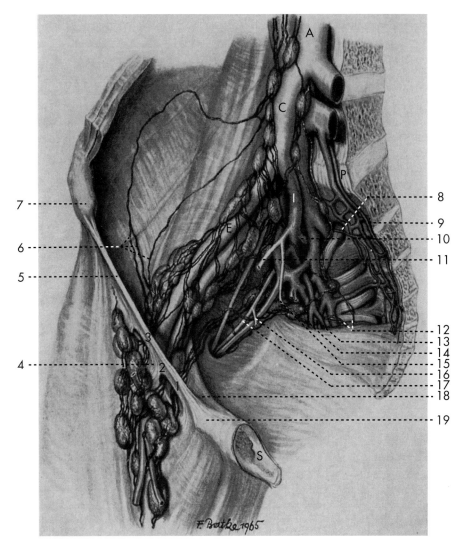

Fig. 2-20 Three groups of draining lymph vessels from the horizontal tract of inguinal lymph nodes to the pelvic lymph nodes. *3,* Lateral pathway to the lateral external iliac lymph nodes and the common iliac lymph nodes; *2,* median, or midline, pathway of the medial external iliac lymph nodes and the hypogastric lymph nodes; *1,* medial pathway to the obturator and inferior gluteal lymph nodes; *4,* connective tissue of the blood vessel canal fascia (interlacunar ligament); *5,* inguinal ligament; *6,* bypasses from the inguinal external iliac to the common iliac lymph nodes; *7,* anterosuperior iliac spine; *8,* lateral sacral artery; *9,* medial sacral artery; *10,* superior gluteal artery; *11,* lateral umbilical ligament; *12,* lymph vessels to the gluteal region; *13,* inferior gluteal artery; *14,* inferior pudendal artery; *15,* uterine artery; *16,* inferior vesical artery; *17,* obturator artery; *18,* superior ramus of the pubic bone; *19,* tuberosity of the pubic bone. *A,* Aorta; *C,* common iliac artery; *E,* external iliac artery; *I,* internal iliac artery; *P,* promontory; *S,* symphysis. (From Reiffenstuhl G: *Das Lymphknotenproblem beim Carcinoma colli uteri und die Lymphirradiatio pelvis. Direkte Bestrahlung des Beckenlymphsystems mit Isotopen,* Vienna, 1967, Urban-Schwarzenberg.)

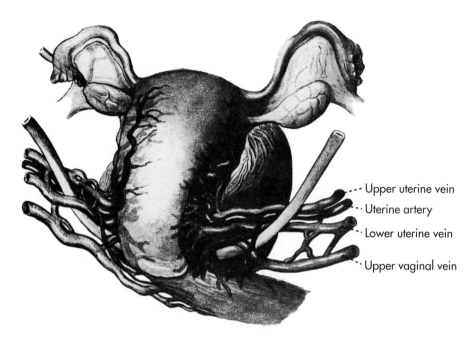

Fig. 2-21   Relation of the ureter to its venous surroundings. On the right side, the ureter runs between the lower uterine vein and upper vaginal vein, ventrally up to the bladder; on the left side, the ureter runs between the uterine artery and the inferior uterine vein. (From Von Peham H, Amreich JA: *Gynaekologische Operationslehre,* Berlin, 1930, S Karger.)

The labels in the figure read:
- Upper uterine vein
- Uterine artery
- Lower uterine vein
- Upper vaginal vein

runs caudal, lying lateral and somewhat medial to the ureter. Near the uterus, the uterine artery crosses over the ureter. The uterine and vaginal veins surround the ureter, crossing and running below and above it, and finally lying lateral to the ureter and making their way to the internal iliac vein (Fig. 2-21).

In the middle of these vessels, the ureter, including its sheath, lies inside a canal running directly through the parametrial connective tissue. The ureteral sheath is loosely connected to the wall of this canal, and it is not difficult to expose the ureter and its sheath if operating in the correct layer. The last segment of the ureter extends from the crossing with the uterine artery ventrally through its orifice into the bladder. At this location the ureter lies in a preformed canal, so it is not fixed to anything surrounding it. The ureter approaches the vaginal wall lateral to the uterine portio and then runs on top of the ventral vaginal wall. But, again, its only connection to the vaginal wall is by loose connective tissue. Cranially, the ureter comes very close to the floor of the vesicouterine cavity, so a fold is formed as soon as the ureter is forced backward. The blood supply of the part of the pelvis containing the ureter is provided by different arteries and is subject to individual variation. A branch of the ovarian artery might reach the ureter, and branches of the common and internal iliac, the iliolumbar, and the superior gluteal and medial rectal arteries might belong to the feeding blood vessels. The ureteral segment near the bladder is supplied by a branch of the uterine artery that leaves the uterine artery and crosses near the ureter (Figs. 2-22 and 2-23). This branch usually is divided into an ascendent and descendent ramus; the descendent one anastomoses with

branches of the superior and inferior vesical arteries that supply the ureter while ascending. Further on, a branch out of the vaginal artery very often leads into this net. Because of the rich blood supply, it is possible to ligate one of the branches in radical procedures, but the blood supply and the adventitial tissue of the ureter must not be destroyed or damaged. The venous drainage of the ureter is performed by the vesical vein plexus to the uterine plexus and indirectly to the ovarian and internal iliac vein.

For locating and sometimes exposing the ureter in the connective tissue matrix (Fig. 2-24, p. 56), the pelvic ureter begins at the terminal on both sides at the sacroiliac articulation. The pelvic ureter first traverses the rectal pillar, then Mackenrodt's ligament, and finally the bladder pillar to reach forward to the bladder. Therefore it is also subdivided in the small pelvis into three sections: (1) pars posterior in the rectouterine ligament, (2) pars intermedia in Mackenrodt's ligament, and (3) pars anterior in the vesicouterine ligament.

Clinical Remarks

The 15-cm segment of the ureter inside the pelvis consists of a descending part, describing a laterally convex turn, and an ascending urethrovesical (or juxtavesical) part, beginning at the so-called knee of the ureter. The ascending juxtavesical segment changes its course if the inner genitalia change position (Fig. 2-25, p. 57). In a person who has cystocele, for example, the ureter approaches the bladder only at the lateral edge, whereas with a higher grade cystocele or a prolapse, it approaches the bladder laterally and from above (Fig. 2-26, p. 57).

During radical vaginal hysterectomy, the uterus is pulled

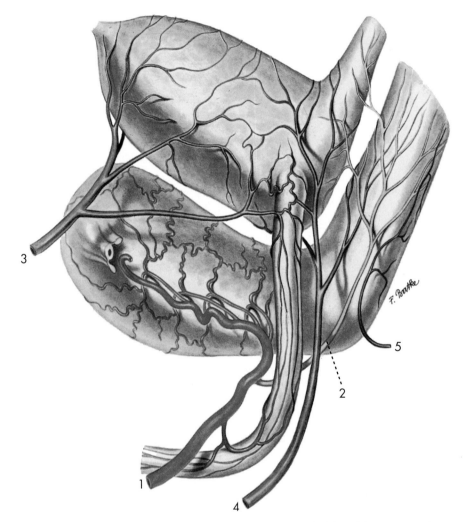

Fig. 2-22 Blood supply of the portion of the ureter near the bladder of the uterus in this area, of the more central parts of the urethra, and of the vagina, as seen from the side. *1,* Uterine artery; *2,* vaginal artery; *3,* superior vesical artery; *4,* inferior vesical artery; *5,* branch of the inferior rectal artery. (From Reiffenstuhl G, Platzer W: *Die Vaginalen Operationen: Chirurgie, Anatomie und Operationslehre,* Berlin, 1974, Urban-Schwarzenberg.)

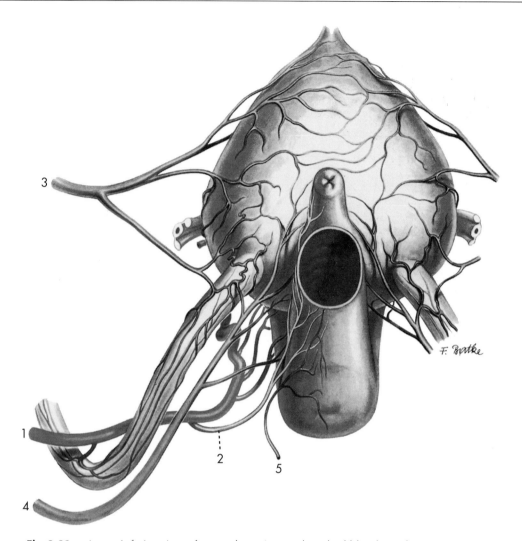

Fig. 2-23 Anteroinferior view of ureteral, uterine, and urethral blood supply. *1* to *5,* see Fig. 2-22. (From Reiffenstuhl G, Platzer W: *Die Vaginalen Operationen: Chirurgie, Anatomie und Operationslehre,* Berlin, 1974, Urban-Schwarzenberg.)

downward with the portio and vaginal cuff. The uterine vessels, the vessels feeding and surrounding the ureter, and the ureter itself (by the uterine artery at the crossing) also are pulled downward, thus changing the course of the ureter. The pelvic knee of the ureter is transformed into a more or less sharp, angular loop. After the uterine vessels are cut and the vessels are divided from the uterus, the ureter fits back into its former position. Then a radical excision of the paraspaces or parametrial spaces is possible without endangering the ureter. A second important point concerning ureter fixation by a vascular framework that appears when the ureter is exposed for modified vaginal radical hysterectomy is as follows: usually the surgeon looks for the ureter inside the vesicouterine ligament. However, if the surgeon does not find the correct layer between vesical and vaginal fascia at the beginning of the operation when loosening the bladder, the operative field is almost always too close to the vagina and cervix. When the vesicouterine ligament is cut, the ureter does not become visible but remains covered by connective tissue (vaginal and cervical fascia). The surgeon

must then dissect along the uterine vessels cranially until reaching the vessels; the ureter is fixed and can always be found there.

Damage to the ureter is more likely to occur during abdominal rather than vaginal hysterectomy. In the vaginal procedure, when the bladder is lifted up after dissection of the supravaginal septum (the condensed connective tissue separating the vesicovaginal space from the vesicocervical space), the ureter is stretched and therefore withdraws from the cervix, which it approaches in the normal anatomic position at about 1.5 cm (Fig. 2-27, p. 58). In addition, the ureter can be forced laterally out of the operative field by the surgeon's finger, forcing the bladder column laterally (Fig. 2-28, p. 59). This procedure removes the knee of the ureter another 2 cm away from the cervix. In comparison, in an abdominal procedure, the ureter is dissectable after exposure of the bladder, which has to be performed strictly in the midline to prevent damage to blood vessels in the bladder column and after forcing the bladder column laterally, best done with a smooth swab. The ureter, which crosses inside the bladder

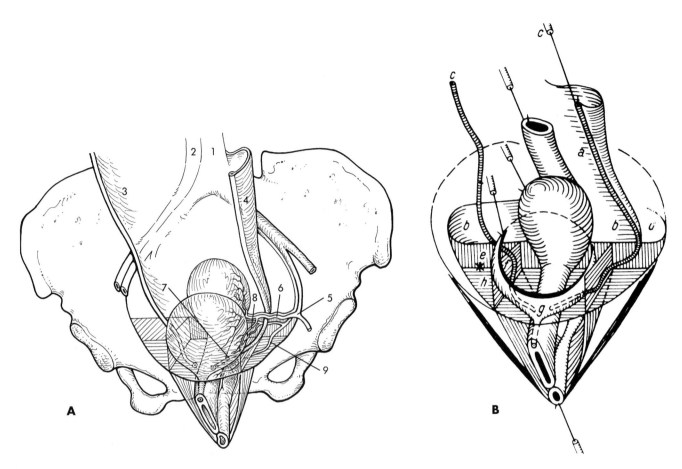

Fig. 2-24 **A,** Schematic representation of the connective tissue of the pelvis according to Amreich. Relative position of the ureter to the blood vessels. On the right side of the pelvis, the ureter and its associated ureteral leaf *(3)* are left in place; on the left, the ureter and its leaf *(4)* are folded medially. In the course of the ureter in the pelvis, one can differentiate posterior, intermediate, and anterior parts. The intermediate part of the ureter uses the middle portion of Mackenrodt's ligament in its course and is crossed there by the uterine artery *(5),* which runs along the upper edge of the ligament and, as a rule, by one of its accompanying veins *(6)* as well. The anterior part *(7)* of the ureter follows a somewhat ascending course that tends toward the medial in the bladder pillar. The efferent veins of the vesical plexus and the superior vesical artery *(8)* lie cranially to the ureter; the vaginal veins *(9)* lie caudal to it. *1,* Aorta; *2,* inferior vena cava, *3;* ureteral leaf (anterior aspect); *4,* ureteral leaf (posterior aspect); *5,* uterine artery; *6,* uterine veins; *7,* ureter (anterior part); *8,* superior vesical artery and vein; and *9,* vaginal vein. **B,** Course of the ureter in the pelvic connective tissue. On the right side, the ureter *(c)* lies in place against the pelvic wall; on the left, with its leaf (the ureteral leaf *[a]* is an upward continuation of the sagittal rectal pillar *[b]).* It is detached from the pelvic wall and folded medially. Thereby a portion of an artificially produced cavity—the pararectal space *(d) (upper level)*—comes into view. The medial boundary of the space is formed by the rectal pillar *(b),* now standing truly sagittally, with its ureteral leaf. The lateral boundary is formed by the pelvic wall. The ureter first runs in the ureteral leaf and the sagittal rectal pillar *(b)* and then uses the middle portion of Mackenrodt's ligament *(e)* and runs forward in the sagittal portion of the bladder pillar *(f)* until it reaches the bladder *(g).* The paravesical space *(asterisk)* is bounded medially by the bladder pillar *(f),* laterally by the pelvic wall, dorsally by Mackenrodt's ligament *(e),* caudally by the horizontal connective tissue foundation *(h),* and cranially by the umbilical ligamental layers (a delicate leaf of connective tissue not shown here). *a,* Ureteral leaf; *b,* sagittal rectal pillar; *c,* ureter; *d,* pararectal space; *e,* Mackenrodt's ligament; *f,* sagittal bladder pillar; *g,* urinary bladder; *h,* horizontal connective tissue foundation; *asterisk,* paravesical space. (From Reiffenstuhl G: *The lymphatics of the female genital organs,* Philadelphia, 1964, JB Lippincott.)

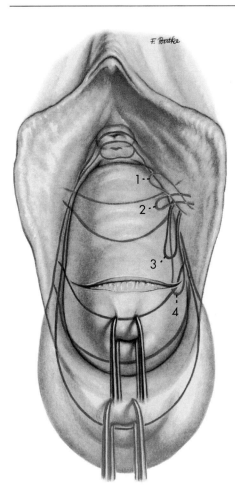

Fig. 2-25   Postion of the ureters and the bladder in uterine prolapse. The ascending ureter in its normal, original state *(1)* becomes almost horizontal *(2)* when the bladder sinks anteriorly. In more extensive cases with moderate *(3)* or severe *(4)* descensus uteri, the ureter descends vertically. (From Reiffenstuhl G, Platzer W: *Die Vaginalen Operationen. Chirurgie, Anatomie und Operationslehre,* Berlin, 1974, Urban-Schwarzenberg.)

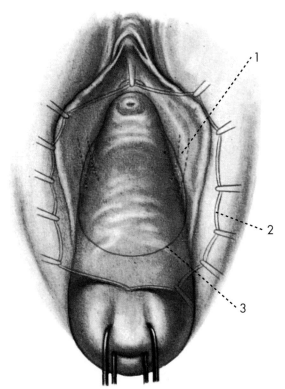

Fig. 2-26   Schematic view of the operative field in prolapse of the bladder and the vagina, showing a section of the ureter near the bladder, the cut edge of the vaginal wall, and the operative margins diagrammatically. *1,* Ureteral course near the bladder; *2,* separated vaginal wall; *3,* edge of operative field. (From Reiffenstuhl G, Platzer W: *Die Vaginalen Operationen. Chirurgie, Anatomie und Operationslehre,* Berlin, 1974, Urban-Schwarzenberg.)

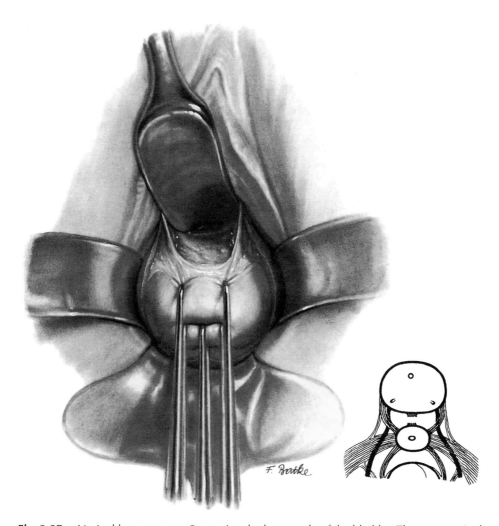

Fig. 2-27   Vaginal hysterectomy. Separating the lower pole of the bladder. The supravaginal septum is divided, and the vesicocervical space is opened. The lower bladder pole is separated upward to the peritoneal reflection, being advanced with a spatula inserted in the vesicocervical space. Laterally, the bladder pillars (ligamentum vesicouterina), coursing from the bladder to the cervix, are stretched. The uterine arteries are medial to the bladder pillars at the edge of the cervix. The diagram shows the anatomic relationships more clearly. (From Reiffenstuhl G, Platzer W: *Die Vaginalen Operationen. Chirurgie, Anatomie und Operationslehre,* Berlin, 1974, Urban-Schwarzenberg.)

column, can be removed from the cervix approximately 1 to 2 cm away by forcing the bladder column laterally. Then it is no longer a risk to clamp the ureter with a parametrial clamp. Also, it is not necessary to clamp the parametrium, which is extended deep down to the upper part of the vagina, because a later clamp placed in the lateral vaginal fornix—after opening the ventral fornix of the vagina—also clamps the rest of the parametrium. If this interaction is being followed and the most caudal clamp is not placed too far caudally, there is nothing to worry about. Possible ureteral damage is the most dangerous aspect of abdominal hysterectomy.

The relationships between ureter and uterus change during pregnancy (Fig. 2-29, p. 60). As the uterus fills out almost all of the pelvis, the ureter becomes closely attached to the lower uterus from the linea terminalis to the orifice into

the bladder, leaving no distance between cervix and uterus in pregnant women.

Liberation of the Ureter

Serious inflammation of the inner genitalia can considerably change the topography of the pelvic ureter. Frequently, the ureter has to be liberated before an adnexal tumor or large myoma is excised. The easiest place to find the ureter according to pelvic anatomy is at the base of the infundibulopelvic ligament. For this procedure, the adnexa is lifted up with a ring forceps, and the peritoneum is lifted up from the pelvic wall by forceps and cut close caudally to the ovarian vessels (Fig. 2-30, p. 61). A smooth, closed scissors is introduced into the peritoneal gap, and the peritoneum is pulled away from the abdominal wall. The peritoneal cut can be

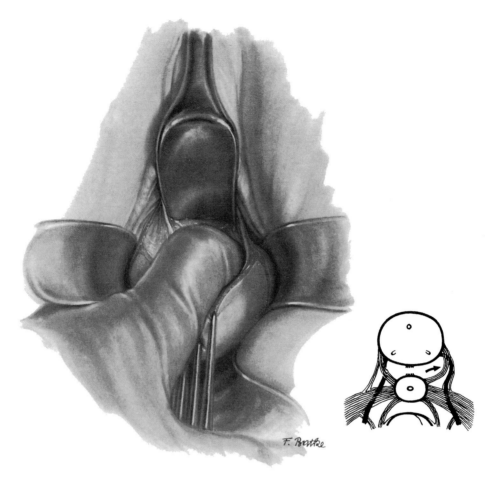

Fig. 2-28 Vaginal hysterectomy. Advancing the bladder. The bladder is held up with an anterior spatula inserted in the vesicocervical space. The surgeon pushes the fibers of the left bladder pillar laterally with the left index finger, thereby displacing the ureter, which courses in the bladder pillar, out of the operative field, as shown in the schema. (From Reiffenstuhl G, Platzer W: *Die Vaginalen Operationen. Chirurgie, Anatomie und Operationslehre,* Berlin, 1974, Urban-Schwarzenberg.)

enlarged caudally without damaging the blood vessels of the pelvic wall (Fig. 2-31, p. 61).

The ureter can be found medially in the depth of the peritoneal gap. In this area, the ureter has a close relationship to the peritoneum and is easily palpated by picking it up with the second and third fingers. In very difficult cases, as with adhesions and concretions, the ureter can be recognized by its peristaltic waves. The ureter should be further liberated with closed scissors until it enters the lateral parametrium (Fig. 2-32, p. 61). The ureter can be forced caudally quite easily.

In severe change caused by adnexal inflammation, the ureter can become fixed onto the lesion and must be dissected very closely. Caution must be exercised so that the ureteral adventitia is not damaged.

PELVIC FLOOR—PERINEAL REGION

The borders of the perineal region are the angle of symphysis, the inferior rami of the pubic bone, the ascendent ramus of the ischiatic bone, the lower edge of the sacrum, and the coccyx (Fig. 2-33, p. 62). The pelvic floor is formed by two layers of muscle and connective tissue. The pelvic and urogenital diaphragms are shown in Fig. 2-34 on p. 63. Each is an incomplete seal of the pelvis, but this deficiency is corrected by shifting the two layers against each other.

Pelvic Diaphragm

The muscular part of the pelvic diaphragm consists of the levator ani and coccygeal muscles and has the form of a funnel. The levator ani muscle originates at the dorsal side of the pubic bone and at the transverse perineal ligament. It inserts at the tendineus arcus of the obturator fascia to the ischial spine, then along the sacrospinous ligament to the coccyx (see Fig. 2-33). The levator ani muscle can be divided into three parts corresponding to its course. The puborectal muscle is shown in Fig. 2-33, *D.* The fibers forming the so-called levator pillars, or columns, have been considered by some gynecologists as the most important part of the levator muscle. These strong parts of the muscle cross caudally and dorsally along the sides of the urethra, vagina, and rectum, making a strong connection with the connective tissue of these organs. Certain fibers of the levator muscle cover the lateral and dorsal

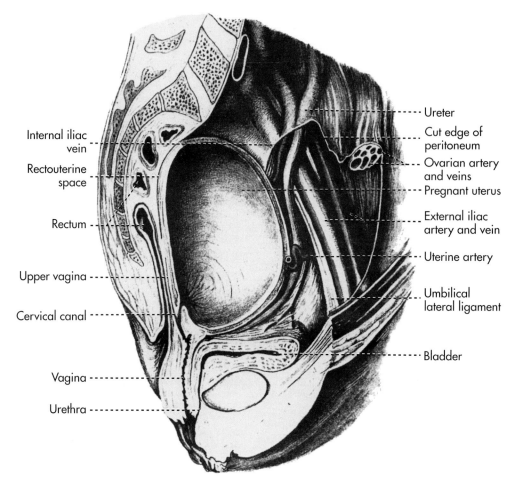

Internal iliac vein

Rectouterine space

Rectum

Upper vagina

Cervical canal

Vagina

Urethra

Ureter

Cut edge of peritoneum

Ovarian artery and veins

Pregnant uterus

External iliac artery and vein

Uterine artery

Umbilical lateral ligament

Bladder

Fig. 2-29   Topography of the ureter in pregnant women. (From Tandler J, Halban J: *Topography of the female ureter,* Vienna, 1901.)

parts of the rectum and, after surrounding the rectum and coming around to the front and joining the internal sphincter ani muscle, they support the rectum by making a muscle loop. Certain parts of the puborectal muscle are called *prerectal fibers* (see Fig. 2-33, *C*) because of their crossing of the ventral wall of the rectum. Together with the perineal wedge (see Fig. 2-34), they divide the levator opening, the *hiatus urogenitalis,* from the anal hiatus.

Starting from the levator columns, smooth and striated fibers of the muscle join the perineal wedge, forming a loop around the vagina. The so-called levator vaginal muscle contractions of the levator columns stretch their arcuate course and reduce the genital hiatus and the diameter of the vagina. The remaining fibers can be described as pubococcygeal and iliococcygeal (see Fig. 2-33, *F*) muscle. They reach out to the top of the coccygeus, passing the rectal coccygeal aponeurosis. The iliococcygeal muscle is a little weaker than the pubococcygeal muscle. The iliococcygeus originates at the fascia of the internal obturator muscle on the tendinous arc of the levator muscle and inserts at the coccyx and the lower parts of the sacrum. The pelvic diaphragm is completed dorsally by the coccygeus muscle (see Fig. 2-33, *G*). The coccygeus muscle extends from ischiatic spine to the coccygeal and sacral bone. The sacrospinous

ligament courses within the coccygeus muscle as its aponeurosis. Usually the pelvic diaphragm is innervated by a long branch of the sacral plexus (sacral nerve no. 4). The anatomic position of the pelvic diaphragm is limited by the orifice of the rectum (anus).

The different parts of the levator muscle combine, which is referred to as a *levator sheet.* Berglas and Rubin studied the levator sheet in living women and described it as a horizontal sheet with an opening near the symphysis (urogenital hiatus). The urethra, rectum, and vagina pass through this aperture. The levator plate is formed by fusion of the pubococcygeal muscles posterior to the rectum. The vagina creates an especially weak point in the pelvic floor, and consequently the incidence of hernias (cystoceles and rectoceles) and prolapse in this area is high. The levator ani muscle antagonizes the muscles of the abdominal wall and is responsible not only for support of the content of pelvis and abdomen, but also for maintenance and compensation of intraabdominal pressure. Whenever one of the two components (muscle systems) is weakened or inactive over a certain period (e.g., splinted by very narrow and strong corsetry), the opposite component compensates by not contracting for a longer period, potentially resulting in genital prolapse.

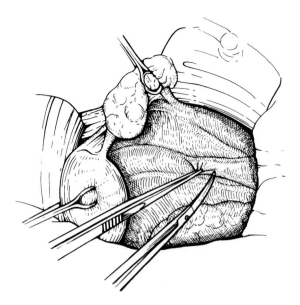

Fig. 2-30 Dissection of liberation of the ureter. Incision of the peritoneum of the pelvic wall. The adnexa is being lifted up by a forceps; the pelvic peritoneum is being pulled away from the pelvic wall by a forceps. The surgeon uses a smooth scissors to incise close and caudally to the ovarian vessels. (From Reiffenstuhl G: Dringliche gynäkologische und gebhurtshilfe Operationen. In Breitner, Kraus, Zuckschwerdt: *Chirurgie Operationslehre,* Bd VI, Berlin, 1977, Urban & Schwarzenberg.)

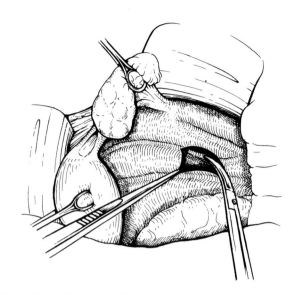

Fig. 2-32 Dissection of the ureter, liberation of the ureter. The pelvic peritoneum is incised; in the depth of the peritoneal gap, the ureter can be seen. With closed scissors, it is being dissected further caudally. (From Reiffenstuhl G: Dringliche gynäkologische und gebhurtshilfe Operationen. In Breitner, Kraus, Zuckschwerdt: *Chirurgie Operationslehre,* Bd VI, Berlin, 1977, Urban & Schwarzenberg.)

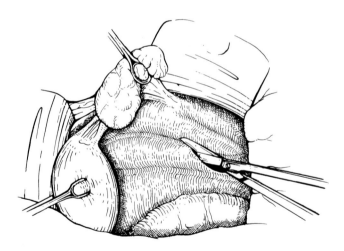

Fig. 2-31 Liberation of the ureter. Enlargement of the peritoneal gap. After pulling of the peritoneum away from the pelvic wall by closed scissors, the peritoneal cut is being enlarged in a caudal direction. (From Reiffenstuhl G: Dringliche gynäkologische und gebhurtshilfe Operationen. In Breitner, Kraus, Zuckschwerdt: *Chirurgie Operationslehre,* Bd VI, Berlin, 1977, Urban & Schwarzenberg.)

When the vesicourethral junction is dislocated from the pelvic cavity, descensus of the vagina and urinary incontinence can result.

Urogenital Diaphragm

The urogenital diaphragm extends inside the pubic angle and protects the wide levator aperture. Openings exist for the vagina, urethra, and the dorsal clitoral vein (Fig. 2-35, p. 63). The urogenital diaphragm includes the deep transverse muscle of the perineum (see Fig. 2-33), which ends in the perineal wedge (centrum tendineum).

The deep transverse muscle of the perineum originates from the ischiatic or pubic bone and, being invaded by connective tissue, crosses the urogenital hiatus. The deep transverse muscle of the perineum encircles the urogenital hiatus, bringing about a urogenital sphincter (urethral vaginal muscle). Frontally, the muscle fibers join the transverse perineal ligament (urethral ligament; see Fig. 2-33, *7*), which forms the ventral part of the urogenital diaphragm together with the arcuate pubic ligament. The free dorsal edge of the diaphragm is supported by the superficial transverse muscle of the perineum (see Fig. 2-34, *5*), which originates from the ischiatic tuberosity and inserts into the perineal wedge. The bulbocavernous and the ischiocavernous muscles (see Fig. 2-34, *4* and *9*) lie directly on the urogenital diaphragm. The two bulbocavernous muscles can close this aperture by contraction. The bulbi vestibuli are superficial to the urogenital diaphragm, as are the major vestibular glands (Bartholin's glands) (see Fig. 2-35). The ducts perforate the urogenital diaphragm and course ventrally around the vaginal aperture to their orifices into the urogenital sinus near the hymen. In inflammatory disease of the vagina, these glands are very likely to be involved by forming an intraglandular abscess above the urogenital diaphragm. The pudendal nerve innervates the urogenital diaphragm. The vaginal, urethral, and urogenital diaphragms are firmly grown together. This is the principal cause of prolapse of the

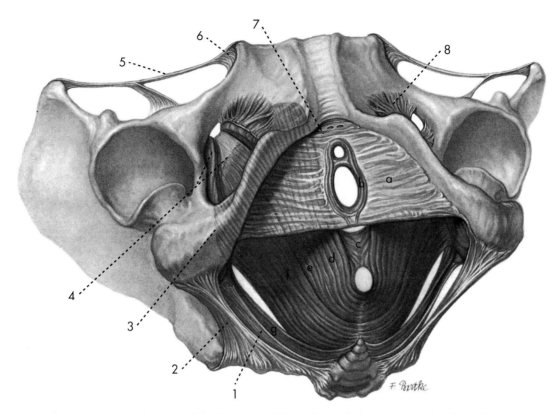

Fig. 2-33 Representation of the ligaments of the pelvis and of the urogenital and pelvic diaphragms. *1,* Sacrospinous ligament; *2,* sacrotuberous ligament; *3,* arcus tendineus of the obturator fascia (levator ani muscle); *4,* obturator internus muscle (cross section) and the arcus tendineus fasciae obturatoriae; *5,* inguinal ligament, arcus iliopectineus; *6,* lacunar ligament; *7,* transverse perineal ligament; *8,* obturator membrane; *a,* deep transverse perineal muscle; *b,* urethrovaginal muscle; *c,* prerectal fibers; *d,* puborectal muscle; *e,* pubococcygeus muscle; *f,* iliococcygeus muscle; *g,* coccygeus muscle. (From Reiffenstuhl G, Platzer W: *Die Vaginalen Operationen. Chirurgie, Anatomie und Operationslehre,* Berlin, 1974, Urban-Schwarzenberg.)

pelvic organs, vagina, bladder, and uterus in cases of pelvic floor damage.

PERINEUM

Knowledge of the anatomic structures of the perineum is essential in colpoperineoplasty, episiotomy, and rupture of the perineum. The area between the anus and the vaginal orifice is of great importance in women. This region, the *perineum,* is about 2.5 cm. The rectovaginal septum meets the pelvic floor and perineal body and increases its muscle strength (see Fig. 2-38). Fibers of many muscles join the rectovaginal septum and form a mass of muscle and connective tissue that builds up the central tendon of the perineum. Therefore the central tendon is created by the connection of many connective tissue and muscle fibers. The following structures belong to the central tendon of the perineum (Fig. 2-36): bulbocavernous muscle (originating bilaterally from the perineal wedge), superficial and deep transverse perineal muscle, some prerectal fibers of the levator ani muscle, fibers of the rectal wall, and superficial parts and fascia of the three parts of the external anal sphincter muscles (see Chap-

ters 22 and 28). Also, the medial muscle fibers of the urethrovaginal muscle (see Fig. 2-36) join the central tendon of the perineum. Some smooth muscle bundles, called *rectovaginal muscles* (see Fig. 2-36), extending from the rectum to the vagina help to construct the perineal wedge. When present, smooth muscle fibers of the rectococcygeal muscle connecting to the levator fascia, containing smooth muscles and the urogenital diaphragm, help form the perineal wedge. A massive, firm connective tissue wedge containing numerous muscle fibers is created. Also called the *perineal wedge* or *perineal body,* it is the base for the perineum. The back of the wedge faces caudally; the other side, facing cranially, is fused with the rectovaginal septum (Fig. 2-37, p. 65).

The vagina is enlarged and the perineum is stretched extensively during delivery. In a sudden increase in tension, the elasticity of the tissue might be inadequate, leading to ruptures of the central tendon of the perineum. These ruptures might extend cranially along the rectovaginal septum and cause dissection of the vaginal wall from the rectal wall and may rupture the fusion between the perineal body and the rectovaginal septum. They might even affect the anal sphincter muscles and the rectal wall. The perineal body and

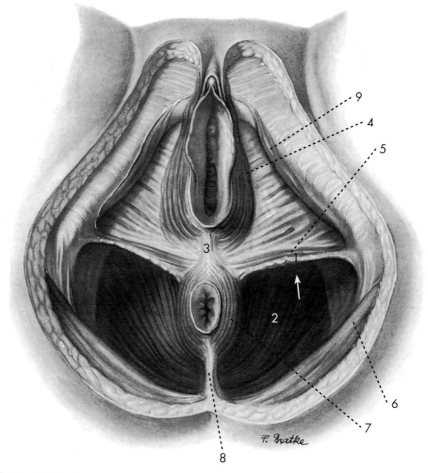

Fig. 2-34 Pelvic floor as seen from below with the urogenital diaphragm and the pelvic diaphragm in situ. *1,* Ischiorectal fossa *(arrow); 2,* levator ani muscle; *3,* perineum; *4,* bulbocavernosus muscle; *5,* superficial transverse perineal muscle; *6,* edge of the gluteus maximus muscle; *7,* external anal sphincter muscle; *8,* anococcygeal ligament; *9,* ischiocavernosus muscle. (From Reiffenstuhl G, Platzer W: *Die Vaginalen Operationen. Chirurgie, Anatomie und Operationslehre,* Berlin, 1974, Urban-Schwarzenberg.)

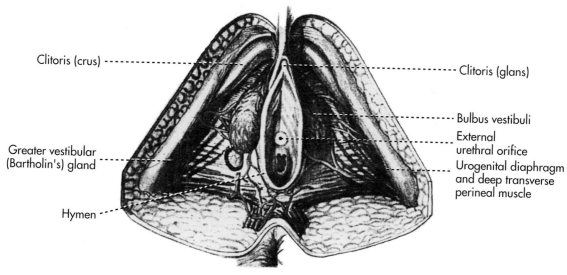

Clitoris (crus)

Greater vestibular (Bartholin's) gland

Hymen

Clitoris (glans)

Bulbus vestibuli

External urethral orifice

Urogenital diaphragm and deep transverse perineal muscle

Fig. 2-35 The female urogenital diaphragm seen from below. Also illustrated are the swelling bodies, or cavernosus bodies. On the right side the urogenital diaphragm is cut to show the major vestibular gland. (From Hafferl A: *Lehrbuch der Topographischen Anatomie,* Berlin, 1957, Springer-Verlag.)

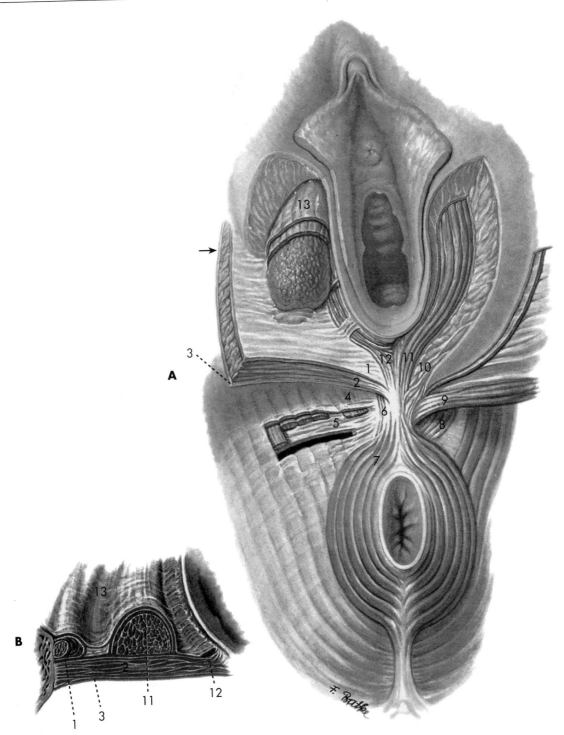

Fig. 2-36 **A,** Architecture of the perineum: diagonally striated musculature; smooth muscle, connective tissue, adipose tissue. *1,* Inferior urogenital fascia; *2,* deep transverse perineal muscle; *3,* superior urogenital fascia; *4,* inferior fascia of the pelvic diaphragm with smooth muscle fibers; *5,* superior fascia of the pelvic diaphragm with the smooth muscle fibers; *6,* rectovaginal muscle; *7,* external and sphincter muscle; *8,* prerectal fibers of the levator ani muscle; *9,* superficial transverse perineal muscle; *10,* deep transverse perineal muscle; *11,* bulbocavernosus muscle; *12,* urethrovaginal muscle; *13,* perineal muscle (superficial); *14,* ischiocavernosus muscle. **B,** Section through the urogenital diaphragm (compare arrow in **A**). (From Reiffenstuhl G, Platzer W: *Die Vaginalen Operationen. Chirurgie, Anatomie und Operationslehre,* Berlin, 1974, Urban-Schwarzenberg.)

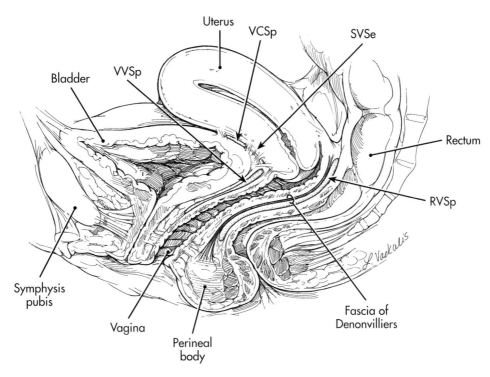

Fig. 2-37 The pelvic connective tissue spaces in median sagittal view. The vesicocervical space *(VCSp)* is separated from the vesicovaginal space *(VVSp)* by fusion between the adventitia of the cervix and bladder, called the *supravaginal septum (SVSe)*. The rectovaginal space *(RVSp)* is shown between the rectum and vagina, extending from the perineal body to the bottom of the cul-de-sac of Douglas. The fascia of Denonvilliers (rectovaginal septum) is a condensation of tissue attached to the undersurface of the posterior vaginal wall along the full length of the rectovaginal space. Note its fusion to the cranial margin of the perineal body. (From Nichols DH, Randall CL: *Vaginal surgery,* ed 4, Baltimore, 1996, Williams & Wilkins.)

wedge are clinically important because they not only divide the urogenital tract from gut, but also maintain the normal topography of the lower pelvic organs. This topic is discussed in Chapters 22 and 28.

FUNCTIONAL AND CLINICAL IMPORTANCE OF PELVIC FLOOR AND PELVIC CONNECTIVE TISSUE

The distal rectum and the lower vagina lie caudally to the levator plate and the coccyx. The portio and the upper part of the vagina, however, usually lie on the levator plate and near the sacrum owing to the perineal turn of the vagina.

The proximal part of the vagina has a horizontal course while a woman is standing. This phenomenon can be shown with casts of the vagina and lateral radiographs.[68-70] The upper part of the vaginal portio and uterus lie posterior to the levator aperture. The inner genitals are kept in their position by the strong cardinal ligaments, which hold the position of the portio and the cranial vagina near the sacrum, on top of an intact and horizontally inclined levator plate.

The vagina is kept in its position by two systems, one from above (cardinal ligament, or parametrium, along with the connective tissue attachment between the vaginal sulci

and the arci tendineus) and one from below (levator muscle or pelvic diaphragm). Genital prolapse can render either one or both mechanisms ineffective.

Zacharin,[79] Milley, and Nichols[35] were able to demonstrate that the urethra is held in position at the back side of the pubic bone by the pubourethral ligaments, which are continuous with the fascia of the urogenital diaphragm and can become pathologically stretched[78] (Fig. 2-38). The pubourethral ligaments contain some striated muscle fibers and smooth muscle fibers and contractile elements that are controlled by the autonomic nervous system. A hypermobile and symptomatic urethra should be surgically repaired by suspension, transvaginal support, or both. According to Nichols,[39,40] different anatomic systems are responsible for support of the birth canal. These systems might be destroyed either individually or in combination, but in reconstructive surgery each anatomic weakness must be considered.

Pelvic Bones

The osseous pelvis is the fixation point for the muscular connective tissue. If operative repair is being considered, it is important to keep in mind that congenital abnormalities, fractures, ruptures, or previous surgery potentially can change the structures of bone and joints.

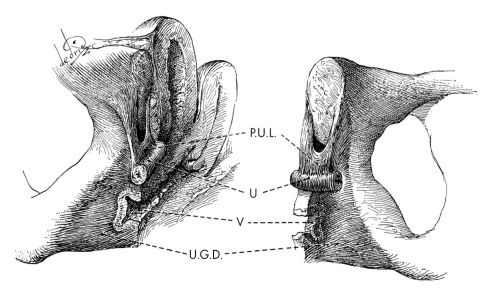

Fig. 2-38 Sagittal view shows the relationship between the pubourethral ligament *(PUL)* and urogenital diaphragm *(UGD)* in the human female. The urethra *(U)* and vagina *(V)* are shown in their relationship to the urogenital diaphragm. Note the bladder sketched into the drawing at the left. (From Milley PS, Nichols DH: *Anat Rec* 170:281, 1971.)

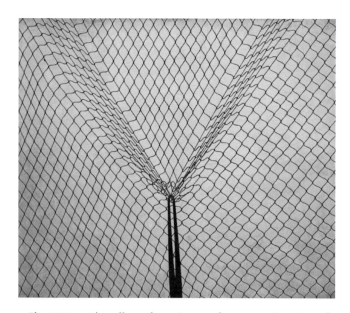

Fig. 2-39 The effect of traction on the connective tissue fibers of the cardinal and uterosacral ligaments is demonstrated. A forceps has been applied to the center of a piece of plastic net, and traction has been applied, demonstrating the distortion of the pelvic tissues resulting from traction on the cervix. Condensation and obliteration of intraareolar spaces account for "ligaments" apparent at operation, reinforced by blood vessels, lymphatics, and nerves and their sheaths, both of which enter and exit along the lateral margin of the upper vagina. (From Nichols DH, Milley PS: Clinical anatomy of the vulva, vagina, lower pelvis and perineum. In Sciarra J, editor: *Gynecology and obstetrics*, Philadelphia, 1992, JB Lippincott.)

Pelvic Connective Tissue

Fibrotic changes of the pelvic connective tissue might prevent a descensus. The connective tissue can be shortened by chronic inflammation, endometriosis, previous radiation, previous surgery, or chronic tension. The round ligament, extending from the uterine fundus to the inguinal canal as an arc, does not play a significant role in supporting the uterus[20] but is partially responsible for anteversion of the uterus (in a low grade). Helping to maintain fixation of the uterus during childbirth may be its most important function. The cardinal ligament (Mackenrodt's) keeps the cervix and the proximal part of the vagina above the levator muscles in their position supported by the uterosacral ligaments. Tension on these ligaments may concentrate their connective tissue into strong bands (Fig. 2-39).

Elasticity of the Central Tendon

During delivery, when the baby's head moves deeper into the pelvis and the enlargement of the vagina begins, the central tendon, being the most elastic part of the perineum, is stretched longitudinally. The rectovaginal septum is also stretched. The dilation of the perineum would be almost impossible without the extreme elasticity of the central tendon. The size of the perineum, normally 2 to 3 cm, can be enlarged to 10 to 15 cm during delivery.

Smooth muscles in this area maintain tone but allow an extension of the tissue until the limits of its elasticity. If this is the case, smooth muscle fibers behave like concentrated connective tissue and help keep the internal genitalia in their position.

Striated muscles react very quickly and maintain both tone and balance, but they are not able to perform rhythmic contractions. The contracted muscles remain a constant length, and balance and tone are maintained as a subsidiary tissue.

Elastic tissue consists of an irregular net, which antagonizes tension similar to an elastic band. With increasing age, elasticity decreases, which may cause the typical complication of descensus of the vagina or uterus in elderly women. Lost or decreased elasticity of the central tendon can be caused by (1) poorly healed injury and their scars, (2) shrinking of the connective tissue and loss of the elastic fibers in old age, or (3) induration and shrinkage of the perineum in kraurosis vulvae or dyspareunia in the climacterium.[27]

REFERENCES AND SUGGESTED READING

1. Averette HE Jr, Viamonte MI, Ferguson JH: Lymphangioadenography as a guide to lymphadenectomy, *Obstet Gynecol* 21:682, 1963.
2. Baden WF: Personal communication, 1996.
3. Brunschwig A: Die Technik der Lymphadenektomie im Becken in Verbindung mit der radikalen Hysterektomie als Behandlung des Collumcarcinoms, *Presse Méd* 1955, p 724.
4. Collette JM: Envahissements ganglionnaires inguino-ilio-pelviens par lymphographie, *Acta Radiol* 49:154, 1958.
5. Corning HK: *Lehrbuch der topographischen Anatomie,* Wiesbaden, 1913, JF Bergmann.
6. Dargent M, Guillemin G: The treatment of operable cancer of the cervix by the combination of radiation and surgery, *Cancer* 8:53, 1955.
7. Dolan PA, Hughes RR: Lymphography in genital cancer, *Surg Gynecol Obstet* 118:1286, 1964.
8. Frankenhauser: *Die Nerven der Gebärmutter,* Jena, 1867, W Braumüller.
9. Fuchs WA: *Lymphographie und Tumordiagnostik,* Heidelberg, 1965, Springer.
10. Fuchs WA, Böök-Hederström G: Inguinal and pelvic lymphography: a preliminary report, *Acta Radiol* 56:340, 1961.
11. Gerteis W: Die Lymphographie beim Genitalcarcinom der Frau, *Arch Gynäkol* 200:109, 1964.
12. Gitsch E: *Radioisotope in Geburtshilfe Gynäkologe,* Berlin, 1977, Walter de Gruyter.
13. Gitsch E: Personal communication, 1990.
14. Gitsch E, Janisch H, Leodolter S: *Neue Erkenntnisse zum Problem einer radioaktiven Markierung der tiefen Lymphabflußgebiete des Beckens.* In Pabst, editor: *Nuklearmedizin,* Stuttgart, 1974, Schattauer.
15. Gitsch E, Janisch H, Leodolter S: Zur Problematik der endolymphatischen P32 Applikation bei der Radioisotopen-Radikaloperation des Kollumkarzinoms vom Typ II, *Gynäkol Geburtshilfe Rundsch* 14:210, 1974.
16. Gitsch E, Janisch H, Tulzer H: Die Radikaloperation des Carcinoma colli uteri mit Radioisotopen vom Typ I, *Z Geburtshilfe Gynäkol* 175:253, 1971.
17. Gitsch E, Janisch H, Tulzer H: Die Isotopen-Radikaloperation des Kollumkarzinoms vom Typ II, *Schweiz Z Gynäkol Geburtshilfe* 3:121, 1972.
18. Gitsch E, Janisch H, Tulzer H: Progress in the radioisotope surgery of the cervical carcinoma, *Eur J Gynaecol Oncol* 1:1, 1980.
19. Gulland GL: The development of lymphatic glands, *J Pathol* 2:447, 1894.
20. Hafferl A: *Lehrbuch der topographischen Anatomie,* Berlin, 1957, Springer.
21. Heinen G: Personal communication, 1965.
22. Hellmann T: Studien über das lymphoide Gewebe: Die Bedeutung der Sekundärfollikel, *Beitr Pathol Anat* 68:333, 1921.
23. Hellmann T: *Lymphgefäß, Lymphknötchen und Lymphknoten.* In Möllendorf V: *Handbuch der mikroskopischen Anatomie der Menschen,* Bd VI, Berlin, 1930, Springer.
24. Hillemanns GH: Die Reaktion des reg. Lymphknoten auf die therapeutische Ra-Rö-Bestrahlung beim Collumcarcinom, *Z Geburtshilfe Gynäkol* 149:156, 1957.
25. Hohenfellner R, Janisch H, Ludvik W: Die Lymphographie bei malignen Erkrankungen des Urogenitalsystems, *Geburtshilfe Frauenheilkd* 25:298, 1965.
26. Janisch H: Zur Frage der Lymphgefäß und Lymphknotenregeneration nach Werteimscher Radikaloperation: eine lymphographische Studie, *Geburtshilfe Frauenheilkd* 28:646, 1968.
27. Janisch H, Leodolter S: On radioactive labelling of the lymph drainage regions of the pelvis, *Lymphology* 9:5, 1976.
28. Joachimovits R: *Das Beckenausgangsgebiet und Perineum des Weibes: eine anatomische und klinische Studie,* Wien, 1969, Wilhelm Maudrich.
29. Kinmonth JB: Lymphangiography in man, *Clin Sci* 11:13, 1952.
30. Kownatzki: *Die Venen des weiblichen Beckens,* Wiesbaden, 1907, JF Bergmann.
31. Latzko W, Schiffmann J: Klinisches und Anatomisches zur Radikaloperation des Gebärmutterkrebses, *Zentralbl Gynäkol* 43:689, 1919.
32. Meigs JV: *Surgical treatment of cancer of the cervix,* New York, 1954, Grune & Stratton.
33. Meigs JV, Sturgis SH: *Progress in gynecology,* vol I, New York, 1950, Grune & Stratton.
34. Milley PS, Nichols DH: A correlative investigation of the human rectovaginal septum, *Anat Rec* 163:443, 1969.
35. Milley PS, Nichols DH: The relationship between the pubourethral ligaments and the urogenital diaphragm in the human female, *Anat Rec* 170:281, 1971.
36. Mitra S: Extraperitoneal lymphadenectomy and radical vaginal hysterectomy for cancer of the cervix (Mitra technique), *Am J Obstet Gynecol* 78:191, 1959.
37. Nathanson IT: Extraperitoneal iliac lymphadenectomy in the treatment of cancer of the cervix. In Meigs JV, Sturgis SH, editors: *Progress in gynecology,* vol I, New York, 1950, Grune & Stratton,.
38. Navratil E: The Schauta-Amreich operation with and without lymphadenectomy. In Meigs JV, Sturgis SH, editors: *Progress in gynecology,* vol IV, New York, 1963, Grune & Stratton.
39. Nichols DH: International perspectives on vaginal surgery. In *Clinical obstetrics and gynecology,* New York, 1982, Harper & Row.
40. Nichols DH, Randall CL: *Vaginal surgery,* ed 4, Baltimore, 1996, William & Wilkins.
41. Noda K: Mitteilung am Weltkrongreß Geburtshilfe, *Gynäkologe,* 1985.
42. Okabayashi H: Radical abdominal hysterectomy for cancer of the cervix uteri, *Surg Gynecol Obstet* 33:335, 1921.
43. Pernkopf E: *Topographische Anatomie des Menschen: Lehrbuch und Atlas,* Berlin, 1941, Urban & Schwarzenberg.
44. Poppi A: L'apparato linfoglandolare nella pubertà, *Riv Clin Pediatr* 34:429, 1936.
45. Reiffenstuhl G: *Anwendung von radioaktiven Isotopen beim Collum-Carcinom der Frau auf Grund neuer anatomischer Kenntnisse,* Wien, 1955, Akademie der Wissenschaften.
46. Reiffenstuhl G: Lymphsystem der Gebärmutter und Scheide. In Seitz, Amreich: *Biologie und Pathologie des Weibes: Handbuch der Frauenheilkunde und Geburtshilfe,* Bd IV, Berlin, 1955, Urban & Schwarzenberg.
47. Reiffenstuhl G: Die Beckenlymphknoten eines Falles von Mycloma plasmocellulare, *Z Gynäkol* 78:75, 1956.
48. Reiffenstuhl G: Zur Frage der Nomenklatur der Beckenlymphknoten, *Klin Wochenschr* 68:247, 1956.
49. Reiffenstuhl G: Über Involution und Neubildung von Lymphknoten, *Arch Gynäkol* 187:375, 1956.
50. Reiffenstuhl G: *Das Lymphsystem des weiblichen Genitale,* Berlin, 1957, Urban & Schwarzenberg.
51. Reiffenstuhl G: Vergleichende klinisch-anatomische Untersuchungen des Lymphsystems vom Neugeborenen und von Erwachsenen, *Geburtshilfe Frauenheilkd* 18:1180, 1958.

52. Reiffenstuhl G: Zum Lymphknotenproblem des Carcinoma colli uteri: Häufigkeitsbefall der Lymphknoten und Radikalisierung der Lymphonodektomie, *Wien Med Wochenschr* 109:294, 1959.

53. Reiffenstuhl G: *Das Lymphgefäßsystem des Affen.* In Hofer H, Schultz AH, Starck D: *Handbuch der Primatenkunde,* Bd III/2, Basel, 1960, S Karger.

54. Reiffenstuhl G: *Lymphatic system of the ureter, bladder and urethra.* In Youssef AF: *Gynecological urology,* Springfield, Ill, 1960, Charles C Thomas.

55. Reiffenstuhl G: Analyse von 60 Lymphonodektonomien bei der Wertheimschen Radikalop Berichte III, *Weltkongreßder Gynäkologie und Geburtshilfe,* 1961.

56. Reiffenstuhl G: Über das Vorkommen von Lymphcysten nach der Lymphonodektomie, *Wien Med Wochenschr* 112:539, 1962.

57. Reiffenstuhl G: Über die Lokalisation der lymphogenen Aussaaten des Carcinoma colli uteri, *Wien Med Wochenschr* 112:751, 1962.

58. Reiffenstuhl G: *The lymphatics of the female genital organs,* Philadelphia, 1964, JB Lippincott.

59. Reiffenstuhl G: The prognostic value of lymphography in carcinoma of the uterine cervix. In Rüttimann A: *Progress in lymphology,* Stuttgart, 1966, Georg Thieme.

60. Reiffenstuhl G: *Das Lymphknotenproblem beim Carcinoma colli uteri und die Lymphirradiatio pelvis: direkte Bestrahlung des Beckenlymphsystems mit Isotopen,* Berlin, 1967, Urban & Schwarzenberg.

61. Reiffenstuhl G: Der prognostische Wert der Lymphographie beim Kollumkarzinom, *Geburtshilfe Frauenheilkd* 27:590, 1967.

62. Reiffenstuhl G: Lymphknotenmetastasen beim Kollumkarzinom und ihre Behandlungsmöglichkeiten, *Z Gynäkol* 90:966, 1967.

63. Reiffenstuhl G: Dringliche gynäkologische und gebhurtshilfe Operationen. In Breitner, Kraus, Zuckschwerdt: *Chirurgie Operationslehre,* Bd VI, Berlin, 1977, Urban & Schwarzenberg.

64. Reiffenstuhl G: The clinical significance of the connective tissue planes and spaces, *Clin Obstet Gynecol* 25:4, 1982.

65. Reiffenstuhl G: Die vaginale Radikaloperation nach Schauter-Amreich zur Behandlung des Collumkarzinoms, *Arch Gynecol Obstet* 242:1, 1987.

66. Reiffenstuhl G, Platzer W: *Die vaginalen Operationen: Chirurgie, Anatomie u Operationslehre,* Berlin, 1974, Urban & Schwarzenberg.

67. Reiffenstuhl G, Platzer W, Knapstein PG: *Vaginal operations: surgical anatomy and technique,* ed 2, Baltimore, 1996, Williams & Wilkins.

68. Richter K: Lebendige Anatomie der Vagina, *Geburtshilfe Frauenheilkd* 26:1213, 1966.

69. Richter K: Die physiologische Topographie des weiblichen Genitale in moderner Sicht, *Z Gynäkol* 34:1258, 1967.

70. Richter K: Die operative Behandlung des prolabierten Scheidengrundes nach Uterusextirpationen: ein Beitrag zur Vaginae fixatio sacrotuberalis nach Amreich, *Geburtshilfe Frauenheilkd* 27:941, 1967.

71. Rüttimann A, del Buono MS, Cocchi U: Neue Fortschritte in der Lymphographie, *Schweiz Med Wochenschr* 91:1460, 1961.

72. Sederl J: Zur Operation des Prolapses der blindendigenden Scheide, *Geburtshilfe Frauenheilkd* 18:824, 1958.

73. Seelig A: *Ausbreitungswege des Gebärmutterkrebses,* Strassburg, 1894, Preisschrift.

74. Seelig A: Pathologisch Anatomische Untersuchungen über die Ausbreitungswege des Uteruscarcinoms im Bereiche des Genitaltractus, *Virchows Arch* 140:80, 1895.

75. Tandler J, Halban H: *Topographie des weiblichen Ureters,* Vienna, 1901, W Braumüller.

76. Uhlenhuth E: *Problems in the anatomy of the pelvis,* Philadelphia, 1953, JB Lippincott.

77. Von Peham H, Amreich JA: *Gynäkologische Operationslehre,* Berlin, 1930, S Karger.

78. Wertheim E: *Die erweiterte abdominale Radikaloperation bei Carcinoma colli uteri,* Berlin, 1911, Urban & Schwarzenberg.

79. Zacharin RF: The suspensory mechanism of the female urethra, *J Anat* 91:423, 1963.

3 The Statics and Dynamics of Pelvic Support

Genital prolapse and urinary incontinence are the most important clinical manifestations that can result from (or co-exist with) functional anatomic deficits of the structures that form the so-called pelvic support mechanism.

Three types of anatomy can be proposed: descriptive, functional, and surgical. Ideally, surgeons need a logical plan for approaching disordered anatomic structures, restoring their specific function, and determining surgical alternatives for repairing structures and restoring previous function. However, surgeons still have a poor understanding of the statics and dynamics of pelvic support. Descriptive anatomy is still imprecise, especially of the supporting structures in the supradiaphragmatic tract of the urethra and vagina.

Functional anatomy does not yet satisfactorily explain either the agonist and antagonist activity of pelvic floor musculature or the important correlations between somatic and vegetative neuromuscular activity. Moreover, the large role of both vascularization and trophism of the paracolpium precludes the use of cadavers for investigating descriptive anatomy.

Concerning surgical anatomy, it is nearly impossible to restore neuromuscular function or a lost reflex activity. Surgical rebuilding of the anatomy does not always reestablish previous function; instead, technical artifices are used to recover function. This is especially true for the surgical treatment of stress incontinence and repair of severe prolapse. In these cases, attempts to rebuild a seriously injured connective tissue or fascial structure or restore a defective neuromuscular reflex function of the pelvic floor are highly unsuccessful. Surgeons must find a compromise between demolition and use of alternative structures or prostheses.

SUSPENSORY AND SUPPORTING SYSTEMS

According to Bonney's studies, pelvic viscera are both suspended from above and supported from below. The suspension system involves the so-called statics of the pelvic floor, whereas the muscular supporting system pertains to the dynamics of the pelvic floor. This distinction is purely formal because the two systems—the suspending static and the supporting dynamic—are complementary and no discontinuity exists between them from either a functional or anatomic perspective.

The static suspension system is located between the peritoneum and the internal fascial aponeuroses of the pelvic floor muscles. The neuromuscular dynamic system includes

the musculofascial structures of both urogenital and pelvic diaphragms.

To understand the pathogenic mechanism, the suspensory and support structures of the pelvic organs must be defined. Abdominal pressure is elevated by a few centimeters of water when changing from a supine to a standing position (with small oscillations synchronous with diaphragmatic movements). In the resting state, even in a standing position, the structures that close the pathway from the pelvis normally are under very little pressure. Walking, running, many forms of work and sports activity, efforts that involve the Valsalva maneuver, coughing, laughing, sneezing, and the like can increase abdominal pressure, which may reach and surpass 100 cm of H_2O. In these situations, the pelvic support system is under strain.

The containment of the genital organs within the pelvis depends on the integrity of at least three systems: muscular, fascial, and neurologic. The pelvic organs—bladder, genital organs, and anorectal canal—are literally suspended to the bony pelvis by a connective tissue apparatus that extends between the peritoneum and the pelvic upper aponeurosis formed by the endopelvic fascia. The pelvic supports are attached to an intact suspensory apparatus that lies on the fascia of the pelvic muscles, which directly supports gravitational weight. It is formed by the internal upper aponeurosis of the levator ani, which fuses at the level of the arcus tendineus with the fascia of the obturator internus, posteriorly with the presacral fascia, and anteriorly with the transversalis abdominal fascia. This fascial structure is continuous with very rich visceral connective fascial structures, in particular the perivaginal fascia.

Underneath the pelvic upper aponeurosis, a complex muscular apparatus that is formed by the muscle of the pelvic diaphragm and the urogenital diaphragm makes up the dynamic support system. This is mediated by a tonic and phasic reflex activity through type I and type II muscle fibers (fast twitch and slow twitch, respectively). This muscular apparatus has important functions integrated by the central nervous system. When abdominal pressure increases as a result of a change in position or because of physical activity, this muscular apparatus modulates its tonic activity. When the increase is sudden (e.g., during an episode of coughing), a series of rapid phasic muscular fiber contractions ensues, and is enhanced for short periods by contractions of fast twitch fibers.

The retroperitoneal connective tissue is organized and condensed in the form of pillars that follow the visceral branches of the hypogastric vessels, thereby constituting pseudoligamentous structures, such as the pubovesicocervical ligaments and the cardinal and uterosacral ligament complex. The uterosacral ligament is the most cranial part of a strong connective tissue and vascular pillar, binding the cervicoisthmic area and the supradiaphragmatic vagina. These pillars maintain the vaginal axis in a dorsal direction, establishing an acute vaginopelvic angle. Moreover, in a standing position the normal arrangement of both uterosacral ligaments and posterior pillars keeps the projection of the cervix oriented toward the centrum tendineum perinei. This projection is important because the vaginopelvic angle becomes more acute under stress, the posterior vaginal fornix is no longer subject to expulsive forces, and, above all, the cervix (or the fundus of the uterus in cases of retroversion) is pushed toward the centrum tendineum perinei, which exerts its supporting function. Moreover, under stress conditions the reflex contraction of the puborectalis muscles reduces the vaginopelvic angle, elevating the centrum perinei. In this way the puborectalis contraction increases both occlusive and supportive functions.

Pelvic dynamics demonstrate the importance of both anatomic integrity and the trophism of endopelvic "fascia," but also of the vascular condition and the neuromuscular integrity of the pelvic floor. It is apparent that the static and dynamic systems are complementary. The perfect function and neuromuscular integrity allow the supporting system to dynamically oppose expulsive forces. The supportive activity of the pelvic floor prevents expulsive forces from causing injury to the relatively stiff and therefore fragile suspension system.

During the filling phase of the bladder, an increase of activity can be detected by electromyogram (EMG), whereas during the micturition phase, there is functional silence on EMG, an expression of muscular relaxation. The integration at the level of the central nervous system allows voluntary muscle contraction during voluntary interruption of micturition, in the initial phase of delay of the stimulus to micturition or defecation, and in numerous other circumstances. This musculofascial system of support dynamically antagonizes the expulsive forces gravitating on pelvic egress, protecting the overlying static suspensory apparatus and intervening directly with the mechanism that guarantees containment and continence of the viscera. Therefore both prolapse and stress urinary incontinence are expressions of a multifactorial disorder that can be caused by traumatic or dystrophic factors that compromise the dynamic and static structures of pelvic support.

THE SUSPENSORY SYSTEMS

The pelvic viscera maintain reciprocal anatomic relations and connections with the bony pelvis by way of a suspensory system formed by a framework of connective tissue extending between the peritoneum and the levator upper aponeurosis—the *endopelvic fascia*. In this structure, "spaces" of loose areolar connective tissue (e.g., the para-

vesical spaces, pararectal spaces, and vesicouterine space) can be recognized. The potential spaces are separated from one another by condensation of connective tissue containing within these septi the course of visceral hypogastric vessels and are called in surgical and anatomic terms the *pillars* that form the true suspensory system. These pillars originate posteriorly and laterally from the presacral and pelvic fascia, course medially and forward, fusing with the perivisceral connective tissue of the rectum, vagina, and bladder, and terminating in the retropubic area. the pillars have pseudoligamentous structures, among which are the uterosacral and cardinal ligaments, which constitute the posterior and lateral attachment systems to the region of the uterine isthmus and cervix, and also the pubovesical ligaments and vesicouterine ligaments, which make up the anterior segment of this suspensory system. This connective tissue architecture can be compared to a double arch. The ends of the points of attachment are the posterior lateral pelvic wall and the retropubic region. The base is wider posteriorly, and the two arches converge, suspending the vagina in its supradiaphragmatic segment included between the pelvic upper aponeurosis and the uterine isthmus region. The uterosacral ligaments are the most cranial and most consistent of this unique structure.

The vagina is fixed laterally, so the anterior and posterior walls touch each other. This fixation is the result of lateral tension, whereas posterior suspension determines the vaginopelvic angle, which is acute posteriorly. This conformation of the vagina is important because it guarantees (1) the occlusive mechanism of the pouch of Douglas during increased abdominal pressure, (2) the proper projection of the cervical isthmus region onto the fibrous center of the perineum, which is necessary for adequate support of the uterus during body movement and expulsive efforts, and (3) the support of the cervical trigonal areas in both static and dynamic situations. The anterior suspensory system of the vesical neck and urethra is often found to be very important in the pathogenesis of stress urinary incontinence. The system, not yet well defined in its anatomic and functional details, forms suspensory structures to the pubic arch (pubourethral "ligaments"), to the anterior vaginal wall, and to the so-called levator vaginal attachments to the arcus tendineus and also the internal upper aponeurosis of the puborectalis muscles. Even in this area, a precise anatomic-functional integration exists between suspensory connective tissue structures and musculofascial support structures formed by the puborectal muscles and the urogenital diaphragm.

Continence in the resting condition is ensured by the following factors:

1. The normal detrusor distention reflex (detrusor compliance)
2. The thickness of the urethral epithelium and its relation to age and endocrine stimulation
3. The presence and size of the subepithelial venous complex
4. The abundance of elastic tissue in all urethral layers
5. The urethral smooth muscle, which is still a subject of

debate not only because of its anatomic and functional independence of the detrusor muscle, but also because of its macroscopic and microscopic description and its innervation

6. The tone of the striated muscle of the external sphincter and of the muscles of the urogenital and pelvic diaphragms

At rest, all these factors normally ensure that urethral pressure is higher than vesical pressure, a condition referred to as the *urethral closing pressure profile.* During episodes of coughing and sudden increases in abdominal pressure, two accessory mechanisms increase this closing pressure to guarantee a positive differential pressure. Because this mechanism is aided by contraction of the striated pelvic muscles, increased pressure occurs at the point of transition from the proximal two thirds to the distal third of the urethra. The second accessory mechanism is closure under stress, which refers to the passive increase of urethral closing pressure due to the transmission of abdominal pressure both on the bladder and on the external wall of the supradiaphragmatic urethra. For these accessory mechanisms to be effective, the following conditions must be present: (1) normal reflex activity of the striated muscles, (2) normal development and function of the striated muscles, (3) usual anatomic relations between the urethra, pelvic diaphragm, and urogenital diaphragm, and (4) closure of the vesical neck during stress. If the bladder neck becomes patent during stress and vesical closure is disrupted, urine penetrates into the proximal urethra and the patient maintains continence only if the underlying muscular tone together with the intrinsic urethral pressure guarantees a positive differential ratio. If this is not present, a loss of urine synchronous with the stress but without participation of the detrusor occurs. For the patient to remain continent, the bladder neck must remain perfectly closed during stress. Patency of the neck and the proximal urethra during stress are necessary conditions for stress urinary incontinence to occur. The integrity of the suspensory structures at the level of the cervical or trigonal regions is essential for the maintenance of closure of the bladder neck under stress.

Some important questions of static and dynamic function and support remain to be clarified. Why is stress incontinence not necessarily related to urogenital prolapse? Why do we observe frequent episodes of severe stress incontinence in the absence of prolapse, or an absence of stress incontinence in the presence of a severe cystourethrocele? One hypothesis is that the maintenance of normal closure of the bladder neck is related not so much to the integrity of the pubourethral ligaments as to the integrity of the anatomic interorgan relationship between the cervical trigonal region and the vaginal wall (i.e., the collective integrity of the suspensory connective tissue structures of the urethra, trigone, and vagina). When the vaginal wall dislocates under stress does not cause a disruption of the trigonal baseplate. Thus various individual or combined lesions affecting the relationships between urethra, trigone, and vagina can explain the presence of stress incontinence even in the absence of an

evident cystourethrocele, whereas the integrity and preservation of the anatomic unity among organs of the system, the bladder neck, trigone, and vagina guarantee closure even in the presence of an obvious dislocation (cystourethrocele). Analysis of cystographic radiographic images while the patient is applying stress substantiates this hypothesis: the radiographic integrity of the baseplate is coincident with continence even in the presence of considerable dislocation and a large cystocele. On the contrary, the radiographic disruption of the baseplate does not always cause urinary stress incontinence because the accessory mechanisms related to the muscles of the pelvic floor may still ensure continence in certain critical conditions.

DYNAMIC SUPPORT STRUCTURES

The musculature that forms the pelvic floor is divided into muscles of the urogenital diaphragm and those of the pelvic diaphragm. Except for the ischiocavernosus muscles, the other muscles that form the pelvic floor insert peripherally to osseous and ligamentous structures of the pelvic girdle. Inferiorly in the midline, they insert to the anococcygeal raphe posteriorly and to the fibrous center of the perineum anteriorly. Two of three perineal superficial muscles (bulbocavernosus and superficial transverse of the perineum) converge on the fibrous center of the perineum and the transverse deep muscle of the perineum and its superficial and deep upper aponeurosis and the anterior and medial bundles of the puborectal muscles with its upper aponeurosis. The fibrous center of the perineum is an important dynamic center of support for the vaginal wall, the cervical trigonal region, and the uterus. Loss of its anatomic integrity can predispose to the disruption of those delicate anatomic functional balances that protect from vaginal prolapse and stress incontinence. Special attention should be given to the surgical reconstruction of defects of this structure in operations to correct uterovaginal prolapse and stress incontinence.

The pelvic diaphragm is formed essentially by the levator ani muscles. A few anatomic considerations about its structure have important functional implications. Contrary to the classic view that defines the puborectal muscle as an integral part of the levator, recent studies show that the puborectalis should be considered as a separate entity, not only because of its histologic characteristics and orientation of the muscle fibers, but also because of its characteristic function. The puborectal muscles therefore form a true muscular arch that surrounds the pelvic viscera and that, when contracting, performs a double sphincteric containment and indirect containment action through the accentuation of the urethrovesical, vaginopelvic, and anorectal angles.

The levator ani is characterized by a fusion posterior to the rectum, called the *levator plate* (Fig. 3-1), and by an anterior part, the *suspensory sling,* that fuses and fixes medially to the perivisceral connective tissues of the rectum, vagina, and urethra. The levator plate occupies a more or less horizontal orientation in the pelvis, centrally fusing with a

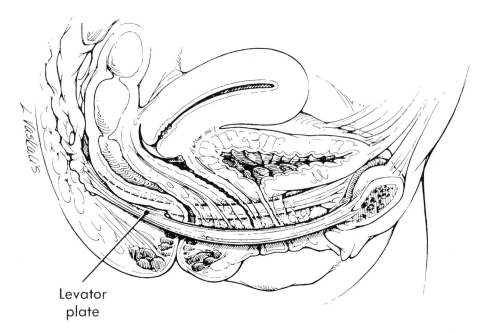

Levator
plate

Fig. 3-1 Sagittal section of the pelvis demonstrates the almost horizontal upper vagina and rectum lying upon and parallel to the levator plate. The latter is formed by fusion of the pubococcygei muscles posterior to the rectum. The anterior limit of the point of fusion is the margin of the genital hiatus, immediately posterior to the rectum. It is the normal position of this levator plate that accounts for the anorectal angle, which is shown.

rectococcygeal raphe posteriorly but with an anterior hiatus circumscribed by bundles of connective tissue that are fixed to the intrahiatal organs by connective tissue forming the so-called hiatal ligament. From a functional point of view, this anatomic interpretation is extremely important because the puborectal muscle is active during the containment phase, whereas the levator plate and the suspensory sling act as an accessory opening mechanism in the evacuation phase.

In summary, the main puborectal muscle bundle that is part of the dynamic system of support fulfills four main functions: (1) it opposes the vector of abdominal thrust to the suspension system, protecting it from dangerous and recurrent pressures; (2) it elevates the fibrous center of the perineum to make it coincide with the cervical and isthmic region of the uterus during sudden increases of abdominal pressure, helping to prevent prolapse of the uterus; (3) it accentuates the urethrovesical and anorectal relationships in the mechanism of continence; and (4) it accentuates the vaginopelvic angle, preventing enterocele.

PATHOGENESIS OF UROGENITAL PROLAPSE

Loss of the correct projection of the cervical isthmic region on the fibrous perineal center (generally caused by a deficit of the uterosacral suspensory structures) represents the first episode of uterine descensus through the genital hiatus. A forward displacement of the uterus with widening of the vaginopelvic angle promotes uterine prolapse or often-associated enterocele. This has been clinically confirmed through frequent observations of subsequent enterocele and

vaginal vault prolapse in patients who have undergone hysteropexy through ventral fixation. Anterior fixation of the uterus exposes the pouch of Douglas to the expulsive forces that, over time, promote the formation of large enterocele. Even the anterior colposuspension performed according to Burch, by passing the normal uterine suspensory mechanism, can promote severe uterine prolapse often in a short time. Defects of the perineal center are a possible cause of anterior prolapse (cystourethrocele), and the insufficiency of the paravaginal connective suspensory tissues and the anterior and posterior septa can cause segmentary prolapse of the vaginal walls (cystourethrocele, paravaginal defect, and rectocele). In the pathogenesis of urogenital prolapse, an important role is played by the musculofascial structures described. The lack of a viable support to the static suspensory structures exposes the internal pelvic organs to a sinking effect.

Biopsies of the puborectal muscles performed in the course of operations for prolapse have demonstrated surprisingly that with predictable dystrophic-type lesions of the muscles, structural changes of neurogenic origin also occur. These observations substantiate the hypothesis that repeated stress on the pelvic floor causes peripheral lesions of muscular innervation, with subsequent neurogenic myopathy and dynamic insufficiency. EMG studies performed in patients with prolapse compared with controlled cases have repeatedly confirmed the presence of tracings supportive of neurogenic myopathy. Also the studies of sacral potential, especially in patients with stress incontinence, have demonstrated prolonged latency in the reflex response to stimuli. Whatever the initial damage—dystrophy or lesion of the suspensory structures, inefficiency of the musculofascial support systems, or primary or secondary deficit of pelvic muscle innervation—the end result is an evolving prolapse of varying degree and severity in which deficits of the suspensory structures and support structures coexist because of the anatomic and functional complementary of these structures.

The pathogenesis of prolapse is therefore multifactorial, and its *primum movens* may be due to (1) traumatic or dystrophic injuries of the suspensory system (menopause, connective tissue disease, and obstetric delivery), (2) primary damage to the supporting muscular system (delivery, senile dystrophic myopathy, and congenital myopathy), (3) neurogenic injuries of the muscular apparatus (spina bifida and peripheral neuropathy), or (4) overstretching of the pelvic floor (delivery, chronic bronchitis, obesity, and chronic constipation). Orthopedic conditions (hip dysplasia, scoliosis, previous fracture, and congenital defect, such as those seen with bladder exstrophy) characterized by an alteration of the normal alignment of the expulsive and restraining lines of force can promote the development of a genital prolapse.

Often several pathogenic factors coexist or follow one another, so a severe genital prolapse can be caused by injury to both the supporting and suspensory systems. In the majority of cases the damage simultaneously involves different compartments; sometimes cystocele is more prevalent than uterine prolapse, enterocele, or rectocele. Rarely a severe prolapse is monosegmentary.

Multiple factors have been incriminated in the pathogenesis of prolapse, including multiparity, dystocia, macrosomia, and traumatic childbearing episodes. Separations and lacerations of upper aponeurotic muscular structures, partial tears of the musculature and its insertion, and lacerations of connective tissue suspension structures by hematomas may be the basis for precocious descensus or can form the basis for the later development of prolapse. No less important are dystrophic factors, including congenital insufficiency or acquired involution, or menopausal or senile atrophy of the musculofascial structures and ligamentous structures. In menopause, a progressive loss of elasticity of connective tissue occurs. More specifically, the subepithelial elastic lamina of the vagina becomes disorganized, with both degenerative changes and fragmentation. These alterations can predispose to prolapse in the nullipara. The studies of Zacharin have documented the existence of racial differences (e.g., more sturdiness of the pelvic floor in Chinese women). Other studies emphasize the predisposition to prolapse in women who have certain pathologic conditions, especially those included in the *joint instability syndrome* (hip dislocation, osteoarthrosis, chondrocalcinosis, and so forth). In other cases, deficit of pelvic muscle innervation and altered neuroendocrine balances (spina bifida and endocrine obesity) are mentioned as primary causes. Chronic medical diseases and all the conditions that may be accompanied by repeated and prolonged increase in abdominal pressure (chronic constipation, chronic lung disease, obesity, and so forth) must be considered. Many of these factors may coexist and synergistically determine prolapse. Effects of iatrogenic factors also must be considered, in particular gynecologic surgical procedures directed to suspension of the anterior vaginal wall and procedures that change the normal anatomic, topographic relationships or vaginal axis.

PATHOGENESIS OF STRESS URINARY INCONTINENCE

Even though stress urinary incontinence may develop in patients with prolapse, more than half of patients with severe genital prolapse are continent and, if asymptomatic, may not need any specific surgical treatment. This can be explained by the following considerations:

1. The often emphasized concept that stress urinary incontinence is caused by the "exit" of the urethrovesical junction from the pelvic manometric girdle is debatable.

2. The opinion that the surgical treatment of stress incontinence must involve the elevation of the urethrovesical junction also is debatable. The female urethra has its own supporting and suspensory systems, and it is the integrity of these systems that allows the closure mechanism to be efficient.

In patients with genuine stress incontinence and detrusor stability, the bladder filling phase is completely normal, and continence at rest is guaranteed. Only under conditions of stress, because of the damage of the specific supporting and suspending structures, does the urethra become momentarily patent and the patient incontinent. A large part of the problem involves ascertaining the location of these damaged structures. By vaginal examination, some studies locate them where the two paraurethral dimples are identified along the anterior vaginal wall, just inside the vaginal introitus. These dimples correspond to the insertion of the anterior pubourethral ligaments, anatomically and embryologically well described, that are located at the level of the mid-portion of the urethra and not at the level of the bladder neck.

All of the supporting and suspending systems (arcus tendineus, urethropelvic ligaments, pubourethral ligaments, retropubic attachment of puborectalis muscle and its sheaths) join in the retropublic space. The urethrocervical junction, surrounded by areolar tissue and supported only from the vaginal "fascia," has fairly good rotational mobility, and at this level the urethral profile shows a very low closure pressure. In videocystourethrography, under stress it is possible to identify two types of continent patients: the first is characterized by a lack of opacification of the entire urethra, the second by a temporary visualization of the proximal portion only, because the closure is ensured at the level of the middle portion of the urethra. The stress continence keystone in the female is therefore represented by the mid-urethral region, where intrinsic and extrinsic closure mechanisms converge and concentrate. From a surgical point of view, these considerations justify the partially obstructive effect of many of the colposuspension and sling procedures and the success of more recent nonobstructive

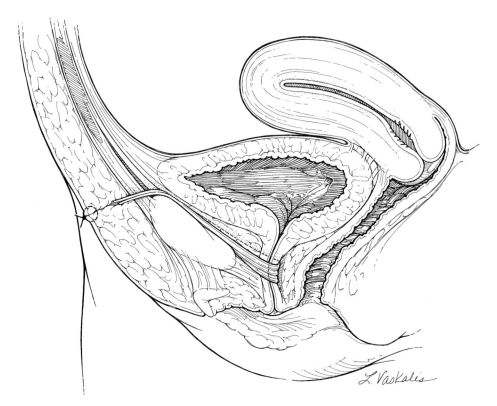

Fig. 3-2 Sagittal section of the pelvis with the tension-free vaginal plastic tape in place. Note the location of the belly of the sling beneath the mid-portion of the urethra. The retropubic ends of the sling are not fixed in place by suture.

procedures supporting the mid-urethra, such as the tension-free vaginal tape (TVT) procedure (Fig. 3-2) and the modified Burch operation. Particularly, the so-called TVT (from Ulf Ulmsten, Uppsala, Sweden) shows that the mini-invasive placement of a suburethral Prolene sling at the level of mid-urethra with no fixation stitches, thus avoiding urethral compression, allows immediate restoration of continence under stress, with no interference with voiding function. Furthermore, it is well known that procedures for the correction of cystocele, such as the transvaginal plication of the pubovesicocervical "fascia," or a paravaginal repair (when a lateral defect is present), are not consistently effective in treating stress urinary incontinence. Moreover, procedures characterized by an anterior *over*correction can cause more or less severe voiding difficulties due to an abnormal fixation of the urethrocervical junction.

RELATIONSHIPS BETWEEN URINARY INCONTINENCE AND PROLAPSE

The clinical observation is frequently made of an association between pathology of micturition and alteration in normal pelvic anatomy. However, the coexistence of incontinence in prolapse must not be considered on the basis of a simple and direct dependence; in fact, stress incontinence in prolapse implies lesions and functional alterations separate from the suspensory apparatus and support apparatus described, and in a clinical situation it must be evaluated sepa-

rately. For example, stress urinary incontinence (1) may be present in the absence of prolapse, (2) may be absent in the presence of prolapse (when an incomplete chronic retention of urine may occur as in some cases of very large cystoceles and in many cases of total uterovaginal prolapse), (3) can accompany vaginal prolapse as an expression of the deterioration of both the suspensory and support system, (4) can be exacerbated by the development of genital prolapse, (5) can be aggravated by procedures for the correction of prolapse (urethrocystopexy, colpoplasty, and so forth), and (6) can be masked by the presence of prolapse. This last possibility (also called *latent incontinence*) is not always easy to document and occurs when a very large cystocele or rectocele or uterine prolapse does not allow opening of the bladder neck, compressing it under stress beneath the pubic arch.

Several aspects regarding the pelvic supporting system statics and dynamics are still unclear, particularly the pathogenesis of prolapse and stress urinary incontinence. A better knowledge of these pathogenetic factors in the future will allow us to optimize, through more rational procedures, some surgical treatment with the ambitious aim to reconstruct and restore extremely delicate and complex functions.

SUGGESTED READING

Al-Rawi ZS: Joint hypermobility in women with genital prolapse, *Lancet* 26:1439, 1982.

Berglas B, Rabin IC: Study of the supportive structures of the uterus by levator myography, *Surg Gynecol Obstet* 97:677, 1953.

Bethoux A, Scali P, Blondon J: Physiopathologie et anatomie pathologique des prolapsus vaginaux, *Rev Prat* 21:1863, 1971.

Blaivus JG: Diagnostic evaluation of urinary incontinence, *Urology* 36:10, 1990.

Burch JC: Cooper's ligament urethrovesical suspension for stress incontinence, *Am J Obstet Gynecol* 100:764, 1968.

Campbell RM: The anatomy and histology of the sacrouterine ligaments, *Am J Obstet Gynecol* 59:1, 1950.

Candiani GB, Ferrari A: *Isterectomia vaginale,* Milano, 1986, Masson.

Candiani GB, Ferrari A: *Le disarmonie statico dinamiche nel-ambito pelvico: la clinica ostetrica e ginecologica,* Milano, 1991, Masson.

Constantinou CE, Govan DE: Spatial distribution and timing of transmitted and reflexly generated urethral pressures in healthy women, *J Urol* 127:964, 1982.

Dickinson VA: Maintenance of anal continence: a review of pelvic floor physiology, *Gut* 19:1163, 1978.

Gilpin SA, Gosling JA, Smith AR, Warrell DW: The pathogenesis of genitourinary prolapse and stress incontinence of urine: a histological and histochemical study, *Br J Obstet Gynaecol* 96:15, 1989.

Gosling F: The structure of the bladder and urethra, *Urology* 87:124, 1979.

Green TH: *Total prolapse of the vagina.* In Hafez ESE, Evans TN, editors: *The human vagina,* Amsterdam, 1978, Biomedical Press.

Herzog AR, Fultz MM: Epidemiology of urinary incontinence: prevalence, incidence and correlates in community populations, *Urology* 36:2, 1990.

Huisman AB: Morfologie van der vrouwelijke urethra, master's thesis, Netherlands, 1979, University of Groningen.

Hutch JA: A new theory of the anatomy of the internal urinary sphincter and the physiology of micturition: the base plate, *J Urol* 96:182, 1966.

Hutch JA: *Anatomy and physiology of the trigone, bladder, and urethra,* New York, 1972, Appleton.

Kamina P: *Anatomia ginecologica ed ostetrica,* Roma, 1975, Marrapese.

Milley PS, Nichols DH: The relationship between the pubourethral ligaments and the urogenital diaphragm in the human female, *Anat Rec* 170:281, 1971.

Netter FH: *Atlante di anatomia fisiopatologica e clinica,* vol 3, *Apparto riproduttivo,* Ciba-Geigy II, 1982.

Nichols DH: Clinical pelvic anatomy: the types of genital prolapse and the choice of operation for repair, *R I Med J* 65:112, 1982.

Nichols DH, Milley PS, Randall CL: Significance of restoration of normal vaginal depth and axis, *Obstet Gynecol* 36:251, 1970.

Nichols DH, Randall CL: *Vaginal surgery,* ed 3, Baltimore, 1989, Williams & Wilkins.

Paramore RH: The supports in chief of the female pelvic viscera, *J Obstet Gynaecol Brit Emp* 30:391, 1908.

Parks AG: Anorectal incontinence, *Proc R Soc* Med 68:21, 1975.

Petros PE: The intravaginal slingplasty operation, a minimally invasive technique for cure of urinary incontinence in the female, *Aust N Z J Obstet Gynecol* 36:453, 1996.

Platze WL: Functional anatomy of the human vagina. In Hafez ESE, Evans TN: *The human vagina,* Amsterdam, 1978, Biomedical Press.

Richardson DA, Ostergard DR: The effect of uterovaginal prolapse on urethrovesical pressure dynamics, *Am J Obstet Gynecol* 146:901, 1982.

Richter K: Gynakologische anatomie des Kleinen Beckens, *Gynakol Rundsch* 19(suppl 1):13, 1979.

Richter K: Massive eversion of the vagina: pathogenesis, diagnosis, and therapy of the "true" prolapse of the vaginal stump, *Clin Obstet Gynecol* 25:897, 1982.

Scali P: *Les prolapsus vaginaux et l' incontinence urinaire chez: la femme,* Paris, 1980, Masson.

Shafik A: Pelvic double-sphincter control complex: theory of pelvic organ continence with clinical application, *Urology* 6:611, 1984.

Smith ARB, Hosker GL, Warrell DW: The role of partial denervation of the pelvic floor in the aetiology of genitourinary prolapse and stress incontinence of urine: a neurophysiological study, *Br J Obstet Gynaecol* 96:24, 1989.

Smith ARB, Hosker GL, Warrell DW: The role of pudendal nerve damage in the aetiology of genuine stress incontinence in women, *Br J Obstet Gynaecol* 96:29, 1989.

Ulmsten U, Henriksson L, Johnson P, Varhos G: An ambulatory surgical procedure under local anesthesia for treatment of female urinary incontinence, *Int Urogynecol J Pelvic Floor Dysfunct* 7:81, 1996.

Wein AJ, Barret DM: *Voiding: function and dysfunction,* St Louis, 1988, Mosby.

Wilson PD, Dixon JS, Brown AD, Gosling JA: Posterior pubourethral ligaments in normal and genuine stress incontinent women, *J Urol* 130:802, 1983.

Wilson PM: Understanding the pelvic floor, *S Afr Med J* 47:1150, 1973.

Zacharin RF: "A Chinese anatomy." The pelvic supporting tissues of the Chinese and occidental female compared and contrasted, *Aust N Z F J Obstet Gynaecol* 17:1, 1977.

Zacharin RF: Pulsion enterocele: review of functional anatomy of the pelvic floor, *Obstet Gynecol* 55:135, 1980.

Zacharin RF: *Pelvic floor anatomy and the surgery of pulsion enterocoele,* New York, 1985, Springer-Verlag.

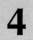

4 Establishing a Diagnosis: The History, Physical Examination, Imaging, and Diagnostic Surgery

DANIEL L. CLARKE-PEARSON

The importance of a thorough preliminary survey of the patient's overall background and current health status cannot be too strongly emphasized. An adequate general medical history, including a careful system review, and a thorough general physical examination are essential to selecting the proper surgical procedure and to achieving the optional surgical outcome. The significant historical and physical findings pertinent to specific surgical conditions are discussed in separate sections of this book. This chapter provides an overview and basis for surgical decision making.

After obtaining the history relevant to the chief complaint, the presence of independent cardiovascular, renal, or pulmonary disease must also be determined, because this information often affects the choice of treatment when more than one alternative is available. The nature and details of past illnesses or operative procedures also are important, and it may be necessary to call, fax, or write to other physicians or hospitals to obtain accurate information on these points. The physician should know if the patient is or has been receiving medications. Certain hormones may cause abnormal bleeding; immunosuppressive chemotherapeutic drugs and broad-spectrum antibiotics may alter vaginal flora, allowing an overgrowth of *Candida* and causing vaginitis; certain cardiovascular medications, thyroid hormones, and cortisone compounds may influence preoperative preparations and choice of anesthesia. A history of allergy or sensitivity to any medications is obviously important.

Social and environmental factors that may affect pelvic symptoms also should be adequately explored. A general understanding of the patient's personality, her mental and emotional attitudes and problems, and the adequacy of her past and present adjustment to various life situations also prove helpful when evaluating pelvic complaints, since nonorganic causes may partially contribute to symptoms arising in relation to the reproductive tract and its function. The gynecologist must make sure to hear not only what the patient says, but also what the patient does not say; nonverbal forms of communication such as body movements, evidence of inner tension or hesitation, and changes in attitude must be noted. All may help in understanding and dealing with the patient's problems.

Finally, the gynecologist should always ask about familial disorders, particularly if there is a family history of malignant disease, diabetes, tuberculosis, or allergies. A strong family history of any of these disorders should alert the physician to watch for similar conditions in the patient.

The gynecologist must approach the care of the patient from a broad viewpoint. Although his or her principal function in the overall care of women has been and undoubtedly should remain that of a highly trained specialist-consultant in the field of gynecology, in practice the gynecologist has long served the important role of a primary care physician for women. For many American women the gynecologist is the principal source of medical supervision, advice, and occasionally initial care for nongynecologic problems. Thus the gynecologist often represents women's initial entrance into the total health care system and provides them continuity of care within this system.

GYNECOLOGIC HISTORY

The patient initially should be allowed to present her chief complaint and the story of her present illness in her own way and words. The patient's age should be noted. If necessary, the physician can eventually guide the conversation to avoid the presentation of repetitious or insignificant material. The following points of information can be elicited by judicious questioning, if they are not spontaneously reported by the patient, to complete the gynecologic history:

1. Menstrual history
   a. Age at menarche
   b. Length of cycle
   c. Regularity of cycle
   d. Premenstrual molimina (e.g., breast pain, tenderness and swelling, skin changes, cramps, headaches, tension, weight gain, edema)
   e. Duration of flow
   f. Associated cramps or pelvic pain and time of occurrence
   g. Description of amount (number of sanitary pads required per day provides a rough index, with three to six as normal) and character of flow
   h. Dysmenorrhea, primary or secondary (characteristics of pain, location of pain, time of onset and subsidence, and effective medications)

i. Dates of the last menstrual period and the previous menstrual period

j. Description of any prior therapy for menstrual disorders

k. If postmenopausal, age at menopause and description of menopausal symptoms

2. Sexual history
   a. Age at first coitus
   b. Frequency of coitus
   c. Dyspareunia
   d. Satisfaction and orgasmic response
   e. Type and duration of contraceptives used

3. Obstetric history
   a. Number of pregnancies and dates (gravidity)
   b. Number of deliveries and dates (parity) and whether births were normal, full term, or presented complications
   c. Type of delivery (spontaneous vaginal, forceps, section)
   d. Episiotomy or other procedure; perineal tears
   e. Birth weight of babies
   f. Postpartum difficulties and complications
   g. Number of miscarriages (duration of pregnancy at the time, complications, need for curettage)

The obstetric profile is recorded as gravida x, para p-q-r-s, where x is the number of pregnancies, p is the number of term pregnancies, q is the number of preterm pregnancies (births), r is the number of aborted pregnancies, and s is the number of living children. Thus gravida 4, para 1-1-1-2 indicates that the patient is having her fourth pregnancy, with one previous term pregnancy, one preterm pregnancy, one abortion, and two living children (one full-term and one preterm birth).

Special inquiries should be made concerning the following:

1. Abnormal bleeding
   a. Character and amount
   b. Any associated symptoms (e.g., pain, discharge)
   c. Relation to periods (premenstrual, postmenstrual, intermenstrual, postmenopausal)
   d. Frequency, duration, and onset (sudden or slow)
   e. If preceded by amenorrhea or other menstrual irregularities

2. Abnormal discharge
   a. Amount, color (yellow, white, brown), odor, and consistency (thin, watery, thick, cheesy, mucoid)
   b. Relation to menstrual cycle (premenstrual or postmenstrual aggravation)
   c. Associated symptoms (vulvovaginal burning and itching, urinary symptoms)

3. Abnormal pelvic or abdominal pain
   a. Type (sharp, dragging, aching, pressure or bearing-down, cramping, colicky, burning)
   b. Sudden or gradual onset
   c. Duration
   d. Whether steady or intermittent
   e. Location and radiation
   f. Relation to menses or to phase of menstrual cycle
   g. Relation to position (upright versus recumbent)
   h. Relation to function of other organ systems (gastrointestinal or urinary tract)
   i. Associated symptoms (abnormal bleeding or discharge, gastrointestinal or bladder disturbances).

Pain referred to the low back or buttocks is commonly associated with disease in the cervix, urethra, bladder neck, or lower rectum and often radiates into one or both legs. Discomfort due to uterine or vaginal disease or associated with inflammatory conditions of the bladder dome usually is localized in the lower abdomen. Ovarian pain and pain due to disease of the fallopian tubes are most often referred to the lower abdominal quadrants just above the groin and often radiate down the medial aspect of the thighs.

4. Back pain: Backache of gynecologic origin is most commonly secondary to endometriosis, chronic pelvic inflammatory disease, large fibroids arising in the posterior uterine wall and wedged in the hollow of the sacrum, or posterolateral extension of carcinoma of the cervix. It is fair to say, however, that most backaches are of musculoskeletal rather than gynecologic origin.

5. Infertility
   a. Duration
   b. Prior use of contraceptives
   c. Type and duration of contraceptives used
   d. Frequency and timing of coitus
   e. Coital habits
   f. Dyspareunia (pain during coitus)
   g. Prior studies
   h. Previous marriages of either partner and any resulting pregnancies

6. Abnormal symptoms of genital relaxation
   a. Feeling of protrusion
   b. Dragging sensation
   c. Pressure
   d. Bearing-down discomfort
   e. Sense of insecurity

7. Associated bladder symptoms
   a. Frequency
   b. Nocturia
   c. Urgency
   d. Dysuria
   e. Difficulty voiding
   f. Incontinence (stress, urgency)

8. Associated bowel symptoms
   a. Constipation
   b. Diarrhea
   c. Pain referred to region of the rectum
   d. Vaginal protrusion on straining during defecation

9. Miscellaneous history of any acute abdominal or pelvic illnesses or operations, especially of the pelvis or of a perforated appendix

10. Psychological and emotional considerations

In a reasonably concise presentation of the gynecologic surgery field, it is impossible even to begin to do justice to the many facets of the various psychosomatic mechanisms and disturbances that may be encountered in the gynecologic patient. Acute or chronic emotional disorders, by interfering with the normal, delicately balanced neuroendocrine control of the cyclic activity of the female reproductive tract, often cause fundamental disturbances in this cyclic function. The result is that distressing symptoms arise on a purely psychosomatic basis. Such psychosomatic mechanisms are almost invariably important in the comprehension and management of many functional gynecologic disorders: so-called hypothalamic amenorrhea, the premenstrual tension syndrome; the "pelvic congestion" syndrome and related types of functional pelvic pain; idiopathic pruritus vulvae; and so on. Undoubtedly, they also play an important etiologic role in many women with recurring functional menstrual irregularities, as well as in some patients suffering from infertility or habitual abortion. Certainly, the significance of psychologic factors in the production of many of the disabling menopausal symptoms experienced by a few women is well recognized.

On the other hand, among the various manifestations of organic disease of the reproductive tract, secondary symptoms may have a psychologic basis. Disturbed function of or complaints localized to the pelvic viscera region invariably cause considerable anxiety. They may raise the specter of premature loss of or failure to completely fulfill childbearing potential, cause concern over possible loss of sexual function, or arouse the fear that cancer or a "shameful social disease" is present. In fact, pelvic symptoms often suggest to the patient a serious threat to her integrity as a female, either as a result of how the disease itself will affect her or as a consequence of the treatment that may be required (e.g., hysterectomy). Thus physicians also must consider emotional factors and sympathetically deal with them by offering explanations and reassurance for patients with obvious organic disease, as well as for those who prove to have functional complaints.

Recognition of women who have significant psychiatric illness or who will likely have difficulty adjusting to surgery and postoperative recovery should lead the gynecologist to seek psychiatric consultation and continued support postoperatively.

GYNECOLOGIC PHYSICAL EXAMINATION

A complete general physical examination should be carried out first, including determination of height, weight, and blood pressure, as well as a survey of the neck, breasts, heart, lungs, abdomen, inguinal and femoral regions, and lower extremities. A nurse or other female attendant should always be present during the physical examination. The presence of another female in the room is comforting to female patients because the examination can be a source of considerable apprehension and embarrassment for some women. Furthermore, it affords the physician some protec-

tion against the possibility that a patient with an unsuspected psychotic tendency or ulterior motive may subsequently allege improper behavior on his or her part in the examining room. The patient should be warm, physically comfortable, and relaxed; she should be properly draped and have had an opportunity to void immediately before examination. The patient's mental ease and relaxation should also be ensured by a conscious effort to gain her confidence and cooperation while obtaining the history and by continued reassurance during the physical examination. If the patient is not comfortable and relaxed, examination is more difficult and maximum information cannot be gained.

The examination conveniently begins with the patient in a sitting position on the edge of the table. The physician first checks the head and neck (including palpation of the thyroid and the cervical and supraclavicular nodes), breasts, axillae, back, and lungs. The patient then lies flat on the table for a further check of the breasts, heart, abdomen, groin, and lower extremities.

Breast Examination

During examination of the breasts, the physician should inspect them first with the patient sitting erect, with her arms at her sides and again raised overhead. This maneuver frequently discloses breast asymmetry, nipple fixation, or a fixed mass underneath the areolar margin, any of which can go unnoticed in the recumbent position. A careful, methodical examination of all quadrants of the breasts and the adjacent axillary regions should then be carried out with the patient in both the erect and supine positions. Palpation is best performed and breast masses most readily appreciated if the flat, palmar surface of the hand and contiguous palmar surfaces of the apposed fingers are employed rather than the actual tips of the fingers. It is important to learn to distinguish the somewhat finely granular, irregular consistency of normal breast tissue from discrete masses that may represent either neoplasm or benign fibrocystic change. It is also important to be aware of the frequent existence of an axillary extension of normal breast tissue, the "axillary tail," and not to mistake it for a tumor; when present, it is almost invariably bilateral and symmetric. Finally, the areolar areas should be compressed gently to demonstrate any abnormal secretion or bloody fluid in the nipple glands and ducts.

Because the patient herself first discovers nearly all breast irregularities or lumps, it is well worth the effort to instruct patients about the proper method of the breast self-examination. Each patient can readily be shown the correct technique during the physician's examination and should be urged to examine her breasts every month, just after completion of the menstrual period, at a time when normal premenstrual breast engorgement and tenderness are not misleading. She should be taught to inspect her breasts in front of a mirror, first with her arms at her side, then with arms overhead, looking for changes in size or contour or for dimpling of the skin. Next, lying flat, she can be shown how to palpate correctly with the right hand all four quadrants of the left breast. With a small pillow under the left shoulder, she should place her left hand under her head while palpating the inner half of the breast, with the left arm down at the side while palpating the outer quadrants. The procedure is then reversed to examine the right breast with the left hand. It is hoped that such instruction in proper self-examination of the breast will enable women to more promptly recognize any changes and hence lead to the earlier detection of breast cancer.

Careful, detailed examination of the abdomen is obviously an integral part of the gynecologic physical examination. It also is particularly important never to neglect examination of both groins, as many gynecologic disorders affecting the vulva and vagina are accompanied by inguinal adenopathy, whether inflammatory or neoplastic.

The patient also should be examined briefly in the standing position, checking for the presence of inguinal or femoral hernias and inspecting the lower extremities for varicosities, edema, or skin lesions.

If there is any question of peripheral arterial insufficiency, the femoral, popliteal, dorsalis pedis, and posterior tibial pulses also should be checked.

Pelvic Examination

The principal portion of the pelvic examination is performed with the patient in the lithotomy position. Rarely, the lateral Sims, knee-chest, or standing position is employed because occasionally it is more suitable than the lithotomy position for determining specific points. The actual pelvic examination begins with inspection; the lower abdomen, the external genitalia (mons veneris, vulvar skin, and labia majora and minora, prepuce and clitoris, introitus, hymeneal or vaginal opening, and visible portions of the anterior and posterior vaginal walls), the urethral meatus, and the anoperineal area are surveyed first for abnormal distribution or character of hair or pigmentation, clitoral hypertrophy, generalized or local skin lesions, visible subcutaneous or submucosal abnormalities (e.g., inflammation, leukoplakia, ulcers, tumors, hernias, cysts, and atrophy). The physician may best recognize gross displacement and relaxations if the patient strains (Valsalva) and the vagina and introitus are seen. The external genitalia, including the labia majora and minora, mons pubis, and perineum, should be palpated next for any masses or swellings. The examiner now sits directly in front of the patient with a suitable flexible lamp and carries out the speculum examination, introducing the previously warmed blades after separating the labia and depressing the perineal body with the opposite hand. (Blades can be warmed by holding them under running warm tap water, warmed in a heated drawer, or under a heating pad.) If the introitus and vagina are dry, it is better to wet the speculum blades with warm water rather than use a lubricant, which can interfere with obtaining cervical and vaginal cytologic smears and specimens for culture of organisms. A Graves bivalve speculum of appropriate size—small (infant), medium ("regular"), medium with narrow blades (Pederson), or large, depending on the size of the introitus and the size and length of the vaginal canal—is in-

serted at the proper angle and with a slight rotary motion. The speculum should be of the proper size to fully evaluate the vagina and cervix while not being so large as to cause the patient pain. In most instances, even in the presence of an intact hymen, the hymeneal opening is sufficient to permit both one-finger bimanual vaginal and speculum examinations (usually employing the narrow-bladed instrument) without difficulty, if they are properly and gently done. (If these examinations are not possible, information obtained by a bimanual rectal examination and with pelvic ultrasound is often sufficient in a young girl; otherwise, examination under anesthesia is necessary.) The speculum is gently but firmly inserted its full length, and the blades are then opened, exposing the cervix for inspection, preparation of a Papanicolaou smear, cervical or endometrial biopsy, or any other office diagnostic procedure required. A little manipulation may be necessary to expose the cervix if the uterus is retroverted or if the vaginal walls are lax and redundant. A cotton pledget grasped at the end of a curved uterine-dressing forceps can be used as a "pusher" to facilitate exposure. As the instrument is withdrawn, the vaginal wall, including the posterior fornix, and any secretions or discharge present are examined for evidence of vaginitis, atrophy, or other lesions.

After the speculum examination, the examiner performs a bimanual vaginal examination. Although it has long been taught that the left hand should be used to perform bimanual examination, it is not mandatory. The hand one is most accustomed to using or with which one feels most natural and proficient during palpatory examination of any body region should be used consistently. The labia are gently separated and one or two well-lubricated fingers of the gloved hand are introduced, depressing the perineum and posterior vaginal wall to avoid undue and uncomfortable pressure against the more sensitive anteriorly placed structures. With the finger(s) depressing the perineum, the perineal body and pubococcygeal (levator) muscles are palpated. The patient is asked to strain or cough, or both, which further reveals any tendency to perineal relaxation, cystocele, rectocele, or prolapse of the uterus or vagina. Abnormalities of the structures at the level of the introitus (urethra, Skene's glands, Bartholin's glands) are searched for between the thumb and forefinger. The fingers are then inserted at the proper angle (approximately 30 to 45 degrees above the horizontal) the length of the vagina, palpating the vaginal wall and exocervix and the external os as this maneuver is carried out.

Bimanual examination of the uterus and adnexal regions is then carefully done, checking the size, outline, consistency, mobility, and position of the uterus, ovaries, and any palpable pelvic masses. The vaginal vaults (lateral fornices or adnexal regions) are then palpated, feeling primarily with the vaginal fingers, the abdominal hand sweeping the adnexa down to them. Anterior and posterior fornices (cul-de-sac, or pouch of Douglas) are then explored bimanually in the same way, and the fingers are then turned and pressed laterally to feel the pelvic walls as well. Normal adnexa are frequently not palpable even under ideal conditions, especially if the patient is unrelaxed or obese. However, under anesthesia, normal-sized ovaries are often palpable even in an obese patient. Unusually mobile adnexa (with relaxed and elongated infundibulopelvic and ovarian ligaments) may result in the ovaries being palpated in the cul-de-sac posteriorly at the time of rectal examination, rather than during vaginal examination. The examiner can expect palpation of "normal-sized" ovaries (e.g., 3.5 × 1.5 cm) in premenopausal women with active ovarian function. However, palpation of "normal-sized" ovaries in a women 3 to 5 years after menopause has not been a normal or expected clinical finding; on the contrary, it suggests that the ovaries are not normal at all and may signify early ovarian cancer, which has its peak incidence between ages 45 and 60.

Finally, the examiner performs a rectovaginal examination (the index finger in the vagina and the middle finger in the rectum) to look for external and internal hemorrhoids, fissures, fistulas, or anorectal polyps or tumors. The uterus is palpated bimanually (only now is the fundus palpable if the uterus is retroverted), together with the ovaries and particularly the cul-de-sac, uterosacral ligaments, and the paracervical and paravaginal regions (so-called anterior parametrium). These areas are best palpated rectovaginally, and herein may lie the diagnostic findings of endometriosis or early spread of cervical carcinoma. The rectal finger also can explore the surface of each pelvic wall in turn, feeling for enlarged nodes or other abnormalities. By having the patient strain or assume the standing position while the examiner maintains two fingers within the rectum and vagina, the examiner may confirm the presence of an enterocele, perhaps suspected but demonstrable in no other way, by feeling the sac with its contents bulging down between the vaginal and rectal fingers. It is important that the rectal finger is not reintroduced into the vagina unless the used glove is discarded and a new glove put on. The stool on the rectal glove finger should be tested for occult blood. When sexually transmitted diseases (e.g., gonorrhea, syphilis, warts) are suspected, the physician should use a new glove after completing the vaginal examination and before beginning the rectovaginal examination. This measure should help to prevent spreading sexually transmitted organisms from the vagina to the rectum.

Patient Consultation

After completion of the physical examination, the patient is allowed to dress in privacy. When the patient returns to the consultation room, the physician reviews the important features of the history and physical findings, explains their significance in easily understood terms, and outlines the suggested plan of further study and treatment, again explaining the need and rationale for the proposed program so that she can readily comprehend its importance and cooperate completely. If the husband, mother, other close relative, or friend has accompanied the patient, it is often wise—but always with the patient's agreement and permission—to invite him or her to sit in on this final summation. In this way, members of the family or friends most vitally interested in and con-

cerned with the patient's welfare can obtain the information about her current medical situation directly and therefore more accurately. This usually guarantees their assistance, if needed, to support her and ensure her understanding of and cooperation with the subsequent course of study and therapy.

DIAGNOSTIC TESTING RELEVANT TO THE EVALUATION OF SURGICAL CONDITIONS

A complete, thoughtfully elicited history and thorough physical examination, with obvious emphasis on the recognition and proper interpretation of significant findings demonstrated by abdominal, pelvic, and rectal examinations, are the two basic and most important elements in the diagnosis of pelvic disorders. The information obtained may be all that is necessary to arrive at an exact diagnosis. At the least, the broad outlines of the clinical problem posed by the chief complaint have been narrowed considerably, so further investigation of a limited number of more likely possibilities may now be effectively undertaken. Only in this way can the wide variety of laboratory tests and special procedures useful for establishing a diagnosis be applied cost-efficiently, avoiding delay in diagnosis and treatment and reducing unnecessary studies to a minimum. A conflict in clinical care arises between the need to reduce and contain health care costs and the medical-legal climate in which the diagnosis and treatment may be questioned without adequate testing or radiographic confirmation. These diagnostic evaluations (which for the purposes of this discussion include laboratory serum evaluation, cultures, radiographs, and diagnostic surgical procedures) are often expensive and, in some instances, invasive procedures. Therefore our emphasis is to delineate the use of these tests, as well as discuss their risks and costs. Special procedures, commonly employed in connection with a specific problem (e.g., urinary incontinence or cervical dysplasia), are described in more detail elsewhere in the text.

Basic Office Diagnostic Techniques

Cytopathology. The diagnosis of gynecologic conditions based on microscopic study of single cell morphology owes its greatest debt to Papanicolaou, who pioneered the recognition of characteristics associated with cervical cancer, as detected by exfoliative cytology of the cervix and vagina. This single diagnostic screening technique has had the largest effect on the reduction of mortality from cervical cancer over the last 5 decades. The Papanicolaou (Pap) smear is now used routinely for screening all sexually active women and all women over age 18. Undoubtedly, the widespread use of cervical cytology screening has decreased the incidence and mortality of invasive cervical cancer. The coincident increase in human papilloma infection of the lower genital tract has resulted in an increasing number of women with "preinvasive" cervical intraepithelial neoplasia. (Chapter 17 discusses appropriate management options.) Genital cytopathologic studies also may suggest endometrial carcinoma or carcinoma arising from the ovary, fallopian tube, or elsewhere in the peritoneal cavity. Cytopathologic specimens obtained from the vulva are less accurate and are not considered a routine screening diagnostic method today. Many times cytopathologic studies of the cervix and vagina also suggest the cause of vaginitis (e.g., *Candida,* herpes, or *Trichomonas*). On the other hand, the Pap smear is not as sensitive or as specific as readily available specific culture techniques for diagnosing these infections.

Key points in performing a Pap smear include the following:
- Good exposure of the cervix with a proper-size speculum
- Sampling of both the ectocervical transformation zone and the endocervical canal
- Preparation of a thin (single cell) layer on the microscope slide (Newer methods of "monolayer" preparations are becoming available, although their use has yet to be fully established.)
- Rapid fixation of the cellular material to avoid air-drying
- Proper labeling of the slide and provision of pertinent clinical information to the laboratory (e.g., last menstrual period, prior history of neoplasm, prior history of pelvic radiation, menopausal status, hormone or oral contraceptive use)

Microscopic Evaluation of Vaginal Smears and Cultures. Vaginitis and cervicitis are the most frequent complaints evaluated by gynecologists. Simple microscopic examination of the vaginal discharge diluted with saline (wet preparation) may identify the offending organism. The addition of a few drops of potassium hydroxide (KOH preparation) makes *Candida* hyphae more easily recognizable. KOH dissolves the epithelial cells and white blood cells, thereby unmasking the hyphae and budding yeast forms.

Culture techniques also are available for identifying offending organism more precisely. They are especially helpful when the clinical diagnosis based on wet preparations and KOH preparations is unclear or in cases resistant to what was thought to be adequate therapy. *Trichomonas* can be cultured on either Feinberg-Whittington medium or Diamond's medium. *Candida* is best cultured on Nickerson's medium. Cultures for herpes and *Chlamydia* must be handled specially with the proper media and transport vials. Gonococcus is best cultured on Thayer-Martin plates. Culture techniques also are available for the routine identification of anaerobes that commonly inhabit the lower genital tract. Cultures of the normal vagina identify several anaerobes and aerobes that are usually found living in symbiosis. Some of these organisms, when grown in excess, can be pathogenic. However, routine bacterial culture of the vagina is many times misleading and of no diagnostic value, since many bacteria are identified. Anaerobic and aerobic cultures therefore should be obtained for abscesses of the vulva, groin, or pelvis or for further delineation of the cause of apparent salpingo-oophoritis. Patients who have vaginitis require appropriate treatment before undergoing elective gynecologic surgery.

Colposcopy. The lower genital tract can be evaluated with the aid of magnification provided by the colposcope. The colposcope is essentially a binocular dissecting microscope, usually used with a magnification power of approximately 15×. Colposcopy is most commonly used to evaluate patients with abnormal Pap smears suggesting cervical intraepithelial neoplasia or invasive carcinoma. Because it is moderately expensive and time-consuming and skill is required to perform it, colposcopy is not a routine screening technique. Nonetheless, when used appropriately in situations requiring further cervical evaluation, colposcopy and directed biopsy may eliminate the need for diagnostic surgical procedures such as cold knife conization. The details of colposcopy technique are discussed in Chapter 17.

Biopsy of the Cervix. Biopsies of suspicious cervical lesions identified with the naked eye or with colposcopic magnification usually can be performed in the office or outpatient setting with little or no anesthesia. Either a punch biopsy instrument or a loop electrosurgical excision device can be used to obtain a directed or excisional biopsy.

Schiller's Test. Schiller's test was used much more extensively before the advent of colposcopy; however, it is still used today in several clinical situations, especially when colposcopy cannot identify an abnormal cervical or vaginal lesion or when correlation with colposcopic findings is advantageous so that surgical biopsies or conization may be performed without the repeated use of the colposcope in the operating room. Schiller's test is based on the observation that glycogenated squamous epithelium (of the cervix and vagina) takes up an iodine-based stain.

Schiller's solution (1 part iodine, 2 parts potassium iodide, 300 parts water) is applied to the vagina and upper cervix with a cotton pledget. Normal squamous epithelium usually takes up the stain, and a homogeneous mahogany-brown color is noted. In many patients with cervical dysplasia, in whom the nuclear/cytoplasmic ratio is increased (and therefore glycogen in the squamous epithelial cytoplasm is diminished), Schiller's stain is not taken up, and the epithelium appears light yellow. This area of unstained epithelium is considered a positive Schiller's test. Unfortunately, a cervix that has undergone trauma that has de-epithelialized the tissue, tissue with cervicitis, and columnar epithelium do not take up the stain, which may lead to a false-positive test. Schiller's test is clearly not as sensitive or specific as colposcopy for identifying cervical intraepithelial neoplasia.

Endocervical Biopsy (Curettage). Endocervical biopsy (curettage) is performed as part of the routine outpatient evaluation of patients with an abnormal Pap smear. It also can be combined with endometrial biopsy for evaluating patients with abnormal uterine bleeding. During a fractional dilation and curettage (D&C), the specimen from the endocervix should be submitted separately from the endometrial specimen to distinguish the pathologic site.

Endocervical curettage is performed with a small, sharp curette that is introduced into the endocervical canal, which is then sampled. Care is taken to avoid trauma to the exocervix, because dysplasia arising in the transformation zone can be scraped off along with the endocervical specimen, thus confusing the true location of the dysplastic squamous epithelium. As with endometrial biopsy, endocervical curettage induces some uterine cramping, which usually can be managed with nonsteroidal antiinflammatory agents. Endocervical curettage should not be performed during pregnancy because of the possibility of rupturing the amniotic membranes.

Vulvar Biopsy. Biopsy of the vulva is critically important to the diagnosis and management of many conditions noted grossly on the vulva. If the lesion is small enough, it can be entirely excised (excisional biopsy). On the other hand, many lesions are too large for excisional biopsy to be carried out in the office, and definitive therapy may require more than excisional biopsy. In this setting, punch biopsy of the vulvar lesion(s) may be performed using the Key's punch and local anesthetic.

After preparation of the vulvar skin with an antiseptic solution such as povidone-iodine, 1% lidocaine is infiltrated into the region to be biopsied. The Key's punch (usually 3 or 4 mm in diameter) is used to obtain a punch biopsy specimen of the skin and superficial subcutaneous tissue. With a rotating motion, the circular punch incises the area of interest, and the base is excised using sharp Iris scissors or a scalpel. The specimen should be oriented on filter paper so that appropriate perpendicular cuts can be made through the tissue at the time of sectioning in the pathology department. Hemostasis is achieved with silver nitrate or a single absorbable suture. This procedure is not associated with any significant major side effect. Because vulvar lesions are not necessarily pathognomonic on general examination, vulvar biopsy is encouraged when any lesion is encountered.

Vaginal Biopsy. Vaginal biopsy usually is performed in the office to evaluate a patient with an abnormal Pap smear in whom a lesion can be seen in the vagina. Colposcopy can aid in locating the vaginal lesion. Dysplasia can occur at any portion of the vagina, although it is frequently located near the vaginal apex. Vaginal biopsy usually can be performed using the same biopsy forceps employed to biopsy the cervix. Local anesthesia with injectable 1% lidocaine or topical analgesia using benzocaine usually is sufficient to allow comfortable biopsy. Hemostasis can be achieved with silver nitrate or a suture.

Endometrial Biopsy. The ease with which a sample of endometrium usually can be obtained for histologic study is of tremendous help in the office evaluation and management of a variety of pelvic disorders. With menstrual disturbances and infertility, two outstanding examples, endometrial biopsy nearly always proves useful and informative. When performing endometrial biopsy, one should ensure that the patient is not pregnant and that she does not have active pelvic inflammatory disease. The biopsy is performed after bimanual examination, which has ascertained the size, shape, and position (anteverted versus midplane or retroverted) of the uterus.

The cervix is exposed by speculum, and the external os is swabbed free of mucus and painted with povidone-iodine (Betadine) solution. The anterior cervical lip is then grasped with a tenaculum a slight distance from the external cervical os. A uterine sound is passed to determine the length and direction of the cervical canal and endometrial cavity. The physician should warn the patient to expect slight discomfort similar to a menstrual cramp. To obviate or reduce the discomfort from the uterine contraction and cramp, a prostaglandin synthetase inhibitor such as ibuprofen 400 mg or sodium naproxen 275 mg orally may be given 15 to 20 minutes before the procedure. The aspiration device (e.g., Pipelle, Vabra aspirator, or Novak Curet) is introduced into the uterus to the top of the fundus. The aspiration device is pressed against the wall of the fundus anteriorly, posteriorly, and laterally and is then withdrawn, removing a sample of endometrium. This sample is then fixed in formalin and processed routinely as a surgical pathology specimen, allowing evaluation of tissue architecture. These endometrial sampling devices function either as a small, sharp curette or as a suction aspirator of endometrial tissue. The two methods are equal in terms of diagnostic accuracy and are similar in potential for risks and complications. Therefore gynecologists usually select one method of endometrial biopsy for their office procedures and perform it routinely.

Details of the recent menstrual history should always accompany the pathology laboratory requisition, which should request endometrial dating if it is for evaluation of infertility. The pathologist's histologic diagnosis of proliferative or secretory endometrium is only partially informative because on the basis of certain histologic criteria the endometrium can be reliably dated during the luteal phase of the cycle. This dating must then be compared against the known day of the patient's current cycle, which should, however, be calculated backward from the actual day of the forthcoming menstrual flow.

Endometrial biopsy is most often used as an index of ovulation and progesterone effect in the course of an infertility investigation or as an aid in the diagnosis and further management of dysfunctional (anovulatory) bleeding. Obviously, biopsy must be performed during the immediate premenstrual phase or on the first day of menstruation to be of any help in either situation. Endometrial biopsy also is diagnostically useful in patients suspected of harboring endometrial cancer; a positive report facilitates the diagnosis, but a negative report is of little value and does not alter the need for diagnostic curettage in women with symptoms suggestive of hyperplasia or malignancy.

Spotting after an endometrial biopsy may occur for a day or so but usually is not severe. A more serious complication of endometrial biopsy is uterine perforation. If the uterus is perforated in the midline, the myometrium of the uterine wall usually contracts and minimizes bleeding. Observation without surgical intervention is usually all that is necessary. Because of the potential for bacteremia induced by endometrial or endocervical biopsy, patients with cardiac valvular disease should receive prophylactic perioperative antibiotics to reduce the possibility of subacute bacterial endocarditis.

Culdocentesis. Access to the peritoneal cavity can be helpful in recognizing intraperitoneal bleeding (which might be associated with an ectopic pregnancy), purulent material from the pelvis associated with tuboovarian abscess or salpingo-oophoritis, or peritoneal fluid that might be studied cytologically to identify malignant cells, as noted with ovarian cancer. The easiest access to the peritoneal cavity to accomplish any of these goals is through the posterior cul-de-sac (pouch of Douglas). The distance between the peritoneum of the posterior cul-de-sac and the vaginal mucosa is less than 1 cm in most women. Therefore it is relatively easy to introduce a needle across the posterior vaginal mucosa just behind the cervix into the pouch of Douglas.

Culdocentesis may be performed using a local (1% lidocaine) or topical (benzocaine) anesthetic. After preparing the vagina with povidone-iodine and obtaining adequate anesthesia, the physician passes a 22-gauge spinal needle attached to a syringe across the mucosa and peritoneum. Blood obtained at culdocentesis (especially if more than 1 ml) suggests intraperitoneal bleeding, especially if blood does not clot after 5 to 10 minutes. (In this setting, especially with a clinical history and symptom complex suggestive of possible ectopic pregnancy, intraperitoneal bleeding must be strongly considered.) Nonclotting blood obtained during culdocentesis is considered a "positive" culdocentesis. On the other hand, obtaining blood that clots may simply mean that the needle at the time of culdocentesis actually performed a venipuncture.

Culdocentesis is neither sensitive nor specific for ectopic pregnancy but can be used in combination with clinical, ultrasound, and laboratory results. Purulent material obtained on culdocentesis should be cultured for anaerobes and aerobes, the results of which may guide specific antibiotic choices for a pelvic infection. In patients treated for ovarian carcinoma, culdocentesis can be performed to obtain a small amount of peritoneal fluid; or if no fluid is present, the cul-de-sac can be lavaged with 10 ml of saline and then aspirated. This fluid should then be submitted for cytopathologic studies to search for malignant cells, which may be an early indicator of recurrent disease.

Tests for Evaluation of Hemorrhagic Tendency. For about 10% to 20% of all serious hemorrhagic disorders in women, the earliest, most significant, or sole manifestation is excessive menstrual flow or prolonged uterine bleeding. Therefore it is important to keep this possibility in mind when studying and treating women with menorrhagia, particularly when there is no response to the usual measures for control of dysfunctional bleeding on a hormonal basis and when local uterine abnormalities that might cause excessive bleeding have been excluded. In this situation, investigation of the possible existence of an abnormal bleeding tendency is clearly indicated.

A useful, simplified approach to the study of these possible hemorrhagic disorders assumes that serious organic disease with secondary hemorrhagic tendencies has been ruled out. The approach is outlined below.

It is therefore appropriate to undertake laboratory testing in a woman with abnormal bleeding when no other organic cause is identified (e.g., cancer, fibroids, polyps). Basic screenings with a platelet count, prothrombin time (PT), partial thromboplastin (PTT), and bleeding time are usually sufficient to identify significant coagulation defects. On the other hand, coagulation testing is not recommended as part of routine preoperative evaluation unless prior history suggests high risk (e.g., alcoholic liver disease, use of anticoagulants, unexplained bleeding; see Chapter 5).

Tumor Markers. A number of tumor markers are particularly useful in the management of women with ovarian cancer or gestational trophoblastic disease (Table 4-1). In the latter condition, hCG may serve as a critical piece of evidence in establishing the diagnosis of malignant sequelae after evacuation of a hydatidiform mole or in establishing the diagnosis of a primary tumor in a young woman with metastatic cancer of unknown origin, which is discussed further in Chapter 64.

On the other hand, the tumor markers commonly found in ovarian cancers should not be used as a diagnostic test because of lack of both sensitivity and specificity. For example, serum CA125 is elevated in 80% of nonmucinous epithelial ovarian cancers; however, it is elevated in only 50% of stage I ovarian cancers. Conversely, CA125 is elevated in a number of benign gynecologic conditions such as endometriosis, uterine fibroids, and pelvic inflammatory disease. Therefore elevated CA125 does not necessarily signal ovarian cancer, and likewise a malignancy cannot be absolutely ruled out in patients with a normal CA125.

Diagnostic Imaging in the Evaluation of Gynecologic Surgical Conditions

Every effort should be made to avoid the unwitting use of elective diagnostic pelvic and abdominal x-ray studies for evaluating an early and unsuspected, normal intrauterine pregnancy. Bearing this point in mind, the following roentgenologic studies are frequently of great value for evaluating many gynecologic disorders (Table 4-2).

Chest Radiograph. As part of the preoperative workup, routine radiographs of the chest are obtained for most patients older than age 50 who are undergoing gynecologic

Table 4-1 Tumor Markers Commonly Useful in the Management of Gynecologic Cancers

Marker	Associated Cancer
hCG	Gestational trophoblastic disease, choriocarcinoma
	Choriocarcinoma of the ovary (ovarian germ cell tumor)
CA125	Epithelial ovarian cancer
α-Fetoprotein (AFP)	Immature teratoma of the ovary
	Endodermal sinus tumor
LDH	Dysgerminoma of the ovary

Table 4-2 Preferred Methods of Imaging Common Gynecologic Conditions

Organ or Tissue and Pathology Suspected	Preferred Method
Ovaries	
Follicle growth	
Tumors	Vaginal ultrasound
Ectopic pregnancy	
Cancer	CT scan
Uterus	
Fibroids	Vaginal ultrasound or MRI
Early pregnancy	Vaginal ultrasound
Congenital anomalies	Hysterosalpingography or possibly vaginal ultrasound
Uterine synechiae	Hysterosalpingography
Carcinoma	MRI
Trophoblastic disease	Ultrasound or MRI
Fallopian Tubes	
Tubal occlusion	Hysterosalpingography
Ectopic pregnancy	Vaginal ultrasound
Cervix	
Incompetent cervix	Hysterosalpingography (cervicogram) or vaginal ultrasound
Carcinoma	CT scan, MRI

CT, Computed tomography; *MRI,* magnetic resonance imaging.

surgery; however, these studies are unnecessary for young, fit patients with no significant past illness who are undergoing uncomplicated surgery. The chest radiograph is important for the initial staging and evaluation of patients with any gynecologic malignancy.

Metastasis may be identified as parenchymal metastasis, pleural effusions, or mediastinal adenopathy. A pleural effusion in association with a pelvic mass and ascites may not necessarily represent advanced ovarian carcinoma but may be Meigs' syndrome. An upright chest radiograph also is the best radiographic method for detecting free air in the peritoneal cavity; air would gather under the diaphragm, suggesting bowel perforation as the cause of pneumoperitoneum. Free air is also noted under the diaphragm for up to 7 to 10 days after abdominal or vaginal surgery. The chest radiograph, on rare occasion, also suggests the cause of pelvic pain and nodularity as evidenced by pulmonary tuberculosis.

Kidney, Ureter, and Bladder. A plain radiograph of the abdomen—kidney, ureter, and bladder (KUB)—may show the following: a pelvic mass, calcified fibroids, a dermoid cyst with recognizable teeth or the characteristic layering pattern of the cyst's contents of liquid sebaceous material, calcified ovarian tumors (occasional psammoma bodies), fetal skeletal structure after 4½ months of pregnancy, lithopedions, or bony changes characteristic of osteoporosis or metastatic cancer. It may reveal or confirm the presence of ascites or intestinal obstruction caused by disease of the pelvic organs.

Intravenous Pyelogram In the past, the intravenous pyelogram (IVP) was frequently used for evaluating patients with gynecologic disorders. This radiographic technique consists of intravenous administration of an iodinated radiographic contrast material excreted from the kidneys. Over the course of excretion, the kidneys and their upper collecting systems can be visualized along with the ureters draining urine to the bladder; the bladder is also outlined. The IVP is particularly helpful for evaluating the kidneys and the course of the ureters. Although information can be gained regarding the shape and position of the bladder, other more specific tests, such as cystoscopy and cystography, are more specific for evaluating the bladder itself. Tomograms can be made through the kidneys during the course of an IVP to assess more fully the upper collecting systems and kidney anatomy.

With regard to the evaluation of common problems associated with gynecologic disease and urologic abnormalities, the following conditions are most commonly studied:

1. Evaluation of a patient with apparent congenital müllerian anomalies should include evaluation of the urologic system. Congenital anomalies of the kidneys or ureters with duplicate or absent collecting systems are frequently found.

2. Before performing gynecologic surgery for benign gynecologic conditions, it is frequently helpful for the surgeon to be sure that the urinary tract is normal or to be able to identify abnormalities. Common abnormalities that might alter the surgical approach include the identification of duplicate collecting systems or absent collecting systems. Furthermore, on rare occasions a pelvic mass is a pelvic kidney. Deviation of the ureter by a pelvic mass or obstruction of the ureter also can be identified. Further evaluation and treatment at the time of gynecologic surgery may be necessary. A pelvic mass arising from the pelvis and attaining the size of a 16-week gestation often causes extrinsic compression of the ureters at the pelvic brim, leading to a variable degree of hydronephroses and proximal hydroureter. Likewise, endometriosis may invade the retroperitoneal space and lead to ureteral deviation or obstruction.

3. During evaluation for gynecologic malignancy, the urinary tract should be inspected as well. Frequently, carcinoma of the cervix deviates or obstructs the ureter in the pelvis, especially if parametrial extension has occurred. Likewise, metastatic disease to the lymph nodes, as is seen with cervical, endometrial, and ovarian carcinomas, may lead to ureteral obstruction or deviation. Abnormalities seen by IVP are incorporated into the staging system for carcinoma of the cervix. Today, it is more common to use a CT scan to stage gynecologic malignancy. CT not only provides images of the urinary tract, but also allows assessment of lymph nodes, liver, and other intraperitoneal organs.

4. IVP may be helpful for evaluating a patient with a possible urinary tract fistula. It is particularly helpful for identifying ureteral injury or ureterovaginal fistula. Other methods for evaluating the bladder and urethra are more specific.

The risks of an IVP are primarily related to reactions noted in patients who have iodine allergies, usually manifested by urticarial reaction or wheezing. More severe reactions can lead to respiratory arrest. Because the contrast material is excreted from the kidneys, patients who have underlying renal disease (e.g., diabetes or hypertensive renal disease) or patients who have taken nephrotoxic drugs (e.g., aminoglycoside antibiotics, cisplatin) are at risk for further renal compromise. Therefore assessment of the patient's history of iodine allergy (e.g., a sensitivity to shellfish or a previous reaction to IVP dye) and an assessment of renal function (serum creatinine) should be undertaken before performing an IVP.

Other methods for assessing the urinary tract, including a retrograde pyelogram, cystogram, and cystourethrogram, are discussed in more detail as they are specifically related to the abnormalities of the lower urinary tract discussed in Chapters 21 and 44 to 49.

Barium Enema. Barium enema is performed primarily to evaluate the colon and terminal ileum. Barium is injected as an enema and observed under fluoroscopic control as it fills the colon and terminal ileum. Radiographs are obtained during the filling and evacuation phases, with detailed films made of areas of interest. Air also can be injected into the colon to obtain more detail of mucosal lesions (air-contrast barium enema). Details of the rectum are poorly evaluated by barium enema and are probably better studied by proctosigmoidoscopy.

Barium enema may reveal involvement of the colon by gynecologic disease. A large pelvic mass may cause extrinsic compression or deviation of the colon. Ovarian carcinoma, in more advanced stages, not only can cause extrinsic compression, but also can actually invade the colon and its mesentery. This situation is most commonly noted in the sigmoid colon, although the cecum and transverse colon also may be involved. Preoperative barium enemas in patients with an adnexal mass may suggest colonic involvement and thereby allow adequate preparation for colonic surgery. Benign conditions, especially endometriosis, also can invade the colon and lead to intestinal obstruction or perforation. Conversely, pelvic disease may have colonic disease as its primary etiology—particularly colon cancer, which may be detected as a pelvic mass either as a palpable rectosigmoid lesion or as an enlarging ovarian metastasis (Krukenberg's tumor). Diverticulitis or a diverticular abscess can be the cause of a pelvic mass, which would be suggested by barium enema. Colonic obstruction, stricture, and fibrosis caused by radiation therapy also can be diagnosed. Rectovaginal fistula often is diagnosed from a barium enema; multiple fistulous tracts, such as those associated with advanced ovarian carcinoma or severe radiation injury, may be more clearly delineated. Barium enema also is indicated in cases of rectal bleeding or a guaiac-positive stool. Colonic carcinoma, polyps, or other associated conditions such as radiation proctitis can cause rectal bleeding.

The primary risks and side effects of barium enema are patient discomfort and exposure to additional radiation. Perforation caused by barium enema is infrequent (probably less than 1 in 1000), although with diverticulitis or colonic carcinoma, perforation may be increased. Barium spilling into the peritoneal cavity can cause barium peritonitis, which can be fatal, unless managed appropriately with prompt evacuation, fecal diversion, and peritoneal lavage. Finally, barium that is allowed to remain in the colon after a barium enema study can become an inspissated hard mass leading to impaction.

Hysterosalpingography. Hysterosalpingography is radiographic delineation of the uterus and fallopian tubes using a contrast material introduced into the uterus through the cervical canal. The contrast outlines the uterine cavity, the lumen of the fallopian tubes and their patency, and the cervical canal. Hysterosalpingography should be carried out under fluoroscopic monitoring, because this method provides maximum information regarding the manner and rate at which the dye fills the uterine cavity and the fallopian tubes, as well as the actual spill of dye from each fallopian tube if it is patent. This dynamic relation between the müllerian tract system and the instilled dye cannot be readily appreciated from the static spot films alone, but the films are taken at the appropriate moment of relevant clinical interest seen by fluoroscopy for subsequent review and reading. The fluoroscopic screening itself can be recorded on videotape and replayed for study purposes.

Hysterosalpingography, a diagnostic procedure commonly used to evaluate female infertility and recurrent abortion, also is helpful for the management and treatment plan of gynecologic disorders such as abnormal uterine bleeding, intrauterine adhesions (Asherman's syndrome), congenital anomalies and diethylstilbestrol exposure in utero and for preoperative evaluation before myomectomy and tubal reconstruction. Hysterosalpingography often is used for postoperative assessment of uterine and tubal integrity, after tubal reconstruction without pregnancy occurring, and after tubal ligation with questionable histologic documentation that the tubes were ligated. Although pregnancies have occurred after hysterosalpingography for evaluation of infertility, proof that the procedure is therapeutic is inconclusive. It is possible that the mechanical flushing effect of the dye instillation may wash out debris in the tube and therefore subsequently facilitate spontaneous pregnancy; however, hysterosalpingography is not best advocated as therapy. The diagnostic value of hysterosalpingography is greatly enhanced by laparoscopy and can sometimes be replaced by the latter procedure. However, for abnormalities within the uterine cavity and the cervical canal, hysterosalpingography provides additional information.

Contraindications to hysterosalpingography include

pregnancy or suspected pregnancy, active uterine bleeding, menstruation, acute pelvic inflammatory disease, and hypersensitivity to iodine or iodine-containing dyes. Complications of hysterosalpingography are relatively infrequent (0.3% to 1.7%). The complication seen most often is pelvic infection following the procedure. Other less frequent complications include allergy to the injected contrast material and vasomotor reactions including flushing, dizziness, and transient hypotension (all of which are self-limiting and not serious). Oil embolism and tubal and peritoneal granulomatous reactions are complications associated with the use of oil-based contrast medium. For these reasons, water-soluble contrast medium is preferable. The risk of radiation exposure to the ovaries is small. The amount of radiation to the ovaries depends on the fluoroscopic unit used, the duration of fluoroscopy (a time limit is set for most machines for this procedure to prevent exceeding the maximum dose of radiation), and the size of the patient. For usual hysterosalpingography examinations, the amount of radiation is small (less than 750 mrad).

Normal Findings. The normal uterine cavity outline is a triangle with the base at the fundus and the apex inferiorly meeting and extending into the endocervical canal. However, many normal variations to this basic simplified outline are seen. The internal os usually is well demonstrated. If there is extreme uterine anteflexion, the fundal part of the uterine cavity is superimposed end-on with the inferior part of the cavity. This problem can be overcome by "straightening" the uterus with tension on the cervical tenaculum or taking an oblique view if the uterus does not straighten. The tubes emerge from the uterine cornua outward and can be identified as the interstitial segment, isthmus, ampulla, and infundibulum.

Abnormal Findings. Abnormalities detectable on hysterosalpingogram include those of the fallopian tubes, uterus, and cervix. Cervical incompetence can be readily demonstrated by the wide internal os and cervical canal. Abnormalities of the fallopian tubes seen on hysterosalpingograms include (1) obstruction with no further filling of the dye beyond the point of obstruction, (2) observation of the fimbrial end with no contrast material spillage, (3) some contrast material spillage with a loculated, confined, well-circumscribed collection, suggestive of adhesions between the distal tube and ovary into a kind of pocket but a fimbrial opening still present, and (4) complete fill and spill of the contrast from the tubes, which, however, show a "fixed" or "rigid" pattern in relation to the uterus suggestive of peritubal adhesions. Obstructed tubes can be caused by pelvic inflammatory disease, endometriosis, previous sterilization, salpingectomy, or previous unsuccessful tubal reconstruction. Salpingitis isthmica nodosa shows a characteristic cricoid, stippling pattern usually present at the isthmal region. Tuberculosis of the tubes may appear similar to salpingitis isthmica nodosa on hysterosalpingograms. Tubal polyps and tumors are also demonstrable. Although an ectopic pregnancy can be localized, hysterosalpingography is not used as a diagnostic imaging technique.

Acquired uterine abnormalities detected by hystersalpingography include (1) myomas, which, if submucous, show distortion or enlargement of the uterine cavity, (2) endometrial polyps, which appear as well-circumscribed filling defects often with a base from the uterine wall, (3) endometrial carcinoma appearing as round filling defects, either single or multiple, (4) uterine synechiae or Asherman's syndrome appearing as filling defects of varying extent, often with a craggy border, and (5) early disruption of a cesarean section scar, appearing as a slight protrusion of dye along the scar line. Congenital anomalies of the uterus identified by hysterosalpingography include (1) arcuate, subseptate, septate, and bicornuate uterus, all of which show changes in the superior aspect of the uterine cavity outline, ranging from a mild heart-shaped intrusion to a complete septum, (2) unicornuate uterus with only one tube emerging from the superior end of a cylindrically shaped uterine cavity, (3) uterus didelphys showing two separate uterine cavities, and (4) T-shaped uterine cavity or a constricted lower segment in women who were exposed to diethylstilbestrol in utero.

Transvaginal and Abdominal Ultrasound. Ultrasound has assumed one of the leading roles as a diagnostic imaging technique for gynecologic disease. Transvaginal sonography has two major advantages over abdominal sonography. First, no acoustic window is required for transvaginal scanning; therefore a full bladder necessary for abdominal sonography is not required. Second, the transvaginal transducer is closer to the pelvic structures than the abdominal probe, thereby increasing the spatial resolution. Because there is little adipose tissue at the vaginal apex, the problem of increased signal attenuation through tissues, with the use of a high-frequency transducer, can be overcome by moving the transducer probe closer to the object. At present, transvaginal transducers have frequencies up to 7.5 MHz compared with abdominal scanning, which usually is carried out with 3.5- or 5.0-MHz transducers.

A transvaginal scan is usually best done with an empty bladder, which also makes the study more comfortable for the patient. A preliminary abdominal scan may infrequently be indicated. Vaginal scanning is carried out with the patient lying in the lithotomy position on a gynecology examination table, slightly in the reverse Trendelenburg position to pool free peritoneal fluid in the pelvis to enhance visualization. The transducer is covered with a condom or a rubber glove into which some sonograph coupling gel has been placed, and more is placed on the outside for lubrication. The probe is then inserted into the vagina up to the vaginal apex, and pelvic structures are visualized in the sagittal or coronal plane. Usually it is helpful to identify the uterus first on the scan so that the adnexal regions can be scanned and structures identified in relation to it. The iliac vein and artery are convenient landmarks for the pelvic sidewalls, and the ovary is usually medial to these vessels. Withdrawing the transducer slightly from the vaginal apex allows the cervix to be scanned. Transvaginal sonography has been employed or is useful for the following gynecologic conditions or situations.

Ovary. Because of its posterolateral location, the normal ovary is difficult to visualize in detail with abdominal scanning. Abdominal scanning of the ovaries requires extensive bladder filling, but even with this maneuver, the ovary sometimes tends to displace deep into the posterior pelvis. Under such circumstances and also with obese patients, the resolution of the sonogram scan is limited. Transvaginal sonography provides a definite improvement in sonographic visualization and scanning of the ovary and has therefore become the method of choice for sonographic scanning of the ovaries. With this technique, visualization of ovarian follicles is improved in as many as 85% to 90% of patients who had suboptimal abdominal ultrasound examination of the ovaries.

Transvaginal sonographic scanning of the ovaries is currently carried out for (1) routine follicle scanning and monitoring of follicle recruitment and rate of growth, (2) ultrasound guidance of follicle aspiration transvaginally for in vitro fertilization, (3) examination of the ovary for ovarian enlargement or adnexal mass, and (4) routine measurement of ovarian size and volume in postmenopausal women to determine its potential value for early detection of ovarian neoplasm. With transvaginal ultrasonically guided oocyte retrieval, fertilization and pregnancy rates are similar to those obtained with laparoscopic recovery, but this method has the added advantages of requiring only local or regional anesthesia, being done readily in the office or clinic, and reducing the cost of in vitro fertilization. Important characteristics of the cyst and mass include evidence of septations, intracystic nodules or excrescences, excrescences on the cyst surface, or solid components. Scoring systems that consider these characteristics predict benign and malignant behavior with a high degree of accuracy.

Tubes. The normal fallopian tube cannot be readily seen on abdominal sonography for a variety of technical reasons, unless the tube is surrounded by or distended with some kind of fluid. Transvaginal sonographic scanning is particularly useful for viewing diseased fallopian tubes and the ovaries. Ectopic pregnancy in the fallopian tubes and ovaries can be readily detected, and any free fluid in the cul-de-sac due to a hemoperitoneum also can be immediately visualized. It then allows culdocentesis to be carried out, if necessary, under vaginal ultrasound guidance. Because of the closeness of a tubal pregnancy examined with a vaginal probe and the high-frequency transducer employed, the image of an ectopic pregnancy has a clearer and better resolution. With an acute disease such as inflamed tubes or a tubal gestation, the walls are widened and the longitudinal endosalpingeal folds can be seen. With ectopic pregnancy, blood clots may fill the tubal cavity, or an unruptured pregnancy sac with or without active heartbeat is seen.

Cervix and Uterus. In the transverse plane, the cervix appears first on the screen if the uterus is anteverted; if the uterus is retroverted, the fundus appears first and is close to the sacrum. The exact position of the uterus and cervix is best displayed when scanning in the longitudinal plane. The internal and external cervical os and the length of the cervi-

cal canal can be measured in the longitudinal views. With this view, cystic structures of the cervical canal, most likely representing endocervical gland structures, must be differentiated from very early ectopic cervical pregnancy. The uterine artery and veins can be recognized together with blood flow at the level of the internal os on a real-time scan. On the exocervix, nabothian cysts are recognized as translucent, thin-walled structures.

The position of the uterus is examined, and common pathologic conditions of the uterine wall (e.g., myomas or polyps) should be sought. Sonographically, myomas display variable echogenicity, arranged in bundlelike, "turbulent" structures interspersed with acoustic shadows produced by the dense fibroid tissues. Unlike ovarian masses, solid masses on the uterus usually move in the direction in which the vaginal probe is pushed; if the sonographic appearance is similar to the uterine texture, the mass is likely to be a fibroid. The postmenopausal uterus tends to be significantly smaller but has a uniform echogenicity if it is not diseased. The uterine cavity and its endometrial lining should be carefully scanned. The appearance of the endometrium changes throughout the menstrual cycle, and an empty uterus shows a regular, thin, obvious "cavity line." If bleeding is present, the blood-filled uterine cavity is readily outlined.

In postmenopausal patients, endometrial thickness, as measured by vaginal sonography, is an accurate predictor of hyperplasia or carcinoma. In nearly all cases of cancer, the endometrial stripe is greater than 5 mm. Despite this, endometrial histologic evaluation (biopsy or dilation and curettage) is required to diagnose pathologic conditions accurately.

Saline Infusion Sonohysterography. Fluid enhances ultrasonographic visualization. When an artificial insemination catheter is inserted into the uterine cavity and saline is injected, the uterine cavity is outlined. This technique allows the examiner to distinguish submucous myomas from polyps. The demonstration of submucous fibroids is useful not only for explaining bleeding but also for planning resection. This technique can also detect intrauterine adhesions. Saline infusion sonohysterography is well tolerated with no need for sedation and may replace the need for hysterosalpingogram in many situations.

Computed Tomography. CT has become increasingly useful for the diagnosis and evaluation of intraabdominal and pelvic lesions, intracranial pathologic conditions, and intrathoracic conditions as they relate to the practice of gynecology. However, the technique is more complex and expensive than sonography and exposes the patient to ionizing radiation. Particularly useful for evaluating pelvic neoplasms, CT offers the ability to assess parietal soft tissue planes, including muscle and fat, as well as bones, vessels, lymph nodes, and other retroperitoneal structures. CT imaging can be further enhanced with the use of contrast medium. If an oral contrast medium is ingested before CT imaging, intraabdominal tumors can be delineated in sharp contrast to the dye-filled loops of bowel. CT scanning is useful for the following conditions: (1) enlarged pelvic and paraaortic lymph nodes, (2) retroperitoneal diseases, (3) assessment of a previously irradiated pelvis, the examination of which is otherwise seriously hampered by extensive fibrosis and scarring, and (4) CT-directed thin-needle biopsies of CT-visible lesions in the pelvis and elsewhere, obviating a major operative procedure to obtain tissue diagnosis.

Because CT can image many organs, it may replace or eliminate the need for several other studies. For example, CT can be used to search for distant metastases in patients with gynecologic malignancies. This single test can be used to evaluate the lungs, liver, upper abdomen, urinary tract, retroperitoneal lymph nodes, and pelvic structures. For staging of gynecologic malignancy, CT may replace chest tomography, liver scanning, pelvic ultrasound, IVP, and lymphangiography.

The broadest application of CT today is for the staging of gynecologic cancers. CT imaging may be helpful for identifying local extension of cervical carcinoma, lymph node involvement, and distant metastases. The identification of metastatic disease in pelvic or paraaortic lymph nodes depends on the size of the lymph node. CT scans cannot differentiate an enlarged lymph node due to hyperplasia from those containing metastases. Lymph nodes of 1.5 to 2.0 cm are considered suspicious, and nodes larger than 2.0 cm are considered abnormal. When evaluating local extension of gynecologic malignancies, such as cervical carcinoma, CT is not entirely accurate and is not necessarily more sensitive or specific than a careful gynecologic pelvic examination. In this setting MRI may be more accurate. CT also may provide information similar to that of an IVP identifying normal kidneys and patent ureters. Detailed evaluation of the urologic system, however, is better performed by IVP.

The role of CT scanning of the pelvis for evaluating pelvic mass is limited. CT cannot distinguish between benign and malignant pelvic masses. The greater resolution of vaginal ultrasound has established ultrasound as the study of choice for ovarian tumors. CT may be helpful for evaluating the characteristics of the mass (solid versus cystic or mixed components) and identifying cyst content, especially if it is fat (such as in a dermoid). Because nearly all cases of a pelvic mass require surgical exploration, excision, and pathologic study, CT scan information does little to help the clinician establish a diagnosis and rarely changes the need for surgical exploration and excision. When evaluating ovarian carcinoma, CT is sensitive for identification of ascites, and it also may identify metastases at other peritoneal sites such as the omentum, liver, or bowel mesentery. However, the sensitivity and specificity of CT scanning for evaluating intraperitoneal disease are limited; rarely are metastases smaller than 2 cm identified, primarily because of the varying consistency of the abdominal cavity, with loops of bowel, omentum, and intestinal mesentery making up parts of the CT cuts.

To identify loops of small bowel, the intestines are usually filled with radiographic contrast material. Likewise, intravenous iodinated contrast material is used to differentiate vessels from retroperitoneal lymph nodes. Without these contrast techniques, CT scanning has a reduced capability to identify intraperitoneal and retroperitoneal disease. Evaluation of depth of invasion of endometrial carcinomas is poorly defined by CT scan; MRI appears to be more accurate.

The CT scan is also helpful in the search for intraabdominal abscesses that may follow gynecologic surgery for patients with pelvic inflammatory disease and lymphocysts after pelvic lymphadenectomy. Abscesses and lymphocysts can be drained using CT-guided needle aspiration and catheter placement. Thus CT scans and CT-guided procedures could be used in place of major surgical procedures in many patients. In a few cases, CT scanning has been helpful for identifying ovarian vein and pelvic vein thrombosis.

Scanning of the abdomen and pelvis takes about 45 minutes; its major risks are exposure to radiation and intravenous contrast material. On the other hand, one of the major advantages of CT scanning is its ability to replace several other diagnostic radiographic techniques.

Magnetic Resonance Imaging. Magnetic resonance imaging (MRI) is becoming an important technique for imaging the female pelvis because it gathers data in multiple planes and produces high contrast of soft tissue. Recently, the addition of intravenously administered contrast agents such as gadolinium (Gd-DPTA) has enhanced soft tissue differentiation.

To obtain magnetic resonance images, the patient is placed inside the bore of a powerful magnet, and a second, oscillating magnetic field is applied to the patient. This second field causes the hydrogen nuclei to move out of alignment with the first, thereby generating the signal.

The technical advantage of MRI includes the ability to obtain images in any dimension; moreover, the absence of magnetic resonance signal by calcium renders bone (with its high calcium content) transparent to the imaging method. Although these characteristics enable good imaging of the brain and spinal cord, absence of a calcium signal renders the technique incapable of picking up calcium deposits in a malignant soft tissue tumor, of which CT is capable. MRI is not hazardous to the patient because it does not use the ionizing radiation of CT. Patients going through MRI studies may feel claustrophobic and anxious as they are delivered into the bore of the powerful magnet.

MRI can be used for imaging the head, thorax, musculoskeletal system, and abdomen and pelvis. MRI continues to undergo evaluation, and its full role, advantages, and limitations for evaluating gynecologic disease have not been defined. Therefore careful study and assessment of MRI scanning in patients should be carried out so that information can be gained concerning its proper role. Because these imaging methods are reasonably expensive and resources are limited, neither MRI nor CT scanning should be used or be considered part of a routine gynecologic evaluation. MRI is currently used to view the abdomen and pelvis in gynecologic practice and probably will be used more in the future because it does not use ionizing radiation.

MRI has been used for imaging the uterus and ovary. The normal uterus appears to have three layers of varying intensity. In the center of the uterus is a high-intensity area consistent with the endometrium. Proceeding outward, a low-intensity "band" thought to be the stratum basale, or innermost myometrium, separates the endometrium from a zone of moderate intensity, which represents the myometrium. The cervix also has three zones identified by MRI. In the center of the cervix is a high-intensity zone correlating with cervical mucus, whereas the stroma and glands of the cervix are of low intensity, and the outer muscularis layer is of intermediate intensity. Studies of the uterus in different phases of the menstrual cycle or in patients receiving oral contraceptives show varying imaging characteristics that reflect fluctuating hormone levels.

MRI appears to be more sensitive than CT in evaluating uterine disease. MRI has been used to detect benign tumors such as fibroids and adenomyosis, as well as malignant tumors such as molar pregnancy, choriocarcinoma, and endometrial cancer, where the tumor location, depth of myometrial invasion, and extent of cervical invasion and myometrial invasion can be readily determined. However, a degenerating myoma may be impossible to distinguish from a uterine sarcoma or other malignancies. Although MRI improves the quality of images and the assessment of myometrial involvement compared to other radiographic techniques, its clinical application remains somewhat limited for *managing* uterine lesions. For example, the depth of myometrial invasion, although of prognostic significance, does not necessarily alter the treatment course, which would include surgical exploration with total abdominal hysterectomy, bilateral salpingo-oophorectomy, and consideration of selective pelvic and paraaortic lymphadenectomy. Likewise, management of a uterine myoma that is symptomatic or that requires surgical resection by myomectomy or hysterectomy would be little influenced by MRI findings. As with other radiographic techniques, MRI does not absolutely confirm histology and may only suggest the distinction between benign and malignant conditions. Whenever malignancy is a serious concern, further diagnostic methods including biopsy must be carried out.

MRI is probably of little more value than CT in evaluating adnexal disease. Normal ovaries are often difficult to identify by MRI because they may not be separated from adjacent loops of small intestine. Small cysts on the ovaries can be seen, and fat included in a dermoid cyst is easily identified. On the other hand, MRI may fail to detect calcification in dermoid cysts. The value of MRI for diagnosing pelvic endometriosis, particularly with nonbleeding or small foci, is not established and may be less promising. MRI may identify implants of endometriosis in the peritoneum and especially in the posterior cul-de-sac, but distinguishing these implants from those of ovarian carcinoma is not yet possible with this imaging technique. MRI may be less accurate than CT for the evaluation of patients with ovarian carcinoma because a longer scan time is necessary for each "cut," and bowel peristalsis, vascular pulsation, and respiration blur the abdominal contents and their images. These technical factors render MRI less sensitive than CT for detection of abdominal carcinomatosis and evaluation of lung lesions. For detection of metastases in lymph nodes, MRI may be as sensitive and specific as CT. Both techniques show enlargement of nodes, with biopsies required to differentiate between enlarged hyperplastic nodes and nodes containing metastatic carcinomas. On the other hand, neither diagnostic technique appears to be sufficiently sensitive for detecting microscopic metastases in normal-sized lymph nodes. Because MRI distinguishes clearly between blood vessels and other retroperitoneal structures, it may be more accurate for detecting lymph nodes, especially when intravenous radiographic contrast material cannot be used at the time of CT imaging.

Pelvic Arteriography. Arteriography of the internal iliac artery, with its myriad collaterals and branches, plays a role in the management of several gynecologic conditions. To perform pelvic arteriography, a catheter must be inserted (usually into the femoral artery) and then the internal iliac trunk cannulated. Selective arteriography of the anterior or posterior division of the internal iliac artery can be accomplished through catheter manipulation and positioning. Arteriogram dye is injected rapidly, and rapid-sequence radiographs are obtained of both the filling and drainage of the arterial and venous systems, respectively.

Pelvic arteriography plays a role in the management of the following conditions:

1. Pelvic arteriography may help locate the site of uncontrolled pelvic bleeding. It is particularly useful in postpartum patients, postoperative patients, patients with a pelvic malignancy, or those infrequent patients who have radionecrosis of the pelvis. In each of these circumstances, arteriography can be used to identify the site of bleeding; in conjunction with arterial embolization, bleeding can be controlled by obstruction of the particular segment of hypogastric artery contributing to the bleeding. Of course, pelvic bleeding can arise from other arteries, such as the inferior mesenteric or the ovarian arteries, neither of which can be visualized or controlled by embolization of the hypogastric artery.

2. Arterial venous malformations can occur congenitally or after gynecologic surgery. The pain, pressure, and potential for hemorrhage have been recognized with arteriovenous malformations, which are best visualized by arteriography. When the specific artery contributing to the vascular malformation is identified, it also can be embolized to partially control symptoms.

3. Patients with gestational trophoblastic disease who have become resistant to therapy may benefit by having a hysterectomy performed to excise a resistant focus of trophoblastic disease invasive to the myometrium. On occasion, arteriography assists in the confirmation of invasive gestational trophoblastic disease of the uterus, thereby verifying potential benefits of hysterectomy in excising occult disease. MRI of

the uterus may be more helpful in identifying invasive disease in the future.

4. Infusion of chemotherapy agents through the pelvic vascular bed is experimental but may have some role in the future treatment of advanced gynecologic malignancy.

Pelvic arteriography requires the skill of a trained vascular radiologist and carries some risk. Aside from the risks associated with the iodinated contrast material previously noted for IVP, complications can arise from cannulation of the femoral and external iliac arteries. Arterial thrombosis and hematoma at the arteriotomy site may occur. Most hematomas resolve spontaneously, although arterial thrombosis may require embolectomy or even arterial bypass surgery. Occasionally, a lower extremity has been lost because of extensive arterial thrombosis.

Diagnostic Surgical Procedures

Examination under Anesthesia. Although a complete pelvic and abdominal examination can identify pelvic disease in most instances, examination under anesthesia occasionally can provide additional information, especially in patients who are uncooperative or in such pain as to not allow a thorough examination. Such patients include some children and adolescents and patients with pelvic pain caused by pelvic inflammatory disease, endometriosis, or malignancy. Patients who are obese also can be difficult to examine while awake. Examination under anesthesia often adds to the diagnostic capabilities for identifying pelvic disease. Before any pelvic surgery is performed, examination should be performed under anesthesia, as the findings may alter surgical technique or strategy.

Examination under anesthesia can be combined with cystoscopy and proctosigmoidoscopy when evaluating patients with gynecologic cancer. In addition, areas of suspicion can be biopsied at this same time using standard punch biopsy forceps or a scalpel or needle biopsy technique.

Fractional Dilation and Curettage. Fractional dilation and curettage (D&C) is the gold standard diagnostic technique for evaluating the endometrium and endocervix. However, with the advent of smaller biopsy devices and the risks and expenses of a surgical procedure requiring anesthesia, most patients can be evaluated and managed based on office endometrial and endocervical biopsies, discussed previously. Fractional D&C should be performed when the biopsy is inconclusive in patients who have not responded to therapy that was based on endometrial biopsy results, or in patients in whom endometrial biopsy could not be performed because of cervical stenosis or a low pain threshold. Hysteroscopy often is performed in conjunction with D&C.

Fractional D&C requires adequate anesthesia levels to perform dilation and sharp curettage of the endocervix and endometrium. It is usually accomplished with general or spinal anesthesia. Some patients tolerate a fractional D&C with only local (paracervical) anesthesia. As the term connotes, fractional D&C obtains a fraction from the endocervix and a sample of the endometrium. These specimens are submitted separately so that the exact location of pathologic process can be more fully identified. This technique is particularly important for distinguishing between endocervical and endometrial adenocarcinoma and for staging endometrial adenocarcinoma.

After adequate anesthesia is achieved, the endocervical canal is curetted sharply. The uterine cavity is then sounded to determine the depth and direction of the canal. The cervix is grasped with a tenaculum to stabilize it and to pull down (and thereby straighten somewhat) the uterine cavity. The cervical canal is dilated with blunt dilating instruments that are graduated in size. The cervix should be dilated only to the size adequate to introduce the appropriate endometrial curette. Thorough curettage of the endometrial cavity is then performed and the tissue submitted to a pathologist. Following sharp curettage, stone forceps are passed into the endometrial cavity, and attempts are made to grasp any endometrial polyp that may not have been removed by the curette.

Complications of fractional D&C include uterine perforation. If the perforation occurs on the lateral aspects of the uterus and a vein or artery is injured, a broad ligament and retroperitoneal hematoma can form. If bleeding is uncontrolled, hysterectomy may be necessary to achieve hemostasis. In most instances, however, uterine perforation occurs in the uterine fundus and is of no consequence. Sharp curettage, especially in an infected uterus, can result in intrauterine synechia with subsequent problems with oligomenorrhea and infertility (Asherman's syndrome).

Hysteroscopy. Hysteroscopy allows transcervical access to the endocervical canal and endometrial cavity. Although it usually is performed in the operating room, newer equipment allows hysteroscopy to be performed in the office. Hysteroscopy is indicated and commonly used for the following conditions:

1. Abnormal uterine bleeding to rule out an organic cause of the endocervical canal or endometrium
2. Suspected submucous leiomyomas or polyps
3. Uterine cavity anomalies due to congenital uterine malformation such as a septate or subseptate uterus
4. If an intrauterine device string is missing and cannot be visualized
5. Postmenopausal bleeding to rule out an organic cause
6. Primary or secondary infertility with hysterosalpingographic abnormalities
7. As a surgical technique for lysis of intrauterine adhesions, septate uterus, or resection of submucous myomas

Diagnostic and operative hysteroscopic techniques are presented in Chapter 41. Potential complications include uterine perforation, hemorrhage, and infection. The medium used to distend the uterus may be absorbed intravascularly and can result in fluid overload, noncardiac pulmonary edema, or intravascular coagulation (DIC).

Cold Knife Conization. A cone-shaped portion of the cervix can be surgically excised and used for diagnosis and treatment of cervical dysplasia. Before conization is considered for diagnosis, patients with an abnormal Pap smear should undergo colposcopy with directed biopsies of the exocervix and endocervical curettage. Most patients with dysplasia can be treated without conization. Cold knife conization is necessary in the following circumstances:

1. The lesion cannot be seen on the exocervix.
2. The lesion extends into the endocervix and cannot be fully evaluated by colposcopy.
3. The endocervical curettage shows dysplasia in the endocervix.
4. Biopsy shows microinvasive carcinoma (less than 3 mm of invasion).
5. The Pap smear suggests invasive carcinoma that cannot be detected by colposcopy and directed biopsies.
6. The Pap smear is two or more grades higher than the dysplasia found on biopsy.

The goal of conization is complete excision of the cervical lesion with an adequate surgical margin. Colposcopic evaluation can be used to individualize the size of the conization so that an excessive amount of normal tissue is not removed. For example, if the exocervix appears normal on colposcopy and disease is suspected in the endocervical canal, a "long, narrow" cone can be designed to excise the cervical canal but not an extensive amount of exocervix. Similarly, when performing a conization during pregnancy for a lesion found to have microinvasion on a colposcopically directed biopsy, a superficial but wide conization around the area detected by colposcopy would be satisfactory for diagnosis, with no attempt made to extend high into the endocervical canal where disease is not suspected. The individualized cone should minimize complications.

Conization usually is performed in an outpatient room under general or spinal anesthesia. After excision of the conization specimen, curettage of the remaining endocervical canal usually is performed. In premenopausal women the addition of a fractional D&C is not necessary or advised unless endometrial disease is suspected.

Immediate complications of conization include intraoperative or postoperative hemorrhage. Bleeding can occur approximately 1 week after surgery when the absorbable suture placed in the surgical bed reabsorbs. Infection of the conization bed may occur, although it infrequently necessitates antibiotic therapy. Long-term complications of conization include cervical stenosis with subsequent infertility or difficult cervical dilation during labor and delivery. Additionally, excessive excision of the cervical stroma can lead to an incompetent cervix, with premature dilation of the cervix during the second trimester or a subsequent pregnancy. Cervical stenosis and incompetent cervix occur in approximately 1% to 2% of patients who undergo conization. Because conization requires operating room time and expense and is associated with some significant complications, it should be avoided unless absolutely necessary. In approximately 90% of evaluated patients with abnormal Pap smears, full treatment is possible without conization.

The carbon dioxide laser can be used in place of cold knife cone biopsy. Laser conization of the cervix is carried out the in the same way as the cold knife procedure. The cervix is injected with vasopressin (Pitressin) to reduce hemorrhage and promote vasoconstriction; laser conization is then performed. Bleeding is minimal both intraoperatively and postoperatively, and the cervix heals well (see Chapter 15).

Diagnostic Laparoscopy. The laparoscope combined with high-resolution video technology now allows the gynecologist to more accurately establish diagnoses and to perform numerous operations that previously required a laparotomy incision. Laparoscopy is the most commonly performed gynecologic surgical procedure in the United States.

There are several indications for gynecologic laparoscopy:

1. Infertility—assessment of tubal factors, such as peritubal adhesions, tubal occlusion, hydrosalpinges, and postoperative evaluation of tuboplasty and appraisal of the ovaries and ovarian function
2. Pelvic pain and dysmenorrhea—searching for causes such as endometriosis, pelvic adhesions, and other responsible pelvic diseases
3. Acute lower abdominal pain—searching for ruptured and unruptured ectopic pregnancy, tubal abortion, leaking corpus luteum, differentiation between these conditions and salpingitis, and translaparoscopic surgical treatment of ectopic pregnancy
4. Pelvic mass—establishing the presence, source, origin, and nature of a mass (fibroids, ovarian cysts, hydrosalpinx, and pelvic malignancy)
5. Known or suspected endometriosis—establishing the diagnosis, extent of disease, suitability of treatment forms, and follow-up of therapy
6. Pelvic cancer—staging and second look to appraise the chemotherapy of ovarian cancer
7. Endocrinopathies and anomalies—evaluation of uterine and ovarian development in primary amenorrhea and premature ovarian failure in secondary amenorrhea
8. Control of vaginal surgery—preventing or evaluating uterine perforation at curettage
9. Foreign bodies and trauma—looking for a displaced intrauterine device or pelvic hematomas

Details of laparoscopic preparation, surgical technique, and potential complications are presented in Chapter 7.

SUGGESTED READING

Bandy L, Clarke-Pearson DL, Silverman PM, Creasman WT: Computed tomography in evaluation of extrapelvic lymphadenopathy in carcinoma of the cervix, *Obstet Gynecol* 65:73, 1985.

Bast RC Jr, Klug TL, St John E, et al: A radioimmunoassay using a monoclonal antibody to monitor the course of epithelial ovarian cancer, *N Engl J Med* 309:883, 1983.

Bohm-Velez M, Mendelson EB, Freimanis MG: Transvaginal sonography in evaluating ectopic pregnancy, *Semin Ultrasound* 11:44, 1990.

Clarke-Pearson DL, Bandy L, Dudzinski M, et al: Computed tomography in evaluation of patients with ovarian carcinoma in complete clinical remission: correlation with surgical-pathologic findings, *JAMA* 255:627, 1986.

Fedele L, Bianchi S, Dorta M, et al: Transvaginal ultrasonography versus hysteroscopy in the diagnosis of uterine submucous myomas, *Obstet Gynecol* 77:745, 1991.

Frates MC, Laing FC: Sonographic evaluation of ectopic pregnancy: an update, *Am J Roentgenol* 165:251, 1995.

Goldstein SR: Saline infusion sonohysterography, *Clin Obstet Gynecol* 39:248, 1996.

Grimes DA: Diagnostic dilatation and curettage: a reappraisal, *Am J Obstet Gynecol* 142:1, 1982.

Mayo-Smith WW, Lee MJ:. MR imaging of the female pelvis, *Clin Radiol* 50:667, 1995.

Pellerito JS, McCarthy SM, Doyle MB, et al: Diagnosis of uterine anomalies: relative accuracy of MR imaging, endovaginal sonography, and hysterosalpingography, *Radiology* 183:795, 1992.

Rucker L, Frey EB, Staten MA: Usefulness of screening chest roentgenograms in preoperative patients, *JAMA* 250:3209, 1983.

Timor-Tritsch IE, Rottem S: *Transvaginal sonography,* New York, 1988, Elsevier.

Twobin NA, Gviazda IM, March CM: Office hysteroscopy versus transvaginal ultrasonography in the evaluation of patients with excessive uterine bleeding, *Am J Obstet Gynecol* 174:1678, 1996.

Valle RF: Diagnostic hysteroscopy. In Keye WR Jr, Chang RJ, Rebar RW, Soules MR, editors: *Infertility: evaluation and treatment,* Philadelphia, 1995, WB Saunders.

Yoder IC: *Hysterosalpingography and pelvic ultrasound: imaging in infertility and gynecology,* Boston, 1988, Little, Brown.

5

Preoperative Evaluation and Preparation for Gynecologic Surgery

DANIEL L. CLARKE-PEARSON

Successful gynecologic surgery is based on thorough evaluation and preoperative preparation of the patient and careful postoperative management. This chapter discusses approaches to the general perioperative management of patients undergoing major gynecologic surgery and discusses specific medical problems that could complicate the surgical outcome.

MEDICAL HISTORY AND PHYSICAL EXAMINATION

Surgery undertaken without a thorough understanding of a patient's medical history and a complete physical examination can result in the development of otherwise preventable complications. The historical information to be obtained includes identifying any significant medical history or medical illnesses that might be aggravated by or that might complicate anesthesia or surgical recovery. Inquiry should be made about current medications being taken, even those discontinued within the previous months before surgery. Specific inquiries should be directed at the possible use of non-prescription drugs and oral contraceptives, because many patients consider these to be a routine part of life rather than a medication. The importance of recognizing such medications is emphasized by the fact that aspirin may lead to intraoperative or postoperative bleeding. Discontinuation of aspirin several weeks before elective surgery is advised to avoid platelet dysfunction. Likewise, oral contraceptives should be discontinued 6 weeks before elective surgery to reduce the risk of postoperative venous thrombosis. Specific instructions must be given to the patient regarding the need to discontinue any other prescription medications before surgery, as well as the recognition of those medications that should be continued (such as cardiac or antihypertensive medications).

The patient should be questioned as to known allergies to medications (most commonly sulfa and penicillin), as well as other allergies to foods or environmental allergens. Because iodinated intravenous (IV) contrast material is used for intravenous pyelogram (IVP), enhanced computed tomography (CT) scan, and venography or arteriography, the patient should be questioned as to her tolerance of other iodinated substances. A history of sensitivity to shellfish may be the only clue to an iodine sensitivity. A history of hypersensitivity to previous intravenously administered iodine-containing compounds should be clearly noted, and the patient should not be further exposed to iodine-containing

compounds unless absolutely mandatory. When IV contrast must be used, corticosteroid preparation should be instituted to prevent life-threatening anaphylactic reactions.

A social history should include use of tobacco, alcohol, and illicit drugs. Smokers should be encouraged to stop smoking 6 weeks preoperatively. In these situations, nicotine patches may help improve the nicotine-dependent patient's pulmonary function. Alcohol abuse may be manifested as nutritional deficiency or bleeding disorders and should lead to further preoperative assessment. Patients who have unusual dietary habits also may be nutritionally deficient, and further evaluation may identify those who would benefit from preoperative nutritional support. The social history should also identify the patient's support system of family, spouse, significant others, and friends who will assist in the patient's recovery from surgery.

Previous surgical procedures, including such minor procedures as dilation and curettage (D&C) or tonsillectomy, should be reviewed, including the patient's course following those surgical procedures; this review can identify potential complications of previous operations, which might be avoided with the current surgery. Reaction and response to anesthetic techniques should be evaluated with the anesthesiologist in charge. Inquiries should be made as to other complications, including excessive bleeding, wound infection, deep vein thrombosis, peritonitis, and bowel obstruction. Previous pelvic surgery should alert the gynecologist to the possibility of distorted surgical anatomy and possible preexisting injury to adjacent organ systems such as small bowel adhesions in the pelvis or ureteral stenosis from previous periureteral scarring. An IVP should be considered in such cases to establish bilateral patency of the ureters or to identify any preexisting abnormality. Operative notes from previous pelvic operations should be obtained and reviewed to precisely determine the prior surgical procedure and surgical findings. Many times, a patient may not be clear on the extent of the procedure or the details of intraoperative findings. This is particularly important in patients who have had surgery for pelvic inflammatory disease, pelvic abscess, endometriosis, or pelvic malignancy.

Family history should be reviewed to minimize the possibility of familial traits that might complicate planned surgery. History of excessive intraoperative or postoperative bleeding, malignant hyperthermia, and other potentially inherited conditions should be sought. General review of systems should also be included in the questioning; searching for any coexisting (GI) and urologic function is particularly important before undertaking pelvic surgery, and many gynecologic diseases also involve adjacent nongynecologic viscera.

A thorough physical examination must be performed preoperatively. Although many women undergoing gynecologic surgical procedures are otherwise healthy, with only pathologic factors identified on pelvic examination, other major organ systems must not be neglected in the physical examination. Identification of abnormalities such as heart murmur or pulmonary compromise should lead the surgeon to obtain additional testing and consultation to minimize intraoperative and postoperative complications.

LABORATORY EVALUATION

Preoperative laboratory studies to be obtained depend on the extent of the anticipated surgical procedure and the patient's general health evaluation. At a minimum for patients undergoing general anesthesia, a blood count including hematocrit, white count, and platelet count should be obtained. Serum chemistry analyses and liver function testing are rarely abnormal in an asymptomatic patient who has no significant medical history and who is not taking medications. Likewise, coagulation studies are of little value unless the patient has a significant medical history.[81] In women younger than age 40, a chest x-ray film and cardiogram are likewise of very low yield in identifying asymptomatic cardiopulmonary disease and may not be necessary.[69,72] On the other hand, women older than age 40 who are undergoing major gynecologic surgical procedures should have a chest x-ray film and cardiogram taken and their serum electrolytes evaluated preoperatively. Even if these studies are normal, they serve as baseline data for comparison to other studies, which might be required in the evaluation of a postoperative complication. Specific studies such as liver function tests, nutritional parameters, arterial blood gases, or pulmonary function tests should be obtained only when there is a significant history or specific risks are anticipated. Further evaluation of adjacent organ systems should be undertaken in individual cases. For example, an intravenous pyelogram helps delineate ureteral patency and course, especially in such cases as a pelvic mass, gynecologic cancer, or congenital müllerian anomaly. However, an IVP is not required for most patients undergoing pelvic surgery.[89]

A barium enema or upper GI series with small bowel follow-through can be of significant value in evaluating some patients before pelvic surgery. Because of the proximity of the female genital tract to the lower gastrointestinal tract, the rectum and sigmoid colon can be affected by benign (endometriosis or pelvic inflammatory disease) or malignant gynecologic conditions. Conversely, a pelvic mass could be of gastrointestinal origin, such as a diverticular abscess or a mass of inflamed small intestines (Crohn's disease). Clearly, any patient with gastrointestinal symptoms should be further evaluated with contrast radiographs, as well as a proctosigmoidoscopy or flexible sigmoidoscopy or

colonoscopy. Other imaging studies, including ultrasonograms, CT scan, or magnetic resonance imaging (MRI), are useful only in selected patients and are not considered helpful as part of the preoperative workup of most patients.

EVALUATION AND PREOPERATIVE MANAGEMENT OF COMMON MEDICAL PROBLEMS
Cardiovascular Diseases

In the past, gynecologic surgeons were relatively free from concerns about cardiovascular disease in their patients undergoing surgery. Over the past 20 years, however, there has been a large increase in the postmenopausal population and in gynecologic surgery patients who have a cardiovascular risk similar to their male counterparts. Despite these factors, the incidence of perioperative cardiovascular complications has decreased markedly owing to improvements in preoperative detection of high-risk patients, preoperative preparation, and surgical and anesthetic techniques.

Preoperative Evaluation. The goal of a preoperative cardiac evaluation is to determine the presence of heart disease and its severity, as well as the potential risk to the patient in the perioperative period. Patients without known symptomatic cardiac atherosclerotic disease, significant dysrhythmias, valvular disease, or congestive heart failure (CHF) are at very low risk of perioperative myocardial infarction or cardiac disease. Every patient should be carefully questioned about symptoms of cardiac disease such as chest pain, dyspnea on exertion, peripheral edema, wheezing, syncope, claudication, or palpitations. Patients with a prior history of cardiac disease should be closely evaluated for worsening of symptoms, which indicates progressive or poorly controlled disease. Old records are indispensable, and every effort should be made to obtain them, particularly if the patient has received treatment at other institutions. Prescriptions for antihypertensive, anticoagulant, antiarrhythmic, antilipid, or antianginal medications may be the only hint of cardiovascular problems. In patients without known heart disease, the presence of diabetes, hyperlipidemia, hypertension, tobacco use, or a strong family history of heart disease identifies a group of patients at higher risk for heart disease who should be more carefully screened.

Physical examination findings such as hypertension, jugular venous distension, laterally displaced point of maximal impulse, irregular pulse, third heart sound, pulmonary rales, heart murmurs, peripheral edema, or vascular bruits should prompt a more complete evaluation. Laboratory evaluation of patients with known or suspected heart disease should include a blood count and serum chemistries. Anemia is poorly tolerated by patients with heart disease, and serum sodium and potassium levels are particularly important in patients taking diuretics and digitalis. Blood urea nitrogen and creatinine values provide information on renal function and hydration status. A chest x-ray study and electrocardiogram are mandatory in the preoperative evaluation and may be particularly helpful when compared with previous studies.

Coronary Artery Disease. Coronary artery disease (CAD) is the primary risk for patients who have cardiac disease and are undergoing gynecologic surgery. The incidence of myocardial infarction following surgery in an adult population is approximately 0.15%.[49] However, in patients who have a prior myocardial infarction, most studies report a reinfarction rate of about 5%.[49,102,108] The risk of reinfarction is inversely proportional to the length of time between infarction and surgery.[102] At 3 months or less, the risk of reinfarction is approximately 30%; from 3 to 6 months, the rate falls to 12%. Six months after myocardial infarction the risk of death due to a perioperative infarction is similar to that in patients with no prior history of ischemic heart disease. Fortunately, it has been demonstrated that careful perioperative management can lower the reinfarction rate even in patients with recent infarctions.[92] This is important because perioperative myocardial infarction is associated with a 50% mortality rate.[108]

Because of the high mortality and morbidity associated with perioperative myocardial infarction, much effort has been made to predict perioperative cardiac risk. Goldman[49] prospectively evaluated preoperative cardiac risk factors and, using a multivariate analysis, identified independent cardiac risk factors (Table 5-1). Using these factors, Goldman created a cardiac risk index that places a patient into one of four risk classes (Table 5-2).

The American College of Cardiology/American Heart Association Task Force guidelines for perioperative cardiovascular evaluation underscore the importance of clinical predictors in preoperative assessment. A stepwise approach divides patients into three groups based on major, intermediate, and minor clinical predictors (Table 5-3). Patients

with major clinical predictors are at high risk of adverse events and require intensive evaluation. Patients with intermediate or minor clinical predictors are further evaluated on the basis of their functional status.

If, after initial clinical evaluation, a patient is thought to be at high risk for coronary artery disease and postoperative myocardial infarction, cardiology consultation should be obtained. Further evaluation can include exercise stress testing, dipyridamole-thallium cardiac perfusion scan, resting gated blood pool study (MUGA), or even cardiac catheterization.

In summary, it is rare for patients younger than age 50 who do not have diabetes, hypertension, hypercholesterolemia, or coronary artery disease to suffer a perioperative myocardial infarction. Conversely, patients with CAD are at increased risk of myocardial infarction in the postoperative period. Careful preoperative evaluation is critically important because myocardial infarctions that occur in the postoperative period are more highly lethal than those that are not associated with surgery, with mortality rates of approximately 50%.

Congestive Heart Failure. Patients with CHF face a substantially increased risk of myocardial infarction during surgery. The postoperative development of pulmonary edema is a grave prognostic sign and results in death in a high percentage of patients. Because patients with heart failure at the time of surgery are significantly more likely to develop pulmonary edema perioperatively, every effort should be made to diagnose and treat CHF before operating. The signs and symptoms of CHF should be sought during the preoperative history and physical examination. Patients able to perform usual daily activities without developing CHF are at limited risk of perioperative heart failure.

To prevent severe postoperative complications, CHF must be corrected preoperatively. Treatment usually involves aggressive diuretic therapy, although care must be taken to prevent dehydration, which may result in hypotension during the induction of anesthesia. Hypokalemia can result from diuretic therapy and is especially deleterious to patients who are also taking digitalis. In addition to diuretics and digitalis, treatment often includes the use of preload

Table 5-1 Risk Factors Associated with Perioperative Myocardial Infarction

Independent Risk Factors	Points*
Jugular venous distension or S_3 gallop immediately preoperatively	11
Myocardial infarction preceding 6 months	10
Presence of premature atrial contractions on preoperative electrocardiogram or any rhythm other than sinus	7
More than five premature ventricular contractions per minute preoperatively	7
Evidence of significant aortic valvular stenosis	3
Age >70	5
Emergency operation	4
Intraperitoneal operation	3
Poor general medical condition	3
PO_2 <60 or PCO_2 >50 mm Hg	
K <3.0 or HCO_3 <20 mEq/L	
Blood urea nitrogen >50 or creatinine >3.0 mg/dl	
Liver disease or debilitated patient	

*Points are assigned to clinical variables and can be totaled to identify risk of postoperative cardiac complications or death (see Table 5-2).

Table 5-2 Risk Class and Occurrence of Perioperative Cardiac Complications

Class	Score*	Total Number of Patients	Patients with Life-Threatening Complications† or Death
I	0-5	537	5 (1%)
II	6-12	316	21 (7%)
III	13-25	130	18 (14%)
IV	≥26	18	14 (78%)

Modified from Goldman L, Caldera DL, Southwick FS, et al: *Medicine* 57:357, 1978.

*Scores derived from factors listed in Table 5-1.

†Life-threatening complications are documented intraoperative or postoperative myocardial infarction, pulmonary edema, or ventricular tachycardia without progression to cardiac death.

Table 5-3 Clinical Predictors of Risk of Perioperative Cardiac Events

Major Clinical Predictors	Intermediate Clinical Predictors	Minor Clinical Predictors
Unstable coronary syndromes	Mild angina pectoris	Advanced age
Decompensated CHF	Prior MI	Abnormal ECG
Significant arrhythmias	Compensated or prior CHF	Rhythm other than sinus
Severe valvular disease	Diabetes mellitus	Low functional capacity
		History of stroke
		Uncontrolled systemic hypertension

CHF, Congestive heart failure; *MI,* myocardial infarction; *ECG,* electrocardiogram.

and afterload reducers. Optimal use of these drugs and correction of CHF may be aided by the consultation of a cardiologist. In general it is preferable for patients to continue following their usual regimen of cardioactive drugs through the perioperative period. In patients with severe or intractable CHF, the perioperative measurement of left ventricular filling (wedge) pressure with a pulmonary artery catheter (Swan-Ganz) may be extremely helpful to guide perioperative fluid management.

Arrhythmias. Nearly all arrhythmias found in otherwise healthy patients are asymptomatic and of limited consequence. However, in patients with underlying cardiac disease, even brief episodes of arrhythmias can cause significant cardiac morbidity and mortality. Preoperative evaluation of arrhythmias by a cardiologist and anesthesiologist is important because surgical stress and many anesthetic agents contribute to the development or worsening of arrhythmias. In patients undergoing continuous cardiographic monitoring during surgery, Kuner et al.[68] reported a 60% incidence of arrhythmias excluding sinus tachycardia. Despite some disagreement, most authors feel that patients with heart disease have an increased risk of arrhythmias, which are commonly ventricular. Conversely, supraventricular arrhythmias are more likely to develop during surgery in patients without cardiac disease. Those patients taking antiarrhythmic medications before surgery should continue taking those drugs during the perioperative period. Initiation of antiarrhythmic medications is rarely indicated preoperatively, but patients in whom arrhythmias are detected before surgery should receive cardiology consultation.

Patients with first degree atrioventricular (AV) block or asymptomatic Mobitz I (Wenckebach) second degree AV block require no preoperative therapy. Conversely, those with symptomatic Mobitz II second degree AV block or third degree AV block should have a permanent pacemaker implanted before undergoing elective surgery. In emergency situations, a pacing pulmonary artery catheter can be used. Before surgery is performed on patients with a permanent pacemaker, the type and location of the pacemaker are important to know because electrocautery units can interfere with demand-type pacemakers. It is preferable to place the electrocautery unit ground plate on the leg to minimize interference when performing gynecologic surgery on patients with pacemakers. In patients with a demand pacemaker in place, the pacemaker should be converted to the fixed-rate mode preoperatively.

Surgery is not contraindicated in patients with bundle branch blocks or hemiblocks. Rarely does complete heart block develop during noncardiac surgical procedures in patients with conduction system disease. However, the presence of left bundle branch block may indicate the presence of aortic stenosis, which can increase surgical mortality if severe.

Valvular Heart Disease. Although there are many forms of valvular heart disease, two types—aortic and mitral stenosis—are primarily associated with significantly increased operative risk. Patients with significant aortic stenosis appear to be at greatest risk, which is further increased if atrial fibrillation, congestive heart failure, or coronary artery disease is also present. In general, patients with significant stenosis of aortic or mitral valves should have them repaired before undergoing elective gynecologic surgery.

Severe valvular heart disease is usually evident during physical examination. Common findings in such patients are listed in the box on p. 97 (top). The classic history presented by patients with severe aortic stenosis includes exercise dyspnea, angina, and syncope, whereas those of mitral stenosis are paroxysmal and effort dyspnea, hemoptysis, and orthopnea. Most patients have a remote history of rheumatic fever. Severe stenosis of either valve is considered when a valvular area is less than 1 cm^2 and diagnosis can be confirmed by echocardiography or cardiac catheterization.

Patients with any valvular abnormality should immediately receive prophylactic antibiotics preoperatively to prevent subacute bacterial endocarditis. The box on p. 97 (bottom) outlines the American Heart Association recommendations for antibiotic valvular prophylaxis. Patients with aortic and mitral stenosis do not easily tolerate sinus tachycardias and other tachyarrhythmias. In patients with aortic stenosis it is important to provide sufficient digitalization to correct preoperative tachyarrhythmias while using propranolol to control sinus tachycardia. Patients with mitral valve stenosis often have atrial fibrillation, and, if present, digitalis should be used to reduce rapid ventricular response.

Patients with mechanical heart valves usually tolerate surgery well. Management of these patients requires antibiotic prophylaxis (see the box on p. 97) and discontinuation of anticoagulant therapy during the perioperative period. Usually, warfarin (Coumadin) is withheld several days before surgery, and anticoagulation is obtained by intravenous

---

SIGNS AND SYMPTOMS OF VALVULAR
HEART DISEASE

AORTIC STENOSIS
Systolic murmur at right sternal border that radiates into
    carotids
Decreased systolic blood pressure
Apical heave
Chest x-ray film with calcified aortic ring, left ventricular
    enlargement
Electrocardiogram with high R waves, depressed T waves
    in lead I, and precordial leads

MITRAL STENOSIS
Precordial heave
Diastolic murmur at apex
Mitral opening snap
Suffused face and lips
Chest x-ray film with left atrial dilation
Electrocardiogram with large P waves and right axis de-
    viation

AMERICAN HEART ASSOCIATION
RECOMMENDATIONS FOR PROPHYLAXIS
OF BACTERIAL ENDOCARDITIS

STANDARD REGIMEN
Ampicillin, 2 g, and gentamicin, 1.5 mg/kg IM or IV 30
    minutes to 1 hour before and 8 hours after

PENICILLIN-ALLERGIC PATIENTS
Vancomycin, 1 g IV slowly over 1 hour, and gentamicin,
    1.5 mg/kg IM or IV 1 hour before; may be repeated
    once in 12 hours if risk of bacteremia is prolonged.

**ORAL REGIMEN FOR MINOR PROCEDURES
IN LOW-RISK PATIENTS**
Amoxicillin, 3 g PO 1 hour before and 1.5 g 6 hours
    later.

---

heparinization. Heparin is discontinued 6 to 8 hours before surgery and resumed a few days postoperatively. Ultimately the patient resumes oral Coumadin maintenance therapy. Alternatively, some authors recommend stopping the warfarin 1 to 3 days preoperatively and restarting it several days postoperatively. Both methods of management did not result in any thromboembolic complications and had similar bleeding complication rates of approximately 15%.

Hypertension. Patients with a history of mild to moderate hypertension alone are apparently at no greater perioperative risk of cardiac morbidity or mortality. However, patients with hypertension and heart disease have a 13% perioperative mortality rate. Therefore the preoperative evaluation of patients with hypertension should emphasize diagnosis of target organ damage. Laboratory studies should include an ECG, chest x-ray, blood count, urinalysis, serum electrolytes, and creatinine. Patients with evidence of coexistent heart disease should undergo cardiac evaluation.

Patients with diastolic pressures greater than 110 mm Hg or systolic pressures greater than 180 mm Hg should have their hypertension controlled before surgery. During surgery, patients with chronic hypertension tend to have increased fluctuations in blood pressure. Chronically hypertensive patients are very susceptible to intraoperative hypotension because of an impaired autoregulation of blood flow to the brain and therefore require a higher mean arterial pressure to maintain adequate perfusion. Additionally, hypertensive patients who also have sweating, palpitations, and headaches should be evaluated for a coexisting pheochromocytoma, as this disease is associated with greatly increased perioperative mortality.

Diabetes Mellitus

Diabetes affects approximately 6% to 7% of all women between ages 20 and 65 and 15% of women between ages 65 and 74.[61] Diabetes can cause problems that affect the cardiovascular, renal, nervous, immune, and gastrointestinal systems. If serum glucose is not controlled at the time of surgery, a twofold increase in morbidity and a threefold increase in postoperative mortality can occur.

Cardiovascular disease in diabetic patients accounts for more than 50% of all deaths.[91] Women with non–insulin dependent diabetes are four times more likely to suffer from myocardial infarction than similar age-adjusted controls and can develop cardiomyopathy or congestive heart failure in absence of coronary artery disease. Therefore the preoperative evaluation should include an investigation of the diabetic's cardiovascular history, especially for symptoms of congestive heart failure. The physical examination must evaluate end organ (cardiac, renal, and ocular) damage to assess the patient's risk for surgical complications and to prevent problems.

Approximately 50% of long-standing diabetics will have nephropathy and 70% will be hypertensive.[91] Strict attention to fluid and electrolytes is necessary in these patients. Diabetics also have an increased risk of acute renal failure after receiving IV iodine contrast, especially if their serum creatinine is ≥2.0 mg/dl, other vascular disease is present, or the onset of diabetes is before age 40.

Complications of diabetes also include defects in the autonomic nervous system, which innervates the esophagus, stomach, and small intestine and can result in decreased esophageal and intestinal motility and delayed gastric emptying. These problems increase the risk of aspiration pneumonitis. Autonomic neuropathy also causes labile changes in pulse and blood pressure, and because of this these patients are known to be at increased risk for intraoperative myocardial infarction.[87]

Diabetes also predisposes postoperative patients to infection. There is a known predisposition to gram-negative and staphylococcal pneumonia and an increased incidence of gram-negative and group B streptococcal sepsis.[111] Diabetics have a sevenfold increase in postoperative gram-negative sepsis compared with the normal population. *Escherichia coli* from the urinary tract most often causes sepsis. On a cellular level, diabetic patients have defects in the ability to mobilize inflammatory cells, phagocytosis function, and bactericidal activity in polymorphonuclear neutrophils. These defects are related to poor glucose control.[93] Decreased amounts of collagen formation, fibroblast growth, and capillary growth also account for the increased incidence of wound dehiscence.[73] Patients with diabetes have approximately a 10% incidence of wound infection compared with 1.8% in those without diabetes.[35]

To complicate management further, surgically related stress is known to increase serum glucose levels and to stimulate increases in insulin antagonists: glucagon, growth hormone, cortisol, norepinephrine, and epinephrine.[48]

Preoperative management of insulin is directed at excellent disease control. Controlled patients should exhibit no glucosuria, infrequent ketoacidosis, and a hemoglobin A_{1c} of 6% or better. Goals include avoiding ketosis, hyperglycemia, and hypoglycemia. Failure to achieve these goals places these patients at risk for fluid and electrolyte disturbances, decreased immune function, osmotic diuresis, and ketoacidosis. The management in the perioperative period is based on whether the patient's disease is controlled by diet, managed with an oral hypoglycemic, or controlled with insulin. If the disease is diet controlled, then this should be continued in the perioperative setting. Approximately 50% of the calories should come from carbohydrates, 35% from fat, and 25% from protein.

Patients taking oral hypoglycemic agents should discontinue their medication the day of surgery and may tolerate a minor operation without insulin. Oral chlorpropamide-like agents need to be stopped the day before surgery because of their long half-life. These patients usually require insulin in the perioperative setting. Insulin does not need to be given unless the serum glucose is above 250 mg/dl. Clearly the most important concept to remember is that patients who have never had insulin administered are usually very sensitive to it, and great care must be taken to prevent significant hypoglycemia. If these patients have major surgery, they most often require a continuous infusion of insulin in 5% dextrose with 0.1 unit of regular insulin/kg/L.

For insulin dependent patients, some authors feel the traditional regimen of giving one third to one half of the patient's total daily requirement of insulin as intermediate-acting insulin (e.g., NPH) the morning of surgery is inadequate.[109] An alternative is to admit the patient 2 days before surgery and begin an insulin drip at 1 to 3 units/hr. Initially, glucose levels are monitored every 1 to 2 hours. After stabilization in the 100 to 200 mg/dl range, glucose monitoring every 4 hours is adequate.

Pulmonary Disease

General Considerations. Patients undergoing abdominal surgery manifest several pulmonary physiologic changes secondary to immobilization, anesthetic irritation of the airways, and the splinting of breathing that inevitably occurs secondary to incisional pain. Pulmonary physiologic changes include a decrease in the functional residual capacity (FRC) and vital capacity (VC), an increase in ventilation perfusion mismatching, and impaired mucociliary clearance of secretions from the tracheobronchial tree. These changes result in transient hypoxemia and atelectasis, which, if untreated, can progress to pneumonia in the postoperative period.[60,76] Postoperative pulmonary dysfunction is more pronounced in patients with advanced age, preexisting lung disease, obesity, a significant smoking history, and upper abdominal surgery.[76]

The majority of postoperative pulmonary complications occur in patients with preexisting pulmonary disease. In these patients, the incidence of pulmonary complications is greater than 70% compared to the low incidence (2% to 5%) in individuals with healthy lungs. The risk of postoperative pulmonary complications is lower in patients who undergo lower abdominal compared to upper abdominal surgery, and nonthoracic, nonabdominal surgery compared to abdominal operations. The presence of chronic obstructive pulmonary disease (COPD) markedly increases the risk for all patients.[76]

Young, healthy patients rarely have abnormal chest x-rays. Therefore chest x-rays should not be obtained routinely in these patients. Most patients with abnormal chest radiographs have history or physical examination findings suggestive of pulmonary disease.[69,72] Chest x-rays should be limited to patients who are over age 40, have a history of smoking or pulmonary disease, and have evidence of cardiopulmonary disease.

In patients at high risk for pulmonary complications, spirometry should be performed with and without bronchodilators to identify patients who may benefit from preoperative treatment with inhaled beta$_2$ agonists and steroids. These include those patients with a history of chronic cough or dyspnea, evidence of pulmonary abnormalities by either physical examination or chest x-ray, a known history of COPD, as well as those patients with a significant smoking history. An arterial blood gas should also be measured.

Chronic Obstructive Pulmonary Disease. Chronic obstructive pulmonary disease is the fourth leading cause of death in North America.[99] Early diagnosis can be difficult because symptoms are usually minimal to absent until late in the course of the disease. Spirometry remains the easiest and most reliable method for detecting changes consistent with COPD, which is heralded by an accelerated deterioration in the forced expiratory volume in one second (FEV$_1$) as compared to baseline.

In contrast to asthma, COPD is characterized by progressive and incompletely irreversible airflow obstruction. Cholinergic agents such as the inhaled quartinary anticholinergic drugs (ipratropium bromide) offer greater bronchodilation than that seen with beta$_2$ agonists. In addition, less than 10% of patients will benefit from steroid therapy in contrast to the majority of patients with asthma who will benefit from the antiinflammatory effects of steroidal therapy. Cessation of smoking decreases the accelerated rate of lung deterioration in patients with COPD. Other preventive measures include the use of pneumococcal and influenza vaccines and the initiation of bronchodilator therapy.

The term *COPD* has been used to encompass both chronic bronchitis and emphysema disease entities that often occur in tandem.[40] Chronic bronchitis has been defined as the presence of productive cough on most days for at least 3 months per year and for at least 2 successive years. It is characterized by chronic airway inflammation and by excessive mucus production. The histologic changes of emphysema include destruction of the alveolar septa and distention of air spaces distal to terminal alveoli. The destruction of alveolar septa is most likely caused by serine elastase, released by neutrophils exposed to cigarette smoke.[40] The destruction of alveoli results in air trapping, loss of pulmonary elastic recoil, collapse of the airways in expiration, increased work of breathing, significant ventilation-perfusion mismatching, and, most important, ineffective cough.[13] The impaired ability for effective cough and clearance of secretions predisposes patients with COPD to atelectasis and pneumonia in the postoperative period.

Pulmonary function testing can be used to quantify the severity of obstructive disease.[76] Patients with COPD typically demonstrate impaired expiratory flow, manifested by diminished FEV_1, FVC, FEV_1/FVC, and MEFR (maximal expiratory flow rate). Arterial blood gases should be obtained preoperatively and may show varying degrees of hypoxemia or hypercapnia. PaO_2 less than 70 mm Hg and a $PaCO_2$ greater than 45 mm Hg is associated with a marked increase in the risk of postoperative pulmonary complications and an increased risk of requirement for postoperative mechanical ventilation.[74]

In gynecologic surgical patients, the risk of postoperative pulmonary complications is confined mainly to those patients with a heavy smoking history and those with COPD. In these patients, prophylactic pulmonary measures should be instituted preoperatively and continued postoperatively to minimize the incidence of atelectasis and pneumonia. Several studies have suggested that preoperative pulmonary preparation of patients with preexisting lung disease can significantly decrease the incidence of postoperative pulmonary complications. Finally, the timing of administration of perioperative prophylactic pulmonary measures is important in that measures instituted preoperatively and continued postoperatively are more effective in reducing the incidence of postoperative pulmonary complications than measures instituted solely in the postoperative period.[19]

The authors' approach to the preoperative preparation of the patient at high risk for postoperative pulmonary complications includes cessation of smoking for as long as possible. Two days of smoking abstinence is sufficient for returning carboxyhemoglobin levels to normal.[4] However, 2 months of smoking abstinence is necessary to significantly lower the risk of postoperative pulmonary complications.[110] Therefore patients undergoing elective surgery should optimally attempt cessation of smoking for as long as possible. Pulmonary function should be optimized with the use of inhaler therapy preoperatively. The anticholinergic inhaled agents should form the mainstay of therapy for patients with COPD. Inhaled $beta_2$-adrenergic agonists can also provide additive effects. These agents should be started at least 72 hours preoperatively, particularly in those patients who have demonstrated clinical or spirometric improvement with bronchodilators. Approximately 10% of patients with COPD benefit from steroid therapy, and these patients can be identified with a steroid challenge (prednisone or its equivalent, 0.5 mg/kg for 2 or 3 weeks).[20] In patients with a suppurative cough and positive sputum culture, a full course of antibiotic therapy can be instituted preoperatively whenever possible. The antibiotics used should cover the most likely etiologic organisms, *Streptococcus pneumoniae* and *Haemophilus influenzae*. Surgery should be delayed if possible in patients with acute upper respiratory tract infections. Finally, instruction in deep breathing, maneuvers, and chest physical therapy are simple to institute and can be started the evening before surgery.[60]

Asthma. Approximately 5% of the U.S. population suffers from asthma.[13] The disease is a chronic inflammatory condition of the airways and is associated with hyperresponsiveness of the tracheobronchial tree and variable, reversible obstruction airways. Multiple triggers are known to precipitate or exacerbate asthma, including inflammatory factors (upper respiratory tract infections, allergens, and chemical sensitizers), and bronchospastic factors, which include exercise, cold air, emotional stress, beta airway adrenergic blockers, and aspirin.[31] The management of asthma requires antiinflammatory therapy for all but those patients with the mildest asthma to address the inflammatory component of the disease and remove inciting stimuli in individuals in whom triggers can be identified. Despite the advances in the pharmacotherapeutic management of asthma over the past 10 years, morbidity and mortality from asthma have been increasing.[47,71]

The preoperative workup of asthmatic patients should direct particular attention to the pulmonary examination, chest x-ray film, arterial blood gas values, and pulmonary function testing. Pulmonary function testing should be performed with and without inhaled bronchodilators. This workup is necessary to assess the current state of the airways and to reveal the presence of any underlying obstructive pulmonary disease. Although pulmonary function testing may be normal in patients who truly have mild asthma, patients with moderate to severe asthma may exhibit peak expiratory flow rates that are 60% to 80% of normal or lower.[71]

The pathophysiology of asthma involves a chronic inflammatory reaction in the airways that is caused by various mediators released in the lungs by eosinophiles or macrophages. These induce microvascular leakage, bronchoconstriction, and epithelial damage, which blocks the distal airways. Mast cell degranulation is not involved in this inflammatory component but with the bronchoconstriction associated with the early response to allergen. Histologic examination of the airways reveals epithelial cell injury, mucosal edema, smooth muscle hypertrophy, and hyperplasia of submucosal mucus glands.

In the past, bronchodilator therapy was the mainstay in first-line pharmacotherapy for asthma. However, the growing appreciation of asthma as a chronic inflammatory disease has led to the use of antiinflammatory therapy as the mainstay of treatment. Current guidelines for asthma management recommend that antiinflammatory treatment be initiated for all patients except those with the mildest forms of asthma. The primary component of antiinflammatory therapy is inhaled corticosteroids, and for moderate to severe asthmatics, these agents are to be used chronically. Corticosteroids inhibit mediator release from eosinophiles and macrophages, inhibit the late response to allergens, and reduce hyperresponsiveness of bronchioles.[9] Adequate control can be achieved with low-dose, inhaled steroids (less than 500 g/day) in most asthmatic patients. Up to 2 mg/day can be inhaled without clinically significant adrenal suppression or significant adverse systemic effects. The onset of action is slow (several hours), and up to 3 months of steroid therapy may be necessary to improve bronchial hyperresponsiveness. For patients with acute exacerbations of asthma, a short course of oral steroids (prednisone 40 to 60 mg/day) may be necessary. Patients with chronic asthma rarely require chronic oral steroid therapy. Those patients who are taking oral steroids should receive a steroid preparation perioperatively for stress coverage.

Until recently, β_2-adrenergic agonists were considered the first-line drugs for asthma. These drugs, inhaled four to six times daily, rapidly relax smooth muscle in the airways and are effective for up to 6 hours. Studies of β_2 agonists in chronic asthma, however, have failed to show any influence on the inflammatory component of asthma. Furthermore, some have suggested that the long-term use of this class of drugs can lead to a worsening of asthma. Thus β_2 agonists are now recommended for short-term relief of bronchospasm or as first-line treatment for patients with very infrequent symptoms or symptoms provoked solely by exercise.

Methylxanthines, such as theophylline, have been relegated to third-line status in asthma management. It is questionable whether these drugs provide any benefit in patients who are on maximal inhaler therapy. The xanthines are limited by their narrow therapeutic window. It is necessary to achieve a serum concentration of at least 10 g/ml, but significant toxicity, including nausea, tremor, and central nervous system excitation, develops at levels greater than 20 g/ml. Xanthines have a limited antiinflammatory effect and have no effect on bronchial hyperresponsiveness or eosinophilic degranulation. It also is important to note that drugs or environmental factors can alter plasma concentrations, thus requiring an adjustment in the theophylline dose. Smoking and phenobarbital, for example, increase clearance of theophylline by the liver, whereas clearance of theophylline is decreased with hepatic disease, cardiac failure, or with the concomitant use of certain drugs, including ciprofloxacin, cimetidine, erythromycin, and troleandomycin.

Cromolyn sodium is highly active in the treatment of seasonal allergic asthma in children and young adults. It usually is not as effective in older patients or in patients in whom asthma is not allergic in character. The drug is taken by inhalation but has a relatively short duration of action (3 to 4 hours). It has a mild antiinflammatory effect but is less effective than inhaled corticosteroids; its role as a single agent is limited.

In asthmatics, elective surgery should be postponed whenever possible until pulmonary function and pharmacotherapeutic management are optimized. For the mild asthmatic, this may simply require the use of inhaled β-adrenergic agonists preoperatively. For the chronic asthmatic, optimization of steroid therapy greatly decreases alveolar inflammation and bronchiolar hyperresponsiveness. Each drug prescribed should be used in maximal dosage before adding another agent. For patients undergoing emergent surgery who have significant bronchoconstriction, a multimodal approach should be instituted, including aggressive bronchodilator inhalation therapy, intravenous methylxanthines, and steroid therapy. Ideally, the steroid therapy can be instituted 3 to 6 days preoperatively. In all asthmatics, pharmacotherapeutic response can be monitored with pulmonary function testing as demonstrated by an improvement in the peak expiratory flow rate.

Anemia

The presence of moderate anemia in itself should not be a contraindication to surgery because it can be readily rectified by transfusion. However, if possible, surgery should be postponed until the cause of the anemia can be identified and the anemia corrected without resorting to the potential risks and expense of blood transfusion. Current anesthetic and surgical practice usually mandates a hemoglobin of 10 g/dl or more or a hematocrit 30% or more volume. Rather than strictly adhering to these levels, it is important to individualize application of these parameters for several reasons. First, more precisely, it is the circulating blood volume that provides oxygen-carrying capacity and tissue oxygenation. Although hemoglobin or hematocrit values may accurately reflect this capacity in most individuals, these values are not always completely accurate. If there has been a recent blood loss, as in severe anovulatory bleeding or a ruptured ectopic pregnancy, the hematocrit can remain normal while blood volume is very low (until the lost volume is replaced with extracellular fluid, which then results in a drop in hematocrit). Conversely, overly hydrated patients can exhibit low hematocrits or hemoglobins but can have a normal red cell mass.

Second, the patient's general physical condition determines her ability to tolerate anemia. The effects of anemia depend on the oxygen requirement of the patient, the rate at which the red cell mass decreases, the magnitude of the anemia, and the ability of compensatory physiologic mechanisms. To maintain the same cardiac output, a patient with a hemoglobin of 10 g/dl requires twice as much coronary blood flow as a patient with a hemoglobin of 14 g/dl. Clearly, a patient with ischemic heart disease will not tolerate anemia as well as a healthy young patient. Therefore the presence of cardiac, pulmonary, or other serious illness justifies a more conservative approach to the management of anemia. Conversely, patients with long-standing anemia can have normal blood volumes and tolerate surgical procedures well. According to the NIH Consensus Group,[82] no evidence has shown that mild to moderate anemia increases perioperative morbidity or mortality.

If large perioperative blood losses are anticipated, patients with normal hematocrit values are generally able to store at least three units of autologous blood preoperatively. Additionally, the use of recombinant human erythropoietin therapy and oral iron and folate can increase the amount of blood an autologous donor may store without developing anemia.[50] Planning for intraoperative red cell recovery and reuse also can be useful in eliminating or reducing the need for homologous transfusions in selected patients.

The Elderly Patient

An ever-increasing number of elderly women are undergoing gynecologic surgery. This is explained by the expanding elderly population and the increasing advances in surgical and anesthetic techniques, which make surgery safer and more available for improving the quality of life for older patients. According to the Bureau of Census, there were 25.2 million women in the United States between age 45 and 65 in 1990. This population is expected to increase to 41.8 million by 2010. Furthermore, it is estimated that half of Americans older than 65 will have an operation.[66,98] In patients over age 80, preoperative medical conditions likely to complicate surgery include the following: (1) more than 50% have hypertension, cardiomegaly, or atherosclerotic heart disease, (2) 80% have ECG abnormalities, (3) over 25% have acute or chronic lung disease, and (4) approximately one third are malnourished, 15% are anemic, and 25% require preoperative blood transfusion. The preoperative assessment of elderly women is often more complex and often benefits from collaboration and consultation with internal medicine and anesthesia colleagues. All the medical problems outlined in this chapter are more likely to occur in elderly gynecologic surgery patients. For this reason, additional care should be given to the preoperative history, physical examination, and laboratory evaluation of elderly women. This should include preoperative chest x-ray, ECG, and metabolic panel to assess renal, hepatic, and nutritional status. Thoughtful preoperative preparation and attention to postoperative care will reduce the incidence of the most common postoperative complications in the elderly, which include respiratory failure, congestive heart failure, thromboembolism, and delirium.

PREPARATION FOR SUCCESSFUL SURGICAL OUTCOME
Nutrition

Women having gynecologic surgery should be in an adequate nutritional state, and an accurate assessment of nutritional status should be made preoperatively. The significance of weight loss and its negative effect on surgical outcome has been recognized for decades. Clinical experience indicates that if nutritional deficits are corrected before surgery, then a quicker recovery, fewer postoperative infections, and more rapid wound healing can occur.[12,107] The preoperative goal is to quantify the malnutrition and provide appropriate preoperative nutritional supplementation.

Energy use varies dramatically with the fasting-feeding cycle and is influenced by every organ system and by hypermetabolic states, such as sepsis, burns, surgery, gastrointestinal disorders, and malignancy. To approximate caloric needs, the patient's height, weight, sex, age, activity level, type of required surgery, and disease state must be considered. Chronic illnesses such as renal, endocrine, and cardiovascular abnormalities can alter nutritional needs.[1] Gastrointestinal problems, including short bowel syndrome, obstruction, fistulas, emesis, gastric suctioning, and diarrhea,[2,67] as well as cancer-related problems including chemotherapy, radiation enteritis, and extensive surgery, also account for increased nutritional requirements.[8,33,101]

Preoperative nutritional assessment is essential. The most important measurement is body weight. When recorded serially as a percentage of the ideal body weight, it is the single most influential reflection of energy and protein reserve; however, extracellular fluid or fluid overload may give a false impression that nutritional stores are unaffected.

Anthropometry is the study of the measurement of size, weight, and proportions of the human body. Triceps skin fold thickness can be used to derive a mid-arm fat area (MAFA), which is the simplest index to measure body fat stores.[17]

The creatinine/height index is the most sensitive indicator of protein-calorie nutrition.[84] The body's total protein reserve is estimated clinically by calculating the approximate muscle mass and visceral protein reserve. Muscle mass can be estimated from a 24-hour urine collection from which a creatinine/height index may be calculated. Visceral protein reserve is estimated by serum albumin and transferrin levels.[17] In general, hypoalbuminemia (2.5 mg/dl or less) coupled with weight loss (10% or more) is associated with significant surgical morbidity and mortality.[6,8]

Some women need additional nutritional support in the perioperative period. The route of administration chosen to deliver the nutritional support must be decided on an individual basis and can include the enteral route, peripheral parenteral nutrition (PPN), or total parenteral nutrition (TPN).

Total parenteral nutrition has gained wide acceptance as a means of providing nutritional support for patients with a variety of medical and surgical problems. The gynecologic literature has focused attention on central hyperalimentation in the setting of advanced gynecologic malignancies or in patients receiving chemotherapy. TPN is given when other routes have not met or cannot meet the patient's nutritional needs. TPN must be delivered through the subclavian or internal jugular vein. This line must be placed following meticulous sterile techniques, and proper daily care must be given to prevent infection. Complications associated with TPN range from metabolic or electrolyte abnormalities, to sepsis, pneumothorax, hemothorax, or air/catheter embolism. In experienced hands, the most frequent, serious problem, catheter infection, has been reduced to around 7%.[58]

The role of TPN in the preoperative setting remains controversial because of its risks, costs, and the difficulty in selecting patients who might benefit from it. A predictive model of nutritional status, designed and validated by Mullen,[77] predicts patients at high risk for operative morbidity or mortality. The prognostic nutritional index (PNI) is calculated using the following formula:

$$PNI = 158 - 16.6 \, [Alb] - 0.78 \, [TSF] - 0.2 \, [TFN] - 5.8 \, [DH]$$

where *Alb* is serum albumin (mg/ml), *TSF* is triceps skin fold thickness (cm), *TFN* is serum transferrin (mg/ml), and *DH* is delayed skin hypersensitivity (scale 0 to 2). Patients with a PNI score greater than 30% are at high risk for postoperative complications.

Four prospective, randomized, controlled studies indicate that the administration of preoperative TPN in selected high-risk patients for 7 to 20 days decreases the frequency of early septic events postoperatively.[42,53,79,100] Improvement in survival was also shown by Mullen.[78] However, because of the small number of patients, changing and improving surgical techniques, better antibiotics, and improvements in specific cancer and critical care treatments, all of the improvement in survival may not be due to preoperative TPN. Similarly, it has been impossible to prove or disprove the cost effectiveness of TPN. Two contemporary trials (Veterans Affairs Cooperative Study Group,[106] and Brennan[15]) critically evaluated the role of perioperative TPN in a prospective, randomized fashion. Both studies found an increase in infectious morbidity in patients who received TPN with no difference in length of hospital stay or mortality. The only group to benefit were those patients who were severely malnourished (less than 5% of the study group); they had fewer noninfectious complications.

In general, it is our opinion that because of the expense and potential complications, perioperative TPN should be given only to severely malnourished patients. Although common sense would suggest that TPN would help many patients, especially those with gynecologic malignancies, the available data would indicate otherwise in the majority of situations.

Fluid and Electrolytes

Pathophysiologic changes that occur in the perioperative period place the surgical patient at risk of developing fluid, electrolyte, and metabolic imbalances that can lead to numerous complications both intraoperatively and postoperatively. It is not unusual for surgical patients to suffer severe preexisting fluid and electrolyte derangements due to inadequate oral intake, nausea and vomiting, and nasogastric suction. In addition, the perioperative period is associated with an increase in circulating levels of catecholamines, ACTH, and aldosterone, which may lead to both metabolic changes and fluid retention. Proper assessment and management of fluid and electrolyte status must begin preoperatively and continue postoperatively. Knowledge of the physiologic changes that occur perioperatively, combined with appropriate correction of deficits, is imperative for minimizing the morbidity and mortality of anesthesia and surgery.

In an average woman, water constitutes approximately 50% to 55% of body weight. Two thirds of this water is contained in the intracellular compartment. One third is in the extracellular compartment, of which one fourth is contained in plasma, and the remaining three quarters is in the interstitium.

Osmolarity, or tonicity, is a property derived from the number of particles in a solution. Sodium and chloride are the primary electrolytes contributing to the osmolarity in the extracellular fluid compartment. Potassium, and to a lesser extent magnesium and phosphate, are the major intracellular electrolytes. Water flows freely between the intracellular and extracellular spaces to maintain osmotic neutrality throughout the body. Any shifts in osmolarity in any fluid spaces within the body will be accompanied by corresponding shifts in free water from spaces of lower to higher osmolarity, thus maintaining a balance in equilibrium.

The daily fluid maintenance requirement for an average adult is approximately 30 ml/kg/day, or 2000 to 3000 ml/day.[88] This is offset partially by insensible losses of 1200 ml/day, which include losses from the lungs (600 ml), skin (400 ml), and gastrointestinal tract (200 ml). Urinary output from the kidney makes up the remainder of the fluid loss, and this output varies depending on total body intake of water and sodium. The kidneys excrete approximately 600 to 800 mOsm of solute/day. Healthy kidneys can concentrate urine up to approximately 1200 mOsm, and therefore minimum output can range between 500 and 700 ml/day. The maximal urinary output capability of the kidney can be as high as 20 L/day, which is common in patients with diabetes insipidus. In a healthy patient, the normal kidney will adjust urine output commensurate with the daily fluid intake. The major extracellular buffer used in acid-base balance is the bicarbonate–carbonic acid system: $CO_2 + H_2O \rightleftharpoons H_2CO_3 \rightleftharpoons H^+ + HCO_3^-$.[75] Typically the body will maintain a bicarbonate/carbonic acid ratio of 20/1 to maintain an extracellular pH of 7.4. Both the lung and kidney play integral roles in maintaining normal extracellular pH through retention or excretion of carbon dioxide and bicarbonate. Under conditions of alkalosis, minute ventilation decreases and renal excretion of bicarbonate increases to restore the normal bicarbonate/carbonic acid ratio. The opposite occurs with acidosis.

Ultimately, the kidney plays the most important role in fluid and electrolyte balance through excretion and retention of water and solute. Circulating antidiuretic hormone (ADH) and aldosterone help modulate the process. Hypothalamic release of ADH is sensitive to serum osmolarity, and aldosterone secretion is responsive to renal perfusion. Under states of dehydration or hypovolemia, serum ADH levels increase, leading to increased resorption of water in the distal tubule of the kidney. In addition, increased aldosterone release promotes increased renal sodium and water retention. The opposite occurs in states of fluid excess. As a result, an individual with normal renal function, as well as normal circulating ADH and aldosterone levels, maintains normal serum osmolarity and electrolyte composition despite daily fluctuation of fluid and electrolyte intake.

Various disease states can alter the normal fluid and electrolyte homeostatic mechanisms, making perioperative fluid and electrolyte management more difficult. Patients with intrinsic renal disease are unable to excrete solute and to maintain acid-base balance. Patients under the stress of chronic starvation or severe illness may have an inappropriately high level of circulating ADH and aldosterone, resulting in fluid and sodium retention. With severe cardiac disease, secondary renal hypoperfusion can lead to increased aldosterone synthesis and therefore increased sodium and water retention by the kidney. Patients with severe diabetes can have a significant osmotic diuresis and have acid-base dysfunction secondary to circulating ketoacids. Correction and optimization of renal, cardiac, or endocrinologic disorders preoperatively are imperative and will often rectify fluid and electrolyte abnormalities.

Fluid and electrolyte management in the perioperative period requires knowledge of the daily fluid and electrolyte requirements for maintenance, replacement of ongoing fluid and electrolyte losses, and correction of any existing abnormalities. Each of these is considered separately.

Fluid and Electrolyte Maintenance Requirements.
Normal daily fluid requirements in an average adult are 2000 to 3000 ml. The body can and does adjust to higher and lower volumes of intake through changes in plasma tonicity. Alterations in plasma tonicity induce adjustments in circulating ADH, which ultimately regulates the amount of water retained in the distal tubule of the kidney. The daily requirement for various electrolytes is shown in Table 5-4. In the preoperative and the early postoperative patient, it usually is necessary to replace only sodium and potassium. Chloride is automatically replaced because it is the usual anion used to balance sodium (NaCl) and potassium (KCl) in electrolyte solutions. Various commercially available solutions contain 40 mmol of sodium chloride, with smaller amounts of potassium, calcium, and magnesium, designed to meet the requirements of a patient receiving 3 L of IV fluids per day. The daily requirement, however, can be met by any combination of IV fluid orders. For example, 2 L of D5.45 normal saline (77 mEq sodium chloride each), supplemented with 20 mEq of potassium chloride, followed by 1 L of D_5W with 20 mEq of potassium chloride would suffice.

Correction of Existing Fluid and Electrolyte Abnormalities. Patients with preoperative fluid or electrolyte abnormalities can pose a diagnostic challenge. The correct diagnosis and therapy are contingent on a correct assessment of total body fluid and electrolyte status. The management of hyponatremia, for example, can be either fluid restriction or fluid replacement, depending on whether there is an over-

Table 5-4 Daily Maintenance Parenteral Requirements

Electrolyte	Requirements
Sodium	100-140 mEq
Potassium	40-60 mEq
Magnesium	30 mEq
Calcium	15 mEq
Carbohydrate	100-150 g
Water	1500 ml/m^2 body surface area

Modified from Magrina JF: *Clin Obstet Gynecol* 31:686, 1988.

all extracellular fluid excess and normal body sodium stores or decreased overall total body sodium stores and extracellular fluid. A detailed history is necessary for documentation of any underlying medical illness and for assessment of the amount and duration of any abnormal fluid losses or intake. Initial evaluation should include an assessment of hemodynamic, clinical, and urinary parameters to determine the overall level of hydration systemically, as well as the fluid status of the extracellular fluid compartment. A well-hydrated patient has good skin turgor, moist mucosa, stable vital signs, and good urinary output. Nonpitting edema is indicative of extracellular fluid excess, whereas a patient who has orthostasis, sunken eyes, parched mouth, and decreased skin turgor clearly has extracellular volume contraction. On a cautionary note, a patient's overall extracellular fluid status does not always reflect the hydration status of the intravascular compartment. A patient can have increased interstitial fluid, yet be intravascularly dry, requiring replacement with isotonic fluid.

Laboratory workup for patients who may have preexisting fluid problems should include blood hematocrit, serum chemistries, glucose, BUN and creatinine, urine osmolarity, and urine electrolytes. Serum osmolarity is mainly a function of the concentration of sodium and is given by the following equation:

$$2 \times \frac{NA^+ + glucose\ (mg/dl) + BUN\ (mg/dl)/2.8}{18}$$

Normal serum osmolarity is typically 290 to 300 mOsm. Blood hematocrit can be used to estimate volume deficit according to the following equation:

Plasma deficit (ml) =
$$\frac{Normal\ blood\ volume - Normal\ blood\ volume \times Normal\ Hct}{Measured\ Hct}$$

Normally, blood hematocrit will rise or fall inversely at a rate of approximately 1%/500 ml alteration of extracellular fluid volume. The BUN/creatinine ratio is typically 10/1 but will rise to a ratio greater than 20/1 under conditions of extracellular fluid contraction. Under conditions of extracellular fluid deficit, urine osmolarity will typically be high (greater than 400 mOsm), whereas urine sodium concentration is low (less than 15 mEq/L), which indicates the kidney's attempt to conserve sodium. Under conditions of extracellular fluid excess, or in cases of renal disease in which the kidney is unable to retain sodium and water, urine osmolarity will be low and urine sodium high (greater than 30 mEq/L). Finally, changes in sodium can indicate the degree of extracellular fluid excess or deficit. In an average person, serum sodium rises by 3 mmol/L for every liter of water deficit and falls by 3 mmol/L for each liter of water excess. One must, however, be careful in making these estimates, because the patient with prolonged water and electrolyte loss may have low serum sodium and marked water deficit.

Specific Electrolyte Disorders

Hypokalemia. Hypokalemia is the most frequently encountered electrolyte disturbance in postoperative patients. Hypokalemia is caused by significant gastrointestinal fluid loss (prolonged emesis, diarrhea, nasogastric suction, and intestinal fistulas), marked urinary potassium loss as a result of renal tubular disorders (renal tubular acidosis, acute tubular necrosis, hyperaldosteronism, and, most commonly, prolonged diuretic use), or prolonged administration of potassium-free parenteral fluids in patients who are NPO. The symptoms associated with hypokalemia include neuromuscular disturbances ranging from muscle weakness to flaccid paralysis and cardiovascular abnormalities including hypotension, bradycardia, arrhythmias, and enhancement of digitalis toxicity. These symptoms rarely occur unless serum potassium is below 3 mEq/L. Treatment consists of potassium replacement, with oral therapy preferable in patients following an oral diet. If necessary, potassium replacement can be given intravenously in doses that should not exceed 10 mEq/hr.

Hyperkalemia. Hyperkalemia is infrequently encountered in patients preoperatively. It usually is associated with renal impairment but also can be associated with adrenal insufficiency, with the use of potassium-sparing diuretics, and with marked tissue breakdown (e.g., in patients with crush injuries, massive gastrointestinal bleeds, or hemolysis). The clinical manifestations are mainly cardiovascular. Marked hyperkalemia (potassium greater than 7 mEq/L) can result in bradycardia, ventricular fibrillation, and cardiac arrest. The treatment chosen depends on the severity of the hyperkalemia and whether other associated cardiac or electrocardiogram abnormalities are present. Calcium gluconate (10 ml of a 10% solution) given intravenously can offset the toxic effects of hyperkalemia on the heart. One ampule each of sodium bicarbonate and D50 with or without insulin causes rapid shift of potassium into cells. Longer-term, cation exchange resins such as sodium polystyrene sulfonate (Kayexalate), taken either orally or by enema, bind and decrease total body potassium. Hemodialysis is reserved for critical conditions for which other measures were not sufficient or have failed.

Hyponatremia. Because sodium is the major extracellular cation, shifts in serum sodium usually are inversely correlated with the hydration state of the extracellular fluid compartment. The pathophysiology of hyponatremia, then, is usually expansion of body fluids leading to excess total body water.[75] The symptoms of hyponatremia are related to both the serum sodium level and the rapidity of its fall. Acute hyponatremia usually becomes symptomatic when the serum sodium falls below 120 to 125 mEq/L, whereas in chronic hyponatremia, symptoms may not occur until the serum sodium falls below 110 mEq/L. Symptoms of hyponatremia can include anorexia, nausea, vomiting, lethargy, headaches, weakness, change in mental status, and seizures.

Hyponatremia due to extracellular fluid excess can be seen in patients with renal or cardiac failure, as well as in conditions such as nephrotic syndrome, in which total body salt, and particularly water, are increased. Administration of hypertonic saline to correct the hyponatremia would be inappropriate in this setting. The treatment should include water restriction with diuretic therapy in addition to correcting the underlying disease process.

Inappropriate secretion of ADH can occur with head trauma, pulmonary or cerebral tumors, and under states of stress. The abnormally elevated ADH results in excess water retention. Treatment includes water restriction and, if possible, correction of the underlying cause. Demeclocycline has been shown to be effective in this disorder through its action in the kidney.

Inappropriate replacement of body salt losses with water alone results in hyponatremia. This typically occurs in patients losing large amounts of electrolytes (as a result of vomiting, nasogastric suction, diarrhea, or gastrointestinal fistulas) that are replaced with hypotonic solutions. Simple replacement with isotonic fluids and potassium usually corrects the abnormality. Rarely will rapid correction of the hyponatremia be necessary, in which case hypertonic saline (3%) can be administered. Hypertonic saline should be very cautiously administered to avoid a rapid shift in serum sodium, which induces central nervous system dysfunction. Common causes of preoperative hyponatremia are shown in the box on p. 105 (top left).

Hypernatremia. Hypernatremia is an uncommon condition that can be life-threatening if severe. Symptoms usually do not develop until the serum sodium exceeds 160 mEq/L and the serum osmolarity reaches 320 to 330 mOsm/kg. The pathophysiology is one of severe extracellular fluid deficit. The consequent hyperosmolar state results in decreased water volume in cells in the central nervous system, which, if severe, can result in disorientation, seizures, intracranial bleed, and death. The causes include excessive extrarenal water loss as seen in patients with high fever, tracheostomy in a dry environment, extensive thermal injuries, diabetes insipidus (either central or nephrogenic), and iatrogenic salt loading. The treatment involves correction of the underlying cause (correction of fever, humidification of the tracheostomy, vasopressin [Pitressin] for control of central diabetes insipidus) and replacement with free water either orally or intravenously with D_5W. As with severe hyponatremia, marked hypernatremia should be corrected slowly.

Acid-Base Disorders. A variety of metabolic, respiratory, and electrolyte abnormalities can result in an imbalance in normal acid-base homeostasis, leading to alkalosis

---

PREOPERATIVE CAUSES OF HYPONATREMIA

DECREASED BODY SODIUM
Diuretics
Salt losing nephropathy

EXCESS VOLUME
Oral or intravenous fluid overload

MEDICAL
Congestive heart failure
Renal failure
Cirrhosis
Nephrotic syndrome
Hypothyroidism
Addison's disease

PHARMACOLOGIC
Antidepressants
Phenothiazines

SULFONYLUREAS
Carbamazepine

SYNDROME OF INAPPROPRIATE ADH

BACTERIA INDIGENOUS TO THE LOWER GENITAL TRACT

Lactobacillus	*Enterobacter agglomerans*
Diphtheroids	*Klebsiella pneumoniae*
Staphylococcus aureus	*Proteus mirabilis*
Staphylococcus epidermidis	*Proteus vulgaris*
Streptococcus agalactiae	*Morganella morganii*
α-Hemolytic streptococci	
Group D streptococci	*Bacteroides species*
Peptostreptococcus	*B. bivius*
Peptococcus	*B. disiens*
Clostridium	*B. fragilis*
Gaffkya anaerobic	*B. melaninogenicus*
Escherichia coli	
Fusobacterium	
Enterobacter cloacae	

KEY ELEMENTS FOR ANTIBIOTIC PROPHYLAXIS IN GYNECOLOGIC SURGERY

1. The procedure should carry a significant risk of post-operative infection.
2. The surgery should involve considerable bacterial contamination.
3. The antibiotic chosen for prophylaxis should be effective against most contaminating organisms.
4. The antibiotic should be present in the tissues at the time of contamination.
5. The shortest possible course of antibiotic prophylaxis should be given.
6. The prophylactic antibiotic chosen should not be one considered for treatment should postoperative infection occur.
7. The risk of complications from the prophylactic antibiotic should be low.

---

or acidosis. Because most of these problems occur postoperatively, they are discussed in Chapter 10.

Antibiotic Prophylaxis

Bacteria that contaminate the gynecologic surgical field are indigenous to the lower genital tract, including both gram-positive and gram-negative aerobes and anaerobes (see the box top right). The primary pathogenic bacteria include the coliforms, *Streptococci, Fusobacterium,* and *Bacteroides.* Gynecologic operations that carry a significant risk of post-operative infection include vaginal hysterectomy, abdominal hysterectomy, cases involving pelvic abscess or inflammation, select cases of pregnancy termination, and radical surgery for gynecologic cancers. Most other gynecologic procedures are considered "clean" and have a low risk (5%) of postoperative wound infection.[41] These include procedures confined to the abdomen, space of Retzius, perineum, and vagina. The box on the right outlines the key elements for antibiotic prophylaxis in gynecologic surgery.[70]

The literature uniformly supports the use of prophylactic antibiotics for vaginal hysterectomy, although their use is controversial in patients undergoing abdominal hysterectomy. Hirsch[59] reviewed the placebo-controlled trials in the English and non-English literature regarding antibiotic prophylaxis in vaginal and abdominal hysterectomy. Included in the review were 48 studies involving 5524 patients who underwent vaginal hysterectomy, and 30 studies involving 3752 patients who underwent abdominal hysterectomy. In vaginal hysterectomy, prophylactic antibiotics decreased febrile morbidity from 40% in control patients to 15% in treated patients and lowered the pelvic infection rate from 25% in control patients to 5% in treated patients. The benefits of antibiotic prophylaxis were less pronounced in the abdominal hysterectomy series; febrile morbidity was reduced in 57% of studies, whereas wound infections and pelvic infections were reduced in a minority of the studies. Overall, antibiotic prophylaxis for abdominal hysterectomy reduced febrile morbidity from 28% in control patients to 16% in treated patients, pelvic infections from 10% to 5%, and wound infections from 8% to 3%, respectively. This analysis is further complicated by a lack of series-to-series uniformity regarding criteria for fever or for diagnosis of infection requiring antibiotic therapy. Nonetheless, we believe that antibiotic prophylaxis should be used in all patients who undergo vaginal hysterectomy and in selected high-risk patients who undergo abdominal hysterectomy. Factors that have been identified as placing patients at high risk for post-hysterectomy infection have included low socioeconomic status, duration of surgery greater than 2 hours, presence of malignancy, and increased number of surgical procedures performed. Obesity, menopausal status, and estimated blood loss have not been shown to be risk factors for postoperative infection when evaluated by multivariate analysis.[52,97]

The antibiotic chosen for prophylaxis for gynecologic surgery should have activity against the broad range of vaginal organisms. The first- and second-generation cephalosporins are well suited, given their activity against grampositive, gram-negative, and anaerobic organisms. Most classes of antibiotics, including the penicillins, tetracyclines, sulfonamides, broad-spectrum penicillins and cephalosporins, and anaerobic drugs (clindamycin/metronidazole), have been shown to be effective as prophylactic antibiotics, although none has been demonstrated to be consistently more effective than first-generation cephalosporins.[21,36,80,94,105]

The timing of administration of the prophylactic antibiotic agent is important. Studies dating back to the work by Burke[16] have demonstrated that antibiotics given for prophylaxis against infection are most active if present in tissues before contamination with an inoculum of bacteria. For patients who undergo hysterectomy, the antibiotic should be present in the tissues before the opening of the vaginal cuff, at which time vaginal organisms gain access to the pelvic cavity. Infusion of an antibiotic, on call to the operating room, within 30 minutes of surgery is ideal for this purpose. For long surgical procedures, particularly when blood loss is significant or when an antibiotic agent with short half-life is used, a second antibiotic dose should be given intraoperatively.

Many prospective studies have documented that short courses of prophylactic antibiotics (24 hours or less) are as efficacious as longer ones, and several clinical trials have found that one perioperative dose of prophylactic antibiotic is sufficient.[45,56,57,80,86] One dose of prophylactic antibiotic has many advantages, including decreased cost, decreased toxicity, minimal alteration of host flora, and subsequent selection of resistant pathogens.

Despite the advantages of using prophylactic antibiotics, the importance of good surgical technique must be emphasized. Antibiotics should not be used in lieu of correct surgical principles such as delicate handling of tissues, good hemostasis, adequate drainage, and avoidance of unnecessarily large pedicles of tissue in ligatures.

Gastrointestinal Preparation

Preparation of the lower gastrointestinal tract before elective gynecologic surgery has several goals. In most gynecologic surgery, when the gastrointestinal tract is not entered, mechanical preparation of the bowel reduces gastrointestinal contents, thus allowing more room in the abdomen and pelvis, facilitating the surgical procedure. Further, even if there is a rectosigmoid colon enterotomy during surgery, the mechanical bowel preparation eliminates formed stool and reduces the bacterial contamination, thus reducing infectious complications. Mechanical bowel preparation can be accomplished by several methods (Table 5-5). The traditional use of laxatives and enemas requires at least 12 to 24 hours and generally causes moderate abdominal distention and crampy pain. In addition, nursing supervision of enema administration and the need for IV fluid replacement make this regimen relatively expensive. Randomized trials comparing traditional mechanical bowel preparation with oral gut lavage (PEG-3350 and electrolytes for oral solution, or GoLYTELY) have found that the use of approximately 4 L of GoLYTELY (administered until the rectal effluent is clear) provides faster, more complete, and more comfortable bowel preparation.[10] Furthermore, the fluid loss following gut lavage with GoLYTELY appears to be clinically insignificant. Gut lavage usually can be performed at home the day before scheduled surgery. In rare cases when the patient cannot drink the 4 L, the GoLYTELY can be administered through a small caliber nasogastric tube. We recommend mechanical bowel preparation to all patients undergoing major abdominal, pelvic, or vaginal surgery.

High infection rates after colonic surgery have led to investigation of methods aimed at reducing these significant complications. Although mechanical bowel preparation is essential and part of all colonic surgery preparation regimens, it does not reduce the infection rate satisfactorily. Reduction of the number of pathogenic flora in the colon is the primary strategy for reducing infection after colonic surgery. The colon has the greatest concentration of bacteria, including both aerobes and anaerobes, in the body. Anaerobes outnumber aerobes by 1000 to 1.

After reducing the bacterial load by mechanical preparation, antibiotics should be used to further reduce the bacterial count and to prevent infections following intestinal (especially colonic) surgery. Over the past decade, perioperative IV antibiotics have replaced the oral bowel preparation with neomycin and erythromycin.[46] We routinely prescribe mechanical *and* antibiotic prophylaxis for patients likely undergoing colorectal surgery (pelvic exenteration or ovarian cancer debulking) and for those at high risk for rectal injury (such as severe cases of endometriosis or pelvic inflammatory disease).

Table 5-5 Mechanical Bowel Preparation Regimens to Begin Day Before Gynecologic Surgery

Time	Traditional Mechanical Preparation	GoLYTELY
Midnight	Clear liquid diet	Clear liquid diet
Noon	Magnesium citrate 240 ml by mouth	GoLYTELY, 4 L by mouth over 3 hr
8:00 PM	Saline enemas to clear, 5% dextrose in one half normal saline IV with 20 mg potassium chloride at 125 ml per hour	
Midnight	Nothing by mouth	Nothing by mouth

Thromboembolism Prophylaxis

Risk Factors. Deep venous thrombosis and pulmonary embolism, although largely preventable, are significant postoperative complications. The magnitude of this problem is relevant to the gynecologist, because 40% of all deaths following gynecologic surgery can be directly attributed to pulmonary emboli.[62] Pulmonary embolism is the most frequent cause of postoperative death in patients with uterine[22] or cervical[34] carcinoma.

The causal factors of venous thrombosis were first proposed by Virchow in 1858 and include a hypercoagulable state, venous stasis, and vessel intima injury. When the patient undergoing gynecologic surgery is specifically considered, two prospective studies have evaluated risk factors associated with the postoperative occurrence of deep venous thrombosis. Clayton et al.[30] studied the risk factors of 124 patients undergoing vaginal and abdominal surgery for benign gynecologic disease. Logistic regression analysis identified five factors to be associated with postoperative deep venous thrombosis: age, varicose veins, percentage overweight, euglobulin lysis time, and serum fibrin-related antigen. The risk factors associated with venous thromboembolic complications have also been assessed in 411 patients undergoing major abdominal and pelvic surgery.[28] Preoperative risk factors identified in this study include age, nonwhite patients, increasing stage of malignancy, history of deep venous thrombosis, lower extremity edema or venous stasis changes, varicose veins, weight, and a history of radiation therapy. Intraoperative factors associated with postoperative deep venous thrombosis included increased anesthesia time, increased blood loss, and transfusion requirements in the operating room. Based on these risk factors, patients may be categorized into high-, moderate-, or low-risk categories (Table 5-6). The recognition of these

Table 5-6 Prophylactic Techniques Appropriate for the Obstetric and the Gynecologic Surgery Patient

Risk Category	Prophylactic Techniques
Low	Graduated compression stockings (GCS)
Moderate	Intermittent pneumatic compression (IPC) (24 hours)
Age <40 years and other risk factor(s)	
Age ≥40 years and no other risk factor(s)	
	Low-dose heparin (q12h) (LDH)
	Low-molecular-weight heparin (qd)
	Graduated compression stockings
High	Intermittent pneumatic compression (5 days)
Age >60	
Cancer	Low-dose heparin (q8h)
Very high	Combination of methods (e.g., IPC and GCS or IPC and LDH)
Pelvic exenteration	
	Inferior vena cava interruption
Radical vulvectomy	
Prior history of DVT/PE	

DVT, Deep venous thrombosis; *PE,* pulmonary embolism.

factors, which are associated with postoperative venous thromboembolism, should allow the clinician to stratify patients into low-, medium-, and high-risk groups.

Prophylactic Methods. Over the past 2 decades, a number of prophylactic methods have undergone clinical trials showing significant reduction in the incidence of deep venous thrombosis, and a few studies have been completed that demonstrate a reduction in fatal pulmonary emboli. The ideal prophylactic method would be effective, free of significant side effects, well accepted by the patient and nursing staff, widely applicable to most patient groups, and inexpensive.

Low-Dose Heparin. The use of small doses of subcutaneously administered heparin for the prevention of deep venous thrombosis and pulmonary embolism is the most widely studied of all prophylactic methods. More than 25 controlled trials have demonstrated that heparin given subcutaneously 2 hours preoperatively and every 8 to 12 hours postoperatively is effective in reducing the incidence of deep venous thrombosis. The value of low-dose heparin in preventing fatal pulmonary emboli was established by a randomized, controlled, multicenter international trial that demonstrated a reduction in fatal postoperative pulmonary emboli in general surgery patients receiving low-dose heparin every 8 hours postoperatively.[65]

Trials of low-dose heparin in gynecologic surgery patients are limited, and a clear consensus as to the value of low-dose heparin in all groups of patients has not been established because of differences in patient selection and length of follow-up. Three randomized, controlled gynecologic surgery studies used the same regimen of low-dose heparin administration: 5000 units subcutaneously 2 hours preoperatively and every 12 hours for 7 days postoperatively. The trials reported by Ballard et al.[7] and Taberner et al.[103] were conducted in patients with benign gynecologic conditions (98%). All patients were older than age 40, and follow-up was discontinued at the time of discharge from hospital. An American study[23] evaluated a larger group of patients on a gynecologic oncology unit. Only 16% had benign gynecologic conditions, and follow-up included the first 6 weeks postoperatively.

The trial by Taberner et al.[103] showed a 23% incidence of deep venous thrombosis in the control group compared with a 6% incidence in the low-dose heparin-treated patients. This difference was statistically significant ($p <0.05$). Unfortunately, although this was a randomized trial, the control group contained a larger number of patients with malignancy. When the cancer patients were excluded from the trial analysis, no significant value remained for the use of low-dose heparin in patients with benign conditions. Ballard's[7] study also evaluated a group of patients who had benign gynecologic diseases. The nontreated control group had a 29% incidence of deep venous thrombosis as compared with a 3.6% incidence in the low-dose heparin-treated group ($p <0.001$). In contrast, a randomized trial of patients undergoing major abdominal and pelvic surgery on a gynecologic oncology service showed no difference in the incidence of thromboembolic complications between the control group (12.4%) and the low-dose heparin-treated group (14.8%).[23] In summary, with regard to gynecologic surgery, only the trial reported by Ballard has found a beneficial effect of low-dose heparin in patients with benign gynecologic conditions. Taberner, in benign gynecology patients, and Clarke-Pearson, in gynecologic oncology patients, did not find low-dose heparin to be of benefit.

In a subsequent trial,[29] two more intense heparin regimens were evaluated in high-risk gynecologic oncology patients. In this study, heparin was given either in a regimen of 5000 units subcutaneously 2 hours preoperatively and every 8 hours postoperatively, or 5000 units subcutaneously every 8 hours preoperatively (a minimum of three preoperative doses) and every 8 hours postoperatively. Both of these prophylaxis regimens were effective in significantly reducing the incidence of postoperative deep venous thrombosis.

Although low-dose heparin is considered to have no effect on measurable coagulation parameters, most large series have noted an increase in the bleeding complication rate, especially a higher incidence of wound hematoma. A prolonged activated partial thromboplastin time (APTT) developed in up to 10% to 15% of otherwise healthy patients after 5000 units of heparin was given subcutaneously.[24] These transiently anticoagulated patients have also been noted in one carefully monitored trial of low-dose heparin in gynecology. Major bleeding complications were encountered postoperatively in these patients. Dockerty et al.[37] also found that estimated blood loss increased from 246 to 401 ml in low-dose heparin-treated patients undergoing inguinal or pelvic lymphadenectomy. Retrospective studies have suggested that low-dose heparin contributed to an increased occurrence of lymphocysts,[90] and a prospective study demonstrated a twofold increase in retroperitoneal lymph drainage volume in patients treated with low-dose heparin.[24] Finally, although relatively rare, thrombocytopenia is associated with low-dose heparin use and has been found in 6% of patients after gynecologic surgery.[24] Although many authors feel that monitoring coagulation parameters is unnecessary for effective and safe low-dose heparin use, periodic postoperative assessment of activated thromboplastin time and platelet count seems prudent to maximize the identification of the 22% of patients who either had prolonged APTT or thrombocytopenia and who are most at risk for development of major clinical hemorrhagic complications.

Low-Molecular-Weight Heparin. Low-molecular-weight heparins (LMWH) are fragments of unfractionated heparin that vary in size from 4500 to 6500 daltons. When compared to unfractionated heparin, LMWH have more anti-Xa and less antithrombin activity, leading to less effect on partial thromboplastin time. Decreased platelet inhibition and microvascular bleeding have been noted with LMWH, which may also lead to fewer complications with bleeding.[104] An increased half-life of 4 hours (in both intravenous and subcutaneous administrations) leads to increased bioavailability when compared to unfractionated heparin. This may allow once- or twice-a-day dosing. Several commer-

cially available LMWH preparations are internationally available, but only two (enoxaparin and dalteparin) have been approved by the FDA for DVT prophylaxis in the United States.

Four randomized controlled trials in gynecologic surgery have compared LMWH to unfractionated LDH, revealing similar rates of bleeding complications and venous thromboemboli.[14,43,54,64] A subsequent meta-analysis of general and gynecological surgery patients from 32 trials likewise indicated that daily LMWH administration is as effective as unfractionated LDH in DVT prophylaxis without any difference in hemorrhagic complications.[63] Caution should be maintained in interpretation of assimilated data involving LMWH, since different anti-Xa activities are associated with the different preparations.[51] In a comparison of prophylactic methods of DVT treatment, LMWH has been suggested by some investigators to be more cost-effective than LDH in general and in orthopedic surgery patients because of the convenience of once-daily dosing.[11]

Mechanical Methods. Stasis in the veins of the legs has been clearly demonstrated on the operating table and continues postoperatively for varying lengths of time. Many authors believe that the combination of stasis occurring in the capacitance veins of the calf during surgery plus the hypercoagulable state induced by surgery is the primary factor contributing to the development of acute postoperative deep venous thrombosis. Prospective studies of the natural history of postoperative venous thrombosis have shown that the calf veins are the predominant site of thrombi and that most thrombi develop within 24 hours of surgery.[25] A growing body of literature supports the important role that the reduction in stasis by mechanical prophylactic methods plays in the prevention of postoperative deep vein thrombosis.

Although probably of only modest benefit, reduction of stasis by short preoperative hospital stays and early postoperative ambulation should be encouraged for all patients. A 20-degree elevation of the foot of the bed, thus raising the calf above heart level, allows gravity to drain the calf veins and should further reduce stasis. More active forms of mechanical prophylaxis include elastic gradient compression stockings and external pneumatic leg compression.

Graded Compression Stockings. The simplicity of graded elastic stockings and the absence of significant side effects are probably the two most important reasons many surgeons include them in routine postoperative orders.[32] Controlled studies of gradient elastic stockings are limited but do suggest modest benefit when carefully fitted.[96] Poorly fitted stockings can be hazardous to some patients in whom a tourniquet effect develops at the knee or midthigh.[22] Variations in human anatomy do not allow manufactured stocking sizes to perfectly fit all patients.

Although most postoperative DVT occurs in the first 72 hours after surgery, approximately 15% occur 7 to 30 days postoperatively. The practice of earlier hospital discharge after major surgery raises concerns about the effectiveness of prophylaxis if it is discontinued at the time of discharge. Of the prophylactic methods available, graded compression stockings are the most logical prophylactic method to be used by the patient after hospital discharge.

External Pneumatic Compression. The largest body of literature dealing with the reduction of postoperative venous stasis has evaluated intermittent external compression of the leg by pneumatically inflated sleeves placed around the calf or leg during intraoperative and postoperative periods. Various pneumatic compression devices and leg sleeve designs are available, and the current literature has not demonstrated superiority of one system over another. In randomized, controlled trials, compression devices appear to reduce significantly the incidence of deep venous thrombosis on a par with that of low-dose heparin. In addition to increasing venous flow and pulsatile emptying of the calf veins, external pneumatic compression also appears to augment endogenous fibrinolysis, which may result in lysis of very early thrombi before they become clinically significant.[3]

The duration of postoperative external pneumatic compression has varied among trials. Because most cases of deep venous thrombosis occur intraoperatively and in the first 72 hours postoperatively,[25] we believe this time interval should be the minimum duration for external pneumatic compression. Several investigators have found external pneumatic compression to be effective when used only in the operating room and for the first 24 hours postoperatively.[83,95]

External pneumatic compression used in patients undergoing major surgery for gynecologic malignancy has been found to reduce the incidence of postoperative venous thromboembolic complications by nearly threefold.[27] Calf compression was applied intraoperatively and for the first 5 postoperative days. In a subsequent trial of similar patients designed to evaluate whether external pneumatic compression might achieve similar benefits when used only intraoperatively and for the first 24 hours postoperatively, there was no reduction of deep venous thrombosis compared with the control group.[26] It appears that patients with gynecologic malignancies remain at risk because of stasis and hypercoagulable states for a longer time than general surgical patients, and if compression is to be effective, it must be used for a least 5 days postoperatively.

External pneumatic leg compression has no significant side effects or risks, although patient tolerance has been cited as a drawback. In our experience, less than 1% of patients request that the compression sleeves be discontinued because of discomfort. However, to achieve maximal effectiveness, compliance in device use is critical, and nurses and physicians alike should stress the importance of use while in bed. The nursing staff can easily manage the equipment, and although initial capital outlay for external pneumatic compressors may seem large, Salzman and Davies[95] calculated that the cost per patient of this prophylactic method is slightly less than that of low-dose heparin given for 7 days postoperatively.

Finally, when we compared low-dose heparin and pneumatic compression in a randomized trial, we found that both methods were equally effective in preventing DVT, although there was significantly more bleeding and transfu-

sions given to the group who received LDH. For this reason, pneumatic compression is the cornerstone of DVT prophylaxis in our institution.[29]

Blood Product Scheduling

Careful preparation and efficient use of blood products are imperative to decrease the risk of iatrogenic spread of bloodborne viral diseases, avoid transfusion reactions, and contain costs. Blood transfusion carries a risk of not only spreading disease, but also of causing isoimmunization, which can complicate future blood component crossmatching. In general, with the exception of extremely young or old patients, those in poor health, or those with compromised cardiopulmonary status, most surgical patients undergoing elective surgery can tolerate moderate blood loss on the order of one unit. With modest blood loss, hemodynamic stability often can be maintained with crystalloid and colloid fluids. Except for unique circumstances, red blood cell transfusion is rarely necessary unless the transfusion requirement is at least two units of blood.

More than 600 red cell blood group antigens have been identified. Of these, 250 represent important antigenic targets for a humoral immune response than can result in significant hemolysis. Fortunately, most patients (97% to 98%) have negative antibody screening tests and can be safely transfused with blood compatible for ABO and Rh type. For the remaining 2% to 3% of patients, a positive antibody screen dictates additional evaluation to identify all antibodies capable of significant red blood cell lysis in vivo.

A type and screen test determines the patient's ABO and Rh blood type and screens the plasma for presence of circulating atypical red cell antibodies. The test usually can be performed in less than 1 hour if no atypical antibodies are discovered. If atypical antibodies are present, however, results may not be available for 24 hours or more. Although the type and screen does not test for every possible anti–red cell antibody, this test will detect the overwhelming majority of clinically significant anti–red cell antibodies. Oberman et al.[85] found only eight significant antibodies in over 80,000 crossmatches performed on blood from 14,000 patients who had negative antibody screens. Heisto[55] similarly detected only 15 antibodies in over 70,000 crossmatches performed on 24,000 patients with negative antibody screens. It has thus been predicted that the type and screen system prevents incompatible transfusions in over 99.9% of cases.

A type and crossmatch screen includes, in addition to ABO and Rh typing and antibody screen, a crossmatch test, which is essentially a type-specific blood compatibility test. Because the actual type-specific unit of blood to be infused is tested against the blood recipient's serum, rare antibodies not detected by the antibody screening will be noted. Blood can be typed and crossmatched within 15 to 20 minutes in patients who have a negative antibody screen, negating the need for routine type and crossmatching of blood preoperatively in patients in whom the likelihood of transfusion is low. Clearly, if there is a reasonable likelihood that a blood transfusion will be necessary, blood should be typed and crossmatched. Furthermore, if atypical antibodies are discovered in the type and screen, delays in crossmatching are common, and it may be prudent to have blood available and crossmatched preoperatively.

As a result of several retrospective studies performed in the 1970s, it became clear that numerous elective surgical procedures rarely resulted in the requirement for perioperative transfusion.[44] Attempts to minimize wasteful crossmatching of blood for elective surgical procedures resulted in implementation of maximal surgical blood order schedules (MSBOS). The goal of an MSBOS is to increase blood bank efficiency by decreasing the number of units crossmatched but not used. The crossmatch/transfusion ratio (C/T) has been suggested as a way to judge the efficiency of routine crossmatching orders. A C/T ratio of 2/1 or 3/1 is an optimal goal. The ratio indicates that 30% to 50% of blood that is crossmatched is actually used. Retrospective analysis of any institution's crossmatching and transfusing practices can be performed to estimate the C/T ratio for any elective surgical procedure. It is recommended that blood be typed and screened for procedures with a C/T ratio routinely above 3/1, while routine preoperative crossmatching be performed for procedures associated with a greater likelihood of transfusion. Ultimately, the optimal blood order schedule needs to be tailored to an individual surgeon's or institution's experience. The use of a suggested MSBOS for gynecology (Table 5-7) can result in significant cost savings.

Concerns over the hazards of allogenic blood transfusion, especially transmission of hepatitis and HIV, have led to the development of preoperative autologous blood donation programs. More recently, concerns have been expressed over the high rate of autologous blood donation for procedures that rarely require transfusion and thereby result in

wasting donated blood that is never transfused. Others have shown that, for most surgical procedures, the preoperative donation of autologous blood is not cost effective.[39] Although the maximal surgical blood order schedule for elective surgery recommends only type and screen for patients undergoing elective hysterectomy (Table 5-7), others have recommended that women donate two units of autologous blood before hysterectomy.[5] However, a study of the value of autologous blood donation in 263 consecutive patients undergoing elective hysterectomy strongly refutes this recommendation.[18] When compared to patients who did not donate autologous blood preoperatively, those patients who donated blood were more likely to have significantly lower hemoglobin levels at hospital admission and discharge. Furthermore, patients who had donated autologous blood were more likely to receive transfusions postoperatively. When subjected to multivariate analysis, the most significant factor associated with postoperative transfusion was preoperative autologous blood donation! This increase in transfusion rate is most likely the result of iatrogenic anemia caused by preoperative autologous donation and a more liberal threshold for transfusing autologous blood. This liberal threshold will likely result in unnecessary transfusion reactions and errors in administration of the incorrect unit of blood. At present, it appears that for patients who will undergo an uncomplicated elective hysterectomy, preoperative autologous blood donation is not cost effective.

PREOPERATIVE DISCUSSION AND INFORMED CONSENT

The rapport and trust that exist between the patient and her gynecologic surgeon begin on the initial office visit and should be built upon at each subsequent interchange. When surgery is deemed advisable, initial discussion should explain in sufficient detail to the patient the findings on examination and the results of testing, the natural history of the disease process, and the goals of the surgical procedure. This discussion should be held in an unhurried manner and be of sufficient detail so that the patient may decide whether to go ahead with preoperative preparation. Because most gynecologic surgery is elective, the gynecologist has the opportunity to thoroughly evaluate the patient from a medical point of view, allow the patient to develop psychologic coping mechanisms, and answer questions that may not have been initially discussed. The surgeon should make himself or herself available to discuss these questions in person or by the telephone before actual hospital admission.

A few days before the anticipated surgery, another preoperative discussion should be held with the patient and key family members. These may include the spouse, a significant support person of an adult woman, or the parents of a minor. Privacy should be ensured to allow thorough and frank discussion, particularly when delicate questions regarding sexuality and sexual function may be raised. Discussions in hallways or office waiting rooms are not optimal.

Table 5-7 Suggested Maximal Surgical Blood Order Schedule for Elective Gynecologic Procedures

Type and Screen

Simple vaginal or abdominal hysterectomy
Oophorectomy
Tuboplasty, tubal ligation
Laparoscopy
Dilation and curettage
Elective abortion

Type and Cross	No. of Units
Complicated hysterectomy	2
Pelvic mass	2
Ovarian cancer	2-4
Myomectomy	2
Radical hysterectomy	2
Pelvic exenteration	6
Type and screen positive for atypical antibodies	2
Coagulopathy or bleeding disorder	2+

The goals of this preoperative discussion should serve to allay anxiety and fears that the patient may have and to answer any questions that may have arisen in the preoperative period. The discussion should serve to further expand on many issues relative to the surgery and its expected outcome and risks; this discussion is the basis for obtaining the signed informed consent.[38] This is an educational process for the patient and her family, and the physician needs to provide explanation in understandable terms. The topics listed in the box below should be discussed, and the patient and family should be invited to ask questions about each one. A discussion of the nature and the extent of the disease process should explain, in lay terms, the significance of the disease process. Is it life-threatening, or will it likely result in significant disability or dysfunction? To what extent does the disease process alter the patient's daily living? If left untreated, could the disease spontaneously resolve, or could it potentially worsen? What is the time course and natural history of the disease?

The goals of the surgery should be discussed in detail. Some gynecologic surgical procedures are performed purely for diagnostic purposes (e.g., D&C, cold knife conization, a diagnostic laparoscopy, or staging laparotomy), whereas most are clearly aimed at correcting an anatomic defect or a specific disease process. The extent of the surgery should be outlined, including notation of which organs will be removed. Most patients like to be informed about the type of surgical incision and estimated duration of anesthesia.

The expected outcome of the surgical procedure should be explained. If the procedure is being performed for diagnostic purposes, the outcome will depend on surgical or pathologic findings that are not known before surgery. When treating anatomic deformity or disease, the expected success of the operation, as well as the potential for failure, should be discussed. This should include a discussion of the probability of failure of tubal sterilization or the possibility that stress urinary incontinence may not be alleviated. When treating cancer, the possibility of finding more advanced disease and the potential need for adjunctive therapy (such as postoperative radiation therapy or chemotherapy) should

be mentioned. Other issues of importance to the patient include discussion of loss of fertility or ovarian function. The physician should raise these issues to make sure the patient adequately understands the pathophysiologic factors that may result from the surgery and to allow her to express her feelings regarding these emotionally charged matters.

The risks and potential complications of the surgical procedure should be discussed with the patient, including the most frequent complications of the particular surgical procedure. For most major gynecologic surgery, the risks include intraoperative and postoperative hemorrhage, postoperative infection, venous thrombosis, and injury to adjacent viscera. Due to the risks associated with blood transfusion, the patient should be clearly informed that she has the option (in elective cases) to secure autologous or donor directed packed cells for potential transfusion. Although this may not be cost effective, the patient, nonetheless, should be given this information as part of the informed consent process.

Unanticipated findings at the time of surgery should also be mentioned. For example, if the ovaries are unexpectedly found to be diseased, it may be the best surgical judgment to remove them. A discussion of these unanticipated findings and the judgments that the surgeon must make intraoperatively will alleviate many instances of surprises after surgery and unhappiness on the part of the patient or her family.

The usual postoperative course should also be discussed in enough detail so that the patient understands what to expect in the days after surgery. Information regarding the need for a suprapubic catheter or prolonged central venous monitoring helps the patient accept her postoperative course and avoids surprises that may be very disconcerting. The expected duration of the recovery period, both in and out of the hospital, should be noted.

Alternative methods of therapy are also to be mentioned as part of the preoperative discussion. Other medical management or other surgical approaches should be discussed along with their potential benefits and complications. Finally, the patient should have an understanding of the outcome of the disease should nothing be done. It should be clear to the patient following this discussion why the proposed surgery is the appropriate next step in her care. We believe that the preoperative informed consent discussion should be initiated by the responsible surgeon and not delegated to nursing staff or house staff, who may not have full understanding of the patient's disease process, or the rapport or responsibility for her ultimate care. The informed consent discussion detailing the information given the patient should be documented in the patient's chart.

The anesthesiologist responsible for the surgical procedure also should have the opportunity to examine the patient, review her laboratory findings, and discuss the proposed anesthetic method with the patient. In many institutions, the consent to the administration of anesthetic is included in the surgical consent form, whereas in others it is a separate form that should be obtained by the anesthesiologist after preoperative discussion.

KEY ELEMENTS OF THE PREOPERATIVE DISCUSSION

1. The nature and extent of the disease process
2. The extent of the actual operation proposed and potential modifications of this operation, depending on unexpected intraoperative findings
3. The anticipated benefits of the operation, with a conservative estimate of successful outcome
4. The risks and potential complications of the surgery
5. Alternative methods of therapy and their risks and results
6. The likely results if the patient remains untreated

REFERENCES

1. Abel RM: Nutritional support in the patient with acute renal failure, *J Am Coll Nutr* 2:33, 1983.

2. Aguirre A, Fischer JE, Welch CE: The role of surgery and hyperalimentation in therapy of gastrointestinal-cutaneous fistulae, *Ann Surg* 180:393, 1974.

3. Allenby F, Boardman L, Pflug JJ, Calnan JS: Effects of external pneumatic intermittent compression on fibrinolysis in man, *Lancet* 2:1412, 1973.

4. Anderson ME, Belani KG: Short-term preoperative smoking abstinence, *Am Fam Physician* 41:1191, 1990.

5. Axelrod FB, Pepkowitz SH, Goldfinger D: Establishment of a schedule of optimal preoperative collection of autologous blood, *Transfusion* 29:677, 1989.

6. Baker JP, Detsky AS, Wesson DE, et al: Nutritional assessment: a comparison of clinical judgment and objective measurements, *N Engl J Med* 306:969, 1982.

7. Ballard RM, Bradley-Watson PJ, Johnstone FD, et al: Low doses of subcutaneous heparin in the prevention of deep vein thrombosis after gynaecological surgery, *J Obstet Gynaecol Br Commonw* 80:469, 1973.

8. Bandy LC, Chin N, Soper JT, et al: Total parenteral nutrition in poor prognosis gestational trophoblastic disease, *Gynecol Oncol* 28:305, 1987.

9. Barnes PJ: A new approach to the treatment of asthma, *N Engl J Med* 321:1517, 1989.

10. Beck DE, Harford FJ, DiPalma JA: Comparison of cleansing methods in preparation for colonic surgery, *Dis Colon Rectum* 28:491, 1985.

11. Bergqvist D, Lindgren B, Matzsch T: Comparison of the cost of preventing postoperative deep vein thrombosis with either unfractionated or low molecular weight heparin, *Br J Surg* 83:1548, 1996.

12. Blackburn GL, Bistrian BR: Nutritional care of the injured and/or septic patient, *Surg Clin North Am* 56:1195, 1976.

13. Blosser SA, Rock P: Asthma and chronic obstructive lung disease. In Breslow MJ, Miller CJ, Rogers MC, editors: *Perioperative management,* St Louis, 1989, Mosby.

14. Borstad E, Urdal K, Handeland G, Abildgaard U: Comparison of low molecular weight heparin vs unfractionated heparin in gynecological surgery. II. Reduced dose of low molecular weight heparin, *Acta Obstet Gynecol Scand* 71:471, 1992.

15. Brennan MF, Pisters PW, Posner M, et al: A prospective randomized trial of total parenteral nutrition after major pancreatic resection for malignancy, *Ann Surg* 220:436, 1994.

16. Burke JF: The effective period of preventive antibiotic action in experimental incisions and dermal lesions, *Surgery* 50:161, 1961.

17. Butterworth CE, Blackburn GL: Hospital malnutrition and how to assess the nutritional status of a patient, *Nutr Today* 9:1, 1974.

18. Canter MH, van Maanen D, Anders KH, et al: Preoperative autologous blood donations before elective hysterectomy, *JAMA* 276:798, 1996.

19. Castillo R, Haas A: Chest physical therapy: comparative efficacy of preoperative and postoperative in the elderly, *Arch Phys Med Rehabil* 66:376, 1985.

20. Chapman KR: Therapeutic approaches to chronic obstructive pulmonary disease: an emerging consensus, *Am J Med* 100:1, 1996.

21. Chodak GW, Plaut ME: Use of systemic antibiotics for prophylaxis in surgery: a critical review, *Arch Surg* 112:326, 1977.

22. Clarke-Pearson DL, Jelovsek FR, Creasman WT: Thromboembolism complicating surgery for cervical and uterine malignancy: incidence, risk factors, and prophylaxis, *Obstet Gynecol* 61:87, 1983.

23. Clarke-Pearson DL, Coleman RE, Synan IS, et al: Venous thromboembolism prophylaxis in gynecologic oncology: a prospective controlled trial of low-dose heparin, *Am J Obstet Gynecol* 145:606, 1983.

24. Clarke-Pearson DL, DeLong ER, Synan IS, Creasman WT: Complications of low-dose heparin prophylaxis in gynecologic oncology surgery, *Obstet Gynecol* 64:689, 1984.

25. Clarke-Pearson DL, Synan IS, Coleman RE, et al: The natural history of postoperative venous thromboemboli in gynecologic oncology: a prospective study of 382 patients, *Am J Obstet Gynecol* 148:1051, 1984.

26. Clarke-Pearson DL, Creasman WT, Coleman RE, et al: Perioperative external pneumatic calf compression as thromboembolism prophylaxis in gynecologic oncology: report of a randomized controlled trial, *Gynecol Oncol* 18:226, 1984.

27. Clarke-Pearson DL, Synan IS, Hinshaw WM, et al: Prevention of postoperative venous thromboembolism by external pneumatic calf compression in patients with gynecologic malignancy, *Obstet Gynecol* 63:92, 1984.

28. Clarke-Pearson DL, DeLong E, Synan IS, et al: Variables associated with postoperative deep venous thrombosis: a prospective study of 411 gynecology patients, *Obstet Gynecol* 69:146, 1987.

29. Clarke-Pearson DL, DeLong E, Synan IS, et al: A controlled trial of two low-dose heparin regimens for the prevention of postoperative deep vein thrombosis, *Obstet Gynecol* 75:684, 1990.

30. Clayton JK, Anderson JA, McNicol GP: Preoperative prediction of postoperative deep vein thrombosis, *Br Med J* 2:910, 1976.

31. Cockroft DW: Hyperresponsiveness in asthma, *Hosp Pract* 25:111, 1990.

32. Conti S, Daschbach M: Venous thromboembolism prophylaxis: a survey of its use in the United States, *Arch Surg* 117:1036, 1982.

33. Copeland EM III, MacFadyen BV Jr, Lanzotti VJ, Dudrick SJ: Intravenous hyperalimentation as an adjunct to cancer chemotherapy, *Am J Surg* 129:167, 1975.

34. Creasman WT, Weed JC Jr: Radical hysterectomy. In Schaefer G, Graber EA, editors: *Complications in obstetrics and gynecologic surgery,* Hagerstown, Md, 1981, Harper & Row.

35. Cruse PJ, Foord R: A five-year prospective study of 23,649 surgical wounds, *Arch Surg* 107:206, 1973.

36. Davey PG, Duncan ID, Edward D, Scott AC: Cost-benefit analysis of cephradine and mezlocillin prophylaxis for abdominal and vaginal hysterectomy, *Br J Obstet Gynaecol* 95:1170, 1988.

37. Docherty PW, Goodman JD, Hill JG, et al: The effect of low-dose heparin on blood loss at abdominal hysterectomy, *Br J Obstet Gynaecol* 90:759, 1983.

38. Easley HA Hammond CB: Informed consent in obstetrics and gynecology, *Postgrad Obstet Gynecol* 10:1, 1986.

39. Etchason J, Petz L, Keeler E, et al: The cost effectiveness of preoperative autologous blood donations, *N Engl J Med* 332:719, 1995.

40. Flenley DC: Chronic obstructive pulmonary disease, *Disease of the Month* 34:537, 1988.

41. Flynn, NM: Reducing the risk of infection in surgical patients. In Bolt RJ, editor: *Medical evaluation of the surgical patient,* Mt Kisco, NY, 1987, Futura Publishing.

42. Foschi D, Cavagna G, Callioni F, et al: Hyperalimentation of jaundiced patients on percutaneous transhepatic biliary drainage, *Br J Surg* 73:716, 1986.

43. Fricker JP, Vergnes Y, Schach R, et al: Low dose heparin versus low molecular weight heparin (Kabi 2165, Fragmin) in the prophylaxis of thromboembolic complications of abdominal oncological surgery. *Eur J Clin Invest* 18:561, 1988.

44. Friedman BA, Oberman HA, Chadwick AR, Kingdon KI: The maximum surgical blood order schedule and surgical blood use in the United States, *Transfusion* 16:380, 1976.

45. Friese S, Willems FT, Loriaux SM, Meewis JM: Prophylaxis in gynaecological surgery: a prospective randomized comparison between single dose prophylaxis with amoxicillin/clavulanate and the combination of cefuroxime and metronidazole, *J Antimicrob Chemother* 24:213, 1989.

46. Fry DE: Antibiotics in surgery: an overview, *Am J Surg* 155:11, 1988.

47. Galant SP: Treatment of asthma: new and time-tested strategies, *Postgrad Med* 87:229, 1990.

48. Goldberg NJ, Wingert TD, Levin SR, et al: Insulin therapy in the diabetic surgical patient: metabolic and hormone response to low dose insulin infusion, *Diabetes Care* 4:279, 1981.

49. Goldman L, Caldera DL, Southwick FS, et al: Cardiac risk factors and complications in non-cardiac surgery, *Medicine* 57:357, 1978.

50. Goodnough LT: Autologous blood donation, *JAMA* 260:65, 1988.

51. Haas S, Haas P: Efficacy of low molecular weight heparins: an overview, *Semin Thromb Hemost* 19:101, 1993.

52. Haley RW, Culver DH, Morgan WM, et al: Identifying patients at high risk of surgical wound infection: a simple multivariate index of patient susceptibility and wound contamination, *Am J Epidemiol* 121:206, 1985.

53. Heatley RV, Williams RH, Lewis MH: Preoperative intravenous feeding—a controlled trial, *Postgrad Med J* 55:541, 1979.

54. Heilmann L, Kruck M, Schindler AE: Prevention of thrombosis in gynecology: double-blind comparison of low molecular weight heparin and unfractionated heparin, *Geburtshilfe Frauenheilkd* 49:803, 1989.

55. Heisto H: Pretransfusion blood group serology: limited value of the antiglobulin phase of the crossmatch when a careful screening test for unexpected antibodies is performed, *Transfusion* 19:761, 1979.

56. Hemsell DL, Martin JN Jr, Pastorek JG II, et al: Single-dose antimicrobial prophylaxis at abdominal hysterectomy: cefamandole vs. cefotaxime, *J Repro Med* 33:939, 1988.

57. Hemsell DL, Johnson ER, Heard MC, et al: Single-dose piperacillin versus triple-dose cefoxitin prophylaxis at vaginal and abdominal hysterectomy, *South Med J* 82:438, 1989.

58. Heymsfield SB, Horowitz J, Lawson DH: Enteral hyperalimentation. In Berk JE, editor: *Developments in digestive diseases,* vol 3, Philadelphia, 1980, Lea & Febiger.

59. Hirsch HA: Prophylactic antibiotics in obstetrics and gynecology, *Am J Med* 78:170, 1985.

60. Hotchkiss RS: Perioperative management of patient with chronic obstructive pulmonary disease, *Int Anesthesiol Clin* 26:134, 1988.

61. Jarrett RJ: Descriptive epidemiology in diabetes types 1 and 2. In Diabetes mellitus, Littleton, Mass, 1986, PSG Publishing.

62. Jeffcoate TN, Tindall VR: Venous thrombosis and embolism in obstetrics and gynaecology, *Aust N Z J Obstet Gynaecol* 5:119, 1965.

63. Jorgensen LN, Wille-Jorgensen P, Hauch O: Prophylaxis of postoperative thromboembolism with low molecular weight heparins, *Br J Surg* 80:689, 1993.

64. Kaaja R, Lehtovirta P, Venesmaa P, et al: Comparison of enoxaparin, a low-molecular-weight heparin, and unfractionated heparin, with or without dihydroergotamine, in abdominal hysterectomy, *Eur J Obstet Gynecol Reprod Biol* 47:141, 1992.

65. Kakkar VV: Prevention of fatal postoperative pulmonary embolism by low dose heparin: an international multicenter trial, *Lancet* 2:145, 1975.

66. Keating HJ III: Preoperative considerations in the geriatric patient, *Med Clin North Am* 71:569, 1987.

67. Kinney JM, Long CL, Gump FE, Duke JH: Tissue composition of weight loss in surgical patients. I. Elective operation, *Ann Surg* 168:459, 1968.

68. Kuner J, Enescu V, Utsu F, et al: Cardiac arrhythmias during anesthesia, *Dis Chest* 52:580, 1967.

69. Lamers RJ, van Engelshoven JM, Pfaff A: Once again, the routine preoperative thorax photo, *Ned Tijdschr Geneeskd* 133:2288, 1989.

70. Ledger WJ, Gee C, Lewis WP: Guidelines for antibiotic prophylaxis in gynecology, *Am J Obstet Gynecol* 121:1038, 1975.

71. Li JT: Three steps toward better management of asthma, *Compr Ther* 22:345, 1996.

72. Loder RE: Routine preoperative chest radiography, *Anesthesiology* 66:195, 1987.

73. McMurry JF Jr.: Wound healing with diabetes mellitus, *Surg Clin North Am* 64:35, 1985.

74. Milledge JS, Nunn JF: Criteria of fitness for anaesthesia in patients with chronic obstructive lung disease, *Br Med J* 3:670, 1975.

75. Miller TA, Duke JH: Fluid and electrolyte management. In Dudrick SJ, Baue AE, Eiseman B, et al, editors: *Manual of preoperative and postoperative care,* Philadelphia, 1983, WB Saunders.

76. Mohr DN, Jett JR: Clinical reviews: preoperative evaluation of pulmonary risk factors, *J Gen Intern Med* 3:277, 1988.

77. Mullen JL, Buzby GP, Waldman MT, et al: Prediction of operative morbidity and mortality by preoperative nutritional assessment, *Surg Forum* 30:80, 1979.

78. Mullen JL, Buzby GP, Matthews DC, et al: Reduction of operative morbidity and mortality by combined preoperative and postoperative nutritional support, *Ann Surg* 192:604, 1980.

79. Muller JM, Keller HW, Brenner U, et al: Indications and effects of preoperative parenteral nutrition, *World J Surg* 10:53, 1986.

80. Munck AM, Jensen HK: Preoperative clindamycin treatment and vaginal drainage in hysterectomy, *Acta Obstet Gynecol Scand* 68:241, 1989.

81. Myers ER, Clarke-Pearson DL, Olt GJ, et al: Preoperative coagulation testing on a gynecologic oncology service, *Obstet Gynecol* 83:483, 1994.

82. National Institutes of Health Consensus Group: Summary of NIH Consensus Development Conference on Perioperative Red Cell Transfusion, *Am J Hematol* 31:144, 1989.

83. Nicolaides AN, Fernandes e Fernandes J, Pollock AV: Intermittent sequential pneumatic compression of the legs in the prevention of venous stasis and postoperative deep venous thrombosis, *Surgery* 87:69, 1980.

84. Nixon DW, Heymsfield SB, Cohen AE, et al: Protein-calorie undernutrition in hospitalized cancer patients, *Am J Med* 68:683, 1980.

85. Oberman HA, Barnes BA, Friedman BA: The risk of abbreviating the major crossmatch in urgent or massive transfusion, *Transfusion* 18:137, 1978.

86. Orr JW Jr, Sisson PF, Patsner B, et al: Single-dose antibiotic prophylaxis for patients undergoing extended pelvic surgery for gynecologic malignancy, *Am J Obstet Gynecol* 162:718, 1990.

87. Page MM, Watkins PJ: Cardiorespiratory arrest and diabetic autonomic neuropathy, *Lancet* 1:14, 1978.

88. Pestana C: *Fluids and electrolytes in the surgical patient,* ed 4, Baltimore, 1989, Williams & Wilkins.

89. Piscitelli, JT, Simel DL, Addison WA: Who should have intravenous pyelograms before hysterectomy for benign disease? *Obstet Gynecol* 69:541, 1987.

90. Piver MS, Malfetano JH, Lele SB, Moore RH: Prophylactic anticoagulation as a possible cause of inguinal lymphocyst after radical vulvectomy and inguinal lymphadenectomy, *Obstet Gynecol* 62:17, 1983.

91. Porte D, Halter JB: The endocrine pancreas and diabetes mellitus. In Williams RH, editor: *Textbook of endocrinology,* Philadelphia, 1981, WB Saunders.

92. Rao TL, Jacobs KH, El-Etr AA: Reinfarction following anesthesia in patients with myocardial infarction, *Anesthesiology* 59:499, 1983.

93. Rayfield EJ, Ault MJ, Keusch GT, et al: Infection and diabetes: the case for glucose control, *Am J Med* 72:439, 1982.

94. Roy S, Wilkins J, Galaif E, Azen C: Comparative efficacy and safety of cefmetazole or cefoxitin in the prevention of postoperative infection following vaginal and abdominal hysterectomy, *J Antimicrob Chemo* 23:109, 1989.

95. Salzman EW, Davies GC: Prophylaxis of venous thromboembolism: analysis of cost effectiveness, *Ann Surg* 191:207, 1980.

96. Scurr JH, Ibrahim SZ, Faber RG, Le Quesne LP: The efficacy of graduated compression stockings in the prevention of deep vein thrombosis, *Br J Surg* 64:371, 1977.

97. Shapiro M, Munoz A, Tager IB, et al: Risk factors for infection at the operative site after abdominal or vaginal hysterectomy, *N Engl J Med* 307:1661, 1982.

98. Shipton EA: The peri-operative care of the geriatric patient, *S Afr Med J* 63:855, 1983.

99. Siafakas NM, Vermeire P, Pride NB, et al: Optimal assessment and management of chronic obstructive pulmonary disease (COPD). The European Respiratory Society Task Force, *Eur Respir J* 8:1398, 1995.

100. Smith RC, Hartemink R: Improvement of nutritional measures during preoperative parenteral nutrition in patients selected by the prognostic nutritional index: a randomized controlled trial, *J Parenter Enteral Nutr* 12:587, 1988.

101. Soper JT, Berchuck A, Creasman WT, Clarke-Pearson DL: Pelvic exenteration: factors associated with major surgical morbidity, *Gynecol Oncol* 35:93, 1989.

102. Steen PA, Tinker JH, Tarhan S: Myocardial reinfarction after anesthesia and surgery, *JAMA* 239:2566, 1978.

103. Taberner DA, Poller L, Burslem RW, Jones JB: Oral anticoagulants controlled by British comparative thromboplastin versus low-dose heparin in prophylaxis of deep vein thrombosis, *Br Med J* 1:272, 1978.

104. Tapson VF, Hull RD: Management of venous thromboembolic disease: the impact of low-molecular-weight heparin, *Clin Chest Med* 16:281, 1995.

105. Trimbos JB, van Lindert AC, Heintz AP, et al: Piperacillin for prophylaxis in gynecological surgery, *Eur J Obstet Gynecol Reprod Biol* 30:141, 1989.

106. Veterans Affairs Total Parenteral Nutrition Cooperative Study Group: perioperative total parenteral nutrition in surgical patients, *N Engl J Med* 325:525, 1991.

107. Vogel CM, Kingsbury RJ, Baue AE: Intravenous hyperalimentation: a review of two and one-half years' experience, *Arch Surg* 105:414, 1972.

108. von Knorring J: Postoperative myocardial infarction: a prospective study in a risk group of surgical patients, *Surgery* 90:55, 1981.

109. Walts LF, Miller J, Davidson MB, Brown J: Perioperative management of diabetes mellitus, *Anesthesiology* 55:104, 1981.

110. Warner MA, Offord KP, Warner ME, et al: Role of preoperative cessation of smoking and other factors in postoperative pulmonary complications: a blinded prospective study of coronary artery bypass patients, *Mayo Clin Proc* 64:609, 1989.

111. Wheat LJ: Infection and diabetes mellitus, *Diabetes Care* 3:187, 1980.

6 Surgical Instrumentation and the Operating Room Team

DAVID H. NICHOLS

INSTRUMENTS AND SUTURES

Although the success of surgery depends more on the surgeon's judgment and technical competence than on the design of the instruments or the quality of the sutures used, the right choices of equipment and materials enable the surgeon to accomplish the best of which he or she is capable with greater ease and efficiency. Furthermore, ensuring that the special instruments or sutures that may be needed are on hand before the start of surgery avoids delays and permits the effective use of each minute of operative time.

OPERATING ROOM AND EQUIPMENT

The operating room should be in a quiet location and should be large enough to provide not only elbow room and moving space for the surgeon and assistants, the anesthesiologist, and the nursing staff, but also convenient access to equipment and instrument tables (Figs. 6-1 and 6-2). Appropriate amounts of suture material, any special instruments that might be used, and sterile supplies, including any packing that may be needed, should be immediately at hand. Modern anesthesia equipment that permits continuous monitoring of the patient's pulmonary and cardiac status should also be in the operating room. Continuous suction equipment, including one weighted speculum equipped with a suction tip, is desirable. A separate suction apparatus with a hand-held tube should be available. A trap for each suction device permits a quick and accurate estimate of the amount of blood lost during surgery.

Lighting

Because most operating room lighting has been designed to illuminate the operative field during procedures such as a laparotomy, it does not always adequately illuminate the horizontal axis of a relatively deep pelvic cavity such as the vagina. Lighting directed over the right-handed surgeon's left shoulder (and vice versa) should provide shadow-free illumination. When the overhead lighting cannot be adapted for vaginal surgery, movable spotlights are necessary; however, these often have an annoying tendency to move or slide out of focus as a result of the movements of operating room personnel. A surgeon may find it advantageous to wear a fiberoptic or tungsten headlight, which provides a shadowless spot of 2 to 4 inches of very bright light in the center of the operative field (Fig. 6-3). Because the wearer is in control of the position of the light at all times, it can be quite helpful. Lighted retractors are occasionally useful.

Operating Table

For vaginal surgery, the operating table should be equipped with "candy cane" stirrups that can be extended at least a foot so that they can be adjusted to the length of the patient's legs. These should be placed so that when the patient's ankles are suspended from the stirrups, acute angulation of the legs does not obstruct venous return. The patient should be positioned on the operating table so that an imaginary line drawn between the two stirrups will intersect each acetabulum, or hip socket. When it is anticipated that the patient will be in the lithotomy position for longer than 2½ hours, Allen universal supports should be used instead to lessen the chance for postoperative femoral neuropathy. The operating table should also permit rapid adjustment into varying degrees of Trendelenburg and reverse Trendelenburg positions, as needed for individual and emergency circumstances. The table height should be sufficiently adjustable to permit the operator either to stand or to sit during the operative procedure.

A lithotomy sheet should have ample casings for the feet so that it can be placed in position readily even though the patient's legs are placed somewhat vertically in the extended leg holders or stirrups. Alternatively, the patient and her legs can be draped with sterile sheets. Thigh-high elastic stockings or pneumatic compression boots for the patient are advisable, and they should be in place before administration of the anesthesia. Their usefulness in significantly decreasing the risk of postoperative pulmonary embolism is well established, and they certainly provide venous compression and thus reduce the rapid pooling of blood into the large venous beds of the patient's legs that occurs when the legs are taken out of the stirrups and lowered into the horizontal recumbent position at the end of the procedure. Lowering the legs without such compression can cause a precipitous and major drop in blood pressure because of what, in effect, is a sudden increase in the size of the venous pool into which a fixed volume of blood is circulating. Intermittent compression boots are useful when there are extensive varicosities or a history of previous thrombophlebitis or of pulmonary embolus.

Special Instruments

Vaginal surgeons usually prefer a few special instruments that are well designed for vaginal procedures. Instruments available for vaginal surgery in standard operating room setups often include the following:

Sharpened curved Mayo scissors
Narrow Deaver retractors

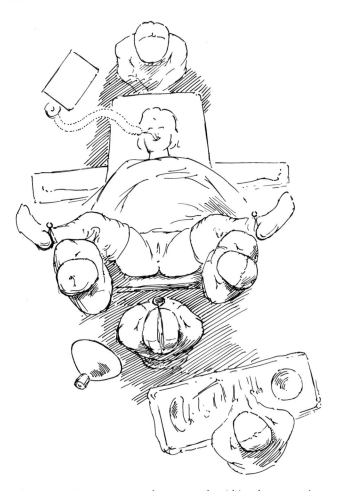

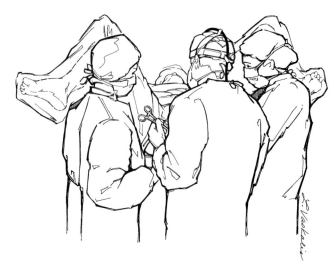

Fig. 6-2   The positions of the surgeons, standing, in relation to the patient. The surgeon is at the center, the first assistant to the surgeon's left, the second assistant to the right. In this arrangement all surgeons are free to move without risking a troublesome back strain. Small, movable platforms should be available to accommodate significant differences in height of members of the operative team. (From Nichols DH, Randall CL: *Vaginal surgery*, ed 4, Baltimore, 1996, Williams & Wilkins.)

Fig. 6-1   Arrangement of personnel within the operating room when a transvaginal surgical route has been chosen. Surgeon in central position at the foot of the operating table with the second assistant to the right and the first assistant to the left. A spotlight over a right-handed surgeon's left shoulder illuminates the perineum. Instrument table to the surgeon's back and somewhat to the right. Instrument nurse behind the instrument table, facing surgeon's back and sharing a full view of operative field so as to follow progress of the surgical procedure visually. Positions of spotlight, nurse, and instrument table are reversed if surgeon is left-handed. (From Instruments and sutures. In Nichols DH, Randall CL: *Vaginal surgery*, ed 4, Baltimore, 1996, Williams & Wilkins.)

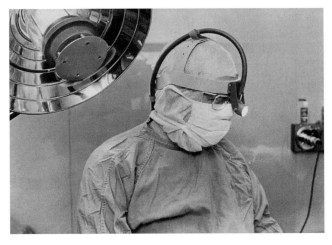

Fig. 6-3   Fiberoptic headlight, which will provide literally shadow-free bright illumination into the depths of a body cavity, even in a horizontal plane. (From Instruments and sutures. In Nichols DH, Randall CL: *Vaginal surgery*, ed 4, Baltimore, 1996, Williams & Wilkins.)

Curved and straight Kocher's forceps
Allis clamps
Rochester or curved Kelly hemostats
Crile hemostats
Lahey thyroid or Gordon uterine vulsella
Double-toothed Jacobs-type tenacula

In addition to the standard instruments, the setup for vaginal hysterectomy should include several Heaney-type hysterectomy forceps and a Heaney-type needle-holder. Bonney and Russian forceps are desirable. Long straight-bladed retractors are useful, such as the Breisky-Navratil in various sizes.

Although ideal, it is not always possible for the surgeon who is performing a vaginal operation to have two assis-

tants. When the surgeon must work with a single assistant, a large Rigby retractor (Fig. 6-4, *H*) is useful because it frees the assistant's hands for knot cutting, sponging, and holding the movable retractors. A weighted speculum is usually quite helpful when, as often happens, the surgeon must accomplish virtually all the surgical dissection within the vagina. A modification of the standard weighted speculum permits continuous suction (see Fig. 6-4, *A*). The suction tubing may be built into the retractor blade, further increasing op-

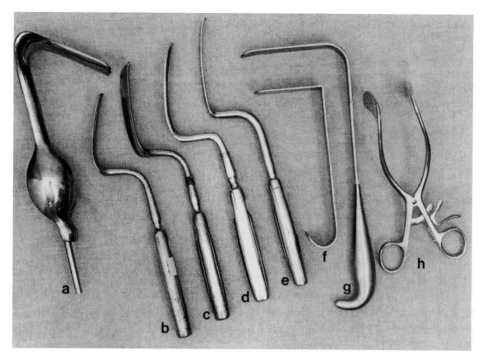

Fig. 6-4 Various retractors. *a,* Remine weighted suction speculum; *b* to *e,* various shapes and sizes of Briesky-Navratil vaginal retractors; *f,* small Heaney retractor; *g,* long-handled Heaney retractor; *h,* large-sized Rigby self-retaining retractor. (From Nichols DH, Randall CL: *Vaginal surgery,* ed 4, Baltimore, 1996, Williams & Wilkins.)

erative exposure (Fig. 6-5). A wall-mounted trap on the suction apparatus makes it possible to estimate at a glance the blood loss collected during surgery.

The instruments of N. Sproat Heaney were especially designed for use within the vagina. The Heaney needle-holder is particularly valuable because the considerable range of angles at which the needle can be grasped permits the surgeon to place curved needles and sutures deep within the pelvis at almost any conceivable angle with relative ease (Figs. 6-6, *C,* and 6-7). The Heaney hemostats have a "pelvic curve" that ensures proper placement and a secure grip on tissues with minimal risk of slippage. For use in a hysterectomy in which the prolapse may not be severe at the start of the operation, the Heaney-Glenner hysterectomy forceps is valuable (see Fig. 6-6, *A*); this instrument has both an upward curve and a lateral curve adapted to the right and left sides of the patient, as stamped on the forceps. The Heaney-Ballantine hysterectomy forceps also is useful (see Fig. 6-6, *B*), as are the Masterson and the Maingot forceps. The latter is useful for clamping the mesovarium during oophorectomy because it neither slips nor tears tissue, even when traction is needed.

During the performance of a vaginectomy or a Schauta radical vaginal hysterectomy, the long mouse-toothed forceps of Krobach is effective in occluding the vagina temporarily (see Fig. 6-6, *D*). Once the operator is familiar with the use of this instrument, one or two of them can be of considerable help during a perineorrhaphy and posterior colporrhaphy.

The Bonney forceps is highly recommended (Fig. 6-8)

because it has both a rat tooth for holding the tissues and occlusive serrated edges for grasping a needle that is deeply placed in tissues. The long Singley forceps is particularly useful for handling the peritoneum and intraabdominal organs with minimal trauma (see Fig. 6-8). The so-called Russian forceps is an excellent choice for use on the vaginal surface of the bladder during anterior colporrhaphy because it distributes the compression of the tissue within its grasp equally over a wide area (see Fig. 6-8).

Most surgeons find it easier to hold a small Heaney retractor (see Fig. 6-4, *F*) than the narrower Deaver retractor. The small Heaney retractor is lightweight, has a short, unobtrusive handle, and can be very helpful during colporrhaphy. However, the long-handled Heaney retractor can be particularly helpful during vaginal hysterectomy in holding the bladder safely out of harm's way after the anterior vesicouterine peritoneal fold has been identified and opened (see Fig. 6-4, *G*).

Breisky-Navratil retractors come in an almost infinite assortment of sizes (see Fig. 6-4, *B* to *E*). In Europe they are commonly used for vaginal surgery but are not as well known in the United States. Having an assortment of these retractors in varying widths and depths immediately available helps to ensure effective retraction in a wide variety of clinical circumstances.

When the handle of a retractor is parallel to the blade, it may be grasped easily and securely, much like a dagger. Moreover, such a grasp is comfortable, reduces the tendency toward retractor slippage or wandering, and does not obstruct the surgical team's view of the operative field. The

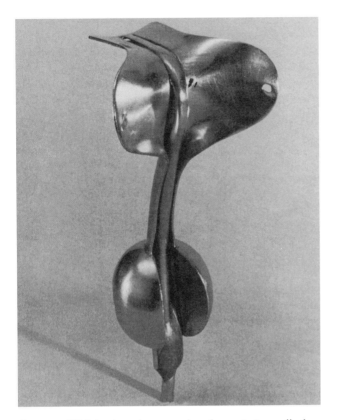

Fig. 6-5   Weighted suction speculum for posterior wall of vagina. Suction tubing has been buried in retractor's posterior blade, improving exposure in the operative field. Available from BEI/Zinnanti Surgical Instruments, Chatsworth, CA 91311, or the custom order department, Mr. William Merz, Baxter V. Mueller, Chicago, IL 60648. (From Instruments and sutures. In Nichols DH, Randall CL: *Vaginal surgery,* ed 4, Baltimore, 1996, Williams & Wilkins.)

use of a flat-bladed retractor, which should be held as shown in Fig. 6-9, may provide even greater exposure into the depths of the wound (Fig. 6-10).

Although the 28-cm Deschamps ligature carrier for the right hand is particularly useful during a right sacrospinous colpopexy procedure, it is also useful during oophorectomy. Its tip curves in a clockwise direction. The tip of a left-handed Deschamps carrier, useful for a left sacrospinous colpopexy, curves in a counterclockwise direction. The blunt point tends to push adjacent blood vessels to one side and is less likely to cause lacerations than is a sharp-pointed needle. It is wise to have as an accessory a long hook to grasp the suture after it has penetrated the tissue. Other ligature carriers and instruments designed for use with specific surgical procedures are described in the respective chapters.

Like the tips of a pair of scissors, the blade of the scalpel should function as if it were an extension of the operator's fingers. A proper position for holding the scalpel to make an incision is noted in Fig. 6-11. For fine dissection, in contrast, the scalpel can be held between the thumb and the first and second fingers, similar to how a pencil is held. Delicacy in applying the scalpel blade to the tissue being dissected requires that the cutting surface of the blade be passed over the tissue many times until the precise separation between tissues has been achieved.

Because the average operating room setup is far more likely to have right-handed surgeons and therefore right-handed scissors than it is to have left-handed surgeons and scissors, it is more important for the left-handed surgeon to learn to cut with right-handed scissors, which are always available, than for the right-handed surgeon to learn to cut with left-handed scissors, which are rarely available.

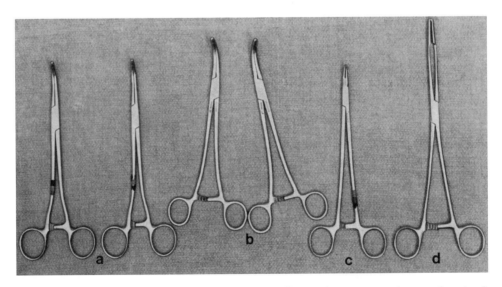

Fig. 6-6   Clamps and needle-holders. ***a,*** Heaney-Ballantine hysterectomy forceps; ***b,*** pair of Heaney-Glenner hysterectomy forceps, with right and left curve; ***c,*** Heaney needle-holder; ***d,*** Krobach mouse-toothed clamp. (From Instruments and sutures. In Nichols DH, Randall CL: *Vaginal surgery,* ed 4, Baltimore, 1996, Williams & Wilkins.)

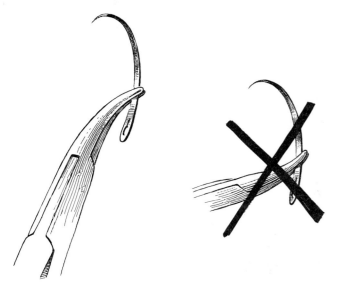

Fig. 6-7   Correct *(left)* and incorrect *(right)* ways to grasp the needle with a Heaney needle-holder. (From Instruments and sutures. In Nichols DH, Randall CL: *Vaginal surgery,* ed 4, Baltimore, 1996, Williams & Wilkins.)

SUTURES

Hermann[8] described the basic requirements for sutures to be used in the closing of surgical wounds as follows:

> The purpose of a surgical suture is to maintain approximation of tissues until the healing process has progressed to the point where artificial support is no longer necessary for the wound to resist normal stresses. Beyond this point, the sutures serve no useful purpose, and may, in fact, be the source of irritation or serve as a nidus for persistent infection. Thus the ideal suture should persist and maintain tensile strength until the tissue has healed sufficiently, and then disappear.

Suture Materials

Chromic catgut, made from the strong submucosal layer of animal intestine, had been the traditional choice for suture material in the past, but the delayed absorption of the new synthetic suture materials (e.g., polyglycolic acid [Dexon] and polyglactin [Vicryl]) makes them clearly superior to similar sizes of chromic catgut. The newer synthetic sutures are strong, which enables the surgeon to use smaller sizes, and they appear to remain stable, even when infection occurs. Braided polyglycolic acid-type sutures, as well as the monofilament poliglecaprone (Monocryl), retain much of their tensile strength for up to a month postoperatively, and the even newer, longer-lasting absorbable sutures (e.g., monofilament polydioxanone [PDS] or polyglyconate [Maxon]) seem to remain strong for up to 3 months. Because these synthetic sutures remain strong longer than catgut does in the tissue in which they are placed, wound healing progresses further before they are absorbed. In addition, there is less tissue reaction to synthetic suture during healing, resulting in a stronger scar. Finally, the formation of

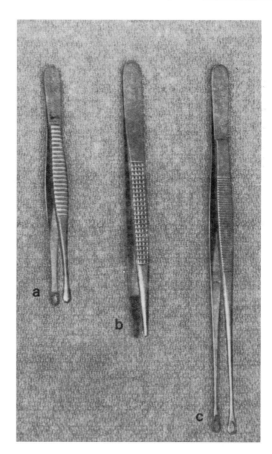

Fig. 6-8   Tissue forceps. *a,* Russian; *b,* Bonney; *c,* Single. (From Instruments and sutures. In Nichols DH, Randall CL: *Vaginal surgery,* ed 4, Baltimore, 1996, Williams & Wilkins.)

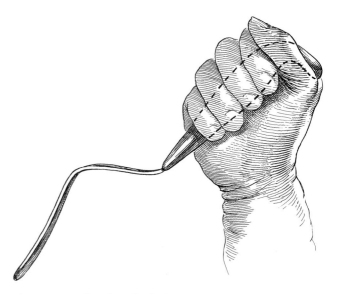

Fig. 6-9   Preferred method of holding a flat-bladed retractor, which keeps the assistant's hand out of the operator's field of view. (From Instruments and sutures. In Nichols DH, Randall CL: *Vaginal surgery,* ed 4, Baltimore, 1996, Williams & Wilkins.)

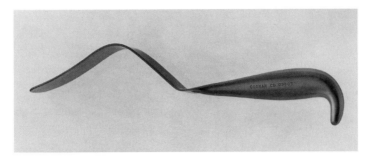

Fig. 6-10 Flat-bladed vaginal retractor CD 1106 or 098034, available in various sizes from BEI/Zinnanti Surgical Instruments, Chatsworth, CA 91311, or from the custom order department, Codman-Shurtleff, New Bedford, MA 02745. (From Instruments and sutures. In Nichols DH, Randall CL: *Vaginal surgery,* ed 4, Baltimore, 1996, Williams & Wilkins.)

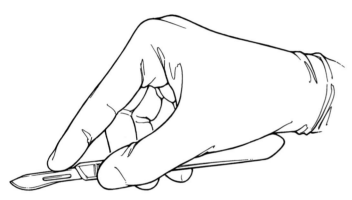

Fig. 6-11 A proper position for holding the scalpel to make an incision is identified. The index finger applies pressure against the blade.

postoperative vaginal granulation tissue is reduced markedly when synthetic sutures are used.

Polybutester (Novafil) is a unique copolymer monofilament nonabsorbable synthetic suture material that has the unique qualities of high breaking strength, similar to that of similar-sized nylon, combined with stretchability proportional to the force applied, and prompt elastic recovery. It is twice as flexible as nylon or polypropylene of similar size, yet secure knots can be formed with three or four throws. These qualities, particularly that of elastic stretching once it is in place, make it ideal for wound closure, especially when a single buried layer technique is chosen. As postoperative edema and swelling develop in the tissues in which the suture is placed, the suture stretches temporarily up to 10% to 15% of its length to lessen the chance that it will tear or strangulate the tissues in which it has been placed. As postoperative edema and swelling subside, the suture stretching contracts, taking up any slack that was produced and holding the tissues in approximation during their long healing phase. This should lessen the chance of postoperative wound dehiscence. Dehiscence unrelated to suture breakage

occurs not at the suture site itself, but lateral to the suture line.[15,16] As Wantz has noted,[19] Gore-Tex is an impervious pliable material made from Teflon. Exceedingly tiny and complex channels pass completely through the material. Fibroblasts and collagen fibers penetrate these crevices. The material is intolerant of infection, and in its presence the material should be removed because bacteria can occupy the microscopic crevices in the suture too small for phagocytes, which are too large to enter. Because the material is inert and does not incite fibroplasia, adhesions between Gore-Tex and the intestine are unlikely when the material is placed intraperitoneally.

The knot pull strength of suture material is important (Fig. 6-12) because it takes valuable time to replace sutures that break while being tied. Routine use of the larger, stronger sizes of suture material has distinct disadvantages, however. Not only does its greater strength increase the risk of tissue injury—because it permits the knots to be tied too tightly without breaking—but also its larger size incites more intensive phagocytic activity because it may not retain its tensile strength any longer than smaller sutures. Thus the use of larger sizes of suture can actually result in a weaker scar than that associated with the use of smaller sizes. In most situations, 0 or 2-0 suture is sufficient, although 3-0 or 4-0 suture is occasionally preferable, particularly in fistula repair.

Technique of Suturing

Various methods can be used to bring two edges together for suture placement. The surgeon can use either a curved needle or a straight needle. The choice depends both on the tension to which the layer is likely to be subjected and on the importance of the layer in providing essential wound support. Some methods clearly take up greater tissue slack than others and thus influence vaginal size when used during colporrhaphy.

When a curved needle has been passed through the patient's tissue, it should be grasped proximal to the point with a tissue forceps or hemostat. If the needle is curved, it

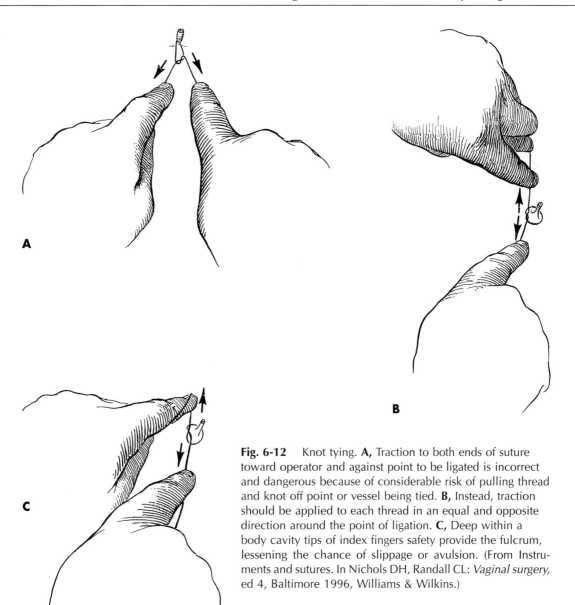

Fig. 6-12 Knot tying. **A,** Traction to both ends of suture toward operator and against point to be ligated is incorrect and dangerous because of considerable risk of pulling thread and knot off point or vessel being tied. **B,** Instead, traction should be applied to each thread in an equal and opposite direction around the point of ligation. **C,** Deep within a body cavity tips of index fingers safety provide the fulcrum, lessening the chance of slippage or avulsion. (From Instruments and sutures. In Nichols DH, Randall CL: *Vaginal surgery,* ed 4, Baltimore 1996, Williams & Wilkins.)

should not be pulled straight through, but rather pulled in the direction of the curve of the needle. This avoids bending or breaking the needle and, equally important, avoids inflicting unnecessary damage or testing of the soft tissue through which the needle has been placed. This pull-through in a curve is accomplished by a twist of the wrist in the direction of the curve, a maneuver similar in concept to that of the follow through of the arm following a golf or tennis swing.

Perforations through the surgical glove place the surgeon at risk for bloodborne infectious diseases. In one study[18] the overall perforation rate was measured at 13.3%, 62% of which were unrecognized during the surgical procedure. Most perforations occurred in the gloved fingers of the non-dominant hand, suggesting perforation due to direct grasping of the needle. More frequent use of tissue forceps to

grasp the needle should reduce this incidence. Among 2166 operations in another study,[9] the incidence of inadvertent injuries was 5.5%, 95% of which were a result of needle sticks. Most occurred at the time of wound closing, and 72.3% occurred on the left hand. Visible blood has been reported found on the hands of 38% of gynecologic surgeons wearing single gloves, but on only 2% of double-gloved surgeons.[3] Double gloving does offer significantly increased protection against needle puncture during surgery and thus offers some measure of protection against exposure to HIV or hepatitis infection. When double gloves are worn it is more comfortable for the surgeon if one of the pairs is a half size larger than that regularly worn. The larger-sized glove is donned first, over which the surgeon puts on the glove of the usual size.

A cut-resistant glove liner made of extended-chain

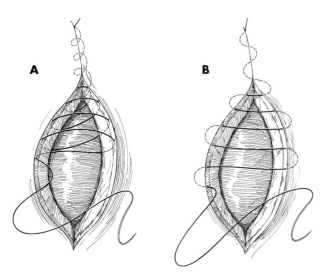

Fig. 6-13 Two methods of subcuticular closure. **A,** The full thickness of the subepithelial layer is used by a spiral-type suture placement. This is particularly useful within the walls of the vagina, where maximum strength of this fibromuscular layer will provide essential support to a healing colporrhaphy. **B,** A snakelike or zigzag suture placement is used immediately beneath the epithelial layer, which produces a superior cosmetic result. This is useful when subepithelial tissue layer strength is not a specific requirement and is particularly helpful in closing perineal skin or epithelial incisions elsewhere in the body. To prevent overlaps or wrinkling of skin edges, make each point of entry beneath the epithelial layer accurately opposite of the point of emergence of the last suture on the opposite side of the incision. (From Instruments and sutures. In Nichols DH, Randall CL: *Vaginal surgery,* ed 4, Baltimore, 1996, Williams & Wilkins.)

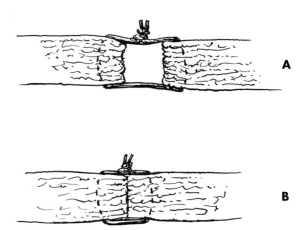

Fig. 6-14 Failure to approximate tissue layers directly during reconstruction gives rise to a suture bridge, often productive of a weak scar, particularly when there is tension on the layers being approximated **(A). B,** Desirable result of layer approximation, which provides opportunity for strong scar development between edges of closely approximated tissues. (From Instruments and sutures. In Nichols DH, Randall CL: *Vaginal surgery,* ed 4, Baltimore, 1996, Williams & Wilkins.)

polyethylene has been developed to be worn between two layers of sterile latex gloves and has been recommended for surgeons who are at high risk of injury from cuts and abrasions, although the liner did not provide protection against needle puncture.[4]

The epithelial trauma of through-and-through suture placement, which penetrates the full thickness of the wound, may release collagenase and interfere with healing.[17] Ascorbic acid antagonizes the elaboration of collagenase, so the systemic administration of vitamin C will favor healing and strong wound scarring. The subepithelial placement of sutures probably reduces this trauma, which is one reason that subcuticular closure of the vaginal wall and of the perineal skin is recommended. Another reason is that subcuticular sutures are less likely to be associated with postoperative granulation tissue than are through-and-through sutures. There are two methods of subcuticular suture placement (Fig. 6-l3); the method chosen depends on whether the full thickness of the subepithelial tissue is to be used to provide maximum strength or whether the goal is close approximation of the most superficial layer for the best cosmetic effect.

It is important to pull up the slack in the suture before tying the knot so that precise apposition of the tissues can be ensured. Any failure to approximate the tissues properly creates a suture bridge and greatly weakens the scar (Fig. 6-14). The knots must be tied square, beginning with the first cast, or the suture may fray and break. In tying a square knot, the first cast may loosen, but the second cast will slide down and remain in place if the operator applies tension on one end of the suture while tying.

In a surgeon's knot, a double turn with the first cast will remain in place; after the second cast the knot will slide down no farther. A third cast for safety is common. Learning to use the newer synthetic sutures may require some knot-tying practice. For example, monofilament sutures need an extra turn to the first cast for knot security, plus three or four additional standard casts.

When closing a hollow viscus such as the bladder or the bowel, the surgeon can place sutures either into or through the wall and can tie the knots either outside (bladder) or inside (rectum) the lumen. A second intramural layer of suture serves to reduce tension on the first layer. The mucosal layer can be included or excluded. Separate sutures can be used in the mucosa if mucosal hemostasis is required.

A pulley stitch is appropriate when it is necessary to bring one fixed tissue and one movable tissue together within a cavity or confined space (Fig. 6-15). Traction on the free end of the pulley stitch, which must be through the fixed tissue, will bring the movable tissue (through which the suture has been passed and tied) to the fixed tissue. Bringing the tissues into direct contact with one another results in a firm, strong scar.

There are several methods for the suture ligation of a pedicle (Fig. 6-16). The contents of the pedicle, the risk of

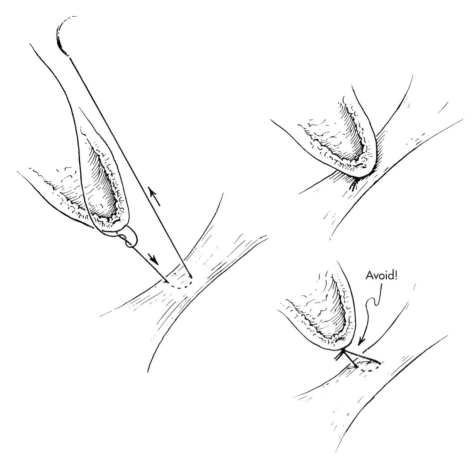

Fig. 6-15 Pulley stitch. Suture has been passed through and tied to a tissue previously mobilized, which is to be brought and fixed to the surface of an immovable structure. Traction on free end of suture after it has been passed through the immovable tissue will bring the mobilized tissue against its surface, where the suture is to be tied. (From Instruments and sutures. In Nichols DH, Randall CL: *Vaginal surgery,* ed 4, Baltimore, 1996, Williams & Wilkins.)

slippage, the tension to which the suture will be subject, and its surgical accessibility determine the method most appropriate for the situation.

Surgeons improve their technical facility in surgery if they learn to use both hands equally well. An acquired skill that requires frequent practice, this technical ambidexterity is especially helpful in the placement of sutures, the application and removal of hemostatic forceps, and knot tying.

Relationship of Sutures to Wound Healing

Although tissue reaction to suture material is proportional to the bulk of the suture material in the wound, this reaction does not determine the strength of a surgical wound closure. The strength of closure is equal to the strength of the scar plus the strength of the suture material. Immediately after closure of the wound and for the next 3 or 4 days, however, the suture material provides all the strength. This strength is approximately 40% of the strength of the tissues before surgery. As healing continues and scar tissue forms, strength increases. The suture material becomes superfluous when the wound has healed and a strong scar has formed.

A wound that does not become infected is approximately one third healed by the sixth postoperative day, two thirds by the tenth. The remaining one third of healing may require several months. Many factors, including the degree of tension applied to the margins of the wound, the biochemistry and physical condition of the particular patient, and the type of suture material used, may produce variances from these generalizations.[17]

If infection occurs, sutures can be absorbed with unusual speed; in fact, they can be absorbed so quickly that they fail to provide adequate support during the initial, critical healing period. When the suture material is nonabsorbable, infection can lead to postoperative formation of a sinus. The suture behaves as in infected foreign body, and the sinus closes only after the suture is extruded or surgically removed.

ROLE OF SURGICAL ASSISTANTS

To some, the handling of tools and tissues comes easily—almost without their conscious realization. Others must laboriously learn the many subtle ways that surgeons use their

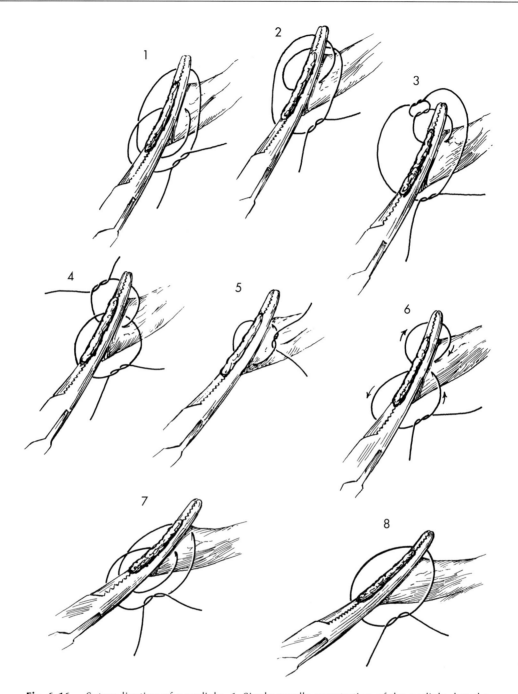

Fig. 6-16 Suture ligation of a pedicle. *1,* Single needle penetration of the pedicle, but the base is doubly ligated; *2,* toe is doubly ligated (recommended for the infundibulopelvic ligament, reinforced by a free tie); *3,* after a small loop over toe of hemostat has been tied, a second loop goes around entire pedicle; *4,* interlocking loops provide security but require a double penetration of pedicle by needle; *5,* double penetration leaves a small portion unligated; *6,* provides security but also requires a double penetration; *7,* the Heaney stitch fixes the suture at two points—the stitch is especially useful for the cardinal or uterosacral ligament and is unlikely to slip but requires a double penetration of the pedicle; *8,* a single free tie, which is most likely to slip under certain circumstances. (From American College of Surgeons. From Nichols DH: *Surg Gynecol Obstet* 147:765, 1978.)

hands to support, expose, remove, manipulate, and repair the tissues of the human body. These movements must be efficient, time-saving, and gentle enough to avoid undue damage to living cells. They require the almost unconscious integration of rather complex movements of both hands.

The hands of the principal surgeon are usually engaged in accomplishing the primary objectives of the operation. The hands of the assistant surgeons must expedite that surgeon's work. This interplay of cooperating hands can produce a flowing and beautiful pattern of teamwork—or, if done badly, it can result in a rough, halting, awkward, and time-consuming exercise.

Good surgical teamwork requires that assistants be constantly alert. They must anticipate the sequence of surgical steps and try to stay ahead of the surgeon in planning the next phase of the operation. They should take pride in seeing how often they can be in position and ready to facilitate the operation without being given specific instructions. When surgeons work together over a period of time, teamwork becomes more efficient and few words need to be spoken. The key words are to *anticipate* and *facilitate.* There is no place at the operating table for an assistant who periodically develops the glazed look of someone in a "catatonic trance." An assistant should feel embarrassed if the surgeon frequently needs to take the initiative in many of these support maneuvers.

Assistants would do well to read about the operation the night before if they are unfamiliar with the condition or planned operation. They should always review the regional anatomy before each procedure. Alert and informed assistants usually are given more operative responsibilities at an early stage of their training than those who are only "doing their job."[6]

Working with a good team of surgical assistants can be one of the great joys of a surgeon's life. The smoothness and precision of a surgical operation directly depend on the individual attention, resourcefulness, experience, and skill of the surgeon's assistants. Each member of the surgical team must know and understand his or her individual role, as well as that of every other member of the team. Experience and knowledge of the operative principles to be followed ensure that unexpected surgical events are rare; conscientious anticipation makes it possible to predict each operative step with accuracy. Advances in modern surgical technology have made this harmony among the surgical team even more important than it has been in the past. Each step during an operation should be performed correctly the first time if the patient is to obtain maximum benefit.

The patient deserves the best assistant available—one who at that moment is more interested in assisting at this particular operation than in superseding the surgeon. A retractor should remain exactly where the surgeon has placed it, the assistant resisting any temptation to move it to get a better view, lest the retractor become an unexpected weapon to the disadvantage of the operation and the patient. Surgery should be efficient, knowledgeable, and technically graceful. As Monaghan[11] has noted, "speed and ease of operating are the product of accuracy and safety. Accuracy and skill come from assiduous practice and analysis of technique. Surgery should be one smooth continuous flowing movement, without undue stops and starts or alarms and excursions."

In the large metropolitan hospitals of Europe, as well as in the small hospitals of the United States, a surgeon may have the privilege of working with the same first assistant or operative team for many years. In the large teaching hospitals of the United States, however, the academic rotation of their training programs makes it necessary for many house officers to seek in succession a maximum exposure to the art

and craft of each attending surgeon's operating room activity. This approach to training places a great burden on the senior members of the operating team to ensure that the operation not only is well performed, but also has been a learning experience for each member of the team, regardless of level of experience. "To the mature surgeon, the teaching of the minutiae of surgical technique can become tedious, with the lingering hope that trainees may have a natural sixth sense or an inherent prompt grasp without repeated admonitions."[1] Although the teaching of assistants is an essential additional responsibility for surgeons in the clinical environment, such training leads inevitably to an academic model of surgical perfection that becomes a major part of the heritage of the next generation of surgeons. The consequence of any break, accidental or intentional, in the continuity of this careful system destroys its harmony and compromises the end result.

Most books on surgical technique make operations look easy. Those who are not part of a progressive training program that exposes them to a considerable volume of surgery will not see a surgeon in trouble often enough to know how to avoid problems nor how to resolve the problems that do occur.[5] Experience with many operations makes it possible for surgeons and their assistants to think clearly and to make correct decisions under pressure. Like the surgeon, the surgical assistant must be aware that most serious postoperative complications in otherwise low-risk patients have their genesis in errors of commission or omission during the operative procedure.[7] Both must note countless details, including the patient's general condition and the readiness of suitable equipment. "A good first assistant can make a clumsy surgeon look great, but a poor first assistant can make a competent surgeon look bad."

Before Surgery

The assistant should know the surgeon's protocol for preoperative and postoperative care and should discuss with the surgeon any possible deviation to be followed in a particular case. If the planned operation is an uncommon one, the surgical assistant should describe to the scrub nurse well ahead of time the goals of the operation and any unusual technical features so that the nurse can locate and prepare rarely used instruments and sutures. "A good scrub nurse must have a flair for organization and be well trained, fast thinking and meticulous."[12] Like every other member of the operative team, the scrub nurse should be calm and not easily "rattled." Furthermore, team members including the surgeon should be well rested, if possible, and in good physical condition.

Before using a scrubbing brush, all members of the surgical team should wash their hands and forearms with soap and water to remove superficial dirt and grease that would contaminate the brush. Scrubbing should include the forearms, and the fingernails require particular attention. After scrubbing, the team should rinse their hands and forearms thoroughly, holding the hands above the level of the elbow so that water does not run from the elbows toward the hands. When the hands are being dried, no part of the towel that has touched the forearm should touch the hand, and there should never be a stroke from the forearm to the hand.

In the operating room before the surgery begins, the assistants and each member of the surgical team should maintain some distance from the others. The nurse should apply the gloves; after the final application, the surgeon may adjust the fingers and wrists. Powder should now be rinsed from the gloves with sterile water.

The assistant should look at the instrument table, observing the instruments on it and the placement of each. In an emergency, an awareness of this layout can be valuable.

During Surgery

The duty of the assistants during surgery is to help the operating surgeon. The first assistant's functions are to anticipate the needs and moves of the surgeon, try to facilitate them, and help to create maximum exposure of the operative site with proper retraction and a clear field of unobstructed vision. The second assistant carries out the wishes of the first assistant and the surgeon, restricting activities to holding instruments or retractors as instructed.

The first assistant has the responsibility of providing hemostasis with the least possible interruption as the operation proceeds. Therefore the assistant should have suction devices, clamps, scissors, ties, or the electrocautery ready for use. Tamponade of any bleeding surfaces with simple pressure should be an almost reflex motion. Sponging, which should be concentrated at the actual site of cutting, clamping, or sewing, should be by quick blotting rather than by dabbing or wiping. Suction is useful in removing blood or secretions that have accumulated away from the center of the operative site.

In clamping vessels that the surgeon has transacted by the incision, the assistant should place hemostatic clamps quickly, but carefully, to include only the vessel and a minimum of its surrounding tissues. As vessels are ligated, the clamps holding them should be opened slowly while the ligature is tightened. Generally, clamped vessels are tied off or coagulated beginning with the last one clamped. When the surgeon ties off a clamped vessel, the assistant holds up the handle of the hemostat so that the surgeon can pass the ligature around it, then drops the hand and elevates the tip of the hemostat. As soon as the hemostat has been taken off and the knot has been tied, the assistant cuts the long ends of the ligature.

In general, suture ends are cut ½ to 1 cm from the knot, as the surgeon instructs. Knots are usually square, requiring three throws if a synthetic suture is used or six if a monofilament suture is used. If the ends of a tie or suture are cut too short, the knot may slip; if the ends are left too long, they become the risk of a foreign body. If able to "palm" the suture scissors when the operation is in a phase that requires suture cutting, the assistant can continue to use the hand holding the scissors and save time (Fig. 6-17). It is also helpful if the assistant can clamp, cut, and tie with either hand.

"What might be called timing is learned only by experience. A good assistant will so time his sponging that the op-

erator experienced the minimum of interference."[5] When vessels are cut, the assistant should wait until the surgeon's hand goes back before sponging. The assistant should not grab for bleeders, but should apply pressure with the sponge and apply the hemostat to the bleeding point accurately as the sponge is removed. As far as possible, only the tip of the hemostat should be applied. When the tie keeps slipping from beneath the tip of the hemostat, another hemostat may be applied from the opposite direction just underneath the tip. The suture should be tied around both, and the second hemostat should be removed first.

It is not necessary for one assistant to do all the clamping, another to do all the tying, and a third to do all the cutting. As a rule, it is easier for the assistant to tie off hemostats on the operator's side, and vice versa. Usually, the one who holds the hemostat can cut sutures much faster and more accurately than can a second assistant who must come into the operative field at arm's length. The handle of a retractor should generally be low, and the assistant should always know where the tip of the retractor is. Assistants should not move refractors without the surgeon's request or permission because the refractors not only may fail to provide sustained exposure of the operative field, but also may cause considerable damage to the structures with which they were in contact.

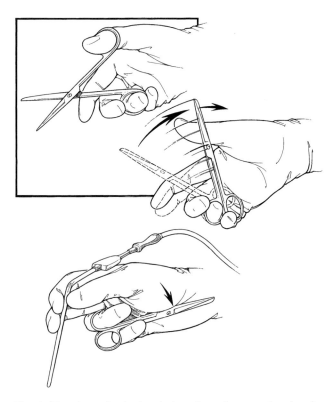

Fig. 6-17   A method of palming the scissors, whereby the scissors, grasped by the fourth finger and thumb as shown, can be quickly flipped back and forth, as indicated in the drawing. When these have been palmed, the medial three fingers of the hand are available for other purposes, such as holding a suction device, as shown, or perhaps tying knots.

Instruments should be passed in a firm and decisive manner. The scrub nurse who is watching the operative field will probably know what the surgeon is likely to want next and will be prepared for the surgeon's request. Hand signals are particularly useful both for avoiding unnecessary conversation and for saving time. Some of the widely accepted hand signals in operating rooms are illustrated in Figs. 6-18 through 6-23.

As dissection proceeds to the deeper tissues, the assistant can often provide helpful countertraction. It is often necessary to redirect the surgical spotlights at different angles to better illuminate the wound; this can be the responsibility of the assistant. As the operation proceeds, the surgeon may wish to shift or reposition the second assistant's retractors.

Surgical assistants should keep their hands as low as possible and well back from the incision when not in use. Furthermore, an assistant who must reach to the other side of any incision should reach to the side of the operative field rather than across it so as not to obstruct the surgeon's view. It is also essential for the assistant to avoid becoming so interested in the operation that he or she bends over and obstructs the surgeon's view of the operative field. However, the assistant should not take his or her eyes off the wound any more than absolutely necessary especially when holding

some piece of tissue or instrument with which the surgeon is working.

Both the surgeon and the assistant learn with experience the importance of gentleness in handling tissues. Roughness can prolong the operation by causing organ damage that requires repair; it can cause an injury that subsequently reveals itself in postoperative complications or sluggish convalescence; it can render anastomoses less than perfect; and it can precipitate immediate or delayed hemorrhage, which is perennially a major cause of avoidable morbidity.

The surgical assistant must be careful not to lean on the patient. Shifting the weight frequently and keeping the lumbar spine as straight as possible prevent the fatigue that leads to carelessness. When tying sutures, the assistant braces the arms, elbows, forearms, and wrists to prevent the hand holding one end of a tie from jerking in the opposite direction should the tie break.

The operative field must be kept orderly and neat; sponges, loose instruments, and cut suture ends should not be left lying about, but should be removed from the field whenever a pause permits. Noise is distracting to a surgical team in the operating room, and unnecessary noise can be counterproductive. Silence encourages a high level of concentration, and there is less chance of inoculating the surgical wound with the team's respiratory bacteria if they refrain from talking. Important observations concerning the operative plan or changes should be verbalized especially when the more experienced surgeon is serving as assistant to the junior, but unimportant observations are best left for another time.

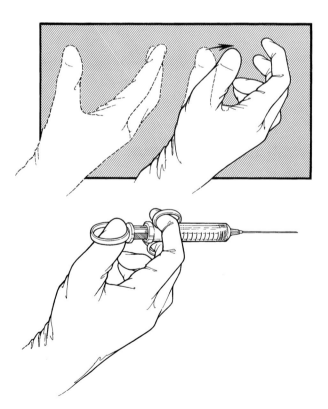

Fig. 6-18 The hand signal for requesting a hand syringe is identified, as if the syringe were already present in the empty hand. The index and middle finger fit the rings of the pressure syringe, and the thumb fits the end of the barrel; as the thumb moves toward the index finger, the injection of a solution is suggested.

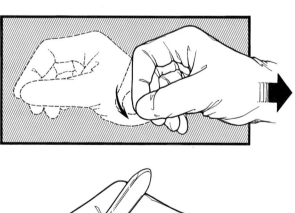

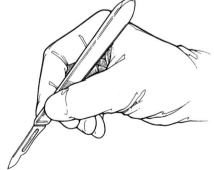

Fig. 6-19 A proper hand signal for requesting a scalpel. The fingers are in the position in which the scalpel would normally be held, and the act of cutting is indicated by bending the wrist and thumb and forefinger.

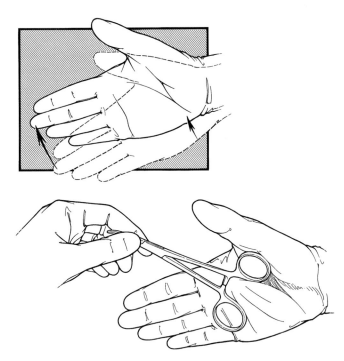

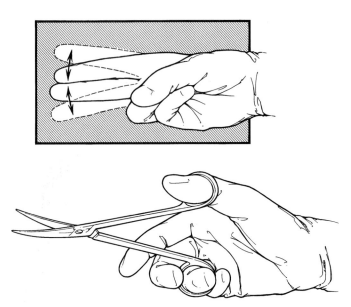

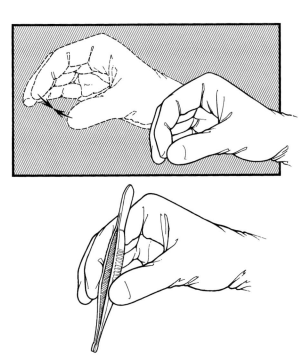

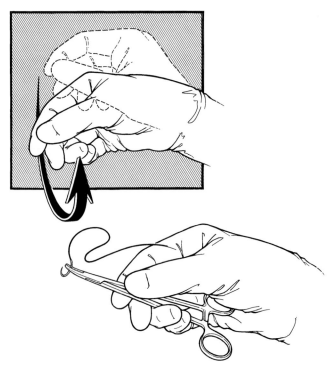

Fig. 6-20 A hand signal for requesting a hemostatic forceps. The operator extends the hand with open palm, moving it up and down so that the forceps can be placed with the rings in the palm of the hand.

Fig. 6-21 A maneuver for requesting scissors, whereby the index and middle fingers are spread in a scissorlike fashion, following which the palm is opened to receive the scissors that have been placed within it.

Fig. 6-22 The figure for requesting a thumb forceps. The hand is positioned as if it had a forceps within it and, by bringing the thumb and index finger together, the movement or motion of the forceps is suggested. The hand is then opened to receive the forceps.

Fig. 6-23 A hand signal for requesting a needle-holder and suture. The hand is poised as if it held a ligature carrier, and, with a rotary motion of the wrist in a clockwise direction, the path of the needle is indicated, and then the palm is flattened to receive the ligature carrier.

Excellence in the performance of one's duties must receive one's undivided concentration. Usually the best of surgeons were formerly the best of assistants. While the wound is being closed, the assistant should review with the surgeon the plans for postoperative care and any special routines to be implemented. In a surgical training program, the surgeon may turn a case over to the assistant, particularly if the assistant has demonstrated interest and ability while assisting the surgeon on similar cases in the past. Expecting the assistant to be aware of the patient's clinical circumstances and the details of the technique to be followed, the surgeon generally plans to become the first assistant in such a delegated case, although he or she must remain acutely observant, highly helpful, and constructively critical. The assistant should never hesitate to ask questions concerning any phase of the operation and the appropriate aftercare.

If problems arise that the assistant doing the surgery feels are beyond his or her ability to handle without compromising patient care, the assistant must immediately convey this concern to the surgeon; if the assistant would like the surgeon to take over the operation or any portion thereof, he or she must not hesitate to say so. Often, the surgeon takes care of the presumably difficult steps and, if still confident of the assistant's ability, permits the latter to resume the surgical operation. When the senior surgeon perceives that a particular maneuver is not going well and asks the assistant who is operating to stop, the assistant must obey instantly—with the hands literally frozen in mid-air, not after the movement or incision in progress has been completed. A scheduled assistant who has been invited to operate on the patient of a private attending surgeon must always remember that such an opportunity is a privilege, not a right.

After Surgery

Even when surgical assistants are tired from having been up the night before, a shower and a clean uniform do a lot to revive their spirit. Male house officers should be freshly shaven each morning. On postoperative rounds, the surgical assistant should check the patient for sweating and pallor, which may indicate internal hemorrhage; restlessness and disorientation, which may suggest cyanosis of hypoxia; and an anxious facies, which may reflect serious sepsis.

The patient's costovertebral angles should be gently jabbed, and asymmetry of discomfort should be noted and brought to the surgeon's attention lest any possible compromise of ureteral patency go undetected. Auscultation and percussion of the chest help exclude atelectasis. Auscultation of the abdomen, listening for bowel sounds, should be routine, as should palpation of the patient's calves; any departure from normal should be noted and monitored. Records of fluid intake, urinary output, and the patient's temperature should be examined.

The patient's questions and complaints should be listened to patiently and attentively, and it should be determined that all of the postoperative orders have been followed and that new ones have been written as healing progresses. Every patient should be seen at least once each day, preferably in the morning, and any difficult questions or clinical departure from normal should be discussed with the senior house officer or the attending surgeon. Patients who are ill or are not doing well should be seen more frequently during the day; when the house officer is going off duty, a report should be given personally to the incoming house officer. A legible note should be written after each visit.

Training

There is a conceptual difference between an assistant who is a fully trained professional associate and an assistant who is participating in an operation as part of a postgraduate training program. Both must have a detailed knowledge of the surgical details of the anticipated procedure and its possible complications. The professional associate, however, also is expected to be familiar by personal experience with the particular operation and to know the operator's preferential or usual approach to this surgical remedy; the individual patient may be preoperatively unknown to this assistant. In contrast, the trainee is expected to have learned the history and clinical findings that have led to surgery, to have grasped the details of the decision-making process for this particular patient, and to understand the specific reasons that this operation was chosen for this patient over alternative procedures. Furthermore, the trainee follows the patient's progress postoperatively.

Surgical Internship*

The purpose of a surgical internship is to provide interns with the opportunity to learn firsthand the surgical methods and techniques of dealing with patients employed by the most respected surgeons in the community. The intern should respond promptly to all calls regarding patients within the hospital, no matter how trivial they may seem, even if he or she is not on duty at the time. The intern should make every effort to understand all the procedures that are employed, taking care to read or inquire about those that are unfamiliar. Tact is as essential as is good judgment. Interns can acquire the latter by continually anticipating all types of situations that may arise.

If possible, an intern who is to assist a surgeon should arrive in the operating room slightly ahead of time to review the patient's chart, introduce one's self to the patient, and supervise the transport of the patient to the operating table, to have the patient prepared and draped for the start of the operation, and to become familiar with the instruments lying on the instrument stand. When the operation begins, the intern should take a place opposite the surgeon. If there is a second intern, he or she should be at the right hand of the first intern; if there is a third intern, he or she takes a position at the surgeon's left hand or between the patient's legs, depending on the patient's position on the operating table.

---

* From Christopher F: *Minor surgery,* ed 5, Philadelphia, 1944, WB Saunders.

The attending surgeon's first duty to the intern is to provide systematic instructions. Every patient in the [teaching] hospital should be accessible to the intern. The surgeon should make it a point to show the intern interesting pathologic conditions and to explain fully the reasons for the various therapeutic measures employed. The surgeon should try to have the intern perform all the operations that he or she is capable of handling and should take pains to guide and encourage the intern's first surgical efforts. A surgeon working at high tension may be unjustly impatient with the surgical team, however, and the intern should strive to be patient and self-contained under such circumstances. In no event can the surgeon subordinate the patient's welfare.

Outside the operating room, the surgeon should use questions to stimulate the intern's interests and should encourage the intern to undertake collateral reading, to attend conferences, and to conduct original investigations. The surgeon should strive to set a good example for the intern in an intellectual approach to surgical problems and in a compassionate attitude toward patients. The attending surgeon should endeavor to delegate responsibilities as far as possible and should introduce the intern to patients as a colleague. It is important for the surgeon to take the time to read all the records and orders that the intern has written and criticize them, if necessary. Above all, the surgeon must remember that the intern is human, subject to all the natural human frailties, and, therefore, susceptible to fatigue.

The intern should be loyal to the attending surgeon, even though their opinions about patient care may differ. These differences can be resolved privately—never within earshot of the patient or nurses. In addition, the intern should be loyal to the hospital, particularly in conversation with the patients, and should endeavor to explain satisfactorily circumstances, that the patient does not understand.

It is to an intern's benefit to be uniformly courteous and respectful to nurses and to address them by name. Treatment suggestions made by older, experienced nurses may well deserve careful consideration; when certain that the orders given are appropriate, however, the intern should maintain authority and not modify the orders to suit the nurse. An intern should never criticize a nurse within hearing distance of a patient.

The intern should make rounds in the evening and write orders that are consistent with patient comfort and safety and with the intern's understanding of the ideas of the attending surgeon. The intern should anticipate the needs of the patient during the night as far as possible. Inexperienced nurses may call an intern needlessly in the middle of the night, based on what the nurse considers to be a serious responsibility to the patient; interns should answer such calls patiently and courteously—never sarcastically.

Surgical Residency*

The surgical resident usually aspires to become an outstanding clinical surgeon. He may begin by acquiring a solid and

---

* From Hardy JD: The superior clinical surgeon, *Surg Gynecol Obstet* 124:1075, 1967.

wide base of knowledge and understanding of basic surgical philosophy and facts. Concurrently, he should develop strong compassion for the sick and a strong surgical conscience. Compassion does not replace the need for an accurate knowledge and application of modern technique, physiology and biochemistry . . . but in the long run, compassion does much for the total human experience, for the young surgeon's personal growth and for the general stature of the profession. A strong surgical conscience will prevent the resident from embarking unaided upon operations with which he is unprepared to cope. The resident will bear in mind that his senior surgeon is held accountable for all complications or deaths. Often the senior surgeon will silently share the responsibility for a resident's error made entirely without his presence or knowledge. Not only does a staff surgeon have a responsibility to support the resident, but the resident has a responsibility to support his surgical senior. The resident should learn early on to accept responsibility for the patients' welfares and survival. It should be assumed that a junior resident will take longer to perform a given operation than his chief, but when the operation is completed, it must be first-class. If at any point the operation is proceeding unsatisfactorily, the resident with the proper surgical conscience will consult his superior at once, before the clinical situation has been damaged or deteriorated. To do this may require a high order of courage and interpersonal relationships. It definitely requires a combination of objective honesty and genuine humility. Thus, the trainee will strive to achieve nothing less than perfection in each instance, for he will come to realize that in accepting anything less than the perfection possible under the circumstances is to subtract something from another person's life.

The residency program must last several years if it is to provide the extended experience necessary for the development of a degree of surgical maturity. In a year, a bright high school graduate can learn to perform most of the common operations expeditiously in the animal laboratory and to achieve an acceptable mortality in dogs. Such a person knows nothing of diagnosis, operative risks, alternatives, the physiologic management of complications, the exercise of sound surgical judgment, and the management of worried human beings, however. Senior residents finish their years of formative experience with a lifetime of learning ahead, confident because of their operative experience, but clearly aware of their limitations. These residents have established a firm foundation toward becoming superior clinical surgeons.

BLOOD EXPOSURE IN THE OPERATING ROOM

No member of the surgical team can afford to be indifferent to the possibility of exposure to transmissible infections in the operating room. Of surgeons, 25% have been infected with hepatitis B, and nearly 50% are at risk of infection because they have not received the highly effective hepatitis B vaccine.[13] The uniformly fatal outcome of clinical AIDS mandates the development of a line of defense against blood exposure that includes strong barriers to contact with patient blood and body fluids, improved operating room techniques, and prompt response to a blood contact or exposure event.

Surgical techniques in which it is necessary to pass the curved surgical needle through tissues require constant vigilance; blind suturing techniques in which the tip of the needle must be palpated for localization should be avoided. The passage of sharp instruments and needle-loaded ligature carriers back and forth between the instrument technician and the surgeon is hazardous. Stapled anastomoses and the use of the cautery instead of the sharp scalpel may be helpful.

A 1991 study showed that a blood contact event took place in 28% of 684 operations, involving a total of 293 operating room personnel.[14] One third of these blood contact events involved percutaneous injury, mucous membrane contact, or blood contact with nonintact skin. Most incidents were preventable. Precautions should be selected according to procedure variables such as anticipated blood loss and length of operation.

Punctures and tears of surgical gloves are the most common reasons for blood contact in the operating room. Double gloving has been shown to reduce blood contact with the hands.[10,14] Placing a glove that is a half size larger than needed over the hand with the correct size glove as a second, outer glove seems to optimize dexterity and minimize constriction of the hand. A lightweight apron worn under the gown minimizes blood contact with the operator's trunk that results from barrier failure associated with major abdominal operations such as cesarean sections. Wearing a protective eye shield also reduces the risk of blood exposure. When blood contact does occur, the application of isopropyl alcohol or povidone-iodine solution and regloving seem useful, given the virucidal effects of these two solutions.

REFERENCES

1. Cannon B: Foreword. In Edgerton MT: *The art of surgical technique,* Baltimore, 1988, Williams & Wilkins.
2. Christopher F: *Minor surgery,* ed 5, Philadelphia, 1944, WB Saunders.
3. Cohn GM, Seifer DB: Blood exposure in single versus double gloving during pelvic surgery, *Am J Obstet Gynecol* 162:715, 1990.
4. Diaz-Buxo JA: Cut-resistant glove liner for medical use, *Surg Gynecol Obstet* 172:312, 1991.
5. Dudley DG: The surgical assistant, *Surg Gynecol Obstet* 115:245, 1962.
6. Edgerton MT: *The art of surgical technique,* Baltimore, 1988, Williams & Wilkins.
7. Hardy JD: The superior clinical surgeon, *Surg Gynecol Obstet* 124:1075, 1967.
8. Hermann JB: Changes in tensile strength and knot security of surgical procedures in vivo, *Arch Surg* 106:707, 1973.
9. Hussain SA, Latif ABA, Choudhary AA: Risks to surgeons: a survey of accidental injuries during operations, *Br J Surg* 75:324, 1988.
10. Matta H, Thompson AM, Rainey JB: Does wearing two pairs of gloves protect operating theatre staff from skin contamination? *Br J Med* 297:597, 1988.
11. Monaghan TM: *Bonney's gynecological surgery,* ed 9, London, 1986, Baillière Tindall.
12. Novak F: *Surgical gynecologic techniques,* New York, 1978, John Wiley & Sons.
13. Palmer D, Barash M, King R, Neil F: Hepatitis among hospital employees, *West J Med* 138:519, 1983.
14. Popejoy SL, Fry DE: Blood contact and exposure in the operating room, *Surg Gynecol Obstet* 172:480, 1991.
15. Rodeheaver GT, Nesbit WS, Edlich RF: Novafil—a dynamic suture for wound closure, *Ann Surg* 204:193, 1986.
16. Rodeheaver GT, Borzelleca DC, Thacker JG, Edlich RF: Unique performance characteristics of Novafil, *Surg Gynecol Obstet* 164:230, 1987.
17. Sanz L, Smith S: Mechanisms of wound healing, suture material, and wound closure. In Sanz LE, editor: *Gynecologic surgery,* Oradell, NJ, 1988, Medical Economics Books.
18. Serrano CW, Wright JW, Newton ER: Surgical glove perforation in obstetrics, *Obstet Gynecol* 77:525, 1991.
19. Wantz G: Open repair of hernias of the abdominal wall. In Wilmore, Cheung, Harkers, et al, editors: *Scientific American Surgery Surgical Techniques* 6:8, Scientific American, 1995, New York.

Laparoscopic Instruments and Techniques

DAN C. MARTIN

Laparoscopy is useful for diagnosing disease and for treating gynecologic patients. The diversity of uses is reflected in the many names that have been applied to this technique, such as pelviscopy,[64] operative laparoscopy,[23,52,66] laser laparoscopy,[42] videolaseroscopy,[53] and therapeutic laparoscopy.[44] Although a distinction is often made between diagnostic and therapeutic procedures, a proper diagnosis can be beneficial to therapy.

Although this chapter covers specific complications, more complete coverage is available elsewhere.[5,38,43] Sterilizations are discussed in Chapter 34.

TISSUE EFFECTS

An important concept in laparoscopy is the tissue effect produced by various types of equipment. Four terms are generally used to describe this effect: coagulation, fulguration, vaporization, and excision.[23,33,45,46] Coagulation generally encompasses tissue heating, desiccation, cautery, denaturation, and cellular death. These effects are basically the result of heat, which can be produced by several techniques including conversion of laser light, conversion of electricity, conduction from a heat probe, and conduction from the heated tissue itself. Vaporization is produced by high-power density energy lasers or electrosurgical tips.[38,39,45] The power density must be above the vaporization threshold so that liquid and solid tissue instantaneously convert into a plume of water vapor and solid remnant. Excision can be performed with any of the various types of equipment. In the most basic form, scissors are used to excise tissue, and hemostasis is achieved with coagulation. Precise dissection has been accomplished with scissors, CO_2 lasers, sapphire-tip YAG lasers, and fine electrosurgical tips.

EQUIPMENT

Equipment can be divided into four categories: electrosurgical, mechanical, thermal, and laser. Although each of these technologies has its proponents, most gynecologists currently use many methods to individualize the approach to specific problems. Coagulators and mechanical devices appear to be the easiest to use and also the most useful for hemostasis, whereas lasers and monopolar electrosurgery can add precision.

Operating Room Setup

Regardless of which type of equipment is chosen, the operating room must be set up adequately to facilitate laparoscopic surgery. Although our operating room commonly uses one monitor placed between the patient's legs for use by both the assistant and the surgeon, other operating rooms use up to three monitors; others do not use any.

An assistant stands on the side of the patient opposite the surgeon. Two or more tables are accessible to the circulator. For procedures such as tubal cannulation, in which both laparoscopy and hysteroscopy are performed simultaneously, two complete camera systems are used. Cameras are electronically routed through a recording device such as a VHS recorder or a Polaroid camera on the electrical path to the monitor. These records are used for documentation.

Mechanical Instruments

Basic mechanical instruments that can be used in many endoscopic procedures are needles, trocars, blunt probes, irrigators, aspirators, scissors, and graspers. The probes used to manipulate and push equipment are smooth to lessen the chance of pulling tissue into the hinges of grasping forceps or scissors. These generally have centimeter markings for measuring structures in the pelvis and can be roughened or blackened for use with lasers. Some instruments have a hinge 2 to 5 cm from the end so that the probe can be angled. This increases the ability to manipulate structures and to measure tissue that is tangential to the viewing angle.

Irrigation and aspiration systems change constantly. High-pressure irrigation systems may be needed for dissection techniques. Nezhat[54] has used this type of dissection to place water barriers between targeted endometriosis and the underlying structures. An incision is made into the peritoneum, and then fluid solutions are injected under pressure into the loose connective tissue. This increases the distance between peritoneal endometriosis and the lateral vessels and ureter. Reich[61] has described the use of similar techniques to dissect organs, in which adnexa are freed from the broad ligament and cysts are dissected. Campo[7] demonstrated that the use of dissection techniques to shell a dermoid from the ovary and remove it with use of endobags decreased spill and saved time.

In addition to specifically designed systems, a standard blood pressure cuff can be used to produce pressure for irrigation. Wall suction for aspiration systems can be used to remove fluid. When the aspiration system also is used for laser or electrosurgical plume, protective filters are placed in the line to prevent the hydrocarbons in the plume from being deposited in the wall pipes. If hydrocarbons accumulate in the pipes, the pipes can become occluded and require major repair.

Different sizes of scissors and grasping forceps have been specially designed for various procedures, ranging from delicate lysis of peritubal adhesions to gross morselization of large tissue. Although one set of scissors and graspers can be used for all procedures, a combination of two or more sizes appears more useful (Figs. 7-1 and 7-2).

The development by Clarke[10] of suturing techniques and loops and the subsequent adaptation of the Roeder loop by Semm[65] preceded the development of other mechanical occlusive devices (Figs. 7-3 and 7-4). Semm subsequently developed a series of instruments including morselizers to fragment and remove large tissue masses (Fig. 7-5). Although catgut was the only suture available in the past, various sutures are now available, including polyglactin (Vicryl) and polydioxanon (PDS). In addition, small and modified needles have been developed for facilitating placement during laparoscopy (Fig. 7-6). Dissolvable clips and stapling devices have been used for laparoscopic hysterectomy, adnexal surgery, appendectomy, laparoscopic bowel resection, and thoracoscopic segmental pneumonectomy (Figs. 7-7 and 7-8).

Donnez[14] in France and Adamyan[2] have worked with fibrin-related glues, which are used within the ovary to hold the capsule together without sutures. However, results are mixed.

Transabdominal suturing of the specimen can be helpful in holding specimens toward the anterior wall for better visualization. The operator passes a 3-0 Vicryl suture on a Keith needle into the abdomen while being careful to avoid vessels. The end is held out of the abdomen. This is then used to suture the specimen, and the needle is reversed and pushed out of the abdomen and cut off. The tension on the sutures is controlled by clamping the two free ends at the abdominal surface. The suture is pulled through at the end of the procedure.

Biopsy forceps that obtain small areas of tissue for analysis also are available. However, excision using scissors, laser, or electrosurgery has been more accurate for diagnosis.[49,51]

Ring forceps, with or without a sponge, are commonly used in the vagina for mobilization. End-to-end anastomotic (EEA) dilators (20 or 25 mm), rectal probes, and the no. 4 Sims' blunt curette have been used to aid in rectal identification.

Bags designed to contain tissue decrease both the chance of contamination with cancer[34] and the operating time.[7] These bags can be commercially designed for laparoscopy, adapted for other surgical uses, or sterilized from modified sandwich bags from home. For large cysts between 8 and 10 cm, sandwich bags can be sterilized and the locking section cut off. If the locking section is left on the bags within the abdomen, the bags can lock down and be difficult to open. Once large tissue specimens are contained in the bag, the neck of the bag is pulled through a slightly enlarged incision; the cyst is visualized and then drained through the external bag before removal.

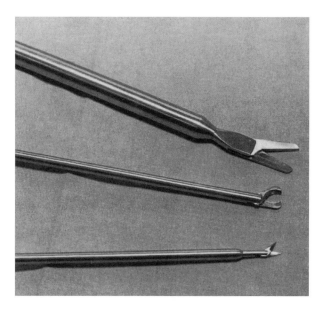

Fig. 7-1 The availability of scissors ranges from microscissors with delicate tips to heavy scissors designed to go through an 11-mm trocar.

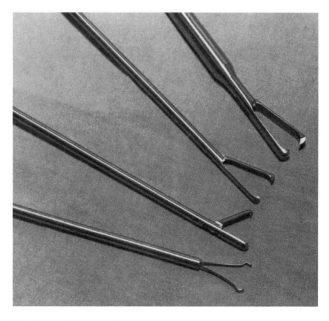

Fig. 7-2 Graspers have been designed for carrying out operations on various pelvic organs.

Robotics

Robotically assisted models are becoming increasingly sophisticated. They increase accuracy by decreasing excursions through mechanical advantage. They may decrease fatigue and pain in the neck, shoulder, and back compared with standard laparoscopic surgery. However, they do increase operating time. In one study of tubal anastomosis, the average time for conventional laparoscopic suturing was 33 minutes per tube; the average time for robotic-assisted suturing was 50 minutes per tube. This is compared to standard suturing of 15 minutes per tube.[41]

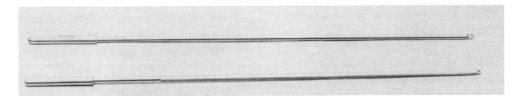

Fig. 7-3   Suturing techniques can be aided by extracorporeal ties with the knot pushed by ligature devices, such as Clarke-Reich ligators (Marlow Surgical Technologies, Inc., Willoughby, Ohio).

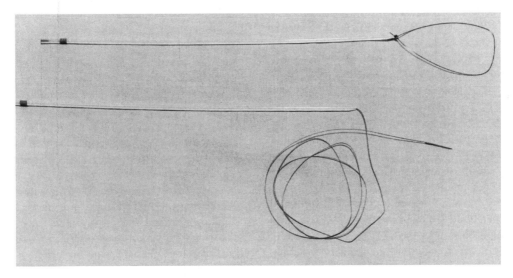

Fig. 7-4   Endoloops and Endoknots (Ethicon Endo-Surgery, Inc., Cincinnati, Ohio) have been very easy to place and use during laparoscopy.

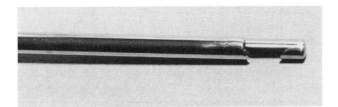

Fig. 7-5   The tissue morselizer (WISAP, Inc., Lenexa, Kan) is used to remove large fragments of tissue by slowly fragmenting the tissue with the jaws and loading it into the barrel of the morselizer.

Electrosurgical Equipment

Electrosurgical equipment consists of unipolar (Fig. 7-9) and bipolar (Fig. 7-10) modes of delivery.[38,46] For both, the tissue effect is produced by converting electrical energy into heat. At low power, this desiccates, denatures, coagulates, and destroys tissue while leaving it in place, generally referred to as *coagulation*. If the current is applied until the tissue is sufficiently heated, thermal spread by conduction occurs and the instrument acts like a cautery tip. Coagulation and cautery are the general effects of bipolar electrosurgical units. Most hospitals have bipolar electrosurgical units designed for sterilization, and newer units have smaller jaws for more precise use (Fig. 7-11). Sterilization units are broader and wider than the smaller bipolar units developed for operative procedures.

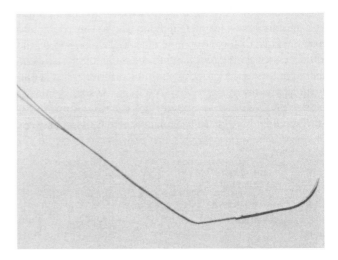

Fig. 7-6   In addition to an ever-increasing line of suture material, sutures specifically designed for use during laparoscopy are available. This ski-slope needle (Ethicon Endo-Surgery, Inc., Cincinnati, Ohio) is designed so that the straight portion can be grasped with the laparoscopic needle holder while maintaining a curved tip.

The electrical waveform has a significant influence on the tissue effect. If the peak power and the delivery unit are constant, a damped waveform has less electrical driving force and appears better for coagulation. On the other hand, an undamped waveform has more electrical driving force

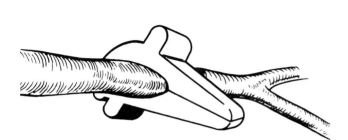

Fig. 7-7 Polydioxanon absorbable clips (Ethicon Endo-Surgery, Inc., Cincinnati, Ohio) can be used by surgeons who wish to avoid permanent devices.

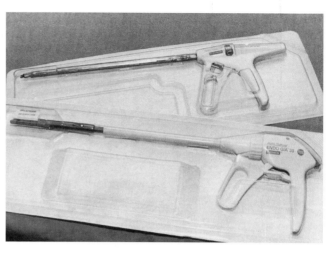

Fig. 7-8 A complete line of Endo GIA and Endo Clip (U.S. Surgical, Norwalk, Conn) instruments has been designed to aid in the removal of larger structures.

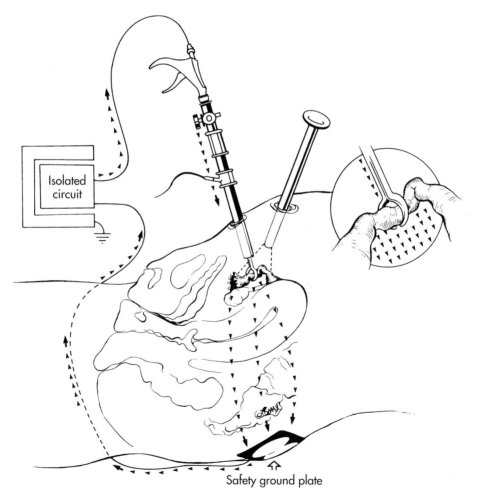

Fig. 7-9 Unipolar techniques use a single pole instrument with the action at the interaction level of a grounded patient. At high-power density, this produces vaporization; at low-power density, this produces coagulation.

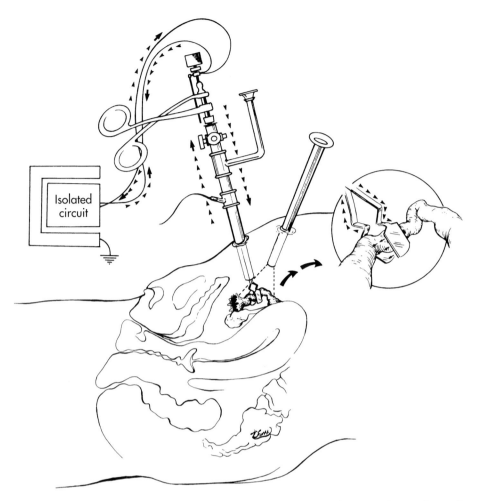

Fig. 7-10 Bipolar coagulation places both the active pole and the grounding pole on the same piece of equipment. In this arrangement, electrical flow occurs between the poles of the equipment and avoids deeper electrical damage to the patient.

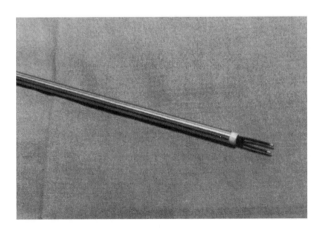

Fig. 7-11 Small, bipolar electrical tips are available for discrete bipolar coagulation (WISAP, Inc., Lenexa, Kan).

and is better for vaporization (cutting) or fulguration. Although these functions are useful for unipolar units, they do not always apply to bipolar units. A bipolar system generally works better with an undamped ("cutting") driving waveform to ensure rapid and adequate coagulation of the tissue between the jaws.

Unipolar delivery can be of low or high power. At low power, these units behave in a fashion similar to bipolar coagulation, but penetration is determined by the amount of energy delivered. On the other hand, energy transfer in bipolar coagulation occurs between the jaws of the coagulator. In addition, at high power the electrosurgical units are capable of vaporization of tissue similar to that of lasers. At power densities of approximately 60,000 W/cm^2, thermal damage from an electrosurgical unit approximates that of a CO_2 laser unit.[39]

Dangers of Electrosurgical Burn

The potential danger of any equipment causes concern. Unipolar electrosurgical burns have been caused by the equipment itself and by misuse.[3,37,71] Although deep and extensive bowel burns can be related to electrical sparking,[74] similar areas of the bowel have been banded with the Falope ring when this equipment was used to replace electrosurgery.[35] In addition, of the 11 cases reported by Thompson and Wheeless,[71] one was recognized as traumatic and five involved direct bowel burns recognized at the time of surgery. The remaining five may have been caused by the needle, the trocar, direct contact, or sparking. Borten[5]

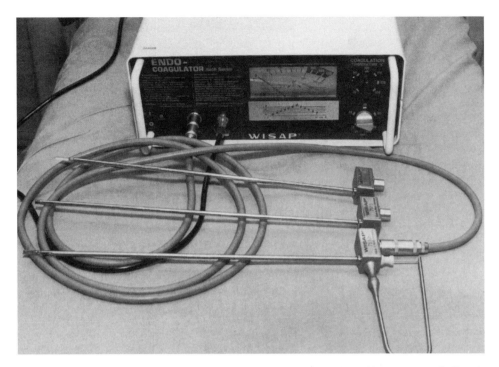

Fig. 7-12 The Endocoagulator (WISAP, Inc., Lenexa, Kan) developed by Semm is a hallmark of pelviscopy.

states that the blind spot of the single-puncture technique may be responsible for unseen accidents. It appears that all equipment can be dangerous when not used safely. Unipolar electrosurgery is safe when appropriately used. Redwine[60] has used electrosurgery to perform extensive excision of endometriosis.

Diagnosing these burns is difficult because their occurrence may go unnoticed. This is similar to cutting the bowel with scissors or lasers during adhesiolysis. When scissors are used, laparotomy may be necessary to determine if the bowel has actually been cut. Determining a burn with electrosurgery can be more difficult because the exact extent of burn may not be evident until after necrosis has occurred.[74] A patient who has progressive abdominal pain, distention, and signs of peritoneal irritation should be evaluated for the possibility of bowel perforation. This is true for all trocar insertion techniques and all types of equipment. Bowel perforation has been reported with the use of all equipment and techniques.

Endocoagulation

Endocoagulation (Fig. 7-12) is one of the hallmarks of pelviscopy[65] and is used instead of electrosurgery to avoid the potential for electrosurgical burns. Although it is possible to inadvertently produce a thermal burn, endocoagulation may be safer because of its slow mechanism of action when compared with electrosurgical or laser techniques. Although thermal units have grasping forceps, which would imply spread from both grasping jaws, the equipment frequently produces a thermal effect from one jaw only. This is used to great advantage with the thermal wedge (Fig. 7-13), which

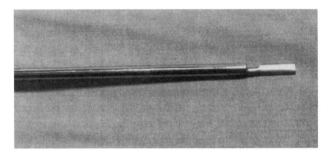

Fig. 7-13 The myoma enucleator is used to provide hemostasis at the depth of a myoma even when this cannot be seen during surgery. This helps prevent inappropriate tearing and hemorrhage from vessels coagulating them before they are seen.

can be placed behind myomas to coagulate vessels before shelling the myomas out of the uterus. On the other hand, thermal coagulation is a slow technique that can increase operating time. In addition, coagulation distorts tissue, can obscure disease, and may render treatment incomplete.

Lasers

The four lasers (Table 7-1) most commonly used in gynecology are the CO_2, argon, potassium-titanyl-phosphate (KTP), and neodymium:yttrium-aluminum-garnet (Nd:YAG).[48] The CO_2 laser produces the most predictable, "what-you-see-is-what-you-get" effect. In addition, no-touch techniques and the ability to avoid blind spots with single puncture make this a very useful and safe laser. However, mirror alignment and smoke plume can be difficult to control. This is probably

Table 7-1 Laser Wavelengths

Carbon dioxide	Infrared	10,600 nm
Nd:YAG	Infrared	1,064 nm
Helium neon	Red	632 nm
KTP	Green	532 nm
Argon	Green	515 nm
	Blue	488 nm
KrCl excimer	Ultraviolet	222 nm

the most commonly used laser for both external and internal gynecologic use.

Although thermal damage from a CO_2 laser can be limited to 100 to 500 μ, this is adequate to achieve hemostasis in most operations for infertility. The fine coagulation line created with this laser does not interfere significantly with identification of tissue planes, but coagulation or occlusive devices are needed for some vessels.

Argon, KTP, and Nd:YAG lasers can be directed down quartz fibers. All three of these lasers have a greater intrinsic depth of penetration than the CO_2 laser; the Nd:YAG laser has the greatest penetration. However, the depth of penetration is most apparent at the low-power densities used for coagulation. On the other hand, high-power densities are created with small fibers and artificial tips. These higher-power densities are associated with decreased thermal coagulation. Very small tips and high-power density can create a thermal coagulation zone similar to that of the CO_2 laser.[29,67]

As with any equipment or technique that is closely monitored, laser use is associated with complications, including hypothermia, emphysema, hemorrhage, transfusion, laparotomy, colostomy, urinary leak, and death.[47] Complication rates for laparoscopy appear to be lower than those associated with laparotomy. Furthermore, many complications occur in the initial learning phase, as was previously discussed for bowel burns.

One logistical problem that arises with the use of lasers is the variation in electrical and water requirements. Different types of equipment require a range of 110 to 240 volts, 5 to 50 amps, and up to 4 gallons per minute of water at 60 pounds per square inch. The specific requirements for setting up a laser in any operating room need to be known. Many operating rooms need to be altered to meet the requirements for water and for 220-volt single-phase current necessary for specific equipment.

INSERTION TECHNIQUES

The proponents of minilaparotomy, open trocar insertion, safety trocars, and needle insertion techniques claim a reduced risk of complications. However, these claims are based on data from small groups of patients. Of note, the Food and Drug Administration (FDA) has published a letter stating that no data are available to conclude that safety trocars are in fact safe.[13]

Any technique can be used to cut the bowel. One potential advantage of open techniques is that when the bowel is

entered it will be noted as the front wall is opened. When closed techniques are used, it is possible to penetrate both the front and back wall of bowel in one motion. Cases have been reported in which the trocar completely penetrated the bowel throughout the case. This was not noted until the equipment was removed.

The Veress needle is designed so that a mechanical hub pushes down against loose tissue and retracts against fibrous and fixed tissue. The needle is held so that the moveable hub can move. If the hub itself is held, then the apparatus does not work as designed. In addition, the air and fluid inlet valve are left open. If the abdomen is lifted as the needle is inserted, entrance into the cavity frequently meets negative pressure and allows bowel to fall away as air is sucked in. Although inserting the needle at an angle oriented toward the uterine fundus or anterior peritoneum is useful in a thin patient with the abdominal wall lifted, this may not be useful in obese patients. In obese patients, aiming the needle directly down can increase the success rate without increasing danger.[26-28]

The following insertion techniques are believed to increase safety:

- Percussion of the gas in the stomach with use of nasogastric tubes for decompression when needed
- Percussion of liver dullness
- Listening for the needle to click
- Listening for air sucked in by negative pressure on lifting the abdomen
- Using intraabdominal negative pressure to pull saline through the hub
- Injecting 10 ml of saline through the needle followed by aspiration to check for contents
- Rotating the needle to check for free motion

None of these has been completely successful.[62]

In a case of mine, the needle was directly in the middle of the transverse colon. Suction worked, water distributed and did not aspirate, and air distributed to both lateral sides because the needle was directly in the middle of the transverse colon.[1]

MARCAINE-MORPHINE BLOCKS

As outpatient procedures become increasingly complex, with multiple incisions created at laparoscopy and with minilaparotomy being used, deadening of incisional pain helps patients feel more comfortable after discharge. These blocks also have increased the sense of well-being postoperatively. A solution of 2 mg of morphine in 10 ml of 0.25% bupivacaine hydrochloride (Marcaine) is injected into the incision. The total amount used is generally 2 to 6 mg in 10 to 30 ml. This is very similar to the Marcaine blocks used by anesthesiologists for long-term pain therapy.[50]

COMPLICATIONS

Although loops increase the ease of certain surgical procedures, they are associated with specific complications. These have been associated with delayed bleeding and with ovarian remnant when salpingo-oophorectomies were performed. Bipolar cautery may be safer than loops in terms of hemostasis.[22] Furthermore, placing loops across both the proximal and distal pedicles of the tube and ovary can result in ovarian remnant.[22,55]

The dangers of insertion techniques and electrosurgical burns were discussed previously. More than 400 endoscopy-related incident reports were recorded by the FDA's Med-Watch program in 1994. An increase also was noted by the FDA's Medical Device Reporting (MDR) system. Med-Watch reported 130 incidents in 1995, which were summarized in a 1996 FDA report.[18] Many of those published incidents reported patient injury or even death. This report includes examples of vascular damage caused by an illuminator controlled by laparotomy, fire produced by placing the fiberoptic cable on a drape, fire originating in the bulb housing of a light source, which delayed the case, and electrical arc injury to a medical assistant standing next to a light source, resulting in burn and ECG changes. An air embolism occurred on insufflation through a Veress needle. Bowel laceration and vascular damage occurred with multiple instruments.[18]

Blades failed to retract and instruments were fractured, thus requiring laparotomy; some of these procedures were delayed due to nonrecognition of the complication at the time of surgery. Retroperitoneal bleeding and puncture of the ureter, liver, stomach, and pancreas were individually reported. External sparking at the metal knob of a stopcock was associated with use of a plastic threaded sleeve. A second-degree burn was noted at the junction of the light cable and laparoscope. A needle ligator misfired and lodged itself into the urethra. Bleeding from the liver was not noticed at the time of surgery because of a malfunctioning camera that had gone green, then red; no replacement was available.[18] These reports were part of the FDA's decision to issue a voluntary call for rewording of shielded trocar marketing material to eliminate any reference to safety.[13]

Surgeons' gowns were burned by sparking, and nurses' hands were lacerated by sharp equipment. A patient's leg was burned when the foot switch was activated while the instrument was resting on the drapes. Multiple small bowel burns and perforations were associated with use of bipolar forceps. Carbon dioxide embolus occurred at hysteroscopy. About twice as many incidents have been reported, covering the same material.[17] An additional 53 incidences were reported under the MDR system. Complications are much the same as in the MedWatch article.[17]

Most complications of laparoscopy appear to be clustered in the early learning phase. This clustering has been documented by the early American Association of Gynecologic Laparoscopists (AAGL) safety surveys[56,57] and more recently by the Southern Surgeons Club (SSC) in studying cholecystectomy.[69] The AAGL showed the highest incidence in the first 25 cases with a significant decline after the first 250 cases. The SSC study demonstrated that 71% of bile duct injuries occurred in the first 13 cases. This resulted in an overall incidence of 2.2% in the first 13 cases and 0.1% thereafter. Through additional training, attending

courses with a partner, group practice, and using the same assistants, 6 cases over the first 3 months or 14 cases over the first year had lower complication rates.[63] Learning time decreased between 1975 and 1991; this appears related to the current use of videoendoscopy as a teaching aid.[57,69]

A specific concern with the use of laparoscopic instruments is the possibility of dissemination of ovarian cancer. An environment rich in carbon dioxide[72] or the small incisions used in laparoscopy* may contribute to an increased rate of tumor implantation. Bags to limit spill and spread can be used for tumors up to 12 cm.[59] However, only 7% of stage I cancers were removed with any type of bag in one review.[34]

ECONOMIC IMPACT

Studies of laparoscopy often demonstrate cost savings and quicker return to normal activities.[11,12,36] This can be particularly true if both direct and indirect costs are analyzed.[16] However, this may be related to expectation rather than biology; endoscopy can increase rather than decrease cost.[24,31,70,73] Current expansion into increasingly complex procedures can add to the time and cost rather than decrease it.[41]

One other area of concern and cost is the increased use of disposable equipment. Although some contend that replacing permanent equipment with disposable is economical, until this happens, hospitals will still place both the permanent and disposable equipment on the table. The net effect at cholecystectomy is an increase of $425 when compared with nondisposable equipment. When this was added to the use of a laser and the routine use of cholangiography, there was an increase of $1271 per case compared with the cost of electrosurgery, permanent sutures, and selective cholangiography.[73]

A second area of concern is that much of our history of hospitalizing patients is based on tradition rather than need. Outpatient laparotomy for tubal anastomosis, myomectomy, ovarian cystectomy, salpingoneostomy, tubouterine implantation, partial or total salpingectomy or oophorectomy, adhesiolysis, ectopic pregnancy, vaginal hysterectomy, and laparoscopically assisted hysterectomy has been used successfully.† Even open appendectomy is less expensive, and return to work is not significantly affected when compared with laparoscopy for appendectomy.[75] Patients who pay for expenses out of pocket use outpatient services more commonly than others.[6]

Bipolar coagulators, unipolar electrosurgery, thermal cautery, and lasers can be used to coagulate, vaporize, or excise tissue. Combining these techniques can be better than concentrating on any one of them. Changes in the use of this equipment have been rapid, and attending quality update courses appears essential in the development and maintenance of optimal techniques.

---

*References 8, 9, 21, 32, 34, 40.
†References 4, 15, 19, 20, 25, 30, 58, 68, 70.

REFERENCES

1. Adamson GD, Martin DC: *Endoscopic management of gynecologic disease,* Philadelphia, 1996, Lippincott-Raven.
2. Adamyan LV, Myinbayev OA, Kulakov VI: Use of fibrin glue in obstetrics and gynecology: a review of the literature, *Int J Fertil* 36:76, 1991.
3. Baumann H, Jaeger P, Huch A: Ureteral injury after laparoscopic tubal sterilization by bipolar electrocoagulation, *Obstet Gynecol* 71:483, 1988.
4. Berger GS: Outpatient pelvic laparotomy, *J Reprod Med* 39:569, 1994.
5. Borten M, Freidman EA: *Laparoscopic complications: prevention and management,* Philadelphia, 1986, BC Decker.
6. Browne DS, Frazer MI: Hysterectomy revisited, *Aust N Z J Obstet Gynaecol* 31:148, 1991.
7. Campo S, Garcea N: Laparoscopic conservative excision of ovarian dermoid cysts with and without an endobag, *J Am Assoc Gynecol Laparosc* 5:165, 1998.
8. Canis M, Botchorishvili R, Wattiez A, et al: Tumor growth and dissemination after laparotomy and CO_2 pneumoperitoneum: a rat ovarian cancer model, *Obstet Gynecol* 92:104, 1998.
9. Childers JM, Aqua KA, Surwit EA, et al: Abdominal-wall tumor implantation after laparoscopy for malignant conditions, *Obstet Gynecol* 84:765, 1994.
10. Clarke HC: Laparoscopy—new instruments for suturing and ligation, *Fertil Steril* 23:274, 1972.
11. Demco LA: Cost comparison of Canadian and US abdominal and laparoscopic hysterectomy and cholecystectomy surgery, *Gynaecol Endosc* 6:177, 1997.
12. Demco L, Culham B: Cost analysis of gynaecological endoscopy, *Gynaecol Endosc* 6:173, 1997.
13. Department of Health and Human Services: Food and Drug Administration letter to Manufacturers of Laparoscopic Trocars, Rockville, Md, Aug 23, 1996.
14. Donnez J, Nisolle M, Karaman Y, et al: CO_2 laser laparoscopy in peritoneal endometriosis and in ovarian endometrial cyst, *J Gynecol Surg* 5:361, 1989.
15. Dorsey JH, Holtz PM, Griffiths RI, et al: Costs and charges associated with three alternative techniques of hysterectomy, *N Engl J Med* 335:476, 1996.
16. Ellstrom M, Ferraz-Nunes J, Hahlin M, Olsson JH: A randomized trial with a cost-consequence analysis after laparoscopic and abdominal hysterectomy, *Obstet Gynecol* 91:30, 1998.
17. Food and Drug Administration: Incident report revisited: focus on the medical device reporting system, *Minim Invasive Surg Nurs* 10:80, 1996.
18. Food and Drug Administration, MedWatch: Number of MedWatch incident reports jumps, *Minim Invasive Surg Nurs* 10:44, 1996.
19. Foulk RA, Steiger RM: Operative management of ectopic pregnancy: a cost analysis, *Am J Obstet Gynecol* 175:90, 1996.
20. Frishman GN, Seifer DB: Laparoscopic-assisted tubal anastomosis, *J Am Assoc Gynecol Laparosc* 2:411, 1995.
21. Gleeson NC, Nicosia SV, Mark JE, et al: Abdominal wall metastases from ovarian cancer after laparoscopy, *Am J Obstet Gynecol* 169:522, 1993.
22. Goldberg J: Complications of laparoscopic salpingo-oophorectomy, *J Gynecol Surg* 11:51, 1995.
23. Gomel V: Operative laparoscopy: time for acceptance, *Fertil Steril* 52:1, 1989.
24. Grimes DA: Technology follies: the uncritical acceptance of medical innovation, *JAMA* 269:3030, 1993.
25. Hunt R: Personal communication on outpatient laparotomy for microsurgical anastomosis, 1987.
26. Hurd WH, Pearl ML: Avoiding and recognizing blood vessel injuries during laparoscopy, *The Female Patient* 19:33, 1994.
27. Hurd WH, Bude RO, DeLancey JO, et al: Abdominal wall characterization with magnetic resonance imaging and computed tomography: the effect of obesity on the laparoscopic approach, *J Reprod Med* 36:473, 1991.
28. Hurd WW, Bude RO, DeLancey JO, Pearl ML: The relationship of the umbilicus to the aortic bifurcation: implications for laparoscopic technique, *Obstet Gynecol* 80:48, 1992.
29. Joffe SN, Brackett KA, Sankar MY, Daikuzono N: Resection of the liver with the Nd:YAG laser, *Surg Gynecol Obstet* 163:437, 1986.
30. Johns DA, Carrera B, Jones J, et al: The medical and economic impact of laparoscopically assisted vaginal hysterectomy in a large, metropolitan not-for-profit hospital, *Am J Obstet Gynecol* 172:1709, 1995.
31. Jordan AM: Hospital charges for laparoscopic and open cholecystectomy, *JAMA* 266:3425, 1991.
32. Kadar N: Laparoscopic management of gynaecological malignancies: time to quit? I. *Gynaecol Endosc* 6:135, 1997.
33. Kelly HA, Ward GE: *Electrosurgery,* Philadelphia, 1932, WB Saunders.
34. Kindermann G, Maassen V, Kuhn W: Laparoscopic management of ovarian tumors subsequently diagnosed as malignant, *J Pelvic Surg* 2:245, 1996.
35. King T: Appendiceal and bowel applications of Falope rings occurred, personal communication, Nov 20, 1986.
36. Levine RL: Economic impact of pelviscopic surgery, *J Reprod Med* 30:655, 1985.
37. Levy BS, Soderstrom RM, Dail DH: Bowel injuries during laparoscopy: gross anatomy and histology, *J Reprod Med* 30:168, 1985.
38. Luciano AA, Soderstrom RM, Martin DC: Essential principles of electrosurgery in operative laparoscopy, *J Am Assoc Gynecol Laparosc* 1:189, 1994.
39. Luciano AA, Whitman G, Maier DB, et al: A comparison of thermal injury, healing patterns, and postoperative adhesion formation following CO_2 laser and electromicrosurgery, *Fertil Steril* 48:1025, 1987.
40. Maiman M, Seltzer V, Boyce J: Laparoscopic excision of ovarian neoplasms subsequently found to be malignant, *Obstet Gynecol* 77:563, 1991.
41. Margossian H, Garcia-Ruiz A, Falcone T, et al: Robotically assisted laparoscopic tubal anastomosis in a porcine model: a pilot study, *J Laparoendosc Adv Surg Tech* 8:69, 1998.
42. Martin DC: CO_2 laser laparoscopy for endometriosis associated with infertility, *J Reprod Med* 31:1089, 1986.
43. Martin DC: *Manual of endoscopy,* Santa Fe Springs, 1990, AAGL.
44. Martin DC: Therapeutic laparoscopy. In Martin DC, editor: *Laparoscopic appearance of endometriosis,* Memphis, 1990, Resurge Press.
45. Martin DC: Tissue effects of lasers, *Semin Reprod Endocrinol* 9:127, 1991.
46. Martin DC: Tissue effects of lasers and electrosurgery. In Vitale GC, Sanfilippo JS, Perissat J, editors: *Laparoscopic surgery: an atlas for general surgeons,* Philadelphia, 1995, JB Lippincott.
47. Martin DC, Diamond MP: Operative laparoscopy: comparison of lasers with other techniques, *Curr Probl Obstet Gynecol Fertil* 9:563, 1986.
48. Martin DC, Diamond MP, Yussman MA: Laser laparoscopy for infertility surgery. In Sanfilippo JS, Levine RL, editors: *Operative gynecologic endoscopy,* New York, 1989, Springer-Verlag.
49. Martin DC, Hubert GD, Vander Zwaag R, El-Zeky FA: Laparoscopic appearances of peritoneal endometriosis, *Fertil Steril* 51:63, 1989.
50. Martin DC, Mays KS: Anesthetic/analgesic block for focal tenderness. In Coutinho EM, Spinola P, de Moura LH, editors: *Progress in the management of endometriosis,* London, 1995, Parthenon Publishing.
51. Martin DC, Vander Zwagg R: Excisional techniques for endometriosis with the CO_2 laser laparoscope, *J Reprod Med* 32:753, 1987.
52. Murphy AA: Operative laparoscopy, *Fertil Steril* 47:1, 1987.
53. Nezhat C, Crowgey SR, Nezhat F: Videolaseroscopy for the treatment of endometriosis associated with infertility, *Fertil Steril* 51:237, 1989.
54. Nezhat C, Nezhat FR: Safe laser endoscopic excision or vaporization of peritoneal endometriosis, *Fertil Steril* 52:149, 1989.
55. Nezhat F, Nezhat C: Operative laparoscopy for the treatment of ovarian remnant syndrome, *Fertil Steril* 57:1003, 1992.
56. Phillips J, Hulka J, Keith D, et al: Laparoscopic procedures: a national survey for 1975, *J Reprod Med* 18:219, 1977.

57. Phillips J, Keith D, Keith L, et al: Survey of gynecologic laparoscopy for 1974, *J Reprod Med* 15:45, 1975.

58. Powers TW, Goodno JA Jr, Harris VD: The outpatient vaginal hysterectomy, *Am J Obstet Gynecol* 168:1875, 1993.

59. Quinlan D, Townsend DE, Johnson GH: Safe and cost-effective laparoscopic removal of adnexal masses, *J Am Assoc Gynecol Laparosc* 4:215, 1997.

60. Redwine DB: Laparoscopic excision of endometriosis with 3-mm scissors: comparison of operating times between sharp excision and electro-excision, *J Am Assoc Gynecol Laparosc* 1:24, 1993.

61. Reich H: Laparoscopic treatment of extensive pelvic adhesions, including hydrosalpinx, *J Reprod Med* 32:736, 1987.

62. Rosen DM, Lam AM, Chapman M, et al: Methods of creating pneumoperitoneum: a review of techniques and complications, *Obstet Gynecol Surv* 53:167, 1998.

63. See WA, Cooper CS, Fisher RJ: Predictors of laparoscopic complications after formal training in laparoscopic surgery, *JAMA* 270:2689, 1993.

64. Semm K: New methods of pelviscopy (gynecologic laparoscopy) for myomectomy, ovariectomy, tubectomy, and adnectomy, *Endoscopy* 2:85, 1979.

65. Semm K, Friedrich ER: *Operative manual for endoscopic abdominal surgery,* Chicago, 1987, Mosby.

66. Semm K, Mettler L: Technical progress in pelvic surgery via operative laparoscopy, *Am J Obstet Gynecol* 138:121, 1980.

67. Shirk GJ: Use of the Nd:YAG laser for the treatment of endometriosis, *Am J Obstet Gynecol* 160:1344, 1989.

68. Slowey MJ, Coddington CC: Microsurgical tubal anastomoses performed as an outpatient procedure by minilaparotomy are less expensive and as safe as those performed as an inpatient procedure, *Fertil Steril* 69:492, 1998.

69. Southern Surgeons Club: A prospective analysis of 1518 laparoscopic cholecystectomies, *N Engl J Med* 324:1073, 1991.

70. Summitt RL Jr, Stovall TG, Lipscomb GH, Ling FW: Randomized comparison of laparoscopy-assisted vaginal hysterectomy with standard vaginal hysterectomy in an outpatient setting, *Obstet Gynecol* 80:895, 1992.

71. Thompson BH, Wheeless CR Jr: Gastrointestinal complications of laparoscopy sterilization, *Obstet Gynecol* 41:669, 1973.

72. Volz J, Koster S, Schaeff B, Paolucci V: Laparoscopic surgery: the effects of insufflation gas on tumor-induced lethality in nude mice, *Am J Obstet Gynecol* 178:793, 1998.

73. Voyles CR, Petro AB, Meena AL, et al: A practical approach to laparoscopic cholecystectomy, *Am J Surg* 161:365, 1991.

74. Wheeless CR: *Thermal gastrointestinal injuries.* In Phillips JM, editor: *Laparoscopy,* Baltimore, 1977, Williams & Wilkins.

75. Williams MD, Collins JN, Wright TF, Fenoglio ME: Laparoscopic versus open appendectomy, *South Med J* 89:668, 1996.

8 Cystoscopy

NEIL D. JACKSON

For far too long the female pelvis has been artificially compartmentalized into anterior, posterior, and intermediate zones of specialized interest. These artificial compartments of primary interest have left the patient with complex problems involving more than one pelvic zone and have resulted in receiving less than comprehensive care from attending physicians. Consequently, a patient with complex problems of pelvic support and function has been compelled to go from physician to physician to address all the elements of her problem. This frequently has led to more than one operation and more than one anesthetic to ultimately treat all her problems.

A look into the past often demonstrates the habit of relearning what was prior practice. For example, over the past 2 decades, specialists who treat the female pelvis have expressed an increased appreciation and understanding of the diagnostic techniques and tools of our fellow colleagues. Howard Kelly,[7] often referred to as the father of modern gynecology, employed an early cystoscope and wrote frequently in the urology literature. A classic lesion in identifying patients with interstitial cystitis is Hunner's ulcer; few of us remember that Guy Hunner was a gynecologist and was visualizing the bladder with a rudimentary air cystoscope. An air cystoscope with illumination provided by a head mirror and a candle was an early instrument used by another early pioneer in gynecology, J. Marion Sims.

HISTORY

The early development of the cystoscope is credited to Philipp Bozzini of Frankfort, Germany.[2] In 1806 he designed the first cystoscope, which was a series of funnels supported by a light stand. The funnels were inserted into the urethra, and a candle served as the illumination source, with a mirror reflecting the light down the hollow of the funnel. Twenty years later Pierre Segalas simplified the handling of the instrument by adding a rubber stylet for introduction into the urethra and further modifying the instrument so that the light source was less likely to burn the investigator. However, Antonin Desormeaux developed the first practical instrument, adapting both straight and bent tubes with varying angulation to facilitate inspection of more of the bladder surface.

Later in the nineteenth century Max Nitze developed a lens system that further increased the field of vision. Utilizing prismatic physics he was able to invert the image seen through the scope, turning the previously inverted image to an upright view.[20] With the introduction of the electric lamp for illumination, Hopkins added a lens system in 1954 consisting of long glass blocks interspersed by short air locks that improved visual clarity—a principle of the lens systems used in the rigid cystoscopes of today.[5]

INSTRUMENTATION

The cystoscope is an important and valuable instrument for viewing the bladder, urethra, and ureteral orifices. In simplest terms, it is a tube with a series of lenses and a light-conducting medium for illumination and visualization. The arrangement of the lenses can provide for direct vision or varied angulation for observation of all recesses of the bladder and urethra. Illumination is provided by a fiber-optic light source connected to the rod-lens conducting bundle within the scope, thereby providing "cool light" within the bladder[6] (Fig. 8-1).

The basic cystoscope consists of an outer sheath with a sliding removable inner obturator for introduction, a bridge, and a telescope with terminal eyepiece. The outer sheath provides a port for introduction of distending fluids and for surgical instruments. The bridge may be fitted with a moveable lever (Albarran lever) at the working end for manipulation of ureteral catheters or other instruments. There are two types of cystoscopes—rigid and flexible. The difference between the two is the internal fiber-optic bundle in the flexible scope as opposed to the rod-lens system in the rigid scope. The rigid scope provides sharper optics, a larger diameter for water flow, a larger working channel that permits the use of a greater range of accessory medical instruments, and greater stability and ease of orientation during cystoscopic perusal of the bladder.[1] With the rigid rod-lens cystoscope, separate lens scopes of 30 degrees, 70 degrees, and 120 degree retroview lens may be necessary for viewing the entire surface of the bladder. In most instances, however, the 30 degree lens may be sufficient, particularly for an experienced observer.

In 1973 Tsuchida reported on the development of a flexible fiber-optic cystoscope. This optical system consisted of a single image-bearing fiber-optic bundle of coated parallel optical fibers and two light-bearing fiber-optic bundles that can transmit light even when bent. The flexible scope is smaller and more comfortable for the patient than the rigid scope. It can be used with the patient in the supine position and has greater maneuverability past a partial obstruction.[19] The tip of the flexible scope can be moved 180 to 220 degrees by a thumb control located adjacent to the eyepiece. It

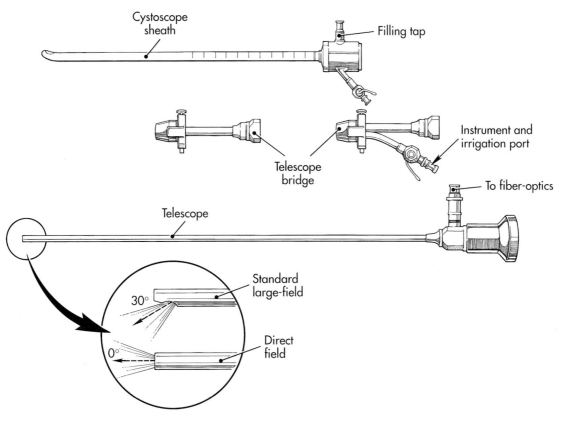

Fig. 8-1   Standard irrigating cystoscope.

has an irrigating port and allows for the introduction of guide wires, dilators, and so forth. For the most part, examination of women is comprehensive and well tolerated with the rigid scope.

The eyepiece of either type of scope can be connected to a small television camera and television monitor for educational purposes. Videotaping and Polaroid still-photography can be captured for documentation and later review.

The lens system within the rigid telescope can be set at 0 degrees, which provides straight-on viewing and is especially adapted for urethral inspection. The 30-degree angled lens telescope provides easy inspection of the bladder base and trigone, whereas the 70- and 120-degree scopes facilitate inspection of the sidewalls, dome of the bladder, and urethrovesical neck in a retroview fashion. However, in most instances the bladder and urethra can be completely inspected with a 0-degree and 30-degree telescope, particularly with television monitoring, rotation, and angling of the telescope while holding the television camera steady.

Cystoscopes are made in a variety of sizes from 6 to 25 Fr. The smaller 6 to 8 Fr is suitable for pediatric patients. For office outpatient cystoscopy, 18 to 22 Fr satisfies most purposes.

CYSTOSCOPY

The thought of any invasive procedure weighs heavily in the mind of the patient whose only knowledge of the procedure may have been from a less than accurate, but well-meaning nonprofessional source. A careful and gentle description of the intended procedure, in the comfort of the consultation room before moving to the examining room and disrobing, can go a long way in diffusing patient anxiety.

Cystoscopy is conducted in the lithotomy position with the legs abducted and supported. This may be conducted in specially designed cystoscopy chairs or a birthing chair. A distention medium is necessary for viewing the periphery of the urethra and bladder. Sterile water, normal saline, or lactated Ringer's solution may be used. *If electrocoagulation is likely, one should not use electrolyte solutions.* After antiseptic preparation of the skin, the sheath with the obturator is introduced past the meatus. The tip of the sheath has an anterior angulation or slight J-shape configuration that should be introduced first by elevating the opposite end, thereby creating the least potential for trauma to the urethral mucosa (Fig. 8-2).

The obturator is removed and the 0 angle telescope fixed in position. With the urethral lumen centered in the field, the scope is advanced with the distention medium running until the entire urethra has been visualized. At the urethrovesical junction, anterior finger pressure from the vagina can occlude the entrance to the bladder, and a panoramic view of the urethra can uncover inflammation, polyps, fronds, diverticulum deformity, or breaks in mucosal integrity (Fig. 8-3).

The opening to a urethral diverticulum may be hidden in a mucosal fold. Compression of the urethra with the finger in the vagina may create an efflux of secretion from a urethral diverticulum, which in turn will be seen through the scope, a technique proposed by Robertson[13] using an air or carbon dioxide distention medium. Withdrawal of the scope to the mid-urethra while the patient strains indicates the degree of mobility of the proximal urethra and, when compared to the Q-tip test, may further confirm the degree of mobility of the bladder neck. With the flow of the distention medium turned off and the telescope in the midurethra, the neck of the bladder should be closed or nearly so and remain so when the patient is asked to cough. Failure to remain closed suggests intrinsic urethral sphincter deficiency.[15] Assessment of the effectiveness of Kegel's squeezes can be made and viewed by the patient if television monitoring is employed, providing a great opportunity for biofeedback of this important exercise. Seeing the results of one's own efforts provides positive comprehensive understanding of the merit of such exercises.

Any discomfort can be modified by intraurethral instillation of 1% lidocaine (Xylocaine) gel at the start of the procedure, although this can alter the appearance of the urethral mucosa and may be omitted if the unadulterated appearance of the urethral epithelium is desired. In patients with meatal stenosis, dilation of the stenosis may be necessary to pass the cystoscope. To achieve dilation, the base of the bladder and bladder pillar can be infiltrated with local anesthetic to provide patient comfort.[11] A 30-degree telescope is satisfactory for inspection of the bladder. The base of the bladder is comprised of granular-appearing epithelium at the trigone—the triangular area bordered by the two ureters and the urethra. The granular appearance is due to squamous metaplasia. A raised ridge of epithelium (interureteric ridge) extends between the ureteral ostia. Since urine is delivered to the bladder from the kidneys in peristaltic waves, one can wait a few moments with the ureteral os in view and observe the os open and an eddy current of urine being ejected into the bladder (Figs. 8-4 and 8-5). The time interval between peristaltic spurts varies according to the degree of patient hydration at the time of examination.

If one is particularly interested in confirming the patency of the ureters or is in doubt as to identification of the ureteral ostia, intravenous injection of methylene blue or indigo carmine is easily done. The dye is excreted by the kidneys and appears as a blue stream ejected from the ureteral openings. Asymptomatic congenital abnormalities of the urinary tract are common, second only to the circulatory system in frequency of occurrence. Absence of one ureteral opening, un-

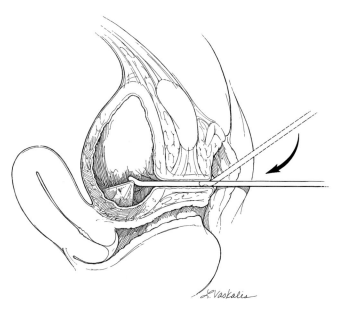

Fig. 8-2   Method of introducing a cystoscope.

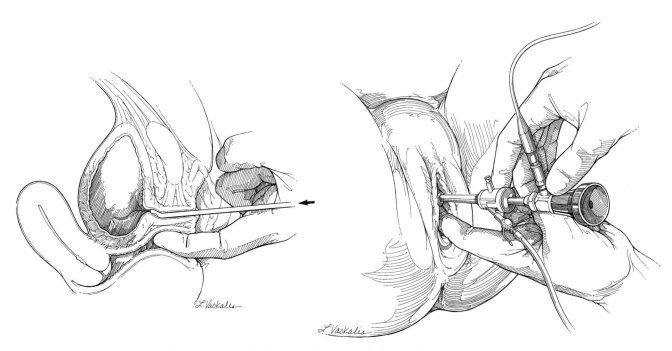

Fig. 8-3   Use of a finger in the vagina helps guide the cystoscope.

usual placement of the opening, or more than two openings may indicate a congenital abnormality and thus warrants further documentation by imaging studies.

A thorough examination of the bladder should include all bladder surfaces. This may require more than one telescope with different mirror angulations, particularly for examining the anterior dome of the bladder. Systematic perusal around the clock ensures total inclusion. The dome is marked by an air bubble that accompanies each cystoscopy. Complete examination is achieved by rotating the telescope and changing the long axis angle that the scope makes with the long axis of the patient.

The position of the bladder base at rest and with the patient straining provides accurate assessment of the integrity of bladder support. Attention to the epithelium, its vascularity, continuity, smoothness, and the presence of any polyps, stones, areas of friability, bleeding, or foreign bodies should be noted in size and location. Further documentation with videotaping or photographs aids subsequent examiners in locating the area under investigation. Certainly one is not going to become an expert cystoscopist without long apprenticed, supervised training, but an appreciation of the normal is attainable with supervised practice. Departures from the normal can serve a basis for referral to a trained urologist, which benefits the patient.

In patients who have undergone previous surgery, particularly for incontinence or reconstructive pelvic surgery, the possible infiltration of suture material in the bladder must be kept in mind (Fig. 8-6).

Generally, bladder tumors occur less frequently in women than in men. They can occur at any age, but most often develop in those 65 to 70 years of age.[3,10] Bladder cancer is the eighth most common cancer in women, accounting for 4% of cancers in women. The majority of transitional cell tumors occur at the base of the bladder. Many have a papillary, pedunculated, or polypoid appearance. Early lesions such as carcinoma in situ may be difficult to distinguish from normal epithelium, at best appearing as

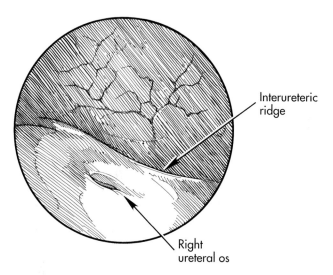

Interureteric ridge

Right ureteral os

Fig. 8-4   Cystoscopic view of normal ureter.

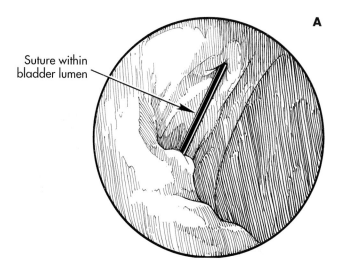

A

Suture within bladder lumen

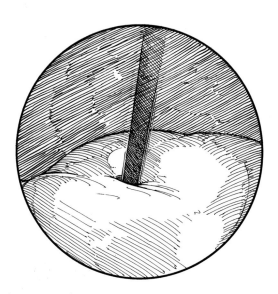

Fig. 8-5   Indigo carmine reflux from a normal ureter.

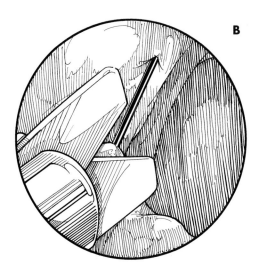

B

Fig. 8-6   **A-B,** Suture within bladder lumen.

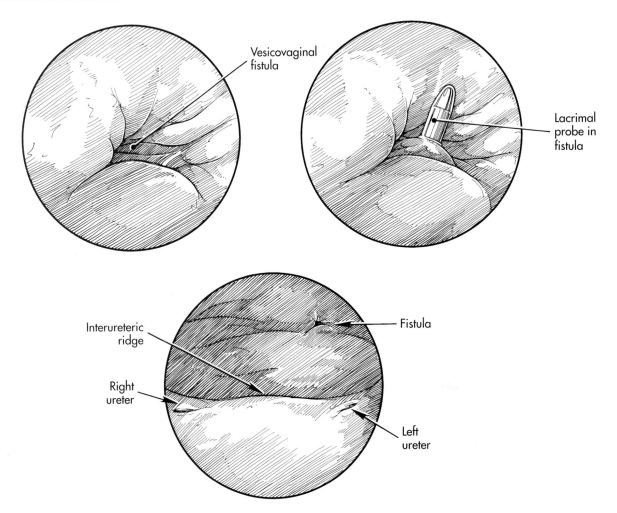

Vesicovaginal
fistula

Lacrimal
probe in
fistula

Interureteric
ridge

Fistula

Right
ureter

Left
ureter

Fig. 8-7   Vesicovaginal fistula.

velvety erythematous lesions. Discovery of any such abnormalities or of abnormal urine cytology should be referred for urologic consultation. In the past 2 decades the occurrence of bladder cancer has increased, but at the same time the death rate from bladder cancer has steadily declined, likely attributable to improved early detection.

Vesicovaginal fistula in the United States most commonly is the result of operative trauma. The bladder has a great propensity for healing, and when entered and subsequently repaired it often heals completely. The most common reason for fistula formation is *unrecognized injury* to the bladder.[9] Those fistulas that occur after hysterectomy frequently are found at the bladder base above the trigone[8,14] (Fig. 8-7).

Cystoscopically, the proximity of the ureters to the bladder is an important determination in examining for repair. Close proximity may require stenting of the ureters to avoid ureteral compromise during the repair. When one fistula is found, more may be present, so careful cystoscopic examination is a key to discovery of all defects.[17]

With the close proximity of the bladder during surgery for incontinence and pelvic reconstruction, discovery of any sutures in the bladder at the time of surgery is extremely important.[16] Even in the most experienced hands, an unintended bladder suture placement may occur, occasionally as the result of the constraint of scarring and concurrent pathology. Careful cystoscopic examination of the bladder leads to its discovery and timely removal.

In abdominal operations it is possible to perform cystoscopy even before closing the abdomen. An alternative is to examine the bladder from above with the cystoscopic or laparoscopic telescope.[18] A purse-string suture is placed in the dome of the bladder, and a telescope is introduced through a small incision in the bladder dome. With the purse-string suture tightened and closed by clamping it to prevent leakage, the bladder can be distended with fluid through an indwelling transurethral catheter and inspected for errant sutures. At the completion of this *telescopic examination,* the bladder is drained through the Foley catheter, the telescope removed, and the purse-string suture securely tied.

COMPLICATIONS

Cautious introduction of the cystoscope with prompt attention to resistance will avoid trauma to the urethra and bladder. Resistance to passage of the scope may be caused by false passages within the urethra and by urethral stricture and stenosis. Use of a smaller-caliber rigid scope or flexible scope helps to uncover the source of resistance, and once the cause is uncovered, appropriate therapy can be instituted.

Extreme carelessness during introduction of the scope can lead to bladder perforation. Inability to maintain adequate distention of the bladder may be an indication of a bladder perforation and should alert the cystoscopist to look for such an occurrence.

The incidence of bladder infection after cystoscopy is a subject of considerable debate. Colonization of the vagina and distal urethra would seem to provide a source for introduction of organisms into the bladder with the introduction of the scope.[4,12] Prevention of infection with short-term (24 hours) nitrofurantoin or sulfa therapy has been used with success in our facility for the past several years.

SUMMARY

Cystoscopy is a valuable tool with many applications for the surgeon performing pelvic surgery. Its incorporation and utilization can lead to discovery of a number of conditions. Facility with its use can often avert delay in diagnosis and sharpen the dependability of diagnosis in other circumstances. Recognition of unsuspected urologic problems and early referral to a urologic specialist will leave the patient the beneficiary in our goal toward improved comprehensive care of female patients.

REFERENCES

1. Clayman RV, Reddy P, Lange PH: Flexible fiberoptic and rigid rod-lens endoscopy of the lower urinary tract: a prospective controlled comparison, *J Urol* 131:715, 1984.
2. Desnos E: The nineteenth century. In Murphy LJT, editor: *The history of urology*, Springfield, Ill, 1972, Charles C Thomas.
3. Edwards PD, Hurm RA, Jaeschke WH: Conversion of cystitis glandularis to adenocarcinoma, *J Urol* 108:568, 1972.
4. Hares MM: A double-blind trial of half-strength Polybactrin-soluble GU bladder irrigation in cystoscopy, *Br J Urol* 53:62, 1981.
5. Hopkins HH, Kopany NS: A flexible fiberscope, using static scanning, *Nature* 179:39, 1954.
6. Kavoussi LR, Clayman RV: Office flexible cystoscopy, *Urol Clin North Am* 15:601, 1988.
7. Kelly HA: The direct examination of the female bladder with elevated pelvis—the catheterization of the ureters under direct inspection, with and without elevation of the pelvis, *Am J Dis Wom Child* 25:1, 1894.
8. Lee RA, Symmonds RE, Williams TJ: Current status of genitourinary fistula, *Obstet Gynecol* 72:313, 1988.
9. McAninch JW: Vesical trauma and hemorrhage. In Glenn JF, editor: *Urologic surgery*, ed 4, Philadelphia, 1991, JB Lippincott.
10. Melicos MM: Tumors of the urinary bladder: a clinicopathological analysis of over 2500 specimens and biopsies, *J Urol* 74:498, 1955.
11. Ostergard DR: Bladder pillar block anesthesia for urethral dilatation, *Am J Obstet Gynecol* 136:187, 1980.
12. Richards B, Bastable JRG: Bacteriuria after outpatient cystoscopy, *Br J Urol* 49:561, 1977.
13. Robertson JR: Air cystoscopy, *J Obstet Gynecol* 32:328, 1968.
14. Robertson JR: Endoscopic examination of the urethra and bladder, *Clin Obstet Gynecol* 26:347, 1983.
15. Robertson JR: Urethral diverticula. In Ostergard DR, Bent AE, editors: *Urogynecology and urodynamics: theory and practice*, ed 3, Baltimore, 1991, Williams & Wilkins.
16. Stamey TA: Endoscopic suspension of the vesical neck for urinary incontinence, *Surg Gynecol Obstet* 6:547, 1973.
17. Staskin DR: Vesicovaginal fistula. In Glenn JR, editor: *Urologic surgery*, ed 4, Philadelphia, 1991, JP Lippincott.
18. Timmons MC, Addison WA: Suprapubic teloscopy: extraperitoneal intraoperative technique to demonstrate ureteral patency, *Obstet Gynecol* 75:137, 1990.
19. Tsuchida S, Sugawara H: A new flexible fibercystoscope for visualization of the bladder neck, *J Urol* 109:830, 1973.
20. Wickham JEA, Miller RA: Nephroscopy: endoscopic instruments and their accessories. In Wickham JEA, Miller RA, editors: *Percutaneous renal surgery*, New York, 1983, Churchill Livingstone.

9 Central Venous and Intraperitoneal Catheters

DANIEL L. CLARKE-PEARSON

Access to the central venous system and to a lesser extent the peritoneal cavity has gained importance in the management of many patients undergoing gynecologic and obstetric surgery. Certainly, the safe placement of catheters for venous access (e.g., central venous monitoring, replacement of blood products, chronic antibiotic therapy, administration of chemotherapy, and total parenteral nutrition) is of significant benefit to gynecologic and obstetric surgeons. The use of central venous catheters was first reported in 1952 by Aubaniac,[2] who initially described placement of an infraclavicular catheter for blood volume replacement. A decade later, Wilson reported the use of a similar catheter for the measurement of central venous pressure. Subsequent improvements in catheter placement technique and equipment have led to the safe placement and use of both short- and long-term catheters, some of which may be used for up to several years. In most oncology services and for the management of other critically ill surgery patients, central venous monitoring and central venous access for rapid blood product replacement are common. In the current context, it is almost impossible to fathom that our predecessors undertook radical hysterectomy and even pelvic exenteration without this support, which we consider so fundamental in our surgical practice.

Long-term access to the peritoneal cavity is significantly less important yet holds potential benefits in the treatment of some gynecologic malignancies with intraperitoneal chemotherapy and for the relief of symptomatic malignant ascites. Although intraperitoneal access has been commonly used for peritoneal dialysis in patients with renal failure, recent clinical trials appear to demonstrate that intraperitoneally administered chemotherapy may result in an improved response rate and survival in carefully selected women with advanced ovarian carcinoma.

CENTRAL VENOUS ACCESS
Indications

Central venous catheterization, including Swan-Ganz catheters are commonly used in the management of critically ill surgical and nonsurgical patients. These catheters, which are often placed and left for several days, are considered temporary. In this context the common indications for central venous catheter placement include poor or inadequate peripheral venous access, rapid or large volume fluid and blood product replacement, total parenteral nutrition, and administration of other agents such as chemotherapy or an-

tibiotics. Central venous catheters are often used to measure central venous pressure or to allow Swan-Ganz catheter placement for perioperative hemodynamic monitoring.

Permanent central venous catheters are considered in patients who need long-term venous access for multiple courses of intravenous chemotherapy or total parenteral nutrition. Permanent central venous catheters also provide access for the administration of antibiotics, blood transfusions, and fluids and also allow for frequent blood sampling.

Regarding both temporary and permanent venous access, several different types of catheters may be selected for use. Each has distinct advantages and disadvantages, and some may be selected predominantly based on the surgeon's personal choice. The temporary venous catheters are most commonly placed either into the subclavian vein or through the internal jugular vein. Both approaches are discussed subsequently, since it is important for a surgeon to have the skills to place both types of catheters. The subclavian vein catheterization allows the patient more freedom of neck movement and is particularly useful and appropriate in patients who have an obese neck or who have had surgery that might have deformed or distorted neck anatomy. Compared with the subclavian vein approach, internal jugular vein catheterization results in a significantly lower risk of pneumothorax. Since the internal jugular vein is more accessible to the anesthesiologist during surgery, it is frequently chosen when a central venous catheter is inserted intraoperatively. An internal jugular vein approach also may be more accessible in the middle of cardiopulmonary resuscitation, during which chest compression may make subclavian vein access difficult.

Permanent catheters can be divided into those that are passed percutaneously and have a portion of the catheter exposed (Hickman, Broviac, and Groshong catheters) and those that are placed completely subcutaneously, such as the Port-A-Cath.[9] Catheters that are placed externally are easily accessed, since special needles and equipment are not required, and are immediately available for use. Most of the external catheters come supplied as both single- and double-lumen catheters. Double-lumen catheters allow for simultaneous infusion of blood products, total parenteral nutrition, and antibiotics. Patients with external catheters may shower and bathe, but swimming and the use of hot tubs are contraindicated. Most external catheters also require flushing with heparin solution up to three times a week, and many patients are unhappy with having a catheter exposed on their chest surface. The subcutaneous catheters are ideal for patients who will receive chronic and frequent infusions in an outpatient setting. The Port-A-Cath systems are easy to care for, result in improved body image of the patient, and have a decreased risk for infection. Minimum maintenance is required; they need to be flushed only once a month, and there are no dressings to be changed. Finally, patients may participate in all activities including swimming. In general, the Port-A-Cath systems have a small catheter lumen, thereby somewhat limiting the infusion rate, and require a special needle (Huber needle) for accessing the Port-A-Cath safely.

Techniques

Internal Jugular Vein Catheterization

Anatomy. From the base of the skull the internal jugular vein takes a posterolateral course in relationship to the internal carotid artery and the common carotid artery until the vein unites with the subclavian vein, thus forming the brachiocephalic vein. At the point the internal jugular vein meets the subclavian vein, the internal jugular vein is lateral and anterior to the common carotid artery. On the right, the internal jugular vein, the brachiocephalic vein, and the superior vena cava almost feed directly into the right atrium. For this reason, the right internal jugular vein is a better choice for cannulization, as compared to the left, where the

brachiocephalic vein is longer and enters the subclavian vein at an angle. In addition, the cupula of the right lung is lower than that on the left. The thoracic duct, which is only on the left, is more likely to be injured during catheterization on the left side. The superior segments of the internal jugular vein are overlapped by the posterior belly of the digastric muscle and is medial to the sternocleidomastoid muscle. In its mid portion, where the vein is cannulated, it is located in the depression between the sternal and clavicular heads of the sternocleidomastoid muscle (Fig. 9-1, *A*). The most distal portion of the internal jugular vein lies behind the clavicle. These anatomic relationships are important to recognize and use in the course of cannulating the internal jugular vein. Adjacent to the internal jugular vein is the carotid artery and cranial nerves IX, X, and XII. On the left, the thoracic duct opens near the union of the left subclavian and left internal jugular vein. On the right, a smaller lymphatic duct joins the venous system at the same location. As noted above, the internal jugular vein also passes close to the apex of the lung, and this is more so on the left.

Technique

1. The patient is placed in the Trendelenburg position, which facilitates distention of the neck veins and also re-

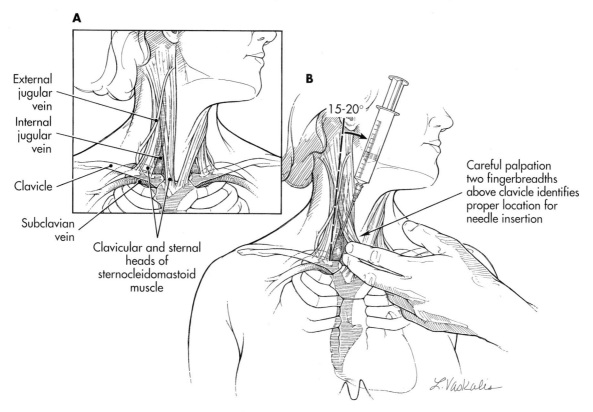

Fig. 9-1 **A,** Anatomic location and orientation of the internal jugular vein in the triangle formed by the sternal and clavicular heads of the sternocleidomastoid muscle and the clavicle. **B,** Placement of the internal jugular vein catheter. The carotid artery is retracted medially with two fingers just above the clavicle. At the apex of the triangle formed by the two heads of the sternocleidomastoid muscle, the needle is inserted in a caudal direction at a 15- to 20-degree angle from the axis of the carotid artery and internal jugular vein.

duces the risk of air embolism. In the approach to the right internal jugular vein, the patient's head is turned to the opposite side, which stretches the vein and further accentuates the muscular landmarks.

2. As shown in Fig. 9-1, *A*, the internal jugular vein lies in a triangle formed by the sternal and clavicle heads of the sternocleidomastoid muscle and the clavicle. These landmarks must be identified. The carotid artery also should be identified, as it lies just medial to the internal jugular vein in this triangle. The neck and shoulder are prepared and draped as a sterile field. Using sterile gloves, the operator palpates the carotid artery and retracts the artery medially using two fingers.

3. A 22-gauge needle attached to a 5- to 10-ml syringe is inserted at the apex of the triangle formed by the two heads of the sternocleidomastoid muscle (see Fig. 9-1, *B*).

4. A slight negative pressure is maintained on the syringe as the needle is directed caudally, parallel to the medial border of the clavicular head and at a 45-degree angle to the frontal plane. The vein should be cannulated after the needle has been advanced a few centimeters. If this approach is not successful, the needle should be withdrawn completely and redirected 5 to 10 degrees more laterally. The operator should not direct the needle medially because this likely will result in carotid artery cannulization. Once the location of the vessel has been identified with a small gauge needle, a larger (usually 14 to 16 gauge)

Intracath needle is then inserted in the same angle and position. When the vein is cannulated, the syringe is removed and the gloved finger is placed over the opening of the Intracath to prevent air embolism. A guidewire is then introduced into the needle and advanced. The needle is withdrawn and an introducer with dilator is placed over the guidewire. A 3- to 5-mm incision must be made in the skin of the neck to facilitate passage of the dilator. The guidewire and dilator are removed, and the catheter is then advanced through the introducer. Once the catheter is located in the proper position, the introducer is peeled away and the catheter is sutured to the skin to maintain its proper position. A chest x-ray should be obtained to ensure proper positioning and to rule out pneumothorax. If the internal jugular line was inserted intraoperatively, a chest x-ray should be obtained in the recovery room.

Subclavian Vein Catheterization

Anatomy. The subclavian vein begins at the lateral border of the first rib and arches behind the clavicle and over the first rib anterior to the insertion of the anterior scalene muscle. Just medial to the anterior scalene muscle, the subclavian vein joins the internal jugular vein to form the brachiocephalic vein. The subclavian vein anteriorly is covered by the clavicle. As the subclavian vein crosses the first rib, it is separated from the subclavian artery by the anterior scalene muscle, which is about 1 cm thick (Fig. 9-2). Other

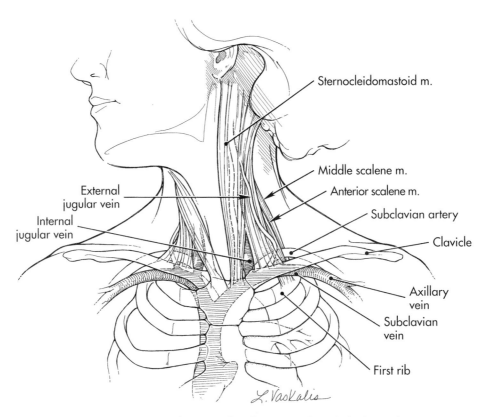

Fig. 9-2 Anatomy relevant to the placement of a subclavian catheter.

vital structures in this region include the thoracic duct, which enters the internal jugular vein near its junction with the subclavian vein, passing anterior to the subclavian artery and posterior to the internal jugular vein. Medial to the attachment of the anterior scalene muscle to the first rib, the apical pleura is in contact with the inferior portion of the subclavian vein. A clear understanding of these anatomic relationships is critical to reduce the risk of injury to the pleura, lung, thoracic duct, and subclavian artery.

Technique. Several techniques have been described elsewhere in the literature. The technique we use has been described by Grant[6] and is outlined here.

1. The patient should be positioned supine on the operating table with the arms drawn toward her feet and secured at her side. If the shoulders rest in a shrugged position the vein takes a more variable course and may be more difficult to locate. The skin should be prepared with sterile preparation solution from the midneck to below the nipple line and from the anterior axillary line to just across the sternum.

2. The patient should be placed in approximately 15 degrees of Trendelenburg position and the junction of the middle and medial thirds of the clavicle located. The left subclavian vein is the preferred site of insertion because of its straighter course to the superior vena cava and right atrium. The target for subclavian vein catheterization is a 2 × 2 cm area bounded inferiorly by the first rib, poste-

riorly by the anterior scalene muscle as it inserts on the tubercle of the first rib, anteriorly by the clavicle and superiorly by the upper edge of the clavicle. A 16-gauge needle is attached to a 10-ml syringe and the barrel of the syringe placed in the deltopectoral grove. The tip of the needle is withdrawn approximately 2 cm away from the inferior edge of the clavicle just lateral to the 2-cm target zone. One percent lidocaine is injected at this site with a 25-gauge needle. The needle is then slowly advanced toward the "target" area with the syringe held against the patient's shoulder and horizontal to the floor (Fig. 9-3). Frequent small aspirations are applied to the syringe as the needle is advanced. The vein usually is entered after 4 to 6 cm of needle insertion and is easily identified by the free flow of venous blood into the syringe. If the vein is not entered, the needle should be removed slowly and completely with intermittent aspiration (as on occasion the vein has been punctured through-and-through and would be located upon withdrawing the needle). If no blood is aspirated, the needle should be completely removed and any plugs of tissue or blood clot flushed from the syringe and needle before reinsertion. In performing a second pass, the target area should be re-evaluated and a point slightly more cephalad on the anterior scalene muscle should be selected. Insertion more posteriorly should be avoided because the vein does not lie behind the anterior scalene muscle and the needle di-

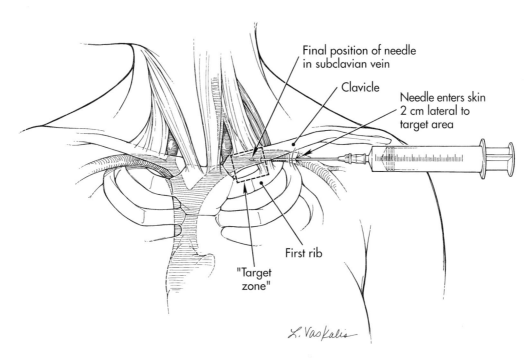

Fig. 9-3 Placement of a subclavian catheter. The needle is inserted in the skin about 2 cm lateral to the "target zone" and beneath the clavicle. The target zone is bounded by the first rib inferiorly, the anterior scalene muscle as it inserts on the tubercle of the first rib posteriorly, the clavicle anteriorly, and superiorly by the upper edge of the clavicle. The needle should be inserted with the bevel directed anteriorly.

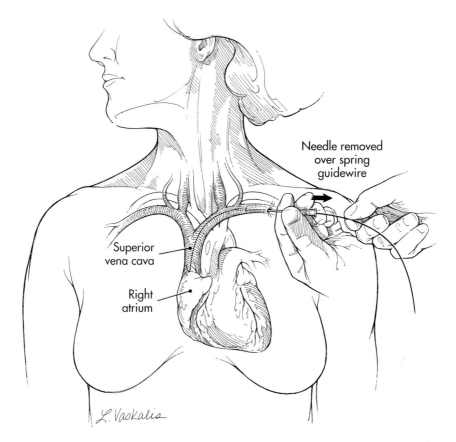

Fig. 9-4   Placement of spring guidewire. Once the needle has punctured the subclavian vein, it should be advanced another 0.5 cm. A spring guidewire is passed through the needle and advanced into the superior vena cava or right atrium. The needle is withdrawn over the guidewire.

rected in this fashion is more likely to injure the subclavian artery and the cupula of the lung. The level of the needle should be directed anteriorly.

3. Once free flow of blood is obtained, the needle should be advanced approximately 0.5 cm, and then a guidewire is advanced through the needle (Fig. 9-4). The needle is then removed.

4. A 1 cm skin incision is then made at the puncture site. We prefer to use the Cook introducer kit. The Cook introducer is fed over the guidewire and advanced into the subclavian vein. The introducer has an inner catheter (dilator) and an outer sheath (Fig. 9-5, *A*).

5. After insertion, the dilator is removed and catheter is threaded through the outer sheath and into the right atrium (see Fig. 9-5, *B*).

6. The outer sheath is withdrawn by splitting it, and the correct position of the catheter tip is confirmed by injection of contrast material under fluoroscopic observation (see Fig. 9-5, *C*).

Variations in the subsequent steps depend on whether the catheter will remain external (such as Hickman, Broviac, or Groshong catheter) or will be totally implanted (such as a Port-A-Cath). External catheters are further prepared by tunneling underneath the skin of the chest wall. In this technique, before insertion of the semi-permanent catheter into the subclavian vein, a tunnel is created between an incision in the medial chest wall above the breast. Using a tunneler between this chest wall incision and the subclavicular incision, the catheter is drawn cephalad through the tunnel (see Fig. 9-5, *D*). Subsequently the catheter is inserted into the subclavian vein (steps 5 and 6 above) (see Fig. 9-5, *A* to *C*). Once the tip of the catheter is located properly in the right atrium, the remainder of the catheter is withdrawn and cut to proper length. A Dacron cuff attached to the catheter remains in the subcutaneous tract. The subclavicular incision and the chest wall tunneling incision are closed, and the distal end of the catheter is secured to the skin with a suture wrapped about the catheter (see Fig. 9-5, *E*). Sterile dressing is applied, and a chest x-ray is obtained to confirm catheter tip location and to ensure that no pneumothorax has occurred.

If a subcutaneous Port-A-Cath is used, an incision is made in the chest wall above the breast in approximately the midclavicular line. A subcutaneous pocket is created with blunt dissection just above the chest wall fascia, and a tunnel is created between the pocket and the subclavicular incision. The subclavian catheter is then withdrawn through

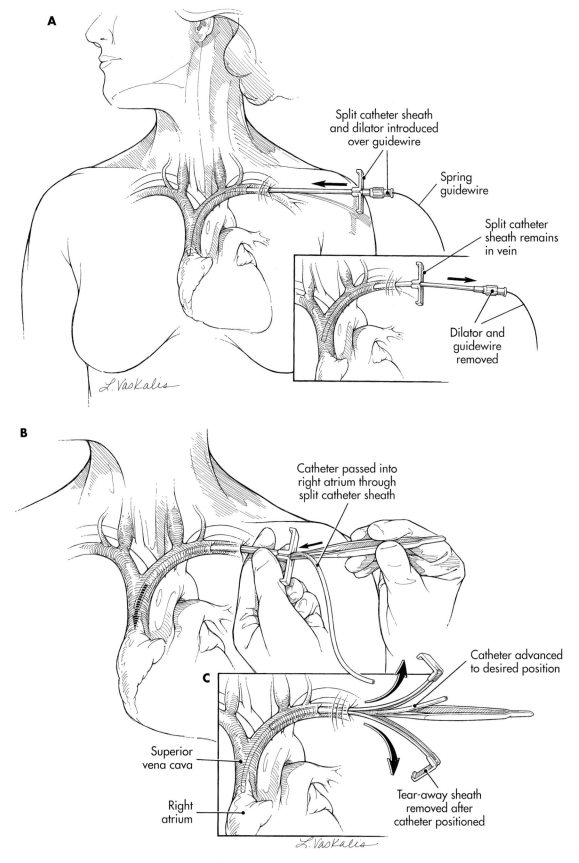

Fig. 9-5 **A,** A split catheter sheath and vein dilator are passed over the guidewire and inserted into the subclavian vein. The guidewire and dilator are withdrawn, leaving the split catheter sheath in the vein. **B,** The catheter is inserted through the split catheter sheath and passed into the right atrium. Proper placement is confirmed by fluoroscopy and dye injection. **C,** The split catheter sheath is withdrawn while the catheter is pushed forward using DeBakey forceps.

Continued

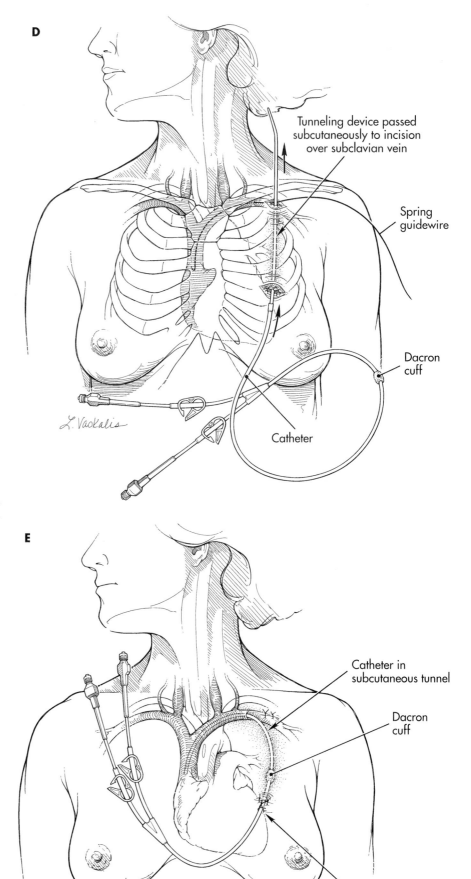

Fig. 9-5, cont'd   D, Placement of an external catheter. An incision is made in the chest wall in the midclavicular line. A tunnel is made between this incision and the incision through which the subclavian guidewire has been passed. The tunneling device with the catheter attached is passed through the subcutaneous tunnel. **E,** The catheter is pulled back into the subcutaneous tunnel, locating a Dacron cuff within the subcutaneous tissue. The skin incision sites are closed, and the catheter is sutured to the skin.

D

Tunneling device passed subcutaneously to incision over subclavian vein

Spring guidewire

Dacron cuff

Catheter

L. Vaokalis

E

Catheter in subcutaneous tunnel

Dacron cuff

Suture securing catheter to skin

L. Vaokalis

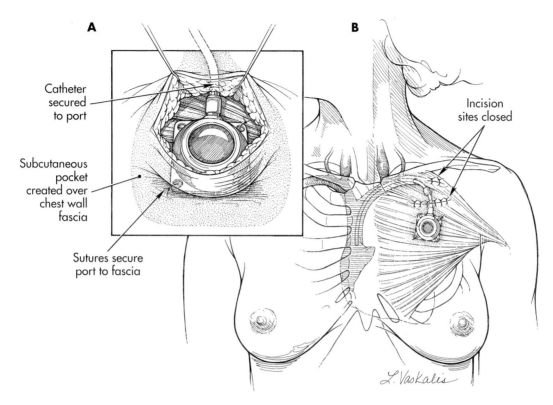

Fig. 9-6   **A,** Placement of a subclavian Port-A-Cath. Following steps Figure 9-5, *A* to *E,* a subcutaneous "pocket" is formed over the chest wall fascia. The catheter is cut to proper length and secured to the port. The port is then sutured to the chest wall fascia with 2-0 Prolene. **B,** The skin incisions are closed over the port site and the subclavian incision.

the tunnel and cut to proper length and securely attached to the Port (Fig. 9-6, *A*). The Port is placed in the pocket and secured to the chest wall using two or three 2-0 Prolene sutures. The incision for the subcutaneous pocket and the subclavicular incisions are both closed, and the Port is flushed with heparinized saline (see Fig. 9-6, *B*). A chest x-ray should be obtained to confirm proper catheter tip location and to ensure that no pneumothorax has occurred.

Complications

Complications associated with the placement of central venous access catheters occur in approximately 3% to 6% of all patients. These complications include infection, pneumothorax, hemothorax, air embolism, venous thrombosis, and perforation of the subclavian or carotid arteries. The risk of complication is influenced somewhat by the vein selected and is clearly related to the technical expertise of the surgeon and by patient-related factors such as anatomy and patient habitus. Of the more acute and serious complications, pneumothorax is the most frequent and should always be considered and evaluated by use of immediate chest x-ray. If a pneumothorax is encountered, a chest tube is required in approximately half the cases, although many small pneumothoraces can be managed expectantly.

To reduce the risk of thrombosis at the catheter tip, many surgeons prescribe 1 mg of oral warfarin daily.[3] If a thrombus does develop at the catheter tip, urokinase, 5000 units/

ml, should be instilled into the catheter and repeated 1 hour later if the catheter appears to remain obstructed.[8]

Catheter site infection occurs in 1% to 2% of cases, whereas sepsis associated with infection of the central line may occur slightly more frequently. Infection of the line clearly depends on the duration of use, the care in maintaining the catheter, and the patient's susceptibility to infection. The most common organism is *Staphylococcus aureus,* which should initially be treated with intravenous antibiotics. A central line should be removed if antibiotic therapy fails.[4] Occlusive plastic dressing applied over catheter insertion sites is associated with a higher degree of moisture retention and subsequent infections. For this reason, occlusive nonpermeable dressings are discouraged. Topical antibiotics such as polymyxins/neomycin applied at the entry site of external semi-permanent or permanent catheters may decrease the rate of skin infection.

Catheter Maintenance

Catheters that are not being continuously used should be flushed biweekly or weekly using 5 ml of heparinized saline (100 units of heparin per milliliter of saline). Ports that are not in use should be flushed in a similar fashion once a month. External catheters should be cared for using aseptic technique. The site is cleansed and dressed with antibiotic ointment at least once or twice a week. Ports are accessed using a special noncoring needle called a Huber needle

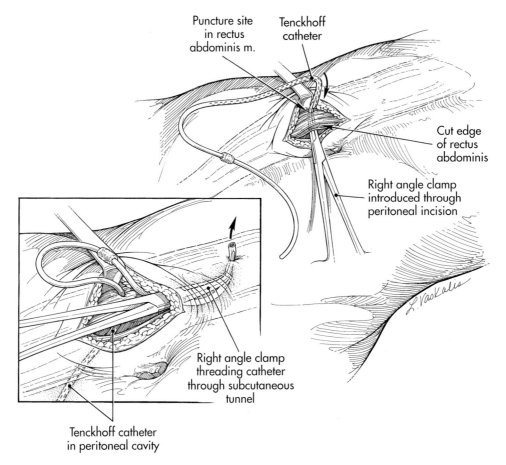

Puncture site
in rectus
abdominis m.

Tenckhoff
catheter

Cut edge
of rectus
abdominis

Right angle clamp
introduced through
peritoneal incision

Right angle clamp
threading catheter
through subcutaneous
tunnel

Tenckhoff catheter
in peritoneal cavity

Fig. 9-7   Placement of an intraperitoneal Tenckhoff catheter. An incision is made lateral to the umbilicus into the peritoneal cavity. Using a right angle clamp, the peritoneum, muscle, and fascia are punctured and the catheter drawn into the peritoneal cavity. The catheter is tunneled subcutaneously about 5 cm and exits through the skin. A Dacron cuff on the catheter is located in the subcutaneous tissue. The peritoneum, fascia, and skin are closed, and the catheter flushed with heparinized saline.

inserted through the skin until it punctures the septum and accesses the Port. These noncoring needles allow up to 2000 punctures of a Port.

INTRAPERITONEAL ACCESS

The use of catheters placed into the peritoneal cavity has gained popularity over the past decade because of evidence suggesting that the administration of intraperitoneal chemotherapy may be of therapeutic advantage in patients with advanced ovarian cancer who have minimal intraperitoneal disease.[1,7] Administration of chemotherapy into the peritoneal cavity results in a substantial increase in concentration of the selected drug (usually Cisplatin). As with central venous catheters, peritoneal catheters may be extrinsic and exit through the skin (Tenckhoff catheter) or be totally implanted (Port-A-Cath). The obvious advantage to the totally implanted catheter is that the patient has no external catheter to manipulate or deal with and her activity such as bathing or swimming is not limited. The Tenckhoff catheter requires additional care and sterile technique and is associated with a slightly higher risk of peritonitis. The Tenckhoff catheter

is more likely to allow aspiration of fluid from the peritoneal cavity such as in patients with recurrent ascites requiring frequent paracentesis for symptomatic relief.

Techniques

Tenckhoff Catheter Insertion. The Tenckhoff catheter is usually inserted into the peritoneal cavity just lateral to the umbilicus. We usually perform this procedure under general anesthesia or MAC anesthesia with local infiltration of the incision site. An incision site lateral to the umbilicus is selected and an approximately 3 cm incision is made through the skin, subcutaneous tissue, fascia, rectus muscle, and peritoneum. The peritoneal cavity should be assessed for adjacent adhesions, and if extensive adhesions are apparent, the procedure should be abandoned. If intraperitoneal access can be achieved, a site is selected lateral to the primary peritoneal incision and a right angle clamp is passed through the peritoneum, muscle belly, and fascia grasping the catheter and pulling it into the peritoneal cavity. The catheter is then directed toward the pelvis. A subcutaneous tunnel above the rectus fascia is created and the catheter exited through that tunnel and through a separate

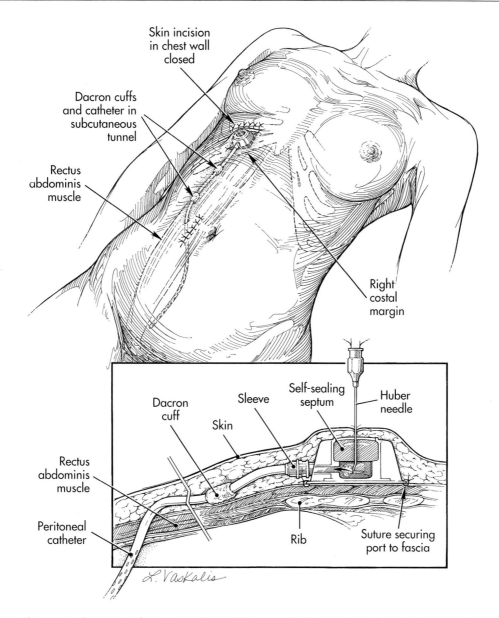

Fig. 9-8 Placement of an intraperitoneal Port-A-Cath. The peritoneal cavity is accessed as described in Fig. 9-7. Parallel to and 4 cm above the right costal margin the skin and subcutaneous layers are incised and a pocket is created above the chest wall fascia. The catheter is introduced into the peritoneal cavity and tunneled to the costal pocket. The catheter is cut to proper length and attached to the port. The port is secured to the chest wall fascia with 2-0 Prolene sutures. The skin over all incisions is closed. *Inset,* The port is accessed with a noncoring Huber needle.

skin incision (Fig. 9-7). A Dacron cuff on the catheter remains in the subcutaneous tissue layer that will ultimately have ingrowth of fibroblast securing the catheter in place. The catheter is not sutured to the skin but is flushed with heparinized saline. The fascial incision is closed as is the subcutaneous tissue and skin. The catheter should be maintained in a sterile fashion for at least 1 month but thereafter may be managed by a clean technique.

Intraperitoneal Port-A-Cath. The intraperitoneal Port-A-Cath is most commonly selected for the administration of intraperitoneal chemotherapy. This allows a totally implanted device that requires no specific care or maintenance by the patient and only requires flushing of the cath-

eter on a monthly basis with heparinized saline. Similar to a Tenckhoff catheter, an incision is made just lateral to the umbilicus, and if free access to the peritoneal cavity is achieved, a catheter is inserted into the peritoneal cavity. A subcutaneous tunnel is directed toward the costal margin. A subcutaneous pocket is then created beneath a second incision usually approximately 4 cm above the right costal margin. The catheter is cut to the proper length and secured to the Port. The Port is then secured to the chest wall fascia with 2-0 Prolene sutures. As with the central venous Port-A-Caths, a Huber noncoring needle is used to access the Port and the Port is flushed before wound closure (Fig. 9-8).

Complications

Reported complications for both intraperitoneal catheters include intestinal injury, catheter blockage and infections of the peritoneal cavity or the abdominal wall.[10] The implanted subcutaneous Port-A-Cath systems appear to have a lower risk of infection and better patient acceptance. Catheter blockage with either system is reported to occur in approximately 8% to 10% of cases with infection in approximately 8% of cases.[5] In order to reduce infection it is recommended that catheters not be placed at the time of intestinal surgery and clearly should not be placed when there is ongoing intraperitoneal infection. Strict aseptic technique should be used when catheters are accessed. The most vexing problem with intraperitoneal catheters is blockage, and to date no clear cut optimal method has been identified in order to prevent deposition of fibrin around the catheter. Because of potential for late erosion into the intestine, catheters should be removed at the completion of the patient's chemotherapy course.

REFERENCES

1. Alberts DS, Liu PY, Hannigan EV, et al: Intraperitoneal cisplatin plus intravenous cyclophosphamide versus intravenous cisplatin plus intravenous cyclophosphamide in stage III ovarian cancer, *N Engl J Med* 335:1950, 1996.

2. Aubaniac R: L'injection intraveineuse sons-claviculaire: advantages et techniques, *Presse Med* 60:1456, 1952.

3. Bern MM, Lokish JJ, Wallach SR: Very low doses of warfarin can prevent thrombosis in central venous catheters, *Ann Int Med* 1112:423, 1990.

4. Corona ML, Narr BJ, Thompson RL: Infections related to central venous catheters, *Mayo Clin Proc* 65:979, 1990.

5. Davidson SA, Rubin SC, Markman M, et al: Intraperitoneal chemotherapy: analysis of complications with an implanted subcutaneous Port and catheter system, *Gynecol Oncol* 41:101, 1991.

6. Grant JP: Insertion of right atrial catheters for chemotherapy, antibiotics, and hyperalimentation. In Sabiston D, editor: *Atlas of general surgery*, Philadelphia, 1994, WB Saunders.

7. Howell SB, Zimm S, Markman M, et al: Long-term survival of advanced refractory ovarian carcinoma patients with small volume disease treated with intraperitoneal chemotherapy, *J Clin Oncol* 5:1607, 1987.

8. Lawson M, Bottino JC, Hurtubise MR: The use of urokinase to restore the patency of occluded central venous catheters, *Am J Intravenous Ther Clin Nutr* 41:29, 1982.

9. Nelson BE, Mayer AR, Tseng PC: Experience with the totally implanted ports in patients with gynecologic malignancies, *Gynecol Oncol* 53:98, 1994.

10. Rubin SC, Hoskins WJ, Markman M, Hakes T, Lewis JJ: Long-term access to the peritoneal cavity in ovarian cancer patients, *Gynecol Oncol* 33:46, 1989.

11. Wilson NJ, Grow JB, Demong CV, Prevedel AE, Owens JC: Central venous pressures in optimal blood volume maintenance, *Arch Surg* 85:563, 1962.

10 Postoperative Care and Management of Complications

DANIEL L. CLARKE-PEARSON and DAVID H. NICHOLS

Efforts to prevent intraoperative and postoperative complications must begin preoperatively. They include the many issues in establishing the diagnosis and in preoperative evaluation and preparation (see Chapters 4 and 5). Immediately before a surgical procedure, the surgeon should review the patient's record to refresh his or her memory about significant points in the patient's history, preoperative laboratory findings, and the recommendations of consultants. This review should include the findings of medical students, house officers, fellows, and referring physicians. When specific changes in the usual preoperative preparation of the patient are indicated, the surgeon should confirm that they have been performed.

MANAGEMENT OF INTRAOPERATIVE COMPLICATIONS

Complications during surgery can be divided into those associated with anesthesia (e.g., aspiration, drug reactions, and malignant hyperthermia) or those occurring as a result of surgical care. Of the intraoperative surgical complications, hemorrhage and injury to adjacent organs are the most common. Each of these complications is discussed in detail in specific chapters of this text and are not reiterated here (see Chapters 15, 46, 48, and 51).

It is worthwhile to discuss the key elements to the successful management of intraoperative complications: prevention, recognition, and proper repair. The avoidance of complications is the surgeon's ultimate goal. This results from proper preoperative and intraoperative prevention. The surgeon should recognize high-risk patients and make additional allowances. The most important clinical factors associated with intraoperative complications include obesity, large pelvic mass, adhesions, cancer, and prior radiation therapy.

Recognizing these factors in a patient should lead the surgeon to prepare for a difficult case, which poses an increased risk for complications. In difficult cases the surgeon would likely want an aggressive mechanical and antibiotic bowel preparation and would want to position the patient in Allen stirrups so that cystoscopy and proctoscopy can be performed easily. The surgeon would obtain deep retractors, secure additional skilled surgical assistance, and schedule additional operating time.

Prevention of complications, of course, depends greatly on surgical skill and technique. One of the most important keys to this is the careful establishment and recognition of anatomy. In difficult cases, anatomy is often distorted or obscured by a large mass, adhesions, obesity, and so forth. Skilled surgeons can recognize and establish the proper anatomic relationships to avoid intraoperative complications. For example, injury to the ureter is rare if it has been identified. Further, if the pathologic condition is adjacent to the ureter, skilled surgeons will mobilize the ureter and protect it from injury. Careful tissue handling and sharp dissection result in less tissue injury and fewer complications.

Immediate recognition of complications is extremely important, because an injury that is not recognized until postoperatively is always a more serious complication. Although intraoperative hemorrhage is not difficult to recognize, injuries to the small bowel, colon, bladder, and ureter may go unrecognized for days. The delay in recognizing the injury results in the most frequent source of medical malpractice claims associated with a surgical procedure. It is therefore imperative that the surgeon have a high degree of suspicion that an injury may have occurred and then pursue immediate evaluation. When ureteral injury is possible, for example, the surgeon should identify the ureter, inject intravenous indigo carmine to check for a ureteric leak, perform cystoscopy to confirm ureteral patency, and pass a ureteral stint if necessary. Other techniques can be used to evaluate gastrointestinal injury (see Chapters 50 and 51).

Repair of the injury is the final step in successfully managing intraoperative complications. Intraoperative consultation with other surgical colleagues should be liberally sought. Immediate discussion with the patient and family regarding the complication and the expected outcome is critical. Clear and timely documentation of the injury and intraoperative management are important for potential medicolegal defense.

Finally, postoperative care of patients with complications is critical to achieve the desired outcome. The surgeon, who is embarrassed that he or she has a patient with a complication, may wish to "forget" it and handle the postoperative recovery as if the patient does not have a complication. It is a huge mistake to remove the Foley catheter too early from the injured bladder or to begin a diet prematurely in a patient who has had a gastrointestinal injury. Even if another surgical consultant managed the complication, the primary gynecologist should remain closely involved with the patient daily throughout her postoperative recovery. Embarrassment or guilt (or assuming that another physician is now in charge of the patient) has led some surgeons to abandon patients with complications; this is a grave error in management that will likely result in a poor outcome and increase the probability of legal action.

POSTOPERATIVE CARE AND MANAGEMENT OF POSTOPERATIVE COMPLICATIONS
Fluid and Electrolytes

General Considerations. In an average woman, total water constitutes approximately 50% to 55% of body weight. Two thirds of this water is contained in the intracellular compartment. One third is contained in the extracellular compartment, of which one fourth is contained in plasma and the remaining three quarters in the interstitium.

Osmolarity, or tonicity, is a property derived from the number of particles in a solution. Sodium and chloride are the primary electrolytes contributing to the osmolarity in the extracellular fluid compartment. Potassium, and to a lesser extent magnesium and phosphate, are the major intracellular electrolytes. Water flows freely between the intracellular and extracellular spaces to maintain osmotic neutrality throughout the body. Any shifts in osmolarity in any fluid space within the body are accompanied by corresponding shifts in free water from spaces of lower to higher osmolarity, thus maintaining a balance in equilibrium.

The daily fluid maintenance requirement for the average adult is approximately 30 ml/kg/day, or 2000 to 3000 ml/day.[17] This is offset partially by insensible losses of 1200 ml/day, which include losses from the lungs (600 ml), skin (400 ml), and gastrointestinal tract (200 ml). Urinary output from the kidney provides the remainder of the fluid loss, and this output varies depending on total body intake of water and sodium. The kidney excretes approximately 600 to 800 mOsm of solute per day. Healthy kidneys can concentrate urine up to approximately 1200 mOsm, and therefore minimum output can range between 500 and 700 ml/day. Maximal urinary output capability of the kidney can be as high as 20 L/day, as seen in patients with diabetes insipidus. In healthy patients, the normal kidney adjusts urine output commensurate with daily fluid intake.

The major extracellular buffer used in acid-base balance is the bicarbonate–carbonic acid system: $CO_2 + H_2O \rightleftharpoons H_2CO_3 \rightleftharpoons H^+ + HCO_3^-$.[14] Typically the body maintains a bicarbonate/carbonic acid ratio of 20/1 to maintain an extracellular pH of 7.4. Both the lung and kidney play integral roles in maintaining normal extracellular pH through retention or excretion of carbon dioxide and bicarbonate. Under conditions of alkalosis, minute ventilation decreases and renal excretion of bicarbonate increases to restore the normal bicarbonate/carbonic acid ratio. The opposite occurs with acidosis.

Ultimately, the kidney plays the most important role in fluid and electrolyte balance through excretion and retention of water and solute. Circulating antidiuretic hormone and aldosterone help modulate the process. Hypothalamic release of antidiuretic hormone is sensitive to serum osmolarity, and aldosterone secretion is responsive to renal perfusion. Under states of dehydration or hypovolemia,

serum antidiuretic hormone levels increase, leading to increased resorption of water in the distal tubule of the kidney. In addition, increased aldosterone release promotes increased renal sodium and water retention. The opposite occurs in states of fluid excess. As a result, an individual with normal renal function, as well as normal circulating antidiuretic hormone and aldosterone levels, maintains normal serum osmolarity and electrolyte composition despite daily fluctuation of fluid and electrolyte intake.

Various disease states can alter the normal fluid and electrolyte homeostatic mechanisms, making perioperative fluid and electrolyte management more difficult. Patients with intrinsic renal disease are unable to excrete solute and to maintain acid-base balance. In patients with the stress of chronic starvation or severe illness, the level of circulating antidiuretic hormone and aldosterone may be inappropriately high, resulting in fluid and sodium retention. With severe cardiac disease, secondary renal hypoperfusion can lead to increased aldosterone synthesis and therefore increased sodium and water retention by the kidney. And finally, a patient with severe diabetes can have a significant osmotic diuresis and have acid-base dysfunction secondary to circulating ketoacids. Correction and optimization of renal, cardiac, or endocrinologic disorders preoperatively are imperative and often rectify fluid and electrolyte abnormalities.

Fluid and electrolyte management in the preoperative and perioperative periods requires a knowledge of the daily fluid and electrolyte requirements for maintenance, replacement of ongoing fluid and electrolyte losses, and correction of any existing abnormalities. Each of these three is considered separately.

Fluid and Electrolyte Maintenance Requirements. The normal daily fluid requirement in an average adult is 2000 to 3000 ml. The body can and does adjust to higher and lower volumes of intake through changes in plasma tonicity. Alterations in plasma tonicity induce adjustments in circulating antidiuretic hormone, which ultimately regulates the amount of water retained in the distal tubule of the kidney. In the preoperative and the early postoperative patient, it is usually necessary to replace only sodium and potassium. Chloride is automatically replaced, concomitant with sodium and potassium, because chloride is the usual anion used to balance sodium and potassium in electrolyte solutions. Various solutions are commercially available that contain 40 mmol of sodium chloride, with smaller amounts of potassium, calcium, and magnesium, designed to meet the requirements of a patient who is receiving 3 L of IV fluids per day. The daily requirement, however, can be met by any combination of IV fluid orders. For example, 2 L of D5.45 normal saline (77 mEq sodium chloride each), supplemented with 20 mEq of potassium chloride, followed by 1 L of D_5W with 20 mEq of potassium chloride would suffice.

Fluid and Electrolyte Replacement. Fluid and electrolyte losses beyond the daily average must be replaced by appropriate solutions. The choice of solutions for replacement depends on the composition of the fluids lost. Often, it is difficult to measure free water loss, particularly in patients who have high "insensible" losses from the lungs or skin, or into the GI tract. Procurement of daily weights in these patients can be very useful. Up to 300 g of weight loss daily can be attributable to weight loss from catabolism of protein and fat in a patient who is taking nothing by mouth.[17] Anything beyond this, however, would be due to fluid loss and should be replaced accordingly.

A patient with a high fever can have increased pulmonary and skin loss of free water, sometimes in excess of 2 to 3 L/day. These losses should be replaced with free water in the form of D_5W. Perspiration typically has one third the osmolarity of plasma and can be replaced with D_5W or, if excessive, with D5.25 normal saline.

A patient with acute blood loss needs replacement with appropriate isotonic fluid, blood, or both. A wide range of plasma volume expanders, including albumin, dextran, and hetastarch solutions, contain large-molecular-weight particles (greater than 50,000 molecular weight). These particles are slow to exit the intravascular space, with about half of them remaining after 24 hours. These solutions are expensive, however, and for most cases, simple replacement with 0.9 normal saline or lactated Ringer solution will suffice. One third of the volume of lactated Ringer or normal saline typically remains in the intravascular space with the remainder going to the interstitium.

Appropriate replacement of gastrointestinal fluid loss depends on the source of fluid loss in the GI tract. Gastrointestinal secretions beyond the stomach, and up to the colon, are typically isotonic with plasma (Table 10-1), with similar amounts of sodium, slightly lower amounts of chloride, slightly alkaline pH, and with more potassium, in the range of 5 to 10 mEq/L.[20] Under normal conditions, stool is hypotonic; however, under conditions of increased flow (e.g. severe diarrhea), stool contents are isotonic with a composition similar to that of the small bowel. Gastric contents are typically hypotonic, with one third the sodium of plasma, increased amounts of hydrogen ion, and low pH.

In a patient with gastric outlet obstruction, nausea and vomiting, or nasogastric suction, appropriate replacement of gastric secretions can be provided with a solution such as D5.45 normal saline with 20 mEq/L of potassium. Potassium supplementation is particularly important to prevent hypokalemia in these patients, whose kidneys attempt to conserve hydrogen ion in the distal tubule of the kidney in exchange for potassium ion.

In patients with bowel obstruction, 1 to 3 L of fluid can be sequestered daily in the gastrointestinal tract. This fluid should be replaced with isotonic saline or lactated Ringer solution. Patients with enterocutaneous fistulas or new ileostomies should have fluid replaced with isotonic fluids.

Postoperative Fluids and Electrolyte Management. Several hormonal and physiologic alterations in the postoperative period can complicate fluid and electrolyte management. The stress of surgery induces an inappropriately high level of circulating ADH. Circulating aldosterone levels also are increased, especially if sustained episodes of hypotension have occurred either intraoperatively or postoperatively. The elevated levels of circulating ADH and aldosterone make the postoperative patient prone to sodium and water retention.

Total body fluid volume may be significantly altered postoperatively. First, 1 ml of free water is released for each gram of catabolized fat or tissue, and, in the postoperative period, several hundred milliliters of free water is released daily from tissue breakdown, particularly in a patient who has undergone extensive intraabdominal dissection and who is NPO. This free water is often retained, secondary to the altered levels of ADH and aldosterone. Second, fluid retention is further enhanced by "third spacing," or sequestration of fluid in the surgical field. The development of an ileus can result in an additional 1 to 3 L of fluid per day being sequestered in the bowel lumen, bowel wall, and peritoneal cavity.

In contrast to renal sodium homeostasis, the kidney lacks the capacity for retention of potassium. In the postoperative

Table 10-1 Composition of Gastrointestinal Secretions

	Volume (ml/24 hr)	Na (mEq/L)	K (mEq/L)	Cl (mEq/L)	HCO$_3$ (mEq/L)
Salivary	1500 (500-2000)	10 (2-10)	26 (20-30)	10 (8-18)	30
Stomach	1500 (100-4000)	60 (9-116)	10 (0-32)	130 (8-154)	—
Duodenum	1000 (100-2000)	140	5	80	—
Ileum	3000 (100-9000)	140 (80-150)	5 (2-8)	104 (43-137)	30
Colon	—	60	30	40	—
Pancreas	500 (100-800)	140 (113-185)	5 (3-7)	75 (54-95)	115
Bile	200 (50-800)	145 (131-164)	5 (3-12)	100 (89-180)	35

From Shires GT, Canizaro P: Fluid and electrolyte management of the surgical patient. In Sabiston DC Jr, editor: *Textbook of surgery,* ed 14, Philadelphia, 1991, WB Saunders.

period, the kidneys continue to excrete a minimum of 30 to 60 mEq/L of potassium daily, irrespective of the serum potassium level and total body potassium stores. If this potassium loss is not replaced, hypokalemia may develop. Tissue damage and catabolism during the first postoperative day usually result in the release of sufficient intracellular potassium to meet the daily requirements. However, beyond the first postoperative day, potassium supplementation is necessary.

Correct maintenance of fluid and electrolyte balance in the postoperative period starts with the preoperative assessment, with emphasis on establishing normal fluid and electrolyte parameters before surgery. Postoperatively, close monitoring of daily weight, urine output, hematocrit, serum electrolytes, and hemodynamic parameters will yield the necessary information to make correct adjustments in crystalloid replacement. The normal daily fluid and electrolyte requirements must be met, and any unusual fluid and electrolyte losses, such as from the gastrointestinal tract, lungs, or skin, must be replaced. After the first few postoperative days, third-spaced fluid begins to mobilize back into the intravascular space, and ADH and aldosterone levels revert to normal. The excess fluid retained perioperatively is thus mobilized and excreted through the kidneys, and exogenous fluid requirements decrease. The patient with inadequate cardiovascular or renal reserve is prone to fluid overload during this time of third-space resorption, especially if intravenous fluids are not appropriately reduced.

The most common fluid and electrolyte disorder in the postoperative period is fluid overload. Fluid excess can occur concomitant with normal or decreased serum sodium. Large amounts of isotonic fluids usually are infused intraoperatively and postoperatively to maintain blood pressure and urine output. Because the infused fluid is often isotonic with plasma, it remains in the extracellular space. Under such conditions, serum sodium remains within normal levels. Fluid excess with hypotonicity (decreased serum sodium) can occur if large amounts of isotonic fluid losses (e.g., blood and gastrointestinal tract) are inappropriately replaced with hypotonic fluids. Again, the predisposition toward retention of free water in the immediate postoperative period compounds the problem. An increase in body weight occurs concomitantly with fluid expansion. In a patient who is NPO, catabolism should induce a daily weight loss as great as 300 g/day. Clearly, a patient who is gaining weight in excess of 150 g/day is in a state of fluid expansion. Simple fluid restriction corrects the abnormality. When necessary, diuretics can be employed to increase urinary water excretion.

States of fluid dehydration are uncommon but occur in a patient who has large daily fluid losses that are not replaced. Gastrointestinal losses should be replaced with the appropriate fluids. Patients with high fevers should be given appropriate free water replacement, in that up to 2 L/day of free water can be lost through perspiration and hyperventilation. Although these increased insensible losses are diffi-

cult to monitor, a reliable estimate can be obtained through the trend in body weight.

Specific Electrolyte Disorders

Hyponatremia. Because sodium is the major extracellular cation, shifts in serum sodium usually are inversely correlated with the hydration state of the extracellular fluid compartment. The pathophysiology of hyponatremia, then, usually is expansion of body fluids leading to excess total body water.[14] The symptoms of hyponatremia are related to both the serum sodium level and the rapidity of its fall. Acute hyponatremia usually becomes symptomatic when the serum sodium falls below 120 to 125 mEq/L, whereas in chronic hyponatremia, symptoms may not occur until the serum sodium falls below 110 mEq/L. Symptoms of hyponatremia can include anorexia, nausea, vomiting, lethargy, headaches, weakness, change in mental status, and seizures.

Hyponatremia in the state of extracellular fluid excess can be seen in patients with renal or cardiac failure as well as in conditions such as nephrotic syndrome, where total body salt, and particularly water, are increased. Administration of hypertonic saline to correct the hyponatremia would be inappropriate in this setting. The treatment should include water restriction with diuretic therapy in addition to correction of the underlying disease process.

Inappropriate secretion of ADH can occur with head trauma, pulmonary or cerebral tumors, and under states of stress. The abnormally elevated ADH results in excess water retention. Treatment includes water restriction and, if possible, correction of the underlying cause. Demeclocycline has been shown to be effective in this disorder through its action in the kidney.

Inappropriate replacement of body salt losses with water alone results in hyponatremia. This typically occurs in patients losing large amounts of electrolytes (secondary to vomiting, nasogastric suction, diarrhea, or gastrointestinal fistulas) that are replaced with hypotonic solutions. Simple replacement with isotonic fluids and potassium usually corrects the abnormality. Rarely will rapid correction of the hyponatremia be necessary, in which case hypertonic saline (3%) can be administered. Hypertonic saline should be very cautiously administered to avoid a rapid shift in serum sodium, which induces central nervous system dysfunction.

Hypernatremia. Hypernatremia is an uncommon condition that can be life threatening if severe (serum sodium greater than 160 mEq/L). The pathophysiology is one of severe extracellular fluid deficit. The consequent hyperosmolar state results in decreased water volume in cells in the central nervous system, which, if severe, can result in disorientation, seizures, intracranial bleed, and death. The causes include excessive extrarenal water loss, as seen in patients with high fever, tracheostomy in a dry environment, extensive thermal injuries, diabetes insipidus (either central or nephrogenic), and iatrogenic salt loading. Treatment consists of correction of the underlying cause (correction of fever, humidification of the tracheostomy, pitressin for control of central diabetes insipidus) and replacement with free water either orally or intravenously with D_5W. As with severe hyponatremia, marked hypernatremia should be corrected slowly.

Hypokalemia. Hypokalemia may be encountered postoperatively in patients with significant gastrointestinal fluid loss (prolonged emesis, diarrhea, nasogastric suction, intestinal fistulas), marked urinary potassium loss secondary to renal tubular disorders (renal tubular acidosis, ATN, hyperaldosteronism, prolonged diuretic use), or from prolonged administration of potassium-free parenteral fluids in patients who are NPO. The symptoms associated with hypokalemia include neuromuscular disturbances ranging from muscle weakness to flaccid paralysis and cardiovascular abnormalities including hypotension, bradycardia, arrhythmias, and enhancement of digitalis toxicity. These symptoms rarely occur unless the serum potassium is below 3 mEq/L. The treatment is potassium replacement. Oral therapy is preferable in patients on an oral diet. If necessary, potassium replacement can be given intravenously in doses that should not exceed 10 mEq/hr.

Hyperkalemia. Hyperkalemia is infrequently encountered in postoperative patients. It usually is associated with renal impairment but also can be seen in patients with adrenal insufficiency, with the use of potassium-sparing diuretics, and with marked tissue breakdown, as seen in patients with crush injuries, massive GI bleeding, or hemolysis. The clinical manifestations are mainly cardiovascular. Marked hyperkalemia (potassium greater than 7 mEq/L) can result in bradycardia, ventricular fibrillation, and cardiac arrest. The treatment chosen depends on the severity of the hyperkalemia and whether there are associated cardiac or electrocardiogram abnormalities. Calcium gluconate (10 ml of a 10% solution) given intravenously can offset the toxic effects of hyperkalemia on the heart. One ampule each of sodium bicarbonate and D50 with or without insulin causes a rapid shift of potassium into cells. Longer term, cation exchange resins such as Kayexalate, taken either orally or by enema, bind and decrease total body potassium. Hemodialysis is reserved for emergent conditions for which other measures are not sufficient or have failed.

Acid-Base Disorders. A variety of metabolic, respiratory, and electrolyte abnormalities can result in an imbalance in normal acid-base homeostasis, leading to alkalosis or acidosis. Changes in the respiratory rate directly affect the amount of carbon dioxide exhaled. Respiratory acidosis is caused by carbon dioxide retention in patients with hypoventilation from central nervous system depression; this can be seen under conditions of oversedation from narcotics, particularly in the presence of concurrent severe chronic obstructive pulmonary disease. Respiratory alkalosis results from hyperventilation either due to excitation of the central nervous system from drugs or pain or iatrogenically from excess ventilator support. Numerous metabolic derangements can result in alkalosis or acidosis, and these are discussed further in this section. Fortunately, proper fluid and electrolyte replacement and maintenance of adequate tissue perfusion help to prevent most acid-base disorders postoperatively.

Alkalosis. The most common acid-base disorder encountered in the postoperative period is alkalosis, which usually is of no clinical significance and resolves spontaneously. Alkalosis can be caused by the following factors:

1. Hyperventilation associated with pain
2. Posttraumatic transient hyperaldosteronism, which results in decreased renal bicarbonate excretion
3. Nasogastric suction, which removes hydrogen ions
4. Infused bicarbonate during blood transfusions in the form of citrate, which is converted to bicarbonates
5. Administration of exogenous alkali
6. Use of diuretics

Correction of the alkalosis can usually be easily achieved with removal of the inciting cause, as well as with correction of extracellular fluid and potassium deficits (Table 10-2). Full correction can usually be safely achieved over 1 to 2 days.

Marked alkalosis, with serum pH greater than 7.55, can result in serious cardiac arrhythmias or central nervous system seizures. Myocardial excitability is particularly pronounced with concurrent hypokalemia. Under such conditions, fluid and electrolyte replacement may not be sufficient to rapidly correct the alkalosis. Acetazolamide (250 to 500 mg) orally or intravenously can be given two to four times daily to induce renal bicarbonate diuresis. Treatment with an acidifying agent is rarely necessary and should be reserved for acutely symptomatic patients (cardiac or CNS dysfunction) or for patients with advanced renal dis-

Table 10-2 Metabolic Alkalosis

Disorder	Source of Alkali	Cause of Renal HCO_3 Retention
Gastric alkalosis		
Nasogastric suction	Gastric mucosa	↓ ECF, ↓ K
Vomiting		
Renal alkalosis		
Diuretics	Renal epithelium	↓ ECF, ↓ K
Respiratory acidosis and diuretics		↓ ECF, ↓ K, ↑ PCO_2
Exogenous base	$NaHCO_3$, Na citrate, Na lactate	Coexisting disorder of ECF, K, PCO_2

↓ *ECF,* Extracellular fluid depletion; ↓ *K,* potassium depletion; ↑ *PCO_2,* carbon dioxide retention.

ease. Under such conditions, HCl (5 mEq/hr to 10 mEq/hr of a 100 mmol solution) can be given through a central line. Ammonium chloride also can be given orally or intravenously but should not be given to patients with hepatic disease.

Acidosis. Metabolic acidosis can be potentially serious as a result of its effect on the cardiovascular system. Under conditions of acidosis, effects include decreased myocardial contractibility, a propensity for vasodilatation of the peripheral vasculature leading to hypotension, and refractoriness of the fibrillating heart to defibrillation. These effects promote decompensation of the cardiovascular system and can hinder attempts at resuscitation.

The primary pathophysiology of metabolic acidosis involves a decrease in serum bicarbonate level as a result of consumption and replacement of bicarbonate by circulating acids or owing to replacement by other anions, such as chloride. The proper workup includes a measurement of the anion gap:

$$\text{Anion gap} = Na^+ - (Cl^- + HCO_3^-) =$$
$$10 \text{ to } 14 \text{ mEq/L (normal)}$$

The anion gap is composed of circulating protein, sulfate, phosphate, citrate, and lactate.

Patients with metabolic acidosis can be divided into two groups based on the anion gap (increased vs. normal anion gap). An increase in circulating acids will consume and replace bicarbonate ion, thus increasing the anion gap. The causes include an increase in circulating lactic acid secondary to anaerobic glycolysis, as seen under conditions of poor tissue perfusion; increased ketoacids, as seen in cases of severe diabetes or starvation; exogenous toxins; and renal dysfunction, which leads to increased circulating sulfates and phosphates. The diagnosis can be established through a thorough history and measurement of serum lactate (normally less than 2 mmol/L), serum glucose, and renal function parameters. Metabolic acidosis in the face of a normal anion gap usually is the result of an imbalance of the ions chloride and bicarbonate, under conditions leading to excess chloride and decreased bicarbonate. Hyperchloremic acidosis can be seen in patients who have undergone saline loading. Bicarbonate loss is seen in patients with small bowel fistula, new ileostomies, severe diarrhea, or renal tubular acidosis. Finally, in patients with marked extracellular volume expansion, commonly seen postoperatively, the relative decrease in serum sodium and bicarbonate results in a mild acidosis. Table 10-3 summarizes the various causes of metabolic acidosis.

The treatment of metabolic acidosis depends on the cause. In patients with lactic acidosis, restoration of tissue perfusion is imperative and can be carried out through cardiovascular and pulmonary support, as needed, oxygen therapy, and aggressive treatment of systemic infection when appropriate. Ketosis from diabetes can be corrected gradually with insulin therapy. Ketosis resulting from chronic starvation or from lack of caloric support postoperatively can be corrected with nutrition. In patients with

Table 10-3 Causes of Metabolic Acidosis

High Anion Gap	Normal Anion Gap	
	Hyperkalemic	Hypokalemic
Uremia	Hyporeninism	Diarrhea
Ketoacidosis	Primary adrenal failure	Renal tubular acidosis
Lactic acidosis	NH_4Cl	Ileal and sigmoid bladders
Aspirin	Sulfur poisoning	
Paraldehyde	Early chronic renal failure	Hyperalimentation
Methanol	Obstructive uropathy	
Ethylene glycol		
Methylmalonic aciduria		

normal anion gap acidosis, bicarbonate losses from the gastrointestinal tract should be replaced, excess chloride administration curtailed, and, when necessary, a loop diuretic used to induce renal clearance of chloride. Dilutional acidosis can be corrected with mild fluid restriction.

Bicarbonates should not be given unless serum pH is less than 7.2 or unless acidosis has caused severe cardiac complications. Furthermore, close monitoring of serum potassium is mandatory. Under states of acidosis, potassium exits the cell and enters the circulation. A patient with a normal potassium concentration and metabolic acidosis actually is intracellularly potassium depleted. Treatment of acidosis without potassium replacement results in severe hypokalemia and its associated risks.

Postoperative Infections

Evaluation. Infections are a major cause of morbidity in the postoperative period. Risk factors of infectious morbidity include lack of perioperative antibiotic prophylaxis, contamination of the surgical field, either from infected tissues or from spillage of large bowel contents, an immunocompromised host, poor nutrition, chronic and debilitating severe illness, poor surgical technique, and preexisting focal or systemic infection. Sources of postoperative infection include the lung, urinary tract, surgical site, pelvic sidewall, vaginal cuff, abdominal wound, and sites of indwelling intravenous catheters. Early identification and treatment of infections result in the best outcome for patients with these potentially serious complications.

The standard definition of febrile morbidity for surgical patients is temperature 100.4° F (38° C) or higher on two occasions at least 4 hours apart in the postoperative period, excluding the first 24 hours. Febrile morbidity is common after gynecologic surgery and has been estimated to occur in as much as one half of patients. Febrile morbidity, when it occurs within the first 2 postoperative days, is usually self-limited and resolves without therapy. Although fever is a sign of infection, the diagnosis of infection is based on the combination of fever and clinical and laboratory evidence of an infected focus.

The workup of the febrile surgical patient should include a review of the patient's history with regard to risk factors and potential sites for infection, as well as thorough physi-

POSTHYSTERECTOMY INFECTIONS

OPERATIVE SITE	NONOPERATIVE SITE
Vaginal cuff	Urinary tract
Pelvic cellulitis	Asymptomatic bacteriuria
Pelvic abscess	Cystitis
Supravaginal, extraperi-	Pyelonephritis
toneal	Respiratory
Intraperitoneal	Atelectasis
Adnexa	Pneumonia
Cellulitis	Vascular
Abscess	Phlebitis
Abdominal incision	Septic pelvic thrombo-
Cellulitis	phlebitis
Simple	
Progressive bacterial	
synergistic	
Necrotizing fasciitis	
Myonecrosis	

From Hemsell DL: *Obstet Gynecol Clin North Am* 16:381, 1989.

cal examination with particular emphasis on the potential sites for infection (see the box above). This should include inspection of the pharynx, a thorough pulmonary examination, percussion of the costovertebral angles for tenderness, inspection and palpation of the abdominal incisions, examination of sites of intravenous catheters, and an examination of the extremities for evidence of deep venous thrombosis or thrombophlebitis. In gynecologic patients, appropriate workup also may include inspection and palpation of the vaginal cuff for signs of induration, tenderness, or purulent drainage. A pelvic examination also should be performed to identify a mass consistent with a pelvic hematoma or abscess and to look for signs of pelvic cellulitis.

The laboratory and radiologic evaluation may include a white blood cell count with differential, a catheterized urinalysis and culture, and a chest x-ray for patients with signs and symptoms localizing to the lung. Blood cultures also can be obtained but most likely will yield little unless the patient has a high fever (greater than 102° F). In patients with costovertebral angle tenderness, an intravenous pyelogram may be indicated to rule out ureteral damage or obstruction from surgery, particularly in the absence of laboratory evidence of urinary tract infection. Patients who have persistent fevers without a clear localizing source should have a CT scan of the abdomen and pelvis to rule out the presence of an intraabdominal abscess. Finally, in patients who have undergone gastrointestinal surgery, a barium enema or upper GI series with small bowel follow-through may be indicated late in the course of the first postoperative week if fevers persist to rule out an anastomotic leak or fistula.

Urinary Tract Infections. The urinary tract has historically been the most common site of infection in gynecologic surgical patients. However, the incidence reported in the more recent gynecologic literature has been less than 4%. This decrease in urinary tract infections has most likely

been due to the increased use of perioperative prophylactic antibiotics. The incidence of postoperative urinary tract infection in gynecologic surgical patients not receiving prophylactic antibiotics has been confirmed to be as high as 40%, and even a single dose of perioperative prophylactic antibiotic has been shown to decrease the incidence of postoperative urinary tract infection from 35% to 4%.[10]

Although the urinary tract is one of the more common sites of postoperative infection, few of these are serious. Most infections are confined to the lower urinary tract. Pyelonephritis is a rare complication postoperatively. Catheterization of the urinary tract, either intermittently or continuously through an indwelling catheter, has been implicated as a main cause of urinary tract contamination. Therefore the use of urinary catheters should be minimized or avoided when possible.

Symptoms of a urinary tract infection include urinary frequency, urgency, and dysuria. In patients with pyelonephritis, other symptoms have commonly included headache, malaise, nausea, and vomiting. The diagnosis of urinary tract infection is made microbiologically and is defined as the growth of greater than 10^5 organisms per milliliter of urine cultured. The majority of the infections are caused by coliforms, with *Escherichia coli* being the most common pathogen. Other pathogens include *Klebsiella, Proteus,* and *Enterobacter* spp. *Staphylococcus* spp. are the causative bacteria in fewer than 10% of cases.

The treatment of urinary tract infection includes hydration and antibiotic therapy. Commonly prescribed and effective antibiotics have included penicillins, sulfonamides, cephalosporins, and nitrofurantoin. The choice of antibiotic for treatment should be made with knowledge of the susceptibility of organisms cultured at each institution. In some institutions, for example, more than 40% of *E. coli* strains are resistant to ampicillin. For uncomplicated urinary tract infections, an antibiotic should be chosen that is effective against *E. coli* while awaiting the urine culture and sensitivity data. Patients who have a history of recurrent urinary tract infections, those with chronic indwelling catheters (Foley catheters or ureteral stents), and those who have urinary conduits should begin a regimen of antibiotics that will be effective against the less common urinary pathogens such as *Klebsiella.* More resistant organisms, such as *Pseudomonas,* may also be encountered in these patients.

Pulmonary Infections. The respiratory tract is an uncommon site for infectious complications in gynecologic surgical patients. Hemsell[8] noted only 6 cases of pneumonia in more than 4000 women who underwent elective hysterectomy. This low incidence is probably a reflection of the young age and good health status of gynecologic patients in general. In acute care facilities, pneumonia is a frequent nosocomial infection, particularly in the elderly. Risk factors include extensive or prolonged atelectasis, preexistent chronic obstructive pulmonary disease, severe or debilitating illness, central neurologic disease causing an inability to clear oropharyngeal secretions effectively, and nasogastric suction. In surgical patients, early ambulation and aggressive management of atelectasis are the most important preventive measures. The role of prophylactic antibiotics remains unclear.

Gram-negative organisms account for a significant proportion (40% to 50%) of hospital-acquired pneumonias. These organisms gain access to the respiratory tract from the oral pharynx. Gram-negative colonization of the oral pharynx has been shown to be increased in patients in acute care facilities; it has been associated with the presence of nasogastric tubes, preexisting respiratory disease, mechanical ventilation, tracheal intubation, and paralytic ileus, which is associated with an increase in the microbial overgrowth in the stomach. Interestingly, antimicrobial drugs seem to significantly increase the frequency of colonization of the oral pharynx with gram-negative bacteria.

A thorough lung examination should be included in the workup of all febrile surgical patients. In the absence of significant lung findings, a chest x-ray is probably of little benefit in patients at low risk for postoperative pulmonary complications. A chest x-ray should be obtained in patients with pulmonary findings or with risk factors for pulmonary complications. A sputum sample also should be obtained for gram stain and culture. Treatment includes postural drainage, aggressive pulmonary toilet, and antibiotics. The antibiotic chosen should be effective against both gram-positive and gram-negative organisms.

Phlebitis. Intravenous catheter–related infections are common, with a reported incidence of 25% to 35%.[22] The intravenous site should be inspected daily and the catheter removed if there is any associated pain, redness, or induration. Unfortunately, phlebitis can occur even if the intravenous site is monitored closely. In one study, more than 50% of the cases of phlebitis became evident more than 12 hours after discontinuation of IV catheters. In addition, less than one third of patients had symptoms related to the intravenous catheter site 24 hours before the diagnosis of phlebitis.

Intravenous catheters should be inserted using careful, sterile technique, and they should be changed frequently. The incidence of catheter-related phlebitis rises significantly after 72 hours; therefore intravenous catheters should be changed at least every 3 days. The institution of intravenous therapy teams has resulted in a decreased incidence of phlebitis by as much as 50%. This decrease was thought to be due not so much to surveillance of the intravenous catheter site by the intravenous therapy teams, but rather to frequent changing of intravenous catheters.

The diagnosis of phlebitis can be made in the presence of fever, pain, redness, induration, or a palpable venous cord. Occasionally, suppuration is present. Phlebitis is usually self-limiting and resolves within 3 to 4 days. The treatment includes application of warm, moist compresses and prompt removal of any catheters from the infected vein. Antibiotic therapy with antistaphylococcal agents should be instituted for catheter-related sepsis. Excision or drainage of an infected vein is rarely necessary.

Wound Infections. Cruse[3] studied the epidemiology of wound infections in more than 62,000 patients. In this study, the wound infection rate varied markedly, depending on the extent of contamination of the surgical field. The wound infection rate for clean surgical cases (infection not present in the surgical field, no break in aseptic technique, and no hollow viscus entered) was less than 2%, whereas the incidence of wound infections with dirty, infected cases was 40% or greater. Preoperative showers with hexachlorophene slightly lowered the infection rate for clean wounds, whereas preoperative shaving of the wound site with a razor increased the infection rate. A 5-minute wound preparation immediately preoperatively was as effective as a 10-minute preparation. The wound infection rate increased with increasing length of preoperative hospital stay and with longer duration of surgery. In addition, incidental appendectomy increased the risk of wound infection in patients undergoing clean surgical procedures. The study concluded that the incidence of wound infections could be decreased by the institution of short preoperative hospital stays, hexachlorophene showers before surgery, minimizing shaving of the wound site, use of meticulous surgical technique, decreasing operative time as much as possible, bringing drains out through sites other than the wound, and through dissemination of information to each surgeon of his or her wound infection rate. A program instituting these conclusions helped to decrease the clean wound infection rate from 2.5% to 0.6% over an 8-year period.

In general, the wound infection rate in obstetric and gynecologic services has been less than 5%, reflective of the clean nature of most gynecologic operations. The symptoms of wound infection often occur late in the postoperative period, usually after the fourth postoperative day, and can include fever, erythema, tenderness, induration, and purulent drainage. The management is mostly mechanical and involves opening the infected portion of the wound above the fascia, with cleansing and debridement of the wound edges as necessary. Wound care, consisting of debridement and dressing changes two or three times daily with mesh gauze, promotes growth of granulation tissue, with gradual filling in of the wound defect by secondary intention. The authors prefer to pack wounds with dry rather than wet gauze because better debridement of the wound edges is achieved upon the removal of dry gauze. Clean, granulating wounds can often be secondarily closed successfully, shortening the time required for complete wound healing.

The technique of delayed primary wound closure can be used in infected surgical cases to lower the incidence of wound infection. Briefly, the technique involves leaving the wound open above the fascia during the initial surgical procedure. Vertical interrupted mattress sutures through the skin and subcutaneous layers are placed 3 cm apart but are not tied. Wound care is instituted immediately after surgery and continued until the wound is noted to be granulating well. Sutures then can be tied and the skin edges further approximated using staples. With this technique of delayed primary wound closure, the overall wound infection rate has been shown to decrease from 23% to 2.1% in high-risk patients.[2]

Pelvic Cellulitis. Vaginal cuff cellulitis is present to some extent in most patients who have undergone hysterectomy and is characterized by erythema, induration, and tenderness at the vaginal cuff. Occasionally, a purulent discharge from the apex of the vagina is present. The cellulitis is often self-limited and does not require any treatment. Fever, leukocytosis, and pain localized to the pelvis may accompany a severe cuff cellulitis and most often signifies extension of the cellulitis to adjacent pelvic tissues. In such cases, broad-spectrum antibiotic therapy should be instituted with coverage for gram-negative, gram-positive, and anaerobic organisms. If purulence at the vaginal cuff is excessive, or a fluctuance or a mass is noted at the vaginal cuff, the vaginal cuff should be gently probed and opened with a blunt instrument. The cuff can then be left open for dependent drainage or, alternatively, a drain can be placed into the lower pelvis through the cuff and removed when drainage, fever, and lower pelvic symptoms have resolved.

Intraabdominal and Pelvic Abscess. The development of an abscess in the surgical field or elsewhere in the abdominal cavity is an uncommon severe complication after gynecologic surgery. It is most likely to occur in contaminated cases in which the surgical site is not adequately drained or as a secondary complication of hematomas. The causative pathogens recovered in patients who have intraabdominal abscess are usually polymicrobial in nature. The aerobes most commonly identified include *E. coli, Klebsiella, Streptococcus, Proteus,* and *Enterobacter.* Anaerobic isolates are also common, usually from the *Bacteroides* spp. These pathogens mainly come from the vagina but also can be derived from the gastrointestinal tract, particularly when the colon has been entered during surgery.

The diagnosis of intraabdominal abscess is sometimes difficult to make. The evolving clinical picture is often one of persistent febrile episodes with a rising white blood cell count. Findings on abdominal examination may be equivocal. An abscess located deep in the pelvis may be palpable by pelvic or rectal examination. Diagnosis for abscesses above the pelvis depends on radiologic confirmation.

Ultrasound can occasionally delineate fluid collections in the upper abdomen and pelvis. However, bowel gas interference makes visualization of fluid collections or abscesses in the mid-abdomen difficult. CT scanning is therefore much more sensitive and specific for diagnosing intraabdominal abscesses and is often the radiologic procedure of choice. Occasionally, if conventional radiologic methods fail to identify an abscess and the index of suspicion for an abscess remains high, an indium-labeled leukocyte scan may be useful for locating the infected focus.

Standard therapy for intraabdominal abscess is surgical evacuation and drainage combined with appropriate parenteral antibiotics. Abscesses low in the pelvis, particularly in the area of the vaginal cuff, can often be reached through a vaginal approach. In many patients, the ability to drain an abscess by placement of a drain percutaneously under CT guidance has obviated the need for a surgical exploration. With CT guidance, a pigtail catheter is placed into an ab-

scess cavity and left in place until drainage decreases. Gram stain and anaerobic and aerobic cultures should be obtained to guide antibiotic selection. The "gold standard" of initial antibiotic therapy has been the combination of ampicillin, gentamicin, and clindamycin. Adequate treatment also can be achieved with currently available broad-spectrum single agents, including broad-spectrum penicillin, second- and third-generation cephalosporins, and sulbactam, clavulanic acid–containing preparations.

Necrotizing Fasciitis. Necrotizing fasciitis is an uncommon infectious disorder, with approximately 1000 cases occurring annually in the United States. The disorder is characterized by a rapidly progressive bacterial infection involving the subcutaneous tissues and fascia, while characteristically sparing underlying muscle. Systemic toxicity is a frequent feature of this disease, as manifested by the presence of dehydration, septic shock, disseminated intravascular coagulation, and multiorgan system failure.

The pathogenesis of necrotizing fasciitis involves a polymicrobial infection of the dermis and subcutaneous tissue. Hemolytic streptococcus was initially thought to be the primary pathogen responsible for the infection in necrotizing fasciitis. However, it is now evident that numerous other organisms are often cultured in addition to *Streptococcus,* including other gram-positive organisms, coliforms, and anaerobes. Bacterial enzymes such as hyaluronidase and lipase released in the subcutaneous space destroy the fascia and adipose tissue and induce a liquefactive necrosis. In addition, noninflammatory intravascular coagulation or thrombosis subsequently occurs. Intravascular coagulation results in ischemia and necrosis of the subcutaneous tissues and skin. Late in the course of the infection, destruction of the superficial nerves produces anesthesia in the involved skin. The release of bacteria and bacterial toxins into the systemic circulation can cause septic shock, acid-base disturbances, and multiorgan impairment.

The diagnostic criteria for necrotizing fasciitis have been defined by Fisher.[5] These include extensive necrosis of the superficial fascia and subcutaneous tissue with peripheral undermining of the normal skin, a moderate to severe systemic toxic reaction, the absence of muscle involvement, the absence of *Clostridia* in wound and blood culture, the absence of major vascular occlusion, intensive leukocytic infiltration, and necrosis of subcutaneous tissue.

Most patients are in pain, which in the early stages of the disease is often disproportionately greater than that expected from the degree of cellulitis present. Late in the course of the infection, the involved skin may actually be anesthetized secondary to necrosis of superficial nerves. Temperature abnormalities, both hyperthermia and hypothermia, are common, concomitant with the release of bacterial toxins, as well as with bacterial sepsis, which can be present in up to 40% of patients. The involved skin is initially tender, erythematous, and warm. Edema develops and the erythema spreads diffusely, fading into normal skin, characteristically without distinct margins or induration. Subcutaneous microvascular thrombosis induces ischemia in the skin, which becomes cyanotic and blistered. Eventually, as necrosis develops, the skin becomes gangrenous and may spontaneously slough. Most patients have leukocytosis and acid-base abnormalities. Finally, subcutaneous gas may develop, which can be identified by palpation and x-ray. The finding of subcutaneous gas by x-ray is often indicative of clostridial infection, although it is not a specific finding and may be due to other organisms. These organisms include *Enterobacter, Pseudomonas,* anaerobic *Streptococci,* and *Bacteroides,* which, unlike clostridial infections, spare the muscles underlying the affected area. A tissue biopsy specimen for gram stain and aerobic and anaerobic culture should be obtained from the necrotic center of the lesion to identify the etiologic organisms. Although a diagnosis of necrotizing fasciitis is often made at surgery, a high index of suspicion and liberal use of frozen section biopsy can often provide an early lifesaving diagnosis and minimize morbidity.

Predisposing risk factors for necrotizing fasciitis include diabetes mellitus, trauma, alcoholism, an immunocompromised state, hypertension, peripheral vascular disease, intravenous drug abuse, and obesity. The extremities are the most frequent site of infection, but infection can occur anywhere in the subcutaneous tissues, including the head and neck, trunk, and perineum. Necrotizing fasciitis has been known to occur after trauma, surgery, burns, and lacerations, as a secondary complication in perirectal infections or Bartholin's abscesses, and de novo. Increased age, delay in diagnosis, inadequate debridement at initial operation, extent of disease on initial presentation, and diabetes mellitus are all factors that have been associated with an increased likelihood of mortality from necrotizing fasciitis. Clearly, early diagnosis and aggressive management of this lethal disease have led to improved chances of survival. In an earlier series, mortality was consistently over 30%; in more recent series, the mortality has decreased to less than 10%.

Successful management of necrotizing fasciitis involves early recognition, immediate initiation of resuscitative measures (including correction of fluid, acid-base, electrolyte, and hematologic abnormalities), aggressive surgical debridement and redebridement as necessary, and broad-spectrum antibiotic therapy. Many patients benefit from central venous monitoring and high caloric nutritional support.

At surgery, the incision should be made through the infected tissue down to the fascia. An ability to undermine the skin and subcutaneous tissues with digital palpation often will confirm the diagnosis. Multiple incisions can be made sequentially toward the periphery of the affected tissue until well-vascularized, healthy, resistant tissue is reached at all margins. The remaining affected tissue must be excised. The wound can then be packed and sequentially debrided on a daily basis as necessary until it displays healthy tissue at all margins. Hyperbaric oxygen therapy can be of some benefit, particularly in patients whose cultures are positive for anaerobic organisms. The primary concern after the initial resuscitative efforts and surgical debridement is the management of the open wound. Allograft and xenograft skin can be used to cover open wounds, thus decreasing heat and evaporative water loss. Interestingly, temporary biologic closure of open wounds also seems to decrease bacterial growth. Finally, skin flaps can be mobilized to help cover open wounds once the wound infections have resolved and granulation has begun.

Postoperative Nutrition and Gastrointestinal Complications

Postoperative Nutritional Requirements and Parenteral Support. Most patients have adequate nutrition before gynecologic surgery and reestablish dietary intake soon postoperatively. However, some patients (e.g., those with cancer) may need additional nutritional support. A number of retrospective surgical studies have demonstrated that nutritional support improves postoperative outcome in a variety of categories including surgical complications, sepsis, wound infections, and mortality. The Veterans Affairs Cooperative Study Group best evaluated the role of total parenteral nutrition (TPN) in a multiinstitutional prospective, randomized trial that reported a series of 395 malnourished patients randomly assigned to receive TPN for 7 to 15 days before surgery and 3 days postoperatively (treatment arm) or no perioperative TPN at all (control arm). The patients were then followed for 90 days after the surgery and were evaluated in terms of morbidity and mortality. Major complications during the first 30 days, as well as the overall 90-day mortality rates, were similar in both the treated and control arms. The only advantage to TPN was in a small group of patients with extremely severe malnutrition where the incidence of noninfectious complications was significantly less common. The study defined severe malnutrition as any patient with a nutritional risk index score of less than 83. The authors of that study concluded that preoperative TPN should be limited to patients who were severely malnourished unless there were other specific indications.[23]

When the patient has only mild or moderate malnutrition preoperatively or is nutritionally normal biochemically, but the proposed surgery is likely to require a prolonged catabolic period of more than 7 to 10 days, then TPN should be instituted in the early postoperative period as soon as the patient is hemodynamically stable. This type of management should be strongly considered in patients undergoing pelvic exenterations, urinary diversions, or multiple enterectomies.

In patients who need additional nutritional support and who have an intact, functioning GI tract, enteral nutrition should be instituted because it is the easiest and least expensive method of delivery associated with the fewest complications. Contraindications to this route of delivery include intestinal obstruction, gastrointestinal bleeding, and diarrhea. Many different types of enteral support are commercially available and can be chosen based on their caloric content, fat content, protein content, osmolality, viscosity, and price. Depending on the patient's particular problem, the route of delivery may be through a Dobbhoff feeding tube, a gastrostomy tube, or a feeding jejunostomy tube.

Overall, TPN has been widely accepted as a way to provide nutritional support in surgically ill patients. TPN must be delivered through a subclavian or internal jugular vein, and the placement of this catheter must be made using meticulous sterile surgical technique. Proper daily care must be given to avoid infectious complications, and a eumetabolic state may be obtained if multivitamins, including folate, B_{12}, and trace metals (cobalt, iodine, manganese, and zinc), are used to supplement the 2 to 3 L/day TPN solution. Essential fatty acids are supplied weekly, and iron may be added if hyperalimentation is prolonged and bone marrow stores have become depleted. Appropriate adjustments in TPN contents must be made in patients with liver, renal, or cardiac dysfunction. The most frequent complication, infection, occurs in only 5% to 10% of patients when managed by an experienced team.

Ileus. After abdominal or pelvic surgery, most patients have a component of intestinal ileus. The exact mechanism by which this arrest and disorganization of gastrointestinal motility occurs is unknown, but it appears to be associated with the opening of the peritoneal cavity and is aggravated by more extensive manipulation of the intestinal tract and prolonged surgical procedures. Infection, peritonitis, and electrolyte disturbances can also result in an ileus. For most patients undergoing common gynecologic operations, the degree of ileus is minimal and gastrointestinal function returns relatively rapidly, allowing for the resumption of oral intake within a few days of surgery. On the other hand, the patient who has persistently diminished bowel sounds, abdominal distention, and nausea and vomiting requires further evaluation and more aggressive management.

Ileus usually is manifested by abdominal distention and initially should be evaluated by physical examination. Pertinent points of the abdominal examination include assessment of the quality of bowel sounds and palpation to search for tenderness or rebound. The possibility that a patient's signs and symptoms may be associated with a more serious intestinal obstruction or other intestinal complication also must be considered. Pelvic examination should be performed to evaluate the possibility of a pelvic abscess or hematoma that may be contributing to the ileus. Abdominal x-ray films of the abdomen in the flat (supine) and upright positions usually aid in the diagnosis of an ileus. The most common radiographic findings include dilated loops of small and large bowel, as well as air-fluid levels in the upright position. Massive dilation of the colon or stomach sometimes is noted. Rectal examination, proctosigmoidoscopy, or barium enema should exclude the remote possibility of distal colonic obstruction suggested by a dilated cecum. The flat plate of the abdomen in the postoperative gynecology patient, especially in the upright position, also may show evidence of free air. This is a common finding after surgery and lasts from 7 to 10 days in some instances; it is not indicative of a perforated viscus in the majority of patients.

The initial management of a postoperative ileus is aimed at gastrointestinal tract decompression and maintenance of appropriate intravenous replacement of fluids and electrolytes. A well-positioned and properly functioning nasogastric tube should be used to evacuate the stomach of its fluid and gaseous contents. Furthermore, and of great importance, prolonged nasogastric suction continues to remove swallowed air, which is the most common source of air in the small bowel. Some clinicians prefer a longer small intestinal tube (Cantor or Miller-Abbott tube). These tubes, which usually have a mercury-filled bag on their distal tip, may be propelled by peristalsis through the pylorus and into the small bowel, thus allowing a better evacuation of the small bowel. The disadvantages of "long tubes" are that they take a longer time to become positioned and may not enter the small bowel as a result of the decreased intestinal motility associated with ileus. Fluid and electrolyte replacement must be adequate to keep the patient well perfused. Significant amounts of third-space fluid loss occur in the bowel wall, the bowel lumen, and the peritoneal cavity during the acute episode. Further, gastrointestinal fluid losses from the stomach can lead to a metabolic alkalosis and depletion of other electrolytes as well. Careful monitoring of serum chemistries and appropriate replacement are necessary. Most cases of severe ileus begin to improve over several days. In general, this is recognized by reduction in abdominal distention, return of normal bowel sounds, and passage of flatus or stool. Follow-up abdominal x-ray films should be obtained as necessary for further monitoring. When gastrointestinal tract function appears to have returned to normal, the nasogastric tube can be discontinued and a liquid diet instituted. On the other hand, if a patient shows no evidence of improvement over the first 48 to 72 hours of medical management, other causes of ileus should be sought, including ureteral injury, peritonitis from pelvic infection, unrecognized gastrointestinal tract injury with peritoneal spill, or fluid and electrolyte abnormalities such as hypokalemia. It has been suggested that in the evaluation of persistent ileus, water-soluble upper gastrointestinal contrast study can assist in the resolution of the ileus. However, prospective randomized data regarding this therapeutic maneuver are lacking.

Small Bowel Obstruction. Obstruction of the small bowel after major gynecologic surgery occurs in approximately 1% to 2% of patients. Adhesion to the operative site is the most common cause of small bowel obstruction. Should the small bowel become adherent in a twisted position, distention, ileus, and bowel wall edema can lead to partial or complete obstruction. Less common causes of postoperative small bowel obstruction include herniation of the small bowel into an incisional hernia and an unrecognized defect in the small bowel or large bowel mesentery. Early in its clinical course, a postoperative small bowel obstruction may have signs and symptoms identical to those of an ileus. Initial conservative management as outlined for the treatment of an ileus is appropriate. Because of the potential for mesenteric vascular occlusion and resulting ischemia or perforation, worsening symptoms of abdominal pain, progressive distention, fever, leukocytosis, or acidosis should be evaluated carefully because immediate surgery may be necessary. In most cases of small bowel obstruction following gynecologic surgery, the obstruction is only partial and the symptoms usually resolve with conservative management. As with an ileus, further evaluation after several days of conservative management may be necessary. Evaluation of the gastrointestinal tract with barium enema and an upper gastrointestinal series with small bowel follow-through is most appropriate. In most cases, complete obstruction is not documented, although a narrowing or tethering of the segment of small bowel can lead to suspicion of the site of the gastrointestinal problem. Further conservative management with nasogastric decompression and intravenous fluid replacement may allow time for bowel wall edema or torsion of the mesentery to resolve. If this process becomes prolonged, and the patient's nutritional status is marginal, total parenteral nutrition may be necessary. Conservative medical management of postoperative small bowel obstruction usually results in complete resolution. However, if after full evaluation and an adequate trial of medical management persistent evidence of small bowel obstruction remains, an exploratory laparotomy may be necessary to surgically evaluate and manage the obstruction. Most cases just require lysis of adhesions, although a segment of small bowel that is badly damaged or extensively sclerosed from adhesions may require resection and reanastamosis.

Colonic Obstruction. Colonic obstruction following surgery for most gynecologic conditions is exceedingly rare. It is almost always associated with a pelvic malignancy, which in most cases will have been known at the time of the initial operation. Advanced ovarian carcinoma is the most common cause of colonic obstruction in postoperative gynecologic surgery patients. Pelvic malignancy causes extrinsic impingement of the colon. Intrinsic colonic lesions may have gone unrecognized, especially in a patient with some other benign gynecologic condition. When colonic obstruction is manifested by abdominal distention and abdominal radiographs reveal a dilated colon and enlarging cecum, further evaluation of the large bowel with barium enema or colonoscopy is necessary. Dilation of the cecum on abdominal x-ray to greater than 10 to 12 cm in diameter requires immediate evaluation and surgical decompression through a colostomy. This should be performed at the earliest point at which the obstruction is documented. Conservative management of colonic obstruction is not appropriate because the mortality of colonic perforation is exceedingly high.

Diarrhea. Episodes of diarrhea are common after abdominal and pelvic surgery as the gastrointestinal tract returns to its normal function and motility. However, prolonged and multiple episodes may represent a pathologic process such as impending small bowel obstruction, colonic obstruction, or pseudomembranous colitis. Excessive amounts of diarrhea should be evaluated by abdominal x-ray films and stool samples for *Clostridium difficile* toxin, the presence of ova and parasites, and bacterial culture. Proctoscopy and colonoscopy also may be indicated in severe cases. Evidence of intestinal obstruction should be managed as outlined previously. Infectious causes of diarrhea should be managed with appropriate antibiotics and

fluid and electrolyte replacement. *C. difficile* associated with pseudomembranous colitis can result from exposure to any antibiotic. Discontinuation of these antibiotics (unless needed for another severe infection) is advisable, along with the institution of appropriate therapy. Because of the expense of vancomycin, the authors usually institute therapy with metronidazole. This therapy should be continued until the diarrhea abates, and several weeks of oral therapy may be necessary to completely resolve the pseudomembranous colitis.

Fistula. Gastrointestinal fistulas following gynecologic operations also are relatively rare. They most often are associated with malignancy, prior radiation therapy, or surgical injury to the large or small bowel that was improperly repaired or unrecognized. Signs and symptoms of gastrointestinal fistula are often similar to those of small bowel obstruction or ileus, except that a fever usually is a more prominent component of the patient's symptomatology. When fever is associated with gastrointestinal dysfunction postoperatively, evaluation should include early assessment of the gastrointestinal tract for its continuity. When fistula is suspected, water-soluble gastrointestinal contrast material is advised to avoid the complication of barium peritonitis. Evaluation with abdominal pelvic CT scan also may help to identify a fistula and associated abscess. Recognition of an intraperitoneal gastrointestinal leak or fistula requires immediate surgery unless the fistula has drained spontaneously through the abdominal wall or vaginal cuff.

Enterocutaneous fistula arising from the small bowel and draining spontaneously through the abdominal incision can occasionally be managed successfully with medical therapy. This should include nasogastric decompression, replacement of intravenous fluids, total parenteral nutrition, and appropriate antibiotics to treat an associated mixed bacterial infection. If the infection is under control and no other signs of peritonitis are present, the surgeon may consider allowing potential resolution of the fistula over a period of up to 2 weeks. Some authors have suggested the use of somatostatin to decrease intestinal tract secretion and allow for earlier healing of the fistula. In some cases this has resulted in spontaneous closure of the fistula. If, on the other hand, the enterocutaneous fistula does not close with conservative medical management, surgical correction with resection, bypass, or reanastomosis will be necessary in most cases.

A rectovaginal fistula following gynecologic surgery usually is the result of surgical trauma that may have been aggravated by extensive adhesions in the rectovaginal septum associated with endometriosis, pelvic inflammatory disease, or pelvic malignancy. Management of a small rectovaginal fistula can take a conservative medical approach, hoping that decreasing the fecal stream will allow closure of the fistula. In other patients, a small fistula that allows continence except for an occasional leak of flatus can be managed conservatively until the inflammatory process in the pelvis resolves. At that point, usually several months later, correction of the fistula is most appropriate. Large rectovaginal fistulas without hope of closing spontaneously are best managed by initial diverting colostomy followed by repair of the fistula after inflammation has resolved. Once the fistula closure is healed and established to be successful, take-down of the colostomy should be performed.

Other Complications of Pelvic and Vaginal Surgery

Vaginal Vault Evisceration. Dehiscence of the apex of the vagina with extrusion of omentum, intestine, or both generally suggests that the reconstruction of the supports of the vault, or the reconstitution of the levator plate during surgery, was inadequate, resulting in a faulty vaginal axis. Evisceration occurs only rarely after vaginal hysterectomy and seems independent of whether the vaginal vault is left opened or closed. It may be that a pathologically long (greater than 15 cm) small bowel mesentery permits the intraabdominal contents to exert unusual pressure on the surface of the cul-de-sac in the pelvic floor and vaginal vault. On the other hand, it may be that sudden, massive increases in intraabdominal pressure (e.g., violent coughing or postoperative retching) or extreme overexertion (e.g., heavy lifting), in which the entire force of increased intraabdominal pressure is directed to the long axis of the vagina, leads to evisceration.

The viability and integrity of the protruding structure determine the appropriate treatment. Protruding loops of intestine should be cleaned, drawn back into the peritoneal cavity at laparotomy, and fully inspected. If the tissues remain viable, the pelvic defect can be repaired with special care to obliterate the cul-de-sac and any enterocele that may be present. Any question about intestinal viability or the condition of the base of mesentery is an indication for bowel resection. Any necrotic vaginal tissue should be excised. The vaginal vault should be closed.

Foreign Bodies. Seldom are instruments left behind or lost during vaginal surgery. Although uncommon, a sponge or pack may occasionally be left in the cul-de-sac or a tissue plane. A sponge saturated with blood quickly assumes the color of the surrounding tissues and can easily be buried in a line of cleavage or beneath a flap or fold of plicated tissues. Sponges should be counted periodically during the course of a procedure, especially before the peritoneum is closed and again at the conclusion of the operation while the patient is still anesthetized and draped. If a missing sponge is not found in the pelvis or abdomen, vagina, or in the folds of drapes, a roentgenogram of the abdomen and pelvis should be obtained while the patient is still on the operating table. (It may be necessary to obtain separate films of the lower and upper abdomen if the patient is obese.) Only sponges with radiopaque marking should be used in surgery, and they can generally be seen on x-ray films. Under no circumstances should a sponge be cut in half during an operative procedure, lest a missing, unmarked half be invisible on a postoperative roentgenogram. Because they are so easily lost, small pushers or swabs in the surgical field are never separated from their holding forceps. Although foreign bodies have been found incidentally months or years after being left behind, most are found within a few days through clinical infection or intestinal ileus.

A foreign body forgotten during surgery generally causes a septic fever that is unresponsive to any antibiotic combination. An abscess pointing into the vagina can form, and probing the abscess can bring forth a few threads of the offending foreign body. Signs of local peritonitis indicate that foreign body is intraperitoneal; if transvaginal removal cannot be easily accomplished, abdominal laparotomy with drainage and culture of the purulent material may be necessary. When there are signs of extraperitoneal infection, such as localized subepithelial fluctuation, the surgeon should gently open into the tissue planes near the site of the suspected abscess.

A vaginal examination shortly before discharge from the hospital permits the identification of any unsuspected hematoma, the separation of any intravaginal adhesions, and the removal of overlooked intravaginal sponges or packing. A forgotten intravaginal sponge or packing invariably results in a profuse and offensive vaginal discharge that causes the patient considerable distress. Fortunately, a forgotten sponge or packing in the vagina rarely causes any serious damage, and the discharge subsides promptly after removal.

Problems with Postoperative Voiding. The bladder has a triple nerve supply—somatic, sympathetic, and parasympathetic—and the perception of and balance between those sometimes opposing influences vary from patient to patient and from time to time. Even minor physiologic and psychologic events can disturb the harmony of these influences. Therefore difficulty in the resumption of voiding after a major event such as pelvic surgery is a rather common problem, although it is not often predictable with any degree of certainty. Such difficulty may occur after any surgical procedure, but it is most likely to occur after procedures involving the abdomen and pelvis (e.g., episiotomy, colporrhaphy, hysterectomy, herniorrhaphy, hemorrhoidectomy, and laparotomy).

Prevention of Difficulties in Voiding. Facilitating the patient's postoperative resumption of voiding is of primary importance. The circumstances under which the patient is expected to void must be as private and comfortable as possible, and the patient's attendants must be prompt and calm when assisting. Years ago, von Peham and Amreich[24] noted that some patients encounter difficulty when they try to void in the recumbent position. If possible, the patient should be permitted to void while sitting in a natural position, using a nearby toilet if feasible (if not, a portable commode can be used or a bedpan if the patient is confined in bed). Some postoperative patients, however, can void more comfortably at first from a semistanding position, probably because it reduces the likelihood of levator spasm. Others may find manual suprapubic compression over the bladder helpful once voiding has begun, and this technique is more effective when the patient leans somewhat forward during the voiding process.

Overdistention of the bladder (urine volume greater than 500 ml) is to be avoided at all costs. Overdistention not only is painful, but also appears to interfere temporarily with the blood supply of the bladder and thus reduce local resistance to infection. In addition, overdistention can cause a transient paralysis of the detrusor that can require days to overcome.

Synthetic absorbable sutures, such as those made of polyglycolic acid (e.g., Dexon and Vicryl) instead of catgut, appear to decrease postoperative intravaginal adhesions and swelling and edema of pelvic tissues. This is particularly noteworthy after colporrhaphy that includes any reconstructive plication or support of the vesicle neck, where longer lasting monofilament absorbable synthetic sutures of polydioxanone (e.g., PDS) or polyglyconate (e.g., Maxon) are used. The surgeon should instruct patients who have undergone a suprapubic sling procedure and have been accustomed to emptying their bladders by tightening the rectus muscles to increase intraabdominal pressure; patients should not use rectus muscles in the future, since voluntary rectus muscle contraction can tighten the sling sufficiently to occlude the urethra. When transurethral drainage is necessary, a silicone-coated Foley catheter (which is undoubtedly less irritating to the urethral mucosa than is the uncoated rubber of the standard catheter) reduces mucosal edema and thus decreases the risk of urethral obstruction.

If a patient has an extensive history of bladder decompensation (e.g., associated with a long-standing or massive cystocele), some intrinsic detrusor hypotonia can be predicted. Bladder tone can be increased by the judicious administration of bethanechol chloride (Urecholine) initially 10 mg three times daily; depending on the patient's response, it can be increased progressively to 25 mg four times daily before catheter removal and for several days thereafter until the patient can again void comfortably. In obviously anxious patients, preliminary sedation with diazepam-like drugs and judicious use of analgesics in doses tailored to the patient's needs can be very helpful.

Although stimulation of β-adrenergic receptors tends to relax the bladder neck and trigone in the presence of low amounts of noradrenaline, it tends to cause smooth muscle contractions. Because the bladder neck is well supplied with α-adrenergic receptors, α-adrenergic blocking agents, such as phenoxybenzamine hydrochloride (Dibenzyline) in a dose of 10 mg by mouth 4 to 5 hours after surgery and repeated, if necessary, once or twice during the first 24 hours, have been effective. Any β-blockers, such as propranolol hydrochloride (Inderal), may induce not only hypertonia by stimulating detrusor tone, but also some spasm of the bladder neck by selective blocking.

Causes and Treatment of Inability To Void. It is known that postoperative voiding difficulty can result from several causative factors. Additional factors that influence the process of voiding almost certainly exist but cannot yet be predictably or accurately understood or measured, especially the patient's motivation. There are some whose confidence in the function of their bladders is sufficient to overcome almost any disturbance. For those who are having difficulty, however, the calm, optimistic, and serene understanding of their attendants is of utmost importance during the brief time that for them constitutes a disquieting and disabling crisis.

Anxiety. A powerful cause of inability to void is anxiety on the part of the patient or her attendant staff. Sometimes this is preconditioned by fear, conversation with other patients, hearsay, or observation of other patients. Treatment includes appropriate counseling, calmness, cheerful confidence, and empathy from the attendant staff, as well as appropriate sedation and pain relief. Some authorities recommend the administration of tea to induce some detrusor hyperactivity or beer to provide some general body sedation.

Mechanical Interference. Local physical factors, such as the presence of vaginal packing, local edema, rectal fullness, or any obstruction of the urethra or ureters, may interfere with the physiology of voiding in the postoperative patient. Any mechanical factors that interfere with the opening of the internal urethral sphincter during attempts to void may play a role, especially those factors that inhibit the physiologic obliteration of the posterior vesicourethral angle. For example, very few women can void while a tight vaginal packing is in place. In these cases, any mechanical obstruction of the vagina or urethra must be removed; gentle urethral dilation can relieve any urethral stricture that is obstructing normal flow. Overhydration must be avoided when an indwelling catheter is to be removed; it not only exaggerates any difficulties that may be present but also causes rapid and unnecessary overdistention of the bladder.

Reflex Interference. Neurologic reflex interference with the normal physiology of voiding, as often seen after parturition, episiotomy, and hemorrhoidectomy, may be coincident with a levator spasm that causes a reflex spastic contraction in both the internal and external urethral sphincters. Patient nervousness and embarrassment accentuate this problem, of course. Sitz baths, analgesia, and time are the greatest help, because the bladder and urethral sphincters will again begin to relax when the painful but temporary levator spasm has finally been overcome. Similarly, pain in the rectus abdominis muscles as a result of a laparotomy incision often reflexly induces levator spasm, interfering with the physiologic descent of the vesicle neck during the voiding process. Again, patience, analgesia, and the temporary use of an α-adrenergic blocker (e.g., phenoxybenzamine) are often helpful.

As mentioned earlier, overdistention of the bladder can result in a temporary detrusor paralysis and is therefore to be avoided at all costs. It can develop insidiously in an oversedated and overhydrated patient who may fail to perceive or respond to bladder fullness. Once overdistention has become pathologic, the treatment is primarily expectant; bladder tone generally returns several days after continuous decompression by an indwelling catheter. It is essential, however, to prevent additional or future episodes of overdistention.

Neurologic Abnormality. A primary neurologic defect can lead to chronic bladder hypotonia. Because such a defect may be associated with diabetes, central nervous system lues, or multiple sclerosis, the patient's medical history may suggest the correlation. Neuropathy resulting from a herniated intervertebral disk may be evident; in this instance there is coincident constipation and usually a history of sudden onset. Herniated low disks that involve the cauda equina but are too far caudal to be evident on a myelogram may be present. Skillful neurologic evaluation is required for appropriate diagnosis.

Surgeons often recognize hypotonia preoperatively and may plan to stimulate the detrusor subtly by administering bethanechol (Urecholine) postoperatively. The initial dosage may be as low as 10 mg three times a day, but to obtain clinical effectiveness it may be necessary to increase the dosage rapidly to as much as 50 to 75 mg three times daily.

Drug-Induced Detrusor Hypotonia. Coincident and often long-term consumption of common tranquilizing agents may be associated with unexpected and sometimes chronic detrusor hypotonia. Surgeons should suspect this effect in patients who take daily doses of diazepam (Valium), chlordiazepoxide hydrochloride (Librium), thioridazine hydrochloride (Mellaril), chlorpromazine hydrochloride (Thorazine), prochlorperazine maleate (Compazine), and meprobamate (Miltown). In many instances other physicians may have prescribed these drugs, and the patient may have become so accustomed to taking them that she forgets to include them in her medical history. Discontinuation of such a drug, when it is a contributing factor to detrusor hypotonia, can result in a rather prompt reappearance of normal bladder tone.

The induction of detrusor hyperactivity by the deliberate creation of a chemical cystitis (e.g., by instilling merbromin [Mercurochrome] or ether in the bladder) is neither popular nor recommended. Not only are the results unpredictable, but also the procedure may unexpectedly lead to a longstanding chemical cystitis, sometimes of massive degree.

Bladder Management after Removal of the Catheter. After urogynecologic procedures, or whenever the catheter is left in place for more than 48 hours, special considerations should be observed.

Transurethral Catheter. The administration of antibiotics or antibacterials to "cover" the bacteria often associated with a prolonged indwelling bladder catheter need not begin until the day the catheter is removed. A urine culture and sensitivity study should be obtained at this time; if the culture reveals an infection, the most effective antibiotic should be prescribed until a subsequent culture shows the infection has been eradicated. Delaying the administration of antibiotics until this time seems to prevent or retard the development of antibiotic resistance in potential infecting organisms, which often occurs when antibacterial coverage is instituted in the immediate postoperative course. After urinary fistula repair, however, the immediate administration of antibiotics is appropriate to decontaminate the urine and mucosal layer of the freshly repaired bladder wound during the early healing phase.

The surgeon should instruct the nursing staff to catheterize the patient as necessary if she is unable to void after the

indwelling catheter has been removed. (Infinite gentleness is essential in catheterizing these already apprehensive individuals, whose tissues are understandably tender.) An alternative is to catheterize the patient two or three times daily, immediately after she voids but a small amount, until the postvoiding residual volume is no more than 100 ml on two consecutive occasions. The amount the patient voids usually is of prognostic significance, even when the initial residual volume is undesirably high. It is much more encouraging if a patient is voiding 100 to 200 ml with a residual volume of 200 to 250 ml, for example, than if she is voiding only 10 to 20 ml with the same residual volume. The prognosis for early resumption of adequate voiding is good. In the first situation, the amount voided can be expected to increase as the amount of residual urine decreases. In the second situation, it should be expected that resumption of adequate voiding will require a significantly longer time, often several weeks.

A patient who cannot void in adequate amounts after catheter removal may be taught self-catheterization with the soft plastic 14-Fr Mentor female catheter; as an alternative, she may be discharged with a Foley catheter in place and clamped, with the clamp opened and the bladder drained periodically as necessary. The surgeon should clearly explain that the inability to void postoperatively is temporary, that it is by no means rare or unusual, and that it is unlikely to lengthen or change the patient's convalescence in any way. Giving the patient a handout sheet concerning the use of the catheter is often quite helpful (see the box on p. 174, left).

Suprapubic Catheter. Suprapubic catheters are popular for prolonged postoperative bladder drainage or when resumption of normal bladder function is uncertain (such as after a radical hysterectomy). Surgeons may consider using a suprapubic catheter in two particular instances: (1) after repair of a fistula at the vesicle neck, as a means of keeping the catheter away from the site of fistula repair and (2) after the creation of a neovagina that requires the use of a vaginal obturator postoperatively. Should the surgeon be an advocate of suprapubic catheterization, patients may find a handout concerning the use of the suprapubic catheter informative (see the box on p. 174, right).

Prolapse of Fallopian Tube. When the vault of the vagina has been left open or partly open after hysterectomy, there is a watery drainage for the first 2 days postoperatively. Unless there is an unexpected urinary fistula present, the drainage consists of other body fluids such as serum, lymph, pus, or a combination of all three. Should it persist beyond 6 weeks, the possibility of prolapse of one end of a fallopian tube should be investigated.

A rare complication of vaginal and abdominal hysterectomy, prolapse of the fallopian tube through the apex of the vagina results in a peritoneal fistula. Such a prolapse is generally a consequence of (1) leaving the vaginal vault open at the conclusion of a hysterectomy and suturing the cut ends of the tube along a cut edge of the vault or (2) prolapse of the fimbriated end of the tube through the peritoneal opening unexpectedly and undetected as the peritoneum is being

---

PATIENT INFORMATION SHEET: USE OF A TRANSURETHRAL CATHETER

The bladder must be given time to rest so that the swelling and irritation caused by the surgery can subside. The length of time needed for recovery varies from person to person; it may take anywhere from a few days to several weeks. The greater the need for the repair and thus the greater the scope of the repair, the longer the period of recovery of comfortable bladder function.

During this recovery period, a person's kidney system continues to work, of course, and it is necessary to drain the urine from the bladder until functional recovery of the bladder has been completed. This drainage is provided by an indwelling catheter inserted through the urethra, the usual canal between the vulva and the bladder, at the time of surgery. This catheter can be clamped to stop the flow of urine until there is a sufficient amount in the bladder to produce a sense of urgency and a desire to void. At that time, the clamp can be removed, the bladder emptied, and the clamp reapplied.

After approximately 2 weeks of bladder rest, the catheter is removed by cutting it across with clean scissors sometime during the midmorning hours. Please call the office that weekday afternoon to tell us how the bladder is functioning. If you are passing adequate amounts of urine and the intervals between voidings are longer than 2 hours, it is likely that comfortable bladder function has returned. There may be a mild sensation of burning or irritation during voiding until the swelling in the urethra from the catheter has subsided, usually within 1 or 2 days. Should urinary burning and frequency increase instead of decrease, be sure to call the office.

PATIENT INFORMATION SHEET: USE OF A SUPRAPUBIC CATHETER

The physician who wishes to put the recently repaired tissues around the urethra, bladder, and vagina at complete rest while they recover from surgery may place a catheter into the bladder through a tiny incision in the skin of the lower abdomen. This is a temporary way of diverting the urine until the patient's own bladder is able to function again. Furthermore, it saves a patient the nuisance, discomfort, and irritation associated with repeated catheterization during the healing process.

By the time preliminary healing is under way, usually after the fourth postoperative day, this catheter may be fitted with a clamp that, when tightened, stops the flow of urine through the catheter and permits the bladder to fill. When the bladder is full and the patient feels a desire to void, she is encouraged to do so; after she has voided or has tried to void through the urethra, the clamp is opened and the bladder drained through the suprapubic catheter. This procedure is continued on a regular basis until the patient is able to pass most of the urine normally through the urethra and less than 2 ounces is drained from the suprapubic catheter after each voiding. Therefore it is important to keep a running account of the amount of urine voided naturally each time and the amount obtained from the catheter after each voiding.

When the residual volume of urine in the bladder after each voiding has remained less than 2 ounces, the suprapubic catheter clamp should be left firmly applied for a full 1 or 2 days to see whether regular urinary voiding is well established. If so, the catheter is removed by simply cutting across its midpoint. The Foley bulb rapidly decompresses, and the internal portion of the catheter is quietly and easily extracted by gentle traction. The catheter will be removed in your physician's office. The opening left by the catheter usually closes within a day or two, although a small amount of urine often drips from this opening at first, so a small dressing is necessary until the opening has closed.

---

closed. Closing most of the vault in layers is the recommended procedure because it securely buries the transected ends of the tubes beneath the wall of the vagina, well away from all vaginal edges, and prevents the development of a peritoneal fistula. Indications of the uncommon peritoneal fistula include a watery discharge and a friable soft tissue vaginal vault excrescence that bleeds easily and, at first, appears to be granulation tissue but fails to heal after simple cauterization or attempts to curette away the suspected granulations. If local excision fails and discharge persists, salpingectomy may be necessary as a cure; otherwise, the patient is likely to experience intermittent hydrorrhea, and the fistula provides a potential route for ascending infection.

In a useful transvaginal technique of total salpingectomy for a posthysterectomy fallopian tube prolapse, the operator begins by making a horizontal incision through the full thickness of the vagina posterior to the prolapsed tube and the vaginal scar. The operator incises the peritoneal cavity horizontally and carefully inspects the peritoneal side of the prolapsed tube. Mobilizing the tube, the operator makes another horizontal vaginal incision anterior to the prolapsed tube, removes the entire tube and a collar of vagina between the two incisions, and completes the procedure by closing the peritoneum and vagina separately. Alternatively, the salpingectomy may be performed laparoscopically or by laparotomy if there are many adhesions to surrounding tissues.

Neurologic Sequelae. Sciatic, perineal, and femoral nerve injury can occur as a complication of pelvic surgery. Perineal nerve injury is characterized by postoperative foot drop, difficulty walking, and inability to abduct or even lift the foot. The lateral surface of the leg and dorsal surface of the foot may be numb.

Patients with sciatic nerve injury demonstrate weakness of the hamstring muscles coincident with difficulty walking. Treatment consists of physiotherapy, including massage and galvanic electrical stimulation of the perineal nerve. The prognosis for recovery is good, but slow, often requiring several weeks or even months.

Prevention of neuropathy is centered on giving much attention to the proper position of the patient's legs in the stirrups, requiring flexion of the knees and hips and ensuring minimal external rotation of the latter.

Excessive external rotation of the thigh of the patient with legs in "candy-cane" stirrups for operations longer than

1.5 hours invites femoral neuropathy. This is identified post-operatively by the discovery of numbness and paresthesias of the thigh. The knee buckles when the patient stands, and often she cannot walk without assistance.

Treatment of femoral neuropathy is primarily by physiotherapy, including massage, active and passive quadriceps exercises, and a great deal of patience. Femoral neuropathy in a patient having vaginal surgery can be prevented by placement of lateral supports to the thigh of each leg in stirrups, inhibiting excessive abduction and exaggerated external rotation.

Femoral neuropathy also can follow laparotomy, usually in a thin patient in whom a self-retaining retractor had been used and there had been pressure from the lateral retractor blades on the femoral nerve or psoas muscles. The type of abdominal incision used seems to be of no importance.

Prevention of this neuropathy is by most careful placement of the lateral retractor blades, use of the smallest blade that is effective, and placement of a folded laparotomy pad beneath the tip of the blade to cushion the lateral pelvic wall. The prognosis for recovery is good but takes several weeks.

Prolonged gynecologic surgery—usually over three hours—on a patient in the lithotomy position risks compromise of circulation and neurologic function of the legs; this occurs if external pressure to a fascial compartment is sustained by the position of the supporting stirrups, elevating the pressure within the compartment to sufficiently obstruct arteriolar circulation with the contained muscles. Ischemia promotes edema, which further compresses the contained nerves and compromises function. Compression syndrome following prolonged surgery may be suspected if the patient complains of cramping in the lower legs, which appear firm and tense although pulsation of the pedal arteries are palpable. Accentuation of the pain is elicited upon passive stretching of the muscles within the fascial compartment. These symptoms may progress, often rapidly, to numbness, burning, and difficulty moving the legs. This may be followed by foot drop and decreased sensation over the feet.

Prompt consultation with a vascular or orthopedic surgeon is desirable. Muscle pressure measurements should be obtained immediately, and if elevated and within the first 12 hours postoperatively, surgical fasciotomy should be performed promptly to decompress the compartment and inhibit further damage to its contents. After 12 hours the risk of infection in tissue now partially necrotic or with circulatory compromise is accentuated and may outweigh the benefits of decompression. To aid circulation within the compartment, the patient's legs should be positioned at the level of her heart.

Prevention of compartment syndrome in surgical cases of long duration in which stirrups are used requires that padded stirrups carefully support both legs and thighs, paying special attention to position of the patient's feet to avoid passive dorsiflexion of the ankle. Passive repositioning of the legs is recommended during the surgical procedure.

The prognosis for recovery is good if permanent nerve and muscular damage has not occurred, although recovery can take several weeks. Significant neuromuscular damage can be suspected in a patient with compression syndrome who develops foot drop.

Deep Vein Thrombosis and Pulmonary Embolism

Pulmonary embolism accounts for 40% of deaths following gynecologic surgical procedures.[11] To prevent these serious complications, an effective program aimed at identifying high-risk patients and using prophylactic venous thromboembolism regimens should be followed. In addition, the early recognition and immediate treatment of deep vein thrombosis and pulmonary embolism are critical. Most pulmonary emboli arise from the deep venous system of the leg, although following gynecologic surgery, the pelvic veins also are a known source of fatal pulmonary embolus. The diagnosis of lower extremity deep venous thrombosis requires a high level of suspicion and the appropriate use of diagnostic tests. The signs and symptoms of deep vein thrombosis of the lower extremity include pain, edema, erythema, and prominent vascular pattern of the superficial veins. These signs and symptoms are relatively nonspecific in that from somewhere between 50% and 80% of patients with these symptoms do not actually have deep vein thrombosis. Conversely, approximately 80% of patients with symptomatic pulmonary emboli have no signs or symptoms of thrombosis in the lower extremities. Because of the lack of specificity, when the surgeon recognizes signs and symptoms, additional diagnostic tests should be performed to establish the diagnosis of deep vein thrombosis. The "gold standard" for diagnosis of deep vein thrombosis has been a contrast venogram. Unfortunately, this study is modestly uncomfortable, requires the injection of a contrast material that may cause allergic reaction or renal injury, and may result in phlebitis in approximately 5% of patients.

Newer diagnostic tests have been developed that are less invasive yet have a high accuracy rate in most patients. Impedance plethysmography is a noninvasive study that measures the change in electrical impedance of the lower extremity when venous blood flow and volume are altered by an occlusive cuff on the thigh. This study may be performed at the patient's bedside and repeated as often as necessary without any risk to the patient. Correlation with venography in symptomatic patients approaches 95%. The test is very good for the identification of deep venous thrombi in the popliteal, femoral, and external iliac segments. It is less accurate (30%) in identifying calf vein thrombosis and does not identify thrombi occurring in the internal iliac venous system. False-positive results are primarily due to extrinsic venous compression. In gynecology, this might include a large pelvic mass compressing the external iliac or common iliac vein.

Doppler ultrasound also has been used for the noninvasive diagnosis of deep vein thrombosis, although its accuracy is slightly less than that of impedance plethysmography. This is primarily due to the variable interpretation of audible venous flow patterns, which may be somewhat subjective. B-mode duplex Doppler imaging has been found to be more effective in the diagnosis of symptomatic venous thrombosis, especially when it arises in the proximal lower extremity. With duplex Doppler imaging, the femoral vein can be visualized and clots may be seen directly. Compression of the vein with the ultrasound probe tip allows for assessment of venous collapsibility; the presence of a thrombus diminishes vein wall collapsibility. Color flow studies also have been added to this imaging technique. Doppler imaging is less accurate when evaluating the calf venous system and pelvic veins. Magnetic resonance imaging (MRI) can also identify thrombi in the deep venous system quite accurately. The primary drawback to MRI is the time involved in examining the lower extremity and pelvis, as well as the expense of this technology. All of these diagnostic studies are accurate when performed by a skilled technologist and in most patients may replace the need for routine contrast venography.

The treatment of postoperative deep venous thrombosis requires the immediate institution of anticoagulant therapy. Heparin should be initiated giving a bolus of 5000 units intravenously, followed by a continuous intravenous infusion of 1000 units/hr. Approximately 4 hours after initiation of heparin therapy, an activated partial thromboplastin time (APTT) should be obtained to assess the adequacy of the anticoagulant effect. In general, prolongation of the APTT to 1.5 to 2.0 times the control level achieves appropriate anticoagulant therapy. The goals of anticoagulant therapy include the prevention of clot propagation or embolization and prevention of rethrombosis in a high-risk patient; the risks are primarily bleeding complications. Oral maintenance therapy using sodium warfarin (Coumadin) is advised for at least 3 months. Standard treatment regimens called for the use of intravenous heparin for 10 days, followed by continuation of Coumadin for 3 months. However, a randomized trial evaluated a 10-day regimen of heparin compared with a 5-day regimen of heparin and found the 5-day regimen to be equally effective in treating acute thrombosis and preventing rethrombosis.[9] Therefore it is recommended that intravenous heparin be maintained for 5 days and during that time oral Coumadin be initiated. Alternatively, low-molecular-weight heparin may be given subcutaneously as initial therapy. Monitoring of Coumadin should be measured by INR values and obtained on a daily basis until a stable dose of Coumadin is established. Thereafter the INR is checked at intervals of every 1 to 2 weeks for the duration of 3 months' therapy. Anticoagulant therapy may be discontinued in 3 months if the cause of deep vein thrombosis episode (such as an acute surgical event or trauma) has been eliminated.

The major hazard of anticoagulant therapy in a postoperative patient is an increased risk of bleeding complications. Therefore it is important that APTT, PT, INR, platelet count, and hematocrit be monitored carefully and that the anticoagulant does not drastically alter the patient to a hypocoagulable state. Heparin-induced thrombocytopenia is a rare complication and has been reported in association with both low-dose prophylactic heparin and standard anticoagulant doses. Therefore periodic checks of platelet count while the patient is on heparin therapy are advised. Some investigators have advocated thrombolytic therapy (streptokinase or urokinase) for the treatment of acute deep vein thrombosis. However, the risk of bleeding complications in a surgical site contraindicates thrombolytic therapy in postoperative patients.

The diagnosis of pulmonary embolism also requires a high index of suspicion, because many of the signs and symptoms are associated with other, more common pulmonary complications following surgery. The classic findings of pleuritic chest pain, hemoptysis, shortness of breath, tachycardia, and tachypnea should alert the physician to the possibility of a pulmonary embolism. Many times, however, the signs are much subtler and may only be suggested by a persistent tachycardia or a slight elevation in the respiratory rate. Patients suspected of pulmonary embolism should be evaluated initially by chest x-ray, electrocardiogram, and an arterial blood gas. Any evidence of abnormality should be further evaluated by ventilation-perfusion lung scan, searching for evidence of decreased perfusion in areas of adequate ventilation. Unfortunately, a high percentage of lung scans may be interpreted as "indeterminate." In this setting, careful clinical evaluation and judgment are required to decide whether pulmonary arteriography should be obtained to document or exclude the presence of a pulmonary embolism.

Immediate anticoagulant therapy, identical to that outlined for the treatment of deep vein thrombosis, should be initiated. Respiratory support including oxygen and bronchodilators and an intensive care setting may be necessary. Massive pulmonary emboli are usually quickly fatal, although on rare occasion, pulmonary embolectomy has been successfully performed. The use of pulmonary artery catheterization with the administration of thrombolytic agents bears further evaluation and may be important in the patient with massive pulmonary embolism. In situations in which anticoagulant therapy is ineffective in the prevention of rethrombosis and repeated embolization from the lower extremities or pelvis, vena cava interruption may be necessary. This may be accomplished through the percutaneous placement of a vena cava umbrella or filter, or the use of a large clip to obstruct the vena cava above the level of the thrombosis. In most cases, however, anticoagulant therapy is sufficient to prevent repeat thrombosis and embolism and to allow the patient's own endogenous thrombolytic mechanisms to lyse the pulmonary embolus.

Cardiovascular Diseases

In the past, gynecologic surgeons were relatively free from concerns about cardiovascular disease in their patients undergoing surgery. Over the last 20 years, however, there has been a large increase in the postmenopausal population and in gynecologic surgery patients who have a cardiovascular risk similar to their male counterparts. Despite these factors, the incidence of perioperative cardiovascular complications has decreased markedly due to improvements in preoperative detection of high-risk patients, preoperative preparation, and surgical and anesthetic techniques.

Coronary Artery Disease (CAD). Coronary artery disease is the major risk to cardiac patients undergoing abdominal surgery. The incidence of myocardial infarction following surgery in an adult population is approximately 0.15%. However, in patients who have a prior myocardial infarction, most studies report a reinfarction rate of about 5%. The diagnosis of postoperative myocardial infarction is often difficult. Chest pain present in 90% of nonsurgical patients with myocardial infarction may be present in only 50% of patients with postoperative infarction, owing to the masking of myocardial pain by coexisting surgical pain and the use of analgesia.[18] Thus maintenance of a high level of suspicion for postoperative infarction is extremely important in patients with CAD. The presence of arrhythmia, congestive heart failure, hypotension, dyspnea, or elevations of pulmonary artery pressure can indicate infarction and should prompt a thorough cardiac investigation and electrocardiographic monitoring. Measurement of creatinine phosphokinase MB isoenzyme levels is the most sensitive and specific indicator of myocardial infarction and should be obtained in all patients suspected of postoperative infarction.

Despite the high incidence of silent myocardial infarction, routinely obtaining postoperative ECGs for all patients with cardiovascular disease is controversial. Many patients will exhibit P-wave changes that spontaneously resolve and do not represent ischemia or infarction. Conversely, patients with proven myocardial infarctions may show few or no ECG abnormalities. If routine screening of asymptotic patients is desired, ECGs should be obtained 24 hours after surgery, because it has been shown that no significant ECG changes will occur immediately postoperatively that do not persist for 24 hours.[4] Although there are no uniform guidelines, it seems prudent to continue with serial ECGs for at least 3 days postoperatively.

Postoperative management of patients with CAD is based on maximizing delivery of oxygen to the myocardium and decreasing myocardial oxygen utilization. Most patients benefit from supplemental oxygen in the postoperative period, although special care should be exercised in patients with chronic obstructive pulmonary disease (COPD). Oxygenation can be easily monitored by pulse oximetry. Certainly, anemia is detrimental because of loss of oxygen-carrying capacity and resultant tachycardia and should therefore be carefully corrected in high-risk patients.

Patients with CAD may benefit from pharmacologic control of hyperadrenergic states that result from increased postoperative catecholamine production. β-Blockers decrease heart rate, myocardial contractility, and systemic blood pressure, all of which are increased by adrenergic stimulation. Perioperative β-blockers have been shown to significantly reduce arrhythmias and myocardial infarctions. Certainly, patients receiving β blockade therapy before surgery should continue to receive it in the perioperative period, because abrupt withdrawal results in a rebound hyperadrenergic state.

Labetalol, a mixed α- and β-receptor blocker, may be useful in patients with CAD who are also hypertensive because reflex tachycardia is limited. Additionally, labetalol has been shown to have antiarrhythmic effects. The use of osmolal is advantageous in patients with asthma, which can be exacerbated by sympathomimetic β-blockers, because it is a cardioselective β-blocker without intrinsic sympathomimetic activity and thus should not cause bronchoconstriction.

Although prophylactic nitrates have been used in the perioperative period for many years, this practice remains controversial. Nitroglycerin enhances blood flow to ischemic areas, increases collateral flow and myocardial oxygenation, and reduces angina.[6] The route of administration, dosage, and duration of therapy are controversial as well; thus perioperative treatment with nitrates should be initiated in conjunction with consultation with a cardiologist.

Nifedipine, a calcium channel blocker, may be given sublingually in the postoperative period. It lowers blood pressure by selectively dilating arteries and begins to decrease blood pressure in 5 minutes, which plateaus in 30 minutes.[12] The ultimate fall in blood pressure is related to the degree of hypertension initially present because vasodilation is more profound in patients with hypertension. Care must be taken when giving this drug because ischemia and myocardial infarction have been reported following hypotension associated with Nifedipine.

Congestive Heart Failure (CHF). Postoperative CHF results most frequently from excessive administration of intravenous fluids and blood products. Other common postoperative causes are myocardial infarction, systemic infection, pulmonary embolism, and cardiac arrhythmias. It is important to determine the cause of postoperative heart failure because successful treatment is based on simultaneous treatment of the underlying cause.

Diagnosis of postoperative CHF is often more difficult, because the signs and symptoms of CHF listed in the box below are not specific and can result from other causes. The most reliable method of detecting CHF is by chest radiography, in which the presence of cardiomegaly or evidence of pulmonary edema is a helpful diagnostic feature.

Acute postoperative CHF frequently manifests as pulmonary edema. Treatment of pulmonary edema can include intravenous furosemide, supplemental oxygen, intravenous morphine sulfate, and elevation of the head of the bed. In-

---

SIGNS AND SYMPTOMS OF CONGESTIVE HEART FAILURE

Presence of an S_3 gallop
Jugular venous distention
Lateral shift of the point of maximal impulse
Lower extremity edema
Basilar rales
Increased voltage on electrocardiogram
Evidence of pulmonary edema or cardiac enlargement on chest x-ray
Tachycardia

travenous aminophylline may be useful if cardiogenic asthma is present. Laboratory evaluation including an electrocardiogram, arterial blood gases, serum electrolytes, and renal function chemistries should be expediently obtained. If the patient does not rapidly improve, she should be transferred to an intensive care unit.

Hypertension. During surgery, patients with chronic hypertension tend to have increased fluctuations in blood pressure. Chronically hypertensive patients are very susceptible to intraoperative hypotension because of an impaired autoregulation of blood flow to the brain and therefore require a high mean arterial pressure to maintain adequate perfusion.

The treatment of early postoperative hypertension usually is limited to drugs that can be given parentally, because absorption through the gastrointestinal mucosa may be diminished and transdermal absorption may be erratic in patients who are cold and are rewarming. Despite these difficulties, it is generally best to maintain antihypertensive medication postoperatively if blood pressures are elevated. Certainly, patients receiving preoperative beta blockade should be maintained on parenteral therapy to prevent rebound tachycardia, hypercontractility, and hypertension.

Hemodynamic Monitoring. Over the past 25 years, hemodynamic monitoring has become integral to the perioperative management of patients with cardiovascular and pulmonary disease. The major impetus for this advancement resided in the need for the quantitative estimate of cardiac function and resulted in the development of bedside pulmonary artery catheterization. The effect of monitoring of cardiac function is demonstrated by the significant reduction of myocardial infarctions in high-risk patients who are aggressively monitored for 72 to 96 hours postoperatively.

Before the development of the pulmonary artery catheter, central venous pressure (CVP) measurement was used to assess intravascular volume status and cardiac function. To measure the CVP, a catheter is placed into the central venous system, most frequently the superior vena cava. A water manometer or a calibrated pressure transducer is connected to the CVP line, and thus an estimation of right atrial pressure can be obtained. Right atrial pressure is determined by the balance between cardiac output and venous return. Cardiac output is determined by heart rate, myocardial contractility, preload, and afterload. Thus, if the pulmonary vascularity and left ventricular function are normal, the CVP accurately reflects the left ventricular and end-diastolic pressure (LVEDP). LVEDP reflects cardiac output or systemic perfusion and has been considered the standard estimator of left ventricular pump function. Venous return is determined primarily by the mean systemic pressure, which propels blood towards the heart, balanced against resistance to venous return, which acts in the opposite direction. Thus, if right ventricular function is normal, the CVP accurately reflects intravascular volume.

Unfortunately, left and right ventricular function is frequently abnormal or discordant, and therefore the relationship of CVP to cardiac function or intravascular volume is not maintained. When this occurs, measurement of pulmonary artery occlusion pressures is required to accurately assess volume status and cardiovascular function. The use of a pulmonary artery catheter also allows the detection of changes in cardiovascular function with more sensitivity and rapidity than does clinical observation.

In 1970, Swan, Ganz, and colleagues introduced and popularized the use of a balloon-tipped pulmonary artery flotation catheter (Swan-Ganz catheter) that provided measurement of pulmonary artery and pulmonary artery occlusion pressures.[21] Since then, continued refinements have broadened the capabilities of the catheter to measure cardiac output, obtain intracavitary electrocardiograms, and provide temporary cardiac pacing.

The standard pulmonary artery occlusion catheter is a 7-Fr, radiopaque, flexible polyvinyl chloride, 4-lumen catheter with a 1.5-ml latex balloon at its distal tip. Most often, a right internal jugular cannulation is used for placement of the catheter, because this site provides the most direct access into the right atrium. After the catheter is placed into the right atrium, the balloon is inflated and the catheter is "pulled" by blood flow through the right ventricle into the pulmonary artery. The position of the catheter can be identified and followed by the various pressure waveforms generated by the right atrium, right ventricle, and pulmonary artery. As the catheter passes through increasingly smaller branches, the inflated balloon eventually occludes a pulmonary artery. The distal lumen of the catheter, which is beyond the balloon, now measures left atrial pressure (LAP), and in the absence of mitral valvular disease, LAP approximates LVEDP. Thus pulmonary capillary wedge pressure (PCWP) equals the LAP, which equals LVEDP and is normal with 8 to 12 mm Hg. Additionally, because the standard pulmonary artery catheter has an incorporated thermistor, thermodilution studies can be performed to determine cardiac output. This thermodilution method is performed by injection of cold 5% dextrose in water through the proximal port of the catheter, which cools the blood entering the right atrium. The change in temperature measured at the more distal thermometer (4 cm from the catheter tip) generates a curve with an area proportional to cardiac output. Knowledge of the cardiac output is helpful in establishing cardiovascular diagnoses. For example, a patient with hypotension, low to normal wedge pressure, and a cardiac output of 3 L/min is most likely hypovolemic. Conversely, the same patient with a cardiac output of 8 L/min is probably septic with resultant low systemic vascular resistance.

Despite the great benefit in critically ill patients, the use of pulmonary artery catheters is associated with a small but significant complication rate. The complications can be grouped into those occurring during venous cannulation and those resulting from the catheter or its placement. The most common problems encountered during venous access are cannulation of the carotid or subclavian artery and a pneumothorax. Problems resulting from the catheter itself include dysrhythmia, sepsis, and disruption of the pulmonary artery. Clearly, pulmonary artery catheters should be placed under the supervision of experienced personnel and in a setting where complications can be rapidly diagnosed and treated.

Postoperative Hemorrhage

Management of Postoperative Hemorrhage. When postoperative bleeding occurs within the first 24 hours postoperatively, there will be signs of internal hemorrhage with dropping of the hematocrit. External bleeding is obvious, but concealed internal bleeding is from either the ovarian artery or a branch of the internal iliac. The patient should be promptly reoperated on, and the bleeding vessel found and ligated. The surgeon should be especially mindful of the position of the ureter, which may not be in its usual position; it should be separately identified to avoid its ligation.

When evidence of postoperative intraperitoneal bleeding is first found after the initial 24 hours, the patient generally can be treated by careful observation to determine possible progression of the hematoma, and, if necessary, transfused and given antibiotics. A CT scan is a useful method of measuring the size of the hematoma, and an ultrasound evaluation will identify whether the mass is cystic. A persistent cystic mass that is retroperitoneal and has become infected often can be drained percutaneously under real-time ultrasound guidance.

Careful observation of the patient's vital signs during the first 2 postoperative days should reveal any intraperitoneal bleeding. It is important to monitor the patient's hemoglobin and hematocrit. The physician should suspect a coagulation defect if the patient shows unexpected ecchymosis or if a sample of venous blood fails to form a firm clot. A patient whose external blood loss is insignificant, but who seems to be bleeding persistently and is unusually restless, should undergo laparotomy. Bleeding points should be identified and ligated, any hematoma should be evacuated, and the source of bleeding should be sought.

If intraabdominal hemorrhage has stabilized at the end of the first postoperative 24 hours and there is no evidence of further bleeding, operative intervention is seldom necessary unless a presumed hematoma becomes infected and requires drainage. Under unusual circumstances, such as the presence of shock due to blood loss or evidence of massive postoperative hemorrhage within the bases of the cardinal ligaments, aggressive surgery may be required. For example, although bilateral ligation of the hypogastric and ovarian arteries is not usually time-consuming, it can dramatically arrest an alarming rate of hemorrhage.

Every gynecologic surgeon should have experience with the technique of transperitoneal bilateral hypogastric artery ligation, particularly when the technique can be readily learned by isolation of the hypogastric arteries on fresh autopsy material. Once the surgeon finds the arteries, identifies the relevant surgical anatomy, clearly distinguishes the position of the ureter and the hypogastric vein, and excludes these structures from the operative field, he or she places sutures for ligation around the hypogastric artery below the origin of the superior gluteal artery. Practice makes it convenient and easy to learn or teach this procedure so that the operator is ready when such a ligation is necessary in an emergency. Should this fail, percutaneous transcatheter embolization performed by a radiologist experienced in this technique can control massive hemorrhage.

Externally evident hemorrhage after vaginal surgery is usually of extraperitoneal origin. When the blood loss approximates that seen with the menstrual period, firm vaginal packing is usually sufficient to achieve control. Surgical intervention can be necessary if such tamponade is inadequate and blood loss continues or accelerates. If hemorrhage occurs during the first postoperative day, the rapidity of blood loss is a reliable indication of the vessel size involved. Any suspicion that sustained intraperitoneal bleeding comes from an unsecured uterine or ovarian artery mandates a prompt surgical approach. Persistent transvaginal bleeding after a vaginal repair usually arises from a small artery in the edge of a vaginal incision.

When evidence of retroperitoneal bleeding is first noted 10 to 14 days after surgery, the patient generally should be readmitted to the hospital for observation. An examination under anesthesia can be useful. If continued bleeding is evident but time is not of the essence, selective embolization can control the bleeding at its source, or laparotomy may be required.

It is often difficult for the surgeon to accept postoperative bleeding as the result of technical problems, and this may prolong the delay in reoperation for its control. One should limit the number of transfusions for a given period while hematologic causes are ruled out. The decision to reoperate is best made during daylight hours.

Blood loss from the sixth to perhaps the fourteenth postoperative day most commonly results from a local infection that has hastened suture absorption or an abscess under pressure that has eroded into an adjacent vascular bed. At this stage, tissues are edematous and friable, and any additional sutures placed will not be secure. Dissection destroys tissue planes and breaks up established barriers of "inflammatory membrane," thereby both disseminating the infection and increasing its clinical virulence. The possibility of undiagnosed diabetes should be investigated, and appropriate measures should be employed if the disease is found. Tight vaginal packing may control such bleeding, even in the presence of infection, and broad-spectrum antibiotics should be administered.

Local applications of the microfibrillar collagen Avitene may be effective. It exerts its hemostatic effect by attracting functioning blood platelets that adhere to the microfibrils, triggering the formation of thrombi in the adjacent tissue. Because it can cause fibrosis that leads to ureteral obstruction, Avitene should not be used near the ureter. The bladder should be put at rest by the insertion of an indwelling catheter. If vaginal packing is not effective and a coagulopathy has been excluded, the patient should be returned to the operating room.

Hematomas may form intraperitoneally or extraperitoneally. The occasional retroperitoneal hematoma is ominous, however, because it affords an excellent culture medium in proximity to the vaginal or rectal flora and is likely to account for postoperative abscess formation. A palpable hematoma that is increasing significantly in size should probably be evacuated. Again, a coagulopathy must be excluded.

Small hematomas in the vault of the vagina or beneath a reapproximated tissue plane generally liquefy, and, although they may become infected, they usually drain spontaneously through the vaginal suture line. Because these hematomas are common in the vaginal vault, many surgeons leave a small opening in the center of the vault for drainage after hysterectomy.

Blood Component Replacement. Nearly all postoperative hematologic problems are related to perioperative bleeding and blood component replacement. The magnitude of the problem is underscored by the fact that two thirds of all blood transfused in the United States is administered to surgical patients. Although the primary cause of postoperative bleeding, lack of surgical hemostasis, is well known to gynecologic surgeons, other, less-appreciated, nonmechanical factors may compound the problem.

Many patients who are massively transfused (more than 1 blood volume) are noted to develop a coagulopathy. Some theories attribute this coagulopathy to dilution of platelets and labile coagulation factors by the use of platelet and factor poor packed red blood cells (PRBCs), fibrinolysis, or disseminated intravascular coagulation (DIC). Acceptance of these theories has frequently resulted in the use of dogmatic schemes of replacement of fresh-frozen plasma (FFP) and platelets, depending on the number of units of PRBCs given. It is the authors' opinion, however, that it is preferable to use both clinical and laboratory evaluation to individualize blood replacement rather than adhering to a set replacement recipe.

Studies on trauma victims who receive massive transfusion report that those who developed thrombocytopenia following red blood cell replacement manifested bleeding diatheses that responded to infusion of fresh blood but not FFP.[15] The investigators concluded that dilutional thrombocytopenia is a major cause of posttransfusion bleeding. However, more recently in a prospective, randomized, double-blind study, prophylactic platelet administration during massive transfusion was not helpful.[19] Although it seems that these studies are contradictory, they demonstrate the need for obtaining platelet counts during transfusion of large amounts of blood. If clinical evidence of excessive bleeding exists and the platelet count is less than 100,000/mm^3, platelets should be transfused, because platelets are consumed during surgery and higher levels are required to maintain hemostasis following surgery.

Most clotting factors are stable for long periods with the exception of factors V and VIII, which decrease to 15% and 50% of normal, respectively. Despite this loss, factors V and VIII rarely decrease below the levels required for hemostasis. In 1985, the National Institute of Health Consensus Conference on the use of FFP concluded that there was little or no scientific evidence to support the use of FFP for bleeding diatheses following multiple blood transfusions. FFP should be given, however, if there is clinical bleeding, platelet count greater than 100,000/mm^3, and a partial thromboplastin time greater than 1.5 times control.

It appears that the volume of blood transfused does not correlate with the occurrence of postoperative bleeding diatheses. Rather, it has been shown that the magnitude of abnormalities in coagulation testing correlates with the duration of hypovolemic shock. Also, patients in hypovolemic shock frequently develop DIC, which may compound the bleeding. Thus most of the problems associated with massive transfusion are the result of inadequate replacement administered too late.

Donor blood is prevented from coagulating by the addition of citrate, which chelates calcium, thus blocking calcium-dependent steps in the coagulation cascade. Therefore hypocalcemia following transfusion of large amounts of stored blood that contains excess citrate is a theoretical danger. Indeed, it has been shown that at high transfusion rates, ionized calcium levels will transiently fall but return toward baseline levels at the completion of transfusion. Citrate is metabolized at the equivalent rate of 20 units of blood per hour, and therefore routine supplemental calcium is not warranted. However, hypothermia, liver disease, and hyperventilation slow the metabolism of citrate, requiring close monitoring of ionized calcium levels when these conditions prevail.

As donor blood is stored, potassium leaches from the red cells and plasma levels may reach as high as 30 mEq/L. Despite this large potassium load, rarely are serum potassium levels elevated even in patients receiving massive transfusions. Indeed, patients often are hypokalemic as a result of the metabolic alkalosis that follows transfusion, which is caused by the hepatic metabolism of citrate to bicarbonate.

Pulmonary Disease

General Considerations. Patients undergoing abdominal surgery manifest several pulmonary physiologic changes secondary to immobilization, anesthetic irritation of the airways, and the splinting of breathing that inevitably occurs secondary to incisional pain. Pulmonary physiologic changes include a decrease in the functional residual capacity (FRC) and vital capacity (VC), an increase in ventilation perfusion mismatching, and impaired mucociliary clearance of secretions from the tracheobronchial tree. These changes result in transient hypoxemia and atelectasis, which, if untreated, can progress to pneumonia in the postoperative period. Postoperative pulmonary dysfunction is more pronounced in patients with advanced age, preexisting lung disease, obesity, a significant smoking history, and upper abdominal surgery.

The majority of postoperative pulmonary complications occur in patients who have preexisting pulmonary disease. In these patients, the incidence of pulmonary complications is greater than 70%, as compared to the low incidence (2% to 5%) in individuals with healthy lungs. The risk of postoperative pulmonary complications is lower in patients who undergo lower abdominal compared to upper abdominal surgery, and nonthoracic, nonabdominal surgery compared to abdominal operation. The presence of COPD markedly increases the risk for all patients.

Asthma. In recent years, the recognition of asthma as an inflammatory condition that should be treated with antiinflammatory agents has increasingly led to the use of corticosteroids for treatment. Because corticosteroids inhibit mediator release from eosinophils and macrophages, inhibit the late response to allergens, and reduce hyperresponsiveness of the bronchioles, they have become the first-line therapy for chronic asthma.[1] Inhaled steroids are active and have greatly reduced the steroid dose required to achieve optimal results. The steroid effect is dose related, but many asthmatics can be controlled with low-dose inhaled steroids (less than 1000 μg/day). Onset of action is slow (several hours) and up to 3 months of steroid therapy may be required for optimal improvement of bronchial hyperresponsiveness. Even in acute exacerbation of asthma, steroid treatment has been shown to enhance the beneficial effect of β_2-adrenergic treatment.

Occasionally, a short course of oral steroids may be necessary in addition to inhaled steroids during acute exacerbation of asthma. However, for adults with chronic asthma, only a minority require chronic oral steroid therapy. Those patients taking oral steroids should receive intravenous steroid support perioperatively.

Until recently, β_2-adrenergic agonists were considered the first-line drugs for asthma. These drugs, inhaled 4 to 6 times daily, rapidly relax smooth muscle in the airways and are effective for up to 6 hours. Studies of β_2 agonists in chronic asthma, however, have failed to show any influence of these agents on the inflammatory component of asthma. Furthermore, some have suggested that the long-term use of this class of drugs can lead to a worsening of asthma. Thus, beta$_2$ agonists are now recommended for short-term relief of bronchospasm or as first-line treatment for patients with very infrequent symptoms or symptoms provoked solely by exercise.[7]

Methylxanthines, such as theophylline, have been relegated to third line status in the management of asthma. It is questionable whether these drugs add any benefit to patients on maximal inhaler therapy. The xanthines are limited by their narrow therapeutic window. It is necessary to achieve a serum concentration of at least 10 μg/ml, but, significant toxicity, including nausea, tremor, and central nervous system excitation, develops at levels greater than 20 Fg/ml. Xanthines have a limited antiinflammatory effect and have no effect on bronchial hyperresponsiveness or eosinophilic degranulation. It is also important to note that plasma concentrations can be altered by drugs or environmental factors, requiring an adjustment in the theophylline dose. Smoking and phenobarbital, for example, increase clearance of theophylline by the liver; clearance of theophylline is decreased with hepatic disease, cardiac failure, or the concomitant use of certain drugs, including ciprofloxacin, cimetidine, erythromycin, and troleandomycin.

Anticholinergic agents are weak bronchodilators that work through inhibition of muscarinic receptors in the smooth muscle of the airways. The quaternary derivatives such as ipratropium bromide (Atrovent) are available in an inhaled form that is not absorbed systemically. Anticholinergic drugs can provide additional benefit in conjunction with standard steroid and bronchodilator therapy but should not be used as single-agent therapy, because they do not (1) inhibit mast cell degranulation, (2) have any effect on the late response to allergens, and (3) have an antiinflammatory effect.

Cromolyn sodium is highly active in the treatment of seasonal allergic asthma in children and young adults. It is usually not as effective in older patients or in patients in whom asthma is not allergic in character. The drug is taken by inhalation but has a relatively short duration of action (3 to 4 hours). It has a mild antiinflammatory effect but is less effective than inhaled cortical steroids, and its role as a single agent is limited.

Chronic Obstructive Pulmonary Disease. The greatest risk factor for the development of postoperative pulmonary complications is the presence of underlying COPD. The term *COPD* has been used to encompass both chronic bronchitis and emphysema—disease entities that often occur in tandem. Cigarette smoke is implicated in the pathogenesis of both, and any treatment plan must include cessation of smoking. Chronic bronchitis is defined as the presence of productive cough on most days for at least 3 months per year and for at least 2 successive years. It is characterized by chronic airway inflammation and excessive mucus production. The histologic changes of emphysema include destruction of alveolar septa and distention of air spaces distal to terminal alveoli. The destruction of alveolar septa is most likely caused by serine elastase, released by neutrophils exposed to cigarette smoke. The destruction of alveoli results in air trapping, loss of pulmonary elastic recoil, collapse of the airways in expiration, increased work of breathing, significant ventilation-perfusion mismatching, and an ineffective cough. The impaired ability for effective cough and clearance of secretions predisposes patients with COPD to atelectasis and pneumonia in the postoperative period.

In gynecologic surgical patients, the risks of postoperative pulmonary complications are confined mainly to patients with COPD or a history of heavy smoking. In these patients, prophylactic measures should be instituted preoperatively and continued postoperatively to minimize the incidence of atelectasis and pneumonia. Several studies have suggested that preoperative pulmonary preparation of patients with preexisting lung disease can significantly decrease the incidence of postoperative pulmonary complications by 50% to 70%.

Atelectasis. Atelectasis accounts for more than 90% of all postoperative pulmonary complications. The pathophysiology involves a collapse of the alveoli resulting in ventilation-perfusion mismatching, intrapulmonary venous shunting, and a subsequent drop in Pao$_2$. Collapsed alveoli are susceptible to superimposed infection, and if improperly managed, atelectasis progresses to pneumonia. Patients with atelectasis have decreased FRC and lung compliance, which results in greater difficulty breathing. In general, despite the decrease in Pa_{O_2}, the P_{CO_2} remains unaffected unless atelectatic changes progress to large volumes of the lung or unless there is preexisting lung disease.

Physical findings associated with atelectasis can include a low-grade fever. Auscultation of the chest may reveal decreased breath sounds at the bases or dry rales on inspiration. Percussion of the posterior thorax may suggest elevation of the diaphragm. Radiologic findings include the presence of horizontal lines or plates noted on the posteroanterior chest x-rays, occasionally with adjacent areas containing hyperinflation. These changes are most pronounced during the first 3 postoperative days.

Therapy for atelectasis should be aimed at expanding the alveoli and increasing the functional residual capacity. The most important maneuvers are those that promote maximal inspiratory pressure, which is maintained for as long as possible. This promotes not only an expansion of the alveoli but also secretion of surfactant that stabilizes alveoli. This can be achieved with aggressive supervised use of incentive spirometry, deep breathing exercises, coughing, and, in some cases, positive expiratory pressure with a mask (continuous positive airway pressure [CPAP]). Oversedation should be avoided, and patients should be encouraged to ambulate and change positions frequently. Fiberoptic bronchoscopy for removal of mucopurulent plugs should be reserved for patients who fail to improve with the usual measures.

Cardiogenic (High-Pressure) Pulmonary Edema. Cardiogenic pulmonary edema can result from myocardial ischemia, myocardial infarction, or simply from intravascular volume overload, particularly in patients with low cardiac reserve or renal failure. The process usually begins with an increase in the fluid in the alveolar septa and bronchial vascular cuffs, ultimately seeping into the alveoli. Complete filling of the alveoli impairs secretion and production of surfactant. Concomitant with alveolar flooding, there is a decrease in lung compliance, impairment of the oxygen diffusion capacity, and an increase in the arteriolar-alveolar oxygen gradient. Ventilation-perfusion mismatching in the lung results in a decrease in the Pa_{O_2}, eventually resulting in decreased oxygenation of the tissues and impairment of cardiac contractility.

Symptoms may include tachypnea, dyspnea, wheezing, and use of the accessory muscles of respiration. Clinical signs may include distention of the jugular veins, peripheral edema, rales upon auscultation of the lungs, and an enlarged heart. Radiographic findings can include the presence of bronchiolar cuffing and increased interstitial fluid markings extending to the periphery of the lung. The diagnosis can be further confirmed with central hemodynamic monitoring, which will denote an elevated central venous pressure and, more specifically, an elevation in the pulmonary capillary wedge pressure.

A thorough evaluation of the patient's volume status should be made. In addition, myocardial ischemia or infarction should be ruled out by ECG and cardiac enzymes. The management of cardiogenic pulmonary edema includes oxygen support, aggressive diuresis, and afterload reduction to increase the cardiac output. In the absence of myocardial infarction, an inotropic agent may be used. Mechanical ventilation should be reserved for cases of acute respiratory failure.

Noncardiogenic Pulmonary Edema (Adult Respiratory Distress Syndrome [ARDS]). In contrast to cardiogenic pulmonary edema, in which alveolar flooding is a result of an increase in the hydrostatic pressure of the pulmonary capillaries, alveolar flooding in patients with ARDS is the result of an increase in pulmonary capillary permeability. The primary pathophysiologic process is one of damage to the capillary side of the alveolar-capillary membrane. This results in rapid movement of fluid from the capillaries to the pulmonary interstitial space and, thereafter, to the alveoli. Lung compliance decreases, and oxygen diffusion capacity is impaired, resulting in hypoxemia. If not managed aggressively, respiratory failure commonly results.

There are a number of causes of ARDS, and in fact there are several distinct ARDS states. The causes of ARDS include shock, sepsis, massive nonlung trauma as from fractures or burns, multiple red blood cell transfusions, aspiration injury, inhalation injury, pneumonia, pancreatitis, DIC, and fat emboli. Irrespective of the cause, the evolving clinical picture and management are very similar, with the exception that an attempt is made to identify and treat the inciting cause.

The evolving clinical picture of ARDS passes through several stages. Initially, patients develop tachypnea and dyspnea without remarkable findings on clinical evaluation or on chest x-ray. As lung compliance is impaired, functional residual capacity, tidal volume, and vital capacity all decrease. The Pa_{O_2} decreases, and characteristically increases only marginally with oxygen supplementation. During these early stages, the management plan should include a thorough attempt to identify the inciting cause and initiate treatment as indicated. This can include aggressive hemodynamic and circulatory resuscitation in patients with shock, aggressive broad-spectrum antibiotic therapy in patients who are septic, and aggressive replacement with cryoprecipitate or fresh-frozen plasma in patients with DIC. An attempt should be made to maintain the arterial oxygen above 90%. This may be achievable initially through oxygen administered by mask. For patients with severe hypoxemia, endotracheal intubation with positive-pressure ventilation should be instituted.

Hemodynamic monitoring is invaluable and should be initiated early in the course of the disease process. Patients with any evidence of fluid overload should receive aggressive diuresis; others may require fluid resuscitation for maintenance of tissue perfusion while maintaining the pulmonary-capillary wedge pressure below 15 mm Hg. Other measures for general care should include the placement of a nasogastric tube, gastric acid suppression with H_2 blockers, and steroids in patients with the fat emboli syndrome.

With aggressive management, particularly if the inciting cause is identified and treated, ARDS can be reversed during the first 48 hours with few sequelae. Beyond the first 48 hours, however, progression of ARDS causes lung damage that may leave a residual pulmonary fibrosis. With progression beyond 10 days, multiorgan system failure occurs and mortality is greater than 80%. Guidelines for initial ventilatory support can include a respiratory rate greater than 40/min, arterial Po_2 less than 70 mm Hg, Pco_2 greater than 55 mm Hg, or arterial pH less than 7.30.[25]

REFERENCES

1. Barnes PJ: A new approach to the treatment of asthma, *N Engl J Med* 321:1517, 1989.

2. Brown SE, Allen HH, Robins RN: The use of delayed primary wound closure in preventing wound infections, *Am J Obstet Gynecol* 127:713, 1977.

3. Cruse PJ, Foord R: The epidemiology of wound infection: a 10-year prospective study of 62,939 wounds, *Surg Clin North Am* 60:27, 1980.

4. Driscoll AC, Hobika JH, Etsten BE, et al: Clinically unrecognized myocardial infarction following surgery, *N Engl J Med* 264:633, 1961.

5. Fisher JR, Conway MJ, Takeshita RT, et al: Necrotizing fasciitis: importance of roentgenographic studies for soft-tissue gas, *JAMA* 241:803, 1979.

6. Gallagher J, Moore RA, Jose AB, et al: Prophylactic nitroglycerin infusions during coronary artery bypass surgery, *Anesthesiology* 64:785, 1986.

7. Hargreave FE, Dolovich J, Newhouse MT: The assessment and treatment of asthma: a conference report, *J Allergy Clin Immunol* 85:1098, 1990.

8. Hemsell DL: Infections after gynecologic surgery, *Obstet Gynecol Clin North Am* 16:381, 1989.

9. Hull RD, Raskob GE, Rosenbloom D, et al: Heparin for 5 days as compared with 10 days in the initial treatment of proximal venous thrombosis, *N Engl J Med* 322:1260, 1990.

10. Ireland D, Tacchi D, Bint AJ: Effect of single-dose prophylactic co-trimoxazole on the incidence of gynaecological postoperative urinary tract infection, *Br J Obstet Gynaecol* 89:578, 1982.

11. Jeffcoate TNA, Tindall VR: Venous thrombosis and embolism in obstetrics and gynaecology, *Aust N Z J Obstet Gynaecol* 5:119, 1965.

12. Lacche A, Basaglia P: Hypertensive emergencies: effects of therapy by nifedipine administered sublingually, *Curr Ther Res* 34:879, 1983.

13. Leventhal A, Pfau A: Pharmacologic management of postoperative overdistention of the bladder, *Surg Gynecol Obstet* 146:347, 1978.

14. Miller TA, Duke JH: Fluid and electrolyte management. In Dudrick SJ, Bane AE, Eiseman B, et al, editors: *Manual of perioperative and postoperative care,* Philadelphia, 1983, WB Saunders.

15. Miller RD, Robbins TO, Tong MJ, et al: Coagulation defects associated with massive blood transfusions, *Ann Surg* 174:794, 1971.

16. Nichols DH: Getting the postoperative patient to void, *Contemp Obstet Gynecol* 12:41, 1978.

17. Pestana C: *Fluids and electrolytes in the surgical patient,* ed 4, Baltimore, 1989, Williams & Wilkins.

18. Rao TL, Jacobs KH, El-Etr AA: Reinfarction following anesthesia in patients with myocardial infarction, *Anesthesiology* 59:499, 1983.

19. Reed RL, Ciavarella D, Heimbach DM, et al: Prophylactic platelet administration during massive transfusion: a prospective, randomized, double-blind clinical study, *Ann Surg* 203:40, 1986.

20. Shires GT, Canizaro P: Fluid and electrolyte management of the surgical patient. In Sabiston DC Jr, editor: *Textbook of surgery,* ed 14, Philadelphia, 1991, WB Saunders.

21. Swan HJ, Ganz W, Forrester J, et al: Catheterization of the heart in man with the use of a flow-directed balloon-tipped catheter, *N Engl J Med* 283:447, 1970.

22. Tomford JW, Hershey CO, McLaren CE, et al: Intravenous therapy team and peripheral venous catheter-associated complications: a prospective controlled study, *Arch Intern Med* 144:1191, 1984.

23. Veterans Affairs Total Parenteral Nutrition Cooperative Study Group: Perioperative total parenteral nutrition in surgical patients, *N Engl J Med* 325:525, 1991.

24. von Peham H, Amreich J: *Operative gynecology,* Philadelphia, 1934, JB Lippincott.

25. Wellman JJ, Smith BA: Respiratory complications of surgery. In Lubin MF, editor: *Medical management of the surgical patient,* Boston, 1988, Butterworth.

H. ALEXANDER EASLEY III

According to the Harvard Medical Practice Study in New York, a large number of patients treated in hospitals were injured due to negligence, but only a small fraction of them instituted malpractice claims.[8] Furthermore, most of the claims that *were* instituted did not actually involve malpractice.[3] Why so many adverse events? Why this paradox?

Medical malpractice awards in jury verdicts averaged over $500,000 in 1996, an increase of 14% over 1995, and 25% of all verdicts were at or above $1 million.[6] Largely due to a "soft" insurance market aided by favorable investment rates, professional liability carriers have not been under pressure to raise rates.[7]

The origin of medical malpractice cases is paradoxical and complex. Awards are frequent and expensive. Legislatures and courts are not likely to single out medical negligence for change in citizens' rights under the tort system. Tort reform is increasingly unlikely. Under these contemporary adverse conditions, what can the gynecologic surgeon do to lower the risk of being charged with malpractice?

WHAT IS MALPRACTICE?

Negligence was scarcely recognized as a separate tort before the nineteenth century, when the Industrial Revolution gave rise to a dramatic increase in the number of accidents.[15] Medical malpractice is a particular type of negligence. Negligence is a tort, or a civil wrong for which a court provides a remedy in the form of a legal action for damages.[15] Negligence is a tort committed unintentionally. It provides redress for damages incurred because of the unreasonable conduct of another. To sustain a cause of action for negligence, the plaintiff must prove that:

1. The defendant owed a *duty* to the plaintiff to conform to a certain standard of conduct to protect him from unreasonable risks
2. The defendant *breached* that duty by failing to conduct himself according to the required standard
3. The defendant's breach *caused* an injury to the plaintiff
4. The defendant experienced actual damages

The specific conduct that constitutes malpractice involves the second element just listed. In every medical malpractice case the defendant physician must have breached the duty he or she owed to act as a reasonably prudent physician having standard professional skill and knowledge under the same or similar circumstances.[15] If the physician is a specialist, his or her duty is to exercise the special skill of a similarly trained* physician.

The failure of a physician to obtain informed consent is *not* a separate tort. The patient is owed a duty to be informed of the risks of medical treatment or surgery. Thus breach of this duty also constitutes negligence. A separate discussion of informed consent appears later.

A *mistake,* if it is not unreasonable, is not negligence. An error in the exercise of judgment, as long as it is not unreasonable, is not negligence. However, the standard of conduct is an external one imposed by society on the physician. So a mistaken belief that a certain treatment or failure to treat is reasonable, while not intentional, immoral, or unethical, may nevertheless constitute negligence.

SOURCE OF STANDARD OF CARE

How is the standard of care established? What is well accepted by reasonably trained gynecologists who are board certified or eligible should prevail as the standard of care applicable to any circumstance encountered. Textbooks commonly used as guidelines by the gynecologist in training and practice, while not authoritative or controlling authority, should reflect well-accepted standards of practice as of the time of their writing. Peer-reviewed studies and reviews published in the periodical literature may constitute standards if the treatments proposed therein are well accepted in practice. Thus new therapies and procedures, even when they are proposed by leading investigators in the specialty, need some time before they become the customary standard.

In medical malpractice, litigation "experts" are required to explain the standard of care to juries because jurors are laypersons who are not expected to know it. These experts, of course, are physicians usually in the same specialty as the defendant physician-gynecologists, including subspecialty reproductive endocrinologists, oncologists, and maternal-fetal medicine specialists, as indicated by the facts of the case. Testimony is elicited in the form of an opinion from the gynecologist of whether, given the facts of the case, the

---

*A physician who treats a patient with a procedure usually performed by a physician with a specialty different from the treating physician can be held to the same standard as the specialty physician. The determining factors are the extent of overlap in the usual practice areas and the availability of specialists in the locality.

defendant physician's conduct met the requisite standard of care under the circumstances. This testimony is a *crucial* requirement in all cases. Gynecologists possess tremendous influence in determining whether another gynecologist has been negligent. Consequently, any physician asked to provide service as an expert witness should seriously consider the importance of giving an opinion about the standard of care and whether the defendant met the standard. Those well-trained gynecologists who practice the specialty daily are uniquely qualified to state clearly the care appropriate under the circumstances of a particular case. Only with participation by physicians as expert witnesses can the integrity of standards in the practice of gynecologic surgery be maintained and protected from attack by unscrupulous physicians willing to modify the standards to effect an outcome in a malpractice case.

In an effort to prevent erosion of the standards by testimony from such physicians, many states have legislated various qualifications for expert witnesses.[10] However, except for moderate requirements for active clinical practice, none of the statutes precludes a plaintiff's use of a professional witness, or a physician seeking expert witness work as a significant income source.

INFORMED CONSENT

As stated previously, failure to obtain adequate informed consent from a patient is negligence. True informed consent requires that a patient have an opportunity to knowledgeably evaluate the options available regarding her care and the risks associated with each.[4]

Theories

Two theories control the legal principle of informed consent. The first is the *reasonable physician* rule. Under this theory, the adequacy of consent is determined by what information a reasonable physician under similar circumstances would give to the patient to fully inform her of the risks and benefits of the proposed procedure or therapy. The second theory is the *reasonable patient* rule. Under this theory, the adequacy of consent depends on what a patient needs to make an intelligent choice. Although the *reasonable patient* rule prevails only in a minority of jurisdictions, the most prudent and safe approach for the gynecologic surgeon is this rule. To satisfy the standard, the surgeon must answer this question: "What would a reasonable patient need to know to make a fully informed decision whether to undergo the proposed procedure?"

Requisites

To obtain legally adequate informed consent, the patient must be told the following[1]:
1. The nature of the procedure (i.e., what is the patient going to have done to her)
2. The alternatives to the procedure that the patient could choose for treatment, even though they may be less effective

3. The significant risks of the procedure. What is significant depends on the likelihood of injury and the degree of harm. This balance dictates disclosure of the following:
   a. The common but less serious risks, such as infection, voiding problems, and discomfort
   b. The less common but serious risks, including major bleeding and damage to the bowel, bladder, or ureters
   c. The possibility that the procedure may not correct the condition
   d. The possibility that intraoperative problems could necessitate additional surgery to correct abnormal conditions already existing or developing during the procedure

The patient's signature on a consent form is evidence of informed consent, but the law requires the physician to explain the information to her. Explanations vary depending on the sophistication of the patient. Some patients can read a form, ask questions, and be adequately informed. Others need a simple explanation and careful attention. In many settings a nurse or office secretary presents the patient with an unintelligible "consent" form, which the patient signs. Clearly this signed form *alone* does not constitute legally adequate informed consent. The interactive "PACE" program sold by the American College of Obstetricians and Gynecologists is an excellent informed consent transaction. It clearly satisfies the legal requirements, but currently its scope is limited to much less than the gynecologic surgeon needs to cover the full range of surgical procedures; it is also expensive.

A sample informed consent form is shown in Fig. 11-1.

Special Situations

There are several exceptions to the above rules. Minors, emergencies, and certain procedures may involve special rules in most jurisdictions.

Minors. Generally, a minor is incompetent to give consent to medical treatment. At the age of majority, 18 years in North Carolina,[11] for example, the patient can give consent as an adult. Before then the patient's parent or guardian must consent for her unless the minor meets three specific exceptions:
1. The minor is an emancipated or mature minor.
2. The minor is seeking the prevention, diagnosis, or treatment of pregnancy, sexually transmitted disease, other reportable disease, substance abuse, and emotional disturbance.
3. The parent cannot be located, there is insufficient time to contact the parent, or the parent refuses to consent and delay would endanger or be fatal to the child.

A minor is emancipated when she is married, a member of the armed forces, or ruled emancipated by court order in North Carolina. Only an emancipated minor can consent to abortion in North Carolina without parental consent or involvement unless a judicial decree waives this require-

CONSENT FOR ABDOMINAL HYSTERECTOMY

TO: Dr._____ and _____.

(hospital)

I have a condition called_____

(use medical term with description)

1. **What I consent to have done:**

   I agree to allow my doctor and his assistants to perform an operation on me called **ABDOMINAL HYSTERECTOMY**. My doctor will make an incision in my lower abdomen. He will remove my uterus (womb).

2. **Why I am having this operation:**

   I am having this operation because_____

(patient to write here)

   _____

   _____

   _____

3. **What my doctor has explained to me:**
   - The operation to be performed
   - The reason why I need this operation
   - The risks of the operation
   - The discomforts that I might have
   - That a perfect result is not guaranteed

4. **How I could treat my condition without surgery:**

   I know I do not have to have this operation to save my life but it will improve my health. I have either tried medication to help my condition or I could not take the medication. I think this operation is the best treatment for my condition.

5. **Risks explained to me:**
   - Damage to a vein or artery that could cause serious bleeding
   - Making a hole in my bladder that could cause a tract (fistula) between my vagina and bladder
   - That I may have difficulty emptying my bladder
   - That I may develop bulging in my rectum (rectocele) or my vagina (vaginal vault eversion)
   - That I may develop infection in my incision or in my pelvis

   I know that these problems are not likely to occur. I know that other complications that are even less likely could occur, such as blood clots, nerve problems, or even death. Knowing all these risks, I have decided to have this operation.

6. **Other surgery that may be necessary:**

   If any of the complications listed above should occur during my operation, other surgery may be necessary. My doctor could discover during my operation other conditions such as abnormalities with my appendix, fallopian tubes, and ovaries or bulging in the rectum or vagina. I will allow my doctor to correct these conditions and others to improve the results of this operation or prevent my having to have another operation in the future. I will allow my doctor to decide what is necessary. If my doctor removes my ovaries, then I may have to take estrogen to avoid symptoms such as hot flashes and vaginal dryness.

7. **Complications of anesthesia:**

   My anesthesiologist is responsible for explaining to me the risks of anesthesia.

SIGNED:_____

(patient or person authorized to consent)

DATE: _____

WITNESS:_____

Fig. 11-1   Sample of informed consent form.

ment.[12] Prevention of pregnancy does *not* include sterilization procedures for minors.[13]

Informed consent is largely a communication issue with specific requirements for information content. The encounter with the patient and her family during the transaction is an excellent opportunity for education and building rapport and trust. These latter two positive emotions immeasurably strengthen the physician-patient relationship.

HOW TO PREVENT MALPRACTICE

As mentioned earlier, the Harvard Medical Practice Study found that most patients who had adverse outcomes from negligence in hospitals did not bring malpractice claims, but most malpractice claims that were brought did not constitute negligence. These cases are typical of those litigated in the United States in the past decade. What could explain this discrepancy and paradox?

Some years ago a university researcher found that patients who eventually institute a malpractice claim might do so from social and emotional predispositions that evolve during their contact with the health care system.[5] Such patients experience injury, surprise, disappointment, and humiliation and finally develop intense hostility. Out of retribution and preservation of self-esteem, they feel the need to strike out against the people who caused their injury.

Why do patients develop this pattern of thought? The health care system is powerful and can be impersonal. When, for example, adequate informed consent is not obtained, sufficient rapport is not established through the informed consent transaction or other contacts. Patients' expectations are unreasonable. Patients' families, who could be incorporated into rapport building, engender suspicion and need for accountability into the patients' thought processes. Any one or more of these factors can be operable in pushing the patient into becoming litigious after an adverse outcome. Remember, *incidents don't sue, people do.*

Prevention of a malpractice suit begins *prospectively* before the surgical procedure. Then, when complications occur, the gynecologic surgeon must aggressively treat the complication, communicate in a compassionate and caring way with the patient and her family, and pay close attention to her in the postoperative period, even if physicians from other specialties assume primary responsibility for treating the complication. There is no need to admit guilt. If adequate informed consent was obtained before surgery, the gynecologic surgeon should remind the patient and family that the complication was a foreseeable risk and did not occur because of substandard or unreasonable care, if that is true. Remind the patient that *recognition* of a complication and prudent treatment of it are the elements of the standard of care in the postoperative period.

PRACTICE PATTERNS

The gynecologic surgeon learns the standard of care during rigorous study and training in residency and fel-

lowship. Other sources of well-accepted, customary standard treatment are available for guidance. The American College of Obstetricians and Gynecologists (ACOG) has published Technical Bulletins, now called Educational Bulletins, for many years. Many of these excellent consensus monographs include topics relating to gynecologic surgery. Although the College specifically disclaims that these bulletins are intended to constitute standards of care, they are used widely by both plaintiff and defense attorneys as strong evidence of such standards. The ACOG Criteria Sets cover specific indications and prerequisites for many procedures in gynecologic surgery. Adherence to such criteria clearly shows compliance with well-accepted indications for these procedures and the appropriate preoperative work-up. Other materials that should be incorporated into a complete understanding of standards of care are the ACOG Committee Opinions and Practice Patterns that cover gynecologic surgery and the Guidelines for Practice of the American Society for Reproductive Medicine.

It is vitally important to think *prospectively in retrospect.* This means that the gynecologic surgeon should attempt to analyze especially difficult decision-making scenarios as if he or she were rendering an opinion about another gynecologist's conduct under the circumstances. In other words, would other reasonable gynecologists conclude that the surgeon is adhering to the requisite standard of care under the circumstances? For example, in a difficult endometriosis case in which dissection of the ureter is required but it is not visualized optimally, should the surgeon perform a postoperative cystoscopy to ensure patency of the ureter? Thinking *prospectively in retrospect* in this circumstance would probably dictate that the surgeon make an effort to ensure ureteral integrity.

SUGGESTED ACTIONS TO AVOID MALPRACTICE

There are a number of advisory sources for legal risk management that include abstracts of actual litigated cases and commentary thereon.[14] Following is a list of suggested actions for specific situations to avoid malpractice in gynecologic surgery.

Informed Consent

- Use a form (see Fig. 11-1) that contains simple language but is very inclusive.
- Give the form to the patient and ask her to take it home and discuss it with her family and to return it at a preoperative visit when you can answer questions.
- Explain to the patient the purpose of the form and *what it says.*
- When describing the complications, tell the patient that you will do everything possible to correct them and obtain the services of other specialists as necessary.

The Written Chart

- The chart should be neat and succinct.
- The indications for surgery should be clearly stated and consistent with published, accepted criteria such as ACOG Educational Bulletins, Criteria Sets, Committee Opinions, and Practice Patterns and the published or known criteria in effect for the patient's managed care organization.
- Include in the operative note a specific section "Indications for Surgery" in which you reiterate the indications and summarize succinctly your efforts at obtaining informed consent.

Preoperative Evaluation

- Obtain complete past medical history, social history, family history, and review of systems.
- Order mechanical and antibiotic bowel preparation for large masses, expected adhesions, or endometriosis.
- Specifically mention that there is no history of cardiac disease, angina, asthma, liver, renal or intestinal disease or seek consultation as appropriate.
- Teach patients about wound care and catheter care.

Intraoperative Protocol

Abdominal Cases

- Always place a Foley catheter in the bladder.
- Identify the ureter, preferably by a retroperitoneal approach.
- Ensure ureteral integrity in cases involving difficult dissection of the ureter.
- Use prophylactic antibiotics.

Vaginal Cases

- Use a Foley catheter in the bladder or instill dye solution.
- Perform cytoscopy for extensive anterior colporrhaphy.
- Perform rectal examination after posterior colporrhaphy.
- Perform culdoplasty with vaginal hysterectomy to prevent later vault prolapse.

Laparoscopy Cases

- Enter the abdomen above or beside old midline incisions, especially if using closed technique.
- Use a technique such as passive loss of saline through the Veress needle to ensure intraperitoneal placement of CO_2.
- Place accessory trocars under direct visualization of inferior epigastric vessels or 8 cm lateral to midline and observe the sites for bleeding after removal.[2]
- Identify the ureter for any adnexal surgery and LAVH.
- Ensure cautery devices do not touch bowel.
- Perform difficult or extensive operative laparoscopy only after strict credentialing or significant experience without complications or poor outcomes.
- Be as familiar as possible with all equipment, especially electrosurgical generators, insufflation devices, and irrigation equipment.
- In the laparoscopic sterilization operative note describe findings that substantiate complete occlusion of the tubes; if one method is not exact, use a secondary method of occlusion.
- Perform pregnancy testing on patients with delayed menses and offer it to any patient using unreliable contraception before procedures, especially sterilization procedures.

Hysteroscopy Procedures

- Perform operative hysteroscopy only after strict credentialing or significant experience without complications or poor outcomes.
- Have an excellent understanding of the equipment used.
- If uterine perforation occurs, observe and test patient for a reasonable period of time for evidence of intraabdominal bleeding.

Postoperative Care

- Consider the diagnosis of hyponatremia especially after hysterectomy in a patient with lethargy and nausea and after hysteroscopy for imbalance of irrigation fluid.
- Do not delay opening an incision with indicia of necrotizing fasciitis.
- Remember small bowel obstruction is more common after total abdominal hysterectomy than any other gynecologic surgery.[9]
- Consider using appropriate adhesion barriers after extensive dissection.
- Respond expediently to patients' complaints after discharge home and consider having the office nurse call the patient soon after the discharge.

NEW TECHNOLOGY

New surgical techniques, particularly so-called minimally invasive laparoscopy and hysteroscopy, have assumed a prominent place in the armamentarium of gynecologic surgeons. Much of the impetus for this development is attributable to surgical instrument manufacturers and salespersons. Many surgeons are not experienced or trained well enough to control the enhanced level of risk inherent in these techniques. Furthermore the efficacy of many of these techniques in producing optimal outcomes for the patient has not been demonstrated in well-designed studies. Not only are the adverse outcomes and surgical complications of major concern, but also the role of adequate informed consent to the procedures assumes a new dimension. Strict credentialing, monitoring outcomes and complications, and expedient withdrawal of surgical privileges when appropriate should minimize injury and the potential malpractice litigation that follows.

CONCLUSION

Since malpractice cases do not occur unless there is a poor outcome, gynecologic surgeons must be well trained, meticulous, and endowed with excellent judgment to avoid a bad outcome. However, all bad outcomes do not result from negligence. Mistakes, if reasonable, are not negligence. The exercise of surgical judgment, if reasonable, affords the gynecologic surgeon flexibility in his or her approach in the operating room. But many plaintiffs bring lawsuits for bad outcomes that do not eventuate from negligence, and many patients injured by medical negligence do not bring lawsuits. Adequate informed consent, strong patient rapport, and the gynecologic surgeon's demonstration of concern and a caring and professional attitude, especially when complications occur, will go far toward prevention of a malpractice claim. The specialty must be proactive in requiring strict credentialing and monitoring outcomes and complications. When litigation does occur, gynecologic surgeons must participate as expert witnesses to ensure the standard of care is accurately and honestly presented to jurors.

REFERENCES

1. ACOG Criteria Set, no 26, Aug 1997.
2. ACOG Educational Bulletin, no 239, Operative laparoscopy, Aug 1997.
3. Brennan TA, Sox CM, Burstin HR: Relation between negligent adverse events and the outcomes of medical-malpractice litigation, *N Engl J Med* 335:1963, 1996.
4. Easley HA, Hammond CB: Informed consent in obstetrics and gynecology, *Postgrad Obstet Gynecol* 7:1, 1987.
5. Easley HA, Hammond CB: Management of malpractice risk, *Postgrad Obstet Gynecol* 6:4, 1986.
6. Liability Reform, *AMA News,* Aug 4, 1997, p 35 (cites 1997 data from *Jury Verdict Research*).
7. Liability Reform, *AMA News,* Aug 4, 1997, p 3 (cites 1997 data from *Jury Verdict Research*).
8. Localio AR, Lawthers AG, Brennan TA, et al: Relation between malpractice claims and adverse events due ot negligence, *N Engl J Med* 325:245, 1991.
9. Malinak, LR, Young AE: Peritoneal closure: when and why, *Contemp Obstet Gynecol* July 1997, p 102.
10. N.C. Gen. Stat. Secs. 1A-1, Rule 9 and 8C, Rule 702.
11. N.C. Gen. Stat. Sec. 48A-2.
12. N.C. Gen. Stat. Sec. 90-21.6.
13. N.C. Gen. Stat. Sec. 90-271.
14. *OB-GYN Malpractice prevention,* Baltimore, Williams & Wilkins.
15. Prosser W: *Law of torts,* ed 4, St Paul, 1971, West Publishing.

12 Ethics in Gynecologic Surgery

THOMAS E. ELKINS and DOUGLAS BROWN

Advances in scientific technology (e.g., increased information from genetic testing, new breakthroughs in fetal surgery, and additional life-sustaining interventions) continue to expand medicine's ability to affect the process of birth, life, and death. The introduction of managed care and a greater emphasis on primary care are redesigning the way health care is delivered. The questions raised by such advances should not be addressed with medical knowledge alone.

APPROACHING BIOMEDICAL ETHICS[1]

Many theories, philosophic traditions, and cultural adaptations influence decision-making in medicine and provide context for gynecologic surgeons as they consider three basic issues about ethical decision-making. First, what distinguishes values, morals, and ethics? Second, what distinguishes extrinsic and intrinsic decision-making? Third, is patient-centered decision-making a realistic goal?

What Distinguishes Values, Morals, and Ethics?

Each individual forms a personal sense of what is of ultimate value and what is of lesser value. These core values serve as a prism through which information is interpreted before being applied to life's decisions. Thus certain relationships, experiences, circumstances, and objects are so important to an individual that he or she is prepared to suffer great loss rather than violate them.

Morals are common conceptions about what is right or wrong, what ought to or ought not to be done. Such views are taken for granted in daily activities and can usually be safely acted on without conflict. However, some situations require a collective judgment from individuals with competing goals or diverging viewpoints. A reflective approach to decision-making (e.g., ethics) is necessary to avoid situations involving a harmful abuse of power, such as a physician attempting to manipulate the transfer of information to steer a patient into agreement or to avoid patient malpractice suits.

Ethics essentially deals with determining what ought to be done in a given situation with all things considered. Some differences in judgment can be traced to variations in reasoning patterns. For instance, one person may be very logical, deductive, and abstract. Another person may be more intuitive, pragmatic, and affective. Other differences in judgment can be traced to variations in what is taken into consideration and the value given to that. For instance, one physician may support a woman in her desire to receive treatment for her infertility, whereas another

physician—the "gatekeeper" for the patient's health maintenance organization—may be most concerned with providing cost-effective primary care for a large number of patients. Before all options can be analyzed thoroughly, the participants in the decision-making process must respect (re- + spectare, to look again) each other enough to listen carefully to recognize and understand these differences.

An ethical dilemma arises when compelling value-based justifications exist for two or more conflicting courses of action. On initial examination, the possible choices may appear equally strong. For example, a physician caring for a patient who is refusing surgical treatment of a large pelvic mass may be torn between promoting what may be the patient's best medical interests and respecting the patient's personal choice to refuse treatment.

Ethics, as a discipline within medicine, involves three steps. First, a framework is established for analyzing differing points of view. Second, a determination is made as to whose interests are most critical in the situation. Third, a course of action is adopted that promotes those interests with the least imposition of compromise on those affected by the decision.

What Distinguishes Extrinsic and Intrinsic Decision-Making?

By primarily using objective or dispassionate reasoning, extrinsic decision-making is well suited for discussion and debate about case-specific ethical dilemmas, public policy issues, research protocols, and surgical procedures characteristic of modern medicine. Ethics committees (both hospital based and national), institutional research review boards, and departmental quality improvement programs more often than not promote an extrinsic process for decision-making.

This approach to decision-making—the foundation on which medical ethics has been established as a modern discipline—can be further divided into formalist and consequentialist decision-making.[3] Formalists draw their conclusions separate from and before the circumstances being faced. Consequentialists establish their conclusions within the circumstances being faced and look to outcomes for verification.

Intrinsic (or virtue-based) decision-making focuses on the character of the decision-maker(s); it is well suited for providing stability when facing multiple and often subtle decisions for which there is little (if any) time for research, reflection, or discussion. Many physicians and other health care professionals at the front lines of delivering medical care make ethical choices based on their value systems.

Intrinsic decision-making has received increasing attention in the past decade. Alasdair MacIntyre,[12] in *After Virtue,* argued that Aristotle's[2] *Nicomachean Ethics* remains a reliable foundation for ethical decision-making. Aristotle analyzed virtue in terms of courage, moderation, loyalty, wisdom, and integrity. MacIntyre, recognizing the influence of Jewish and Christian traditions, added humility and gratitude to the Aristotelian list of virtues. Pellegrino and Thomasma,[15] in *The Virtues in Medical Practice,* have presented a forceful interpretation of intrinsic decision-making in the delivery of health care.

Is Patient-Centered Decision-Making a Realistic Goal?

Gynecologic surgery directly affects sexual function, urinary and anal continence, and reproductive capacity. Drawing on the strengths of extrinsic and intrinsic approaches to patient care, gynecologic surgeons ought to be sensitive to the emotions, goals, and feelings of their patients. Surgeons are not properly trained if they are not adequately informed about depression, loss of self-esteem, and anxiety. The importance of sensitivity to the patient should be self-evident to surgeons performing bilateral oophorectomies for younger patients or hysterectomies with certain medical indications at any age. In the words of such a patient:

> Something is wrong. I sit here and the tears stream down my cheek uninvited. It hits me. I am losing a friend. They tell me it is no longer good . . . useless . . . dried up . . . gone. Yet it once held life. It gave life. It brought forth life. . . . It carried, supported, nurtured and gave me five children. It hurts to hear them say, "It's dried up and useless." What a thing to say about something that brought forth so much life! I feel bad for it to hear it being talked about in such a "throw it away" mode.

DECISION-MAKING OBLIGATIONS

When ethical concerns require careful analysis, the decision-making process and the soundness of the decision should be measured by reflection on a least six obligations:

1. Does sufficient trust exist among the involved parties for truthful and adequate information to be exchanged?
2. Is the patient's right to self-determination protected?
3. Is the patient's consent truly informed?
4. Does the decision promote the well-being of the patient?
5. Is the decision just?
6. Is confidentiality ensured?

Does Sufficient Trust Exist Among the Involved Parties for Truthful and Adequate Information To Be Exchanged?

A sound decision necessitates that truthful and adequate information pass between patients and their physicians. Physicians must focus on their patients, listen with interest for insightful comments, and avoid steering their patients toward predetermined conclusions. A physician's responsibil-

---

TO THE UTERUS WITHIN ME

Once you were vibrant—beautiful, full of life. You were
   filled with life-giving fluids and you were able to
   caress and hold a child within you.
You cradled each one until it was time to let them go
   . . . some sooner than others. You served me well.
I thank you for the role that you played in that special
   time of my life. You were created to be ready at a
   certain time when I called upon you.
And carry life you did! Five times. Each pregnancy so
   different. Remember?
Heavenly Father—Lord of Life—Spirit of Life—Thank
   you.
Thank you for all the parts of my body. All the parts that
   have gone together to create the whole of who I am
   encased in this shell of mine and called "Janice."
Some parts are hurting more than others. Some have
   dried up and are no longer needed. They have served
   me well. My appendix went a long time ago . . . never
   even missed that. I've had many haircuts—finger nails
   clipped—warts removed—teeth pulled. Parts of my
   body have gone by the wayside down thru the years.
Lord, I want to give you thanks for creating me as a
   woman with all the capabilities for giving birth. Thank
   you for the gift of my uterus that carried five lives to
   fruition. Thank you for a job well done.

From McCarthy J. Printed with permission.

ity is to recognize when competing demands for his or her attention weaken the ability to listen and prevent hearing important information.

Both patient and physician should be free to express concern that adequate information has not been shared. A physician should not assume that he or she, rather than the patient, knows what information needs to be shared. In general, a patient benefits from an understanding of her medical condition, its prognosis, and the treatment(s) available. A perception that essential information has been concealed or distorted undermines trust.

The ability to establish trust is central to practicing medicine. For a variety of reasons, trust cannot be established with some patients, even after considerable effort. In such cases, the physician should assist the patient in transferring her care to another qualified medical professional.

Is the Patient's Right to Self-Determination Protected?

A sound decision requires respect for a patient's right to self-determination. This right derives from her broader societal liberty to set personal values of conduct and to choose voluntarily a course of action consistent with those values. Such freedom necessitates that others avoid interfering, except when the individual is not competent to make decisions or when the chosen course of action infringes on the freedom and interests of others. It is a purpose of law to clarify the boundaries within which individuals exercise their autonomy (*auto* + *nomos*, self-law or self-rule).

It is the physician's responsibility to maximize his or her patient's liberty to choose the direction, nature, and consequence of her health care. To do so requires restraint. A physician may have to consider an alternative management plan if the patient rejects the course of treatment that the physician judges to be in the best medical interests for the patient. For instance, a physician is restricted from removing ovaries or the uterus from a patient who objects, except for emergency reasons, even when the physician thinks it is advisable.

Is the Patient's Consent Truly Informed?

A sound decision necessitates the patient's *informed* consent to the course of action. Informed consent is generally defined as the willing and uncoerced acceptance of a medical intervention, its risks and benefits, and alternatives with their risks and benefits.[17] The ethics argument for the informed consent process in medical practice focuses on the protection of a patient's right to self-determination, with legal protection for the physician being a *secondary* purpose.

A patient's right to make her own decision about medical interventions extends to her the liberty to refuse recommended medical treatment. In 1914 Judge Benjamin Cardozo pointed to the future when he argued that "every human being of adult years and sound mind has a right to determine what shall be done with his own body."[18] The meaning of consent—itself still a novelty in 1914—expanded to informed consent by the 1950s and informed choice by the 1970s.

At times, a patient's capacity to comprehend and process the information presented to her can be in doubt. Through consultation and further discussion with the patient, the physician should attempt to clarify the patient's capacity to consent. If the patient is unable to consent, the physician should seek a substitute decision-maker.

Does the Decision Promote the Well-Being of the Patient?

A sound decision entails a concerted effort to promote the well-being of the patient. Since the formation of the Hippocratic traditions, beneficence (*bene* + *facto*, to do good for another) has been central to the motivations and purposes of medicine. The most basic form of beneficence is nonmaleficence (i.e., "do no harm"). This reminder is certainly relevant to the practice of medicine. Even though technologic advances continue to improve a physician's ability to repair injuries and cure diseases, the most important expression of beneficence remains to "do no harm." "Can" does not imply "should." The disadvantages to be balanced with benefits include intentional harm and harm that can arise despite the best intentions (e.g., unwanted side effects of medication or complications of surgical treatment).

Is the Decision Just?

A sound decision involves consideration of the implications a course of action has on third parties immediately affected and on the interests of the larger society. A democratic society is committed to freedom and justice. Accordingly, individuals are free to claim what they are due based on specified personal properties or characteristics. It is important for all members of society to participate in the ongoing responsibility to select criteria relevant to the benefits and burdens being assigned. For instance, in our society, ethnicity, gender, and religious persuasion are not considered to be legitimate criteria by which to determine the distribution of such benefits as housing, education, employment, or health care.

Individuals equally concerned about justice may use different theories of justice to determine what would be a fair distribution of benefits and burdens. Some might argue that the distribution should correlate with need, effort, contribution, merit, or ability to pay. Others might argue that benefits and burdens should be distributed equally or randomly. The approach taken in a given situation should be relevant to the benefits and burdens being assigned. Commitment to a just decision creates an obligation to treat fairly those who are alike according to the selected criteria. No one should receive unequal treatment unless it is demonstrated that he or she differs significantly from others in a relevant way.

Achieving fairness is most difficult when constraints, such as scarcity of resources, force judgments about competing claims that appear equal based on existing distribution criteria. For instance, a critically ill patient needs intensive care, but the intensive care unit is full. All the patients in the unit meet the medical criteria for intensive care. If the available resources cannot be redistributed to accommodate another patient, additional criteria must be used to decide which patients should receive intensive care and which should be transferred to a less intensive setting. The selection of additional criteria (e.g., the increased risk if transferred or the likelihood of successful recovery) is itself an ethical issue.

Is Confidentiality Ensured?

A sound decision depends on the confidential handling of sensitive information. A patient's freedom to make decisions about her health care includes the right to decide how and to whom personal medical information is communicated. Carelessness about patient privacy undermines patient trust. This hazard is especially acute when many professionals are involved in patient care, when patient care is delivered in an educational setting, or when insurance companies and HMOs are involved. In the near future, the increasing availability of genetic information will make confidentiality even more difficult to maintain.

In general, protecting a patient's privacy takes precedence over other obligations. In some situations, however, maintaining confidentiality can result in harm to a third party immediately affected by the patient's choice. In other situations, maintaining confidentiality may conflict with being accountable to society; for confidentiality to be breached, however, the magnitude of risk to others must be actual and grave. Ethical judgment and legal regulations about reporting communicable diseases may not coincide.

In the rare instances when breaking confidence is deemed justifiable, the physician should attempt to explain the circumstances to the patient, solicit the patient's approval, and remain committed to the patient's care.

PRINCIPLES OF BIOMEDICAL ETHICS

Over the centuries, certain principles of biomedical ethics have become almost standardized. A clinical list might include only autonomy, justice, and beneficence. An extended list may include nonmaleficence, truth telling, contract (covenant or promise) keeping, and respect for life.

As illustrated by the evolution of thought in the ACOG Ethics Committee's bulletins, substantial debate has in recent years surrounded the meaning and use of these principles for decision-making in obstetrics and gynecology. Beneficence had been the anchoring ethical principle in the history of medicine for generations. However, autonomy became for many the most important of these principles in the rights-oriented 1970s and 1980s, when the emphasis on informed consent became paramount in surgery.[13] Some advocates of the principle of autonomy virtually equated beneficence and paternalism. Since the 1980s, the principle of beneficence has been reemphasized, with texts such as Pellegrino's and Thomasma's[14] *For the Patient's Good: The Restoration of Beneficence in Health Care.* With the advent of managed health care and welfare reforms, concerns about justice are now receiving more attention.

Many would argue that throughout these recent decades the concern for a basic respect for life (whether expressed as the sanctity of life, relative sanctity of life, or quality of life) has overwhelmed all others. Certainly, the debates over abortion, prenatal testing, end-of-life management, and the management of handicapped newborns attest to this assessment. Our society is divided over the basic issue of human value or worth. Some regard human value or worth to be a reflection of the creative spirit of a loving God and therefore inherent within all persons, including the young, old, or disabled. Others link human value or worth to the capacity of persons to function in society. Surgeons making decisions must respect these concerns, especially when dealing with disabled or marginalized patients and their families.

Most of our educational efforts in residency training programs have focused on imparting information about these age-old principles. They remain useful in clarifying ethical issues and categorizing our responses to them. They are readily applicable to a case presentation method of learning ethics, which makes them especially helpful to the gynecologic surgeon.

CONTEMPORARY PRAGMATIC CONCERNS
The Ethical Challenge of Managed Care

More than 10 years ago in New Orleans, Louisiana, at one of the first national ethics conferences sponsored by the American Medical Association, someone stated that economics would soon drive the ethics of medical care more than any principle, theory, or ideal could ever have achieved.[9] It was noted that research-oriented care for patients was then being restricted by economic concerns, and it was predicted that even routine health care would be restricted in America by the year 2000. This development has happened sooner than expected.

Examples are endless. Scheduling a patient for a hysterectomy can become a maze of second opinions, mandated presurgical trials of numerous alternative therapies, mounds of paperwork, and billing and coding frustrations. At current reimbursement rates, it becomes almost financially unjustifiable to allow the same level of resident-fellow educational experience. For medically indigent patients, the current health care system must seem frankly hostile to their needs. State medical assistance physician reimbursement rates for general gynecology and gynecologic surgery have reached all-time lows for hysterectomy; similar rates can be found for other comparable procedures. The recent announcement by Medicare that annual examinations would be reimbursed only every 2 to 3 years is a new pinnacle in this thinking.

Perhaps even more worrisome is the trend of HMO-medical advisors to direct patient care management decisions through rigid payment policies that allow few alternatives for unsuspecting patients. The physicians making such decisions are often minimally clinically active or not even gynecologists at all. It has become the nation's strongest "peer review" system, despite a marked absence of peer reviewers and an economic motivation that can be, at times, in harsh contrast with patients' best interests.

As emphasized by Bruce Drukker in his 1998 presidential address at the Society for Gynecologic Surgeons, only the ethical concern for our patients' well-being will ever modify such a pervasive and powerful economic movement in health care.[8] Ethics education and reflection for physicians may soon become a subject of much interest to gynecologic surgeons. To date, it has been sorely neglected in the majority of residency training programs.

Management of Terminally Ill Patients

Current societal debates such as physician-assisted suicide, euthanasia, and terminal sedation highlight the concerns of an aging America. Howard Brody, speaking in 1998 at the Society for Gynecologic Surgeons, emphasized the need for physicians to become more concerned about improving the quality of life and relieving the pain of terminally ill patients.[5] He stressed that these concerns had to be addressed with an understanding of the diversity of cultures within our own society. These goals are made even more difficult by the fear of death, a fear often created by (1) unrealistic expectations of medicine and technology, (2) a deemphasis on religion and an increased emphasis on materialism, and (3) a diminishing family involvement in the dying process. It will be a topic of debate for years to come. Surgeons, especially in gynecologic oncology, will be frequently drawn into such discussions. Concerns over quality of life, avoidance of futile (and possibly harmful) treatments, and the nuances of substituted informed consent in terminal care and analysis are beyond the scope of this chapter and will require increasing attention among surgeons over the next decade.

The Promises and Pitfalls of Evidence-Based Gynecologic Surgery

The shift to evidence-based medicine has the potential to force ethical principles on an unsuspecting specialty. All procedures may eventually require statistically justifiable outcomes to receive reimbursement coding. "Do it right, and do it well, doctor; or something else!" Only the best procedures, those with lasting benefit to patients, will survive. The problem of endless procedures without clearly positive outcomes should diminish as evidence-based medicine becomes a reality.

Our own specialty's forays into surgical innovation without prior documentation of success have helped to create the need for such a change. Examples of the problem are myriad. Over 60 different procedures for the surgical correction of stress urinary incontinence now exist, with less than five randomized, prospective, controlled studies having been conducted to verify the claims.

Procedures with such a history are numerous. The answer for the purist in research is to mandate a change in the entire process. Many are doing just that in a slow but steady way. Annual research meetings sponsored by the American Urogynecology Society (AUGS) and over 20 years of effort by the Gynecologic Oncology Group (GOG), for example, promote this kind of change. Such research integrity is an example of ethical analysis applied to a surgical specialty, and it should be applauded.

Such a system, of course, has pitfalls. Outcome-based, or evidence-based, medical practice downplays the wisdom of experience in surgery, "evidence" that defies statistical validity while providing lifesaving expertise to younger surgeons. Some anecdotes must never be forgotten, lest they become a series of "commonly encountered problems" in a particular surgical procedure. Surgery is one field in which the "case report" should never be ignored as material lacking sufficient data and therefore unsuitable for consideration in peer-reviewed publications. Anatomic and physiologic variations require a freedom of surgical innovation that cannot always be predicted or programmed for study purposes.

Finally, evidence-based medicine, without close scrutiny, can become a classic example of an "end" that justifies any "means." This risk is similar to the extremes presented by William James[11] in his classic work *Pragmatism*. Evidence-based medicine will be appropriate only if great care is taken to broaden the parameters of evaluation to include economic costs as well as clinical cure rates, morbidity as well as mortality, depression as well as cardiac function, self-esteem as well as "successful" surgical excisions, and availability and access to reasonable care for all as well as the provision of outstanding care that can be achieved only by a few.

Surgical Training Issues in Gynecology

Residency training in gynecologic surgery in America is sometimes limited to only a few months of a 4-year program.[16] Surgical anatomy relevant to the contemporary pelvic surgeon is not formally taught in medical school or residency programs. In gynecology, initial knot-tying skills, clamp placement skills, management of hemorrhage, and bowel-bladder-ureteral injuries usually are taught in the operating room with live, human patients. Laboratory efforts are minimal in most gynecologic training programs; the programs usually are industry sponsored and teach the use of a company's particular equipment as much as basic surgical skills. The training "ground," even for basics, becomes the living, human patient.

The 4-year curriculum is now crowded with primary care rotations, as well as much more knowledge to master in obstetrics, infertility, and oncology. Money is not available to sponsor anatomy courses or surgical skill training laboratory experiences. Many times, gross anatomy takes a back seat in medical school to molecular biology in the quest for cellular-based knowledge. Some wonder if acceptable surgery can still be mastered within such a crowded residency period. With this in mind, the move to develop new educational tracts and subspecialties to ensure the presence of highly trained, markedly skillful, advanced gynecologic pelvic floor urogynecologic surgeons has a great ethical impetus. To do otherwise, in light of our current residency curriculums, would be an ethical problem.

As with other issues, however, this response can be corrupted by physicians' failure of motivational integrity. A certificate of "fellowship" in pelvic reconstructive surgery, for example, is not a license to charge higher fees than nearby colleagues or shirk educational and research responsibilities that should accompany such societal investment in a physician and should not serve merely as a means to market one's skills.

The Relationship of Surgical Research to Profit-Oriented Industry

With the diminishing availability of governmental research and clinical support funds, pilot studies of new procedures or new technologies often are supportable only with the help of commercial industry. The potential for conflicts of interest on the part of surgeons is clear and potentially dangerous. Financially benefiting from the use of an industry's equipment or advertising for them has become so widespread that the American College of Obstetricians and Gynecologists published a recent statement offering guidelines for physicians and surgeons facing such issues.[10]

Evolving Issues in Informed Consent

Informed consent for surgery has undergone many revisions in different states over the past 5 to 10 years. Many states have adopted lengthy, comprehensive documents for patients to read and sign before surgery. The essence of informed consent, however, remains the conversation between two persons who share a covenant relationship that should transcend the contracted document of "informed consent."[7]

Many questions appear almost "nonanswerable" in America's pluralist society. Concerns about whether human life begins at conception, implantation, fetal individualization (14 to 21 days), or at birth will probably never be answered with a solid consensus. The "answers" to such questions lead to very restrictive or very supportive attitudes toward in vitro fertilization and associated new reproductive technologies. For society, answers will be sought in policy and legislation. For the individual surgeon and patient, answers will be found in honesty, informed consent, and mutual respect for each individual's personal limitations.

Other questions find "answers" within honesty and informed consent. Whether or not residents in training assist actively or passively, for example, is not nearly as important as the patient's understanding of the resident's role in her case and the clear discussion of this role by the attending physician in any training program.

CONCLUSIONS AND PERSONAL REFLECTIONS

The following conclusions are personal reflections and defining comments about ethics. They relate gynecologic surgery and its ethics to a cross-cultural, transcontinental view of women's health and surgical innovation. Some terms in gynecologic surgery—*ethics, motivation, compassion, wisdom, integrity*— are found globally. In more desperate areas of the world, such as rural West Africa, they may simply be more readily recognizable. They must not be forgotten now in America.

The Individual Patient: The Motivational Force for Ethical Innovation in Gynecologic Surgery

Baba Rachia, or "Rachel," is still leaking from her obstetrics fistula in remote Northern Ghana. She came to a hospital over 6 years ago. Several months before, she had survived 5 to 6 days of obstructed labor. The macerated, dead fetus had passed, and her sepsis had resolved. She did not die, unlike 40 to 70 other women per 1000 who delivered in remote, rural West Africa in 1987; however, her vagina was left with gaping holes (each greater than 5 cm) adjacent to her bladder and rectum. Six years and five operations later, she still leaks. Her need, and that of the many underserved women like her, is a driving, motivating force. The same can be said for patients with pelvic prolapse and incontinence whose problems remain despite several procedures, cancer patients who have been unresectable, or patients with complications from procedures we have done. Our inadequacy as surgeons is highlighted by the patients representing our failures. They serve as reminders in our careers so that we never forget that we must improve. They prompt our humility and provide a motivation for us that overpowers all "conflicts of interest." They give meaning to the terms *beneficence, justice,* and *autonomy.* They demand a covenantal response.

The Capacity for Compassion: An Essential Companion to Reasoning in Medical Ethics

Catherine Hamlin, Martha Hagood, Ann Ward, and Martha Gilleland-Stewart are all pioneer women who, as obstetricians and gynecologists, went with many others to develop

ing countries in the service of women with extreme health care needs. Their contribution to our world began with the journey—"the courage to go." Bonhoeffer described it as the vacating of our "comfortable pews," or our "comfort zones," to be face to face with our world.[4] It is the deeply personal analogue of the theologic concept of "costly grace." It may be, as in the case of the women listed above, a geographic change. However, this may not be required. It is the willingness to provide care for those in need, beyond the complexity of concerns for personal incomes, lifestyles, and career enhancement. As business interests become more overpowering in American medicine, this capacity to lessen our own personal benefits for the benefit of our patients will separate medicine from other professions and preserve quality in women's health care. The compassion of doctors that drives them to meet the needs of underprivileged women throughout the world, despite the many financial constraints that make such thoughts seen unreasonable, will enhance the core of integrity essential to women's health care now and in the future.

Competency: Establishing Systems of Training and Innovation To Bring Excellence with Relevance to Gynecologic Surgery

In a similar way, gynecologic surgery in America must be willing to establish new levels of excellence with a special relevance for our setting. For example, this focus entails increasing the knowledge and skill required to meet the needs of a female population that is aging both remarkably and well. Minimally invasive and radically extensive procedures will be required, and only innovations driven by the purity of patient needs will be both helpful and reasonable. Similarly, it will soon become unethical not to consider the financial burden that surgery presents to the minimally insured patient "supported" only in a small part by contemporary "managed care," or to ignore the psychosocial effects of surgery in an era of evidence-based medicine.

The Virtue of Ageless Enthusiasm and Wisdom in Surgery

Many are in our midst today who fit in a specialized category of gynecologic surgery. For them, "ethics" has been defined in their vision of surgery as an art form forever still to be mastered. "Virtue" has been clarified by the knowledge gained from vast experience, and the wisdom to know that it is still incomplete. "Integrity" in surgery has been the stabilizing factor in careers buffeted by stressful changes in surgical technology, legal interactions, reimbursement of patterns, training emphases, chaotic institutional administrations, and patient population needs. They serve as role models for gynecologic surgeons and need to be encouraged as teachers, often even beyond retirement requirements. Experience in surgery is a priceless gem that cannot be obtained quickly. The best young surgical hands become problematic with overdissection in a sacrospinous suspension, or too little dissection in fistula repair. With experience comes knowledge and steadily improving surgical skills.

Ethics: Ideals Dependent Today on Integrity and Courage

As economic forces and corporate mentalities increasingly override American "managed care," the response of physicians and surgeons to hold tightly to their salaries and possessions is both predictable and worrisome. The plight of poverty is relative, with sharp declines in income (currently being seen among many American physicians groups) often being as stressful as continuous lifetime poverty. When the protection or accumulation of wealth becomes a motivating goal, there is no end point to greed. Such lessons are learned quickly when working for long periods in developing regions of our world, where resources are scarce, and even basic health care is a struggle to provide. Patients become increasingly vulnerable as the health care industry becomes increasingly driven by the desire for difficult-to-achieve profit margins and as health care institutions' providers become associated with available or accessible wealth. In such times, innovative surgery may become merely another marketing tool, with advertising and business administration skills becoming far more important than basic science in the minds of some surgeons and surgical institutions. It is a time ripe for marketing scams, business schemes, and lucrative medical dishonesty in America.

Oversight of a system with such potential for abuse is a growing interest of hospital ethics committees, performance improvement programs, quality assurance boards, federal medical fraud task forces, and legal prosecutors. Policing our own profession will no longer be an option for physicians and surgeons unless we begin to prove to Americans that we are willing to stand for ethically supportable positions that have historically made medicine an honored and trusted profession.

The words of this chapter are neither original nor outdated. In the presidential address of the American Urogynecology Society in October 1997, Shull[20] bluntly stated that American physicians must learn to make appropriate decisions, not only in surgery and clinic, but in their domestic and spiritual lives as well, to reestablish the integrity and joy of our profession. Scott,[19] in the 1997 presidential address to the American Gynecologic and Obstetrics Society, was even more direct in his comments. He quoted extensively from the recent text of Yale Law Professor Stephen Carter,[6] who defined *integrity* as (1) making a decision about what is right or wrong in a given situation, (2) standing up for what is right regardless of the personal costs, and (3) openly stating the reason for making the decision. Scott further concluded that to reemphasize integrity in today's American health care setting will at times require extreme courage for individuals within our profession to make certain that medicine remains focused on the patients' best interests and well-being.

David Nichols contributed greatly to this chapter, both in its formulation and its editing. His conclusions were those one would expect from someone with his wisdom and integrity; there has never been a more appropriate time for gynecologic surgeons to place at the core of their concerns the desire "to do unto others as we would like for others to do unto us." It has never been more of a challenge in our profession to represent such a simple proposition.

REFERENCES

1. American College of Obstetricians and Gynecologists Technical Bulletin Committee: *Ethical decision-making in obstetrics and gynecology,* bulletin no 136, Washington, DC, 1989.
2. Aristotle: *Nicomachean ethics,* Indianapolis, Ind, 1985, Hackett Publishing (Translated by Terence Irwin).
3. Beauchamp TL, Childress JF: *Principles of biomedical ethics,* ed 4, New York, 1994, Oxford Press.
4. Bonhoeffer D: *The cost of discipleship,* New York, 1974, Macmillan (Originally published in 1937).
5. Brody H: Euthanasia and physician-assisted suicide. Paper presented at the Society for Gynecologic Surgeons, Orlando, Fla, March 1, 1998.
6. Carter S: *Integrity,* New York, 1996, Harper Collins.
7. Cassell E: *Talking with patients,* Cambridge, Mass, 1985, MIT Press.
8. Drukker B: Presidential address presented to Society for Gynecologic Surgeons, Orlando, Fla, March 1, 1998.
9. Epps CH: Economic constraints and ethical decision-making symposium: a new ethic for a new medicine? Presented at AMA Hastings Center Sponsor Conference, New Orleans, March 16, 1986.
10. American College of Obstetrics and Gynecologists Ethics Committee.
11. James W: *Pragmatism,* Indianapolis, 1981, Hackett Publishing (Originally published in 1907).
12. MacIntyre A: *After virtue: a study in moral theory,* ed 2, Notre Dame, 1984, University of Notre Dame Press.
13. McCullough LB, Chervenak FA: *Ethics in obstetrics and gynecology,* New York, 1994, Oxford University Press.
14. Pellegrino ED, Thomasma DC: For the patient's good: the restoration of beneficence in health care, New York, 1988, Oxford University Press.
15. Pellegrino ED, Thomasma DC: *The virtues in medical practice,* New York, 1993, Oxford University Press.
16. Podratz KC: Gynecologic surgery: an imperiled ballet. Presidential address to Central Association of OB/GYN, Scottsdale, Ariz, Nov 1, 1997, *Am J Obstet Gynecol* 178:1229, 1998.
17. Rosoff AJ: *Informed consent: a guide for health care providers,* Rockville, Md, 1981, Aspen Systems.
18. *Schloendorff v. Society of New York Hospital,* 211 NY 125, 105 NE 92, 93 (1914).
19. Scott J: Presidential address presented to American Gynecologic and Obstetrics Society Annual Meeting, Vancouver, 1997.
20. Shull R: Presidential address presented to American Gynecologic and Obstetrics Society Annual Meeting, Vancouver, 1997.

13 Incisions

DAVID H. NICHOLS

Although a wide range of abdominal incisions is available to the gynecologic surgeon, the fundamental guiding precept is ensuring adequate exposure of the entire operative field. This must take into account the many likely ramifications of extension of the original planned surgery. For example, surgery performed on a postmenopausal woman to remove a 5 cm adnexal mass, although quickly performed through a cosmetically attractive Pfannenstiel's incision, may reveal that the lesion is malignant; a thorough exploration of the abdomen is indicated in the course of staging the disease, including the possibility of paraaortic node dissection, further pelvic surgery, and occasionally omentectomy. Similarly, the incision for total abdominal hysterectomy in a patient being treated for adenocarcinoma of the endometrium should permit adequate exposure for pelvic node sampling if the latter is desired consequent to an unexpectedly greater depth of myometrial invasion by the tumor. An incision that is most effective surgically may not be the one that is most attractive cosmetically. If the latter consideration is critical for the patient requiring hysterectomy, perhaps hysterectomy by the vaginal route should be done safely, avoiding an abdominal incision altogether.

Operative exposure for abdominal surgery involving the anterior surface of the sacrum, such as sacral colpopexy or presacral neurectomy, must provide sufficient exposure for surgery to be done safely.

The tiny incisions used with laparoscopy are considered in the appropriate chapters.[55,61]

GENERAL PRINCIPLES

The surgeon should be able to extend the chosen incision if circumstances discovered during the course of operation necessitate a larger operative exposure. Most pelvic surgery can be performed effectively through a lower midline incision. This can be easily extended if necessary, often alongside the umbilicus, and repaired effectively with a minimal risk of postoperative development of evisceration or wound hernia.

The Maylard, or transverse, incision provides excellent exposure of the pelvis, although it does take a little longer to perform and to repair. The exposure for coincident surgery of the upper abdomen may be compromised (e.g.,

hepatic or diaphragmatic biopsy, omentectomy, or paraaortic node dissection), so the surgeon should have carefully evaluated the potential for this need preoperatively. The Cherney incision, which avoids transecting the rectus muscles by temporarily detaching them from their insertion on the pubis, provides effective exposure of the pelvis and retropubic areas, but not as broad an exposure as that provided by the Maylard or midline incision. It can be used to convert a Pfannenstiel's incision into a more effective surgical exposure should circumstances require.

Pfannenstiel's incision is the most cosmetically attractive abdominal incision, but provides access for the least amount of exposure of the pelvis when compared to the midline or Maylard transverse incision. Pfannenstiel's incision is least likely to present a risk of postoperative wound herniation and is suitable for tubal ligation, hysterectomy for benign disease when the uterus is small, ovarian cystectomy, and certain instances of tubal or adnexal reconstructive surgery.

ANATOMY OF THE ANTERIOR ABDOMINAL WALL

The muscular layers of the anterior abdominal wall must be considered individually because of the differences in the direction in which their fibers run; an incision should traverse each layer separately. The most superficial muscular layer is that of the external oblique (Fig. 13-1). The underlying internal oblique, with fibers almost at right angles to those of the external oblique, is shown in Fig. 13-2; the deepest layer, the transversus abdominis, is shown in both frontal and side view in Fig. 13-3. Because these muscles function synergistically, a cutaway drawing of their positions relative to one another is shown in Fig. 13-4. The cutaneous nerves arise from the seventh to twelfth thoracic nerves, the anterior cutaneous branch of the iliohypogastric nerve, and the ilioinguinal nerve. These nerves curve forward and downward between the internal oblique and transversalis muscles. The anterior cutaneous branch of the iliohypogastric nerve terminates after piercing the aponeurosis of the external oblique muscle just above the subcutaneous inguinal ring. The ilioinguinal nerve passes through the subcutaneous ring to innervate the skin of the labia majora and me-

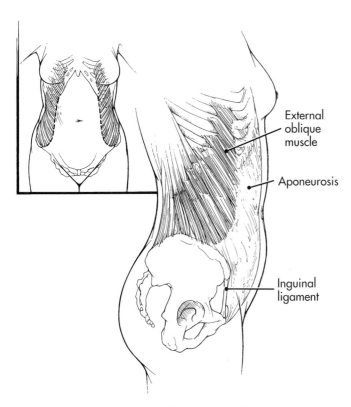

Fig. 13-1 Sagittal view of the external oblique muscle and its aponeurosis in the adult female. Frontal view is shown in the inset.

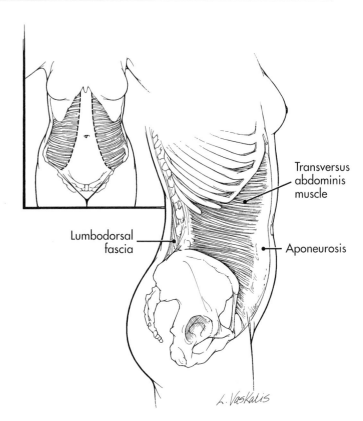

Fig. 13-3 Sagittal view of the transversus abdominis muscle in the adult female. Frontal view is shown in the inset.

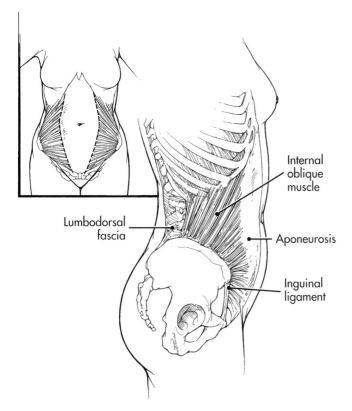

Fig. 13-2 Sagittal view of the internal oblique muscle and its aponeurosis in the adult female. Frontal view is shown in the inset.

dial aspect of the thigh. The anterior branches supply the internal oblique and transverse abdominal muscles as they pass forward between them, and the terminal anterior cutaneous branches supply the rectus muscles, entering from their lateral side.

The superficial and deep nerves of the anterior abdominal wall enter the muscles laterally (Fig. 13-5). If an incision can spare transection of these nerves, muscular function will be preserved, but the surgeon must be careful not to include entrapped nerve tissue in a suture line, which can cause severe postoperative pain. The latter phenomenon is poorly understood because it resembles the response pattern of receptor fiber subjected to chronic stimulation. Sippo and Gomez[60] hypothesize that, unlike other sensory receptors, pain receptors are nonadaptive to continuous or repeated stimulation and can even lower their threshold for excitation when continuously stimulated, as by entrapment in an incisional closure. Until this stimulation is removed by either interruption using local anesthetic infiltration of the site of nerve trauma or, failing this, resection of the nerve, the cascade of transmissions from the receptor continues and the perceived intensity of the pain increases.[27,48,61] The mechanism of this pain relief after local anesthetic injection is not well understood, but it has been hypothesized that the nerve block allows the threshold of stimulation to reset to its original level at a time when ongoing stimulation is subliminal. Although the stimulation is still present, it does not trigger the conduction of a pain impulse.

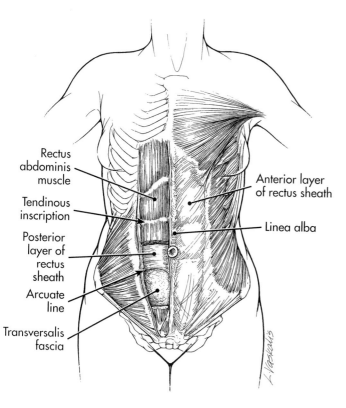

Rectus
abdominis
muscle

Tendinous
inscription

Posterior
layer of
rectus
sheath

Arcuate
line

Transversalis
fascia

Anterior layer
of rectus sheath

Linea alba

Fig. 13-4   A composite of the muscles of the anterior abdominal wall of the adult female. The superficial muscles are shown on the left. In the illustration to the right of the drawing, the rectus abdominis muscle, external and internal oblique muscles, and lower half of the rectus abdominis have been removed to show the structures underneath. Notice the position of the arcuate line. Above the arcuate line, the posterior leaf of the internal oblique aponeurosis and the aponeurosis of the transversalis unite to form the posterior wall of the rectus sheath. Below the arcuate line, a posterior wall of the rectus sheath is formed only by the muscular plate of the transversalis.

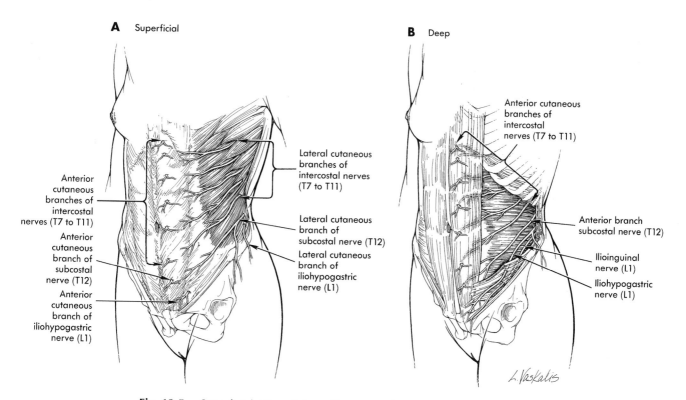

A Superficial

B Deep

Anterior
cutaneous
branches of
intercostal
nerves (T7 to T11)

Anterior
cutaneous
branch of
subcostal
nerve (T12)

Anterior
cutaneous
branch of
iliohypogastric
nerve (L1)

Lateral cutaneous
branches of
intercostal nerves
(T7 to T11)

Lateral cutaneous
branch of
subcostal nerve (T12)

Lateral cutaneous
branch of
iliohypogastric
nerve (L1)

Anterior cutaneous
branches of
intercostal
nerves (T7 to T11)

Anterior branch
subcostal nerve (T12)

Ilioinguinal
nerve (L1)

Iliohypogastric
nerve (L1)

Fig. 13-5   Superficial **(A)** and deep **(B)** nerves of the anterior abdominal wall.

The arterial blood supply of the anterior abdominal wall to its various layers is shown in Fig. 13-6. Although the superior and inferior epigastric arteries are continuous with one another in 50% of people, individual variation in this relationship is significant, and in many people no common pathway between these vessels exists. In the presence of obliterative disease of the femoral artery, it is possible for blood in the inferior epigastric artery to flow in the opposite direction, and it may supply considerable collateral circulation to the lower extremity. In such patients, it is important

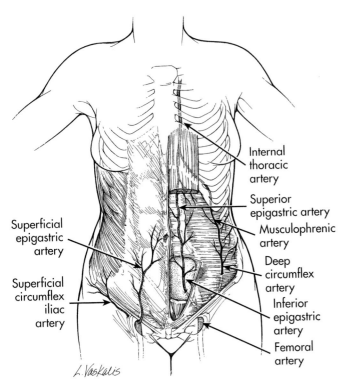

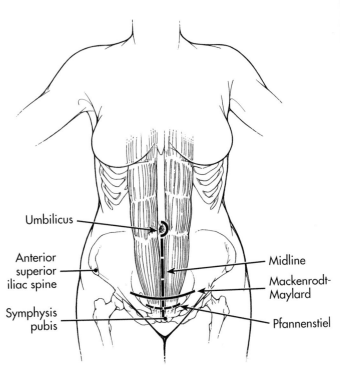

Fig. 13-6   Arterial blood supply of the anterior abdominal wall. The superficial arteries should be noted to the left of the drawing, the deep arteries to the right. Although there is frequently direct continuity between the superior and inferior epigastric artery, it is subject to considerable variation, and at times no anastomosis exists between the two.

Fig. 13-7   The frequent incisions of the anterior abdominal wall are shown in relation to the anterior superior iliac spines.

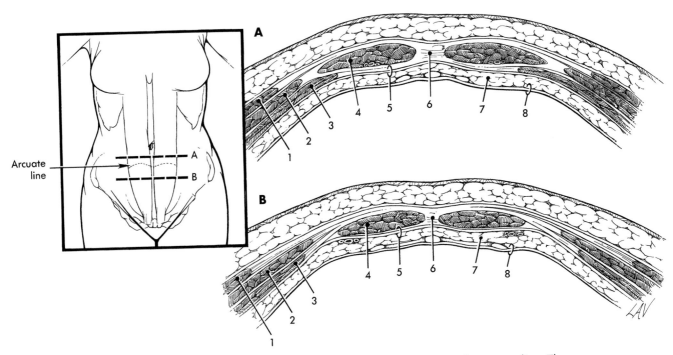

Fig. 13-8   **A,** Transverse section of the anterior abdominal wall above the arcuate line. The posterior leaf of the aponeurosis of the internal oblique muscle and the aponeurosis of the transversus abdominis muscle unite to form the posterior wall of the rectus sheath. **B,** Transverse section through the anterior abdominal wall below the arcuate line; the posterior wall of the rectus sheath is formed only by the transversalis fascia. *1,* External oblique muscle; *2,* internal oblique muscle; *3,* transversus abdominis muscle; *4,* rectus abdominis muscle; *5,* transversalis fascia; *6,* linea alba; *7,* extraperitoneal tissue (fat); *8,* peritoneum.

to palpate the pulsations of the dorsalis pedis artery after the inferior epigastric artery has been temporarily occluded but before it is transected so that the circulation of the lower extremity is not jeopardized.

The basic bony landmarks are shown, along with the site for the principal incisions used in transabdominal pelvic surgery: midline, the Mackenrodt-Maylard, and Pfannenstiel's. The muscular components involve the rectus abdominis, the external oblique, the internal oblique, and the transversus abdominis muscles; the fibers of each run in a different direction.[14] Tendinous inscriptions of the muscle can be identified, and the blood supply is from the superior and inferior epigastric artery on each side. These arteries anastomose on each side in 50% of patients. The nerve supply enters the muscles laterally, as shown.

The sites of the usual incisions in the lower anterior abdominal wall are shown in Fig. 13-7, particularly as they relate to the bony landmarks of the pelvis, the symphysis pubis and the anterior superior iliac spine, and to the rectus abdominis muscle and umbilicus.

Cranial to the arcuate line, there is a useful posterior fascia to the rectus sheath, but caudal to the arcuate line, this fascia disappears, leaving only a relatively weak transversalis fascia in its place.[67] This is shown in transverse section of the anterior abdominal wall in Fig. 13-8. Internal access to the organs of the pelvis is affected by the patient's position on the operating table (Fig. 13-9). Exposure of the pelvis during laparotomy is improved by tilting the head of the operating table downward 30 degrees.[38]

PREPARATION FOR THE OPERATION

In preparing for surgery, the operator scrubs the hands thoroughly with povidone-iodine solution. Because most glove puncture sites are at the fingertip, the surgeon should shorten and clean the fingernails preoperatively. The iodophors and chlorhexidine gluconate solution are stable and nontoxic. Chlorhexidine has shown continued disinfection of hands gloved for 3 hours, whereas 10% povidone-iodine detergent has demonstrated a less persistent effect.[3] Although the Centers for Disease Control and Prevention recommend a 5-minute scrub from the hands and arms to elbows before each operation, 2 to 5 minutes of scrubbing seems adequate between operations.[42] Lowbury reported a 98% reduction in skin bacterial counts after a 2-minute scrub.[40] After surgery, the hands should be washed to remove blood and other contaminants, with particular attention to the area beneath the fingernails.[42] An alcohol solution (46% to 70% ethyl or isopropyl alcohol) appears to be virucidal.

To lessen trauma to the skin and reduce the incidence of incisional infection, any hair that may interfere with making an incision should be removed either with scissors or occasionally an electric trimmer. Leaving the skin of the vulva unshaved does not increase the incidence of wound infection and makes the patient more comfortable postoperatively. If necessary, the site of the incision may be shaved or clipped in the operating room immediately before surgery.

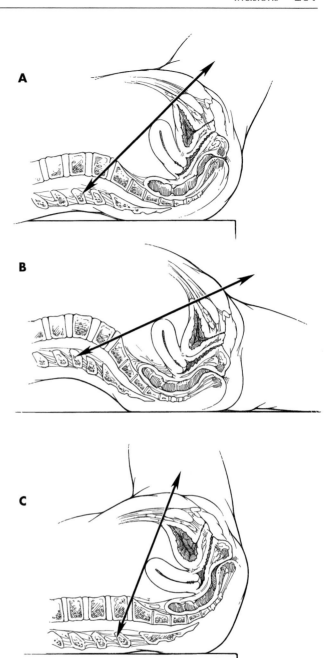

Fig. 13-9 The axis of the pelvic inlet is shown in relation to the various surgical positions. These have a relation to the operative exposure that can be expected during transabdominal surgery according to the position of the patient and her legs on the operating table. When the legs are supported at an angle of 45 degrees in relation to that of the body, as during laparoscopy or combined abdominal-pelvic surgery, the transabdominal exposure of the pelvic organs is as shown in **A.** When the body axis and the legs are both horizontal and parallel to the surface of the operating table, as during laparotomy, the transabdominal view is as shown in **B.** When the legs are in stirrups, as during transvaginal surgery, and the thighs are at about right angles to the horizontal axis of the body and the operating table, the relationship is shown in **C.** Note the differences in arching of the lower back in relation to the three positions.

Because iodine is a broad-spectrum antimicrobial, the iodophor complex with the nonsurfactant polyvinyl pyrrolidine (Betadine) is appropriate for use on intact skin; it is not suitable for use in an open wound, however, because it could be absorbed and its high molecular weight would make it difficult for the kidneys to excrete.[18] After any foreign material has been scrubbed from the incisional site, the skin is painted with povidone-iodine solution and allowed to dry. Traditionally, the vagina is similarly painted with the same antiseptic solution, although Amstey and Jones[1] found no benefits from this procedure beyond those obtained by washing the vagina with saline preoperatively, provided the patient received prophylactic antibiotic.

CHOICE OF SUTURE FOR CLOSING THE WOUND

Sanz et al.[56] reported that polyglyconate (Maxon) and polyglactin (Vicryl) consistently exhibited better tensile strength than polydioxanone (PDS) and chromic catgut during the late postoperative period; they thought this to be beneficial when wound healing might be delayed, as in corticosteroid therapy, infection, chemotherapy, and in diabetic patients. Bourne et al.[7] determined that the in vivo half-life tensile strength of polyglycolic acid (Dexon Plus) and polyglactin 9, 10 (Vicryl) is 2 weeks, whereas those of polyglyconate (Maxon) and polydioxanone (PDS) are 3 and 6 weeks, respectively. For low-risk patients, continuous fascia closure with a no. 0 polyglactin suture has been reported to be effective. Leaper, Pollack, and Evans[37] showed that 1 cm bites have a suture-holding capacity twice as strong as 0.5 cm bites. When a continuous suture is used and the bites are 1 cm from the cut edge of the fascia and placed at 1 cm intervals, a suture length four times the length of the incision is recommended.

A study of Smead-Jones closure comparing no. 1 polyglycolic acid suture (Dexon) to continuous muscular fascial closure using no. 1 Prolene demonstrated that the permanent suture group had one third of the frequency of incisional hernias on follow-up as the absorbable suture group. As Morrow[46] and Colombo et al.[15] point out, vertical subumbilical incisions at risk for dehiscence or delayed healing should be closed with a mass running permanent suture. Those at risk include women who are elderly, diabetic, or malnourished, those who have pulmonary disease, take steroids, have ascites, will receive postoperative radiation or chemotherapy, are very muscular, or have never been pregnant.[39]

Polybutester (Novafil) is a unique copolymer monofilament nonabsorbable synthetic suture material that has the unique qualities of high breaking strength, similar to that of nylon of the same suture size, combined with stretchable elasticity proportional to the force applied, and exhibiting prompt elastic recovery. It is twice as flexible as nylon or polypropylene of similar size, and yet secure knots can be formed with three or four throws. These qualities, particularly that of elastic stretching once it is in place, make it ideal for wound closure, especially when a single layer technique is chosen. As postoperative edema and swelling develop in the tissues in which the suture has been placed, the suture stretches temporarily up to 10% or 15% of its length to lessen the chance of tearing or strangulating the tissues in which it has been placed. As postoperative edema and swelling subside, the suture contracts to the degree that it had been stretched, taking up any slack that was produced and holding the tissues in approximation during their long healing phase. This should lessen the chance of postoperative wound dehiscence. Dehiscence unrelated to suture breakage occurs not at the suture site, but lateral to the suture line.[53,54]

The use of permanent monofilament absorbable suture is recommended for the closure of most midline incisions. In a very thin patient, however, the suture knots at the ends and midpoint of the fascial closure may remain permanently palpable, to the distress of the patient. Therefore in thin patients the use of a monofilament delayed absorption suture material such as polydioxanone (PDS) or polyglyconate (Maxon) should be employed. Metz et al.[45] reported that polydioxanone (PDS) retained its integrity in the wound for at least 35 days but found that glycolic acid–trimethylene carbonate (Maxon) became fragile and disintegrated easily 14 days after implantation.

Loosely applied sutures, not intended for hemostasis, promote stronger wound formation because they do not unnecessarily disturb tissue vascularity. However, the knot should be tied snugly. Although polyglycolic acid sutures are strong and recommended for incisional closure, catgut is most useful for tying smaller bleeders because it is supple and easy to handle. When using synthetic sutures, the surgeon must be careful not to puncture the outer surface of the suture by using forceps, needle tips, or ligature carriers, because trauma to the suture may inhibit its strength considerably or cause it to fracture or break.[43] Synthetic sutures should be tied with multiple casts, usually a surgeon's knot followed by three square knots. Subcutaneous sutures are used frequently in a thin abdomen but never in a fat one. A few interrupted stitches placed subcutaneously in Camper's fascia of a thin woman prevent postoperative scar depression during and after the healing phase.[13]

EXCISION OF OLD SCAR

Careful excision of scars is important in approaching the peritoneal cavity through a previous surgical incision. The excision of unsightly scars with subsequent meticulous closure of the skin by subcutaneous sutures ensures a better cosmetic appearance. Consideration should be given to making the new incision away from the scar of the previous operation when there is reason to suspect the presence of underlying attached intestine. However, reopening a previous incision may be appropriate if it is placed to ensure adequate exposure for the management of the anticipated diagnosis or if a postoperative hernia, which should be repaired, weakens it. It has been reported that an upper midline incision is more uncomfortable during the first 24 postoperative hours than a transverse incision.[2]

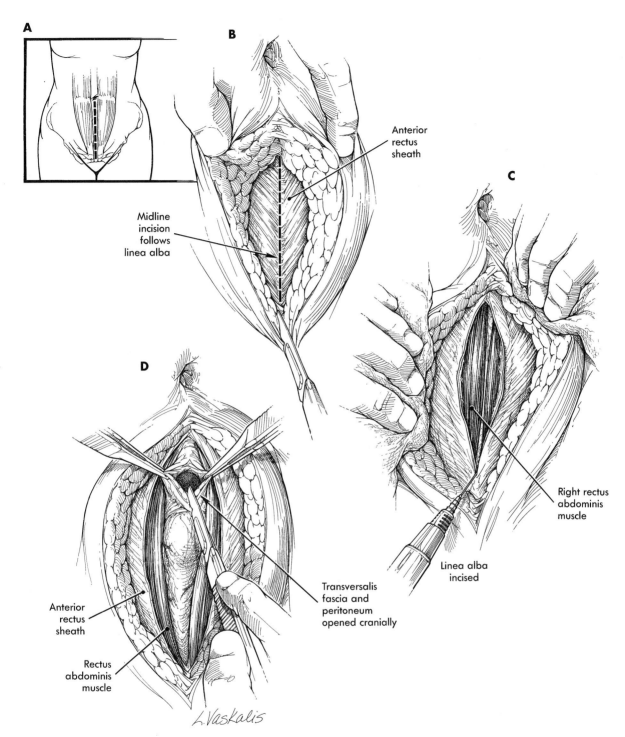

Fig. 13-10   The technique of a midline incision in the lower abdomen. **A,** Site of the incision between the umbilicus and pubis. **B,** The midline incision continues through the subcutaneous tissue to expose the linea alba of the anterior rectus sheath. **C,** This sheath is incised, and, **D,** the transversalis fascia and peritoneum are grasped between forceps and opened at the cranial end of the incision.   *Continued*

MIDLINE INCISION

Using a scalpel, the operator incises the skin exactly in the midline from a point below the umbilicus to a point just caudal to the upper margin of the symphysis pubis (Fig. 13-10, *A*). If the incision is ended earlier, the lateral retraction of the skin margins pull the lower end of the incision above

the pubis, limiting exposure. Making the incision quickly tends to put the smaller arteriolar blood vessels in spasm and therefore reduce blood loss during the procedure.[30]

After quickly incising the subcutaneous tissue, the operator identifies the linea alba in the midline between the rectus abdominis muscles (see Fig. 13-10, *B*) and incises it

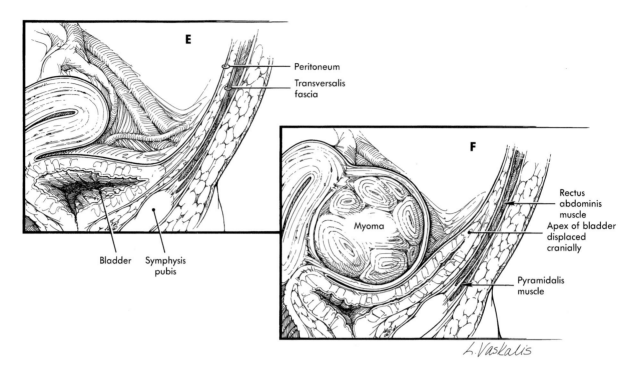

Fig. 13-10, cont'd **E,** The usual position of the apex of the bladder within the anterior abdominal wall extends just above the superior margin of the symphysis pubis. **F,** Not infrequently, and particularly when there is a leiomyoma in the anterior portion of the uterus, the apex of the bladder may be displaced cranially.

either with scissors or with the needlepoint tip of the electrosurgical scalpel (see Fig. 13-10, *C*). The underlying peritoneum is identified and picked up between two forceps at the cranial end of the incision to avoid any inadvertent penetration of the bladder (see Fig. 13-10, *D*). Usually, the dome of the bladder lies behind the pubis (see Fig. 13-10, *E*), but some intraabdominal pathologic conditions (e.g., a retropubic leiomyoma [see Figs. 13-10, *F,* and 13-11] or adhesion from previous surgery) occasionally displaces it cranially.

While small Richardson retractors hold the edges of the rectus muscles apart, the operator and the first assistant each insert an index finger into the peritoneal cavity to elevate the peritoneum so that it can be cut between the two fingers (see Fig. 13-10, *G*). The thickness of the layer can be estimated by transillumination against the overhead surgical spotlight, which outlines the upper pole of the bladder beneath the peritoneum. As the incision approaches the bladder, the number of blood vessels transacted increases, indicating the proximity of the bladder; great caution is essential to prevent accidental cystotomy.

Peritoneal washings are taken, if desired, and the abdomen is explored. A Bookwalter or Balfour self-retaining retractor is inserted. If the patient is unusually thin, the lateral margins of the retractor blades are padded to protect the underlying femoral nerve and lessen the risk of postoperative femoral neuropathy.

If necessary to provide adequate exposure, the incision may be extended cranially to the left of the umbilicus. Angling the incision in this direction makes it possible to avoid the right-sided ligamentum teres (see Fig. 13-10, *H*). The operator may stitch the peritoneum to the cut edge of the incisional skin, if desired, to improve exposure or limit subcutaneous inoculation by bacteria from the pelvis, or may sew wound towels in place to protect the exposed subcutaneous tissue.

At the completion of the procedure, the operator may close the incision in the older, traditional fashion: (1) closing the peritoneum and transversalis fascia with a running absorbable suture, although the need for separate peritoneal closure has been questioned for over 100 years[36] (Recently, surgeons have concluded that a separate closure offers no advantage and some disadvantages.*), (2) closing the fascia with interrupted synthetic absorbable suture (see Fig. 13-10, *I*), and (3) approximating the skin with a running subcuticular suture, staples, or running or interrupted silk mattress sutures. With the current trend toward reduced length of postoperative hospital stay, as well as the inconvenience of removing staples and skin sutures from an incompletely healed incisional wound, it has been found that less postoperative discomfort and a more appealing cosmetic result occur when the skin incision is closed with a 4-0 subcuticular polyglycolic acid suture, which of course need not be removed. Subcutaneous tissues are not regularly approximated by a separate suture layer because the blood supply of this fatty layer is so poor that suture material may induce necrosis and postoperative subcutaneous infection.

Generally speaking, an old abdominal scar should be excised to provide a fresh area of vital tissue during postoperative wound healing, except possibly when there is reason

---

*References 17, 19, 24, 32, 52, 68.

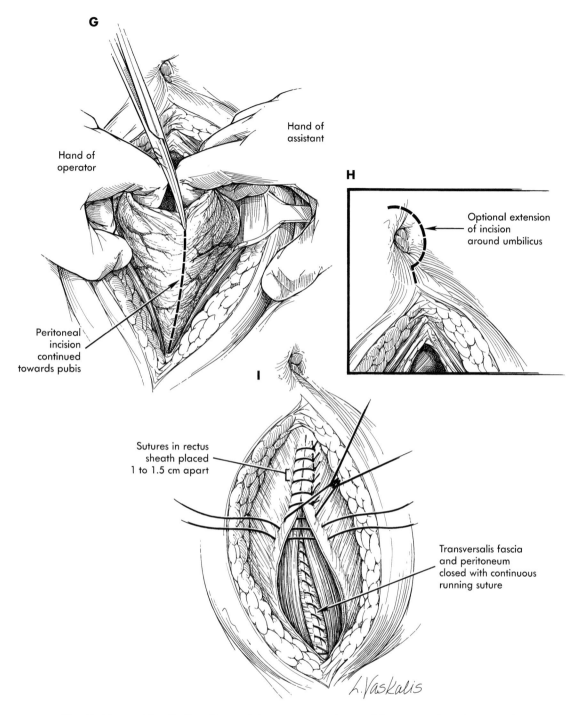

G

Hand of
operator

Hand of
assistant

H

Optional extension
of incision
around umbilicus

Peritoneal
incision
continued
towards pubis

I

Sutures in rectus
sheath placed
1 to 1.5 cm apart

Transversalis fascia
and peritoneum
closed with continuous
running suture

L. Vaskalis

Fig. 13-10, cont'd   G, One finger of the operator and one of the operator's assistant are inserted into the peritoneal cavity, and the incision is carried downward toward the pubis. Transillumination of this flap by looking through its peritoneal side discloses the outline of the apex of the bladder, marking the caudal limit of the pubic peritoneal dissection **(H).** When it is necessary to obtain additional exposure to extend the midline incision cranially, it should be performed around the left side of the umbilicus to avoid the ligamentum teres. **I,** The transversalis fascia and peritoneum may be closed by a continuous suture at the option of the surgeon, and the rectus aponeurosis may be closed by interrupted or running sutures placed 1 to 1.5 cm apart, and 1 to 1.5 cm away from the fascial margin. Stitches are not usually placed in the subcutaneous tissues, and the skin is closed by clips or a running subcuticular suture.

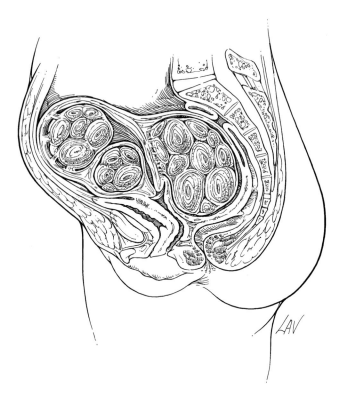

Fig. 13-11   Sagittal section through the pelvis of a patient with multiple myomata. Note the ascent of the bladder fundus onto the anterior abdominal wall, where it must be specifically identified by careful dissection when an incision is made for abdominal hysterectomy.

to suspect that intestine is adherent to the undersurface of an old incision.

It is important to place the stitches in the fascia at least 1 to 1.5 cm lateral to the cut edge of the incision and at least 1 or 1.5 cm distant from one another to reduce the risk of devascularization and necrosis from suture pressure. If the operator decides to use interrupted sutures in the deep musculofascial layer, a Smead-Jones deep-deep-shallow-shallow configuration or a modified deep-shallow-shallow-deep configuration that involves fascia, muscle, and peritoneum may be appropriate (Fig. 13-12).

Alternatively, the operator may close the incision by a single buried through-and-through layer of long-lasting monofilament polyglycolic acid–type suture material[22,31] or a synthetic monofilament permanent suture (Fig. 13-13). The one-layer closure of the deeper tissues makes a special effort to close the parietal peritoneum unnecessary,[17,20] although some surgeons prefer to close this peritoneum. The synthetic nonabsorbable, but slightly elastic, tissue suture polybutester (Novafil) can be used to great advantage in this one-layer full-thickness closure.[53,54] Its capacity to stretch between 10% and 15% postoperatively accommodates wound swelling and edema, yet its inherent elasticity takes up the slack as the swelling and edema subside. As a result, the tension in the tissues in which the suture has been placed remains more constant, theoretically reducing the risk of devascularization, necrosis, and subsequent incisional hernia. In placing these stitches, the operator may find it useful with better exposure to start suturing at each end of the

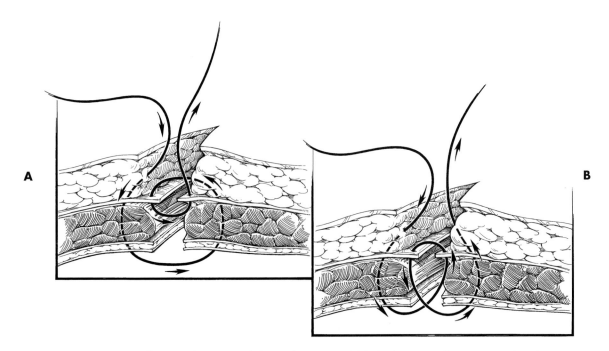

Fig. 13-12   The Smead-Jones single layer closure, in which the interrupted sutures are placed through the full thickness of the rectus fascia, muscle, and peritoneum in a deep-deep-shallow-shallow configuration as shown in **A.** An alternative deep-shallow-shallow-deep placement is illustrated in **B.**

wound and have the stitches ultimately meet in the middle of the incision. These sutures, which may include fascia and muscle, are snugly placed but not so tightly as to devascularize the tissues in which they are located.

Upward extension of a lower abdominal midline incision may be either transumbilical, which unless performed on a patient with a shallow umbilicus may be difficult to repair, or periumbilical, which is simple to close.[16] The technique of Denehy et al. involves grasping the skin at the most lateral aspect of the umbilicus with an Allis clamp and retracting it medially. The straight incision is continued to the rectus fascia, taking care not to perforate the umbilicus. The Allis clamp is removed, and the resultant symmetric, curvilinear incision is nonbeveled and easy to close.

PARAMEDIAN INCISION

Like the midline incision, the paramedian incision avoids the nerve supply of the rectus muscles that enter from the lateral side. Although the paramedian incision transects more blood vessels, it heals well.[26] Should it someday be necessary to reenter the abdomen of a patient who has had a paramedian incision, the surgeon should not make a midline or contralateral paramedian incision, because these incisions may interfere with the blood supply of the tissue being incised and risk wound hernia. The surgeon who reenters a previous paramedian incision will find that the muscle is adherent to its sheath and must be split rather than dissected free.

A paramedian incision involves making a vertical incision through the skin and subcutaneous tissue 1 inch lateral to the midline (Fig. 13-14, *A*). The rectus sheath is in-

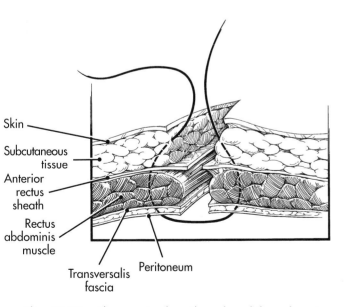

Skin
Subcutaneous tissue
Anterior rectus sheath
Rectus abdominis muscle
Transversalis fascia
Peritoneum

Fig. 13-13 Placement of a through-and-through suture through the rectus fascia, muscle, and transversalis fascia and peritoneum. The sutures are placed 1.5 cm lateral to the fascial incision, and 1.5 cm apart. Inclusion of the peritoneum and transversalis fascia, as shown, is optional. This suture can be of interrupted stitches or over-end-over technique, according to the surgeon's preference.

cised 1 inch lateral to the midline (see Fig. 13-14, *B*). The operator reflects the medial flap of the rectus sheath from the muscle and retracts the muscle laterally, separating it from the midline (see Fig. 13-14, *C*). Then the operator incises the transversalis fascia and peritoneum beneath the muscle 1 inch lateral to the midline (see Fig. 13-14, *D*).

The pararectus incision, in which the muscle is retracted medially, is not regularly used because of damage to the nerve supply of the muscle that enters from its lateral border. For the same reason, a transrectus incision is not recommended.

TRANSVERSE INCISIONS

Because they are made in the direction of Langer's lines, transverse incisions produce cosmetically more attractive scars. Wound herniation is rare after transverse incisions, and the incisions seldom cause any permanent damage to the strategic nerve or blood supply of the musculature of the anterior abdominal wall.[9]

Pfannenstiel's Incision

The principal disadvantage of Pfannenstiel's incision is that exposure is limited when compared with the midline or Maylard incision and is not useful when upper abdominal exposure may be anticipated. Similarly, because it opens more tissue planes at a larger exposed surface area of subcutaneous tissue, it should not be used if infection or abscess formation is present, since any infectious condition may inoculate the subcutaneous tissue and invite wound abscess. Because Pfannenstiel's incision takes longer to make, it is contraindicated when speed is necessary. If, after Pfannenstiel's incision has been made, it becomes clear that better operative exposure is required, the incision can be converted to a Cherney incision.

Turner-Warwick[63-66] developed a "supra-pubic-cross" incision that enabled him to repair the great majority of abdominal approach fistulas through the original horizontal Pfannenstiel's skin incision. The upper and lower skin flaps were appropriately mobilized to allow a midline abdominal wall incision to be made up to the level of the umbilicus, leaving the original horizontal Pfannenstiel's rectus sheath closure intact. For the same reason, a transrectus incision is not recommended.

In performing Pfannenstiel's incision,[49] the operator places a transverse incision, convex curve downward, in the skinfold two fingerbreadths above the upper margin of the symphysis pubis and carries it through skin and subcutaneous tissue to the rectus sheath (Fig. 13-15, *A*). Incising the sheath transversely over the belly of each rectus muscle, the operator continues laterally beyond the lateral margins of the rectus muscle and the medial borders of the external and internal oblique muscles. The two incisions in the rectus fascia join in the middle (see Fig. 13-15, *B*). A Kocher clamp is placed on each side, and, with traction applied anteriorly, the rectus aponeurosis is separated from the underlying rectus muscle by sharp and blunt dissection. Usually, the

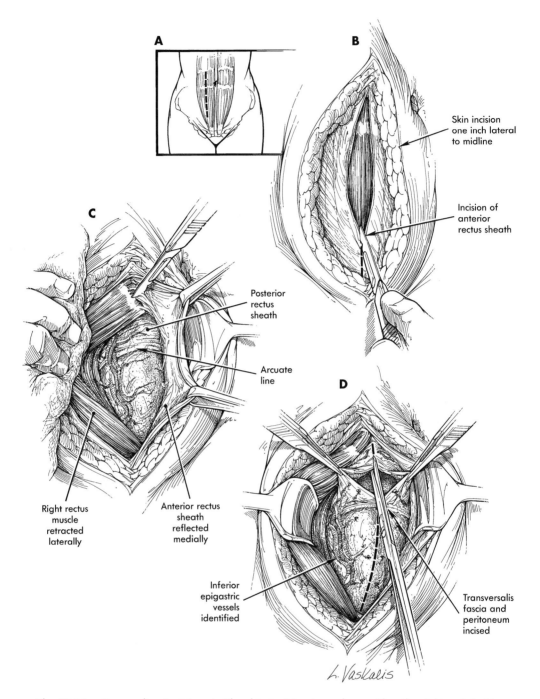

Fig. 13-14   Paramedian incision. **A,** The skin incision is made on either the right or left side of the abdomen along the path of the dashed line, 1 inch lateral to the midline. The anterior rectus sheath is incised over the midportion of the underlying rectus muscle **(B),** and retracted laterally, while the anterior rectus sheath is reflected medially **(C). D,** The posterior rectus sheath, transversalis fascia, and peritoneum are incised in the bed temporarily vacated by the muscle.

pyramidalis remains firmly attached to the underside of the aponeurosis (see Fig. 13-15, *C*). At this point, the operator removes the Kocher clamps from their original placement, applies them to the upper cut edge of fascia, and similarly dissects the fascia from the muscle far enough to permit a midline incision of adequate length through the parietal peritoneum at the cranial end of the exposure (see Fig. 13-15, *D*). Picking up the peritoneum between two he-

mostats, the operator opens it in the midline (see Fig. 13-15, *E* and *F*). The incision is extended cranially, between the operator's fingers. Caudal transillumination of the thickness of the peritoneal flap will avoid penetration of the fundus of the attached bladder.

In closing Pfannenstiel's incision, it appears to make little difference whether the parietal peritoneum is closed or not. The operator can bring the central bellies of the rectus

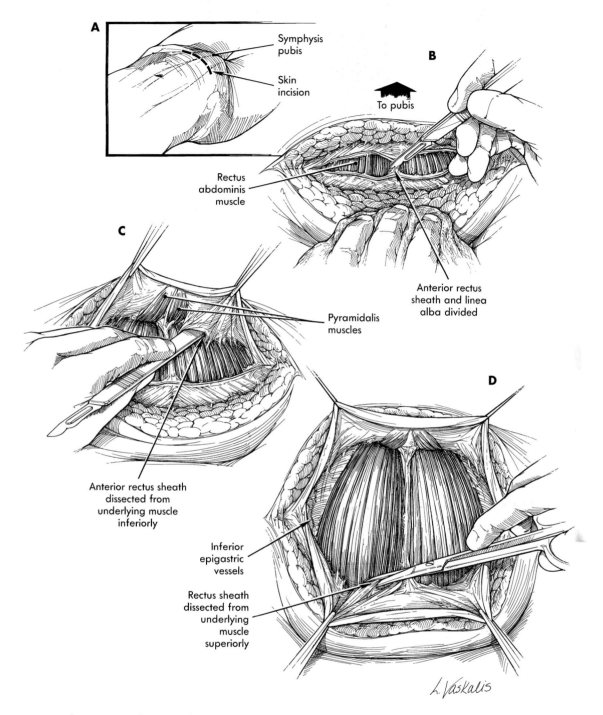

Fig. 13-15 Pfannenstiel's incision. **A,** A transverse elliptical skin incision is made in the suprapubic area. **B,** Subcutaneous tissue is incised, exposing the anterior rectus sheath, which is incised exposing the underlying rectus abdominis muscle. The anterior sheath is separated from the muscle by sharp and blunt dissection **(C),** first in the caudal portion of the incision and then beneath the cranial portion of the anterior rectus sheath **(D).**

Continued

muscles together with a few loosely tied interrupted sutures of polyglycolic acid if any diastasis is present[51] (see Fig. 13-15, *G*) and can close the transverse fascial incision with a 2-0 or 1-0 synthetic absorbable suture (polyglycolic acid–type). Subcutaneous tissues are not approximated, and the skin is closed with either staples (see Fig. 13-15, *H*), which

are left in place for 5 postoperative days, or a subcuticular closure with 4-0 undyed polyglycolic acid–type sutures. The latter is particularly useful if the patient must be discharged before the fifth postoperative day.[23,55]

For the patient in whom a minimally visible, cosmetically attractive skin incision is essential, the surgeon may

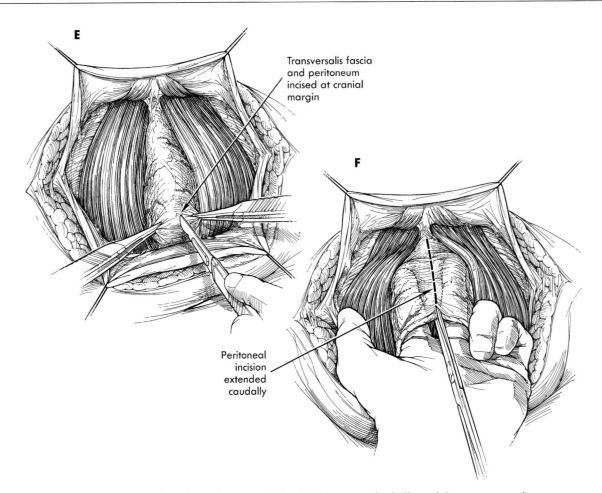

Transversalis fascia
and peritoneum
incised at cranial
margin

Peritoneal
incision
extended
caudally

Fig. 13-15, cont'd   The peritoneum is identified between the bellies of the rectus muscles, and the transversalis fascia and peritoneum are grasped with forceps and incised in the midline at the cranial margin of the exposure **(E). F,** The operator's fingertips are inserted caudally beneath the peritoneum, and the incision is extended downward between the operator's fingers, with care being taken to recognize and avoid the cranial margin of the apex of the bladder at the inferior pole of the incision. At the completion of surgery, closing the parietal peritoneum and transversalis fascia is optional.

elect the "low" Pfannenstiel's incision. Here, the transverse skin incision is made a fingerbreadth below the pubic hairline, and the abdominal wall and subcutaneous tissue are dissected cranially from the rectus fascia, which can then be opened transversely in classic Pfannenstiel fashion (Fig. 13-16).

Küstner's incision[34,35] is not often recommended. It differs from Pfannenstiel's incision in that the skin and subcutaneous tissue are dissected from the anterior rectus sheath, which is then opened in the midline, but does not reduce the risk of postoperative wound herniation. Küstner's incision can be considered in a patient who has had a previous Pfannenstiel's incision when, for cosmetic appearance of the skin of the lower abdomen, reoperation requiring the greater exposure made possible by a midline incision is required, as suggested by Turner-Warwick. If, after Pfannenstiel's incision has been made, it becomes clear that better operative exposure is required, the incision can be converted to a Cherney incision.

One should not convert a Pfannenstiel's incision to a Maylard incision. With Pfannenstiel's incision the anterior surface of the rectus muscle has been dissected from the undersurface of the rectus fascia, and after a secondary Maylard muscle transection, the cut ends of the muscle no longer come together with simple reapproximation of the rectus fascial layer. For this reason, converting an inadequately exposing Pfannenstiel's incision to a Cherney incision is a better choice, because healing after the Cherney does not require that the muscle be firmly adherent to the underside of the rectus fascia.[62]

Cherney Incision

In 1940, Cherney[10] described a transverse incision in the fold above the pubis. The tendons of the rectus abdominis muscles, provided that they are well developed, are bluntly dissected from the underlying bladder and vesicouterine fold of the peritoneum and transacted near their insertion on the pubic symphysis (Fig. 13-17, *A*). When the tendons have been reflected cranially, the transversalis fascia and peritoneum can be incised transversely beneath them (see

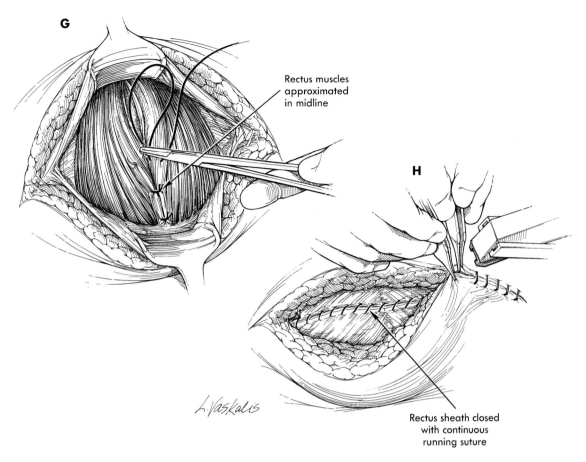

Fig. 13-15, cont'd   G, The rectus muscles are approximated by a series of loosely tied interrupted stitches to relieve any diastasis. **H,** The rectus aponeurosis is closed with a continuous running suture, and the skin incision is closed with staples or a subcuticular suture.

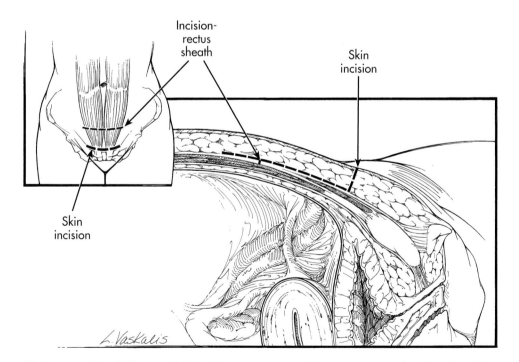

Fig. 13-16   "Low" Pfannenstiel's incision. A transverse skin incision is made a fingerbreadth beneath the upper border of the pubic hairline, and the skin and subcutaneous tissue are dissected from the anterior rectus aponeurosis, as shown in the path of the broken line and reflected cranially. A transverse incision in the rectus sheath is made at a more cranial level as shown.

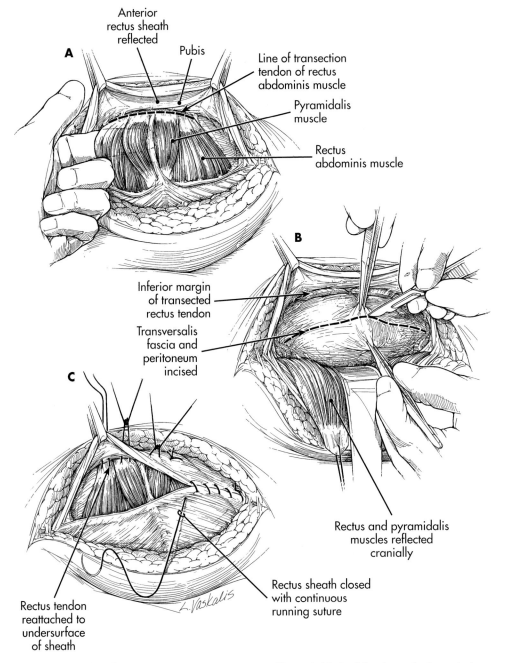

Fig. 13-17 The Cherney incision. **A,** A transverse elliptical skin incision is made through the skin and subcutaneous tissue. The tendon of the rectus abdominis muscle and pyramidalis is transected on each side, as shown by the broken line. **B,** The muscles are reflected cranially, and the peritoneum and transversalis fascia are picked up between forceps and incised transversely. **C,** At the conclusion of surgery, the tendon of the rectus muscle is attached to the undersurface of the rectus sheath by several interrupted stitches, and the original incision in the rectus aponeurosis is closed with a continuous running suture. The skin incision is closed with staples or a subcuticular closure.

Fig. 13-17, *B*). The Cherney incision requires less time to perform than the Maylard and does not require drainage because there is no bleeding from the transected tendon. Poor development of the tendon, however, contraindicates this incision.[8]

At the conclusion of the operation, the surgeon carefully reattaches the transacted ends of the tendinous sheath to the undersurface of the rectus sheath and pubic periosteum with interrupted sutures and closes the transverse incision in the rectus aponeurosis with a running suture similar to that used in a Pfannenstiel's closure (see Fig. 13-17, *C*). The Cherney incision supplies better exposure than does Pfannenstiel's incision, and it is particularly useful when some of the surgery must be performed in the space of Retzius.

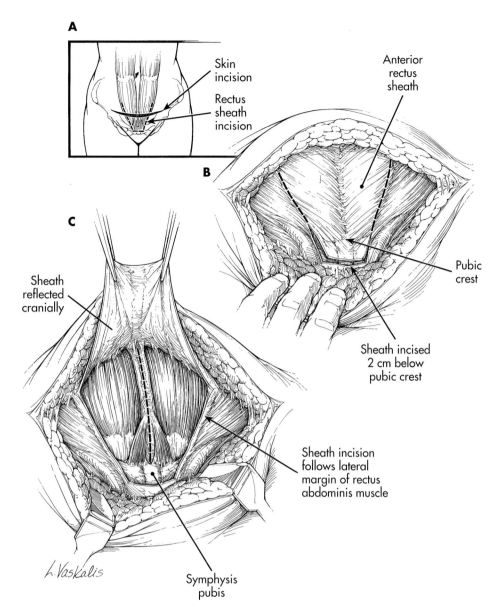

Fig. 13-18 The suprapubic "V" incision. **A,** Excellent exposure of the space of Retzius is provided when a transverse skin incision is made just above the pubic hairline. **B,** The skin and subcutaneous tissues are dissected from the anterior rectus sheath, which is incised 2 cm below the pubic crest and along the path of the broken line. **C,** The rectus sheath is reflected cranially, and the transversalis fascia and peritoneum are incised in the midline, as shown by the broken line.

V-Shaped Incision

Turner-Warwick[66] described a V-shaped 4 cm horizontal incision in the rectus sheath 2 cm *below* the upper margin of the pubis (Fig. 13-18, *A* and *B*). The operator angles this V-shaped incision sharply upward so that the edges of the consequent flap remain within the lateral margins of the rectus muscle. The rectus sheath is reflected cranially, and the abdomen is opened in the midline between the rectus muscles (see Fig. 13-18, *C*). Because there is no distal rectus sheath margin to retract, the exposure of the retropubic space is unusually good.

For the patient who is concerned with the cosmetic appearance of the scar, the surgeon can make the initial skin incision as if it were to be a low Pfannenstiel's modification. The lateral extension of the rectus sheath incision without transaction of the rectus muscle provides additional operative exposure, if necessary.

Mackenrodt-Maylard Incision

In 1901, Mackenrodt[41] developed the transverse muscle-cutting abdominal incision that Maylard[44] modified in 1907 by restricting it to the area below the umbilicus. Because the incision is transverse, it does not disturb the innervation of the abdominal musculature. Furthermore, because the tension from the lateral abdominal muscles is parallel to the line of incision, there is no unusual tension on the suture line. It provides excellent exposure of the pelvis, but not of the upper abdomen. The incidence of postoperative incisional hernia is increased in the patient with chronic respiratory disease. The transverse Maylard incision, which is similar to the elliptical transverse incision of Bardenheuer,[6] is a better choice for such a patient than is the midline incision because the resultant incisional scar will be stronger.

Beginning approximately 2 inches above the upper border of the symphysis pubis and using a scalpel,[25] the operator makes a suprapubic transverse skin incision down to the anterior rectus sheath, incises the sheath transversely over the belly of each rectus muscle, unites the two incisions in the rectus sheath (Fig. 13-19, A and B), and cuts across the muscle bellies of each rectus abdominis muscle with an electrosurgical scalpel[12,13] (see Fig. 13-19, C). If the patient has any obstruction of the common iliac vessels, the direction of blood flow in the inferior epigastric arteries may be cranial instead of caudal. In such a circumstance, ligation of these vessels could interfere with the circulation to the patient's legs.[33] To obviate this misfortune, the operator should make certain to palpate the dorsalis pedis artery and determine the direction of blood flow before clamping and

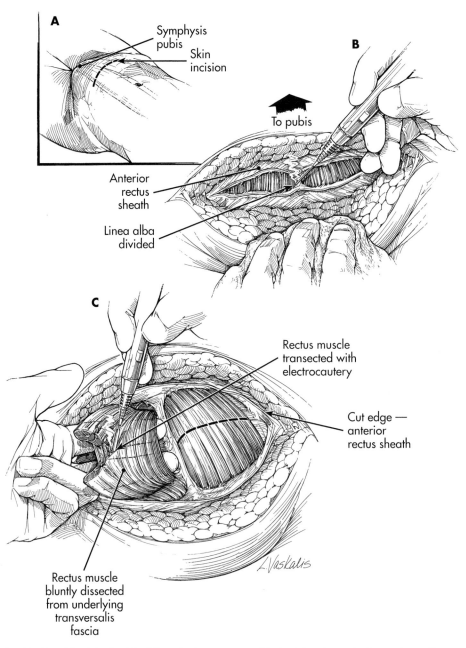

Fig. 13-19   The Maylard incision. **A,** A transverse skin incision is made 5 cm above the superior border of the pubis. **B,** The anterior rectus sheath is incised in the same line, exposing the bellies of the rectus abdominis muscles. The muscle is bluntly dissected from the underlying transversalis fascia and incised transversely on each side, along the path of the broken side, using an electrosurgical scalpel **(C).**

cutting the epigastric vessels. Any blood vessels encountered are clamped and tied. As there is no sheath at this level, the operator attaches the transected muscle by interrupted mattress stitches to the rectus sheath at the upper margin of the incision to keep the transected muscle from retracting beneath the incision (see Fig. 13-19, *D*). Then, picking up the peritoneum, the operator incises it transversely. If additional exposure is necessary, the operator identifies, clamps, cuts, and ligates the inferior epigastric vessels (see Fig. 13-19, *E*).

In closure, because of the raw surfaces offered by the transected bellies of the rectus muscles, the parietal peritoneum beneath them should be closed as a separate layer (see Fig. 13-19, *F*). The possibility of oozing from the transected

rectus muscles under the fascia makes it necessary to place a subfascial 10-mm flat Jackson-Pratt drain (see Fig. 13-19, *G*). Making traction that the mattress sutures previously placed through the muscle and fascia of the upper wound, the operator places an additional mattress stitch from upper fascia through upper muscle, lower muscle, and lower fascial edge on one side and the same structures in reverse order on the opposite side. Finally, the operator closes the fascial layers with either interrupted or continuous sutures of 1-0 synthetic material and the skin with either running subcuticular sutures of 3-0 or 4-0 polyglycolic acid–type material (see Fig. 13-19, *H*), or staples. If a nonabsorbable monofilament suture is chosen, polybutester (Novafil) has been

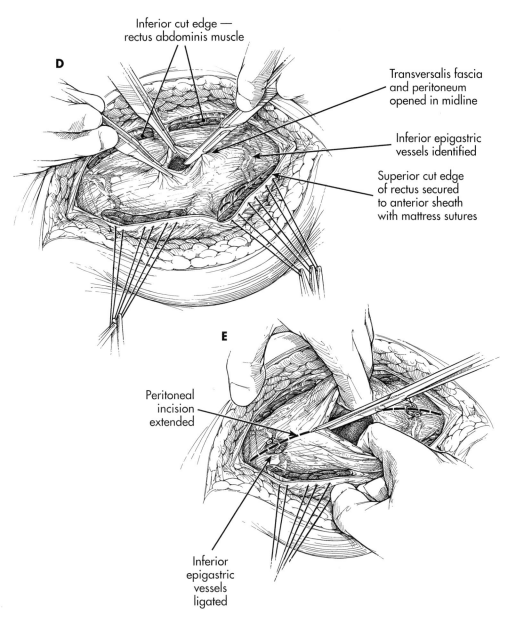

Fig. 13-19, cont'd   D, The transversalis fascia and peritoneum are opened, and the superior cut edge of the rectus abdominis is secured to the anterior sheath with mattress sutures. **E,** The peritoneal incision is extended laterally, and the inferior epigastric vessels must usually be ligated and cut.

Continued

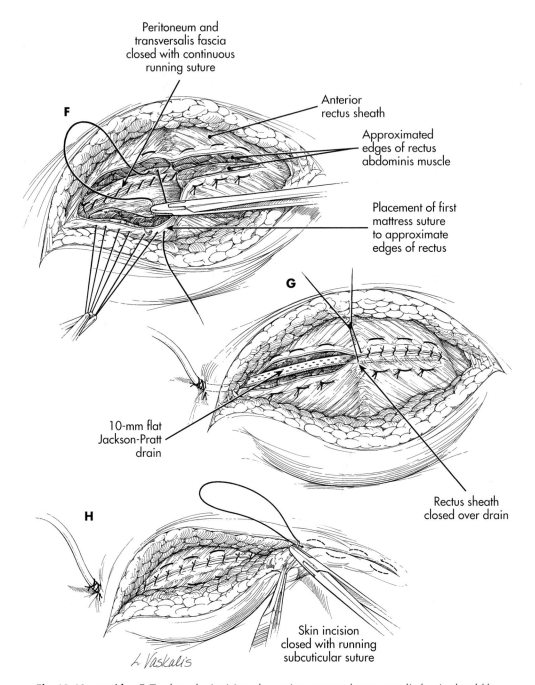

Peritoneum and
transversalis fascia
closed with continuous
running suture

Anterior
rectus sheath

Approximated
edges of rectus
abdominis muscle

Placement of first
mattress suture
to approximate
edges of rectus

10-mm flat
Jackson-Pratt
drain

Rectus sheath
closed over drain

Skin incision
closed with running
subcuticular suture

L. Vaskalis

Fig. 13-19, cont'd   F, To close the incision, the peritoneum and transversalis fascia should be approximated with a continuous running suture, and the gap between the edges of fascia and muscle is approximated by a series of mattress stitches placed as shown. **G,** A Jackson-Pratt drain is placed beneath the fascial edges, and the rectus sheath is closed with interrupted sutures. The skin incision is closed with either a running subcuticular suture (**H**) or staples.

reported to be superior to polypropylene (Prolene) in handling characteristics and in providing a cosmetically better-looking scar.[5,43]

Muscle-Splitting Incisions

The gridiron incision is used primarily for uncomplicated appendectomy, although it can be used to drain a large pelvic or abdominal abscess that does not point into the cul-de-sac or anterior wall of the rectum.[28] The operator first makes

an incision over McBurney's point to expose the aponeurosis of the external oblique muscle, incises the muscle parallel to its fibers, and retracts it (Fig. 13-20, *A* and *B*). The fibers of the internal oblique and transversalis muscles run perpendicular to the incision, and the operator divides these muscles along their axis (see Fig. 13-20, *C*). This exposes the transversalis fascia and peritoneum, which are incised (see Fig. 13-20, *D*). After completing the surgical procedure required, the operator closes the incision in layers.

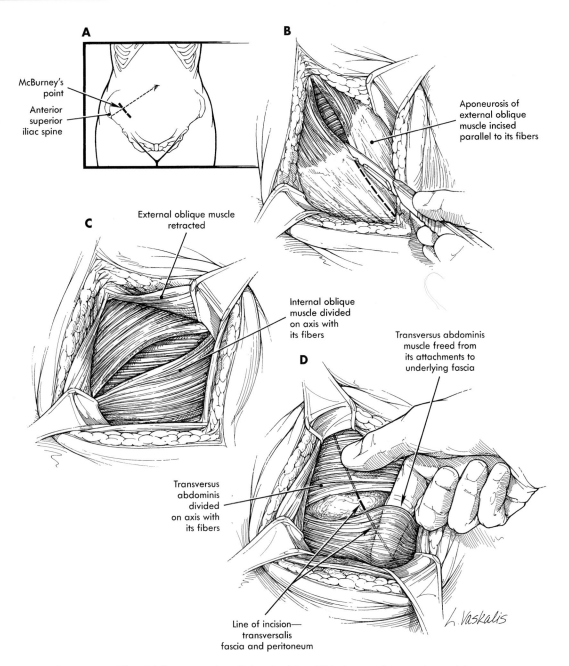

A

McBurney's point

Anterior superior iliac spine

B

Aponeurosis of external oblique muscle incised parallel to its fibers

C

External oblique muscle retracted

Internal oblique muscle divided on axis with its fibers

Transversus abdominis muscle freed from its attachments to underlying fascia

D

Transversus abdominis divided on axis with its fibers

Line of incision— transversalis fascia and peritoneum

L. Vaskalis

Fig. 13-20   The Gridiron muscle-splitting incision. This is most frequently used for appendectomy or for drainage of a pelvic abscess that is pointed to the inguinal area. McBurney's point for locating the appendix is noted by the dashed line in **A,** which intersects a line between the umbilicus and the anterior superior iliac spine, as shown by the dotted line. The skin incision is made along the path of the dashed line. The subcutaneous tissue is incised similarly, and the aponeurosis of the external oblique muscle is incised parallel to its fibers **(B).** The external oblique muscle is retracted, exposing the underlying internal oblique muscle, which is divided on an axis parallel with its fibers **(C).** This, in turn, exposes the underlying transversus abdominis, which is divided on an axis in the direction of its fibers, and the muscle is freed from its attachments to the underlying transversalis fascia and peritoneum, as shown in **D.** The muscle is retracted, exposing the underlying peritoneum, which is incised along the site of the dashed line in **D.**

MANAGEMENT OF OBESE PATIENTS

Abdominal incisions in an obese patient generally need drainage. As mentioned earlier, a Maylard incision generally requires the placement of a subfascial drain, which prevents the development of a hematoma from the cut edge of the rectus muscle. An obese patient who has had a midline incision needs a subcutaneous, self-contained suction apparatus to inhibit the development of a postoperative seroma to which she is predisposed because of the larger subcutaneous surface area.

Morrow et al.[47] pointed out the dangers of making a transverse incision under the panniculus. They demonstrated that better exposure can be obtained by a midline vertical incision, providing the panniculus is drawn downward below the superior margin of pubis, which can be palpated as the incision is made. This avoids buttonholing the skin beneath the panniculus. Shepherd et al.[57] demonstrated the strength of a continuous one-layer closure for midline incisions using a nonabsorbable single-layer technique.

Gallup et al.[23] emphasize the importance of subcutaneous drainage by a closed system for the first 72 hours postoperatively or until the drainage is less than 50 ml for 24 hours.

Subcutaneous tissue of a markedly obese patient should be drained by a self-contained suction apparatus (Jackson-Pratt, not a Penrose drain), which should be removed in about 72 hours.

In a very obese woman with a large pendulous panniculus, the operator may sometimes make an incision above the umbilicus, away from the panniculus, and use a Bookwalter retractor secured to the operating room table to displace the incision inferiorly and provide adequate exposure[25] (Fig. 13-21). Gallup[22] advocated making a midline incision in these patients, usually extended around the umbilicus rather than passed through it, closing the fascia with a nonabsorbable monofilament suture, and using a suprafascial closed drainage system.[21] The drain should remain in place for 72 hours or until the drainage is less than 50 ml during a 24-hour period. In obese patients, the skin staples should remain in place for 2 weeks postoperatively.[11] Although surgeons may be tempted to perform a panniculectomy on the disfigured woman, they seldom do so. This cosmetic addition to laparotomy not only may involve considerations of salvage, sacrifice, or physical relocation of the umbilicus, but also may result in considerable blood loss and a remarkably longer period of convalescence. In the multipara, the procedure often coincidentally stretches and weakens the fascia of the anterior abdominal wall and causes some significant diastases of the rectus muscle. Not uncommonly, there is an associated umbilical hernia. As alternatives to panniculectomy, rigid dietary discretion or liposuction can dissipate subcutaneous fat, but they may only accentuate a faulty appearance, which is the consequence of fascial weakness.

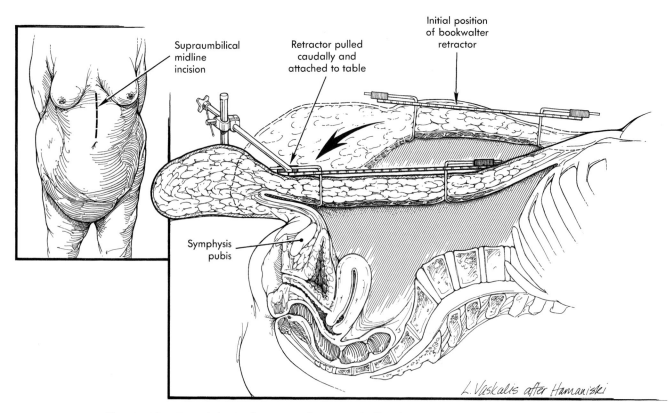

Fig. 13-21   Transabdominal incision for a morbidly obese patient. The panniculus is reflected downward, and a supraumbilical midline incision is shown along the path of the dashed line. The Bookwalter retractor is inserted into the peritoneal cavity as shown, displacing the panniculus caudally.

Panniculectomy

Coincident panniculectomy may provide better operative visualization in some patients and does favor improved patient satisfaction.[29,50] When the surgeon and patient have decided on a panniculectomy, the next decision necessary is whether to use a midline subumbilical skin incision or a transverse one; the former does not usually require umbilical relocation, but the latter generally does if the umbilicus is to be preserved (Fig. 13-22). Fascial "pants over vest" layering[51] reinforces the deeper weakness of the anterior abdominal wall (Fig. 13-23). Precise surgical hemostasis is essential; the residual subcutaneous fat layer must be dissected free of the underlying fascia, and the wound must be drained through a separate stab wound.

When a great deal of postoperative overdistention, coughing, or nausea and vomiting is anticipated, midline incisions can be supported temporarily by retention stitches. A maximum of strength can be given to the approximation of the fascial layers by sutures of monofilament nonabsorbable material placed lateral to the incision, through each side of the fascial incision, and brought back adjacent to the original incision (Fig. 13-24). Usually three sets can be placed on each side, and, at the conclusion of repair of the incision, they are tied against the bolster of a 4 × 4 rolled compress.

COINCIDENT HERNIA

When the abdominal cavity has been opened for surgery through an incision in the anterior abdominal wall, any symptomatic hernia of the abdominal wall or pelvis should be repaired before the abdomen is closed.[4] The repair of enterocele and prolapse of the vaginal vault are discussed in Chapters 23 and 26, respectively. The repair of umbilical hernia is discussed in Chapter 14. It is possible to repair inguinal and femoral hernias intraabdominally, if surgical exposure can be obtained at the site of weakness, by using an appropriate initial surgical incision. Techniques for intraabdominal indirect inguinal herniorrhaphy and intraabdominal femoral herniorrhaphy are shown in Fig. 13-25 (p. 222). A direct inguinal hernia also can be repaired intraabdominally. It represents a congenital defect or weakness at the medial edge at the line of origin of the transversalis and internal oblique muscles. The hernia is reduced and the sac inverted and excised in the same manner as the indirect hernia. The transversalis fascia and the edges of the transversalis and internal oblique muscles are sutured to the inguinal ligament or the superior pubic ligament, which is the extension of the inguinal ligament toward the symphysis. An unusually weak or difficult internal hernial orifice may be occluded by sewing a synthetic plastic patch in place beneath the peritoneal incision.

POSTOPERATIVE CARE

In the course of normal healing, the skin incision becomes watertight 48 hours after surgery. It is best kept dry during that initial period so that bacteria that can cause postoperative infection do not enter the incision. The patient can obtain the soothing effects of heat with a heat lamp or a blow-type hair dryer.

Ultrasound examination, if not clinical findings, can confirm postoperative incisional sepsis. The appropriate investigation of an abscess cavity includes incision, drainage, and culture of the cavity contents.[28] The incision, which communicates with the abscess cavity, can be packed open, and the skin incision can be loosely closed by a series of interrupted sutures placed approximately 4 inches apart. Between these stitches, some additional sutures can be placed approximately 1 inch apart, but not tied. The wound will heal more rapidly if the operator waits until the purulence of the abscess has subsided and a layer of healthy granulation tissue has covered the base of the raw wound, usually about 4 days, before tying these sutures.

The entrapment of the iliohypogastric nerve during the closure of Pfannenstiel's incision can give rise to a most disabling postoperative pain that runs from the incisional site down into the labia or inner aspect of the thigh. Occasionally, a neuroma is palpable, or reexploration of the wound reveals the nerve trapped within the scar; if so, the surgeon excises the nerve and ligates the ends.[59] This injury is more likely to occur when the transverse fascial incision extends beyond the lateral edge of the rectus sheath into the substance of the internal oblique muscle or when the sutures at the corners of this fascial incision are so widely placed that they incorporate branches of the nerve in the closure.

In consideration of nerve entrapment after Pfannenstiel's incision, Sippo[58] has found in his patients that the right side is most often involved and occasionally more than one nerve is involved. When the iliohypogastric nerve is entrapped, pain management may require an ilioinguinal or iliohypogastric nerve block established by infiltrating the tissue with 10 ml of a 2:1 mixture of 0.5% bupivacaine (Marcaine) and 1% lidocaine (Xylocaine) without epinephrine. The operator inserts the tip of a 3-inch 25-gauge spinal needle beneath the external oblique aponeurosis at a point 1 inch medial and 1 inch inferior to the anterior superior iliac spine, advances the needle toward the pubic tubercle, and injects the solution with steady, even pressure. Without removing the needle, the operator redirects it in a fan-shaped fashion to inject the solution in increments, making the last deposition almost perpendicular to the midline. The surgeon can repeat the injection weekly two or three times; if symptoms recur after a third injection, however, surgical exploration of the wound may be necessary.

If the patient is taking corticosteroids, the daily administration of 50,000 U of vitamin A postoperatively decreases the risk of premature suture absorption. Dermal injury apparently stimulates the elaboration of collagenase, which is hostile to the development of a strong scar. The daily postoperative administration of 500 mg of vitamin C, at least theoretically, can inhibit this collagenase elaboration. Most patients are willing to continue taking vitamin C for 2 or 3 months postoperatively.

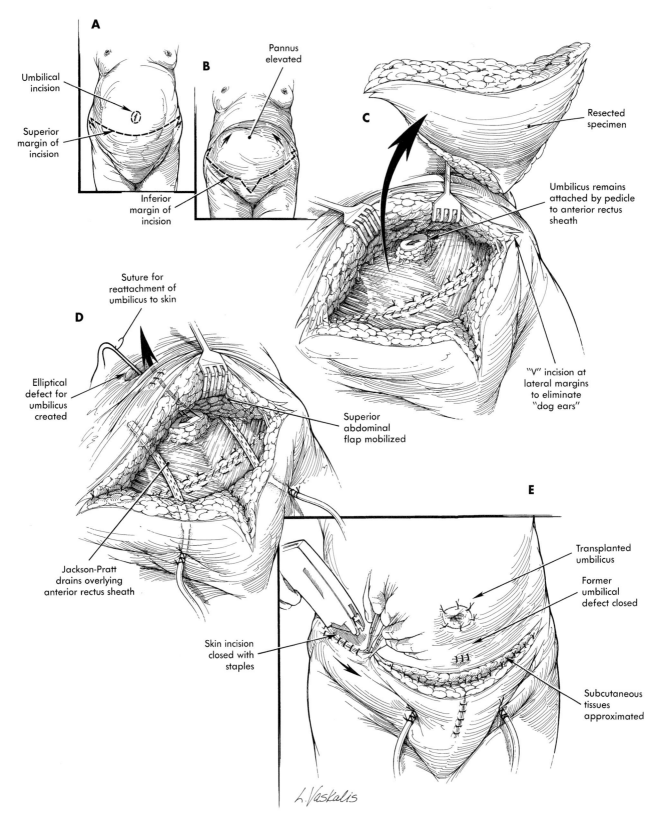

A, Umbilical incision

Superior margin of incision

Inferior margin of incision

B, Pannus elevated

C, Resected specimen

Umbilicus remains attached by pedicle to anterior rectus sheath

"V" incision at lateral margins to eliminate "dog ears"

D, Suture for reattachment of umbilicus to skin

Elliptical defect for umbilicus created

Superior abdominal flap mobilized

Jackson-Pratt drains overlying anterior rectus sheath

E, Transplanted umbilicus

Former umbilical defect closed

Subcutaneous tissues approximated

Skin incision closed with staples

L. Vaskalis

Fig. 13-22 Panniculectomy performed using a transverse elliptical incision. **A,** The skin and subcutaneous tissues are incised along the path of the dashed line, and an incision is made around the umbilicus as shown. **B,** The pannus is elevated, and the inferior margin of the incision is made as shown, with a V-shaped extension in the center. **C,** The specimen is removed, and V incisions to eliminate "dog ears" are made at the lateral margins of the incision. **D,** Hemostasis is obtained, an elliptical incision is made for reimplantation of the umbilicus, subcutaneous drains are placed on each side, and closure of the skin incision is begun. **E,** The umbilicus is fixed in its new position by some interrupted sutures, the former umbilical defect is closed, and the skin incision is closed with staples.

SCHUCHARDT'S PERINEAL INCISION

Schuchardt's incision—a deep incision through the skin of the vulva, vagina, and perineum—markedly increases the surgical access to the vaginal vault when it has been compromised. The tissue in this area is intensely vascular, but a preliminary infiltration of the site by bupivacaine (Marcaine) or lidocaine (Xylocaine), 0.5% in 1:200,000 epinephrine solution, suppresses the blood loss (Fig. 13-26). This "liquid tourniquet" is not a substitute for surgical hemostasis, but a complement to it. Although the transected blood vessels still bleed, they do not bleed as much, and the operator can readily grasp and tie or coagulate them with the electrosurgical unit.

Schuchardt's incision is unilateral. If the patient's left side is to be the site of the incision, the operator should begin at approximately the 4-o'clock position on the hymenal ring. The perineal skin incision is made on a line from the 4-o'clock position on the vulva to a point midway between the anus and the left ischial tuberosity. To increase exposure, the right-handed operator may insert the index finger of the left hand into the wound, establishing traction to the patient's right, while the first assistant may use an index finger to establish countertraction to the patient's left; this maneuver effectively stretches the tissues to be incised (Fig. 13-27, A, p. 224). The vaginal incision is made similarly in the 4-o'clock position (see Fig. 13-27, B). The levator ani often appears in the depths of the wound. The distal portion of the levator may be incised to aid in the exposure of the vaginal vault.

Using a series of temporary interrupted sutures, the operator can sew a sterile towel or sponge to the upper cut edge of the incision to isolate the raw surfaces of the incision temporarily from the remaining surgery (see Fig. 13-27, C). At the conclusion of the intended surgery, the

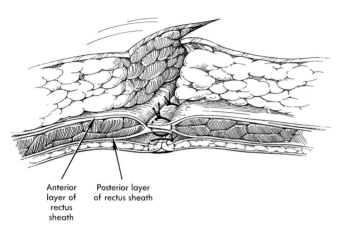

Anterior layer of rectus sheath   Posterior layer of rectus sheath

Fig. 13-23 When there is marked diastases between the rectus muscles, they may be brought closer together and the incision can be made stronger by a "pants-over-vest" closure using interrupted stitches as shown. It is optional whether the peritoneum should be closed.

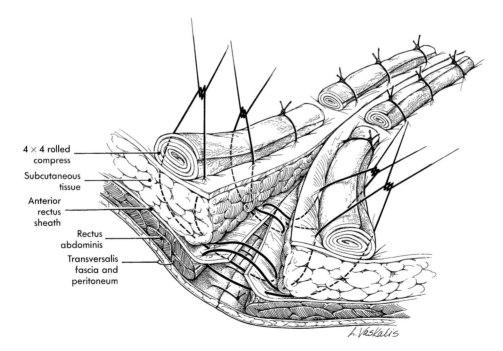

4 × 4 rolled compress
Subcutaneous tissue
Anterior rectus sheath
Rectus abdominis
Transversalis fascia and peritoneum

L. Vaskalis

Fig. 13-24 Retention sutures. Anticipated excess of postoperative overdistention, coughing, or vomiting may put additional strain on a midline incision, and retention stitches may give additional support. A maximum of this strength can be given to the approximation of the fascial layers by placing monofilament nonabsorbable sutures lateral to the incision, through each side of the fascial incision, and brought back adjacent to the original incision, as shown. Usually, three sets can be placed on each side. After the fascia and skin incisions have been separately repaired, these retention sutures are tied against the bolsters of 4 × 4 rolled compresses as shown.

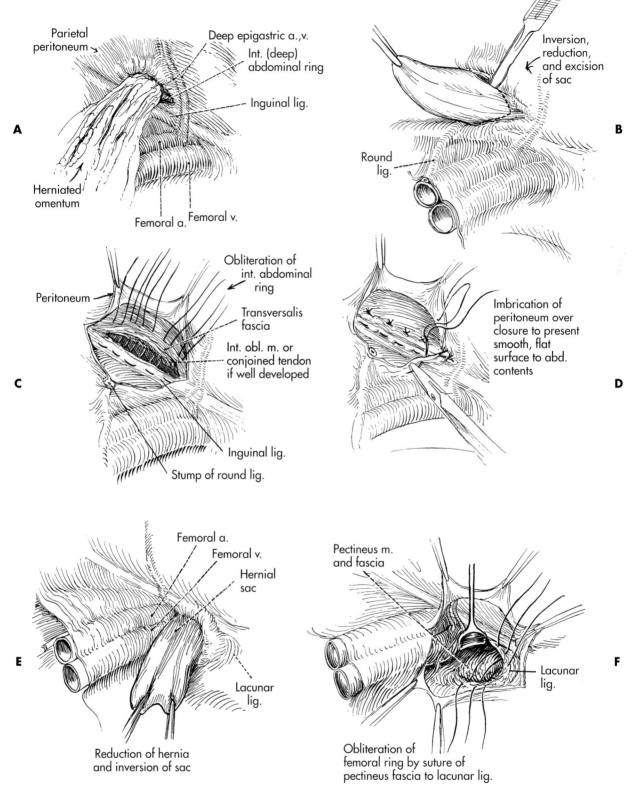

Fig. 13-25   See legend on opposite page.

Fig. 13-25, cont'd   The anatomy for intraabdominal inguinal and femoral herniorrhaphy. **A,** Abdominal view of the inguinal hernia and its contents are noted as a defect in the parietal peritoneum between the inguinal ligament and the deep epigastric artery and vein. The contents are reduced by gentle traction, and the sac is inverted into the abdominal cavity. An incision is made through the peritoneum at the base of the sac in the direction noted by the dashed line **(B). C,** The round ligament is ligated, permitting the internal ring to be closed completely. The inguinal ligament is sewn to the internal oblique muscle or conjoined tendon and transversalis fascia using permanent suture material or staples. **D,** The peritoneum is closed over the inguinal ligament, if desired. **E** and **F,** The details of intraabdominal femoral herniorrhaphy are shown. Notice that the hernia displaces the femoral artery and vein somewhat laterally. **E,** The hernia is reduced, the sac is inverted into the abdomen, and the sac is excised. **F,** The lacunar ligament is sutured to the pectineus fascia to obliterate the femoral canal. The sutures are started medially and continued toward the femoral vein until the femoral ring is obliterated except for an adequate exit for the femoral vessels and nerve. It may be necessary to remove some of the deep inguinal lymphatics, nodes, and areolar tissue to ensure a secure closure. (From Ball TL: *Gynecologic surgery and urology,* ed 2, St Louis, 1963, Mosby.)

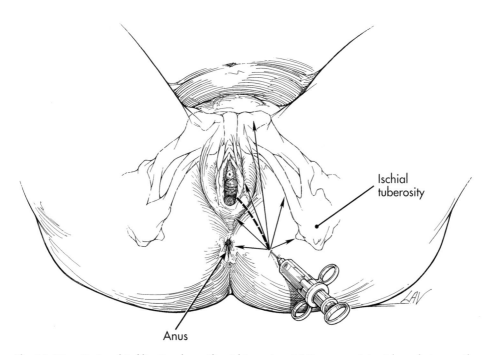

Fig. 13-26   Perineal infiltration by a "liquid tourniquet." From a point midway between the anus and the ischial tuberosity, a no. 22 spinal needle is used to thoroughly infiltrate the tissues along the pathways *(arrows)* with a solution of dilute epinephrine (1 : 200,000). Dashed line shows the path of Schuchardt's incision.

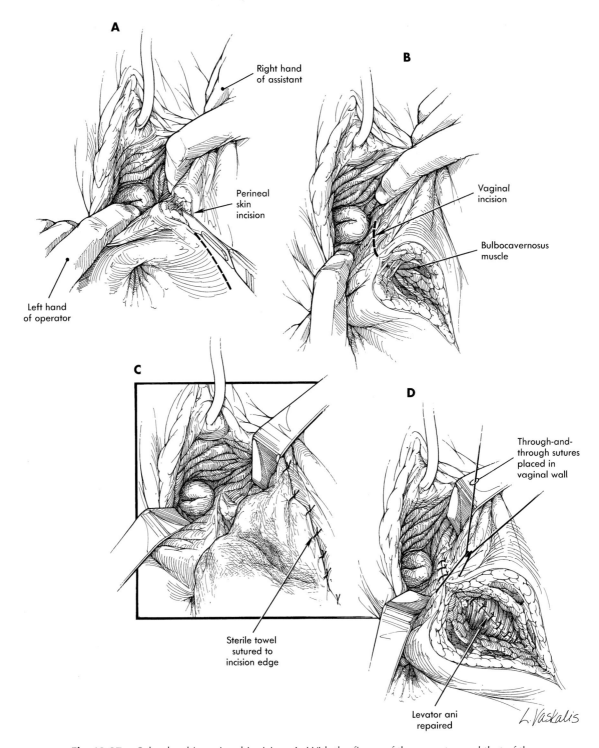

Fig. 13-27 Schuchardt's perineal incision. **A,** With the finger of the operator and that of the operator's assistant making traction in opposite directions, a skin incision is made along the path of the dashed line, midway between the anus and the ischial tuberosity. **B,** The incision is carried into the vagina. The cut edges of the bulbocavernosus are seen in the depths of the wound. **C,** A sterile towel may be sutured to the upper edge of the Schuchardt's incision. The incision is closed by interrupted sutures through the vaginal wall. **D,** The edges of the levator ani are approximated with interrupted sutures, as are those of the bulbocavernosus muscle, and the perineal skin is closed with interrupted sutures.

operator cuts the towel free and closes the incision with a series of interrupted absorbable through-and-through sutures placed in the full thickness of the vaginal wall (Fig. 13-27, D). The incision in the levator ani can be closed by separate interrupted stitches, or the cut edges of the levator can be included with the stitches placed through the wall of the vagina in its depth. The perineal skin is similarly closed with interrupted absorbable sutures.

REFERENCES

1. Amstey MS, Jones AP: Preparation of the vagina for surgery, *JAMA* 245:839, 1981.
2. Armstrong PJ, Burgess RW: Choice of incision and pain following gallbladder surgery, *Br J Surg* 77:746, 1990.
3. Ayliffe GAJ: Surgical scrub and skin disinfection, *Infect Control* 5:23, 1984.
4. Ball TL: *Gynecologic surgery and urology,* ed 2, St Louis, 1963, Mosby.
5. Bang RL, Mustafa MD: Comparative study of skin wound closure with polybutester (Novafil) and polypropylene, *J R Coll Surg Edinburgh* 34:205, 1989.
6. Bardenheuer's incision. In Graves WP: *Gynecology,* ed 4, Philadelphia, 1928, WB Saunders.
7. Bourne RB, Bitar H, Andreae PR, et al: In-vivo comparison of four absorbable sutures: Vicryl, Dexon Plus, Maxon, and PDS, *Can J Surg* 31:43, 1988.
8. Brand E: Letter to the editor, *Am J Obstet Gynecol* 165:235, 1991.
9. Breen JL: Transverse incisions and the total abdominal hysterectomy, Gynecol Surg Film Festival, New York, Sept 1987.
10. Cherney LS: A modified transverse incision for low abdominal operations, *Surg Gynecol Obstet* 72:92, 1940.
11. Chez RA, Gallup DG: Mass midline closure to avoid wound disruption, *Contemp Obstet Gynecol,* Oct 1989, p 62.
12. Chez RA, Krebs HB: Steps in performing the Maylard incision, *Contemp Obstet Gynecol,* Sept 1991, p 39.
13. Chez RA, McDuff HC: The Pfannenstiel incision, *Contemp Obstet Gynecol* 7:55, 1976.
14. Christopherson WA: Surgical incisions and their anatomic basis. In Buchsbaum HJ, Walton LA, editors: *Strategies in gynecologic surgery,* New York, 1986, Springer-Verlag.
15. Colombo M, Maggioni A, Parma G, et al: A randomized comparison of continuous versus interrupted mass closure of midline incisions in patients with gynecologic cancer, *Obstet Gynecol* 89:684, 1997.
16. Denehy TR, Einstein M, Gregori CA, Breen JL: Symmetrical periumbilical extension of a midline incision: a simple technique, *Obstet Gynecol* 91:293, 1998.
17. Duffy DM, DiZereta GS: Is peritoneal closure necessary? *Obstet Gynecol Surv* 49:817, 1994.
18. Edgerton MT: *Fundamentals of wound management in surgery: technical factors in wound management,* South Plainfield, NJ, 1977, Chirurgecom.
19. Ellis H, Heddle R: Does the peritoneum need to be closed at laparotomy? *Br J Surg* 64:733, 1977.
20. Franchi M, Ghezzi F, Zanaboni F, et al: Nonclosure of peritoneum at radical abdominal hysterectomy and pelvic node dissection: a randomized study, *Obstet Gynecol* 90:622, 1997.
21. Gallup DC, Gallup DG, Nolan TE, et al: Use of subcutaneous closed drainage system and antibiotics in obese gynecologic patients, *Am J Obstet Gynecol* 175:358, 1996.
22. Gallup DG, Nolan TE: How to reduce surgery risks, *Contemp Obstet Gynecol,* 1990, p 172.
23. Gallup DG, Talledo OE, King LA: Primary mass closure of midline incisions with a continuous running monofilament suture in gynecologic patients, *Obstet Gynecol* 73:675, 1989.
24. Gilbert JM, Ellis H, Foweraker S: Peritoneal closure after lateral paramedian incision, *Br J Surg* 74:113, 1987.
25. Greer BE, Cain JM, Figge DC, et al: Supraumbilical upper abdominal midline incision for pelvic surgery in the morbidly obese patient, *Obstet Gynecol* 76:471, 1990.
26. Guillou PJ, Hall TJ, Donaldson DR, et al: Vertical abdominal incisions: a choice? *Br J Surg* 67:395, 1980.
27. Guyton AC: *Textbook of medical physiology,* Philadelphia, 1976, WB Saunders.
28. Hajj SN, Mercer LJ, Ismail MA: Surgical approaches to pelvic infections in women, *J Reprod Med* 33:159, 1988.
29. Hallum A, et al: Panniculectomy combined with major pelvic surgery in morbidly obese women with gynecologic cancer, *J Gynecol Tech* 3:9, 1997.
30. Hambley R, et al: Wound healing of skin incisions produced by ultrasonically vibrating knife, scalpel, electrosurgery, and carbon dioxide laser, *J Dermatol Surg Oncol* 14:1213, 1988.
31. Hoffman MS, Villa A, Roberts WS, et al: Mass closure of the abdominal wound with delayed absorbable suture in surgery for gynecologic cancer, *J Reprod Med* 36:356, 1991.
32. Hugh TB, Nankivell C, Meagher AP, Li B: Is closure of the peritoneal layer necessary in the repair of midline surgical abdominal wounds? *World J Surg* 14:231, 1990.
33. Krupski WC, Sumchai A, Effeney DJ, Ehrenfeld WK: The importance of abdominal wall collateral blood vessels, *Arch Surg* 119:854, 1984.
34. Kustner O: Der suprasymphysare kreuzschnitt, eine methode der coeliotomie bei wenig umfanglichen affektioen der weiblichen beckenorgane, *Monatsschr Geburtshilfe Gynäkol* 4:197, 1896.
35. Küstner O: Methodik der gynaekologischen Laparotomie, *Verh Dtsch Ges Gynäkol* (9 Kongr) 9:580, 1901.
36. Landau L, Landau T: The history and technique of the vaginal radical operation (Translated by Eastman & Giles), New York, 1897, William Wood.
37. Leaper DJ, Pollack AV, Evans M: Abdominal wound closure: a trial of nylon, polyglycolic acid and steel sutures, *Br J Surg* 64:603, 1977.
38. Lee RA: *Atlas of gynecologic surgery,* Philadelphia, 1992, WB Saunders.
39. Lewis RT, Wiegand FM: Natural history of vertical abdominal parietal closure: Prolene versus Dexon, *Can J Surg* 32:196, 1989.
40. Lowbury EJL: Skin disinfection, *J Clin Pathol* 14:85, 1961.
41. Mackenrodt A: Die Radikaloperation de Gebärmutterscheidenkrebses mit. Ausräumung des Beckens, *Verh Dtsch Gynäkol* 9:139, 1901.
42. Masterson BJ: Skin preparation, *Clin Obstet Gynecol* 31:736, 1988.
43. Masterson BJ: Selection of incisions for gynecologic procedures, *Surg Clin North Am* 71:1041, 1991.
44. Maylard AE: Direction of abdominal incisions, *Br Med J* 2:895, 1907.
45. Metz SA, Chenqini N, Masterson BJ: In-vivo tissue reactivity and degradation of suture materials: a comparison of Maxon and PDS, *J Gynecol Surg* 5:37, 1989.
46. Morrow CP: Discussion of Lewis RT, et al: *Year Book of obstetrics and gynecology,* St Louis, 1991, Mosby.
47. Morrow CP, Hernandez WL, Townsend DE, Disaia PJ: Pelvic celiotomy in the obese patient, *Am J Obstet Gynecol* 127:335, 1977.
48. Mountcastle VB: *Medical physiology,* ed 13, St Louis, 1974, Mosby.
49. Pfannenstiel J: Ueber die Vortheile des suprasymphysaren fascienquerschnitts für die gynäkologischen Koliotomien zugleich ein Beitrag zu der Indikationsstellung der Operationswege, *Samml Klin Vortr (Leipsig),* 268:1735, 1900.
50. Ramani L, Rock JA, Horowitz IR: Abdominal incisions in the obese, *J Gynecol Tech* 3:133, 1997.
51. Ranney B: Diastasis recti and umbilical hernia: causes, recognition, and repair, *So Dakota J Med* 43:5, 1990.
52. Robbins GF, Brunschwig A, Foote FW: Deperitonealization: clinical and experimental observations, *Ann Surg* 130:466, 1949.
53. Rodeheaver GT, Borzelleca DC, Thacker JG, Edlich RF: Unique performance characteristics of Novafil, *Surg Gynecol Obstet* 164:230, 1987.

54. Rodeheaver GT, Nesbit WS, Edlich RF: Novafil—a dynamic suture for wound closure, *Ann Surg* 204:193, l986.
55. Ronaboldo CJ, Rowe-Jones DC: Closure of laparotomy wounds: skin staples versus sutures, *Br J Surg* 79:1172, 1992.
56. Sanz LE, Patterson JA, Kamath R, et al: Comparison of Maxon suture with Vicryl, chromic catgut, and PDS in fascial closure in rats, *Obstet Gynecol* 71:418, 1988.
57. Shepherd JH, Cavanagh D, Riggs D, et al: Abdominal wound closure using a nonabsorbable single-layer technique, *Obstet Gynecol* 61:248, 1983.
58. Sippo WC: Personal communication, March 1990.
59. Sippo WC, Burghardt A, Gomez AC: Nerve entrapment after Pfannenstiel incision, *Am J Obstet Gynecol* 157:420, 1987.
60. Sippo WC, Gomez A: Nerve-entrapment syndromes from lower abdominal surgery, *J Fam Pract* 25:585, 1987.
61. Sola AE: Myofascial trigger point therapy, *Res Staff Physic,* Aug 1981, p 38.
62. Thompson JD: Incisions for gynecologic surgery. In Thompson JD, Rock JA, editors: *Te Linde's operative gynecology,* ed 7, Philadelphia, 1992, JB Lippincott.
63. Turner-Warwick R: Vesico-vaginal fistula: the resolution of the frozen pelvis by caeco-vaginoplasty. In Rob C, Smith R, editors: *Operative surgery,* London, 1986, Butterworths.
64. Turner-Warwick R: The functional anatomy of the urethra. In Droller MJ, editor: *The surgical management of urologic disease,* St Louis, 1992, Mosby.
65. Turner-Warwick R: Obstetric and gynaecological injuries of the urinary tract—their prevention and management. In Bonnar J, editor: *Recent advances in obstetrics and gynaecology,* 18, London, Churchill Livingstone (in press).
66. Turner-Warwick R, Worth P, Milroy E, Duckett J: The suprapubic V incision, *Br J Urol* 46:39, 1974.
67. von Peham H, Amreich J: *Operative gynecology* (Translated by LK Ferguson), Philadelphia, 1934, JB Lippincott.
68. Williams DC: The peritoneum: a plea for a change in attitude towards this membrane, *Br J Surg* 42:401, 1953.

14 Eviseration and Repair of Ventral Hernias

DONALD G. GALLUP

Wound infections and their sequelae, dehiscence, eviseration, and abdominal wall hernias result in significant emotional and financial problems for patients who have undergone operations using a transabdominal or transvaginal approach. The purpose of this chapter is to supply guidelines for preventing wound infections and their sequelae, to identify at-risk patients and modify incision techniques for these patients, and to outline management strategies for those patients who have wound complications.

DEHISCENCE AND EVISERATION

Technically, wound dehiscence is separation of the layers of an abdominal incision. Incomplete or partial dehiscence is separation of the layers posterior to the skin, sometimes including the fascia. If the peritoneum is included in the disruption, the dehiscence is considered complete. If the intestine protrudes through the wound, the term *eviseration,* also referred to as *burst abdomen,*[25] is used. Eviseration also can present vaginally as a result of vaginal operations, trauma, or severe prolapse. A superficial wound dehiscence implies that the wound has separated down to, but not through, the fascial layer.

Superficial Dehiscence

Certain patients are at greater risk for abdominal wound infection and seroma and resulting superficial separation.[14,38,42] Large series, such as those by Cruse and Foord,[8] have noted decreased wound infection rates with the use of preoperative hexachlorophene showers and the avoidance of chromic catgut for subcutaneous closure. They and others[4] have noted a decrease in wound infections when abdominal and pubic hair is clipped rather than shaved the evening before surgery. Some researchers have advocated depilatories, but these are expensive and have almost equal efficacy in preventing wound infections as no shaving.[52] Whenever it is feasible, the author prefers an electric razor in the operating room to remove hair from the incision site.

Other methods to decrease incision complications include avoiding closely approximated parallel incisions and using laser or cautery to incise the skin. In general, closure should be delayed for contaminated or dirty wounds such as enterotomy in unprepared bowel or rupture of an abscess cavity. In one series of perforating appendicitis, researchers noted a reduction in wound infection rate from 34.17% to 2.3% with a delayed closure method.[19] Others have used delayed closure and successfully reduced wound infections

in obese patients and those with cancer, with intraabdominal infection, or bowel content contaminations.[5] After closure of the fascia, the author uses copious amounts of saline to irrigate the wound. Antibiotic solutions are avoided. Horizontal mattress sutures of 3-0 nylon or 3-0 monofilament polypropylene are placed 2 to 3 cm apart and loosely tied over gauze saturated with a diluted povidone-iodine solution. These 4×8 dressing sponges are changed every 8 hours with a wet-to-dry technique, using sterile saline. Some surgeons use bridges, consisting of rolled gauze on the lateral borders of the incision.[35] In 4 or 5 days, depending on the appearance of the subcutaneous tissues, the previously placed sutures are tied to approximate the skin edges. Steri-strips can be used to approximate uneven skin edges.

Two other issues for prevention, particularly in high-risk patients, include the use of prophylactic antibiotics and closed drainage systems. Although prophylactic antibiotics have been shown to be effective in patients having vaginal surgery or radical hysterectomy,[53] no randomized, prospective studies have proven their efficacy in high-risk patients having abdominal hysterectomy.[11] Moreover, prophylactic antibiotics have not proven to be effective in obese patients, as alluded to in 1995 by Perlow.[41] Cephalosporins are the most popular antibiotics used for prophylaxis. Coverage for anaerobes and enterococci should be ensured in patients when bowel surgery is anticipated.

Since obese patients are at high risk for superficial wound separation, prophylactic subcutaneous drains have been suggested, but their use remains controversial. As noted by Cruse and Foord,[8] a Penrose-type drain, particularly when exited through the incision, can increase the risk of superficial wound infection. Prophylactic drainage of the subcutaneous tissues should be accomplished with a *closed* drainage system such as a Blake or Jackson-Pratt. In over 360 obese patients who had a subcutaneous closed drainage system placed, the author and his associate have reported a superficial wound infection rate of 2.8% to 3.1% in three separate series of patients.[14-16]

In the series of obese patients reported by Morrow,[38] none of the obese patients who developed wound infections had subcutaneous drains. Those opposing subcutaneous drains in obese patients suggest they may act as a wick and increase wound infection rates, and Scott[51] reported operating on 56 patients whose panniculi thickness measured 6 to 11 cm. They used prophylactic antibiotics, and subcutaneous drains were not used. Wound infection developed in only one patient. A time-honored surgical principle is to eliminate dead space. Subcutaneous areas in obese patients rarely contain adequate supportive tissues to approximate subcutaneous tissues. Someone wishing to use subcutaneous sutures should choose a running technique with a fine, polyglycolic acid suture. An alternative technique for obese patients is the use of subcutaneous retention suture, as reported by Soisson (1993).[55] The effort to resolve the continued debate about the use of subcutaneous drains in obese patients was recently addressed in a publication from the Medical College of Georgia.[14] Obese gynecologic patients with midline incisions were divided into four groups: (1) no subcutaneous drain, no antibiotics; (2) no subcutaneous drain, antibiotics; (3) subcutaneous drain, no antibiotics; and (4) subcutaneous drain, antibiotics. In this prospective study of 197 patients, a trend for fewer superficial wound complications was noted in the subcutaneous drain, prophylactic antibiotic group. The wound breakdown rate was 14% in the no drain, no antibiotic group, compared with 2% in the drain, antibiotic group. Because of the low rates of wound infections and numbers of patients in each group, these differences were not statistically significant. A power analysis revealed a minimum of 800 patients would be needed to show a significant difference.

Management. Superficial separation of layers anterior to the fascia usually is associated with wound infections or seromas. Many surgeons suggest opening the entire length of the wound, although this decision should be individualized. Often, a separation due to a seroma or hematoma can be managed by opening only a portion of the affected area. Cultures for aerobic and anaerobic bacteria should be obtained, and the opening should always be gently probed with a sterile gloved finger to ensure the fascia and peritoneum are intact. In the presence of gross contamination, the wound is packed open with sterile saline–soaked gauze, which should be changed every 8 hours. Dakin's solution, hydrogen peroxide, or povidone-iodine adds little to wound healing in these situations and may adversely affect wound healing because of cytotoxic effects on fibroblasts.[34] The author concurs with a time-honored clinical practice of never placing something in a wound that one would not want placed in his or her eye.

Once wet to dry dressings are initiated, the surgeon may choose one of two methods for further management: (1) secondary closure in 2 to 5 days or (2) allowing the wound to heal by second intention. A number of studies over the past decade have shown the efficacy of the former by reducing healing time, reducing patient inconvenience, and resulting in success rates of 88% to 95%.[10,23,63] Some used antibiotics and an en bloc closure technique. A 1996 study from Tulane compared reclosure with an en bloc technique to a second intention group.[47] Secondary closure not only resulted in a significant reduction in healing time, but also a calculated cost savings of $850.00 per patient.

At our institution, we use a technique similar to that of the University of Mississippi report.[10] After opening the wound to the fascia, the subcutaneous tissues are sharply debrided daily, and wet-to-dry saline-soaked dressings are applied every 8 hours. Unless the patient has a concomitant infection, such as cellulitis or cuff infection, antibiotics are not used. When the healing bed of granulation tissue is beefy-red and without exudate or necrotic debris, the wound is closed in a treatment room on the ward under local 1% lidocaine anesthesia. Patients may be premedicated with 50 mg of meperidine hydrochloride intramuscularly. An aseptic technique is used. We also do not use an en bloc technique, but use mattress sutures of no. 0 polypropylene sutures though the skin, 1 cm from the skin edge and 2 cm apart.

Evisceration

Prevention of evisceration is related to management of the fascial closure, particularly in high-risk patients (see the box below). Additionally, ascites, vomiting, or coughing can result in evisceration in some high-risk patients.[18] The choice of sutures in fascial closure is important and is thoroughly discussed in the Chapter 13. We concur that midline incisions in high-risk patients should be closed with a large bore (no. 0 to no. 2) monofilament suture. The choice of incision is a factor to consider, and older studies have suggested that evisceration was three to five times more common when vertical incisions were used compared to transverse incisions.[22,58,59] These studies concluded that eviscerations with midline incisions could be due to poorly chosen suture materials or use of inappropriate fascial closure techniques. At least one study noted less of a problem with dehiscence in patients with midline incisions compared to those with transverse incisions. Chromic catgut sutures should never be used for fascial closure. In closing midline incisions, many surgeons continue to prefer a layered closure, an un-

---

PREDISPOSING RISK FACTORS FOR WOUND COMPLICATIONS

1. Anemia
2. Ascites
3. Cancer
4. Chemotherapy
5. Coagulation abnormalities
6. Corticosteroid use
7. Diabetes
8. Immunoincompetence: human immunodeficiency virus (HIV), renal transplant patients
9. Intraabdominal infections: appendicitis, enterotomy in unprepared bowel, diverticular abscess or rupture, ruptured tuboovarian abscess
10. Obesity
11. Older patient age
12. Other systemic disease (e.g., lupus)
13. Poor nutrition, including alcoholism
14. Prior abdominal irradiation
15. Prior abdominal surgery
16. Prolonged operative procedure
17. Prolonged preoperative hospitalization
18. Pulmonary disease, chronic

necessary technique for the vast majority of gynecologic patients. If this technique is used, sutures should always be loosely tied. The major cause of wound evisceration is use of too many sutures, placed too close to the fascial edge and too close together, and tied too tightly.[27] Often at reoperation for evisceration, the sutures and knots are intact, but the suture has torn through the fascia.

In recent years, some have advocated a Smead-Jones technique as the traditional closure of midline incisions in high-risk patients.[62] A no. 1 nylon or monofilament polypropylene suture is used in this far-far, near-near suturing technique (Fig. 14-1). This closure is time consuming. Based on earlier reports from general surgeons and trauma surgeons, this author and his associates began using a running mass closure for high-risk patients with midline incisions in the early 1980s. In our first report, we used no. 2 polypropylene in 210 patients. No eviscerations occurred.[17] When older and more recent series of running mass closure are tabulated, the fascial dehiscence rate is only 0.34% (Table 14-1). Most of the recent reported series are from large gynecologic cancer services.* To use this running mass closure, closely spaced bites are taken and placed 1.5 to 2 cm from the fascial edge (Fig. 14-2). These sutures should not be tied too tightly. Some use loop sutures, and only a single knot is required. The major advantage of this closure is that tension is equally distributed over a continuous line. The technique also is faster and cost-efficient compared to interrupted closures.

The rare problem with wound sinus formation using this closure has been largely alleviated with the use of delayed

---

*References 3, 7, 14, 16, 17, 30, 36, 39, 40, 48, 54, 56.

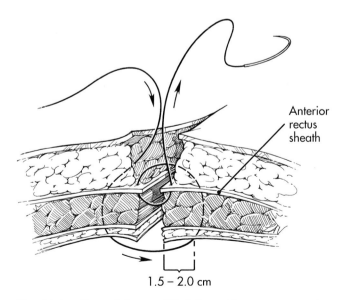

Anterior rectus sheath

1.5 – 2.0 cm

Fig. 14-1 One of the modified Smead-Jones suture techniques. Using a no. 0 or no. 1 monofilament delayed absorbable material, the suture is widely placed through anterior sheath, muscle, posterior sheath, and peritoneum, if available. On the second pass, only the anterior sheath is included. Sutures should be tied loosely.

absorbable suture instead of permanent suture. Long-term follow-up for incisional hernia formation after this closure is rarely reported in any of the published series. Colombo et al.[7] did have follow-up from 6 months to 3 years in their randomized series. Incisional hernias occurred in 10.4% of patients with continuous closure and in 14.7% with interrupted Smead-Jones closure. These differences were not statistically different, but no. 1 polyglycolic acid was used in the Smead-Jones group.

Diagnosis. Evisceration is one of the most dangerous postoperative complications. The mortality associated with evisceration ranges from 10% to 35% in several reported series.[2,29,43,46] This rate usually is associated with other complications such as sepsis and major organ failures. Mortality can be reduced by early diagnosis and prompt, aggressive management, and Helmkamp's[22] 10-year study noted a mortality of only 2.9%. Evisceration is less likely in gynecologic patients than in general surgical patients. Evisceration usually occurs from 5 to 14 days postoperatively, with a mean of 8 days. Conceivably, the low mortality rates achieved in the past could be in jeopardy as the push to care for postsurgical patients at home increases.

One of the early signs of complete dehiscence and impending evisceration is the seepage of serosanguineous pink discharge from an apparently intact wound. It may be present several days before evisceration occurs. The patient is frequently conscious of something giving away. Although occult hematomas can be the cause of such discharge, these patients' wounds should be examined at every 6 to 8 hours. With seepage, the wound can be partially opened and gently explored with a sterile gloved finger to determine whether the fascia and peritoneum are intact. The use of clamps, cotton-tipped applicators, or other instruments is dangerous and not as informative. Occasionally, obesity, poor condition of tissues, or presence of exudative infection can make bedside diagnosis difficult. Both ultrasound and computed tomography (CT) have been used to confirm the diagnosis. These tests require moving the patient and can increase the risk of evisceration.

Management. If suspicion of impending evisceration is entertained, the appropriate place for reclosure is the operating room. With very few exceptions, eviscerations should be closed as soon as they are recognized. Bowel usually will protrude from the opened incision (Fig. 14-3). When a delay of several hours is anticipated because of a recent meal, the bowel can be replaced using sterile gloves and gently packed in place with lap pads soaked in diluted povidone-iodine. A sterile plastic drape can be added.[37] An abdominal binder should be placed over these layers. After cultures are obtained, prophylactic broad-spectrum antibiotics should be initiated. Baseline blood counts and serum electrolytes should be obtained.

When the patient is under general anesthesia in the operating room, the wound should be meticulously explored to determine the extent of dehiscence. All necrotic tissue, clots, and suture material should be removed. Aerobic and anaerobic cultures should be obtained, if not done so previously.

Table 14-1   Running Mass Closure in Midline Incisions

Authors	No. Patients	Materials	No. Patients with Fascial Dehiscence
Murray and Blaisdell (1978)	255	PGA (no. 1)	1
Archie and Feldman (1981)	120	MFPP (no. 1)	1
Shepherd et al. (1983)	200	MFPP (no. 2)	0
Knight and Griffen (1983)	419	MFPP (no. 1)	4
Gallup et al. (1989)	210	MFPP (no. 2)	0
Gallup et al. (1990)	285	MFPG (no. 1)	1
Orr et al. (1990)	129	MFPG (no. 1)	0
Montz et al.(1991)*	231	MFPG (no. 0)	0
Sutton et al. (1992)†	154	MFPB (no. 0)	1
Rodrigues et al. (1996)*	115	MFPD (no. 0)	0
Gallup et al. (1996)	197	MFPG (no. 1)	0
Columbo et al. (1997)†	308	MFPG (no. 1)	1
TOTALS	2623		9 (0.34%)

PGA, Polyglycolic acid; *MFPP*, monofilament polypropylene; *MFPG*, monofilament polyglyconate; *MFPB*, monofilament polybutester; *MFPD*, monofilament polydioxanone.
*Looped suture with running Smead-Jones technique.
†Looped suture.

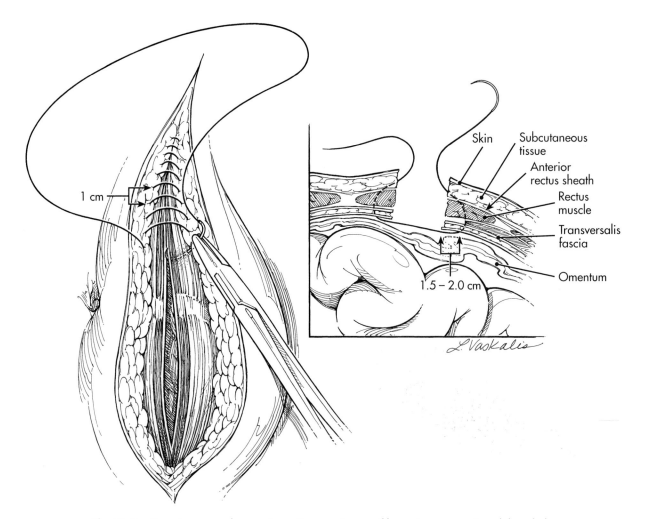

Fig. 14-2   Running mass closure. A no. 0 or no. 1 monofilament permanent or delayed absorbable suture is initiated from the cephalad end of the incision. Another is started from the lower end of the incision. They are loosely tied together at the mid portion of the vertical incision. Note the wide (1.5 to 2 cm from the fascial edge) bites. All knots are buried. The peritoneum is included if easily available.

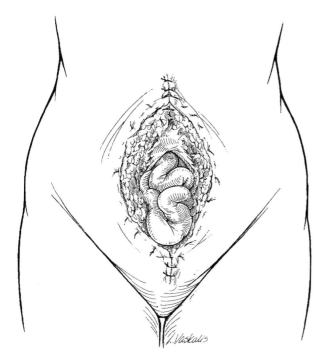

Fig. 14-3 Wound evisceration. The skin, fascia, and peritoneum have separated along most of the wound, exposing the underlying small intestine.

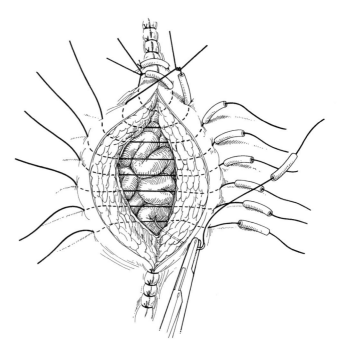

Fig. 14-4 Through-and-through closure of a wound evisceration using a no. 2 monofilament permanent suture. If fascial edges are not widely separated or necrotic, a Smead-Jones closure can be used.

The bowel and omentum should be inspected and cleansed with several liters of warm normal saline.

Closure of evisceration can be done with through-and-through stay sutures (Fig. 14-4). A no. 2 nylon or polypropylene suture is used, and the sutures are placed 2.5 to 3 cm from the skin edges. The sutures pass through all layers and should be placed 2 cm apart to allow for edema. This technique is of particular value when the wound edges are ragged or the patient's condition is poor. Debridement of grossly infected or devitalized skin, subcutaneous tissue, muscle, and fascia should be accomplished before closure is attempted (Fig. 14-5). Skin edges unopposed between these large sutures can be approximated with 3-0 interrupted polypropylene. Sutures should be left in for at least 2 weeks.

If the fascial margins can be located and are not ragged, a Smead-Jones closure with no. 1 polypropylene suture can be used (see Fig. 14-1). If gross infection is evident, the wound should be packed open, using a delayed closure technique. In clean or clean-contaminated wounds, the author prefers to close the skin. The skin may be the ultimate layer protecting the patient if the fascia separates again. Some use metal clips, but in this instance, the author prefers interrupted horizontal mattress sutures using a 2-0 monofilament permanent suture such as polypropylene. Subcutaneous closed drainage usually is used.

Often the fascia does not come together, or the tissue is too friable to hold sutures. Marlex or Gore-Tex mesh should be used only in clean abdominal wall defects because of the high rate of enteric fistulas, subsequent hernia, and extrusion in the contaminated or infected wound.[26] When a

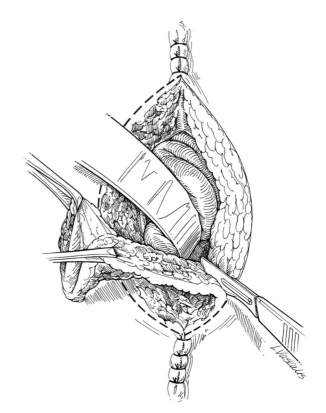

Fig. 14-5 Before closure with the through-and-through technique, devitalized tissue is resected. During closure, bowel is protected with a retractor, or "fish." Hemostasis is ensured before placement of the large-bore sutures.

through-and-through closure is not needed, further support to fascial edges that cannot be approximated is achieved by using an absorbable polyglycolic acid mesh (Dexon), which is ideal for contaminated wounds, although postoperative hernia is likely.[9] Another option is the use of Silastic Sheeting (Dow Corning Corp., Midland, Mich). This temporary abdominal wall closure has been used successfully in catastrophic situations by trauma surgeons. The sheeting is sutured to the edge of the fascial wound. If the visceral edema resolves rapidly, and when infection has subsided, primary fascial closure can often be accomplished during the same hospitalization.[65]

Postoperative care should include the insertion of a nasogastric tube. Ileus is likely, even if the bowel is not distended at the time of reclosure. The tube should be left in until bowel function returns. To promote healing, serum proteins must be augmented by total parental nutrition when the patient is unable to tolerate an adequate diet. Many of these patients spend several days in an intensive care unit. If the wound is packed open, wet-to-dry saline dressing should be used as previously noted, and secondary closure should be considered. Broad-spectrum antibiotics should be modified according to culture sensitivity.

Vaginal Evisceration

Protrusion of large or small bowel through the vagina has been reported after trauma, surgery, vigorous coitus, and insertion of foreign bodies, and this rare form of evisceration can occur spontaneously in postmenopausal women with preexisting enteroceles.[13,20,28,49,64] These eviscerations often are associated with loss of vaginal integrity because of prior irradiation and have been noted to occur after sacrospinous fixation of the prolapsed vagina.[12] Vaginal lacerations during coitus can occur as a "colpotomy" in patients with an intact uterus and often are caused by coital positions that permit deep penetration or coitus performed while inebriated.[13] Emetic-inducing chemotherapy has led to vaginal evisceration in patients who have had ovarian cancer debulking surgery.[66]

Diagnosis. Most patients with vaginal evisceration have lower abdominal or rectal pain, followed by a serosanguineous or bloody discharge. An obvious sign is prolapse of the bowel beyond the introitus (Fig. 14-6). Careful history may elicit one of the previously noted causes. If the blood supply to the prolapsed bowel has been compromised, signs of obstruction or an acute abdominal condition may be present.

Management. Although many investigators are adamant about a transabdominal approach to evaluate patients with vaginal evisceration, selected patients can be managed transvaginally.[20] A transvaginal approach is reasonable if (1) the time from protrusion is less than 6 hours, (2) the bowel is viable and easily reduced, (3) the bowel is intact without evidence of instrumentation, and (4) abdominal findings are normal. In this situation, the bowel is irrigated with several liters of warm saline and gently pushed into the cavity with the patient in the Trendelenburg position. The bladder can be evaluated for intactness by transurethral in-

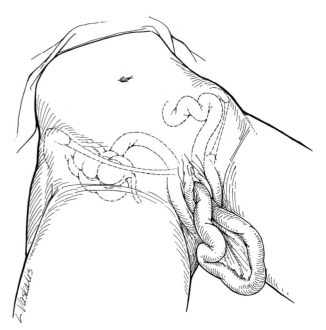

Fig. 14-6   Vaginal evisceration. Rupture of an enterocele can occur in postmenopausal women, resulting in ileum protruding through the vagina. This also can occur after vigorous coitus in younger women.

sertion of methylene blue solution. The rectosigmoid can be evaluated by intraoperative proctosigmoidoscopy. If these tests reveal no defects, the vagina can be closed in two layers with absorbable suture. Broad-spectrum antibiotic coverage should be initiated before surgery. If the aforementioned conditions are not met, or if the patient has had penetration with some type of blunt or jagged device, a transabdominal approach is indicated. Once the bowel is brought into the abdominal cavity, it should be carefully run and injuries repaired. Nonviable bowel should be resected. The vaginal defect can be repaired from above or below. Ideally, these patients should be operated on using adjustable laparoscopy stirrups. Obliteration of the cul-de-sac by a Halban technique should be considered.

Protrusion of Intestines Through Uterus and Vagina

A rare form of vaginal evisceration occurs during abortion procedures in which the uterus is perforated and the intestine is brought through the dilated cervix by the suction device or grasping forceps (Fig. 14-7).

The surgical approach in this scenario should be transabdominal to adequately reduce the bowel and to carefully evaluate the usually large uterine lacerations associated with the evisceration. Prophylactic antibiotics should be initiated, and the patient should be counseled about the possibility of hysterectomy. The "above and below" approach, as noted previously, should be used and can facilitate removal of any remaining intrauterine products of conception. Once products have been removed, attention should be directed to the uterine injury. Most of these can be repaired primarily. The

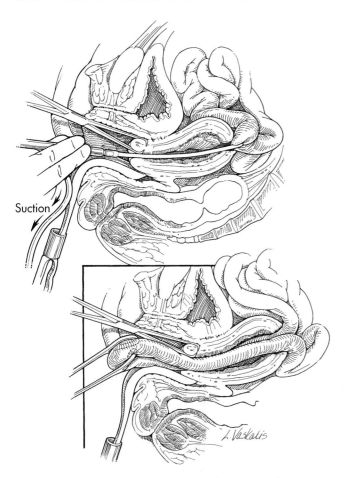

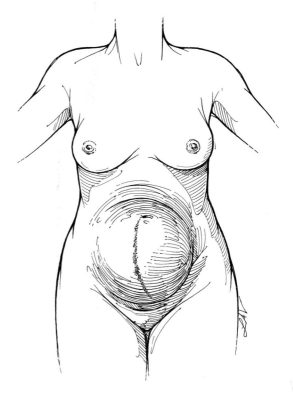

Fig. 14-8   A large ventral hernia occurring in a lower midline incision.

Fig. 14-7   Uterine perforation during therapeutic abortion. A suction curette has perforated the uterus and trapped a loop of ileum. Insert shows placental forceps grasping the trapped loop and pulling it through the dilated cervix.

bladder and rectum should be evaluated for any associated injuries. After these steps have been completed, the bowel should be run and carefully evaluated for injuries. Irrigation of the abdominal cavity with several liters of warm saline should be done before abdominal closure.

VENTRAL HERNIA

Gynecologic patients have a lower risk of postoperative hernia than general surgical patients. The frequency of hernia formation is higher in patients with midline incisions than in those with transverse incisions. Hernia formation in general gynecologic patients is estimated to be a little over 3% when a midline incision is used.[60] The factors noted in the box on p. 228 often predispose patients to ventral hernia formation. Other factors include coughing or vomiting, which increase abdominal pressure, and postoperative hematoma formation or infection in the wound area. The rate of hernia formation in a gynecologic cancer population is slightly increased at about 5%.[24,54] It is similar to ventral hernias reported on a general surgical population.[6,31,50] Ventral hernias may appear years later, particularly if absorbable suture is used for closure.[33]

Diagnosis

Hernias in most patients can be diagnosed by history and physical examination. The patient complains of abdominal pressure and may even notice a protuberance after standing for extended periods of time or when straining or coughing. These symptoms frequently abate when she is lying supine. The symptoms may gradually worsen, and the patient may palpate a mass, which disappears when she is recumbent. The smaller the defect through which the bowel has herniated, the greater the chance of incarceration, obstruction, and infarction. In such rare instances, patients have symptoms and signs of an acute abdominal condition. Patients with large hernias may note bowel peristalsis beneath the skin. Although the size of the initial defect may be small, the size of the resultant hernia can assume varying proportions. A large amount of small bowel and omentum can escape from a small fascial defect into the easily expandable subcutaneous space.

On physical examination, careful palpation of the abdominal wall reveals a distinct fascial defect, and the edges are easily palpable. Having the patient cough or raise her head from the table often easily demonstrates the defect. Alternatively, having the patient stand and cough often demonstrates the defect, large or small (Fig. 14-8). In obese patients or patients with diastasis of the recti (usually associated with multiparity), differentiating between a ventral hernia or simply thin and attenuated fascia is often difficult. In such instances, abdominal CT or ultrasound can often establish the diagnosis.

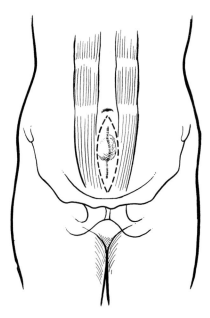

Fig. 14-9 An elliptical incision is used to excise redundant skin and previous scar over the hernia. (From Mitchell GW: Incisional hernia. In Nichols DH, editor: *Reoperative gynecologic surgery,* ed 2, St Louis, 1997, Mosby.)

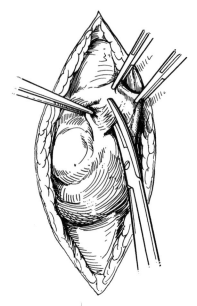

Fig. 14-10 To dissect the hernia sac, tooth clamps (e.g., Kocher) are placed for traction on the fascial edge. Using countertraction, the peritoneal edge is cut from the undersurface of the fascia. (From Mitchell GW: Incisional hernia. In Nichols DH, editor: *Reoperative gynecologic surgery,* ed 2, St Louis, 1997, Mosby.)

Management

The surgical management of hernias must follow the basic principle of hemostasis and closure without tension. If a primary closure can be accomplished, fascia should be approximated to fascia after all scar has been excised. Dissection of the hernial sac from fat, rectus muscles, and peritoneal margins should be done, and the entire sac should be resected.

Not all hernias require surgical repair. Elderly, obese patients with multiple medical problems may be candidates for a more conservative approach. Patients with prior radiation therapy and several prior repair attempts are often in this category. In such patients, a change in lifestyle, use of abdominal binders, and trusses tailored to the anatomic defect can often give palliative, safe relief of major symptoms.

Preoperative Care for Hernia Repair. With the rare exception of bowel incarceration or obstruction, ventral hernia repair is an elective procedure. All patients should be instructed in meticulous cleansing of the abdomen at home the evening before surgery. Abdominal hair encroaching on the proposed operative field should be removed in the operating room, preferably by clip preparation. A modified bowel preparation is indicated (see the box above). Outpatient bowel preparation can be safely used, even in patients undergoing colon resection. It is less expensive and more easily tolerated by the vast majority of patients.[1,32] Because the rectosigmoid area is rarely involved, enemas the morning before surgery are unnecessary. Diabetes and other systemic problems should be controlled for optimal surgical results. For patients unable to tolerate polyethylene glycol–electrolyte solution, magnesium citrate, one half bottle every 6 to 8 hours can be substituted. We no longer use oral

---

BOWEL PREPARATION FOR HERNIA REPAIR

1. Clear liquid diet 24 hours before surgery
2. Chilled oral polyethylene glycol electrolyte solution (PEG-ELS, GoLYTELY) day before surgery
   a. One liter per hour or until rectal effluent clear
   b. Do not continue oral intake >4 hr
   c. Total volume should be <4 L
3. Intravenous antibiotics in a prophylactic dose just before surgery, effective against anaerobes
   a. Cefoxitin—2 g
   b. Ceftizoxime—1 g
   c. Cefotetan—1 g
   d. Ampicillin/sulbactam—3 g

---

neomycin or erythromycin in these usually older patients.

Surgical Management of Small Hernias. Regardless of the size of the hernia, the previous skin scar and subcutaneous tissue should be removed posterior to the level of the hernia sac and fascia (Fig. 14-9). The entire sac is freed from its attachments to the subcutaneous tissue above and the fascia below to visualize the full extent of the defect (Fig. 14-10). The sac is then opened, and finger exploration can help in the decision regarding further opening of the peritoneum (Fig. 14-11). The incised peritoneum is then grasped with multiple clamps, countertraction is applied by the protective fingers of the surgeon, and intestinal adhesions are sharply incised to safely release adherent bowel loops (Fig. 14-12). After releasing the omentum and bowel, it is important to determine whether the hernial defect can

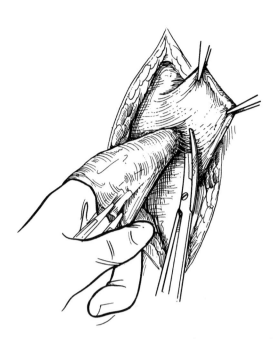

Fig. 14-11   The hernia sac is opened. A finger is inserted into the sac, allowing dissection downward to the origination of the hernia. Countertraction is maintained. (From Mitchell GW: Incisional hernia. In Nichols DH, editor: *Reoperative gynecologic surgery,* ed 2, St Louis, 1997, Mosby.)

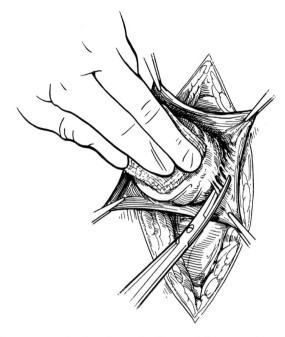

Fig. 14-12   The hernia sac is dissected from any intestinal adhesions by the traction-countertraction technique. (From Mitchell GW: Incisional hernia. In Nichols DH, editor: *Reoperative gynecologic surgery,* ed 2, St Louis, 1997, Mosby.)

be adequately closed, using the available fascia, before excising the sac. In such situations, a layer for layer fascial closure or an overlap fascial closure should be done. If fascia is deemed inadequate for primary closure, the defect must be bridged with a nonabsorbable mesh or some type of fascial partition, and release technique can be used.

Small hernias in the area of the umbilicus often are more suitable for the transverse repair. After excision of the usually small peritoneal sac, which often includes omentum, the defect is closed with a Smead-Jones technique (see Fig. 14-1). All sutures are placed before tying to avoid inclusion of bowel when "blind" suturing is used. A permanent monofilament suture should be used, and subcutaneous tissue should be mobilized cephalad and caudad to allow for adequate wide suture placement.

Small or large vertical hernia defects require wide mobilization (at least 4 to 5 cm) of the subcutaneous tissue from the underlying fascia (Fig. 14-13). Once this is accomplished, many small hernias can be closed with a Smead-Jones technique. Some prefer to close the peritoneum, if available, in a separate layer. Again, large bore monofilament suture should be used. In the rare cases when abundant viable fascia is available, an imbricated overlapping technique can be used (Fig. 14-14). Theoretically, this vest-over-pants technique provides a relatively stronger closure, but it is time consuming. Due to the wide mobilization of subcutaneous tissue, the use of closed drainage systems in the subcutaneous spaces should be strongly considered (Fig. 14-15). These drains should always exit through the skin, several centimeters from the primary incision. Drains may be removed by postoperative day 5 but must be left in place until any drainage

from the incision has ceased. An abdominal binder is placed over the closed incision. Staples or 2-0 polypropylene horizontal mattress sutures can be used for skin closure.

Surgical Management of Large Hernias. Large fascial defects or hernias associated with attenuated and weak fascia often require closure with aid of polypropylene mesh or Gore-Tex. These materials are inert, usually retain tensile strength until the wound has matured, and allow growth of connective tissue in the wound area. The implanted mesh should completely bridge the usually oval defect. The hemostasis must be meticulous, and all foreign bodies, such as sutures, should be removed before suturing. Before inserting the mesh, wide dissection of the subcutaneous tissue from the underlying fascia must be done, as previously discussed (see Fig. 14-13). The peritoneum can be preserved to permit its primary closure. As Fig. 14-16 (p. 238) shows, the mesh is inserted posterior to the rectus muscles on one side. Use of permanent mesh is reserved for uncontaminated wounds. Alternatively, the tailored mesh can be sutured anterior to the fascia with the same "U" suture technique. In the former situation the rectus muscles and any remaining fascia can be closed over the mesh with a Smead-Jones technique (see Fig. 14-16, *C*). Permanent polypropylene sutures are always used to anchor the mesh. Closed suction drainage is placed (see Fig. 14-15), and the subcutaneous tissue can be closed with a running 3-0 polyglycolic acid suture over the drains. Options for skin closure are staples or sutures. When mesh is unavailable or has previously failed, autologous tensor fascia lata has been advocated.[21] This technique has led to thigh wound hematomas, seromas, or infection in obese, diabetic, or smoking patients. To avoid

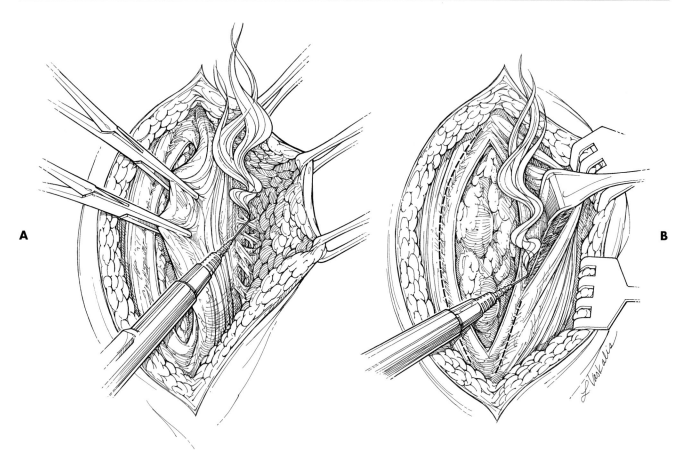

Fig. 14-13 Whether a primary closure or a synthetic mesh is used, the subcutaneous tissue must be separated from the anterior fascia, as noted in **A,** by using a needle tip Bovie. The rectus muscles are widely separated from the underlying fused posterior fascia and peritoneum. The rectus margins are noted by the dashed line **(B).** A knife can be used instead of a Bovie. This step is particularly useful when a mesh is required.

these problems, Tucker et al.[61] have successfully used videoscopically assisted fascia lata harvest. This minimally invasive technique can reduce thigh complications and has an obvious cosmetic advantage.

The author often manages large ventral hernias by use of muscle component separation techniques. These sliding flap techniques have been advocated since the early 1990s, and defects as large as 15 × 25 cm have been successfully closed.[44,45,57] One concern over the use of this repair is weakness in the lateral aspect of the wound where some type of relaxing incision is used, resulting in a late occurring spigelian hernia. Contraindications to this technique include presence of an abdominal stoma or presence of multiple different abdominal incisions. These relaxing incisions achieve a "tensionless" coaptation of the linea alba.

Several techniques are described. In the component separation or fascial position/release, incisions are placed lateral to the rectus muscles and separately in the transversus. The neurovascular bundle of the rectus must be preserved[57] (Fig. 14-17, p. 239). We prefer a sliding myofascial flap, where only one incision, 2 cm lateral to the rectus muscle and through only the external oblique, is used. The external oblique must be bluntly dissected off the underlying internal

oblique through the entire length of this parasagittal incision[44] (Fig. 14-18, p. 239). Hemostasis is mandatory after separation. The rectus muscle with the overlying rectus sheath and its attached internal oblique-transversus muscles can be advanced about 5 cm in the epigastrium, 10 cm around the umbilicus and 3 cm in the suprapubic region. Thus bilateral advancement is available at 10, 20, and 6 cm, respectively. In both techniques, wide separation of the subcutaneous tissue from the fascia is needed before parasagittal incisions (see Fig. 14-13). The "new" midline fascial edges are reunited with a Smead-Jones technique with large bore polypropylene suture. The repair can be reinforced with polypropylene mesh, sutured anterior to the fascia. Subcutaneous drainage, as previously described, and abdominal binders are used.

Postoperative Care. General guidelines for postoperative care should be considered for small or large hernias. Preoperative heparin plus compression boots should be continued until the patient is fully ambulating, because these patients are at risk for thromboembolic complications. Patients are kept at bed rest for the first 24 hours and then ambulated with assistance. We also remove the intraoperatively inserted nasogastric tube at 24 hours, although some prefer

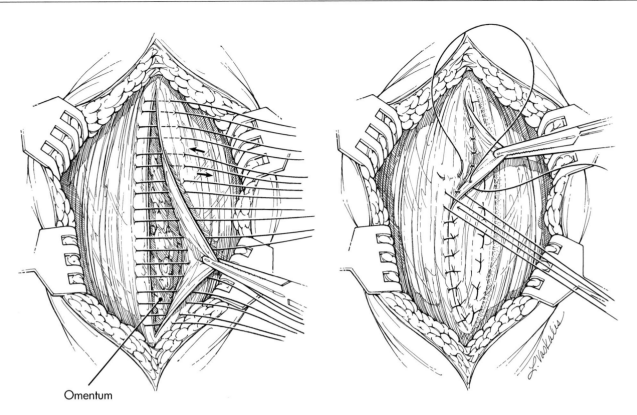

Omentum

Fig. 14-14   Vest-over-pants closure for hernias with adequate fascial margins and good strength. After the subcutaneous tissue has been widely dissected (see Fig. 14-13), horizontal mattress ("U") sutures are placed distal from one fascial edge and passed through the opposite fascial margin **(A).** All sutures are tied, and the opposite fascial margin is reapproximated to the distal portion of the fascia using interrupted sutures **(B).** Permanent no. 0 or no. 1 monofilament sutures are used for hernia repairs.

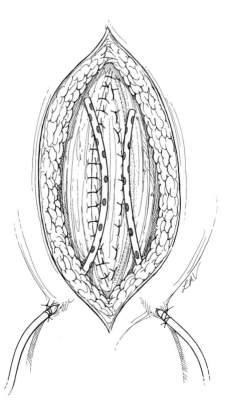

Fig. 14-15   Because of the wide dissection, bilateral Jackson-Pratt (shown here) or Blake drains are placed anterior to the closed fascia.

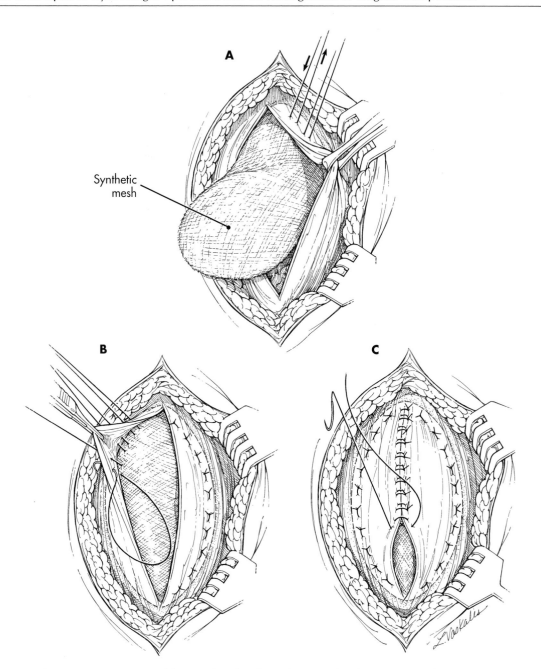

Fig. 14-16   Large ventral hernia closed with synthetic mesh. The rectus muscles have been separated from the underlying posterior fascia and peritoneum (see Fig. 14-13, *B*). Often the peritoneum can be closed. The mesh is tailored to the wound and inserted posterior to the rectus muscles and fascia. It is fixed using a horizontal mattress suture passing from fascia through the mesh and back out through the fascia **(A).** After uniting the fascia to one side, the opposite fascial edge is sutured in a similar manner **(B).** Closure of the rectus muscle or fascia is accomplished with a modified Smead-Jones technique **(C).**

to leave it in place until the patient passes flatus. A liquid diet is initiated after return of bowel function is assessed by the usual parameters of active bowel sounds and lack of abdominal distention. If abdominal distention or vomiting ensues, the tube is reinserted. The abdominal binder and dressings are removed at 24 hours, and the wound is inspected at least twice a day. Prophylactic antibiotics, as noted in the box on p. 234, are switched to maintenance antibiotics in patients who have had a mesh inserted. Based on our previous studies on obese patients, we leave drains in for 72 hours or until drainage is less than 50 ml/24 hr.[14,15]

Upon discharge, patients are instructed to avoid strenuous physical activity, particularly not lifting anything over 5 pounds, for 6 weeks. One occasional long-term bothersome complication is persistent accumulation of fluid in the suprafascial space. When this occurs, periodic aspiration or reinsertion of a drain, plus a binder, is indicated. If the aspiration is suspect for infection, cultures should be obtained.

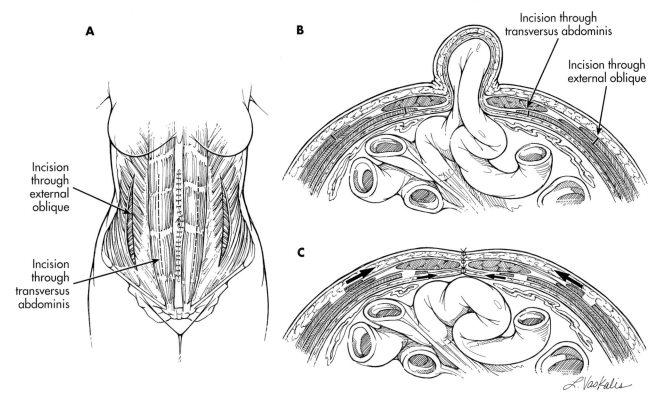

Fig. 14-17 Fascial partition. Parasagittal relaxing incisions are placed through the external oblique (gap), lateral to the rectus muscles, after wide mobilization of the skin and subcutaneous tissues **(A).** A schematic transverse representation shows the placement of these incisions **(B).** These two incisions allow wide mobilization of the fascia to allow reapproximation in the midline **(C).** A Smead-Jones suture technique can accomplish this closure instead of interrupted sutures.

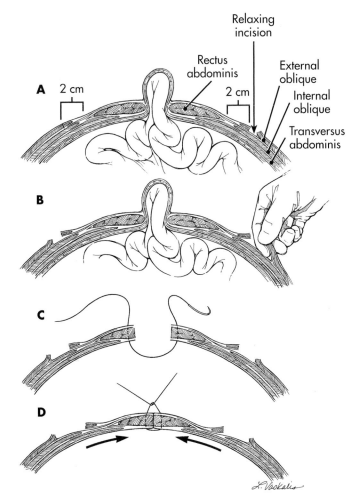

Fig. 14-18 Sliding myofascial flap, using component separations. After wide mobilization of the skin and subcutaneous layers, a relaxing vertical incision is made 2 cm lateral to the rectus muscle through the external oblique **(A).** The flap is further mobilized laterally by blunt dissection **(B).** An interrupted or Smead-Jones placement of no. 1 monofilament permanent suture is placed at least 1.5 cm from the fascial edge **(C).** When the suture is tied, these bilateral relaxing incisions allow closure of large ventral hernias **(D).**

Wounds associated with hernia repair deserve frequent evaluations during the 6-week convalescence. This can be accomplished in the office or by various home health care agencies. Patients and agencies are instructed that swelling or discharge from the wound mandates immediate reevaluation.

REFERENCES

1. ACOG educational bulletin: Antibiotics and gynecologic infections, American College of Obstetricians and Gynecologists, no 237, June 1997, *Int J Gynaecol Obstet* 58:333, 1997.
2. Alexander HC, Prudden JF: The causes of abdominal wound disruption, *Surg Gynecol Obstet* 122: 1223, 1966.
3. Archie JP Jr, Feldtman RW: Primary abdominal wound closure with permanent continuous running monofilament sutures, *Surg Gynecol Obstet* 153:721, 1981.
4. Balthazar ER, Colt JD, Nichols RL: Preoperative hair removal: a random prospective study of shaving versus clipping, *South Med J* 75:799, 1982.
5. Brown SE, Allen HH, Robins RN: The use of delayed primary wound closure in preventing wound infections, *Am J Obstet Gynecol* 127:713, 1977.
6. Carlson MA, Ludwig KA, Condon RE: Ventral hernia and other complications of 1000 midline incisions, *South Med J* 88:450, 1995.
7. Colombo M, Maggioni A, Parma G, et al: A randomized comparison of continuous versus interrupted mass closure of midline incisions in patients with gynecologic cancer, *Obstet Gynecol* 89:684, 1997.
8. Cruse PJ, Foord R: The epidemiology of wound infection: a 10-year prospective study of 62,939 wounds, *Surg Clin North Am* 60:27, 1980.
9. Dayton MT, Buchele BA, Shirazi SS, Hunt LB: Use of an absorbable mesh to repair contaminated abdominal-wall defects, *Arch Surg* 121:954, 1986.
10. Dodson MK, Magann EF, Sullivan DL, Meeks GR: Extrafascial wound dehiscence: deep en bloc closure versus superficial skin closure, *Obstet Gynecol* 83:142, 1994.
11. Duff P: Antibiotic prophylaxis for abdominal hysterectomy, *Obstet Gynecol* 60:25, 1982.
12. Farrell SA, Scotti RJ, Ostergard DR, Bent AE: Massive evisceration: a complication following sacrospinous vaginal vault fixation, *Obstet Gynecol* 73:560, 1991.
13. Friedel W, Kaiser IH: Vaginal evisceration, *Obstet Gynecol* 45:315, 1975.
14. Gallup DC, Gallup DG, Nolan TE, et al: Use of a subcutaneous closed drainage system and antibiotics in obese gynecologic patients, *Am J Obstet Gynecol* 175:358, 1996.
15. Gallup DG: Modifications of celiotomy techniques to decrease morbidity in obese gynecologic patients, *Am J Obstet Gynecol* 150:171, 1984.
16. Gallup DG, Nolan TE, Smith RP: Primary mass closure of midline incisions with a continuous polyglyconate monofilament absorbable suture, *Obstet Gynecol* 76:872, 1990.
17. Gallup DG, Talledo OE, King LA: Primary mass closure of midline incisions with a continuous running monofilament suture in gynecologic patients, *Obstet Gynecol* 73:675, 1989.
18. Reference deleted in proofs.
19. Grosfeld JL, Solit RW: Prevention of wound infection in perforated appendicitis: experience with delayed primary wound closure, *Ann Surg* 168:891, 1968.
20. Hall BD, Phelan JP, Pruyn SC, Gallup DG: Vaginal evisceration during coitus: a case review, *Am J Obstet Gynecol* 131:115, 1978.
21. Hamilton JE: The repair of large of difficult hernias with mattressed onlay grafts of fascia lata, *Ann Surg* 167:85, 1968.
22. Helmkamp BF: Abdominal wound dehiscence, *Am J Obstet Gynecol* 128:803, 1977.
23. Hermann GG, Bagi P, Cristoffersen I: Early secondary suture versus healing by second intention of incisional abscesses, *Surg Gynecol Obstet* 167:16, 1988.
24. Hoffman MS, Villa A, Roberts WS, et al: Mass closure of the abdominal wound with delayed absorbable suture in surgery for gynecologic cancer, *J Reprod Med* 36:356, 1991.
25. Jenkins TP: The burst abdominal wound: a mechanical approach, *Br J Surg* 63:873, 1976.
26. Jones JW, Jurkovich GJ: Polypropylene mesh closure of infected abdominal wounds, *Am Surg* 55:73, 1989.
27. Jurkiewicz MJ, Morales L: Wound healing, operative incisions, and skin crafts. In Hardy JD, editor: *Hardy's textbook of surgery,* Philadelphia, 1983, JB Lippincott.
28. Kambouris AA, Drukker BH, Barron J: Vaginal evisceration: a case report and a brief review of the literature, *Arch Surg* 116:949, 1981.
29. Keill RH, Keitzer WF, Nichols WK, et al: Abdominal wound dehiscence, *Arch Surg* 106:573, 1973.
30. Knight CD, Griffen FD: Abdominal wound closure with a continuous monofilament polypropylene suture, *Arch Surg* 118:1305, 1983.
31. Krukowski ZH, Cusick EL, Engeset J, Matheson NA: Polydioxanone or polypropylene for closure of midline abdominal incisions: a prospective comparative clinical trail, *Br J Surg* 74:828, 1987.
32. Le TH, Timmcke AE, Gathsight JB Jr: Outpatient bowel preparation for elective colon resection, *South Med J* 90:526, 1997.
33. Lewis RT, Wiegand FM: Natural history of vertical abdominal parietal closure: Prolene versus Dexon, *Can J Surg* 32:196, 1989.
34. Lineaweaver W, Howard R, Soucy D, et al: Topical antimicrobial toxicity, *Arch Surg* 120:267, 1985.
35. Mendenez MA: The contaminated wound. In O'Leary JP, Watering EA, editors: *Techniques for surgeons,* New York, 1985, John Wiley & Sons.
36. Reference deleted in proofs.
37. Morris DM: Preoperative management of patients with evisceration, *Dis Colon Rectum* 25:249, 1982.
38. Morrow CP, Hernandez WL, Townsend DE, Disaia PJ: Pelvic celiotomy in the obese patient, *Am J Obstet Gynecol* 127:335, 1977.
39. Murray DH Jr, Blaisdell FW: Use of synthetic absorbable sutures for abdominal and chest wound closures, *Arch Surg* 113:477, 1978.
40. Orr JW Jr, Orr PF, Barrett JM, et al: Continuous or interrupted fascial closure: a prospective evaluation of no. 1 Maxon suture in 402 gynecologic procedures, *Am J Obstet Gynecol* 163:1485, 1990.
41. Perlow JH: Obstetric management of the obese patient, *Contemp Obstet Gynecol* 40:15, 1995.
42. Pitkin RM: Abdominal hysterectomy in obese women, *Surg Gynecol Obstet* 142:532, 1976.
43. Pratt JH: Wound healing—evisceration, *Clin Obstet Gynecol* 16:126, 1973.
44. Ramirez OM, Ruas E, Dellon AL: "Components separation" method for closure of abdominal-wall defects: an anatomic and clinical study, *Plast Reconstr Surg* 86:519, 1990.
45. Reedy MB, Hoganson N, Tadvick L: Abdominal wall muscle component separation for repair of large ventral hernias, *J Pelvic Surg* 3:91, 1997.
46. Richards PC, Balch CM, Aldrete JS: Abdominal wound closure, *Ann Surg* 197:238, 1983.
47. Robinson WR, Champlin SA: A trial of secondary closure versus second-intention closure in surgical wound separation, *J Gynecol Tech* 2:13, 1996.
48. Rodriguez GC, Clarke-Pearson DL, Ho CM, et al: A comparison of interrupted versus continuous Smead-Jones abdominal closure, *J Gynecol Tech* 2:19, 1996.
49. Rolf BB: Vaginal evisceration, *Am J Obstet Gynecol* 107:369, 1970.
50. Sahlin S, Ahlberg J, Granstrom L, Ljungstrom KG: Monofilament versus multifilament absorbable sutures for abdominal closure. *Br J Surg* 80:322, 1993.
51. Scott HW Jr, Law DH IV, Sandstead HH, et al: Jejunoileal shunt in surgical treatment of morbid obesity, *Ann Surg* 171:770, 1970.

52. Seropian R, Reynolds BM: Wound infections after preoperative depilatory versus razor preparation, *Am J Surg* 121:251, 1971.

53. Sevin BU, Ramos R, Gerhardt RT, et al: Comparative efficacy of short-term versus long-term cefoxitin prophylaxis against postoperative infection after radical hysterectomy: a prospective study, *Obstet Gynecol* 77:729, 1991.

54. Shepherd JH, Cavanagh D, Riggs D, et al: Abdominal wound closure using a nonabsorbable single-layer technique, *Obstet Gynecol* 61:248, 1983.

55. Soisson AP, Olt G, Soper JT, Berchuck A, et al: Prevention of superficial wound separation with subcutaneous retention sutures, *Gynecol Oncol* 51:330, 1993.

56. Sutton G, Morgan S: Abdominal wound closure using a running, looped monofilament polybutester suture: comparison to Smead-Jones closure in historic controls, *Obstet Gynecol* 80:650, 1992.

57. Thomas WO III, Parry SW, Rodning CB: Ventral/incisional abdominal herniorrhaphy by fascial partition/release, *Plast Reconstr Surg* 91:1080, 1993.

58. Thompson JB, Mclean KF, Collier FA: Role of the transverse abdominal incision and early ambulation in the reduction of postoperative complications, *Arch Surg* 59:1267, 1949.

59. Tollefson DG, Russell KP: The transverse incision in pelvic surgery, *Am J Obstet Gynecol* 68:10, 1954.

60. Trimbos JB, Smit IB, Holm JP, Hermans J: A randomized clinical trial comparing two methods of fascia closure following midline laparotomy, *Arch Surg* 127:1232, 1992.

61. Tucker JG, Choat D, Zubowicz VN: Videoscopically assisted fascia lata harvest for the correction of recurrent ventral hernia, *South Med J* 90:399, 1997.

62. Wallace D, Hernandez W, Schlaerth JB, et al: Prevention of abdominal wound disruption utilizing the Smead-Jones closure technique, *Obstet Gynecol* 56:226, 1980.

63. Walters MD, Dombroski RA, Davidson SA, et al: Reclosure of disrupted abdominal incisions, *Obstet Gynecol* 76:597, 1990.

64. Wilson F, Swartz DP: Coital injuries of the vagina, *Obstet Gynecol* 39:182, 1972.

65. Yeh KA, Saltz R, Howdieshell TR: Abdominal wall reconstruction after temporary abdominal wall closure in trauma patients, *South Med J* 89:497, 1996.

66. Zanetta G, Colombo M, Cormio G, Gabriele A: Vaginal evisceration after surgery in patients receiving chemotherapy for advanced ovarian cancer, *J Pelvic Surg* 3:159, 1997.

15 Hemorrhage and Shock

BETH E. NELSON and PETER E. SCHWARTZ

Massive hemorrhage and its attendant complications occur predominately in the intraoperative or postpartum state in gynecology and obstetrics. Hemorrhage accounts for 13% of maternal deaths in the United States.[35] The best preventive measures are anticipation of situations in which hemorrhage can occur and use of meticulous surgical technique. Obtaining careful medical histories to identify patients with coagulopathies, reviewing prior operative reports to identify difficult sites of dissection, and assessing prior obstetric complications allow preparation for potential bleeding complications. Immediate action at the initial occurrence of significant bleeding can prevent the escalation of its severity. The steps to control hemorrhage depend on the individual situation. This chapter reviews the management of bleeding complications in obstetrics and gynecology and describes techniques used by the authors to control massive hemorrhage.

PREOPERATIVE EVALUATION
Coagulopathies

A history of easy bruising or coagulation difficulties, particularly at a prior operation, or a known coagulopathy in a preoperative surgical patient requires a hematologic evaluation before surgery, because simple measures may prevent significant intraoperative bleeding.[65] A simple bleeding history in every preoperative patient should include a listing of all prescribed and over-the-counter medications, inquiries about any family history of excessive bleeding, and questions regarding excessive bleeding following trauma or surgery.[59] Coagulation factor deficiencies or platelet dysfunction can be a contributing factor in the etiology of hemorrhage, and replacement therapy may obviate severe complications. Knowledge of the coagulation system with its intrinsic and extrinsic pathways is important in instituting appropriate preventive therapy.[4,52] The coagulation system is shown in Fig. 15-1. The intrinsic system requires no extravascular component for initiation, whereas the extrinsic pathway is activated by tissue factor (thromboplastin) found only when vascular integrity has been violated. The two pathways have been shown to have multiple sites of interaction.

In patients with platelet abnormalities, a platelet count should be obtained to assess quantitative defects. Abnormal intraoperative bleeding rarely occurs when the platelet count is greater than 50,000.[67] The bleeding time has been used to evaluate platelet function; however, its usefulness in predicting surgical blood loss has been disputed.[16,54] The bleeding time is elevated in thrombocytopenia, after aspirin or nonsteroidal antiinflammatory drug ingestion, after use of some penicillins and cephalosporins, and in cyclooxygenase deficiency, factor V or VIII deficiency, uremia, liver failure, congenital afibrinogenemia, and Bernard-Soulier syndrome.[15,30,56] Patients with these conditions may be asymptomatic until intraoperative or postoperative bleeding occurs.

The prothrombin time (PT) and partial thromboplastin time (PTT) are usually irregular in patients with a coagulation factor deficiency, and specific factor levels can be measured in the workup of such patients.[61] Elevations of PT and PTT are predictive of a coagulation abnormality only when elevated more than 1.3 times control levels.[67] Factor VIII deficiency is the most common hereditary hemorrhagic disorder.[4] Absence of factor VIII, an X-linked genetic disorder, and therefore rarely seen in women, causes hemophilia A. Deficient von Willebrand's factor, closely related to factor VIII levels, results in decreased factor VIII and platelet dysfunction. Patients with von Willebrand's disease usually experience immediate hemorrhage after injury. In contrast, hemophiliacs have delayed bleeding and develop spontaneous, deep tissue hemorrhage. In both diseases, the PT is normal and the PTT is increased. Specific factor levels and the clinical picture allow differentiation.[61] Factor IX deficiency, an X-linked trait known as hemophilia B, is less common than hemophilia A.[4] Carriers may exhibit deficiency states. Factor XI deficiency occurs most commonly in patients of Ashkenazi Jewish backgrounds, and levels are further decreased in pregnancy.[60] Inheritance is autosomal recessive, and the bleeding defect is usually mild. The PTT is elevated in patients with deficiency of factors IX and XI, and patients with hemophilia B may have an increased PT as well.[4,61] Factors II (prothrombin), VII, IX, and X are synthesized in the liver. An elevated PT occurs in factor VII deficiency, vitamin K deficiency, and mild liver dysfunction. In the setting of severe vitamin K deficiency or liver disease, the PTT also can become abnormal. Because vitamin K is produced in the intestine, deficiency should be considered in patients with obstructive jaundice, malnutrition, malabsorption, and short gut syndromes.[67] Subcutaneous or intravenous replacement of vitamin K usually reverses the deficiency and results in normalization of the PT within 12 to 24 hours.[28] Inherited deficiencies of factors II, V, and X, while unusual, also result in elevated PT and PTT.[65] Acquired coagulation factor inhibitors also can contribute to hemorrhage.[53]

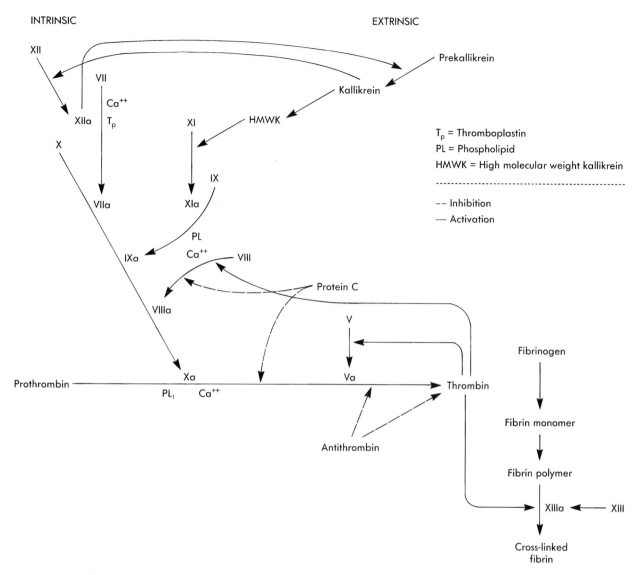

Fig. 15-1   Coagulation system, demonstrating multiple interactions of the intrinsic and extrinsic pathways.

Desmopressin (DDAVP), a synthetic analogue of vasopressin with no vasoactive effects, is useful for obtaining hemostasis in several pathologic states.[28,38] Intravenous, subcutaneous, or intranasal administration of DDAVP results in increased levels of factor VIII, von Willebrand's factor, tissue plasminogen activator, and increased platelet adhesiveness. It has proven useful in decreasing blood loss when used perioperatively in patients with hemophilia A, von Willebrand's disease, and platelet dysfunction resulting from uremia or pharmacologic agents. Some patients with excessive bleeding of unknown cause also can benefit.

Antifibrinolytic agents, such as tranexamic acid and epsilon aminocaproic acid, are useful in prophylaxis and treatment of hemorrhage, primarily in cardiac and oral surgery.[28] Estrogen also may prove beneficial in patients with renal failure or von Willebrand's disease.[28] Factor XII, factor VII, and von Willebrand's factor are all increased by estrogen ad-

ministration, whereas antithrombin III and protein S levels are decreased.

Disseminated intravascular coagulation (DIC) can develop as a result of intraoperative or postoperative hemorrhage or as a complication of abruptio placentae. Preeclampsia, sepsis, surgery for malignancy, and amniotic fluid embolism also can precede DIC. DIC is initially characterized by thrombosis in the microvasculature, followed by fibrinolysis and consumptive coagulopathy with resultant bleeding.[6] The operative site and the venous or arterial punctures can ooze. A laboratory profile typically reveals a falling platelet count and fibrinogen and elevated fibrin split products. Because fibrinogen is elevated in pregnancy, hypofibrinogenemia may not always be evident. Correction of the underlying problem, such as evacuation of retained fetal or placental tissue or treatment of gram-negative sepsis, reverses the process. Replacement of coagulation factors with fresh-frozen plasma (FFP), repletion of fibrinogen with cryoprecipitate, and platelet transfusions are necessary to support the patient.[20] Therapy with blood products is often massive but must be tailored to the specific deficit.

SUPPORTIVE CARE OF A HEMORRHAGING PATIENT

The initial evaluation and supportive therapy of any patient experiencing massive hemorrhage must begin by attaining suitable intravenous access with multiple large-bore catheters. A test tube of fresh uncitrated patient's blood can be taped to an IV pole, thus permitting the operative team a firsthand observation of initial clotting and clot behavior of the patient's blood. The quality of the initial clot and its occasional dissolution, which suggests coagulopathy, can be seen at a glance. Laboratory data, including hemoglobin and hematocrit, platelet count, PT and PTT, fibrinogen, fibrin split products, and serum calcium, should be obtained to guide appropriate replacement. Blood bank personnel should be notified of the nature of the situation so that adequate supplies of blood products can be obtained and cross-matched. Invasive hemodynamic monitoring including Swan-Ganz catheterization should be instituted. A Foley catheter should be placed in the urinary bladder, and urine output should be carefully monitored. Large volumes of crystalloid and blood expanders are often required in addition to packed red blood cells, FFP, and other blood products. Normal saline or lactated Ringer's solution should be infused at a ratio of 3 ml of crystalloid per 1 ml of blood lost. Stored blood is deficient in platelets and coagulation factors, particularly factors V and VII. The need for platelet transfusion in the setting of massive hemorrhage is best assessed by following the platelet count, but generally a patient must lose more than 15 units of blood before experiencing thrombocytopenia.[67] Repletion of coagulation factors with FFP has been advocated at a ratio of 1 unit FFP to 6 units packed red blood cells. However, support for this traditional approach lack supporting data, and it appears that even after loss of the entire circulating blood volume, coagulation factors may not be significantly depleted.[31,67] It is believed that repletion of coagulation factors occurs from storage sites in the interstitial space.

Gynecologic Hemorrhage

Intraoperative Hemorrhage. In our experience, intraoperative hemorrhage during gynecologic surgery is most frequently encountered in the region of the ureter or infundibulopelvic ligament and the venous plexus along the pelvic sidewall deep to the uterosacral ligaments. Bleeding most often occurs during difficult pelvic surgery for conditions such as extensive endometriosis or broad ligament leiomyomata. However, hemorrhage can also occur with routine cases. Preventive techniques include use of small tissue pedicles and double ligatures for ovarian and uterine vascular pedicles.

The key to controlling pelvic sidewall hemorrhage intraoperatively often involves exposing the ureter to avoid ureteric injury. The ureter can be readily exposed as it crosses the common iliac artery and descends into the pelvis by opening the peritoneum lateral to the infundibulopelvic ligament and sweeping the medial leaf of the broad ligament with a tonsil suction (Fig. 15-2). The ureter is freed along its course in the broad and cardinal ligaments by applying gentle traction to the areolar tissue surrounding the ureter and dissecting in the ureteric plane with a Mixter clamp. Care must be taken to avoid dissection perpendicular to the ureter to prevent injury to the external or internal iliac vein. In a patient who is bleeding after complications from a hysterectomy, it may be helpful to redivide the round ligament closer to the pelvic sidewall, if the ovary and fallopian tube have been left in place, before attempting to expose the ureter. Once the course of the ureter is delineated, it can be retracted to provide improved exposure of the bleeding vessels for ligature placement.

Arterial ligation may be required for control of hemorrhage during pelvic surgery. Ligation of the anterior division of the hypogastric (internal iliac) artery is a classic surgical technique; uterine or ovarian arterial ligature, however, may be more appropriate at times, particularly in obstetric hemorrhage.[13,14,18,49] Fig. 15-3 demonstrates the site of ligature in each of these instances. The anterior division of the hypogastric artery encompasses the uterine, vaginal, superior vesical, and middle hemorrhoidal arteries. A position 2.5 to 3 cm distal to the bifurcation of the common iliac artery should be chosen to preserve the posterior division of the hypogastric artery.

The hypogastric artery maybe readily exposed by incising the pelvic sidewall peritoneum. This is accomplished by dividing the round ligament (Fig. 15-4) and extending the peritoneal incision cephalad and parallel to the infundibulopelvic ligament (Fig. 15-5). The soft tissue of the pelvic sidewall is swept away with the tonsil suction exposing the hypogastric artery. A Mixter clamp is gently placed around the hypogastric artery, starting from the lateral side and progressing medially (Fig. 15-6). Lesser-angled clamps should not be used because they may perforate the underlying hypogastric vein, resulting in massive bleeding. The artery is then doubly ligated but not divided. Ligation of the hypogastric artery rarely stops all bleeding because of collateral vessels.[11] It usually reduces the flow of blood so that identification of the bleeding site is possible. In addition, by reducing pulse pressure, thrombosis more readily occurs. The success of hypogastric artery ligation in controlling uterine bleeding has been reported to vary from 40% to 100%.[11,12,18,39,63] Complications include lower extremity paresis, inadvertent ligation of a common iliac artery, wound infection, ureteral injuries, and cardiac arrests.

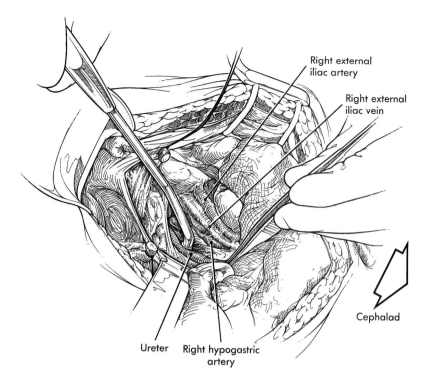

Fig. 15-2   Sweeping the medial leaf of the broad ligament with a tonsil sucker to expose the ureter.

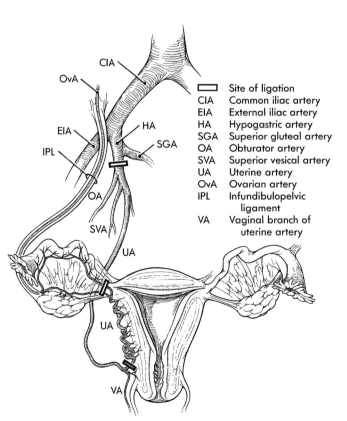

☐	Site of ligation
CIA	Common iliac artery
EIA	External iliac artery
HA	Hypogastric artery
SGA	Superior gluteal artery
OA	Obturator artery
SVA	Superior vesical artery
UA	Uterine artery
OvA	Ovarian artery
IPL	Infundibulopelvic ligament
VA	Vaginal branch of uterine artery

Fig. 15-3   Site of ligation of the hypogastric, uterine, and uteroovarian arteries.

Uterine artery ligation is carried out by taking large "bites" through the uterine wall to encompass the artery at the cervical isthmus just above the bladder flap and near the anastomosis between the uterine and ovarian blood supplies at the ovarian ligament.[19] Selective ligation of the uterine artery at its origin from the hypogastric artery usually is not practical owing to the hypervascularity in this area associated with pregnancy.

Massive gynecologic hemorrhage also can be encountered with arteriovenous malformations, in gestational trophoblastic disease, and in extensive malignancies, particularly when the lateral pelvic wall is invaded.[5,21,23,57,58] Occasionally, intraligamentous leiomyomata, ovarian remnants, or endometriomas can extend to the pelvic sidewall, and venous injury can occur lateral to the hypogastric artery. In such an event it may be necessary to resect a segment of the anterior division of the artery to expose the bleeding site. If uncontrollable bleeding occurs, particularly with hemorrhage resulting from a malignancy infiltrating the pelvic sidewall, it is possible to pack the sidewall with large operating room sponges to control the bleeding. The tails of the sponges are removed through the abdominal wall through a separate incision. The sponges can be removed when the patient is stable.

A new approach to the management of persistent bleeding in gynecologic patients—fibrin glue—was reported to be successful in two patients with gynecologic malignancies and in a postpartum patient.[40] Fibrin glue is composed of equal parts of cryoprecipitate and bovine thrombin (1000 U/ml) simultaneously sprayed from plastic syringes onto the

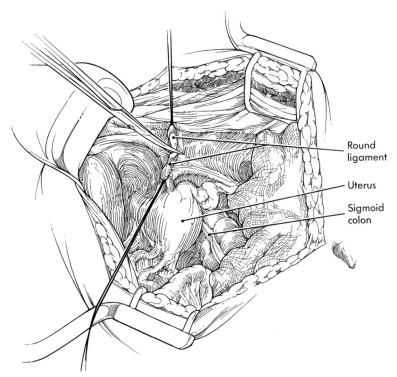

Fig. 15-4   In preparation for exposing the pelvic sidewall vascular structures, the round ligament has been doubly suture ligated and then divided.

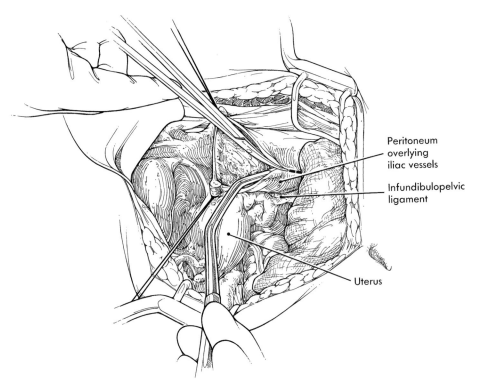

Fig. 15-5   After division of the round ligament, the incision in the pelvic sidewall peritoneum is extended cephalad and parallel to the infundibulopelvic ligament. The tonsil suction is placed parallel to the lateral surface of the infundibulopelvic vessels to avoid vascular injury by the scissors.

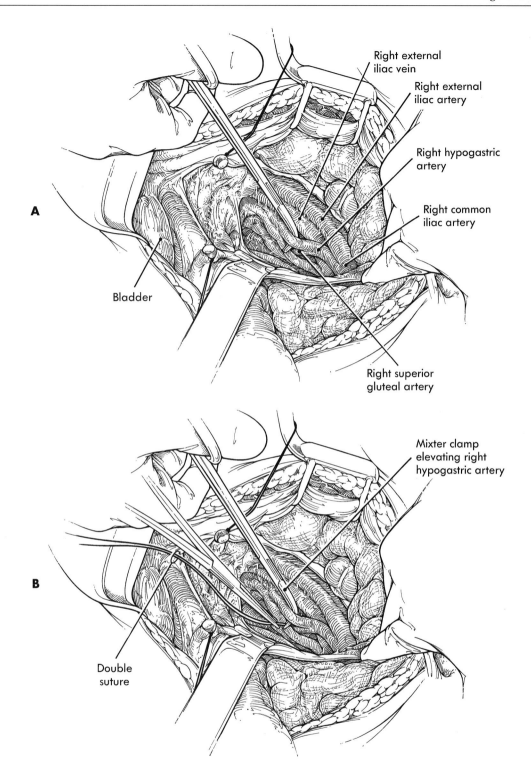

Right external
iliac vein

Right external
iliac artery

Right hypogastric
artery

Right common
iliac artery

A

Bladder

Right superior
gluteal artery

Mixter clamp
elevating right
hypogastric artery

B

Double
suture

Fig. 15-6   **A,** A Mixter clamp has been gently placed from the superolateral surface of the hypogastric artery to the inferomedial aspect. **B,** A double suture is placed in the jaws of the clamp, and the clamp is withdrawn to ligate the hypogastric artery.

bleeding site. It is extremely important to have the surgical field as dry as possible. Fibrin glue can be applied in a wet field in conjunction with an absorbable surgical gelatin sponge (Gelfoam) or collagen hemostat (Avitene). The biochemical principle of the fibrin glue approach is that thrombin converts the fibrinogen in cryoprecipitate into fibrin monomer. Factor XIII then converts the fibrin monomer into a fibrin polymer that acts as a hemostatic mesh. The process takes approximately 2 minutes. Use of cryoprecipitate prepared from pooled human blood sources carries the risk of infectious complications, including hepatitis B and acquired immunodeficiency syndrome (AIDS). Infectious complications can be obviated through the use of autologous blood if one preoperatively anticipates a strong likelihood for hemorrhagic complications.[62] Unfortunately, one cannot routinely anticipate this complication. Fibrin glue is not a substitute for meticulous surgical techniques.

Postoperative Hemorrhage. Postoperative patients who have undergone gynecologic surgery most commonly develop hemorrhage from bleeding sites at the vaginal cuff or from retroperitoneal hematomas. The latter can be an occult site of massive blood loss. After hysterectomy, significant bleeding occurs in 0.3% to 2.9% of cases.[27,68] Careful inspection of the vaginal cuff with appropriate suturing under anesthesia often controls bleeding. If bleeding persists, angiographic embolization often is successful and avoids a return to the operating room.[29,55] Surgical exploration with evacuation and arterial ligation may be required if interventional angiographic techniques are unsuccessful.

Intraoperative Obstetric Hemorrhage

Intraoperative obstetric hemorrhage is most often related to cervical or vaginal lacerations, abnormal placentation, or uterine atony. Cesarean section performed for placenta previa can precede the development of massive intraoperative hemorrhage during placental removal. Placenta accreta, increta, or percreta, in the setting of multiple previous cesarean sections, can likewise lead to hemorrhage. McShane et al.[43] reported on 147 patients with placenta previa of whom 11 had placenta accreta. Five required hysterectomy to control hemorrhaging. In this study, 27% of women with placenta previa who had previously undergone cesarean section had placenta accreta.

When hemorrhage is anticipated, placental removal manipulations to correct uterine atony should be immediately instituted. Uterine massage, intravenous infusion of oxytocin (Pitocin), intravenous or intramuscular methylergonovine, and intramuscular or intramyometrial prostaglandin $F_{2\alpha}$ analogs (PGF$_2$) can be used. Inspection for lacerations into the uterine vasculature or extension into the lower uterine segment should be performed. When these measures fail, bilateral hypogastric artery ligation has been considered as the next step.

In our experience, many obstetricians are uncomfortable performing hypogastric artery ligations during cesarean section to control massive hemorrhage. They often prefer to perform a supracervical or total abdominal hysterectomy to achieve this goal. However, a hysterectomy does not always achieve hemostasis. When we have been asked to assist in controlling massive bleeding after the latter surgeries, bilateral hypogastric artery ligations are promptly performed to reduce the amount of blood flow to identify sites of active bleeding, which then can be controlled by mechanical techniques. Normally, the clot must first be removed from a blood-filled pelvis using large sponges. After bilateral hypogastric artery ligation,

meticulous inspection must be used to identify bleeding sites that can be controlled with sutures or surgical clips. The technique of ligation is discussed in the preceding section.

An alternative to hypogastric artery ligation for the management of uterine bleeding during cesarean section is a bilateral uterine artery ligation, which is done to save the uterus. If bleeding persists after uterine artery ligation, the ovarian arterial supply may be ligated at the uteroovarian ligament (see Fig. 15-3). By selecting the uteroovarian ligament rather than the infundibulopelvic ligament, ovarian function is not disturbed. Indeed, a successful pregnancy has been reported in a woman in whom postpartum hemorrhage was controlled during a previous cesarean section by bilateral uterine and ovarian artery ligations.[44]

AbdRabbo[1] has described a stepwise uterine devascularization for management of uncontrollable postpartum hemorrhage with preservation of the uterus in 103 women that included sequential unilateral or bilateral uterine artery ligation, lower uterine vessel ligation, and then sequential unilateral or bilateral ovarian artery ligation. The entire protocol was successful in controlling hemorrhage in 100% of patients. No hysterectomies were performed in this series. Unilateral or bilateral uterine artery ligation alone was effective in 83% of patients. The high success rate may reflect earlier intervention as the author's experience developed in the management of postpartum hemorrhages. An additional innovative method to control focal hemorrhage using excision and layered closure of an atonic placental implantation site has been reported.[42]

Diffuse oozing from cut tissue edges usually is due to a coagulopathy accompanying the massive hemorrhage and associated massive transfusions. Because of the massive blood loss commonly incurred during an obstetric hemorrhage, the development of DIC is always a possibility and should be treated immediately. Once the surgeon attends to mechanically controllable bleeding, he or she should close the abdomen and manage the coagulopathy with blood replacement products.

Some physicians have advocated uterine packing to control bleeding during cesarean section. However, this is a measure of last resort and has generally been abandoned.[70] Packing can obscure continued hemorrhage and delay definitive therapy. Control of postpartum hemorrhage from a placental implantation site in the lower uterine segment following packing with thrombin-soaked gauze has been reported.[7] Case reports in 1996 suggested that uterine tamponade can be achieved using one or more Foley catheters to control hemorrhage secondary to postpartum atony, cervical hemorrhage caused by a low-lying placenta, or bleeding secondary to a cone biopsy.[17] The intrauterine Foley catheters were distended with up to 80 ml of saline in the postpartum hemorrhage cases, after standard therapy failed to control the bleeding. Transcatheter arterial embolization techniques may be required if mechanical measures are unsuccessful in managing uterine hemorrhage. These techniques are discussed later.

Postpartum Hemorrhage

Postpartum hemorrhage is most often related to uterine atony.[2] Predisposing conditions of atony include hydramnios, multiple gestation, macrosomia, high parity, intrauterine infection, precipitous or prolonged labor, preeclampsia, and use of halogenated anesthetics and uterine relaxants such as magnesium sulfate or tocolytics. Hemorrhage immediately after vaginal delivery should prompt an assessment of uterine tone. Bimanual massage of the uterus with simultaneous administration of oxytocics or prostaglandin analogs often controls uterine atony and should be promptly initiated. Postpartum hemorrhage was controlled in 22 of 26 patients receiving intramuscular 15-methyl-prostaglandin F_2.[10] Side effects include fever, nausea, vomiting, diarrhea, and hypertension. Prostaglandin E_2 (PGE_2) intravaginal suppositories also have been used to treat postpartum hemorrhage.[33] Continuous intrauterine irrigation with PGE_2 has recently been reported in 22 women, with success in all.[51]

Uterine atony can result from retained placental fragments or products of conception. Manual exploration of the uterus should be routinely performed in instances of postpartum hemorrhage. The placenta should be inspected at each delivery to ensure placental fragments or succenturiate lobes are not retained in the uterus. Placental implantation in the noncontractile lower uterine segment can result in hemorrhage nonresponsive to oxytocics. Tamponade of this area using a large Foley catheter balloon has been successful.[9] Even if ultimately unsuccessful, this maneuver may allow preparation of the patient for transarterial catheter embolization or surgery. Hypogastric artery ligation usually is unsuccessful when the cause of postpartum hemorrhage is uterine atony.

Pelvic ultrasound can be useful in evaluating uterine contents and identifying intraperitoneal free fluid, suggesting uterine rupture.[37] The ultrasound examination also can delineate an intrauterine clot or retained placental fragments. Gentle sharp curettage of the uterus is the next step if placenta remnants are present, but great care must be taken not to perforate the uterine wall.

If atony is not present, a careful inspection of the cervix and vagina to identify mucosal lacerations should be carried out. Rapid delivery, macrosomia, and forceps delivery are factors associated with occurrence of lacerations. Cervical and vaginal lacerations should be repaired with a running absorbable suture. Uterine rupture should be considered, particularly in women who have undergone vaginal delivery after cesarean section or after uterine surgery such as myomectomy. Uterine inversion can also result in postpartum hemorrhage. After abortion, similar causes of hemorrhage must be considered, including uterine atony, vaginal or cervical lacerations, and uterine perforation. Arterial embolization in the angiography suite may avert surgical exploration. Arterial ligation or hysterectomy may be required if less invasive techniques are unsuccessful. Alternative therapies, such as local infusions of vasopressors through fluoroscopically placed arterial catheters, have been described.[46,58]

MANAGEMENT OF MASSIVE HEMORRHAGE
Treatment Options

Interventional Radiology. Interventional radiologic techniques were first used in the management of massive hemorrhage in desperately ill gynecologic cancer patients.[57,58] These patients often had suppressed bone marrow or had previously been irradiated in the region of the bleeding and were not amenable to immediate operation to control the hemorrhage because of cardiovascular instability. Interventional radiologic techniques were not initially recognized as valuable in benign gynecology or obstetrics because massive hemorrhage was an uncommon complication. However, during the past two decades angiographic techniques have been introduced into the successful management of massive postpartum hemorrhage and into benign gynecologic processes that have led to such hemorrhage.* The application of these techniques may allow women to avoid hysterectomy and preserve reproductive function.

Selective Arteriography. Selective arteriography initially was used to identify bleeding sites so that surgical strategies could be used to control the hemorrhage. Subsequently, it was recognized that the same arterial catheters placed into the vessels that led to the bleeding site could also deliver vasoactive agents to control the bleeding. Vasopressin became the most commonly used vasoactive agent and was infused through selective arterial catheter techniques to control bleeding secondary to esophageal varices, gastric ulcers, and intestinal anastomosis sites.[66] The complications from vasopressin infusion included systemic effects from the pharmacologic agent and ischemic damage to bowel. Thrombosis or infection at the catheter site occurred because these catheters often had to be left in place several days with the infusion running to control the bleeding. The combination of regional intraarterial infusion of a vasoconstrictor (dopamine, norepinephrine) with transcatheter embolization and use of a military antishock trousers (MAST) suit has been applied recently with successful control of pelvic hemorrhage.

Catheterization. Balloon catheters that could be inserted into larger blood vessels under fluoroscopic guidance were subsequently developed. Inflation of the balloon obstructed the vessel proximal to the bleeding site and controlled the hemorrhage.[58,69] This technique has had little use in gynecologic oncology. Stainless steel coils (e.g., Gianturco coils) also have been developed and can be placed through selective arterial catheterization techniques into bleeding vessels. The stainless steel coils are most valuable when the vessel is short (e.g., the renal vessels); this situation makes arterial embolization techniques dangerous to carry out because embolized material might reflux into the aorta and lead to distant embolization and ischemic complications. Finally, liquid tissue adhesives have been developed that can be passed through arterial catheters and that congeal on entry into the bloodstream. Liquid tissue adhe-

---

*References 24, 25, 29, 34, 50, 64, 71.

sives have had limited application in the management of hemorrhage secondary to obstetric and gynecologic processes.

Transcatheter Embolization. The most frequently used technique for the management of massive hemorrhage in obstetrics and gynecology has been transcatheter embolization of synthetic material. This technique initially began with embolization of autologous tissue or autologous blood clot for management of massive hemorrhage.[26,58] Because patients with massive hemorrhage frequently have an associated coagulopathy, it was necessary to add pharmacologic agents to make the blood clot rapidly.[8] The development of an absorbable surgical gelatin sponge (Gelfoam) shows that synthetic material can be safely used in the transcatheter management of massive hemorrhage. At Yale–New Haven Hospital, Gelfoam particles formed by dicing Gelfoam pads into small pieces are routinely used rather than Gelfoam powder because the latter may obstruct the vasa nervorum, causing nerve injury.[29]

SELECTIVE ARTERIOGRAPHY AND EMBOLIZATION TECHNIQUES

For selective arteriography to identify a bleeding site, it is necessary that the patient bleed at a rate greater than 0.5 ml/min.[47] If the patient is not actively bleeding during arteriography, the bleeding site will not be recognized. The performance of arteriography is based on the Seldinger technique. A hollow needle with a stent is placed in a major artery. The stent is then removed and a flexible stainless steel guidewire is advanced through the needle into the artery. For obstetric and gynecologic patients, the femoral artery is commonly accessed. The guidewire is advanced into the abdominal aorta under fluoroscopic control. The needle is removed over the guidewire, and a flexible polyethylene catheter is inserted over the guidewire and advanced into the aorta. Usually the tip of the catheter is preformed so that it can be guided into divisions of the abdominal aorta. Once the guidewire is removed, a lower abdominal arteriogram is performed to identify the bleeding sites in the pelvis.

After the aortogram has identified the most likely bleeding sites, the arterial catheter is selectively inserted under fluoroscopy into one of the major arteries supplying the bleeding site. In the authors' experience, the most common sources for bleeding in the pelvis have been the hypogastric arteries, the fourth lumbar artery, and the median circumflex femoral artery. The bleeding less commonly originates from the ovarian artery or the inferior epigastric artery. It is always necessary to consider dual blood supply to bleeding sites.[11] Certainly, the intact uterus has multiple sources of blood supply including two uterine and ovarian arteries. In dealing with complications in gynecologic cancer management, the dual blood supply of the stomach and the duodenum must also be considered.

One limitation of selective arteriography to determine the arterial source for bleeding is massive hemorrhage

which leads to severe volume depletion and resultant arterial spasm, producing a false-negative result on arteriographic examination. It may be necessary to give glucagon intraarterially to dilate the vessels to establish the bleeding source.

Individual physician experience in performing selective arteriography and transcatheter embolization of synthetic material is critical for success.[29,64] The circumstances of massive hemorrhage require that the most experienced personnel be actively involved in the selective arteriography and embolization techniques. Unilateral embolization of pelvic sidewall vessels, including the hypogastric artery, is insufficient for the successful control of massive hemorrhage in the pelvis. One must evaluate arteriographically the blood supply to both pelvic sidewalls and routinely embolize both hypogastric arteries, when intact, to stop the bleeding. The procedure must not be abandoned if no obvious bleeding site is identified after a cursory arteriographic examination has been performed. The source of the massive bleeding is frequently small vessels that require selective arteriographic approaches.[48] The fourth lumbar and the medium circumflex arteries, and at times accessory obturator vessels arising from the inferior epigastric artery, may be injured and may not be associated with obvious bleeding on a screening aortogram.

Patient support during the procedure must be extensive. At Yale–New Haven Hospital, a shock team that includes anesthesiologists, interventional radiologists, and gynecologic oncologists actively participates in the management of massive hemorrhage in obstetric or gynecologic patients. A team effort is required to successfully take the very sick patient in hemorrhagic shock through interventional radiologic techniques.

Case Studies

Some examples of our successful use of this technique to control massive bleeding in gynecologic surgical situations include a patient who underwent a cone biopsy for evaluation of a carcinoma in situ of the cervix. She hemorrhaged during the biopsy; the hemorrhage was apparently controlled with suture ligatures, but the patient developed recurrent postoperative bleeding twice during the ensuing month and required suture ligation in the operating room. A hysterectomy appeared to be the next appropriate step to control the massive bleeding, because it was not permanently controllable by suture ligation on the two prior occasions. Fig. 15-7, *A,* shows a selective hypogastric arteriogram revealing that the source of this patient's bleeding was the left uterine artery. After selective embolization of that vessel (see Fig. 15-7, *B*), the bleeding was completely controlled. The patient subsequently had a normal term pregnancy.

This technique also was successfully used for a bicycle straddle injury in a 27-year-old woman. The patient had a 15 cm right labial hematoma. Fig. 15-8 shows the source of the bleeding: a branch of the right pudendal artery. Rather than performing an evacuation in the operating room and packing this extensive hematoma, the patient underwent a Gel-

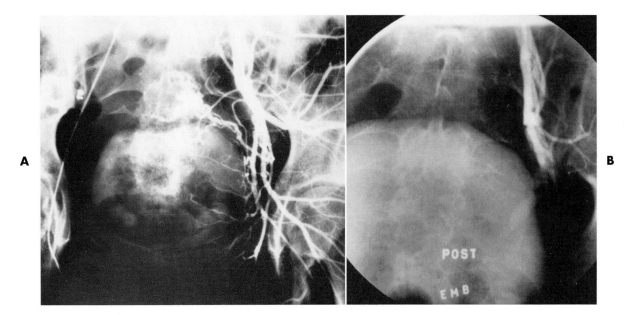

Fig. 15-7 **A,** Selective left hypogastric arteriogram, demonstrating that the source of uterine bleeding after a cone biopsy is the left uterine artery. **B,** Complete control of bleeding achieved after transcatheter embolization of Gelfoam.

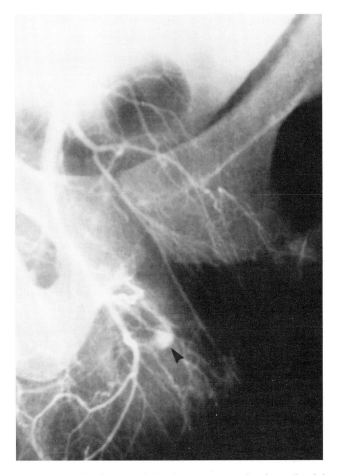

Fig. 15-8 Bleeding into labia from an injured right pudendal artery after a bicycle straddle injury. The *arrow* indicates the bleeding site.

foam embolization of the right internal pudendal artery with no untoward effects.

A patient with von Willebrand's disease underwent an elective pregnancy termination at 8 weeks' gestation.[32] The patient received preoperative and postoperative cryoprecipitate at the time of suction dilation and curettage (D&C). However, massive hemorrhage occurred 16 days later and was unresponsive to cryoprecipitate, D&C, uterine packing, antibiotics, and oxytocin administration. This patient underwent bilateral hypogastric arterial embolization, and the bleeding was completely controlled.

These approaches have been used in the management of massive postpartum hemorrhage. Fig. 15-9 shows a lower abdominal aortogram revealing a ligated left hypogastric artery. The patient had undergone a laparotomy for what proved to be an unsuspected intraabdominal pregnancy. When the pregnancy was recognized to be intraabdominal, a hysterectomy and removal of the placenta from the left pelvic sidewall were performed. Because of massive hemorrhage, a vascular surgeon was asked to ligate the left hypogastric artery. The ligation initially controlled the bleeding, but the patient subsequently required 33 units of blood to replace intraabdominal blood loss. The patient was taken to the interventional radiography suite rather than the operating room because she was hemodynamically unstable. An aortogram confirmed that the patient was bleeding from the hypogastric artery distal to the ligation site. The patient first underwent an embolization of the right hypogastric artery. Subsequent selective arteriography revealed a communication between the left fourth lumbar artery and the left hypogastric vessels (see Fig. 15-9). This vessel was embolized. A subsequent selective arteriogram identified the presence of collateral circulation to the left pelvic sidewall through the

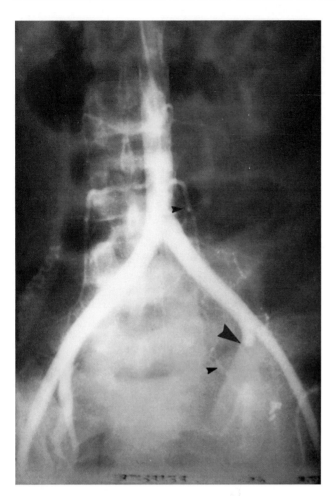

Fig. 15-9 A lower abdominal aortogram revealing a ligated left hypogastric artery *(large arrow)* in a patient massively bleeding intraabdominally after removal of an intraabdominal pregnancy, the placenta having implanted on the left pelvic sidewall. A unilateral hypogastric artery ligation was performed at the time of surgery to control bleeding. Collateral circulation between the left fourth lumbar artery *(small arrows)* and the left hypogastric vessels *(large arrow)* was controlled by selective arteriography and Gelfoam embolization of the lumbar artery.

left median circumflex femoral artery, which also was embolized, and all bleeding ceased.

Abnormal placentation is the most common reason for massive hemorrhage in obstetric patients. A patient underwent an elective cesarean hysterectomy for delivery of her third child after having two pregnancies complicated by placenta accreta. The patient underwent an uncomplicated cesarean hysterectomy but went into shock in the recovery room. She remained hemodynamically unstable despite 10 units of blood replacement. The patient was taken to the angiography suite where a hypogastric arteriogram revealed abnormal venous structures involving the right (Fig. 15-10, A) and left pelvic sidewalls (see Fig. 15-10, B). After having bilateral hypogastric artery embolization, the patient stopped bleeding and required no further blood replacement. Her postoperative course was uncomplicated.

Hypogastric artery ligation to control bleeding during surgery can be very effective. However, once a hypogastric artery ligation has been performed and bleeding persists, the opportunity to rapidly perform selective arteriography and transcatheter embolization is limited because alternative access through the rich collateral circulation of the postpartum pelvis must be sought. For example, a 24-year-old primigravida underwent a cesarean section for failure to progress.[29] The cesarean section was complicated by a uterine artery laceration at surgery and a subsequent vaginal hemorrhage and fever 6 days postoperatively. The patient was hospitalized and responded to the transfusions of 2 units of blood and 3 days of intravenous antibiotics. She was discharged and went into hypovolemic shock on the twelfth postoperative day. The patient returned to the hospital and underwent a prompt exploratory laparotomy, subtotal hysterectomy, and bilateral hypogastric artery legations because of persistent bleeding. However, she continued to bleed "briskly." She received 10 units of blood and 4 units of FFP, at which point the community hospital's blood bank reported to the surgeon that all blood had been exhausted. The patient was transferred to Yale–New Haven Hospital in a MAST suit. She was stable on admission, and an initial emergency arteriogram revealed no active bleeding. However, 2 hours later, the patient hemorrhaged. The preembolization arteriogram (Fig. 15-11, A) shows no obvious site of bleeding. A late-phase arteriogram (see Fig. 15-11, B) revealed bleeding from the right pelvic sidewall. Selective arteriography confirmed the right median circumflex femoral artery as the source of hemorrhage (see Fig. 15-11, C). Following embolization of this vessel, all bleeding stopped.

OTHER INDICATIONS FOR SELECTIVE ARTERIOGRAPHY AND EMBOLOTHERAPY

Selective arteriography and embolotherapy have been applied to the management of bleeding in four women with abdominal pregnancies and four women bleeding from cervical ectopic pregnancies.[22,24,36,41,45] Bleeding in all eight ectopic pregnancy patients was successfully managed using this technique. The cervical pregnancies required curettages to complete the treatment.

ADVANTAGES AND DISADVANTAGES OF SELECTIVE ARTERIOGRAPHY AND EMBOLOTHERAPY
Advantages

1. The bleeding site is often extremely difficult or impossible to identify at surgery. Huge clots can be present in the pelvis and in the retroperitoneum after massive hemorrhage, making it extraordinarily difficult to identify normal anatomic structures.
2. Injury to the ureters, bladder, or bowel can occur during a surgical attempt to identify the site of bleeding.

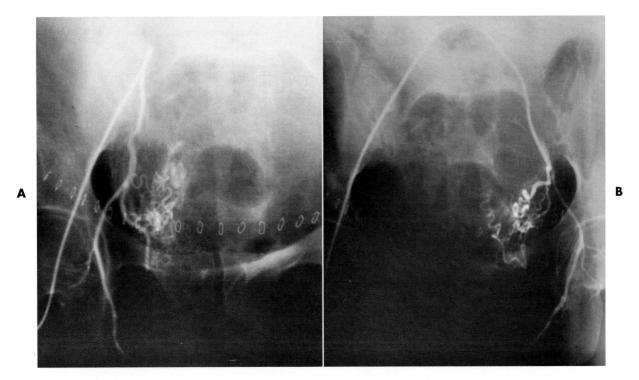

Fig. 15-10   **A,** Abnormal vascular pattern involving the right pelvic sidewall in a patient hemorrhaging after a cesarean hysterectomy. **B,** Abnormal vascular pattern involving the left pelvic sidewall.

3. The rich collateral circulation associated with pregnancy can negate the effects of hypogastric ligation in that circumstance.

4. A hysterectomy can be avoided and fertility can be preserved with successful selective arterial embolization techniques.

5. It is much easier to identify and embolize branches of the hypogastric artery before surgical intervention than after hypogastric artery ligation has failed to control the bleeding. The tiny Gelfoam particles that are embolized through the arterial catheter travel farther down the arterial tree than the site where the hypogastric artery is routinely ligated surgically. These particles often go beyond the sites where the collateral circulation enters into the arterial tree. Thus a transcatheter hypogastric artery Gelfoam particle embolization is far more effective in most circumstances.[3]

Disadvantages

1. It may take from 1 to 6 hours to be accomplished successfully.

2. The embolized material might be dislodged, embolize further into other parts of the arterial tree, and cause complications.[29] However, the long length of the hypogastric artery and most of the other vessels involved in routine pelvic hemorrhage are such that the problem of secondary particle embolization is unlikely.

3. Necrosis of normal tissue may occur,[34] but more likely as a result of embolizing vessels that supply the intestine.

The rich vascular supply of the postpartum pelvis and, indeed, the blood to the pelvis in general are such that necrosis of normal tissue is not a routine complication when embolotherapy controls bleeding from pelvic sites.

Selective arteriography and embolization techniques can be performed in community hospital diagnostic imaging departments. Most departments have angiographers routinely performing these techniques in the management of trauma patients and evaluation of cardiac and other disorders. The technical development of digital substraction angiograms makes identification of bleeding sites easier to recognize.[64] Gynecologists and obstetricians should alert the angiographer to be on standby when a patient is likely to have massive hemorrhage. Interventional radiologic techniques can avert significant complications associated with surgery in a hemodynamically unstable patient in whom one is trying to control massive hemorrhage.

Methods for control of hemorrhage in the obstetric and gynecologic patient have been reviewed. The best of these is prevention. Preparation in anticipation of hemorrhagic complications can minimize the severity of bleeding and allow preservation of reproductive ability in selected patients.

Prompt action to control hemorrhage must be instituted in each instance. The cause of bleeding, whether anatomic or hematologic, must be sought and corrected. Knowledge of the broad armamentarium available to the practitioner and of the facilities and individual consultants in one's own institution is vital when facing a hemorrhagic complication.

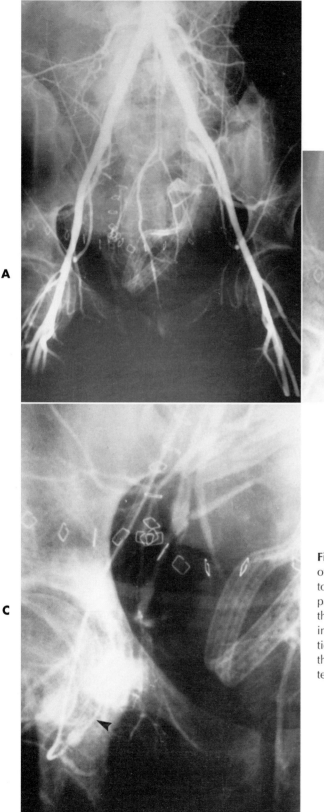

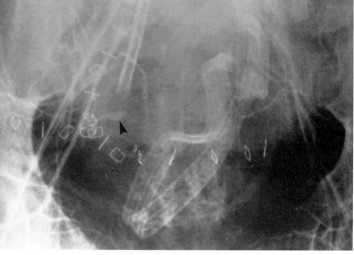

Fig. 15-11   A, Aortogram revealing no evidence of extravasation of contrast in a patient who had undergone a subtotal hysterectomy and bilateral hypogastric artery ligations for massive postpartum hemorrhage. No active bleeding was clinically evident at the time of this study. **B,** A late-phase arteriogram revealing bleeding from the right pelvic sidewall *(arrow)* 2 hours after **A.** The patient was now vigorously bleeding per vagina. **C,** The source of the bleeding *(arrow)* was the right median circumflex femoral artery, which was then embolized to control the bleeding.

REFERENCES

1. AbdRabbo SA: Stepwise uterine devascularization: a novel technique for management of uncontrollable postpartum hemorrhage with preservation of the uterus, *Am J Obstet Gynecol* 171:694, 1994.

2. American College of Obstetricians and Gynecologists: Diagnosis and management of postpartum hemorrhage, technical bulletin no 143, July 1990.

3. Athanasoulis CA: Therapeutic applications of angiography, *N Engl J Med* 302:1117, 1980.

4. Beck WS, editor: *Hematology,* ed 4, Cambridge, Mass, 1985, MIT Press.

5. Beller U, Rosen RJ, Beckman EM, et al: Congenital arteriovenous malformation of the female pelvis: a gynecologic perspective, *Am J Obstet Gynecol* 159:1153, 1988.

6. Bick RL: *Disseminated intravascular coagulation and related syndrome,* Boca Raton, Fla, 1983, CRC Press.

7. Bobrowski RA, Jones TB: A thrombogenic uterine pack for postpartum hemorrhage, *Obstet Gynecol* 85:836, 1995.

8. Bookstein JJ, Chlosta EM, Foley D, Walter JF: Transcatheter hemostasis of gastrointestinal bleeding using modified autogenous clot, *Radiology* 113:277, 1974.

9. Bowen LW, Beeson JH: Use of a large Foley catheter balloon to control postpartum hemorrhage resulting from a low placental implantation, *J Reprod Med* 30:623, 1985.

10. Buttino L Jr, Garite TJ: The use of 15 methyl F$_2$ alpha prostaglandin (Prostin 15M) for the control of postpartum hemorrhage, *Am J Perinatol* 3:241, 1986.

11. Chait A, Moltz A, Nelson JH Jr: The collateral arterial circulation in the pelvis: an angiographic study, *Am J Roentgenol* 102:392, 1968.

12. Chattopadhyay SK, Deb Roy B, Edrees YB: Surgical control of obstetric hemorrhage: hypogastric artery ligation or hysterectomy? *Int J Gynaecol Obstet* 32:345, 1990.

13. Clark SL, Phelan JP, Yeh SY, et al: Hypogastric artery ligation for obstetric hemorrhage, *Obstet Gynecol* 66:353, 1985.

14. Cruikshank SH, Stoelk EM: Surgical control of pelvic hemorrhage: bilateral hypogastric artery ligation and method of ovarian artery ligation, *South Med J* 78:539, 1985.

15. Day HJ, Rao AK: Evaluation of platelet function, *Semin Hematol* 23:89, 1986.

16. De Caterina R, Lanza M, Manca G, et al: Bleeding time and bleeding: an analysis of the relationship of the bleeding time test with parameters of surgical bleeding, *Blood* 84:3363, 1994.

17. De Loor JA, van Dam PA: Foley catheters for uncontrollable obstetric or gynecologic hemorrhage, *Obstet Gynecol* 88:737, 1996.

18. Evans S, McShane P: The efficacy of internal iliac artery ligation in obstetric hemorrhage, *Surg Gynecol Obstet* 160:250, 1985.

19. Fahmy K: Uterine artery ligation to control postpartum hemorrhage, *Int J Gynaecol Obstet* 25:363, 1987.

20. Feinstein DI: Diagnosis and management of disseminated intravascular coagulation: the role of heparin therapy, *Blood* 60:284, 1982.

21. Forssman L, Lundberg J, Schersten T: Conservative treatment of uterine arteriovenous fistula, *Acta Obstet Gynecol Scand* 61:85, 1982.

22. Frates MC, Benson CB, Doubilet PM, et al: Cervical ectopic pregnancy: results of conservative treatment, *Radiology* 191:773, 1994.

23. Ghosh TK: Arteriovenous malformation of the uterus and pelvis, *Obstet Gynecol* 68:40, 1986.

24. Gilbert WM, Moore, TR, Resnik R, et al: Angiographic embolization in the management of hemorrhagic complications of pregnancy, *Am J Obstet Gynecol* 166:493, 1992.

25. Glickman MG: Pelvic artery embolization. In Berkowitz RL, editor: *Critical care of the obstetric patient,* New York, 1983, Churchill Livingstone.

26. Goldstein HM, Medellin H, Ben-Menachem Y, Wallace S: Transcatheter arterial embolization in the management of bleeding in the cancer patient, *Radiology* 115:603, 1975.

27. Gray LA: Open cuff method of abdominal hysterectomy, *Obstet Gynecol* 46:42, 1975.

28. Green D, Wong CA, Twardowski P: Efficacy of hemostatic agents in improving surgical hemostasis, *Transfus Med Rev* 10:171, 1996.

29. Greenwood LH, Glickman MG, Schwartz PE, et al: Obstetric and nonmalignant gynecologic bleeding: treatment with angiographic embolization, *Radiology* 164:155, 1987.

30. Harker LA, Slichter SJ: The bleeding time as a screening test for evaluation of platelet function, *N Engl J Med* 287:155, 1972.

31. Harrigan C, Lucas CE, Ledgerwood AM, Mammen EF: Primary hemostasis after massive transfusion for injury, *Am Surg* 48:393, 1992.

32. Haseltine FP, Glickman MG, Marchesi S, et al: Uterine embolization in a patient with postabortal hemorrhage, *Obstet Gynecol* 63(suppl):78, 1984.

33. Hertz RH, Sokol RJ, Dierker LJ: Treatment of postpartum uterine atony with prostaglandin E2 vaginal suppositories, *Obstet Gynecol* 56:129, 1980.

34. Jander HP, Russinovich NA: Transcatheter Gelfoam embolization in abdominal, retroperitoneal, and pelvic hemorrhage, *Radiology* 136:337, 1980.

35. Kaunitz AM, Hughes JM, Grimes DA, et al: Causes of maternal mortality in the United States, *Obstet Gynecol* 65:605, 1985.

36. Kivikoski AI, Martin C, Weyman P, et al: Angiographic arterial embolization to control hemorrhage in abdominal pregnancy: a case report, *Obstet Gynecol* 71:456, 1988.

37. Lee CY, Madrazo B, Drukker BH: Ultrasonic evaluation of the postpartum uterus in the management of postpartum bleeding, *Obstet Gynecol* 58:227, 1981.

38. Lethagen S: Desmopressin (DDAVP) and hemostasis, *Ann Hematol* 69:173, 1994.

39. Likeman RK: The boldest procedure possible for checking the bleeding—a new look at an old operation, and a series of 13 cases from an Australian hospital, *Aust N Z J Obstet Gynaecol* 32:256, 1992.

40. Malviya VK, Deppe G: Control of intraoperative hemorrhage in gynecology with the use of fibrin glue, *Obstet Gynecol* 73:284, 1989.

41. Martin JN, Ridgway LE, Connors JJ, et al: Angiographic arterial embolization and computed tomography–directed drainage for the management of hemorrhage and infection with abdominal pregnancy, *Obstet Gynecol* 76:941, 1990.

42. McGuinness TB, Jackson JR, Schnapf DJ: Conservative surgical management of placental implantation site hemorrhage, *Obstet Gynecol* 81:830, 1993.

43. McShane PM, Heyl PS, Epstein MF: Maternal and perinatal morbidity resulting from placenta previa, *Obstet Gynecol* 65:176, 1985.

44. Mengert WF, Burchell RC, Blumstein RW, Daskal JL: Pregnancy after bilateral ligation of the internal iliac and ovarian arteries, *Obstet Gynecol* 34:664, 1969.

45. Mitty HA, Sterling KM, Alvarez M, Gendler R: Obstetric hemorrhage: prophylactic and emergency arterial catheterization and embolotherapy, *Radiology* 188:183, 1993.

46. Mud HJ, Schattenkerk ME, de Vries JE, Bruining HA: Nonsurgical treatment of pelvic hemorrhage in obstetric and gynecologic patients, *Crit Care Med* 15:534, 1987.

47. Nusbaum M, Baum S: Radiographic demonstration of unknown sites gastrointestinal bleeding, *Surg Forum* 14:374, 1963.

48. O'Hanlan KA, Trambert J, Rodriguez-Rodriguez L, et al: Arterial embolization in the management of abdominal and retroperitoneal hemorrhage, *Gynecol Oncol* 34:131, 1989.

49. O'Leary JA. Uterine artery ligation in the control of postcesarean hemorrhage, *J Reprod Med* 40:189, 1995.

50. Pais SO, Glickman M, Schwartz PE, Pingoud E, Berkowitz R. Embolization of pelvic arteries for control of postpartum hemorrhage, *Obstet Gynecol* 55:754, 1980.

51. Peyser MR, Kupfermine MJ: Management of severe postpartum hemorrhage by intrauterine irrigation with prostaglandin E2, *Am J Obstet Gynecol* 162:694, 1990.

52. Prydz H: Triggering of the extrinsic blood coagulation system. In Thornsom JM, editor: *Blood coagulation and haemostasis,* ed 3, New York, 1985, Churchill Livingstone.

53. Reece EA, Foik HE, Rappaport F: Factor VIII inhibitor: a cause of severe postpartum hemorrhage, *Am J Obstet Gynecol* 144:985, 1982.

54. Rodgers RP, Levin J. A critical reappraisal of the bleeding time, *Semin Thromb Hemost* 16:1, 1990.

55. Rosenthal DM, Colapinto R: Angiographic arterial embolization in the management of postoperative vaginal hemorrhage, *Am J Obstet Gynecol* 151:227, 1985.

56. Sattler FR, Weitekamp MR, Ballard JO: Potential for bleeding with the new beta-lactam antibiotics, *Ann Intern Med* 105:924, 1986.

57. Schwartz PE: Arterial hemorrhage in gynecologic malignancies. In Delgado G, Smith JP, editors: *Management of complications in gynecologic oncology,* New York, 1982, John Wiley.

58. Schwartz PE, Goldstein HM, Wallace S, Rutledge FN: Control of arterial hemorrhage using percutaneous arterial catheter techniques in patients with gynecologic malignancies, *Gynecol Oncol* 3:276, 1975.

59. Sramek A, Eikenboom JC, Briet E, et al: Usefulness of patient interview in bleeding disorders, *Arch Intern Med* 155:1409, 1995.

60. Steinberg MH, Saletan S, Funt M, et al: Management of factor XI deficiency in gynecologic and obstetric patients, *Obstet Gynecol* 68:130, 1986.

61. Suchman AL, Griner PF: Diagnostic uses of the activated partial thromboplastin time and prothrombin time, *Ann Intern Med* 104:810, 1986.

62. Tawes RL Jr, Sydorak GR, DuVall TB: Autologous fibrin glue: the last step in operative hemostasis, *Am J Surg* 168:120, 1994.

63. Thavarasah AS, Sivalingam N, Almohdzar SA: Internal iliac and ovarian artery ligation in the control of pelvic hemorrhage, *Aust N Z J Obstet Gynaecol* 29:22, 1989.

64. Vedantham S, Goodwin SC, McLucas B, Mohr G. Uterine artery embolization: an underused method of controlling pelvic hemorrhage, *Am J Obstet Gynecol* 176:938, 1997.

65. Wallerstein RO Jr: Laboratory evaluation of a bleeding patient, *West J Med* 150:51, 1989.

66. Waltman AC, Greenfield AJ, Novelline RA, Athanasoulis CA: Pyloroduodenal bleeding and intraarterial vasopressin: clinical results, *Am J Roentgenol* 133:643, 1979.

67. Weaver DW: Differential diagnosis and management of unexplained bleeding, *Surg Clin North Am* 73:353, 1993.

68. White SC, Wartel L, Wade ME: Comparison of abdominal and vaginal hysterectomies: a review of 600 operations, *Obstet Gynecol* 37:530, 1971.

69. Wholey MH, Stockdale R, Hung TK: A percutaneous balloon catheter for the immediate control of hemorrhage, *Radiology* 95:65, 1970.

70. Wittich AC, Salminen ER, Hardin EL, Desantis RA: Uterine packing in the combined management of obstetrical hemorrhage, *Mil Med* 161:180, 1996.

71. Yamashita Y, Harada M, Yamamoto H, et al: Transcatheter arterial embolization of obstetric and gynaecological bleeding: efficacy and clinical outcome, *Br J Radiol* 67:530, 1994.

16 Minor and Ambulatory Surgery

DAVID H. NICHOLS

Surgeons regularly perform minor gynecologic surgery in an office setting, although they generally perform procedures that require any significant surgical dissection in the operating room of an ambulatory care center or a hospital. Patients may not need an anesthetic for the simplest maneuvers, such as endometrial biopsy, but they should receive effective anesthesia, often by local infiltration, if the discomfort is likely to be severe or more than momentary.

BIOPSY OF THE VULVA

Local anesthesia is appropriate for a patient undergoing biopsy of a suspicious lesion of the vulva. The surgeon can obtain a sample of the full thickness of the vulvar skin by using the Keyes skin biopsy drill (Fig. 16-1). Alternatively, a sharp biopsy punch can be used to obtain one or more specimens. Then the base of the biopsy site should be coagulated to minimize bleeding.

SURGERY OF BARTHOLIN'S GLAND

Although a Bartholin's cyst usually compresses Bartholin's gland around its deep periphery, making the gland invisible to the naked eye, the cyst is actually of the duct rather than of the gland. The surgical excision of such a cyst is often a formidable procedure because the vascularity of the tissues in this area can result in an unexpectedly high blood loss. Unless there is an opening to the external skin, the future secretions of the remaining buried but functional glandular tissue can reaccumulate and create a new and often symptomatic cyst requiring reexcision.

An acute Bartholin's abscess can be treated initially by aspiration with a no. 19 needle and syringe. The aspirate should be sent for bacteriologic identification, culture, and sensitivity testing. Cultures may show pure anaerobic, aerobic, or mixed bacteria. Bacteroides of various groups and *Peptostreptococci* are the most common anaerobes, whereas *Escherichia coli* and *Neisseria gonorrhoea* are predominant aerobes. Meanwhile, the patient should begin a 7-day regimen of 400 mg of metronidazole two times daily and 250 mg of penicillin four times daily. If the infecting organism is found to be *N. gonorrhoea,* the patient should be given 1 g of probenecid and 3.5 g of ampicillin. When tissue edema subsides, the patency and function of the duct return to normal in approximately 80% of cases.[9]

Incision and drainage of a Bartholin's abscess can be performed in the vestibular area close to the hymen through an area of fluctuation. The surgeon should make a 1- to 2-inch incision and insert a drain or wick, which should remain in place for 24 hours. Because the skin heals and seals itself rapidly, recurrence is not uncommon, particularly if the infection has damaged the duct.

A simple, alternative treatment of a Bartholin's cyst is to create a new duct by inserting a Word catheter through a stab wound into the cyst cavity, inflating the bulb with saline, and allowing it to remain in place for 3 to 4 weeks until the track of the wound has become epithelialized, thus forming the new duct (Fig. 16-2).[27] The surgeon should always inflate the bulb with saline rather than air because the latter may permit premature deflation. While the small catheter is in place, the protruding proximal end can be tucked out of the way into the vagina. At the end of the 3- to 4-week period, the bulb on the catheter is deflated and the catheter removed. This procedure is particularly useful when infection is present.

A small Foley catheter also can be used to create a new duct. The surgeon inflates the bulb and tightly ligates the entire catheter approximately 3 inches from the site at which it enters the skin. The catheter can be transected just distal to the point of ligation, which should occlude both the central and side lumina. Again, the free end of the catheter can be tucked into the vagina.

A noninfected Bartholin's cyst that is recurrent following previous marsupialization can be treated by laser or excision. If the gynecologist is comfortable with the use of the CO_2 laser, it is an effective and quick method of creating a new duct into a Bartholin's cyst.[25] A 1.5-cm oval defect is created by a circular incision with the laser from the vulvar skin into the cyst cavity at the site of the original duct tract. Antibiotics are not necessary, and healing is complete in about a month.[10] Retreatment can be offered, if necessary, and the cyst wall can be vaporized with a defocused laser beam.[22]

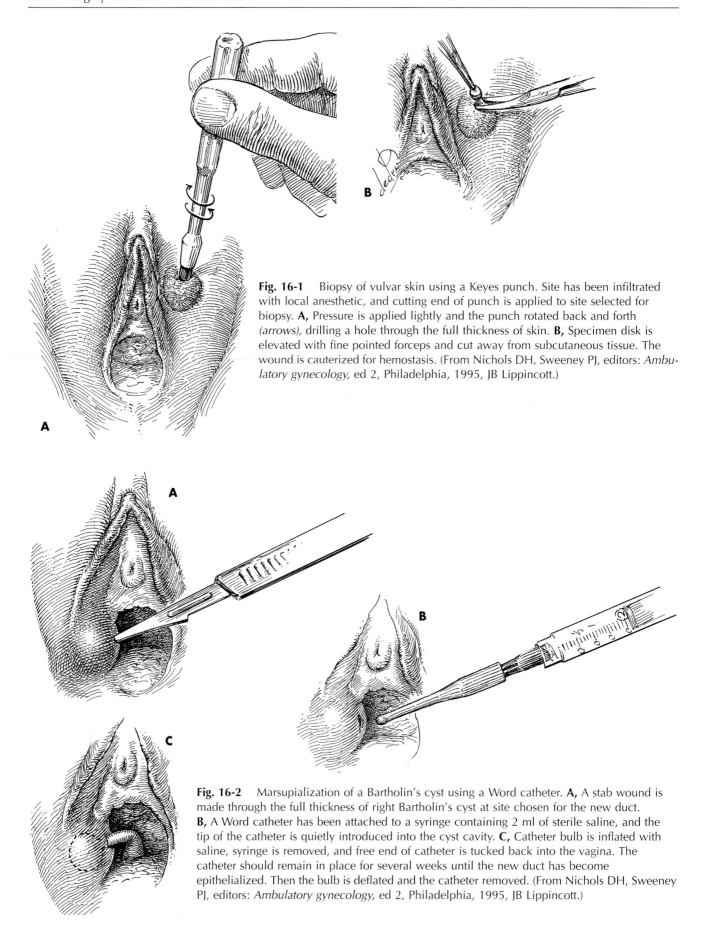

Fig. 16-1   Biopsy of vulvar skin using a Keyes punch. Site has been infiltrated with local anesthetic, and cutting end of punch is applied to site selected for biopsy. **A,** Pressure is applied lightly and the punch rotated back and forth *(arrows),* drilling a hole through the full thickness of skin. **B,** Specimen disk is elevated with fine pointed forceps and cut away from subcutaneous tissue. The wound is cauterized for hemostasis. (From Nichols DH, Sweeney PJ, editors: *Ambulatory gynecology,* ed 2, Philadelphia, 1995, JB Lippincott.)

Fig. 16-2   Marsupialization of a Bartholin's cyst using a Word catheter. **A,** A stab wound is made through the full thickness of right Bartholin's cyst at site chosen for the new duct. **B,** A Word catheter has been attached to a syringe containing 2 ml of sterile saline, and the tip of the catheter is quietly introduced into the cyst cavity. **C,** Catheter bulb is inflated with saline, syringe is removed, and free end of catheter is tucked back into the vagina. The catheter should remain in place for several weeks until the new duct has become epithelialized. Then the bulb is deflated and the catheter removed. (From Nichols DH, Sweeney PJ, editors: *Ambulatory gynecology,* ed 2, Philadelphia, 1995, JB Lippincott.)

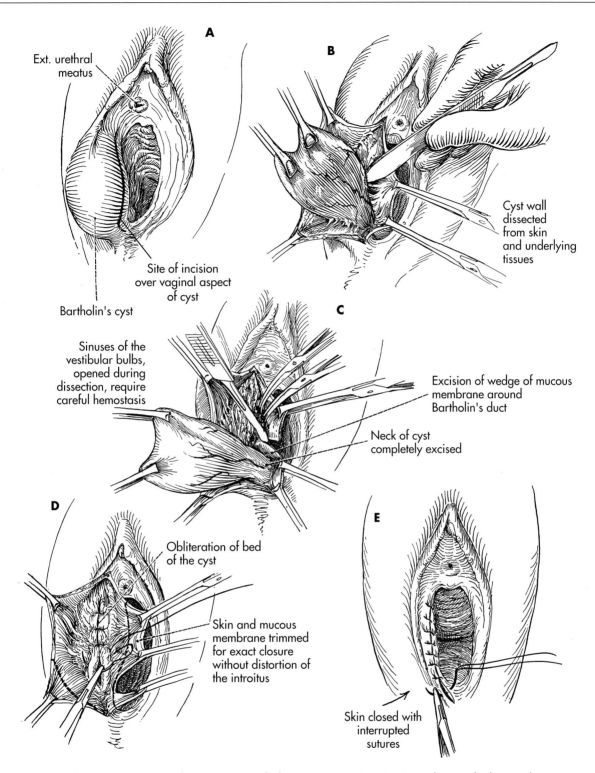

Fig. 16-3 Excision of a recurrent Bartholin's cyst. **A,** An incision is made near the hymenal margin. **B,** The cyst is dissected from the skin and underlying tissues, leaving the flattened gland attached to the cyst wall **(C). D,** Excess skin is trimmed and the deeper tissues approximated with interrupted stitches. **E,** The skin is also closed with interrupted sutures. (From Ball TL: *Gynecologic surgery and urology,* ed 2, St Louis, 1963, Mosby.)

Surgical excision of the cyst should be accomplished under general anesthesia, with great care taken to extirpate the Bartholin's gland itself. The gland usually is compressed beneath the wall of the cyst. It is flattened by the adjacent cyst and can be difficult to distinguish from the surrounding tissue. However, if any fragment of gland remains behind, it ultimately begins to secrete mucus, which, lacking a duct to the skin, will accumulate and form another cyst that may have to be retreated. The operation of excision is shown in Fig. 16-3.

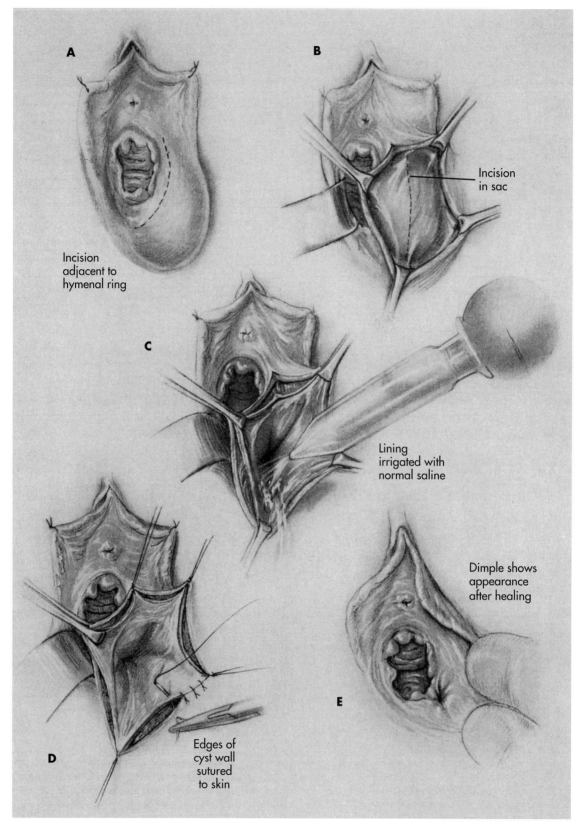

Fig. 16-4 Marsupialization of a Bartholin's cyst. **A,** An incision is made near the site of Bartholin's duct. The wall of the cyst is incised **(B)** and irrigated **(C). D,** The edges of the cyst wall are sutured to the skin. **E,** The new orifice contracts with healing and is represented as a dimple at the site of the original duct. (From Ball TL: *Gynecologic surgery and urology,* ed 2, St Louis, 1963, Mosby.)

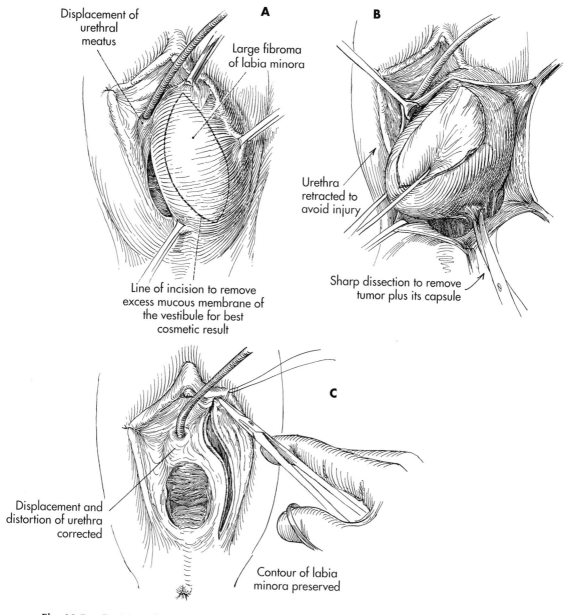

A

Displacement of urethral meatus

Large fibroma of labia minora

Line of incision to remove excess mucous membrane of the vestibule for best cosmetic result

B

Urethra retracted to avoid injury

Sharp dissection to remove tumor plus its capsule

C

Displacement and distortion of urethra corrected

Contour of labia minora preserved

Fig. 16-5 Excision of a vulvar fibroma. **A,** A large fibroma beneath the left labia is shown. It displaces the urethra to the patient's right. The skin incision to be made is shown by the dashed line. **B,** The tumor is removed using sharp dissection. **C,** The incision is closed using interrupted stitches. (From Ball TL: *Gynecologic surgery and urology,* ed 2, St Louis, 1963, Mosby.)

A large, uninfected Bartholin's cyst can be marsupialized. The surgeon cuts a window from the vestibular skin that includes the cyst wall and then sews the edge of the residual cyst lining to the vestibular skin by using a series of interrupted through-and-through stitches. Healing leaves a permanent fistula between the cyst cavity and the skin, which essentially becomes a new duct. The ostium gradually contracts over a period of months, so over time it is scarcely visible but continues to be functional (Fig. 16-4). Bartholin's cyst or abscess also can be treated rapidly with chemicals when alternative treatments or facilities are not available; these include outpatient incision into the cavity using minimal local anesthetic to evacuate it and insertion for 48 hours of a stick of silver nitrate, which coagulates and destroys the lining of the cyst.[48]

A solid lesion within Bartholin's gland requires needle biopsy or surgical excision to exclude malignancy.[1] A tumor of the gland may be adenocarcinoma; a tumor of the duct may be transitional or squamous cell carcinoma. Bartholin's carcinoma is serious and is generally treated by radical vulvectomy and bilateral groin dissection. Excision of a benign vulvar fibroma is illustrated in Fig. 16-5.

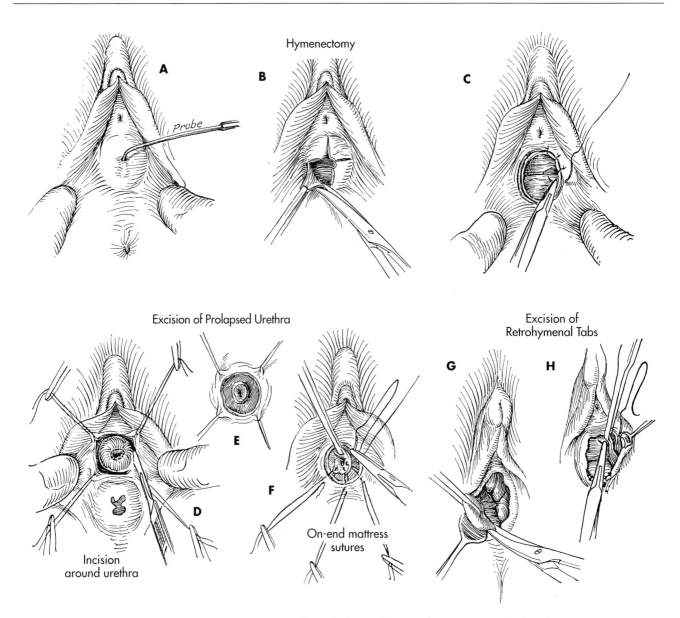

Hymenectomy

Excision of Prolapsed Urethra

Excision of Retrohymenal Tabs

Incision around urethra

On-end mattress sutures

Fig. 16-6   **A** to **C,** Hymenectomy. **A,** The pinhole-sized hymenal opening is probed to determine the presence of a vaginal canal. A cruciate incision is made, and the hymen excised in quadrants **(B)** and the new edges approximated by interrupted sutures **(C). D** to **F,** Excision of prolapsed urethra. **D,** Guide sutures are placed and a circular incision made around the prolapsed urethra. **E,** The prolapsed mucosa is excised. **F,** Interrupted mattress sutures are placed as shown (sewing the urethral mucosa to the skin of the vestibule). **G** and **H,** Excision of retrohymenal tabs. **G,** Painful retrohymenal tabs are grasped and excised at their base. **H,** Interrupted sutures bring the vaginal wall to the hymenal margin. Examination assures the surgeon that there is no postoperative introital obstruction. (From Ball TL: *Gynecologic surgery and urology,* ed 2, St Louis, 1963, Mosby.)

LESIONS OF THE URETHRA

Prolapse of the urethra is common, particularly in postmenopausal women and occasionally in newborns. It rarely causes bleeding and need not be treated if asymptomatic. Should it begin to bother the patient, it can be treated by excising the circular area and sewing the cut edge of wall of the urethra to the cut edge of the circumferential skin of the vulva by a series of interrupted sutures (Fig. 16-6, *D* to *F*).

When a lesion of the distal urethra causes bleeding, it is essential to differentiate the benign and relatively harmless urethral caruncle from the more ominous and invasive carcinoma of the urethra. The carcinoma tends to be somewhat more friable and harder when palpated, but histologic examination of biopsy material is necessary to confirm the diagnosis. The treatment of caruncle is simple excision, but the treatment of carcinoma varies between interstitial radia-

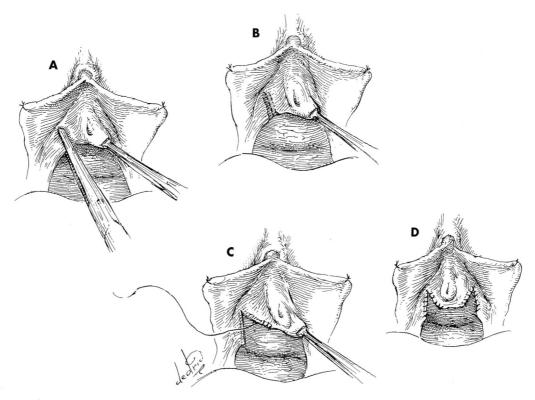

Fig. 16-7   Urethrolysis. **A,** Site of hymenal attachment to urethra is crushed in a forceps, first on one side and then the other. **B,** Incision to be made through crushed tissue is shown by dashed line. **C,** Cut edge of incision is overcast by a running linked suture. **D,** End result. (After C Wood, Mason Clinic, Seattle, Wash.)

tion and radical surgery, depending on the circumstances of the particular case.

SURGERY OF THE HYMEN

Incision and hymenectomy are curative for an imperforate hymen (see Fig. 16-6, *A* to *C*). A small but rigid hymen that obstructs the vagina can be treated by hymenotomy at the 4- and 8-o'clock positions; digital stretching by the patient maintains the opening during the healing phase. Midline perineotomy, sufficient to admit three fingerbreadths into the vagina, is the treatment of choice for a rigid, inelastic perineum. The edges of the incision should be sewn to the perineal skin transversely, at right angles to the original incision.

A patient who has recurrent postcoital cystitis may have a congenital anomaly of thick lateral bands connecting the urethral meatus to the hymenal margin. Urethrolysis at this site is curative (Fig. 16-7). Perineotomy does not always relieve introital stenosis (Fig. 16-8), which occurs most often in postmenopausal women, but Z-plasty is curative (Fig. 16-9).

VULVAR VESTIBULAR SYNDROME (VULVAR VESTIBULITIS, FOCAL VULVITIS)

The vulvar vestibule, which is located between the hymen and the inner margin of the labia minora, is a most unusual epithelial area. It is of endodermal embryologic origin and is not acetowhite (i.e., does not appear temporarily white when moistened with 3% acetic acid). It can become the site of a painful condition called by various names—*vulvar vestibular syndrome, vulvar vestibulitis,* and *focal vulvitis*—and a specific causal agent is not known. It is more frequent between the ages of 18 and 45, is seen predominantly in white women, and in some way may be causally related to oral contraceptive use. The condition can be of sudden onset, and after some months will occasionally undergo spontaneous remission. Focal, well-demarcated areas in the tissues of the vestibule are exquisitely painful when touched with the moistened tip of a cotton swab.

Weström and Willén[41] histologically demonstrated neural hyperplasia in the vestibular specimen of the majority of their patients with vulvar vestibulitis treated by vestibulectomy. An intense inflammatory reaction dominated by lymphocytes and plasma cells is a common coincidental finding. The neural hyperplasia may provide a morphologic explanation of the characteristic pain of this syndrome and, by surgical removal of this tissue, explain the higher success of symptomatic relief by vestibulectomy[4] in contrast to the inconsistent symptomatic relief by simple undercutting.[6]

The tissues appear normal under gross inspection, although occasionally they are erythematous and at times have a slightly granular surface. It is not acetowhite, suggesting a lack of any relationship with human papillomavi-

Plastic Repair of Constricted Introitus

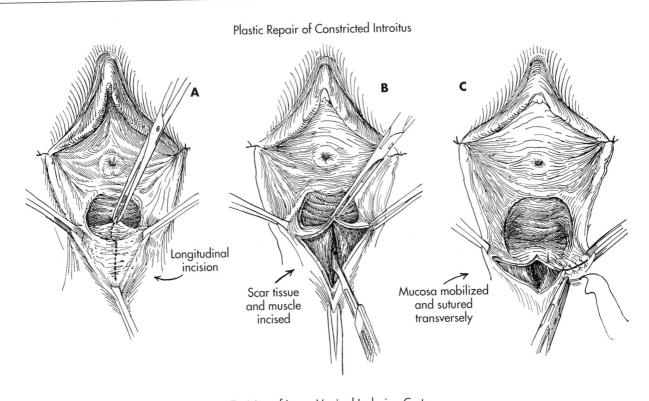

Excision of Large Vaginal Inclusion Cyst

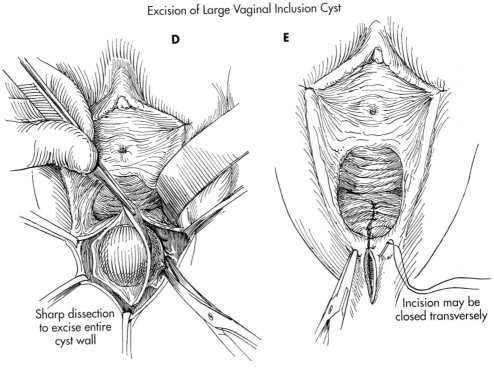

Fig. 16-8 **A to C,** Plastic repair of constricted introitus. **A,** A midline incision is made in the skin of the perineum, and the extent of the subepithelial fibrosis is determined. **B,** Obstructive scar tissue, muscle, and fibrosis are incised, the flaps undermined, and the incision closed transversely using interrupted stitches **(C). D** and **E,** Excision of large vaginal inclusion cyst. When an inclusion cyst is the source of obstructive dyspareunia, it should be excised. **D,** A midline longitudinal incision is made, and the cyst and its complete squamous epithelial lining are removed by sharp dissection. **E,** The incision is closed, but if the perineum is still obstructive, it can be closed transversely. (From Ball TL: *Gynecologic surgery and urology,* ed 2, St Louis, 1963, Mosby.)

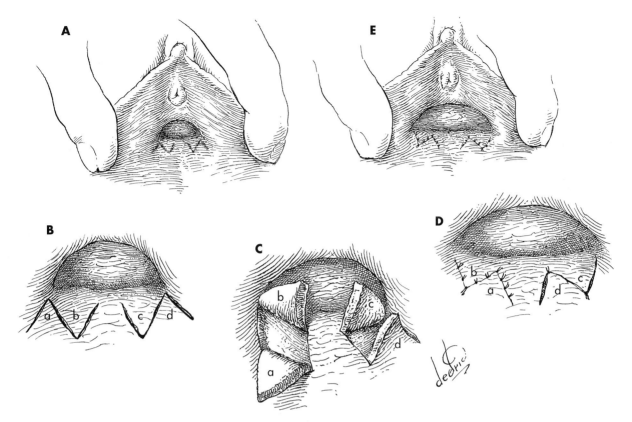

Fig. 16-9 Z-plasty. **A,** Preoperative introital stenosis, showing lines of incision. **B** to **D,** Full-thickness flaps are undermined, rotated, and sewn in place. **E,** Introital enlargement at conclusion of procedure. (From Nichols DH, Randall CL: *Vaginal surgery,* ed 4, Baltimore, 1996, Williams & Wilkins.)

rus (HPV); conversely, if the area appears acetowhite after it has been moistened with acetic acid, such a positive finding may indicate a distinctly dissimilar but painful condition related to HPV. The latter acetowhite areas often can be eliminated by laser vaporization with good symptomatic relief. The condition has been identified from time to time for more than 100 years,[36] but it has received increased attention since 1981.*

The gynecologist may suggest alternative or noncoital means of sexual gratification for the couple, but applying a cotton ball saturated with 4% aqueous lidocaine (Xylocaine) to the vestibular area some 15 minutes before coitus often provides sufficient temporary anesthesia for sexual relations. For a non-acetowhite lesion not associated with coincident human papillomavirus infection, a course of treatment can be initiated using 15 minute applications of these lidocaine-soaked cotton balls four times daily for 6 months, if relief of symptoms is obtained. Xylocaine ointment can be applied to the area for temporary relief during the day. For unknown reasons, oral contraceptives can exacerbate the condition, so the patient should stop taking them for at least 6 months. Remission occurs in approximately 50% of cases.

If the syndrome persists after 6 months of observation and treatment, vestibulectomy and perineoplasty provide re-

lief in most cases. The gynecologic surgeon should reconfirm the diagnosis preoperatively by examining the vestibule with a magnifying glass or low-power colposcope. A cluster of raised, pinkish or yellowish papules in the area of pain is often present, and this specific site of pain can be carefully delineated with a marking pen immediately before the administration of anesthesia to ensure complete excision of the affected area (Fig. 16-10). The full epithelial thickness, including the adjacent hymen of this sensitive area within the vestibule, should be excised. The full thickness of the posterior vaginal wall should be mobilized for 2 or 3 cm so that it can be brought down to cover this raw area at the conclusion of the operation; it is attached to the skin of the perineum by two layers of interrupted sutures.[43] Because postoperative oozing at this site is common, the patient may be kept in the hospital for a day or two after surgery. The prognosis for postsurgical pain relief seems better for those patients whose pain is present *only* when the tissue is touched, in contrast to those whose pain is constant regardless of whether the tissues are touched.

TREATMENT OF AN OBSTRUCTED VAGINA

A hemivagina associated with a didelphic uterus, or a bicornuate or septate vagina, may be totally or partially obstructed. When the obstruction is complete, the patient

---

*References 4, 15, 16, 18, 26, 30, 41, 43-45.

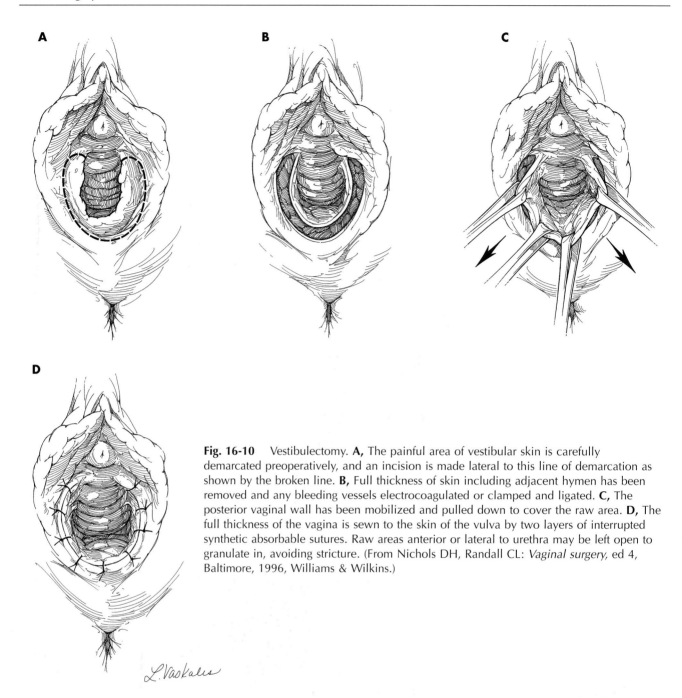

A

B

C

D

Fig. 16-10   Vestibulectomy. **A,** The painful area of vestibular skin is carefully demarcated preoperatively, and an incision is made lateral to this line of demarcation as shown by the broken line. **B,** Full thickness of skin including adjacent hymen has been removed and any bleeding vessels electrocoagulated or clamped and ligated. **C,** The posterior vaginal wall has been mobilized and pulled down to cover the raw area. **D,** The full thickness of the vagina is sewn to the skin of the vulva by two layers of interrupted synthetic absorbable sutures. Raw areas anterior or lateral to urethra may be left open to granulate in, avoiding stricture. (From Nichols DH, Randall CL: *Vaginal surgery,* ed 4, Baltimore, 1996, Williams & Wilkins.)

has dysmenorrhea, and the monthly blood accumulates as a palpable mass in the lateral wall of the vagina.[42] The patient also can have congenital abnormalities of the urinary tract. The gynecologist can confirm the diagnosis by aspiration of old blood from the mass. Treatment consists of prompt marsupialization to create a large vaginal window that connects the two vaginal cavities.

EXCISION OF THE VAGINAL APEX

A precancerous lesion of the vaginal apex can be treated by full-thickness excisional biopsy (Fig. 16-11). This lesion may indicate vaginal intraepithelial neoplasia in a patient who had cervical intraepithelial neoplasia previously treated

by hysterectomy, but the tissue must be studied in the laboratory to exclude possible unexpected invasion of subepithelial tissues.

CULDOCENTESIS AND COLPOTOMY

Culdocentesis, usually performed at a site in the midline of the upper posterior vaginal wall between the uterosacral ligaments, is useful for identifying the nature and character of any fluid that is distending the cul-de-sac of Douglas (Fig. 16-12). With the unanesthetized patient in the lithotomy position and the cul-de-sac exposed, the needle with syringe attached is positioned against the cul-de-sac, and the patient is asked to cough. At the moment of the

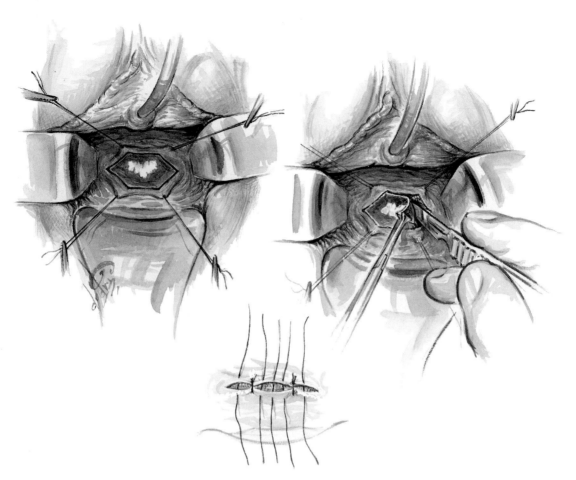

Fig. 16-11 Excision of vaginal apex. Lesion is carefully demarcated by Schiller's stain, and four guide sutures are inserted as shown. Subepithelial tissue may be infiltrated by 0.5% lidocaine in 1:200,000 epinephrine solution for hemostasis. The tissue to be excised is indicated by an incision through the full thickness of the vaginal wal. This is excised by sharp dissection, and vaginal edges are brought together by a series of interrupted polyglycolic acid sutures placed as shown. If there is concern about preserving vaginal depth, closure can be made vertically rather than horizontally. (From Nichols DH, Randall CL: *Vaginal surgery*, ed 4, Baltimore, 1996, Williams & Wilkins.)

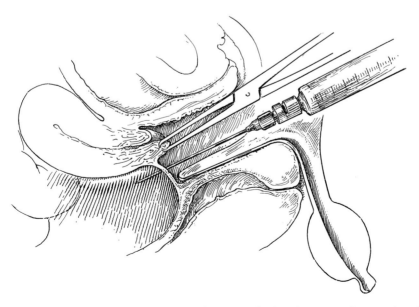

Fig. 16-12 Culdocentesis. The cervix has been steadied with a tenaculum, and a sharp pointed no. 18 needle attached to a syringe is inserted directly into the bulging cul-de-sac. The fluid is then aspirated and examined. (From Nichols DH, Sweeney PJ, editors: *Ambulatory gynecology*, ed 2, Philadelphia, 1995, JB Lippincott.)

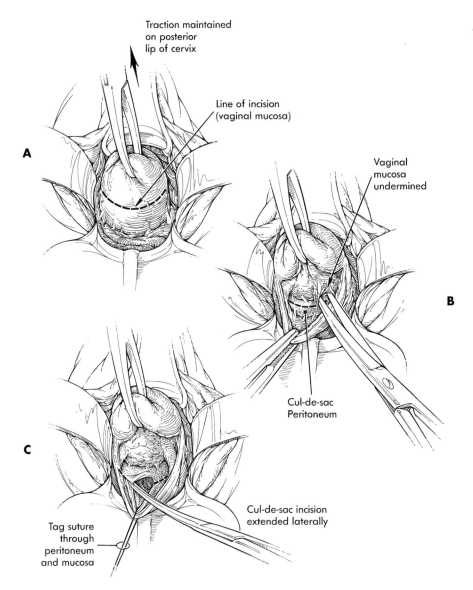

Traction maintained
on posterior
lip of cervix

Line of incision
(vaginal mucosa)

A

Vaginal
mucosa
undermined

B

Cul-de-sac
Peritoneum

C

Cul-de-sac incision
extended laterally

Tag suture
through
peritoneum
and mucosa

Fig. 16-13 Posterior colpotomy. **A,** Traction by a tenaculum applied to the posterior lip of the cervix *(arrow)*. The site for transverse incision through the posterior vaginal wall overlying the cul-de-sac is indicated by the dashed line. The vaginal mucosa is undermined (**B**) by sharp dissection, exposing the peritoneum of the cul-de-sac. **C,** The peritoneum is picked up and incised, and a tag suture is placed through peritoneal edge and vaginal wall.

cough, the tip of the needle is quickly thrust through the vaginal wall into the cul-de-sac, and a sample of fluid aspirated. Blood-tinged serous fluid may represent a follicle cyst, but pure, unclotted blood may indicate an ectopic pregnancy.

When an abscess is suspected, culdocentesis should be performed in an operating room, and the needle should be inserted at the site of fluctuation, as determined by bimanual abdominal-rectal-vaginal palpation. If the fluid distending the cul-de-sac of Douglas is purulent, the surgeon should leave the needle in place, enlarge the entry into the cavity by surgical colpotomy, and promptly institute drainage. The abscess contents require prompt bacterial identification, culture, and sensitivity testing. Other aspirates are treated appropriately. Posterior colpotomy may permit direct exam-

ination and treatment of the adnexa. The technique is shown in Fig. 16-13 and in sagittal section in Fig. 16-14. If central dysmenorrhea is a significant complaint, the uterosacral ligaments can be clamped, and a segment resected to interrupt the nerve supply that runs through them to the uterus. A fold of peritoneum should be interposed between the cut ends of each ligament to prevent nerve regeneration, and then the tissues should be reunited[12] (Fig. 16-15).

EXCISION OF AN ENDOMETRIAL OR ENDOCERVICAL POLYP

The surgeon should excise in its entirety any polyp that protrudes through the external cervix and send it for prompt laboratory study. If the polyp is small, its base

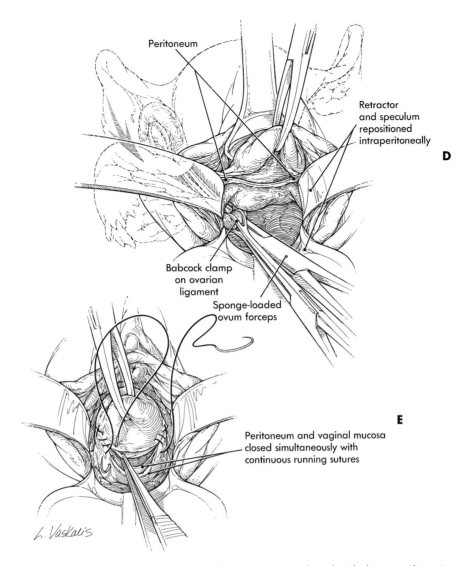

Peritoneum

Retractor
and speculum
repositioned
intraperitoneally

D

Babcock clamp
on ovarian
ligament

Sponge-loaded
ovum forceps

E

Peritoneum and vaginal mucosa
closed simultaneously with
continuous running sutures

L. Vaskalis

Fig. 16-13, cont'd A sponge-loaded ovum forceps is inserted, and with downward traction, will bring the adnexa into the operative field **(D).** The ovarian ligament can be grasped by a Babcock clamp for traction. The pelvis is inspected, and any surgery is accomplished. **E,** The incision is closed by a running through-and-through suture.

can be grasped within the jaws of a small hemostat and the polyp twisted off; it is better to remove a larger polyp by excision of its entire stalk. Because the site of the larger polyp's origin and attachment to the endocervix or endometrium is not usually visible, the following steps can be performed: the polyp can be fed through the loop of a tonsil snare, the loop advanced within the endocervical or endometrial cavity until its progress stops, and the snare then slowly tightened to crush and transect the pedicle of the polyp (Fig. 16-16, *A* to *E*). If the stalk is so firm that it resists cutting, electrosurgical cautery can be applied to the snare at the same time pressure to the snare is made, and this will transect the stalk. A prolapsed submucous myoma or adenomyoma can be similarly excised. The procedure is simple and quick and, since the prolapsed tissue usually is infected, safer than hysterectomy.[5] Rarely, anterior vaginal hysterotomy can be em-

ployed (see Fig. 16-16, *F* and *G*). A vaginal fibroma can be excised by sharp dissection (Fig. 16-17, *A* to *D*). The patient should be reexamined after a month to determine whether she has other polyps that should also be removed and studied.

TREATMENT OF A WOLFFIAN DUCT CYST

Large wolffian duct cysts occasionally appear along the sidewalls or beneath the lateral surface of the vaginal apex. Filled with clear mucus,[32] they are anatomically separate from the urethra and bladder. If they are enlarging or causing dyspareunia, they should be treated, preferably by marsupialization. Excision sometimes leads to unexpectedly profuse bleeding, and ureteral ligation is possible when deep sutures are placed at the base of the cyst cavity to control the bleeding (see Fig.16-17, *E* to *G*).

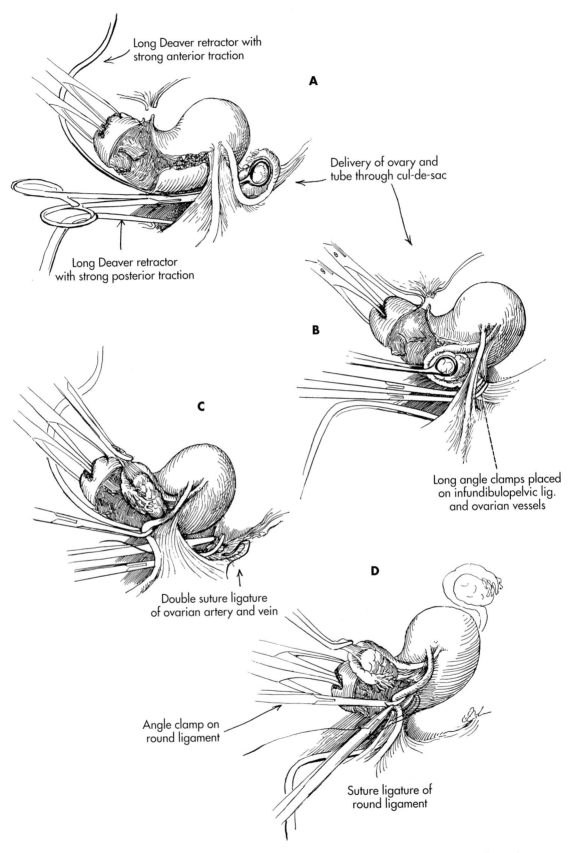

Fig. 16-14 Posterior colpotomy seen in sagittal section. A colpotomy has been made, and the left ovary grasped by a ring forceps **(A).** If ovary and the tube are to be removed, the infundibular pelvic ligament is clamped **(B)** and cut **(C).** Transfixion sutures replace the clamps. **D,** The round ligament may be clamped and ligated for additional exposure if necessary. (From Ball TL: *Gynecologic surgery and urology,* ed 2, St Louis, 1963, Mosby.)

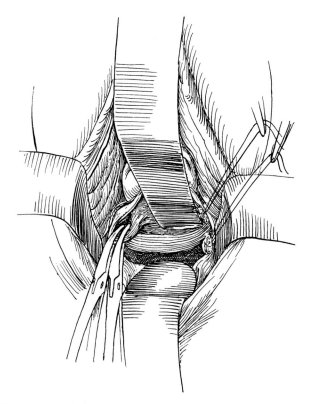

Fig. 16-15 The Doyle procedure for lysis of uterosacral ligaments. The posterior cul-de-sac has been opened. The uterosacral ligaments can be clamped, cut, and tied. A fold of peritoneum is placed between the cut ends of each ligament, and they are reattached to the vagina and the incision closed. (From Ball TL: *Gynecologic surgery and urology*, ed 2, St Louis, 1963, Mosby.)

TREATMENT OF CERVICAL INTRAEPITHELIAL NEOPLASIA

Coincident with careful cytologic interpretation of the screening Papanicolaou smear, colposcopy permits gynecologists to locate the exact site of any epithelial abnormalities of the cervix, vagina, or vulva and to perform a biopsy on these suspicious areas for histologic study. Obviously invasive malignancy should be confirmed by the examination of tissue obtained by punch biopsy.

Cryosurgery and Laser Therapy

When the surgeon has identified a premalignant condition and can visualize the entire lesion colposcopically, a spectrum of definitive treatment is available to the patient. For example, premalignant lesions can be treated by cryosurgery[29,37,39] or laser vaporization* as alternatives to surgical excision. This subject is discussed fully in Chapters 17 and 18.

When a patient with cervical intraepithelial neoplasia wishes to preserve her uterus so that she can become preg-

nant, among the options for treatment of her condition are (1) cryosurgery, (2) laser surgery, (3) electrodissection (LEEP), and (4) conization. However, a treatment other than conization is permissible, only if the following conditions are met:

1. The surgeon must be able to completely visualize the abnormal epithelium.
2. The result of endocervical curettage must be negative.
3. The findings of cytology must be consistent with the findings of colposcopy.
4. The patient must be willing to participate in long-term follow-up.

Conization of the Cervix

Conization becomes necessary for study of the entire lesion when it is not possible to estimate the endocervical extent of a lesion with certainty and the findings of endocervical curettage are inconclusive or when a colposcopically directed biopsy shows microinvasion (or possible microinvasion) of a malignancy. When this condition is discovered during pregnancy (when the squamocolumnar junction everts), a shallow "coin biopsy"–type conization avoids the potentially dangerous excision of the endocervix.[11] The placement of six purse-string sutures close to the vaginal reflection reduces eversion of the squamocolumnar junction and prevents excessive blood loss.[12]

Although diagnostic conization has been largely replaced by colposcopically directed biopsy, conization continues to be valuable when a microinvasive lesion is discovered and for investigating an abnormal Pap smear result when the squamocolumnar junction is so high that it cannot be visualized and a biopsy cannot be performed. The procedure is primarily diagnostic, but it can be therapeutic under certain circumstances (e.g., when the gynecologist can visualize the entire lesion and can include it within the surgical specimen). However, excision of the entire lesion does not preclude future development of other areas of dysplasia or carcinoma in situ, and continued Pap smear surveillance is mandatory.

Technique of Conization. Most gynecologists have recently discontinued the practice of routine preoperative shaving of vulvar and suprapubic hair before a conization, although it is sometimes helpful to clip long hair to keep it out of the way.[40]

A simple technique of conization that provides adequate hemostasis consists of infiltration of the cervical stroma with not more than 50 ml of 0.5% lidocaine (Xylocaine) in 1:200,000 epinephrine solution. This causes a marked spasm of cervical blood vessels that produces a visible blanching of the cervix. With a no. 11 pointed scalpel, a cone of proper-sized tissue is removed, up to but not including the internal cervical os. (Although some gynecologists prefer laser conization, the so-called cold-knife conization is entirely effective.) It is absolutely essential that the axis of the cone parallel the axis of the cervix; perfora-

*References 2, 3, 7, 8, 24, 31, 34, 38, 39, 47.

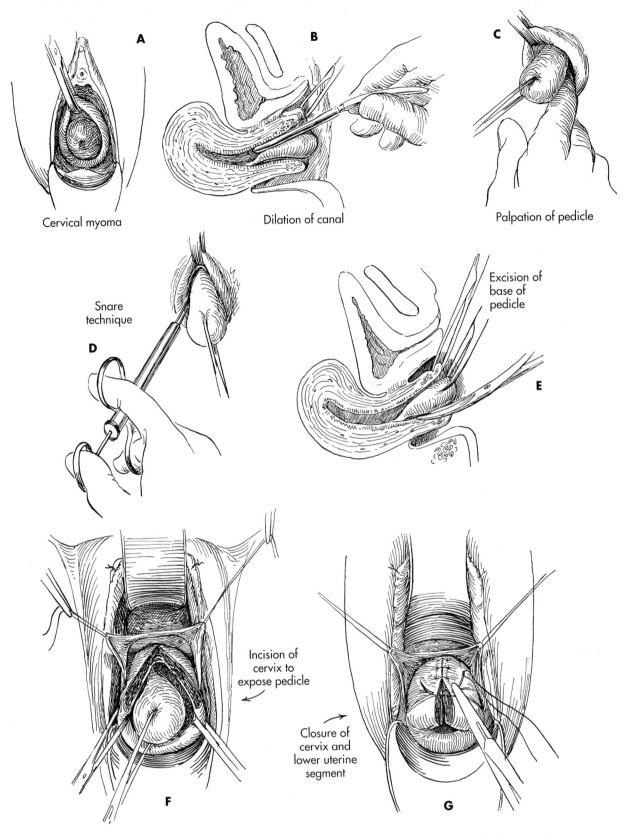

A

Cervical myoma

B

Dilation of canal

C

Palpation of pedicle

Snare
technique

D

E

Excision of
base of
pedicle

F

Incision of
cervix to
expose pedicle

G

Closure of
cervix and
lower uterine
segment

Fig. 16-16 **A** to **E,** Pedunculated cervical myoma. **A,** The prolapsed cervical myoma is shown protruding through the external cervical os. The canal is dilated **(B),** and the pedicle is palpated **(C). D,** The loop of a tonsil snare is passed around the myoma or polyp and advanced as far as it will go; the base is then crushed and transected by tightening the wire snare, and the lesion removed. **E,** Alternatively, the pedicle may be transected with scissors. **F** and **G,** Anterior vaginal hysterotomy. When the prolapsed polyp or fibroid is too large to be delivered, a transverse incision can be made in the anterior vaginal wall, the bladder dissected from the cervix and retracted out of harm's way, and a longitudinal incision made in the cervix anteriorly **(F).** The myoma is removed, the incision in the cervix is closed by interrupted sutures **(G),** and the transverse vaginal incision is closed separately. (From Ball TL: *Gynecologic surgery and urology,* ed 2, St Louis, 1963, Mosby.)

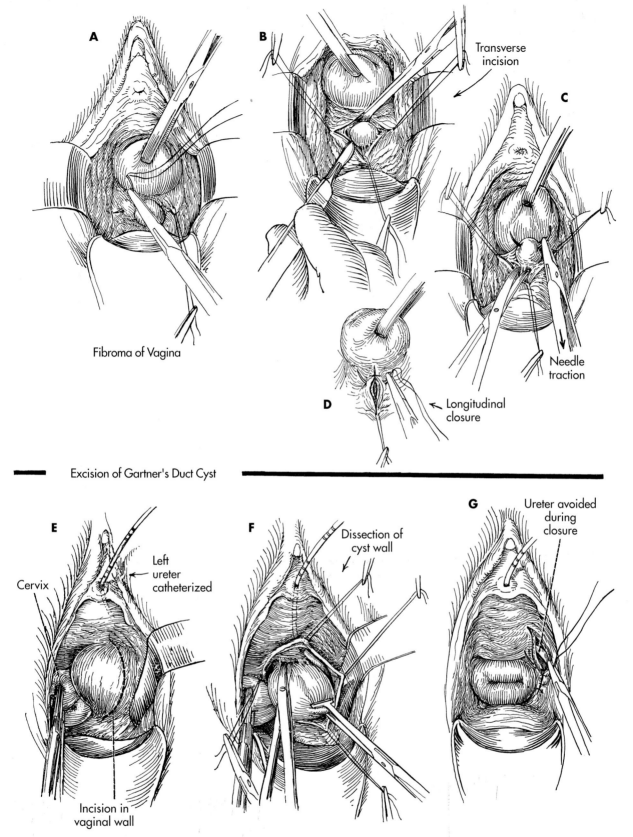

Fibroma of Vagina

Transverse incision

Needle traction

Longitudinal closure

Excision of Gartner's Duct Cyst

Ureter avoided during closure

Left ureter catheterized

Cervix

Dissection of cyst wall

Incision in vaginal wall

Fig. 16-17 **A** to **D,** Excision of a vaginal fibroma. **A,** Guide sutures are placed lateral to each side of the fibroma. **B,** A transverse incision through the vagina is made between them, exposing the fibroma. It can be fixed with a needle for traction and removed by sharp dissection **(C),** and the vaginal incision can be closed longitudinally **(D). E** to **G,** Excision of Gartner's duct cyst. **E,** An incision is made as shown by the dashed line overlying the cyst. A ureteral catheter has been placed in the left ureter to aid in its identification during the operation. **F,** The cyst is removed by sharp dissection. **G,** The incision is closed after hemostasis has been obtained; the ureter is avoided scrupulously. The catheter is then removed. (From Ball TL: *Gynecologic surgery and urology,* ed 2, St Louis, 1963, Mosby.)

tion of the uterus at the apex of the cone can damage the neighboring organs and tissues.

The 12-o'clock position on the surgical specimen may be marked by a suture. Bleeding or oozing points should be coagulated with the electrosurgical unit. As an alternative procedure for preliminary hemostasis, deep hemostatic sutures of absorbable material can be placed in the 3- and 9-o'clock positions. If significant oozing occurs immediately, which happens only rarely, a more hemostatic "hot" electroconization may follow. This procedure is not performed routinely, because if the initial conization does not remove the entire lesion, electroconization leaves no fresh adjacent tissue to study by immediate biopsy. In addition, the tissue destruction causes significant postoperative cervical scarring. Once the cone of cervical tissue has been obtained and the numerous bleeding points coagulated, the cervix is packed for 24 to 48 hours with ¼-inch iodoform gauze. The subject of conization is discussed in considerable detail in Chapters 17 and 18.

Complications of Conization. Hemorrhage can occur either at the time of conization or within the first postoperative weeks. Visible bleeding points should be electrocoagulated; if there is a general ooze, the area should be suture-ligated. Mild bleeding can be stopped by application of the tip of a silver nitrate stick or a cotton applicator soaked in negatol (Negatan) or Monsel's solution. If this is not successful, packing the affected area with microfibrillar collagen (Avitene) is generally effective. (Avitene attracts functioning blood platelets, which adhere to the microfibrils and thus trigger the formation of thrombi in the adjacent tissue. Although more expensive, it is more effective than either Gelfoam or Surgicel.) A "pulsating" ooze should be treated by a carefully placed suture. If bleeding recurs, bilateral transvaginal ligation of the uterine artery may be required. Hysterectomy or internal iliac ligation may be required, although rarely, to control excessive recurrent postoperative bleeding, particularly if the conization has transacted a major branch of the uterine artery and the artery has retracted into the substance of the cervix or lower uterine segment.

Cervical stenosis is the principal long-range complication of inadvertent resection or trauma to the internal cervical os. After conization, the cervix heals by scar formation; contraction of the scar tissue can reduce the diameter of the canal and lead to a stenosis or stricture. The gynecologist who performs a conization of the cervix must make certain that the patient's cervical canal does not become stenotic after the operation because stenosis can progress to occlusion and then to amenorrhea, hematometra, and possibly endometriosis. The patient must be advised to return for postoperative examinations at regular intervals for at least 6 months. At each visit, the gynecologist should test the patency of the cervical canal by carefully passing a small dilator or sound through the canal and inner os.

The cervix tending to stenosis cannot always be dilated sufficiently without anesthesia to alter the progressive tightening of scar tissue. In this case, the use of a laminaria tent for 24 hours has been recommended.[20] The operator must

not allow the laminaria tent to slip into the uterine cavity, however, for it will swell, making it difficult to remove from the uterus without the insertion of a second laminaria tent to dilate the cervix. If a stenosis does develop, dilating the canal while the patient is under anesthesia and suturing an old-fashioned stem pessary into the canal to be worn for several months (or until it falls out) may be preferable to occasional, usually futile, sounding or dilation in the office or clinic. A stenosis may require long-term treatment by periodic endocervical dilation until the surface of the cervix has been reepithelialized, the scar stabilized, and healing completed.

"Hot" conization has little place in the treatment of chronic cervicitis. The procedure is not cost effective in such cases. Moreover, it carries additional risks, including the formation of scar tissue and its troublesome sequelae. When endocervicitis causes chronic leukorrhea that distresses the patient enough to require treatment, strip cauterization or electrocoagulation of the affected area of the cervix may be the procedure of choice. Because infection often involves the depths of the endocervical glands, superficial cauterization of the cervix by local applications of a caustic or silver nitrate is not indicated.

Conization and Curettage: Preferred Sequence. The indications for conization and fractional curettage do not often coexist, but the procedures are not mutually exclusive. If the conization that precedes curettage is carefully done, the results of the fractional curettage can be satisfactory.[23] However, identification of the source of the tissue specimens is generally better if the conization takes place after the cervix and uterus have been sounded but before the curette is used in the canal or uterine cavity. An external mucocutaneous junction around the margin of an erosion can be removed, of course, with a large biopsy loop without coagulating the endocervix. Even when the conization involves the excision of 1 or 2 cm of the endocervix, as it usually does, the gynecologist can use the small, sharp curette to determine the presence of any friable tissue or a softened area in the lower uterine segment adjacent to the inner os that suggests malignancy. When such curettage of the endocervix does not suggest carcinoma, it probably will be necessary to dilate the inner os to admit a larger curette and polyp forceps to the uterine cavity.

When a dilation and curettage (D&C) and conization are to be performed on the same patient at the same time, the D&C is done immediately *after*—never before—the conization.

DILATION AND CURETTAGE

A frequently performed surgical procedure in gynecology is cervical dilation and uterine curettage. Referred to universally as D&C, this operation is often the first surgical procedure to be undertaken by the physician who is preparing to specialize in obstetrics or gynecology. The technique of D&C is not difficult to learn; in fact, few surgical procedures are as straightforward or routine.[19]

Conventional D&C of the uterus is performed for the following reasons:

1. To evaluate abnormal uterine bleeding when the cervical os is so tight that an endometrial biopsy cannot be performed
2. To evaluate and diagnose the cause of postmenopausal uterine bleeding when endometrial biopsy has not established the diagnosis
3. Immediately preceding hysterectomy in a patient with abnormal uterine bleeding to uncover positive or suspicious endometrial findings that may influence the operative decision
4. To empty the uterus of its contents when unwanted products of conception remain, such as after an incomplete abortion
5. In a patient with intractable menorrhagia and an enlarged uterus to distinguish between adenomyosis interna and uterine leiomyomata, particularly submucous leiomyomata, and thus to determine appropriate treatment
6. To complete the workup of an infertility patient with leiomyomata when a hysterogram has not revealed the location and types of leiomyomata present (e.g., submucous)
7. To evaluate the condition of a patient with an abnormal Pap smear when there is no gross or colposcopically visible lesion of the cervix
8. To free adhesions and possibly insert an intrauterine device to keep the walls of the uterine cavity apart during the healing process in a patient with known or suspected intrauterine synechiae (Asherman's syndrome)

Transvaginal ultrasonography can be useful in the management of spontaneous abortion and aids significantly in determining which patients require D&C. If tissue has been passed and transvaginal ultrasound shows the diameter of retained products to be less than 50 mm, an outpatient expectant nonsurgical treatment can be applied with considerable savings of both cost and time. Nielsen and Hahlin[28] found that repeat transvaginal ultrasound of these expectantly treated patients 3 days later demonstrated disappearance of the products of conception in 79% of their cases. If the diameter of the retained products of conception exceeds 15 mm, D&C should be performed.

Routine D&C for investigation of abnormal uterine bleeding results in a low yield of cancer diagnosis in women younger than 70 years of age.[33] Transcervical hysteroscopy, even in the office, is a better method for diagnosing persistent abnormal bleeding,[46] and often the underlying disease is found to be an endometrial polyp or submucous myoma, which may have gone undetected by D&C.[4,13,14] The diagnostic accuracy of hysteroscopy over D&C is unquestioned,[17] and even as an operative procedure and under anesthesia it can be used in an appropriately well-equipped office setting.[46] The subject of hysteroscopy is considered in detail in Chapter 41.

Although a D&C can be performed with the patient under analgesia only or under local anesthesia (e.g., paracervical block), it is generally performed with the patient under brief general or regional anesthesia so that the gynecologist can carefully examine the internal genitalia without causing any discomfort to the patient.

Operating room procedure manuals create both dogma and confusion regarding the degree of surgical preparation that a patient needs for a D&C. Recommendations seem to be based principally on the site at which the procedure will take place. In all instances, cleansing or bacteriostatic douches, pubic shaving, and enemas are not only unnecessary but add to the patient's discomfort.

Setting

A D&C is ideally suited to an ambulatory setting. In this setting, the vagina and cervix are painted with a solution of povidone-iodine (Betadine). Instruments are sterile, draping is minimal, and the surgeon, whose hands have been washed but not necessarily scrubbed, wears sterile gloves.

In the hospital operating room, a D&C is generally done under maximum aseptic techniques, because the gravid, atrophic, or cancerous uterus is easily perforated under anesthesia and can become infected. After the patient has been prepared with nonabrasive perineal and vaginal wash, the operative area is painted with povidone-iodine. The patient is fully draped, and instruments are sterile. The surgeon is fully gowned, masked, capped, and gloved.[21]

Technique

Suction curettage can be used to complete an abortion (see Chapter 56). If suction curettage is not available, conventional curettage can be used to remove retained products of conception (Fig. 16-18). When curettage is to be performed on a recently pregnant uterus, an oxytocic should be administered either intramuscularly or intravenously; such an injection produces a firm contraction of the myometrium, thus increasing its resistance to perforation. Often a *dull* curettage is used in the pregnant uterus to avoid the removal of too much endometrium.

Outpatient curettage of the nonpregnant uterus with the Vabra suction apparatus can be preceded by the administration of analgesia or a paracervical block. In the majority of diagnostic cases, uterine curettage should be done fractionally with a sharp curette.

When the patient is under anesthesia, the gynecologist should first perform a careful examination. This always provides vital, sometimes unexpected, information useful in diagnosis and future clinical management. It also can provide valuable information about the appropriate route and technical details of a possible future hysterectomy. The following should be noted: the size, shape, and mobility of the uterus, the location and size of the cul-de-sac, and the strength and elasticity of the uterosacral ligaments, the cardinal ligaments, and the urogenital diaphragm.

After determining the axis and size of the uterus, the operator grasps the anterior cervical lip with a tenaculum for

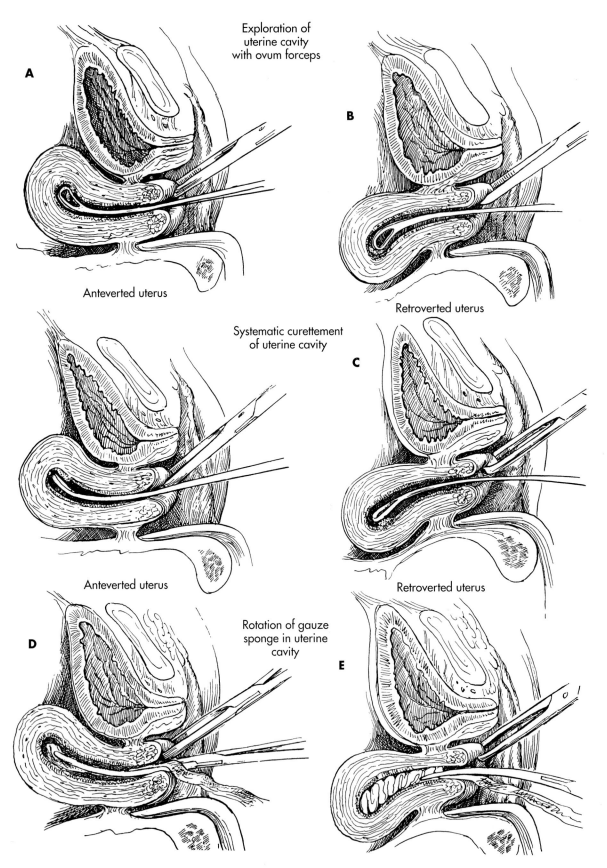

Fig. 16-18 Dilation and curettage for incomplete abortion. The cervix is grasped with a clamp and the canal gently and progressively dilated. If the uterus is retroverted, the curve of the dilation is reversed. The uterine cavity can be explored digitally, and the retained products of conception extracted by an ovum forceps **(A),** introduced in reverse direction if the uterus is retroverted **(B).** Other fragments are gently removed. The uterine cavity may be *lightly* curetted by a large dull curette **(C),** and the cavity packed with a saline soaked sponge, which is rotated and extracted **(D** and **E).** (From Ball TL: *Gynecologic surgery and urology,* ed 2, St Louis, 1963, Mosby.)

traction and carefully scrapes the endocervical canal with a small, sharp curette (e.g., the Duncan) up to, but not beyond, the internal cervical os. Curettage may begin at the 12-o'clock position and proceed in a careful clockwise or counterclockwise direction around the circumference of the cavity. The curettings are saved on a piece of gauze (e.g., Telfa) to be examined separately from the curettings obtained later from the endometrial cavity.

A blunt-tipped, malleable Simpson uterine sound should then be bent to accommodate the anteflexion, anteversion, retroflexion, or retroversion of the uterus. It is best to grasp the sound at its round shaft. Holding it firmly by the flat part of the end impedes the tendency of the sound to follow the path of least resistance, the axis of the uterus. The force exerted on both sound and curette during their introduction into the uterine cavity should be minimal, similar to that required to hold a pencil for writing; forceful insertion increases the risk of perforation.

After the sound has been gently inserted into the uterine cavity, the depth of the cavity from the external cervical os to the top of the fundus should be carefully measured. The size of the endometrial cavity tells the operator the precise depth to which the curette may be passed during the curettage. The cervical canal and internal cervical os are then expanded by the passage of graduated dilators until they are large enough to permit introduction of the largest size curette or polyp forceps to be used during the procedure. Gradual dilation with the patient under anesthesia markedly reduces the risk of rupture or permanent damage to the musculature of the cervix.

While gently introducing a sharp curette into the endometrial cavity until it reaches the top of the fundus, the operator grasps the handle firmly and, by traction against the resisting uterus, scrapes the endometrial cavity with the curette down to, but not through, the presumed basal layer. In an orderly clockwise or counterclockwise direction, the operator scrapes all segments and quadrants of the endometrium. The operator stops scraping when the passage of the sharp edge of the curette across the surface of the endometrium produces the delicate sensation of a "grating" resistance, characteristic of the basal layer.

The endometrium has been curetted in this orderly fashion, and any submucous irregularities, diverticula, or septa in the uterine cavity have been noted. The separate curettings of the endometrium and the endocervix (which have been saved on a separate piece of gauze) are now carefully examined and palpated. The experienced clinician often recognizes the difference between malignancy and endocrine dysfunction by the gross appearance of the endometrial fragments. (No therapy should be initiated, however, before histologic confirmation.) Benign tissue is soft and spongy; when squeezed, it is somewhat elastic and resists shattering. Fragments of normal endometrium, both proliferative and premenstrual, or secretory, can usually be smoothed out on a sponge, where they appear to be fragments of relatively thin or thick membrane. In contrast, malignant tissue tends to be hard and rather fragile; if squeezed gently, it fragments and shatters. When placed on a sponge, these fragments appear to be bits of tissue that have more texture and substance and are unlikely to smooth out as a membrane would.

The operator should then use polyp or kidney stone forceps to explore the cavity of the uterus, because the curette can miss an endometrial polyp of almost any size, particularly if the polyp has a narrow base. After the polyp forceps has been introduced, the jaws are opened and then closed in various quadrants of the uterine cavity; after each closing, a tug is made to see if any resistance is encountered. If this procedure locates a narrow-based polyp of a size that permits it to negotiate the dilated cervical canal, it can be removed safely by twisting the forceps.

After the removal of all instruments, the operator should carefully inspect the uterus and cervix. If there is much fresh bleeding from the endometrial cavity, the uterine cavity should be carefully sounded to ensure that the uterus was not perforated nor the endocervix lacerated. Should either of these events have occurred, appropriate observation and treatment should be instituted. Excessive bleeding from tenaculum marks on the cervix can be cauterized, or a gentle and temporary packing can be placed against the face of the cervix.

The operative report should be dictated immediately while all the details of each procedure are fresh in the surgeon's mind. A plan should be made for the removal of any packing that was used. The patient or her family should be informed of the operative findings and discharge instructions, and arrangements should be made for postoperative evaluation and follow-up.

Complications

Although a minor surgical procedure, a D&C must be performed with delicacy and precision if it is to be effective. Done carelessly, forcefully, or thoughtlessly, the procedure can cause serious harm to the patient.

Uterine Perforation. If the length of the sound or curette that has passed into the uterine cavity is longer than the measured length of that cavity, the uterine wall has been perforated. When such a perforation occurs, the instrument can be introduced all the way to its handle without any resistance. Uterine perforation generally results from a failure to identify the axis of the cavity of the uterus, which may often be in anteflexion or retroflexion; it also results from the subsequent use of force in introducing the instrument into the uterine cavity, often on the presumption that it is negotiating a somewhat stenotic internal os. The myometrium that is soft because of pregnancy or invasion by malignant tumor can be perforated quite easily (Fig. 16-19).

When the *sound* has perforated the uterus, the operator should promptly withdraw the instrument. Little of consequence will usually follow. The position of the uterus should be carefully determined by bimanual examination and the sound bent to negotiate the uterine cavity safely. If the sound has been reinserted along the axis of the uterine cavity, the insertion generally stops when the tip of the instru-

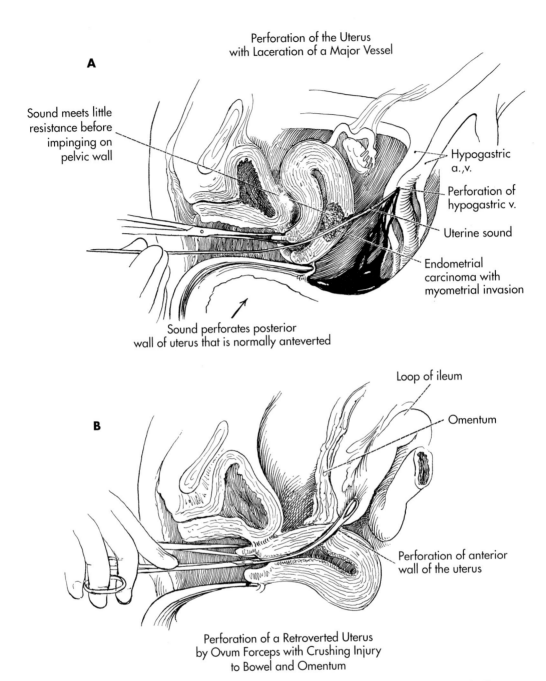

Perforation of the Uterus
with Laceration of a Major Vessel

A

Sound meets little
resistance before
impinging on
pelvic wall

Hypogastric
a.,v.

Perforation of
hypogastric v.

Uterine sound

Endometrial
carcinoma with
myometrial invasion

Sound perforates posterior
wall of uterus that is normally anteverted

Loop of ileum

Omentum

B

Perforation of anterior
wall of the uterus

Perforation of a Retroverted Uterus
by Ovum Forceps with Crushing Injury
to Bowel and Omentum

Fig. 16-19   Perforation of uterus at curettage. **A,** Failure to recognize axis of a markedly anteflexed uterus can lead the curette to perforate the posterior wall of the uterus. **B,** Similarly, perforation of the anterior wall of the uterus can occur when retroflexion is present. (From Ball TL:
Gynecologic surgery and urology, ed 2, St Louis, 1963, Mosby.)

ment has reached the fundus of the uterus. The operator can then complete the procedure.

If, following perforation of the uterine wall with the sound, the proper axis of the uterus cannot be determined, it is best to discontinue the procedure and reschedule later, at which time the myometrium will have had an opportunity to heal. The patient should be told postoperatively of the perforation and should be watched for tachycardia, hypotension, abdominal tenderness, fever, and other signs of intraperitoneal bleeding or of uterine or pelvic infection. Any of these signs become evident within 24 hours.

If the tip of the sharp curette has perforated the uterus and the surgeon does not realize it, curettage can cause serious damage to the visceral contents of the pelvis. If the curettings contain evidence of perforation (e.g., intestinal epithelium, bowel wall tissue, or bowel contents), immediate laparotomy is essential to repair the damage. If the operator strongly suspects that the intestine has been damaged, but the character of the curettings fails to confirm this suspicion, a preliminary diagnostic laparoscopy can be of value. If it appears that the bowel has not been damaged, the patient may be observed only.

Curettage and Asherman's Syndrome. In carefully, thoroughly, and systematically removing the tissue that lines the uterine cavity, the operator always must be mindful of the possibility that an overthorough curettage can literally remove all the endometrium and result in amenorrhea. This most unfortunate result of a curettage, known as Asherman's syndrome, most commonly occurs after a particularly thorough cleaning out of an aborting uterus.

It is not the technique of curetting as much as the status of the myometrium that largely determines the risk of removing too much endometrium. The deeper invaginations of endometrial tissue into the myometrium usually are not removed even during a thorough curettage of the nonpregnant uterus, and these undisturbed portions of endometrium generally proliferate rapidly after a curettage. Because the myometrium of the pregnant or aborting uterus is relatively soft and relaxed, however, the curette tends to spread the myometrial fibers more readily; as a result, curetting removes endometrial tissue at a much greater depth than it would if the myometrial tone was that of a nonpregnant uterus. Therefore when curettage of an aborting uterus is indicated, an operator should avoid overvigorous curettage to decrease the risk of removing too much endometrium. Intravenous or intramuscular injection of an oxytocic (e.g., Ergotrate, Methergine, Pitocin) 2 or 3 minutes before curettage of the uterine cavity should ensure firm contraction of the myometrium.

Endocervical Stenosis. If endocervical stenosis in a patient about to undergo a D&C is so severe that it is possible to insert only a small and very narrow sound or probe and not possible to significantly dilate the endocervical canal, the surgeon can insert a small laminaria tent along the path of the sound and reschedule the D&C 24 hours later. At that time the laminaria tent can be removed; the cervix will be sufficiently dilated to permit insertion of a small curette. For the diagnosis of abnormal uterine bleeding, aspiration biopsy is a faster and less costly alternative to D&C.[33]

OFFICE ENDOMETRIAL BIOPSY FOR AMBULATORY PATIENTS

Endometrial biopsy done as an office procedure on a fully ambulatory patient often identifies a malignancy in the endocervix or in the uterine cavity. However, it is best to depend on the result of biopsy and to plan therapy for endocervical or endometrial malignancy only when the pathology report identifies it. As the first step of therapy, the gynecologist should make a careful appraisal of the clinical stage of the malignancy based on findings on examination under anesthesia and during a prehysterectomy fractional curettage of the cervix and uterine cavity.

It is equally important to perform operating room fractional curettage when the results of biopsies taken in the office or clinic are negative and there is a clinical suspicion of malignancy. Preliminary hysteroscopy can help to identify and localize any suspicious areas or sites of the endometrium. First the endocervical canal and then the uterine cavity must be thoroughly explored. In the uterus, the use of both the polyp forceps and a curette, usually larger than that used in the cervix, ensures detection of a pedunculated polyp or an infiltrating malignancy. When a patient has recurrent abnormal or postmenopausal bleeding despite a benign or negative sampling, hysteroscopy can help establish the diagnosis.

Many gynecologists are no longer using rigid, hollow steel curettes of varying sizes for endometrial biopsy; instead they are using a flexible plastic Pipelle- or Curelle-type curette, which is an inexpensive and disposable unit (Fig. 16-20). Because it is only 3.1 mm in outer diameter, its insertion is virtually painless and can be done without preliminary dilation or anesthesia. After the insertion of its tip into the uterine cavity, suction is applied by traction on a built-in plunger, and the tip is moved back and forth several times within the cavity as the hollow tube is rotated. In this way, the four quadrants of the endometrial cavity are sampled quickly. The plastic curette is removed from the uterus and the tip is cut off. By pushing the plunger to its original position, the undamaged contents of the hollow tube are expressed into a specimen jar containing an appropriate fixative. When a sample of tissue adequate for histologic analysis has been obtained, the procedure has become a most cost-effective substitute for formal dilation and curettage.[14,35]

When an inadequate sample of tissue has been obtained, or symptoms of abnormal bleeding persist, diagnostic and operative hysteroscopy can provide the diagnosis. The experienced hysteroscopist with adequate equipment should be able to provide the service quickly and safely and often in a properly equipped office.[2,46] The subject is fully discussed in Chapter 41.

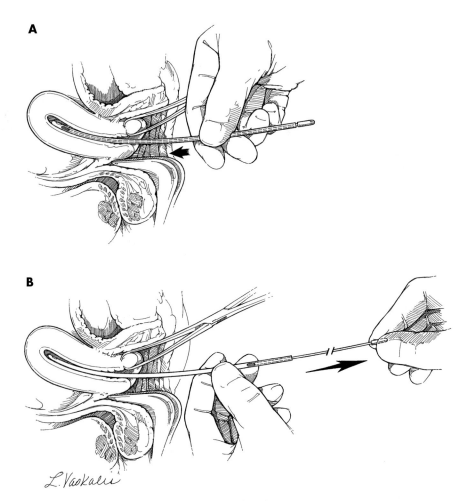

Fig. 16-20 Endometrial biopsy using the Pipelle or Curelle. **A,** A plastic curette with sheath fully advanced is inserted through cervix into full depth of endometrial cavity. A tenaculum may be used to steady the cervix if necessary. **B,** While holding sheath, piston is quickly and fully withdrawn from it until it is stopped and linked in position. Sheath is rotated as it is moved back and forth several times to sample the endometrium. Then it is withdrawn and the tip cut off and discarded. Contents of the hollow tube are expressed into a specimen jar by pushing plunger to its original position. (From Nichols DH, Randall CL: *Vaginal surgery,* ed 4, Baltimore, 1996, Williams & Wilkins.)

REFERENCES

1. Axe S, Parmley T, Woodruff JD, Hlopak B: Adenomas in minor vestibular glands, *Obstet Gynecol* 68:16, 1986.
2. Baggish MS: Management of cervical intraepithelial neoplasia by carbon dioxide laser, *Obstet Gynecol* 60:378, 1982.
3. Baggish MS, Dorsey JH: CO_2 laser for the treatment of vulvar carcinoma in situ, *Obstet Gynecol* 57:371, 1981.
4. Bazin S, Bouchard C, Brisson J, et al: Vulvar vestibulitis syndrome: an exploratory case-control study, *Obstet Gynecol* 83:47, 1994.
5. Ben-Baruch G, Schiff E, Menashe Y, Menczer J: Immediate and late outcome of vaginal myomectomy for prolapsed pedunculated submucous myoma, *Obstet Gynecol* 72:858, 1988.
6. Bornstein J, Zarfati D, Goldik Z, Abramovici H: Perineoplasty compared with vestibuloplasty for severe vulvar vestibulitis, *Br J Obstet Gynaecol* 102:652, 1995.
7. Burke L: The use of the carbon dioxide laser in the therapy of cervical intraepithelial neoplasia, *Am J Obstet Gynecol* 144:337, 1982.
8. Capen CV, Masterson BJ, Magrina JF, Calkins JW: Laser therapy of vaginal intraepithelial neoplasia, *Am J Obstet Gynecol* 142:973, 1982.
9. Cheetham DR: Bartholin's cyst: marsupialization or aspiration? *Am J Obstet Gynecol* 152:569, 1985.
10. Davis GD: Management of Bartholin duct cysts with the carbon dioxide laser, *Obstet Gynecol* 65:279, 1985.
11. DiSaia PJ: Microinvasive cancer of the cervix in pregnancy. In Nichols DH, DeLancey JOL, editors: *Clinical problems, injuries, and complications of gynecologic and obstetric surgery,* ed 3, Baltimore, 1995, Williams & Wilkins.
12. DiSaia PJ, Creasman WT: *Clinical gynecologic oncology,* ed 2, St Louis, 1984, Mosby.
13. Doyle JB: Paracervical uterine denervation of the cervical plexus for relief of dysmenorrhea, *Am J Obstet Gynecol* 70:1, 1955.
14. Emanuel MH, Wamsteker K, Lammes FB: Is dilatation and curettage obsolete for diagnosing intrauterine disorders in premenopausal women with persistent abnormal uterine bleeding? *Acta Obstet Gynecol Scand* 76:65, 1997.
15. Friedrich EG Jr: The vulvar vestibule, *J Reprod Med* 28:773, 1983.
16. Friedrich EG Jr: Vulvar vestibulitis syndrome, *J Reprod Med* 32:110, 1987.

17. Gimpelson RJ, Rappold HO: A comparative study between panoramic hysteroscopy with directed biopsies and dilatation and curettage: a review of 276 cases, *Am J Obstet Gynecol* 158:489, 1988.

18. Goetsch MF: Vulvar vestibulitis: prevalence and historic features in a general gynecologic practice population, *Am J Obstet Gynecol* 164:1609, 1991.

19. Grimes DA: Diagnostic dilation and curettage: a reappraisal, *Am J Obstet Gynecol* 142:1, 1982.

20. Hale RW, Pion RJ: Laminaria: an underutilized clinical adjunct, *Clin Obstet Gynecol* 15:829, 1972.

21. Haskins A: Sterile techniques for dilitation and curettage, *JAMA* 241:623, 1979.

22. Heah J: Methods of treatment for cysts and abscesses of Bartholin's gland, *Br J Obstet Gynaecol* 95:321, 1988.

23. Helmkamp BF, Denslow BL, Bonfiglio TA, Beecham JB: Cervical conization: when is uterine dilatation and curettage also indicated? *Am J Obstet Gynecol* 146:893, 1983.

24. Kaufman RH, Friedrich EG Jr: The carbon dioxide laser in the treatment of vulvar disease, *Clin Obstet Gynecol* 28:220, 1985.

25. Lashgari M, Keene M: Excision of Bartholin duct cysts using the CO_2 laser, *Obstet Gynecol* 67:735, 1986.

26. McKay M, Frankman O, Horowitz BJ, et al: Vulvar vestibulitis and vestibular papillomatosis—report of the ISSVD Committee on Vulvodynia, *J Reprod Med* 36:413, 1991.

27. Nichols DH, McGoldrick KL: Minor and ambulatory surgery. In Nichols DH, Sweeney PJ, editors: *Ambulatory gynecology*, ed 2, Philadelphia, 1995, JB Lippincott.

28. Nielsen S, Hahlin M: Expectant management of first-trimester spontaneous abortion, *Lancet* 345:84, 1995.

29. Ostergard DR: Cryosurgical treatment of cervical intraepithelial neoplasia, *Obstet Gynecol* 56:231, 1980.

30. Peckham BM, Maki DG, Patterson JJ, Hafez GR: Focal vulvitis: a characteristic syndrome and cause of dyspareunia, *Am J Obstet Gynecol* 154:855, 1986.

31. Raphael SI, Burke L: Laser and cryosurgery. In Nichols DH, Evrard JR, editors: *Ambulatory gynecology*, Philadelphia, 1985, Harper & Row.

32. Rock JA, Azziz R: Wolffian duct cyst at the vaginal vault. In Nichols DH, editor: *Clinical problems, injuries, and complications of gynecologic surgery*, ed 2, Baltimore, 1988, Williams & Wilkins.

33. Smith JJ, Schulman H: Current dilatation and curettage practice: a need for revision, *Obstet Gynecol* 65:516, 1985.

34. Stafl A, Wilkinson EJ, Mattingly RF: Laser treatment of cervical and vaginal neoplasia, *Am J Obstet Gynecol* 128:128, 1977.

35. Teale GR, Dunster GD: The Pipelle endometrial suction curette: how useful is it in clinical practice? *J Obstet Gynaecol* 18:53, 1998.

36. Thomas TG: Hyperaesthesia of the vulva. In *The diseases of women*, Philadelphia, 1880, Henry C Lea.

37. Townsend DE: Cryosurgery for cervical intraepithelial neoplasia, *Obstet Gynecol Surv* 34:828, 1979.

38. Townsend DE, Richart RM: Cryotherapy and the carbon dioxide laser management of cervical intraepithelial neoplasia: a controlled comparison, *Obstet Gynecol* 61:75, 1983.

39. Townsend DE, Levine RU, Crum CP, Richart RM: Treatment of vaginal carcinoma in situ with the carbon dioxide laser, *Am J Obstet Gynecol* 143:565, 1982.

40. Walton LA, Baker VV: Mechanical and chemical preparation of the abdomen and vagina. In Buchsbaum HJ, Walton LA, editors: *Strategies in gynecologic surgery*, New York, 1986, Springer-Verlag.

41. Weström LV, Willén R: Vestibular nerve fiber proliferation in vulvar vestibulitis syndrome, *Obstet Gynecol* 91:572, 1998.

42. Wiser WL: Mass in the lateral wall of the vagina. In Nichols DH, DeLancey JOL, editors: *Clinical problems, injuries, and complications of gynecologic and obstetric surgery*, ed 3, Baltimore, 1995, Williams & Wilkins.

43. Woodruff JD, Friedrich EG Jr: The vestibule, *Clin Obstet Gynecol* 28:134, 1985.

44. Woodruff JD, Genadry R, Poliakoff S: Treatment of dyspareunia and vaginal outlet distortions by perineoplasty, *Obstet Gynecol* 57:750, 1981.

45. Woodruff JD, Parmley TH: Infection of the minor vestibular gland, *Obstet Gynecol* 62:609, 1993.

46. Wortman M: Diagnostic and operative hysteroscopy. In Penfield AJ, editor: *Outpatient surgery*, Baltimore, 1997, Williams & Wilkins.

47. Wright VC, Davies E, Riopelle MA: Laser surgery for cervical intraepithelial neoplasia: principles and results, *Am J Obstet Gynecol* 145:181, 1983.

48. Yüce K, Zeyneloglu HB, Bukulmez O, Kisnisci HA: Outpatient management of Bartholin gland abscesses and cysts with silver nitrate, *Aust N Z J Obstet Gynaecol* 34:93, 1994.

17 Management of Cervical Intraepithelial Neoplasm

FREDERICK J. MONTZ

One of the great successes in the history of cancer control and prevention is the result of widespread cervical and upper vaginal exfoliative cytology screening and the direct decrease in the incidence and associated morbidity and mortality of cervical cancer. Over the decades that have ensued following the first reports by Papanicolaou and Traut[75] of a proposed screening technique for cervical cancer and its precursors, cervical cancer death rates have decreased manyfold. Cervical cancer, once the most common cause of cancer death in American women in the 1950s, is now a distant eighth in the late 1990s.[78] As opposed to endometrial and ovarian cancer, cervical cancer is an entity sometimes neglected by the general public. Unfortunately, cervical cancer remains a life-threatening disease for a significant percentage of North Americans[76] and is the leading cause of cancer death in developing countries, claiming almost 500,000 lives per year.[76] American women with financial, cultural, linguistic, geographic, temporal, or other barriers to health care, particularly if they are recent immigrants from "developing" communities, are at the highest risk for this disease.[69] For a subset of women without traditional risk factors but in whom adenodysplasias and malignancies develop, screening is difficult and optimal therapy is controversial.[79]

Today's clinician must continue to be adroit at the evaluation and surgical management of the full range of cervical precancers. It is the goal of this chapter to succinctly outline standards for cervical cancer screening and evaluation of the abnormal Papanicolaou (Pap) smear, although it is beyond the author's intent to offer an all-inclusive review. The major focus of this discussion is on the actual surgical techniques used and the reality of associated complications and outcomes.

PAPANICOLAOU SMEAR CLASSIFICATION

Papanicolaou and Traut's discoveries of the value of exfoliative cytology in cervical cancer prevention, which were first reported in the 1940s,[75] have led to one of the great success stories in cancer prevention and control. Although the Papanicolaou classification was used for almost 50 years, the system had significant shortcomings, particularly regarding the lack of quantification of adequacy of the smear for interpretation and difficulty with interobserver variability. These difficulties served as an impetus for the development of a new classification system[14,68] According to some of the most important contributors to the develop-

ment of the so-called Bethesda System, its merits include (1) the elimination of the numerical Papanicolaou class designations, (2) the evaluation of specimen adequacy as an integral part of the diagnostic report, and (3) the use of precise diagnostic terms to facilitate unambiguous communication between cytopathologists and clinicians.[50] Although much controversy surrounded the initial application of the Bethesda System, it has now become the standard for reporting exfoliative cervical and vaginal cytology results (see the box on p. 283). The Bethesda System introduced the cytologic diagnosis of "low grade" and "high grade" squamous intraepithelial lesions (LGSIL and HGSIL). One should remember that the Bethesda System is not meant to replace the "CIN" histologic classification put forth by Richart[83]; it should be used only for reporting the results of exfoliative cytology.

EVALUATION AND MANAGEMENT OF AN ABNORMAL PAP SMEAR
Squamous Dysplasias

Controversy exists regarding the optimal screening frequency in selected low-risk populations with a confirmed history of normal Pap smears. We prefer to follow the screening guidelines provided by the American Cancer Society[4] and American College of Obstetricians and Gynecologists,[5] which are combined below:

1. Screening should begin at age of first coital experience or 18 years old, whichever comes first.
2. Screening should be repeated yearly as long as the cervix is in situ.
3. Posthysterectomy vaginal cytology is not cost effective except in individuals with a history of prior cervical or vaginal dysplasia.[77]
4. Selected low-risk women may participate in a screening program every 3 years if they are not subject to changes in risk factors and have had three annual Pap smears that are satisfactory for interpretation and assessed as being normal.

Regardless of the controversies, we strongly encourage our primary care colleagues to modify their screening protocols based on individual risk factors and probability of compliance.

Adenodysplasias

Exfoliative cytology, predominantly because it samples the "exposed" cervix and not the most cephalic aspects of

THE BETHESDA SYSTEM, WITH 1991 MODIFICATIONS

FORMAT OF THE REPORT
Statement on Adequacy of the Specimen for Evaluation
General Categorization that may be used to assist with clerical triage (optional)
Descriptive Diagnoses

ADEQUACY OF THE SPECIMEN
Satisfactory for evaluation
Satisfactory for evaluation but limited by (specify reason)
Unsatisfactory for evaluation (specify reason)

GENERAL CATEGORIZATION (OPTIONAL)
Within normal limits
Benign cellular changes: see Descriptive Diagnoses
Epithelial cell abnormality: see Descriptive Diagnoses

DESCRIPTIVE DIAGNOSES
Benign Cellular Changes
Infection
Trichomonas vaginalis
Fungal organisms morphologically consistent with *Candida* spp.
Predominance of coccobacilli consistent with shift in vaginal flora
Bacteria morphologically consistent with *Actinomyces* spp.
Cellular changes associated with herpes simplex virus
Other

Reactive Changes
Reactive cellular changes associated with:
 Inflammation (includes typical repair)
 Atrophy with inflammation ("atrophic vaginitis")

Radiation
Intrauterine contraceptive device (IUD)
Other

Epithelial Cell Abnormalities
Squamous Cell
 Atypical squamous cells of undetermined significance: qualify*
Low-grade squamous intraepithelial lesion encompassing:
 HPV+
 Mild dysplasia/CIN 1
High-grade squamous intraepithelial lesion encompassing:
 Moderate and severe dysplasia
 CIS/CIN 2 and CIN 3
Squamous cell carcinoma
Glandular Cell
 Endometrial cells, cytologically benign, in a postmenopausal woman
 Atypical glandular cells of undetermined significance: qualify*
 Endocervical adenocarcinoma
 Endometrial adenocarcinoma
 Extrauterine adenocarcinoma
 Adenocarcinoma, not otherwise specified (NOS)
Other Malignant Neoplasms: Specify
Hormonal Evaluation (applied to vaginal smears only)
 Hormonal pattern compatible with age and history
 Hormonal pattern incompatible with age and history: specify
 Hormonal evaluation not possible due to: specify

*Atypical squamous or glandular cells of undetermined significance should be further qualified as to whether a reactive or a premalignant or malignant process is favored.
†Cellular changes or human papillomavirus (HPV)—previously termed *koilocytosis atypia*, or *condylomatous atypia*—are included in the category of low-grade squamous intraepithelial lesion.

the endocervical canal, appears to be less effective at screening for adenodysplasias and early endocervical cancers than for similar squamous lesions.[9,18] However, because these disease processes are relatively rare, the widespread use of a more "aggressive" screening than simple brush sampling of the distal endocervical canal proximate to the squamocolumnar junction (SCJ) is not indicated. In that subset of women for whom there is an inordinate concern about the possibility that an endocervical dysplasia is extant, actual endocervical cell harvesting (endocervical curettage, or ECC) as a means of screening may be justifiable.[79,101] However, this high-risk subpopulation of women is not well defined, therefore a more aggressive approach is far from universally accepted. Unquestionably, women who have a screening Pap smear that demonstrates changes of atypical glandular cells of undetermined significance or worse are deserving of thorough endocervical, endometrial, and even other, more distal site sampling and evaluation, since the rate of

underlying adenocarcinoma in these women may be as high as 4%.[42]

SPECIFIC MANAGEMENT TECHNIQUES
Technique Selection

Today's clinician has a plethora of therapeutic options available to him or her for treating a cervical cancer precursor. Generally, we base our decision regarding therapy on the answers to the following questions:

1. What is the probability that the cervical lesion will progress to invasive cancer if left untreated?
2. What is the probability of there being a concomitant invasive cancer that has not been appreciated?
3. What are the patient's stated desires regarding future childbearing (with this response being interpreted in light of the patient's age and prior pregnancy history)?

Two case scenarios serve to demonstrate the guidance value of the responses.

CASE 1

A 23-year-old G0 medical student is referred for evaluation of a persistently abnormal Pap smear. She started undergoing exfoliative cytology screening shortly after coitarche at age 17 and has had annual examinations thereafter. One year before referral, during the process of her annual well-woman evaluation and oral contraceptive renewal, she was noted to have a Pap smear satisfactory for evaluation and interpreted as atypical squamous cells of undetermined significance (ASCUS) by a cytopathology laboratory that is not only known to you, but whose evaluations you trust. She did not undergo further evaluation at that time (e.g., colposcopy with directed biopsies), since her primary care physician recommended that the Pap smear be repeated in 6 months, with which she was compliant. This repeat Pap smear also demonstrated ASCUS. Her physician again believed that any further evaluation was unnecessary and that she would be best served by a repeat Pap smear in 6 months (that is, 12 months from the time of the first abnormal Pap). This repeat screening, her Pap smear, interpreted by the same cytopathology laboratory, again was satisfactory for evaluation and demonstrated findings consistent with ASCUS. This medical student is now referred to you for evaluation and therapy recommendations. The review of her symptoms and past history is truly unremarkable and noncontributory, because she has no other cervical cancer "high-risk lifestyle" factors. Colposcopic evaluation is satisfactory and demonstrates a dominant acetowhite lesion with a regular mosaic pattern between 4 and 6 o'clock located at the SCJ. No associated abnormal vascular changes exist. Numerous, small microcondyloma are noted distant from the SCJ. A biopsy of the ectocervical lesion and an ECC are performed. Final pathology, which you personally review, demonstrates CIN I with HPV effect. The ECC shows normal endocervical cells. What therapy would you select? ▲

CASE 2

A 43-year-old G4 P3 SAB1 is referred by her internist because of an abnormal Pap smear noted on annual screening. The Pap smear results were made available to the patient 4 months ago, but she has been "too busy" to come in for her appointment. The fact that she had an abnormal smear in the late 1980s stands out. This allegedly demonstrated a "precancerous" change, and she remembers undergoing a "microscopic biopsy." She also states that her cervix was "frozen" by her gynecologist after he had reviewed the biopsy results. The results of her most recent Pap smear are available; a reliable laboratory processed the specimen, and a colleague well known to you reviewed the slide. Results demonstrating a high-grade squamous intraepithelial lesion (HGSIL) cannot rule out invasive cancer. The completion of her review of symptoms is unremarkable except for symptoms of loss of urine with physically stressful activity, pelvic heaviness worsening at the end of the day, coital laxity, and the need to splint for defecation. Past medical history is remarkable for gestational diabetes with her terminal pregnancy. All of her children weighed over 3500 g (the last was 4250 g) and were successfully delivered vaginally. She has no underlying or ongoing medical diseases and has not had surgery except for a postpartum tubal ligation after the birth of her last child 7 years ago. Physical examination demonstrated a hypermobile urethra with an associated cystocele that descended to the introitus with Valsalva. The cervix descended to 2 cm from the introitus. With elevation of the cystocele, it was evident that the patient had a concomitant rectocele and breakdown of the perineal body. No enterocele was appreciated distinct from the rectocele. Loss of urine with a full bladder after coughing was confirmed with the patient in a supine position. Colposcopic evaluation was unsatisfactory because the acetowhite lesion extended into the endocervical canal and demonstrated acetowhite changes extending from 2 to 10 o'clock (in a clockwise manner). Associated with these changes were coarse mosaicism and abnormal, "punctuation mark"–like vessels. What would be your next step in managing this patient? ▲

Although these two cases represent the extremes of the cervical preinvasive disease spectrum and aggressiveness of therapy, they also serve to highlight the fact that not only do multiple appropriate treatment protocols exist, but also many appropriate, potential treatment methods for managing these women are available. The author's preference would be to not treat the first patient at all, because it is highly unlikely (less than 15% chance) that a significant precancer will ever develop and even less likely (less than 5% chance) that cancer will ever develop.[73] Progression of disease, if it occurs, usually takes years, unless a new, underlying immune dysfunction (e.g., AIDS) develops. Annual follow-up Pap smears are probably adequate. Similarly, should she suffer a side effect of therapy for her "nondisease," she would unquestionably have the lowest risk-benefit ratio. If we would treat the patient in Case 1 for some reason (patient anxiety, concern about the ability to access the health care system, and so forth), cryotherapy would be preferred.

In Case 2, we would recommend a "see and treat" loop electrosurgical excision procedure (LEEP). As described later in this chapter, this treatment offers the advantages of obtaining diagnosis and therapy at a single outpatient setting while minimizing the need for repeat clinic visits by a patient who has already demonstrated a degree of noncompliance. To us, other potential options would be colposcopic-directed biopsy followed by a LEEP or cold-knife conization (CKC), assuming that the specimen from the directed biopsy did not demonstrate anything worse than early FIGO stage IA disease. The final option would be to proceed directly to a CKC, thus avoiding the interval step of colposcopic-directed biopsy. Hysterectomy, even if indicated for other medical reasons, should not be performed until a LEEP or CKC is completed along with a final pathologic evaluation demonstrating clear surgical margins.

Although a thorough and intricate discussion of the evaluation and treatment of the breadth and depth of cervical dysplasias showing abnormal Pap smears is beyond the scope of this chapter and text, the reader needs to have a basic understanding of the general tenets followed by the author. Therefore we would recommend that the following guidelines be followed based on the Pap smear result (Table 17-1).

Cryotherapy

Indications. Cryotherapy is widely used when (1) satisfactory colposcopic evaluation could be obtained and the collected ECC fails to demonstrate extension of dysplasia to the endocervical locale; (2) the dysplastic lesion envelopes two quadrants of the cervix or less and, if two quadrants are involved, they are adjacent; and (3) there is minimal concern that an underlying microinvasive cancer has been missed.[26] It has been demonstrated that the more significant the dysplastic lesion, regarding both surface area and degree of dysplasia, the less likely that cryotherapy will be successful at clearing the cervical intraepithelial neoplasia.[27,89] We generally reserve cryotherapy for only the lowest grades of HPV-related dysplasias that have failed to regress over time or occur in women who have a low probability that the lesion will ever spontaneously regress (e.g., chronic immune compromised).

Technique. We prefer to perform cryotherapy during the early follicular phase. This timing minimizes the chance of cryotherapy being performed in women who are pregnant and also lessens the chance after the procedure of mistaking

Table 17-1   Guidelines for Management of Abnormal Pap Smear

Pap Smear Report	Intervention	Time to Follow-Up Pap Smear
ASCUS: unclassified or "favor inflammation"	Identify source of inflammation and treat such; if no evident source, simply follow up	6 months × 2
ASCUS: as above but persistent or with concerns regarding capacity to comply with follow-up recommendations	1. Colposcopy and biopsy: treat based on degree of dysplasia (all CIN II or worse: LEEP) and probability that patient will be compliant with follow-up (CIN I with these concerns: cryotherapy) 2. Consider automated rescreening or HPV typing	6 months after evaluation and treatment
ASCUS: favor dysplasia	As per persistent ASCUS	6 months after evaluation and treatment
Low-grade squamous intraepithelial lesion (LGSIL)	As per persistent ASCUS	As per persistent ASCUS
High-grade squamous intraepithelial lesion (HGSIL)	Colposcopy and loop electrical excision procedure. In those settings where there is concern at the time of the colposcopy that an underlying malignancy is present, a punch biopsy should be obtained before LEEP or equivalent procedure	Every 3 months for 2 years and then every 6 months for 3 years. If all Pap smears have remained normal throughout the 5-year follow-up, annual screening can be undertaken.
Invasive cancer	1. Gross lesion evident: biopsy 2. No grossly evident lesion: colposcopy with biopsy; if this fails to identify invasive disease, LEEP if skilled with this procedure and appropriate pathologist for consultation is available; if both of these criteria are not fulfilled: cold knife conization	Individualized based on final diagnosis and treatment
Atypical glandular cells of undetermined significance (AGCUS)	1. Colposcopy with directed biopsies 2. Endocervical curettage 3. Endometrial biopsy/curettage 4. If these fail to explain the source of the AGCUS cells and they persist on repeat Pap smear, consideration should be given to a cold knife cone and diagnostic laparoscopy	Individualized based on final diagnosis and treatment
Adenodysplasia or "adenocarcinoma in situ"	1. Colposcopy with directed biopsy, ECC, and, if patient is at risk for endometrial pathologic changes, EMC 2. Cold knife cone; if no cancer identified at time of initial biopsy 3. If no invasive cancer is diagnosed at CKC review and childbearing is completed: type I hysterectomy (vaginal or abdominal) with attention given to ensure that the entire cervix is removed 4. As per number 3 but desire future childbearing: consideration can be given to conservative follow-up, although the patient must fully understand the potential risks and the deficiencies in our understanding of the natural history of this disease process	

any discharge for menses; this obviates the need to place a tampon in the vagina, which we would rather avoid while the cervix is healing. Before arriving at our consultation suite to have the cryotherapy performed, the patient should take a low-dose NSAID (e.g., 400-mg ibuprofen) to minimize any significant cramping during the cryotherapy. After informed consent is obtained, the largest speculum that does not cause laceration or remarkable discomfort is inserted into the vagina. Colposcopy is repeated to demonstrate the extent of the lesion and to confirm that a more severe change is not evident. Thereafter the largest probe available is used to maximize the chance for obtaining an adequate ice ball. The probe should extend past the lesion by 3 mm or more. If this is not possible, we do not perform repeated, overlapping freezes, but prefer to proceed to an excision procedure (e.g., LEEP) or laser for ablation (see discussion of these techniques later in this chapter). After ensuring that the lesion will be encompassed, we coat the cryo tip with a water-soluble lubricant and apply it to the lesion, guaranteeing that it does not touch any of the nearby vagina. The goal with cryotherapy is to ensure that an adequate ice ball forms so that an area at least 7 mm beyond the evident lesion is frozen (and therefore subsequently sloughed off). Unquestionably, the longer that the liquid nitrogen flows and the cryo probe tip remains at −60° F, the more likely it is that such a degree of freeze will occur. Whether the freeze takes 3 minutes, 5 minutes, or multiple applications is not the point; the degree of cryo destruction is. We prefer to actu-

ally measure 7 mm lateral to the margins of the lesions using a reusable microruler and mark this parameter with a surgical pen (Fig. 17-1). Once the ice ball has reached this margin, we stop the cryotherapy (Figs. 17-2 and 17-3). Rarely does this occur in less than 3 minutes, and in most cases 5 to 7 minutes is the rule. If we have not been able to obtain an adequate ice ball after 10 minutes, our experience shows that it is unlikely to occur with further freezing. In this situation we stop the procedure, document the noted results, and follow the patient as per our routine. We do not have any data regarding failure rates in these relatively rare settings. There are data regarding the use of a multiple short freeze-thaw-freeze technique versus a single, longer freeze, with the former potentially being preferable.[28] However, as previously stated, the total length of freeze is probably most important, not whether a multifreeze technique is used.[40]

Complications
Immediate Complications. Patients must be made aware of two universal side effects of cryotherapy: cramping and a watery serosanguineous discharge. As noted previously, we encourage our patients to take some form of analgesic, preferentially an NSAID, approximately 30 minutes before undergoing cryotherapy. Using this approach, our pa-

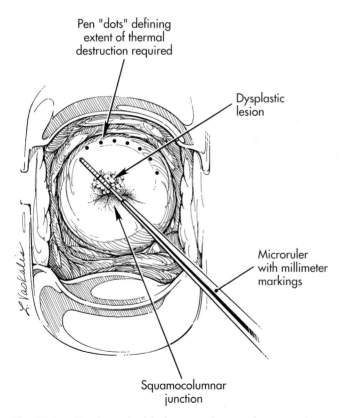

Fig. 17-1 Cervix marked before cryotherapy demonstrating the extent of thermal destruction needed.

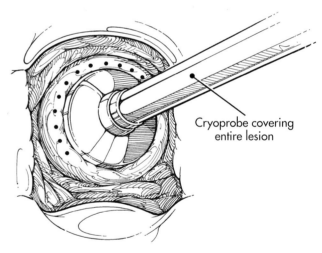

Fig. 17-2 Application of cryo tip to cervix.

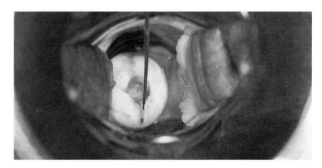

Fig. 17-3 "Ice ball" following cryotherapy.

tients rarely have had significant intraprocedural discomfort, although all have some cramping. Similarly, discomfort after cryotherapy occurs but rarely is significant and usually is easily managed with oral, nonnarcotic analgesics. The watery discharge that follows the thawing of the frozen cervix can range from a transparent gray fluid to an opaque pink if an associated vaginitis has occurred. Significant associated bleeding is rare, although the discharge is almost always heavy enough to require a panty liner to prevent outerwear staining. In most cases, the discharge abates within 2 to 3 weeks; however, it may persist if infectious process is present. We reserve further evaluation and antimicrobial therapy for women who have concomitant symptoms (e.g., pain, burning, pruritus) or in whom the discharge has persisted for more than 3 weeks. Should that rare case of salpingo-oophoritis occur, the physician must ensure that an associated cervical stenosis with pyometra has not developed. If this is demonstrated ultrasonographically, a gentle cervical dilation under appropriate antibiotic coverage should be adequate. Theoretically, microintramural abscesses could develop that would be refractory to antibiotic therapy. If these occur, a hysterectomy may be necessary.

Delayed Complications. Although cervical stenosis can be a permanent anatomic record of cryotherapy[99] and a rare cause of mucometra,[34] no significant data have supported that this causes infertility or iatrogenic perversion of normal labor.[38,58,101] In contradistinction, data have supported the hypothesis that cryotherapy actually can improve the "quality" of the cervical mucus and the probability of fecundity.[10] Similarly, we have been unable to identify data supporting the belief that cryotherapy affects adequacy of subsequent Pap smears or colposcopy.

Outcome. As summarized above, most investigators believe a direct relationship exists between the probability of adequately destroying a cervical dysplastic lesion with cryotherapy and the degree and extent of the underlying cellular abnormality.[18,36,72,96] Generally it can be assumed that durable 5-year or more cure rates in the 80% to 90% range can be obtained when the dysplasia is not full thickness and accompanies only two or less adjacent quadrants, although some authors have achieved equal success rates even when lesions that are at high risk for failure are treated with cryotherapy.[12] However, in many individuals' experience, cure rates may fall as low as 50% to 60% when the disease is more extensive.[18] It also is important to define what is implied by the word *cure*. It is not uncommon in these settings for the actual dysplasia to be destroyed when it is the result of an underlying viral and probably persistent infectious process. Any recurrence simply may be a remanifestation of the HPV infection, lacking an associated dysplasia.

Laser Vaporization and Laser Cone

After their introduction in the late 1970s and early reports of their usefulness,[93] lasers have been widely used in the management of cervical dysplasias, with the first clinical series being published in the early 1980s.[13,24,55] These and subsequent series demonstrated that the effectiveness of the CO_2 laser in the treatment of cervical dysplasias when used as a replacement for cryotherapy[87,96] or CKC biopsy.[6,91,95] Following a burst of excitement and use in our own institution, as in many others, laser vaporization and laser cone have fallen out of favor as the preferred method for managing most patients with cervical dysplasia, although they still are an important part of the armamentarium of the physician managing vaginal and vulvar dysplasias (see Chapter 18). Some skilled surgeons still have lasers readily available to them as a first-line treatment for cervical dysplasia. We acknowledge that these are acceptable regimens in unique environments. Our preference not to use this group of instruments arises from our opinion that lasers are both costly to purchase and maintain and difficult for the "casual" user to master. Therefore they lack the necessary "cost-effectiveness" ratio needed to recommend them as the preferred treatment, especially in an era when measures of efficiency have become an important, if not the preeminent, outcome measure.

By acknowledging the above realities, we believe the laser, when used for vaporization, is probably the preferred method of management of cervical dysplasia in the following patients: (1) those with a topographically large lesion involving three or more quadrants but isolated to the ectocervix, and (2) those in whom the dysplastic lesion is fully visualized but extends, in continuity, from the ectocervix onto the adjacent vagina. In our opinion, laser is the preferred method of treatment in these two settings because it allows for treatment of the lesions without destruction or removal of the underlying tissues, and it achieves an acceptable cosmetic and functional outcome. As with any ablative technique, one caveat must always be followed: multiple, colposcopically directed biopsies of the microscopically worst-appearing areas have to be collected and pathologically reviewed before lesion destruction. This ensures that an early invasive lesion is not inappropriately ablated and therefore inadequately treated.

Technique

1. After obtaining informed consent, a thorough repeat colposcopic examination of the cervix and upper vagina is performed using an acetic acid bath. This is performed usifg a nonreflective speculum that is as large as the patient can comfortably tolerate. A cannula, through which smoke can be removed with a surgical plume evacuator, must be attached to the speculum. Any newly appreciated, potentially malignant lesions are biopsied and sent for pathologic evaluation. If the colposcopic criteria are such that the cancer concerns are overwhelming, we recommend delaying the vaporization until the biopsy results are returned and do not demonstrate an underlying malignancy.
2. Lugol's solution should be liberally applied to the upper vagina and cervix to outline the dysplastic lesions.
3. With 1% lidocaine with 1:100,000 units of epinephrine, a circumferential intracervical block is performed using a 25-gauge spinal needle. A further description and illus-

tration of this technique is given under the discussion on LEEP. If the lesion to be vaporized extends onto the vagina, a similar, infraepithelial infiltration of local anesthetic must be administered. When injected into the subepithelial tissues, the local anesthetic actually acts as a fluid "safety shield" to help limit vaporization from an excessive depth.

4. The laser must be set to an appropriate power setting and spot size. The general rule is to use the highest power density that can be safely employed (much of which is based on the individual surgeon's experience and skill). We prefer a 2-mm spot size with a power density of 1000 W/cm^2. This allows for rapid destruction with minimal lateral thermal spread and associated pain.

5. After the plume evacuator is activated, the area to be destroyed is outlined to mark a distance 6 to 7 mm lateral to the lesion on the cervix and 2 to 3 mm lateral to the lesion on the vagina. The entire transformation zone should be destroyed. With a microruler, the depth of destruction is carried to 6 to 7 mm on the cervix (to ensure destruction of any involved cervical gland crypts), while only to the second epithelial surgical plane of the vagina. This depth of vaporization of the vaginal epithelium is an extension of Reid's work describing the appropriate depth of epithelial destruction on the vulva.[82] By vaporizing only the superficial papillary dermis while allowing for thermal necrosis of the deep papillary dermis, one guarantees adequate destruction of any full-thickness vaginal dysplasias while allowing for rapid and cosmetically and functionally acceptable healing.

6. The base of the defect on either the cervix or vagina is not routinely treated with any hemostatic agent, because the thermal energy of the laser itself usually is sufficient. When bleeding is evident, we prefer to apply mature Monsel's solution and associated pressure with a rectal swab. Usually, 30 seconds of pressure with the Monsel's-soaked swab will be adequate to control any bleeding. In those extremely rare instances, continued bleeding may necessitate a directed suture placed in a figure-of-eight fashion.

7. After treatment, we recommend that the patient abstain from intercourse for 2 weeks after the vaporization and avoid the use of vaginal tampons (see below).

Complications. The laser vaporization side effects—a malodorous discharge and mild spotting or bleeding while the crater at the site of vaporization heals—are ubiquitous, occurring to a greater or lesser extent in all patients. The significant and potentially life-threatening side effects of heavy bleeding that requires active intervention or a true soft tissue infection with associated hyperpyrexia are uncommon, occurring in less than 2% of treated individuals in large combined series.[87,96] We recommend that our patients refrain from the use of vaginal tampons to control any discharge or bleeding, because toxic shock syndrome following vaginal vaporization has been reported.[19]

Outcome. In skilled hands, laser vaporization is highly successful at ablating even high-grade dysplasias with re-

currence rates in the 2% to 10% range depending on the author and study.[6,91,95] These numbers are comparable to those reported for other ablative and resective techniques.

Loop Electrical Excision Procedure

Indications. Following the introduction of the use of thin, metal wire loops and diathermy electric energy in the management of cervical lesions by Cartier[25] and the advances put forth by Prendiville and colleagues in 1986[81] and 1989,[80] loop electrical excision techniques have become a mainstay in the evaluation and management of cervical and other lower genital tract precancer changes. Due to the extensive use of these techniques over the intervening years, the clinician by the late 1990s has a large volume of data on which to base clinical management decisions. The advantages of this procedure are numerous with limited disadvantages (see the box below).

Despite the tens of thousands of LEEPs performed worldwide each year for numerous indications, controversy remains regarding the full extent of indications for this procedure. One of these controversies surrounds the use of a "see and treat" protocol that incorporates LEEP.

Use of LEEP in a "See and Treat" Setting. The traditional protocols for the screening and management of cervical precancers use a three-step technique. In step one, the screening Pap smear is obtained and processed. If the Pap smear is deemed significantly abnormal as described previously, the patient is called back for step two. In step two, the patient undergoes colposcopy with the appropriately directed biopsies and endocervical or endometrial samples as

---

ADVANTAGES AND DISADVANTAGES OF LEEP

ADVANTAGES
1. Inexpensive with durable equipment
2. Easily mastered technique, even by non-physicians
3. Pathologic confirmation of cytologic, pathologic, or clinical impression
4. Capacity to tailor procedure to meet the extent of the lesion and the goals of the resection
5. When used in a "see and treat" setting, allows for single visit evaluation and therapy of a significantly abnormal Pap smear
6. Performed quickly, under local anesthesia, and in an office setting

DISADVANTAGES
1. Potential for excessive thermal destruction and specimen morselization if performed incorrectly
2. Thermal injury to vagina and site of ground pad
3. Postprocedural bleeding at site of resection
4. Postprocedural local soft tissue infection

indicated. Following the review of the histologic specimens, a decision is made regarding therapy or further evaluation, which leads to step three. In this step, the patient undergoes either an attempt at definitive therapy of the cervical dysplasias (e.g., cryotherapy, LEEP) or further diagnostic evaluation (e.g., LEEP or cone biopsy). This three-step protocol requires repeated visits by the patient and makes inefficient use of both the patient's and health care provider's time. It has been proposed that evaluation and therapy can be more efficiently completed by compressing these three steps into two (step one: screening Pap smear; step two: "see and treat" [i.e., colposcopy and immediate therapy before obtaining a histologic diagnosis or, potentially, a diagnostic cone biopsy]) or even one ("one-stop shopping," in which rapid cytology interpretation before the patient leaves the screening site is followed by immediate colposcopy and therapy or diagnostic cone[21]).

Three fact-based beliefs are espoused to support the use of a "see and treat" LEEP technique for evaluation and treatment of a significantly abnormal Pap smear.

1. The Pap smear and colposcopically directed biopsies poorly predict the actual status of underlying cervical dysplasia. For high-grade dysplasias and microinvasive cancer colposcopically directed biopsies have an "undercall" rate of as high as 50%.[17,39,54] This undercall, when patients are treated with ablative techniques, has led to an increase in the rates of inappropriately treated invasive cancers.[7,90]

2. High-grade cervical dysplasias that have a 30% or more chance of advancing to cancer often develop in those patients whose socioeconomic and situational barriers to adequate treatment and follow-up are the greatest.[66,71] These barriers include language, logistics, costs, and the lack of a culturally sensitive screening and treatment environment.[67] The magnitude of these barriers is demonstrated by the fact that between 27%[92] to 70%[88] of women who have biopsy-proven high-grade dysplasias will be lost to follow-up during initial evaluation and never undergo definitive therapy.

3. When compared with traditional evaluation and therapy-critical pathways, the "see and treat" technique can offer a cost savings of as much as 31% over traditional triage and treatment protocols when state-of-the-art accounting techniques are used for cost

analysis.[60] This cost savings can be realized because of the low rates of complications, untoward side effects, and disease recurrence associated with LEEP when it is performed by an experienced health care professional.[3,30]

However, some have expressed concern that "see and treat" will lead to overtreatment of many patients who either do not need any treatment or could be treated with a less-expensive modality (e.g., cryotherapy). Overtreatment is associated with an increase in cost of evaluation and treatment and an increase in rates of serious and costly complications. It has been proposed that immediate LEEP of all patients with an abnormal Pap smear would cost approximately $120.00 (1994 U.S. dollars) more per patient compared with the traditional three-step algorithm and lead to an overtreatment rate of almost 50%.[85]

Data published in recent peer review literature help to resolve these questions regarding the value of "see and treat" LEEP. The initial study presenting the use of LEEP in a "see and treat" protocol came from Bigrigg and associates at the Gloucestershire Royal Hospital.[15] Their experience is unique in that clinical (i.e., non-MD) assistants were trained to provide colposcopic assessment and treatment with the LEEP. A standard colposcopic examination was performed at the time of evaluation of an abnormal Pap smear. A LEEP was immediately performed in those patients in whom the entire transformation zone was visible and an abnormality identified. Patients with unsatisfactory colposcopy were referred for cold knife cone under general anesthesia. Bigrigg's data demonstrated that 32% of patients referred with an essentially negative screening smear (i.e., inflammatory changes or ASCUS) but for whom a repeat Pap smear was requested had no dysplasia evident on the LEEP. The same was true for 16% of patients with mild, 3% with moderate, and 1% with severe dysplasia/rule out invasion (Table 17-2). The corollary was that 32% of the same group of women referred for reevaluation of inflammatory or ASCUS Paps demonstrated high-grade dysplasia or worse at the time of the LEEP. Excellent correlation existed between referring Pap smear and LEEP pathology in the groups of patients that had the more severe squamous changes (HGSIL or rule out invasive disease) (Table 17-2). In this large population-based study, 90% of women required only a single visit to the clinic for therapy. The majority of those requiring more than a single visit returned because of pathologic consider-

Table 17-2   Cytologic Findings and LEEP Histologic Results

	Histology				
Cytology	No dysplasia	CIN I	CIN II	CIN III or worse	Total
Negative; repeat (e.g., inflammatory changes, ASCUS)	16 (32%)	18 (36%)	10 (20%)	6 (12%)	50
Mild dyskaryosis	15 (16%)	108 (44%)	65 (26%)	59 (24%)	247
Moderate dyskaryosis	14 (3%)	79 (19%)	169 (41%)	150 (36%)	412
Severe dyskaryosis, invasive	2 (1%)	22 (8%)	57 (21%)	191 (70%)	272
Total	47	227	301	206	981

Data from Bigrigg MA, Codling BW, Pearson P, et al: *Lancet* 336:229, 1990.

ations with only six patients (1%) needing further evaluation because of complications following the LEEP. Pathologic interpretation was acceptable with positive margin rates (44 of 981, or 4%) and rates of unusable material (3 of 981, or <1%) that are superior to what has been noted in randomized trials of LEEP compared with cold knife cone.

Following Bigrigg's report, numerous reviews of varying quality have reported data, in part or in whole, regarding the use of "see and treat." Of these, three are worthy of summary because the authors posed the majority of the appropriate questions and included adequate information in their manuscripts in a way that allows clinicians to interpret the authors' experience and arrive at independent conclusions. A summary of two of these three articles, plus data from Bigrigg et al., is given in Table 17-3.

When reviewing the combined experience from almost 2000 patients,[19,82,87,91] certain phenomena become evident:

1. "See and treat" LEEP can be performed with minimal associated complications.
2. The success rate with a single treatment and the associated ability to limit the number of patient visits for colposcopic evaluation and treatment is approximately 90%.
3. In patients in whom the referring Pap smear was consistent with a high-grade dysplasia, the rates of histologic concordance are high and justify the use of "see and treat" LEEP.
4. Young patients who have minimal cytologic abnormalities on the Pap smear have the highest risk for a negative "see and treat" LEEP.

The data supporting the use of "see and treat" LEEP in the evaluation of patients with Pap smear findings consistent with high squamous-grade intraepithelial lesions or worse are generally convincing. Less data support the universal application of this method when evaluating patients, particularly those under the age of 40 who have minimal (AS-CUS) or low-grade (LGSIL) abnormalities. With the complementary use of other markers for high-risk disease (e.g., HPV DNA types), perhaps a subset of women with low-grade changes can be identified that would have such a high probability of harboring a high-grade dysplasia that "see and treat" LEEP could be justified. Similarly, when barriers to care are nearly insurmountable for a significant percentage of the population (e.g., developing countries and underserved communities in the United States), perhaps the attempt to decrease the rates of both high-grade dysplasias and cervical cancer justifies the risk of overtreatment-related complications These latter hypotheses remain to be proven.

Technique (Fig. 17-4). When one selects a LEEP in the management of CIN, it is important that the resection matches the evident or feared lesion. For example, when a previous colposcopy was determined "satisfactory," a biopsy demonstrated a high-grade dysplasia, and an ECC collected at the time of the colposcopically directed biopsy did not show any underlying dysplasia, a simple resection of the visible lesion and the squamocolumnar junction would be adequate. In contradistinction, when a lesion extended into the canal and its limits were not fully visible, a "sombrero"-type LEEP should be performed. In this technique, a further resection of the endocervical glands is completed using a narrower

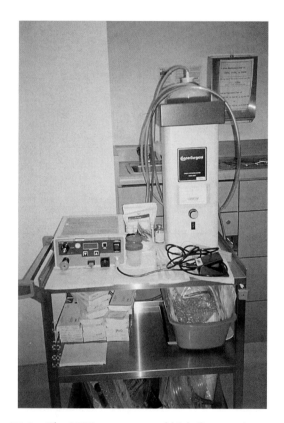

Fig. 17-4   The LEEP generator and high-flow smoke evacuator. Note that these are both located on a single, mobile cart to facilitate movement to multiple rooms to maximize equipment use in an efficient manner.

Table 17-3   Comparison of Three Major Trials of "See and Treat" LEEP

Author	Negative LEEPS in Low-Grade Paps	LEEPs for Low-Grade Paps That Showed High-Grade Dysplasia	Negative LEEPs in High-Grade Paps	LEEPs for High-Grade Paps That Showed Low-Grade Dysplasia	Percentage of Patients Treated at a Single Visit	Major Complication Rate
Bigrigg[61]	31/297 (10%)	140/297 (47%)	16/684 (2%)	101/684 (15%)	897/981 (90%)	6/981 (<1%)
Keijser[41]	5/20 (25%)	8/20 (40%)	24/393 (6%)	19/393 (5%)	386/424 (91%)	32/424 (8%)
Alvarez[3]	60/98 (62%)	27/98 (27%)	29% of CIN 2; 10% of CIN 3*	29% of CIN 2; 9% of CIN 3*	Not stated	2/98 (1%)

*Actual numbers not listed in text.

loop. To reemphasize, the critical point of these illustrations is that the degree of resection must match the disease.

We follow a standard protocol in performing our LEEPs, regardless of the extent of the intended resection:

1. The LEEP is preferentially performed in the follicular phase of the cycle for the reasons listed in the discussion of cryotherapy. This luxury is not always an option in the "see and treat" setting.

2. We do not routinely "premedicate" our patients, because discomfort is almost uniformly minimized with appropriate administration of local anesthesia. For the very rare patient who has demonstrated a level of anxiety that will interfere with the performance of the LEEP, we suggest that they have either a glass or two of their favorite alcoholic beverage or a very low dose of a short-acting anxiolytic just before arriving at our offices. Of course, should the patient choose either of these two "premedications," she will need to be accompanied by a designated driver.

3. Except in those cases where premedication is used, informed consent is obtained, and a review of potential complications and management recommendations following the LEEP is completed. Patients requiring premedication must have informed consent obtained at a separate prior visit.

4. A plastic or insulated speculum that is as large as is comfortable for the patient is placed in the vagina, fully exposing the cervix.

5. The colposcopy is either performed (in the "see and treat" setting) or repeated using our routine protocol of 3% acetic acid bathing of the cervix. We repeat the colposcopy to ensure that a more severe (i.e., invasive) lesion has not been missed and to thoroughly assess the anatomy of the cervix to tailor the LEEP to match both the abnormality and the cervical architecture.

6. The cervix and upper vagina are bathed in Lugol's solution to facilitate resection of the entire lesion and squamocolumnar junction (Fig. 17-5).

7. With 1% lidocaine with 1 : 100,000 units of epinephrine, a circumferential intracervical block is performed using a 25-gauge spinal needle (see Color Plate 1 following p. 304).To facilitate the establishment of the block without inducing undue pain, we request that the patient "cough" at the moment we slide the needle into the cervix, literally allowing the patient to inadvertently push the cervix against the needle. The cervix is injected at four different sites (12-, 3-, 6-, and 9-o'clock positions) with the needle being inserted 2 cm and withdrawn as pressure is placed on the plunger. A total of 8 to 10 ml of local anesthesia is usually all that is needed to obtain excellent analgesia.

8. While waiting for the anesthetic effect to be maximized, we complete the necessary placement of the electric ground pad and the safety checks. These also

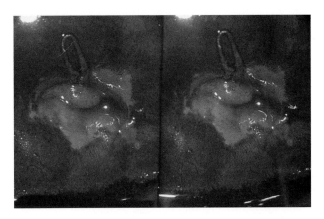

Fig. 17-5   Lugol's bathing of the cervix to demonstrate pathologic (i.e., nonstaining) areas.

are performed later using the preset ground loop setting on the most commonly used electrical generators and must be performed in both the cut and coagulation mode.

9. Using a loop that encompasses the entire lesion and the squamocolumnar junction, we perform an excision of the ectocervix. Depending on the loop size, a power setting from 40 to 55 W of pure cutting current is used for excision. Pure cutting decreases coagulation artifact on the specimen margin without increasing the risk of bleeding. Every attempt is made to remove the entire lesion in a single specimen and with a single pass (Color Plates 2 to 4). When the lesion is too large to be incorporated into a single pass, it should be removed in two equal specimens. The specimens must be labeled and inked in so that the processing pathologist understands the orientation.

10. Should an endocervical excision be deemed necessary, a smaller loop (usually 0.8 cm wide) is used for the second, endocervical pass (Figs. 17-6 and 17-7). The power setting must be lower when using the smaller loop (e.g., 40 W, pure cutting). Again, all attempts to remove the specimen in one piece and in a single pass should be made (Fig. 17-8). Similarly, one should attempt to center the endocervical canal in the middle of the specimen to prevent removing excessive cervical stroma on one side of the specimen while compromising a margin on the contralateral side. As with the ectocervical specimen, the tissue must be marked to facilitate optimal interpretation.

11. After obtaining the endocervical loop specimen, we prefer to collect an endocervical curettage, because we believe that information is beneficial in stratifying patient follow-up triage.[44]

12. Once all specimens have been collected, bleeding vessels are cauterized using the ball electrode and a pure coagulation current of 60 W (Fig. 17-9). We do not coagulate the entire base of the surgical defect,

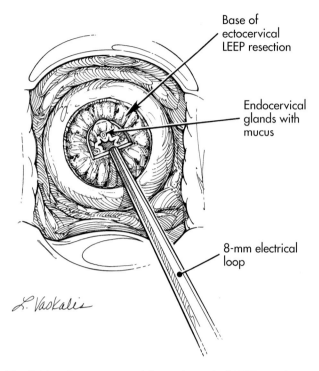

Base of
ectocervical
LEEP resection

Endocervical
glands with
mucus

8-mm electrical
loop

L. Vaskalis

Fig. 17-6   Procurement of the endocervical LEEP specimen.

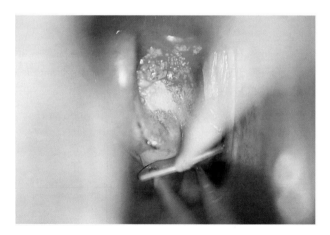

Fig. 17-7   The cervical defect after excision of the endocervical specimen.

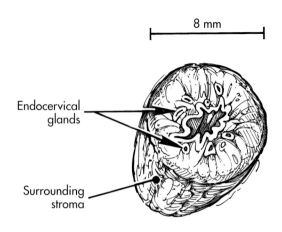

8 mm

Endocervical
glands

Surrounding
stroma

Fig. 17-8   The intact endocervical LEEP "donut" specimen.

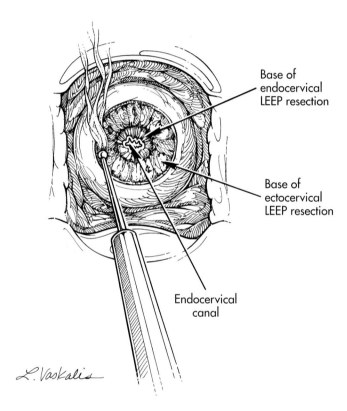

Base of
endocervical
LEEP resection

Base of
ectocervical
LEEP resection

Endocervical
canal

L. Vaskalis

Fig. 17-9   Directed cauterization of isolated bleeding points using the ball electrode.

because we believe this potentiates thermal necrosis with subsequent infection and scarring. Similarly, we do not perform any sophisticated "spot welding" in an attempt to evert what will become the new ectocervical os, because we prefer to simply allow the defect to heal with the least amount of additional trauma. Before removing the speculum from the vagina, we coat the surgical defect with "mature" Monsel's solution (thickened to the consistency of a high-quality paste) to ensure hemostasis once the vasoconstrictive effect of the injected epinephrine has worn off (Fig. 17-10).

13. The vagina is inspected for any inadvertent thermal injury while the speculum is being removed, and the ground pad is removed from the patient's leg with the site inspected to ensure no cutaneous trauma has occurred. The patient is queried about the degree of pain suffered and whether she has any other questions.

14. We routinely schedule a return visit approximately 10 days after the LEEP. At that visit, the LEEP site is inspected, the pathology from the specimens reviewed, a follow-up program outlined, and further questions answered. At this point in the patient's care, we would refer her back to her primary care

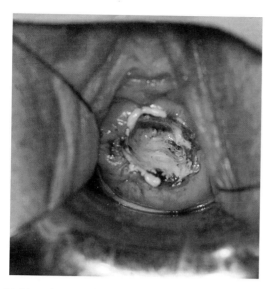

Fig. 17-10   Coating the final cervical defect with Monsel's solution after obtaining adequate hemostasis with the ball cautery and before removing the vaginal speculum.

physician (PCP) for the completion of the follow-up, because most of our patients have been referred by their PCPs for evaluation and management (see Table 17-1).

Complications. One of the great advantages of LEEP, particularly when compared with CKC, is the marked decrease in both short- and long-term complication rates. Most large clinical experiences have noted a 2% post-LEEP bleed rate that requires some form of intervention and a rate of infection that is even less than 2%.* Although post-LEEP infection is uncommon, the dysplasia being treated in many cases represents the effect of a sexually transmitted disease. Therefore in those individuals at high risk for a concomitant gonorrhea or chlamydia infection, or who have symptoms or findings consistent with these infections, we delay the LEEP until cultures or assays are returned negative or satisfactory treatment has been completed. Long-term effects, specifically those that can impair fertility, seem to be uncommon, with most studies failing to identify any LEEP-associated pejorative effects.[59,97]

Outcome. All the credible data to date support the claim that LEEP is as successful at removing cervical precancers and at the same low rate of recrudescence (less than 5%) as the data associated with CKC.[56,74,80] The knowledgeable clinician can predict with a certain degree of accuracy which patients are going to manifest persistence of significant dysplasia after LEEP. A recent article from one of the pioneering investigators in this field has confirmed what others had previously reported[29]: persistence or early recurrence of CIN III is statistically more common in individuals in whom the margins of resection demonstrate dysplasia (16.5%) compared with similar patients with negative resection margins (1.9%, $p < .001$).[31] Although not all investigations have supported this finding,[65] we have found anecdotally that such is the case, and we triage our patients' follow-up based on a combination of margin interpretation and ECC. In those individuals in whom the margin and the ECC is negative, we subsequently screen the patients with Pap smears every 6 months. Patients in whom the ECC is negative and the deep LEEP margins are positive undergo more aggressive follow-up with Pap smears every 3 months for 2 years followed by Pap smears every 6 months for 3 years. Similar patients with an ECC demonstrating dysplasia are either followed in the same manner but with the addition of serial ECCs, or undergo a repeat excisional procedure if any significant concern exists about an extant, unappreciated cervical cancer.[7]

Cold Knife Cone

Indications. The traditional indications for CKC in the management of cervical precancers are illustrated in the box above. These indications have been brought into question because of two new developments or realities. First, our understanding of the oncogenic potential of a minimally abnormal Pap smear has remarkably changed. It is now understood that a cervical malignancy has little chance of developing in the majority of women with a minimally abnormal Pap smear even if left untreated and that the vast majority of these cellular changes resolves spontaneously.[62,94] Therefore the appreciation that the treatment in most cases is worse than the underlying disease has led to a hesitancy to apply criteria numbers 1 and 2 in the box above when the cytologic and colposcopic findings represent only HPV and LGSIL.

The second major event that has led to the decreased use of CKC is the development and wide acceptance of LEEP in the medical community. As outlined previously, LEEP is a highly effective tool that is potentially less costly and has lower rates of associated significant complications.

Therefore we believe only two indications exist for performing a CKC: adenodysplasias of the endocervix and a biopsy consistent with microinvasive cancer. We favor CKC in both of these settings because the specimen submitted to the pathologist for interpretation is guaranteed to be a single piece of tissue. Therefore the difficulties with orientation and "reconstruction" that may occur when a multispecimen LEEP is performed can be avoided. A second rationale for using CKC in these settings, where margin and specimen interpretability is at a premium, is that with less-skilled

---

COLD KNIFE CONE INDICATIONS

1. Unsatisfactory colposcopy
2. Positive endocervical curettage
3. Biopsy consistent with microinvasive cancer
4. Pap smear results that are discordant from colposcopically directed biopsy findings
5. Adenodysplasia

---

*References 6, 19, 25, 33, 82, 87, 91, 95, 96.

"LEEPologists" the incidence of thermal destruction of the margin or the entire specimen in the most flagrant instances of thermal abuse is high.[61] However, LEEP, when performed by a competent and adroit surgeon employing a large enough loop to incorporate the entire ectocervical and endocervical specimen in a single pass and in a single piece of intact tissue, is to be preferred to the not uncommon reality of the morselized, disoriented CKC.[70] The tool or technique does not matter in the special settings of endocervical adenodysplasias and microinvasive squamous carcinomas, but the quality of the specimen does.

Technique. It has been our experience that, regardless of the individual surgeon, CKCs are generally performed in a similar manner with only minor personal variations.

1. After obtaining informed consent and preoperative internal medicine and anesthesia consultation as necessary, the patient is taken to the outpatient surgery center and the procedure performed under sterile conditions.

2. Because of the volume of cervix to be resected and the potential for significant bleeding at the time of resection, we prefer to perform the procedure under systemic analgesia with a protected airway and apply local anesthesia with the associated vasoconstrictive (e.g., epinephrine) into the cervix. The administration of the local anesthetic in the cervix allows the anesthesiologist to use less anesthetic agent and therefore facilitate rapid reversal and early release. Epinephrine decreases intraoperative bleeding, which speeds up the procedure performance. We believe that performing the procedure with an electric cautery is simply an extension of a LEEP and therefore should be performed in the office setting using only local anesthesia. We note one exception to this latter recommendation: when exposure and manipulation of the cervix and upper vagina is impaired because of perverted anatomy. In such a setting, we perform the procedure in a monitored setting where systemic analgesics and relaxants can be administered while relying on locally injected agents for an important percentage of cervical anesthesia.

3. After the patient has been prepared and draped in the dorsal lithotomy position, the vagina and cervix are bathed in Lugol's solution to ensure that all nonstaining areas are resected.

4. A single-tooth tenaculum is placed on the anterior cervix adjacent to the fornix of the vagina. Care should be taken to ensure that the cervix itself is not traumatized by the tenaculum in a way that would lead to difficulties with specimen interpretation.

5. The cervix is manipulated and a figure-of-eight stitch of delayed absorbable suture is placed at the cervical vaginal junction bilaterally at the 3- to 4-o'clock and 8- to 9-o'clock positions (Color Plate 5). Care is taken to place the suture deeply enough into the paracervical and cervical tissue in an attempt to ligate the cervical branch of the uterine artery without deviating laterally into the environs of the ureter and the bladder. Whether the placement of these two sutures is truly valuable in decreasing blood loss at the time of CKC is debatable. Regardless, we leave the sutures long after they have been tied; they serve as a valuable adjunct in manipulating the cervix during the course of the CKC.

6. The tenaculum is removed from the anterior cervix, and a small uterine sound is placed into the endocervical canal. We have found that placing this sound facilitates the appropriate angulation of the excision from the ectocervix toward the endocervical margin and directs the depth of the cone resection.

7. With a no. 11 scalpel blade, the ectocervix is incised lateral to the Lugol's solution nonstaining area and any previously documented lesions (Color Plate 6).

8. We believe in the importance of tailoring the degree and shape of cervical resection so that it correlates with the disease process being treated. For treatment of a squamous lesion, the angle of resection is advanced to obtain a "cone"-like specimen (hence the name) while ensuring an adequate endocervical margin. We aim for a transection of the endocervix at 2 cm above the ectocervical os to remove the entire site at risk and guarantee an adequate margin of clearance. If the cone is being performed for diagnosis or therapy of an adenodysplasia, the cone is more cylindrical. It should extend approximately 7 mm lateral from the canal and all the way to the endocervical endometrial junction (approximately 3 cm). Although microhysteroscopy has been proposed as a method to ascertain the site of the endocervical-endometrial junction, we have not found this to be practical. During the cutting of the cone, care should be taken to avoid unnecessary traumatization of the specimen that is to be resected. We prefer to place an Allis clamp at the site of ectocervical incision closest to the plane of the cervical stroma being cut. We try to limit repeated placements of this clamp because that only leads to specimen trauma and hindering of optimal pathologic evaluation.

9. After the specimen has been removed from the operative field, we are precise in our attempts to ensure proper marking to facilitate orientation by the pathologist. We accomplish this by (1) not opening the specimen and (2) placing a suture at the ectocervix incision site at the 12-o'clock position (Color Plate 7). We do not ink the specimen in the operating room because the pathologist does this at the time of "grossing in" the tissue (see later discussion on specimen processing).

10. An endocervical curettage is collected and sent as a separate specimen. We, like our colleagues at Los Angeles County Womens and Childrens Hospital, have found that the ECC results are a valuable post-cone triage tool.[81] We do not routinely perform an endometrial curettage; its use is limited to patients with specific indications for an endometrial evaluation.[37,86]

11. The base of the cone defect is cauterized at those sites where bleeding is evident (Color Plate 8). Per our description of the LEEP, we do not cauterize the entire defect base, because we believe this increases tissue necrosis, infection, and scarring.

12. We attempt to avoid the use of sutures (such as the Sturmdorf method) to induce hemostasis, because we believe this use increases the risk of both short- and long-term complications.[32] When brisk bleeding persists despite directed cautery, we place interrupted figure-of-eight sutures using no. 0 chromic sutures and incorporating the bleeding site. We specifically use chromic suture because we believe delayed absorbable suture may potentiate local cervical stroma infection with associated delayed bleeding.

13. After adequate hemostasis is obtained, the cone defect site is bathed in Monsel's solution, the retracting sutures are cut so that they just extend to the introitus (to be an easily available "retractor" should the patient bleed after the procedure), and the retractors and speculum are removed from the vagina. When the patient returns for her 10-day postoperative visit, we cut these mobility sutures.

Cone Biopsy in Pregnancy

Because of the wide availability of colposcopy, cone biopsy in pregnancy has become a rare event. It usually is reserved for those settings in which a colposcopically directed biopsy has demonstrated an invasive cancer for which the depth or other associated high-risk criteria for spread cannot be discerned on the specimen supplied or when colposcopic biopsies cannot explain cervical cytologic findings strongly suggestive of invasive cancer.[35]

Because of the remarkably high rate of associated complications, many are greatly hesitant about performing cone biopsies during pregnancy. From a maternal perspective, the risk of bleeding has contributed to this hesitancy. Mean blood losses as high as 500 ml have been reported when cone biopsies were performed in the third trimester, with less blood loss occurring when these same procedures were performed earlier in pregnancy.[8,84] There are other, allegedly potential, maternal complications of cones in pregnancy (e.g., cervical infection, stenosis, DVT and pulmonary emboli, cervical laceration during labor), although we were unable to identify data supporting that these events occurred more often after cone biopsies. Fetal complications are probably more of a concern, with reported increases in first trimester abortion rates and preterm labor, with the latter occurring in as many as 15% of patients.[32] Averette et al.,[8] however, failed to identify an increase in abortion and premature birth rates when comparing their selected data with a similar general pregnant population.

Much of the discussion regarding the use of CKC in pregnancy is moot in light of the wide availability of LEEP. Because of the hemostatic effect of the electrical energy transmitted through the metal loop, we believe this is the preferred method for the rare instance when a pregnant women requires excision for diagnostic purposes. We prefer

to observe what may be early cervical cancers throughout pregnancy without instituting therapy until fetal maturity has been confirmed. At that time, when any diagnostic resection-related induction of labor would have a minimally negative effect, we proceed with obtaining the definitive diagnosis or exclusion of invasive cancer. We prefer to perform a LEEP per our routine, but in the operating room setting with the full range of anesthetic and instrument options. We perform a colposcopically directed segmental resection of the most concerning area while avoiding any attempts to remove the full squamocolumnar junction and transformation zone. The procedure is performed to rule out cancer, not to treat dysplasia, which can be delayed until the postpartum period, when complete involution of the pregnant cervix has occurred.

Complications. Postcone complications can be generally categorized as immediate (within the first few weeks) and delayed. The two most common immediate complications are bleeding and infection. We believe the latter often facilitates the former.

The historical literature has reported significant postcone bleeding in 10% to 15% of CKCs,[2,11] with larger resections more likely to have significant postcone bleeding.[53] Numerous technique modifications have been proposed over the years in an attempt to further decrease the incidence of this potentially life-threatening complication; the majority of literature from the past decade reports a lower rate of postprocedural hemorrhage,[46,95] although this improvement has not been universal.[47] We believe that excessive use of cautery and suture both potentiate this complication by increasing the necrosis and foreign material in the cervix and therefore increasing the probability of a local infection. As the base of the defect is infected, the tissue becomes necrotic and sloughs off, exposing uncoagulated blood vessels. In those patients with bleeding, we immediately institute antibiotic therapy, employ the remnant of the stay sutures for manipulation, remove all previously applied sutures from the cervix, and attempt directed electrocautery while reserving limited suture placement for that very uncommon setting when cautery is unsuccessful.

Infection is a relatively rare complication of CKC, although postcone soft tissue infections, PID, and even pyometra have occurred. As with LEEP, patient selection and precone cervical cultures in the high-risk setting can be valuable.

The most worrisome long-term complications of CKC, in our era of delayed childbearing, are those that negatively affect fecundity. A valuable reservoir of data exists from which to obtain factual information to help counsel our patients about these potentially important side effects. In general, these data demonstrate the following:

1. The larger the cone (in both volume and depth) the more potential for difficulty with fecundity.[52]
2. No proven increase in secondary infertility exists in women who have undergone CKC compared with similar patients.[20,49]
3. The data generally support the belief that CKC increases the probability of a second trimester preg-

nancy wastage, preterm birth, and decreased birth weight, although it is less clear what effect CKC has on the length of labor.[48,51,57,98]

Outcome. When attempting to intelligently assess outcome information that reflects cone effectiveness rates, it is important to stratify results based on the setting in which the cone was performed. In general, CKC is remarkably successful treating preinvasive squamous diseases, with commonly reported success rates in the high-90% range in the larger studies.[1,15,43,85] It is more difficult to accurately grasp the data regarding the effectiveness of CKC in the management of the two diseases for which we are most likely to use it. CKC is probably a highly effective method, approximating hysterectomy in managing FIGO stage Ia1 and early Ia2 disease, with a growing clinical experience to support this belief.[16,23,45,63] We echo the opinions of Morrow et al.[64] and Gilbert et al.[32] that stage Ia cancers can be separated into two groups. One group includes those with less than 3 mm of invasion and no high-risk findings who are adequately managed with CKC. Type I hysterectomy offers little, if any, advantage and has the potential for increased morbidity and cost. Those in a second group, with more deeply invasive disease or high-risk criteria for extracervical spread, need to have the entire cervix with a margin of surrounding tissue resected and the "at-risk" lymph nodes removed and microscopically evaluated. This is best accomplished with a modified radical hysterectomy and pelvic lymphadenectomy.

The difficulty with CKC and the management of adeno-dysplasias of the endocervix, particularly adenocarcinoma in situ, has more to do with the anatomy of the endocervical gland ducts than with the technique itself. Although some controversy exists surrounding the issues, numerous studies from reputable institutions have repeatedly demonstrated a high rate of both persistent disease (approximately 40%) and unappreciated underlying malignancies (nearly 15%) in those cases where a cone biopsy is performed for adeno-CIS and margins are interpreted as disease-free.[5,79,100] These data have led leaders in our discipline to propose that a cone biopsy is inadequate as definitive therapy for women with adeno-CIS and that a simple, extrafascial hysterectomy should be considered the minimal standard. If cone margins are positive for adeno-CIS, we would recommend either a repeat resection, when maintenance of fertility is a high priority, or the performance of a type II hysterectomy, to ensure adequate removal of the entire cervix.

Specimen Processing. Numerous instances exist in which the results of the histologic evaluation of a LEEP or CKC cone specimen modify the anticipated clinical course. Therefore the value of appropriate specimen handling, processing, and interpretation must be emphasized. In the case of a LEEP, as discussed above, the appropriate selection of loop size, power setting, and current type, as well as skill of the clinician, all play a role in the degree of thermal artifact and specimen morselization and whether these interfere with pathologic interpretation. Once the specimens have been resected, appropriate tissue orientation can be valuable to the pathologist charged with specimen processing

and interpretation. We still prefer to mark the ectocervical margin at the 12-o'clock position with a single suture. This is extremely difficult if the specimen has been divided into numerous parts as a result of a transection of the ideal "donut"-shaped (as in a LEEP) or "cone"-shaped specimen. We do not ink the surgical margins in the office or operating room; the evaluating pathologist does this while completing the gross description of the specimen, although completing this at the bedside can be valuable. All collected specimens are immediately placed in fixative before drying occurs. Although selected individuals have proposed an added value of step-serial sections of the entire specimen at 300-μm intervals to produce 60 to 80 sections per cone,[22] we do not believe this offers a significant advantage over standard specimen processing. The donut (or cone) is opened at the 12-o'clock position and laid flat. Twelve blocks (correlating to the "hours of the clock") are obtained by cutting the original specimen in what is functionally a radial manner. Each of these blocks is embedded separately. Initially, a single level section is obtained from each of the 12 blocks. Therefore a total of 12 unique sections to be evaluated microscopically are generated. However, more levels (e.g., "deeper cuts") would be obtained when a discordance exists between anticipated results and final results, or special concerns about the existence of a more aggressive lesion that has not be appreciated are extant.

With the persistence and, in selected communities, the increasing importance of cervical precancers as a source of disease-related morbidity, the active clinician must master the essentials of the diagnosis and treatment of these disease processes. Fortunately, with attention to triage, technique, and follow-up, the worst possible sequelae of cervical dysplasia (e.g., invasive cancer) usually can be easily avoided with minimal treatment-related short- or long-term morbidity. In most environments, it is not an actual "treatment" failure that leads to the development of invasive cancer, but a "system" failure resulting from inadequate screening pretreatment evaluation or follow-up.

REFERENCES

1. Abdul-Karim FW, Nunez C: Cervical intraepithelial neoplasia after conization: a study of 522 consecutive cervical cones, *Obstet Gynecol* 65:77, 1985.
2. Ahlgren M, Ingemarsson I, Lindberg LG, Nordqvist RB: Conization as treatment of carcinoma in situ of the uterine cervix, *Obstet Gynecol* 46:135, 1975.
3. Alvarez RD, Helm CW, Edwards RP, et al: Prospective randomized trial of LLETZ versus laser ablation in patients with cervical intraepithelial neoplasia, *Gynecol Oncol* 52:175, 1994.
4. American Cancer Society: Update January 1992: The American Cancer Society guidelines for the cancer-related checkup, *CA Cancer J Clin* 42:44, 1992.
5. American College of Obstetricians and Gynecologists: *Cervical cytology: evaluation and management of abnormalities,* ACOG technical bulletin, no 183, Washington, DC, 1993.
6. Andersen ES, Pedersen B, Nielsen K: Laser conization: the results of treatment of cervical intraepithelial neoplasia, *Gynecol Oncol* 54:201, 1994.

7. Anderson MC: Invasive carcinoma of the cervix following local destructive treatment for cervical intraepithelial neoplasia, *Br J Obstet Gynaecol* 100:657, 1993.

8. Averette HE, Nasser N, Yankow SL, Little WA: Cervical conization in pregnancy: analysis of 180 operations, *Am J Obstet Gynecol* 106:543, 1970.

9. Ayer B, Pacey F, Greenberg M, Bousfield L: The cytologic diagnosis of adenocarcinoma in situ of the cervix uteri and related lesions. I. Adenocarcinoma in situ, *Acta Cytol* 31:397, 1987.

10. Baram A, Paz GF, Peyser MR, et al: Treatment of cervical ectropion by cryosurgery: effect on cervical mucus characteristics, *Fertil Steril* 43:86, 1985.

11. Benedet JL, Anderson GH, Simpson ML, Shaw D: Colposcopy, conization, and hysterectomy practices: a current perspective, *Obstet Gynecol* 60:539,1982.

12. Benedet JL, Miller DM, Nickerson KG, Anderson GH: The results of cryosurgical treatment of cervical intraepithelial neoplasia at one, five, and ten years, *Am J Obstet Gynecol* 157:268, 1987.

13. Benedet JL, Nickerson KG, White GW: Laser therapy for cervical intraepithelial neoplasia, *Obstet Gynecol* 58:188, 1981.

14. The Bethesda system for reporting cervical/vaginal cytologic diagnoses—report of the 1991 Bethesda Workshop, *JAMA* 267:1892, 1992.

15. Bigrigg MA, Codling BW, Pearson P, et al: Colposcopic diagnosis and treatment of cervical dysplasia at a single clinic visit: experience of low-voltage diathermy loop in 1000 patients, *Lancet* 336:229, 1990.

16. Bissett D, Lamont DW, Nwabineli NJ, et al: The treatment of stage I carcinoma of the cervix in the west of Scotland 1980-1987, *Br J Obstet Gynaecol* 101:615, 1994.

17. Bonardi R, Cecchini S, Grazzini G, Ciatto S: Loop electrosurgical excision procedure of the transformation zone and colposcopically directed punch biopsy in the diagnosis of cervical lesions, *Obstet Gynecol* 80:1020, 1992.

18. Boon ME, de Graaff Guilloud JC, Kok LP, et al: Efficacy of screening for cervical squamous and adenocarcinoma: the Dutch experience, *Cancer* 59:862, 1987.

19. Bowen LW, Sand PK, Ostergard DR: Toxic shock syndrome following carbon dioxide laser treatment of genital tract condyloma acuminatum, *Am J Obstet Gynecol* 154:145, 1986.

20. Buller RE, Jones HW III: Pregnancy following cervical conization, *Am J Obstet Gynecol* 142:506, 1982.

21. Burger RA, Monk BJ, Van Nostrand KM, et al: Single-visit program for cervical cancer prevention in a high-risk population, *Obstet Gynecol* 86:491, 1995.

22. Burghardt E: *Colposcopy and cervical pathology: textbook and atlas,* ed 2, Stuttgart, 1991, Georg Thieme Verlag.

23. Burghardt E, Girardi F, Lahousen M, et al: Microinvasive carcinoma of the uterine cervix (International Federation of Gynecology and Obstetrics stage IA), *Cancer* 67:1037, 1991.

24. Burke L, Covell L, Antonioli D: Carbon dioxide laser therapy of cervical intraepithelial neoplasia: factors determining success rate, *Lasers Surg Med* 1:113, 1980.

25. Cartier R: *Practical colposcopy,* Basel, 1977, S Karger.

26. Charles EH, Savage EW: Cryosurgical treatment of cervical intraepithelial neoplasia, *Obstet Gynecol Surv* 35:539, 1980.

27. Creasman WT, Hinshaw WM, Clarke-Pearson DL: Cryosurgery in the management of cervical intraepithelial neoplasia, *Obstet Gynecol* 63:145, 1984.

28. Creasman WT, Weed JC Jr, Curry SL, et al: Efficacy of cryosurgical treatment of severe cervical intraepithelial neoplasia, *Obstet Gynecol* 41:501, 1973.

29. Felix JC, Muderspach LI, Duggan BD, Roman LD: The significance of positive margins in loop electrosurgical cone biopsies, *Obstet Gynecol* 84:996,1994.

30. Ferenczy A, Choukroun D, Arseneau J: Loop electrosurgical excision procedure for squamous intraepithelial lesions of the cervix: advantages and potential pitfalls, *Obstet Gynecol* 87:332, 1996.

31. Gardeil F, Barry-Walsh C, Prendiville W, et al: Persistent intraepithelial neoplasia after excision for cervical intraepithelial neoplasia grade III, *Obstet Gynecol* 89:419, 1997.

32. Gilbert L, Saunders NJ, Stringer R, Sharp F: Hemostasis and cold knife cone biopsy: a prospective randomized trial comparing a suture versus non-suture technique, *Obstet Gynecol* 74:640, 1989.

33. Girardi F, Heydarfadai M, Koroschetz F, et al: Cold-knife conization versus loop excision: histopathologic and clinical results of a randomized trial, *Gynecol Oncol* 55:368, 1994.

34. Guijon FB: Mucometria: a rare complication of cryosurgery, *Am J Obstet Gynecol* 159:26, 1988.

35. Hannigan EV, Whitehouse HH III, Atkinson WD, Becker SN: Cone biopsy during pregnancy, *Obstet Gynecol* 60:450, 1982.

36. Hatch KD, Shingleton HM, Austin JM Jr, et al: Cryosurgery of cervical intraepithelial neoplasia, *Obstet Gynecol* 57:692, 1981.

37. Helmkamp BF, Denslow BL, Bonfiglio TA, Beecham JB: Cervical conization: when is uterine dilatation and curettage also indicated? *Am J Obstet Gynecol* 146:893, 1983.

38. Hemmingsson E: Outcome of third trimester pregnancies after cryotherapy of the uterine cervix, *Br J Obstet Gynaecol* 89:675, 1982.

39. Higgins RV, Hall JB, McGee JA, et al: Appraisal of modalities used to evaluate an initial abnormal Papanicolaou smear, *Obstet Gynecol* 84:174, 1994.

40. Kaufman RH, Conner JS: Cryosurgical treatment of cervical dysplasia, *Am J Obstet Gynecol* 109:1167, 1971.

41. Keijser KG, Kenemans P, van der Zanden PH, et al: Diathermy loop excision in the management of cervical intraepithelial neoplasia: diagnosis and treatment in one procedure, *Am J Obstet Gynecol* 166:1281, 1992.

42. Kennedy AW, Salmieri SS, Wirth SL, et al: Results of the clinical evaluation of atypical glandular cells of undetermined significance (AGCUS) detected on cervical cytology screening, *Gynecol Oncol* 63:14, 1996.

43. Killackey MA, Jones WB, Lewis JL Jr: Diagnostic conization of the cervix: review of 460 consecutive cases, *Obstet Gynecol* 67:766, 1986.

44. Kobak WH, Roman LD, Felix JC, et al: The role of endocervical curettage at cervical conization for high-grade dysplasia, *Obstet Gynecol* 85:197, 1995.

45. Kolstad P: Follow-up study of 232 patients with stage Ia1 and 411 patients with stage Ia2 squamous cell carcinoma of the cervix (microinvasive carcinoma), *Gynecol Oncol* 33:265, 1989.

46. Krebs HB: Outpatient cervical conization, *Obstet Gynecol* 63:430, 1984.

47. Kristensen GB, Jensen LK, Holund B: A randomized trial comparing two methods of cold knife conization with laser conization, *Obstet Gynecol* 76:1009,1990.

48. Kristensen J, Langhoff-Roos J, Kristensen FB: Increased risk of preterm birth in women with cervical conization, *Obstet Gynecol* 81:1005, 1993.

49. Kullander S, Sjoberg NO: Treatment of carcinoma in situ of the cervix uteri by conization, *Acta Obstet Gynecol Scand* 50:153, 1971.

50. Kurman RJ, Malkasian GD Jr, Sedlis A, Solomon D: From Papanicolaou to Bethesda: the rationale for a new cervical cytologic classification, *Obstet Gynecol* 77:779, 1991.

51. Lee NH: The effect of cone biopsy on subsequent pregnancy outcome, *Gynecol Oncol* 6:1, 1978.

52. Leiman G, Harrison NA, Rubin A: Pregnancy following conization of the cervix: complications related to cone size, *Am J Obstet Gynecol* 136:14, 1980.

53. Luesley DM, McCrum A, Wade-Evans T, et al: Complications of cone biopsy related to the dimensions of the cone and the influence of prior colposcopic assessment, *Br J Obstet Gynaecol* 92:158, 1985.

54. Massad LS, Halperin CJ, Bitterman P: Correlation between colposcopically directed biopsy and cervical loop excision, *Gynecol Oncol* 60:400, 1996.

55. Masterson BJ, Krantz KE, Calkins JW, et al: The carbon dioxide laser in cervical intraepithelial neoplasia: a five-year experience in treating 230 patients, *Am J Obstet Gynecol* 139:565, 1981.

56. Mathevet P, Dargent D, Roy M, Beau G: A randomized prospective study comparing three techniques of conization: cold knife, laser, and LEEP, *Gynecol Oncol* 54:175, 1994.

57. McLaren HC, Jordan JA, Glover M, Attwood ME: Pregnancy after cone biopsy of the cervix, *J Obstet Gynaecol Br Commonw* 81:383, 1974.

58. Monaghan JM, Kirkup W, Davis JA, Edington PT: Treatment of cervical intraepithelial neoplasia by colposcopically directed cryosurgery and subsequent pregnancy experience, *Br J Obstet Gynaecol* 89:387, 1982.

59. Montz FJ: Impact of therapy for cervical intraepithelial neoplasia on fertility, *Am J Obstet Gynecol* 175:1129, 1996.

60. Montz FJ, Holschneider CH, Ghosh K, et al: See and treat loop electrical excision procedure: a resource analysis using activity based costing (abstract), *Gynecol Oncol* 64:362, 1997.

61. Montz FJ, Holschneider CH, Thompson LD: Large-loop excision of the transformation zone: effect on the pathologic interpretation of resection margins, *Obstet Gynecol* 81:976, 1993.

62. Montz FJ, Monk BJ, Fowler JM, Nguyen L: Natural history of the minimally abnormal Papanicolaou smear, *Obstet Gynecol* 80:385, 1992.

63. Morris M, Mitchell MF, Silva EG, et al: Cervical conization as definitive therapy for early invasive squamous carcinoma of the cervix, *Gynecol Oncol* 51:193, 1993.

64. Morrow CP, Curtin JP, Townsend DE, editors: *Synopsis of gynecologic oncology,* ed 4, New York, 1993, Churchill Livingstone.

65. Murdoch JB, Morgan PR, Lopes A, Monaghan JM: Histological incomplete excision of CIN after large loop excision of the transformation zone (LLETZ) merits careful follow-up, not retreatment, *Br J Obstet Gynaecol* 99:990, 1992.

66. National Cancer Institute: *Healthy People 2000,* US Department of Health and Human Services, DHHS pub no (PHS) 91-50212, Bethesda, Md, 1990.

67. National Cancer Institute Cancer Screening Consortium for Underserved Women: Breast and cervical cancer screening among underserved women: baseline survey results from six states, *Arch Fam Med* 4:617, 1995.

68. National Cancer Institute Workshop: The 1988 Bethesda system for reporting cervical/vaginal cytologic diagnoses, *JAMA* 262:931, 1989.

69. National Center for Health Statistics: *Healthy People 2000 Review,* Hyattsville, Md, 1993, US Public Health Service.

70. Naumann RW, Bell MC, Alvarez RD, et al: LLETZ is an acceptable alternative to diagnostic cold-knife conization, *Gynecol Oncol* 55:224, 1994.

71. Orbell S, Crombie I, Robertson A, et al: Assessing the effectiveness of a screening campaign: who is missed by 80% cervical screening coverage? *J R Soc Med* 88:389, 1995.

72. Ostergard DR: Cryosurgical treatment of cervical intraepithelial neoplasia, *Obstet Gynecol* 56:231, 1980.

73. Ostor AG: Natural history of cervical intraepithelial neoplasia: a critical review, *Int J Gynecol Pathol* 12:186, 1993.

74. Oyesanya OA, Amersasinghe C, Manning EA: A comparison between loop diathermy conization and cold-knife conization for management of cervical dysplasia associated with unsatisfactory colposcopy, *Gynecol Oncol* 50:84,1993.

75. Papanicolaou GN, Traut HF: *Diagnosis of uterine cancer by the vaginal smear,* New York, 1943, Commonwealth Fund.

76. Parkin DM, Muir CS, Whelan SL, et al: *Cancer incidence in five continents,* International Agency for Research on Cancer (WHO) and International Association of Cancer Registries, no 120, vol VI, Geneva, 1992.

77. Pearce KF, Haefner HK, Sarwar SF, Nolan TE: Cytopathological findings on vaginal Papanicolaou smears after hysterectomy for benign gynecologic disease, *N Engl J Med* 335:1559, 1996.

78. Platz CE, Benda JA: Female genital tract cancer, *Cancer* 75:270, 1995.

79. Poynor EA, Barakat RR, Hoskins WJ: Management and follow-up of patients with adenocarcinoma in situ of the uterine cervix, *Gynecol Oncol* 57:158, 1995.

80. Prendiville W, Cullimore J, Norman S: Large loop excision of the transformation zone (LLETZ): a new method of management for women with cervical intraepithelial neoplasia, *Br J Obstet Gynaecol* 96:1054, 1989.

81. Prendiville W, Davies R, Berry PJ: A low voltage diathermy loop for taking cervical biopsies: a qualitative comparison with punch biopsy forceps, *Br J Obstet Gynaecol* 93:773, 1986.

82. Reid R: Superficial laser vulvectomy. III. A new surgical technique for appendage-conserving ablation of refractory condylomas and vulvar intraepithelial neoplasia, *Am J Obstet Gynecol* 152:504, 1985.

83. Richart RM. Cervical intraepithelial neoplasia: a review. In Sommers SC, editor: *Pathology annual,* New York, 1973, Appleton-Century-Crofts.

84. Rogers RS III, Williams JH: The impact of the suspicious Papanicolaou smear on pregnancy: a study of nationwide attitudes and maternal and perinatal complications, *Am J Obstet Gynecol* 98:488, 1967.

85. Roland PY, Naumann RW, Alvarez RD, et al: A decision analysis of practice patterns used in evaluating and treating abnormal Pap smears, *Gynecol Oncol* 59:75, 1995.

86. Rubin SC, Battistini M: Endometrial curettage at the time of cervical conization, *Obstet Gynecol* 67:663, 1986.

87. Rylander E, Isberg A, Joelson I: Laser vaporization of cervical intraepithelial neoplasia: a five-year follow-up, *Acta Obstet Gynecol Scand Suppl* 125:33, 1984.

88. Santos C, Galdos R, Alvarez M, et al: One-session management of cervical intraepithelial neoplasia: a solution for developing countries. A prospective, randomized trial of LEEP versus laser excisional conization, *Gynecol Oncol* 61:11, 1996.

89. Schmidt C, Pretorius RG, Bonin M, et al: Invasive cervical cancer following cryotherapy for cervical intraepithelial neoplasia or human papillomavirus infection, *Obstet Gynecol* 80:797, 1992.

90. Shumsky AG, Stuart GC, Nation J: Carcinoma of the cervix following conservative management of cervical intraepithelial neoplasia, *Gynecol Oncol* 53:50, 1994.

91. Skjeldestad FE, Hagen B, Lie AK, Isaksen C: Residual and recurrent disease after laser conization for cervical intraepithelial neoplasia, *Obstet Gynecol* 90:428, 1997.

92. Spitzer M, Chernys AE, Seltzer VL: The use of large-loop excision of the transformation zone in an inner-city population, *Obstet Gynecol* 82:731, 1993.

93. Stafl A, Wilkinson EJ, Mattingly RF: Laser treatment of cervical and vaginal neoplasia, *Am J Obstet Gynecol* 128:128, 1977.

94. Syrjanen K, Kataja V, Yliskoski M, et al: Natural history of cervical human papillomavirus lesions does not substantiate the biologic relevance of the Bethesda System, *Obstet Gynecol* 79:675, 1992.

95. Tabor A, Berget A: Cold-knife and laser conization for cervical intraepithelial neoplasia, *Obstet Gynecol* 76:633, 1990.

96. Townsend DE, Richart RM: Cryotherapy and carbon dioxide laser management of cervical intraepithelial neoplasia: a controlled comparison, *Obstet Gynecol* 61:75, 1983.

97. Turlington WT, Wright BD, Powell JL: Impact of the loop electrosurgical excision procedure on future fertility, *J Reprod Med* 41:815,1996.

98. Weber T, Obel E: Pregnancy complications following conization of the uterine cervix, *Acta Obstet Gynecol Scand* 58:259, 1979.

99. Weed JC Jr, Curry SL, Duncan ID, et al: Fertility after cryosurgery of the cervix, *Obstet Gynecol* 52:245, 1978.

100. Widrich T, Kennedy AW, Myers TM, et al: Adenocarcinoma in situ of the uterine cervix: management and outcome, *Gynecol Oncol* 61:304, 1996.

101. Wolf JK, Levenback C, Malpica A, et al: Adenocarcinoma in situ of the cervix: significance of cone biopsy margins, *Obstet Gynecol* 88:82, 1996.

18 Lower Genital Tract Laser Surgery

MICHAEL S. BAGGISH

CERVIX

Cervical Intraepithelial Neoplasia

The carbon dioxide (CO_2) laser, the dominant method for treating cervical intraepithelial neoplasia (CIN) during the 1980s, has now been displaced by large loop electrical excision.[23,50,55]

Compared with other ablative techniques, the laser had the advantage of producing conelike defects precisely and rapidly. The therapeutic results of laser vaporization performed from 1982 to 1992 demonstrated a high degree of efficacy, with cure rates for high-grade lesions ranging from 90% to 96%, preservation of the anatomic integrity of the cervix, and a visible squamocolumnar junction postoperatively.[2,7,22,31] The series of Baggish, Dorsey, and Adelson[17] reported 10-year results in more than 3000 women, with elimination of CIN in all grade categories using a single laser treatment in 94% of cases. Nevertheless, the major overriding disadvantage dogging all ablation techniques is the absence of a histologic specimen for pathologic evaluation. Clearly, it is always better to obtain a suitable specimen to determine the adequacy of resection margins and whether invasive disease is present.

Laser vaporization is an easily learned operation performed through the colposcope. The laser micromanipulator is coupled to the objective of the colposcope, rendering both lenses identically focused. Vaporization is guided by the following facts:

1. Endocervical glands (clefts) may plunge into the underlying stroma to a depth of up to 6 to 7 mm, but involvement of the cleft with extension of CIN rarely exceeds a depth of 3 mm.[2,3]
2. Advanced grades of CIN tend to spread out not only onto the portio but upward into the canal. CIN rarely extends beyond 1 cm (measured from the squamocolumnar junction).[37,42,56]

Using these data, vaporization is performed by marking a 3-mm peripheral margin beyond the atypical transformation zone and vaporizing down to a *maximal* depth of 1 cm (10 mm) (Fig. 18-1). The deepest part of the vaporization zone is in juxtaposition to the endocervical canal. The defect is gently graded to produce a funnel-shaped crater (Fig. 18-2). The finished product is identical to a small cone. This operation, performed at 30 to 40 W of power with a 2-mm spot (beam diameter), should be completed in 5 minutes with or without local anesthesia. Ten percent or fewer patients have some bleeding postoperatively, usually occurring 4 to 7 days.[5] The bleeding is self-limited and usually stops

spontaneously. Only a small minority of patients require treatment, typically an application of Monsel's paste. If arteriolar bleeding occurs, the bleeding vessel should be sutured. Vaginal discharge ceases within a week or two, and healing is complete within 4 weeks with a visible squamocolumnar junction located at the anatomic external os (Figs. 18-3 and 18-4).

Compared with laser vaporization, the laser excisional cone requires excellent hand-eye coordination and skill. The laser cone employs a manipulating hook to place traction on the tissue as it is cut to obtain sharp margins and to limit thermal artifact. The specifications for laser cone include a beam diameter of 1.0 mm or less, a power density of at least 4000 W/cm² to 16,000 W/cm², and special handling of the endocervical margin (superpulse resection or sharp section). Properly trained personnel should complete the cone within 10 to 12 minutes, with a mean blood loss of less than 10 ml.[10,11] When the procedure is skillfully performed, tissue margins show thermal injury of less than 160 μm. Excessive thermal injury to the specimen can only be attributed to faulty technique.[34] The loop electrical excision procedure (LEEP) requires less technical skill and cuts through tissue by identical methodology (i.e., vaporization). Because the 0.2-mm wire electrode ranges from 5 mm to 2.0 cm in diameter, vaporization is rapid compared with the 0.3- to 0.5-mm spot obtained by the laser, which, in turn, must be connected by sweeping across the tissue field to produce an incision.

Baggish et al.[14] compared thermal injury zones between electrical loop and superpulsed laser (Table 18-1). Accurate measurement showed that thermal artifact was not significantly different between the two techniques. The tissue margins were acceptable from the standpoint of pathologic interpretation (see Table 18-1).

Baggish, Dorsey, and Adelson[17] reported a series of 954 laser excisional cones, with 97% showing no evidence of persistent or recurrent disease. Four cases of invasive carcinoma were detected, which otherwise might have been missed if an ablative procedure had been performed. Seventy-three women had disease extending to the margin; of these, 44 had no further treatment and remained free of disease. Twenty-five women with persisting atypia underwent repeat cone or hysterectomy. Comparing morbidity, time to complete the operation, and healing results, there is no rational reason *not* to perform an excisional operation.

The lessons learned with laser excisional cone can be directly applied to LEEP. The operations are performed under local anesthesia. Hemostasis is acquired by combining a va-

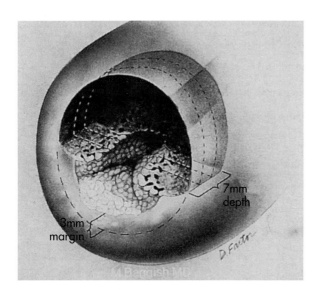

Fig. 18-1   Vaporization is carried out plane after plane to a maximum central depth of 10 mm. The margin around the atypical transformation zone is 3 mm.

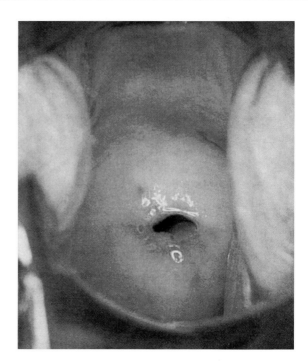

Fig. 18-3   Postoperative multiparous cervix.

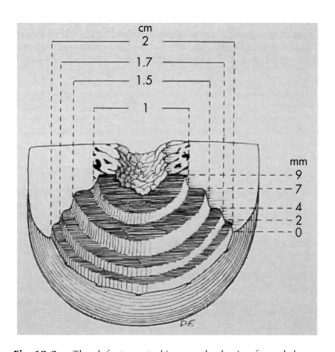

Fig. 18-2   The defect created is a gently sloping funnel shape.

Table 18-1   Mean Measured Depth of Thermal Damage Secondary to Cervical Excision

Technique	Ectocervical Margin (mm)	Endocervical Margin (mm)
Carbon dioxide laser	0.187	0.295
Electrosurgical loop	0.164	0.137

soconstrictor with local anesthesia. Mixing 0.5 ml of vasopressin with 50 ml of 1% Xylocaine produces 1:100 diluted solution. Between 10 and 12 ml of this solution injected with a 25- to 27-gauge needle directly into the cervix produces excellent anesthesia and vasospasm. The objective is to place the needle just beneath the mucosa, inject under pressure, and blanch the cervix white (Fig. 18-5). When the needle is removed, no bleeding is seen. Injecting circumferentially with a 2- to 3-mm margin outside the abnormal transformation zone produces a visible landmark demarcating the peripheral extent of the cone.[19]

Loop electrical excision is now the preferred technique for elimination of both low-grade and high-grade squamous intraepithelial neoplasia.[54,57]

Simple excision of the transformation zone to a depth (height) of 5 to 9 mm is adequate treatment of CIN I (low-grade squamous intraepithelial lesions). The peripheral extent of the loop excision depends on the size and geography of the transformation zone (Fig. 18-6).

The skill of the surgeon, the electrosurgical generator, and the selection of the appropriate loop determine the degree of thermal injury and the readability of the specimen (Table 18-2). Similar variability relates to laser excisional procedures and includes the type of laser (superpulsed versus continuous wave output) and the skill of the surgeon.

The author prefers a constant-voltage electrosurgical generator, a tungsten steel loop sized to the transformation zone, and a pure cut waveform at a power of 40 to 50 W

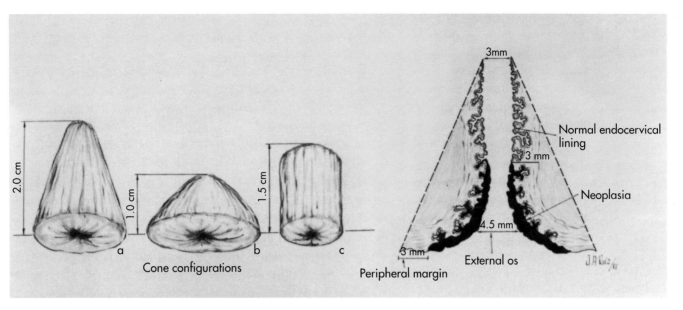

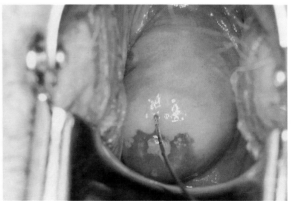

Fig. 18-4   Cone configurations based on laser geography of the atypical transformation zone.

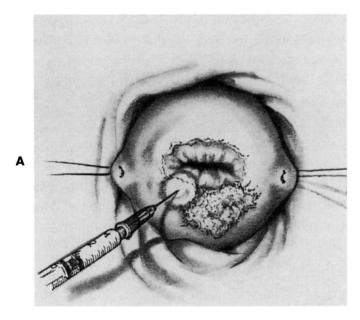

Fig. 18-5   **A,** A diluted vasopressin solution (mixed with 1% lidocaine) is injected just beneath the mucosa. The injection sites are placed peripheral to the atypical transformation zone. **B,** A 26-gauge needle is inserted just beneath the mucosa, and 1:100 vasopressin is injected under pressure (note blanching).

(Fig. 18-7). The operation can be completed in 3 to 6 seconds. The key aspect to this surgery is to activate the electrode on contact with the tissue to guide, not push, the electrode and to exit the tissue quickly on completion of excision.

The author prefers the technique of selective double excision for high-grade disease, again depending on the geography of the abnormal transformation zone.[19] After excision of the transformation zone as described above, a second, small loop is selected, measuring 5 mm in height and 8 mm in width. A 5 mm high supplemental excision is taken in the immediate vicinity of the endocervical canal (Color Plate 9). Power for this portion is reduced to 35 to 40 W. On completion of the excisional portion of the operation, a ball electrode is selected for spray coagulation of any bleeding sites

Table 18-2   Specifications for Loop Electrical Excision of the Transformation Zone*

Peripheral margin	3.0 mm
Height	8 to 10 mm*
Power setting	50 W pure cut
Generator type	Constant voltage

*Supplemental 5 mm excision of the endocervical canal (SDE) for high-grade lesions.

(Fig. 18-8). Forty watts of spray coagulation effectively controls the small bleeding vessels and results only in superficial thermal injury to the tissue (Color Plate 10).

Many reports have been published documenting the effectiveness of loop excisional procedures.[41,45,53,74]

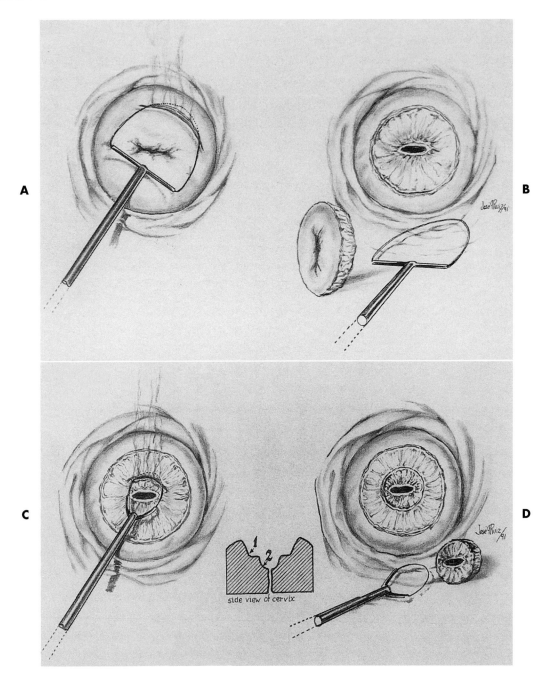

Fig. 18-6   **A,** The 0.2-mm loop electrode vaporizes the cervix across a 10 mm × 20 mm front. **B,** The transformation zone is resected with a 3-mm peripheral margin. A disclike specimen is obtained. **C,** For a high-grade lesion, selective double excision (SDE) is performed with a 5 mm × 6 mm electrode. **D,** A conical-type defect is produced measuring 1.5 cm in height.

Recently, cold conization and electrical loop conization were compared from the standpoint of pathologic interpretation[38,66] (Color Plate 11).

Complications after laser and loop operations to the cervix have been acceptably low compared with other techniques.[43,47] Cervical stenosis has been reported in 1.3% of cases. Cervical incompetence is a rarity, as is pelvic inflammatory disease (0.05%).[17] Excessively large excisional cones effectively remove a substantial volume of cervical stroma and endocervical mucosa and result in cervical ste-

nosis and infertility. Cervical substance also can be removed to some degree by performing multiple cervical operative procedures over time.[20] The additive result is a shrunken, stenotic, functionless remnant flush with the vaginal vault. Table 18-2 lists the specifications for excisional conization performed by loop electrical excision for high-grade squamous neoplasia (CIN 2 or 3).

Perhaps the single operation for which the CO_2 laser maintains an advantage over the electrical loop is the combination cone. The technique for the laser combination cone

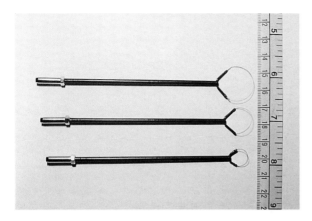

Fig. 18-7 Three loop electrodes that allow the gynecologist to tailor the particular loop to the size of the abnormal transformation zone.

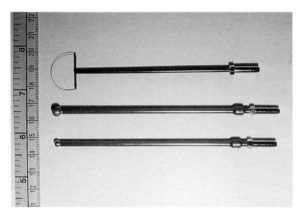

Fig. 18-8 Two ball electrodes (2 mm and 4 mm) are illustrated. The ball electrode is held off the tissue, and the ESU is set for spray coagulation.

has been amply described in the literature.[16,29,76] This technique is ideally suited for geographically extensive CIN (i.e., involving three or four quadrants and extending into the vaginal fornices). Briefly, the ectocervical portion of the lesion is vaporized to sculpted depths (e.g., less than 1 mm in the vagina, 1 to 2 mm on the ectocervix, and 3 to 4 mm in proximity to the canal). A narrow (1 cm or less) cylindrical excisional cone removes the portion of the lesion extending into the endocervical canal (Fig. 18-9). The advantages of the combination cone versus a conventional excisional cone are apparent by measuring the volume of tissue removed with each procedure. The combination cone conserves at least twice as much cervical stroma compared with a large excisional cone.[1]

Reproductive Outcome after Laser or Electrical Loop Excision of the Cervix

Several studies have evaluated the long-term effects of cervical excision or ablation on reproductive function. One study observed 1000 women who had large loop excision of the transformation zone.[40] Of the 192 subsequent pregnan-

cies, 7% had first-trimester miscarriages, and 1.5% had second-trimester losses. Of the latter, one was a missed abortion at 14 weeks; the other two delivered at 16 and 22 weeks. Both followed a prolonged period of painful contractions, that is, no cervical incompetence. Deliveries after 24 weeks were matched with controls and showed no significant differences, with the single exception of the study group having a 2½ times greater incidence of smoking.

A recent controlled study (1997) evaluated 64 women who had laser conizations versus 64 women in a control group.[58] No difference was observed in the rates of preterm delivery and duration of pregnancy with cone heights less than 10 mm. Those having cones greater than 10 mm had an increased risk of preterm delivery and shortened duration of pregnancy.

A Canadian consecutive of study 574 women treated by electrical loop surgery determined that excision of the cervix to a maximal depth of 1.5 cm and a mean frontal diameter of 1.8 cm did not appear to adversely affect subsequent pregnancy outcome and parturition.[35] Premature delivery was not observed in this study. Two stillbirths and three first-trimester spontaneous abortions were recorded.

Another report from the Netherlands based on a total of 424 patients and 96 subsequent pregnancies determined that diathermy loop excision did not affect fertility nor pregnancy outcome.[45]

Finally, a 10-year study of 3070 patients who underwent laser excision, conization, or a combination of the two reported a 1.3% incidence of stenosis and no instance of incompetent cervix.[17]

Cervical Stenosis

Regardless of its cause, cervical stenosis is best treated with a CO_2 laser. *Only* lasers equipped with superpulse are acceptable instruments for this operation. Superpulsing delivers laser energy to tissue in intermittent bursts with very high peak powers (Fig. 18-10). The peak powers exceed the highest continuous power output of the laser by a factor of 5 to 10 times. The duty cycles of such lasers are very low (i.e., 10%, which translates into laser time off tissue of 0.9 second and on tissue of 0.1 second). During the pulse interval, the tissue cools down sufficiently to reduce thermal damage significantly. The operative principle for alleviation of cervical stenosis consists of careful, layer by layer vaporization of the fibrotic tissue constricting the cervical canal until visible (reddish) endocervical tissue is identified. A baby Hegar sound is then placed into the canal. The beam diameter is narrowed from 1.5 mm to less than 0.5 mm by adjusting the variable focusing mechanism located on the laser micromanipulator. The remnant on the endocervical canal is cut along a single axis. After this maneuver, an immediate relief of stenosis allows progressively larger dilators to be placed through the canal. The procedure is completed by everting the endocervical mucosa by enlarging the beam to 1 mm and gently placing it just peripheral to the mucosal margin (buttoning; Fig. 18-11). This operation is the only reliable method for relieving cervical stenosis. If

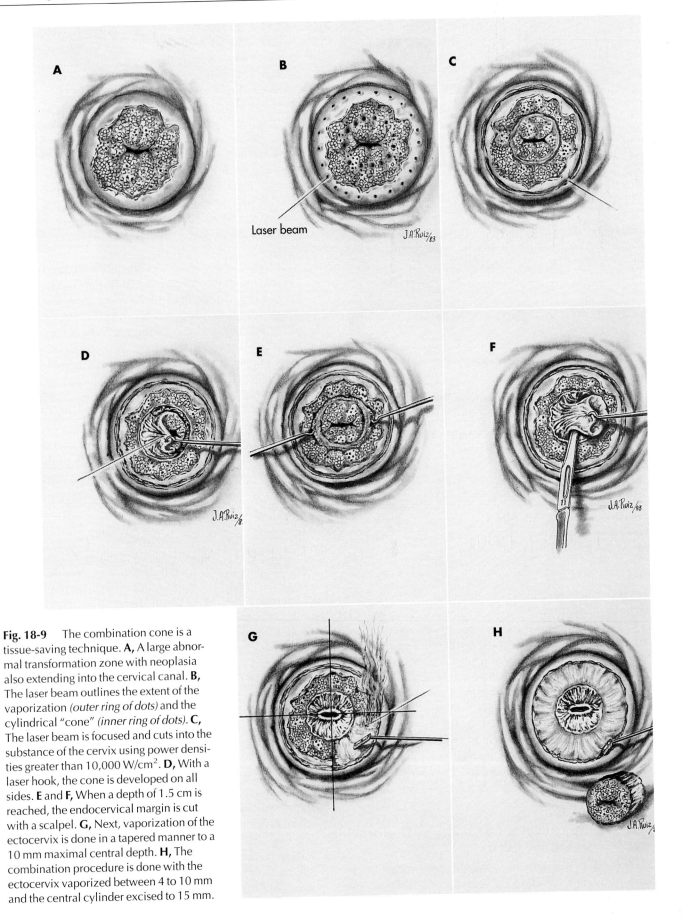

Fig. 18-9 The combination cone is a tissue-saving technique. **A,** A large abnormal transformation zone with neoplasia also extending into the cervical canal. **B,** The laser beam outlines the extent of the vaporization *(outer ring of dots)* and the cylindrical "cone" *(inner ring of dots).* **C,** The laser beam is focused and cuts into the substance of the cervix using power densities greater than 10,000 W/cm². **D,** With a laser hook, the cone is developed on all sides. **E** and **F,** When a depth of 1.5 cm is reached, the endocervical margin is cut with a scalpel. **G,** Next, vaporization of the ectocervix is done in a tapered manner to a 10 mm maximal central depth. **H,** The combination procedure is done with the ectocervix vaporized between 4 to 10 mm and the central cylinder excised to 15 mm.

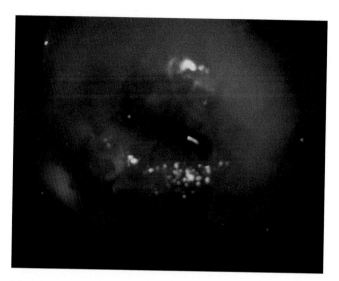

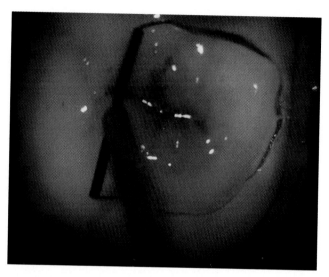

Plate 1 Injection of local anesthesia (1% lidocaine with epinephrine 1:100,000 dilution) directly into the cervical stroma.

Plate 2 Passage of adequate sized loop through the cervix in a manner that completely excises the evident abnormality and the squamocolumnar junction en bloc.

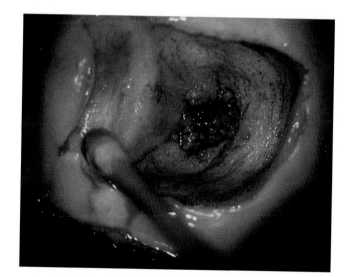

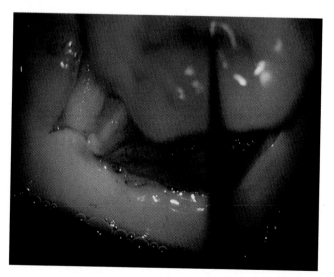

Plate 3 The cervical defect after excision of the ectocervical specimen.

Plate 4 The intact ectocervical LEEP "donut" specimen.

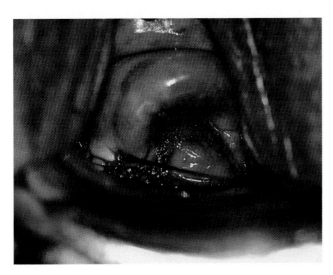

Plate 5 Placement of the CKC retention sutures at the cervical-vaginal reflection at 3- to 4- and 8- to 9-o'clock.

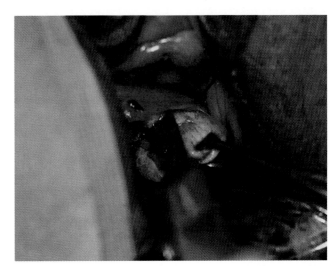

Plate 6 Incision into the ectocervix in a circumferential manner, lateral to the non–Lugol's staining lesions and the squamocolumnar junction.

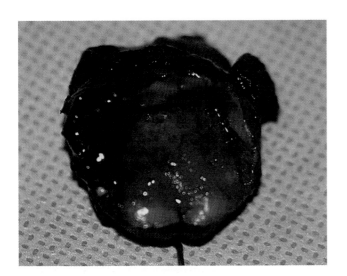

Plate 7 The intact ectocervical CKC "cone" specimen.

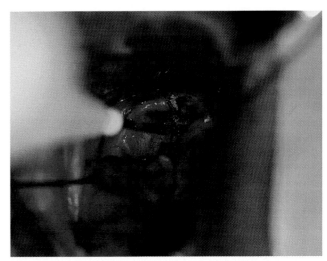

Plate 8 The post-CKC defect after directed cauterization of isolated bleeding points using the cautery.

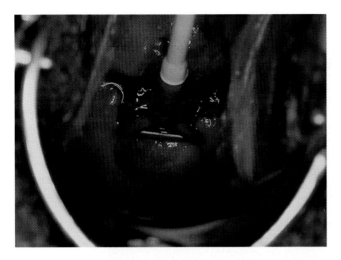

Plate 9   A, Under colposcopic guidance, the loop electrode makes contact with the cervix.

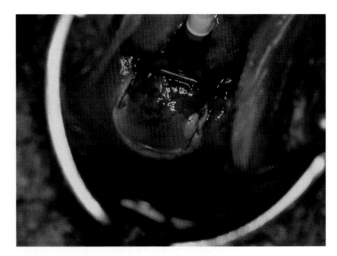

Plate 9   B, The electric current is activated (closed circuit) and the loop is guided upward.

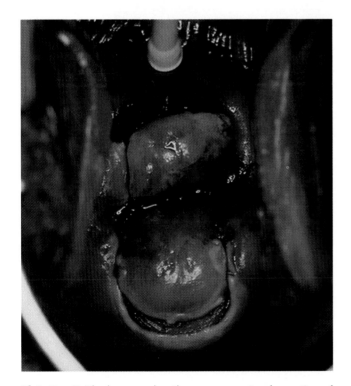

Plate 9   C, The loop reaches the upper margin of resection of the T-zone.

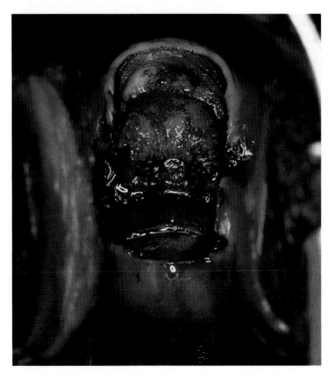

Plate 9   D, The specimen is removed, leaving an 8- to 10-mm defect and light bleeding.

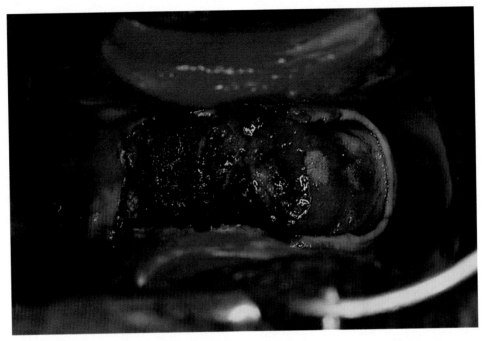

Plate 10   Same cervix as in Plate 9 after spray coagulation of bleeding vessels.

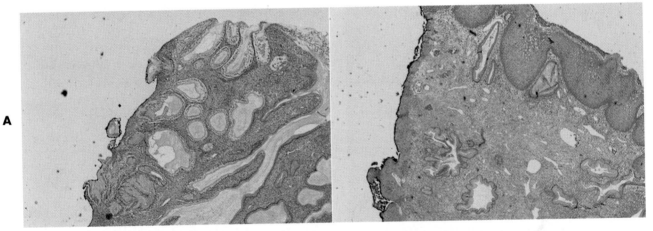

Plate 11   Note the clean endocervical (**A**) and ectocervical (**B**) margins after a properly performed LEEP. The fine black line shows carbon formation and the deeper pink tissue also demonstrates thermal injury.

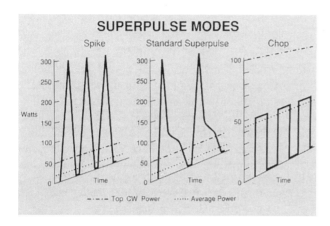

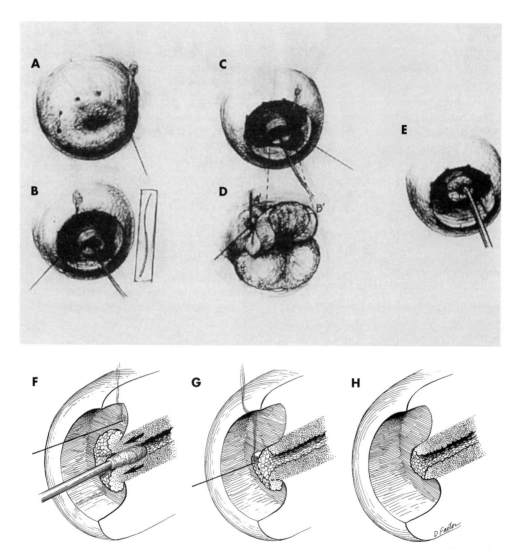

Fig. 18-10 Superpulsing produces very high peaks of power for an instantaneous part of a second followed by a refractory interval. During the latter, tissue cools and diminishes thermal injury.

Fig. 18-11 **A** to **E,** Scar tissue is vaporized away; then the endocervical canal is split by a superpulsed beam. The remaining endocervical canal is everted. **F** and **H,** The technique of laser eversion of the endocervix is shown (buttoning).

any endocervical mucosa is present, the degree of success for this operation is 80%.[13,49] Postoperatively, conjugated estrogen is administered in doses of 5 mg daily. The patient is seen weekly to keep the canal dilated. This combination should be continued for 6 to 8 weeks postoperatively; invariably some rescarring occurs.

Cervical Myoma

Cervical myomas of any size can be excised by a CO_2 laser using a superpulsed beam. The aim of this operation is to preserve the structural integrity of the cervix and to spare more or less completely normal cervical tissue. The greatest risk of this operation is cervical incompetence, which results from inexact excision. The margin of the myoma is identified, and a 1:100 vasopressin solution is injected into the periphery of the myoma. The myoma is cut along the line where it joins normal cervix either on the anterior or posterior cervical lip. A laser hook device is placed into the myoma, placing tension on the tissue. The laser sharply excises the myoma free. This is repeated at all attached margins. To gain exposure for large myomas, the cervix can be split along its anterior or posterior axis. After the myoma has been removed, the cervical wound is sewn with 3-0 polyglycolic acid–type (Dexon or Vicryl) suture. Rosenzweig et al.[64] reported eight excisions of moderate and large cervical tumors with restoration of normal anatomy in every case. No immediate or delayed bleeding was observed.

VULVA

Vulvar Intraepithelial Neoplasia

In recent years, vulvar intraepithelial neoplasia (VIN) has become more frequent in a younger population.[67] The peak age of this disorder is now 35 to 54 years.[68] Vulvar intraepithelial neoplasia can be classified together with cervical intraepithelial neoplasia and vaginal intraepithelial neoplasia to constitute a triad of disorders known as *intraepithelial neoplasia of the lower genital tract.* Several articles have recorded a coexistence of VIN and human papillomavirus (HPV) infections, particularly HPV types 16 and 18.[24,71] Several series of cases involving CO_2 laser treatment have been reported in the literature during the past 10 years.[15,32,48,69,72]

Although the natural history of this disorder, particularly its relationship to invasive squamous cell carcinoma, is by no means clear, recent data suggest that VIN may be two distinct diseases—that occurring in the population below the age of 40 and a more aggressive entity occurring after the age of 50.[10] In the latter group, a more linear relationship seems to exist between intraepithelial disease and subsequent invasive cancer. In the below-40 group, spontaneous remissions have been reported, and progression from the intraepithelial stage to invasive disease is uncommon. Therapy for VIN emphasizes conservative versus radical treatment. Although in the past, simple vulvectomy and skinning vulvectomy have been standards of therapy, these have largely been replaced by local excision and ablative

procedures. The difficulty encountered with ablative procedures in the treatment of this disorder relate, again, to the lack of a tissue specimen for the pathologist and the determination of whether invasive disease is present or whether margins of excision are involved with intraepithelial neoplasia. Regardless of the therapeutic regimen, conservative or radical, a substantial number of cases persist or recur.

The CO_2 laser has proved to be as efficacious as more radical procedures for the treatment of VIN. New therapeutic techniques employing this device and obtaining a tissue specimen for the pathologist effectively blunt the objections to laser vaporization, particularly relating to missing invasive cancer.

Any treatment regimen must emphasize the principle that VIN is part of a regional disease rather than a focal disorder. Careful evaluation of both the vagina and the cervix is imperative to the therapeutic regimen. Additionally, with any conservative therapy, follow-up is extremely important. This must include colposcopic examination of the vulva after the application of 4% acetic acid and the acquisition of directed biopsies when suspicious skin changes are seen.

Baggish et al.[21] have quantified the depth of involvement of epidermis, as well as skin appendages, associated with VIN. Any therapeutic program that does not consider the contiguous spread of neoplasia to skin appendages will fail to remove the disease completely. In an evaluation of over 1000 specimens, skin appendages were involved in 38% of patients with vulvar carcinoma in situ. The appendages most frequently involved were the pilosebaceous apparatus, hair follicles, and sebaceous glands (Fig. 18-12). Clearly, a differential depth of treatment must be considered in any schema that seeks to preserve normal anatomy while eliminating VIN. Treatment in hair-bearing areas of the labia majora, the perineum, and perianal areas requires vaporization to a depth of 2.5 mm (Fig. 18-13). Treatment of the labia minora requires treatment to a depth not exceeding 1 mm. Treatment of periclitoral skin should be tailored individually and based on biopsy measurement of the depth of the neoplasia. Equally important to depth of treatment are the peripheral margins. A minimum circumferential boundary of 3 mm beyond any single or contiguous lesion is required. Wide peripheral margins and adequate depth are the key elements to eliminating disease with a single treatment; multiple-stage treatment may be necessary for geographically extensive disorders. Diagnosis must be made with the aid of magnification in a fashion analogous to CIN. Colposcopic examination and organized mapping of all lesions followed by multiple biopsies must precede any treatment program. Depending on the extent of disease, therapy may be performed under local or general anesthesia.

The CO_2 laser is the most appropriate device to use for vulvar intraepithelial disease, primarily because it is heavily absorbed by water, is primarily a vaporizing laser, and creates mainly surface injury rather than deep coagulative injury. All vulvar laser treatments should be performed with a superpulsed beam, since superpulsing minimizes thermal injury. Baggish et al.[21] and Reid et al.[28,59,60] have identified

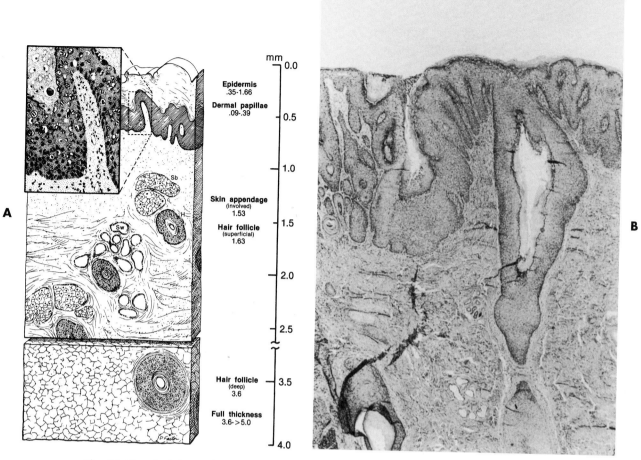

Fig. 18-12 **A,** Schema for epithelial thickening with vulvar carcinoma in situ and involvement of skin appendages (mean depth 1.53 mm). **B,** Carcinoma in situ extending down hair shaft.

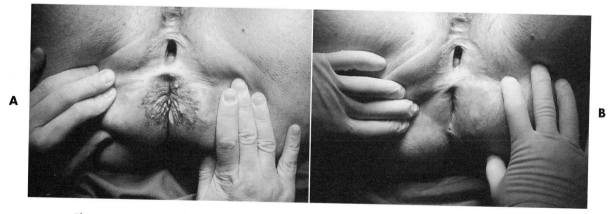

Fig. 18-13 **A,** This woman had a prior "simple" vulvectomy for vulvar CIS. She was referred for CO_2 laser treatment because of perianal CIS. **B,** Eight weeks after laser treatment to the perianal skin and anal mucosa.

the various anatomic layers of vulvar skin on the basis of gross, colposcopic evaluation. Thermal artifact always occurs with laser vaporization because of its heating action. This creates an identifiable yellowish hue to the dermis. (The normal appearance of vulvar dermis is rosy pink.) With su-

perpulse beams, this pink appearance is frequently seen because thermal artifact is diminished. Thermal artifact injury in skin may penetrate to a depth of approximately 500 μm. This zone of thermal injury, which will subsequently slough, should be included in any specification for treatment.

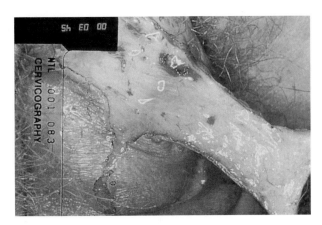

Fig. 18-14 CO_2 laser thin section peals away neoplastic epithelium. The 1- to 2-mm deep sample provides the pathologist with a sample of tissue and at the same time removes the diseased epithelium and dermis.

All laser treatment of the vulva requires some form of anesthesia. For extensive disease, which will be either ablated or excised in a single sitting, general anesthesia is indicated. When local anesthesia is used, treatment can be staged depending on the extent of the disease. The main disadvantage to local anesthesia is pain at the anesthetic injection site. The volume of local anesthesia injected must be carefully limited to avoid toxicity.

Once the appropriate anesthetic has been administered, the laser beam should be adjusted to deliver a spot of approximately 0.5 mm. Trace spots outline the extent of vaporization or excision to be done. This is most conveniently carried out by setting the timing interval at approximately 0.2 second and setting the power meter to approximately 10 W. If a superpulsed beam is to be used, the most convenient setting is 300 pulses per second at a 0.3 msec pulse width. Tracing may be carried out either with the free hand piece using magnifying loops or directing the laser by a micromanipulator attached to a colposcope. The optical loops should deliver a magnification of approximately 2.5 to 3 times.

The preferred method of treating VIN is by laser thin section (Fig. 18-14). This permits intradermal removal of strips of vulvar skin so that the tissue can be analyzed by the pathologist for both the presence of invasive disease and adequacy of surgical margins.[20] Thin section is carried out in the following manner: using a 27 gauge needle, an intradermal injection of either saline or local anesthesia plus 1:100 diluted vasopressin is placed within the area to be treated. Several injections may be required. The purpose of the injection is to create a heat sink within the dermis to absorb heat and minimize thermal damage. The laser beam diameter is set at 0.5 mm or less. An average superpulse power of approximately 22 W is obtained. The previously marked trace spots are connected by making a slow, sweeping movement of the laser beam. A laser hook is placed at a margin of the incision, and a tissue plane is developed in the superficial reticular dermis. With constant traction being placed upward, the thin section is completed by removing

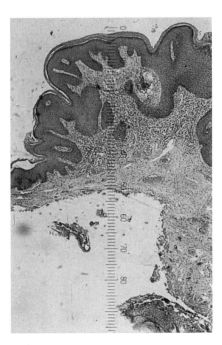

Fig. 18-15   Section of vulvar skin removed by thin section.

strips of epithelium to depths ranging between 1 and 2 mm (Fig. 18-15). No sutures or grafting is required. The laser-treated area will heal in a manner analogous to a laser vaporization. After excision, but still using the superpulse setting previously noted, the laser beam's diameter is increased to 1 to 1.5 mm. Superficial vaporization is carried out to a 3-mm peripheral margin. The char material is swabbed away with 4% acetic acid.

Although vaporization has more disadvantages than thin section, it occasionally is indicated, especially in strategic locations such as the clitoris and labia minora, which have been previously adequately biopsied. Vaporization should be carried out to the appropriate skin level depending on the location of the lesion. Vaporization is best done with a superpulsed beam using a beam diameter of approximately 1.5 to 2 mm. When the perianal skin is involved, a laser speculum should be placed into the anus and the rectal mucosa swabbed with 4% acetic acid. A moist 4 × 4 sponge should be placed in the anus above the intraepithelial lesion to prevent methane gas explosion during laser treatment. Vaporization in the anus should be carried to a depth not exceeding 0.5 mm (Fig. 18-16).

All skin wounds created by laser vaporization or excision are painful. Frequently, this pain is delayed, with maximal discomfort coming 3 to 4 days after laser treatment. Covering the wounds ameliorates the severity of the pain. Bio-occlusive dressings should be applied immediately after surgery if possible. When these wounds are covered, they are virtually painless. Covered wounds also heal more rapidly than undressed wounds because they retain moisture. Dressings are allowed to fall off, which usually occurs several days after treatment. For extensive laser wounds, patients are asked to take sitz baths using Instant Ocean (Fig. 18-17).

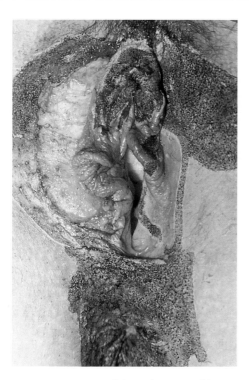

Fig. 18-16 Extensive CIS of the vulva treated by a combination of laser thin-section excision and vaporization.

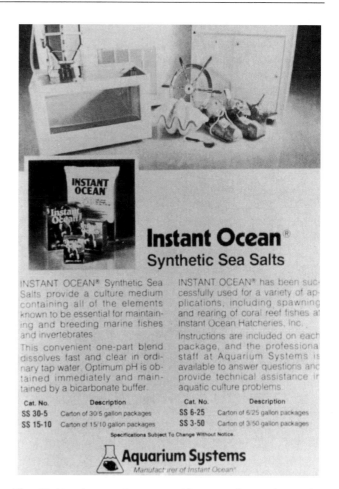

Fig. 18-17 Instant Ocean provides a soothing solution for patients to diminish their discomfort after vulvar laser surgery. It additionally debrides the wounds.

Ocean water can be reconstituted by dissolving Instant Ocean (sea salts) in tap water. Ocean water is more comfortable for patients than are saline sitz baths and tend to debride the wounds, thereby enhancing healing.[52] Patients should take seawater sitz baths approximately four to six times daily. A 1:4 diluted solution of Betadine provided in a plastic bottle is squirted on the perineum after urination or defecation. After bathing or irrigation, the areas are dried using an electric hair dryer on the air cycle. Alternatively, the skin may be thoroughly covered with Silvadene cream, which is reapplied several times a day. All patients are instructed to wear oversized cotton pants to provide adequate circulation of air to the vulva and also to provide a barrier for the Silvadene cream. Healing usually is complete in approximately 6 weeks. The patient should be seen at approximately 2-week intervals until healing is complete and thereafter every 6 months.

Most patients have little immediate pain, mainly because the nerve-sealing action of the laser causes a clublike nerve ending, compared with the shaving brush pattern seen after a knife cut. Delayed bleeding is rare after laser vaporization or thin section. When full-thickness excision occurs, scarring invariably results. Great care must be taken during any excision or vaporization treatment to avoid extension beyond the reticular dermis. Deeper vaporization is made evident by fine, white subvulvar fat. In our series of 51 cases, no infections have occurred. Another concern is coaptation of the labia, which may be avoided by having patients manually separate the labia during sitz baths.

Several series in the literature report cure rates of approximately 80%.[15,69,75] With the thin section, these cure

rates may exceed 90%. Careful long-term follow-up is imperative.

Because vulvar carcinoma in situ is a disease predominantly of younger women, conservative methods of treatment that preserve functional anatomy should be offered to every patient. Even with extensive lesions, laser therapy compares favorably to other methods of treatment. Paget's disease may be the exception; recurrent disease is quite common after laser therapy.

Condylomata Acuminata

The single most frequent indication for CO_2 laser surgery in the lower genital tract during the past decade was condylomata acuminata.[4,6] Unfortunately, the greatest abuse of the laser as a therapeutic tool involved attempts to eliminate condylomata acuminata. The recent history of this disease has been hallmarked by overdiagnosis, overtreatment, and overreaction by the gynecologic community. The acme of this frenzy to treat human papillomavirus was reached when a group of unfortunate women were submitted to more or less total ablation of the vulva, vagina, and cervix.[63] The results of this type of unsubstantiated therapeutic adventurism are predictable: the subclinical HPV infection was not eliminated, the number of complications was excessive, and the postoperative pain inflicted on the patient was unnecessary.

Genital warts are ugly and may cause some discomfort. They spread principally by autoinoculation and may undergo spontaneous regression. HPV is an opportunistic invader that preys on an immunocompromised host. Several factors provide ample opportunity for accelerated growth of genital warts, including immunosuppressive drugs, corticosteroids, oral contraceptives, pregnancy, diabetes mellitus, cigarette smoking, and human immunodeficiency virus infections. The only potentially significant danger associated with warts occurs in children and young adults who are afflicted with laryngeal papillomas. Genital warts by themselves are associated with no significant risk, with the possible exception of misdiagnosis.[12] For this reason, a representative biopsy or even multiple biopsies should be performed before any laser operation.

CO_2 laser ablation of genital warts is indicated for gross disease. Subclinical HPV infections, koilocytosis, and papillosis are not indications for laser treatment. Other than for research purposes, HPV typing is not advantageous and adds unnecessary expense to the workup. It is prudent to reserve laser vaporization for severe disease and attempt to eliminate mild infections with less draconian measures.

The goal of laser vaporization is to eliminate all visible condylomata. The colposcope should be used in all cases to pick up small warts not visible to the naked eye and to provide the best means to examine the anal canal, vestibule, urethra, vagina, and cervix properly. Every patient should have extragenital sites examined for the presence of warts. Although the role of males in the transmission of this disease to female partners is not clear, nevertheless, they should be examined and treated if warts are present on genitalia.[34]

Although local anesthesia may be used, most patients require general or regional anesthesia to permit laser vaporization. Skill and precision result in the removal of warts while preserving normal surrounding tissues. In this circumstance, depth of vaporization does not improve results. In fact, no wart should be vaporized deeper than the level of the surrounding skin surface (Fig. 18-18). Power levels should be set at 40 to 60 W, and beam diameter should be set at 3 mm. Experienced surgeons may use even higher powers to shorten the laser exposure. When vaporization has been completed, the laser beam should be defocused and the power should be dropped to less than 10 W. The defocused beam is carried across the surrounding skin, blanching it white but producing no vaporization or charring. This technique raises surface skin temperatures to approximately 50° C and results in sloughing of the epidermis while preserving undisturbed the underlying papillary dermis. This peripheral blanching or brushing should take in skin to a radius of 1 to 2 cm around to the vaporized warts.[9,36] Anal warts are vaporized by inserting a laser speculum into the anus in a manner analogous to the technique described for VIN except vaporization is more superficial (i.e., to the level

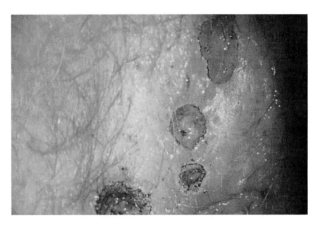

Fig. 18-18 Genital warts are vaporized no deeper than to a level of the surrounding normal skin.

of the surrounding anal mucosa). A nasal speculum is inserted into the urethra, and the laser beam is directed to vaporize urethral warts superficially at a power setting of 10 to 15 W, beam diameter 1.5 mm. Finally, a speculum is placed into the vagina, a laser hook is used to provide exposure, and all visible warts are eliminated; similarly, the cervix is inspected and treated as necessary. All treated areas are thoroughly swabbed with 4% acetic acid to clean off all carbon. A pudendal nerve block is done to eliminate immediate postoperative pain. Silvadene cream is liberally applied to the treated area. Oral contraceptives should be discontinued. Patients should be advised to use condoms for a minimum of 6 months after surgery.

The postoperative treatment regimen is identical to that described for VIN. It is preferable to see these patients within 1 week after surgery. The labia should be separated to prevent coaptation. The operative site should be irrigated with saline, and Silvadene cream should be reapplied. Several studies following the above routine have reported elimination of warts after one or two laser treatments in over 90% of patients. For those patients who are immunologically compromised, supplemental and chronic applications of 5-fluorouracil cream have been recommended.[46] Long-term data about this routine are lacking, and possible mutagenic effects of these applications on surrounding tissues are unknown. Recently, Reid et al.[61] have diminished recurrent warts after laser debulking by administering recombinant interferon.

Laser vaporization of warts during pregnancy has produced varying results.[8,33] High numbers of failures are uniformly observed in early pregnancy. Treatment during the third trimester produces better results, but the elimination of warts also may relate to the subsequent termination of the pregnancy state. The author prefers not to treat beyond 34 gestational weeks because of the increased risk of bleeding and also to allow sufficient time for healing of the operative site before delivery.

The laser does not remove all viable HPV from the lower genital tract. It is likely that large volumes of replicating virus are destroyed as the warts are vaporized; however,

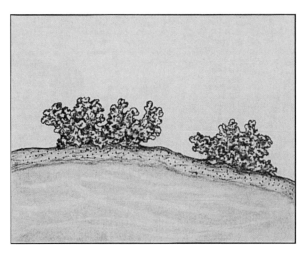

Fig. 18-19 Human papillomavirus is present in both the gross wart and the normal-appearing surrounding skin.

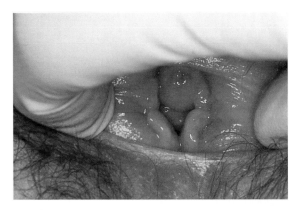

Fig. 18-20 Vulvar vestibulitis exposed characteristic vestibulitis configuration. Extensive erythema and ectasia around Bartholin's gland-duct area.

the patient's own immune system probably plays an important role in the final outcome (Fig. 18-19).

VULVAR VESTIBULITIS (VULVODYNIA)

A recent application of laser technology is for the treatment of vulvar vestibulitis (vulvodynia, vulvar pain syndrome).[39] Vulvar vestibulitis is a condition of unknown etiology associated with burning pain, erythema, and vascular ectasia limited to the vestibule—more specifically, to the skin around Bartholin's glands, the minor vestibular glands, and Skene's glands (Figs. 18-20 and 18-21). Patients typically can date the onset of the problem, describing initial symptoms of pruritis, dryness, painful intercourse, and burning discomfort. The pruritis and concomitant burning lead both the patient and her gynecologist to believe that she has a fungal vaginitis; hence 99% of women are treated with topical antifungals that either have no effect on the patient's symptoms or make them worse.[18,51] Unfortunately, most of the "fungal infections" are diagnosed over the telephone. Those evaluated in the office are uncommonly diagnosed objectively and seldom, if ever, cultured. The patient's itch-

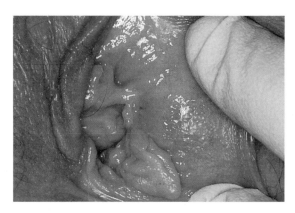

Fig. 18-21 Bartholin's duct opening juxtaposition to the hymenal ring.

ing disappears, leaving her with significant burning pain whenever intercourse is attempted.

The Vulvar Disorders Clinic currently has 285 women with vulvar vestibulitis, of whom 80% historically stopped intercourse or had intercourse less than six times a year because of pain during and after. Tampon insertion, close-fitting jeans, tight underwear, certain exercise, and urination also may be painful for these women.

All patients diagnosed with vulvar vestibulitis should be thoroughly evaluated to rule out infections (fungal, bacterial, and parasitic), as well as other causes of discomfort. The initial treatment is medical and includes avoidance of intercourse, treatment of superficial secondary infections, elimination of all topical medications, distilled water irrigation of the vestibule after voiding, administration of amitriptyline, biofeedback, and calcium citrate. The conservative regimen is attempted for 3 to 4 months. Patients who fail to improve are offered surgical options.

Hexascan Laser Treatment

Hexascan laser or flash lamp–excited dye laser has been reported to be an effective technique for treating vulvar vestibulitis in selected patients.[18,62] The basis for the treatment revolves on the findings of erythema and ectasia, that is, dilated inflammatory capillaries. The hypothesis for the associated pain contends that a causalgia-like condition is produced by the stimulation of the nerves around the distended vessels. The photocoagulative visible light laser emits beams (e.g., KTP-532) that are selectively absorbed by hemoglobin and are likewise selectively reflected by the surrounding skin. Hence the blood-filled, dilated capillaries are selectively coagulated and collapsed. Patients who respond best to this treatment have significant erythema (8 to 10/10) and minimal or no deep Bartholin tenderness. The treatments are performed under local anesthesia supplemented with conscious sedation. The author recommends a series of three treatments at monthly intervals. The dosage on the KTP-532 laser is set at 4 W, and the pulse width is 40 msec (treatment one), 50 msec (treatment two), and 60 msec (treatment three) (Fig. 18-22, *A* and *B*). The procedure begins at the posterior fourchette and works upward adjacent

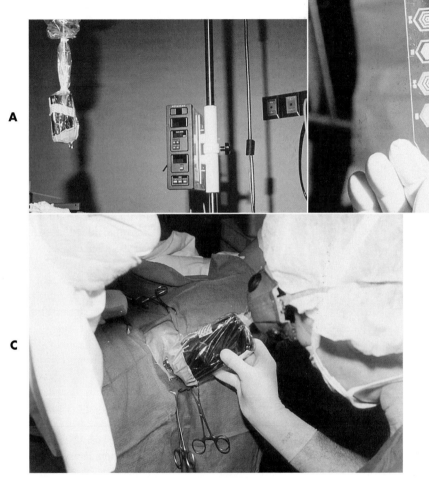

Fig. 18-22 **A,** The Hexascan computer and handpiece (draped). **B,** Patterns that can be selected by the Hexascan computer. **C,** The handpiece is applied to the vestibular skin.

to the hymenal ring on each side to the urethra. The handpiece of the Hexascan is positioned perpendicular to and flattening out the underlying skin (see Fig. 18-22, *C*); 120 pulses are delivered with each handpiece application (Fig. 18-23). When the entire vestibule has been treated, the patient is transferred to a recovery area for 1 to 2 hours and then goes home. Postoperatively, she is given Motrin 800 mg tid for 72 hours.

The penetration of the KTP-532 Hexascan laser beam is measured in fractions of millimeters; the beam does not penetrate beyond the dermis. The flash lamp dye laser penetrates deeper and beyond the dermis and potentially can result in scar formation. Approximately 40% of patients who receive this therapy are "cured," that is, able to have

pain-free intercourse, and do not have recrudescence of symptoms.

The KTP-532 Hexascan laser also is exceedingly useful for treating lower genital tract hemangiomas and vulvar varicosities. The results of treatment are immediately visible (i.e., the lesions are virtually erased). The author prefers staged treatment, that is, dividing the area of treatment of large lesions into zones and spacing treatment at 6 week intervals to access skin color, elasticity, and subdermal scarring (if any). For these lesions, 60 to 80 msec pulse widths have given the best results. Upon completion of treatment, patients are prescribed Instant Ocean baths twice daily for 1 week and Silvadene cream tid and hs for 3 to 4 weeks (Fig. 18-24).

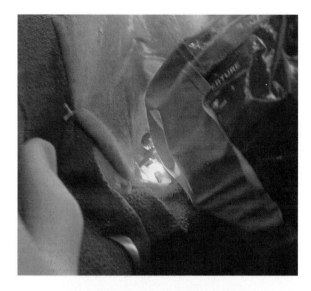

Fig. 18-23 The laser is activated, creating a bright green light.

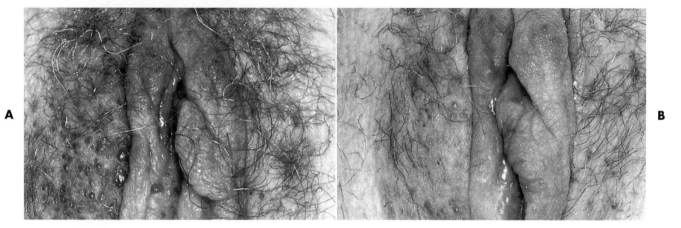

Fig. 18-24 **A,** Woman with extensive vulvar hemangioma bilaterally. **B,** Four weeks after Hexascan treatment.

Excision of Bartholin's Glands and Vestibular Skin and Advancement of the Vagina

The best treatment results for vulvar vestibulitis syndrome, insofar as normal, pain-free intercourse, are observed after surgical excision. Although the initial results after the surgery described by Woodruff and Parmley[73] were quite good, failures occurred after 12 to 18 months. One obvious deficiency of that procedure became apparent: the vestibular skin was removed including a portion of Bartholin's duct. The underlying gland was left behind with either no duct or one that was defective. This oversight is corrected by removing the gland and duct, and excellent results are seen with follow-ups at more than 1 year. Approximately 95% of treated women have pain-free intercourse and another 5% have no vestibular or introital pain but complain of an intermittent "discomfort" in the lower portion of the one labium majus (75% on the left side).

The carbon dioxide laser coupled to a Ziess Opmi One microscope mounted on an S-2 stand is used as a light-scalpel for this procedure (Fig. 18-25, *A*). A Coherent Ultrapulse laser serves this purpose flawlessly. In fact, the laser is uniquely able to perform this fine cutting; no other instrument or device offers the surgeon this sort of excellent advantage. Although gynecologists are typically not experienced with fine, precision surgery, in many instances it proves highly beneficial to wound healing and limitation of scarring.

The Bartholin duct opening is located with a microscope at the lower external margin of the hymenal ring (see Fig. 18-25, *B*).[18] The gland is located deep and slightly lateral to the duct. A 1:100 diluted solution of vasopressin is injected into the operative site with a 25- or 26-gauge needle. A 1.5- to 2.0-cm incision is made into the vestibule over the gland and carried down approximately 1 cm to the bulbocavernosus muscle. The gland is dissected free from the vaginal wall medially and from the ischiorectal fossa laterally (see Fig. 18-25, *C*). In actuality, the gland can be identified only with the operating microscope. The blood supply is secured with mosquito clamps and suture ligated with 4-0 Vicryl. The gland is carefully separated from the bulb of the vestibule and excised with Stephen's scissors (see Fig. 18-25, *D*). The defect is closed with 3-0 Vicryl. The hymenal ring

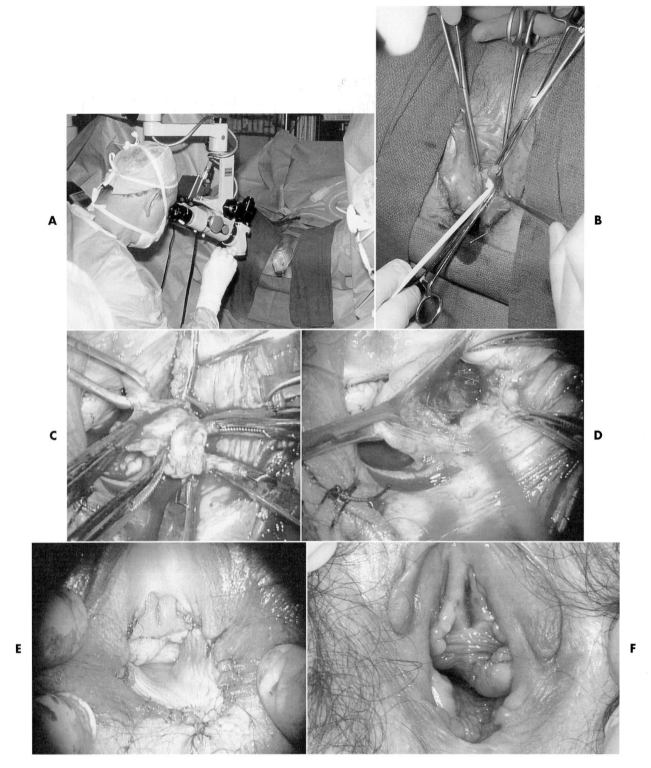

Fig. 18-25 **A,** The surgeon focuses the operating microscope and CO_2 ultrapulse laser on the operative site. **B,** An incision has been made into the left vestibule just lateral to Bartholin's duct. **C,** Bartholin's gland is isolated and its vascular supply clamped. **D,** The gland is removed and the vascular pedicals are suture ligated with 4-0 Vicryl. The vagina is to the right of the medial Allis clamp. **E,** The vestibule has been excised and the vagina advanced. **F,** Eight weeks after Bartholin gland excision, vestibule excision, and vaginal advancement.

and vestibular skin are removed including the skin of the fossa navicularis to the margin of the perineal skin. The cut margin of the lower vagina is undermined after infiltration with 1:100 vasopressin and advanced to the margin of the labun minus and perineum, where it is sutured into place with 4-0 Vicryl (see Fig. 18-25, *E*). The operation from start to finish is performed under microscopic control coupled to a video (the latter for the benefit of the assistants).

Upon completion of the surgery, the patient spends 6 to 8 hours in the recovery area and is discharged home. Silvadene cream is applied to the wound tid and hs. Instant Ocean baths are started 24 hours after completion of the surgery. All patients are seen weekly to inspect and clean the operative site. At 4 weeks, a silicone-rubber vaginal form is fitted, and the patient places this in her vagina daily for 10 to 15 minutes until she resumes intercourse (see Fig. 18-25, *F*).

VAGINA
Vaginal Intraepithelial Neoplasia

The vagina is more difficult to treat than either the vulva or cervix because of its large surface area, its numerous folds and fornices, its limited maneuvering space, and its laborious exposure. Most women find stretching of the vagina extremely uncomfortable and reflexly resist this by contracting their levator ani muscles, which in turn increases the pain. Because of the aforementioned factors, conventional surgery is difficult to perform and good assistance is problematical to render. The operating microscope with multiple magnification options and consistently bright light is the most useful tool for facilitating vaginal surgery. An 11-inch-long titanium laser hook permits examination of vaginal folds and the posthysterectomy vaginal tunnels located at the vaginal vault (Fig. 18-26). Control of bleeding in the vagina is crucial because, as previously stated, the view of the operative site, particularly in the upper and middle thirds of the vagina, is tenuous under the best circumstances. As with other locations in the lower genital tract, the CO_2 laser is best suited for vaginal surgery. The ability to operate without directly touching the tissue and at the same time to obtain thermally based hemostasis are real advantages in this location. Electrosurgical cutting and cryosurgical instruments are ill-suited and even hazardous to use in the vagina.[27]

The vaginal mucosa in a menstruating woman is less than 500 μm in thickness. A postmenopausal women's epithelium is 100 to 200 μm deep, and the entire wall may be only 2 to 3 mm thick. With the exception of girls and women with adenosis, the vagina does not contain glands or crypts; therefore intraepithelial neoplasia is limited to the vaginal mucous membrane; the neoplastic process does not project into the underlying stroma unless invasion is present.

Vaginal intraepithelial neoplasia (VAIN) is the least common of the group of lower genital tract premalignancies (i.e., an annual incidence of 0.2 per 100,000 women).[26] It is more common in women who have had CIN or VIN. The disorder most often is located in the upper third of the va-

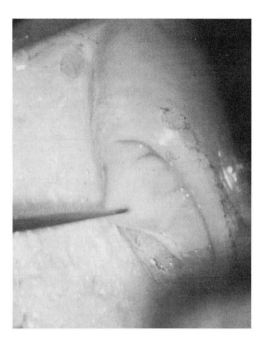

Fig. 18-26 A titanium laser hook exposes a vaginal vault tunnel in a woman who has previously undergone hysterectomy.

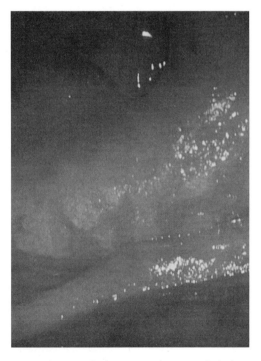

Fig. 18-27 Plaques of white vaginal intraepithelial neoplasia located in the upper, posterior third of the vagina.

gina and is multifocal. The lesions are best identified by colposcopic examination after generous swabbing of the vagina with 4% acetic acid. The VAIN appears as white, flat or raised foci usually devoid of abnormal vessels (Fig. 18-27). Occasionally, a pigskinlike punctuation is visualized, but mosaic patterns are a rarity. Confluent papillomatous growths also may be seen, particularly in the anterior and posterior fornices. These wartlike lesions are difficult to grade on the basis of colposcopic appearance alone and should be plentifully biopsied before undertaking laser treatment. Typically, these lesions are initially detected as a result of routine cytology. Patients who have undergone hysterectomy should continue to undergo annual cytologic sampling of the vagina for this reason.

Adequate examination and mapping of the vagina is not an easy task and will not be completed in 5 or 10 minutes. This examination takes about 30 minutes to perform adequately (Fig. 18-28). Most failures of therapy are related to inadequate preoperative evaluation. Invasive cancer after treatment for intraepithelial neoplasia invariably was present at the time of the initial treatment.[72] Women who develop VAIN after hysterectomy demand scrupulous attention to diagnosis and sampling before embarking on laser treatment. Elderly women who show cytologic atypia and who have confirmation of VAIN on directed biopsy should be given a 30-day course of estrogen cream into the vagina and then be reevaluated by cytology and colposcopy. It is not uncommon for such women to have normal findings after intensive local steroid therapy. Additionally, if no reversion to normal is observed, the vagina is in much better condition to undergo laser surgery and heals infinitely better than an unprepared, atrophic vagina. We have witnessed this fact time and again and now routinely prepare all postmenopausal women with topical estrogen.

The key to laser vaporization of the vagina is to use power densities of approximately 500 W/cm² and a beam diameter of 2 mm. All laser treatments *must* be performed with the aid of a laser hook, otherwise a significant area of the vagina will be missed and disease will persist. Vaporization should be carried to a depth of 1 mm or less. Deeper vaporization adds nothing to cure rates but will surely increase complications. Very wide peripheral margins are required to eliminate this multifocal disease. Disease in the upper third of the vagina should be treated by vaporizing the entire upper third of the vagina. If the disease spreads into the middle third, then the entire upper two thirds are vapor-

ized. When VAIN is found to involve upper, middle, and lower thirds of the vagina, the entire vagina should be vaporized in two planned, staged sessions. It is preferred to carry out the operation using a superpulsed laser at settings varying from 100 to 300 pulses per second with pulse interval at 0.1 to 0.3 msec (Fig. 18-29). This preserves underlying stromal tissue and shortens healing time. Properly performed laser vaporization results in no scar formation, rapid healing, and no reduction in vaginal capacity. As stated previously, all surgery should be done with a CO_2 laser coupled to an operating microscope (colposcope) under general or regional anesthesia. Attempting this surgery under local block is the shortest route to therapeutic failure. After the vaporization, the treated area is thoroughly swabbed with 4% acetic acid, and the vagina is flushed two times with sterile chilled water. This water irrigation is accomplished by means of an asepto syringe. Finally, using a vaginal applicator, the vagina is filled with triple sulfa cream. The vaginal cream is employed mainly as a vehicle to prevent the opposing vaginal walls from coapting during the healing phase.

Postoperative bleeding is not a problem after vaginal laser vaporization, and it makes no sense to apply routinely caustic solution such as ferric subsulfate (Monsel's solution).

Results with laser treatment of VAIN have varied from 65% elimination of disease up to 90%.[25,70] More than one treatment may be required. Jobson and Homesley[44] treated the entire vagina at a single setting and achieved cures above 90%. The group in Birmingham, England, reported high failure rates and a number of invasive carcinomas after laser vaporization in women who had previous hysterecto-

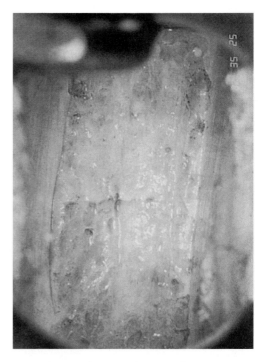

Fig. 18-29 Superpulse vaporization of upper vagina. Note the clean appearance of the superficial ablation of the vagina (less than 1 mm depth).

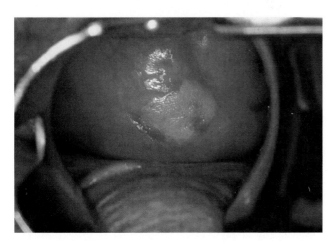

Fig. 18-28 Typical papillomavirus (VAIN) lesion of the vagina.

mies.[72] A report from the United States advocates excision of the vaginal vault in such cases.[42] The question again arises as to the accuracy of preoperative diagnosis and whether similar advocated techniques were used, accessory hooks, and extensiveness of peripheral vaporization. Sharp and Saunders[65] reported a technique in the vagina analogous to the laser thin section used in the vulva. These same authors reported 24 cases of VAIN, 16 of which were treated by CO_2 laser ablation. Four have required other therapy to deal with recurrent VAIN.

Dorsey and Baggish[30] reported 11 cases of VAIN, of which 83 were treated by laser only, 6 by laser plus excision, and 5 by laser plus 5-fluorouracil cream. The remaining 17 cases were treated by total vaginectomy or partial vaginectomy. The cure rates using laser in this large series was 80%; however, 40% of the cases required more than one laser exposure.[30]

The CO_2 laser remains an exceedingly precise and useful instrument for the treatment of lower genital tract disease. In this period of rising medical costs, instruments with such diversified uses, particularly by more than one surgical specialty, are cost effective and worthy of maximal usage.

REFERENCES

1. Anderson ES, Pedersen B: Combination laser conization: early and late complications, *J Gynecol Surg* 13:51, 1997.
2. Anderson MC: Treatment of cervical intraepithelial neoplasia with the carbon dioxide laser: report of 543 patients, *Obstet Gynecol* 59:720, 1982.
3. Anderson MC, Hartley RB: Cervical crypt involvement by intraepithelial neoplasia, *Obstet Gynecol* 55:546, 1980.
4. Baggish MS: Carbon dioxide laser treatment for condylomata acuminata venereal infections, *Obstet Gynecol* 55:711, 1980.
5. Baggish MS: Complications associated with carbon dioxide laser surgery in gynecology, *Am J Obstet Gynecol* 139:568, 1981.
6. Baggish MS: Treating viral venereal infections with the CO_2 laser, *J Reprod Med* 27:737, 1982.
7. Baggish MS: Laser management of cervical intraepithelial neoplasia, *Clin Obstet Gynecol* 26:980, 1983.
8. Baggish MS: Condylomata acuminata genital infections treated by the CO_2 laser. In Baggish MS, editor: *Basic and advanced laser surgery in gynecology,* Norwalk, Conn, 1985, Appleton-Crofts-Century.
9. Baggish MS: Improved laser techniques for the elimination of genital and extragenital warts, *Am J Obstet Gynecol* 153:545, 1985.
10. Baggish MS: Laser for the treatment of vulvar intraepithelial neoplasia. In Baggish MS, editor: *Basic and advanced laser surgery in gynecology,* Norwalk, Conn, 1985, Appleton-Crofts-Century.
11. Baggish MS: A comparison between laser excisional conization and laser vaporization for the treatment of cervical intraepithelial neoplasia, *Am J Obstet Gynecol* 155:39, 1986.
12. Baggish MS: Laser therapy for genital warts. In Winkler B, Richart RM, editors: *Clinical practice of gynecology: human papillomavirus infections,* New York, 1989, Elsevier.
13. Baggish MS, Baltoyannis P: Carbon dioxide laser treatment of cervical stenosis, *Fertil Steril* 48:24, 1987.
14. Baggish MS, Barash F, Noel Y, Brooks M: Comparison of thermal injury zones in loop electrical and laser cervical excisional conization, *Am J Obstet Gynecol* 166:545, 1992.
15. Baggish MS, Dorsey JH: CO_2 laser for the treatment of vulvar carcinoma in situ, *Obstet Gynecol* 57:371, 1981.
16. Baggish MS, Dorsey JH: Carbon dioxide laser for combination excisional vaporization conization, *Am J Obstet Gynecol* 151:23, 1985.
17. Baggish MS, Dorsey JH, Adelson M: A ten-year experience treating intraepithelial neoplasia with the CO_2 laser, *Am J Obstet Gynecol* 161:60, 1989.
18. Baggish MS, Miklos JR: Vulvar pain syndrome, *Obstet Gynecol Surv* 50:618, 1995.
19. Baggish MS, Noel Y, Brooks M: Electrosurgical thin loop conization by selective double excision, *J Gynecol Surg* 7:83, 1991.
20. Baggish MS, Richart R, Ferenczy A, Gerbie M: Potential complications of loop excision, *Contemp Obstet Gynecol* 39:93, 1994.
21. Baggish MS, Sze EH, Adelson MD, et al: Quantitative evaluation of the skin and accessory appendages in vulvar carcinoma-in-situ, *Obstet Gynecol* 74:169, 1989.
22. Benedet JL, Miller DM, Nickerson KG: Results of conservative management of cervical intraepithelial neoplasia, *Obstet Gynecol* 79:105, 1992.
23. Bigrigg MA, Codling BW, Pearson P, et al: Colposcopic diagnosis and treatment of cervical dysplasia at a single clinic visit, *Lancet* 366:229, 1990.
24. Buscema J, Woodruff JD, Parmley TH, Genadry R: Carcinoma in situ of the vulva, *Obstet Gynecol* 55:225, 1980.
25. Capen CV, Masterson BJ, Magrina JF, Calkins JW: Laser therapy of vaginal intraepithelial neoplasia, *Am J Obstet Gynecol* 42:973, 1982.
26. Cramer DN, Cutler SJ: Incidence and histopathology of malignancies of the female genital organs in the US, *Am J Obstet Gynecol* 118:443, 1976.
27. Dini MM, Jajag K: Iliovaginal fistula following cryosurgery for vaginal dysplasia, *Am J Obstet Gynecol* 136:692, 1980.
28. Dorsey JH: Understanding CO_2 laser surgery of the vulva, *Colpo Gynecol Laser Surg* 1:205, 1984.
29. Dorsey JH: Excisional conization of the cervix by CO_2 laser. In Baggish MS, editor: *Basic and advanced laser surgery in gynecology,* Norwalk, Conn, 1985, Appleton-Crofts-Century.
30. Dorsey JH, Baggish MS: Multifocal vaginal intraepithelial neoplasia with uterus in situ. In Sharp F, Jordan J, editors: *Gynecological laser surgery. Proceedings of the Fifteenth Study Group of the Royal College of Obstetricians and Gynecologists,* Ithaca, NY, 1986, Perinatology Press.
31. Evans AS, Monaghan JM: Treatment of cervical intraepithelial neoplasia using the carbon dioxide laser, *Br J Obstet Gynaecol* 90:553, 1983.
32. Ferenczy A: Using the laser to treat vulvar condylomata acuminata and intraepithelial neoplasia, *Can Med Assoc J* 128:135, 1983.
33. Ferenczy A: Treating genital condyloma during pregnancy with the carbon dioxide laser, *Am J Obstet Gynecol* 148:9, 1984.
34. Ferenczy A: Evaluation and management of male partners of condyloma patients, *Colpo Gynecol Laser Surg* 2:15, 1986.
35. Ferenczy A, Choukroun D, Falcone T, Franco E: The effect of cervical loop electrosurgical excision on subsequent pregnancy outcome: North American experience, *Am J Obstet Gynecol* 172:1246, 1995.
36. Ferenczy A, Mitao M, Silverstein SP: Latent papillomavirus and its relationship to recurrence of genital warts following laser surgery, *N Engl J Med* 313:784, 1985.
37. Fluhmann FC: *The cervix uteri and its disease,* Philadelphia, 1961, WB Saunders.
38. Fowler JM, Davos I, Leuchter RS, Lagasse LD: Effect of CO_2 laser conization of the uterine cervix on pathological interpretation of cervical intraepithelial neoplasia, *Obstet Gynecol* 79:693, 1992.
39. Friedrich EG: Vulvar vestibulitis syndrome, *J Reprod Med* 32:110, 1987.
40. Haffenden DK, Bigrigg A, Codling BW, Read MD: Pregnancy following large loop excision of the transformation zone, *Br J Obstet Gynaecol* 100:1059, 1993.
41. Hallam N, West J, Harper C, et al: Large loop excision of the cervical transformation zone (LLETZ) as an alternative to both local ablative and cone biopsy treatment: a series of 1000 patients, *J Gynecol Surg* 9:77, 1993.
42. Hoffman MS, Roberts WS, LaPolla JP, et al: Laser vaporization of grade 3 vaginal intraepithelial neoplasia, *Am J Obstet Gynecol* 165:1342, 1991.

43. Indman PD, Arndt BC: Laser treatment of cervical intraepithelial neoplasia in an office setting, *Am J Obstet Gynecol* 152:674, 1985.

44. Jobson VW, Homesley HD: Treatment of vaginal intraepithelial neoplasia with the carbon dioxide laser, *Obstet Gynecol* 62:90, 1983.

45. Keijser KGG, Kenemans P, Retromella H, et al: Diathermy loop excision in the management of cervical intraepithelial neoplasia: diagnosis and treatment in one procedure, *Am J Obstet Gynecol* 166:1281, 1992.

46. Krebs HB: Prophylactic topical 5-fluorouracil for the treatment of human papillomavirus–associated lesions of the vulva and vagina, *Obstet Gynecol* 68:837, 1989.

47. Larsson G, Gullberg B, Grundsell H: A comparison of complication of laser and cold knife conization, *Obstet Gynecol* 62:213, 1983.

48. Leuchter RS, Townsend DE, Hacker NF, et al: Treatment of vulvar carcinoma in situ with the CO_2 laser, *Gynecol Oncol* 19:314, 1984.

49. Luesley DM, Williams DR, Gee H, et al: Management of postconization cervical stenosis by laser vaporization, *Obstet Gynecol* 67:126, 1986.

50. Luesley DM, Cullimore J, Redman CW, et al: Loop diathermy excision of the cervical transformation zone in patients with abnormal cervical smears, *Br Med J* 300:1690, 1990.

51. Marinoff SC, Turner MLC: Vulvar vestibulitis syndrome: an overview, *Am J Obstet Gynecol* 165:1228, 1991.

52. McCullough AM, MacLean AB: Healing of the vulvar epithelium after laser treatment, *J Gynecol Surg* 6:33, 1990.

53. Paraskevaidis E, Jandial L, Mann EMF, et al: Pattern of treatment failure following laser for cervical intraepithelial neoplasia: implications for follow-up, *Protocol Obstet Gynecol* 78:80, 1991.

54. Prendiville W: Large loop excision of the transformation zone in diagnosis and treatment of cervical intraepithelial neoplasia. In Prendiville W, editor: *Clin Obstet Gynecol* 38:622, 1995.

55. Prendiville W, Cullimore J, Norman S: Large loop excision of the transformation zone (LLETZ): a new method of management for women with cervical intraepithelial neoplasia, *Br J Obstet Gynaecol* 96:1054, 1989.

56. Przybora LA, Plutowa A: Histological topography of carcinoma in situ of the cervix uteri, *Cancer* 12:263, 1959.

57. Oyesanya OA, Amerasinghe CN, Manning EAD: Outpatient excisional management of cervical intraepithelial neoplasia, *Am J Obstet Gynecol* 168:485, 1993.

58. Raio L, Ghezzi F, Dinaro E, et al: Duration of pregnancy after carbon dioxide laser conization of the cervix: influence of cone height, *Obstet Gynecol* 90:978, 1997.

59. Reid R: Superficial laser vulvectomy. III. A new surgical technique for appendage-preserving ablation of refractory condylomas and vulvar intraepithelial neoplasia, *Am J Obstet Gynecol* 152:504, 1985.

60. Reid R, Elfont EA, Zirkin RM, Fuller TA: Superficial laser vulvectomy. II. The anatomic and biophysical principles permitting accurate control over the depth of dermal destruction with the carbon dioxide laser, *Am J Obstet Gynecol* 152:261, 1985.

61. Reid R, Greenberg MD, Pizzuti DJ, et al: Superficial laser vulvectomy. V. Surgical debulking is enhanced by adjuvant systemic interferon, *Am J Obstet Gynecol* 166:815, 1992.

62. Reid R, Rutledge LH, Preop S, et al: Flashlamp excited dye laser therapy of idiopathic vulvodynia is safe and efficacious, *Am J Obstet Gynecol* 172:1684, 1995.

63. Riva JM, Sedlacek TV, Cunnane MF, Mangan CE: Extended carbon dioxide laser vaporization in the treatment of subclinical papillomavirus infection of the lower genital tract, *Obstet Gynecol* 73:25, 1989.

64. Rosenzweig BA, Baggish MS, Sze EHM: Carbon dioxide laser therapy for benign cervical tumors, *J Gynecol Surg* 6:97, 1990.

65. Sharp F, Saunders N: The treatment of vaginal premalignancy, *Clin Pract Gynecol* 2:211, 1990.

66. Sideri M, Schettino F, Spolti N, et al: Loop diathermy to replace conization in the conservative treatment of in situ cancer of the uterine cervix, *J Gynecol Surg* 10:235, 1994.

67. Singer A: The treatment of vulvar premalignancy, *Clin Pract Gynecol* 2:231, 1990.

68. Sturgeon SR, Brinton LA, Devesa SS, Kurman RJ: In situ and invasive vulvar cancer incidence trends (1973-1987), *Am J Obstet Gynecol* 166:1482, 1992.

69. Townsend DE, Levine RU, Richart RM, et al: Management of vulvar intraepithelial neoplasia by carbon dioxide laser, *Obstet Gynecol* 60:49, 1982.

70. Townsend DE, Levine RU, Crum CP, Richart RM: Treatment of vaginal carcinoma in situ of the vagina, *Am J Obstet Gynecol* 43:565, 1982.

71. Wolcott HD, Gallup DG: Wide local excision in the treatment of vulvar carcinoma in situ: a reappraisal, *Am J Obstet Gynecol* 150:695, 1984.

72. Woodman CBJ, Jordan JA, Wade-Evan T: The management of VAIN after hysterectomy, *Br J Obstet Gynaecol* 91:707, 1984.

73. Woodruff JD, Parmley TH: Infection of the minor vestibular glands, *Obstet Gynecol* 62:609, 1983.

74. Wright TC, Gagnon S, Richart RM, Ferenczy A: Treatment of cervical intraepithelial neoplasia using the loop electrosurgical excision procedure, *Obstet Gynecol* 79:173, 1992.

75. Wright VC, Davies E: Laser surgery for vulvar intraepithelial neoplasia: principles and results, *Am J Obstet Gynecol* 156:374, 1987.

76. Wright VC, Davies E, Riopelle MA: Laser cylindrical excision to replace conization, *Am J Obstet Gynecol* 150:704, 1984.

19 Vaginal Hysterectomy

DAVID H. NICHOLS

About 650,000 hysterectomies are performed annually in the United States, a somewhat lower number compared with previous years.[67] About 70% of these are performed transabdominally and 30% transvaginally.[41] Welch and Randall[83] reported in 1958 that 50% of the hysterectomies at the Mayo Clinic were done vaginally; currently, less than one third of hysterectomies are performed this way.[8] A similar figure was obtained at the Lahey Clinic,[10,11] and 60.9% of 9967 hysterectomies were performed vaginally at the University of Vienna.[23]

The complications of 1851 abdominal and vaginal hysterectomies performed between September 1978 and August 1981 were studied in detail at nine institutions by the Collaborative Review of Sterilization, an observational study coordinated by the Centers for Disease Control and Prevention. This review concluded that "women who underwent vaginal hysterectomy experienced significantly fewer complications than women who had undergone abdominal hysterectomy" and went on to recommend that "vaginal hysterectomy with prophylactic antibiotics should be 'strongly considered' for those women of reproductive age for whom either surgical approach is clinically appropriate."[14]

Surgical histrionics or dogmatic pronouncements should not be involved in the selection of an operative procedure for hysterectomy. The gynecologic surgeon should try to gain equal competence in the transabdominal, transvaginal, and laparoscopic techniques for hysterectomy. The surgeon can then confidently choose the particular approach that seems to be in the best interests of each patient.

The performance of hysterectomy requires the following of the surgeon:
1. Proper and effective training and experience
2. Awareness of possible complications, including intraoperative ones, and their treatment
3. Three-dimensional thinking[36] and the necessary psychomotor skills

Following the initial careful preoperative pelvic examination (supine and standing) and the decision that hysterectomy is in the patient's best interests, this conclusion and the alternatives should be thoughtfully given to the patient with abundant opportunity for the patient to discuss any questions or details. She should be made aware of the possible complications of surgery and the details of the usual convalescence, and she should be given the opportunity to formulate and express her views about what has been proposed. The surgeon should know how the patient perceives her problem, its proposed remedy, and the likely effects on her future life and relationships.

The indications for abdominal hysterectomy can ultimately evolve as the contraindications for vaginal hysterectomy (e.g., presence of a suspicious adnexal mass, uterine immobility, invasive cancer, very large uterine leiomyomata, or lack of operator experience, enthusiasm, and confidence). Indications relating to the choice of operative route are listed in Table 19-1.

The goals of reconstructive surgery, whether performed transvaginally, transabdominally, or translaparoscopically, are as follows:
1. Relief of symptoms
2. Restoration of normal anatomic relationships
3. Restoration of function

These goals should be achievable with any of the operation choices for a particular patient.

The professional may encounter conflict and controversy with the second of these goals. Standard anatomic texts describe in detail a cadaver's anatomic and organ relationships, but these observations can sharply contrast with those of a living human in whom voluntary muscle tone permits the vagina to lie upon a normally empty rectum, which in turn lies upon an intact levator plate[58,69] (see Chapter 3). The normal upper vaginal axis of a woman who is standing is thus horizontal and not vertical as shown in textbook descriptions of cadaver anatomy. If a vaginal hysterectomy patient has previously sustained a vesicourethral pinup operation, this will have changed the axis of the anterior vaginal wall to a more anterior position. In this circumstance, assurance of support of the posthysterectomy vaginal vault assumes special significance. If the uterosacral ligaments are palpably strong, a culdoplasty[52] using long-lasting synthetic suture is effective, but if the ligaments are weak, a coincident colpopexy, preferably transvaginal, may be indicated. Restoration, support, and suspension of the vaginal vault into the hollow of the sacrum and over an intact levator plate are major goals of reconstruction if the vault is to remain postoperatively where it is intended to be. The transvaginal approach can best accomplish this because a New Orleans or McCall-type culdeplasty[52] can be easily added. A deep cul-de-sac should be sought and excised or obliterated if found. If the anatomic support of the vault is found wanting, it should be provided by coincident colpopexy, either transvaginal or transabdominal. The surgeon should be familiar and experienced with the techniques of each (see Chapter 26). Reduction in operative time and surgical blood loss depends directly on precise knowledge of each patient's connective tissue septa, planes, and potential spaces. The blood vessels run within the septa; the vessels should be

Table 19-1   Vaginal versus Abdominal Approach to Possible Hysterectomy

		Approach	
Indication	Vaginal	Laparoscopically Assisted Vaginal Hysterectomy	Abdominal
Myomata uteri	Occasionally	Occasionally	Usually
Pelvic inflammatory disease	Rarely	Occasionally	Almost always, except for posterior colpotomy
Recurrent dysfunctional uterine bleeding	Usually	Occasionally	Occasionally
Endometriosis	Rarely	Occasionally	Usually
Adenomyosis	Usually	Occasionally	Occasionally
Symptomatic pelvic relaxation	Usually	Occasionally	Occasionally
Adnexal mass	Rarely	Occasionally	Always
Pelvic pain	Rarely	Occasionally	Usually
Cancer of cervix			
Stages 0 and Ia	Usually	Rarely	Occasionally
Corpus cancer	Occasionally	Occasionally	Usually

Modified from Thompson JD: *Clin Obstet Gynecol* 24:1245, 1981.

clamped and cut before blood is lost. The patient's convalescence is generally more comfortable after a vaginal than after an abdominal hysterectomy. Moreover, during a vaginal operative procedure, the surgeon can correct any problems of pelvic relaxation, which are often present in a patient whose condition requires a hysterectomy.[58,75]

The gynecoid pelvis provides the most room for successful transvaginal hysterectomy, whereas the android type can compromise exposure. The slant that the vulva makes with the body axis frequently suggests the type of pelvis. A slant perpendicular to the body axis is characteristic of an android or anthropoid pelvis. The operator can determine whether the width of the vaginal outlet is adequate for transvaginal hysterectomy by inserting a closed fist between the ischial tuberosities during the pelvic examination; if the fist fits comfortably, the width of the bony pelvis is adequate.[57]

The most important single observation in evaluating the feasibility of vaginal rather than abdominal hysterectomy is the demonstrable mobility of the uterus. A movable uterus generally can be readily removed by a vaginal procedure. Conversely, a uterus that is not movable should rarely be approached transvaginally, even when the vaginal operation seems otherwise indicated, as when the patient is extremely obese or a vaginal or perineal repair is necessary. The phenomenon of pseudoprolapse can demonstrate the degree of uterine mobility; when the pelvic musculature is effectively relaxed under anesthesia, if moderate traction brings an ordinarily well-supported cervix nearly to the introitus, the uterus is sufficiently mobile to permit a vaginal hysterectomy.

TEMPORARILY SHRINKING A FIBROID UTERUS WITH LEUPROLIDE ACETATE

Leuprolide acetate (Lupron Depot), a powerful synthetic analog of naturally occurring gonadotropin-releasing hormone, can be given intramuscularly as a 3.75-mg dose once a month for 3 to 6 months. It temporarily decreases uterine and myoma volume by about a third in most patients. In many instances this sufficiently reduces the size of a myomatous uterus to permit vaginal hysterectomy instead of an abdominal one.[70]

VAGINAL HYSTERECTOMY FOR A PATIENT WITHOUT PROLAPSE

The vagina is often the appropriate route for hysterectomy when the uterus is movable, whether prolapsed or not.[58,65] Vaginal hysterectomies are the easiest to perform because the anatomy of the uterine supports is constant and unaltered by disease. Hospitalization can be shortened,[63,80] and the patient is often home by the first or second postoperative day. Vaginal hysterectomy can be performed easily on a nulligravida patient.

Provided that the uterus is movable, the less the prolapse, the easier the hysterectomy; the greater the prolapse, the more difficult the hysterectomy. Anatomic differences are fewer in patients without prolapse and greater and less predictable in patients with some degree of prolapse. In fact, massive vaginal eversion with procidentia can be among the most challenging of all gynecologic surgical cases, because each progressive step requires precise surgical judgment and the resolution of the problems that arise requires creative resourcefulness. In 100 such operations in which a significant degree of prolapse exists, the anatomic challenges, findings, and solutions will never be identical in any two procedures.

In some cases the anus seems to be the most dependent portion of the perineum, and the patient literally sits on her anus. This uncommon finding usually indicates a major defect in the integrity of the levator ani. Such a defect may be associated with postmenopausal estrogen deficiency and loss of tissue tone, but it is more likely to result from major trauma to the levator ani and pelvic diaphragm, an acquired or congenital deficiency of innervation, or a degenerative neurologic disease. This syndrome is discussed further in Chapter 29.

CONSERVATION VERSUS PROPHYLACTIC REMOVAL OF THE OVARIES

From a theoretical standpoint, the criteria that determine the choice of removing the ovaries at the time of vaginal hysterectomy are the same as those that apply during an abdominal operation[4,74] Prophylactic ovarian removal, however, is less common when hysterectomy is accomplished by the vaginal approach, because the ovaries are not technically as readily accessible during a vaginal hysterectomy as during an abdominal laparotomy. They may be removed, however, by coincident operative laparoscopy.

Indications for Oophorectomy

When evaluating the indications for oophorectomy, the surgeon should balance the results of removing the ovaries with the relatively low risk (in most cases) that the patient may later develop an ovarian neoplasm if the ovaries are preserved.[38,64,66] For example, a patient who has a family history of ovarian cancer may be considered a candidate for prophylactic oophorectomy at the time of vaginal hysterectomy. She should be told that oophorectomy would reduce but not eliminate her risk of developing carcinoma of the ovary, because the disease seems to have certain potential general coelomic manifestations. Elective oophorectomy in the premenopausal patient is a preoperative decision in which the patient should participate.

In their studies of steroidogenesis in the postmenopausal ovary, Mattingly and Huang[51] demonstrated that stromal steroid production persists for a long time after menopause, even though estrogen production falls precipitously when menstruation ceases; therefore the postmenopausal ovary continues to have an important metabolic function. The authors noted that in reported studies of 7765 patients whose ovaries had been conserved at the time of hysterectomy (and presumably inspected and found to be grossly normal) and who had been followed for varying intervals after surgery, only 12 women were known to have developed cancer in the preserved ovaries, an incidence of only 0.15%. The overall general incidence of ovarian malignancy suggests that the eventual frequency of ovarian cancer is approximately 1 per 70 patients; however, this estimate includes the whole population, most of whose ovaries had never been previously inspected.

Although castration should not be routine at any age, it appears that so-called prophylactic oophorectomy should be considered after the age of true ovarian senescence, whether demonstrable at 40 or 70 years of age; the tendency of the ovaries to neoplasia does not disappear when steroidogenesis ceases. As a general rule, transvaginal removal of a grossly normal ovary may be encouraged in a patient older than 55 and discouraged in a patient younger than 40; the operator's advice to those patients in between may be somewhat flexible, depending more on the present degree

of ovarian activity than on the chronologic age of the patient. The surgeon must take into account that oophorectomy in a younger patient will accelerate the onset of osteoporosis and other degenerative changes.[79] Because there seems to be no particular age at which all ovaries must be removed, the view of the surgeon who elects not to perform routine oophorectomy is defensible, although the patient should actively participate in the preoperative decision.

Vaginal Hysterectomy Laparoscopically Assisted

If the uterus is movable and of less than 16 weeks' gestational size, it generally can be removed transvaginally. In many such cases, ovarian tissue can be removed transvaginally, saving the patient the additional discomfort and expense of coincident laparoscopy. But if the infundibulopelvic ligament is short, or the ovaries adhere to the pelvic sidewall, thus precluding safe transvaginal extirpation, they usually can be retrieved by operative laparoscopy *following* the vaginal hysterectomy and closure of the peritoneal cavity (VHLA). When VHLA is scheduled, the operative team will know that the vaginal hysterectomy is to be done *first*. They also will know that if a planned oophorectomy can be accomplished transvaginally, as is usually possible, the optional laparoscopy can be eliminated; this saves operating time and expense, patient discomfort, and extra equipment charges. Laparoscopic hysterectomy is discussed in Chapter 20.

Estrogen Replacement Therapy

Sluijmer et al.[77] have demonstrated that the postmenopausal ovary produces substantial amounts of androstenedione and testosterone, as well as some estrone and β estradiol. Although estrogen can be readily replaced after oophorectomy, many authors argue that the usual replacement therapy only relieves the subjective vasomotor symptoms of menopause and, unless continued over time, does not prevent the degenerative changes that may follow castration. Furthermore, Randall[66] and Nichols and Randall[57] noted that patients for whom estrogen supplementation or replacement had been prescribed after a surgical menopause tended to discontinue the medication after 1 or 2 years. He suggested that because the more significant degenerative effects that may follow estrogen withdrawal may not appear for years, patients do not immediately associate cause and effect.

To be effective, estrogen replacement therapy must be administered prophylactically. The particularly undesirable body changes are preventable but apparently are irreversible once they develop. Moreover, as Robinson, Cohen, and Higano[71] pointed out, the standard postmenopausal daily dose of 1.25 mg of conjugated estrogen is only partially successful in altering postmenopausal blood serum lipid levels. A dose of 2.5 mg/day is somewhat more effective. The optimal effect may necessitate 5 mg/day or more, however, and this dosage is likely to produce such distressing secondary effects as breast tenderness, fluid retention, and weight gain.

PROCEDURE FOR VAGINAL HYSTERECTOMY

As surgeons develop their own techniques through personal experience and comparisons with the procedures described by other operators, they usually identify and embrace many fundamental principles. They do not merely memorize the sequence of operative steps. Step four need not follow step three; it may follow step six or seven or even be skipped, completely depending on the characteristics of a particular patient's tissues and the operator's development of tissue relationships. The "whys" of doing something are every bit as important as the "whats." Illustrations enhanced by sagittal drawings can help surgeons visualize important operative details by adding a three-dimensional or spatial geometric concept to their surgical thinking; for example, they can show that only in cases of advanced prolapse does the surgery start in tissues that actually protrude from the pelvis.

Obstetrician-gynecologists who prefer to stand while they do episiotomy repairs are likely to prefer to stand during vaginal hysterectomy and repair. This position seems to give the operator desirable mobility with minimal muscle tension. If the operator chooses to stand, the operating table should be raised almost to its maximum height. Regardless of operative technique, some operators prefer to be seated.

Horizontal light sources are always desirable for surgical procedures within the pelvis. Because operating room spotlights tend to wander during the course of a procedure, some operators use a fiberoptic forehead lamp, which provides a readily directed, shadowless illumination into the depths of the wound and into the hollow of the sacrum. Illuminated retractors may be useful deep in the pelvis. The operator and all assistants must keep their visual attention on the operative field; no one needs to watch the nurse, clock, technician, or one another. A retractor can cause an injury if held by an uninterested assistant who allows it to wander, or it can obscure the telltale spurt of a small, unsecured artery. When tension on a pedicle or adjacent structure is relaxed, bleeding from a momentarily exposed vessel can remain undetected if the operator and assistants have not been closely watching the operative field.

Initial Procedures

A liquid diet is desirable for the day preceding surgery. The day before surgery the rectum should be carefully cleansed by an oral electrolyte bowel preparation (GoLYTELY, NuLYTELY, Colyte) or enema. The patient should be instructed to void just before coming to the operating room. A single dose of a "prophylactic" antibiotic,[53] usually a cephalosporin, is given either intramuscularly or intravenously when the patient is ready for transit to the operating room.[26,27,78] The bladder must be catheterized at the beginning of surgery only if it is palpably distended, because a bladder that contains a little urine is easier to identify during surgery than one that is empty. If desired, 60 ml of dilute indigo carmine, methylene blue solution, or sterile evaporated milk can be instilled into the bladder preoperatively to facilitate recognition of any unanticipated bladder opening, which occasionally occurs during the course of a gyneco-logic operative procedure. This should be done routinely for every patient who has undergone a cesarean section in the past.

As soon as the patient is under anesthesia, the surgeon should perform a careful preoperative bimanual pelvic reexamination to decide whether to proceed with the hysterectomy vaginally or to perform it abdominally. The size, position, shape, and especially the mobility of the uterus should be carefully assessed. The freedom and position of the cul-de-sac should be noted and the thickness and length of the uterosacral ligaments evaluated. Elongation of the cervix should be noted because any cervical elongation affects the spot where the incision through the vagina should begin. The direction and depth of the vaginal axis at rest also should be noted.

A preliminary fractional dilation and curettage (D&C) should be performed if the patient has a history of abnormal bleeding. This procedure usually suggests the cause of the bleeding. If the curettings are grossly suspicious of malignant disease, an immediate frozen section can be requested for clarification. Furthermore, it provides additional information about the size, mobility, consistency, position, and internal architecture of the uterus. The position of the uterus is particularly important. A prolapsed uterus is rarely in anteversion unless a suspension or fixation procedure was performed earlier. A retroverted uterus usually is accompanied by pathologic elongation of the infundibulopelvic ligaments; in this case, the ovaries are generally in the cul-de-sac, which makes them much more accessible if they are to be removed through the vaginal incision during the operation.

Following examination under anesthesia and preliminary curettage of the uterus, traction is established by applying a Jacob's clamp or a double-toothed tenaculum to the anterior lip of the cervix, and the integrity of the urogenital diaphragm and the anterior vaginal wall is assessed. In looking at the anterior vaginal wall, the examiner should note any cystocele, or paravaginal defect, and observe whether it disappears when the vault is temporarily replaced in the sacral hollow.

This evaluation indicates whether suspension or support of the urethra and lower vagina should accompany the repair and whether the planned reconstruction is likely to restore the normal vaginal axis and depth. Another Jacob's clamp or tenaculum is applied to the posterior lip of the cervix and used to evaluate the location and size of the cul-de-sac of Douglas and the strength and size of the uterosacral ligaments, which become more readily demonstrable as they are stretched by traction (Fig. 19-1). The attachment of the cul-de-sac to the cervix then usually becomes more obvious, which helps the operator determine the appropriate site for the initial incision to circumscribe the cervix. Having been grasped anteriorly and posteriorly with two Jacob's clamps, the cervix is drawn downward so that both the cervix and the upper vagina can be adequately exposed with the use of vaginal refractors. (If the labia minora are large enough to obstruct exposure of the vagina, they should be

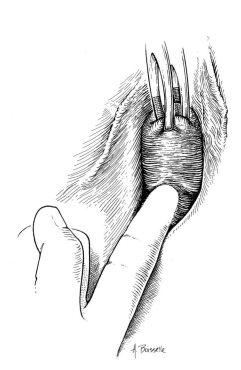

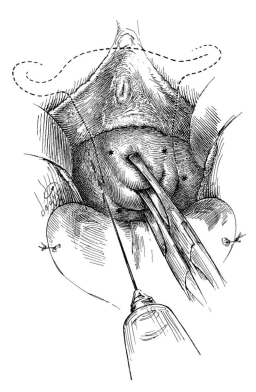

Fig. 19-1 Traction is made to a tenaculum applied to the posterior lip of the cervix and site of cul-de-sac of Douglas, palpated as shown. The length and strength of uterosacral ligaments are noted. (From Nichols DH, Randall CL: *Vaginal surgery,* ed 4, Baltimore, 1996, Williams & Wilkins.)

Fig. 19-2 The cervix is grasped with two double-toothed tenacula, one anterior and one posterior to the external os, and downward traction is applied. Vaginal retractors of adequate length and proper design then provide satisfactory exposure of the cervix and upper vagina. In a premenopausal patient who has received preventive antibiotics, the circumference of the cervix, along a line where a circumcision-like incision is about to be made, may be first carefully infiltrated with a mixture of 1:200,000 epinephrine (Adrenalin) and 0.5% lidocaine (Xylocaine) or bupivacaine (Marcaine). This is readily accomplished using a pressure syringe and a long 22-gauge spinal needle. Before injecting solution at each puncture site, traction is applied to the plunger of the syringe to make certain no blood is obtained, thus preventing intravenous or intraarterial injection of the solution. If a bloody aspirate is obtained, the needle is repositioned. The cervical insertions of the uterosacral ligaments, or paracervical portions of the cardinal ligaments, and the bladder pillars (as noted by asterisks) should be the objectives of this infiltration. About 50 ml of this solution, half into either side and 8 ml at each injection site, usually provides adequate infiltration. (From Nichols DH, Randall CL: *Vaginal surgery,* ed 4, Baltimore, 1996, Williams & Wilkins.)

temporarily fixed to the skin lateral to the labia majora by one or two sutures on each side.)

The selective paracervical infiltration of not more than 50 ml of 0.5% lidocaine (Xylocaine) or bupivacaine (Marcaine) in 1:200,000 epinephrine (Adrenalin) solution,[24,58] or vasopressin, a so-called liquid tourniquet, considerably decreases blood loss during surgery, particularly in premenopausal, nonhypertensive women. In addition, the use of this agent seems to lessen the amount of additional anesthesia and reduce the need for immediate postoperative analgesia, and it facilitates the identification of cleavage planes as they are developed and separated. Because it produces a temporary ischemia, the infiltration of lidocaine can reduce the immediate resistance to infection,[17] but since prophylactic antibiotics have been started preoperatively, a therapeutic concentration should already have been disseminated within the pelvic tissues, and there should be no increase in morbidity. When a patient is receiving halothane or cyclopropane anesthesia, has been taking a β-blocker (e.g., propranolol), or has unstable or severe hypertension or coronary heart disease, normal saline solutions may be substituted for the epinephrine solution. However, a much larger volume of fluid is needed, which may tend to slightly distort the anatomy.

The anesthetist should be informed as the injection is given. The actual infiltration is most easily accomplished with the use of a pressure syringe and a 22-gauge spinal

needle (Fig. 19-2). Before injecting the solution, the operator should pull and release the plunger of the syringe to make certain that no blood is obtained; if there is blood in the aspirate, the operator must reposition the needle to avoid intravenous or intraarterial injection of the solution. The solution is not injected into the cervical tissue itself but into the tissues to which the cervix is attached and the tissues around the cervix, such as the bladder pillars, the lower cardinal ligaments, and the insertions of the uterosacral ligaments. A wait of 15 minutes from the time of completion of the injection until the start of surgery permits wider dissemination of the fluid into the intercellular connective tissue,[59] but this time is a luxury that not all operating room schedules permit. Although the use of the "liquid tourniquet" may reduce blood loss significantly, it is only a complement and not a substitute for careful dissection and meticulous surgical hemostasis.

Operative Technique

Making the Initial Incision. The correct spot for circumcision of the vagina before hysterectomy is often at some distance from the external cervical os.[22] As Bandler[2] pointed out, the closer the initial incision to the external cervical os, the greater the bleeding and the more dissection of the cervical branches of the uterine blood vessels is required to reach the cul-de-sac. Conversely, less bleeding occurs when the incision is made farther above the external cervical os, but the risk of inadvertently opening the bladder or rectum is greater. Most surgeons compromise, based in large part on their estimate of the length of the cervix and the palpable level of the peritoneum of the posterior cul-de-sac. Traction is made to the cervix against countertraction provided by suitable retractors. The initial incision should be at the level of the base of the cul-de-sac of Douglas (Fig. 19-3).

Using either curved Mayo scissors or a scalpel, the operator opens the vagina by making a circumcision-like incision around the cervix through the full thickness of the vaginal membrane along the grooved depression noticeable in the transverse rugae (Fig. 19-3). At the upper limits of the vagina, there are fewer rugae as the vagina blends with the epithelial layer of the cervix, which has no rugae. Posteriorly the incision exposes the uterosacral ligaments and peritoneum of the cul-de-sac, but the initial incision should not cut the ligaments nor actually open through the peritoneum into the cul-de-sac (Fig. 19-4).

Dissecting the Vagina. After making the initial incision around the cervix, the operator removes the Jacob's clamps or the double-toothed tenacula and reapplies them to pull the cut edge of the vagina toward the lower cervix and external os. With continued cervical traction against retractor-provided countertraction, it is critical for the operator to continue the dissection in the correct cleavage plane because dissection in the wrong plane greatly increases blood loss; even more important, an incorrect dissection jeopardizes the blood supply of the tissue flaps on which the success of the repair partly depends. The full thickness of the vaginal wall should be peeled back from all underlying connective tissue, but only for a short distance unless the uterosacral ligaments are markedly elongated. In this case, the tips of only partially opened scissors may be used in a "cut and push" maneuver to "skin" the vagina over a considerable distance from the external surfaces of the connective tissue plane that covers these ligaments.

If unexpected infection is observed in the cervix, the operator can free the cervix from the surrounding tissues to the level of the internal os and then amputate it from the fundus before opening the peritoneum either anteriorly or posteriorly, thereby reducing the risk of contamination and postop-

erative peritonitis. Shortening the cervix in this manner occasionally makes it easier for the operator to hook a finger around the fundus of the uterus to facilitate opening the anterior peritoneum.

Opening the Posterior Peritoneum. The operator usually can identify the cul-de-sac of Douglas readily after pulling the subvaginal tissue layer taut with forceps. If the peritoneum is not evident, the full thickness of the posterior vaginal membrane is undermined for several centimeters and then incised vertically to expose the peritoneum of the cul-de-sac of Douglas, which can then be entered under direct vision (Fig. 19-5).

If the dissection has been in the wrong plane or if adhesions have obliterated the cul-de-sac of Douglas, the operator may be unable to identify the posterior peritoneal fold, which lines the cul-de-sac, after circumcising the cervix and stripping back the wall of the vagina. In this event, the operator should begin the hysterectomy extraperitoneally by clamping and ligating the uterosacral and caudal portions of the cardinal ligaments close to the cervix (Fig. 19-6). Unless abnormally restrained (e.g., by adhesions), the uterus will be brought closer to the operator and will bring with it both its posterior and anterior peritoneal attachments. Later in the procedure, the peritoneum can be identified and opened under direct vision.[3,39,58] This procedure, the same as the "climb-up" maneuver recommended by Krige,[43] is infinitely preferable to stabbing blindly in the hope of opening into the peritoneum, which involves considerable risk of inadvertent penetration of any adherent bowel or the rectum and enhances bleeding.

The operator can easily open the peritoneum but should open it no more than is necessary to admit an examining finger or two. Keeping the opening as small as possible not only reduces unnecessary bleeding but also prevents an incision that could detach an unsecured uterosacral ligament from the uterus. The operator then explores the interior intraabdominal surface of the cul-de-sac with one or two fingers to identify any enterocele or potential enterocele for later excision. Any pathologic adhesions or cul-de-sac irregularity, as well as the nature of any intraperitoneal fluid, should be noted. The operator should also sweep the posterior surface of the uterus with an index finger superiorly to ensure that the uterus is free, confirm the size of the uterus, and determine the position of any fibroids or other disease. Although the uterosacral ligaments should not be included in this preliminary incision into the cul-de-sac of Douglas, their thickness and possible elongation should be noted at this time.

If possible, it is preferable to avoid joining the peritoneum to the vaginal cuff at this stage by placing interrupted sutures for hemostasis, even when oozing persists. Such sutures increase the risk of future enterocele if later in the procedure the operator fails to resect any excess of peritoneum in the cul-de-sac before placing the purse-string closure of peritoneum cranial to these sutures.

Cutting the Uterosacral Ligaments. The uterosacral ligaments are clamped and, if elongated and strong,

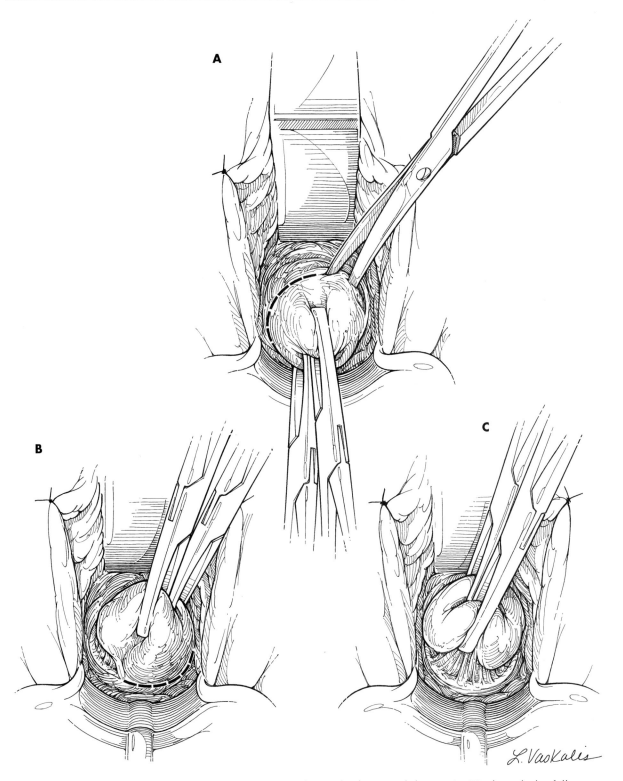

Fig. 19-3 The incision is now carried completely around the cervix **(A)**, through the full thickness of the vagina **(B)**, and the Jacob's clamps repositioned so that the external teeth are in the cut edge of the incision **(C).** The full thickness of the rim of vaginal wall is freed by sharp and blunt dissection exposing the underlying paracolpium.

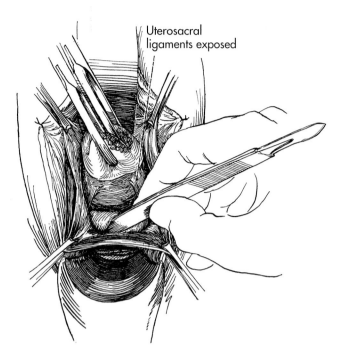

Uterosacral
ligaments exposed

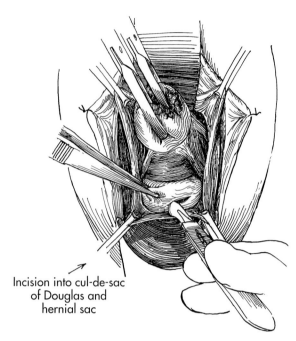

Incision into cul-de-sac
of Douglas and
hernial sac

Fig. 19-4 The posterior vaginal wall may be grasped with Allis clamps, the uterosacral ligaments identified, and the dissection continued until the peritoneum of the cul-de-sac is evident. The degree of herniation of the cul-de-sac varies but almost inevitably exists coincident with prolapse. The larger the herniation, the more extensive the dissection and exposure at this time. (From Ball TL: *Gynecologic surgery and urology,* ed 2, St Louis, 1963, Mosby.)

Fig. 19-5 The cul-de-sac peritoneum is now picked up with a thumb forceps and the peritoneal cavity entered. An exploration of the pelvis is carried out with one finger while strong traction is made on the uterus in an anterior direction. The status of the ovaries and tubes, as well as the presence of any bowel or omentum adhesions to the uterus, is determined. (From Ball TL: *Gynecologic surgery and urology,* ed 2, St Louis, 1963, Mosby.)

shortened, after which they are cut from the uterus. (Double-clamping "for safety" is elective, according to the surgeon's preference.) The tip of the clamp should include the uterosacral and the lower portion of the cardinal ligaments. In placing a suture around this pedicle, the flexibility of the operator's wrist is important because it permits the operator to push and pull the needle through the tissues along the course of the needle's curved direction; this prevents the laceration of tissue that is more likely to occur when the needle is pushed through in a straight line. Just as the follow-through of a golfer's swing affects the accuracy of the ball's flight, the flexibility of the surgeon's wrist minimizes the size of the opening and the trauma to tissues that can result from each placement of a hemostatic suture around each pedicle.

The uterosacral ligaments are secured by transfixion ligature to the posterolateral surface of the vagina at approximately the 4- and 8-o'clock positions. These sutures should include the full thickness of the vaginal wall so that the ligaments will be firmly and permanently reattached to the vagina at this point (Fig. 19-7). These uterosacral sutures should not yet be cut so that they can be used for later identification of the ligaments, which possibly will be included in the repair.

Entering the Vesicovaginal Space. Anteriorly the full thickness of the cut edge of the vagina can be identified between forceps at either side of the 12-o'clock position. Using Mayo scissors—with the points directed away from the bladder—the operator makes an inverted T-shaped incision in the anterior vaginal wall, having entered the vesicovaginal space (Fig. 19-8). The opening can be enlarged by spreading the tips of the Mayo scissors, which are then withdrawn without being closed.

The full thickness of the vaginal wall is now separated from the bladder (Fig. 19-9). If the position of the cervix at this point suggests that the prolapse is not as great as the operator had suspected, the inverted T-incision becomes especially advantageous in exposing the undersurface of the bladder. On the other hand, if the prolapse appears to be greater than the operator had expected (because the hold of the uterosacral ligaments on the uterus has been released), a horizontal vaginal incision alone may be sufficient to permit dissection of bladder from cervix because the vesicouterine peritoneal fold becomes closer to the surgeon's hand and vision.

The bladder, readily identified by its looseness, can be picked up in the midline with forceps and gentle tension placed on it. The supravaginal septum is incised and entered

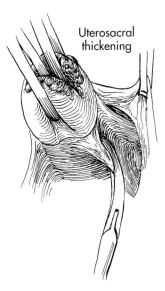

Uterosacral thickening

Fig. 19-6   The uterosacral thickenings are cut. This connective tissue is useful in reestablishing the vaginal obturator, obliterating the cul-de-sac, and suspending the vaginal vault. As with any hernia, tissue useful in the herniorrhaphy should not be sacrificed. A curved Heaney or Kocher clamp is used to grasp the tissue. The uterosacral ligaments are ligated and the ends of the ligatures left long and tagged. Resection of the uterosacral thickenings permits further descensus of the uterus. Palpation of the cul-de-sac can be carried higher in the pelvis and the size of the fundus more accurately determined. The operator may start planning for the correction of the cul-de-sac hernia and resection of excess peritoneum that will be part of the posterior repair. (From Ball TL: *Gynecologic surgery and urology,* ed 2, St Louis, 1963, Mosby.)

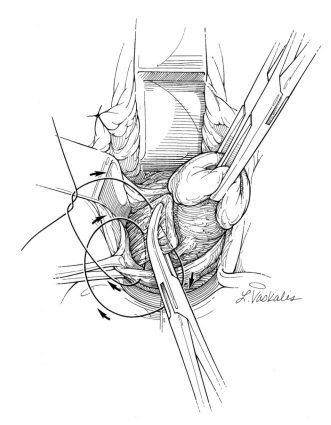

Fig. 19-7   Cut ends of uterosacral ligaments are secured to the posterolateral surface of vagina by transfixion ligature at about the 4- and 8-o'clock positions. These sutures include the full thickness of the vaginal wall; the now-shortened ligaments should be firmly and permanently reattached to the vagina at this point. Ends of these uterosacral sutures are left long to facilitate later identification and probable involvement of the ligaments in closure of the repair. (From Nichols DH, Randall CL: *Vaginal surgery,* ed 4, Baltimore, 1996, Williams & Wilkins.)

in the midline with the points of the curved Mayo scissors pointing downward or posteriorly. The plane of separation follows the line of fusion between the posterior layer of the connective tissue of the anterior vaginal wall and the encapsulation of the cervix. The operator should elevate the handles of the Mayo scissors during this maneuver to ensure that the scissor tips are pointed away from the undersurface of the bladder. The operator separates the bladder from the cervix by meticulously snipping the fine fibers that bind the connective tissue capsule of the bladder to that of the cervix. This sharp dissection is much safer than bluntly stripping the bladder away from the cervix, either with the finger or a sponge, because blunt stripping can lacerate the lowest section of the bladder fundus.[34]

Dissecting along the Proper Cleavage Plane. As the scissors approach the vesicouterine peritoneal fold, the tissues usually become readily distinguishable. The operator can generally ensure a bloodless and safe entry into the proper cleavage plane by pressing firmly against the cervix with the closed curved tips of the Mayo scissors pointing toward the cervix and, while elevating the handles of the scissors above the horizontal, spreading apart the tips of the

scissors and withdraw them while maintaining pressure of the scissor tips against the cervix. After this maneuver, the opening may be readily enlarged. This dissection is carried upward until the anterior vesicouterine peritoneal fold is free. The fold is recognized by its almost frictionless smoothness to palpation or visualized as the white line of a double fold of peritoneum. Once the desired opening has been established along the proper cleavage plane, a retractor is placed beneath the bladder to hold it away from the cervix (Fig. 19-10). The anterior vesicouterine peritoneal fold may be opened at this time (Figs. 19-11 and 19-12) and a long-handled retractor inserted.

Either immediately before or after retraction of the bladder superiorly, the so-called bladder pillars can be clamped, cut, and ligated near their attachments to the cervix. These pillars are never as strong as they may appear, and they usually contain portions of the cervical capsule. This surgical maneuver provides considerable protection to

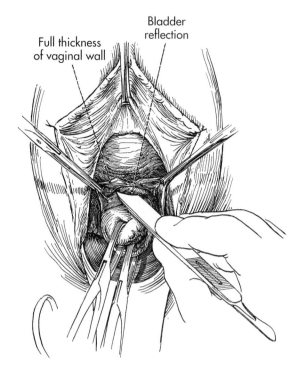

Full thickness
of vaginal wall

Bladder
reflection

Fig. 19-8 An inverted T-incision is made anteriorly through the full thickness of the vaginal wall entering the vesicovaginal space. The fusion between the connective tissue capsule of the bladder and that of the vagina is separated by sharp dissection through the supravaginal septum. The bladder is pushed off the cervix by the knife handle entering the fragile areolar tissue between these organs. The vesicouterine reflection of the peritoneum appears between the bladder and upper part of the cervix. Cautery or ties can control any active bleeding. The remainder of the anterior vaginal wall will be opened after the hysterectomy. This sequence in the steps of the operation avoids unnecessary bleeding from the incised anterior vaginal wall during the hysterectomy. The extent of this first incision is shown in this figure. (From Ball TL: *Gynecologic surgery and urology,* ed 2, St Louis, 1963, Mosby.)

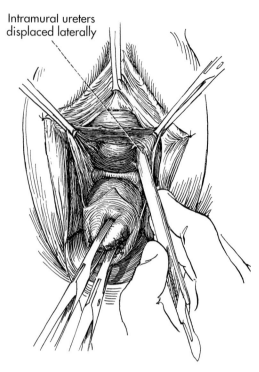

Intramural ureters
displaced laterally

Fig. 19-9 This shows the dissection carried farther and the landmarks of importance. The bladder base, vesicouterine peritoneal fold, and cervix should be clearly evident if the correct tissue plane was entered. Previous surgery or scarring occasionally can make this difficult. A sound placed in the bladder can help differentiate the tissue of the bladder base from the cervix when they are unusually adherent. (From Ball TL: *Gynecologic surgery and urology,* ed 2, St Louis, 1963, Mosby.)

the ureters by ensuring that the subsequent dissection will be closer to the cervix and relatively distant from the ureteral knees.

Although a gauze-covered thumb can strip the bladder capsule from that of the cervix along a cleavage plane up to the anterior peritoneal fold, this procedure risks tearing the bladder if the operator has not entered the correct plane. Adhesions and fibrosis following previous low cervical cesarean section may have obscured the proper plane, and careful sharp dissection reduces the risk of bladder penetration. Occasionally the operator's readiness to dissect and desire to avoid penetrating the bladder causes him or her to incise within or beneath the connective tissue capsule of the cervix, particularly if the initial incision around the cervix was too close to the external cervical os. Because the operator did not enter the anatomic plane between the bladder and

the cervix, continuing sharp dissection can lead beneath the peritoneum that covers the anterior uterine segment. The smooth undersurface of the peritoneum can be recognized by palpation, but it should not be opened yet if it is not readily and actually visualized; it is difficult to determine the actual site of the peritoneal reflection from the superior surface of the bladder unless the area is under direct vision. Failure to proceed with caution at this stage is one of the most common reasons for unintentional bladder penetration. Fortunately, any bladder injury that occurs at this point will be well above the bladder trigone and relatively easy to repair transvaginally after the uterus has been removed.

Opening the Anterior Peritoneal Fold. The proper time to open the peritoneum during the course of mobilization and identification of the bladder is soon after the smooth, thin layer of peritoneum has been visualized; it usually appears as a fold or double reflection after the cardinal and uterosacral ligaments and the bladder pillars have all been separated from the uterus. Because all pedicles have been cut close to the cervix, the uterus has further descended, bringing the peritoneum down with it. After the anterior peritoneal fold has been recognized by palpation

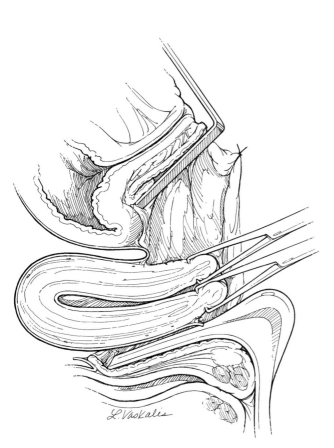

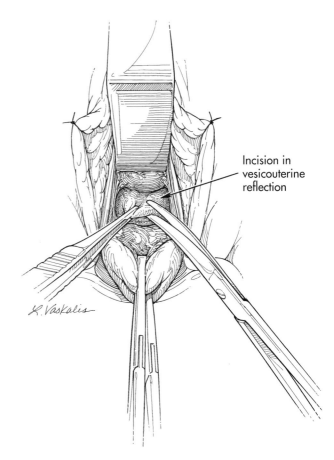

Incision in vesicouterine reflection

Fig. 19-10 Exposure of the anterior peritoneum is now facilitated by displacing the bladder anteriorly and holding it out of harm's way with a retractor. The anterior vesicouterine peritoneal fold is now much easier to observe, and it can be brought closer to the operator after detachment of the cardinal ligaments. Usually it can be identified by a somewhat frictionless sensation imparted to the operator's examining finger, or it may appear as a whitish fold of tissue because of the doubled thickness of peritoneum where it folds back upon itself to extend over the bladder. (Modified from Nichols DH, Randall CL: *Vaginal surgery*, ed 4, Baltimore, 1996, Williams & Wilkins.)

Fig. 19-11 Attention is directed toward opening anteriorly into the peritoneal cavity. To this end the uterus is now drawn strongly downward. Assistants who can anticipate and sense the steps of this operation can make matters easy by drawing the uterus in just the right direction. A retractor can be used to retract the bladder if it seems to facilitate the exposure of the peritoneum. The bulge of the vesicouterine fold of peritoneum is picked up with thumb forceps and sharply incised. Frequently this is not as simple as illustrated, and the surgeon finds himself or herself too close to the cervix and lower uterine segment of the uterus, with the cleavage plane entering the superficial layers of fibromuscular tissue. An excessive amount of bleeding indicates that the wrong cleavage plane has been entered, so the surgeon should try dissecting closer to the bladder. In elderly patients the bladder wall is thin, and in a procidentia the musculature is further attenuated. In such patients the bladder may be inadvertently entered, but this is not a serious complication. If it does happen, the bladder should be closed in two layers with interrupted 4-0 or 3-0 polyglycolic acid–type sutures either immediately, if adequate exposure exists, or after the hysterectomy, and the operation continued.

and visualized but not yet opened, the portion of the bladder pillars closest to the cervix can be included in the clamp across the adjacent portion of the cardinal ligament. However, a small, rather superficial artery in the bladder pillar often bleeds as the vaginal membrane is reflected from the midline over the cervix. When such bleeding occurs, it is advisable to clamp and ligate or coagulate the vessel and adjacent bladder pillar separately on each side close to the cervix. Similarly, the surgeon should identify the cardinal ligament tissue to each side of the cervix and clamp, cut, and ligate that structure without picking up the uterine vessels separately.

Clamping and Ligating the Uterine Vessels. In a vaginal hysterectomy, one nonslipping clamp at a time can be used on each cardinal ligament. With the vaginal approach,

traction applied to the cervix brings down the uterine artery, which pulls down the ureter. The use of a second clamp decreases the distance of safety between the clamp and the ureter, thus putting the ureter at risk. With a total abdominal hysterectomy, however, two clamps may be used simultaneously on each portion of the cardinal ligament detached

Fig. 19-12   Both index fingers are passed within the peritoneal cavity, and, with a lateral rolling motion, the opening is enlarged; at the same time, the ureters and their surrounding areolar tissue are displaced laterally. This maneuver aids in keeping the ureters out of the field of operation and simulates the same method used to displace the ureters during an abdominal hysterectomy.

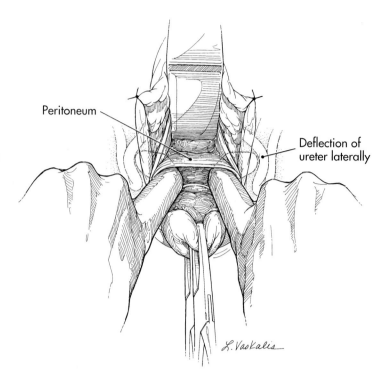

from the uterus, because upward traction on the uterus pulls the uterine artery *away* from the ureter.

An intermediate or advanced degree of uterine prolapse may occasionally allow the surgeon to use a clampless technique, in which uterine pedicles are ligated by primary passage of the needle without preliminary clamping. The operator who uses this technique must be careful *not* to cut the pedicle until after the first cast of the stitch has been placed and tightened. Then the pedicle of the ligated tissue should be cut, the first cast of the knot tightened *again,* and the second cast placed and tightened.

If separately identified, the uterine vessels should be safety clamped and ligated with a tie that is cut 1 cm from the knot to prevent its use for subsequent traction (Fig. 19-13). However, when the uterus is large or when an irregular or intraligamentous fibroid has distorted the usual anatomic relationships, it can be more difficult to locate the uterine artery and adjacent veins in the cardinal ligament tissue caught in the initial clamp. At this point, a cautious, deliberate push or pull on the clamped tissues along the axis of the ascending branch of the uterine artery invariably separates the anterior and posterior layers of ligament attached to the lower uterine segment sufficiently to disclose an underlying segment of the uterine vessels; usually these vessels promptly and literally bulge into the operator's view. (This maneuver may tear a small vein, but the vein can easily be clamped along with the uterine artery.) The uterine vessels can then be clamped (extraperitoneally, without including the peritoneum either anteriorly or posteriorly), cut, and ligated with a minimal amount of ligamentous tissue. After the uterine vessels have been ligated, the remaining superior portions of the broad ligament, including the adja-

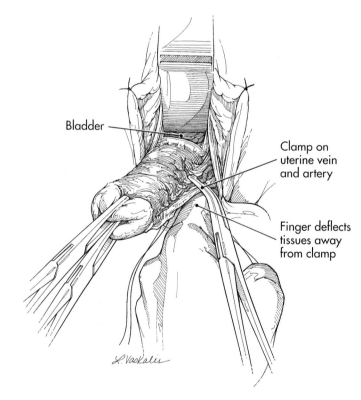

Fig. 19-13   The left uterine artery is now clamped as shown. The index finger in the peritoneal cavity pushes laterally as the clamps are applied. Suture ligatures are placed around the vessels. This procedure is repeated for the right uterine artery and veins.

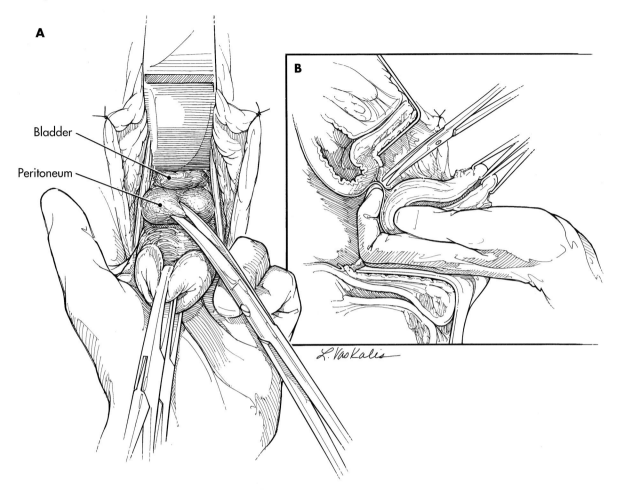

Fig. 19-14   An alternative method of opening the anterior peritoneal fold. **A,** The first and second fingers of the operator's left hand have been inserted through the opening of the posterior cul-de-sac and flexed above the uterine fundus. The anterior vesicouterine peritoneal fold, now identified and distended by the tips of the operator's fingers as shown, may be opened safely under direct vision. A long-handled Heaney or Deaver retractor may then be inserted to hold the bladder anteriorly while the uterus is removed. **B,** Sagittal section shows flexing of the operator's fingers over the fundus of the uterus to visualize the anterior vesicouterine peritoneal fold.

cent peritoneum both anteriorly and posteriorly, can be clamped and caught in a transfixing ligature without disturbing or jeopardizing the ligation of the uterine vessels.

Delayed Entry into the Peritoneal Cavity. A variety of techniques permits safe entry into the peritoneal cavity through the anterior vesicouterine peritoneal fold. In selecting the appropriate technique, the operator must consider the specific degree and type of prolapse involved, the presence of a coexistent cystocele that the operator intends to repair, the size of that cystocele, the extent of cervical descent, the degree of cervical motility (i.e., whether the cervix can be brought closer to the operator by traction on the tenaculum), and the length of the cervix. Often the site of the anterior vesicouterine peritoneal reflection is at the same level as the site of the posterior peritoneal reflection (within the cul-de-sac of Douglas) to the uterus.

The anterior peritoneal fold should be opened only under direct vision—never blindly—because a blind entry could easily damage the bladder. If the operator was previously unable to identify the anterior peritoneal plication with certainty and postponed further attempts at an anterior opening into the peritoneal cavity, a point of safe opening can now be positively identified either by longitudinal section of the cervix or by inserting the operator's first and second left fingertips through the posterior peritoneal opening over the fundus of the uterus[11,39,57] and spreading them beneath the vesicouterine peritoneal fold, thus making it both palpable and visible (Fig. 19-14). If identification of the peritoneum is still uncertain, particularly if the uterus is longer or larger than average, a Sims uterine sound may be bent in the shape of a large U and inserted through the posterior peritoneal opening over the top of the fundus, and the tip made to distend the anterior cul-de-sac, which may be dissected beneath the tip and opened under direct vision[28] (Fig. 19-15). Grasped with forceps and tented as a vertical fold, the peritoneum can be opened with the scissors safely and readily. To

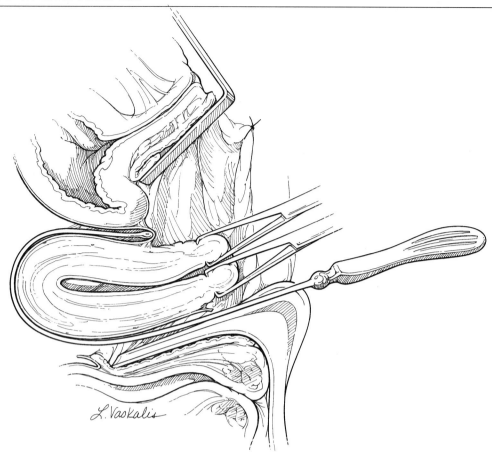

L. Vaskalis

Fig. 19-15 When the anterior cul-de-sac is difficult to identify, particularly in a patient with previous cesarean section or with a greater-than-average uterine length, a Sims uterine sound bent in the shape of a U may be inserted through the posterior peritoneal opening and over the uterine fundus, as shown. The tip can be palpated, and dissection *beneath* the tip will expose the peritoneum of the anterior cul-de-sac, which can be safely opened.

facilitate later identification of the edges of the peritoneum, some surgeons tag the midline of both the anterior and the posterior edges with a suture left long for easy retrievability when it is time to close the peritoneum (Fig. 19-16).

The operator explores the anterior cul-de-sac with an index finger, noting any disease or adhesions and making certain that the incision has properly entered the peritoneal cavity anteriorly. The operator can then insert both index fingers into this anterior peritoneal opening, enlarging it by spreading the fingers laterally. A long-handled Heaney or Deaver retractor can be inserted to keep the bladder up and out of the operative field. The relationship of the ureter to the uterine artery during hysterectomy is shown in Fig. 19-17.

Ligating the Cardinal–Uterosacral Ligament Complex. With the peritoneum opened both posterior and anterior to the uterine fundus, the operator clamps, cuts, and ligates the upper cardinal and lower broad ligaments. Clamps should be applied from the cornual angles downward, and the tips of the hemostats should be placed so that each is within the peritoneal cavity, both anteriorly and posteriorly. This placement seals off the broad ligament by compressing both its anterior and posterior peritoneal leaves between the jaws of the hemostat. This step effectively pre-

vents the extension of any laceration into the very vascular venous plexus located within layers of the broad ligaments. The hemostats should be immediately replaced by transfixing ligatures.

Removing the Uterus

Failure of the Uterus to Descend. After the cardinal-uterosacral ligament complex has been ligated and the cul-de-sac opened both anteriorly and posteriorly, the operator may find that traction applied to the cervix fails to move the uterus any further down. This event requires investigation, for under normal circumstances the broad ligament and its contents, including both round and ovarian ligaments, offer little resistance to downward traction. The operator should suspect and must determine with certainty if the patient has in the past undergone a ventral fixation or Gilliam-type uterine suspension or if adhesions are binding the uterus to other intraabdominal organs. Any one or more of the following conditions also could interfere with the descent of the uterus: (1) parametrial and broad ligament fibrosis from previous or chronic infection, (2) pelvic endometriosis, or (3) undiagnosed pelvic carcinoma, extending either from the uterus or from an extrauterine site.

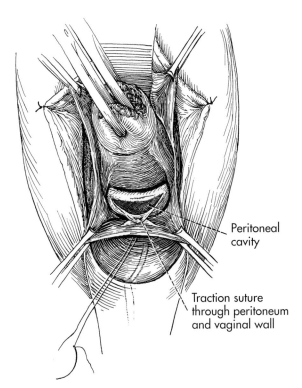

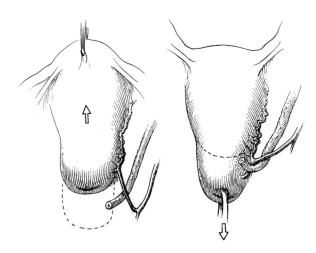

Fig. 19-17 Relationship of ureter to uterine artery during hysterectomy. Dashed line represents a usual position of the uterus. *Left,* Relationship between uterine artery and ureter when upward traction is applied to uterine fundus as in abdominal hysterectomy. *Right,* Change in this relationship when downward traction is applied as during vaginal hysterectomy. (From Nichols DH, Randall CL: *Vaginal surgery,* ed 4, Baltimore, 1996, Williams & Wilkins.)

Fig. 19-16 An absorbable suture can be used to tag the peritoneum to the posterior vaginal wall. The posterior thickenings or uterosacral ligaments contain blood vessels that can be a troublesome source of bleeding from the posterior flap. These vessels should be systematically ligated. They are vaginal branches of the hypogastric artery that in males are called the *inferior vesical arteries.* Furthermore, if the cul-de-sac hernia is large, the dissection must be more complete, and the vessels originating from the superior and middle hemorrhoidal vessels may be encountered. (From Ball TL: *Gynecologic surgery and urology,* ed 2, St Louis, 1963, Mosby.)

Another possibility is a mechanical obstruction to the further descent of the uterus. For example, the patient may have significant adenomyosis or a large fibroid uterus, with its leiomyomata interfering with the delivery of the uterus. The operator then must choose one of several alternative procedures. The first is to abandon the vaginal approach to hysterectomy at this point and finish the operation transabdominally. As Allen[1] cautioned,

I do not believe that large tumors should be attacked through the vagina. How large a tumor one should attack depends on one's experience and skill, but also on the location of the tumor in the uterus. Relatively small tumors immediately beneath the bladder or extending out into the broad ligament, where the uterine blood supply is reached with difficulty, are much more important as contraindications than large tumors if they are in the fundus. Once the lower blood supply is secured, these upper tumors can be reached and morcellated with, shall I say, impunity.

A possible alternative is amputation of the cervix and of any fibroid tumors of the uterus (Fig. 19-18), provided that

they can be grasped safely through the vagina.[21,38] Werner and Sederl,[84] and other authorities, have recommended bisection of the noncancerous uterus and removal of first one side and then the other. The operator should choose the option that is consistent with the patient's best interests and the operator's confidence, experience, and technical ability.

Delivery of the Uterus. If there is no interference with the descent of the uterus, the operator continues to apply traction on the cervix, drawing it further down. It may be necessary in avoiding hematoma to clamp, cut, and ligate the middle portion of the broad ligament separately, again with care to ensure that both the anterior and posterior leaves of the broad ligament peritoneum are included within the grasp of the hemostat on either side. By now transfixion ligatures on the uterine blood vessels, including both the ascending and descending branches of the uterine artery, should have secured the blood supply to the uterus.

When the fundus of the uterus is low in the pelvis, the operator can deliver it through either the anterior or the posterior peritoneal opening (Fig. 19-19). If the fundus is freely movable and readily visualized, however, it need not be "flipped" either anteriorly or posteriorly for delivery. Hemostats are applied to the cornual angle of the uterus on either side, and the uterus is removed. The cavity is opened immediately and the endometrium and endocervical canal carefully inspected to determine if there is any grossly visible but unsuspected pathology present that might alter the surgical plan. Immediate frozen section is requested if the possibility of malignancy is uncertain.

Removing the uterus without flipping it decreases the risk of contaminating the peritoneal surfaces through contact with a bacteriologically dirty cervix. Retroperitoneal infection in the cellular tissues is responsible for posthyster-

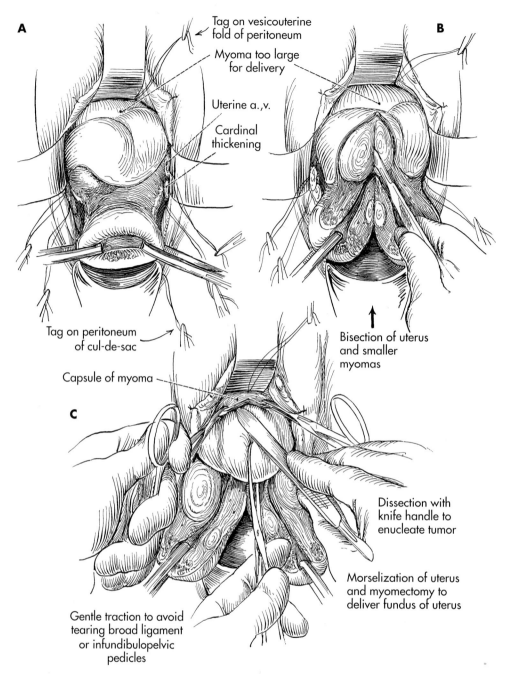

A

Tag on vesicouterine fold of peritoneum

Myoma too large for delivery

Uterine a.,v.

Cardinal thickening

B

Tag on peritoneum of cul-de-sac

Bisection of uterus and smaller myomas

Capsule of myoma

C

Dissection with knife handle to enucleate tumor

Morselization of uterus and myomectomy to deliver fundus of uterus

Gentle traction to avoid tearing broad ligament or infundibulopelvic pedicles

Fig. 19-18   The operation proceeds as in any vaginal hysterectomy until the uterine artery and veins have been identified, doubly clamped, cut, and ligated. At this time the vesicouterine fold of peritoneum and the peritoneum of the cul-de-sac will have been entered. Both of the peritoneal reflections have been tagged with a suture ligature. The cardinal thickenings and the uterosacral thickenings will have been cut, clamped, and ligated and appropriately identified for closure of the vaginal vault at the conclusion of the operation. **A,** Two Jacobs tenacula are placed on the cervix at the lateral angles in preparation for dissecting the uterus.

   B, Strong traction is made downward and outward, and a knife is used to bisect the cervix in the midsagittal plane. Small fibroids that are encountered can be bisected together with the uterus itself rather than performing a myomectomy.

   C, A large myoma that could not be delivered under the symphysis is grasped with a tenaculum. A vaginal myomectomy is performed by grasping the capsule of the myoma with Allis clamps. The operator cautions the assistants to exert only gentle traction from now on, because with the delivery of the uterus, considerable strain is placed on the infundibulopelvic pedicles. They may be torn and the ovarian vessels ruptured. The myoma is enucleated either by the knife handle technique **(C)** or by the use of scissors, thus leaving the capsule intact. After removing the large myoma, the remainder of the uterus is delivered to the outside and the bisection continued. (From Ball TL: *Gynecologic surgery and urology,* ed 3, St Louis, 1963, Mosby.)

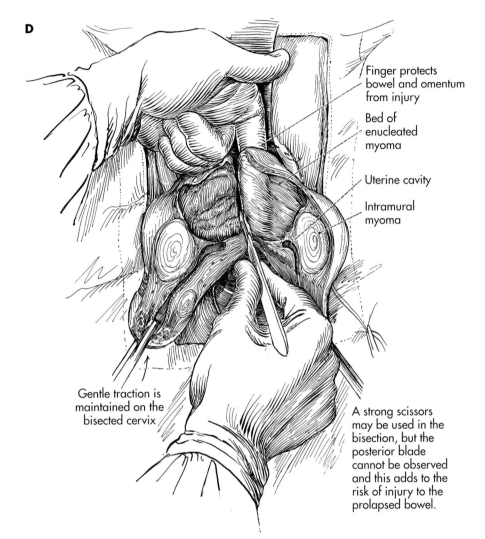

D

Finger protects
bowel and omentum
from injury

Bed of
enucleated
myoma

Uterine cavity

Intramural
myoma

Gentle traction is
maintained on the
bisected cervix

A strong scissors
may be used in the
bisection, but the
posterior blade
cannot be observed
and this adds to the
risk of injury to the
prolapsed bowel.

The myomectomized uterus can now be delivered
and the bisection completed

Fig. 19-18, cont'd   The bisection is continued by cutting through the remainder of the posterior portion of the capsule of the myoma that was removed. **D,** A finger should be placed behind the uterus to protect bowel or omentum from injury. Small laparotomy pads are used to
pack off the bowel and omentum. In performing the bisection a strong scissors may be used;
a crushing instrument, particularly when the posterior blade cannot be observed, adds to the
risk of injury to prolapsed bowel or omentum. (From Ball TL: *Gynecologic surgery and urology,* ed 3, St Louis, 1963, Mosby.)   *Continued*

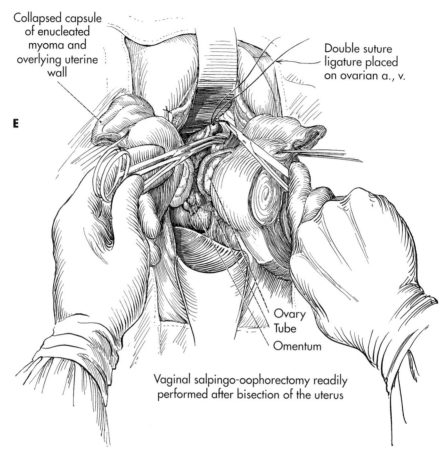

Collapsed capsule
of enucleated
myoma and
overlying uterine
wall

Double suture
ligature placed
on ovarian a., v.

E

Ovary
Tube
Omentum

Vaginal salpingo-oophorectomy readily
performed after bisection of the uterus

Fig. 19-18, cont'd   The two halves of the bisected uterus, together with tubes and ovaries, are delivered out of the pelvis. Traction is made on the capsule of the enucleated myoma and, together with gentle traction on the cervix, the infundibulopelvic pedicles are visualized. Angle clamps are used to clamp the infundibulopelvic pedicle, and this is double ligated with a 0-PGA suture (**E**). The round ligament is double clamped, cut, and ligated, and the left half of the uterus is removed together with the tube and ovary on that side attached to the specimen. An identical procedure is carried out on the right side, completing the removal of the uterus, tubes, and ovaries. The surgeon further explores the pelvis for other pelvic disease. The closure of the vaginal vault and the anterior and posterior colporrhaphies is completed in the same manner as a routine vaginal hysterectomy.

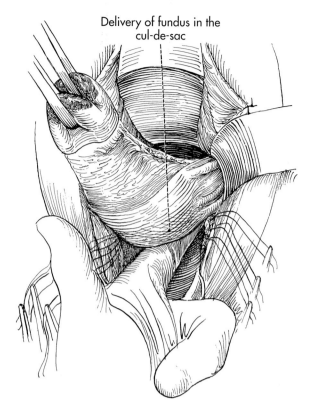

Delivery of fundus in the
cul-de-sac

Fig. 19-19 The vesicouterine reflection of the peritoneum is smaller in all dimensions than the rectovaginal reflection or pouch of Douglas. The fundus of the uterus is thus more easily delivered posteriorly than by forcibly extracting it through a hiatus artificially created between the vagina and bladder. Some local disease may cause a variation in this rule. In this type of surgery one does not create bigger openings when such can be avoided. The basic objectives (namely, to decrease the size of the genital hiatus and to strengthen the obturators filling this outlet) make logical the delivery of the items posteriorly.

The uterus is now mobile except for the resistance offered by the round ligaments, tubes, and infundibulopelvic vessels and their connective tissue thickenings. The fundus is now delivered through the posterior route by applying bullet tenacula alternately along the posterior aspect of the uterus. This sometimes is accomplished by a finger alone. If it does not come out without difficulty, make traction on the fundus and push the cervix back up under the symphysis; this has the effect of rotating the organ about its last remaining attachments. This maneuver usually is successful unless abnormal attachments exist. In this event the anterior Deaver retractor is manipulated to see the reason for resistance and any structures adherent to the uterus or adnexa. Failure to deliver the uterus by this technique is rare.

Following this dissection the bladder neck is plicated prophylactically and the vaginal wall appropriately resected to correct any cystocele. The incision is carried toward the vault to meet the upper incision. Any posterior colporrhaphy is completed and a high perineorrhaphy is done to complete the reconstruction of the pelvic floor as necessary. (From Ball TL: *Gynecologic surgery and urology,* ed 2, St Louis, 1963, Mosby.)

ectomy morbidity much more frequently than is peritonitis; therefore, prophylactic amputation of the external cervix may be indicated whenever the size or relative immobility of the uterus seems likely to necessitate more than the usual manipulation of the uterus as the fundus is being freed and removed.

If the body of the uterus is movable but too large to permit comfortable delivery through either the anterior or posterior peritoneal opening, and piecemeal morselization is not desired, the operator can incise the myometrium circumferentially. Such an incision should be carried symmetrically around the full circumference of the uterus, into the myometrium, parallel to the axis of the uterine cavity and just beneath the serosa, the so-called Lash incision.[42,56,58] The uterus is freed by this procedure much as a banana is peeled by turning the skin inside out. The procedure brings the cervix closer to the operator but does not violate the integrity of the endometrial cavity (Fig. 19-20). Incision of the lateral portions of myometrium medial to the remaining attachment of the broad ligament results in considerable additional descent and mobility of the as yet unremoved fundus (Fig. 19-21). Alternatively as when further uterine descent is compromised at this point by adnexal adhesive disease, the uterus can be bisected, and as one half is displaced upward, the opposite half is removed separately, adnexa last.[29]

At this point the operator replaces the cornual angle hemostats with transfixion ligatures. After these are tied, an additional bite is taken through the round ligament on each side, and the suture is tied again. Any traction on the adnexal pedicles will then be borne principally by the round ligament, which has been ligated higher than the infundibulopelvic ligament by virtue of the extra bite. This leaves the residual ovaries at a higher level within the pelvis postoperatively, away from direct attachment to the vaginal cuff, markedly lessening the risk of postoperative dyspareunia.

Performing an Oophorectomy. The adnexa should be carefully inspected on each side. If they are to be removed, particular care must be taken to ensure ligation of the ovarian vessels (Figs. 19-22 and 19-23).* When performing a vaginal oophorectomy of an obviously benign ovarian tumor, the operator should first doubly clamp the mesovarium, cut between the clamps, and then remove the ovary, using the clamp on the mesovarium as a handle so that the ovarian tumor does not fill the vagina and obstruct the operator's vision of its pedicle. One occasionally encounters a large, smooth, surfaced, and apparently benign ovarian tumor, too large to be safely removed through the vagina without risk of rupture. The size can be reduced by trocar following hysterectomy, and oophorectomy or salpingo-oophorectomy easily accomplished in the usual transvaginal manner. Alternatively, if the ovaries appear to be reasonably accessible, but removal by clamp technique is not feasible, oophorectomy using the Endoloop technique can be used after the hysterectomy.[25,28] The ovary is grasped with a long Babcock clamp and pulled into the vagina. The Endoloop suture

---

*References 4, 57, 58, 59, 61, 74.

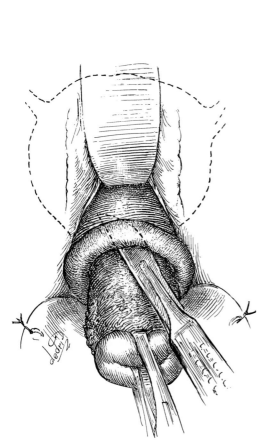

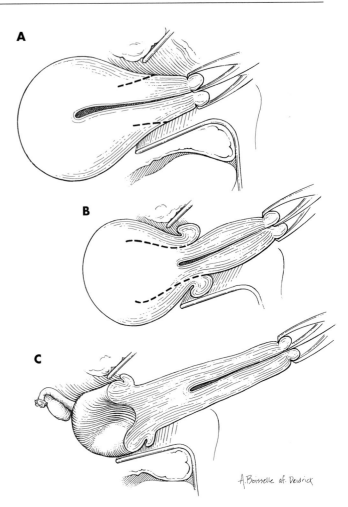

A.Boisselle af. Deidrick

Fig. 19-20 Lash incision into the myometrium. The operator has already secured by transfixion ligature inferior and major blood supply of uterus (ascending and descending branches of uterine artery) and has determined that the uterus is not being deviated or fixed by any previously unsuspected adhesions. If it is now determined that the body of uterus is too big to permit delivery, outer superficial myometrium can be incised circumferentially. If circumferential incision has been properly placed, the bulk of the uterus can be enucleated without transgressing the endocervical or endometrial cavity. The large, bulky uterus is thereby increased in length and decreased in width, which in essence "makes the cork smaller than the neck of the bottle." (From Nichols DH, Randall CL: *Vaginal surgery,* ed 4, Baltimore, 1996, Williams & Wilkins.)

Fig. 19-21 **A,** Sagittal drawing of a large, bulky uterus. Cardinal and uterosacral ligaments have been separated from sides of uterus, but delivery of the body is difficult because of its size. The pathway for the incision into the myometrium parallel to axis of the uterus is identified by the *dashed line.* **B,** Incision has been deepened, as traction further exteriorizes the cervix. Myometrial incision will be extended further as indicated by the *dashed line.* **C,** The uterus can now be delivered outside the pelvis. Its length has increased as its diameter has decreased, as shown. The cornual angle now can be clamped under direct visualization and the uterus cut free. (Modified from Nichols DH, Randall CL: *Vaginal surgery,* ed 4, Baltimore, 1996, Williams & Wilkins.)

is brought around the clamp and ovary and tightened at the mesovarium, and a second loop fixed close to the first. The ovary is then excised under direct vision and the process repeated on the opposite side.

The operator may decide to spare the tube and mesosalpinx, which can appreciably aid in subsequent peritonealization of the intraperitoneal mesovarium stump. In this case, the operator must be careful to preserve the tubal blood supply when ligating the ovarian pedicle. When the tube and ovary are to be removed, the round ligament is clamped, cut, and ligated.[3,74] The slanted Deschamps' ligature carrier with its blunt point is good for ligation of the in-

fundibulopelvic ligament. After the cornual angle stitches have been tied, the uncut ends of the sutures can be secured in a clamp and kept long for later use in the procedure. If there are many adhesions, the leaves of the broad ligament can be spread by tunneling with the scissor tips for mobilization of the components that have been ligated separately.[3]

Adnexectomy en bloc with vaginal hysterectomy can be accomplished using the technique of Candiani and Ferrari.[3] The uterus is exteriorized, and the round ligament on the left is clamped and divided. The two leaves (sheets) of the broad ligament are visualized, and a tunnel is dissected between the leaves of the left mesosalpinx.

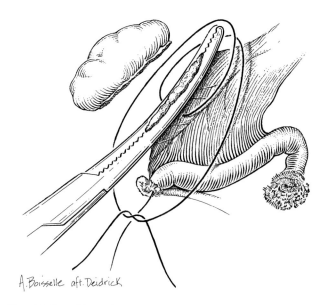

A. Boisselle aft. Deidrick

Fig. 19-22 Vaginal oophorectomy. When the infundibulopelvic ligament is short, transvaginal oophorectomy can be accomplished as shown. The mesovarium has been clamped and the ovary removed. There is a single penetration of the mesovarium at its midpoint, and each end of the suture is passed around the distal tip of the hemostat and tied beneath the heel of the clamp. (From Nichols DH, Randall CL: *Vaginal surgery*, ed 4, Baltimore, 1996, Williams & Wilkins.)

After the left ovary and tube are clamped together, the adnexum is pulled forward and medially, and the two leaves of the mesosalpinx are cut separately. The mesosalpinx is opened completely, and the left adnexum is separated from the infundibulopelvic ligament. The infundibulopelvic ligament is clamped and the specimen cut free 1 cm from the cranial pole of the ovary. The infundibulopelvic pedicle is transfixed with a PGA suture, and a second suture is applied as a free tie. The three pedicles can be separately identified from top to bottom: round ligament, infundibulopelvic ligament, and cardinal uterosacral ligament. A similar dissection is performed on the opposite side.

Recognizing and Preventing an Enterocele. The operator may identify an enterocele, enterocele sac, or potential enterocele at this time by exploring the cul-de-sac with a finger (Fig. 19-24). At times, packing the interior of the sac with a moistened gauze sponge facilitates identification and aids dissection. Because the patient should already be in a 5- or 10-degree Trendelenburg position, the contents of the abdomen usually can be readily packed away from the operative field with some gauze packing. An enterocele sac can easily be separated from the surrounding connective tissue by alternating sharp and blunt dissection as far down as the anterior surface of the rectum, which is identified by the small condensations of fat adherent to the peritoneum and by the noticeably longitudinal muscle layer of the outer rectal wall.

Inspecting the anterior or vesicouterine peritoneum, the operator should excise any excess or redundant peritoneum

left after the opening and dissection of the anterior peritoneal cul-de-sac to decrease the possibility of an anterior postoperative enterocele. The bladder, if at all distended, should now be emptied of urine by catheter because this seems to facilitate reperitonealization by making the anterior cut edge of the peritoneum more readily visible and accessible. Should it be difficult to locate the anterior peritoneum, the operator can lightly grasp the tissues inferior to the anterior peritoneum with successive gentle bites of an unlocked hemostat so as to "walk" or roll these tissues toward the operator until the anterior peritoneal edge can be identified. When unmistakably visible, the peritoneal edge is grasped by a hemostat, and sutures are placed to close the peritoneal opening.

Closing the Peritoneum. The primary purpose of peritoneal closure following vaginal hysterectomy is to incorporate the strength of the subperitoneal connective tissue retinaculum into a firm scar at the bottom of the pelvis that will resist increases in intraabdominal pressure. The mesothelial lining of the peritoneal cavity per se has little supportive value. Attaching the shortened uterosacral–cardinal ligament stumps to the vaginal vault at hysterectomy aids significantly in support of the vault postoperatively. Although this tends to pull the sides of the vault laterally, theoretically increasing the risk of future enterocele, this risk is overcome by the firm purse-string closure of the peritoneum; this closure incorporates the more proximal part of each uterosacral ligament, thus bringing them together in the midline at the 6-o'clock position of the purse-string when it has been snugly tied.

The operator begins peritoneal closure with a full length of suture: polydioxanone absorbable 0 suture. Traction on the previously clamped and held transfixion ligature readily identifies the uterosacral ligament. After placing a stitch through the peritoneal surface and into the peritoneal side of the left uterosacral ligament, the operator reefs the posterior peritoneum in a linear fashion by a series of bites until the same level on the opposite uterosacral ligament location is reached. This posterior peritoneal reefing should be along the level of the reflection of the peritoneum from the anterior wall of the rectum. Reefing sutures placed any higher than this would displace an excessive amount of rectum into the vaginal space.

The purse-string sutures[11,43,58] placed to close the peritoneum, and any suture placed to bring the uterosacral or infundibulopelvic and round ligaments together, should be above or proximal to the ligature on the pedicles. The purpose of the suture that brings the ligamentous structures together is twofold: to promote a firm tissue union and to ensure that all ligated pedicles will be extraperitonealized. The ligatures on the uterine vessels are not caught up on an approximating suture. Although the vessels will retract into the parametria, their ligated pedicles remain extraperitonealized.

After passing the peritoneal closure stitch through the uterosacral ligament and adjacent peritoneum (Fig. 19-25), first on one side and then on the other, the operator relaxes traction on the previously held uterosacral transfixing

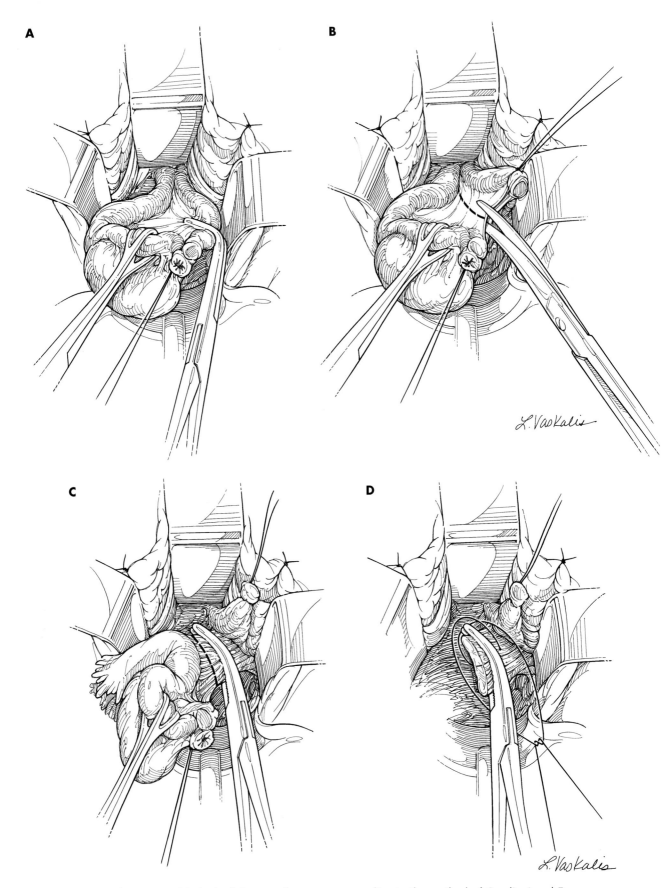

Fig. 19-23 Vaginal salpingo-oophorectomy according to the method of Candiani and Ferrari.[3] The uterus has already been removed. **A,** The round ligament has been clamped, cut, and tied and is clamped again proximal to the tie. **B,** The broad ligament has been opened by tunneling with the closed scissor tips, and the anterior leaf incised along the path of the *dashed line.* **C,** The adnexa are pulled medially and the infundibulopelvic ligament clamped as shown and transected along the path of the *dashed line.* **D,** The clamp across the infundibulopelvic ligament is replaced by a transfixion ligature.

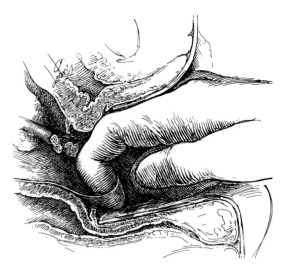

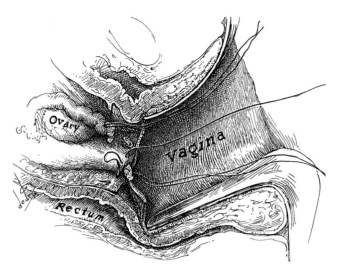

Fig. 19-24   The importance of recognizing evidence of a potential enterocele or an existing enterocele sac always warrants careful exploration of the cul-de-sac by the operator's fingers, as shown in this sagittal section. For demonstration or identification purposes, a suspected sac can be packed with a gauze sponge to facilitate demonstration of excess peritoneal connective tissue, which is mobilized by both sharp and blunt dissection down to a point where yellow fat indicates the site of the rectum. Excision of this excess peritoneum extends downward and across the anterior surface of the rectum. Any fat that is present belongs on the rectal side of the dissection. The rectum should be recognized promptly during this dissection either by characteristic condensations of fat or by the longitudinal muscle fibers of the outer layer of the rectal wall. In the same manner, the anterior residual peritoneum should be inspected. If there is excessive redundant peritoneum anteriorly, it should be excised at this time, lessening the postoperative possibility of an anterior enterocele. (From Nichols DH, Randall CL: *Vaginal surgery,* ed 4, Baltimore, 1996, Williams & Wilkins.)

Fig. 19-25   Beginning of a high peritoneal closure stitch through the peritoneal surface of the uterosacral ligament; the posterior peritoneum is just above its cut edge. (From Nichols DH, Randall CL: *Vaginal surgery,* ed 4, Baltimore, 1996, Williams & Wilkins.)

ligatures. Grasping the ipsilateral adnexal pedicle suture on the patient's right side, the operator again applies gentle traction to bring the round ligament into view. The operator then passes the peritoneal closure stitch through the round ligament proximal and medial to the previously placed pedicle ligation. The round ligaments do not support the vagina; they are incorporated in the purse-string stitch only to enhance peritonealization of the pelvis. The anterior peritoneum is then identified, any excess is excised, and the remainder reefed by a series of bites that continue to and through the opposite round ligament. At this point the operator has continued the stitch entirely around the peritoneal opening, through the round and uterosacral ligaments on each side (Fig. 19-26).

After carefully removing all intraabdominal, intraperitoneal packing, the operator takes up all slack in the purse-string peritoneal suture[11,43,58] by reefing the tissues fairly snugly along the suture, both anteriorly and posteriorly. Only after such reefing should the operator tie the purse-string suture to close the peritoneal cavity; to be effective,

all reefing should be accomplished before—not as—this stitch is tied. This plication of tissues at the bases of the uterosacral ligaments actually draws the pubococcygei and their fasciae together,[16,46,47] narrowing the genital hiatus. After the purse-string peritoneal closure stitch has been tied, both ends of the stitch should be left long and held for possible later use.

Because the uterosacral ligaments are relatively fixed in position, this suturing technique brings the movable round ligaments that are also included in the purse-string suture to the semifixed uterosacral ligaments. This technique tends to reestablish the horizontal axis of the upper vagina[35,58] and appreciably decreases the likelihood of a postoperative enterocele.

Closing the Vaginal Wall.   The round ligament pedicle stitches can be tied together beneath the base of the bladder to provide auxiliary support to the intraabdominal contents should the peritoneal sutures be broken or come untied. The retracting sutures in the labia minora may now be cut and the vagina prepared for closure. If a colporrhaphy is not being performed and maximal vaginal depth is to be preserved, the vagina is closed in a sagittal direction[10,11,57,58] (Fig. 19-27).

After completing any anterior colporrhaphy, the operator begins closing the anterior vaginal wall. He or she passes the needle on one end of the preserved peritoneal closure stitch through each side of the uppermost portion of the anterior vaginal wall, from the inside out on one side and the outside in on the other, at precisely the level of the vault that corresponds to the previous sutures in the uterosacral ligaments, which were held for tying later. The operator then ties the end of the previously tied peritoneal closure stitch (sewn beneath the anterior vaginal wall at its apex, as noted earlier) to its other held end. He or she should take care (as

Fig. 19-26 If a marking suture has not been placed and locating the anterior peritoneum is difficult, tissue caudal to the anterior peritoneum is lightly grasped with successive gentle bites of an unlocked hemostat in such fashion as to "walk up" this area until the anterior peritoneum is recognized and grasped in forceps. Peritonealization is accomplished using a full length of absorbable synthetic 0 or 2-0 suture held in a light hemostat for later identification. I prefer to begin this stitch on the peritoneal side of the left uterosacral ligament. Traction is made on the previously clamped and held transfixion ligature of the uterosacral ligament, but the ligament is readily identified by putting it on tension. Proceeding in a clockwise fashion, the posterior peritoneum is reefed by a series of bites until the opposite uterosacral ligament location is reached. A suture passes through the right round ligament, anterior peritoneum, and left round ligament and is then ready to be tied. (From Nichols DH, Randall CL: *Vaginal surgery,* ed 4, Baltimore, 1996, Williams & Wilkins.)

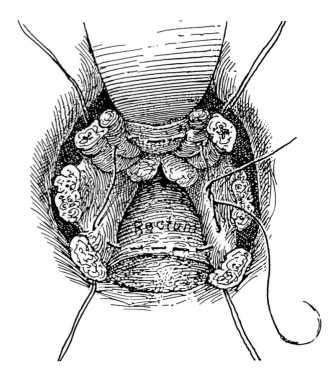

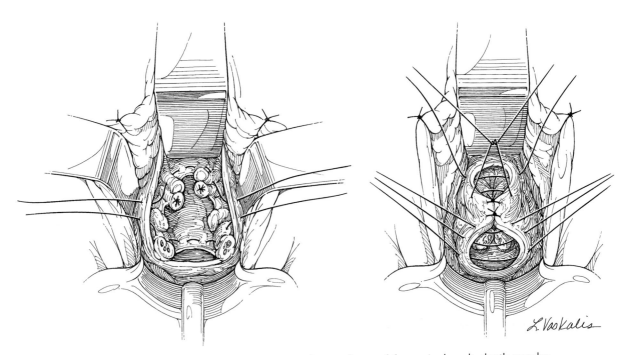

Fig. 19-27 When there has been no coincident prolapse of the vaginal vault, depth may be preserved by closure from side to side. A stitch of polyglycolic acid–type suture is passed through the full thickness of the lateral vaginal wall and peritoneum, the round ligament portion of the adnexal pedicle, a reefing of the anterior peritoneum, and the same structures in reverse order on the opposite side. A second stitch is placed through the full thickness of the posterolateral vaginal wall, uterosacral ligament stump, a reefing of posterior peritoneum, and the same structures in reverse order on the opposite side. Any remaining gaps in the vaginal wall can be closed by interrupted sutures.

when preparing to tie the peritoneal purse-string suture) to reef the tissues to be tied rather snugly together before seating and tying the knot. This suture fixes the anterior vault to the edge and level of the peritoneal purse-string suture, effectively lengthening the anterior vaginal wall and aiding in the support of the vaginal vault.

By tying the held end of the peritoneal closure stitch to an uppermost stitch in the anterior vaginal wall, with a bite or two to either side of the midline, the operator effectively unites the anterior connective tissue capsule of the vagina to the area where the peritoneal stitch brought the uterosacral ligaments together. Because each uterosacral ligament has in effect been joined to the posterolateral surface of the vaginal wall, this unites the tissue capsule of the anterior vaginal wall to that of the posterior vaginal wall.[22]

The anterior vaginal wall is closed by either running or interrupted subcuticular sutures placed from side to side. A subcuticular closure provides a more exact, smoother approximation of the subepithelial layers. This alignment not only reduces postoperative development of foci of granulation tissue in the suture line, and thus the likelihood of future development of an enterocele, but also appreciably strengthens the vault.[3,58,61] Closing the vagina from side to side in a longitudinal direction rather than from front to back provides an additional 2 or 3 cm of vaginal length, which at times can mean the difference between a depth that contains the sexual partner and a depth that does not.

Performing a Culdeplasty. When the cardinal-uterosacral ligaments are elongated but strong, as is usual with uterovaginal prolapse, and the vagina is obviously shortened or telescoped, the operator can increase the vaginal depth by fixing the vagina posterior to this ligament complex. One method of doing this is to use the McCall[52,58,62] culdeplasty or a modification of it. In one modification the operator excises most of the peritoneum of any coexistent enterocele before placing the polyglycolic acid–type culdeplasty stitches, thus repairing the enterocele while reducing the size of the subsequent cul-de-sac (Fig. 19-28). If the vault is unusually wide, an appropriate wedge should be removed and the edges approximated. The culdoplasty stitch should be tied under direct vision to eliminate the chance that the now buried proximal end of a fallopian tube will prolapse postoperatively into the line of the vaginal incision, creating an annoying problem.

If the posterior vault is wide, as may occur after an enterocele repair, the operator can dissect a V-shaped wedge of excess vaginal membrane free, remove it, and sew the cut edges of the V together from side to side (Fig. 19-29). This maneuver brings the vaginal attachments of the uterosacral ligaments still closer together toward the midline and is entirely consistent with the purse-string peritonealization and surgical narrowing or V-shaped wedging of a voluminous vaginal vault, as described. The operator should tie the purse-string peritonealization stitch under direct visualization to avoid the possibility of trapping any intraabdominal structure, such as an ovary, a knuckle of tube, or bowel, in the stitch.

Elkins et al.[16] have demonstrated by cadaver dissection that the uterosacral ligaments attach not only the base of the cervix, but also have a broad attachment along the posterior surface of the cervix, in some cases extending almost to the uterine isthmus (Fig. 19-30).

When strong but elongated uterosacral ligaments are noted in a patient with moderately severe uterine prolapse undergoing transvaginal colpopexy, a high McCall culdeplasty[52] can restore a normal axis of the vagina. While the uterus is still present, an attachment between the uterosacral ligaments can be made before the hysterectomy, and if the cervix is to be preserved, bringing them together and attaching the most distal plication stitches to the posterior surface of the cervix is most helpful. Coincident vaginal hysterectomy then can be performed, as by the Döderlein-Krönig technique through the anterior colpotomy.[15,16,19] Occasionally a lowest uterosacral plicating stitch will be included in the hysterectomy specimen. The higher the plication of the uterosacral ligaments within the pelvis, the farther away the ureters. This brings some safety to the procedure, as well as creating a longer postoperative vaginal depth.

When hysterectomy is being performed on a patient with long and strong uterosacral ligaments, use of the Döderlein-Krönig technique permits access, careful definition, and safe plication of the uterosacral ligaments before their transection and before completion of the hysterectomy if the hysterectomy is accomplished by the Döderlein-Krönig technique in which the uterine fundus is rotated forward through an anterior colpotomy incision until it is clearly beyond the introitus.

Anterior rotation of the uterine fundus through the anterior colpotomy during a Döderlein-Krönig (D-K) vaginal hysterectomy places the uterosacral ligaments on a greater and more identifiable stretch during this hysterectomy than is possible during conventional Heaney-type hysterectomy, thus enhancing their surgical usefulness.[16]

THE DÖDERLEIN-KRÖNIG VAGINAL HYSTERECTOMY

The revival of interest in the Döderlein-Krönig technique for vaginal hysterectomy[16,19,20,37,72] has been stimulated by four factors: its applicability to laparoscopically assisted hysterectomy, a useful place for surgical students to start with the confidence to learn the technique for vaginal hysterectomy, a safe method for vaginal hysterectomy by an experienced vaginal operator in a patient with adhesive obliteration of the cul-de-sac precluding safe posterior entry early in the operation, and last, it provides an additional opportunity to use a patient's strong uterosacral ligaments in posthysterectomy support of the vaginal vault. The transvaginal technique essentially follows.

Technique

A Jacobs clamp or vulsellum is placed on the anterior lip of the cervix, which is incised anteriorly from the 9- to the 3-o'clock positions. The connective tissue of the bladder is

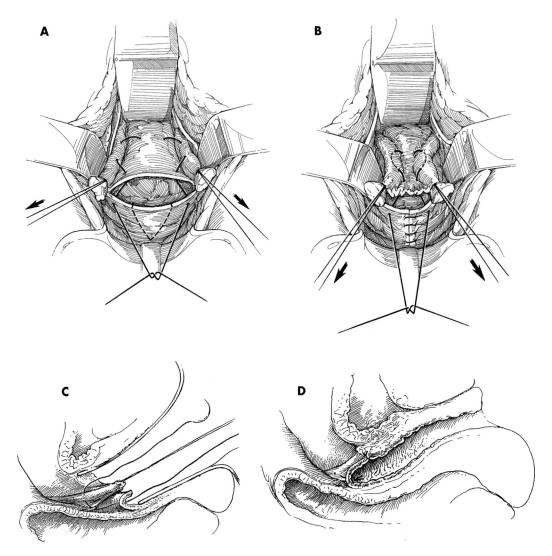

Fig. 19-28 The modified McCall culdeplasty. **A,** Any enterocele sac has been resected, and using a long-lasting polyglycolic acid suture, the stitches are placed through the vaginal wall, through the cut edge of the peritoneum, and high on the medial surface of the uterosacral ligament; a bite is taken in the peritoneum overlying the anterior surface of the rectum. The same structures are stitched in reverse order on the opposite side. When using a monofilament suture, it is wise to place a second McCall stitch approximately 1 cm cranial to the first. In the event of unexpected breakage of one of the sutures during the tying process, one unbroken suture still remains to support the vault of the vagina. A very wide posterior vault may be narrowed by excising an appropriately sized wedge as shown by the *dashed line.* **B,** The sides of the V-shaped wound in the posterior vaginal wall are closed with interrupted polyglycolic acid sutures. This closure not only narrows the vault but also brings the uterosacral ligaments fixed to the vault closer together. After the peritoneum is closed, the McCall stitches are tied. **C,** The first half of the modified culdoplasty stitch is shown in sagittal section before tying and closure of the peritoneal cavity and vaginal vault. **D,** The stitch is shown after tying and subsequent closure of the peritoneal cavity and vaginal vault. The apex of the vagina is now cranial and posterior to the new peritoneal cul-de-sac. (From Nichols DH, Randall CL: *Vaginal surgery,* ed 4, Baltimore, 1996, Williams & Wilkins.)

separated from the connective tissue of the cervix by sharp dissection up to the anterior vesicouterine peritoneal fold, and a long-handled Heaney retractor is inserted to hold the bladder from harm's way. The vesicouterine peritoneal fold is incised, and the Heaney retractor is slipped into the peritoneal cavity. Strong upward traction to the retractor is made in the 12-o'clock position. A vulsellum or a Lahey thyroid

clamp is placed in the midline of the lower uterine segment, traction is applied, and the second clamp is placed cranial to the first. The Jacobs clamp on the cervix is pushed back into the hollow of the sacrum, and additional successive bites of the thyroid clamp "walk up" the anterior wall of the fundus, until it can be delivered through the anterior peritoneal opening. The Jacobs clamp on the cervix is released, and

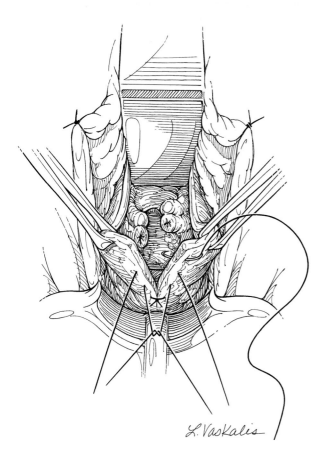

Fig. 19-29 Whenever the vaginal vault is excessively wide, it can be easily narrowed by excision of a V-shaped wedge and the defect closed by interrupted through-and-through suture, as shown.

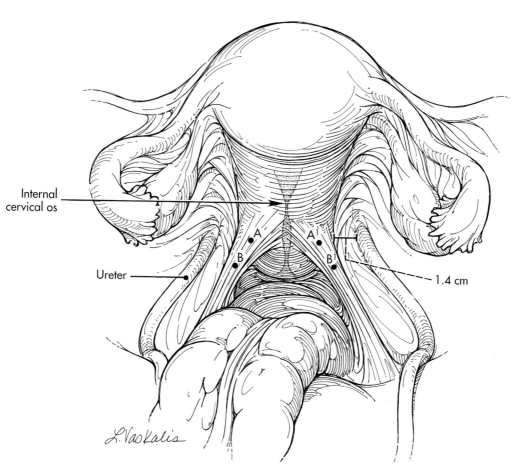

Internal cervical os

Ureter

A

B

A¹

B¹

1.4 cm

Fig. 19-30 The uterosacral ligaments insert normally on the back of the cervix, not into its base.[16] Plicating sutures should unite A to A¹ and B to B¹ and be placed in the medial halves of the ligaments safely away from the ureters, which are but 1.4 cm away from the lateral surfaces of the ligaments.

each cornual angle of the uterus is clamped with Heaney hemostats, which may each include the round ligament and tube. These pedicles are cut from the uterus, and the clamps are replaced with transfixion ligatures that are held. Successive bites of the clamp continue downward toward the cervix, and the cardinal ligaments including the uterine artery are clamped and cut on each side close to the cervix. The lowermost clamp on each side includes the uterosacral ligament, posterior vaginal wall, rectovaginal septum, and peritoneum. These clamps are replaced with transfixion ligatures. Any residual midline vaginal wall is transected and the vaginal cuff closed by suturing each uterosacral ligament to the cuff and to each other, and the posterior cuff is closed with a running locked suture. The anterior cuff is sutured to the posterior cuff with interrupted sutures, uniting the anterior vaginal connective tissue with that of the upper posterior vaginal wall.

Rarely, and usually in a patient with procidentia, the uterosacral ligament may have no palpable, usable strength. In this circumstance, the operator must find an alternate method of fixing and stabilizing the vaginal vault; otherwise the unfixed vault may later telescope and evert. In such a patient the operator can sew the vault to the sacrospinous[58] or sacrotuberous ligament, or to the fascia of the pelvic diaphragm,[33] after the peritoneal cavity has been closed (see Chapter 27).

THE MANCHESTER OPERATION

When a patient with symptomatic prolapse desires surgical treatment that will preserve her uterus or her fertility and has the combination of cervical elongation coincident with strong though elongated cardinal-uterosacral ligaments, cystocele, and rectocele, the Manchester[73] (or Fothergill's) operation can be considered. In the previous generation it was the surgical treatment of choice for most patients with symptomatic uterine prolapse, but with the more widespread use of postmenopausal estrogen replacement therapy and its tendency to prolong the years of uterine bleeding, the operation has lost much of its favor and has largely been replaced by vaginal hysterectomy with colporrhaphy. The latter operation, of course, removes the uterus as a source for future bleeding.

Additional potential difficulties exist concerning the Manchester operation for which the surgeon must be prepared. If the cardinal–uterosacral ligament complex is of unusually poor quality, it may be inadequate to support the vaginal vault postoperatively. If there is no significant elongation of the cervix, amputation of a normal-sized cervix as a means of mobilizing the cardinal-uterosacral ligaments may disturb the integrity of the internal cervical os, precipitating a risk of postoperative cervical incompetence.[18] The diminished size or caliber of the vagina following colporrhaphy will interfere with vaginal dilation during subsequent labor and delivery damaging the vaginal repair, which will make future re-repair more difficult by virtue of the scarring already present from the colporrhaphy. Post-

Manchester cervical stenosis can lead to mechanical dysmenorrhea and to secondary infertility.

All things considered, the Manchester operation is a worthy one provided that the patient knows and is willing to accept the risks and disadvantages and the surgeon who chooses to perform it is equally adept at vaginal hysterectomy in case the operative change becomes necessary during the procedure. Coincident enterocele is often present and should be sought; if found, it should be corrected to avoid future progression or recurrence of the prolapse.

The technique is illustrated and described in Fig. 19-31.

Trachelectomy

The cervix remaining after a subtotal or supracervical hysterectomy occasionally requires surgical removal, or trachelectomy. Most frequently this is required as part of the reparative surgery to relieve a symptomatic prolapse, and because cystocele and rectocele usually coexist, a coincident anterior and posterior colporrhaphy are performed.

Occasionally, the remaining cervix will be the site of severe dysplasia or intraepithelial neoplasia, for which trachelectomy would be an appropriate remedy—with or without coincident colporrhaphy, depending on the presence of cystocele and rectocele. Trachelectomy is most easily accomplished transvaginally, but there is little indication for "prophylactic" removal of the retained cervix[60]; however, any patient with a retained cervix should have it evaluated regularly with cytologic study and colposcopy as necessary, because any cervix may harbor future neoplasia.

Ikedife[32] reported a high incidence of primary infertility in women with a long (4 to 6.5 cm) cervix in the absence of uterine or vault prolapse with no other explanation for their lack of fertility. Removal of a markedly elongated cervix should accompany transabdominal construction of a sacrocervical ligament (see Chapter 26).

Laparoscopy and Hysterectomy

For the hysterectomy candidate in whom the condition of the adnexa is uncertain, and adnexal or pelvic adhesions that might compromise the ability to safely perform vaginal hysterectomy, a preliminary diagnostic laparoscopy should clarify whether it is safe to perform vaginal hysterectomy. This is the diagnostic contribution of laparoscopy to the planned surgery.

When troublesome adhesions have been identified before hysterectomy, they can be severed during preliminary laparoscopy and the adnexa freed or removed, thus making vaginal hysterectomy safely possible in this particular patient and permitting surgical attention to support of the vault postoperatively; coincident repair of any other features of pelvic relaxation through the same transvaginal operative exposure also is possible. This, then, is laparoscopically assisted vaginal hysterectomy. Portions of the hysterectomy can be added to what is done laparoscopically (e.g., transaction of the round ligaments, broad ligaments, preparation of the bladder flap). The entire hysterectomy occasionally can be done through the laparoscope,[68] the so-called

Text continued on p. 351

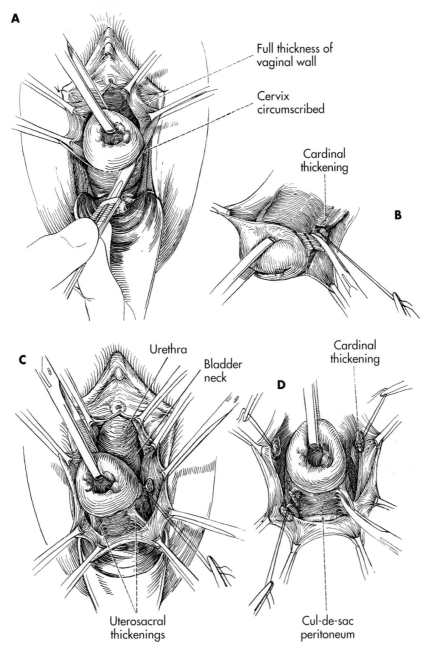

A

Full thickness of
vaginal wall

Cervix
circumscribed

Cardinal
thickening

B

C

Urethra

Bladder
neck

Cardinal
thickening

D

Uterosacral
thickenings

Cul-de-sac
peritoneum

Fig. 19-31   The Manchester operation. Dilation and curettage (D&C) is done. The cervix should be dilated
to a no. 10 Hegar dilator and the length of the cervical canal measured.

The full thickness of the vaginal wall is opened from the bladder reflection with an inverted V incision, and
then the incision is continued to the urethral meatus in the same manner as illustrated for a simple anterior
repair. The bladder is dissected then at its natural line of cleavage, and the urethra mobilized for future placation. Bleeding points are ligated or cauterized, and then attention is directed to the cervical amputation. The
inverted V incision at the bladder reflection is now extended around the cervix **(A).** The degree of hypertrophy
of the cervix, the extent of the prolapse, and the elongation of the visceral connective tissue determine the site
of amputation of the cervix. The internal os is the guiding landmark in describing descensus. In general, 2 cm
from the internal os to the point of amputation will allow for shortening of the ligaments and correction of the
cystocele and rectocele, both of which strengthen the vagina as an obturator and contribute to correction of
the prolapse.

The flaps are now developed laterally and posteriorly to demonstrate the cardinal and uterosacral ligaments. The extent of this dissection is governed by the amount of cervix to be amputated. The ligaments
should be cut, clamped, and tied close to the cervix to permit suture in the midline **(B).** By suture of these
thickenings, anterior to the amputated cervix for the cardinal structures and posterior for the uterosacral thickenings, the vagina is restored as a competent obturator.

The cardinal ligaments, which at this level contain the descending branch of the uterine artery, are secured
with two suture ligatures of 0-PGA **(B).** They are mobilized to a sufficient length to be brought together in the
midline after the cervical amputation **(C).**

The posterior thickenings, the uterosacral ligaments, are cut, clamped, and tied **(D).** These thickenings
contain vaginal branches of the inferior vesical arteries, and failure to respect this fact can cause postoperative
bleeding and a hematoma of the rectovaginal septum.

Continued

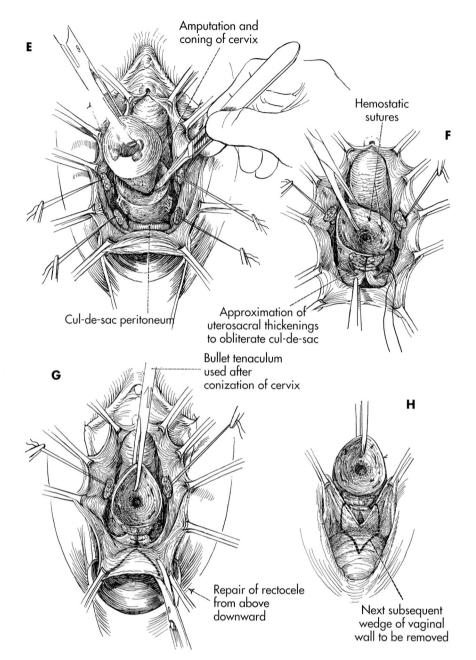

E

Amputation and
coning of cervix

Hemostatic
sutures

F

Cul-de-sac peritoneum

Approximation of
uterosacral thickenings
to obliterate cul-de-sac

Bullet tenaculum
used after
conization of cervix

G

H

Repair of rectocele
from above
downward

Next subsequent
wedge of vaginal
wall to be removed

Fig. 19-31—cont'd   The cervix is amputated and coned **(E).** Active bleeding points are secured and ligated or cauterized. A bullet tenaculum is attached to the anterior lip of the cervix, which is drawn anteriorly **(F).**

Following the principle of correcting the pelvic floor as a whole, attention is now directed to obliteration of the cul-de-sac; some degree of herniation inevitably exists because of the nature of uterine prolapse **(E and F).** This is done by dissecting the full thickness of the vaginal wall from the cul-de-sac peritoneum and subsequently from the rectum in retrograde fashion. It is continued until the posterior thickenings (uterosacral ligaments) fan out and lose their identity as their vessels approach their origins from the hypogastric artery. Hemostasis is important as the ligaments are approximated. The operator should realize the proximity of the ureters so that they are neither ligated nor distorted.

The uterosacral ligaments are now united in the midline **(F).** If a definitive hernial sac is evident, the peritoneum is opened before this and the neck of the sac transfixed and amputated. Retrograde dissection is continued, stopping periodically to unite the uterosacral thickenings and control bleeding. (From Ball TL: *Gynecologic surgery and urology,* ed 2, St Louis, 1963, Mosby.)

Depending on the size of the cul-de-sac herniation, the rectovaginal septum is soon reached. The dissection goes remarkably well if it is in the right plane. Simultaneous correction of the upper portion of the rectocele is started. No part of the composite picture of the pathologic anatomy of prolapse is thus neglected **(F and G).**

G, Retrograde method of dissection. Consecutive wedge-shaped sections of the posterior vaginal wall are removed, the uterosacral thickenings approximated, and the field kept free of active bleeding. The connective tissue fanning out toward the sacrum gradually thins, and its identity is lost in the perirectal connective tissue.

H, Appearance of this dissection and line of trimming if folded back and seen from the vaginal aspect. This line of incision will be met from below upward when the perineorrhaphy is done and the lower part of the rectocele is corrected.

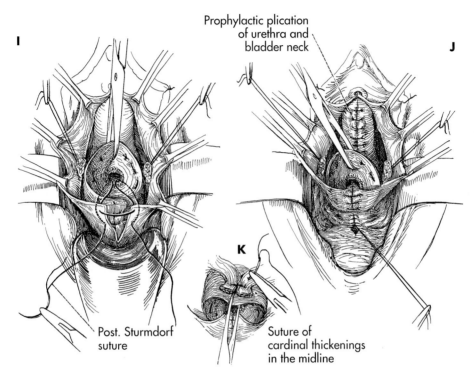

I

Prophylactic plication
of urethra and
bladder neck

J

K

Post. Sturmdorf
suture

Suture of
cardinal thickenings
in the midline

Fig. 19-31—cont'd   An inverting suture, commonly known as a Sturmdorf, is used to slide the flaps of the vagina over the raw fibromuscular tissue of the cervix **(I).** As illustrated, this has the effect of drawing the edges into the new external os and re-creating the posterior fornix.

Interrupted sutures of 2-0 PGA are now inserted to approximate the posterior wall. The last suture is left long and is tagged as a landmark for later use when the reconstruction of the perineal body and completion of the rectocele repair are done from below upward **(J).**

A full-length plication of the urethra, bladder neck, and bladder base is done in the same manner as illustrated for a simple anterior repair **(E to L).** This plication is done regardless of the preexistence of stress incontinence. The anatomic arrangement that results in incontinence can easily be fabricated in repair of the anterior wall by the surgeon intent upon curing the protuberances of a cystocele and rectocele but neglecting a prophylactic plication of the bladder neck. Once again, the importance of attacking the herniation as a whole is apparent **(J).**

The cardinal thickenings are then sutured in the midline by several interrupted sutures **(K).** This feature of the operation shortens these extensions of the parietal connective tissue and enhances their contribution to the support of the pelvic floor.

Continued

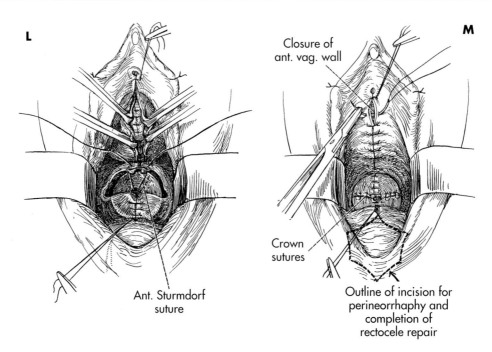

Fig. 19-31—cont'd An anterior Sturmdorf-type suture is placed and left untied pending a study of the flaps of the anterior wall **(L).** The original inverted **V** incision will have reconstructed a few centimeters of the anterior vaginal wall comprising the anterior fornix. The remainder of the walls is developed by the following method: (1) push the cervix toward the sacrum with the tenaculum and observe the flaps of the anterior vaginal wall, (2) cross the Allis clamps so that one flap overlaps the other, and (3) observe the amount of vaginal wall to be resected on each side and then do the resection with the Metzenbaum scissors as done in a simple anterior repair.

The anterior vaginal wall is now closed with interrupted sutures of 2-0 PGA suture, beginning at the anterior fornix. As the walls are approximated, more vaginal wall can be resected if this seems indicated. The anterior Sturmdorf suture, when tied, will complete the reconstruction of the anterior vaginal wall **(M).**

The lateral or crown sutures that bring together the vaginal wall in the lateral fornices are placed as shown in **M.** These sutures should include some of the superficial layers of the fibromuscular structure of the cervix, since their purpose is to epithelize all raw areas. (From Ball TL: *Gynecologic surgery and urology,* ed 2, St Louis, 1963, Mosby.)

As in the posterior repair previously illustrated for a simple vaginal plastic operation, a butterfly section of skin and mucous membrane is outlined on the perineum **(M).** The landmarks are the skin just anterior to the anus, the mucocutaneous junction laterally, and above this the hymenal ring or its remnants **(M).** The genital hiatus must now be closed at one of its crucial areas. Its anteroposterior length must be decreased and the width of its transverse slit narrowed. This cannot be done by a routine method of placing sutures in the hiatus. Descriptions of the placing of "levator sutures" are as unrealistic as the frequent illustrations of this anatomic forgery. The levator muscles (specifically, the puborectali) are centimeters away from the perineum. One should not place heavy sutures and forcibly draw the insertions of a group of paired, laterally placed muscles to an abnormal position in the midline. The plastic reconstruction of the genital aperture requires more selective surgery if a functional vagina is desired.

From the hymenal ring the butterfly pattern is advanced by incisions up to the traction suture left from the retrograde dissection and repair of the rectocele **(M).** This proceeds without the usual difficulty in locating the proper line of cleavage between vagina and rectum, since this has already been identified from above.

The last phase of this operation, the formation of a strong obturator and a narrow hiatus, is now begun. The musculature of the perineum is built up by using interrupted sutures of 0-PGA suture. Multiple sutures are placed without strangulation to build up the perineum so that the approximation of the bulbocavernosi and remnants of the transverse perineal muscles decreases the genital aperture and adds to the support of the pelvic viscera. The anterior edges of the puborectalis can be drawn to the midline to decrease the pelvic aperture, but this must be done with caution or a stricture will result despite the fact that adequate vaginal wall remains. Repeated palpation of the lower third of the vagina is necessary during the reconstruction of the perineum. The operator should individualize each operation, because the depth of the pelvic floor varies, as does the extent of the musculature support remaining in each patient. The vaginal wall is closed with interrupted sutures of 2-0 PGA suture. (From Ball TL: *Gynecologic surgery and urology,* ed 2, St Louis, 1963, Mosby.)

laparoscopic hysterectomy, although even then the specimen usually is removed through the vagina rather than by morselization through the laparoscope.

One difficulty with a totally laparoscopic hysterectomy concept is that little or no provision is made for effectively reattaching the transacted ligamentous supports of the uterus to the vagina to aid in vaginal support after hysterectomy. Now that it has been shown that total laparoscopic hysterectomy is possible in the hands of a very experienced laparoscopist, it must be proven that the method is as safe as or safer than the traditional approach and is cost-effective.

Laparoscopically *assisted* vaginal hysterectomy, on the other hand, is a substitute for abdominal hysterectomy and may increase the number of patients who can safely enjoy the reduced pain and shorter hospitalization afforded by vaginal hysterectomy. The subject is discussed in considerable detail in Chapter 20.

Final Procedures

After surgery the bladder is emptied by catheter, and observational cystoscopy can be performed to ensure bilateral ureteral patency. The vaginal cavity can be lightly packed for 24 hours with 2-inch plain or iodoform gauze, and if so, a silicone-coated transurethral Foley catheter can be inserted. Packing not only provides hemostatic pressure and obliterates potential spaces, but also bolsters the new sutures in the vaginal vault against the strains of recovery room coughing or emesis and soaks up secretions to remove blood and serum and prevent pooling.[43] Unless there is considerable oozing, it is usually unnecessary to pack the vagina, however, and the presence of vaginal packing makes it difficult for patients to void. Routine insertion of an indwelling transurethral catheter is not recommended if colporrhaphy has not been done and packing was not used, because the risk of subsequent cystitis appears to be much less if the patient is able to void by herself.

Before completing the operation, the surgeon should perform a rectal examination to check for anal stricture and to confirm rectal integrity. If a stitch passes through the rectal mucosa, it should be visualized on the rectal side and cut and the ends permitted to retract into the perirectal tissues.

VAGINAL HYSTERECTOMY AND PARTIAL VAGINECTOMY

In the hands of a surgeon experienced in the procedures, vaginal hysterectomy with partial vaginectomy seems to have several advantages for the definitive treatment of in situ carcinoma of the uterine cervix when the disease has extended to or involves the vagina, as determined by preoperative colposcopically directed biopsy.[81] For example, this approach permits specific preoperative and intraoperative delineation of the lesion to be removed, which is not possible with other techniques. The operation itself consists of vaginal hysterectomy and removal of a predetermined amount of vaginal cuff. Simon et al.[76] have suggested that vaginal hysterec-

tomy can be performed for the cervix cancer patient with microinvasion (i.e., less than 3 mm).

In preparation for surgery, the vagina is lightly painted with tincture of iodine or freshly prepared Schiller's solution. The nonglycogen-containing areas of the cervix and vagina, which should be removed because of their pathologic and precancerous nature, are then clearly visualized because they do not take up the iodine stain. Furthermore, the multicentric origin of the disease can be appreciated. With this type of visualization, the operator can readily determine the level at which the cuff, along with a comfortable margin of uninvolved tissue, should be amputated—a determination that can be estimated or surmised only during an abdominal hysterectomy.

Because a vaginal hysterectomy is essentially an extrafascial procedure, it permits additional mobilization of the parametrium and the removal of more tissue with the operative specimen than does the standard intrafascial total abdominal hysterectomy. This can be a particular advantage if the pathology report discloses superficial unsuspected microinvasion of the carcinoma to a depth less than 3 mm (which by probability has not yet progressed to the point of lymphatic extension).

Measuring the amount of vagina being removed is easier during a vaginal hysterectomy than during an abdominal hysterectomy. In the vaginal operation, the operator cuts the cardinal ligament support system from the uterus *after* the vagina has been "measured and cut," before the vagina has been stretched. However, during an abdominal hysterectomy the stretch of the vagina is greater because the cardinal ligaments are cut *before* the vagina is measured and cut, and traction on the uterus during its removal stretches the vagina. An apparent 1-inch cuff of (stretched) vagina with a uterus removed abdominally may, as the previously stretched tissue contracts, prove to be only one third or one half inch of vagina.

Finally, as mentioned earlier, a patient who has undergone vaginal surgery generally has a distinctly less complicated, more comfortable postoperative course and a shorter recovery period than does a patient who has undergone abdominal surgery.

Schuchardt Perineal Incision

When transvaginal exposure is awkward and accessibility seems limited, the operator may use the Schuchardt perineal incision for vaginal hysterectomy or fistula repair. It is usually desirable for the right-handed operator to make the incision on the patient's left side and vice versa. When the case is difficult or the operator is not yet experienced in this procedure, instillation of 60 ml of sterile evaporated milk or a solution of methylene blue into the bladder before the procedure permits prompt recognition of any inadvertent bladder penetration.

The tissues to be incised may be infiltrated thoroughly with a solution of 0.5% lidocaine (Xylocaine) or bupivacaine (Marcaine) in 1 : 200,000 epinephrine (Adrenaline) in a fanlike fashion by inserting a 22-gauge spinal needle

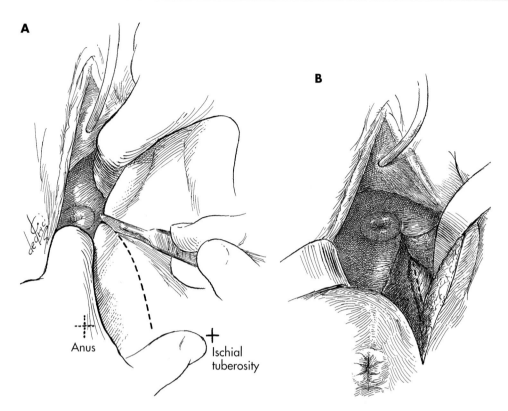

Anus

Ischial
tuberosity

Fig. 19-32 Schuchardt incision. **A,** The incision is started immediately behind site of hymenal margin and continued posterolaterally in a gentle curve around the anus to end at a point midway between the anus and left ischial tuberosity. The surgeon and assistant introduce their index fingers deeper into the vagina, maintaining tension, and the vaginal portion of the incision is continued in a posterolateral direction as high as is necessary to provide the desired exposure of the vaginal vault. **B,** Lowermost fat tissue of ischiorectal fossa has been divided, and the medial portion of the pubococcygeus muscle is visible in depths of the wound. A portion of this can be divided if necessary *(dashed line)*. Bleeding points are clamped as they are encountered and coagulated with an electrosurgical unit, with care being taken to not coagulate the surface of the rectum if it is visible within the wound. At the conclusion of the operation, the Schuchardt incision is closed in layers. (From Nichols DH, Randall CL: *Vaginal surgery,* ed 4, Baltimore, 1996, Williams & Wilkins.)

through the skin of the perineum midway between the anus and the left ischial tuberosity.[43] To further reduce blood loss, the operator should use the electrosurgical scalpel to make the incision. The skin incision follows a curved line from the 4-o'clock position at the hymenal margin to a point halfway between the anus and the ischial tuberosity (Fig. 19-32).

To protect the nearby rectum from damage during this incision, the right-handed operator inserts the left index finger into the vagina and depresses the perineum and rectum; the assistant on the right simultaneously inserts an index finger into the vagina to provide pressure in an anterolateral direction and keep the tissues taut. The operator begins the incision immediately behind the site of the hymenal margin and continues it posterolaterally in a gentle curve around the anus, ending it at a point midway between the anus and the left ischial tuberosity. To maintain tension, the surgeon and the assistant insert their index fingers more deeply into the vagina, and the surgeon continues the vaginal portion of the

incision in a posterolateral direction as high as is necessary to provide the desired exposure of the vaginal vault. This incision divides the lowermost fatty tissue of the ischiorectal fossa.

In the depths of the wound, the medial portion of the pubococcygeus muscle is visible, and a portion of it can be divided if necessary for better exposure. Bleeding points are clamped as they are encountered and are coagulated with the electrosurgical unit; care must be taken not to coagulate the surface of the rectum, however, as it tends to remain prominently in the wound. At the conclusion of the operation, the Schuchardt incision is closed in layers. The vaginal stitches may include and unite any severed portions of the pubococcygeus muscle, bringing them together beneath the edges of the vaginal incision (see Chapter 13).

If an incision of this depth is not necessary, the operator may make a classic mediolateral episiotomy incision on one or both sides, which later should be carefully closed by reapproximation of all incised tissue layers.

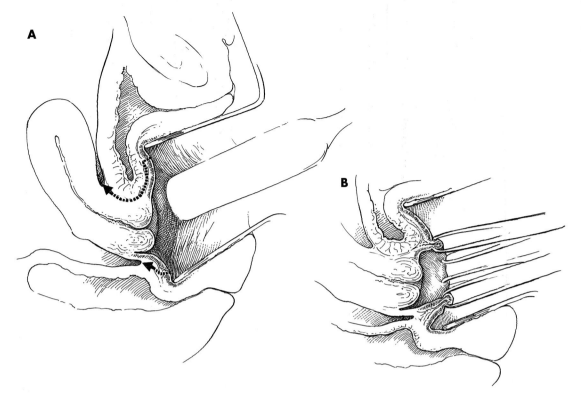

Fig. 19-33   Partial vaginectomy with hysterectomy. The vagina and cervix are carefully exposed and thoroughly examined, and the amount of the vagina to be removed with specimen is determined with precision. **A,** Lines of proposed dissection are shown in sagittal drawing. Infiltration here by 1:200,000 epinephrine (Adrenaline) in 0.5% lidocaine (Xylocaine) solution aids hemostasis and later identification of connective tissue planes and spaces. **B,** Distal to this point, the vagina is grasped circumferentially by a series of single-toothed tenacula. (From Nichols DH, Randall CL: *Vaginal surgery,* ed 4, Baltimore, 1996, Williams & Wilkins.)

Procedure for Partial Vaginectomy with Hysterectomy

The first step in performing a partial vaginectomy with hysterectomy is to apply an appropriate iodine solution to the cervix and upper half of the vagina and to note any areas that do not take the stain. The operator then applies a rim of colpohemostats to a fold of the vagina at least 1.5 inches away from the lateral margin of the cervix and lateral to any nonstained tissue within the vagina (Fig. 19-33), tucks the cervix into this fold, and makes an incision through the full thickness of the vagina with Mayo scissors or an electrosurgical scalpel (Fig. 19-34). The counterpressure from anterior, posterior, and lateral retractors permits the bladder and its fascia to recede promptly from the point at which the vagina was held by the colpohemostats. After establishing the vaginal flap circumferentially and carefully noting the position of the ureters, the operator clamps, cuts, and ligates the lateral fascial bundles on either side. The operator then separates the rectum from the tissues to be removed by gentle dissection, identifies the posterior cul-de-sac, makes an opening into it, and clamps, cuts, and ligates the posterior and lateral portions of the uterosacral ligaments.

The fundus of the uterus can be brought through either the anterior or the posterior colpotomy. The adnexa are then in-spected and, if necessary, removed. Hemostats are applied over the cornual angles of the uterus, and the uterus, cervix, and parametrial tissues are removed en masse, after which the hemostats are replaced by transfixion ligatures. There may be areas of venous oozing around the base of the bladder, but there should be no active bleeding. The vaginal vault then can be closed with an absorbable suture on each side that goes through the anterior vault, round ligament, and anterior peritoneum on each side. A second set of sutures is placed through the posterolateral vault, uterosacral ligament pedicle, posterior peritoneum, and the same structures on the opposite side, as suggested by Durfee (see Fig. 19-27).

If, after hysterectomy, the vagina seems too short for sexual intercourse, a sheath of mobilized peritoneum can be sewn to the distal cut edge of the vagina and the peritoneal cavity closed at a higher level. The patient should wear an obturator postoperatively during the period of vaginal reepithelialization. The operator can perform an anterior or posterior colporrhaphy before closing the Schuchardt incision. Distal vaginal length can be added by using the Williams' vulvovaginoplasty or a perineorrhaphy if the perineum is inadequate.

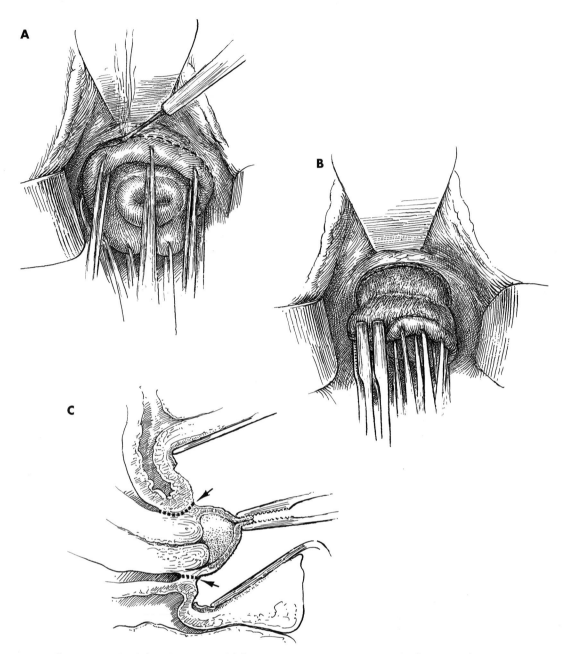

Fig. 19-34 Partial vaginectomy with hysterectomy. **A,** Traction is applied to tenacula against countertraction supplied by retractors. Incision is made by electrosurgical knife, scissors, or scalpel through the full thickness of the vagina. **B,** The vagina is inverted as a sleeve over the cervix. An alcohol-soaked sponge is applied against the face of the cervix, single-toothed tenacula are removed, and the anterior and posterior walls of vagina are brought together by a series of Krobach mouse-toothed clamps, straight Kocher hemostats, or heavy sutures. **C,** Sagittal section further illustrates line of sharp dissection to be followed to gain both anterior and posterior entry to the peritoneal cavity. (From Nichols DH, Randall CL: *Vaginal surgery,* ed 4, Baltimore, 1996, Williams & Wilkins.)

THE SCHAUTA-AMREICH RADICAL VAGINAL HYSTERECTOMY

An enthusiastic position for this operation for the treatment of invasive cervix cancer has been championed by several American enthusiasts, including McCall, Barclay, Smale, Hatch, and Crisp.[10] (Stages IA, IB, and IIA with no evidence of lymphatic or vascular penetration, and with negative

lymphography, or negative pelvic nodes obtained by extraperitoneal transabdominal section.) It has been kept alive in Europe by the clinics of Navratil,[55] Carenza,[5-7] Novak,[59] Högler,[30] Reiffenstuhl,[69] Massi,[48-50] and Dargent,[13] among others. It is an especially useful operation for a young patient with early stage invasive cervical cancer who wishes to preserve her ovarian function, a very obese patient in whom

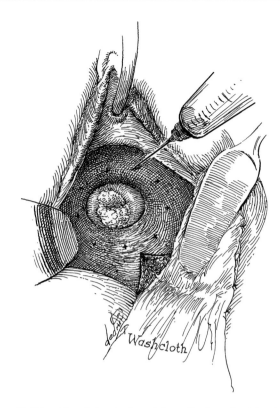

Fig. 19-35 The Schauta-Amreich radical vaginal hysterectomy. A Schuchardt incision has been made and a gauze pack temporarily sewn into the incision. The vagina is being infiltrated by 0.5% lidocaine in 1:200,000 epinephrine solution. The small crosses mark the site of each needle penetration. (From Nichols DH, Randall CL: *Vaginal surgery*, ed 4, Baltimore, Williams & Wilkins, 1996.)

exposure for radical abdominal hysterectomy might be difficult, a patient at higher than average medical risk, and a cancer patient with genital prolapse and a coincident large and symptomatic cystocele and rectocele. A place exists for preliminary or coincident transabdominal or laparoscopic pelvic lymphadenectomy, as discussed and described in Chapters 37, 38, and 66, to which the reader is referred for technical advice and assistance. Occasions exist where the radical vaginal hysterectomy with pelvic lymphadenectomy can be accomplished as a combined vaginal-abdominal procedure, which can involve two separate operative teams working simultaneously to save time.

Technique of the Schauta-Amreich Radical Vaginal Operation[44]

A Schuchardt incision can be used if necessary for better operative exposure and would be performed as described above. The circumference of the vagina, at which the vaginal circumcision will be made, is thoroughly infiltrated by a solution of 0.5% lidocaine in 1:200,000 epinephrine (Fig. 19-35), and the vagina grasped circumferentially by a series of single-toothed forceps or tenacula (Fig. 19-36). The vagina is then circumscribed by an incision opening di-

rectly into the vesicovaginal and rectovaginal spaces. Traction and counterpressure are made between appropriate intravaginal retractors, and traction to the tenacula on the specimen is made to obtain the best cleavage plane; the cut edges of the mobilized vagina are grasped from front to back with Krobach or Kocher clamps (Fig. 19-37, p. 357) or sewn together by a series of interrupted mattress-type traction sutures. Sharp and blunt dissection, performed very carefully, exposes both anterior and posterior cul-de-sacs. The left paravesical space is entered and made to communicate with the left pararectal space. The ureter is palpated in the "bladder pillar" between the paravesical space and the vesicovaginal space (Fig. 19-38, p. 358). Högler[30] has pointed out that the larger any coexistent cystocele, the more lateral the axis and location of the ureters.

The left ureter is palpated within the bladder pillar. The bladder pillar is incised along its lateral edge superficial to the ureter, the ureter is exposed (Fig. 19-39, p. 358), and its tunnel explored with the tips of the closed scissors. The left uterine artery is skeletonized and ligated. A similar procedure is carried out on the patient's right side (Fig. 19-40, p. 358). The bladder pillar is cut from the cardinal ligament at an appropriate spot (the pararectal and paravaginal spaces having been joined) and the cul-de-sac of Douglas opened. The peritoneum is carefully dissected from the medial side of the rectal pillar (Fig. 19-41, p. 358), and each rectal pillar and uterosacral ligament carefully cut from its attachment to the rectum. The anterior peritoneal cul-de-sac is opened and appropriate retractors are inserted. Each cardinal ligament is clamped and cut close to the pelvic sidewall (Fig. 19-42), and the clamps replaced with transfixion ligatures. The adnexa are examined and excised if necessary. The broad and round ligament of each side is clamped and cut and the specimen removed from the operative field. The peritoneum is closed, and the exposed undersurface of the bladder reduced in size by gathering it in a series of transversely placed interrupted sutures that cover the ureter at the ureterovesical junction and burying this junction in a fold of the bladder wall. If a cystocele is present, it is repaired (see Chapter 21). If the operator wants to lengthen a shortened vagina, the peritoneum may be mobilized for a Davyoff vaginal lengthening procedure (Fig. 19-43, p. 359) as described previously, and the peritoneal cavity closed at a higher level by a purse-string suture. Any posterior repair and perineorrhaphy can be performed if planned, and the Schuchardt incision is closed.

If the operator wants to control oozing, the subperitoneal lateral spaces can be packed with gauze, which is completely removed 24 hours after surgery. The urethral catheter is removed on the seventh to tenth day, and the patient is taught intermittent self-catheterization to determine postvoiding residual volume and relieve bladder distention until complete function is restored. Bethanechol can be useful for a maximum of 3 months postoperatively in restoring bladder tone during the long healing phase in the presence of partial, but absence of complete, bladder denervation.[40]

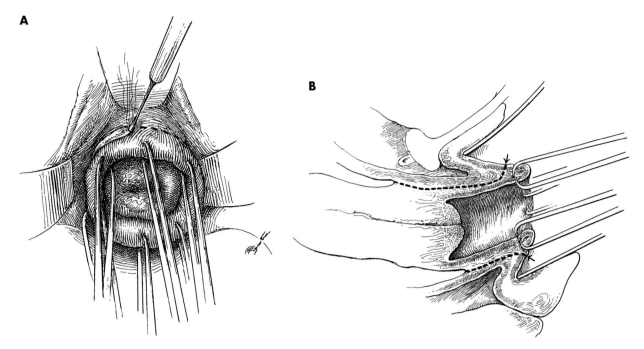

Fig. 19-36   A, The circumference of the vagina has been grasped with single-toothed tenacula and an incision made directly into the vesicovaginal space. **B,** Sagittal view shows the cuff of vagina held by single-toothed tenacula. The *dashed line* shows the pathway of incision and dissection. (From Nichols DH, Randall CL: *Vaginal surgery,* ed 4, Baltimore, Williams & Wilkins, 1996.)

Radical Trachelectomy

Dargent (see Chapter 66) has described in detail his experience with radical trachelectomy, which may provide an important alternative to radical hysterectomy for some women who have invasive cervical cancer and wish to have children. In all cases, a laparoscopic pelvic lymphadenectomy precedes the trachelectomy to ensure the nodes are negative.

Combined Abdominovaginal Procedures

For those women in whom vascular or lymphatic penetration has been established preoperatively by biopsy study or lymphography, a combined vaginal-abdominal hysterocolpectomy, including lymphadenectomy,[9,13] can have certain advantages. The surgeon can plan an operative procedure for these patients that combines the best features of both the vaginal and the abdominal operations into a single or composite operative procedures. To shorten operating time, minimize the risks to the patient as much as possible, and promote surgical efficiency, such a composite procedure may best be performed with the simultaneous use of two operating teams.

The vaginal portion of the operation permits the widest possible excision of parametrium, rectal pillars, and uterosacral ligaments and the removal of a predetermined amount of vagina or vaginal cuff at the time of the initial operative procedure, under the direct vision and control of the operator. The vaginal approach ensures vastly improved dissection of the paracolpium, the inferior portion of the horizon

tal connective tissue ground bundle, the inferior portion ofthe rectal pillars, and the vesicouterine ligaments. Ureteral exposure and dissection can best be accomplished during the vaginal portion of the operation. Meanwhile, through an appropriate incision, the abdominal team will have begun the bilateral extraperitoneal or intraperitoneal lymphadenectomy, which may be completed while the vaginal team is closing the Schuchardt incision. Combined synchronous operation has been reported by Mitra,[54] Howkins,[31] and Vidakovic,[82] among others, in various sequential modifications. The combined operation should be of particular value for those in whom vascular or lymphatic penetration has been established preoperatively by biopsy study or lymphography. However, whether such a combined operation will provide an improved prognosis remains to be proven.

POSTHYSTERECTOMY FALLOPIAN TUBE PROLAPSE

Posthysterectomy prolapse of the fallopian tube is sporadically encountered. At first it is mistaken for some granulation tissue at the vaginal vault, but its true nature becomes evident when it fails to heal after curettement and office cauterization. Because it is a source of chronic and often blood-tinged vaginal discharge, it requires surgical treatment by salpingectomy (preferably total) to reduce longterm postoperative pain.

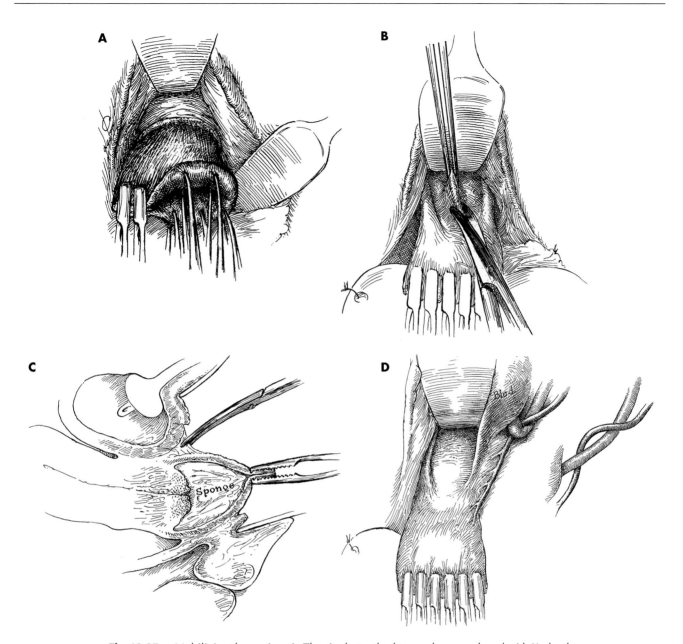

Fig. 19-37 Mobilizing the vagina. **A,** The single-toothed tenacula are replaced with Krobach mouse-toothed forceps. **B,** The connective tissue septum between the bladder and cervix is cut by sharp dissection. **C,** Sagittal view shows sharp dissection of the connective tissue beneath the bladder and cervix. The handles of the scissors are elevated, directing the incision away from the bladder. **D,** Phantom view shows the relationship between the ureter, bladder *(Blad),* and uterine artery. When downward traction is applied *(left),* the uterine artery brings with it the "knee" of the ureter. The relationship without traction is shown to the *right.* (From Nichols DH, Randall CL: *Vaginal surgery,* ed 4, Baltimore, Williams & Wilkins, 1996.)

Although salpingectomy can be performed by laparotomy, a less formidable approach can be either by operative laparoscopy[45] or as an office procedure by transvaginal excision, after applying a benzocaine spray and applying an Endoloop of 2-0 plain catgut tightly around the base of the mass. Wetchler and Hurt[85] have described an excellent operative technique. Allis clamps are placed just below the lateral angle of the cuff, and a transverse incision is made in the vault just posterior to the prolapsed tube and vaginal scar. By sharp and blunt dissection the vaginal wall is freed from the underlying peritoneum, which is opened, and the cul-de-sac is explored. Adhesions are freed and a separate horizontal incision is made in the vagina *anterior* to the prolapsed tube and vaginal cuff to remove a portion of the vagina wall around the prolapsed tube. The mesosalpinx is clamped and cut, the specimen removed, pedicles are ligated, and the peritoneum and vaginal cuff closed separately.

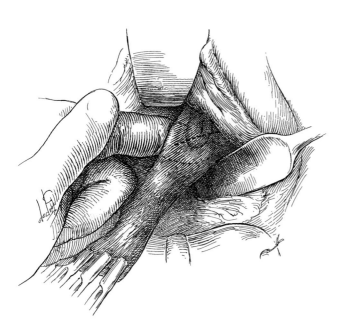

Fig. 19-38 Palpation of the ureter. The paravesical and vesi-covaginal spaces have been opened, and the ureter is palpated within the bladder pillar on the patient's left. An incision is made in the lateral margin of the bladder pillar along the side of the *dashed line.* (From Nichols DH, Randall CL: *Vaginal surgery,* ed 4, Baltimore, Williams & Wilkins, 1996.)

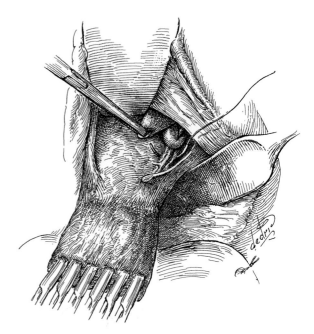

Fig. 19-39 Exposure of the ureter. The left ureter has been exposed in the bladder pillar and the uterine artery skeletonized, preparatory to its ligation. (From Nichols DH, Randall CL: *Vaginal surgery,* ed 4, Baltimore, Williams & Wilkins, 1996.)

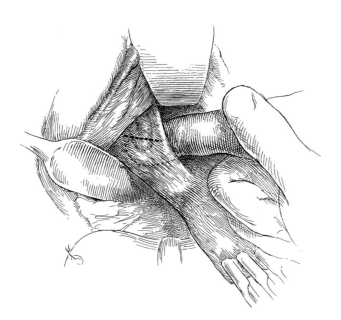

Fig. 19-40 Palpation of the opposite ureter. The right ureter is palpated, and the bladder pillar will be incised in its lateral margin as shown by the *dashed line.* (From Nichols DH, Randall CL: *Vaginal surgery,* ed 4, Baltimore, Williams & Wilkins, 1996.)

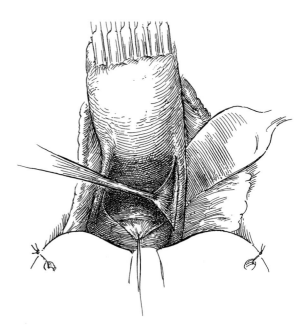

Fig. 19-41 Dissection of the rectal pillars. Both anterior and posterior cul-de-sacs have been opened. The peritoneum medial to the left rectal pillar is dissected free in preparation for ligation of the pillar close to the rectum. (From Nichols DH, Randall CL: *Vaginal surgery,* ed 4, Baltimore, Williams & Wilkins, 1996.)

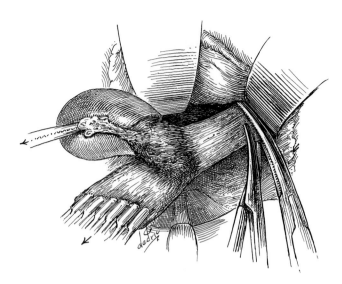

Fig. 19-42 Transection of the parametrium close to the pelvic wall. The uterine fundus has been brought through the anterior peritoneal opening and the vaginal cuff and cervix drawn sharply down. The cardinal ligament (parametrium) has been clamped close to the pelvic sidewall and will be cut free, as shown, first on one side and then on the other. The peritoneum will then be approximated and the Schuchardt incision closed. (From Nichols DH, Randall CL: *Vaginal surgery,* ed 4, Baltimore, Williams & Wilkins, 1996.)

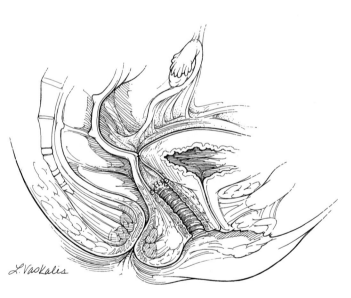

Fig. 19-43 Lengthening of the vagina by Davyoff procedure. Proximal length can be added to a shortened vagina by attaching its cut edges to the margins of previously freed peritoneal flaps. The peritoneal cavity is securely closed by a separate cranially placed suture, as shown. Squamous epithelium will migrate beneath the "vaginal" peritoneum from the cut edges of the vagina.

REFERENCES

1. Allen E: Discussion, *Am J Obstet Gynecol* 6l(suppl):219, 1951.
2. Bandler SW: *Vaginal celiotomy,* Philadelphia, 1911, WB Saunders.
3. Candiani GB, Ferrari AG: *Isterectomia vaginale,* Milano, 1986, Italia Editori.
4. Capen CV, Irwin H, Magrina J, Masterson BJ: Vaginal removal of the ovaries in association with vaginal hysterectomy, *J Reprod Med* 28:589, 1983.
5. Carenza L: Attuali indicazioni alla colpoisterectomia allargata nel trattamento del cervico-carcinoma, *Patol Clin Ostet Ginecol* l:3, 1973.
6. Carenza L, Nobili F, Lukic A: The Schauta-Amreich radical vaginal hysterectomy. In Nichols DH, editor: *Gynecologic and obstetric surgery,* St Louis, 1993, Mosby.
7. Carenza L, Villani C: Schauta radical vaginal hysterectomy, *Clin Obstet Gynecol* 25:913, 1982.
8. Carlson KJ, Nichols DH, Schiff I: Indications for hysterectomy, *N Engl J Med* 328:856, 1993.
9. Childers JM, Hatch KD, Tran AN, Surwit EA: Laparoscopic para-aortic lymphadenectomy in gynecologic malignancies, *Obstet Gynecol* 82:741, 1993.
10. Copenhaver EH: Vaginal hysterectomy: an analysis of indications and complications among 1000 operations, *Am J Obstet Gynecol* 84:123, 1962.
11. Copenhaver EH: Hysterectomy: vaginal versus abdominal, *Surg Clin North Am* 45:751, 1965.
12. Crisp WE: The Schauta operation, *Obstet Gynecol* 33:453, 1969.
13. Dargent D, Arnould P: Percutaneous pelvic lymphadenectomy under laparoscopic guidance. In Nichols DH, editor: *Gynecologic and obstetric surgery,* St Louis, 1993, Mosby.
14. Dicker RC, Greenspan JR, Strauss LT, et al: Complications of abdominal and vaginal hysterectomy among women of reproductive age in the United States. The Collaborative Review of Sterilization, *Am J Obstet Gynecol* 144:841, 1982.
15. Döderlein A, Krönig S: Die technik der vaginalen Bauch-Holen-operationen, Leipzig, 1906, Verlag von S Hirzel.
16. Elkins TE et al: Initial report of anatomic and clinical comparison of the sacrospinous ligament fixation to the high McCall culdoplasty for vaginal cuff fixation at hysterectomy for uterine prolapse, *J Pelvic Surg* 1:12, 1995.
17. England GT, Randall HW, Graves WL: Impairment of tissue defenses by vasoconstrictors in vaginal hysterectomies, *Obstet Gynecol* 61:271, 1983.
18. Fisher JJ: The effect of amputation of the cervix uteri upon subsequent parturition, *Am J Obstet Gynecol* 62:644, 1951.
19. Gallup DG, Welham RT: Vaginal hysterectomy by anterior colpotomy technic, *South Med J* 69:752, 1976.
20. Garry R, Hercz P: Initial experience with laparoscopic-assisted Döderlein hysterectomy, *Br J Obstet Gynaecol* 102:307, 1995.
21. Gigliotti B: Isterectomia vaginale per morecellement. Considerazion di tecnica chirurgica e casistics personale, *Riv di Ostetrics e Ginecologia* II 1:18, 1989.
22. Gitsch E, Palmrich AH: *Gynecological operative anatomy,* Berlin, 1977, Walter de Gruyter.
23. Gitsch G, Berger E, Tatra G: Trends in thirty years of vaginal hysterectomy, *Surg Gynecol Obstet* 172:207, 1991.
24. Gray LA: *Vaginal hysterectomy,* ed 3, Springfield, Ill, 1983, Charles C Thomas.
25. Hefni MA, Davies AE: Vaginal endoscopic oophorectomy with vaginal hysterectomy: a simple minimal access surgery technique, *Br J Obstet Gynaecol* 104:621, 1997.
26. Hemsell DL, Bawdon RE, Hemsell PG, et al: Single-dose cephalosporin for prevention of major pelvic infection after vaginal hysterectomy: cefazolin versus cefoxitin versus cefotaxime, *Am J Obstet Gynecol* 156:1201, 1987.
27. Hemsell DL, Johnson ER, Hemsell PG, et al: Cefazolin for hysterectomy prophylaxis, *Obstet Gynecol* 76:603, 1990.

28. Hoffman MS: Transvaginal removal of ovaries with endoloop sutures at the time of vaginal hysterectomy, *Am J Obstet Gynecol* 165:407, 1991.

29. Hoffman MS, DeCesare S, Kalter C: Abdominal hysterectomy versus transvaginal morcellation for the removal of enlarged uteri, *Am J Obstet Gynecol* 171:309, 1994.

30. Högler H: *Schauta-Amreich's radical vaginal operation of cancer of the cervix,* Springfield, Ill, 1963, Charles C Thomas.

31. Howkins J: Synchronous combined abdomino-vaginal hysterocolpectomy for cancer of the cervix: a report of fifty patients, *J Obstet Gynecol Br Emp* 66:212, 1959.

32. Ikedife D: Long vaginal cervix: a clinical entity, *J Obstet Gynecol* 10:333, 1990.

33. Inmon WB: Pelvic relaxation and repair including prolapse of vagina following hysterectomy, *South Med J* 56:577, 1963.

34. Janisch H, Palmrich AH, Pecherstorfer M: *Selected urologic operations in gynecology,* Berlin, 1979, Walter de Gruyter.

35. Jaszczak SE, Evans TN: Vaginal morphology following hysterectomy, *Int J Gynaecol Obstet* 19:41, 1981.

36. Kamina P: From the anatomy to the technic of vaginal hysterectomy, *Rev Fr Gynecol Obstet* 85:434, 1990.

37. Kaminski PF et al: The Döderlein vaginal hysterectomy: a useful approach for the neophyte vaginal surgeon, *J Gynecol Surg* 6:123, 1990.

38. Kammerer-Doak D, Mao J: Vaginal hysterectomy with and without morcellation: The University of New Mexico hospital's experience, *Obstet Gynecol* 88:560, 1996.

39. Käser O, Iklé FA, Hirsch HH: *Atlas of gynecologic surgery,* ed 2, New York, 1985, Thieme-Stratton.

40. Kemp Birgit: Personal communication, Aachen, 1998.

41. Kjerulff KH et al: Hysterectomy: An examination of a common surgical procedure, *J Wom Health* 1:141, 1992.

42. Kovac SR: Intramyometrial coring as an adjunct to vaginal hysterectomy, *Obstet Gynecol* 67:131, 1986.

43. Krige CF: *Vaginal hysterectomy and genital prolapse repair,* Johannesburg, 1965, Witwatersrand University Press.

44. Landau L, Landau T: *The history and technique of the vaginal radical operation,* New York, 1897, Wm Wood (Translated by BL Eastman and AE Giles).

45. Letterie GS, Byron J, Salminen ER, Miyazawa K: Laparoscopic management of fallopian tube prolapse, *Obstet Gynecol* 72:508, 1988.

46. Malpas P: The choice of operation for genital prolapse. In Meigs JV, Sturgis SH, editors: *Progress in gynecology,* vol 3, New York, 1957, Grune & Stratton.

47. Malpas P: Genital prolapse. In Claye A, Bourne A, editors: *British obstetric and gynaecological practice,* ed 3, London, 1963, William Heinemann.

48. Massi G: Alcune riflessioni in tema de radicalita nella churgia vaginale, *Riv Ostet Ginecol* 4-5:123, 1992.

49. Massi G, Savino L, Susini T: Schauta-Amreich vaginal hysterectomy and Wertheim-Meigs abdominal hysterectomy in the treatment of cervical cancer: a retrospective analysis, *Am J Obstet Gynecol* 168:928, 1993.

50. Massi G, Savino L, Susini T: Reply to letter of Than, *Am J Obstet Gynecol* 171:287, 1994

51. Mattingly RF, Huang WY: Steroidogenesis of the menopausal and postmenopausal ovary, *Am J Obstet Gynecol* 103:679, 1969.

52. McCall ML: Posterior culdeplasty: surgical correction of enterocele during vaginal hysterectomy: a preliminary report, *Obstet Gynecol* 10:595, 1957.

53. McGregor JA, Phillips LE, Roy S, et al: Results of a double-blind, placebo-controlled clinical trial program of single-dose ceftizoxime versus multiple-dose cefoxitin as prophylaxis for patients undergoing vaginal and abdominal hysterectomy, *J Am Coll Surg* 178:123, 1994.

54. Mitra S: *Mitra operation for cancer of the cervix,* Springfield, Ill, 1960, Charles C Thomas.

55. Navratil E: Radical vaginal hysterectomy (Schauta-Amreich operation), *Clin Obstet Gynecol* 8:676, 1965.

56. Nichols DH: Vaginal hysterectomy. In Nichols DH, editor, *Gynecologic and obstetric surgery,* St Louis, 1993, Mosby.

57. Nichols DH, Randall CL: Vaginal hysterectomy. In *Vaginal surgery,* ed 3, Baltimore, 1989, Williams & Wilkins.

58. Nichols DH, Randall CL: *Vaginal surgery,* ed 4, Baltimore, 1996, Williams & Wilkins.

59. Novak F: *Surgical gynecologic techniques,* New York, 1978, John Wiley & Sons.

60. Pasley WW, Leigh RW: Trachelectomy: a review of fifty-five cases, *Am J Obstet Gynecol* 159:728, 1988.

61. Philipp K: Ergebnisse der routinemaBigen entfernung der Ovarien und/oder Tuben im Rahmen der vaginalen Hysterektomie, *Geburtshilfe Frauenheilkd* 40:159, 1980.

62. Piura B: Prophylactic posterior culdoplasty, *Am J Obstet Gynecol* 155:685, 1986 (letter).

63. Powers TW, Goodno JA Jr, Harris VD: The outpatient vaginal hysterectomy, *Am J Obstet Gynecol* 168:1875, 1993.

64. Pratt JH: Technique of vaginal hysterectomy, *Clin Obstet Gynecol* 2:1125, 1959.

65. Pratt JH, Daikoku NH: Obesity and vaginal hysterectomy, *J Reprod Med* 35:945, 1990.

66. Randall CL: The risks of gynecologic malignancies in older women, *Clin Obstet Gynecol* 7:545, 1964.

67. Ranney B: Decreasing numbers for vaginal hysterectomy and plasty, *S D J Med* 43:7, 1990.

68. Reich H, DeCaprio J, McGlynn F: Laparoscopic hysterectomy, *J Gynecol Surg* 5:213, 1989.

69. Reiffenstuhl G, Platzer W: *Atlas of vaginal surgery,* Philadelphia, 1975, WB Saunders.

70. Rein MS, Friedman AJ, Stuart JM, MacLaughlin DT: Fibroid and myometrial steroid receptors in women treated with gonadotropin-releasing hormone agonist leuprolide acetate, *Fertil Steril* 53:1018, 1990.

71. Robinson RW, Cohen WD, Higano N: Estrogen replacement therapy in women with coronary atherosclerosis, *Ann Intern Med* 48:95, 1958.

72. Saye WB, Espy GB III, Bishop MR, et al: Laparoscopic Döderlein hysterectomy: a rational alternative to traditional abdominal hysterectomy, *Surg Laparosc Endosc* 3:88, 1993.

73. Shaw WF: Plastic vaginal surgery. In Kerr JMM, Johnstone RW, Phillips MH, editors: *Historical review of British obstetrics and gynecology,* Edinburgh, 1954, Livingstone.

74. Sheth SS: The place of oophorectomy at vaginal hysterectomy, *Br Obstet Gynaecol* 98:662, 1991.

75. Shull BL, Capen CV, Riggs MW, Kuehl TJ: Preoperative and postoperative analysis of site-specific pelvic support defects in 81 women treated with sacrospinous ligament suspension and pelvic reconstruction, *Am J Obstet Gynecol* 166:1764, 1992.

76. Simon NL, Gore H, Shingleton HM, et al: Study of superficially invasive carcinoma of the cervix, *Obstet Gynecol* 68:19, 1986.

77. Sluijmer AV, Heineman MJ, De Jong FH, Evers JL: Endocrine activity of the postmenopausal ovary: the effects of pituitary down-regulation and oophorectomy, *J Clin Endocrinol Metab* 80:2163, 1995.

78. Soper DE, Yarwood RL: Single-dose antibiotic prophylaxis in women undergoing vaginal hysterectomy, *Obstet Gynecol* 69:879, 1987.

79. Speroff T, Dawson NV, Speroff L, Haber RJ: A risk-benefit analysis of elective bilateral oophorectomy: effect of changes in compliance with estrogen therapy on outcome, *Am J Obstet Gynecol* 164:165, 1991.

80. Stovall TG, Summitt RL Jr, Bran DF, Ling FW: Outpatient vaginal hysterectomy: a pilot study, *Obstet Gynecol* 80:145, 1992.

81. Thompson JD, Lyon JB: Vaginal hysterectomy, *Clin Obstet Gynecol* 9:1033, 1964.

82. Vidakovic S: The vagino-abdominal approach to the extended operation, *Arch Gynakol* 186:420, 1955.

83. Welch JS, Randall LM: Vaginal hysterectomy at the Mayo Clinic, *Obstet Gynecol* 4:199, 1961.

84. Werner P, Sederl J: *Abdominal operations by the vaginal route,* Philadelphia, 1958, JB Lippincott.

85. Wetchler SJ, Hurt WG: A technique for surgical correction of fallopian tube prolapse, *Obstet Gynecol* 67:747, 1986.

20 Laparoscopic Hysterectomy

THOMAS G. STOVALL and ROBERT L. SUMMITT, JR.

More than any other operation, hysterectomy has been the subject of considerable public scrutiny. With the explosion in laparoscopic instrumentation, expanding interest in laparoscopic surgical techniques, a push to reduce hospital stay, and patient interest in minimally invasive surgery, a natural evolution has occurred between hysterectomy and laparoscopy. Since the first report,[32,51] laparoscopically assisted hysterectomy has become a widely accepted and practiced surgical technique. Despite its use and acceptance by many gynecologic surgeons, little if any consensus exists on its most efficient use. In fact, some gynecologic surgeons claim the technique is virtually useless and believe it offers little if any advantage. Others believe that laparoscopically assisted hysterectomy is a remarkable technique that offers significant advantages to patients.

RATIONALE FOR ITS USE

The use of laparoscopy to perform a hysterectomy or to assist with its accomplishment should be viewed as a surgical technique rather than a radical departure from the past. As with any advancement, the goal is to reduce the morbidity or mortality associated with hysterectomy, improve patient convenience, or reduce the cost incurred while maintaining the current outcome parameters. In fact, the procedure could be viewed as being cost effective even if the costs were significantly increased as long as the improved outcome warranted the additional expense.

Unfortunately, the use of laparoscopic techniques has been exploited and therefore has preceded scientific study. We are now forced to draw conclusions from literature that is less than ideal and from studies with less than perfect designs.

No one argues that hysterectomy should be done only when more conservative and less morbid attempts to control the patient's condition have failed. Also, no one argues, and the literature is clear, that vaginal hysterectomy offers significant and real advantages compared to abdominal hysterectomy.[12,28] Thus, if laparoscopic assistance is to have a role in hysterectomy, it should allow for conversion from an abdominal to vaginal approach for hysterectomy; this conversion must be associated with no greater risks, no greater total cost, no greater patient charges, or unquestionable benefits that can be easily documented. If this is not the case, then the use of the technique must be questioned and possibly abandoned altogether.

EQUIPMENT

A discussion of all the instruments developed to assist with the accomplishment of this procedure is beyond the scope of this text. The array of equipment depends on whether the primary technique chosen is electrosurgical, stapling, laser, or suture use. The choice of equipment also depends somewhat on whether the operator chooses an assisted, total, or subtotal procedure.

Few studies have compared one technique to another or one instrument to another. This generally has been considered less important and left to the discretion of the surgeon. Disposable versus nondisposable instrumentation also has met with controversy. While some authors have suggested that disposable instrumentation offers the advantage of ready accessibility, others have suggested that its increased cost is unwarranted. No studies have yet to show that disposable instrumentation is less expensive, nor have studies demonstrated its safety. Therefore it appears reasonable to conclude that the use of disposable instrumentation offers little or no advantage and should be avoided because of its increased cost.

Daniell et al.[10] reported on a series of 62 patients who underwent laparoscopically assisted vaginal hysterectomy (LAVH). Stapling was used in 49 patients, with bipolar cautery in 11 and a combination in 2 patients. No difference was apparent in hospital stay between the stapling (2.53 days) and the cautery (2.75 days) groups. However, the stapling group required significantly shorter operating times (117 versus 223 minutes). This time savings in the operating room did not translate to overall savings in patient hospital charges. The mean hospital charge in the stapling group was $9310 versus $6227 in the electrosurgery group. Carter and Bailey[5] have reported on the use of the Nd:YAG laser in combination with laparoscopic stapling. No advantages over more conventional electrosurgical techniques were demonstrated with this technique. Disadvantages included the high capital of the equipment and ongoing maintenance cost. The same logic also can be applied to the use of the carbon dioxide laser.

The various instruments used for laparoscopic hysterectomy are listed in the box on p. 362. The type and number of trocars used depend on the specific operative technique. For example, when using a stapling device, larger trocar diameters are required. Most LAVHs can be accomplished with a 10-mm periumbilical port and two additional 5-mm suprapubic ports. The video system, including the lapa-

---

**INSTRUMENTATION COMMONLY USED
FOR LAPAROSCOPIC HYSTERECTOMY**

PELVISCOPY EQUIPMENT
1. Telescopes
   a. 10-mm diameter, 0-degree lens
   b. 10-mm diameter, 45-degree lens (optional)
2. Endoscopic trocars
   a. 12 mm (for laser/staples)
   b. 10 mm or 5 mm
3. Operating instruments
   a. 5-mm hook scissors
   b. 5-mm atraumatic graspers
   c. 5-mm traumatic graspers
4. Endoscopic trocar converters—depends on type of trocars used
5. Unipolar electroscope
6. Suction/irrigating system
7. Uterine manipulator
8. Video system

VAGINAL HYSTERECTOMY EQUIPMENT
1. No specialized vaginal surgery instruments are required
2. Candy-cane or Allen stirrups
3. Stapling devices
4. Bipolar electrosurgical unit with forceps
5. Nd:YAG laser
6. CO_2 laser

---

roscope, light source, camera, monitor, and insufflator, is the same used for other types of operative laparoscopies. The irrigator/aspirator, scissors, and other accessory instrumentation also are similar. A variety of instruments are available for uterine manipulation. The Hulka tenaculum is generally acceptable for most patients, but several "specialized" instruments have been designed for this purpose. The remainder of the instruments depends on the technique chosen to ligate the various tissue pedicles. To date, stapling has no clear advantage over suture or electrocautery, although some authors have suggested that electrosurgery is faster than suture placement and ligation. Again, the specific instrumentation and technique are probably best left to the discretion of the surgeon.

PATIENT SELECTION

Much has been written about patient selection for vaginal, abdominal, and laparoscopically assisted vaginal hysterectomy. Unfortunately, many issues and variables preclude a simple or standardized approach. Studies have shown that LAVH is more expensive and requires more operative time, resources, and surgical expertise. Thus, although vaginal hysterectomy is the procedure of choice if it can be performed, each surgeon must rely on his or her own training

and expertise until a standardized approach can be developed and validated.*

Because of the advantages of vaginal hysterectomy, most surgeons now state that LAVH should be performed only if the surgeon would otherwise perform an abdominal hysterectomy. Although this statement seems appropriate on the surface, it is still complicated by considerable bias on the part of the operating surgeon and a lack of standardization regarding patient selection. Richardson et al.[53] studied 98 women who had relative contraindications for vaginal surgery. Of these, 75 underwent LAVH and 23 elected vaginal hysterectomy. Five (6.7%) in the LAVH group required laparotomy, as did two (8.7%) in the vaginal hysterectomy group. The authors concluded that most hysterectomies could be performed vaginally, if attempted. In other words, it is very difficult to perform a vaginal hysterectomy if one does not attempt a vaginal hysterectomy. Daniell et al.[10] further demonstrated the confusion over hysterectomy approaches. Patients enrolled in this study had "indications for LAVH similar to those for conventional abdominal hysterectomy." However, when the indication for hysterectomy is examined more closely, the majority of patients had indications that normally would be considered appropriate for a vaginal approach, such as uterovaginal relaxation, menorrhagia, sterilization, dysplasia, and adenomyosis.

In a different approach, Kovac[25] performed laparoscopy on 46 women whose referring gynecologists had advised an abdominal hysterectomy. These patients were considered poor candidates for vaginal hysterectomy. Laparoscopy was used to judge if a vaginal hysterectomy was possible; 42 of 46 (91%) patients underwent an uncomplicated vaginal hysterectomy.

In another approach, Han[16] reported on a series of 306 (87.7%) patients from his private practice who underwent vaginal hysterectomy. Five patients were converted to a vaginal route with the assistance of a laparoscope. The author stated that a vaginal route was selected for every patient except those who had a universally accepted indication for laparotomy or who posed predictable technical difficulties. Han concluded that the proportion of vaginal hysterectomies in the total number of hysterectomies should be greater than 80%, perhaps closer to 90%, instead of the current 25% to 30%. He believes that laparoscopy would assist in converting a potential abdominal hysterectomy case to a vaginal one in very limited cases (2% to 3%).

Although each of these studies is different, collectively they demonstrate that much confusion exists about who is and who is not a candidate for a vaginal, an abdominal, or a laparoscopically assisted approach.

SURGICAL PROCEDURE

As with most gynecologic procedures, a number of techniques have been described.[26,42-44,47,54,62] A generic description of the procedures that can be used to safely ac-

---

*References 2, 18, 19, 38, 45, 48.

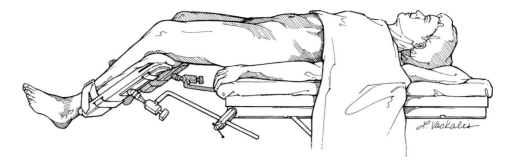

Fig. 20-1 Patient postioning for the laparoscopic portion of the procedure.

complish an LAVH follows. Patient positioning for laparoscopic and vaginal surgery is critical. Inadequate or improper positioning can complicate the procedure, frustrate the surgical team, and result in intraoperative or postoperative complications. Many surgeons have found that it is best to use one position for the laparoscopic portion of the case and another for the vaginal portion. For the endoscopic portion of the case, the patient is placed in the dorsal lithotomy position with the thighs at the level of the abdominal wall and the lower leg placed low with the knee bent (Fig. 20-1). For the vaginal portion, candy-cane stirrups are used to position the legs high and lateral (Fig. 20-2).

Following an examination under anesthesia, the perineum, vagina, and lower abdomen are prepared with diluted povidone-iodine solution. The operator attaches a uterine manipulator to the cervix through a side-opening Graves speculum, making certain to antevert the uterus. A variety of uterine manipulators have been described, and some are manufactured specifically for LAVH. A Foley catheter is inserted and the patient is draped using standard laparoscopy drapes. A trocar is inserted periumbilically. Following correct placement and gas insufflation of the abdomen, either two 12-mm trocars (if endoscopic staples are used) or two 5-mm trocars are placed in the right and left lower quadrants, 6 to 8 cm above the pubic rami and lateral to the inferior epigastric vessels (Fig. 20-3). If endoscopic staples are used, three 12-mm trocars allow maximum flexibility for insertion and direction of the endoscopic stapling device. Once the trocars are in place, an intraabdominal survey that includes examination of the uterus, tubes, ovaries, and cul-de-sac should be performed.

Once the abdominal and pelvic surveys are complete, the pelvic anatomy should be normalized and any adhesions lysed. The round ligaments are desiccated or ligated and then incised. Beginning at the left round ligament, the peritoneum of the vesicouterine fold is incised with the hook scissors. Attachment of the unipolar cautery to the scissors allows for dissection and desiccation of peritoneal vessels and maximizes visualization. The incision is continued across the lower uterine segment to the opposite round ligament (Fig. 20-4). On completion of the incision, the bladder is sharply dissected off the lower uterine segment and cervix. This is best accomplished by lifting the lower peritoneal edge with graspers and using curved scissors to incise and

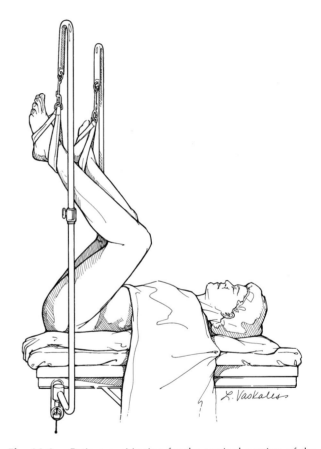

Fig. 20-2 Patient positioning for the vaginal portion of the procedure.

dissect the loose areolar tissue and bladder from the uterus. To maintain good hemostasis, the electrocautery is activated before cutting. Some surgeons prefer to use a contact-tip Nd:YAG laser for dissection. As previously noted, this extremely expensive instrument has not been shown to be superior to cautery. Once the bladder flap has been developed, the ureters are identified by incision of the medial leaf of the broad ligament and dissection of the retroperitoneal space, similar to an abdominal hysterectomy.

If staples are to be used, the proper staple size is chosen and the staples inserted through one of the lower abdominal ports on the same side of the uterus to be stapled. If electrosurgery is to be used, the bipolar coagulation instrument is inserted. When ovaries are to be removed, the infundibu-

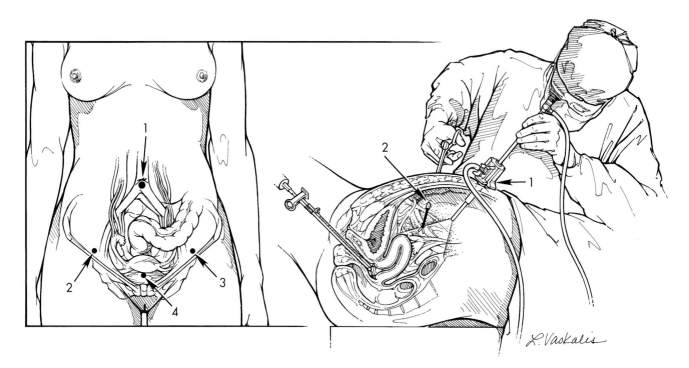

Fig. 20-3   Trocar placement.

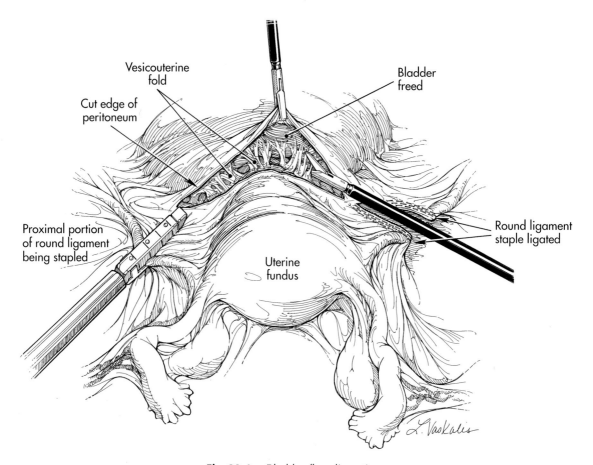

Fig. 20-4   Bladder flap dissection.

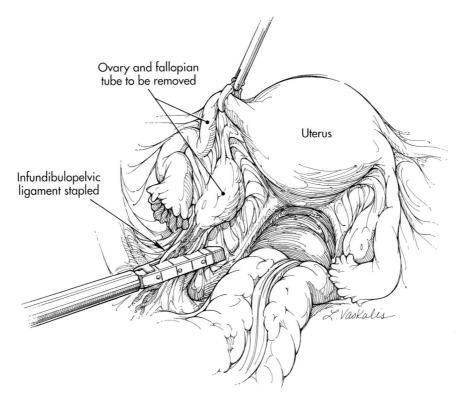

Fig. 20-5   Ligation of the infundibulopelvic ligament.

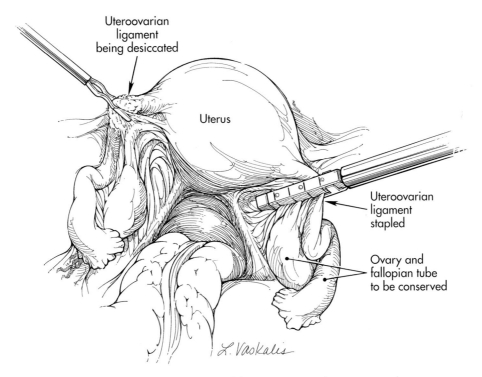

Fig. 20-6   Ligation of the uteroovarian ligament.

lopelvic ligament is ligated or desiccated lateral to the ovary (Fig. 20-5). If the ovary is not removed, the same procedure is completed medial to the ovary. The tip of the stapler should be past the cut edge of the anterior peritoneum (Fig. 20-6). Once positioned, the stapling unit is closed and locked in place. The closed position is inspected, ensuring that no bowel is enclosed and that the ureter is visualized and free. The safety is released, and the stapling unit is activated. After removal of the stapling unit, the cut and stapled edges are inspected for hemostasis and proper staple alignment (Fig. 20-7). If satisfactory, the same procedure is performed on the opposite side. Some surgeons stop the laparoscopic portion of the procedure at this point, and others proceed with ligation or desiccation of the uterine vasculature.

With the ureter under direct vision, the uterine vasculature is desiccated and cut. If staple-ligation is used, the uterus is again pushed upward and to the opposite side from the one being stapled. The endoscopic staples are opened and aligned along the uterus, incorporating the uterine artery. The open stapling device is pushed down to the apex of the previously cut pedicle, the stapler is closed, and again the position of the ureter is inspected (Fig. 20-8). If satisfactory, the stapler is fired and removed slowly while the sur-

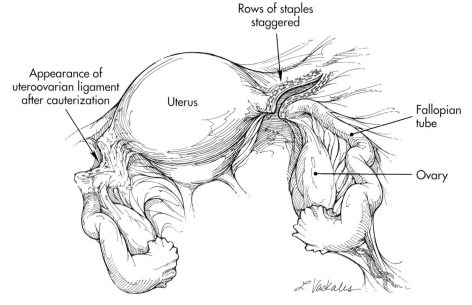

Fig. 20-7   Appearance of staple line after transsection.

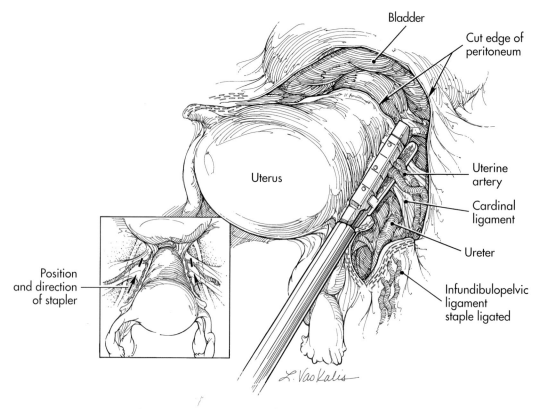

Fig. 20-8   Ligation of the uterine vasculature.

geon checks for hemostasis. The procedure is repeated on the opposite side. Again, some surgeons stop the laparoscopic portion of the procedure at this point, and others proceed with ligation of the cardinal ligaments with or without opening the anterior or posterior cul-de-sac.

Before any further surgery, the level of the bladder must be well mobilized. The cardinal ligaments can either be staple-ligated or desiccated with electrocautery. It is extremely important to visualize and avoid the ureter during this step. Once this is completed, the vagina can be entered through an anterior colpotomy incision. A posterior colpotomy incision also can be made, although it is not necessary and can be made much more easily during the vaginal portion of the surgical procedure.

Once the endoscopic dissection is complete, the vaginal approach is begun as in any traditional vaginal hysterectomy. Adequate exposure is obtained, and the uterine manipulator is removed. A tenaculum is applied to the cervix, and the vaginal hysterectomy is begun in standard fashion through a posterior cul-de-sac incision, as previously described. Following uterine removal and closure of the vagina, it is suggested that a pneumoperitoneum be reestablished for inspection of the surgical pedicles and irrigation of the pelvis and to confirm hemostasis. The trocars are removed, and the skin incisions closed in standard fashion. The patient is then taken to the recovery room. It has been our practice to discharge patients on the afternoon of surgery.

LITERATURE SUMMARY

Numerous case reports and case series of LAVH have been published since 1989, when the laparoscope was first used to perform the initial operative portion of the hysterectomy.[51] However, despite the volumes of literature that have been written and the hours of debate devoted to this subject, little agreement remains on the indications and contraindications of this surgical approach. Much of this confusion stems from the methods that were used to develop and introduce the technique. That is, from the beginning only a few well-designed clinical trials compared laparoscopic assistance to the more traditional surgical approaches. Similar phenomena occurred with the introduction of laparoscopic cholecystectomy. Stoney[58] suggested that if laparoscopic cholecystitis had originated in an academic setting and subsequently spread to community hospitals, more importance would have been given to the publication and analysis of results. In an effort to summarize the current status of the literature on laparoscopically assisted vaginal hysterectomy, a number of published reports have been selected. Although it is impossible to include all published reports, an effort has been made to be as inclusive as possible.

Nezhat et al.[35] prospectively randomized 20 patients with a uterine size of less than 14 weeks who were considered candidates for abdominal hysterectomy. Seven of ten patients in the abdominal hysterectomy group were operated for leiomyomata, two of whom had a history of previous

surgery. The mean uterine weight was 213 g (60 to 534 g). Although some of these patients had previous stage III or IV endometriosis, no mention was made in the report regarding the status of the endometriosis at the time of hysterectomy. In the 10 patients randomized to laparoscopically assisted hysterectomy, 2 were operated for leiomyomata, whereas 7 were operated for stage III or IV endometriosis. Again, the current stage of endometriosis in these patients was not reported. Although not part of this study protocol, 96 laparoscopic hysterectomies were reported by the authors as an addendum to this study. These cases help to further establish the safety and feasibility of the operative approach when performed by experienced laparoscopic surgeons. However, they do not establish any benefit to this approach over vaginal hysterectomy or abdominal hysterectomy. Only rigorously controlled randomized trials can accomplish this.

Liu[29] reviewed his experience with 72 women who underwent laparoscopic hysterectomy using a combination of bipolar electrocoagulation, CO_2 laser, and operative laparoscopy. No complications were reported in this series. Indications for surgery included adenomyosis, pelvic pain with proven or suspected endometriosis, adhesive disease, and leiomyoma; 29 patients had undergone previous pelvic surgery. Concomitant surgical procedures included salpingo-oophorectomy (49), vaporizations or excision of endometriosis implants (26), adhesiolysis (45), and appendectomy (14). Liu[29] reported an average hospitalization cost of $3772. This report again confirms the feasibility of performing the procedure, but no further conclusions can be drawn without specific preoperative selection criteria controls and a comparison group. Other statements made in this chapter cannot be substantiated, such as greater comfort compared to abdominal hysterectomy as a result of tissue desiccation rather than suturing, decreased adhesion formation, and decreased pulmonary problems. These questions can be answered only in properly designed prospective randomized trials. This trial was subsequently expanded with similar results reported.[30]

Padial et al.[39] reported 75 patients following laparoscopically assisted vaginal hysterectomy, 40 of whom underwent bilateral or unilateral salpingo-oophorectomy. The mean uterine weight was 159 g (41 to 462 g), with an average estimated blood loss of 295 ml (25 to 1300 ml). The mean postoperative hospital stay was 2.37 days. These authors retrospectively compared these patients to the first 100 consecutive vaginal and abdominal hysterectomies over the same period. Although no data were reported in the comparison group, the authors stated that those patients who had a laparoscopic approach reported less discomfort, required less postoperative analgesia, and were able to ambulate earlier than other patients who had traditional vaginal or abdominal hysterectomy over the same time period.

Boike et al.[1] reported 82 cases of LAVH. Fifty cases were selected and matched with 50 vaginal and 50 abdominal hysterectomies. Indications for LAVH included uterine leiomyomas, pelvic relaxation, cervical dysplasia, abnormal bleeding, and family history of ovarian cancer. The mean postoperative stay following LVAH was 2.5 days compared with 3.8 days and 4.5 days in the vaginal and abdominal hysterectomy group, respectively. The calculated cost of the procedure was higher for the laparoscopically assisted group ($12,469 ± $1750) when compared with either the vaginal hysterectomy group ($9355 ± $2440) or abdominal hysterectomy group ($10,626 ± $1424). The authors stated that the majority of women in this series would have undergone abdominal hysterectomy before the advent of laparoscopically assisted vaginal hysterectomy. However, one must question the need for abdominal hysterectomy when the indication for the surgical procedure is nulliparity, prior pelvic surgery,[9] or the need to guarantee ovarian removal (preoperative decision for prophylactic oophorectomy).

Howard and Sanchez[22] compared the results of 15 patients assigned to undergo laparoscopically assisted vaginal hysterectomy or total abdominal hysterectomy. The assignment to one of the two groups was based on the attending physician present for the case. Patients enrolled in this study were thought to have a contraindication to vaginal hysterectomy, such as endometriosis, chronic pelvic pain, adnexal disease, uterus size of 12 to 18 weeks, prior pelvic surgery, or adhesive disease. The time of hospital discharge was at the discretion of the resident physician involved in the case management. Mean anesthesia (201 ± 36 versus 147 ± 26) and operating time (169 ± 36 versus 119 ± 25) were significantly longer in the LAVH group than in the TAH group, but no difference was demonstrated in uterine weight, estimated blood loss, hematocrit change, or complication rates. The patients undergoing LAVH had less postoperative pain than those having TAH, as reflected by less narcotic analgesia use and lower visual analog scale scores. The mean duration of hospital stay was shorter for the LAVH group than in the TAH group (3.7 ± 1.7 days versus 5.2 ± 3.1 days). However, total cost of the procedure was not significantly different for TAH and LAVH ($4524 ± $1234 versus $3926 ± $1096, respectively). Therefore it appears that the decreased cost of hospital stay is offset by the additional operating time and equipment cost of laparoscopically assisted hysterectomy.

Daniell et al.[10] have reported a review of 68 patients who underwent LVAH. The indications for hysterectomy are not well defined because the report states that the majority of patients had more than one indication. As an example, 13 patients underwent LAVH for uterovaginal relaxation. One can certainly question the need for a laparoscopic approach in these patients. Six (8.8%) patients required conversion to a laparotomy. This report provides some comparative information on the use of endoscopic staples versus cautery. Stapling was used in 49 patients and bipolar cautery in 11 with a combination in 2. No difference was noted in hospital stay between the stapling (2.53 days) and cautery (2.75 days) groups. The stapling group required significantly shorter operating times (117 versus 223 minutes). In this study the time saved in the operating room did not translate to an overall cost savings in total hospital cost. The mean hospital cost in the stapling group was $9310 versus $6227 in the cautery group.

Davis[11] reviewed the experience in 46 patients undergoing LAVH for stage III or IV endometriosis. The procedure was completed in 40 patients, with the remaining 6 patients being converted to laparotomy. Two patients required transfusion, one required ureteral stent placement, and one had an unrecognized bowel injury. Abdominal wall hematomas also occurred, with eight patients having apical vaginal strictures, two of whom subsequently required repeat surgical procedures. The mean operating time was 191 minutes. This trial demonstrates the feasibility of completing a laparoscopic vaginal hysterectomy in the presence of extensive endometriosis and demonstrates that some patients normally requiring an abdominal approach can have laparoscopically assisted hysterectomy performed. However, it also demonstrates a high complication rate even when experienced laparoscopic surgeons perform the surgery.

Richardson et al.[53] studied 98 women who had relative contraindications for vaginal surgery by traditional criteria. They found that most hysterectomies could be performed vaginally and that LAVH is a much slower procedure. If LAVH is done, it should be converted to a vaginal procedure as early as possible to reduce the overall operating time.

Carter et al.[6] reported a case-controlled study in which patients were selected from a group of 81 women undergoing hysterectomy for pelvic pain. Nineteen patients were chosen from the TAH group and 19 from the LAVH group. The average surgery time for LAVH was 144 minutes and for TAH 98 minutes ($p < 0.005$). No differences were found in blood loss and change in hemoglobin from preoperative levels between the two groups. The TAH group used an average of 436 mg meperidine during their hospital stay, significantly more than the 197 mg used by the LAVH group ($p < 0.005$). The length of stay was 2.1 days for the LAVH group and 3.5 days for the TAH group ($p < 0.001$). On a scale of 1 to 10 (10 being complete normal activity) the activity level of women undergoing LAVH was 9.2 by day 24 compared with 6.4 for those having TAH ($p < 0.005$).

Summitt et al.[61] reported the results of a prospective randomized trial that included 56 women scheduled for vaginal hysterectomy. Patients scheduled for vaginal hysterectomy were randomly assigned to undergo either a laparoscopically assisted vaginal hysterectomy with endoscopic staples ($N = 29$) or a standard vaginal hysterectomy ($N = 27$). The most common indication in these groups of patients was leiomyomata uteri; the second most common indication was pelvic pain of uterine origin unresponsive to conservative therapy. The mean operative time in the laparoscopically assisted group (120.1 ± 28.5 minutes) was approximately twice that of the standard vaginal hysterectomy group (64.7 ± 27.0 minutes). No statistical difference existed in the mean uterine weight in the laparoscopically assisted group, which conformed to the standard vaginal hysterectomy group (162.6 ± 89.5 g versus 203.7 ± 143.0 g). The estimated blood loss in the LAVH group (203.8 ± 130.5) was statistically less than in the standard hysterectomy group (376.1 ± 261.5). However, the postoperative hematocrits were statistically higher in the vaginal hysterectomy group than in the laparoscopically assisted group. Oophorectomies were successfully completed in all cases in which they were indicated. All procedures were performed on an outpatient basis with the mean hospital cost being $4891 ± $355 ($4311 to $5247) for vaginal hysterectomy and $7905 ± $501 ($7197 to $8289) for laparoscopically assisted vaginal hysterectomy. Postoperative pain and antiemetic medication required was the same in both groups, except on the second postoperative day, in which patients undergoing LVAH required significantly more pain medication than patients undergoing standard hysterectomy.

Redwine[50] reviewed hysterectomies performed in a community hospital. This study is important because it reconfirms the benefits of vaginal hysterectomy. In this study, vaginal hysterectomy was faster and less expensive than any other form of hysterectomy, including LAVH.

DIAGNOSTIC LAPAROSCOPY BEFORE HYSTERECTOMY

Johns et al.[23] retrospectively reviewed 2563 hysterectomies performed by 37 gynecologists in a metropolitan hospital. Disposable laparoscopic instruments and stapling devices were never used in the study. During the study period, the number of LAVH procedures increased, the number of abdominal procedures decreased, and the number of vaginal hysterectomies remained relatively constant. The study is one of the only ones to report a cost savings with LAVH compared with an abdominal approach ($6431 versus $6552). The cost of vaginal hysterectomy was still the lowest at $5869. The author concluded that LAVH was cost-effective by using reusable instruments and avoiding staples.[23]

Two studies[25,50] have addressed the question of whether laparoscopy is beneficial before planned hysterectomy. Cartwright[34] reported a small series of patients who were candidates for vaginal hysterectomy, except they had undergone prior pelvic surgery. A laparotomy was performed before the hysterectomy to eliminate the possibility of adhesions. All patients underwent successful vaginal hysterectomy. Kovac et al.[25] reported a series of patients who were referred and told they needed an abdominal hysterectomy. Following laparoscopy, the majority of these patients underwent a successful vaginal hysterectomy. Although both authors agree that laparoscopy before hysterectomy can aid in selection of operative approach, there are no guidelines to suggest which patients and under what circumstances this would be helpful. Although laparoscopy has been suggested for use in patients who are suspected of having adhesive disease, it has been demonstrated that the presence or absence of pelvic adhesions cannot be predicted preoperatively.[59] Studies also have been reported in which laparoscopic assistance was used to accomplish hysterectomy for endometrial cancer and radical hysterectomy. Ongoing prospective, randomized trials currently under way will be useful to determine the role of laparoscopy for the treatment of gynecologic malignancy.[8,24,33,34,46]

COMPLICATIONS

The true incidence of complications with LAVH, laparoscopic hysterectomy, or laparoscopic supracervical hysterectomy is unknown. Initial case reports highlighted a specific complication.[3,17,37,63] Few complications have been reported to date, and investigators are possibly reluctant to report complications.

Schwartz[55,56] reported a retrospective analysis of complications from 45 consecutive patients; 40 had laparoscopic supracervical hysterectomies, and 5 were laparoscopically assisted vaginal hysterectomies. Five (11%) had operative complications, one of which was a bladder injury. Three (7%) had anesthetic complications from fluid overload. Seven (16%) had postoperative complications, and a 4% rate of nursing complications as a result transient nerve injuries was reported. There were also 25 (56%) equipment complications, the most frequent being dysfunction of the bipolar cautery. This report demonstrates the high complication rate seen with the introduction of laparoscopically assisted hysterectomy.

Hill et al.[20] reported a series of 220 women undergoing LAVH at the Melbourne Gynoscopy Centre. Complications occurred in 35 (15.9%). Among these were anterior abdominal wall vessel injury in 5 patients, bladder injury in 5, febrile illness in 13, secondary hemorrhage in 4, temporary ureteral obstruction in 4, and Richter hernia in 1. In this series ureteral catheterization was performed in 68 patients, and cystoscopy was performed in 79.

Nezhat et al.[36] reviewed 361 hysterectomies performed at laparoscopy for benign gynecologic disease in which bipolar electrodesiccation was used; carbon dioxide laser also was used for cutting and treatment of associated pelvic disease. The procedure included desiccation and transection of the cardinal–uterosacral ligament complex along with an anterior and posterior colpotomy incision. Some patients had subtotal hysterectomy, and others had total laparoscopic hysterectomy. Some had genital prolapse repair, and others had laparoscopic Burch retropubic urethropexy. Eleven patients had colon resection. Uterine size ranged from 4 to 26 weeks with a weight of 36 to 1530 g; 186 uteri weighed less than 150 g. The patients suffered inferior epigastric vessel injury, one bladder injury, and two small bowel injuries. No febrile morbidity was reported. Two patients required transfusion. A total of 40 (11.1%) complications were reported.

Meikle et al.[31] reviewed 3112 LAVH procedures—1618 TAH and 690 vaginal hysterectomies. LAVH was associated with significantly more bladder injuries and longer operating times than TAH but shorter hospitalization. Similar findings were noted in the review of the Finnish National Register of LAVH.

A national register for laparoscopic hysterectomies was founded at the beginning of 1993.[20] During a 2-year period, 1165 laparoscopic hysterectomies were reported. The mean operating time was 132 minutes, with an average hospital stay of 3.3 days and a mean convalescence period of 17.9 days. Complications occurred in 10.2% of the procedures. Of the 10.2%, infection occurred in 5.6%, vascular complications in 1.2%, urinary tract complications in 2.7%, and bowel complications in 0.4%. This report provides a good perspective on the complications associated with laparoscopic hysterectomy, but because the inclusion criteria for using this approach were not controlled, it does not provide guidance with respect to who should undergo the procedure.

PROPOSED INDICATIONS FOR LAPAROSCOPICALLY ASSISTED VAGINAL HYSTERECTOMY

The proposed indications for LAVH are as numerous as the authors who publish them, because few agree on the indication for hysterectomy and even more disagree on the indication for LAVH. The more commonly debated indications for LAVH are listed in the box below.

For the patient with chronic pelvic pain not responding to medical or conservative surgical therapy, hysterectomy can be considered. Before the hysterectomy, a multidisciplinary team approach, including physical therapy, has been shown to be beneficial.[14,49,52] Following hysterectomy, Carlson et al.[4] found significant reduction in symptoms, which was associated with an improvement in the patient's life quality. Stovall et al.[60] reviewed 104 patients who underwent hysterectomy for chronic pelvic pain thought to be of uterine origin. Patients were followed for a mean of 21.6 months, with 78% of patients showing significant reduction in their pain. However, 22% of patients had no pain relief or had an exacerbation of pain. These findings suggest that hysterectomy should be done only in those patients who do not respond to nonsurgical treatment and in those with pain of uterine origin.

Hysterectomy is often done concurrently when a patient requires surgical intervention for a benign but persistent ovarian tumor. As with other benign conditions, the uterus should not be removed if the patient desires future fertility. Gambone et al.[15] reviewed the records of 100 patients who underwent adnexectomy and incidental hysterectomy for benign adnexal disease and compared these to a group of risk-matched women who underwent adnexectomy without hysterectomy for similar conditions. These authors found a significant increase in operative and perioperative morbidity, estimated blood loss, and longer hospital stay in patients who underwent an incidental hysterectomy at the time of adnexectomy. The long-term effects of this practice are not known.

It has been suggested that a laparoscopic approach can be helpful when prophylactic oophorectomy is planned at the time of hysterectomy. The current data do not support this supposition. Recent studies suggest that the overwhelming percentage of oophorectomies can be accomplished at the time of vaginal hysterectomy.[21,57]

Leiomyomata uteri is the most common indication for hysterectomy and should be considered only for patients who do not desire future fertility. Hysterectomy can be used to manage the symptoms commonly associated with myomas, including abnormal uterine bleeding, pelvic pressure, and pain. Other indications for hysterectomy in a patient with myomas include rapid uterine enlargement, ureteral compression, or growth following menopause. Rapid uterine enlargement (more than 6 weeks' increase in gestational size in less than 12 months) previously has been thought to be associated with a higher incidence of sarcomatous change. A recent study did not confirm this, and patients with rapid uterine enlargement did not have an increased incidence of leiomyosarcomas.[27,40] Some gynecologists suggest removal of the uterus, even if asymptomatic, when it reaches 12 gestational weeks in size. They base their judgment on the possibility of malignancy, inability to palpate the ovaries on bimanual examination, and the suggestion that, as the uterus enlarges, the morbidity for hysterectomy increases. However, one must remember that the incidence of leiomyosarcomas is rare; adnexal palpation is not possible in up to 20% of patients, and even if palpable, this practice has not been shown to decrease the morbidity of ovarian cancer or lead to earlier detection. Studies also suggest no difference in surgical morbidity between patients with a 12-week-size uterus and those with a 20-week-size uterus if both procedures are done abdominally. However, most uteri that are 12 weeks in size can best be removed through the vagina.[13,41] Thus when all of this is considered, hysterectomy should probably be considered only in a symptomatic patient who does not desire future fertility.

Although endometriosis is a common cause of infertility, it is an uncommon reason for hysterectomy because generally it can be treated with medical or conservative surgical approaches. Most patients with endometriosis who require hysterectomy do so because of pelvic pain or dysmenorrhea. Less common reasons include endometriosis involving other organ systems such as the urinary or gastrointestinal tract.

With limited data available, what then is the role of laparoscopy before or as part of a vaginal hysterectomy? If one adds laparoscopy to a large number of patients before hysterectomy, one loses or diminishes several of the advantages of vaginal hysterectomy, namely decreased operative and anesthesia time. Also, one adds cost to the procedure and the risk and morbidity of laparoscopy. If this view is modified

---

> **PROPOSED INDICATIONS FOR LAPAROSCOPICALLY ASSISTED VAGINAL HYSTERECTOMY**
>
> Chronic pelvic pain unresponsive to conservative therapy
> Leiomyomata uteri
> Endometriosis (either recent or prior history)
> Pelvic adhesive disease
> Potential benign adnexal disease
> Poor uterine mobility

to include laparoscopic assessment for only those patients with risk factors for endometriosis or pelvic adhesive disease, fewer patients will require laparoscopy. However, not all patients with historical or pelvic examination predictors of adhesions are actually found to have adhesions, and, even if these predictors are present, it does not necessarily preclude a vaginal approach to hysterectomy. Therefore laparoscopy before vaginal hysterectomy does not appear practical on a widespread basis.

The use of operative laparoscopic techniques to ligate the infundibulopelvic ligaments or utero-ovarian ligaments, uterine arteries, and cardinal ligaments is proposed to increase the use of the vaginal approach. Various techniques, advantages, disadvantages, and preoperative indications have been suggested. No consensus exists on the proper circumstances under which operative laparoscopic techniques would be helpful. We do know that when standard vaginal hysterectomy can be performed, adding the laparoscopic approach shows no advantage. In fact, the data by Summitt et al.[61] show several disadvantages to this approach. To date, no available data show that an intended abdominal hysterectomy can be converted to a vaginal approach. Because this procedure is new, operator experience and well-defined indications are lacking.

In the absence of well-defined indications for this technique, proposed reasons for performing LAVH relate to conditions that might require abdominal surgery or contraindicate a vaginal approach. Some examples include chronic pelvic pain that has not responded to conservative therapy, leiomyomata uteri, endometriosis (or a prior history of endometriosis), pelvic adhesive disease, potentially benign adnexal disease, and poor uterine mobility. Currently, no data support the supposition that patients undergoing hysterectomy for pelvic pain or a prior history of endometriosis are not candidates for a vaginal approach. No current way standardizes the preoperative assessment of these patients, which must be done before determining if abdominal hysterectomy can be replaced in some instances with a laparoscopically assisted approach.

Others have said that if the ovaries were to be removed (age over 40 years), the laparoscopic approach offers the advantage of being able to remove the ovaries. In our experience, it is very unusual not to be able to remove the ovaries during a vaginal approach. In our view, a laparoscopically assisted approach should not be used by the surgeon not already well trained in vaginal surgery.

Laparoscopy does not necessarily simplify the procedure, but in many instances complicates it. It may be possible in the future to use these techniques on patients with early-stage endometrial or ovarian cancer. The approach in these patients would include laparoscopy with cytology, assisted vaginal hysterectomy, bilateral salpingo-oophorectomy, and lymph node sampling. This is a potentially promising technique. However, larger series with multicenter randomized trials are mandatory to fairly assess the complications.

REFERENCES

1. Boike GM, Elfstrand EP, Delpriore G, et al: Laparoscopically assisted vaginal hysterectomy in a university hospital: report of 82 cases and comparison with abdominal and vaginal hysterectomy, *Am J Obstet Gynecol* 168:1690, 1993.
2. Bornstein SJ, Shaber RE: Laparoscopically assisted vaginal hysterectomy at a health maintenance organization: cost-effectiveness and comparison with total abdominal hysterectomy, *J Reprod Med* 40:435, 1995.
3. Bronitsky C, Stuckey SJ: Complications of laparoscopic-assisted vaginal hysterectomy, *J Am Assoc Gynecol Laparosc* 2:345, 1995.
4. Carlson KJ, Miller BA, Fowler FJ Jr: The Maine women's health study. I. Outcomes of hysterectomy, *Obstet Gynecol* 83:556, 1994.
5. Carter JE, Bailey TS: Laparoscopic-assisted vaginal hysterectomy utilising the contact-tip Nd:YAG laser: a review of 67 cases, *Ann Acad Med Singapore* 23:13, 1994.
6. Carter JE, Ryoo J, Katz A: Laparoscopic-assisted vaginal hysterectomy: a case control comparative study with total abdominal hysterectomy, *J Am Assoc Gynecol Laparosc* 2:116, 1994.
7. Cartwright DS: Diagnostic laparoscopy immediately preceding elective hysterectomy, *AAGL 18th Annual Meeting Proceedings,* 1992, p 88.
8. Childers JM, Surwit EA: Case report: combined laparoscopic and vaginal surgery for the management of two cases of stage I endometrial cancer, *Gynecol Oncol* 45:46, 1992.
9. Coulam CB, Pratt JH: Vaginal hysterectomy: is previous pelvic operation a contraindication? *Am J Obstet Gynecol* 116:252, 1973.
10. Daniell JF, Kurtz BR, McTavish G, et al: Laparoscopically assisted vaginal hysterectomy. the initial Nashville, Tennessee experience, *J Reprod Med* 38:537, 1993.
11. Davis GO, Wolgamott G, Moon J: Laparoscopically assisted vaginal hysterectomy as definitive therapy for stage III and IV endometriosis, *J Reprod Med* 38:577, 1993.
12. Dicker RC, Greenspan JR, Strauss LT, et al: Complications of abdominal and vaginal hysterectomy of reproductive age in the United States. The Collaborative Review of Sterilization, *Am J Obstet Gynecol* 144:841, 1982.
13. Friedman AJ, Haas ST: Should uterine size be an indication for surgical intervention in women with myomas? *Am J Obstet Gynecol* 168:751, 1993.
14. Gambone JC, Reiter RC: Nonsurgical management of chronic pelvic pain: a multidisciplinary approach, *Clin Obstet Gynecol* 33:205, 1990.
15. Gambone JC, Reiter RC, Lench JB: Short-term outcome of incidental hysterectomy at the time of adnexectomy for benign disease, *J Womens Health* 1:197, 1992.
16. Han GS: Assessing the role of laparoscopically assisted vaginal hysterectomy in the everyday practice of gynecology, *J Reprod Med* 41:521, 1996.
17. Härkki-Sirén P, Sjöberg J, Mäkinen J, et al: Finnish national register of laparoscopic hysterectomies: a review and complications of 1165 operations, *Am J Obstet Gynecol* 176:118, 1997.
18. Harris MB, Olive DL: Changing hysterectomy patterns after introduction of laparoscopically assisted vaginal hysterectomy, *Am J Obstet Gynecol* 171:340, 1994.
19. Hidlebaugh D, O'Mara P, Conboy E: Clinical and financial analyses of laparoscopically assisted vaginal hysterectomy versus abdominal hysterectomy, *J Am Assoc Gynecol Laparosc* 1:357, 1994.
20. Hill DJ, Maher PJ, Wood CE: Complication of laparoscopic hysterectomy, *J Am Assoc Gynecol Laparosc* 1:159, 1994.
21. Hoffman MS: Transvaginal removal of ovaries with Endoloop sutures at the time of transvaginal hysterectomy, *Am J Obstet Gynecol* 165:407, 1991.
22. Howard FM, Sanchez R: A comparison of laparoscopically assisted vaginal hysterectomy and abdominal hysterectomy, *J Gynecol Surg* 9:83, 1993.

23. Johns DA, Carrera B, Jones J, et al: The medical and economic impact of laparoscopically assisted vaginal hysterectomy in a large, metropolitan, not-for-profit hospital, *Am J Obstet Gynecol* 172:1709, 1995.

24. Kadar N, Lemmerling L: Urinary tract injuries during laparoscopically assisted hysterectomy: causes and prevention, *Am J Obstet Gynecol* 170:47, 1994.

25. Kovac SR, Cruikshank SH, Retto WF: Laparoscopic-assisted vaginal hysterectomy, *J Gynecol Surg* 6:185, 1990.

26. Lee CL, Soong YK: Laparoscopic hysterectomy with the Endo GIA 30 Stapler, *J Reprod Med* 38:582, 1993.

27. Leibsohn S, d'Ablaing G, Mishell DR Jr, Schlaerth JB: Leiomyosarcoma in a series of hysterectomies performed for presumed uterine leiomyomas, *Am J Obstet Gynecol* 162:968, 1990.

28. Leventhal ML, Lazarus ML: Total abdominal and vaginal hysterectomy: a comparison, *Am J Obstet Gynecol* 61:289, 1951.

29. Liu CY: Laparoscopic hysterectomy: a review of 72 cases, *J Reprod Med* 37:351, 1992.

30. Liu CY: Laparoscopic hysterectomy: report of 215 cases, *Gynaecol Endo* 1:73, 1992.

31. Meikle SF, Nugent EW, Orlean M: Complication and recovery from laparoscopic-assisted vaginal hysterectomy compared with abdominal and vaginal hysterectomy, *Obstet Gynecol* 89:304, 1997.

32. Nezhat C, Nezhat F, Silfen SL: Laparoscopic hysterectomy and bilateral salpingo-oophorectomy using multifire GIA surgical stapler, *J Gynecol Surg* 6:287, 1990.

33. Nezhat CR, Burrell MO, Nezhat FR, et al: Laparoscopic radical hysterectomy with paraaortic and pelvic node dissection, *Am J Obstet Gynecol* 168:864, 1992.

34. Nezhat CR, Nezhat FR, Burrell MO, et al: Laparoscopic radical hysterectomy and laparoscopically assisted vaginal radical hysterectomy with pelvic and para-aortic node dissection, *J Gynecol Surg* 9:105, 1993.

35. Nezhat F, Nezhat C, Gordon S, Wilkins E: Laparoscopic versus abdominal hysterectomy, *J Reprod Med* 37:247, 1992.

36. Nezhat F, Nezhat CH, Admon D, et al: Complications and results of 361 hysterectomies performed at laparoscopy, *J Am Coll Surg* 180:307, 1995.

37. Ostrenski A: Endoscopic bladder repair during total modified laparoscopic hysterectomy: a case report, *J Reprod Med* 38:558, 1993.

38. Ou CS, Beadle E, Presthus J, Smith M: A multicenter review of 839 laparoscopic-assisted vaginal hysterectomies, *J Am Assoc Gynecol Laparosc* 1:417, 1994.

39. Padial JG, Sotolongo J, Casey MJ, et al: Laparoscopy-assisted vaginal hysterectomy: report of seventy-five consecutive cases, *J Gynecol Surg* 8:81, 1992.

40. Parker WH, Fu YS, Berek JS: Uterine sarcoma in patients operated on for presumed leiomyoma and rapidly growing leiomyoma, *Obstet Gynecol* 83:414, 1994.

41. Peiter RC, Wagner PL, Gambone JC: Routine hysterectomy for large asymptomatic uterine leiomyomata: a reappraisal, *Obstet Gynecol* 79:481, 1992.

42. Pelosi MA, Pelosi MA III: Laparoscopic hysterectomy with bilateral salpingo-oophorectomy using a single umbilical puncture, *New Jersey Med* 88:721, 1991.

43. Pelosi MA, Pelosi MA III: Laparoscopic supracervical hysterectomy using a single umbilical puncture (mini-laparoscopy), *J Reprod Med* 37:777, 1992.

44. Pelosi MA, Villalona E: Laparoscopic hysterectomy, appendectomy, and cholecystectomy, *New Jersey Med* 90:207, 1993.

45. Phipps JH, John M, Hassanaien M, Saeed M: Laparoscopic- and laparoscopically assisted vaginal hysterectomy: a series of 114 cases, *Gynaecol Endo* 2:7, 1993.

46. Photopulos GJ, Stovall TG, Summitt RL Jr: Laparoscopic-assisted vaginal hysterectomy, bilateral salpingo-oophorectomy, and pelvic lymph node sampling for endometrial cancer, *J Gynecol Surg* 8:91, 1992.

47. Pruitt AB, Stafford RH: Laparoscopic-assisted vaginal hysterectomy: a continuing evolution of surgical technique, *J S C Med Assoc* 88:433, 1992.

48. Raju KS, Auld BJ: A randomized prospective study of laparoscopic vaginal hysterectomy versus abdominal hysterectomy each with bilateral salpingo-oophorectomy, *Br J Obstet Gynaecol* 101:1068, 1994.

49. Rapkin AJ, Kames LD: The pain management approach to chronic pelvic pain. *J Reprod Med* 32:323, 1987.

50. Redwine DB: Laparoscopic-hysterectomy compared with abdominal and vaginal hysterectomy in a community hospital, *J Am Assoc Gynecol Laparosc* 2:305, 1995.

51. Reich H, DeCaprio J, McGlynn F: Laparoscopic-hysterectomy, *J Gynecol Surg* 5:213, 1989.

52. Reiter RC, Gambone JC: Demographic and historic variables in women with idiopathic chronic pelvic pain, *Obstet Gynecol* 75:428, 1990.

53. Richardson RE, Bournas N, Magos AL: Is laparoscopic hysterectomy a waste of time? *Lancet* 345:36, 1995.

54. Saye WB, Espy GB III, Bishop MR, et al: Laparoscopic Doderlein hysterectomy: a rational alternative to traditional abdominal hysterectomy, *Surg Laparosc Endosc* 3:88, 1993.

55. Schwartz RO: Complications of laparoscopic hysterectomy, *Obstet Gynecol* 81:1022, 1993.

56. Schwartz RO: Laparoscopic hysterectomy: supracervical vs assisted vaginal, *J Reprod Med* 39:625, 1994.

57. Sheth SS: The place of oophorectomy at vaginal hysterectomy, *Br J Obstet Gynaecol* 98:662, 1991.

58. Stoney WS: Laparoscopic cholecystitis: problem of rapid growth, *South Med J* 84:681, 1991.

59. Stovall TG, Elder RE, Ling FW: Predictors of pelvic adhesions, *J Reprod Med* 34:345, 1989.

60. Stovall TG, Ling FW, Crawford DA: Hysterectomy for chronic pelvic pain of presumed uterine etiology, *Obstet Gynecol* 75:676, 1990.

61. Summitt RL Jr, Stovall TG, Lipscomb GH, Ling FW: Randomized comparison of laparoscopic-assisted vaginal hysterectomy versus standard vaginal hysterectomy in an outpatient setting, *Obstet Gynecol* 80:895, 1992.

62. Vietz PF, Ahn TS: A new approach to hysterectomy without colpotomy: pelviscopic intrafascial hysterectomy, *Am J Obstet Gynecol* 170:609, 1994.

63. Woodland MB: Ureter injury during laparoscopy-assisted vaginal hysterectomy with the endoscopic linear stapling, *Am J Obstet Gynecol* 167:756, 1992.

21 Cystocele

DAVID H. NICHOLS

When considering the indications for surgical repair of damage to the anterior vaginal wall, the gynecologist must first correlate the damage with the patient's symptoms. It is necessary both to investigate the patient's history, including any urinary incontinence or recurrent or chronic cystitis, and to check carefully for evidence of coexistent prolapse of the uterus, vaginal vault, or rectum and for signs of enterocele. Chronic constipation relieved by severe straining may favor progression or recurrence of cystocele.

Any history of urinary stress incontinence, which may have been relieved as the prolapse progressed, is important.[55] The supports of the urethra, even though attenuated, may have more strength than do those of the bladder because of their continuity with the urogenital diaphragm. Predictably, the degree of bladder descent when the prolapse is advanced usually exceeds the degree of accompanying urethral descent, resulting in an angulation or kinking of the urethra at its junction with the bladder.

Relative contraindications to transvaginal surgery for urinary stress incontinence include the following:
1. Chronic respiratory disease
2. Socially disabling recurrent urinary stress incontinence
3. Lifestyle that involves regular heavy lifting (e.g., nurses in nursing homes)
4. A fundamental error in diagnosis (e.g., detrusor instability)

Although the bladder itself is not suspended, it receives support from the vagina and its attachments[27] (Fig. 21-1). Thus damage to the vaginal wall itself, the connective tissue to which the vagina is attached, or both may affect the bladder supports and lead to cystocele.[72] When a cystocele is large, increases in intraabdominal and intravesical pressure are greater in the dependent portion of the cystocele than in the attenuated urethrovesical junction. Hodgkinson[30] observed that the hydrostatic pressure within the bladder is always greater at the bottom of this column of fluid than midway up or at the top. A coexistent defect in the posterior vaginal wall, of course, aggravates this tendency toward bladder distention. Because of the absence of adequate posterior vaginal or perineal support, the elasticity of the sagging bladder when filling is relatively unrestrained.

Preoperative evaluation of the presence or absence of urinary stress incontinence generally indicates whether the anterior genital segment has been damaged. Because various types of incontinence exist and often occur simultaneously in a single patient, it is essential to determine the precise nature of the problem in each patient—whether the problem is primarily one of stress, overflow, urgency incontinence, or a combination of these. A proper urodynamic diagnosis is required for the identification and selection of an appropriate surgical remedy[31,42] (see Chapter 45).

The gynecologist who is selecting an operation for the repair of the anterior vaginal wall must consider the future functions and strains to which that wall may be subjected—not only coitus but also future pregnancy and parturition and not infrequently heavy physical work. All these factors must be correlated with current findings, which may partially be the result of earlier attempts at surgical repair. Furthermore, allowances must be made for any atrophic changes that have occurred or are expected to occur after the patient's menopause.

ASYMPTOMATIC CYSTOCELE

Repair of an asymptomatic cystocele is seldom indicated *unless* it is coincident with pelvic repair performed for other reasons or unless the gynecologist has observed unmistakable evidence of the cystocele's progressive protrusion into the vagina over time. Within limitations, the larger the cystocele and the more advanced its progression, the more complicated its repair and the less certain the restoration of normal bladder function because some permanent impairment to a properly balanced nerve supply may be present.[9] The primary advantage of reexamination by the same gynecologist over a period of years is that of following evidence of progression to a degree that requires operative repair and being able to make that recommendation before increased medical risks associated with the patient's advancing age preclude elective surgery. At each examination the gynecologist should record his or her impression of the size of the lesion in a manner that permits reliable comparison with findings on subsequent reexaminations.

Should the gynecologist and the patient decide that surgery is indicated for an asymptomatic cystocele, a primary objective is the restoration of normal anatomic relationships, with attention to contributing causative factors, all in a conscious effort to reduce the risks of recurrence in later years.

The degree of vaginal cornification demonstrable on visual or cytologic examination often indicates the extent of postmenopausal atrophy. This index should correlate at least roughly with the persistence of lateral wall rugal folds. If there is little cornification, an estrogen deficiency should be

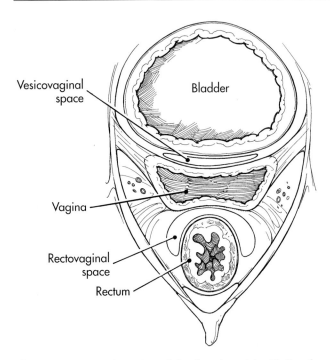

Fig. 21-1 Coronal section of the female pelvis. Notice the tissue condensations, which extend from each anterior vaginal sulcus to the pelvic sidewall. These, plus the vaginal wall between them, form a hammock for the bladder, which is separated from the vagina by the vesicovaginal space. However, the paravesical and pararectal "spaces" are filled with loose areolar tissue.

suspected. The gynecologist should estimate the relevance of this deficiency to the development of the cystocele and should consider the advisability of vaginal or systemic estrogen replacement.

Low urethral closure pressure is one cause of postoperative urinary incontinence.[7,10] It may be present but unidentified, particularly in postmenopausal patients, especially those with massive eversion of the vagina.[66] A simple method of detecting low urethral closure pressure consists of inserting a pediatric-sized Foley catheter (no. 8 or 10 with a 3-ml bulb), partly inflating the bulb with 1 ml of saline, and applying gentle traction to the catheter to see whether it can be drawn easily through the urethra. If the catheter is drawn readily through, the urethra should be tightened by appropriate placation to the extent that the partly inflated bulb can no longer be drawn through the urethra. Marking the catheter at 1-cm intervals from the bulb provides a "ruler" to measure urethral length and the area of low urethral pressure.[5] If the partly inflated Foley bulb can be drawn only into the proximal urethra, funneling should be expected and can be surgically remedied.

SYMPTOMS OF CYSTOCELE

Cystocele is often asymptomatic, and coincident urinary stress incontinence is infrequent. Patients may describe a sense of pelvic pressure and "falling out," sensations often related to a coexistent uterine or vault prolapse. Descent of the uterus or bladder seem to annoy patients to a degree proportional to the time it takes the condition to develop. Patients appear to notice a rapidly developing prolapse fairly quickly and to make an early request for reconstruction and relief, but they may accept a slowly progressive descensus without comment or complaint. A patient with a large cystocele may or may not be aware of a mass protruding from the vagina associated with a bearing-down sensation, but she generally notices a sense of pelvic heaviness after she has been standing for a time, the effect of gravitational pull.

Some patients have learned to elevate a large cystocele manually to facilitate voiding. Surprisingly, only the larger cystoceles are associated with any significant amount of residual urine.[26] The large dumbbell-shaped bladder that is often evident with complete procidentia, for example, frequently leads to a degree of persistent urinary stasis that contributes both to infection and to stone formation. Presumptive chronic cystitis is not the inevitable result of supposedly "stagnant urine," however. Women with residual urine often complain that when they stand after apparently emptying their bladders, they immediately feel a desire to void again, but they find that they can void very little additional urine when they sit down the second time. A reason for these sensations is that the hydrodynamics associated with the standing position differ from those of the sitting position. When the bladder contains a great volume of residual urine, some overflow incontinence may occur.

Urinary stress incontinence is not a characteristic or even frequent experience of a majority of women with cystocele, unless there has been a rotational descent of the bladder neck.[25] Urinary stress incontinence usually requires colporrhaphy including coincident and specific repair of coexistent damage to both midline and lateral supports of the bladder neck and urethra.

Some patients with cystocele may have coincident urinary dysfunction that can be assessed urodynamically but is clinically masked by the vesicourethral kinking coincident with cystocele. This dysfunction sometimes includes the potential for urinary stress incontinence,[18] and if anterior colporrhaphy fails to include specific surgical steps to provide adequate support or elevation of the vesicourethral junction, postoperative urinary stress incontinence may become evident,[39] to the distress of both patient and surgeon. Prevention of this unwelcome development requires full vaginal length anterior colporrhaphy that includes special attention to restoring the supports of the vesical neck. Coincident funneling should be reduced by appropriate Kelly-type stitches. Hypermobility of the vesicourethral junction can be reduced by plication of the urogenital diaphragm (pubourethral ligaments) beneath the vesicourethral junction. With *full-length* anterior colporrhaphy, regardless whether the patient has had preoperative urodynamic studies, the incidence of postoperative urinary stress incontinence will be reduced.[6,7] A large cystocele with significant volume of residual urine may, from the stagnation of urine, promote chronic or recurrent cystitis.

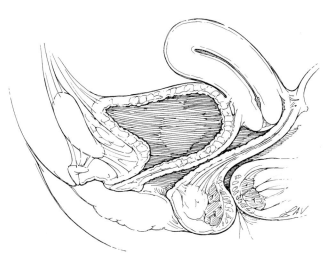

Fig. 21-2 The partly filled bladder is shown in the center of this sagittal drawing of the pelvis. There is both rotational descent of the vesicourethral junction and funneling of the urethra. This is an "anterior" cystocele, since it is located anterior to the interureteric ridge (Mercier's bar).

TYPES AND CAUSES OF CYSTOCELE

Two anatomic systems maintain the vesicourethral junction and urethra in position. The pubourethral "ligament" portion of the urogenital diaphragm suspends it, and the vaginal wall and its attachments support it. Damage to either or both systems can alter the pelvic location of the urethra and affect its function.[13,15,48,51,72]

Cystocele has been described according to its position anterior to the interureteric ridge or posterior to it.[4] These conditions may coexist, and both must be recognized and corrected if surgery is to be effective.

Anterior Cystocele (Pseudocystocele)

In patients who have only an anterior cystocele (pseudocystocele or pseudourethrocele), a straining effort causes the downward bulging or rotational descent of the urethra. This descent is permitted by the separation of the urethra from the urogenital diaphragm and the pubourethral ligament portion of the urogenital diaphragm that binds it to the pubis,[44,48,51] or separation of the vagina from its intermediate connective tissue attachment to the arcus tendineus.[57,74] The degree of rotational descent of the urethrovesical junction is variable, and the bladder may or may not herniate behind the urethrovesical junction. The condition is often associated with urinary stress incontinence. This type of damage is usually postobstetric and is often associated with a wide subpubic arch.

With anterior cystocele, the diameter of the urethra is unchanged except at its proximal end, where the diameter may be increased if funneling or vesicalization of the urethra has occurred (Fig. 21-2). Pathologic dilation of the midportion or distal urethra (true urethrocele) is quite uncommon, but it can result from pathologic stretching

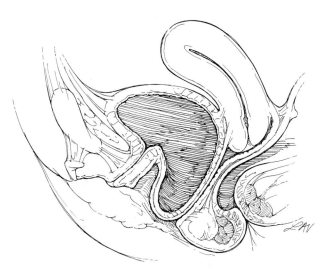

Fig. 21-3 A large cystocele is seen *posterior* to Mercier's bar.

from within the urethra, occasionally digital or manipulative, or, rarely, from necrosis of the internal wall of a preexisting infected urethral diverticulum. However, a *routine* full-length plication of a normal, *undilated* urethral wall may itself be followed by later stricture and "postmenopausal stenosis," creating an iatrogenic obstructive uropathy that sometimes requires a lifetime of troublesome periodic urethral dilation.

True or Posterior Cystocele (Distention Cystocele)

Almost without exception, a true cystocele results either from a stretching of the anterior vaginal wall during parturition beyond its ability to involute postpartum, possible even during "normal" vaginal delivery, or from the atrophic changes of aging and of pelvic straining on the intrinsic structural components of the vaginal wall, even if they have not been damaged earlier[71] (Fig. 21-3). The most common type of cystocele is the late result of an overstretching and subsequent eversion of the wall of the vagina. Rugal folds of the anterior vaginal epithelium decrease and may disappear as the weakness within the vaginal wall allows the bladder to bulge into the vagina. The lateral attachments of the vagina and bladder may be relatively undamaged if they are merely compressed against the side wall of the pelvis during labor.

Usually, the cystocele does not become clinically evident until after menopause. With the postmenopausal loss of estrogen-related elastic tissue and smooth muscle tone, the relaxation and redundancy associated with weakened connective tissue support increase, and symptoms develop. In such instances, the vaginal walls, especially the anterior and posterior walls, may remain pathologically thinned. Later, as a result of circulatory stasis and chronic hyperemia, the vagina may appear hypertrophic. Some women appear to have a basic congenital defect in the elastic tissue and smooth muscle components of the vagina that contributes to the condition.

Displacement Cystocele

Because it results from a primary and pathologic elongation of the lateral or "ligamentous" attachment and support of the vagina, a displacement cystocele is quite different from that produced by simple overstretching of the connective tissues within a previously normal vaginal wall. Damage to the lateral vaginal supporting tissues may be the result of either of two mechanisms: (1) damage to attached tissues, such as the supports of the cervix, and (2) damage to the lateral supports of the vaginal wall itself resulting from the forces of labor.

The cervix is attached to the upper anterior vaginal wall, and the tissues that support both the vagina and the cervix are component parts of the cardinal ligaments. Because these tissues tend to function as an anatomic unit, the displacement of one component often leads to similar displacement of the other. Like eversion or prolapse of the upper vagina, a displacement cystocele may develop rapidly when it is the result of obstetric injury to the cardinal–uterosacral ligament complex, or it may occur more insidiously in older women as a result of long-standing increased intraabdominal pressure.

When, because of inadequate dilation during parturition, a segment of the vaginal wall becomes a soft tissue obstruction to the passage of a rapidly descending presenting part, slowing the descent until the segment gives way, the supporting tissues attached to the rolled-up, telescoping segment of the vagina become overstretched and avulsed as the presenting part descends. This mechanism may not have damaged the integrity of the vaginal wall itself, however, so eventual repair should shorten the lateral attachments of the vagina and cervix and reestablish the vaginal length either by colpopexy or full length paravaginal repair. In its pure form, this type of cystocele is an eversion of the vagina with relatively well-preserved rugal folds, although the sulci disappear to some extent.

Rugae of comparable size on both the anterior and lateral vaginal walls suggest displacement cystocele, whereas diminished rugae on the anterior wall along with more clearly defined rugae on the lateral walls suggest distention cystocele. The surgeon must identify the cause of the recurrent cystocele as displacement, overdistention, or a combination of the two—with demonstrable defects in the midline supporting structures, the lateral supporting structures, or both—and must note the relationship of the cystocele to the urethrovesical junction or urogenital diaphragm.

If one has determined that a cystocele should be repaired, to achieve the best optimal result it is essential to decide whether the vaginal vault is partially prolapsed so that this element also can be surgically corrected during the same operative procedure. Examination of the patient when she is standing and reexamination under anesthesia is important, with traction applied to the vaginal vault when the pelvis muscles are relaxed and pain is absent. Displacement cystocele especially should be considered when considering a repair of a recurrent cystocele, or one that is seen in a nullipara.

Postmenopausal bladder urgency may be associated with an atrophic "urethritis and trigonitis." The atrophic changes that occur after menopause result in significant thinning of the epithelial and subepithelial layers of the urethra and the bladder trigone, making them oversusceptible to stimulation and irritation. When this can be demonstrated or is even suspected, vaginal or systemic estrogen replacement therapy is likely to reduce the patient's symptoms promptly. If the therapy is effective, surgical repair should be deferred for a month or two until the beneficial results and symptomatology have stabilized and long-term response can be reevaluated.

Cystocele Caused by Multiple Factors

Sometimes a cystocele results from a combination of the factors. The importance of each component may be noticeable at different levels within the vagina. The gynecologist who is contemplating a repair must consider the mechanism or combination of mechanisms that accounts for the pathology demonstrable in an individual patient.

In at least one fourth of the instances of symptomatic genital prolapse, both the upper and the lower vagina are everted. Because the relative significance of these factors differs from patient to patient, the technique selected for repair must be based on an appraisal of the relative importance of the etiologic factors in each patient.[43]

Paravaginal Defect

When anterior sulci are absent, the gynecologist should examine the patient for lateral detachment of the urethral paravaginal tissues. According to Baden and Walker,[2] such a detachment should be suspected when the anterior vaginal wall is relaxed. If the anterior vaginal wall is not elevated when the patient squeezes her pelvic muscles tightly (i.e., in a "holding" position), the connective tissue and vascular supports of the anterior vaginal wall may have been detached from the arcus tendineus, on one but usually both sides.

The vagina itself is not attached directly to the arcus tendineus,[14,18,29,54,67] but the anterior vaginal fornix is attached to the arcus tendineus by a meshwork or bridge of intervening connective tissue that may be subject to various strains and stretching or even partial avulsion. Because this type of strain usually is a consequence of trauma during labor and delivery, detachment of these tissues is more common in parous patients. It also may be related to lifestyle, however, and occasionally may follow the pull of massive vaginal eversion, even in the nullipara. Therefore direct surgical attachment of the vaginal sulcus to the arcus tendineus may to some extent correct the widening of the anterior vaginal wall that occurs with certain types of cystocele.[18,57,74,75] Bilateral attachment is generally necessary when stretching or avulsion of the lateral supports has resulted in a cystocele.[60,74] Large midline defects of the vaginal wall are much more common and are remedied by the standard midline plications and colporrhaphy. The existence or coexistence of the less common lateral defects should be determined preoperatively for appropriate planning of surgical technique. Paravaginal repair is discussed at some length in Chapter 27.

RECURRENT CYSTOCELE

When a cystocele has recurred after an initial repair, the gynecologist who is contemplating reoperation must first try to determine why the earlier surgery was unsatisfactory. The gynecologist should review the hospital surgical dictation of the previous operation, relate the earlier procedure to the current findings, and then weigh these factors when choosing the technique and sutures for a reoperation.

During the physical examination of a patient with recurrent cystocele, the gynecologist should check the position of the vaginal vault when the patient is standing and bearing down, as by a Valsalva maneuver. This procedure discloses any coincident partial eversion of the vaginal vault that brings the bladder with it. It is essential to determine and surgically remedy any coincident prolapse of the vaginal vault.

Voluntary isometric pubococcygeal perineal resistance exercises (fifteen 3-second squeezes six times a day) may be recommended preoperatively if a patient has coincident urinary stress incontinence or has weak voluntary contractions of her pubococcygei. The program may be resumed with benefit starting the day after surgery and continued for 6 months postoperatively to aid in reestablishment of continence. A program of voluntary pubococcygeal resistance exercises greatly helps the patient.[17,36,53] If she is unable to voluntarily contract her pubococcygei, a course of biofeedback training may be useful in safeguarding against recurrence.[11,32,59]

TECHNIQUES OF COLPORRHAPHY

If the gynecologist has determined that a cystocele repair is necessary, it is essential to determine whether the vaginal vault is partially prolapsed so that this condition can be surgically corrected during the same operative procedure. Examination of the patient while she is *standing,* and preoperative reexamination while she is in the lithotomy position (after the administration of anesthesia, when the pelvic muscles are relaxed and the patient has no pain) are confirmatory, and appropriate surgical steps can then be planned to restore vaginal length (e.g., sacrospinous colpopexy—see Chapter 26). Examination under anesthesia with traction to the vault will demonstrate a partial or complete eversion that might otherwise be unsuspected. The preoperative consent and informed consent for colporrhaphy might well include the expression "with possible colpopexy." It is especially important to consider vaginal vault descent, sometimes quite unexpected and not obvious to casual inspection, when planning the repair of a recurrent cystocele or of a cystocele in a nullipara.

In a postmenopausal patient with greater than usual atrophic changes, surgery may be preceded and followed by estrogen replacement therapy to restore the vascularity, elasticity, thickness, and cellular integrity of the vaginal wall.

Because cystocele results primarily from damage to the vagina—either to its supports or to the vaginal wall itself—the primary site for reconstructive surgery for cystocele must be the vagina. Many operations designed to restore a defective posterior urethrovesical angle also elevate the proximal urethra to a position that once again permits a normal response to changes in intraabdominal pressure. Only when these surgical changes affect the proximal urethra, as well as the bladder, is this important aid to continence restored.[22]

The technique appropriate for dissection and repair of the anterior vaginal wall in an individual patient depends on many factors, including the presence of vaginal telescoping or coexistent vault eversion. A short vagina due to telescoping may be surgically lengthened by a coincident procedure, such as vaginal hysterectomy or a Manchester operation (see Chapter 19), by shortening of the cardinal or uterosacral supports, by a transvaginal sacrospinous colpopexy, or by transabdominal sacrocolpopexy (see Chapter 26). Restoration of vaginal depth by returning the vagina, with the bladder, to the pelvis is the essence of surgical treatment of a displacement cystocele.

In procidentia, as defined by Ricci and Thom,[56] the entire uterus protrudes from the pelvis. As a rule, the eversion of the vagina is complete and an enterocele is present, and only a minimal or secondary rectocele may be present. The supporting vaginal and uterine portions of the cardinal ligaments are markedly elongated and often attenuated. Therefore the displacement is greatest and most apparent in relation to the anterior vaginal wall and cervix, which function as an anatomic unit because they are attached by continuity to each other and to the pelvic sidewalls.

With massive prolapse, both suffer severe circulatory changes, resulting not only from stasis due to their compression against the sides of the genital hiatus, but also from congestion aggravated by gravity. The degree of chronic congestion apparently stimulates corresponding lymphangiectasia, which in turn stimulates considerable fibroblastic proliferation within the vaginal wall. Chronic edema leads to hypertrophy and fibrosis, which thicken the anterior vaginal wall. These tissues elongate with advancing age and sag noticeably because they are deficient and defective in other components, especially elastic tissue.[43]

After mobilizing the full thickness of the anterior vaginal wall, including the epithelium and the underlying fibromuscular connective tissue layer, the gynecologic surgeon can enter the desired plane most readily by opening directly into the vesicovaginal space.[61] Sharp dissection should be used to enter the proper pelvic spaces, although the spaces can be developed safely by blunt dissection after they have been entered. It takes longer to locate the correct plane after an initial dissection in the wrong plane than to find it correctly the first time. This initial direct approach to the vesicovaginal space is equally useful for anterior colporrhaphy when a cystocele is to be repaired without coincident hysterectomy or cervical amputation and when there has been previous hysterectomy or cervical amputation. Ricci and Thom[56]

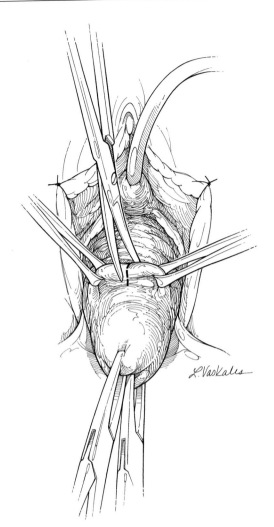

Fig. 21-4   A means of entering the vesicovaginal space of the patient not receiving coincident hysterectomy. The anterior vaginal wall is grasped between two Allis clamps overlying the vesicovaginal space, and an incision is made between them directly into the vesicovaginal space.

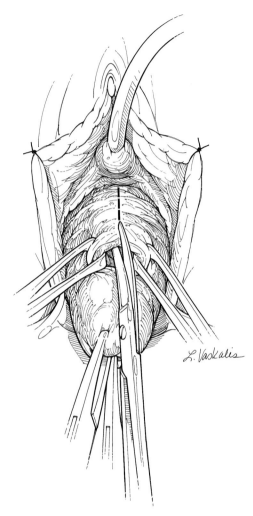

Fig. 21-5   The incision directly into the vesicovaginal space is extended along the path of the dashed line after the full thickness of the vaginal wall has been grasped by repositioning the Allis clamps as shown. The incision is continued both cranially and caudally.

described a useful technique for exposing the bladder, essentially as follows:

> The most dependent portion of the vaginal wall is grasped between two Allis clamps (Fig. 21-4). The anterior vaginal wall is rolled or massaged between the index finger and thumb several times to accentuate the planes of separation between bladder and vaginal wall. The full thickness of the vaginal wall is cut between these two instruments with a curved scissors, the tip of the scissors pointing perpendicular to the axis of the vagina, exposing an avascular space and bringing the bladder musculature into view (see Fig. 21-4). The full thickness of the cut surfaces of the vaginal wall are grasped with Allis clamps now turned 90 degrees, and with scissors the vaginal wall is cut upward exactly in midline (Figs. 21-5 and 21-6). This incision is continued beyond the urethrovaginal junction where the cleavage plane ends. The bladder wall is displaced from both lateral flaps of the incised vaginal wall and cut from the cervix, exposing the vesicouterine peritoneal fold, which may be incised, the index finger introduced, and the pelvis explored.

Reconstruction of the Anterior Vaginal Wall

Cystocele is commonly associated with a degree of uterine prolapse less than procidentia. A transurethral Foley catheter, preferably silicone coated, is inserted, and the bladder is emptied. Any resistance to the passage of the catheter suggests a urethral stricture. Under this circumstance, the surgeon must be careful to avoid urethral plication at this point, which would only make the stricture worse. In fact it may be wise to dilate this urethra postoperatively in the operating room while the patient is still anesthetized.

Alternatively, the avascular space may be entered through the full thickness of the anterior vaginal wall by means of an inverted T-shaped incision at the point where the vagina meets the cervix.[3] The midpoint of the anterior vaginal cuff incision is grasped between two forceps and incised exactly in the midline and directly into the avascular vesicovaginal space (Figs. 21-7 and 21-8). The incision is then carried superiorly to the point of fusion of urethra with vagina, and a plane is carefully dissected between the ure-

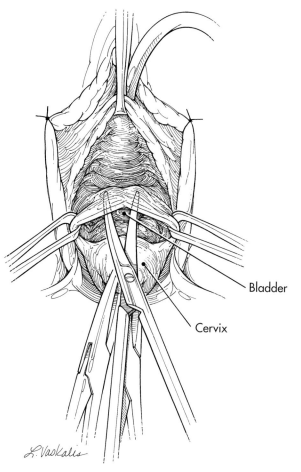

Bladder

Cervix

Fig. 21-6   To avoid cutting a viscus, the closed tips of the dissecting scissors are inserted beneath the vaginal wall and advanced, establishing a cleavage plane. The tips of the scissors are *then* spread apart, and while so spread are withdrawn, widening the plane of dissection in the vesicovaginal space.

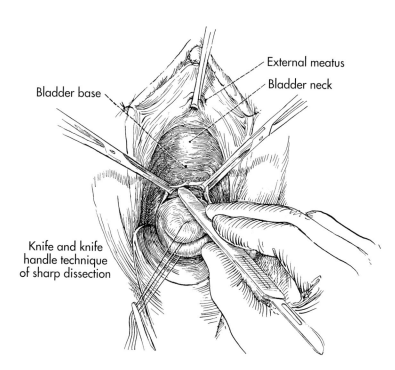

External meatus

Bladder neck

Bladder base

Knife and knife handle technique of sharp dissection

Fig. 21-7   A circumferential incision has been made at the junction between the cervix and the anterior vaginal wall, two Allis clamps 1 cm apart are placed as shown, and a short midline incision is made through the full thickness of the anterior vaginal wall, creating an inverted T-incision. By blunt dissection the tissues are separated from the underside of the vagina. (From Ball TL: *Gynecologic surgery and urology,* ed 2, St Louis, 1963, Mosby.)

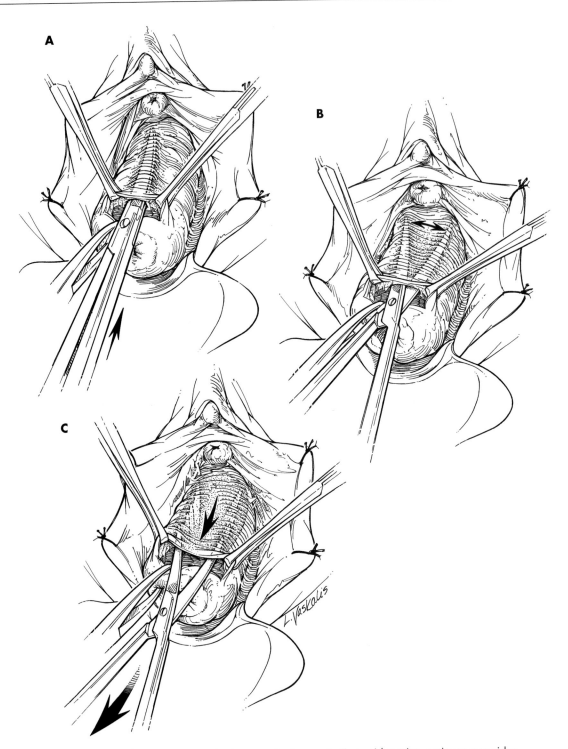

Fig. 21-8 Hilton's maneuver in the use of scissors. **A,** To avoid cutting a viscus or unidentified blood vessel, the closed tip of the dissecting scissors can be used to establish a plane. Once the scissors have been inserted, the tips may be spread **(B)** and the opened scissors withdrawn **(C).** Thus the connective tissue plane is successfully widened without risk to the underlying viscus.

thra and vaginal wall. The remainder of the suburethral anterior vaginal wall is incised in the midline to within 1 or 1.5 cm of the external urethral meatus (Fig. 21-9).

The extent of the earlier damage to the supports of the urethrovesical junction, the degree of attenuation, and the integrity of the tissue available for plication determine the amount of bolstering necessary for the urethrovesical junction.

In performing an anterior colporrhaphy, the surgeon should reconstruct the full length of the anterior vaginal wall, including the urethrovesical junction and the supports of the

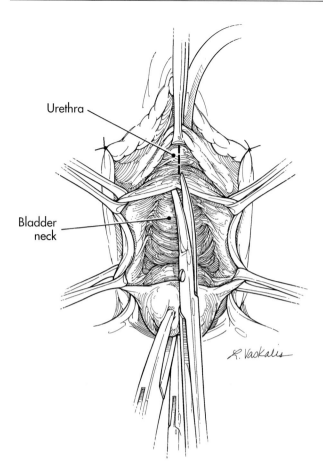

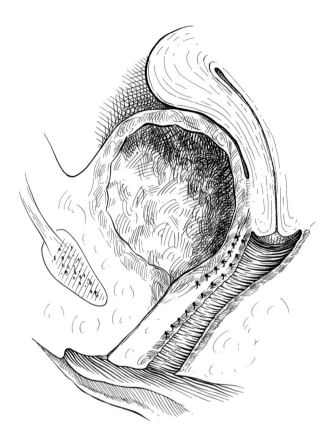

Fig. 21-9 The incision in the anterior vaginal wall is continued to the external urethral meatus.

Fig. 21-10 Sagittal section of a partly filled bladder following anterior colporrhaphy in which insufficient attention was paid to re-creation of a vesicourethral angle. Flattening of this angle occurs in such patients, which is conducive to postoperative urinary incontinence.

urethra. This involves separating the urogenital diaphragm from the vagina, plicating it beneath the urethra, and reattaching it to the vagina. This procedure is sometimes associated with temporary postoperative difficulty in voiding, but it is far preferable to straightening the neck of the bladder and obliterating the urethrovesical angle, which may provoke iatrogenic urinary stress incontinence (Fig. 21-10).

Because the patient being operated on is in the lithotomy position and under anesthesia, the tissue relationships that prevail differ from those that prevail when she is conscious and standing. Vulnerability to urinary continence is greatest when the fully conscious patient is in the standing position. Surgical repair of a large hypotonic "decompensated" cystocele probably restores some intravesical pressure, reducing the incontinence. Surgical support of the urethrovesical junction should strengthen the anatomic and physiologic factors that contribute to postoperative continence. Temporary stimulation by bethanechol (Urecholine) may stimulate postoperative bladder function in this special circumstance.

By sharp dissection with either scissors or scalpel (Fig. 21-11) the operator separates the full thickness of the anterior vaginal wall from the bladder laterally and anteriorly as far as the lateral limits of the vesicovaginal space, sometimes almost to the pubic rami, in a line of cleavage that preserves the attachment between the subepi-

thelial fibromuscular connective tissue layer and the vaginal epithelium. As the dissection proceeds laterally, a possibly incomplete but identifiable musculoconnective tissue may be freed between the connective tissue left attached to the vaginal epithelium and the predominantly muscular bladder wall. Ideally it is possible to establish such lines of cleavage without compromising the blood supply of these supporting tissues; great care must be taken to open along tissue planes because simply slicing tissue into arbitrary layers is likely to damage the tissue planes that usually harbor blood supply.

The simple Sims technique does not require lateral dissection and therefore does not disturb the vaginal blood supply, leaving the entire thickness of the vaginal wall intact and retaining the attachment of all musculoconnective tissue to the vaginal epithelium. In this technique the surgeon excises a carefully measured ovoid or wedge of the redundant full thickness of thinned vaginal wall.[61] Unless the entire full thickness of the anterior vaginal wall has been correctly mobilized, however, only the superficial epithelial layer may be excised, and such an operative procedure would be as inadequate in the treatment of cystocele as the simple

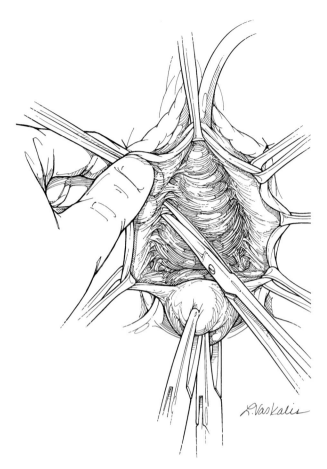

Fig. 21-11 The tissues of the urogenital diaphragm are separated from the underside of the anterior vaginal wall by sharp dissection using either scissors or scalpel. Pressure of the scissor tips against the fingertips of the surgeon's opposite hand protects against "buttonholing."

excision of an ellipse of overlying skin would be in the treatment of an inguinal hernia.

Urethrovesical Junction. Funneling of the vesical neck physiologically shortens the urethra to a degree equal to the lengthening of the physiologic bladder neck. As a result the effective urethrovesical junction is often displaced to a more distal segment of the urethra, where it is further removed from and less responsive to changes in intraabdominal pressure. When the location of the junction is below the inferior margin of the pubis, there is a disturbing tendency toward urinary stress incontinence. Such a development is not surprising, however, because funneling of the vesical neck usually reflects damage to the supports of both the bladder and urethra and contributes markedly toward a functional break in the "bladder base plate" of Uhlenhuth[63] and Hutch.[33] A pathologically widened urethra should be narrowed by plication, with a catheter in the urethra to guarantee against iatrogenic stricture (Figs. 21-12 and 21-13).

Although Green[28] noted the importance of both the posterior urethrovesical angle and the urethral inclination, others have emphasized vesicourethral funneling as an anatomic defect that, by physiologically "shortening" the effective urethral length, favors the direct hydrostatic transmission of bladder pressure to the urine inside the funnel (see Fig. 21-2). Such funneling should be corrected by the placement of a number of Kelly-type mattress sutures in a way that plicates the funnel and restores the normal tone, configuration, and caliber of the urethral segment (Fig. 21-14). Kelly[38] stitches are subvesicourethral plication stitches that correct funneling with its associated stress incontinence, even though originally they were developed to strengthen a presumed internal urethral sphincter.

Some elongation of the bladder trigone and some lateral displacement of the ureterovesical orifices are likely to occur with massive cystocele.[64,65] This condition disturbs the physiology of continence and may be remedied by the insertion of a U-shaped suture, which is intended not only to shorten the trigone but also to narrow it.[58]

Urethral Supports. Studies[44,76,77] have shown that the urethra is normally suspended from or supported by the pubic bone by means of bilaterally symmetric, anterior, posterior, and intermediate pubourethral "ligaments." Because these bands of muscle and connective tissues pass from the pubic bone to the urethra—not to the bladder—they are comparable to the puboprostatic ligaments in the male. It has been established[44] that these ligamentous supports are continuous with the urogenital diaphragm. Although the posterior "ligament" elongates physiologically during the normal voiding process (Fig. 21-15), any defect or injury that lengthens or loosens the pubourethral ligaments contributes strongly to the occurrence and persistence of urinary stress incontinence.

The posterior urethral wall may be pulled downward and descend more than the anterior urethral wall, giving rise to vesicalization or funneling of the urethra.* This generally can be remedied by sewing the pubourethral ligament portions of the urogenital diaphragm *together beneath* the vesicourethral junction rather than *lateral* to it. This is the essence of "pubourethral ligament plication stitches."

With marked degrees of prolapse and with procidentia, the pubourethral ligaments can become significantly elongated, and they sometimes can be found quite far laterally. It is essential to elevate and support the urethrovesical junction to the physiologic position behind the pubis so that normal relationships can be restored and sudden increases in intraabdominal pressure will register in the proximal urethra, as well as in the bladder. It is particularly important to shorten the pubourethral ligaments in a patient with massive prolapse lest the patient suffer a postoperative iatrogenic urinary stress incontinence that is more distressing and disabling than the prolapse for which she originally sought relief.[62]

The vaginal ends of the pubourethral ligament portion of the urogenital diaphragm can be identified transvaginally

---

*Jacek Mostwin, personal communication, 1998.

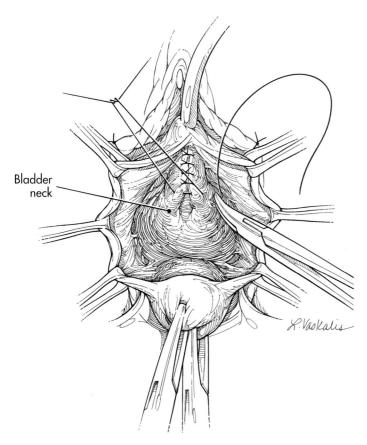

Bladder
neck

Fig. 21-12   If the urethra is pathologically widened, it is plicated for its full length with interrupted absorbable mattress sutures.

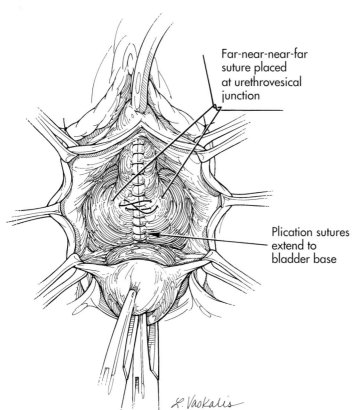

Far-near-near-far
suture placed
at urethrovesical
junction

Plication sutures
extend to
bladder base

Fig. 21-13   Plication extends beyond the vesicourethral junction onto the muscularis of the bladder, if the trigone is widened, as is seen with a large cystocele.

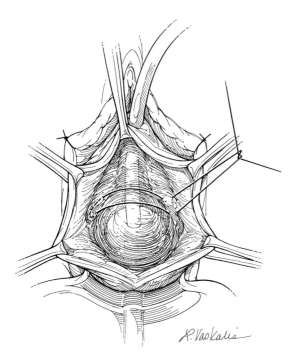

Fig. 21-14 A traditional Kelly stitch for reducing the size of a urethral funnel. It is essentially a three-point mattress stitch placed as indicated. If one stitch is insufficient to relieve urethral funneling, additional stitches can be placed both lateral to the original stitch and cranial and caudal as well. This repair is generally done while an adult-sized Foley catheter is in the bladder to lessen the possibility of creating a urethral stricture. (Modified from Nichols DH, Randall CL: *Vaginal surgery,* ed 4, Baltimore, 1996, Williams & Wilkins.)

and plicated beneath the urethrovesical junction[48] (Fig. 21-16). The operator incises the vagina in the midline and then dissects laterally to the public rami, clearly exposing the tissues of the urethrovesical junction. Although these ligaments are not discrete anatomic structures, they can be recognized as paired tissue condensations or thickenings in the sheetlike tissue of the urogenital diaphragm.

Palpation of the inflated bulb of the transurethral Foley catheter demonstrates the urethrovesical junction, but as Gardiner[24] noted, excessive traction on the catheter may draw the bulb of the Foley catheter into a pathologically widened and funneled urethra. Small, straight Kocher hemostatic forceps are applied to the periurethral tissue 1 to 1.5 cm on either side of its fusion to the urethra, as recommended by Gainey[22] and Frank.[19]

After the ligamentous condensations have been identified, the ligaments can be further shortened by means of a more lateral bite into an often thicker portion. If the retropubic attachments of these ligaments are intact and the Kocher forceps have been properly placed, downward ventral traction on the coccyx *in the direction in which the fibers of the ligament run to the pubis* actually moves the patient slightly on the operating table. The degree of resistance to this pull indicates whether the strength and length of the ligament are sufficient to permit a suburethral plication that will elevate the urethrovesical junction. The tips of the forceps may be brought to the midline to ensure that the tissues can be united and that the plication will indeed elevate the urethra. Mattress-type sutures (2-0 long-lasting synthetic absorbable material, such as polydioxanone [PDS]) or nonabsorbable

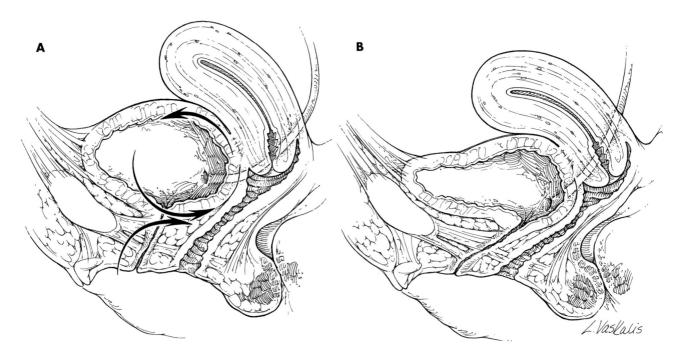

Fig. 21-15 **A,** "Wheeling" of the vesicourethral junction. This occurs physiologically during the voiding process to permit temporary flattening of the urethrovesical angle. **B,** However, when it is present in the patient who is not voiding (as shown in drawing), the anatomic relationship is pathologic and is conducive to the development of urinary stress incontinence.

monofilament synthetic sutures are then placed lateral and medial to the hemostats (see Fig. 21-16).

It usually is possible to achieve the desired retropubic elevation of the urethrovesical junction by means of the essential sutures described. Should these sutures fail to raise the urethrovesical junction cranial to the inferior border of the pubis, the operator should place a second set of pubourethral ligament stitches lateral to the first until a proper degree of elevation has been obtained. Such pubourethral sutures should always be placed *lateral* to the urethra, not in the urethral wall. Because they are placed more laterally than are urethral plication stitches, paraurethral stitches can be inserted directly into the urethral attachment of the pubourethral ligament portion of the urogenital diaphragm,

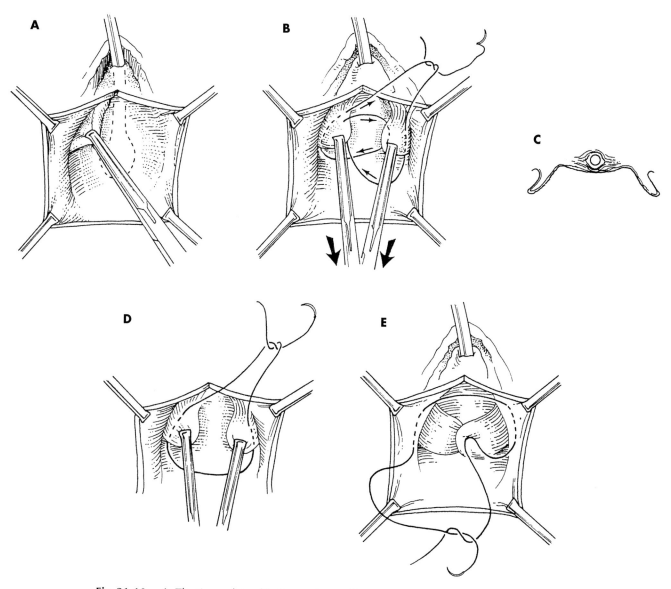

Fig. 21-16   A, The tissues lateral to the urethra and just anterior to the inflated bulb of a Foley catheter are grasped with the tip of a Kocher hemostat, first on one side and then on the other. Traction to the hemostats in the direction of the arrows will move the patient a small amount, confirming their proper placement. **B,** These are plicated with a far-near-near-far suture of polyglycolic acid or nonabsorbable suture. **C,** The depth of the dissection so as to not skeletonize the urethra. When this suture has been tied, effectively elevating the vesicourethral junction but without compromising the lumen of the urethra, the stitch is passed through the underside of the anterior vaginal wall as shown. **E,** When this stitch has been tied, fusion of the anterior vaginal wall and urogenital diaphragm has been restored. When the tissues of the pubourethral portion of the urogenital diaphragm are markedly scarred, a single nonabsorbable mattress stitch may be placed in the tissues lateral to the tips of the Kocher hemostat as shown **(D).** (From Nichols DH, editor: *Reoperative gynecologic and obstetric surgery,* ed 2, St Louis, 1997, Mosby.)

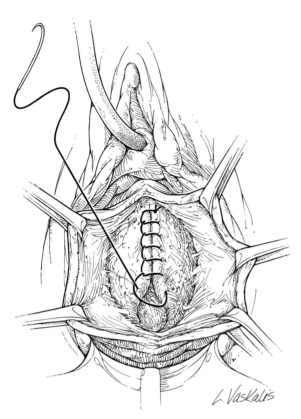

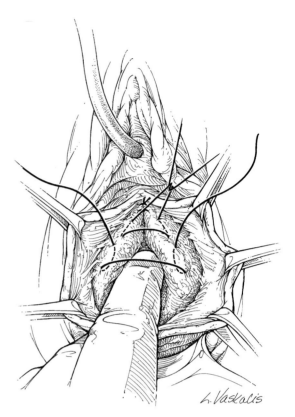

Fig. 21-17 The fibromuscular capsule or adventitia of the bladder of a patient with cystocele is reduced in width by a suture of running locked long-lasting thread placed as shown. Tension on the suture approximates, not strangulates, the tissues.

Fig. 21-18 For the patient with a larger cystocele the operator's index finger depresses the bladder in the midline and the fibromuscular capsule of the bladder is reduced by one or more layers of interrupted mattress sutures placed in a trapezoid configuration. A very large cystocele may receive preliminary reduction by a purse-string suture, the neck of which must be carefully supported by additional side-to-side stitches of absorbable suture material placed in the fibromuscular capsule of the bladder.

which makes them even more effective in elevating the urethrovesical junction. (Any second stitches also bury and reduce the tension of the initial sutures.) The ends of such buried stitches are sewn to the underside of the trimmed anterior vaginal wall to reestablish a normal site of fusion of the vagina to the urogenital diaphragm. After they have been tied, they should neither reduce the urethral diameter nor produce subsequent stricture, which would certainly be accentuated after menopause.

When stress incontinence is the patient's sole problem, a buried, nonabsorbable suture may be used in the plication of pubourethral ligaments. The surgeon must ensure that the suture does not penetrate the lumen of either the urethra or bladder lest it form a nidus for future infection or stone formation. When the urethrovesical junction has been elevated to a spot cranial to the inferior margin of the pubis, any appreciable funneling of the bladder neck or urethra should be corrected by plication with interrupted sutures of 2-0 PGA absorbable or monofilament synthetic nonabsorbable sutures placed directly in the wall of the urethral funnel itself. These can be placed from side to side by the mattress-type suture of Kelly.[38] The stitches of Royston and Rose[58] may be used to shorten a pathologically elongated trigone.

In the presence of a pathologically dilated or funneled urethra, Kelly-type stitches used for urethral plication may be deliberately placed in the wall to reduce its lumen. When Kelly-type plication stitches are placed in the periurethral supporting tissues, they may not only correct funneling but also unintentionally approximate the paraurethral portions of the posterior pubourethral ligaments. The more laterally placed pubourethral ligament sutures, on the other hand, are inserted directly into the urethral attachment of the posterior pubourethral ligament portion of the urogenital diaphragm.[29,41] This placement seems to explain the greater success of this procedure.

Because Kelly plication stitches are particularly useful in the presence of funneling or vesicalization of the urethra and bladder neck, the surgeon may sometimes choose to use *both* pubourethral plication stitches *and* Kelly plication stitches in a particular clinical situation (e.g., rotational descent of the urethrovesical junction with simultaneous urethral funneling). The merits of these techniques for each case must be decided individually.

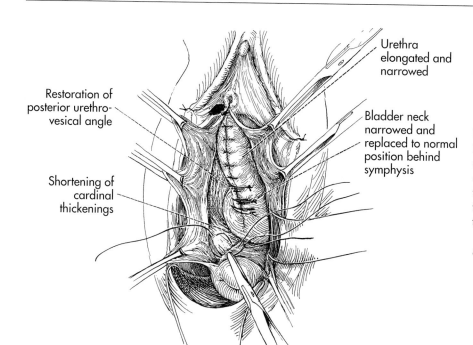

Restoration of posterior urethro-vesical angle

Shortening of cardinal thickenings

Urethra elongated and narrowed

Bladder neck narrowed and replaced to normal position behind symphysis

Fig. 21-19 The urethrovesical angle has been restored as shown, the bladder neck and any funneling have been corrected, and the vesicourethral junction is now near its regular position at the junction of the upper two thirds of the lower third of the back of the pubis. (From Ball TL: *Gynecologic surgery and urology*, ed 2, St Louis, 1963, Mosby.)

Alternative Transvaginal Methods of Support of the Vesicourethral Junction. Obviously several important factors may contribute to urinary stress incontinence. For example, the pubococcygeus muscle may be attached to the lateral paraurethral and paravaginal connective tissues, as has been pointed out by Muellner.[47] Sometimes these factors require the surgeon to use different procedures for anterior colporrhaphy.

When traction on the Kocher hemostatic forceps applied to the paraurethral tissue shows *no* evidence of pubic fixation of the tissue to which the hemostat has been applied (i.e., failure of traction to move the patient a small bit), the paraurethral or paravaginal tissues have been either avulsed or detached on one or both sides of the pelvis, and the pubourethral ligament support is insufficient for reconstruction. In this instance it is necessary to consider alternative methods of support, such as a transplant of the pubococcygeus muscle,[12,20,34] lateral (or paravaginal) fixation sutures, or the use of buried plastic synthetic mesh.

In correcting cystocele, the operator may plicate the entire length of the bladder's fibromuscular connective tissue capsule longitudinally by placing a series of running or interrupted 2-0 or 3-0 long-lasting but absorbable sutures from the connective tissue capsule at the vault of the vagina all the way to the urogenital diaphragm (Figs. 21-17 and 21-18). It is essential to avoid overcorrecting the cystocele because overcorrection may obliterate the posterior urethrovesical angle and, by making the urethra the most dependent portion of the bladder, result in postoperative stress incontinence.[62] A pathologically dilated urethra may be plicated (Fig. 21-19) with special attention to lateral plication of the urethrovesical angle.

Long-term results will be improved by using long-lasting synthetic absorbable suture, such as PDS or poly-glyconate (Maxon), of small diameter in subepithelial layers.

A common error in the performance of anterior colporrhaphy is to separate the vaginal epithelium from the fibromuscular layer of the vagina, plicate the fibromuscular tissue in the midline, trim the vaginal epithelium, and close without ever entering the vesicovaginal space. This repair may damage the vaginal blood supply and can be associated with an increased risk of recurrent cystocele or persistent stress incontinence.

The Gersuny "tobacco pouch" purse-string suture can be used to reduce or invert the bladder wall size of a very large cystocele, but since this stitch provides little intrinsic strength it must always be reinforced by a layer of side-to-side plication stitches. Reconstruction of any defect in the posterior vaginal wall, perineum, and its supporting tissues is desirable.

If it has been determined that the vagina is too long as well as too wide, a not uncommon finding in prolapse of long duration, it may be necessary to shorten the excessive length as well as the width. Failure to shorten this excessive length may precipitate residual as well as recurrent cystocele. This is seen more frequently after sacrospinous fixation than after sacrocolpopexy. To lessen this incidence, usually asymptomatic but nonetheless disconcerting, one can take specific surgical steps to not only shorten the pathologically long vagina and the wall of the bladder beneath it, but also to simultaneously correct any excess vaginal width.[20]

Procedure. A large purse-string suture using either permanent or long-lasting polyglycolic acid–type synthetic suture will simultaneously correct excessive length and width of the bladder wall. The closed neck of the inverted sac of bladder is reinforced with overlying interrupted transverse plication sutures (Fig. 21-20). When it is time to tie the

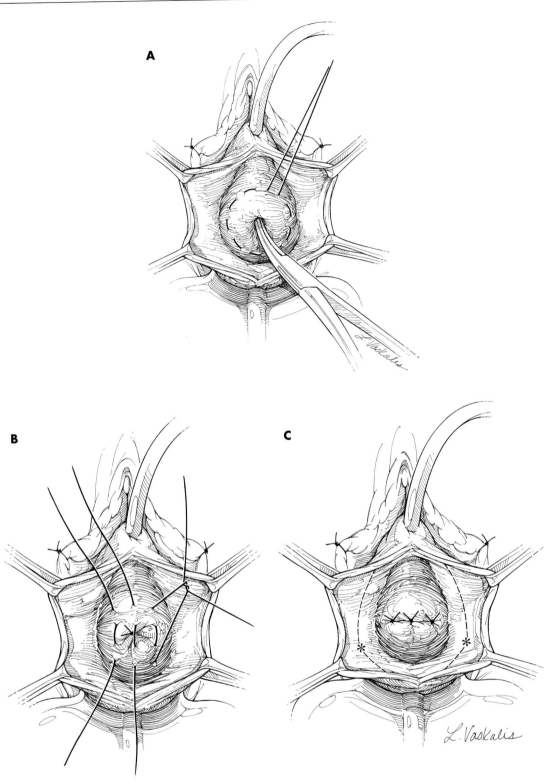

Fig. 21-20 The anterior vaginal wall has been opened, displaying an increase in both vaginal and bladder length as well as width. **A,** The vesicovaginal space is dissected laterally for its full dimension, and a large purse-string suture is placed posterior to the reinforced urogenital diaphragm. **B,** The suture is tied, and the repair reinforced by a series of transversely placed plication stitches. **C,** Sufficient vaginal wall is excised from each flap to both narrow and shorten the vagina as indicated by the *dashed line.* The *asterisks* mark the new cranial position of the vaginal vault. The sides will be brought together at this point and next sewn to the mucosal edge at the apex of the vagina. (From Nichols DH, editor: *Reoperative gynecologic and obstetric surgery,* ed 2, St Louis, 1997, Mosby.)

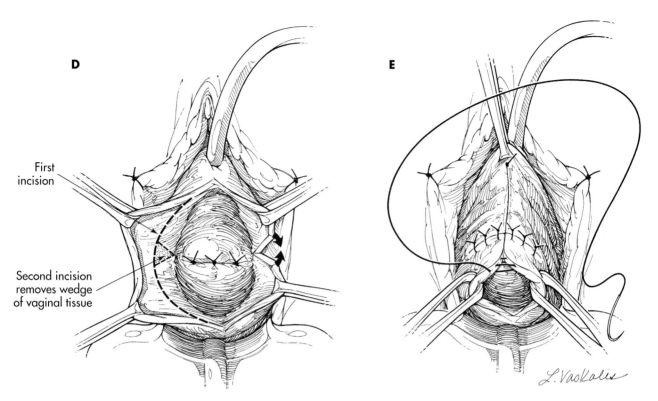

Fig. 21-20, cont'd D, Alternatively, after trimming of the anterior vaginal wall as suggested by the dashed line, a wedge of tissue is excised from each side of the anterior vaginal wall and converted into a linear wound by a series of interrupted stitches. **E,** The remaining anterior vaginal wall is closed with a running subcuticular suture.

purse-string suture, the center of the "circle" should be invaginated gently by the tip of a closed curved Kelly hemostat, and at the last moment as the knot is being tied the hemostat is withdrawn, ensuring an appropriate and desired invagination of the bladder muscularis and mucosa.

Where the defect is of increased length alone, and not width, as in some previously operated patients, one or more layers of transversely placed sutures will achieve a similar good result (Fig. 21-21). The excessive anterior wall is trimmed appropriately before closure to shorten both length and width.

Pubococcygeus Muscle Transplant of Ingelman-Sundberg. The operator isolates the finger-thick medial pedicle of the pubococcygeus on each side by dissection and transects it in the midportion of the vagina at the level of the urethrovesical junction. Sewing the two pedicles together by transfixion suture provides useful vesicourethral junction support after the repair of a cystocele, as after the repair of a urethrovaginal fistula. In fact, failure to provide some such support after the repair of a fistula at the urethrovesical junction is likely to result in postoperative urinary stress incontinence.

The first step in performing a pubococcygeus muscle transplant is to open the vagina in the midline into the vesicovaginal space. The operator then mobilizes the full thickness of the walls laterally almost to the pubic rami, beyond the lateral limits of the vesicovaginal space, if necessary. Palpation of the upper two thirds of the lateral vaginal wall permits identification of the medial borders of the pubococcygei, which can be visualized with a little dissection. Alternatively, some operators prefer to make an inverted U-shaped incision through the full thickness of the anterior vaginal wall to expose the full length of the urethra, most of the bladder, and laterally the pubococcygei at the point where they cross the urethra and the vagina.

The operator mobilizes a finger-sized pedicle of the pubococcygeus muscle on each side and separates it laterally from the remainder of the muscle (Fig. 21-22). When transected posteriorly, this muscle graft is suspended because of its continuity with the superior extremity of the rest of the muscle. The portion mobilized should be long enough to permit it to be joined to the pedicle from the other side snugly, but without tension, by means of a series of transfixion sutures placed in a side-to-side fashion beneath the urethrovesical junction.

To prevent its retraction and loss of support, the free segment of the posterior pubococcygeus from which the upper muscle was cut is now sewn by a mattress suture to the main body of the levator ani on its respective side.

Lateral or Paravaginal Fixation. When midline plication is not an effective treatment of rotational descent of the urethrovesical junction, lateral or paravaginal fixation on one or both sides may be necessary. If a patient has both a lateral defect and a midline lesion that should have been diagnosed preoperatively, a midline incision in the anterior vaginal wall provides operative exposure for the repair of each of these elements (i.e., pubourethral ligament plication with anterior colporrhaphy, and paravaginal fixation). One approach is

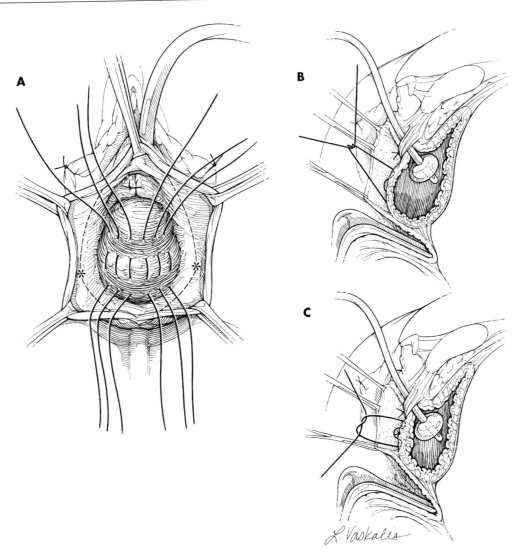

Fig. 21-21   Increased vaginal and bladder length but not width can be corrected by an operation in which an incision is made into the vesicovaginal space, and the vaginal wall separated from the fibromuscular wall of the bladder. **A,** At the midportion of the cystocele, and considerably posterior to the plicated urogenital diaphragm, a series of transverse plication stitches are placed in the fibromuscular wall of the bladder. **B** and **C,** If necessary, a second layer can further imbricate this tissue. (From Nichols DH, editor: *Reoperative gynecologic and obstetric surgery,* ed 2, St Louis, 1997, Mosby.)

to attach the paraurethral connective tissue to the arcus tendineus on the undersurface of the pubis.* This approach is discussed and described thoroughly in Chapter 27.

Plastic Mesh Support. When a large cystocele is associated with an abnormal thinning of the vaginal wall, a single-layered, porous plastic mesh insert can be used to encourage the formation of an adequately strong, satisfactorily functional vaginal wall.[45,49] The operator sews a layer of Mersilene mesh gauze into the vesicovaginal space, covering the entire surface of the exposed bladder surface that had previously been in contact with the anterior vagina. Fibroelastic connective tissue infiltrates and fixes the anterior vaginal wall after implantation. This type of foreign material is best used on postmenopausal or previously sterilized patients because the stretching and dilation of labor in a fertile patient would probably disrupt the attachments and result in avulsion of the mesh.

Mersilene mesh appears to be particularly effective when used to support the anterior vaginal wall because it is flexible, permanent, porous, and only a single layer in thickness. Perhaps most important, connective tissue readily infiltrates it, forming a permanently thickened, pliable tissue layer between the mesh and the undersurface of the vagina. The procedure used to place a Mersilene mesh insert is similar to that used to place a Tantalum patch, introduced for the same purpose by Moore, Armstrong, and Will.[46] Moore has abandoned the use of tantalum, however, because it may fragment in this area where it is subject to repeated bending.

*References 2, 18, 51, 57, 60, 74, 75.

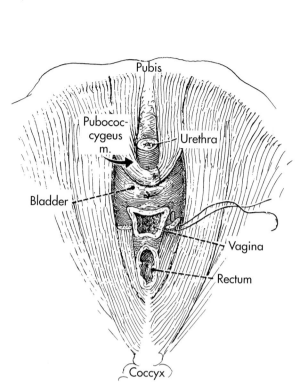

Fig. 21-22 When the tissues of the urogenital diaphragm are pathologically weak at the vesicourethral junction, an alternative method to support this tissue is the pubococcygeus muscle transplant. The dissection in the vesicovaginal space is carried laterally until the pubococcygei are identified. Each pubococcygeus is transected as shown by the *dashed line* and approximated in an overlapping fashion beneath the vesicourethral junction. The posterior cut end of each pubococcygeus is fixed to the adjacent ileococcygeus muscles to inhibit subsequent development of rectocele. (From Nichols DH, Randall CL: *Vaginal surgery*, ed 4, Baltimore, 1996, Williams & Wilkins.)

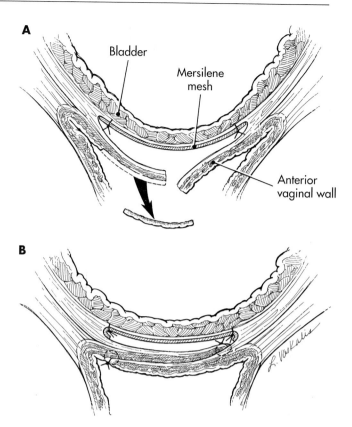

Fig. 21-23 For a very large cystocele and a very thin vagina with which to support its repair, a piece of Mersilene mesh cut to size may be fixed into position to the bladder capsule, but this should be buried beneath the vagina by a vaginal lapping operation. **A,** One flap of vagina is split, separating the epithelium from the underlying fibromuscular layer, and the excess epithelium is excised. **B,** The tip of this fibromuscular layer is then sewn to the underside of the unsplit flap of the opposite side, and the unsplit cut edge of the opposite side sewn to the point from which the epithelium was excised, effectively doubling the thickness of the fibromuscular wall of the vagina at this point. (Modified from Nichols DH, Randall CL: *Vaginal surgery*, ed 4, Baltimore, 1996, Williams & Wilkins.)

(Friedman and Meltzer[21] used a somewhat similar but absorbable collagen mesh prothesis successfully.) Supplemental reinforcement and insulation of this Mersilene mesh patch may be provided by the vaginal lapping operation or by a wide bulbocavernosus fat pad transplant.[41]

After opening the vesicovaginal space and reflecting the full thickness of the anterior vaginal wall from the midline laterally for the full extent of the vesicovaginal space, the operator cuts a pattern of sterile cardboard to fit the estimated size of the defect. From this pattern, a trapezoid-shaped piece of Mersilene gauze is fashioned. The operator then tacks the mesh to the capsular connective tissue underlying the bladder by placing three or four sutures on either side along the lateral margins of the vesicovaginal space, from as high in the vaginal vault as can be reached to the area beneath the urethrovesical junction. (In unusual cases of full length weakness the operator may extend the mesh patch anteriorly to reinforce the urethra as well.) Sutures should also be placed anteriorly into each pubourethral liga-

ment. Laterally the mesh can be attached to the firm tissues of the lateral wall of the perivesical spaces, to the obturator fascia, and to the pelvic diaphragm. The prosthesis should be insulated by the vaginal lapping procedure (Fig. 21-23) or a bulbocavernosus fat pad transplant.

This type of mesh should be used only as a subepithelial prosthesis. Inmon[35] has successfully buttressed the urethrovesical junction when supporting tissues are defective by imbedding a short hammock of Mersilene mesh transvaginally, sewing it to the urethrovesical supporting tissues of first one side and then the other. The material must always be carefully buried beneath a two-layered closure, however, and must not be allowed to come into contact with an epithelial surface.

Necrosis of the covering vaginal flap could result from ischemia; for this reason the cut edges of the vagina must be united without tension. Zacharin[78] has reported success

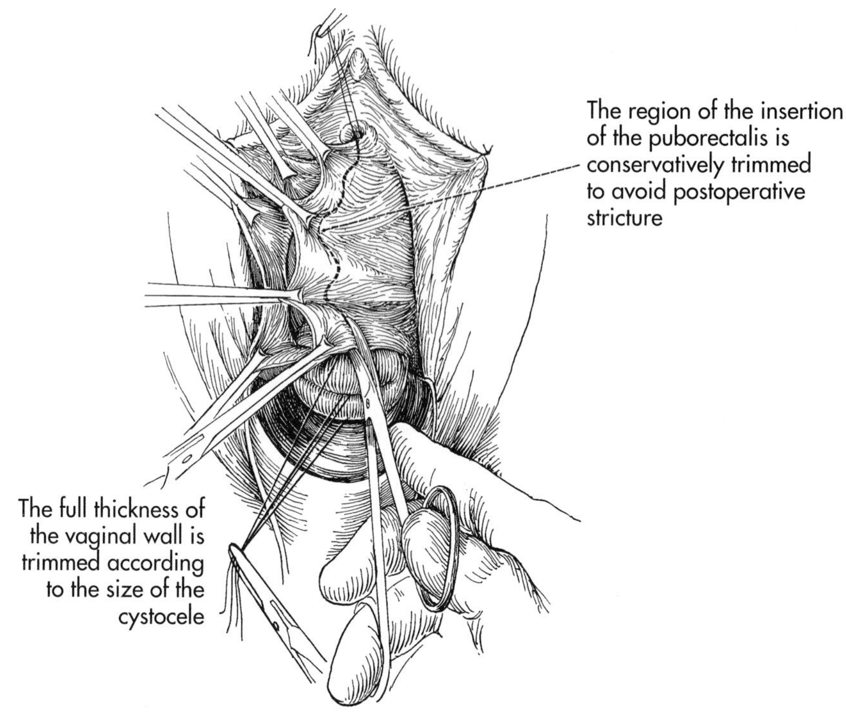

The region of the insertion of the puborectalis is conservatively trimmed to avoid postoperative stricture

Fig. 21-24 Excess but unsplit vaginal wall is trimmed appropriately. (From Ball TL: *Gynecologic surgery and urology,* ed 2, St Louis, 1963, Mosby.)

The full thickness of the vaginal wall is trimmed according to the size of the cystocele

using a free full-thickness patch of excised vaginal skin buried beneath the vaginal flaps, tacked in position in place of the synthetic plastic mesh.

Closure of Vaginal Wall. When vaginal hysterectomy has immediately preceded anterior colporrhaphy, the residual inverted T-shaped flaps of the upper vagina should be carefully trimmed to an inverted V (Figs. 21-24 and 21-25). If a functional vagina is not an objective of surgery, attenuated vaginal walls can effectively support a cystocele repair; the operator can deliberately excise wide flaps of vaginal wall, which is then closed, thereby narrowing the vagina to a fingerbreadth caliber. This does not appreciably improve incontinence, however; it simply narrows the vagina. Correction of increased vaginal length can be separately addressed by excision of an appropriate amount of vaginal wall[50,52] (see Figs. 21-20 and 21-21).

For those patients who wish to preserve a functional vagina, it is essential to avoid the overenthusiastic or careless excision of too much of the anterior vaginal wall. Furthermore, in trimming the vaginal flaps to provide a desirable contour for the vault of the vagina, the operator must remember that the greater the amount of anterior wall flap that is removed, the less the amount of posterior wall flap that can be removed. The operator's failure to make this type of adjustment in procedure also may narrow the vagina unnecessarily, and dyspareunia may follow.

When closed under too much tension, the vaginal membrane may later separate or slough, thereby inviting recurrence. If there is evidence of flap tension, the operator should make simple longitudinal "relaxing incisions" that undermine 1 cm of the full thickness of the lateral vaginal walls at the 3- and 9-o'clock positions to release the tension and increase the caliber of a narrowed vagina (see

Chapter 24). Such lateral relaxing incisions may be left open and the "raw" bases allowed to granulate in, while the patient daily inserts an obturator to retain the desired vaginal circumference, and they usually become reepithelialized within 2 to 3 weeks. The obturator, which can be fashioned from a 50-ml plastic syringe, should be worn at night. In colporrhaphy, it is the reapproximation of the subepithelial fibromuscular tissues that produces the desired repair—not the reapproximation of the superficial vaginal skin.

In some patients, the separation of a thin layer of connective tissue from the undersurface of the vaginal membrane, mobilization, and plication, often by means of multiple, somewhat incomplete rows of fine synthetic absorbable or nonabsorbable sutures, may produce a satisfactory long-term result. The redundant sling of the fibromuscular tissues is shortened and strengthened by duplication because the supporting layer of vaginal membrane fits the newly formed plane of the anterior vaginal wall with much less excision of vaginal membrane than may have been expected.[40]

Aldridge[1] suggested that after the removal of a properly sized, somewhat V-shaped wedge from the vaginal flap beneath the urethra, full-thickness vaginal wall approximation is more important in supporting the urethra than is plication of the urethral wall itself. The operator should close the suburethral vaginal wall with running or interrupted 2-0 absorbable stitches, often placed subcuticularly, through the full thickness of the underlying fibromuscular layer. The first stitch should be near the urethral meatus. If hysterectomy has immediately preceded the repair, the operator should sew the ends of the tied but uncut peritoneal closure stitch to the undersurface of the now trimmed upper vault margins of the anterior vaginal wall near the attachment of the bladder pillars to ensure

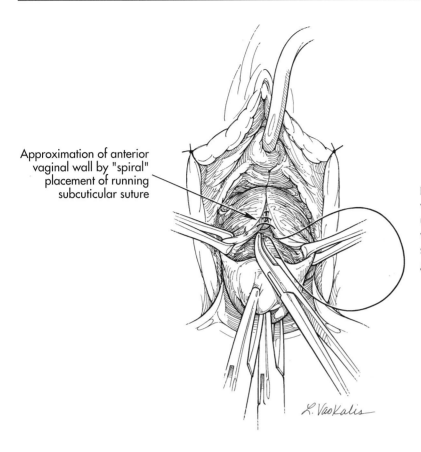

Approximation of anterior vaginal wall by "spiral" placement of running subcuticular suture

Fig. 21-25   The full thickness of the anterior vaginal wall is approximated from side to side, using a running subcuticular suture if the vaginal wall is thick, through-and-through interrupted sutures if it is not. (From Ball TL: *Gynecologic surgery and urology*, ed 2, St Louis, 1963, Mosby.)

maximal elongation of the wall when these stitches have been tied. It is best to slide the index finger down the suture strand of the peritoneal closure stitch to a closure stitch to a point below the knot while bringing the vaginal wall to the point of peritoneal closure. Because the peritoneal closure stitch includes the uterosacral ligaments, this procedure effectively though indirectly attaches the anterior vaginal wall to the uterosacral ligaments, helps lengthen the anterior vaginal wall, and directs the vaginal axis posteriorly. A program of voluntary perineal resistive exercises will enhance the continence mechanism[17,36,37] both preoperatively and for some months postoperatively.

Simultaneous Perineorrhaphy

Because the lower anterior wall rests on the perineal body for the length of the urethra, perineal support also should be provided whenever urethral support has been the major objective of vaginal reconstruction. Coincident perineorrhaphy not only reinforces the external genital sphincter system[79] but also improves the long-term results of repair for the cure of urinary stress incontinence (see Chapter 22).

The Watkins-Wertheim[69,70,73] interposition type of operation in which the uterine fundus is interposed between the bladder and the anterior vaginal wall is not recommended for the treatment of cystocele because of the risk of subsequent bleeding from the retained uterus. In addition, should disease requiring hysterectomy subsequently develop, the extensive adhesions to the uterine fundus and the proximity of the lower ureters and the bladder trigone to the

adherent fundus that result from such an operation make hysterectomy appreciably more difficult. Rarely, if the vaginal wall is very thin and the uterine cervix is well supported, transposition using the Ocejo modification can be used[23] in which the uterus is opened, the entire endometrium excised, and the uterine incision closed.

INABILITY TO VOID POSTOPERATIVELY

Relaxation of the muscular component of the pubourethral ligaments and the urethral attachment to the levator ani (muscular, fascial, or both) is an integral part of the physiologic voiding process, and significant surgical plication of these ligaments beneath the urethrovesical junction may inhibit the normal voiding process until edema has subsided, healing is well under way, and spasms have ceased.[8] A temporary suprapubic cystostomy may be helpful if the surgeon suspects that the patient (e.g., a patient with unusual anxiety or with a very large hypotonic bladder) will be unable to void after anterior colporrhaphy. Suprapubic cystostomy should be used almost routinely after repair of a fistula at the vesical neck (see Chapter 47).

At the time the silicone-coated no. 16 transurethral Foley catheter is removed, the patient may be given a single dose of an α-adrenergic blocker such as phenoxybenzamine (Dibenzyline) 10 mg to relax urethral spasm. An order is left for the patient to be catheterized only if unable to void. If after a day of unsuccessful trying the patient is still unable to void, she may be taught the technique of self-

INSTRUCTIONS FOR INTERMITTENT SELF-CATHETERIZATION

Self-catheterization can be accomplished several times a day, as frequently as someone normally voids. It is important to be sure the bladder never holds more than 500 ml (1 pint) of urine at one time. If the bladder is allowed to hold more than 500 ml for any length of time, the urine can stretch the bladder muscle to the point where it will not function as well as it should, and if the bladder becomes too stretched, it cannot receive a proper blood supply, which can precipitate bladder infection. To avoid these problems make sure that the bladder is emptied every few hours during the day. Some people do the procedure while standing, some sitting on the toilet, and some lying down. Whichever is the easiest for you is the method you should use.

PROCEDURE

1. Wash hands and then wash the perineal area. Spread the labia with one hand, and with the other hand wash the opening from where the urine comes, and the surrounding area, from front to back, using a povidone-iodine (Betadine) packet, or a wash-and-wipe disposable towelette. Use one wipe to wash down the left side of the non–hair bearing inner vaginal lips, then wipe down the inner surface of the right side, and another one to wash down the urethral meatus (the opening from which the urine comes).
2. Hold the labia open with one hand, and grasp the Mentor plastic disposable catheter 2 to 3 inches from the tip, inserting it slowly into the meatus (urethral opening) until the urine begins to drain. Leave it in place until the urine stops coming, and slowly pull the catheter out. If urine begins to drain again, stop and wait until the flow stops before removing the tube. The catheter can be allowed to drain directly into the toilet or container. When the flow of urine is finished, remove the catheter.
3. The catheter should be washed well with soap and water after each rise, and then rinsed with clear water.
4. Each day boil the catheters for 3 to 5 minutes, empty the water, and let them dry. They may be stored in a clean towel, air aluminum foil packet, a Ziplock bag, or a sterilized jar. You should carry a catheter with you whenever you go. Clearly, the catheters can be reused for an almost indefinite period of time if the above procedure is followed. Should you need a new supply, do not hesitate to request this of your physician, who can prescribe a new supply from a surgical supply house.

Adapted from Ebrady SM, Yale-New Haven Hospital, New Haven, Conn.

catheterization, to be used as necessary even after discharge from the hospital. Use of the plastic, flexible "Mentor" 14-Fr female catheter facilitates this procedure considerably. It can be discontinued as soon as the patient is able to void adequate amounts spontaneously and there is but little (less than 60 ml) residual urine obtained. The patient may be given a printed handout of the technique (see the box on the left).

For patients unwilling or unable to learn self-catheterization, a transurethral Foley catheter may be inserted, clamped, and opened and drained as necessary for comfort for 2 weeks and then removed.

REFERENCES

1. Aldridge AH: Personal communication, 1965.
2. Baden WF, Walker TA: Evaluation of the stress incontinent patient. In Cantor EB, editor: *Female urinary stress incontinence,* Springfield, Ill, 1979, Charles C Thomas.
3. Ball TL: *Gynecologic surgery and urology,* St Louis, 1963, Mosby.
4. Ball TL: Anterior and posterior cystocele, *Clin Obstet Gynecol* 9:1062, 1966.
5. Beck RP: Personal communication.
6. Beck RP, McCormick S: Treatment of urinary stress incontinence with anterior colporrhaphy, *Obstet Gynecol* 59:269, 1982.
7. Beck RP, McCormick S, Nordstrom L: A 25-year experience with 519 anterior colporrhaphy procedures, *Obstet Gynecol* 78:1011, 1991.
8. Bhatia NN, Bergman A: Urodynamic predictability of voiding following incontinence surgery, *Obstet Gynecol* 631:85, 1984.
9. Borstad E, Rud T: The risk of developing urinary stress incontinence after vaginal repair in continent women: a clinical and urodynamic follow-up study, *Acta Obstet Gynecol Scand* 68:545, 1989.
10. Bump RC, Fantl JA, Hurt WG: Dynamic urethral pressure profilometry pressure transmission ratio determinations after continence surgery: understanding the mechanism of success, failure, and complications, *Obstet Gynecol* 72:870, 1988.
11. Burgio KL, Robinson JC, Engel BT: The role of biofeedback in Kegel exercise training for stress urinary incontinence, *Am J Obstet Gynecol* 154:58, 1986.
12. Copenhaver EH: *Surgery of the vulva and vagina: a practical guide,* Philadelphia, 1981, WB Saunders.
13. DeLancey JOL: Correlative study of paraurethral anatomy, *Obstet Gynecol* 68:91, 1986.
14. DeLancey JOL: Anatomic aspects of vaginal eversion after hysterectomy, *Am J Obstet Gynecol* 166:1717, 1992.
15. DeLancey JOL: Structural support of the urethra as it relates to stress urinary incontinence: the hammock hypothesis, *Am J Obstet Gynecol* 170:1713, 1994.
16. Dougherty MC et al: Graded pelvic muscle exercises: effect on stress urinary incontinence, *J Reprod Med* 38:684, 1993.
17. Ferguson KL, McKey PL, Bishop KR, et al: Stress urinary incontinence: effect of pelvic muscle exercise, *Obstet Gynecol* 75:671, 1990.
18. Figurnov KM: Surgical treatment of urinary incontinence in women, *Akush Ginekol (Mosk)* 6:7, 1949.
19. Frank RT: Operation for cure of incontinence of urine in the female, *Am J Obstet Gynecol* 55:618, 1947.
20. Franz R: Levator plastik bei relativen Harn inkontinenz, *Gynakologe* 137:393, 1954.
21. Friedman EA, Meltzer RN: Collagen mesh prosthesis for repair of endopelvic fascial defect, *Am J Obstet Gynecol* 106:430, 1970.
22. Gainey HL: Motion picture and personal communication.
23. Gallo D: Ocejo modification of interposition operation. In *Urologica ginecologica,* Guadalajara, 1969, Gallo.
24. Gardiner SH: Vaginal surgery for stress incontinence, *Clin Obstet Gynecol* 6:178, 1963.
25. Gardy M, Kozminski M, DeLancey J, et al: Stress incontinence and cystoceles, *J Urol* 145:1211, 1991.
26. Ghoniem GM, Walters F, Lewis V: The value of the vaginal pack test in large cystoceles, *J Urol* 152:931, 1994.
27. Gosling JA: The structure of the female lower urinary tract and the pelvic floor, *Urol Clin North Am* 12:207, 1985.
28. Green TH: Development of a plan for the diagnosis and treatment of urinary stress incontinence, *Am J Obstet Gynecol* 83:632, 1962.

29. Halban J: *Gynakologische operationslehre,* Berlin, 1932, Urban & Schwarzenberg.

30. Hodgkinson CP: Stress urinary incontinence, *Am J Obstet Gynecol* 108:1141, 1970.

31. Horbach NS, Ostergard DR: Predicting intrinsic sphincter dysfunction in women with stress urinary incontinence, *Obstet Gynecol* 84:188, 1994.

32. Huffman JW, Osborne SL, Sokol JK: Electrical stimulation in the treatment of intractable stress incontinence, *Arch Phys Med* 33:674, 1952.

33. Hutch JA: A new theory of the anatomy of the internal urinary sphincter and the physiology of micturition, *Obstet Gynecol* 30:309, 1967.

34. Ingelman-Sundberg A: Stress incontinence of urine, *J Obstet Gynaecol Br Emp* 59:699, 1952.

35. Inmon WB: Personal communication, 1976.

36. Kegel AH: Progressive resistance exercise in the functional restoration of the perineal muscles, *Am J Obstet Gynecol* 56:238, 1948.

37. Kegel AH: Physiologic therapy for urinary stress incontinence, *JAMA* 146:915, 1951.

38. Kelly HA: Incontinence of urine in women, *Urol Cutan Rev* 1:291, 1913.

39. Krige CF: *Vaginal hysterectomy and genital prolapse repair,* Johannesburg, South Africa, 1965, Witwatersrand Press.

40. Lahodny J: Urethrovesikalsuspension mit autologem Fasziengewebe auf rein vaginalem Weg—Kurzarmschlingenoperation, *Geburtshilfe Frauenheilkd* 44:104, 1984.

41. Martius H: *Martius' gynecological operations,* Boston, 1956, Little, Brown (Translated by M McCall, K Bolten).

42. McGuire EJ: Urodynamics findings in patients after failure of stress incontinence operations, *Prog Clin Biol Res* 78:381, 1981.

43. McGuire EJ, Gardy M, Elkins T, DeLancey JO: Treatment of incontinence with pelvic prolapse, *Urol Clin North Am* 18:349, 1991.

44. Milley PS, Nichols DH: The relationships between the pubourethral ligaments and urogenital diaphragm in the human female, *Anat Rec* 163:433, 1969.

45. Moir JC: The gauze-hammock operation, *J Obstet Gynaecol Br Commonw* 75:1, 1968.

46. Moore J, Armstrong JT, Wills SH: The use of tantalum mesh in cystocele with critical report of ten cases, *Am J Obstet Gynecol* 69:1127, 1955.

47. Muellner SR: The anatomies of the female urethra, *Obstet Gynecol* 14:429, l959.

48. Nichols DH, Milley PS: Identification of pubourethral ligaments and their role in transvaginal surgical correction of stress incontinence, *Am J Obstet Gynecol* 115:123, 1973.

49. Nichols DH: The Mersilene mesh gauze-hammock in repair of severe recurrent urinary stress incontinence. In Taymor ML, Green TH, editors: *Progress in gynecology,* vol 6, New York, 1975, Grune & Stratton.

50. Nichols DH: Anterior colporrhaphy technique to shorten a pathologically long vaginal wall, *Int Surg* 64:69, 1979.

51. Nichols DH, Randall CL: *Vaginal surgery,* ed 4, Baltimore, 1996, Williams & Wilkins.

52. Nichols DH, editor: *Reconstructive gynecologic surgery,* ed 2, St Louis, 1997, Mosby.

53. Peattie AP, Plevnik S, Stanton SL: Vaginal cones: a conservative method for treating genuine stress incontinence, *Br J Obstet Gynaecol* 95:1049, 1988.

54. Reiffenstuhl G: The clinical significance of the connective tissue planes and spaces, *Clin Obstet Gynecol* 25:811, 1982.

55. Resnick NM: Urinary incontinence in the older woman. In Kursh ED, McGuire EJ, editors: *Female urology,* Philadelphia, 1994, JB Lippincott.

56. Ricci JV, Thom CH: Uterovaginal extirpation for procidentia, *Am J Surg* 83:192, 1952.

57. Richardson AC, Lyons JB, Williams NL: A new look at pelvic relaxation, *Am J Obstet Gynecol* 126:568, 1976.

58. Royston GD, Rose DK: A new operation for cystocele, *Am J Obstet Gynecol 33:421, 1937.*

59. Sand PK, Richardson DA, Staskin DR, et al: Pelvic floor electrical stimulation in the treatment of genuine stress incontinence: a multicenter, placebo-controlled trial, *Am J Obstet Gynecol* 173:72, 1995.

60. Shull BL, Baden WF: A six-year experience with paravaginal defect repair for stress urinary incontinence, *Am J Obstet Gynecol* 160:1432, 1989.

61. Sims JM: *Clinical notes on uterine surgery,* London, 1866, Robert Hardwicke.

62. Symmonds RE, Jordan LT: Iatrogenic stress incontinence of urine, *Am J Obstet Gynecol* 82:1231, 1961.

63. Uhlenhuth E, Hunter DT: *Problems in the anatomy of the pelvis,* Philadelphia, 1953, JB Lippincott.

64. Van Duzen RE: The cystoscopic appearance of various types of cystoceles, *South Med J* 23:580, 1930.

65. Van Rooyen AJL, Liebenberg HC: Clinical approach to urinary incontinence in females, *Obstet Gynecol* 53:1, 1979.

66. Veronikis DK, Nichols DH, Wakamatsu MM: The incidence of low-pressure urethra as a function of prolapse-reducing techniques in patients with massive pelvic organ prolapse, *Am J Obstet Gynecol* 177:1305, 1997.

67. Von Peham H, Amreich J: *Operative gynecology,* Philadelphia, 1934, JB Lippincott (Translated by LK Ferguson).

68. Wall LL, Norton PA, DeLancey JOL: *Practical urogynecology,* Baltimore, 1993, Williams & Wilkins.

69. Watkins TJ: The treatment of cystocele and uterine prolapse after the menopause, *Am Gynecol Obstet J* 15:420, 1899.

70. Watkins TJ: Treatment of cases of extensive cystocele and uterine prolapse, *Surg Gynecol Obstet* 2:659, 1906.

71. Watson BP: Imperfect urinary control following childbirth and its surgical treatment, *Br Med J* 11:566, 1924.

72. Weber AM, Walters MD: Anterior vaginal prolapse: review of anatomy on techniques of surgical repair, *Obstet Gynecol* 89:311, 1997.

73. Wertheim E: Zur plastischen Verwendung des Uterus bei Prolapsen, *Centralbl f Gynäk,* 23:369, 1899.

74. White GR: Cystocele—a radical cure by suturing lateral sulci of vagina to the white line of pelvic fascia, *JAMA* 53:1707, 1909.

75. Word BH Jr, Montgomery HA: *Paravaginal fascial repair,* Motion picture and personal communications, 1989.

76. Zacharin RF: The suspensory mechanism of the female urethra, *J Anat* 97:423, 1963.

77. Zacharin RF: A Chinese anatomy—the pelvic supporting tissues of the Chinese and Occidental female compared and contrasted, *Aust N Z J Obstet Gynaecol* 17:11, 1977.

78. Zacharin RF: Free full-thickness vaginal epithelium graft in correction of recurrent genital prolapse, *Aust N Z J Obstet Gynaecol* 32:146, 1992.

79. Zirkovic F, Tamussino K, Haas J: Contribution of the posterior compartment to the urinary continence mechanism, *Obstet Gynecol* 91:229, 1998.

22 Rectocele and Perineal Defect

DAVID H. NICHOLS

Damage to the structures of the posterior vaginal wall or their supporting attachments may result from one or more types of injury. A carefully taken history and a thorough physical examination in the office should clarify the type of injury, the site, and the degree of damage to all demonstrable components of the posterior vaginal wall. The examination should include an evaluation of vaginal caliber, tone, and support with the patient not only prone and relaxed on the examining table, but also erect, both with and without voluntary bearing-down efforts. The strength of voluntary contraction of the pubococcygei and external anal sphincter muscles should be noted. Only by considering the findings under all conditions is it possible for a surgeon to select the operative procedure most likely to restore normal relationships and functions.

Posterior colporrhaphy and perineorrhaphy are separate and distinct surgical operations.[29,36] Some patients require one of the operations, some the other, and many both (Fig. 22-1). Satisfactory correction of only one defect when more than one is present may compound the patient's symptoms and functional problems. Each defect should be recognized and surgically corrected by an appropriate combination of operative procedures to achieve an optimal postoperative result.

The goal of treatment of rectocele is to reduce to normal the size of an overly large and usually asymmetric rectal reservoir, not to eliminate the reservoir altogether. In most instances of rectocele, transvaginal plication of the perirectal fascia, the muscularis of the anterior rectal wall and submucosa, and an appropriate perineal reconstruction will correct the problem.

An unexpectedly shortened and persistently uncomfortable vagina after posterior colporrhaphy can result in dyspareunia. To minimize this complication, a full-length posterior vaginal wall reconstruction may be used in selected cases. Furthermore, if a patient has developed a weakness and thinning throughout the posterior wall of the vagina and the surgeon elects to repair only the lower part of that weakness by standard perineorrhaphy without colporrhaphy, the persistence of disturbed function or an early recurrence, probably with a troublesome exacerbation of symptoms, is predictable; operative treatment by full-length posterior colporrhaphy is necessary in this instance. The normal support that the voluntary pelvic muscles give to the pelvic organs is effectively paralyzed by anesthesia, and pelvic examination under anesthesia may lead to an erroneous diagnosis of rectocele and perineal defect. For this reason, as Jeffcoate[20]

and Porges[33] have noted, the need for and the extent of a posterior vaginal wall repair can best be determined preoperatively by examining the *unanesthetized* patient.

POSTERIOR VAGINAL WALL WEAKNESS

Weakness of the posterior vaginal wall generally is a late effect of the trauma of labor and delivery. Marks[26] described rectocele in terms of postobstetric dehiscence of the rectovaginal septal tissues, permitting overdistention and thinning of the adjacent anterior rectal wall. As the perineal belly and lower rectovaginal fascial supports weaken, the apex of the defect moves inferiorly and anteriorly relative to the sphincter, and abdominal straining during defecation compounds the problem by pushing the bolus of stool farther from the anal opening.[8] This funnel-like distortion of the lower rectum is thus concentrated on the anterior rectal wall.

Rectocele and its associated symptoms of incomplete bowel movements, often requiring manual expression to achieve evacuation, usually becomes worse with the relaxation of pelvic supportive tissues coincident with aging. Aging and loss of hormone support reduce vaginal elasticity, which may lead to damage from overdistention of the vagina. There may be a congenital underdevelopment of the perineal musculature and elastic tissues, often because of associated abnormal innervation (as may be suspected with a coexistent spina bifida occulta). The attachments of the perineal body to the rectovaginal septum may have been avulsed by trauma, or the perineal body, vagina, and rectum may have been separated from the fibrous attachments of the levator ani–pelvic diaphragm complex. Laceration of the rectovaginal septum and Denonvilliers' fascia may obliterate the rectovaginal space, resulting in fusion of the anterior capsule of the rectum to the capsule of the posterior wall of the vagina. In addition, a rectocele (i.e., a herniation or ballooning of the rectum and posterior vaginal wall into the lumen of the vagina) may result from the traction associated with progressive procidentia of a general prolapse.

Sullivan et al.[41] and Capps[8] also have noted that plication of the anal sphincter without correction of coincident and asymptomatic rectocele increases anal outlet resistance and may convert an asymptomatic rectocele to a symptomatic one requiring future secondary repair. Thus, if an anal sphincter plication is to be done, even an asymptomatic rectocele should be repaired simultaneously. Proper repair providing freedom from unexpected rectal outlet obstruction decreases the venous stasis in the terminal hemorrhoidal vessels (coincident to straining at stool), reducing the reformation, progression, and severity of coincident hemorrhoidal disease.

The straining efforts associated with chronic constipation can aggravate minor degrees of damage to the rectal wall and its connective tissue supports. Repeated interference with the progress of the fecal stream may prevent the normal completion of defecation, resulting in physiologic or functional obstruction as the redundant sacculation of the rectum becomes larger and the residual stool stimulates more ineffectual straining. A rectocele may be caused by pulsion or by repeatedly increased intraabdominal pressure, a factor more often evident during a patient's postmenopausal years when atrophic changes decrease the elasticity of the vaginal wall and the integrity of the supporting tissues.

ANORECTAL INCONTINENCE

Definitive avenues of investigation including manometry, continence tests, endorectal ultrasound, and electromyography[7,14,28,30] should be followed for patients who have anorectal incontinence. Colonic transit studies also may be useful. When defecography is employed in the study of patients with defecation disorders, it appears that its main role is to document rectal wall changes during defecation straining as possible causes of evacuation difficulties. Distinct outpocketings of the rectal wall during defecation may be seen along with rectal intussusception, or a combination may be seen.[32] Defecography may demonstrate a pathologic inability of the patient to relax the pelvic floor muscles, creating one cause of obstructed defecation.

Defecography may provide useful information in patients with rectal incontinence and outlet obstruction constipation symptoms. It has little additive value to anorectal manometry in incontinent patients without such symptoms.[34] Defecography is particularly helpful in detecting rectal intussusceptions. However, measurements of anorectal angle and junction in incontinent patients are not significantly different from those in asymptomatic controls. A history of chronic constipation and straining of stool precedes development of fecal incontinence in about half of incontinent patients.

A functional pouch of the *posterior* rectal wall (Fig. 22-2) can be visualized by defecography, and this has been named *posterior rectocele*[9] (Fig. 22-3). Parks[31] notes that "defecography demonstrates abnormalities of the rectal wall. These studies complement, but do not replace, good clinical examination and sound professional judgment." In our present state of knowledge, defecographic measurements cannot be regarded as reliable indicators of the complex physiologic condition of the pelvic floor muscles. Fluoroscopic findings may better demonstrate the ability to evacuate the rectum or to retain rectal content.

It seems likely that postevacuation contraction and closure of the external anal sphincter may be delayed or compromised by the presence of retained rectal stool (as with some symptomatic rectoceles) or anal mucosal or rectal

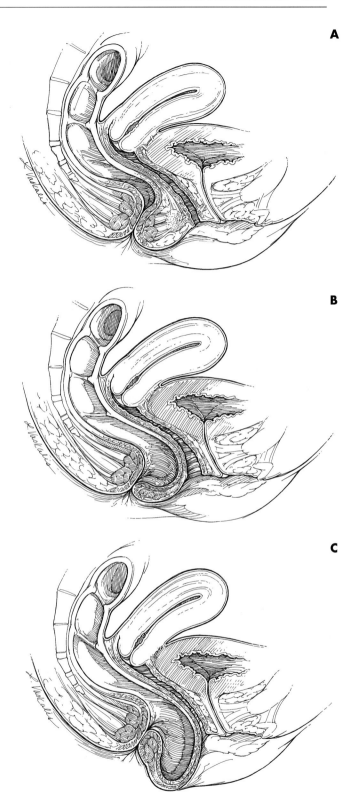

Fig. 22-1   A, Normal relationship between vagina and rectum. **B,** A major perineal defect is seen. There is no rectocele, but restoration of the perineal body is indicated. **C,** A major perineal defect with rectocele. In this circumstance, perineorrhaphy should be accompanied by an appropriate posterior colporrhaphy.

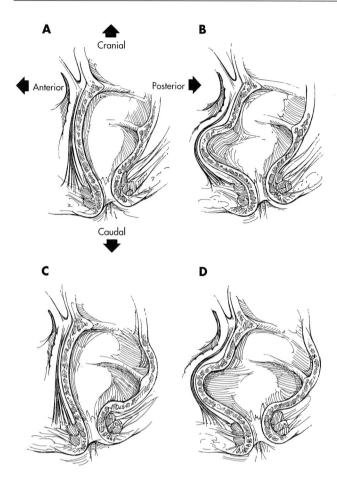

Fig. 22-2 Sagittal views of both anterior and posterior rectocele. **A,** Normal rectum; the vagina is to the left. **B,** Anterior rectocele displacing the vagina. **C,** The rare posterior rectocele. **D,** Combined anterior and posterior rectoceles. (From Nichols DH, Randall CL: *Vaginal surgery,* ed 4, Baltimore, 1966, Williams & Wilkins.)

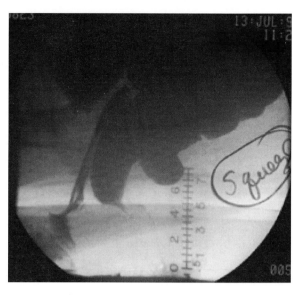

Fig. 22-3 Posterior rectocele. The radiologically opacified vagina is noted to the left of the photograph and the rectum to the right. Notice the rectocele arising from the posterior wall of the rectum. (Courtesy Linda Brubaker, MD.)

prolapse. Perhaps this is part of some anorectal reflex mechanism, and it can result in postevacuation rectal soiling.

When the unanesthetized patient is unable to voluntarily contract her pubococcygei and external anal sphincter during pelvic examination, one should suspect the possibility of causative defective innervation of these muscles. Although occasionally this is of congenital origin (e.g., spina bifida occulta), a more likely explanation is an acquired pudendal neuropathy, as from pathologic stretching of the pudendal nerves during labor and delivery with subsequent atrophy of the damaged nerves.[18,38,39] This can be confirmed by electromyography.[42]

Some report good correlation between noninvasive surface electromyography using an intraanal plug electrode and anal manometry. Tests of pudendal nerve terminal motor latency can reveal unsuspected neuropathy in persons with traumatic fecal incontinence, and combined with anal endosonography can help in the selection of patients for surgery.[13] The thickness and length of the anterior anal sphincters are substantial, as can be demonstrated by endorectal ultrasound and by magnetic resonance imaging. This fact

has an obvious implication in planning and executing the surgical reconstruction of a sphincter defect.[1]

Anatomic Types of Rectocele

Many women who have a rectocele are not constipated, and many women who do not have a rectocele are constipated. The primary symptoms of rectocele, however, are aching after a bowel movement and such difficulty in evacuating the bowel completely that manual expression may be necessary. Effective posterior colporrhaphy should relieve these symptoms but is likely to relieve constipation only if the constipation results from the presence of a pocket of the rectal wall that repeatedly traps stool, precluding complete emptying of the bowel.

The gynecologist who is planning the repair of a rectocele must first determine which type of rectocele is present.[28] The posterior vaginal wall may exhibit three basic types of damage:

1. The full thickness of the vaginal wall may be stretched and attenuated, usually as a result of overdistention during childbirth, and some of the intrinsic elasticity of the fibromuscular vaginal tube may be permanently lost. The damage is greatest where the vaginal wall is farthest removed from its anchoring attachments; damage to the anterior and posterior walls is greater than is damage to the lateral vaginal walls, because the vagina is fixed or attached to the lateral walls. Like cystoceles, a rectocele is associated with the flattening of the rugal folds over its site and is likely to be progressive in its development.

2. The lateral attachments of the vagina to the pelvic sidewall, particularly the vaginal portion of the cardinal ligament, may be stretched as a result of increased intraabdominal pressure or as a result of the vagina's

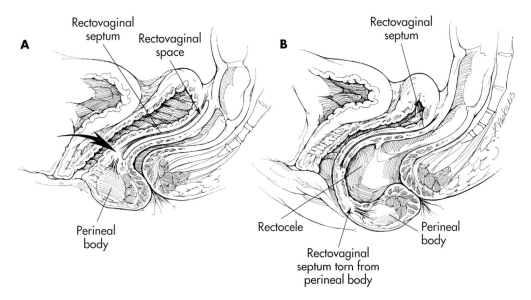

Fig. 22-4 The potential effect of rupture of the rectal vaginal septum. **A,** During childbirth and before hysterectomy, the rectal vaginal septum has been torn from its attachment to the perineal body *(arrow)*. An unrelated abdominal hysterectomy had been performed. **B,** This defect has permitted the development of a large low rectocele between the torn ends, which are now further apart. (From Nichols DH, Randall CL: *Vaginal surgery,* ed 4, Baltimore, Williams & Wilkins, 1996.)

slowness to dilate adequately during labor, causing a roll of undilating vaginal wall to be pushed along during the descent of the presenting part, much as a coat sleeve is turned inside out. Vaginal rugae are generally preserved in the redundant vaginal wall involved in such a rectocele.

3. The lateral attachments of the vagina to the pelvic connective tissue may have been not only stretched, but also torn from the lateral vaginal walls, only to reunite with fusion by scarring and fibrosis at a lower level in the pelvis. Because the refusion is often quite dense and fibrous, this is probably the origin of the nonprogressive, postobstetric prolapse described by Malpas.[25]

All types of damage may coexist in the same patient, producing a combination defect. In addition, each is frequently associated with a defective perineum.

Sites of Damage

Damage may occur to the lower, middle, or upper portions of the posterior vaginal wall in any combination. Damage to the midvagina, which has been referred to as the rectal portion of the posterior vaginal wall, is perhaps the most common. This may be the only lesion that requires repair. Damage in the upper vagina may be noted either as a high rectocele, an enterocele, a potential enterocele, or a widened posterior fornix that may subsequently be narrowed by surgery.

True Low Rectocele. A rather major and inadequately repaired obstetric laceration of the perineum that disrupts the attachments of the levator ani (fascia of the pubococcygeal portion) or the bulbospongiosus muscles to the perineal body and lower vagina may result in a true low rectocele. Either injury may occur without producing a midvaginal or high rectocele. When additional etiologic factors are present, such as a defective or absent Denonvilliers' fascia, as may occur if enterocele has divided its layers, a coexistent middle or high vaginal rectocele may develop.

Most frequently, the injury that produces a low rectocele is a shearing of the lower attachments of the rectovaginal septum and Denonvilliers' fascia from their attachment to the superior portion of the perineal body. A marked gaping or eversion of the introitus usually is evident (Fig. 22-4). Although this causes some loss of support to the sides of the urethra, bladder function is only slightly disturbed unless the urogenital diaphragm also has been torn or the pelvis denervated.[38,39,42] The length of the perineum approximates the length of the urethra, and perineal weakness may disturb the closure mechanism of the proximal urethra.[46] A low rectocele aggravates any tendency to constipation because of the decreased effectiveness and correspondingly increased bearing-down effort during defecation.

Midvaginal Rectocele. Although a midvaginal rectocele also is a late result of obstetric injury, the damage usually does not involve the levator ani; the vaginal attachment and effective support of the pelvic diaphragm are below this area of involvement. The pathologic stretching and laceration of the connective tissues between the vagina and the rectum not only leave these tissues pathologically thin, but also lead to adhesions that fuse the rectal and vaginal capsules to the rectovaginal septum. Such a fusion tends to eliminate the ability of the rectum and the vagina to function independently; the vaginal wall must not only follow the contour of the rectal wall but also must, to some extent, participate in rectal function as well. This is likely to result in persistent difficulties with constipation and defecation. A bearing-down sensation, discomfort after a bowel movement, and inability to empty the bowel completely are the usual symptoms.

A midvaginal rectocele often coexists with a high rectocele, and, if planning to repair one, the surgeon should repair both. As emphasized by Goff,[15] surgery in the midvaginal area should be designed to preserve or restore independent movement of the posterior vaginal and the anterior rectal walls; only at the level of the perineal body should the vaginal and rectal walls be fused in the reconstruction of the posterior vaginal wall. To accomplish this goal, the surgeon must carefully identify and preserve the relatively avascular tissue relationships in the rectovaginal space.

High Rectocele. Like the midvaginal rectocele, a high rectocele usually is the result of a pathologic overstretching of the posterior vaginal wall. In this instance, however, the anterolateral attachments of the cardinal ligaments (hypogastric sheath) bind the vagina and cervix together to such an extent that the cervix functions almost as a part or extension of the anterior vaginal wall.[12,28]

The length of the anterior vaginal wall plus the diameter of the cervix normally equals the length of the posterior vaginal wall. The cranial envelope of the rectovaginal space terminates at the most caudal portion of the pouch of Douglas. This ensures flexibility and mobility but also, with the rectovaginal space, forms a more or less frictionless inclined plane down which the structures anterior to the rectovaginal space can slide without disturbing those primarily rectal structures posterior to the rectovaginal space. Thus, although classic procidentia begins as an eversion of the upper vagina, it usually permits the entire uterus and much of the bladder to extend outside the bony pelvis. An enterocele develops, and the cervix, uterus, and bladder may drop as though in a sliding hernia. (All this often occurs without an accompanying rectocele.)

Such a descensus, noticeably involving the bladder, has been considered evidence of primarily anterior segment damage and usually is the result of chronically increased intraperitoneal pressure. However, it could result from damage sustained during the first stage of labor if bearing-down efforts or attempts to accomplish delivery were made before the cervix was fully dilated. Therefore anterior segment damage per se may not be mechanistically related to damage to the levator ani or its sheath.

In discussing enteroceles, Malpas[25] described prolapse of the vaginal vault with an obvious peritoneal sac, the bulge usually containing omentum or a loop of intestine. The upper rectum forms the posterior wall of the sac, and a high rectocele may coexist with such a prolapse. Because the peritoneal fusion of Denonvilliers' fascia is missing from the posterior vaginal wall that covers an enterocele, support to both the anterior rectal wall and the posterior vaginal wall in this area is lost, and a high rectocele may develop. Similarly, a high rectocele may be associated with a congenital deepening of the pouch of Douglas, because there is no Denonvilliers' fascia to support the anterior rectal wall in this situation either.

On the other hand, a uterovaginal or sliding prolapse does not involve the high rectum, so the peritoneal descent affects only the anterior wall of the pouch of Douglas, usually without dilation of the peritoneal sac. A high posterior colporrhaphy with careful excision of the entire peritoneal pouch is an essential part of the repair of a total vault prolapse, but, because a uterovaginal prolapse may not compromise the integrity of the rectum itself, the major objective of repair is to shorten the cardinal–uterosacral ligament complex and reattach it to the vault of the vagina. When the strength of the cardinal–uterosacral ligament complex is inadequate, coincident sacrospinous or sacral colpopexy may be used to support the vaginal vault (see Chapter 26).

POSTERIOR COLPORRHAPHY AND THE RECTOVAGINAL SEPTUM

When a full-length posterior vaginal reconstruction is performed immediately after vaginal hysterectomy, the progress of blunt finger dissection of the "avascular rectovaginal space" is consistently obstructed at the vaginal apex near the cut edge of the vaginal vault by a thin, but firm, membrane. This membrane usually requires a distinct incision for penetration.

Existence of the Rectovaginal Septum

Tobin and Benjamin[43] concluded that the tissue described by Denonvilliers in the male included two layers: the ventral peritoneal fusion layer and a dorsal or posterior layer composed of rectal fascia. After studying the gynecologic relevance of this information, Ricci and Thom[35] and Uhlenhuth and Nolley[44] reached almost diametrically opposed conclusions; however, their differences in methodology may explain their differences of opinion. The evidence that led Ricci and Thom to deny the existence of "fascial tissue" in the integrity of the vaginal walls was based entirely on the study of hematoxylin and eosin stained histologic preparations and involved no correlation with gross anatomic dissections. The studies of Weber and Walters[45] have demonstrated an abundance of pelvic connective tissue adventitia, but no vaginal "fascia." They describe the adventitia as a "variably discrete connective tissue layer of collagen and elastin between the muscular wall of the vagina and the adjacent paravaginal connective tissue." They have shown that "lateral paravaginal tissue is composed of loose areolar tissue containing blood vessels, lymphatics, and nerves embedded in fat." Uhlenhuth and Nolley, on the other hand, based their conclusion solely on gross dissection and made no attempt at histologic correlation or confirmation.

To reconcile these controversial reports, Milley and Nichols conducted simultaneous studies of both the gross anatomy and related histologic specimens.[27] These studies demonstrated a rectovaginal septum that can be identified as a distinct and relatively strong connective tissue layer between the vagina and the rectal walls (Fig. 22-5). Extending in a curved coronal plane, somewhat in conformity with the curvature of the bony pelvis, this septal structure is attached cranially to the caudal peritoneum and the rectouterine pouch of Douglas and extends inferiorly to its caudal fusion with the perineal body. The tissues of this septum are always adherent to the posterior aspect of the vaginal connective tissue but can easily be separated from it by blunt dissection. The demonstrable dense adherence of the septum to the "vaginal wall" explains, at least partially, why its existence has at times been denied.

In transverse and coronal dissections, this septum was found to curve posterolaterally, paralleling the course of the paracolpium and blending laterally with the parietal layer of the pelvic fascia. It varies it character from a thin, readily perforated translucent membrane to a tougher layer of almost leathery consistency. A septum can be identified during dissection, but only when a definite effort to do so is made.

Histologic studies showed that this septum consists of a fibromuscular elastic tissue, including dense collagen, abundant smooth muscle, and coarse elastic fibers that are all readily separable from the fibromuscular elastic tissue of the posterior vaginal wall. In sections stained by orcein, the elastic fibers in the area of the rectovaginal septum appeared larger and coarser than those in the connective tissue within the vaginal wall proper. It is possible that such differences in elastic tissue fibers give the septum its demonstrable integrity during dissection. Appropriate tissue stains are necessary to demonstrate the presence of a septum. The difficulty of demonstrating a rectovaginal septum histologically with standard hematoxylin-eosin staining may be another reason that the existence of this important structure has often been denied.

These observations are of more than academic interest, because the strength and integrity of this membrane are clinically significant and surgically useful. The rectovaginal septum normally facilitates the independent mobility of the rectal and vaginal walls and, as a result, ensures their functional independence. It also acts as a protective barrier to the spread of neoplasia or infection between the rectum and the vagina, as Uhlenhuth and Nolley suggested.[34]

Surgical Significance of the Rectovaginal Septum

Although not emphasized as an identifiable or significant structural entity, the rectovaginal septum appears to have been recognized and carefully restored in the New York Woman's Hospital type of posterior colporrhaphy described by Goff[15] and later in Bullard's modification of Goff's technique.[28] Uhlenhuth and Nolley suggest an explanation for this lack of emphasis or recognition.[44]

> It has been mentioned that the rectovaginal septum adheres closely to the vagina; it is therefore probable that the surgeon, in performing a posterior colporrhaphy, does not get into the space between the vaginal fascia and rectovaginal septum, but into the space between the rectovaginal septum and rectal fascia.

Generally, the surgeon can easily break down a pathologic thickening of the rectovaginal septum during the preliminary dissection. This thickening is caused by scarring within the posterior avascular rectovaginal space and usually is demonstrable during a preoperative rectovaginal examination to determine whether the posterior vaginal wall can be moved independently of the anterior rectal wall. Rupture of the septum, even in the presence of an apparently intact vagina, may result in adhesions that fix the vaginal wall to the underlying rectal wall. This injury can, in turn, lead to uninhibited distention of the rectum, distention of the posterior vaginal wall, formation of a high or midvaginal rectocele, and symptomatic interference with function.

Because the rectovaginal septum normally curves posterolaterally as it becomes attached to the fascia overlying the levator ani, decreasing the vaginal width by approximating the cut edges after the excision of a midportion of the septum increases the pull on the lateral attachments of the septum that tend to direct the vagina posteriorly toward the sacrum. This tension is likely to restore the original and proper upper horizontal vaginal axis. The excision of an upper vaginal wedge of tissue also may be helpful (Fig. 22-6).

In the repair of an obstetric or surgical episiotomy, restoration of the rectovaginal septum as a distinct layer at the apex of the wound not only provides better support, but also ensures better function and increased comfort. This restoration can be readily accomplished by substituting running subcuticular stitches for the usual through-and-through epithelial stitches. In addition to decreasing the patient's postoperative and postpartum discomfort, this procedure effectively prevents epithelial inclusion cysts.

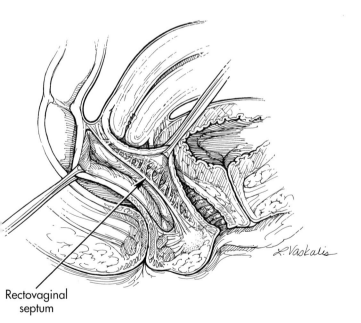

Rectovaginal septum

Fig. 22-5 The rectovaginal septum. It forms the anterior border of the rectovaginal space and has been partly dissected from the underside of the posterior vaginal wall to which it is normally adherent. Note that it is fused to the cranial margin of the perineal body from which it may be torn during labor and delivery.

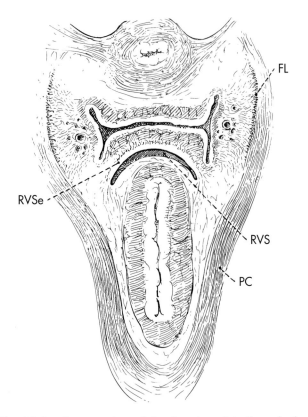

Fig. 22-6 Cross-section of the female pelvis through the lower midportion of the vagina. Note the convex configuration of the pubococcygeus *(PC)*. The rectovaginal space *(RVS)* is indicated between the rectum and vagina, as well as the position of the rectovaginal septum *(RVSe)*. The blood vessels in the connective tissue lateral to the vagina are shown. The fibers of Luschka *(FL)* are shown as they attach the paravaginal connective tissue to the sheaths of the pubococcygei. These connections tend to give the vagina an **H**-shaped configuration. (From Nichols DH, Milley PS: Clinical anatomy of the vulva, vagina, lower pelvis, and perineum. In Sciarra J, editor: *Gynecology and obstetrics,* New York, 1993, Harper & Row.)

The tissues normally supporting the upper third of the vagina are different from those supporting the middle and lower thirds. Harrison and McDonagh[17] wrote that "by far the most commonly neglected step in vaginal plastic procedures is reconstruction of the upper posterior vagina." A low colporrhaphy and perineorrhaphy cannot be expected to provide an anatomically adequate repair of a weakness in the upper third of the vagina. When high rectocele and enterocele coexist, as they frequently do, each must be recognized and repaired separately.

POSTERIOR COLPORRHAPHY WITHOUT PERINEORRHAPHY

When the defect to be repaired involves only the perineal body, reflection and mobilization of the perineal skin and the vaginal membrane should stop at the cranial margin of the perineal body on its vaginal face. When there is a coexistent rectocele of the middle or upper vagina, however, the surgeon should extend the reflection of the vaginal membrane by dissection into the rectovaginal space to a point above the bulge of the rectocele. Any adhesions that bind the anterior wall of the rectum to the full-thickness flap of the posterior vaginal wall should be divided by blunt and, when necessary, sharp dissection.

A patient who has previously undergone an otherwise adequate perineorrhaphy may develop a symptomatic rectocele that may not have been evident at the time of the initial surgery (Fig. 22-7). This herniation may appear to be an enterocele. When the perineal body does not require repair, the surgeon may simply open the posterior vaginal wall directly into the rectovaginal space (Fig. 22-8) through either a transverse (Fig. 22-9) or longitudinal incision into the vagina. This procedure can be performed without denuding or opening the perineum.

With lateral traction on sutures or clamps at the hymenal

Fig. 22-7 A perineorrhaphy may hide an unrepaired midvaginal rectocele. Effective repair must always be *proximal* to the point of weakness.

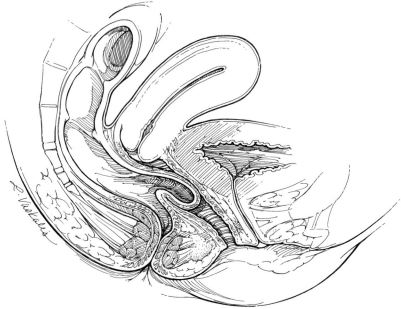

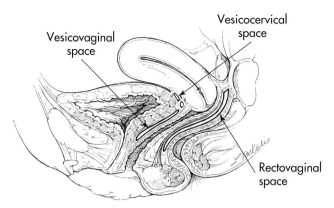

Fig. 22-8 Sagittal section of the normal adult pelvis shows a normal vaginal axis. The fascia of Denonvilliers (the rectovaginal septum) is fused to the undersurface of the posterior vaginal wall and forms the anterior wall of the rectovaginal space. The diagrammatic illustration of continuity between the rectovaginal septum (fascia of Denonvilliers) and the perineal body is shown. Note the rectovaginal, vesicovaginal, and vesicocervical spaces, which permit the organs to function somewhat independently of one another. (From Nichols DH, editor: *Reoperative gynecologic and obstetric surgery*, ed 2, St Louis, 1997, Mosby.)

margin, the surgeon may open the rectovaginal space and establish a line of cleavage between the anterior rectal wall and the connective tissues of the rectovaginal septum, taking care not to open the often attenuated or thinned rectal wall. When episiotomy repairs have resulted in excessive scar tissue, the preliminary insertion of the surgeon's double-gloved finger into the rectum may be advisable for identification and guidance. The surgeon should carry the dissection to free the rectum from the posterior vaginal wall and its adherent septal tissues to a level somewhat superior or cranial to any demonstrable rectocele (Fig. 22-10).

The estimated amount of excess vaginal wall determines the amount of vaginal membrane that should be removed; the excision should involve just enough to permit a normal three-fingerbreadth vaginal introitus and vaginal caliber without demonstrable tightness and stenosis. In deciding the amount of vagina to be removed, the surgeon should take the patient's endocrine age (e.g., future postmenopausal shrinkage and loss of elasticity) into account. DeCosta[11] recommended that the introitus of an older woman be left a little "loose," anticipating that the rigidity of her husband's erection may not be as firm as that in his younger years. In general, it is better to leave too much vaginal skin than too little in a multilayered repair; therefore it is important not to excise any suspected excess vaginal membrane until the repair is essentially complete, at which time the supposed excess of vaginal epithelium often fits surprisingly well over the restored rectovaginal septum.

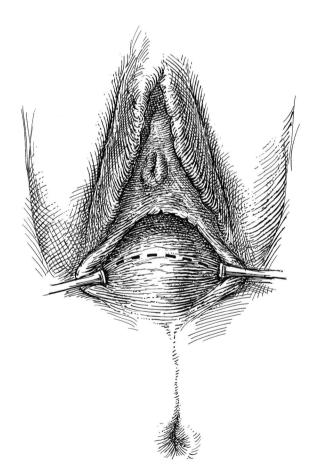

Fig. 22-9 When posterior colporrhaphy without perineorrhaphy is desired, the rectovaginal space may be entered through a transverse incision through the posterior vaginal wall proximal to the perineal body. (Modified from Nichols DH, Randall CL: *Vaginal surgery*, ed 4, Baltimore, 1996, Williams & Wilkins.)

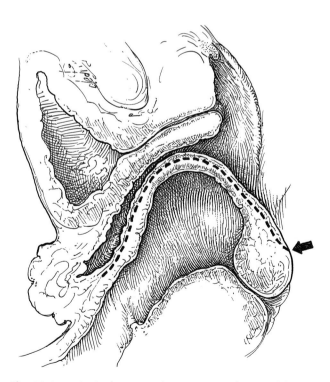

Fig. 22-10 Sagittal section demonstrating the initial line of dissection exposing the full perineum and rectocele. Above the perineum, the dissection enters the rectovaginal space and continues proximal to the highest point of the rectocele. (Modified from Nichols DH, Randall CL: *Vaginal surgery*, ed 4, Baltimore, 1996, Williams & Wilkins.)

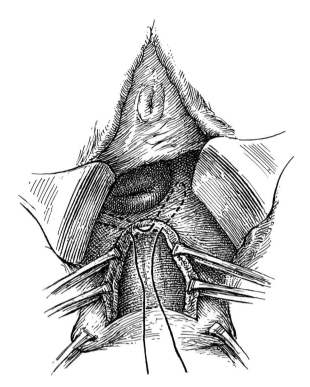

Fig. 22-11 The suture closing the posterior vaginal wall might, at its apex, include a generous bite of the lateral vaginal connective tissue and, when possible, the uterosacral ligaments. (Modified from Nichols DH, Randall CL: *Vaginal surgery*, ed 4, Baltimore, 1996, Williams & Wilkins.)

With a high rectocele, the vaginal incision, as well as the identification and mobilization of the connective tissue that is to become the rectovaginal septum, should be carried to the very apex of the vagina. It may be necessary to cut through the edge of the vaginal cuff to the attachment of the upper portion of the rectovaginal septum to the cul-de-sac. If the upper margin of the portion of the vaginal wall to be removed proves to be higher than the attachment of the rectovaginal septum to the bottom of the pouch of Douglas, the latter is likely to be entered. An open pouch actually is an advantage because it permits the surgeon to identify, shorten, and suture the uterosacral ligaments together under direct vision, incorporating the ligaments in the top of the posterior colporrhaphy. It also provides an opportunity to estimate and excise any excess peritoneum before closure of the pouch, which is particularly appropriate whenever circumstances, such as an excessively wide vault, may predispose the patient to the development of an enterocele.

In the presence of an enterocele, when the posterior vaginal wall has less support from Denonvilliers' fascia, the surgeon often can develop support for the rectovaginal septum by bringing the so-called rectal pillars together in the midline anterior to the rectum. If the uterus has not been removed, the uppermost of the approximating sutures may incorporate the uterosacral ligaments and the posterior aspect of the uterine cervix for additional strength and stability (Fig. 22-11).

Although ballooning of the anterior rectal wall appears to be the result of a rectocele rather than the cause, the surgeon may reduce ballooning by placing one or more layers of running locked 2-0 or 3-0 absorbable suture through the rectal muscularis and the strong submucosal layer[15,23] but *not* including the mucosa, sometimes continuing this downward posterior to the level at which the perineal body is to be reconstructed (see Fig. 22-8). When the correction of ballooning that has increased the size of the rectal reservoir is addressed by a running locked plication, it should be remembered that the submucosa, being the strongest layer of the intestine,[16,19,24] should be included in the stitch. At the same time, the surgeon does not wish the stitch to penetrate the mucous membrane of the rectum. This can be obviated by inserting an overgloved fingertip of the opposite hand into the rectum during the course of this suture placement; this direct palpation will carefully estimate the thickness of the rectal wall and avoid unwelcome penetration of the mucous layer (Fig. 22-12). Then the surgeon closes the full thickness of the posterior vaginal wall from side to side, reconstructs the perineal body, and closes the perineal skin. Even during the performance of a sacrospinous colpopexy, obvious ballooning of the anterior wall of the rectum should be corrected by a running locked stitch of polyglycolic acid suture.

CLASSIC POSTERIOR COLPORRHAPHY

In performing the classic posterior colporrhaphy described by Goff,[15] the surgeon begins by picking up a bite of the hymen and its subcutaneous tissue at approximately the 3- and 9-o'clock positions with a clamp or a suture and anchoring these tissues to the perineal skin lateral to the labia majora to provide lateral traction. (Used only for retraction, these lateral sutures or clamps are removed during the final steps in the reconstruction.) The surgeon then normally makes a narrow V-shaped or wider U-shaped incision through the perineal skin, depending on the size of any perineal defect to be repaired. If an older patient with atrophy and narrowing of the tissues and skin of the perineum wishes to preserve her coital ability, it may be desirable to make only an initial midline skin incision that exposes the subcutaneous tissue of the perineum (Fig. 22-13). Occasionally, an inverted T-shaped incision may be made in the posterior vaginal wall to facilitate access to the rectovaginal space.

After making the initial opening through the perineal skin, the surgeon dissects a segment of skin from the exposed structures of the perineum and perineal body, then continues upward by undermining beneath the full thickness of the posterior wall. Adhesions that thicken the normal attachments of the vaginal membrane may be the result of earlier obstetric damage, and all such attachments should be freed. In addition, in all repairs of a rectocele, it is essential that the vaginal membrane be freed of all appreciable fixation by scar tissue and be separated from all pathologic adhesions to the perineal body and the rectal wall, to a point

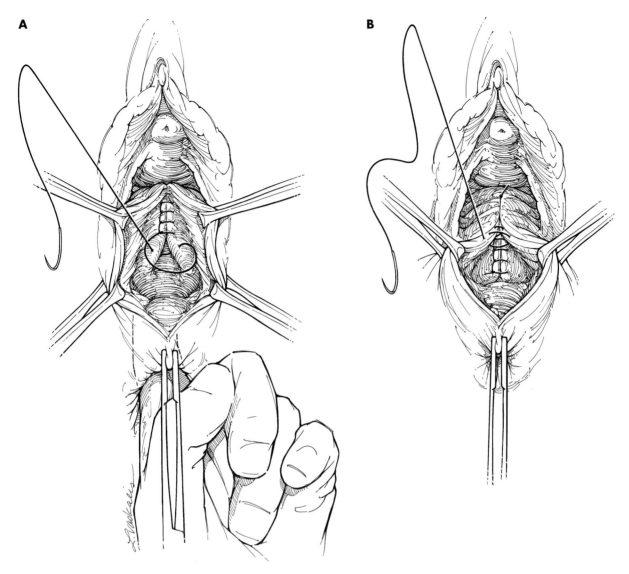

Fig. 22-12   The perirectal fascia, rectal muscularis, and submucosa have been plicated by a running locked stitch. The overgloved finger of the operator, inserted into the rectum, prevents unwanted penetration of the rectal mucosa **(A).** The posterior wall of the vagina is closed by a running subcuticular suture placed in a spiral fashion **(B).**

well above any demonstrable rectocele. The surgeon undermines and frees the perineal skin flaps, exposing the surfaces of what is usually a distorted or irregularly deficient perineum and displaying the defective segments that are to be reconstructed into a more normal perineal body.

After entering the rectovaginal space, the surgeon corrects any anterior ballooning of the rectum as previously described, using one or more layers of running, locked, fine absorbable interrupted sutures placed in the muscularis and connective tissue of the anterior rectal wall, from points both above and below the area of the demonstrable rectocele. An overglove-covered operator's index finger inserted into the patient's rectum during its dissection from perineal body scar tissue, and again during plication of the anterior rectal wall, ensures that good bites will be taken, hopefully

including the submucosa but without penetrating the mucosa itself. This digital maneuver provides a better and more accurate interpretation during surgery of the actual size of the rectal reservoir; any excesses then can be appropriately corrected by suitable plication. Reducing the size of a large rectal reservoir would be expected to improve the efficiency of rectal evacuation.

At the apex, the suture may include a generous bite of the lateral vaginal connective tissue of the paracolpium and, possibly, of the most inferior portion of the uterosacral ligaments, if the incision and dissection were carried into this area.

The rectum may be displaced posteriorly by a retractor; after excision of the estimated excess of vaginal membrane, the cut edges of the full thickness of the posterior

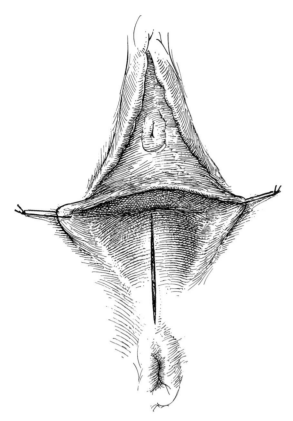

Fig. 22-13 When there is atrophy and narrowing of perineal skin, an initial midline perineal incision may be desirable to expose the base or inferior surface of the perineal body. (Modified from Nichols DH, Randall CL: *Vaginal surgery,* ed 3, Baltimore, 1989, Williams & Wilkins.)

vaginal wall, including the still adherent fibers of the rectovaginal septum, are brought together by a running subcuticular 0 or 2-0 absorbable suture (Fig. 22-14). Carefully and purposefully avoiding attachment to the fascia over the levator ani, the surgeon should continue the running subcuticular suture(s) to the cranial border of the perineal body.

When the use of subcuticular suturing is undesirable because the vaginal wall seems unusually thin, a running locked suture through the full thickness of the posterior vaginal wall, if placed to avoid invagination of the cut edges, may be appropriate to reunite the vaginal membrane in the midline. Although the administration of estrogen for several weeks preoperatively may increase blood loss during the operation, it thickens a vaginal membrane that is noticeably thin (as often occurs after menopause) and facilitates closure and healing. Particularly in the closure of the vaginal membrane, it is important, first, that the sutures bring the tissues together without tension and, second, that the knots be tied loosely enough to avoid blanching the tissues. The risk of tissue strangulation is especially great when interrupted mattress-type sutures are being tied.

In a modification of the frequently used Goff technique, the surgeon may excise a wedge or segment of what is es-

timated to be the proper size and shape from the whole length and full thickness of the posterior vaginal wall, while leaving the septal layer attached.[28] It is important to estimate carefully the amount to be excised, however, if the vaginal circumference is to be sufficient for satisfactory sexual function. The amount of vaginal wall to be retained and therefore the size of the vagina after colporrhaphy vary according to the age of the patient, her parity, and the presence or amount of estrogenic hormones.

The surgeon approximates the lateral cut edges of the vagina, to which the rectovaginal septum has remained fused, by intravaginal subcuticular or interrupted sutures; for the vagina to retain natural independent movement, the rectum and its fascial investments should be uninvolved in this suturing. After this phase of posterior repair, the surgeon should be able to insert a finger between the anterior rectal wall and the reconstituted posterior vaginal wall and rectovaginal septum throughout the full length of the repair, demonstrating that the functional independence of the rectal and vaginal walls has been restored and that there is no iatrogenic fixation of the rectal wall (Fig. 22-15). The attenuated levator fascia may have been united only in the lower half or third of the vagina, which permits a more normal horizontal tilt to the upper vagina. The surgeon finally restores the subvaginal portion of the perineal body by interrupted sutures, continuing the suture line down the vaginal wall, over the perineal body, and back to the hymenal margin.

POSTERIOR COLPORRHAPHY BY LAYERS

The Goff technique of posterior colporrhaphy usually ensures an anatomically acceptable result, but it may not restore the integrity and function of a rectovaginal septum as reliably as the layering technique of Bullard does. Essentially, the layering technique consists of (1) separation of the septal tissues, first from the anterior rectal wall and second from the overlying vaginal membrane, and (2) thickening of the resulting layer of loosely arranged musculoconnective tissue and restoration of an appreciable layer of septum by several plicating stitches of fine suture material. The dissection involves the following steps:

1. The surgeon incises the posterior vaginal wall in the midline to a point well above the rectocele, as far as the apex of the vagina, when a high rectocele or enterocele is present.
2. The surgeon identifies the rectovaginal space and separates the rectal wall by blunt dissection from the over lying connective tissue of the rectovaginal septum, which usually can be done without difficulty.
3. By spreading the points of curved Mayo scissors in demonstrable planes of cleavage, more than by cutting into or through tissue layers, the surgeon reflects the vaginal membrane anteriorly and away from the connective tissue.

These procedures result in (1) a thinned and bulging anterior metal wall that is readily identifiable, (2) a loose and

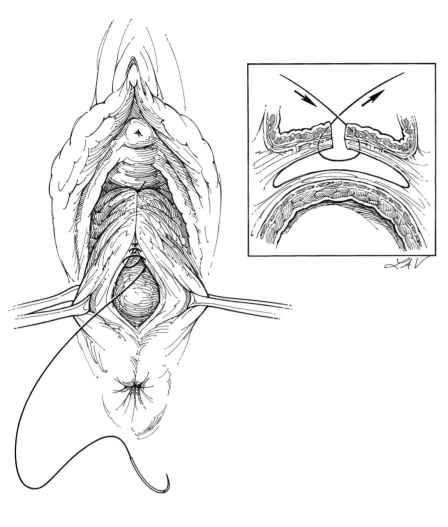

Fig. 22-14   The full thickness of the unsplit but trimmed posterior vaginal wall is brought together by a running subcuticular stitch of 2-0 absorbable suture.

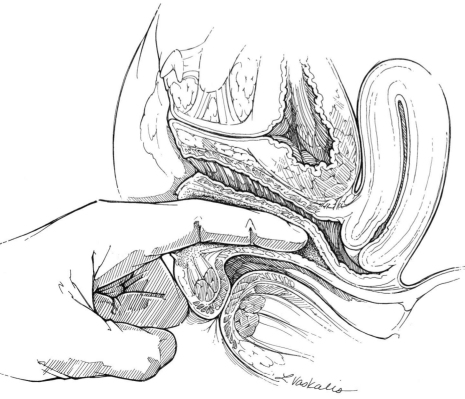

Fig. 22-15   At the completion of the posterior colporrhaphy and before starting the perineorrhaphy, the surgeon should be able to insert an index finger freely between the posterior vaginal wall to which the rectovaginal septum is attached and the anterior surface of the rectum, demonstrating the desired freedom of the plane.

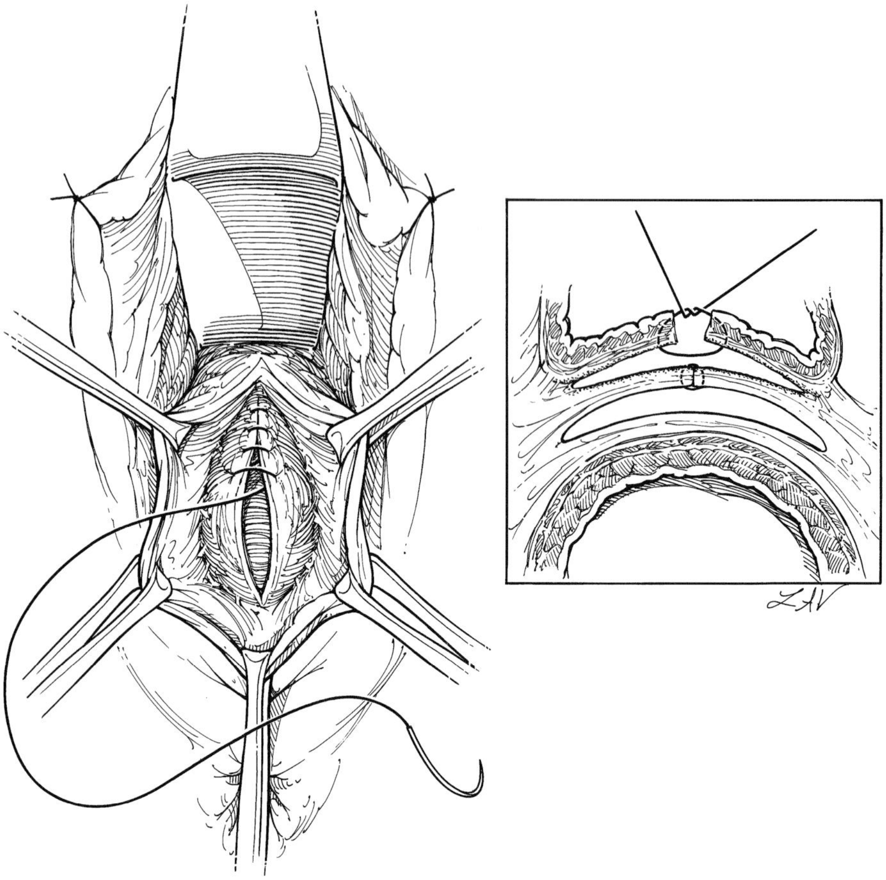

Fig. 22-16 The Bullard modification is shown in which the rectovaginal septum is dissected from the posterior vaginal wall and closed as a separate layer between rectum and vaginal membrane. When this has been accomplished, excess vaginal membrane is trimmed, and the sides are brought by interrupted suture *(inset).* A running subcuticular suture may be used.

somewhat thinned posterior vaginal wall that appears excessive for the caliber of the vagina that is to be restored, and (3) a loosely incomplete, somewhat fragmented, and partially detached layer, often only sections of intervening connective tissues, all of which should be carefully preserved and incorporated by plication with fine suture material into the restoration of a demonstrably stronger rectovaginal septum.

It should be axiomatic that, as a surgeon should not capriciously discard viable tissue that can be incorporated in the repair of a hernia, the gynecologist should not excise tissue that can be used in restoring a rectovaginal septum simply because it is adherent to an assumed excess of posterior vaginal wall that probably will be excised. Rather, the gynecologist should carefully identify a line of cleavage that separates connective tissue from the redundant posterior vaginal membrane and, after thickening by fine plicating sutures, attempt to use this tissue to restore the integrity of a significant rectovaginal septum between the anterior rectal wall and the posterior vaginal membrane. The objective of restoring a recognizable septal layer is the distinctive characteristic of Bullard's modification of Goff's technique of posterior colporrhaphy.

The tissues of the carefully identified rectovaginal septal layer, throughout a width of approximately 3 cm and a length of 5 to 6 cm, are united in the midline. Although thickened by a few plicating sutures, this septum is not at-

tached by suture to either the underlying rectal wall or to the overlying posterior vaginal membrane (Fig. 22-16). It is possible to demonstrate the integrity of this thickened rectovaginal septum and its nonattachment to either the rectal or vaginal walls after the edges of the vagina have been trimmed and reunited in the midline, but before the perineal body has been sutured, by inserting two fingers simultaneously into the space available on either side of the septum, one finger between the septum and vaginal wall and the other between the septum and rectal wall. Reduced adhesion between the layers of repair favors independent mobility of the vagina and the rectum, an important objective of a posterior vaginal repair. A vaginal depth that is too short can be elongated a small amount by incising it transversely and closing it longitudinally.

At the completion of a vaginal repair, an objective evaluation of the result is critical. If the vaginal depth and axis are not satisfactory, it is certainly preferable to make any necessary correction or modification at the time of the initial operation, provided that the patient's condition permits prolongation of the surgery. A vaginal caliber that is tight at the end of surgery will not enlarge after healing is complete. As a matter of fact, if any change occurs, particularly as the patient ages, a tight vagina tends to become even smaller.

If the repair is satisfactory, the surgeon may minimize oozing and collection within the spaces between layers by packing the vagina lightly with 2-inch plain or iodoform gauze, which can be removed the morning of the day after surgery. If the repair has resulted in a vaginal caliber obviously or even suspiciously tight, however, the surgeon may make appropriate relaxing incisions through the thickness of the lateral vaginal walls. When these have been made, the surgeon should pack the vagina rather tightly for a period no longer than 24 hours and an obturator placed in the vaginal cavity to remain in place during the healing process, being removed only during necessary bowel and bladder functions (see Chapter 24). When necessary, full-thickness grafts obtained from the vaginal wall previously resected from either the anterior or the posterior vaginal wall may be cut to size and sewn as a full-thickness patch to fill the defect that has been created. Portions of the vagina that have been excised should be kept wrapped in saline-soaked sponges on the nurse's instrument stand until the conclusion of the operation.

Sutures that are palpated or visualized within the lumen of the rectum should be cut immediately to lessen postoperative pain and the risk of rectovaginal or rectoperineal fistula. The cut ends will promptly retract up and out of the rectal lumen; the loss of that single suture should not jeopardize the effectiveness of the repair.

PERINEORRHAPHY

Historically, one objective of perineorrhaphy was to improve the patient's ability to retain a pessary that could be inserted into the vagina, much as a cork is inserted into the neck of an inverted bottle. Under this unfortunate and incorrect, but popular, concept, a good perineal repair should prevent not only the progression of an upper vaginal prolapse, but also the development of genital prolapse in general. However, the fact that genital prolapse is uncommon among women with unrepaired third- and fourth-degree obstetric lacerations who had long suffered a complete loss of any support that the perineal body would have provided to the uterus, cervix, and upper vagina demonstrates the inadequacy of this concept.

The basic objective of perineorrhaphy is to realign the muscles and connective tissues of the perineal body to a degree that ensures normal relationships and encourages normal, comfortable function. When a patient's perineum is defective or absent, perineorrhaphy increases the vaginal depth (i.e., the length of the posterior vaginal wall; Fig. 22-17).

Defects in the Perineum

A relaxed perineum, which may or may not coexist with a demonstrable rectocele, is rarely caused by inadequate innervation of the muscles that contribute to the support of the components or the perineal body.[38,39,42] More commonly, it is the result of overdistention during parturition or, occasionally, the result of a poorly repaired or unrepaired obstetric laceration of the perineum. When the perineum is the sole or major site of damage, the virtual absence of the perineal body exposes an otherwise normal posterior vaginal wall to a pathologic degree, accounting for the condition

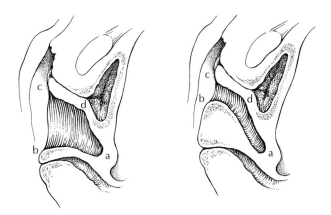

Fig. 22-17 The effect of perineorrhaphy after lengthening the posterior vaginal wall is demonstrated. Sagittal drawing of the pelvis of a patient with a defective perineum is shown on the left. The anterior vaginal wall *(adc)* is longer than the posterior wall *(ab)*. The lengthening of the posterior vagina *(ab)* after perineorrhaphy is shown on the right. The length of the anterior vaginal wall *(adc)* is unchanged. (From Nichols DH, Randall CL: *Vaginal surgery,* ed 4, Baltimore, 1996, Williams & Wilkins.)

known as pseudorectocele. In this case, the insertion of the examining finger into the rectum reveals no abnormality in rectal caliber, angulation, or tone and no irregular distensibility of the anterior rectal wall; in addition, the posterior vaginal and anterior rectal walls are independently mobile. Symptoms are usually minimal, and the patient is often considered a candidate for perineal reconstruction or perineorrhaphy only when other surgery, such as vaginal hysterectomy or anterior colporrhaphy, is indicated.

Congenital absence of the perineum leaves the posterior vaginal wall exposed and simulates the appearance of rectocele, which may not be present. This condition, too, may be termed a pseudorectocele. Proper treatment requires surgical reconstruction of the defective perineum with the use of whatever tissues are available. When an acquired defect is repaired, the tissues to be reapproximated were previously in apposition, and innervation can be expected to be normal; when a congenital defect is repaired, however, connective tissues and muscle must be appropriated from the nearest fibromuscular layers.

An incomplete perineal repair leads to lateral retraction of the muscles that are normally attached to the perineal body. Detachment or interruption of the transverse perineum and the bulbospongiosus muscle must be recognized and corrected. Repair of such a detachment helps to support not only the anterior wall of the rectum, but also the anterior wall of the lower vagina and urethra. In this connection, it should be remembered that the length of the perineal body effectively approximates the length of the female urethra, in part because the medial portion of the pubococcygeal muscle, as it passes along the sides of the vagina, urethra, and rectum, sends slips of connective tissue to fuse with the capsule tissue that invests each of these hollow organs. When indicated, perineorrhaphy effectively complements

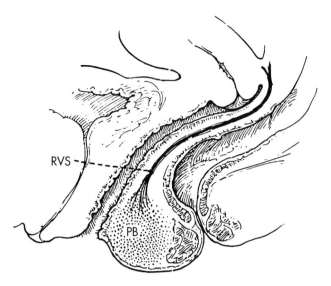

Fig. 22-18   Sagittal section shows the relationship between the rectovaginal septum *(RVS)* and the superior portion of the perineal body *(PB)* with which it blends. (From Nichols DH, Randall CL: *Vaginal surgery,* ed 4, Baltimore, 1996, Williams & Wilkins.)

the support of the anterior vaginal wall and the urethra, improving the continence mechanism.[46]

In examining the patient before perineorrhaphy, it is important to recognize that, as Davies emphasized,[10]

> any perineal laceration which permits the labia minora to retract laterally and expose a gaping vagina harbors the divided and retracted origin of the bulbocavernosus muscle. Such a lesion lowers the efficiency of the voluntary urethral sphincter and should be considered as an etiologic basis for stress incontinence in the female.

The examiner should also carefully note the position of the patient's anus in relation to the most dependent portion of the buttocks, the tip of the coccyx, and the ischial tuberosities. Posterior displacement of the anus strongly suggests that the anal sphincter has been detached from the perineum. This also may occur when a defect of the levator ani is present, either because of an intrinsic fault of the muscle or as a result of defective innervation of this voluntary muscle. In either instance, straining during defecation may, in effect, produce elongation and funneling of the levator ani, with the anus descending to an even more dependent position. The harder the patient strains, the more narrow the stool must become, and the more difficult defecation becomes. Obstipation is often the result. Barrett proposed that this condition be corrected by making an incision *posterior* to the rectum and attaching the separated levators to each other and to the rectal wall[3] (see Chapter 29).

Perineal Body

The perineal body in a woman is a structure of considerable anatomic and physiologic importance. It may be visualized as roughly pyramidal, and a repair must restore the body of the perineum in all three dimensions. The base of the pyra-

mid is situated beneath and parallels the perineal skin. The anterior, posterior, and two lateral surfaces converge superiorly to the most inferior limit of the rectovaginal space, fusing with the lowermost margin of the rectovaginal septum (Fig. 22-18).

STRIATED MUSCLES OF THE PELVIS

The more deeply red striated muscles indicate those capable of considerable contractile strength (e.g., the pubococcygeus) but with a lessened capacity for maintaining residual tone. The lighter pinkish white striated muscle is better adapted for maintaining tone and less adapted for sudden protective contraction.

The principal portion of the levator ani concerned with support of the lower vagina and birth canal attaches to the sides of the vaginal connective tissue through Luschka's fibers rather than to the muscular tissues of the posterior vaginal wall. Although perineal laceration or other obstetric trauma may lengthen, displace laterally, and sometimes detach the levator ani, such damage to the levator ani may produce only a midvaginal rectocele cranial to the perineal body. When examining such a patient, the gynecologist should examine for evidence of external hemorrhoids, because weakness of the perineum and anal sphincter may contribute to their development. When the upper vagina and cervix have prolapsed, however, the distention of the genital hiatus caused by the protrusion may have reduced the tone of the introitus musculature by the same mechanism as the dilating wedge of an enterocele in this area may widen the pelvic outlet. An effective repair restores much of the tone of the lateral vaginal walls, largely as a result of the removal of a major causative factor (i.e., the prolapsing cervix, uterus, or enterocele).

Most so-called levator stitches only increase the approximation of thinned or separated layers of the perineal body and do not usually build up the levator itself. If placed far enough laterally to include the fascia of the pelvic diaphragm, they may reinforce a defective pelvic diaphragm, but if placed directly into the belly of the levator muscle, these sutures may actually destroy portions of the muscle, eventually resulting in a shelflike ridge of nonelastic fibrous tissue within the introitus and immediately beneath the posterior vaginal wall. Superficial, side-to-side stitches are preferable because they usually reconstitute the perineal body and draw the fascia of the pubococcygeal muscles closer to the upper lateral sides of the perineal body. This effectively narrows the widened genital hiatus.

The extent to which reconstruction of a very loose vaginal outlet contributes to coital satisfaction has undoubtedly been overemphasized. Because a noticeable looseness of the vagina is not a common cause of marital incompatibility, prophylactic "tightening up" of the introitus does not necessarily improve marital relations, which are more often frayed by nonanatomic factors. However, indicated correction, but not overcorrection, of a damaged or relaxed peri-

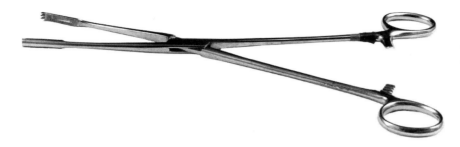

Fig. 22-19 The Krobach (or Chrobach) mouse-toothed clamp is shown. It can be obtained in the United States by special order from BEI Medical Systems/Zinnanti Surgical Instruments, Chatsworth, CA 91311, the custom order department of Codman-Shurtleff, New Bedford, MA 02745, or from Mr. William Merz of Baxter-V Mueller, Chicago, IL 60648.

neal body can improve coital satisfaction within an otherwise compatible domestic relationship.

The elasticity of the premenopausal or estrogen-maintained vagina normally permits it to grasp or contain an erect penis much as an expansible rubber glove grasps a finger. The normal-sized vagina can adapt comfortably and adequately to a large male organ, as well as to a small one. Because the elasticity of the vagina is important in preserving coital harmony, surgeons should avoid unnecessary procedures that tend to result in fibrosis and rigidity in this area.

The argument as to which muscle bundles penetrate the perineal body is, in large part, more academic than practical. The gynecologic surgeon should not regularly attempt to incorporate in the perineal body repair muscle bundles that were not there originally, because displaced bundles are likely to be replaced by fibrosis, resulting in a loss of elasticity and persistent tenderness. The objective of repair should be based on a fairly definite concept of normal fibromuscular attachments and relationships of the perineal body. A successful restoration of the more essential relationships requires a recognition of the function of each component and attachment and allowance for individual variation.

Operative Procedure

Reconstruction begins with uncovering the perineal body along its base beneath the perineal skin and on the vaginal (anterosuperior) side. The usual transverse incision along the posterior hymenal margin is not recommended for perineorrhaphy unless the surgeon is not planning a significant perineal body reconstruction, but rather intends to direct all efforts to the repair of a rectocele well above the perineal body. A transverse incision not only may facilitate the development of the ridgelike, "dashboard" perineum that is often associated with dyspareunia, but also may not provide sufficient exposure of the inferior surface of the base of the perineal body for a complete perineorrhaphy. Without adequate exposure, the surgeon can reconstruct only the anterior and upper portion of the perineal body—the only exposed or denuded area—and cannot involve the equally important middle and posteroinferior portions of the perineal body in the repair. The Krobach clamp, shown in Fig. 22-19, is heavy but relatively atraumatic, providing a good grasp without tearing the tissue to which it is applied. Two of these clamps are useful during perineorrhaphy and posterior colporrhaphy; one is applied to the base of perineal skin that will remain, for which it aids exposure as it

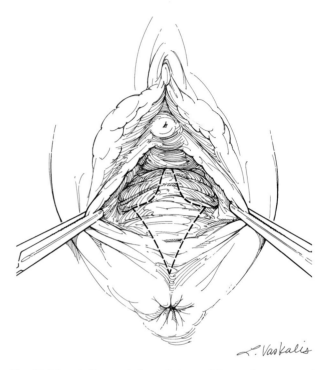

Fig. 22-20 A diamond-shaped piece of tissue of an appropriate width has been carefully estimated. The amount of perineal skin to be removed is determined by the quantity of excess tissue, just enough being excised to permit a normal three-fingerbreadth vaginal introitus without stenosis. It is better to err on the side of leaving a little too much tissue than too little.

will retract by hanging down by itself. The other may be used to grasp in the midline the full thickness of the posterior vaginal wall portion that will be excised.

A V-shaped incision in the perineal skin ensures better access to more of the tissues of the perineal body than is possible with the "standard" transverse incision. Therefore, after applying clamps or traction sutures to the hymenal margin on either side, the surgeon should make a V-shaped incision (Fig. 22-20) in the perineal skin layer (U-shaped for especially large perineal defects). It is important to place the lateral traction sutures or clamps on the hymenal ring rather than on the labia minora (Fig. 22-21); if the placement of the retracting forceps or sutures is too lateral, a superficial transverse ridge, or "dashboard," perineum may develop and subsequently obstruct the vagina.

Scar tissue is carefully freed by sharp dissection to mobilize the tissue from which the perineal body will be reconstructed (Fig. 22-22). The desired size of the vaginal introi-

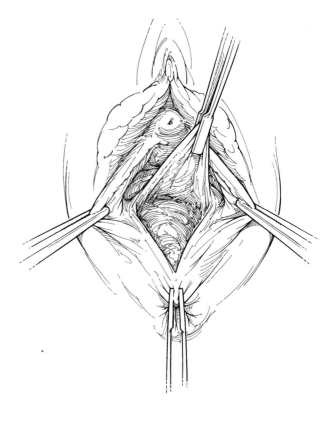

Fig. 22-21   The dissection is carried superiorly into the vagina, exposing the full site of the future perineal body. If rectocele is present, the rectovaginal space is entered, and the dissection freeing rectum from vagina is carried to a level above any rectocele that is present.

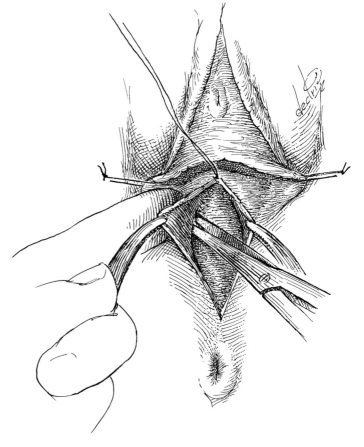

Fig. 22-22   Scar tissue attached to introital skin is carefully freed by sharp dissection so that the tissue from which a perineal body will be built can be mobilized readily. (Modified from Nichols DH, Randall CL: *Vaginal surgery,* ed 4, Baltimore, 1996, Williams & Wilkins.)

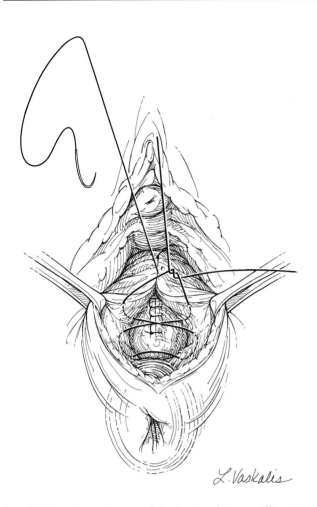

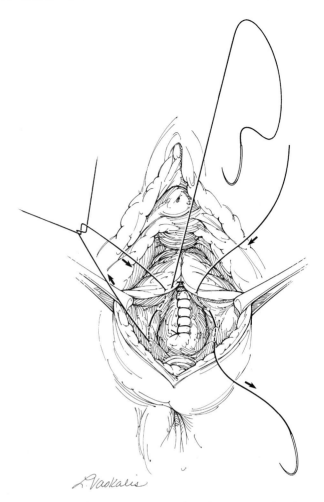

Fig. 22-23 Reattachment of the fascia of Denonvilliers (rectovaginal septum) to the perineal body. Anterior rectal plication has reduced the size of the rectal reservoir for the full limit of the rectocele. A figure-of-eight stitch reattaches the fascia of Denonvilliers to the perineal body. (From Nichols DH, editor: *Reoperative gynecologic and obstetric surgery,* ed 2, St Louis, 1997, Mosby.)

Fig. 22-24 The "11" sutures. When the introitus has been previously narrowed, and occasionally in the presence of a perineal descent syndrome, Denonvilliers' fascia may be reattached to the perineal body by two longitudinal interrupted sutures as shown. After both have been placed, they are tied. This helps to restore the perineum without narrowing the introitus. (From Nichols DH, editor: *Reoperative gynecologic and obstetric surgery,* ed 2, St Louis, 1997, Mosby.)

tus determines the appropriate width for the base of this triangle in relation to the hymenal margin. The greater the amount of epithelium removed, the smaller the caliber of the resulting vaginal orifice.

Any detachment of the connective tissue of the rectovaginal septum from the cranial or uppermost portion of the perineal body (see Fig. 22-4) must be remedied by surgical reattachment to ensure the restoration of normal function, particularly in regard to the role of the perineum and its continuity with the rectovaginal septum during the act of defecation. Because considerable scarring from previous trauma may be present in this vulnerable area, dissection through indistinct cleavage planes should proceed with caution to avoid penetration of the rectum. Reattachment and restoration relieve the problem of incomplete bowel movements, and it is unlikely to recur. To reattach or reinforce the attachment of the fascia of Denonvilliers to the perineal

body, the surgeon should carry the dissection for perineorrhaphy higher than the defect to be repaired, always opening into the rectovaginal space and then attaching or reattaching the underside of the posterior vaginal wall in the rectovaginal space (including the fascia of Denonvilliers) to the perineal body (Figs. 22-23 to 22-25).

After the mobilization and removal of the excess vaginal wall and skin, the reconstruction is often accomplished by side-to-side reapproximation of denuded tissues, both deep and superficial. The upper portion of this side-to-side reapproximation of the perineal body should pull the pubococcygeal muscles closer, although the sutures should not actually include them (Fig. 22-26). This procedure narrows the genital hiatus. Lower placed stitches bring the transverse perinei together, helping to reconstruct the lower portion of the urogenital diaphragm. Similar sutures reattach the bulbospongiosus muscles to the perineal body (Fig. 22-27), and

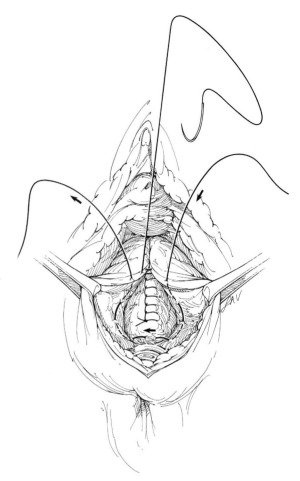

Fig. 22-25   Reconstruction of the long and wide perineum. The full length of the increased rectal reservoir has been reduced by a running locked stitch that ends behind the site at which a new perineal body will be constructed. The underside of the fascia of Denonvilliers (rectovaginal septum) can be reattached to the widened site of the perineal body by a U-shaped suture configuration placed into it as shown. When this stitch has been tied, the perineum will have been reduced in width as well as in length. (From Nichols DH, editor: *Reoperative gynecologic and obstetric surgery,* ed 2, St Louis, 1997, Mosby.)

the perineal skin is closed by a running subcuticular suture (Fig. 22-28).

During reconstruction of the lower third of the vagina when the perineal defect is extreme and little tissue is available for the reconstruction, it may be necessary to provide better support to the rectal ampulla; in this instance, the operator may bring the medial margins of the puborectal or pubococcygeal muscles together by a small series of superficially placed and loosely tied interrupted sutures, which, in turn, may at their insertion be attached to a sagging ampulla[2] (Fig. 22-29). Lee[23] describes his satisfaction with posterior repair that interposes stitches uniting the pubococcygei between the rectum and vagina. In providing such support, it is important to avoid the production of troublesome and inevitably tender ridges beneath the posterior vaginal wall. After placing each stitch and before tying it, the surgeon should cross the ends of the suture and apply traction. If there is a palpable ridge, the operator should promptly remove and replace the stitch, usually closer to the rectum. When perineal surgery is performed under local anesthesia, the voluntary muscle bundles may be more readily identified.

The retracted ends of often long-separated bulbospongiosus muscles should be identified and reattached to the perineal body. Separated segments of the transverse perinei also should be reunited if the medial edge of the levator ani and the puborectal muscle can be identified. In the correction of a low rectocele, the adjacent fascia of the pelvic diaphragm

is attached to the posterolateral surface of the vagina, duplicating the original attachment of Luschka's fibers, fixing and holding the vagina in place. The placement of a few interrupted horizontally placed, loosely tied perineal sutures brings together the smooth muscle of the perineal body, helping reestablish its integrity.

Although not a common result of perineal injury during childbirth, posterior displacement of the anus must be repaired. It is necessary to reattach the capsule of the external sphincter ani to the perineal body, for example, by using a more posteriorly placed figure-of-eight suture (Fig. 22-30, p. 419) as described by Kennedy and Campbell.[21] This step, which stabilizes the perineum, is similar to reattaching spokes to the hub of a wheel (perineal body).

Operative compression of the veins that communicate with hemorrhoids often temporarily aggravates existing hemorrhoids. As postoperative edema subsides, however, a new tissue equilibrium usually develops. The hemorrhoids may undergo involution and improvement, especially if any sphincter weakness has been corrected. For this reason, hemorrhoidectomy should not be done at the same time as a posterior colporrhaphy. The need for hemorrhoidectomy can be evaluated better several months postoperatively.

The superficial perineal fascia may be brought together, and the perineal skin may be closed with running or interrupted sutures. Subcuticular sutures should be used in the closure of both the vaginal epithelium and the perineal skin,

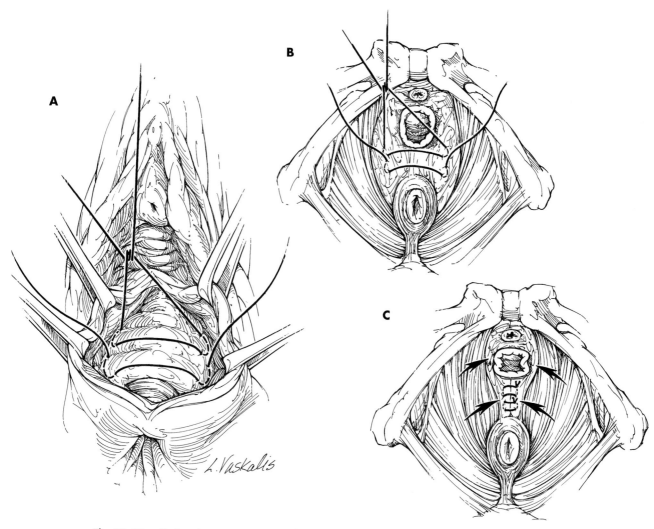

L. Vaskalis

Fig. 22-26   Perineal reconstruction without levator plication. **A,** Perineorrhaphy may be accomplished *without* placing stitches directly into the muscle bellies of the pubococcygei, as shown here with a wide genital hiatus. **B,** Phantom drawing of the wide hiatus. **C,** When the interrupted stitches in the perineal body have been tied, the lateral attachments of this tissue to the fascia of the pubococcygei will bring the latter closer together *(arrows),* narrowing the genital hiatus to a new and normal position. No stitches have been placed directly into the muscular substance of the pubococcygei. (From Nichols DH, Randall CL: *Vaginal surgery,* ed 4, Baltimore, Williams & Wilkins, 1996.)

with care to avoid irregularities in the approximation of the edges being united or in invaginations of epithelial edges. Irregular bulging or invaginations in the suture line are likely to cause granulations and irregularities in healing that may account for persistent tenderness in the scar.

Fig. 22-29, *F,* shows an instrument under study to be used in an attempt to take some of the guesswork out of the repair of the pelvic floor when a functional vagina is desirable. Some of our predecessors sensed the need for such a device if only to impress upon operators the importance of preoperative study in this surgery. Its inclusion in a text of this type is justified when one realizes that in describing a vaginal plastic operation writers find themselves without some standard object that could be used to tell the reader how big to make the vagina. One wonders how long it may take for the

vagina to come into its rightful place among the organs upon which plastic surgery is performed. While moulages are made of future noses, while artists draw ears to guide plastic surgeons, and even simple grafts are planned and plotted days in advance, vaginal plastic surgery is undertaken with a shameful lack of study. Habitually the operators' fingers are unceremoniously poked into the field of operation to determine the ultimate dimensions of the organ. Fat fingers, thin fingers, big fingers, or small fingers—this technique has yet to be replaced by something more esthetic and reliable. While constrictions and dyspareunia, recurrent relaxations and gaping, and scarring and abnormal fixation have been all too frequent results in vaginal surgery, the same postoperative appearance would scarcely be tolerated elsewhere. Should not the guesswork be taken out of this surgery?

Text continued on p. 420

Fig. 22-27   The rectocele had been repaired from the posterior fornix to the perineal body, and the remains of the transverse perineal and bulbocavernosus muscles are being used to build up the perineum.

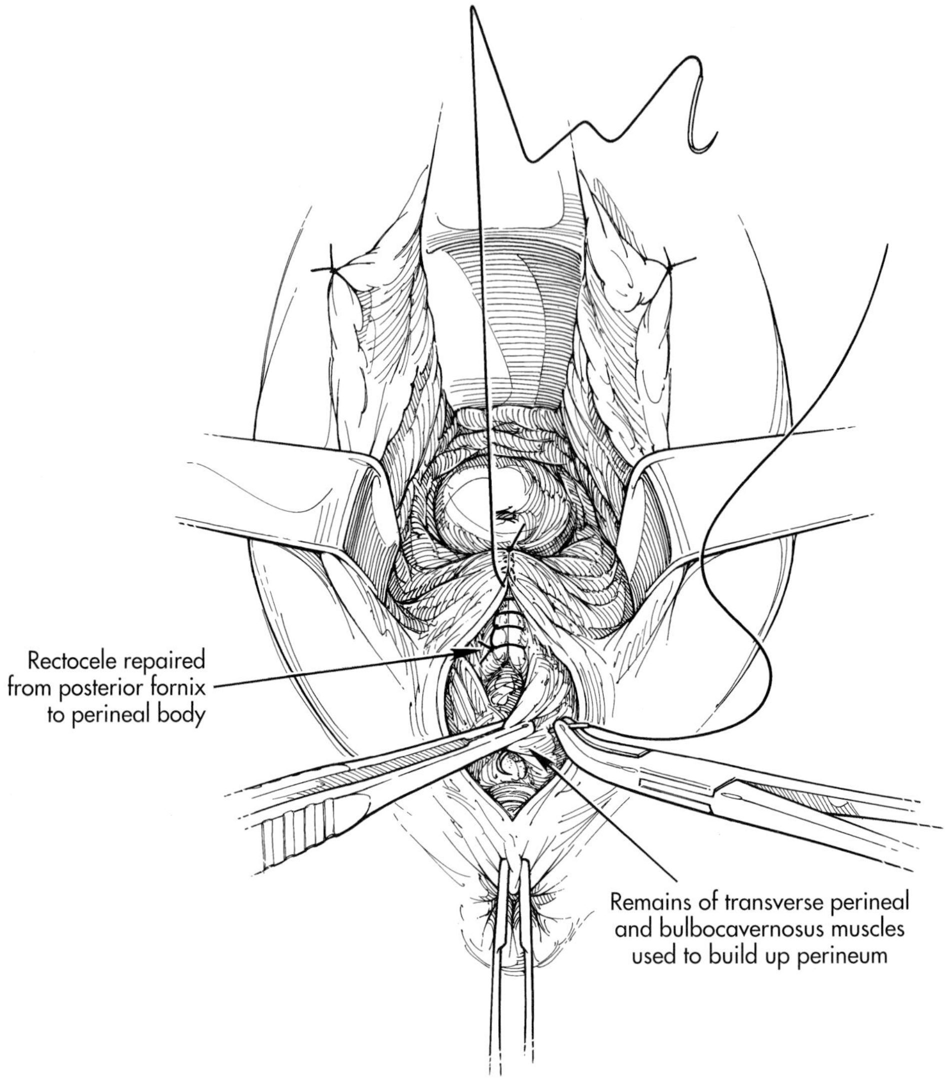

Rectocele repaired from posterior fornix to perineal body

Remains of transverse perineal and bulbocavernosus muscles used to build up perineum

Fig. 22-28   Note that the posterior vaginal wall has been trimmed as necessary and the edges approximated by a "spiral" running subcuticular suture. The perineum is closed by a continuation of the same suture placed in a snakelike fashion.

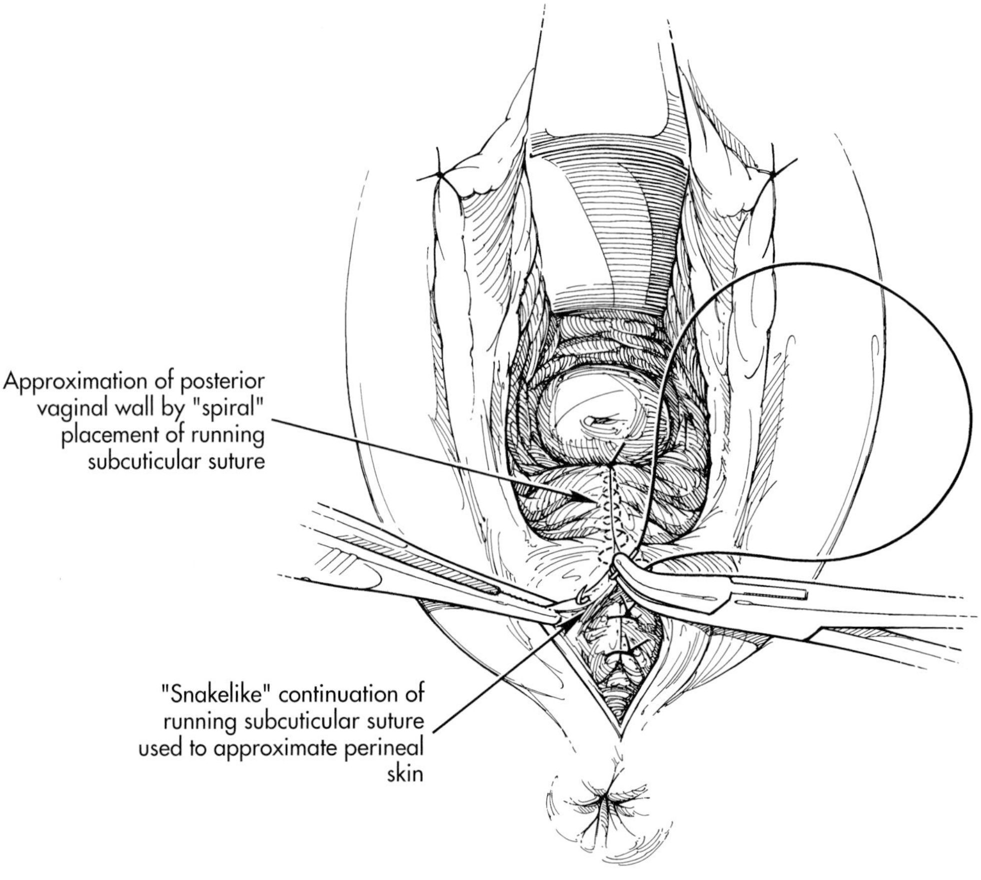

Approximation of posterior vaginal wall by "spiral" placement of running subcuticular suture

"Snakelike" continuation of running subcuticular suture used to approximate perineal skin

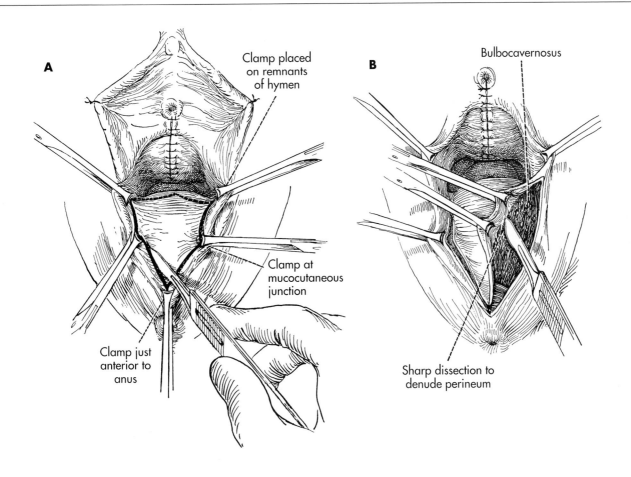

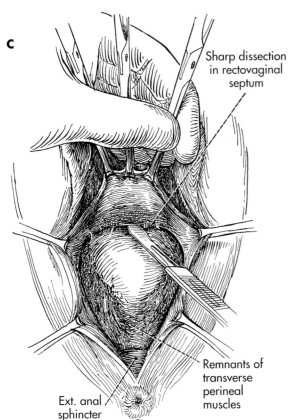

Fig. 22-29 **A,** A V-shaped incision is made between two clamps of the mucocutaneous junction on the posterior vaginal wall as shown, the widths of the V being determined by the extent to which the vagina will be narrowed. This flap is dissected from the underlying perineal body and adjacent scar tissue, and the incision carried in the vagina as indicated by the *dashed line* of an amount appropriate to the degree by which the vagina will be narrowed postoperatively. **B,** This flap is separated by sharp dissection, using either curved Mayo scissors or a scalpel, from the underlying muscle, scar tissue, and connective tissue as shown. **C,** This is carried the full depth of the rectocele, until a point cranial to the rectocele has been reached. If an enterocele is encountered, it is opened and the sac resected and the neck closed. (From Ball TL: *Gynecologic surgery and urology,* ed 2, St Louis, 1963, Mosby.)

Continued

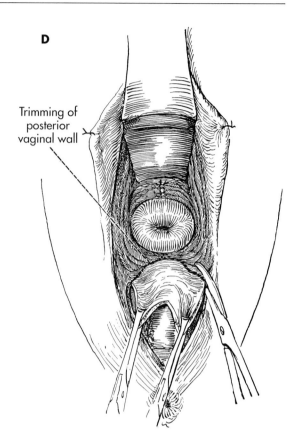

Trimming of posterior vaginal wall

Fig. 22-29, cont'd   D, The excess posterior vaginal wall is trimmed as shown by the *dashed line* and reapproximated using a running subcuticular suture that incorporates the full thickness of the posterior vaginal wall. Any ballooning of the anterior rectal wall is corrected by plication, and the pararectal fascia may be reapproximated by running or interrupted subcuticular sutures. Just before the skin of the perineum is closed, it should be possible for the operator to insert a finger between the undersurface of the posterior vaginal wall and the anterior surface of the rectum, indicating the preservation of the rectovaginal space. **E,** If there is little tissue of substance to be used to support this area, the anterior medial edge of the fascia of the puborectalis may be brought together with interrupted stitches, presuming that they are placed close enough to the rectum that no subvaginal ridges are palpable.

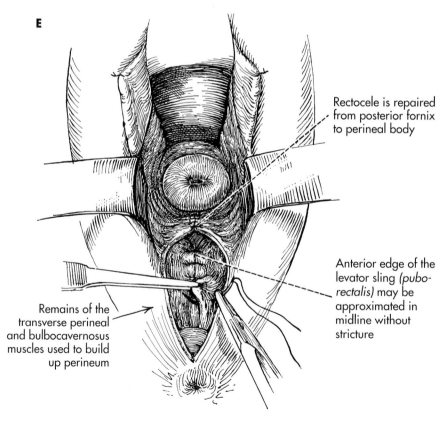

Rectocele is repaired from posterior fornix to perineal body

Anterior edge of the levator sling *(puborectalis)* may be approximated in midline without stricture

Remains of the transverse perineal and bulbocavernosus muscles used to build up perineum

F

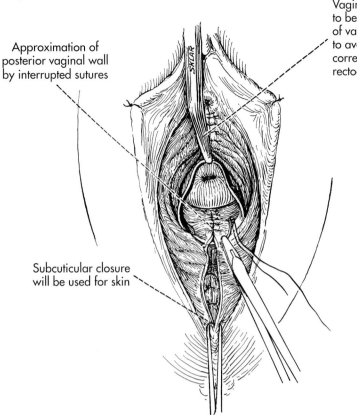

Approximation of
posterior vaginal wall
by interrupted sutures

Vaginal guide *(under study)*
to be used to show the amount
of vaginal wall to be trimmed
to avoid strictures and inadequate
correction of the cystocele and
rectocele

Subcuticular closure
will be used for skin

Fig. 22-29, cont'd   F, The remainder of the posterior vaginal wall is closed, the perineum reconstructed with some interrupted stitches, and the skin closed by a subcuticular suture as shown. (From Ball TL: *Gynecologic surgery and urology,* ed 2, St Louis, 1963, Mosby.)

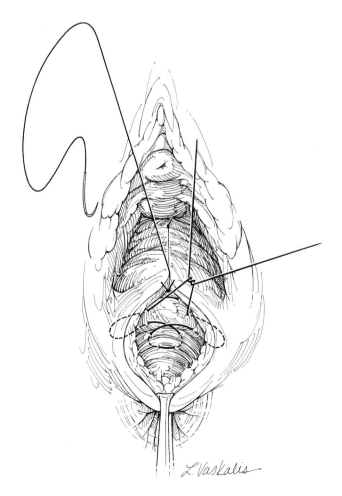

Fig. 22-30   Correction of detachment of the anus from the perineal body. Detachment of the anal sphincter from the perineal body may be corrected by a buried figure-of-eight suture placed as shown. This stabilizes the anus and the perineal body. (From Nichols DH, editor: *Reoperative gynecologic and obstetric surgery,* St Louis, 1997, Mosby.)

L.Vaskalis

While the vaginal surgeon may passionately desire faithfully to restore the virginal dimensions, axis, contour, and markings of his patient, this is not possible. In place of this the objective is resolutely to reconstruct a functional, pain-free, pliable, distensible, and well-supported structure. The dimensions of the instrument under study are based on the studies of Dickinson, who has made some of the most memorable contributions to the human sexual anatomy. He insisted on distinguishing the anatomy of the "quick from the dead," a philosophy vaginal surgeons should devoutly embrace.[2]

When previous trauma, usually obstetric laceration, has damaged the external anal sphincter complex with resultant rectal soiling or anal incontinence, it can be repaired surgically even as part of a posterior repair or perineorrhaphy.

REPAIR OF PREVIOUS FOURTH-DEGREE LACERATION

Successful perineorrhaphy on a patient who has sustained a previous third- or fourth-degree perineal laceration is technically quite different from the "standard" repair in that it must reapproximate the full depth of the external anal sphincter (all three parts) for a distance of about 3 inches. This helps to reduce the size of the rectal reservoir and indirectly improves the gate-keeping function of both external and internal anal sphincters.

It has been emphasized by Aronson and Lee[1] and pointed out by others that because the external anal sphincter consists of contiguous subcutaneous, superficial, and deep portions that extend the better part of 4 cm alongside the lower rectum, the usual "standard" plication of fibers of the subcutaneous external anal sphincter alone does not restore the damage consequent to laceration of the superficial and deep portions. Important and appropriate surgical remedy in light of this observation is described in Chapter 28.

ENDORECTAL REPAIR OF RECTOCELE

Block[5] pointed out that the traditional transvaginal approach to rectocele repair is indispensable when associated with conditions such as cystocele, enterocele, and uterine or vaginal vault prolapse. Sehapayak[37] has emphasized that simultaneous transvaginal posterior repair coincident with endorectal repair of rectocele is contraindicated, since interruption of the natural barriers or mucosal lining on both sides of the rectovaginal septum at the same time may invite infection, abscess formation, and subsequent rectovaginal fistula.

If the size of the rectal reservoir is too large following transvaginal posterior colporrhaphy, and the bowel movements are still incomplete and require manual expression, a surgeon finding conditions and scarring unsuitable for reoperation by the vaginal route, lest the vagina be made too small for coital comfort, may wish to consider endorectal repair.* This is a relatively simple operation to correct low

or midvaginal rectocele designed to reduce the size of the luminal rectal reservoir.

Sullivan[41] first described the endorectal repair of rectocele permitting, after mucosal incision and dissection of flaps, a transanal exposure and plication of the underside of the rectovaginal septum, excision of redundant or prolapsed rectal mucosa, and correction of any coincident anorectal pathology.

Jansen et al.[19] noted the importance of the submucosal layers in intestinal healing, first described by Halsted[16] as the strongest part of the intestinal wall. Lord et al.[24] demonstrated by scanning electron microscopy that it is a honeycomb of collagen fibers forming a strong skeleton-like cylinder through the entire length of the intestine. It contains a plexus of arterial vascularization.[40] They determined that surgical anastomosis with inversion of the intestinal layers with good submucosal approximation resulted in primary intestinal healing and rapid restoration of villous epithelium, but with bad approximation resulted in secondary healing with a predictably weaker scar.

As emphasized by Capps[8] and by Khubchandani[22] and associates, the endorectal repair can be done under local infiltration anesthesia during a short hospitalization. This approach also permits transrectal reattachment of the puborectalis to the perineal body. They report a high rate of success and low incidence of complications.

Preoperative rectal mechanical cleansing, for example, drinking an ice cold electrolyte solution (Nu-Lytely) the day before surgery or giving enemas until clear, adds but a few minutes to the total preparatory time. We perform the endorectal operation as follows.

A Fansler rectal retractor is inserted into the rectum, the obturator removed, and each quadrant of the rectal mucosa carefully examined. The rectal wall at the site of the rectocele and defect in the submucosa is identified and the full thickness of the overlying anterior rectal wall grasped by Allis clamps (Fig. 22-31) and a stitch of absorbable suture material, either 2-0 chromic or PGA, is placed through the full thickness of the rectal wall as shown. This excess rectal wall is incorporated in a tightly drawn running locked stitch (Fig. 22-32), which bridges the weakness in the wall of the rectum in a longitudinal direction cephalad to the initial stitch. As traction is exerted on each stitch as it is placed, the submucosa is tented toward the surgeon, facilitating placement of the succeeding suture. Although the full thickness of the rectal wall is included in this obliterative suture, digital examination of the vagina during the suturing makes certain that attachment to or penetration of the vagina has not occurred. The suture is carried to a point about 1 cm past the upper edge of the rectocele, then tied and returned as a reinforcing lock-stitch to the beginning of the suture line and tied there. Each stitch must be pulled tightly to exert a strangulating effect on the tissue contained within the suture.

Block[6] describes the obliterative suture as "essentially a tightly drawn running lock-stitch which strangulates and causes to slough the tissues in the grip of each stitch, yet preserves the viability and approximates the tissues at the

---

*References 4, 5, 6, 8, 22, 37, 41.

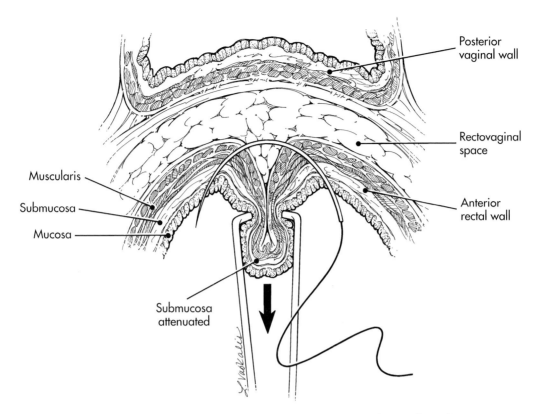

Fig. 22-31 Section showing the endorectal suture placement. The needle and suture are placed through the full thickness of the rectal wall, including the mucosa, submucosa, and muscularis. The unopened and unsewn vaginal wall is shown.

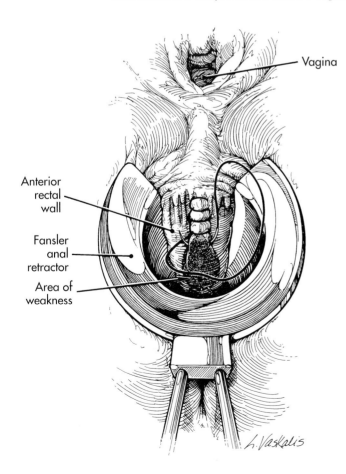

Fig. 22-32 Endorectal repair of rectocele. A Fansler rectal retractor has been inserted into the rectum, and the redundant mucosa and submucosa of the weakened anterior rectal wall have been identified. Starting just proximal to the mucocutaneous junction, a running locked obliterative suture has been started. The suture is placed through both mucosal and submucosal layers and may include the rectal muscularis. With each stitch the suture is tightly drawn. No portion of the intact vaginal wall is included in the suture. When the rectal tissue of the rectocele has been obliterated to a point cranial to the low or midvaginal rectocele, the direction of the suture is reversed and a second obliterative layer is placed reinforcing the initial layer.

base of the suture. This surgical maneuver is peculiarly adapted to rectal surgery, since it cannot be used anywhere else in the body, but in the rectum it is an amazingly versatile tool for the surgeon."

Alternatively, in the techniques of Sullivan,[41] Capps,[8] and Sehapayak,[37] the mucosal and submucosal layers are dissected off the underlying rectal muscularis, which is then plicated and the mucosa closed by a separate layer.

At about the 12-o'clock position, the rectal mucosa may be grasped and incised longitudinally from within the rectum, undermined, and reflected laterally. The rectal side of the rectal muscularis is plicated,[8,22,37,41] excess mucosa is trimmed, and the edges sewn or stapled without tension. If desired, a predetermined full thickness of the rectal wall including the muscularis may be excised in its longitudinal axis following endorectal clamping and suturing or stapling (GIA endo 30 or 60) with excision of this predetermined full-thickness portion of the rectal wall in its longitudinal axis. Coincident endorectal pathology, such as excision of symptomatic hemorrhoids or mucosal prolapse or removal of any rectal polyps, can be undertaken simultaneously if within the operator's area of expertise.

Endorectal repair of rectocele avoids the possibility of vaginal stricture, dyspareunia, or rectovaginal fistula.

REFERENCES

1. Aronson MP, Lee RA, Berquist TH: Anatomy of anal sphincters and related structures in continent women studied with magnetic resonance imaging, *Obstet Gynecol* 76:846, 1990.
2. Ball TL: *Gynecologic surgery and urology,* ed 2, St Louis, 1963, Mosby.
3. Barrett CW: Hernias through the pelvic floor, *Am J Obstet Dis Wom* 59:553, 1909.
4. Bethoux JP: Traitement chirurgical des rectoceles, *Ann Gastroenterol Hepatol* 23:217, 1987.
5. Block IR: Transrectal repair of rectocele using obliterative suture, *Dis Colon Rectum* 29:707, 1986.
6. Block IR: *Dis Colon Rectum* 30:314, 1987 (letter to the editor).
7. Bresler L, Rauch P, Denis B, et al: Traitement des rectoceles sus-levatoriennes par voie endorectale, *J Chir* 130:304, 1993.
8. Capps WF: Rectoplasty and perineoplasty for the symptomatic rectocele, *Dis Colon Rectum* 18:237, 1975.
9. Cavallo G, Salzano A, Grassi R, De Lillo ML: Functional intraperineal pouch of rectal wall, *Dis Colon Rectum* 36:179, 1993.
10. Davies JW: In Ullery JC, editor: *Stress incontinence in the female,* New York, 1953, Grune & Stratton.
11. DeCosta EJ: After office hours—"dance me loose," *Obstet Gynecol* 6:120, 1955.
12. DeLancey JOL: Anatomic aspects of vaginal eversion after hysterectomy, *Am J Obstet Gynecol* 166:1717, 1992.
13. Felt-Bersma RJ, Cuesta MA, Koorevaar M, et al: Anal endosonography: relationship with anal manometry and neurophysiologic tests, *Dis Colon Rectum* 35:944, 1992.
14. Genadry RR, Nichols DH: Recurrent anal incontinence. In Nichols DH editor: *Reoperative gynecologic and obstetric surgery,* St Louis, 1997, Mosby.
15. Goff BM: A practical consideration of the damaged pelvic floor with a technique for its secondary reconstruction, *Surg Gynecol Obstet* 46:866, 1968.
16. Halsted WS: Circular suture of the intestine: an experimental study, *Am J Med Sci* 94:436, 1887.
17. Harrison JE, McDonagh JE: Hernia of Douglas' pouch and high rectocele, *Am J Obstet Gynecol* 60:83, 1950.
18. Jacobs PP, Scheuer M, Kuijpers JH, Vingerhoets MH: Obstetric fecal incontinence: role of pelvic floor denervation and results of delayed sphincter repair, *Dis Colon Rectum* 33:494, 1990.
19. Jansen A, Becker AE, Brummelkamp WH, et al: The importance of the apposition of the submucosal intestinal layers for primary wound healing of intestinal anastomosis, *Surg Gynecol Obstet* 152:51, 1981.
20. Jeffcoate TNA: Posterior colporrhaphy, *Am J Obstet Gynecol* 77:490, 1959.
21. Kennedy JW, Campbell AD: *Vaginal hysterectomy,* Philadelphia, 1942, FA Davis.
22. Khubchandani IT, Sheets JA, Stasik JJ, Hakki AR: Endorectal repair of rectocele, *Dis Colon Rectum* 26:792, 1983.
23. Lee RA: *Atlas of gynecologic surgery,* Philadelphia, 1992, WB Saunders.
24. Lord MG, Valies P, Broughton AC: A morphologic study of submucosa of the large intestine, *Surg Gynecol Obstet* 145:155, 1977.
25. Malpas P: The choice of operation for genital prolapse. In Meigs JV, Sturgis SH: *Progress in gynecology,* vol III, New York, 1957, Grune & Stratton.
26. Marks MM: The rectal side of rectocele, *Dis Colon Rectum* 10:387, 1967.
27. Milley PS, Nichols DH: A corrective investigation of the human rectovaginal septum, *Anat Rec* 163:433, 1968.
28. Nichols DH, Randall CL: *Vaginal surgery,* ed 4, Baltimore, Williams & Wilkins, 1996.
29. Nichols DH: Posterior colporrhaphy and perineorrhaphy: separate and distinct operations, *Am J Obstet Gynecol* 164:714, 1991.
30. Nichols DH, editor: *Reoperative gynecologic and obstetric surgery,* ed 2, St Louis, 1997, Mosby.
31. Parks TG: The usefulness of tests on anorectal disease, *World J Surg* 16:804, 1992.
32. Penninckx F: Fecal incontinence: indications for repairing the anal sphincter, *World J Surg* 16:820, 1992.
33. Porges RF: A practical system of diagnosis and classification of pelvic relaxations, *Surg Gynecol Obstet* 117:769, 1963.
34. Rex DK, Lappas JC: Combined anorectal manometry and defecography in 50 consecutive adults with fecal incontinence, *Dis Colon Rectum* 35:1040, 1992.
35. Ricci JV, Thom CH: The myth of a surgically useful fascia in vaginal plastic reconstructions, *Obstet Gynecol* 7:253, 1954.
36. Richter K: Erkrankungen der Vagina. In Schwalm H, Döderlein G, Wulf KH, editors: *Klinik der Frauenheilkunde und Geburtshilfe,* vol 8, Munich, 1971, Urban & Schwarzenberg.
37. Sehapayak S: Transrectal repair of rectocele: an extended armamentarium of colorectal surgeons, *Dis Colon Rectum* 28:422, 1985.
38. Snooks SJ, Burnes PRH, Swash M: Abnormalities of the innervation of the voluntary anal and urethral sphincters in incontinence: an electrophysiological study, *J Neurol Neurosurg Psychiatry* 47:1269, 1984.
39. Snooks SJ, Swash M, Henry MM, Setchell M: Risk factors in childbirth causing damage to the pelvic floor innervation, *Int J Colorectal Dis* 1:20, 1986.
40. Spjut HJ: Microangiographic study of gastrointestinal lesions, *Am J Roentgenol* 91:1187, 1974.
41. Sullivan ES, Leaverton GH, Hardwick CE: Transrectal perineal repair: an adjunct to improved function after anorectal surgery, *Dis Colon Rectum* 11:106, 1968.
42. Swash M: Electromyography in pelvic floor disorders. In Henry MM, Swash M: *Coloproctology and the pelvic floor,* ed 2, Oxford, 1992, Butterworth-Heinemann.
43. Tobin CE, Benjamin JA: Anatomical and surgical restudy of Denonvilliers' fascia, *Surg Gynecol Obstet* 80:373, 1945.
44. Uhlenhuth E, Nolley GW: Vaginal fascia, a myth? *Obstet Gynecol* 10:349, 1957.
45. Weber AM, Walters MD: Anterior vaginal prolapse: review of anatomy and techniques of surgical repair, *Obstet Gynecol* 89:311, 1997.
46. Zivkovic F, Tamussino K, Haas J: Contribution of the posterior compartment to the urinary continence mechanism, *Obstet Gynecol* 91:229, 1998.

23 Enterocele

DAVID H. NICHOLS

The posterior peritoneal cul-de-sac occasionally extends caudally between the rectum and the vagina to varying depths, even as far as the perineal body.[18,19,33] A deep cul-de-sac becomes an enterocele (a peritoneum-lined sac between the vagina and the rectum) when small bowel mesentery and omentum have lengthened sufficiently to permit them to enter and distend the cul-de-sac. This deep cul-de-sac should be obliterated coincidently whenever it is found at surgery. However, does a long small bowel mesentery precede or follow an enterocele sac?

Because not all deep cul-de-sacs have abdominal content, it is necessary to distinguish between those with bowel content and those without. The former are symptomatic, causing backache and a dragging sensation that is accentuated in the erect position and relieved by lying down; the discomfort is probably the result of omental and mesenteric traction. The latter type, without bowel content, is generally asymptomatic. It is not known whether the two are etiologically different or whether the long intestinal mesentery is the cause or the result of the deep cul-de-sac when the two coexist, although the weight of the bowel with a long mesentery may increase the risk of recurrence of enterocele after treatment.

Despite the frequency with which the vaginal vault is left open at the time of abdominal hysterectomy, postoperative vaginal evisceration is rare.[25] Reported patients generally have been postmenopausal, often with a history of previous operations for vaginal repair. Evisceration coincident with coitus or straining of stool was not uncommon. (Is this because the small bowel mesentery is usually too short[27] to permit routine pressure of the small bowel's weight against the vault of the vagina?) Massive eversion of the vagina may occur with or without enterocele (although the former condition is more common), and enterocele may occur with or without massive eversion (Fig. 23-1). Enterocele and massive eversion often coexist, but they are *separate* anatomic and clinical entities, each requiring separate, specific surgical treatment. The gynecologist must make these distinctions, because the treatments are quite different.

A vagina with previously normal depth may become unexpectedly short and poorly supported after the repair of a challenging enterocele, even though the repair was competently performed. The reason for an unacceptable shortening of the vagina is not always immediately apparent. However, it should be possible to recognize the possibility of such a problem in advance by considering the enterocele's location and cause, which seem to be directly correlated. Taking these factors into account in the selection of the operative procedure not only reduces the likelihood of a recurrence, but also prevents an undesirable degree of vaginal shortening.

TYPES OF ENTEROCELE

Essentially, an enterocele is a herniation of the lining of the peritoneal cavity, with portions of the abdominal viscera within the herniating sac, that extends into areas of the pelvis where the peritoneum is not usually found. Strictly speaking, the term *enterocele* is a misnomer because normally a hernia is named not according to its contents, but according to its location. A better gynecologic term may be *hernia of the cul-de-sac,* but the current use of the term *enterocele* has been accepted for so long that it would be difficult to displace. At any rate, an enterocele that is unrecognized and unrepaired tends to progress and causes increasing discomfort and eventually increasing disability.

An enterocele may be either anterior, posterior, or lateral to the vagina,[31] with or without secondary eversion of the vaginal vault. The surgeon should always distinguish an enterocele with an accompanying vault eversion from one without such a complicating factor[30] because the causes, as well as the objectives and techniques of surgical reconstruction, vary for each type of enterocele and are quite different when vaginal eversion is also present.

There are four basic types of enterocele: congenital, pulsion, traction, and iatrogenic. They may occur either singly or in combination.[17] The progression of each of these types of true prolapse may result in massive eversion of the vagina. Not only are these the most frequently encountered enteroceles, but also each represents one of the basic etiologic factors. The significant relationships in the anatomy of the enteroceles suggest the important differences in etiology.

Congenital Enterocele

An enterocele posterior to the vault of the vagina often is associated with a congenitally deep pouch of Douglas, not generally with eversion of the vaginal vault (Fig. 23-2, *A*). An unusually deep peritoneal pouch generally results from failure of normal fusion of the anterior with the posterior peritoneum of the cul-de-sac during late fetal development. If the soft tissue supports of the pelvis are otherwise intact, this type of posterior enterocele may exist independently of other lesions.

With the congenital type of enterocele related to a pathologically deep pouch of Douglas, the anterior wall of the sac

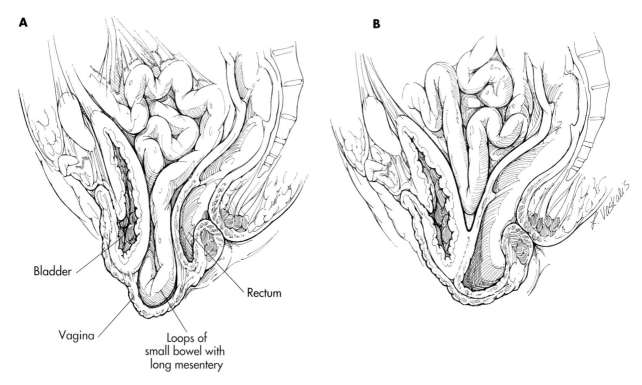

Fig. 23-1   Massive eversion of the vagina. **A,** Massive posthysterectomy eversion of the vagina with enterocele. **B,** The less-frequent massive eversion without enterocele. In this case the connective tissue capsule of the bladder is fused with that of the anterior rectal wall. (Redrawn from Nichols DH, Randall CL: *Vaginal surgery,* ed 4, Baltimore, 1996, Williams & Wilkins.)

is attached to the undersurface of the posterior vaginal wall. This attachment is certainly not present when the descent of the vaginal vault occurs coincidently with general postmenopausal prolapse.

Pulsion versus Traction Enterocele

An enterocele associated with procidentia results from massive anterior segment damage as a result of both pulsion from above and traction from below.[21,33] As the cervix descends, it takes with it the anterior margin of the cul-de-sac, although the posterior peritoneal wall remains in situ and attached to the anterior wall of the rectum. An enterocele that coexists with eversion of the vaginal vault may be the result of *pulsion* from pathologically increased intraabdominal pressure (see Fig. 23-2, *B*). This usually is associated with the uterovaginal or sliding type of genital prolapse. This is a most massive form of damage, and the descent of the entire upper vaginal suspensory apparatus is a secondary effect. Reconstruction of this type of enterocele involves not only excision of the enterocele sac, but also, more important, fixation or suspension of the vaginal vault to some structure capable of supporting it to prevent permanent pathologic shortening of the vagina. Another type of enterocele develops as a result of *traction* on a poorly supported vaginal vault by the other pelvic structures that are already prolapsed (see Fig. 23-2, *C*). Although a traction enterocele is preceded by a cystocele and a rectocele, a pulsion enterocele may be followed by them.

Although pudendal[2,4,5,8] or lateral enteroceles are most uncommon (Figs. 23-3 to 23-5), they may develop in sites of unusual weakness within or alongside the pelvic diaphragm or through the pelvic foramina. There may be a history of sudden traumatic increase in intraabdominal pressure, either from the strain of exceedingly heavy lifting or from sudden massive abdominal compression, as from an explosion or blast. This traumatic increase has been noted in a patient whose abdomen had been run over by the wheel of a car and in a patient on whose abdomen a horse had fallen. The patient with a pudendal or lateral enterocele may notice a mass alongside the vagina, especially when standing. Enteroceles of this type that do not appear externally are likely to be diagnosed at the time of laparotomy for intestinal obstruction, as the neck of the pudendal enterocele is found to be the site of the mechanical obstruction.

UNCOMMON PELVIC FLOOR HERNIAS
Obturator Hernia

An obturator hernia is seen most commonly in elderly women, is associated with a loss of weight, and occurs when the fatty plug that fills the obturator canal becomes atrophied and leaves a potential defect. Any condition that increases intraabdominal pressure will increase the risk of herniation.[26,29,32] The surgeon must remember the relationship of the branches of the obturator artery lest they be cut during the repair of the hernia, resulting in severe

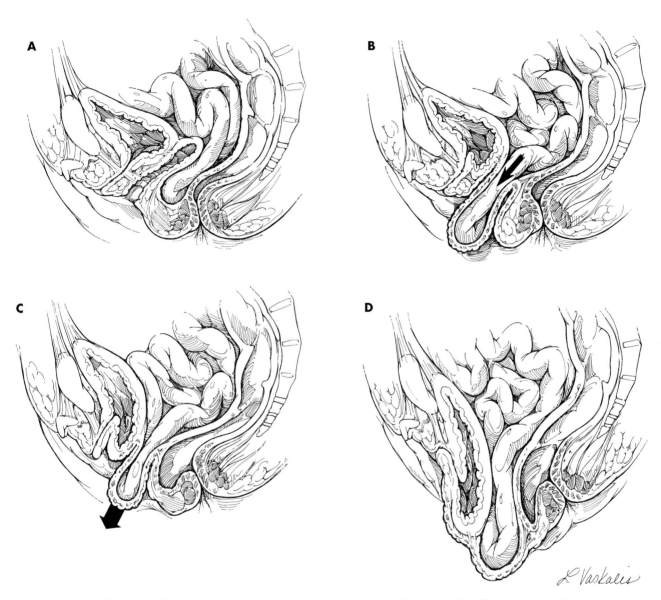

Fig. 23-2 Examples of enterocele. **A,** Posterior "congenital" enterocele without eversion of the vagina. **B,** Pulsion enterocele. The upper vagina is everted, and the enterocele sac follows the everted vault. Cystocele and rectocele are minimal. **C,** Traction enterocele. Eversion of the upper two thirds of the vagina with enterocele, cystocele, and rectocele. **D,** Eversion of the entire vagina, including the tissues distal to the urogenital diaphragm. Notice the change in the urethral axis. (Redrawn from Nichols DH, Randall CL: *Vaginal surgery,* ed 4, Baltimore, 1996, Williams & Wilkins.)

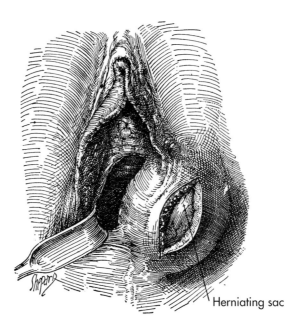

Fig. 23-3 Incision made through the skin overlying a labial or pudendal enterocele, showing the sac of the hernia. (From Watson LF: *Hernia,* St Louis, 1938, Mosby.)

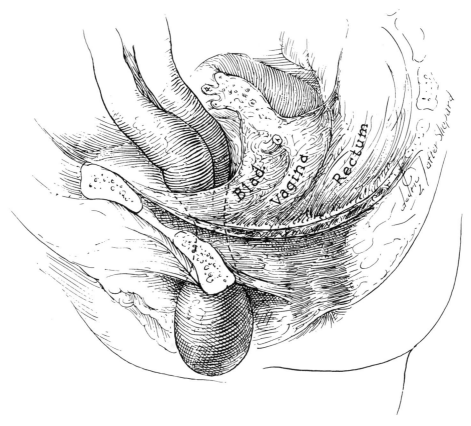

Fig. 23-4 Sagittal view of pudendal or lateral enterocele. (From Nichols DH: *Obstet Gynecol* 40:257, 1972.)

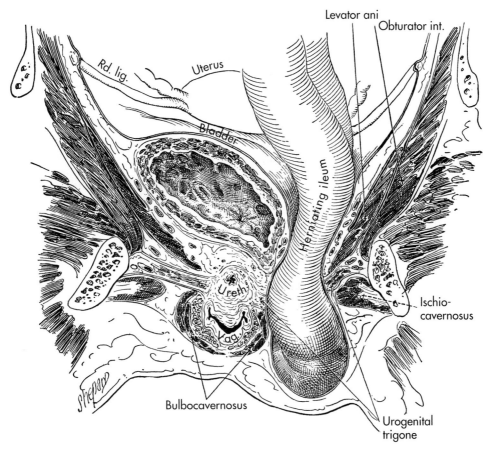

Fig. 23-5   Pudendal hernia. Transverse section showing the relations of the descending sac to the labia majora. (From Watson LF: *Hernia,* St Louis, 1938, Mosby.)

hemorrhage. Because the sac is medial to the neurovascular bundle, the incision should be made posteriorly and medially if the sac cannot be reduced. The opposite side should be examined because there is a 6% incidence of bilaterality.[23] Pressure on the obturator nerve by the hernia may elicit the so-called Howship-Romberg sign, which is characterized by intermittent pain referred to the medial thigh and knee and associated with abdominal pain. It may be of the Richter type (partial herniation only), although if bowel is trapped within the hernia the condition may produce an intestinal obstruction.[32]

Perineal Hernia

A perineal hernia is more common in females than in males, possibly because of attenuation of the pelvic floor during pregnancy. It may be primary (congenitally acquired) or secondary (after exenteration or abdominoperineal resection) and either anterior or posterior to the transverse perineal muscle. It may be seen as a labial mass or a swelling between the anus and the ischial tuberosity[3] and may be associated with difficulty in defecation, although some are asymptomatic, presenting as a soft, reducible perineal mass. Intestinal incarceration and obstruction are uncommon because of the wide neck of the sac. Treatment is always surgical, involving closure of the neck of the sac and reinforce-

ment of tissue defect by fascia transplant, or permanent synthetic fabric is occasionally useful.

Sciatic Hernia

A sciatic is either congenital, resulting from maldevelopment of the piriform muscle, or acquired. Although exceedingly uncommon, it may be one of three types, depending on location: through the greater sciatic foramen, cranial to the piriform muscle, or caudal to the muscle and through the lesser sciatic foramen beneath the sacrospinous ligament. Symptoms, when present, usually are those of intestinal obstruction, which is treated at appropriate laparotomy. Sciatic nerve compression may cause pain that radiates down the posterior thigh. When found, but asymptomatic, these hernias should be treated by obliteration or excision of the sac and tight closure of its neck, most likely transabdominally.

Other Hernias of the Pelvis

Hernias of the broad ligament either above or below the suspensory ligament of the ovary have been described and may cause intraabdominal pain when intestine or omentum has become trapped in the pouch.[8]

Rarely, a rectal hernia may protrude through a defect in the muscles of the pelvic floor, and when extraperitoneal, there is no peritoneal sac. Cali et al.[4] have provided an excellent review of the rare hernias of the pelvic floor.

PUDENDAL HYDROCELE

When a canal persists alongside the round ligament, in the labia majora, and the internal or proximal end of the canal is closed, fluid may collect within the sac, producing a pudendal or labial hydrocele. It differs from labial enterocele in that the neck of the hydrocele sac is closed and the fluid content is not reducible, nor is a cough impulse transmitted. Hydrocele is distinguished from a Bartholin's cyst by its location in the anterocranial portion of the labia majora. Occasionally hydrocele is bilateral.

Pudendal hydrocele is harmless, but when painful it is treated surgically by opening and extirpation of the sac and suture obliteration of the wound. Simple aspiration of the fluid or balloon marsupialization of the sac usually is followed by prompt recurrence. The treatment of pudendal enterocele requires excision of the sac and careful closure of its neck. If the edges of the neck of the sac are crisp and well defined it may be closed from below, but if the edges are rounded or ill defined, transabdominal closure may be more secure and preferable.

Because both pulsion and traction enteroceles are invariably progressive, they tend ultimately to pull with them the organs attached to the sides of the herniating peritoneal sac. As a result, complete eversion of the vaginal vault may occur, usually combined with a degree of lower vaginal eversion. This type of enterocele requires repair.

Iatrogenic Enterocele

Iatrogenic alterations in pelvic anatomy may play a role in the development of an enterocele. For example, an anterior enterocele may develop if an unresected excess of anterior peritoneum was not removed at the time of hysterectomy (Fig. 23-6), or a posterior enterocele may develop if a surgical procedure changed the normally horizontal vaginal axis to a vertical inclination (Fig. 23-7). The failure to recognize and correct an unusually deep cul-de-sac at the time of hysterectomy also may lead to the development of a posterior enterocele.

Burch[3] has suggested that enterocele may follow the urethrovesical "pin-up" operation in 11% to 15% of instances, probably because the operation changes the vaginal axis in a way that may leave the cul-de-sac unprotected and therefore subject to unusual stress from changes in intraabdominal pressure. For this reason, the gynecologic surgeon should take specific intraperitoneal operative steps to obliterate the cul-de-sac at the time of a pin-up operation, thus sparing the patient the risk of the secondary difficulty of subsequent enterocele. Such steps may include the use of Moschcowitz[16] or Halban[6] sutures, or even peritonealization after coincident hysterectomy.

The incidence of enterocele subsequent to vaginal hysterectomy can be determined only by long-term follow-up.

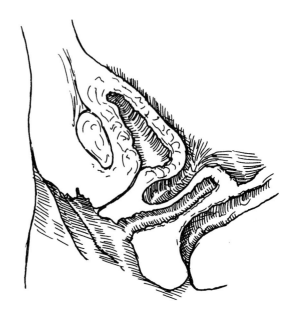

Fig. 23-6   A posthysterectomy anterior enterocele lies between the bladder and the vagina. (Redrawn from Nichols DH: *Obstet Gynecol* 40:257, 1972.)

A postoperative examination at 6 weeks gives no indication of this problem, because it usually is more than 6 months after surgery before an enterocele occurs; often, it is not until after 1 or more years. At 6-week follow-up examinations of 944 patients after vaginal reconstruction, Hawksworth and Roux[7] noted that only 3 had symptoms of enteroceles that required subsequent operation. More than 1 year after surgery, however, 26 of 416 such patients had developed enteroceles that required repair.

Anterior and posterior colporrhaphy should follow vaginal hysterectomy whenever the degree of genital prolapse is significant, as determined by an examination of the unanesthetized patient both while she is supine and while she is standing. Many surgeons elect the vaginal route when hysterectomy is indicated, for example, when there is dysfunctional uterine bleeding, with or without small fibroids. Surgery by this route can often proceed quickly and with a minimum of postoperative discomfort and morbidity. However, an accompanying vaginal prolapse that is demonstrable is likely to subsequently require secondary operative reconstruction. A so-called pseudoprolapse (demonstrated only when traction is applied by a tenaculum to the cervix) may warrant no other attention than recognition at the time of vaginal hysterectomy.

SYMPTOMS OF ENTEROCELE

Patients with an enterocele and vault prolapse often describe a feeling of pelvic heaviness and a bearing-down sensation, especially when standing; these symptoms occur because the pull of gravity stretches the mesentery of the contents of the sac. If the cardinal and uterosacral ligaments are involved in the prolapse, downward traction on the utero-

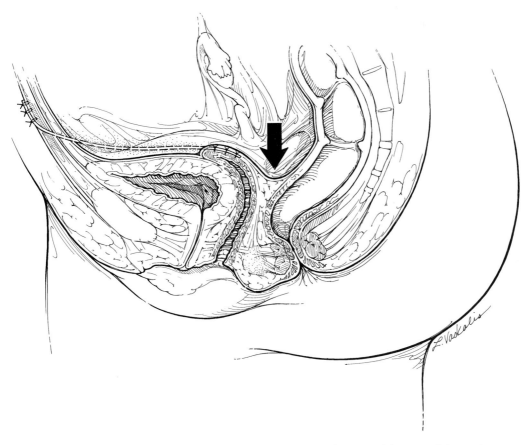

Fig. 23-7 The unprotected cul-de-sac *(arrow)* exposed after ventral fixation of the vagina.

sacral ligaments often causes a backache that may worsen as the day goes on and is quickly relieved by lying down.

The presence of a protruding vulvar mass may cause vaginal discomfort, and coincident dyspareunia, which is accentuated by the dryness of the exteriorized vagina, is common. If the vaginal skin is ulcerated, discharge and bleeding may be troublesome. When rectocele coexists, the patient may have difficulty in emptying the bowel, incomplete movements, and postevacuation discomfort. Urinary complaints are uncommon unless displacement cystocele coexists when there is inability to empty the bladder, resulting in stagnation of urine with overflow incontinence. Thoughtful and appropriate reconstructive genital surgery should relieve the discomfort and distress of all these symptoms.

DIAGNOSIS

The descent of the cul-de-sac without an accompanying enterocele is related primarily to a major defect in the pelvic diaphragm. The descent usually, although not always, is seen in a postmenopausal woman in whom the pelvic diaphragm sags, the levator plate tips, and the horizontal axis of the upper vagina is lost. This condition differs from an enterocele, which is an actual herniation between the rectum

and the vagina, and it is important to distinguish between the two conditions before surgery, since the treatment of each is different (see Chapter 29).

An enterocele can coexist with other manifestations of genital prolapse, but it is likely to be unrecognized when the patient is examined only when relaxed and in the lithotomy position. The proper time to identify an enterocele is before surgery, because damage that is obvious when the patient is awake and straining is less evident when she is anesthetized and in the recumbent position. Preoperative rectovaginal examination of the unanesthetized patient is therefore indicated with the patient both at rest and while straining, in both the lithotomy and standing positions. Contrast radiography occasionally proves helpful.[9-11]

An effective way of distinguishing between enterocele, prolapse of the vaginal vault, rectocele, a defective perineum, and combinations of these weaknesses is by performing a preoperative examination of the standing, unanesthetized patient. With an index finger in the patient's rectum, the gynecologist inserts the thumb into her vagina. The presence of vault prolapse can be established by replacing the vault of the vagina to its highest level within the pelvis and noting what happens when the patient bears down, as by Valsalva maneuver. If a peritoneal sac that contains omentum or a palpable loop of bowel comes down between the

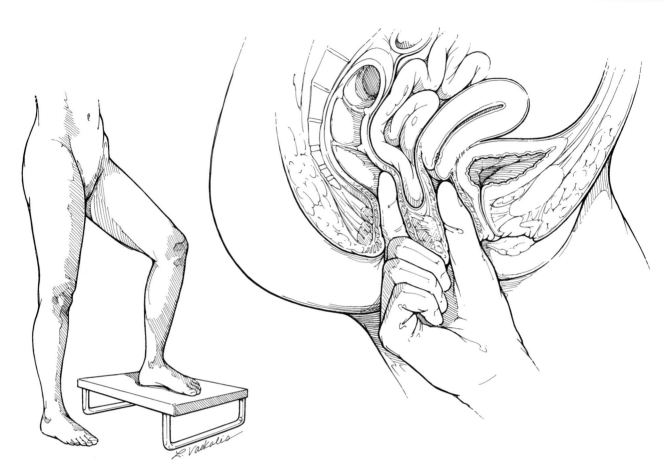

Fig. 23-8 Examination of the patient in a standing position permits the thumb in the vagina to note and replace any descent of the vaginal vault, whereas the index finger introduced into the rectum permits evaluation of any possible rectocele. When the patient strains, any enterocele present is evidenced by palpation of a bowel-filled sac prolapse dissecting the rectovaginal septum.

thumb and the index finger, the woman unquestionably has an enterocele (Fig. 23-8). Because an enterocele splits Denonvilliers' fascia, it weakens the upper posterior vaginal wall. A high rectocele is so often associated with an enterocele that the presence of one should always give rise to a suspicion of the other; the treatment of both should be coincident and often requires a transvaginal, rather than a transabdominal, surgical procedure for optimal success.

The preoperative evaluation is important because many enteroceles thought to have developed after vaginal surgery are actually aggravations of an unrecognized and therefore untreated condition that existed at the time of an original pelvic operation.

MANAGEMENT OF ENTEROCELE

The indicated management of enterocele may be prophylactic, nonsurgical, or surgical.

Prophylaxis

Intraabdominal pressure may be decreased and the development or progression of an enterocele thereby prevented by reducing weight, avoiding tight girdles and corsets, and refraining from smoking cigarettes to decrease smoker's cough.

At the time of a vaginal hysterectomy and repair, the surgeon can do a great deal to prevent postoperative enterocele,[12] even though an existing or potential enterocele may not be obvious in a patient who is anesthetized and in Trendelenburg's position, for example, in which the pull of gravity is toward the head of the table. After removing the uterus and before closing the peritoneum, the surgeon should hook a finger in the cul-de-sac to see if it contains any extra peritoneum that should be excised (Fig. 23-9). If the uterosacral ligaments are strong, they should be shortened and used appropriately to help support the vaginal vault. This procedure may involve a culdeplasty in which stitches are placed into these shortened uterosacral ligaments to draw the vault of the vagina back into the hollow of the sacrum, cranial and posterior to the point at which the peritoneum has been closed[15] (Fig. 23-10). The same type of stitches may be placed immediately after abdominal hysterectomy. Coincident excision and side-to-side approximation of an appropriate wedge from the posterior vaginal vault may be per-

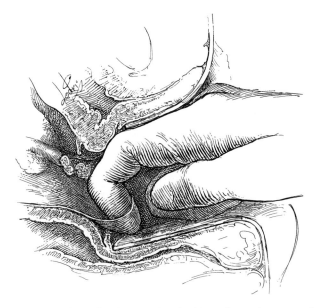

Fig. 23-9 The index finger is hooked into the peritoneum of the cul-de-sac following hysterectomy to identify any enterocele sac that may be present so that it may be excised at this point. (From Nichols DH, Randall CL: *Vaginal surgery*, ed 4, Baltimore, 1996, Williams & Wilkins.)

formed either transvaginally or transabdominally if it is excessively wide (Figs. 23-10 and 23-11).

After vaginal hysterectomy, a high purse-string closure of the peritoneal cavity is often helpful. Taking good bites of both the uterosacral and the round ligaments, but with care to avoid the ureter, the surgeon approximates the connective tissues to which the peritoneum is attached. If a large enterocele has been resected, the surgeon may place two purse-string sutures, one caudal to the other.

Nonsurgical Treatment

Pessaries are occasionally of temporary help in patients with coincident genital prolapse who are not candidates for surgery or whose personal schedule does not permit surgery (e.g., those with small children at home or with an aging relative who requires constant care). Patients are most likely to be able to retain a pessary of the ring type, a rubber doughnut, or sometimes a Gellhorn (see Chapter 26). Isometric pubococcygeal contraction exercises are helpful in restoring muscle tone, but they are not curative.

Surgical Treatment

The goals of the surgical repair of an enterocele are to (1) recognize the entity and its probable cause; (2) expose, dissect, mobilize, and then excise or obliterate the entire sac; (3) occlude the orifice of the sac by ligation as high as possible; and (4) perform all indicated repairs to provide adequate support from below for the occluded orifice of the sac and to reestablish a normal upper vaginal axis, if the axis is defective, so that the area of previous herniation will be held in place over a horizontal levator

plate. The specific objectives of surgical treatment include the following:

1. Restoration of normal anatomy and function
2. Prevention of recurrence as a result of the recognition and consideration of etiologic factors
3. Appropriate surgical treatment of coexistent pelvic disease, when indicated
4. Recognition and treatment of any contributing medical disease

The choice of surgical procedure for the repair of an enterocele is based on several considerations. There is no one standard corrective operation. The etiology, symptoms, and principles of surgical treatment are considerably different for each of the various sites.

Transvaginal procedures involve recognition and excision of the sac (see Fig. 23-11), followed by high ligation of the peritoneum. The transvaginal double purse-string closure of the neck of the sac of an enterocele is essentially a transvaginal Moschcowitz closure. Each of the two purse-string sutures takes some of the strain off the other. In addition, bringing together two areas of peritoneum lining the neck of the sac instead of one produces a stronger scar (Fig. 23-12). This technique is useful if there is a coincident vault prolapse that is to be treated separately.

The problem with the transabdominal Moschcowitz procedure for enterocele is that the operation was originally developed to repair a prolapsed or sliding rectum by attaching it to a fairly strong vagina and cervix. Gynecologists appropriated the operation and reversed the principle by attaching a sliding vagina to the anterior wall of the rectum. The latter has rather poor structural support, however (Fig. 23-13, p. 434).

The Halban or Moschcowitz obliteration of the cul-de-sac helps prevent an enterocele, but it is not an effective treatment for a vault prolapse. Neither the Halban nor the Moschcowitz procedure per se provides adequate support for the vaginal vault. Both obliterate the cul-de-sac, and neither requires skinning out removal of excess peritoneum. There are several problems with this approach. Tying the top stitch at the pelvic brim is difficult, and any central opening that remains can provide access to a loop of small bowel and may cause intestinal obstruction. Furthermore, because it is placed near the ureter, the top stitch may be close enough to pull or displace the tissue to which the ureter is attached, causing a kink in the ureter on either side and leading to urinary obstruction.

Sagittally placed Halban-type stitches (Figs. 23-14 to 23-17, pp. 435 and 436) are literally vertical purse-string or Moschcowitz-type stitches, but they do not disturb the course of the ureter. They are especially useful when the vault has not prolapsed. They can be placed after either transabdominal or transvaginal operations (see Figs. 23-15 and 23-16), but neither type of stitch effectively anchors a poorly supported or unsupported vaginal vault, the latter requiring separate colpopexy. The patient who has a very wide and deep pouch of Douglas and risks chronically increased intraabdominal pressure secondary to obesity or respiratory obstruction from chronic pulmonary disease or vigorous

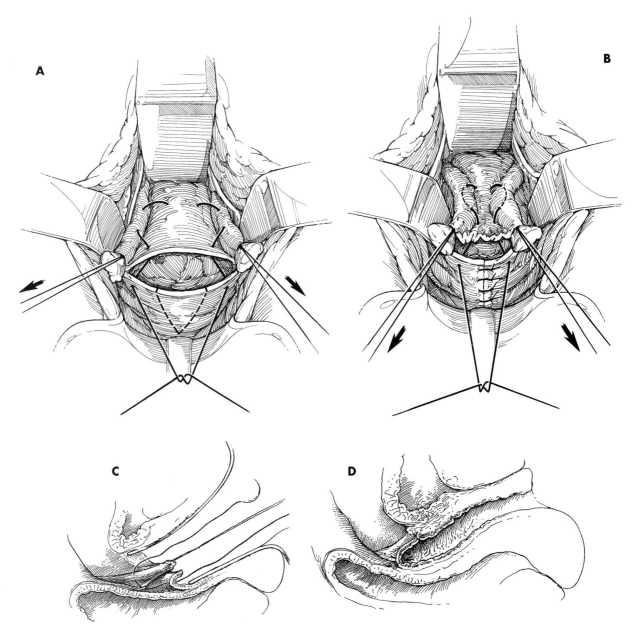

Fig. 23-10   The modified McCall culdeplasty. **A,** Any enterocele sac has been resected, and using a long-lasting polyglycolic acid suture, the stitches are placed through the vaginal wall, through the cut edge of the peritoneum, and high on the medial surface of the uterosacral ligament, and a bite is taken in the peritoneum overlying the anterior surface of the rectum. The same structures are stitched in reverse order on the opposite side. When using a monofilament suture, it is wise to place a second McCall stitch approximately 1 cm cranial to the first. In the event of unexpected breakage of one of the sutures during the tying process, there will still be one unbroken suture left to support the vault of the vagina. A very wide posterior vault may be narrowed by excising an appropriately sized wedge as shown by the *dashed line.* **B,** The sides of the V-shaped wound in the posterior vaginal wall are closed with interrupted polyglycolic acid sutures. This closure not only narrows the vault but also brings the uterosacral ligaments that are fixed to the vault closer together. After the peritoneum is closed, the McCall stitches are tied. **C,** The first half of the modified culdeplasty stitch is shown in sagittal section before tying and closure of the peritoneal cavity and vaginal vault. **D,** The stitch is shown after tying and subsequent closure of the peritoneal cavity and vaginal vault. The apex of the vagina is now cranial and posterior to the new peritoneal cul-de-sac. (From Nichols DH, Randall CL: *Vaginal surgery,* ed 4, Baltimore, 1996, Williams & Wilkins.)

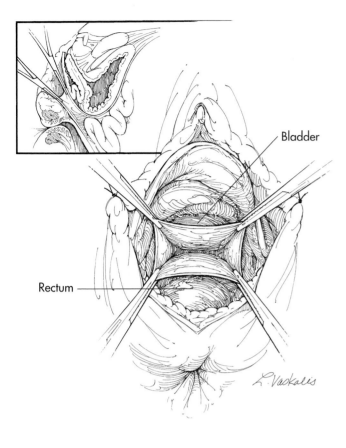

Bladder

Rectum

Fig. 23-11 Transvaginal demonstration of enterocele. An incision has been made through the perineum and into the rectovaginal space. The posterior vaginal wall has been incised in the midline, reaching an enterocele sac that is identified as a double fold of peritoneum attached to the undersurface of the vagina. The sac has been opened, mobilized, and the edges held in hemostats as shown, preparatory to its resection. This is shown in sagittal section in the *inset.* (From Nichols DH, editor: *Reoperative gynecologic and obstetric surgery,* ed 2, St Louis, 1997, Mosby.)

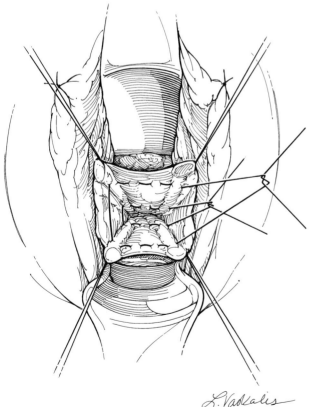

Fig. 23-12 The enterocele has been resected and the peritoneal cavity closed by a purse-string suture that starts on the peritoneal side of the left uterosacral ligament, reefs the posterior peritoneum, the right uterosacral ligament, right round ligament, anterior peritoneum, and left round ligament. After this has been tied, a second purse-string suture is placed 1 cm distal to the first, reinforcing the closure.

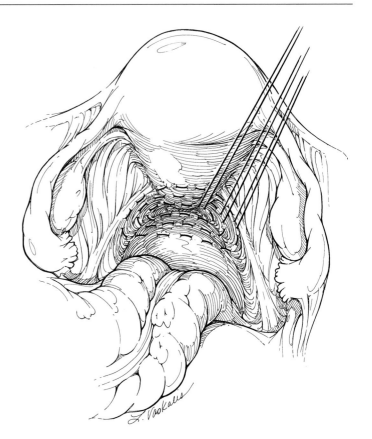

Fig. 23-13   The Moschcowitz procedure. A series of concentric sutures are placed as shown to obliterate the cul-de-sac.

lifestyle, may carry increased risk of reopening a surgically obliterated or fused cul-de-sac. There are two additional surgical methods of obliterating the pouch of Douglas over a wider area. One is to dissect and resect the entire peritoneal lining of the pouch, and after controlling the many areas of oozing and bleeding by ligature or cautery, sew the raw surfaces together by many interrupted sutures. This method is time consuming, usually bloody, and may expose to possible trauma the surfaces of the larger blood vessels and ureters. Another effective, faster, and safer method that does not involve peritoneal resection and is useful when the enterocele is recurrent or has a very wide neck is to obliterate such a wide pouch of Douglas by an initial purse-string suture at its very base, then sewing from front to back a transversely placed continuous nonabsorbable suture that begins at the very bottom of the cavity (Fig. 23-18). By alternate bites 1 cm apart between the interior and the posterior cul-de-sac surfaces, the suture is continued back and forth from one side of the pelvis to the other using a running locked stitch. The stitch is continued by additional rows a centimeter or so cranial to its predecessor until the brim of the pelvis is reached when the suture is tied. A final row of interrupted sutures 1 cm apart is placed at the pelvic brim. During the course of the procedure the site of the vital structures is kept under observation, and trauma to them is avoided. The same technique, but with the steps in reverse order, can be used transvaginally (Fig. 23-19).

An enterocele accompanied by a prolapse of the vault posterior to the cervix in a patient whose uterus has been fixed by a Gilliam suspension or ventral fixation is treated transvaginally by high ligation of the neck of the sac. This includes a deep bite or two into the lower posterior part of the cervix or lower uterine segment, then excision of the sac. If the uterosacral ligaments are strong, they are approximated at the midline and shortened. Any coexistent cystocele or rectocele is repaired, with the rectocele repair including the high, full-length posterior colporrhaphy. If eversion of the upper vagina coexists and the strength of the cardinal and uterosacral ligaments is insufficient to support the vaginal vault securely, the upper vaginal vault may be sewn to the right sacrospinous ligament (see Chapter 26).

Transabdominal procedures that may be used for the repair of an enterocele include excision of redundant cul-de-sac peritoneum with approximation of uterosacral ligaments, transverse obliterative sutures of the Halban type,[6] or circumferential obliterative sutures of the Marion-Moschcowitz type.[13,16] A wide, voluminous posterior vagina should be narrowed by wedging, as suggested by both Waters[28] and Torpin.[24] This procedure, which can be done either transabdominally or transvaginally, tends to approximate the uterosacral ligament attachments closer to the midline. The McCall transvaginal culdeplasty may be useful if there are palpably strong uterosacral ligaments, as with the uterovaginal or "sliding" type of prolapse,[15] and can even be employed transabdominally when surgery is by laparotomy.

If eversion of the vagina coexists with enterocele and the abdomen is open, the surgeon may consider transabdominal colposacropexy (see Chapter 26) to preserve vaginal length; however, any coincident cystocele and rectocele must be repaired by a separate procedure at a later date. Any trans-

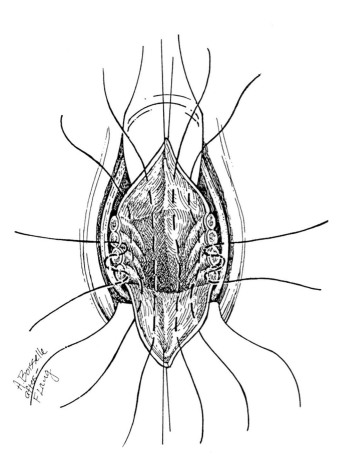

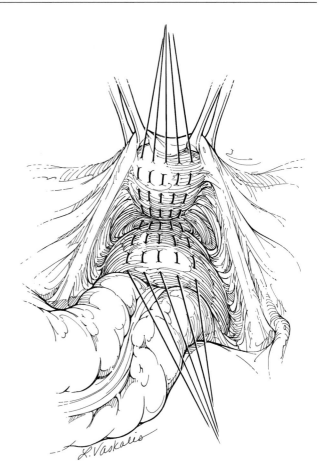

Fig. 23-14 Sagittal obliteration of the cul-de-sac may be performed after vaginal hysterectomy as shown. (From Nichols DH, Randall CL: *Vaginal surgery,* ed 4, Baltimore, 1996, Williams & Wilkins.)

Fig. 23-15 Halban obliteration of the cul-de-sac. The cul-de-sac is being obliterated by a series of interrupted stitches placed from front to back.

abdominal procedure that changes the vaginal axis to a more vertical direction (e.g., the Marshall-Marchetti-Krantz procedure[14] or the Burch procedure,[3] ventral suspension, or fixation) necessitates surgical obliteration of the peritoneum-lined cul-de-sac anterior to the rectum to provide adequate protection for the pouch of Douglas. The increased exposure, vulnerability, and risk of enterocele that result from a failure to obliterate a deep anterior or posterior cul-de-sac should be more widely recognized. An anterior enterocele that develops after hysterectomy is probably best treated by transvaginal resection of the sac and redundant peritoneum, with restoration of the normal upper vaginal axis and correction of any defect in the levator plate.

Anterior enterocele (i.e., anterior to the vagina) rarely can develop following sacrospinous colpopexy if there has been a previous permanent change in the axis of the anterior vaginal wall, for example, from a vaginal "pin-up" procedure such as the Marshall-Marchetti or Burch operation. In this event, the therapeutic approach should be that of obliteration of the peritoneal sac usually transabdominally and possibly incorporating sagittally placed sutures of the Halban type. These sutures recreate the peritoneal fusion of the fascia of Denonvilliers. They should be placed about 1 cm apart.

A pudendal or lateral enterocele may be approached transvaginally if the margins of the neck of the sac can be readily identified. If these margins are ill defined, the surgeon should consider either a combined vaginal-abdominal or an abdominal approach.

The simplest treatment of true rectal prolapse with or without coexistent genital prolapse is the insertion of Thiersch wires to reinforce the anal sphincter. More radical procedures for recurrence are the transperineal resection developed by Altemeier, Hoxworth, and Giuseffi[1] or, better yet, the transabdominal operation developed by Ripstein and Lanter,[22] in which a slinglike pararectal replacement of synthetic plastic material is used to replace or supplement attenuated rectal supports. Coincident genital prolapse should be treated by appropriate surgical reconstruction. Anal prolapse can be treated by retrorectal levatorplasty.

It is essential that the gynecologist recognize an enterocele and any condition likely to result in an enterocele and correlate such a condition with its cause, symptoms, progression, and other coexistent pelvic damage. The possible operative procedures should be chosen on the basis of the correlation between etiology, location, and treatment of various types of enterocele[17] (Table 23-1, p. 438).

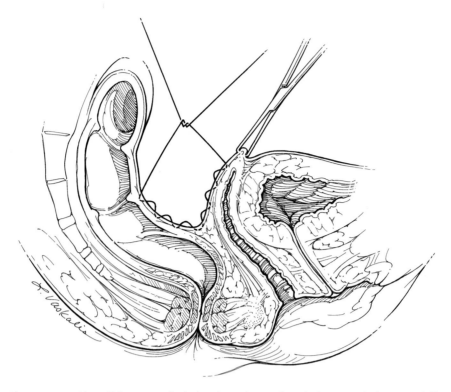

Fig. 23-16   After all interrupted stitches have been placed, they are tied sequentially.

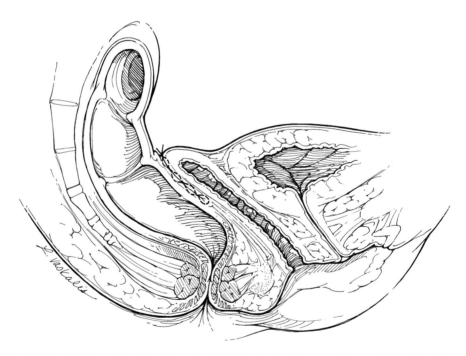

Fig. 23-17   Stitches placed in this sagittal fashion, fusing the posterior vaginal wall and vaginal vault to the anterior surface of the rectum, do not disturb the course of the ureter. An alternative method consists of closing the cul-de-sac from front to back. For the especially deep enterocele the end result of a modification of the Halban sagittal closure that will shorten the cul-de-sac less is shown. Starting at the pelvic brim, stitches are taken alternately in the anterior then posterior wall of the full depth of the cul-de-sac peritoneum, the direction reversed at the bottom, and the suture returned to the site of origin, where it is tied to the free end. Several of these stitches are placed in a sagittal plane.

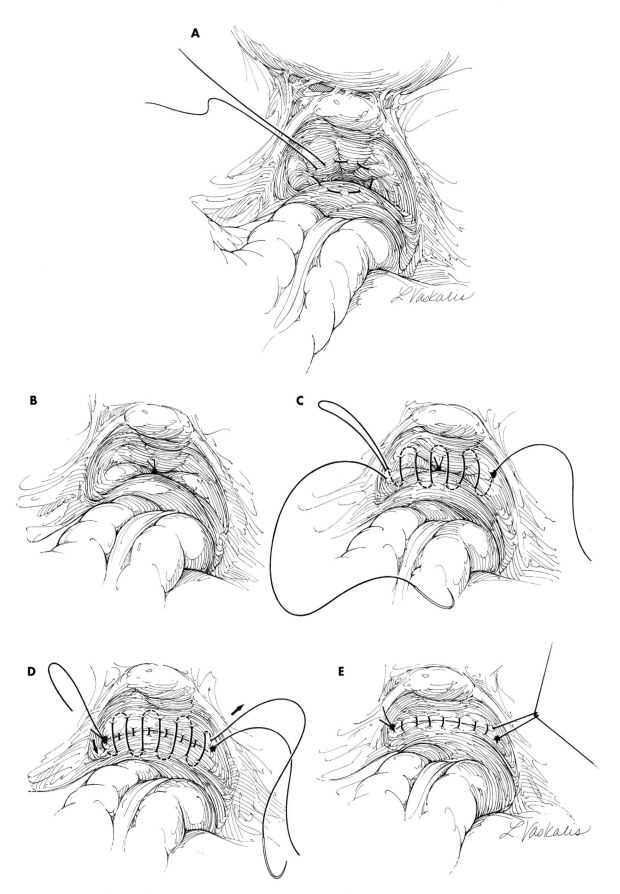

Fig. 23-18 Three-layered transabdominal closure of the cul-de-sac. **A,** A purse-string of synthetic monofilament nonabsorbable suture is placed at the bottom of the cul-de-sac. The suture is tied **(B)**, and a second proximal layer placed from front to back **(C)**, tied, and returned to the opposite side as a third proximal layer **(D)**, and tied again. **E,** A fourth layer can be placed proximal to the third if necessary to completely obliterate the cul-de-sac. (From Nichols DH, editor: *Reoperative gynecologic and obstetric surgery,* ed 2, St Louis, 1997, Mosby.)

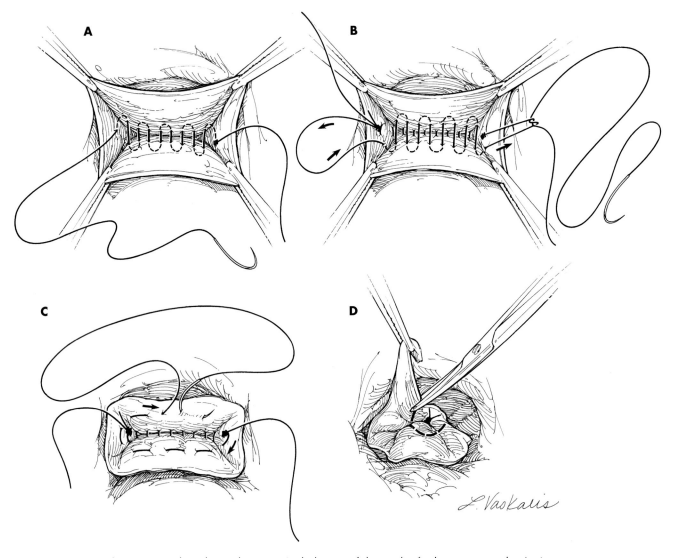

Fig. 23-19 Three-layered transvaginal closure of the neck of a large enterocele. **A,** A synthetic monofilament nonabsorbable suture closes the neck of the sac from front to back. The knot is tied at the 9-o'clock position, the suture loop cut open, and the free end returned as a second slightly distal layer to the starting point, where it is tied to the original stitch end **(B).** A third distal layer is placed as a purse-string **(C),** tied, and the edges of the sac trimmed **(D).** (From Nichols DH, editor: *Reoperative gynecologic and obstetric surgery,* ed 2, St Louis, 1997, Mosby.)

Table 23-1 Correlation between Etiology, Location, and Treatment of Enterocele

Cause	Location	Treatment
Congenital	Sac between posterior vaginal wall and anterior rectal wall	Excision of the sac with high ligation of its neck; approximation of uterosacral ligaments
Pulsion (pushed)	With eversion of vaginal vault	Restore vault depth by shortening cardinal-uterosacral ligaments or culdeplasty if ligaments are strong; if ligaments are of poor quality, sacrospinous fixation or sacrocolpopexy; coincident hysterectomy if desirable
Traction (pulled)	Same as congenital, with lower eversion (cystocele and rectocele) pulling vault into eversion	Same procedure as above plus anterior and posterior colporrhaphy
Iatrogenic	Anterior to vagina, or posterior from change in vaginal axis	Excise or obliterate sac and restore normal vaginal axis if defective

From Nichols DH: *Obstet Gynecol* 40:257, 1972.

REFERENCES

1. Altemeier WA, Hoxworth PI, Giuseffi J: Further experiences with the treatment of prolapse of the rectum, *Surg Clin North Am* 35:1437, 1955.
2. Anderson WR: Pudendal hernia, *Obstet Gynecol* 32:802, 1968.
3. Burch JC: Urethrovaginal fixation to Cooper's ligament for correction of stress incontinence, cystocele, and prolapse, *Am J Obstet Gynecol* 81:281, 1961.
4. Cali RL, Pitsch RM, Blatchford GJ, et al: Rare pelvic floor hernias: report of a case and review of the literature, *Dis Colon Rectum* 35:604, 1992.
5. Chase HC: Levator hernia (pudendal hernia), *Surg Gynecol Obstet* 35:717, 1992.
6. Halban J: *Gynäkologische Operationslehre*, Berlin, 1932, Urban & Schwarzenberg.
7. Hawksworth W, Roux JP: Vaginal hysterectomy, *J Obstet Gynecol Br Commonw* 63:214, 1958.
8. Hunt AB: Fenestrae and pouches in the broad ligament as an actual and potential cause of strangulated intra-abdominal hernia, *Surg Gynecol Obstet* 58:906, 1934.
9. Lash AF, Levin B: Roentgenographic diagnosis of vaginal vault hernia, *Obstet Gynecol* 20:427, 1962.
10. Lenzi E: *L'Ernia vaginale del Douglas o elitrocele*, Pisa, 1959, Edizioni Omnia Medica.
11. Lenzi E, et al: Per una migliore nosografia dellernia del Douglas: elitrocele o enterocele? *Riv Ost Gin Perin* 3:273, 1990.
12. Litschgi M, Käser O: The problem of enterocele, *Geburtshilfe Frauenheilkd* 38:915, 1978.
13. Marion J: Quoted by Read CD: Enterocele, *Am J Obstet Gynecol* 62:743, 1951.
14. Marshall VP, Marchetti AA, Krantz KE: The correction of stress incontinence by simple vesicourethral suspension, *Surg Gynecol Obstet* 88:509, 1949.
15. McCall ML: Posterior culdeplasty: surgical correction of enterocele during vaginal hysterectomy, a preliminary report, *Obstet Gynecol* 10:595, 1957.
16. Moschcowitz AV: The pathogenesis anatomy and cure of prolapse of the rectum, *Surg Gynecol Obstet* 15:7, 1912.
17. Nichols DH: Types of enterocele and principles underlying the choice of operation for repair, *Obstet Gynecol* 40:257, 1972.
18. Nichols DH, Genadry RR: Pelvic relaxation of the posterior compartment, *Curr Opin Obstet Gynecol* 5:458, 1993.
19. Nichols DH, editor: *Reoperative gynecologic and obstetric surgery*, ed 2, St Louis, 1997, Mosby.
20. Pirogoff in Hart DB: *Atlas of female pelvic anatomy*, Edinburgh, 1884, W & AK Johnston.
21. Read CD: Enterocele, *Am J Obstet Gynecol* 62:743, 1951.
22. Ripstein CC, Lanter B: Etiology and surgical therapy of massive prolapse of the rectum, *Am Surg* 157:259, 1963.
23. Rogers FA: Strangulated obturator hernia, *Surgery* 48:394, 1960.
24. Torpin R: Excision of the cul-de-sac of Douglas for the surgical cure of hernias through the female caudal wall: including prolapse of the uterus, *J Med Assoc Ga* 36:396, 1947.
25. Virtanen HS, Ekholm E, Kiilholma PJA: Evisceration after enterocele repair: a rare complication of vaginal surgery, *Int Urogynecol J* 7:344, 1996.
26. Wakeley CPG: Obturator hernia: its aetiology, incidence, and treatment, with two personal operative cases, *Br J Surg* 26:515, 1939.
27. Warwick R, Williams PL: *Gray's anatomy*, ed 35, Philadelphia, 1973, WB Saunders.
28. Waters EG: Vaginal prolapse, *Obstet Gynecol* 8:432, 1956.
29. Watson LF: *Hernia*, ed 2, St Louis, 1938, Mosby.
30. Weed JC, Tyrone C: Enterocele, *Am J Obstet Gynecol* 60:324, 1950.
31. Wilensky AV, Kaufman PA: Vaginal hernia, *Am J Surg* 49:31, 1940.
32. Wilson JM: *Pelvic relaxations and herniations*, Springfield, Ill, 1954, Charles C Thomas.
33. Zacharin RF: *Pelvic floor anatomy and the surgery of pulsion enterocele*, New York, 1985, Springer-Verlag.

24 The Small and Painful Vagina

DAVID H. NICHOLS

Disproportion between the size of a woman's vagina and her partner's penis is a common cause of dyspareunia. Congenital deformities, such as absence of the vagina and uterus, absence of the lower half of the vagina, and obstructive transverse septa at any level, including an imperforate hymen, may result in a vagina that cannot admit or contain the penis comfortably. Some women have a longitudinal vaginal septum that creates a second birth canal that may be coincident with a rudimentary uterine horn, leading to dysmenorrhea as well as dyspareunia. Thick lateral bands connecting the external urethral meatus to the hymenal margin may be a source of dyspareunia. Also, because these bands drag on the meatus during coitus, they may invite recurrent postcoital cystitis.[4] The subject and treatment of vaginal agenesis is discussed in Chapter 43.

Menopausal change may be a factor, especially when a woman has undergone pelvic irradiation or when an unusual degree of progressive atrophy and shrinkage has accompanied the aging process. Some relative flaccidity of the penis of the menopausal woman's partner may compound the coital problem, making vaginal penetration difficult.

There are significant iatrogenic causes of a small vagina. For example, postepisiotomy scarring may decrease the size of the vagina, or hysterectomy, especially radical surgery with partial vaginectomy, may leave the vagina too short. The vaginal diameter may be left too narrow as a consequence of excessive subepithelial placation or the excision of a more than necessary amount of vaginal membrane with colporrhaphy. Subepithelial ridges that form postoperatively may become more tender as the fibrosis of scarring progresses.

Psychosomatic factors also may contribute to dyspareunia associated with a small vagina by inhibiting relaxation of paravaginal muscles. Some women fear being hurt or becoming pregnant, must overcome the psychologic scarring that follows rape, or lack accurate knowledge concerning sexual practices. Some have an unconscious or conscious desire to inflict punishment on themselves or their marital partners.

These factors may be etiologically grouped in any combination. Successful treatment requires identification and proper attention to each contributing factor.

PREVENTION OF A SMALL VAGINA

The best treatment of a small vagina is prevention. If the patient is postmenopausal, particularly if there are signs of mucosal or vulvar atrophy, more or less permanent estrogen replacement therapy will strengthen, restore, and preserve vaginal blood supply and elasticity in estrogen-sensitive pelvic tissues.

Proper techniques of either vaginal or abdominal hysterectomy, particularly in patients who had some degree of genital prolapse, require that elongated cardinal and uterosacral ligaments be shortened and firmly attached to the vault of the vagina. When these ligaments are hypertrophic, culdeplasty is often helpful in preserving or restoring vaginal length. In principle, culdeplasty involves fixing the vaginal vault to the undersurface of strong uterosacral ligaments after bringing them together in front of the vagina, thus reducing any tendency toward enterocele formation (Fig. 24-1). In fact, the surgeon should attempt to identify any actual or potential enterocele and should excise any excess peritoneum before high peritonealization. The excision of any excess width strengthens the vaginal vault. This technique can be successful in conjunction with either vaginal or abdominal hysterectomy, but with the latter the surgeon must be especially careful not to allow a ureteral obstruction.

As Amreich[2] has pointed out a short vagina that ends anterior to the levator plate tends to become even shorter with time, as intraabdominal pressure may then be transmitted in the axis of the vagina. Fixing the vault above the levator plate preserves vaginal depth and lessens any tendency for telescoping, as increases in intraabdominal pressure compress the vagina against the levator plate. If the cardinal-uterosacral ligaments are not strong and surgically useful, the surgeon must use alternative methods of colpopexy to support the vault (see Chapter 26).

When performing colporrhaphy, the surgeon must carefully calculate the amount of the vagina to be excised to ensure an acceptable postoperative vaginal width. There should be suitable allowance for any shrinkage that is likely to occur with aging and hormone withdrawal; all other things being equal, the surgeon should excise less of the vaginal membrane from a premenopausal patient in whom postmenopausal vaginal shrinkage has yet to occur. In addition, the age and genital size of the patient's partner should be considered. In the temporary absence of sexual activity, the periodic insertion of a vaginal obturator is helpful if there is any tendency toward stricture or stenosis.

TREATMENT OF A SMALL VAGINA

With lower vaginal agenesis, the surgeon dissects a tunnel through the vestibular area toward the upper vagina. (If a

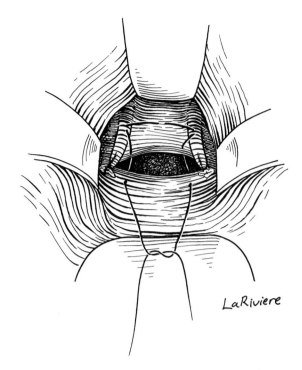

LaRiviere

Fig. 24-1 Modified New Orleans culdeplasty. The enterocele sac has been mobilized, excised, and a synthetic absorbable suture placed high on the uterosacral ligaments.

functional uterus accompanies this condition, a rectal examination reveals a hematocolpos.) The surgeon mobilizes the upper vaginal canal, opens it, and stretches it and sews the upper vaginal skin edge to the skin of the vestibule to cover the raw lower area. It should not be necessary to perform a graft.

A patient with a transverse vaginal septum at any level may have a uterus, which is usually functional. There is no associated urinary tract anomaly, a significant difference from the Rokitansky-Küster-Hauser syndrome. Appropriate excision is the treatment of choice for a vaginal septum or imperforate hymen.

Correction of a Stricture or Stenosis

When the vagina is narrow or constricted at a specific point, the appropriate surgical procedure to provide additional width depends on the site of the constriction. The most common site is the perineum, where constriction often follows overenthusiastic perineorrhaphy or hurried, inadequate reapproximation of an episiotomy, particularly when the pubococcygeal muscles have been approximated anterior to the rectum. A midline perineotomy with a suture of the wound placed at a right angle to the incision may be all that is necessary, although this procedure shortens the vagina slightly (Fig. 24-2). If atrophy is present, a bilateral episiotomy with sliding of the skin margins widens the introitus[14] (Fig. 24-3).

Lateral relaxing incisions through the full thickness of the vagina may relieve a stricture of the midportion of the vagina[13] (Fig. 24-4). The margins of the incision are

undercut, and the vaginal caliber is maintained by a suitable obturator during epithelization and healing. If the vaginal wall has been freshly excised, a patch may be cut of a size sufficient to fill the defect in the lateral vaginal wall and sewn in place as a full-thickness graft. These relaxing incisions can be made in a constricted vagina at any time, even years later, although a brief rehospitalization and anesthetic are necessary. The technique and aftercare are precisely the same as they are in the fresh surgical patient, however.

With moderate constriction of the lower vagina, as seen, for example, in a patient with congenital adrenal hyperplasia, the surgeon may develop a fasciocutaneous flap from the labia and swing it into place to bridge the defect created by a fresh episiotomy[12] (Fig. 24-5, p. 444).

The use of full-thickness skin flaps[9] from the inner thigh, a modification of the Graves operation[7] for construction of a neovagina, may be necessary in patients with extensive constriction of the lower half of the vagina because of either congenital underdevelopment or postoperative stricture. Convalescence requires several weeks of relative rest and several months' use of a vaginal obturator.

Modified Graves Procedure. In the Graves procedure,[7] a method of treating the congenital absence of the vagina, the surgeon creates a tunnel between the bladder and rectum and lines it with four full-thickness flaps of skin. Two of these flaps are raised from the medial surface of the thighs, and two are raised from the full thickness of the skin medial to the labia majora, including the labia minora, which are spatulated. These are all sewn together, inverted into the tunnel of the neovagina, and held there by a glass obturator until they are fixed to the walls of the cavity by healing.

When a stricture or atresia of the lower half of the vagina is so extensive that a simple midline perineotomy with a transverse closure cannot relieve it, a modification of the Graves procedure is useful. After mobilizing two full-thickness flaps from the medial surface of each thigh, the surgeon swings them into the vagina to cover the site of a fresh midline episiotomy. In performing this procedure, the surgeon:

1. Infiltrates the perineum and the medial skin of each thigh subcuticularly with approximately 100 ml of 0.5% lidocaine in 1:200,000 epinephrine solution.
2. Makes a deep midline episiotomy, separating the skin edges enough to establish the desired vaginal diameter.
3. With indelible stain, marks off skin flaps large enough for each to fill half of the space created by the unrepaired episiotomy.
4. Cuts full-thickness flaps, all the way to the underlying fascia, leaving the subcutaneous fat attached to the undersurface of each flap.
5. Undermines the residual skin of the thigh to prepare for its approximation.
6. Swings the flaps medially so that they meet in the midline and approximates their medial edges with interrupted sutures of polyglycolic acid–type material.

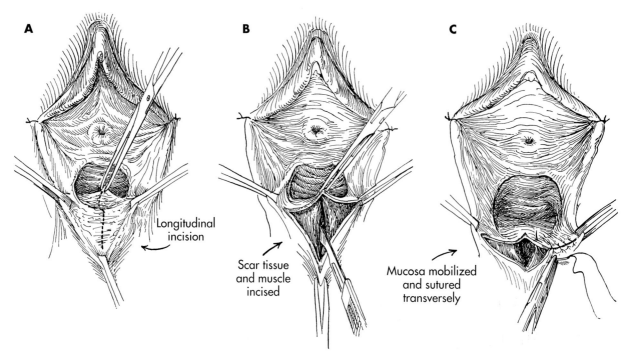

Fig. 24-2 **A,** The area of contraction and scar tissue is outlined by Allis clamps, and a longitudinal incision is made to determine the depth of the scar. **B,** The tissue around the area of contracture is incised. If this extends into the musculature of the perineum or, in the event of a higher stricture, into the musculature of the vaginal wall, the muscle and scar tissue are incised to release the constriction. **C,** The mucosa and skin of the perineum, if the constriction is at the introitus, are then mobilized to permit a transverse closure without tension. The vaginal circumference in this operation is reconstructed larger than normal to allow for some postoperative contracture. The incision is closed with interrupted absorbable sutures, and the sutures are tied just tightly enough to approximate the edges without strangulation of the tissues. (From Ball TL: *Gynecologic surgery and urology,* St Louis, 1963, Mosby.)

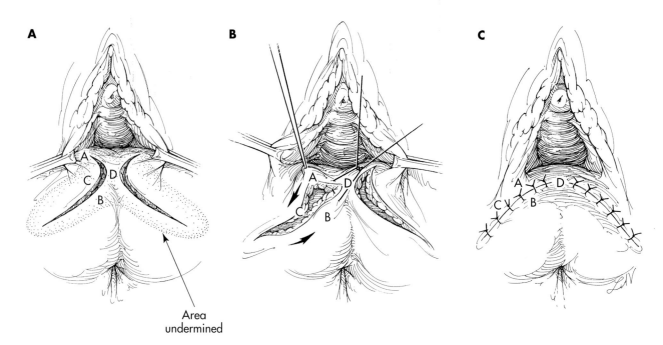

Fig. 24-3 **A,** Bilateral episiotomy is performed with release of contracted tissue by undermining and mobilizing vaginal mucosa and perineal skin. **B,** The incisions are closed by interrupted suture. Point *D* becomes the apex. **C,** Point *A* becomes adjacent to point *B*. Notice that points *A* and *C* have been brought laterally, enlarging the introitus. (From Veronikis DK: The recurrent small and painful vagina. In Nichols DH, editor: *Reoperative gynecologic and obstetric surgery,* ed 2, St Louis, 1997, Mosby.)

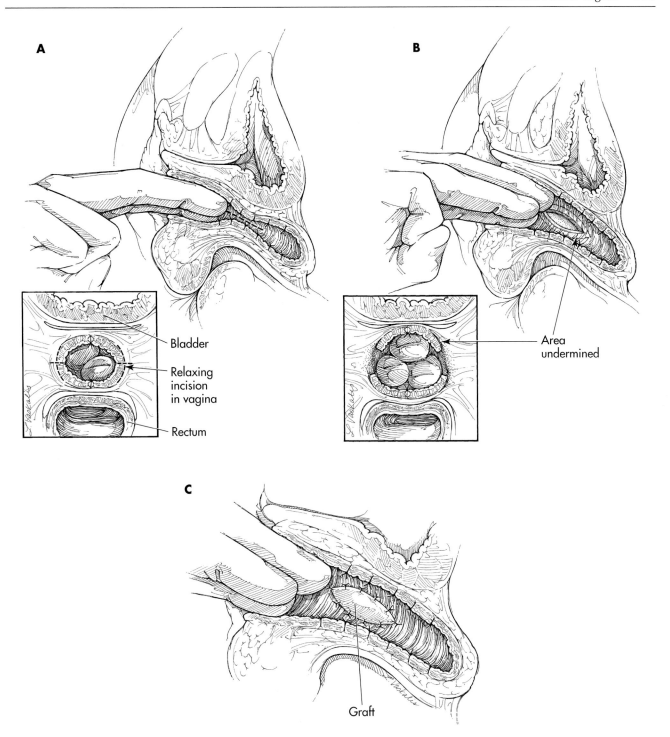

A

Bladder

Relaxing
incision
in vagina

Rectum

B

Area
undermined

C

Graft

Fig. 24-4   **A,** Digital examination of the vagina immediately after colporrhaphy discloses an unexpected stenosis in the middle third that admits only two fingerbreadths. The sites of the lateral relaxing incisions are indicated by the dotted lines. **B,** These incisions are made through the lateral wall of the vagina to a depth sufficient for the vagina to admit comfortably three fingerbreadths. The vagina is undercut for a centimeter in each direction. Any obvious bleeding vessels are clamped and tied, and a firm vaginal packing is inserted. This may be replaced within a day or so by a large vaginal obturator or mold to keep the cut edges of the relaxing incisions apart until healing and epithelialization are well under way, usually by the fifth postoperative day, after which the obturator or dilator may be worn only at night for an additional 2 or 3 weeks. Thus the integrity of the colporrhaphy incisions in the anterior and posterior vaginal walls is not compromised. **C,** A full-thickness graft of tissue saved from the colporrhaphy may be cut to size and sewn in place, if desired. (From Veronikis DK: The recurrent small and painful vagina. In Nichols DH, editor: *Reoperative gynecologic and obstetric surgery,* ed 2, St Louis, 1997, Mosby.)

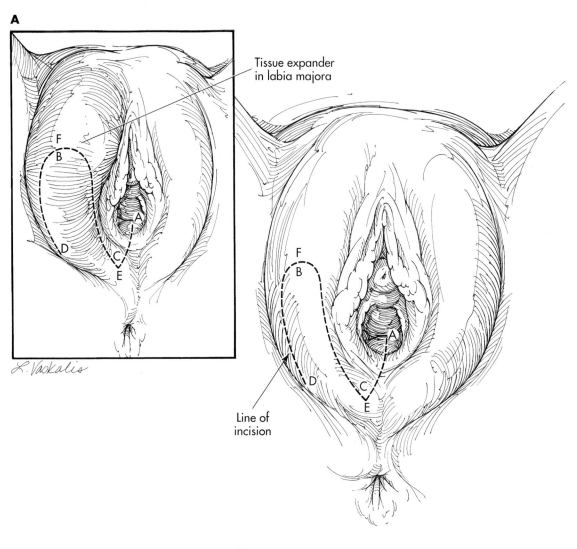

A

Tissue expander
in labia majora

Line of
incision

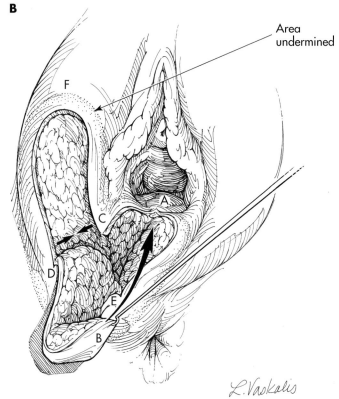

B

Area
undermined

Fig. 24-5 Labial cutaneous flap. At the site of a perineotomy *(A to E),* an incision through the full thickness of the labia skin and subcutaneous fat is made *(broken line).* The base of the flap is wider than the apex, and the flap *DBE* is created and rotated into position as shown. Point *B* is brought to point *A.* The final result after the edges have been approximated is shown in **C.** The introitus has been enlarged by the width of the flap. (From Veronikis DK: The recurrent small and painful vagina. In Nichols DH, editor: *Reoperative gynecologic and obstetric surgery,* ed 2, St Louis, 1997, Mosby.)

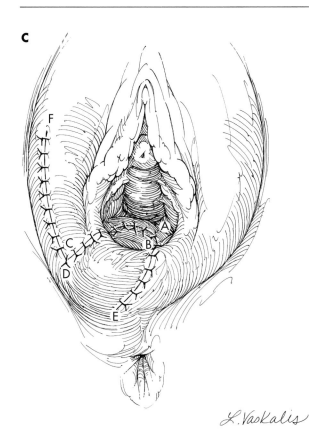

C

L. Vaskalis

Fig. 24-5, cont'd   Labial cutaneous flap. At the site of a perineotomy *(A to E),* an incision through the full thickness of the labia skin and subcutaneous fat is made *(broken line).* The base of the flap is wider than the apex, and the flap *DBE* is created and rotated into position as shown. Point *B* is brought to point *A.* The final result after the edges have been approximated is shown in **C.** The introitus has been enlarged by the width of the flap. (From Veronikis DK: The recurrent small and painful vagina. In Nichols DH, editor: *Reoperative gynecologic and obstetric surgery,* ed 2, St Louis, 1997, Mosby.)

7. Closes the thigh incisions from side to side and sews the apex of the now united flaps to the apex of the episiotomy with polyglycolic-type suture, trimming any excess adipose tissue from the underside of the flaps.
8. Fixes the lateral margins of the flap to the edges of the episiotomy with a few interrupted sutures, again of polyglycolic acid–type material.
9. Inserts a Penrose drain beneath the skin of each thigh, a Foley catheter in the bladder, and a splinting obturator in the vagina.

On the fourth postoperative day, the obturator and the Foley catheter are removed, the flaps and vagina are inspected thoroughly to determine healing, and the obturator is replaced. The patient wears the obturator constantly for 2 or 3 weeks, removing it only when she voids. After this period, she wears the obturator at night for several months until healing has been completed. Long-term postoperative estrogen replacement therapy may be indicated, and frequent wearing of a suitable obturator is often desirable to maintain both vaginal depth and width.

Williams Vulvovaginoplasty. When the vagina is short, for example because of earlier radical pelvic surgery that included partial vaginectomy, the distal vulvovaginoplasty of Williams[15] may add as much as 1 to 2 inches to the length of the vagina if the labia are thick and well developed (Fig. 24-6). As in the Graves procedure, long-term postoperative estrogen replacement therapy and frequent wearing of a suitable obturator are often indicated after a Williams vulvovaginoplasty. If the labia are atrophic and thin, how-

ever, and the atrophic vagina is both narrow and short, vaginectomy followed at the same operation by construction of an Abbe-McIndoe-type[1,10] neovagina is often helpful (see Chapter 25).

In patients who need more depth, the surgeon may use a partial McIndoe procedure to construct a new upper vagina. The use of appropriate vaginal obturators may create and maintain additional depth.[5,8]

Other Methods of Providing Greater Vaginal Depth

When desirable, greater amounts of vaginal depth can be provided by incision in the vaginal vault and dissection of a tunnel of sufficient depth, but preferably extraperitoneal. This raw area can be lined by a full-thickness skin graft (subepithelial fat thoroughly removed) appropriately shaped and sewn in place. It should be held against the raw surface by insertion of a moistened, narrow, vaginal packing. Strict bed rest is necessary for 3 days, and on the fifth postoperative day the packing is removed, the recipient site carefully inspected, and the vagina in its new length fitted with a condom-covered polyurethane foam obturator to be worn constantly for 6 to 8 weeks except during douching or defecation, and then nightly for 3 or 4 months.[11] The procedure is illustrated in Figs. 24-7 and 24-8.

An alternative to the Frank[5]-Ingram[8] method using progressively longer, rigid, Lucite obturators for at least 2 hours daily over a period of 6 to 12 months is the Vecchietti procedure (Fig. 24-9, p. 450),[16-18] which provides transabdominal traction to the vaginal vault around-the-clock for 5 to

Text continued on p. 452

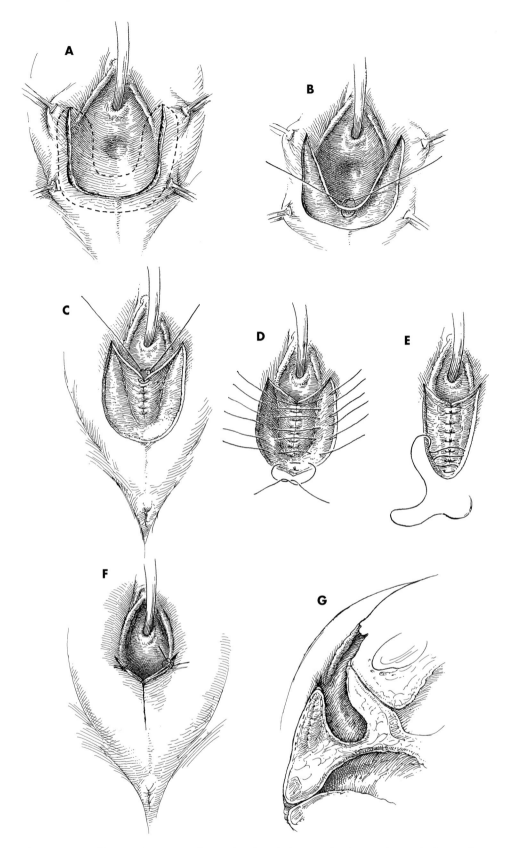

Fig. 24-6   Williams vulvovaginoplasty. The dimpled area of softening beneath the urethra identifies the site of the missing vagina. **A,** Following thorough infiltration with 0.5% lidocaine in 1:200,000 epinephrine solution, a U-shaped incision is made along the inner surface of the labia majora about 4 cm lateral to the urethra and undermined **(B).** The medial margins of the incision are united by interrupted absorbable suture. Notice that the knots are tied on the *inside* of the new vaginal pouch **(C).** The subcutaneous tissue is approximated by a separate layer **(D),** and the lateral margins of the incision are approximated separately. Vulvovaginoplasty at the completion of the operation is shown in frontal view **(F)** and in sagittal drawing **(G).** (After Capraro VJ, Capraro EJ: *Obstet Gynecol* 39:544, 1972; from Nichols DH, Randall CL: *Vaginal surgery,* ed 4, Baltimore, 1996, Williams & Wilkins.)

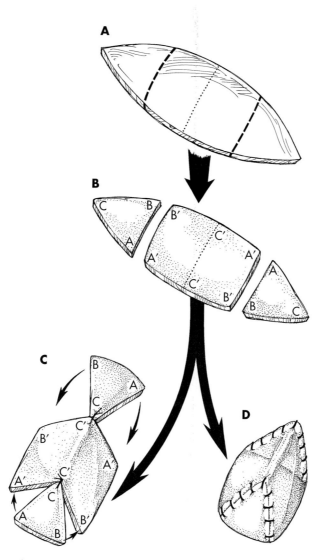

Fig. 24-7   "Tent" full-thickness skin graft for vaginal foreshortening. **A,** A full-thickness piece of skin has been removed from the iliac crest using two elliptical incisions. **B,** All subcutaneous fat is scraped away, and triangles are cut from each end of the ellipse. **C,** The triangles are rotated so that site *C* is sewn to *C'*. **D,** The remainder of the cut edges are brought together by interrupted stitches. This tent will be placed with the rough edge external into the depths of the recipient site in the vaginal wall. The bottom edges may be tacked to the cut margin of the upper edge of the vaginal canal, fixing the graft in place. The cavity is thoroughly packed with sterile cotton balls soaked in saline to obliterate any dead space that may be present. These must be left in place for a minimum of 5 days. (From Nichols DH, Randall, CL: *Vaginal surgery,* ed 4, Baltimore, 1996, Williams & Wilkins.)

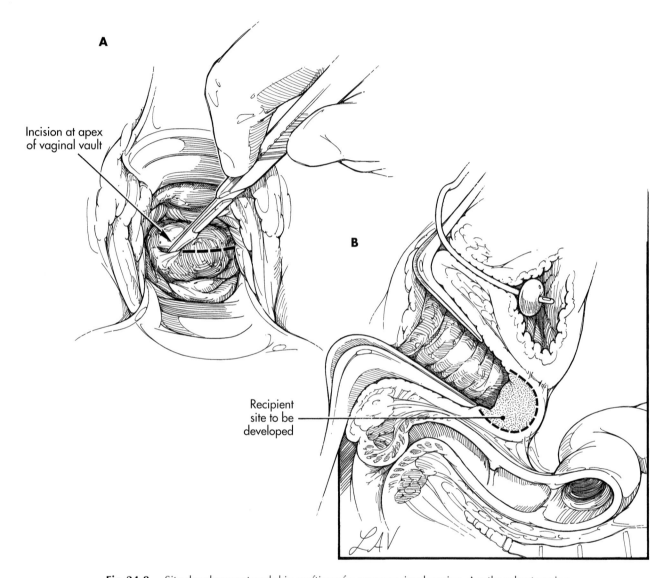

A

Incision at apex
of vaginal vault

B

Recipient
site to be
developed

Fig. 24-8   Site development and skin grafting of a new proximal vagina. A rather short vagina
has been demonstrated following previous surgery and hysterectomy. There is somewhat
dense scar tissue in this area, but it is possible to elongate the vagina by developing an extraperitoneal excavation at the vaginal vault using both sharp and blunt dissection. **A,** A transverse incision is made through the full thickness of the vaginal vault. **B,** Sagittal view of the site
to be developed. (From Nichols DH, Randall CL: *Vaginal surgery,* ed 4, Baltimore, 1996, Williams & Wilkins.)

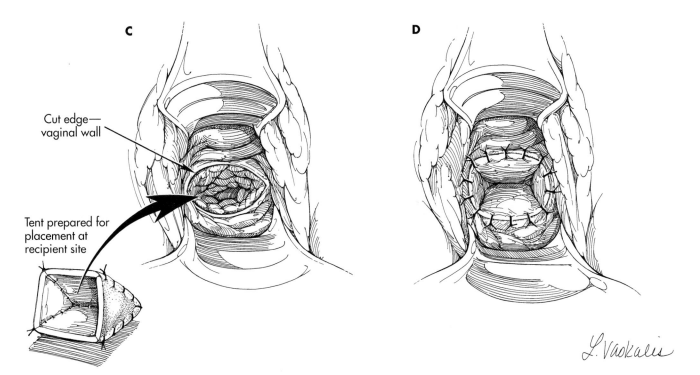

C

Cut edge—
vaginal wall

Tent prepared for
placement at
recipient site

D

L. Vaokalis

Fig. 24-8, cont'd   C, After this cavity has been formed and hemostasis secured, the "tent" of full-thickness skin from the iliac crest is placed into the donor site. **D,** The tent is sewn to the cut edge of the vagina. The tissues are tightly packed with saline-soaked sponges and left to rest for 5 days. The sponges are then removed, the cavity irrigated, and the patient given an obturator to wear until healing is complete.

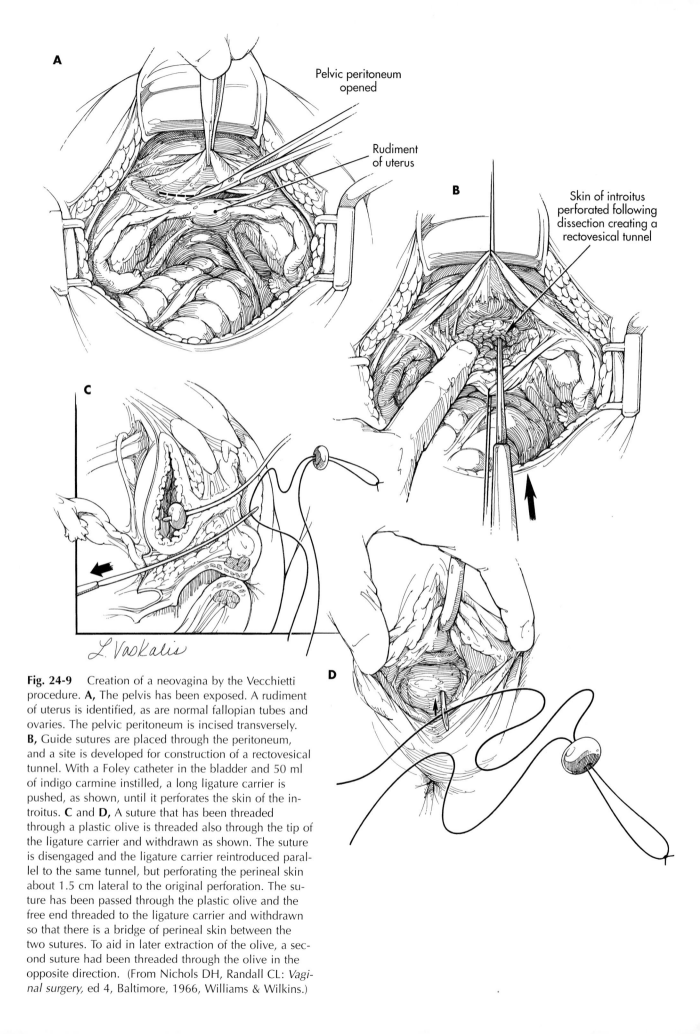

A

Pelvic peritoneum opened

Rudiment of uterus

B

Skin of introitus perforated following dissection creating a rectovesical tunnel

C

L. Vaskalis

D

Fig. 24-9 Creation of a neovagina by the Vecchietti procedure. **A,** The pelvis has been exposed. A rudiment of uterus is identified, as are normal fallopian tubes and ovaries. The pelvic peritoneum is incised transversely. **B,** Guide sutures are placed through the peritoneum, and a site is developed for construction of a rectovesical tunnel. With a Foley catheter in the bladder and 50 ml of indigo carmine instilled, a long ligature carrier is pushed, as shown, until it perforates the skin of the introitus. **C** and **D,** A suture that has been threaded through a plastic olive is threaded also through the tip of the ligature carrier and withdrawn as shown. The suture is disengaged and the ligature carrier reintroduced parallel to the same tunnel, but perforating the perineal skin about 1.5 cm lateral to the original perforation. The suture has been passed through the plastic olive and the free end threaded to the ligature carrier and withdrawn so that there is a bridge of perineal skin between the two sutures. To aid in later extraction of the olive, a second suture had been threaded through the olive in the opposite direction. (From Nichols DH, Randall CL: *Vaginal surgery*, ed 4, Baltimore, 1966, Williams & Wilkins.)

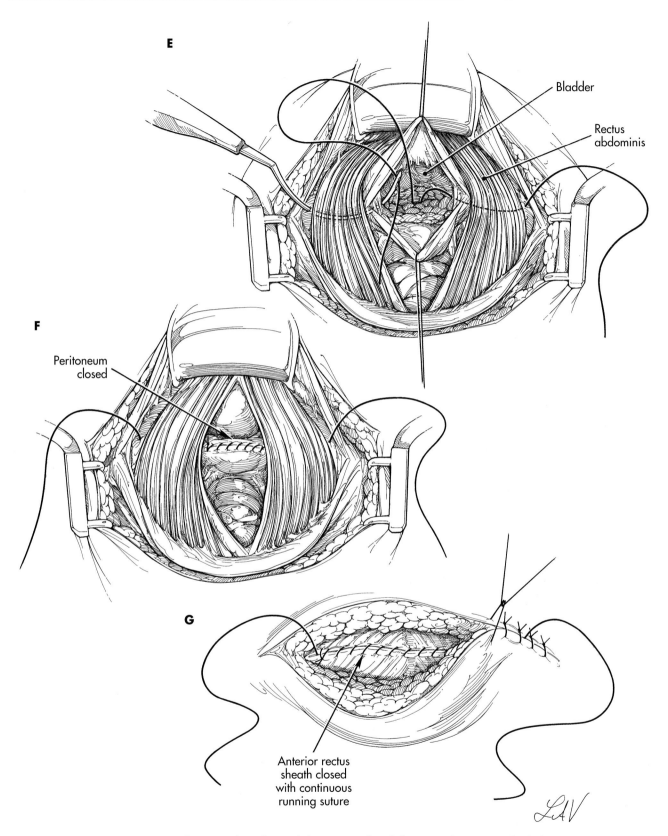

Fig. 24-9, cont'd   E, Each end is withdrawn into the abdomen. A ligature carrier is introduced lateral to the rectus abdominis on each side, following the path of the round ligament, to appear at the peritoneal opening. When the suture has been threaded to it, the carrier is withdrawn and the retroperitoneal sutures exit the abdomen lateral to the rectus sheath on each side. **F,** The initial transverse incision in the pelvic peritoneum is closed, and the abdomen is closed. **G,** The ends of the suture exit the fascia, and the skin is closed. (From Nichols DH, Randall CL: *Vaginal surgery,* ed 4, Baltimore, 1966, Williams & Wilkins.)

Continued

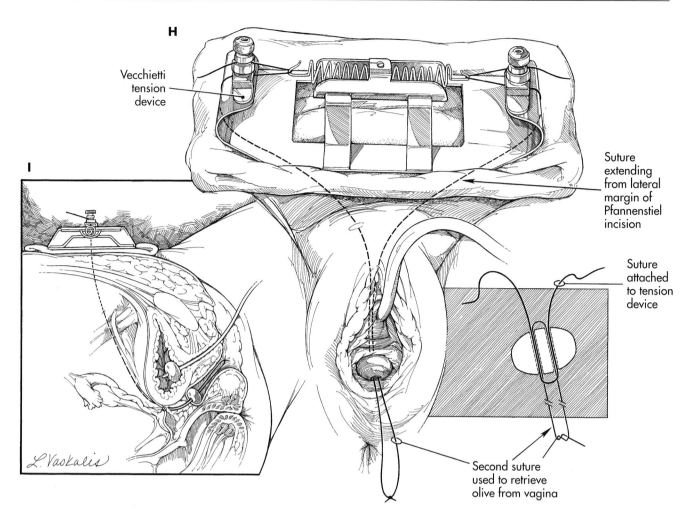

Fig. 24-9, cont'd   H, A sterile padded dressing is placed over the incision, the Vecchietti tension frame placed on the abdomen, and the thread on each side is looped through the spring and fixed in place by a locknut as shown. **I,** With daily traction to the abdominal end of each thread, the tension is adjusted so that the olive will advance along the path of the neovagina about 1 cm per day. After 8 to 10 days, the vagina should measure about 10 cm in depth. The abdominal sutures are cut, flush with the skin surface, the Vecchietti device is removed, and the olive and sutures are withdrawn through the vagina using the looped second suture that had been placed as shown in the *inset.* The patient is given a set of graduated vaginal dilators to apply daily to preserve neovaginal depth. By exchanging them for dilators that are progressively wider, the patient will increase vaginal diameter.

7 days. The unrelenting traction, the tension of which is adjusted daily, rapidly deepens the vagina about 1 cm per day. This is an in-hospital procedure that can be performed by laparotomy or translaparoscopically[3,6,19] depending on the experience of the operator.

Everted and Shortened Vagina

In an occasional patient who has undergone multiple surgical procedures, a shortened vagina—sometimes so short, in fact, that it does not reach the sacrospinous ligament—becomes totally everted. The surgeon has several treatment alternatives from which to choose in this case:

1. The use of Ingram-Frank dilators lubricated with estrogen cream may lengthen the vagina until it reaches the sacrospinous ligament so that the surgeon can perform sacrospinous colpopexy[8] (see Chapter 26).

2. Transabdominal sacrocolpopexy permits the placement of an intermediate bridge using fascia lata or a synthetic plastic material such as Mersilene mesh.

3. Sacrospinous colpopexy (see Chapter 26) allows the surgeon to use deliberate suture bridges of nonabsorbable synthetic monofilament material, such as poly butester (Novofil) or polypropylene (Prolene or Surgilene). If the labia are large enough, the surgeon may also perform a Williams vulvovaginoplasty to increase the depth of the vagina by an additional 1.5 or 2 inches.

OTHER CAUSES OF VAGINAL PAIN

When the vaginal vestibule is exquisitely tender precluding comfortable coitus, and there is no pathologic reduction in the size of the introitus, the possibility of vulvar vestibular syndrome must be considered. This condition and its remedy are discussed in Chapter 16.

For the patient with pathologic sexual psychosocial dynamics, often with a hidden history of childhood sexual abuse or of rape, a vaginismus may be noted. Sexual counseling by a trained therapist may be needed, and sometimes biofeedback may be incorporated.

REFERENCES

1. Abbe R: New method of creating a vagina in a case of congenital absence, *Med Rec* 54:836, 1898.
2. Amreich J: Aëtiologie ünd Operation des Scheidenstumpf Prolases, *Wein Klin Wochenschr* 63:74, 1951.
3. Busacca M, Perino A, Venezia R: Laparoscopic-ultrasonographic combined technique for the creation of a neovagina in Mayer-Rokitansky-Küster-Hauser syndrome, *Fertil Steril* 66:1039, 1996.
4. Cummings KG et al: Scientific exhibit, American College of Obstetricians and Gynecologists, 1976.
5. Frank RT: The formation of an artificial vagina without operation, *Am J Obstet Gynecol* 35:1053, 1938.
6. Gauwerky JFH, Wallwiener D, Bastert G: An endoscopically assisted technique for construction of a neovagina, *Arch Gynecol Obstet* 252:59, 1992.
7. Graves WP: Operative treatment of atresia of the vagina, *Boston Med Surg J* 163:753, 1910.
8. Ingram JM: The bicycle seat stool in the treatment of vaginal agenesis and stenosis, *Am J Obstet Gynecol* 140:807, 1981.
9. Martin LW, Sutorius DS: An improved method for vaginoplasty, *Arch Surg* 98:716, 1969.
10. McIndoe AH, Banister JB: An operation for the cure of congenital absence of the vagina, *J Obstet Gynaecol Br Commonw* 45:490, 1938.
11. Morley GW, DeLancey JOL: Full-thickness graft vaginoplasty for treatment of the stenotic or foreshortened vagina, *Obstet Gynecol* 77:485, 1991.
12. Morton KE, Davies D, Dewhurst J: The use of the fasciocutaneous flap in vaginal reconstruction, *Br J Obstet Gynecol* 93:970, 1986.
13. Nichols DH, Randall CL: *Vaginal surgery,* ed 4, Baltimore, 1996, Williams & Wilkins.
14. West JT, Ketcham AS, Smith RR: Vaginal reconstruction following pelvic exenteration for cancer or postirradiation necrosis, *Surg Gynecol Obstet* 118:788, 1965.
15. Williams EA: Congenital absence of the vagina: a simple operation for its relief, *J Obstet Gynaecol Br Commonw* 71:511, 1964.
16. Vecchietti G: Neovagina nella sindrome di Rokitansky-Küster-Hauser, *Attual Ostet Ginecol* 11:131, 1965.
17. Vecchietti G: Le neo-vagin dans le syndrome de Rokitansky-Küster-Hauser, *Rev Med Suisse Romande* 99:593, 1979.
18. Vecchietti G: Die neovagina beim Rokitansky-Küster-Hauser-Syndrom, *Gynäkologe* 13:112, 1980.
19. Veronikis DK, McClure GB, Nichols DH: The Vecchietti operation for constructing a neovagina: indications, instrumentation, and techniques, *Obstet Gynecol* 90:301, 1997.

25 Vaginectomy

DAVID H. NICHOLS

INDICATIONS FOR VAGINECTOMY

The vagina is surgically removed for many vastly different reasons. When a neovagina has been created, and for one reason or another the patient has failed to keep the vaginal canal open, shrinkage of the neovagina occurs rapidly, with contraction of the scar tissue surrounding the vagina at times producing a rather dense fibrosis. That which seemed to be a vagina of normal depth and caliber at the end of neo-vaginal construction, in the absence of adequate postoperative dilation, may contract both in width and in depth, often to a diameter of less than one fingerwidth, rendering coitus impossible.

Vaginal intraepithelial neoplasia (VAIN) may be suspected from the report of a posthysterectomy Papanicolaou (Pap) smear. This is not only often multifocal, but also may occur in the vault of the vagina at a spot where the surface is poorly visualized, making colposcopy and colposcopically directed biopsy difficult and inconclusive.

Removal of the upper portion of the vagina may be coincident with radical hysterectomy and upper vaginectomy for uterine cancer. The lower portion of the vagina may be removed at the same time as radical vulvectomy for vulvar cancer that involves the vaginal introitus.

One occasionally sees a patient with total posthysterectomy vaginal eversion whose tissues cannot retain a pessary and who suffers a major disability. When such a patient also is a poor medical and surgical risk, a surgical procedure that will solve her prolapse problem swiftly and safely must be performed. LeFort partial colpocleisis has been recommended in the past, but recurrence of the prolapse is sometimes observed along the lateral canals of the vaginal epithelium remaining after the procedure. For many, total transvaginal colpectomy is an acceptable procedure and is followed by extensive scarring and total obliteration of the space formerly occupied by the vagina. Coitus, of course, is impossible. These procedures are discussed at some length in Chapter 26.

TYPES OF VAGINECTOMY AND GOALS

Three types of vaginectomy must be considered by the gynecologist: total, partial, and superficial.

Total Vaginectomy

Total vaginectomy is generally of two types. The first consists of colpectomy without replacement of the vagina, as mentioned above, and usually is part of the treatment of massive genital prolapse in a patient medically and surgically at high risk.

Vaginectomy with Creation of Replacement Neovagina. The second type of total vaginectomy is vaginectomy followed by replacement with a neovagina of sufficient caliber to permit coitus. For this purpose, a wide variety of procedures is available.

Abbe-McIndoe Vagina. The Abbe-McIndoe procedure involves construction of a replacement vagina with a split-thickness skin graft.[1,2] Successful vaginal reconstruction can be achieved even years after initial therapy in patients who have an obliterated vagina from previous radiation or surgery. Stenosis also may be seen after radical hysterectomy and vaginectomy with creation of a neovagina as treatment in patients with cancer of the vagina, or after neovagina formation in patients undergoing pelvic exenteration. The procedure is as follows (Figs. 25-1 to 25-3).

The scarred vagina is excised by scissor dissection beginning lateral and peripheral to the scar, which provides the least chance for inadvertent damage to bowel or bladder.[5,16,17] When this has proceeded close to the vaginal vault, one of the surgeon's fingers is inserted into the rectum to facilitate posterior dissection, which ultimately is made to communicate with the lateral spaces. A Foley catheter is instilled into the bladder, and 100 ml of saline heavily colored with indigo carmine or methylene blue are instilled into the bladder through the Foley catheter and the dissection is carried anteriorly. Hemostasis is achieved, and an obturator covered by harvested split-thickness skin, fresh human amnion,[7,20] or Interceed[11] (Interceed Absorbable Adhesion Barrier, Johnson & Johnson Patient Care, Inc., New Brunswick, NJ) is inserted.

The donor site may be covered by Xeroform or Op-Site. The patient is kept at bedrest and given a low-residue diet with prophylactic medication to curb intestinal activity. For further details of the surgical technique, see Chapter 43.

Williams' Vulvovaginoplasty. If fleshy labia majora are present, the patient may be a candidate for the Williams' vulvovaginoplasty,[26] as described in Chapter 24. This, however, requires infinite patience on the part of both the patient and her sexual companion and a long process of developing postoperative vaginal width and increased depth both by wearing an obturator as necessary and having frequent coitus.

Davydov Peritoneal Transplantation. The Davydov procedure[4] is a transplantation of widely mobilized parietal peritoneum to line the cavity of the neovagina (Fig. 25-4, p. 458). It permits rapid growth of squamous epithelium

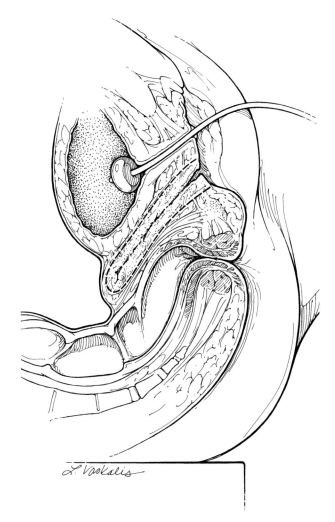

L. Vaskalis

Fig. 25-1   Sagittal section of a massively scarred vagina with a Foley catheter in the bladder, which has been partially distended by saline containing a concentrated indigo carmine solution. The entire vagina is excised by sharp dissection along the sites indicated by the *dashed line*, first on each side, and then posteriorly, and finally anteriorly beneath the urethra and bladder. Dissection from the rectum may be guided by temporarily placing one of the operator's fingers in the rectum during the dissection.

underneath the transplanted peritoneum. This may be accomplished with particular ease when the patient has just received a radical hysterectomy and vaginectomy as treatment for invasive cervical cancer. The technique of laparoscopically assisted Davydov peritoneal transplantation is considered in some detail in Chapter 67.

Follow-Up Procedures. Fresh amnion can be used to cover the neovagina,[7,20] permitting rapid ingrowth of squamous epithelium from the cut edges of the remaining vagina and vulva.

Fresh human amnion is a good biologic dressing, if available. It does not convert to epithelium but most effectively resists infection and permits epithelium to grow upward from established epithelial edges. The popularity of this method may be uncertain because of the prevalence of

AIDS because it is possible to transmit the disease in this fashion. Alternatively, Interceed can be used.[11]

Because of their length, myocutaneous flaps can be transplanted after vaginectomy because of cancer, if the surgeon has scrupulously determined that all active invasive malignant disease has been extirpated. The gracilis myocutaneous flap is good.[18]

It is possible to use a tissue expander buried beneath the labia minora, which, after some weeks of progressive distention, provides a surface area sufficient to line the neovaginal canal.[13] With the patient under general anesthesia, tissue expanders are inserted along a bluntly dissected tract to the internal aspect of the labia minora made from an incision over each groin. These buried expanders are connected by flexible plastic tubing to a valve and reservoir in each groin and the skin is closed. Each expander is initially inflated with 40 ml of sterile saline. Expansion is increased by an increment of 10 to 15 ml each day for the next 2 or 3 weeks to an approximate inflation of 120 ml on each side. At the time of construction of a neovagina, each dilator is inflated to 200 ml for 3 minutes at a time, and this is repeated three times. The large folds of essentially hairless labial skin are identified, the labia minora are incised, and large full-thickness flaps are raised by incision along the inner aspect of each enlarged labia minora and turned into the vagina to line the new cavity. The neovagina is packed for 4 days. The patient is given a vaginal obturator postoperatively to prevent contraction of the neovagina.

There is a place for the transplantation of a loop of sigmoid colon with which to line the neovagina, particularly in a patient who is neither psychologically nor socially able or willing to use dilators of the neovagina regularly in the postoperative period and who is not sexually active at the time of surgery.[3,9] This also may be useful in a patient who has had an exenterative procedure. Because this involves intestinal resection and anastomosis, the patient must be prepared for the possibility of anastomotic leaking and peritonitis and all of its consequences, although the incidence of this complication is low. Sigmoid resection of properly prepared bowel may be performed as described in Chapter 51.

Radical Vaginectomy. Radical vaginectomy may be performed as part of the treatment of invasive cancer involving the vagina.

Technique for a Patient with Previous Hysterectomy. An indwelling Foley catheter is inserted in the bladder, and the vagina is tightly packed. After the abdomen is opened, a traction suture is placed between the residual upper uterosacral ligaments, and the peritoneum is undermined and incised. The bladder is separated from the anterior vagina with gentle sharp dissection, and the posterior dissection divides the peritoneum overlying the psoas muscles to expose the retroperitoneal space and permit identification of the ureter and development of the pararectal and paravesical spaces. The uterine artery is divided at its origin from the internal iliac. The ureter is dissected from the medial leaf of the peritoneum as far as the ureteral tunnel in the anterior

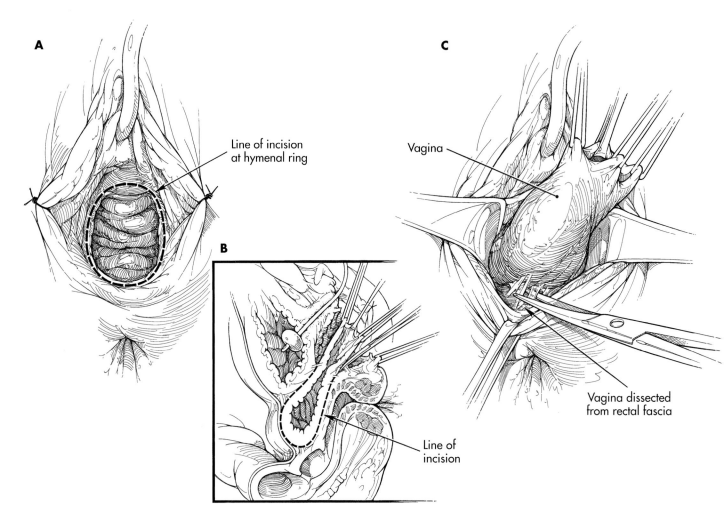

Fig. 25-2   Total transvaginal vaginectomy. This may be particularly valuable as the first step in constructing the neovagina for a patient whose vagina has been occluded by scar tissue. **A,** A Foley catheter is inserted into the bladder and 60 ml of indigo carmine solution instilled. An incision is made circumferentially through the full thickness of the vagina and surrounding scar tissue along the path indicated by the *dashed line.* **B,** By sharp dissection this mobilization of the vagina is carried toward the vault, first on one side of the vagina, then on the other, and finally in the midline. The operator separates the bladder by careful sharp dissection, being mindful of any appearance of violet-stained tissue in the course of the dissection, which would indicate proximity of the bladder. **C,** The posterior midline dissection. This can be best accomplished with the operator's finger in the patient's rectum to identify the latter and avoid unwanted penetration. (From Nichols DH, Randall CL: *Vaginal surgery,* ed 4, Baltimore, 1996, Williams & Wilkins.)

parametrium, after which the peritoneum of the cul-de-sac can be safely divided. The rectovaginal space is developed, and the uterosacral ligaments are divided to the level of the pelvic diaphragm. The vagina is dissected from the anterior vaginal wall as far as possible, and, by placing slight tension on the ureter, the tissue covering the most distal ureter is identified and transacted. The vagina is removed, which may be made easier if a circumferential incision is made around the introitus at the level of planned amputation. A neovagina can be created by lining the cavity with tissue of various sites as described above. The vagina may be removed as part of an exenteration (see Chapter 40).

Partial Vaginectomy. Partial vaginectomy may occur

with radical hysterectomy, either abdominal or vaginal, but, if the cut edge of the peritoneum is sewn to the vaginal cuff, residual depth may be adequate to permit coitus. If this is not true, parietal peritoneum may be mobilized and sewn to the distal cut vaginal edge as a Davydov operation, as described earlier, and the peritoneum separately closed by a purse-string suture within the abdominal cavity as shown. The technique for partial vaginectomy with vaginal hysterectomy is described in Chapter 19.

Partial vaginectomy with hysterectomy, generally done transvaginally, although possible transabdominally, may be used when a severe dysplasia of the upper vagina coexists with carcinoma in situ of the uterine cervix.

Before the vault is closed, if resultant vaginal depth appears insufficient to sustain coitus, the raw surfaces in the upper vagina can be covered by a full-thickness skin graft, amnion, or Interceed. The technique is shown in Fig. 25-5. Fresh amnion can be used to coat the raw area of an upper neovaginal dissection.[7,20] A full-thickness skin graft can be used, which may be obtained from the abdomen or from the skin removed between elliptical skin incisions made over the iliac crest.[15]

When a partial vaginectomy has occurred previously and it is desirable to restore vaginal depth, the following technique is applicable.

Extraperitoneal Construction of a Neovagina
Full or Partial Abbe-McIndoe Operation.[1,14,21,22]

When the vagina is too short for coital comfort and the labia majora are not suitably fleshy for a Williams-type vulvovaginoplasty,[25] depth can be added to the proximal vagina by daily applications of obturators of increasing length (BEI/Zinnanti Surgical Instruments, Chatsworth, CA, 91311, or Faulkner Plastics, 4504 East Hillsborough Ave., Tampa, FL 33610) (the Frank-Ingram[8,10] procedure), which will require an investment of at least 2 hours per day on the part of the patient. Forceful pressure is applied to these vaginal obturators, the length of which is gradually increased until the desired vaginal depth has been achieved. When the amount of discomfort is unacceptable to the patient during this procedure, or when the amount of scar tissue in the vaginal vault prevents effective stretching, an alternative procedure can be used that involves the creation of a cavity at the vault of the vagina, which can be lined with a split-thickness skin graft. The patient must be a given a full description of the procedure and aftercare. The importance of her role in the success of this operation should be discussed. She will be required to wear a vaginal obturator for some months after the operation to prevent unwanted postoperative shrinkage.

The procedure is as follows. A wide strip of split-thickness skin is obtained (Braun electric dermatome set at 0.00018 inch). The author's preference is to use the skin of the suprapubic area of the anterior abdominal wall.[6,19] The surface of the skin is shaved, and multiple subcutaneous injections of sterile saline totaling 200 to 300 ml are made to flatten the skin surface, allowing for a graft of uniform surface dimension and thickness. The skin of the donor site is painted with sterile mineral oil, the graft is removed and wrapped in saline-soaked dressings, and a Xeroform dressing is applied to the donor site. Use of this area of donor skin has the following advantages:

1. Because of its anterior location, the patient is not required to endure the pain and discomfort of sitting or resting on the donor site during the long healing phase.
2. Because the graft is cut superficial to the hair follicles, the hair of the escutcheon covering much of the donor site regrows quickly, thus making the donor site more cosmetically acceptable to the patient (no hair grows within the graft because the hair follicles are not contained in the split-thickness graft).

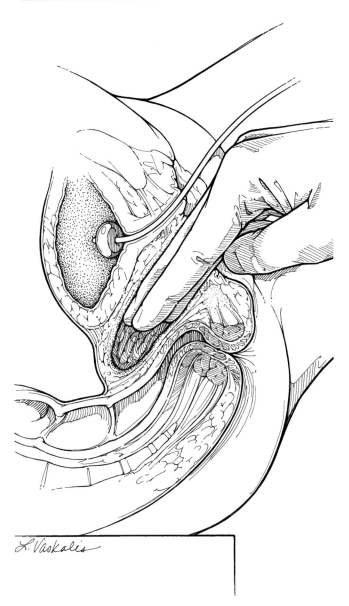

L. Vaskalis

Fig. 25-3 The size and depth remaining after vaginectomy are carefully estimated by insertion of the operator's fingers. The cavity should accommodate at least three and possibly four fingerwidths and demonstrate an adequate vaginal depth. If the width is inadequate, relaxing incisions can be made in the paravaginal scar tissue at the 3- and 9-o'clock positions in the circumference of the vagina.

Technique of Full-Thickness Proximal Vaginectomy.

The area to be excised is carefully identified and four guide sutures placed (Fig. 25-5). With traction to these sutures, circumscribing incisions are made using a scalpel with a no. 11 blade held perpendicular to the surface of the vagina, and the vaginal wall dissected sharply from the underlying tissues. Once a cleavage plane is established, digital fingertip dissection to and beneath the peritoneum is accomplished, aided by Metzenbaum scissor dissection if necessary, until the entire vaginal apex has been freed and removed. Hemostasis is ensured. To preserve depth the vaginal vault is closed vertically.

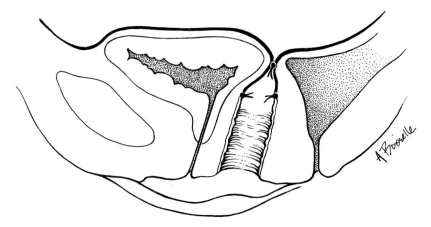

Fig. 25-4   The Davydov operation. Proximal length can be added to a shortened vagina by attaching the margins of the previously dissected parietal peritoneum to the cut edges of the remaining vagina. The peritoneal cavity is securely closed by a separately placed cranial purse-string suture as shown. (From Nichols DH, Randall CL: *Vaginal surgery,* ed 4, Baltimore, 1996, Williams & Wilkins.)

3. Pigmentation of the donor site is minimal, and any that is present is mostly covered by pubic hair regrowth.
4. A thicker split-thickness graft is less likely to shrink postoperatively than a thinner graft.

The surgeon should instill 100 ml of sterile milk or infant formula or of sterile saline deeply colored with indigo carmine into the bladder through an indwelling Foley catheter, which is then clamped. The bladder will be palpable during subsequent dissection of the neovagina. The bulb of the Foley catheter can be palpated, and any unwanted penetration of the bladder is recognized by prompt appearance of dye or milk in the operative field.

In addition, 100 ml of sterile saline is injected beneath the wall of the vaginal vault and upper vagina to compress sites of venous bleeding and make the dissection of the vagina from the surrounding tissues and scar safer, proceeding in a somewhat conical direction to the peritoneum of the cul-de-sac of Douglas, which may be exposed for no more than 1 to 1.5 cm (lessening the chance for future enterocele development as would be risked if the peritoneal exposure were made greater). Such lateral relaxing incisions in the vestibule or medial border of the pubococcygei are made to permit the patient to contain the obturator postoperatively. Bleeding points are clamped and coagulated or tied. Venous oozing can be controlled with a tight vaginal gauze packing placed for a few minutes.

A precut polyethylene foam cylinder, 5 × 15 cm and rounded or tapered at the proximal end, is prepared.[22] The edges of the split-thickness skin (raw side out) are draped over the polyethylene foam obturator (no covering condom is needed). Alternatively, the appropriate-sized Heyer-Schulte "inflatable" obturator can be used. The edges of the graft are approximated with fine absorbable sutures.

The graft-covered obturator is inserted into the neovagina, and the vaginal orifice is closed temporarily by two or three heavy silk sutures, loosely tied, to hold the mold in place for the next 7 to 8 days. The Foley catheter is connected to a drainage system, and the patient is placed on a low-residue diet and bedrest. Between the seventh and tenth postoperative day, the vestibular stitches are cut and removed, the mold is gently removed, under anesthesia if necessary, and the neovagina is inspected.

A transverse incision is made in the full width of the vaginal vault. A new obturator made of firm plastic* or balsa wood covered by rubber measuring 15 cm in length and 12 cm in circumference is inserted. Alternatively, the Heyer-Schulte mold may be reused. The patient is promptly ambulated and instructed in removal and replacement of the obturator, which may be generously lubricated with estrogen cream. The patient is discharged. The mold should be removed only when the patient goes to the toilet, then promptly replaced.

A sanitary napkin worn beneath the patient's underpants may help to hold the obturator in place. The vagina is reinspected in the surgeon's office 1 month after surgery, any granulation tissue is coagulated with silver nitrate, and permission is given to the patient for coital activity, if appropriate. New instructions may be given to the patient to wear the obturator every night during sleep and for a total of 2 additional hours during the day. After 6 postoperative months, if there is no evidence of vaginal stricture, the patient may be asked to wear the obturator nightly three times per week, more frequently if any obstruction to its insertion is observed.

The transvaginal translaparoscopic modification of the Davydov operation using pelvic peritoneum to cover the raw surfaces of the neovagina is described in Chapter 67. Alternatively, cecal or ileocecal segments may be transplanted, although this requires an obligatory bowel resection with its small risk of increased morbidity.[3,9] Length may be added at the distal portion of the vagina by a Williams[25] vulvovaginoplasty as described previously.

Frank-Ingram Vaginal Dilators. For the patient willing to participate actively in achieving additional vaginal length, several months of daily use of lucite vaginal obturators of progressively increasing depth are useful according to the descriptions of Frank[8] and Ingram.[10] The patient must be willing to devote at least 2 hours per day to this endeavor, survive its discomfort, and pursue this program under her gynecologist's guidance for 2 and 6 months. The gynecologist may change the obturator at succeeding visits for a progres-

---

*The Counseller-type silicone plastic obturators are available from Bioteque America, Langhorne, PA 19047.

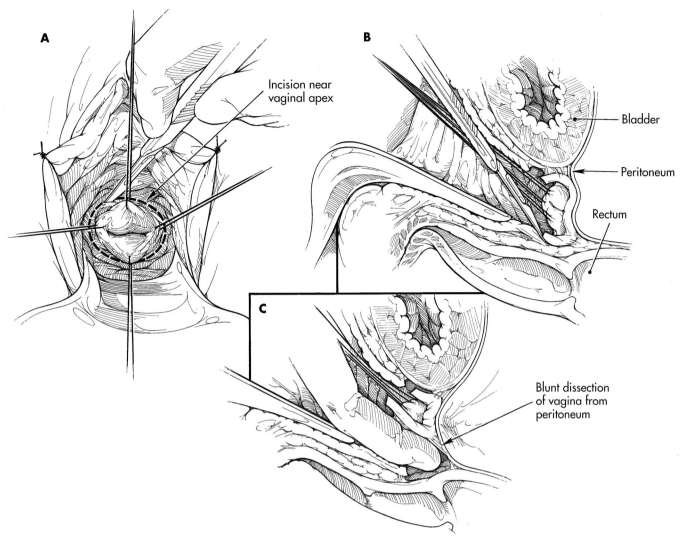

Fig. 25-5 Partial vaginectomy following previous hysterectomy. **A,** View showing the area of the vaginal apex to be removed. Guide sutures are placed as shown, and an incision follows the path of the *dashed line.* **B,** Sagittal section showing sharp dissection extending circumferentially up to the peritoneum. bluntly dissected from the peritoneum. (From Nichols DH, Randall CL: *Vaginal surgery,* ed 4, Baltimore, 1996, Williams & Wilkins.) *Continued*

sively larger size. Regular and frequent coitus aids in the development of increased vaginal depth and ultimate redirection of the vaginal axis toward the hollow of the sacrum.

When the lower half of the vagina needs replacing, full-thickness skin flap transposition as described in Chapter 24 may be employed.

Vecchietti Operation. The Vecchietti operation[16,23,24,25] rapidly develops vaginal depth through round-the-clock traction applied transabdominally to an olive that has been placed within the vaginal vault and threaded to a suture passed from the anterior abdominal wall and attached to a spring supported within a frame that rests on the lower abdomen (see Chapter 24). Additional vaginal length will be evident within a week.

Superficial Vaginectomy Using the CO$_2$ Laser.[12] In a posthysterectomy patient with an abnormal Pap smear, but also in a patient treated by radiation therapy for invasive cervical cancer, an apparent discrepancy may arise between an abnormal cytologic report and the difficulties with effective and decisive vaginal colposcopy. Postmenopausal vaginal atrophy and the vaginal deformities after hysterectomy or radiation therapy, for example, account for some of the disparity. Negative reports obtained on specimens received after random vaginal biopsy are not helpful in the face of persistently positive cytology studies. Traditional cervical vaginectomy often is difficult in such cases and requires grafting and a long period of obturator use to permit preservation or restoration of a coitally useful vagina. Superficial partial vaginectomy using the CO$_2$ laser in the hands of a surgeon experienced in laser surgery and colposcopy has been reported by Julian, O'Connell, and Gosewehr[12] as a most useful procedure. The vagina of a younger patient with a clearly defined small lesion can be studied by direct or colposcopically directed biopsy.

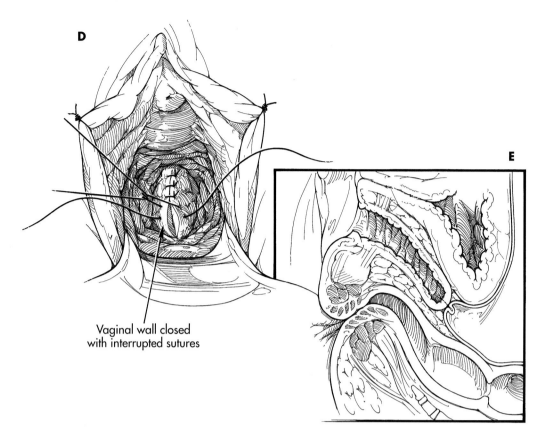

Fig. 25-5, cont'd   **D,** After removal of the vaginal apex, the vaginal incision is closed from side to side by interrupted stitches to help preserve vaginal depth. **E,** Sagittal section of the end result.

Skillfully performed partial superficial vaginectomy provides a surgical specimen for histologic study, helping to discriminate between vaginal intraepithelial neoplasia (VAIN) and cervical intraepithelial neoplasia (CIN), as well as invasive squamous cancer, in contrast to the use of laser vaporization of the area in question, which does not provide a surgical specimen for diagnosis.

Vaginal epithelial regeneration with minimal scarring has been reported after superficial laser excision, and postoperative healing might be hastened in a postmenopausal patient with the use of vaginal obturators and generous, frequent application of intravaginal estrogen cream.

Procedure.[12] After preliminary colposcopy with determination of the amount of vagina to be removed for study, and under general or regional anesthesia, the area is thoroughly infiltrated with a "liquid tourniquet," such as 1:200,000 epinephrine or pitressin solution.

Using the CO_2 laser mounted on a colposcope and employing a sharply focused beam with power density of 750 to 1200 W/cm^2, the surgeon makes an incision just beneath the 3-mm thickness of vaginal epithelium, raising first the posterior flap, then an anterior one, and by traction to an applied Allis clamp, the entire specimen is removed for study. The patient is hospitalized overnight for observation, then discharged with plans for frequent follow-up. Reepithelialization is prompt, but any granulation tissue can be ef-

fectively coagulated with silver nitrate. Obturators, dilators, and vaginal estrogen cream are prescribed as necessary.

PREOPERATIVE AND POSTOPERATIVE CARE

It is important that the patient clearly understand the objectives of treatment. A careful and honest prediction concerning the duration of treatment, the duration of disability, and the degree to which the patient must participate in her care is essential to the success of any of these techniques. With the exception of the nonsurgical Frank-Ingram pressure technique, all the above methods require hospitalization. Most require the wearing of a vaginal obturator postoperatively for varying lengths of time during the day, at night, and for varying weeks or months after surgery, with periodic assessment of residual vaginal size during the interim. Any tendency toward shrinkage or fibrosis of the neovagina must be combated vigorously with reinstitution of dilation and increased number of intervals of wearing the obturator.

For a postmenopausal patient, an adequate dose of estrogen replacement therapy is important in maintaining an adequate vaginal blood supply and vaginal elasticity. The increased thickness it induces in the wall of the vagina acts as a barrier against infection and erosion and improves the patient's coital comfort. The obturators can be generously lubricated with estrogen cream during their use, and, in the interim, 1 g of estrogen cream instilled at bedtime once or twice a week in the neovagina helps to enhance the healing process and maintain good vaginal health postoperatively. This may be used in addition to oral estrogen administration that may be given in adequate dose to retard the development of osteoporosis and protect the patient's cardiovascular system.

REFERENCES

1. Abbe R: New method of creating a vagina in a case of congenital absence, *Med Rec* 54:836, 1898.
2. Berek JS, Hacker NF, Lagasse LD, Smith ML: Delayed vaginal reconstruction in the fibrotic pelvis following radiation or previous reconstruction, *Obstet Gynecol* 61:743, 1983.
3. Burger RA, Riedmiller H, Knapstein PG, et al: Ileocecal vaginal construction, *Am J Obstet Gynecol* 161:162, 1989.
4. Davydov SN: Modifizierte kolpopoese aus peritoneum der excavatio rectouterina, *Obstet Gynecol* (Moscow) 12:55, 1969. Quoted in Käser O, Iklé FA, Hirsch HA: *Atlas der gynäkologischen operationen,* 4 Auflage, Stuttgart, 1983, Georg Thieme Verlag.
5. DiSaia PJ, Rettenmaier MA: Vaginectomy. In Sanz LE, editor: *Gynecologic surgery,* Oradell, NJ, 1988, Med Economics.
6. Dudzinski MR, Rader JS: The mons pubis: an excellent graft donor site in gynecologic surgery, *Am J Obstet Gynecol* 162:722, 1990.
7. Feroze RM, Dewhurst CJ, Welply G: Vaginoplasty at the Chelsea Hospital for Women: a comparison of two techniques, *Br J Obstet Gynecol* 82:536, 1975.
8. Frank RT: The formation of an artificial vagina without operation, *Am J Obstet Gynecol* 35:1053, 1938.
9. Goligher JC: The use of pedicled transplants of sigmoid or other parts of the intestinal tract for vaginal construction, *Ann R Coll Surg Engl* 65:353, 1983.
10. Ingram JM: The bicycle seat in the treatment of vaginal agenesis and stenosis: a preliminary report, *Am J Obstet Gynecol* 1:867, 1981.
11. Jackson ND, Rosenblatt PL: Use of Interceed absorbable adhesion barrier for vaginoplasty, *Obstet Gynecol* 84:1048, 1994.
12. Julian TM, O'Connell BJ, Gosewehr JA: Indications, techniques, and advantages of partial laser vaginectomy, *Obstet Gynecol* 80:140, 1992.
13. Lilford RI, Sharpe DT, Thomas DFM: Use of tissue expansion techniques to create skin flaps for vaginoplasty, *Br J Obstet Gynecol* 95:402, 1988.
14. McIndoe AH, Banister JB: An operation for the cure of congenital absence of the vagina, *J Obstet Gynecol Br Commonw* 45:490, 1938.
15. Morley GW, DeLancey JOL: Full-thickness skin graft vaginoplasty for treatment of the stenotic or foreshortened vagina, *Obstet Gynecol* 77:485, 1991.
16. Nichols DH, Randall CL: *Vaginal surgery,* ed 4, Baltimore, 1996, Williams & Wilkins.
17. Rettenmaier MA, DiSaia PD: Understanding current vaginectomy techniques, *Contemp Obstet Gynecol* 30:109, 1987.
18. Soper JT, Larson D, Hunter VJ, et al: Short gracilis myocutaneous flaps for vulvovaginal reconstruction after radical pelvic surgery, *Obstet Gynecol* 74:823, 1989.
19. Stal S, Spira M: Mons pubis as a donor site for split-thickness skin grafts, *Plast Reconstr Surg* 75:906, 1985.
20. Tancer ML, Katz M, Veridiano NP: Vaginal epithelialization with human amnion, *Obstet Gynecol* 54:345, 1979.
21. Thompson JD, Wharton LR, TeLinde RW: Congenital absence of the vagina, *Am J Obstet Gynecol* 74:397, 1957.
22. Tolhurst DE, van der Helm TWJS: The treatment of vaginal atresia, *Surg Gynecol Obstet* 172:407, 1991.
23. Vecchietti G: Le neo-vagin dams le syndrome de Rokitansky-Kuster-Hauser, *Rev Med Suisse Romande* 99:593, 1979.
24. Veronikis DK: The recurrent small and painful vagina. In Nichols DH, editor: *Reoperative gynecologic and obstetric surgery,* ed 2, St Louis, 1997, Mosby.
25. Veronikis DK, McClure GB, Nichols DH: The Vecchietti operation for constructing a neovagina: indications, instrumentation, and techniques, *Obstet Gynecol* 90:301, 1997.
26. Williams EA: Congenital absence of the vagina: a simple operation for its relief, *J Obstet Gynaecol Br Commonw* 71:511, 1964.

26 Massive Eversion of the Vagina

DAVID H. NICHOLS

More women are living longer, and they are interested in maintaining a self-image of femininity and the capacity for sexual activity beyond the menopause. Few maladies are more disruptive to these goals than is massive eversion of the vagina. It is specific, dramatic, obvious, frustrating, embarrassing, and progressive. It may occur with or without prolapse of the uterus, because uterine prolapse is the result, not the cause, of the eversion. Cystocele, rectocele, or enterocele may coexist, and the distinction is surgically important because each, when present, should be repaired (Fig. 26-1). Clearly, massive eversion of the vagina is a complex disorder, but surgery is curative, relieving symptoms and restoring normal anatomic relationships. It is desirable that the gynecologic surgeon know and be experienced with various operative techniques for repair and that the one selected best fits the need of a particular patient.

Loss of ischiorectal fat from beneath the pelvic diaphragm may occur with massive weight loss, depriving the levator ani of some support from below, and is conducive to development of a genital prolapse.

Although massive eversion of the vagina is more common in postmenopausal patients, it can sometimes also occur in young patients. It is more common in white patients than in black patients for reasons not totally understood. Some cases of massive eversion of the vaginal vault occur in the nullipara—probably related to congenital pelvic tissue weakness, defective innervation, or unusual trauma—but most are seen in parous women. Obstetrically skillful management of labor and delivery reduces the risk of eversion, but postpartum procidentia is the rule in a patient who has survived surgical treatment of her bladder exstrophy. In some childbirth settings, however, persons other than skilled obstetricians deliver babies, and timely, anatomically repaired episiotomy takes place less frequently in these settings. With resurgence of interest in home delivery, an increase in the incidence of genital prolapse, as well as of the other gynecologic consequences of unattended childbirth, can be expected.

That a "dropped uterus" is the result, not the cause, of genital prolapse has not always been appreciated. Surgeons have performed "routine" abdominal hysterectomy for uterine prolapse in the mistaken belief that the removal of a prolapsed uterus will prevent further genital prolapse (i.e., "no uterus, no dropping"). However, the vaginal vault prolapse, which *caused* the uterine prolapse, persists regardless of whether the uterus has been removed. Therefore these patients often may be seen in consultation some time after their primary surgery, frequently referred by their initial surgeon.

PREOPERATIVE HISTORY AND EXAMINATION

In taking the patient's history, the gynecologist should ask whether urinary stress incontinence was a problem when the patient was younger and, if so, if symptoms diminished as the vaginal vault descended. The relief of symptoms under the circumstance of progressive prolapse suggests a kinking of the urethra coincident with the prolapse. Recurrent urinary stress incontinence after the vagina has been repositioned within the pelvis is likely to develop in such patients unless special steps are taken during anterior colporrhaphy to decrease the likelihood of this possibility.

If the patient with massive eversion of the vagina has a history of previous urinary stress incontinence that is no longer present, presumably due to kinking of the urethra coincident with the progression of the prolapse, she should have a urodynamic evaluation, which includes measurement of her urethral pressure profile. If a low urethral closure–pressure closure (less than 20 cm H_2O) is found, the surgeon can plan how the low-pressure urethra should be treated as part of the original primary procedure. A coincident vesicourethral sling procedure is one choice to lessen the chance of postoperative urinary incontinence.

The chronically increased intraabdominal pressure that is so often the cause of massive eversion of the vagina also may lead to the development of a coincident hiatal hernia. Such a patient often gives a history of heartburn when lying down.

The patient should be examined when she is fully awake and standing. The gynecologist should replace the vault and note any possible cystocele, rectocele, or enterocele (Fig. 26-2). Generally, if any weakness is present in these areas, even of a minor degree, it should be repaired simultaneous with the primary procedure. This improves the overall surgical success of a reconstructive procedure and decreases the likelihood that a separate secondary operation will be necessary in the future.

It is sometimes possible to predict with reasonable accuracy the patient with uterine procidentia who will require separate but coincident colpopexy. This can be determined by identifying the primary site of weakness in the upper or the lower vaginal supports. With the patient in the lithotomy position on the examining table the gynecologist should replace the prolapse within the pelvis and have the patient bear down and observe to see which organs appear first. If the cervix and uterus appear first followed by the rest of the vagina and some cystocele and rectocele, the patient has massive primary damage to the upper suspensory supports of the vagina, particularly the cardinal and uterosacral lig-

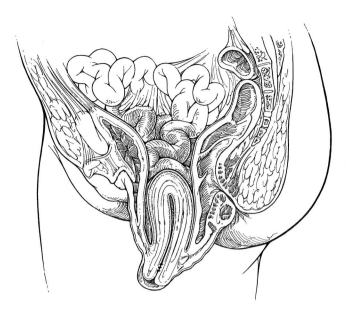

Fig. 26-1   Massive eversion of the vagina and the organs to which it is attached are shown in sagittal section.

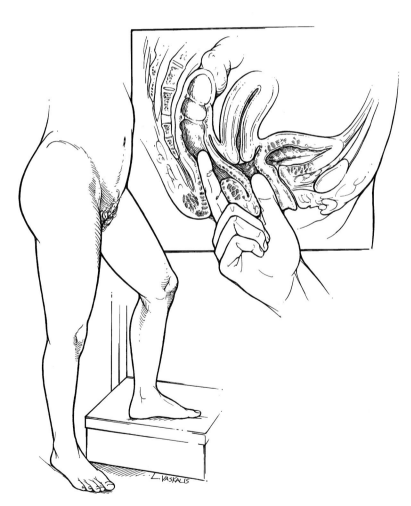

Fig. 26-2   Examination of the patient in the standing position.

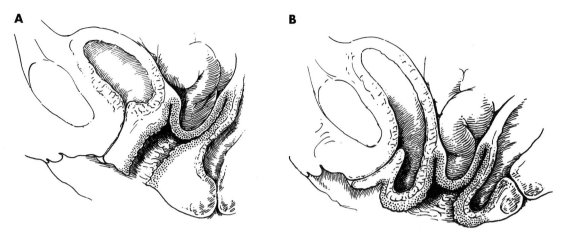

Fig. 26-3 **A,** Partial eversion of the vagina without cystocele and rectocele is noted after hysterectomy. **B,** Partial eversion of the vaginal vault after hysterectomy coexists with obvious cystocele and rectocele. (From Nichols DH, Randall CL: *Vaginal surgery,* ed 4, Baltimore, 1996, Williams & Wilkins.)

aments, and will probably require hysterectomy and colpopexy as part of the primary procedure. If, on the other hand, the cystocele and rectocele appear first followed by the cervix, the primary damage in all likelihood is concentrated on the supports of the lower pelvis, particularly the pelvic and urogenital diaphragms, and the patient will probably be best treated by a skillful vaginal hysterectomy with colporrhaphy and probably will not require planning for a coincident sacrospinous colpopexy.

The gynecologist should beware of the unsuspected anatomic weaknesses of the patient who has been operated on several times previously without lasting success. Often an underlying systemic or generalized connective tissue weakness is present that has been undiagnosed and unappreciated.[48]

PREVENTION OF RECURRENT PROLAPSE

When surgical repair of a genital prolapse is indicated, the skilled surgeon has several techniques from which to choose. Because of the various etiologic factors, different surgical procedures are required for correction. As a surgical maxim, the surgeon "should make the operation fit the patient, not the patient fit the operation." A surgeon tends to use most frequently the operations that he or she performs best, but every surgeon must thoroughly learn the various techniques available to ensure that he or she can perform the procedure that best fits the particular combination of damage in any individual patient. Significant steps can be taken in the operating room to prevent recurrent prolapse.

Posthysterectomy vaginal vault eversion occurs when the support of the vaginal vault is inadequate. During total hysterectomy, the uterosacral–cardinal ligament complex is surgically detached from the uterus and, if not reattached to the vaginal vault, undergoes atrophy. After a few months or years, it may no longer be sufficiently strong to be of much use in surgical reconstruction of any future vault eversion.

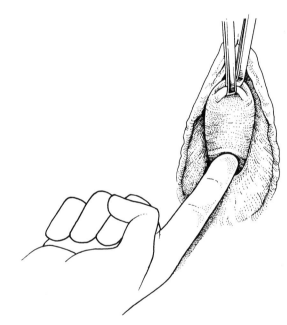

Fig. 26-4 When traction is made to a tenaculum applied to the posterior lip of the cervix, one can palpate both the length and strength of the uterosacral ligaments, as well as the base of the cul-de-sac of Douglas. (Redrawn from Nichols DH, Randall CL: *Vaginal surgery,* ed 4, Baltimore, 1996, Williams & Wilkins.)

Furthermore, even a partial degree of eversion generally will progress if ignored at hysterectomy or otherwise left unattended (Fig. 26-3). To prevent eversion, the surgeon must determine the strength and length of the patient's uterosacral-cardinal ligaments at the time of hysterectomy (Fig. 26-4). If they are strong and long, they should be shortened before they are attached to the vaginal vault (Fig. 26-5). A wide vaginal vault should be surgically narrowed (Fig. 26-6), the cul-de-sac should be obliterated, and any enterocele should be excised. Sewing the uterosacral

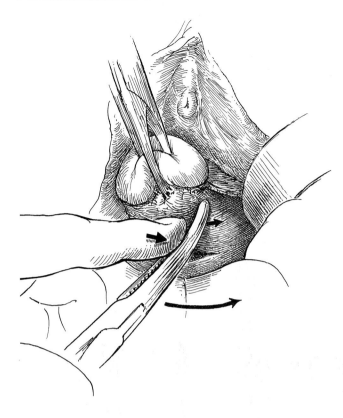

Fig. 26-5 The uterosacral ligaments are identified and clamped, and if these appear elongated and seem strong, the clamps may be placed to ensure some shortening of the ligaments as they are cut from the uterus. The tip of this clamp usually includes the lower portion of the cardinal ligament. Necessary shortening is accomplished by placement of the *unlocked* clamp across the uncut uterosacral ligament. The operator's finger presses the clamp as shown; the heel is moved a further distance than the tip. A lateral retractor displaces the vaginal wall, previously stripped from the surface of the ligament. (From Nichols DH, Randall CL: *Vaginal hysterectomy,* ed 4, Baltimore, 1996, Williams & Wilkins.)

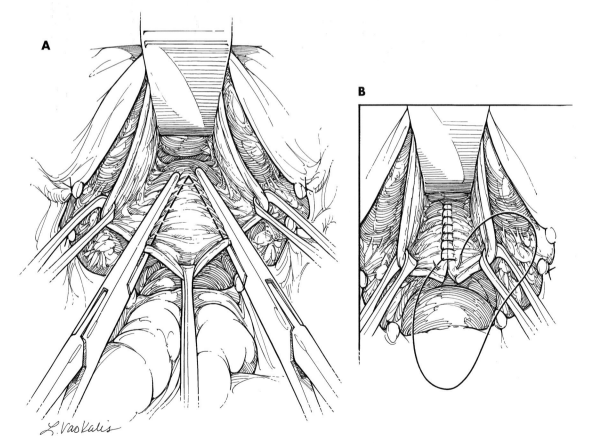

Fig. 26-6 **A,** After hysterectomy, a wide vaginal vault can be narrowed by excising a wedge from the center of the posterior wall *(dashed line).* **B,** The cut edges are united by a running locked stitch.

Continued

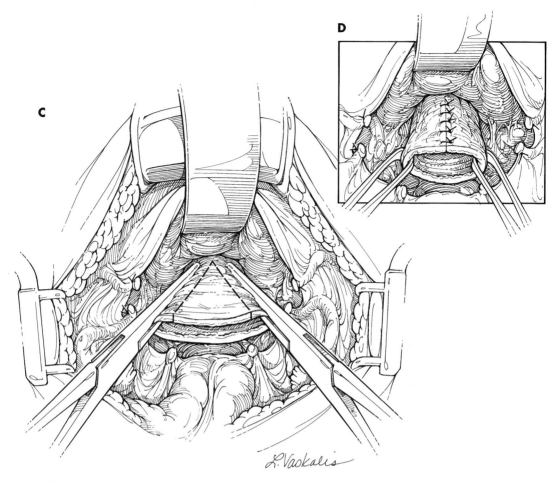

L. Vaokalis

Fig. 26-6, cont'd   C, If it is too wide, the anterior vaginal wall can be narrowed by excising a wedge *(dashed line)* after the bladder has been dissected down and held out of the way as shown. **D,** The cut edges are united by interrupted stitches. This is one form of abdominal cystocele repair.

ligaments together at the time of posthysterectomy reperitonealization is useful, and the New Orleans or McCall culdeplasty can be used.[13,32] When the strength of the uterosacral-cardinal ligaments is insufficient for this technique, as it may be in a patient with total genital procidentia, the surgeon must use an alternative method of colpopexy.

The surgeon should attempt to restore the normal depth and axis of the vagina, particularly after any urethrovesical pin-up operation (such as the Marshall-Marchetti-Krantz[26] or the Burch modification[8]) that pulls the vagina anteriorly. This often can be achieved by an appropriate perineorrhaphy and posterior colporrhaphy. If the uterosacral-cardinal ligaments are *not* strong enough to be surgically usable, colpopexy to a nongynecologic structure (e.g., the sacrospinous ligament or the sacrum) may be required to restore vaginal depth.

Amreich[3] noted the importance of preserving vaginal depth after hysterectomy. If, after removal of the uterus, the vagina is otherwise well supported and sits on an intact levator plate, pressure from the pelvic diaphragm will counter the intraabdominal pressure applied to the vagina; com-

pressed between these two pressures, the vagina remains in place. However, if the vagina is short and ends anterior to the levator plate (Fig. 26-7) after hysterectomy, it may telescope on itself, becoming even shorter as intraabdominal pressure is directed along the axis of the vagina. (This is less likely to occur in a patient who has had a Wertheim or Schauta radical hysterectomy, because the scarring in this area after either of these procedures is so great that very little will disturb it.) Although most cases of massive eversion of the vagina are seen in women who have experienced previous hysterectomy, some women with procidentia and complete eversion of the vagina have never had previous pelvic surgery. Because in this circumstance the uterus serves as a passenger with the prolapse and not the cause, its influence is therefore more or less passive. The primary defect has to do with the integrity of the connective tissue supports of the vaginal vault and vagina, which, in the presence of massive vault eversion, have been seriously compromised. When the uterus is present in a patient with massive eversion of the vagina, the uterosacral–cardinal ligament complex is always extensively elongated. If these supports are strong, they may be used, after sufficient shortening and

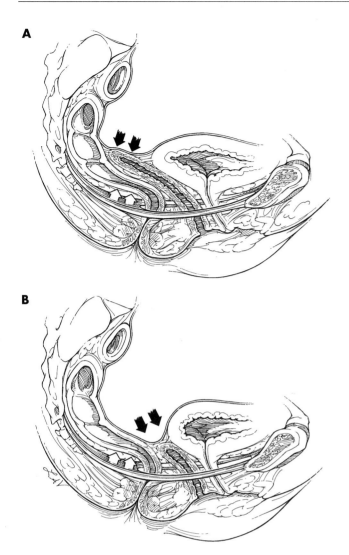

Fig. 26-7 **A,** The long posthysterectomy vagina in which the vaginal vault is supported above the intact levator plate *(white arrows)* and posterior to its anterior margin. Increases in intraabdominal pressure *(black arrows)* tend to squeeze the vagina against the intact levator plate. **B,** The vault of a shorter posthysterectomy vagina ends *anterior* to the intact levator plate *(white arrows),* and increases in intraabdominal pressure *(black arrows)* are exerted in the axis of the vagina, tending to cause it to telescope and to become even shorter. (Redrawn from Amreich J: *Wien Klin Wochenschr* 63:74, 1951.)

culdeplasty, to support the vault and hold it in place back within the pelvis where it belongs.

Elkins has emphasized the good results that can be obtained from high midline plication of the uterosacral ligaments before they have been transected.[13] A Döderlein-Kronig vaginal hysterectomy is required for this, as it brings the uterus through the anterior peritoneal opening, thereby exposing the previously untouched posterior cul-de-sac for surgical attention.

With complete procidentia, even in the presence of an enterocele, the uterosacral ligament complex usually is inef-

fective for postoperative vaginal support; therefore primary coincident colpopexy can be planned as part of the primary surgical operation.[24,32]

Because a "dropped" uterus is the result and not the cause of genital prolapse, eversion of the vaginal vault can be distinctly independent of the presence or absence of the uterus.

Eversion or protrusion of parts or all of the vagina beyond the hymenal ring may involve various levels of the vagina either singly or in any combination, depending on which of the various supporting structures have been damaged. Damage to the vaginal supports at the level of the urogenital diaphragm or below may be associated with perineal defect and urethral hypermobility. Damage to the middle group of supports, including the rectovaginal septum and fibromuscular vaginal wall and its lateral attachments to the pelvic side wall (the levator ani and arcus tendineus in particular), may permit the development of cystocele and rectocele, discussed in their separate chapters, and damage by stretching or avulsion of the uterosacral–cardinal ligament complex may permit eversion of the vaginal vault independent of any coincident enterocele.

The multiplicity of possible anatomic supportive defects that give rise to the combinations of clinically significant damage that may be encountered in examination of a patient with posthysterectomy vaginal eversion were studied and evaluated by DeLancey in 94 cadavers of various ages.[11] He confirmed other studies and opinions, finding that the upper third of the vagina is suspended by vertical fibers of the paracolpium (i.e., cardinal ligament continuations that arise from a broad area on the pelvic sidewalls). Suspension of the midvaginal paracolpium comes from attachment through a connective tissue bridge to the arcus tendineus and of the lower vagina by fusion to the perineal body and its muscular and fibrous attachments. The integrity of the pelvic diaphragm, including the levator ani and its effective innervation, plays a key role in vaginal support. This study supports the concept that damage to the tissue of these levels may occur singly or in any combination, and to achieve an optimal result the gynecologic surgeon should identify each site of damage preoperatively and incorporate suitable remedial steps in the surgical reconstruction. Symptomatic patients in whom other sites of simultaneous weakness are unidentified and untreated may need a future reoperation with its attendant risks, suffering, and expense.

The symptoms of vaginal vault eversion include backache, a feeling of vaginal fullness, and presence of a protruding vaginal mass while the patient is standing, when the pull of gravity aggravates the descent of the parts. Vaginal vault eversion uncommonly can occur as a consequence of an isolated deficiency in genital support, the vault coming down according to the attenuation of the vaginal portion of the uterosacral–cardinal ligament complex. Vaginal vault eversion is seen far more frequently as the consequence, usually progressive, of damage to several levels of genital support.[1,5,11,32]

Reconstructive surgery has the following three goals:

1. Relief of symptoms
2. Restoration of anatomic relationships between the pelvic organs
3. Restoration of function of each component organ system

To achieve a perfect surgical reconstruction, the surgeon must determine preoperatively all specific sites of damage[5,11,32] and, in the operating room, must reaffirm the presence and extent of the damage by a careful examination under anesthesia immediately preceding the operation. Consideration of these observations determines the extent and details of the specific reconstruction. Broad allowances for unexpected changes of surgical plan and extent as the operation evolves should be covered in the informed consent discussed with the patient.

Significant and essential anatomic and pathophysiologic differences exist between *partial* eversion of the vaginal vault to the midpoint of the vagina (often diagnosed by examination of the patient while she is standing and bearing down or straining), *subtotal* eversion (protrusion of the vagina and organs to which it is attached through the hymen but cranial to an intact urogenital diaphragm), and *total* eversion of the vagina, which includes the above plus eversion of all vaginal tissues, including those below or caudal to the urogenital diaphragm.

Urinary incontinence coexists more commonly in a postmenopausal than in a premenopausal patient with total eversion of the vagina. It may be of several types and can be best demonstrated by examination of the awake patient with a partly filled bladder and with the vaginal vault digitally replaced and held in an intrapelvic position, preferably manually or by rectal swabs.[58] The types of incontinence include urinary stress incontinence, overflow incontinence (from a bladder never completely empty), incontinence from significant detrusor or urethral instability, or incontinence resulting from low urethral pressure (a urethral closure pressure less than 20 cm H_2O) or any combination of the above. The causes of the latter, related to decreased urethral tone, are difficult to pinpoint but may include decreased estrogen, decreased urethral wall elasticity, decreased vascularity, decreased muscle contractility, and a decrease in the effective paraurethral tissue support. The consequences of not knowing, however, are usually obvious (e.g., troublesome postoperative urinary incontinence resulting from loss of unrecognized preoperative urethral kinking in spite of coincident anterior colporrhaphy).

Because effective repair of the coincident low-pressure urethra (as by vesicourethral sling, periurethral injections, bulbocavernosus fat pad transplant, or urethral plication) greatly improves patient satisfaction with surgery, its presence should be determined ahead of time. Low urethral closure pressure should be suspected in every instance of total vaginal eversion seen in a postmenopausal patient, especially in women who have not been participating in estrogen replacement therapy (ERT). In the author's experience, a low urethral closure pressure exists in 56% of such patients.[58] Its prevalence in postmenopausal patients is a reason for prescribing biweekly vaginal instillations of 1 to 2 g of estrogen cream for a month or two preoperatively and weekly installations during at least the first year postoperatively.

If sophisticated urodynamic laboratory testing is not available, a simple method of demonstrating probable low urethral closure pressure can be used. Preoperatively, in the examining room and with the patient's bladder partly full, *the vaginal vault is manually replaced,* and the patient, previously incontinent or not, is asked to cough and strain, and one observes whether urine is involuntarily lost. This examination is performed first with the patient in the lithotomy position and then standing.

If incontinence is demonstrated while straining, a condition of low urethral closure pressure is strongly suspected. An inexpensive preliminary screening test consists of passing of a no. 8 pediatric Foley catheter into the bladder, clamping the catheter, partially inflating the Foley bulb with 1 ml of saline, and applying gentle traction on the catheter to draw the partially inflated bulb easily through the urethra. If this can be done, the diagnosis of low urethral closure pressure is likely, and an appropriate surgical remedy should be incorporated in the primary reconstructive repair. If the bulb cannot be pulled through with gentle traction, 0.25 ml of saline is removed from the bulb and traction is reapplied to the catheter, the bulb of which is now partially inflated with the residual 0.75 ml of saline. If the bulb can be drawn through the urethra with minimal resistance, the diagnosis of low urethral closure pressure can be seriously entertained. If the partially inflated Foley bulb can be drawn into only the proximal urethra, funneling of the vesical neck should be seriously suspected. These suspicions should of course be confirmed by more sophisticated laboratory assessment and urethral pressure profile if such a facility is available and is affordable by the patient.

Vaginal prolapse as a complication of pelvic exenteration may be treated by transvaginal sacrospinous colpopexy, but coincident perineal hernia anterior to the colpopexy has been effectively remedied by transvaginal placement of a crescent-shaped piece of plastic mesh sutured between the pubic rami and covered by the anterior vaginal wall.[6]

Simultaneous prolapse of the rectum and vagina occurs occasionally (Fig. 26-8).[54] Surgical treatment of one element will not benefit the other, but it is possible to treat both during the same surgery. One method is transvaginal-transperineal, with colpopexy and repair, and resection of the prolapsed rectum; however, if transabdominal exploration is necessary, surgical treatment of both prolapses can be offered by laparotomy.[54] In this instance, the rectal prolapse should be treated first, often by rectopexy with or without intestinal resection according to the amount of redundant bowel present. Because sacrocolpopexy will be anterior to the rectal suspension, it should be performed as the second procedure, and the cul-de-sac should be obliterated before the abdomen is closed. Any necessary

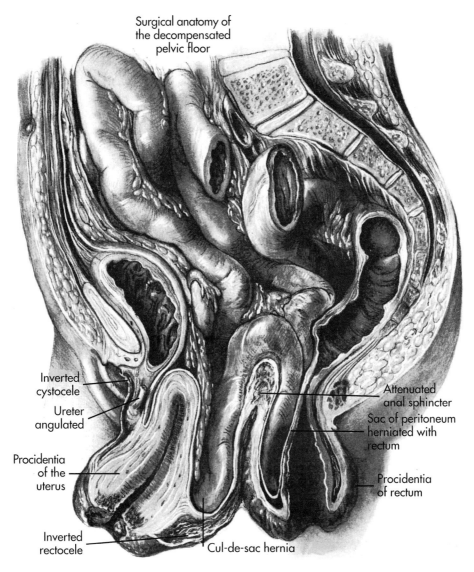

Surgical anatomy of
the decompensated
pelvic floor

Inverted
cystocele

Ureter
angulated

Procidentia
of the
uterus

Inverted
rectocele

Cul-de-sac hernia

Attenuated
anal sphincter

Sac of peritoneum
herniated with
rectum

Procidentia
of rectum

Fig. 26-8   Simultaneous genital prolapse and rectal prolapse are shown in sagittal section. Because they are each of entirely different cause, each must be repaired separately. (From Ball TL: *Gynecologic surgery and urology,* ed 2, St Louis, 1963, Mosby.)

transvaginal repair of cystocele or rectocele should be accomplished separately.

SACROSPINOUS RECTOPEXY AS PART OF THE TREATMENT OF COMBINED GENITAL AND RECTAL PROLAPSE

Chronically increased intraabdominal pressure can precipitate genital prolapse or rectal prolapse, or occasionally both. When these are symptomatic or socially disabling, an appropriate surgical solution should be considered, hopefully one that will repair or address all the areas of weakness during a single surgery. Because this genital prolapse includes descent of the uterus (if present), the vaginal vault, some enterocele, and cystocele and rectocele, each site of weakness must be determined carefully. The rectal prolapse should be differentiated from anal mucosal prolapse, since the surgical treatment is fundamentally different for each.

Procedure

After a thorough mechanical bowel preparation consisting of a liquid diet for 2 days and ingestion the day before surgery of a liter of electrolyte bowel cleanser (NuLYTELY or GoLYTELY) or enemas until clear, the patient is taken to surgery for an appropriate remedy, often under conduction anesthesia. The vaginal treatment of the genital prolapse includes vaginal hysterectomy, excision of any enterocele, colporrhaphy, and colpopexy, if indicated. If strong uterosacral ligaments are present, a McCall or New Orleans culdeplasty is advisable, but if the uterosacral ligaments are judged to be of insufficient strength to support the vaginal vault, a right sacrospinous colpopexy will remedy this weakness.

Transperineal treatment of the rectal prolapse, the latter recognized by the characteristic concentric rings of rectal mucosa covering the extrusion, may be by an Altemeier-Dunphy type: resection of the prolapsed bowel with primary transperineal anastomosis. Since the axis of the resultant bowel often fails to demonstrate an anorectal angle, the latter may be re-created by coincident postanal (retrorectal) levatorplasty. In the latter procedure, the retrorectal space is entered from below, the rectococcygeus muscle transected, and the posterior wall of the new rectum sewn with several interrupted stitches to the periosteum of the lower sacrum. The bellies of the pubococcygei are united in the midline *posterior* to the rectum, effectively lengthening the levator plate and enhancing the anorectal angle. This favors a restoration of continence once the tone of the dilated external and sphincter has been restored. The midline of the anterior surface of the new rectum is stitched to the left sacrospinous ligament by some interrupted stitches placed through the muscularis and submucosa, but not mucosa. The posterior colporrhaphy and perineorrhaphy are then completed.

Postoperative care includes putting the bowel at rest for several days, followed by a liquid diet, daily stool softeners, and appropriate antibiotic coverage. If a nasogastric tube had been inserted during the operation, it is clamped as soon as bowel sounds are heard, and small aliquots of nutrient liquid are given through the tube. If these are retained and there is no nausea and vomiting, the tube is removed and the patient given a full liquid diet for 3 days or until rectal gas has been regularly passed, and then a low-residue diet is added for 1 month postoperatively. Laboratory work includes a periodic hemogram and electrolyte estimations, with correction to normal as necessary. Pulmonary toilet is instituted postoperatively, and the patient begins walking as soon as she is able.

When it is necessary to postpone surgery for a symptomatic genital prolapse, temporary relief of symptoms may be provided by an intravaginal pessary such as the Gellhorn (Fig. 26-9), a ring, or an inflatable pessary.

The surgeon should be familiar with the varying degrees of vaginal vault eversion so that each can be recognized at the initial examination, and again at the beginning of a surgical procedure, and to confirm their disappearance at the conclusion of surgery and at follow-up examinations for at least 2 years. In *partial eversion,* the upper supports are weakened (vaginal portion of the cardinal ligaments and the uterosacral–cardinal ligament complex). This is often but not exclusively associated with a poor or vertically oriented vaginal axis. Enterocele usually is present, but cystocele and rectocele do not always coexist.

In *total eversion,* the entire vagina is inside out, including massive attenuation, stretching or avulsion of the attachments of the vagina to the urogenital diaphragm and the levator ani, and sometimes a considerable amount of attenuation or detachment of paravaginal supports. The latter can be identified by examining the patient in lithotomy position and replacing the vault to its usual position in the hollow of the sacrum and observing the anterior vaginal wall first with the patient at rest and again while straining. A sponge forceps or parallel tongue blades of two tongue depressors or a vaginal elevating forceps can be opened and spread,[5] bringing each anterior vaginal sulcus into contact with the site of the arcus tendineus on the obturator fascia. The gynecologist should carefully evaluate for residual midline cystocele (often demonstrating diminished rugal folds), because this would indicate a significant coincident defect in the midline support of the bladder and anterior vaginal wall, which should be repaired as well.

The patient with *total* prolapse of the vagina (including tissues normally attached to the urogenital diaphragm) must be considered to have a clinically significant paravaginal defect unless proven otherwise, and the surgeon should be prepared to repair it appropriately at the time of the original operation.[5,32] For those patients with a partial genital prolapse that occurs cranial to the vesicourethral junction, and in whom the lower part of the vagina does not descend appreciably with the vault or with traction to the vault, a paravaginal defect requiring repair is less common, but it should be estimated at the time of surgery by replacement of the vault to a position adjacent to the ischial spine and by careful examination of the anterior vaginal wall, first unsupported, and again when supported by a vaginal elevator or sponge forceps.

An element of lateral anterior sulcus and forniceal stretching (or less commonly detachment) often exists with cystocele. When the "lateral" cystocele is sufficiently symptomatic or progressive as to require surgical correction, the operator may elect the transvaginal White paravaginal reattachment operation.[32,60] However, if vaginal vault eversion coexists, the primary surgical goal should be reconstitution of effective support of the vaginal vault by either a transvaginal (sacrospinous colpopexy) or transabdominal (sacrocolpopexy) surgical route. Reconstitution of vaginal vault support often "straightens out the sagging clothesline" of compromised anterior vaginal sulcus support, obviating the need for direct, separate surgical paravaginal reattachment.

TRANSVAGINAL SURGICAL TREATMENT

The vaginal approach is particularly useful if the patient has significant medical risks. Methods of transvaginal surgical treatment include the following:

1. Vaginal hysterectomy and repair,[32] or the Manchester-Fothergill operation
2. Partial (LeFort) colpocleisis or colpectomy[12,32]
3. Transvaginal sacrospinous colpopexy with definitive treatment of cystocele and rectocele through the same operative exposure[13,27,32-34,41,42] or sacrospinous cervicopexy
4. Attachment of vaginal cuff to iliococcygeus fascia[20,35,47]
5. Reattachment of vaginal sulci to the *full length* of each arcus tendineus or to the obturator fascia

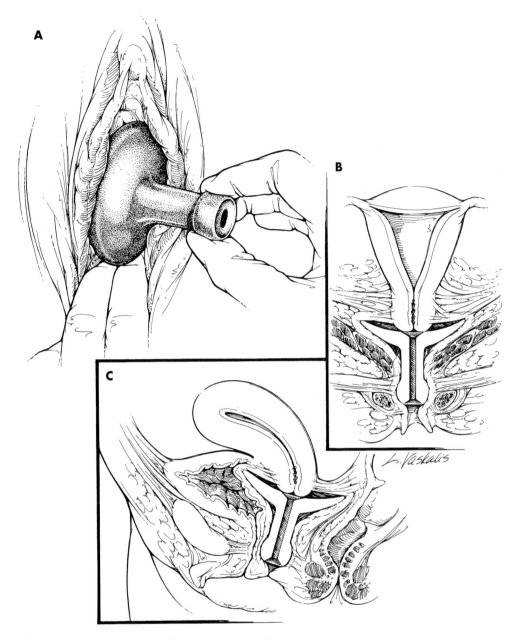

Fig. 26-9 Insertion of a Gellhorn pessary. **A,** The perineum is depressed, and the disc portion of the pessary is inserted. **B,** It should rest comfortably and be retained above the pelvic diaphragm. **C,** Notice in sagittal section that the properly fitted pessary elevated the vaginal vault and uterus to a position once again within the pelvis and, at the same time, relieved some of the distention of the cystocele and rectocele.

Because no single procedure can correct all pathologic conditions that may be present in various types of prolapse, it is often necessary to resourcefully combine several surgical operations.

In the surgical treatment of genital prolapse developing after hemipelvectomy,[21] it is necessary to fix the subvaginal connective tissue to a residual immobile pelvic anchorpoint such as the inguinal ligament on the affected side, combined with appropriate colporrhaphy, colpopexy, or both. Midline plication of the pubococcygei may be necessary to form a useful pelvic floor.

Vaginal Hysterectomy and Repair

Because the pathologic descent of the uterus is the result of genital prolapse, hysterectomy is not as important as the repair itself, nor should it be the prime objective of surgery for genital prolapse. Hysterectomy may be useful as a way to mobilize parametrial tissues for use in reconstructive surgery, but it should be an adjunct to repair. For the patient who wishes to retain the uterus, the surgeon may elect to perform colpopexy without hysterectomy.

Vaginal hysterectomy and repair constitute the correct procedure most often selected for genital prolapse. If the uterosacral-cardinal ligaments are strong, they can be shortened and attached to the vault of the vagina, providing a satisfactory result. When the usual coexisting enterocele is present, it should be excised, and the New Orleans or McCall culdeplasty is helpful. If the patient wishes to retain the uterine fundus, a Manchester-Fothergill operation may be considered; however, the possibility of subsequent pregnancy or abnormal uterine bleeding must be understood. For the same reasons, the Watkins-Wertheim uterine transposition operation is not recommended.

Partial Colpocleisis or Colpectomy

Although partial colpocleisis (LeFort) (Fig. 26-10) or colpectomy has at various times been a popular treatment option in older patients,[12] four problems are specific to this type of operation: (1) it limits or destroys vaginal coital function; (2) because the operation is extraperitoneal, it does not permit the intraperitoneal repair of an enterocele; (3) postoperative urinary stress incontinence may result from fusion of the anterior rectal wall to the base of the bladder, flattening the posterior urethrovesical angle; and (4) if the uterus is retained, the patient may have subsequent bleeding from a number of causes, including carcinoma. In addition, because the uterus and cervix are hidden behind the new vaginal septum, investigation into the source of the bleeding is difficult. Therefore we recommend partial colpocleisis only rarely.

If the uterus is still present, a LeFort partial colpocleisis can be performed (see Fig. 26-10), with appropriate attention directed to any defects of the anterior and posterior subvaginal tissues. If necessary this procedure can be accomplished using local anesthesia.

Total colpectomy can be effective and satisfactory in certain older patients for whom surgery entails greater risks than for most patients and for whom preservation of coital potential may be neither essential nor personally desirable. This is especially true when the tissues are not strong enough to be used effectively in reconstruction.[9,38,55] Colpectomy should be considered a destructive rather than a reconstructive operative approach (Fig. 26-11). Because there is no route for subsequent uterine drainage, colpectomy is inappropriate when the uterus has been retained. To assess the potential for postoperative urinary stress incontinence, preoperative urodynamic evaluation is timely, and if positive findings for stress incontinence are determined, appropriate surgical remedy including coincident colporrhaphy is indicated, including adequate attention to suburethral plication and support by the urogenital diaphragm. Coincident levator plication to narrow the urogenital hiatus is helpful, along with an appropriate perineorrhaphy. Coexistent enterocele should be recognized and excised, lest symptomatic and troublesome vulvar hernias occur in patients who have undergone total colpectomy as a treatment for prolapse of the vaginal vault. Generally these are a result of enteroceles that were unrecognized or recurred and were untreated at the time of the original surgery.

Other Transvaginal Reconstructive Procedures

Although obstetric trauma is the most significant and frequent factor in initiating vaginal eversion, the endocrine and nutritional changes during and after menopause seem to accelerate the progression of vaginal eversion by causing atrophic weakening of muscular and connective tissues. Thus it is not uncommon to encounter an aging but sexually active patient who has vaginal eversion, cystocele, and rectocele, but who, because of poor voluntary pelvic muscle strength, cannot retain a vaginal pessary. Genital prolapse may have

Fig. 26-10 Le Fort partial colpocleisis **A,** An area to be denuded is outlined from the external urinary meatus to the bladder reflection on the cervix. Along the outline, an incision is made that extends through the mucosa and superficial musculature of the vaginal wall. **B,** The area is now denuded of mucosa, leaving as much of the muscular wall as is possible while dissecting in this unnatural line of cleavage. Considerable general oozing may be encountered despite the fact that patients subjected to this procedure are postmenopausal. **C,** A similar area is denuded posteriorly but also including a triangular area of the skin of the perineum. Bilateral strips of mucosa are left. **D,** Using interrupted sutures of 2-0 chromic catgut, the mucosa of the vault is approximated over the cervix. After the anterior wall has been united to the posterior wall, the lateral edges on each side are approximated. **E,** The denuded vaginal wall is approximated anteroposteriorly by a series of mattress sutures in conjunction with the mucosal closure. When the area of the bladder neck is reached, this is plicated not only in the event of stress incontinence, but also for prophylactic purposes. **F,** The musculature of the perineal body is built up with interrupted sutures to aid in the obliteration of the genital aperture. Successive rows of mattress sutures continue the obliteration of the vaginal canal. The skin of the perineum is approximated in the midline by interrupted sutures. **G,** The remainder of the anteroposterior approximation is done, and drains are placed in both of the lateral tunnels of the vagina that result. (From Ball TL: *Gynecologic surgery and urology,* ed 2, St Louis, 1963, Mosby.)

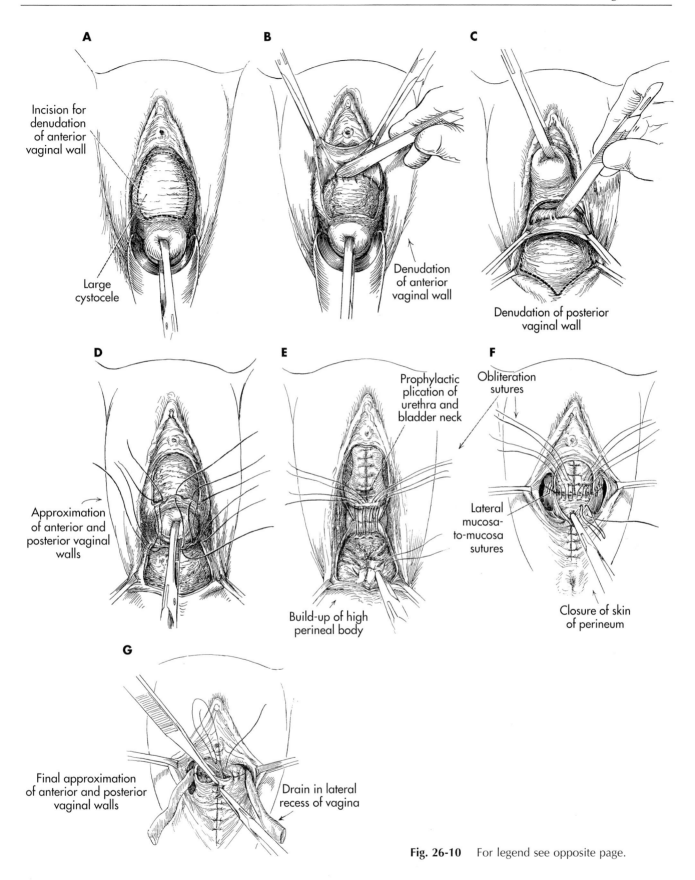

A

Incision for
denudation
of anterior
vaginal wall

Large
cystocele

B

Denudation
of anterior
vaginal wall

C

Denudation of posterior
vaginal wall

D

Approximation
of anterior and
posterior vaginal
walls

E

Prophylactic
plication of
urethra and
bladder neck

Build-up of high
perineal body

F

Obliteration
sutures

Lateral
mucosa-
to-mucosa
sutures

Closure of skin
of perineum

G

Final approximation
of anterior and posterior
vaginal walls

Drain in lateral
recess of vagina

Fig. 26-10   For legend see opposite page.

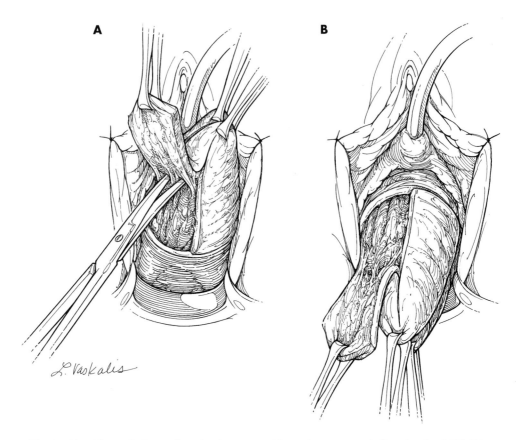

Fig. 26-11   The technique of total colpectomy. After subcutaneous infiltration by 0.5% lidocaine in 1:2000,000 epinephrine solution, the vagina is circumscribed by an incision at the
hymen and marked into quadrants, each of which is separately removed by sharp dissection
(**A** and **B**).

progressed in association with postmenopausal atrophic
changes. The prolapsed uterus can be removed without difficulty, and if the cardinal and uterosacral ligaments are
strong, they should be shortened and used to support the vaginal vault.[32,52] Sometimes, however, these tissues are not
of sufficient strength to support the everted vagina. This
condition, a general prolapse, usually indicates a major
problem with the integrity of *all* endopelvic soft tissues, especially those of the pelvic diaphragm.

The vault descends without a true enterocele in approximately 20% of patients[29] (Fig. 26-12, p. 476). Although
enterocele and massive eversion of the vagina usually
coexist, they are *separate* anatomic and clinical entities,
each requiring definitive, specific surgical treatment. When
eversion of the vagina follows a previous hysterectomy,
enterocele coexists in at least two thirds. This disabling
and uncomfortable outcome suggests that insufficient attention had been paid during surgery to the reinforcement
and correction of weakened genital supports. If strong
uterosacral-cardinal ligaments can be found at the sides of
the everted vaginal vault, they can be shortened and the
vagina can be attached to them for support,[32,52] followed
by excision of any enterocele and by high ligation of the
peritoneum. As mentioned earlier, however, the residual
and unattached uterosacral ligament complex gradually

seems to atrophy after total hysterectomy, and after a
few months or years is no longer sufficiently strong to
offer much usefulness for surgical reconstruction. With
minimal or negligible uterosacral strength, alternative
methods of restoring vaginal depth and axis must be
employed.

A number of alternative techniques have been described.
As early as 1892, Zweifel[63] wrote that by using a parasacral
posterior approach he had attached a prolapsed vagina to the
sacrotuberous ligament. White[62] in 1909 described transvaginal suture of the vagina to the arcus tendineus (White
line). Inmon[20] and later Symmonds et al.[52] reported stitching the vagina to the fascia of the pelvic diaphragm. In
1951, Amreich[3] reported his experience using both a trans-
gluteal (Amreich I) and transvaginal (Amreich II) approach
to attach an everted vagina to the sacrotuberous ligament.
Sederl[44] sewed the vagina to the sacrospinous ligament
(Fig. 26-13, p. 477). More recently, Richter[41,42] enthusiastically described his success with the use of the sacrospinous
ligament, renewing interest in this operation.

Transvaginal sacrospinous colpopexy has specific advantages. First, it permits restoration of a functional vagina with
a more normal, horizontally inclined upper vaginal axis atop
the levator plate,[31] thereby decreasing the risk that vault
eversion will recur. Second, unlike abdominal sacrocol-

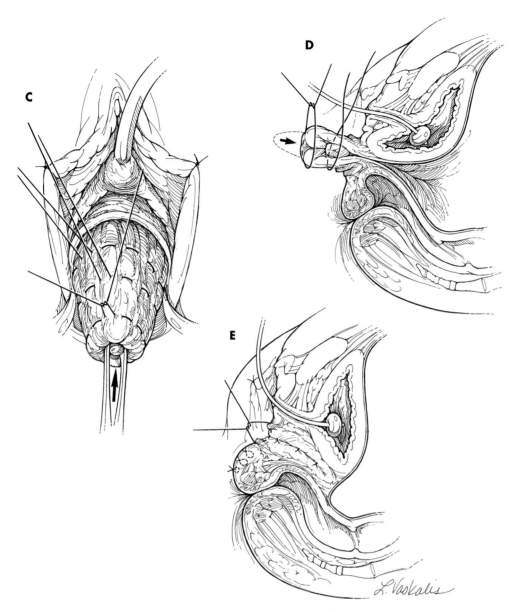

Fig. 26-11, cont'd A series of purse-string, synthetic absorbable sutures are placed **(C)** and tied, with progressive inversion of the soft tissue before tying each suture **(D).** An appropriate perineorrhaphy may complete the operation. **E,** The final result.

popexy, it offers a convenient opportunity to correct cystocele, rectocele, or enterocele simultaneously through the same operative exposure. Third, it is a shorter procedure than the abdominal counterpart and therefore requires less duration and depth of anesthesia. Finally, because it is principally extraperitoneal, there is a reduced risk of atelectasis, peritonitis, postoperative ileus, intestinal obstruction, incisional pain and hernia, and other hazards of transabdominal surgery. For the patient with uterine procidentia and demonstrably weak cardinal-uterosacral ligaments, coincident transvaginal sacrospinous colpopexy can be planned with vaginal hysterectomy and colporrhaphy as part of the primary operative procedure.[10,28,31]

Primary sacrospinous colpopexy, usually bilateral and immediately after vaginal hysterectomy, is surprisingly easy to perform in a patient with extensive prolapse but who has no strong, surgically useful uterosacral–cardinal ligament complex. We agree with Hirsch et al.,[17] who have recommended bilateral sacrospinous colpopexy for the patient with a very relaxed pelvic floor, markedly widened outlet, and vaginal or recurrent prolapse. The fact that the patient has not undergone previous surgery, which would alter tissue planes and spaces, facilitates the procedure. The addition of sacrospinous colpopexy to vaginal hysterectomy with anterior and posterior colporrhaphy (between the steps of peritoneal closure and the posterior repair) extends the operating time for the experienced vaginal surgeon by only approximately 15 to 20 minutes. This

A

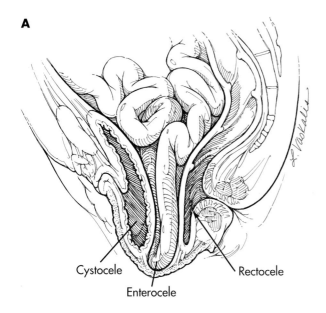

Cystocele

Enterocele

Rectocele

B

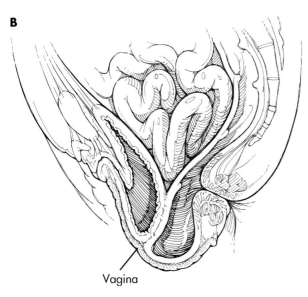

Vagina

Fig. 26-12   Massive eversion of the vagina with or without coincident enterocele. **A,** An enterocele is present in the majority of patients with massive eversion of a posthysterectomy vagina. **B,** Occasionally, however, the connective tissue capsule of the bladder is fused with that of the anterior rectum. It is important to make the distinction during surgery because, in the absence of enterocele, further dissection in this area is unnecessary and hazardous. If enterocele is present, however, identification, opening, excision, and closure of the neck of the enterocele removes it from the operative field. If it is present but undiagnosed and untreated it will progress over time, usually necessitating still another operative procedure. (From Nichols DH: *Reoperative gynecologic and obstetric surgery,* ed 2, St Louis, 1967, Mosby.)

is the time required for penetration of the rectal pillar and identification and placement of the vagina to one sacrospinous ligament or, more recently, to each. By correctly using this procedure, the surgeon can provide adequate support for the vagina, lengthen the well-supported vagina,

restore bladder and rectal function, and preserve normal coital ability.[19,35]

Transvaginal Sacrospinous Fixation

For transvaginal sacrospinous colpopexy, the operator's fingers should be of at least average length to be able to reach the hollow of the sacrum. An operator with short fingers has a distinct handicap for this operation. With the patient under anesthesia, the examiner confirms the sites of the damage, noting any that were previously undetected, and by simultaneously placing the index finger of each hand against each ischial spine and sacrospinous ligament estimates the width of the vaginal vault available for bilateral colpopexy, if this is desired (Fig. 26-14), or if a unilateral colpopexy is planned estimates the amount by which a wide vault should be narrowed. If a known coincident urinary incontinence is associated with a low urethral closure pressure and a hypermobile vesicourethral junction is identified, the operator may have chosen to incorporate a vesicourethral sling procedure as part of the operation.[32] In this case an incision is made in each groin parallel to the inguinal ligament, through the subcutaneous tissue and rectus aponeurosis. With the blunt tips of the curved Mayo scissors (curve directed toward the pubis) the central belly of each rectus muscle is penetrated, the direction of penetration going through the transversalis fascia to the site of the obturator foramen. The tips of the scissors are opened and withdrawn, and the operator's attention directed to the vaginal portion of the operation.

When bilateral sacrospinous colpopexy is planned, it is helpful that the surgeon initially insert absorbable marking sutures on the surface of each corner of the very apex of the everted vagina to identify the site at which the subsequent colpopexy stitches will be attached to the underside of the vagina. An ideal distance between these marking stitches in the everted vaginal vault is about 8 or 9 cm apart, one at the 3- and the other at the 9-o'clock position.

After the completion of any necessary hysterectomy and with the patient in the dorsal lithotomy position, the operator makes a V-shaped incision in the perineum of a width sufficient to create an introital diameter of three fingerbreadths at the conclusion of the operation, dissects the underside of the vagina from any scar tissue, and reflects the skin and the posterior vaginal wall from the perineal body until the avascular rectovaginal space has been entered. Development of this space is continued to the vaginal apex. The posterior vaginal wall is incised longitudinally as necessary, and if the vagina is to be narrowed by planned colporrhaphy, the excess vaginal wall is excised. Any enterocele sac is identified and opened.

When the surgeon opens an enterocele coincident with massive eversion of the vagina after previous total abdominal hysterectomy, the danger of unplanned cystotomy is slightly greater than when the opening and dissection of the enterocele follows previous total vaginal hysterectomy, since the relationship of the vesical peritoneum to the vault after abdominal hysterectomy may be different from its location after vaginal hysterectomy. After total abdominal hysterectomy, a surgeon often brought the bladder per-

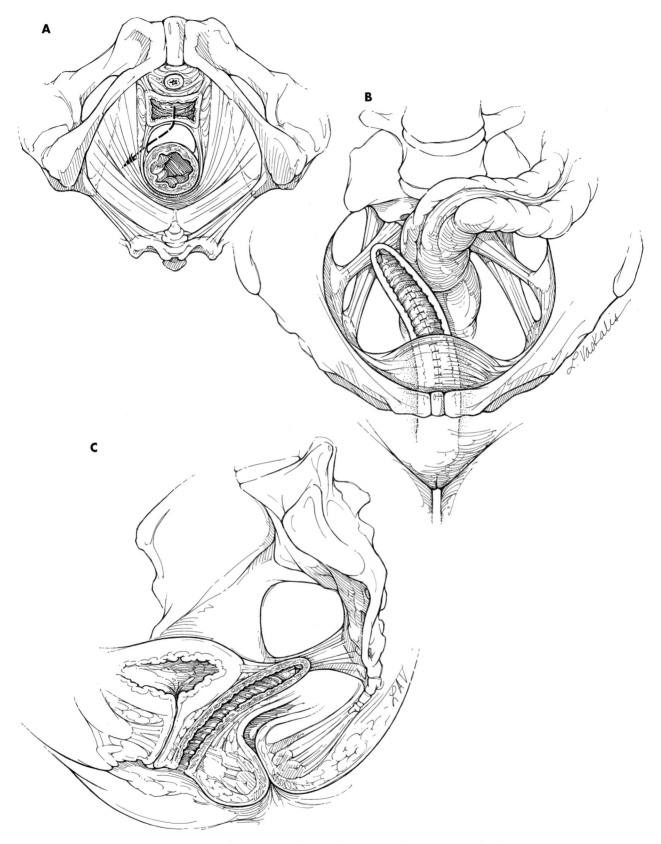

Fig. 26-13 Technique of right sacrospinous colpopexy. **A,** A path of dissection through a the posterior vaginal wall into the rectovaginal space and then through a window in the descending rectal septum into the right pararectal space. The dissection always proceeds toward the ischial spine in the lateral wall of the pararectal space. **B,** The vagina is sewn to the right sacrospinous ligament–coccygeal muscle complex at a point 1½ fingerbreadths medial to the right ischial spine. **C,** After the fixation stitches have been tied, the vagina is attached to the right sacrospinous ligament, indicating a fairly normal vaginal depth and axis after appropriate colporrhaphy.

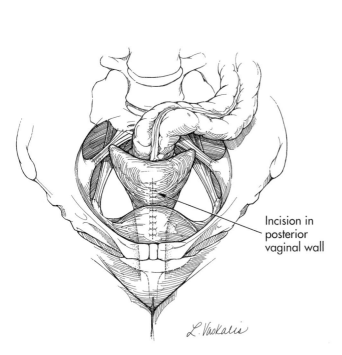

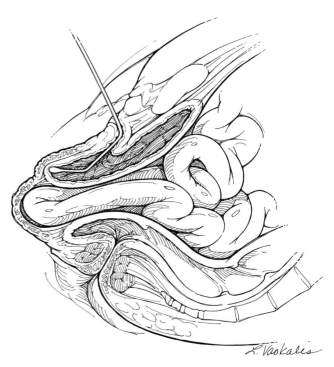

Incision in
posterior
vaginal wall

Fig. 26-14   Bilateral sacrospinous fixation, used when the vaginal vault is wide enough to reach from one side to the other. A phantom drawing shows the effective bilateral sacrospinous colpopexy. This very effectively maintains a widened vaginal vault. The site of the posterior colporrhaphy closure is shown in the midline of the posterior vaginal wall. (From Nichols DH, Randall CL: *Vaginal surgery,* ed 4, Baltimore, 1996, Williams & Wilkins.)

Fig. 26-15   If the limits of a partly filled bladder cannot be determined precisely, palpating the tip of a bent uterine sound can identify at surgery the site where the bladder and the wall of an enterocele sac come together. This will aid the safe dissection of the enterocele from the bladder.

itoneum across the vault of the open or closed vagina by attachment of the peritoneum to the anterior surface of the rectum, which would now place the bladder across the top of the vaginal vault. After vaginal hysterectomy, however, the surgeon commonly performs peritonealization by placing one or more purse-string sutures, and the center of the midline purse-string generally overlies the cut edge of the vaginal vault, away from the bladder.

Identification of the site at which an enterocele sac meets the bladder may be difficult in a patient with previous hysterectomy. Palpation of the tip of a bent blunt uterine sound inserted through the urethra into the bladder can facilitate identification (Fig. 26-15).

Once opened, the enterocele sac is mobilized and resected. After determining by palpation that there is no surgically useful uterosacral-cardinal ligament support, the surgeon closes the sac by high, purse-string reperitonealization and excises the excess peritoneum of the enterocele.

Locating the Sacrospinous Ligament. It is easier for a right-handed operator to use the patient's right sacrospinous ligament, although the left can be used if desired. If bilateral colpopexy is planned, each side is dissected and exposed separately. The sacrospinous ligament is an aponeurosis located within the substance of each coccygeus muscle, which extends from each ischial spine to the lower portion of the sacrum. Therefore, with the right index finger introduced

into the rectovaginal space, the operator seeks first the ischial spine on either side at about the 9- or 3-o'clock position and traces the fingerlike thickening of the sacrospinous ligament that runs posteriorly from this point to the hollow of the sacrum. To find these structures safely, the operator must understand the nature and boundaries of the connective tissue spaces.

Each rectal pillar separates the rectovaginal space from each pararectal space. When penetrating the descending rectal septum or pillar that separates the rectovaginal space and the perirectal space, one observes varying degrees of thickness of this septum between different patients. The ease of exposure of the coccygeus muscle–sacrospinous ligament complex depends on the thickness of the rectal pillar and whether it exists as one fused or two separate and distinct layers. To avoid drawing the rectum into the dissection, it is necessary to penetrate *both* layers in proceeding from the rectovaginal space to the pararectal space, providing safe entry into the pararectal space, lest the presence of the thin rectal wall be undetected and thus traumatized by the tip of the long Allis clamp that will be applied to the coccygeus muscle–sacrospinous ligament complex (risking a tear of the rectum, which must be instantly recognized and repaired using two layers of absorbable suture, or risking a penetration of the rectal wall by the tip of the ligature carrier or needle).

The rectum is particularly vulnerable on the patient's left because of the closeness of the rectum here to the pelvic sidewall. This is especially important during bilateral colpopexy, and the presence of scarring from previous surgery in this area requires vigilant precision in this dissection to avoid rectal trauma.

Following this path toward the ischial spine, the surgeon should penetrate the descending rectal septum by either sharp or blunt dissection *closer to the undersurface of the vagina* than to the rectum; in doing so, the operator should aim directly at the site at which the ischial spine has been palpated. The length and strength of the descending rectal septum seem to vary inversely with the diameter of the rectum, making the septum easier to penetrate in a patient with a large rectocele.

If the operator is the least bit uncertain about whether the rectal wall has been grasped, torn, or penetrated, a change of glove rectal examination should be performed on the spot to confirm proper suture placement before any knots have been tied and to confirm the lack of rectal wall trauma. If sutures have been improperly placed and have penetrated the rectal lumen, they should be immediately withdrawn and replaced in an anatomically proper position. Some surgeons make this rectal examination routine at this point of the operation.

The rectal pillar is perforated at a spot overlying the ischial spine. If the pillar is thin or weak, it often can be penetrated by blunt dissection with the fingertip; if not, the operator can use the tips of the Mayo scissors or a long hemostatic forceps, such as a tonsil or a Varco-Cooley forceps (Fig. 26-16). After their insertion through the new window in the right pillar, the tips of the scissors or forceps may be opened and spread to enlarge the window and expose the superior surface of the pelvic diaphragm. A long, preferably straight, retractor (Fig. 26-17) is inserted into the wound, displacing the rectum to the patient's left; another displaces the cardinal ligament and ureter anteriorly. Similar exposure can be obtained with the use of three narrow Deaver retractors, but they are not as easily applied. (The curve of the Deaver retractors offers no advantage and also poses the risk of the tip of a retractor being pushed across the anterior surface of the sacrum, damaging the sacral veins.)

Direct illumination of this deep area is essential. A spotlight just over the operator's shoulder or a suitable bright fiberoptic forehead lamp or a lighted retractor can provide the necessary illumination.

Blunt dissection proceeds easily to the ischial spine. The superior surface of the coccygeus muscle is readily identified, running posterolaterally from the ischial spine. Areolar tissue may be pushed from the surface of the right coccygeus muscle containing the sacrospinous ligament, if desired, using a "rosebud" or wisp sponge. Bleeding within the pararectal space is uncommon; when it does occur, usually of anomalous venous origin, it is easily controlled by medium-sized vascular clips.

Visualization and concentration of tissue in the coccygeus muscle–sacrospinous ligament complex will be improved by grasping the complex with the tip of a long Allis clamp at a point approximately two fingerwidths medial to the ischial spine.

Selection of Ligature Carrier for Sacrospinous Colpopexy. A number of ligature carriers for sacrospinous colpopexy are available. These include the use of a free

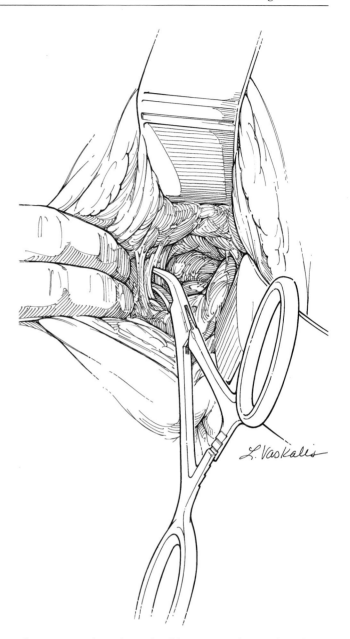

Fig. 26-16 The right cardinal ligament and ureter have been displaced anteriorly by a Breisky-Navratil retractor in the 12-o'clock position, and the rectum has been displaced to the patient's left by a retractor in the 4-o'clock position. An opening is made either bluntly or by using a sharp, pointed hemostat through the descending rectal septum into the right pararectal space, at the site of the ischial spine. This opening is enlarged by spreading the point of the hemostat or the Mayo scissors to permit access to the coccygeus muscle, which lies in the lateral wall of the pararectal space and contains within it the sacrospinous ligament. (From Nichols DH: Surgical correction of defects in pelvic support. In Rock JA, Thompson JD, editors: *Te Linde's operative gynecology,* ed 8, Philadelphia, 1997, JB Lippincott.)

taper-point Mayo needle (never a wedged needle, which is too brittle), the Deschamps ligature carrier (Fig. 26-18) (BEI/Zinnanti Surgical Instruments, Chatsworth, Calif.) of an appropriate size, a Miya hook[27] (Zinnanti Surgical Instruments, Chatsworth, Calif.), the Shutt punch[45]

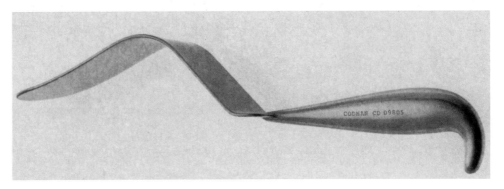

Fig. 26-17   Flat blade retractor is available in various sizes from special order department of BEI/Zinnanti Surgical Instruments, Chatsworth, CA 93311, Codman & Shurtleff, New Bedford, MA 02745, or from Mr. William Metz, Baxter V. Mueller, Chicago, IL 60648.

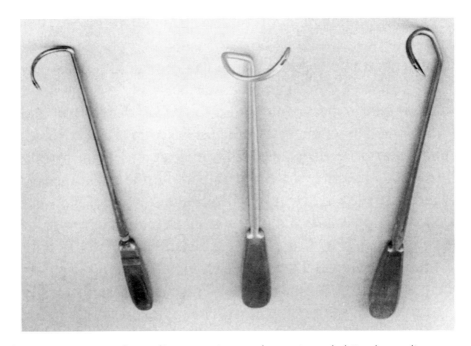

Fig. 26-18   Long Deschamps ligature carriers are shown. An angled Deschamps ligature carrier (modeled after one modified by Rosenshein) noted at the right is useful when the sacrospinous ligament is unusually deep. The handle must be swung through a wide arc. These instruments are available on special order from BEI/Zinnanti Surgical Instruments, Chatsworth, CA 93311, Codman & Shurtleff, Custom Device Dept., New Bedford, MA 02745, or Mr. William Metz, Baxter V. Mueller, Chicago, IL 60648.

(Figs. 26-19 and 26-20) (Linvatec Corporation, Largo, Fla.) an anthroscopic ligature carrier, the Endo Stitch[43,59] (US Surgical Corporation, Norwalk, Conn.), a laparoscopic suturing device, the Laurus needle driver[25] (Laurus Medical Corporation, Irvine, Calif.), and the Nichols-Veronikis (N-V) ligature carrier[57] (BEI/Zinnanti Medical Systems, Chatsworth, Calif.). All can be used to penetrate the substance of a sacrospinous ligament under direct vision during its course within the coccygeus muscle, and it is appropriate for the operator to be familiar with the use of several of these instruments so that the one that best fits the needs of a particular patient's clinical situation may be chosen.

Passage of a sharp-pointed, potentially dangerous free needle may be difficult because of the limited space in which to safely manipulate the needle, and the sharp point risks penetration or laceration of nearby bowel or blood vessel. The blunt-tipped Deschamps ligature carrier should penetrate the sacrospinous ligament from below along a path at a right angle to the direction of the fibers of both muscle and ligament. Comfortable use here of the Deschamps often requires a longer learning curve. It is available in a number of configurations for either the right or left hand, and its needle eye aperture can accommodate two sutures simultaneously, permitting placement of two sutures with but one pass of the ligature carrier (see Fig. 26-18). Suture retrieval from the Miya hook is sometimes difficult, especially in an obese patient, since this carrier penetrates the ligament downward from the top side, tending to bury its

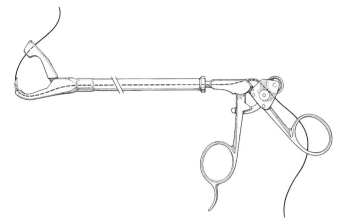

Fig. 26-19   The Shutt suture punch consists of a long hollow tunnel within the body of a forceps that terminates in a hollow needle. Monofilament suture is threaded through the tunnel; the suture passes beneath a friction wheel until it reaches the tip of the hollow needle. Then the direction of movement of the friction wheel is reversed so that the tip of the suture is withdrawn until it is barely within the substance of the hollow needle and no longer projects beyond it. The instrument is available from Linvatec, Largo, FL 34643. (From Nichols DH, Randall CL: *Vaginal surgery,* ed 4, Baltimore, 1996, Williams & Wilkins.)

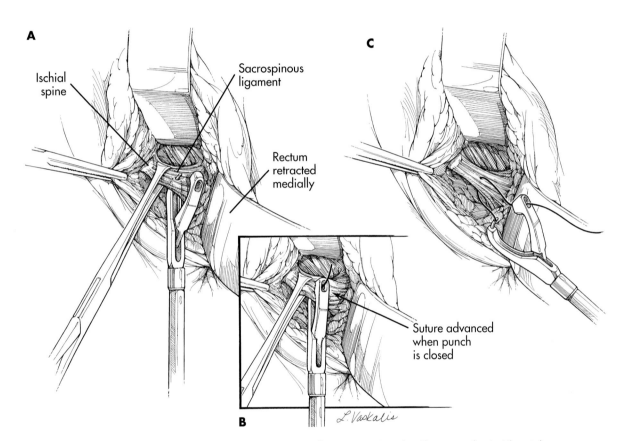

Fig. 26-20   Penetration of the sacrospinous ligament using the Shutt punch. **A,** The right pararectal space has been entered and the ischial spine identified. The coccygeus muscle–sacrospinous ligament complex running posterior medially from the ischial spine to the sacrococcygeal area is exposed and grasped by a long-handled Allis or Babcock clamp. The tip of the Shutt punch is pushed under and through the ligament-muscle complex, the cardinal ligament being held out of harm's way by an anterior retractor and the rectum held medially by a second retractor. **B,** The jaws of the punch are closed, and the friction wheel rotated to propel the suture through the hollow needle in the fenestration in the upper jaw of the punch. **C,** The free end is grasped with a hemostat, the punch opened and removed, and the suture disengaged from the ligature carrier. Additional stitches may be placed as necessary. The long-handled Allis or Babcock clamp is removed. (From Nichols DH, Randall CL: *Vaginal surgery,* ed 4, Baltimore, 1996, Williams & Wilkins.)

emerging tip. The amount of actual ligament encompassed or grasped by the Shutt punch occasionally is less than optimal[24] owing to an unexpected thickness of the overlying coccygeus muscle and a limited maximal aperture of the jaws of the instrument. It may be better suited to those patients in whom the coccygeus muscle–sacrospinous ligament complex is not thickly developed, permitting appropriate penetration of the ligament itself despite the reduced size of the opening of the jaws of the punch. The Endo Stitch and Laurus needle driver are disposable instruments designed originally for other uses, and we have no experience with them for colpopexy.

The N-V ligature carrier[57] was designed expressly for sacrospinous colpopexy, either unilateral or bilateral (Figs. 26-21 to 26-25). The bite aperture of the opened jaws is 2 cm, wider than that of the Shutt punch, and the eye of the blunt needle can accommodate two sutures simultaneously. Suture placement is facilitated by the separate hinge of both upper and lower jaws responsive to squeezing the handle of the device after the sacrospinous ligament–coccygeus

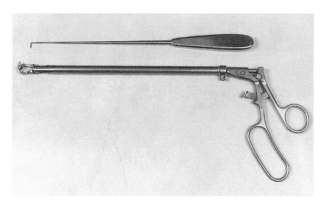

Fig. 26-21 The Nichols-Veronikis ligature carrier is shown with the jaws in the closed position along with the suture-catching hook used to retrieve the suture loops (available from BEI Medical Systems/Zinnanti Surgical Instruments, Chatsworth, CA 91311). (From Nichols DH, editor: *Reoperative gynecologic and obstetric surgery*, ed 2, St Louis, 1997, Mosby.)

muscle complex has been grasped by a long Allis or Babcock clamp, which bunches together the surgically useful tissues including the ligament. It is not necessary to move the handle of the ligature carrier during direct vision suture placement and retrieval of the suspensory sutures. Suture retrieval is facilitated by grasping the suture loops as shown in Fig. 26-23, *C*. Once secured, the N-V ligature carrier is removed. An alternative method for suture placement is shown in Fig. 26-24. We have used it for the majority of our sacrospinous ligament colpopexies since 1995 without complication. Alternatively, the ligament can be penetrated using a free curved Mayo needle (never a swedged-on needle, as the latter is made of relatively brittle extruded wire that is easily broken). The free needle grasped by a standard needle holder is passed *through* the coccygeus muscle–sacrospinous ligament complex from below upward in a path at a right angle to the direction of the fibers of the fibromuscular complex, keeping the needle safely away from the pudendal nerve and vessels. All penetrations are made at least one, and preferably two, fingerwidths medial to the ischial spine on each side of the pelvis.

Placing the Sutures. If using the right sacrospinous ligament, the operator places the middle finger of the left hand on the medial surface of the patient's right ischial spine and under direct vision pushes the tip of the long-handled Deschamps ligature carrier beneath the lower edge of the sacrospinous ligament–coccygeus muscle complex, and then by rotating the handle, pushes the tip of the long-handled Deschamps ligature carrier (see Fig. 26-18) into and through the coccygeal muscle–sacrospinous ligament at a point 1½ to 2 fingerbreadths medial to the ischial spine. The carrier tip must go *through* (not around or under) the ligament. Obvious resistance should be encountered as the tip of the ligature carrier passes through the ligamentous tissue, and the operator must overcome this resistance by persistent forcefulness in the process of rotating the handle of the ligature carrier. Once the ligament has been penetrated, gentle traction on the handle should actually move the patient on the table, confirming proper placement. If there is no resistance, the ligature carrier may be in front of the

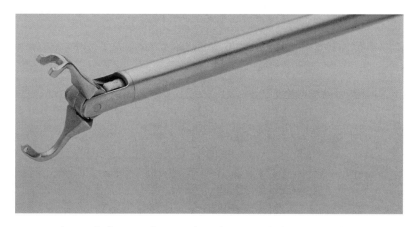

Fig. 26-22 The Nichols-Veronikis punch is shown with the jaws in the open position.

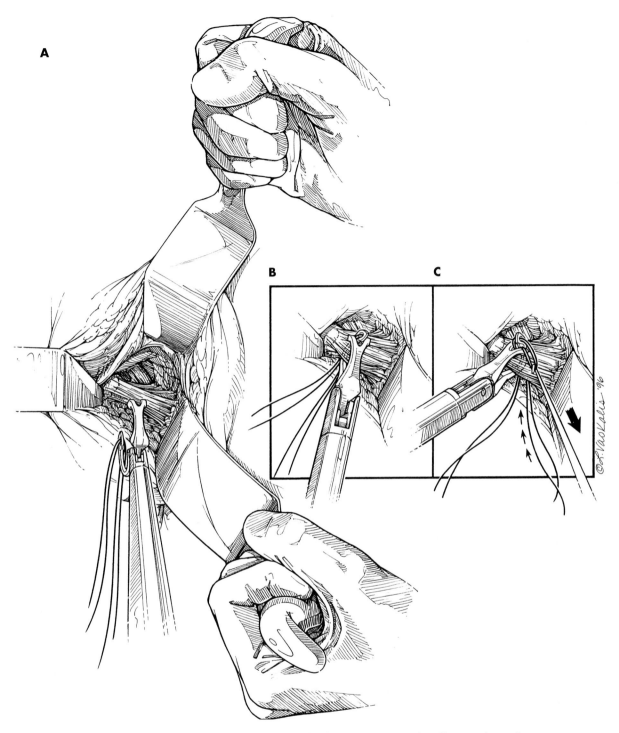

Fig. 26-23 Placement of the Nichols-Veronikis ligature carrier under effective, direct illumination as furnished by a fiber-optic headlight. An opening has been made into the right pararectal space by creation of a window through the right rectal pillar, exposing the surface of the right coccygeus muscle containing the sacrospinous ligament. **A,** Suitable retraction is obtained, and at a point well removed from the ischial spine the muscle-ligament complex may be grasped by a long-handled Allis or Babcock clamp. **B,** At a point at least $1\frac{1}{2}$ fingerbreadths medial to the spine the tip of the lower jaw of the opened ligature carrier is pushed gently beneath the lower margin of the complex, and the jaws of the carrier closed, advancing the needle tip holding *two* sutures through the ligament. The suture loops are grasped by a fine-pointed suture hook. **C,** Traction to the hook brings one end of the pair of sutures through the ligament. The ligature carrier is opened and removed. (From Nichols DH, editor: *Reoperative gynecologic and obstetric surgery,* St Louis, 1997, Mosby.)

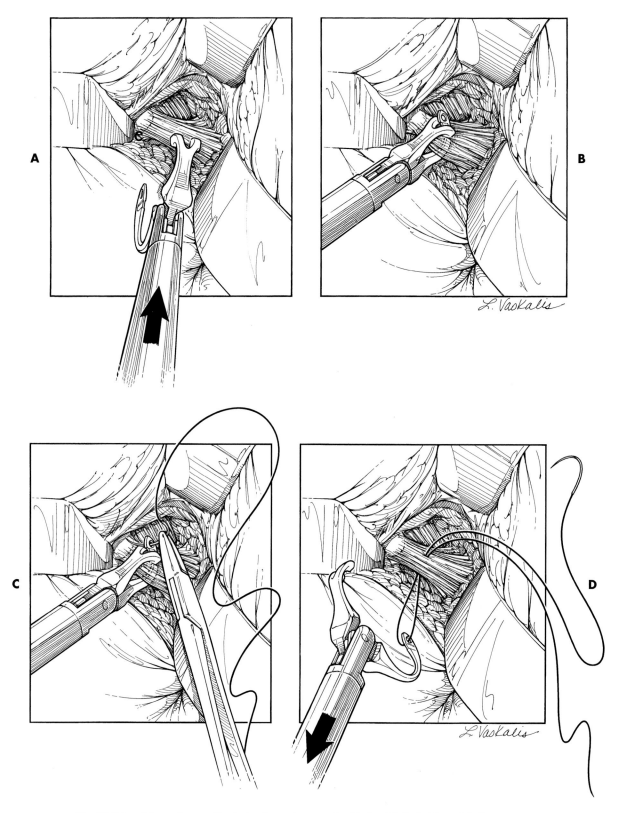

Fig. 26-24 Alternative method of suture placement with the Nichols-Veronikis ligature carrier. **A,** The "unloaded" ligature carrier with jaws opened is advanced toward the exposed right coccygeus muscle–sacrospinous ligament complex. **B,** The jaws are closed, advancing the needle tip as shown, exposing the eye. **C,** A swedged-on needle and suture are placed through the eye of the needle. **D,** The needle is pulled all the way through and retrieved, and the jaws of the ligature carrier opened, pulling the suture through the ligament.

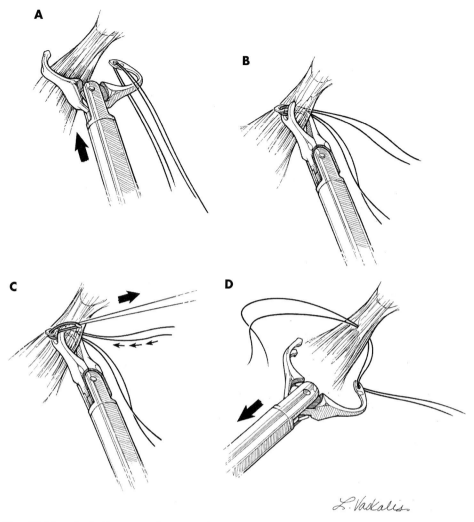

Fig. 26-25 A similar procedure can be employed using the patient's left sacrospinous ligament–coccygeus muscle complex. (From Nichols DH, editor: *Reoperative gynecologic and obstetric surgery*, ed 2, St Louis, 1997, Mosby.)

ligament or it may be around the ligament, exposing the structures behind the ligament to potential injury; in either case the operator should remove the ligature carrier and reinsert it through the substance of the ligament. (Rarely, the nearby sacrotuberous ligament will be found to be stronger and more convenient than the sacrospinous, in which case suture to the sacrotuberous ligament may be substituted.[3,61])

Simultaneous use of both nonabsorbable and absorbable synthetic suture for colpopexy is generally of value. The use of a long-lasting synthetic absorbable suture such as PDS or Maxon permits penetration of the full thickness of a thin vaginal wall at the site of the marking suture. One end of the suture is threaded on a free needle, and the full thickness of the vaginal wall is penetrated from below up, then reinserted in the opposite direction through the vaginal wall 1 to 1.5 cm away, creating a bolster of vaginal wall. When ultimately tied the knot will be located permanently *beneath* the posterior vaginal wall. The totally buried nonabsorbable suture, on the other hand, permits a long-lasting support of the subepithelial tissues once the preliminary scar formation from the absorbable suture has developed.

If the window made through the descending rectal septum is smaller than 3 cm in diameter as a result of excessive and unyielding scar tissue, and the operator is certain that the rectum has been displaced medially, and if it is difficult to expose the surface of the muscle, an alternative approach to the ligament may be taken. The operator inserts the tip of the left middle finger through the window and along the inner surface of the pelvic diaphragm until the tip of the ischial spine and the sacrospinous ligament are identified. Keeping the lateral surface of the tip of the middle finger adjacent to the tip of the spine, the operator directs the tip of the long-handled or the modified Deschamps ligature carrier along the undersurface of the left index finger until it reaches the coccygeus muscle–sacrospinous ligament complex (Fig. 26-26). At a point palpably 1½ to 2 finger-breadths medial to the spine and well away from the underlying pudendal nerve and vessels (to avoid trauma to these

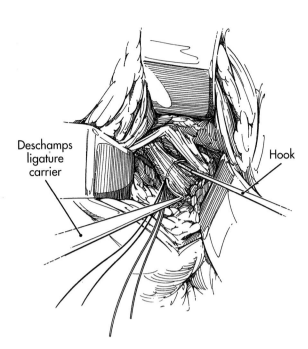

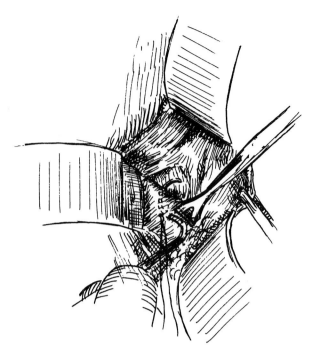

Fig. 26-26   The coccygeus muscle and sacrospinous ligament have been penetrated by the blunt end of a long Deschamps ligature carrier at a point 2 to 3 cm medial to the ischial spine, safely away from the pudendal nerve and vessels and the sciatic nerve. The ligature carrier was previously threaded with a full, uncut length of 54-inch no. 2 synthetic delayed absorbable suture, or a nonabsorbable synthetic suture, or both. Traction to the hook exteriorizes the suture, and the Deschamps ligature carrier is removed. (From Nichols DH. In Rock JA, Thompson JD, editors: *Te Linde's operative gynecology*, ed 8, Philadelphia, 1997, JB Lippincott.)

Fig. 26-27   The opening through the right rectal pillar has been enlarged and the sacrospinous ligament–coccygeal muscle complex has been grasped with a long Babcock clamp. At a point about 1½ fingerbreadths medial to the right ischial spine, the sacrospinous ligament and coccygeal muscle have been penetrated by the suture-bearing tip of a long Deschamps ligature carrier. (From Nichols DH, editor: *Reoperative gynecologic and obstetric surgery*, ed 2, St Louis, 1997, Mosby.)

structures), the operator pushes the tip of the ligature carrier beneath the lower edge of the coccygeus muscle, rotates the tip of the ligature carrier vertically, and penetrates the full thickness of the sacrospinous ligament (Fig. 26-27). The fingers of the left hand are then withdrawn, the retractors are suitably repositioned, the tip of the ligature carrier is visualized, and the suture loop(s) grasped with a hook (Figs. 26-25 to 26-29), and the carrier removed; the operation proceeds in the usual fashion.

The blunt point of the Deschamps ligature carrier is less apt to lacerate nearby blood vessels than is the sharp point of the conventional needle. If desired, a second suture is similarly placed 1 cm medial to the first and is held. Alternatively, after pulling the loop through and removing the ligature carrier, the operator may retain both of the free ends of the suture, cut the loop in its center, pair each end of the cut loop with its respective free suture end, and thus obtain two sutures through the ligament with but one penetration by the Deschamps carrier (Fig. 26-30).

Once the operator is comfortable with surgery in the pararectal space and is able to find the coccygeus muscle–sacrospinous ligament easily, it is not essential to use the special ligature carriers that have been described, and in their place the operator can use a conventional half-curved

strong Mayo needle with a tapered point, through which the suture to be used has been threaded. A swedged needle, being brittle because it is made of extruded wire, may break, and a broken needle tip may not only be hard to find but also may be lost. When the free needle in the grasp of a conventional needle holder has been passed through the muscle-ligament complex at the desired spot, the now-exposed tip is grasped by a Heaney-type needle holder, the original needle holder is removed, and the needle with suture is comfortably extracted following its inherent curve.

The free end of the nonabsorbable sutures through the ligament are sewn to the underside of the vagina, but not yet tied. If unilateral colpopexy has been planned, the sutures are fixed to the midline of the undersurface of the posterior vaginal wall at the very vault of the vagina. Ideally, the operator sews the vagina to the muscle-ligament as a firm tissue-to-tissue approximation. One method of bringing the soft movable vagina to the surface of the coccygeal muscle and ligament is by creating a "pulley" stitch (Fig. 26-31, p. 489) to be tied later, pulling the vagina directly onto the muscle and ligament. After placing the stitch in the ligament, the operator rethreads one end of the suture on a free needle and ties it by a single half-hitch to the full thickness of the fibromuscular layer of the undersurface of the vaginal apex, keeping the free end of the suture long (Fig. 26-32, p. 490). This pulley need be created with only one of the suture pairs. The second, or "safety," stitch can be inserted

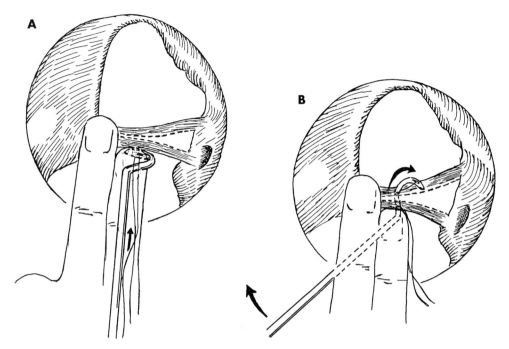

Fig. 26-28 The middle and index fingers of the operator's left hand have been inserted through a "window" in the rectal pillar into the right pararectal space. The lateral side of the tip of the middle finger touches the medial surface of the ischial spine. **A,** The Deschamps ligature carrier is positioned as shown and advanced down the index finger until its tip touches the right coccygeal muscle–sacrospinous ligament complex at a point 1½ fingerbreadths medial to the ischial spine, safely away from the pudendal nerves and vessels. As it penetrates the muscle-ligament complex (the ligament within the muscle is shown by the broken line) by rotation of the handle, the latter is simultaneously swung to the operator's left, *beneath* his or her palm, so that the tip of the ligature carrier penetrates the ligament from below upward at right angles to the axis of the ligament, as shown in **B.** (From Nichols DH, Randall CL: *Vaginal surgery,* ed 4, Baltimore, 1996, Williams & Wilkins.)

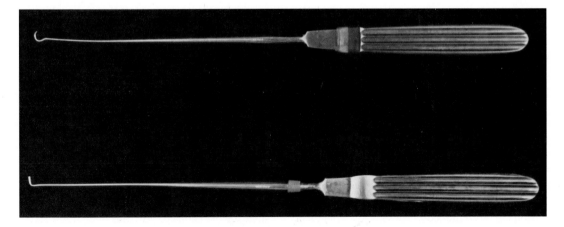

Fig. 26-29 Thread-catching hooks.

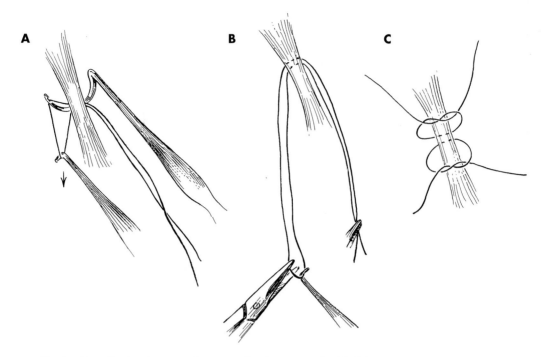

Fig. 26-30   Cutting the suture loop. **A,** After the suture, doubled, has been passed through the ligament and caught by the hook, the ligature carrier is removed. **B,** The loop may be cut in the center and each end paired with its respective free suture. **C,** This results in two sutures through the ligament but with only one penetration by the Deschamps ligature carrier. (From Nichols DH, Randall CL: *Vaginal surgery,* ed 4, Baltimore, 1996, Williams & Wilkins.)

through the muscular wall of the vagina, but not tied until later. If a bilateral colpopexy is to be performed, the colpopexy sutures are fixed to the lateral sides of the vaginal vault at the sites identified by the preliminary marking sutures, and a mirror image of the same procedure is performed separately on the opposite side of the pelvis. Digital rectal examination confirms rectal integrity.

Performing the Colporrhaphy. Because retropubic pin-up operations or needle suspensions pull the vagina in anteriorly and sacrospinous colpopexy pulls the vagina in an almost opposite posterior direction, a lifetime tug-of-war exists between these forceful pulls, predisposing toward failure of one or the other. For this reason, we recommend full-length anterior colporrhaphy instead of needle suspension to accompany sacrospinous colpopexy. In the Sze et al.[53] series, in which colpopexy was performed by using the Miya hook, the prolapse recurrence rate was 33%, an unacceptably high incidence suggesting that sacrospinous colpopexy and needle suspension not be combined in the same patient at the same time. The surgeon should replace the prolapsed vaginal vault to its normal position within the pelvis and carefully examine the anterior vaginal wall to determine the size and extent of a cystocele. If an anterior colporrhaphy has not yet been performed, a full-length repair of the anterior vaginal wall usually is done at this point. Allis clamps can be applied to the vaginal wall at the central portion of the cystocele and approximated in the midline to indicate the maximal extent of vaginal wall that should be resected during the anterior colporrhaphy. These Allis clamps can be replaced with mark-

ing sutures to indicate the lateral margins of the planned excision.[27] If the anterior vaginal wall is excessively and pathologically long, it should be *shortened as well as narrowed.* If a suburethral sling procedure is to be performed (usually because of a low urethral closure pressure), the vaginal portion of placement is now accomplished, and the tails of the sling brought to the abdomen by traction through the retropubic tunnels to be sewn transabdominally to the rectus aponeurosis as the final step of the operation. The operator should now begin the upper part of the posterior colporrhaphy.

The vagina normally is much wider at the vault. This is particularly evident when the vagina has turned inside-out, as from massive posthysterectomy prolapse. If unilateral colpopexy has been performed, a wide vaginal vault should be deliberately narrowed by the excision of excess vagina (Fig. 26-33). The width and length of the vagina determine the width of posterior vaginal wall to be removed. The vaginal length and width may have been modestly shortened after the excisions of previous operations. Excision of a narrower strip may permit an elastic but shortened vagina to be stretched to the region of the ischial spine.

There being no vaginal "fascia" per se,[32,60] anterior and posterior colporrhaphy involves plication of the subepithelial fibromuscular connective tissue and of the bladder and rectal capsule. Coincident demonstrable paravaginal defect should be repaired by reattaching the connective tissue of the vaginal sulci to the connective tissue of the arcus tendineus, or to the underlying obturator fascia, simultaneously with the colporrhaphy.

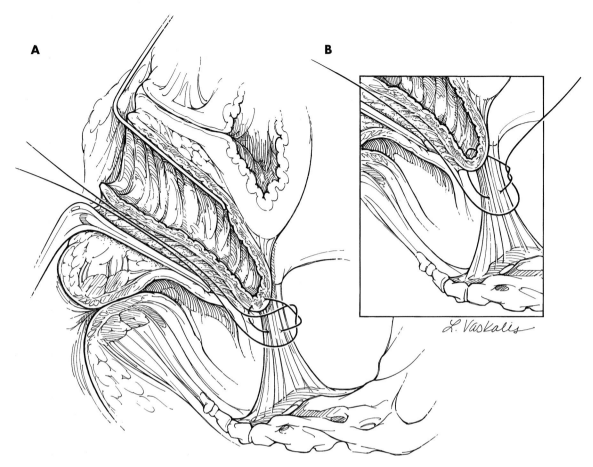

Fig. 26-31   **A,** The "pulley stitch." One end of the suture through the sacrospinous ligament has been sewn to the undersurface of the cut edge of the vaginal vault. Traction to the other end of the suture draws the vagina up and laterally to the surface of the ligament, and the ends are tied together, fixing the vagina to the ligament at this point. **B,** A second "safety" stitch similarly placed through the ligament is sewn to the subepithelial tissues of the vaginal wall and tied. (From Nichols DH, Randal CL: *Vaginal surgery,* ed 4, Baltimore, 1996, Williams & Wilkins.)

When the vagina is thin or greater vaginal length is desired, each end of the absorbable colpopexy stitch may be inserted *through* the vagina (Fig. 26-34). This should be done after an appropriate segment of posterior vaginal wall has been excised as part of the posterior colporrhaphy and after side-to-side approximation with a running subcuticular stitch of polyglycolic acid suture has united the sides of the upper half of the vagina. Tying the fixation stitches before this latter step reduces the visibility of the vaginal vault, making suture of the colporrhaphy more difficult.

Whether a colpopexy can be unilateral or bilateral depends partly on the width of the vaginal vault. If it is wide and the operator intends to keep it that way, the colpopexy should be bilateral; a unilateral colpopexy allows the unattached side of a wide and unnarrowed vault to descend gradually. If the vault is narrow or if the operator has narrowed it, the colpopexy should be unilateral. If a narrow vault is attached bilaterally, the undersurface of the vagina cannot reach the surface of each coccygeal muscle–sacrospinous ligament complex without suture bridges. If

the suture material used in these bridges is absorbable, the scar will be weak, and the prolapse more likely to recur; if the material is nonabsorbable polypropylene (Prolene, Surgilene) or polybutester (Novofil), however, the replaced vault generally will stay in place. The results of a unilateral colpopexy usually are good if a wide vault is resected to convert the shape of the vagina from one resembling a light bulb to that of a cylinder of uniform diameter—because the vagina is now an instrument of coitus, not parturition.

When an obstructive vaginal narrowing was not created after sacrospinous ligament colpopexy with colporrhaphy, sexually active patients have described improvement (or no change) in their sexual function. There should be no need to excessively narrow the vagina by the coincident colporrhaphy, creating an unnecessary barrier to marital comfort.[19,32,35]

Tying the Sacrospinous Fixation Stitches. When the upper 2 inches of posterior vaginal wall have been approximated, traction on the free end of the pulley stitch (opposite to the end that had been fixed to the undersurface of the va-

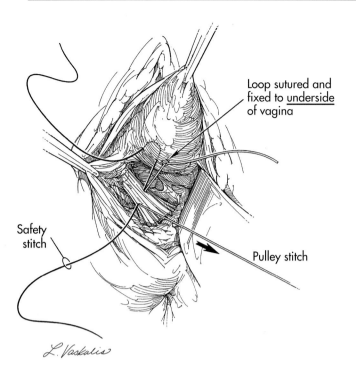

Fig. 26-32 A gentle tug to the ligature carrier or by the suture that has been grasped by the hook should actually move the patient a small degree on the table, indicating proper placement of the suture through the substance the sacrospinous ligament. The ligature carrier is removed. Direct palpation of the suture and of the ischial spine confirms the required distance between the two. If the suture seems too close to the ischial spine, traction is placed on it, and a new suture is added medial to the offending suture, which is then removed. If desired, an additional suture or two can be inserted through the muscle-ligament complex medial to the first suture. In the patient with chronic respiratory disease a suture or two of nonabsorbable synthetic no. 1 Prolene, Novofil, or Surgilene can be added or substituted for the absorbable sutures. The end of one suture is threaded on a free Mayo needle, which is then sewn to the undersurface of the vaginal wall through the full thickness of the fibromuscular layer and fixed in this position by a single half-hitch. The end of the second piece of suture is stitched through the full thickness of the vagina, grasped on the vaginal side, and made to penetrate the full thickness of the vaginal wall a second time 1 cm removed from the first penetration. This permits the knot to be tied ultimately beneath the posterior vaginal wall and gives a bolster or 1 cm of vaginal wall to the stitch for added security (the safety stitch). These sutures are held on hemostats until the upper posterior vaginal wall has been reapproximated for 3 to 5 cm. Then the sacrospinous fixation stitches are tied, fixing the vaginal vault to the surface of the sacrospinous ligament–coccygeus muscle complex, and the remainder of the posterior colporrhaphy and perineorrhaphy are completed. (From Nichols DH: Central compartment defects. In Rock JA, Thompson JD, editors: *Te Linde's operative gynecology,* ed 8, Philadelphia, 1997, JB Lippincott.)

gina) takes up all slack and pulls the vagina directly onto the surface of the coccygeus muscle–sacrospinous ligament complex. The pulley stitch and then the second or safety stitch are tied with surgeon's knots. It is essential to tie the pulley stitch *snugly* so that there is no void or bridge of

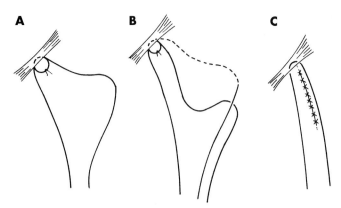

Fig. 26-33 **A,** A wide vaginal vault after sacrospinous colpopexy. **B,** The result of the failure to narrow this wide vault; there may be prolapse of the left side. **C,** The result of narrowing this wide vault by excision of a proper-width tissue from the anterior and posterior vaginal wall, converting the shape of the vagina to that of a cylinder of more or less uniform diameter. It is now an instrument of coitus and not parturition. (Redrawn from Nichols DH, Randall CL: *Vaginal surgery,* ed 4, Baltimore, 1996, Williams & Wilkins.)

absorbable suture between the vagina and the ligament (Fig. 26-35). Absorbable suture bridges hinder the formation of strong scar tissue; thus, once the suture is absorbed, the scar tissue may not be able to hold the vagina to the ligament and the prolapse may recur. Each of the other colpopexy stitches are then tied, fixing the vaginal vault in the hollow of the sacrum. Fig. 26-36 shows an effect on the urethrovesical junction of bringing an everted vault of the vagina back into the hollow of the sacrum.

It is best to use 0 or 1 long-lasting polydioxanone-type suture material (PDS or Maxon) as the nonabsorbable suture in this procedure, because too fine a suture in the sacrospinous ligament may act somewhat like a Gigli saw and with tying actually cut through the ligament. The heavier suture thickness has good knot-tying strength and, because it is of controlled, slow absorbency, will last for several weeks. In contrast, catgut retains its maximal strength and continuity for only 7 to 10 days.

Although the operator must ensure that the knot of any nonabsorbable suture is buried beneath the vagina, permanent sutures such as monofilament synthetic suture (e.g., 0 or 1 polypropylene [Prolene] or polybutester [Novofil]) can be especially recommended as the colpopexy stitches for patients with the following conditions:

1. Recurrent vaginal vault eversion
2. Chronic respiratory disease, which will periodically increase intraabdominal pressure
3. A vagina that is too short to reach the ischial spine (In this circumstance, the operator may create deliberate nonabsorbable suture bridges between the top of the vault of the short vagina and the surface of the coccygeus muscle–sacrospinous ligament.)
4. A predicted need for the patient to perform heavy lifting after convalescence

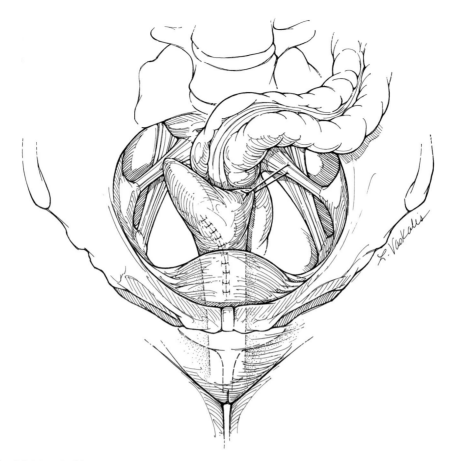

Fig. 26-34 Deliberate creation of a nonabsorbable suture bridge. When the vagina is too short or narrow to reach the ischial spine, a *nonabsorbable* suture bridge may be created on one or both sides, as shown.

The remainder of the posterior colporrhaphy and perineorrhaphy are then completed.

Completing the Procedure. The depth of the vagina after sacrospinous colpopexy depends on the distance from the vulva to the point at which the vagina is fixed to the sacrospinous ligament. In most instances, the distance from the vulva to the ligament and hence the length of the restored vagina is greater than 4 inches; rarely the distance may be only 3 or 3½ inches. When this distance is short, the fixation stitches should be placed closer to the sacrum and a greater effort made to lengthen the vagina by building up the thickness and depth of the perineal body at reconstruction; at times, a Williams vaginoplasty can be used to lengthen the distal end of a short vagina.

The vagina can be packed lightly with iodoform gauze for 24 hours. Postoperatively, the vault of the vagina lies in its normal horizontal axis, although it deviates to one side of the patient if a unilateral attachment was made. Similarly, because the rectal pillar is compressed between the vagina and the sacrospinous ligament to which the vagina was attached, immediate postoperative examination shows the rectum to be pulled to the side of the attachment. Within a few weeks, the pillar must elongate, because by then the rectum is again found to be approximately in the midline.

Postoperatively, many patients notice a transient mild discomfort or pulling sensation deep in the buttock on the side of the attachment, without transmission of discomfort to the thigh. This discomfort regresses within a few days or weeks as the edema subsides.

Postoperative examination usually shows excellent vaginal depth and axis, and increased intraabdominal pressure presses the vagina against the levator plate and accentuates the restored horizontal axis of the vagina. To date, no patient of the author has complained of dyspareunia after this type of vaginal fixation.

Transvaginal Sacrospinous Cervicopexy

Transvaginal sacrospinous cervicopexy or uterine fixation[40] can be employed in young patients with prolapse who wish to preserve their uterus. This can be unilateral, involving a deep stitch to the back of the cervix at the site of the cervical attachment of each uterosacral ligament, or it can be bilateral, creating deliberate suture bridges of a nonabsorbable suture between each uterosacral ligament and the sacrospinous ligament. Subsequent pregnancy usually is uneventful.[24]

Managing Operative Complications. If a sharp needle tip penetrates the lumen of any adjacent viscus (most likely rectum), the needle should be withdrawn and no rectal re-

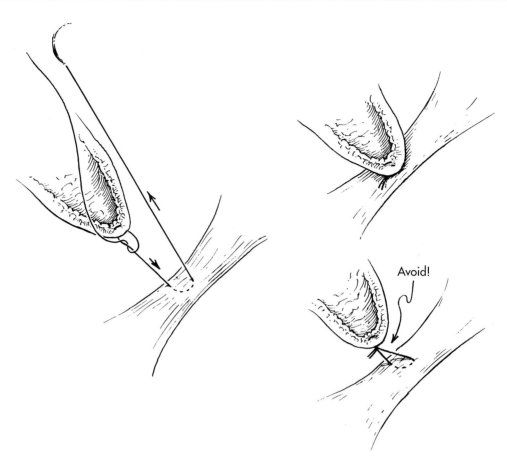

Fig. 26-35 A suture has been passed through the sacrospinous ligament, and a firm bite is taken into the tissues of the vaginal wall to which it is fixed at this point by a single half-hitch as shown on the left. Traction to the opposite free end of the suture will use the point of passage through the firm tissue as a pulley, bringing the movable tissue to this point, where the two tissues are now in direct contact with one another and a conventional knot is tied, fixing the new relationship, seen in the upper right. A suture-bridge, as shown on the lower right, should be avoided unless under certain circumstances a nonabsorbable suture has been used. (From Nichols DH, Randall CL: *Vaginal surgery,* ed 4, Baltimore, 1996, Williams & Wilkins.)

pair is necessary. On the other hand, any laceration should be repaired by a standard two-layered closure. If at any time during the procedure a rectal examination indicates that a suture has transgressed the wall of the rectum, the operator should promptly remove the suture and replace it in a proper position outside the rectal lumen.

Immediate, severe postoperative gluteal pain *running down the posterior surface of the affected leg* would indicate probable pudendal nerve trauma, a rare complication of sacrospinous colpopexy. Sutures placed in error *adjacent* to the ischial spine risk trauma to the pudendal nerve as it bends around the ischial spine, or to the posterior cutaneous nerve of the thigh, which is deep to the spine, or even to the sciatic nerve, which is deep and lateral to the spine. Such a complication would be manifest by immediate postoperative pain running down the posterior surface of the thigh, often accompanied by perineal paresthesia or anesthesia. A treatment of choice is prompt reoperation with removal of the offending suture and repositioning of new colpopexy sutures to the sacrospinous ligament either significantly more

medial to the spine or to a medial position in the ligament of the opposite side.

When persistent severe buttock pain is identified after sacrospinous colpopexy, entrapment of the pudendal nerve on the affected side should be considered, particularly if the pain is transmitted to the posterior surface of the leg and the pain was not present preoperatively. Motor abnormality may be absent, but some perineal anesthesia following the distribution of the affected pudendal nerve might be noted. Transvaginal surgical exploration of the tissues around the ischial spine of the affected side with removal of the offending colpopexy stitch can be effective even as long as 2 years after the initial operation.[2] There may be sufficient residual postoperative scarring in this area between the vagina and the sacrospinous ligament to obviate the need for replacement of the colpopexy stitch, or a fresh sacrospinous colpopexy can be performed at this time on the opposite side of the pelvis.

Although rare, hematoma may occur, usually within the pararectal space, and its presence is suggested by a falling

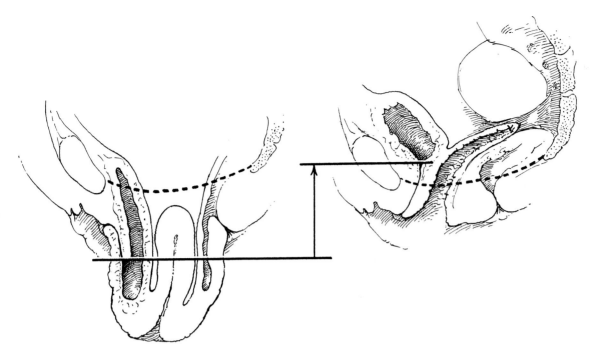

Fig. 26-36   The relationship of the vesicourethral junction to the pubis and pelvis is illustrated in sagittal section. The usual location of the pelvic diaphragm is indicated by the *dashed line.* The vesicourethral junction is indicated by the *solid line.* On the left, advanced genital prolapse is depicted, showing that eversion of the vagina may pull on tissues supporting the vesicourethral junction, exteriorizing the latter. The effects of restoration of vaginal depth and axis are shown on the right. Repositioning of the vagina has provided upward traction to tissues of the vesicourethral junction, helping restore them to a position within the pelvis. (From Nichols DH: *Clin Obstet Gynecol* 21:759, 1978.)

hematocrit. The findings by pelvic and rectal examination may not be confirmative as a result of local postoperative discomfort, but a significant collection of extraperitoneal blood is demonstrated by a pelvic CT scan. Its progress toward liquefaction or absorption can be followed by subsequent CT scans. Once stabilized, and after any necessary transfusion, most are surprisingly asymptomatic and will absorb over a period of several weeks. Infection within such a hematoma is manifested by pain and persistent fever. Drainage of the cystic cavity should be considered, as accomplished by percutaneous placement of a suction drain under real-time ultrasound guidance, using local anesthesia.

A case of postoperative evisceration has been reported in a patient who was straining at stool 3 months after sacrospinous colpopexy and repair,[15] emphasizing the importance of permanently avoiding postoperative constipation. The authors speculated that it may have occurred at the site of a recurrent enterocele to which insufficient attention had been given previously.

Late Complications. In spite of the usual full-length anterior colporrhaphy (with special attention to the support of the vesicourethral junction), mild, generally transient urinary stress incontinence develops in some patients, probably the result of a temporary straightening of the posterior urethrovesical angle. It tends to disappear after several months as a new posterior angle becomes established. Kegel isometric perineal resistive exercises are helpful. Rarely, subsequent suprapubic urethrovesical suspension or periurethral collagen injection may be recommended.

Recurrent but asymptomatic cystocele without stress incontinence has been the most frequent complication of colpopexy.[29,32,46] This type of cystocele generally becomes evident within the first 3 months after surgery but usually does not require treatment. In some cases, cystocele probably results from progression following under-repair at the time of surgery or from *failure to recognize and surgically shorten an anterior vaginal wall that had become pathologically elongated.* In other cases, it may develop from natural progression of the disease; in still other cases, from unrecognized and unrepaired lateral (paravaginal) attenuation or avulsion. The presence and degree of the latter, when recognized preoperatively or intraoperatively, should be repaired as part of the reconstructive surgery.

Rarely, congenitally poor collagen or "protoplasm" may be incriminated. This appears to be an inherited event, suspected by the presence of wide abdominal striae and coincident and often re-recurrent hernias elsewhere in the body. Vaginal recurrences may be recognized as soon as 2 months after surgery in a repair that had seemed "perfect" at the conclusion of the operative procedure. This patient may require interposition of a subepithelial, well-insulated layer of plastic polyester mesh (Mersilene, Johnson & Johnson) cut to size and tacked in place. This also may apply to a patient with severe chronic respiratory disease, such as asthma or bronchitis, whose vaginal wall may benefit from an extra layer of support.

Paraiso et al.[35] have reported a significant recurrence of prolapse of the anterior vaginal segment after 4 or 5 postoperative years, whether or not there had been previous vaginal reconstruction or whether or not there was anterior colporrhaphy at the time of sacrospinous ligament suspension.[18,46]

Because the sacrospinous ligament is thicker and presumably stronger than the iliococcygeal fascia, we rarely use the latter to support the vaginal cuff, nor have we much experience with nor enthusiasm for using the most posterior portion of the arcus tendineus for this purpose. It is our belief that bilateral sacrospinous colpopexy will better accomplish the same goal with more security, because of the extra strength of the sacrospinous ligament compared with the iliococcygeus fascia, lessening the chance of recurrent prolapse and restoring a modestly longer vaginal canal.

TRANSABDOMINAL SURGICAL TREATMENT

Some abdominal approaches have been used to treat massive eversion of the vagina. An abdominal route should certainly be considered if the patient has a history of extensive previous pelvic surgery or if it is necessary to investigate for an adnexal tumor. A transabdominal approach should be strongly considered if massive vaginal eversion is secondary to a previous ventral fixation of the vagina or uterus, because it is difficult to return this type of vaginal axis to normal by a transvaginal operation without freeing the vagina or uterus from its attachment to the anterior abdominal wall. Similarly, after a vesicourethral Marshall-Marchetti-Kranz[26] or Burch[8] pin-up operation, a lifetime tug-of-war will persist between the anterior fixation of the vagina and the posterior pull.

Ventral Fixation

Although ventral fixation of the uterine fundus to the anterior abdominal wall was once popular, it does not relieve the cause of the prolapse. The patient may be reasonably comfortable for awhile, but over time the continued progression of the prolapse becomes evident. Although the uterine fundus may remain fixed to the abdominal wall, the uterus and cervix often elongate until, ultimately, the vagina and those organs to which it is attached again descend. The patient, meanwhile, has often forgotten the nature of her original surgery, which may have taken place many years before; her operative records may be unobtainable or may have been lost; and the previous surgeon may no longer be available. An operator may begin what was expected to be a routine vaginal hysterectomy and repair only to find upon opening the peritoneum that the uterine fundus extends all the way to the anterior abdominal wall (Fig. 26-37). At that point a tug on the cervix produces a confirmatory visible dimpling in the anterior abdominal wall.

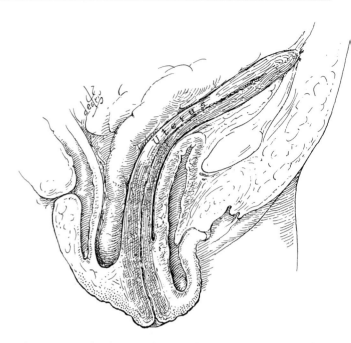

Fig. 26-37 The failure of ventral fixation of the uterus to retard progression of genital prolapse. An enterocele has developed. (From Nichols DH, Randall CL: *Vaginal surgery,* ed 4, Baltimore, 1996, Williams & Wilkins.)

A drawback of ventral fixation of either the uterine fundus or the vaginal vault or midvagina (i.e., after hysterectomy or after a vesicourethral pin-up operation) is that it leaves the cul-de-sac of Douglas exposed. Because the procedure alters the axis of the vagina, the cul-de-sac becomes more directly vulnerable to increases in intraabdominal pressure (Fig. 26-38). This vulnerability of the cul-de-sac may explain the 11% to 15% incidence of enterocele that has been noted after fixation of the vagina to Cooper's ligament in the treatment of stress incontinence, as described by Burch.[8] The cul-de-sac should be clearly obliterated as a separate step in any abdominal surgery that changes the normal horizontal axis of the upper vagina.

Sacropexy

The transabdominal method of retroperitoneal sacropexy is a satisfactory but complex procedure. It is particularly attractive when the vagina is too short to be brought to the ischial spine or when it is necessary to open the abdomen for an unrelated reason (e.g., the removal of an ovarian tumor). The surgeon must remember that a transabdominal sacropexy corrects eversion of the vaginal vault but does not correct eversion of the lower vagina.

Arthur and Savage[4] and Falk[14] attached the fundus of the uterus to the periosteum of the sacrum. It is even more effective to remove the uterus and attach the vagina to the sacrum by a retroperitoneal bridge of polyester (Mersilene) mesh or fascia lata,[32,36] because this reestablishes a somewhat horizontal vaginal axis and the retroperitoneal bridge will not lengthen with time. However, coexistent intestinal diverticulosis is a relative contraindication to the use of synthetic mesh because of the risk of future perforation of a di-

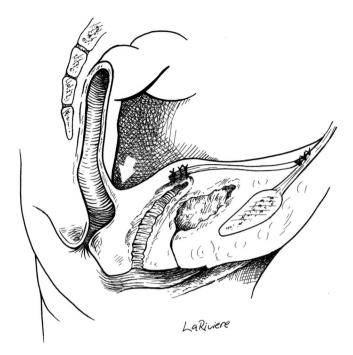

LaRiviere

Fig. 26-38   The unprotected cul-de-sac after ventral fixation of the vagina is noted by the arrow. (Redrawn from Nichols DH: Repair of enterocele and prolapse of the vaginal vault. In Barber H, editor: *Goldsmith's practice of surgery,* Philadelphia, 1981, JB Lippincott.)

verticulum at the site of the mesh. If the mesh bridge becomes infected, it should be removed. The simultaneous correction of cystocele or rectocele is associated with a special risk, since it increases the risk of infection at the site of the nonabsorbable sutures and polyester (Mersilene) mesh, and it is not recommended. It is the author's opinion that any coincident cystocele or rectocele should be repaired at another time.

Massive eversion of the vagina is to be expected after even a single pregnancy in a patient with a history of exstrophy of the bladder, even if the patient's delivery had been by cesarean section. The obvious anatomic weakness of the anterior vaginal wall prevents its use as a basis for surgical support, because so many of these patients have previously undergone a cystectomy. One possibility, should an enormous "cystocele" (i.e., a massive relaxation of the anterior wall of the vagina with bulging accompanied by a subjective feeling of falling out and fullness) appear without uterine descent, is a modification of the Watkins-Wertheim transposition in which the operator sews the fundus of the uterus to the periosteum of the pubic rami.[32] To this may be added the Ocejo modification described by Gallo,* in which the operator amputates the cervix, opens the uterus, and excises the entire endometrial cavity before the transposition. (The limits of the endometrial cavity may be defined by the intrauterine installation of an ampule of indigo carmine, which stains a deep violet color to all the functional tissue

*Personal communication, 1982.

that is to be removed.) The uterine wall is then reunited, and the transposition is finished.

When a procidentia accompanies a prolapse in a patient with a history of bladder exstrophy, the cardinal or uterosacral ligament generally is not strong enough to support the vaginal vault. In this case, one may use an operation mentioned by Howard Jones.[22] The operator obliterates the cul-de-sac of Douglas by a transabdominal approach and attaches the vagina by an intermediate polyester (Mersilene) strip to the periosteum of the pubis. Alternatively, Jones has suggested ventral fixation using the cervical stump remaining in such a patient after deliberate subtotal hysterectomy. Because there is no bladder, there is minimal displacement of the ureterosigmoidostomy that may have been accomplished at the time of the preceding cystectomy, usually in the patient's youth.

For preservation of the uterus and potential fertility in a patient with bladder exstrophy and a symptomatic and severe genital prolapse, a subperitoneal plastic belt may be placed within a tunnel created to encircle the cervix and brought in a retroperitoneal fashion to the rectus aponeurosis.[7] The cul-de-sac should be deliberately obliterated.

Transabdominal Sacropexy. Because of the possibility of contamination of the operative field by microorganisms from the vagina, a patient who is to undergo transabdominal sacropexy should be given a single preoperative dose of an appropriate prophylactic antibiotic. A Foley catheter is inserted into the bladder. The operator opens the lower abdomen through a lower midline incision and explores the abdomen.[14,32,36] Fingers or an obturator elevating the vagina make it easy to identify the vaginal vault (Fig. 26-39, *A* to *C*). The operator makes a transverse incision in the peritoneum covering the uppermost portion of the vagina, reflecting the peritoneum both anteriorly and posteriorly for 2 to 3 cm. This line of cleavage denudes the musculoconnective tissue wall of the vagina. After identifying the bladder, with its attachment to the anterior peritoneal reflection, the operator notes any enterocele. A longitudinal incision is made through the peritoneum over the sacral promontory, and the incision is extended caudally for 5 to 6 cm below the promontory (see Fig. 26-39, *D* to *F*). The peritoneal flaps on either side may be caught in retraction sutures left long enough to permit an adequate exposure of the bifurcation of the aorta and the common iliac veins. The midsacral artery and vein may require ligation or cautery if damaged and bleeding to permit development of a 6 to 8 cm area of clean periosteum over the promontory of the sacrum between the common iliac veins. The exposed area of the anterior longitudinal ligament and periosteum must be freed of all connective tissue, and hemostasis must ensure a dry field where a segment of fascia lata or plastic gauze is to be sutured to the ligament and periosteum. Small blood vessels may be electrocoagulated to ensure a dry operative field.

A 2-0 guide suture is placed on each side of the vaginal apex. Three pairs of 2-0 coated *nonabsorbable* braided synthetic Ethibond (Johnson & Johnson) sutures are placed transversely 1 cm apart in the central portion of the vaginal

Text continued on p. 500

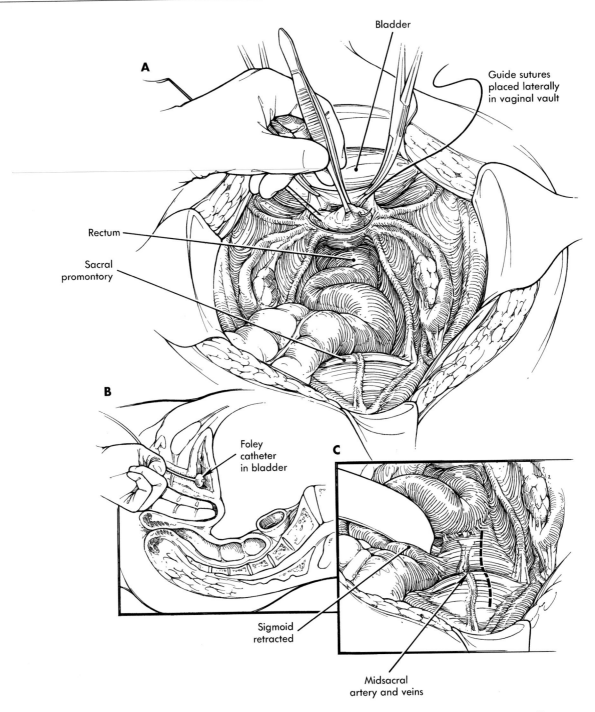

Bladder

Guide sutures placed laterally in vaginal vault

A

Rectum

Sacral promontory

B

Foley catheter in bladder

C

Sigmoid retracted

Midsacral artery and veins

Fig. 26-39 Transabdominal sacrocolpopexy. The abdomen has been opened by a midline incision. The vaginal vault is manually elevated, shown, and the peritoneum covering it is incised transversely **(A).** Bowel is packed out of the way, and the promontory of the sacrum is exposed. **C,** The peritoneum overlying the promontory is incised *(broken line).*

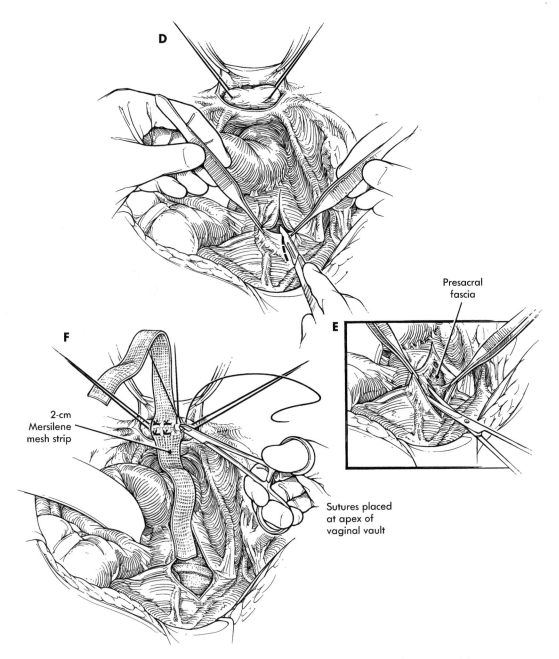

Fig. 26-39, cont'd **D,** The tissues are carefully separated, exposing the presacral fascia **(E).** **F,** The central belly of a precut band of polyester (Mersilene) or fascia lata is sewn to the vaginal vault.

Continued

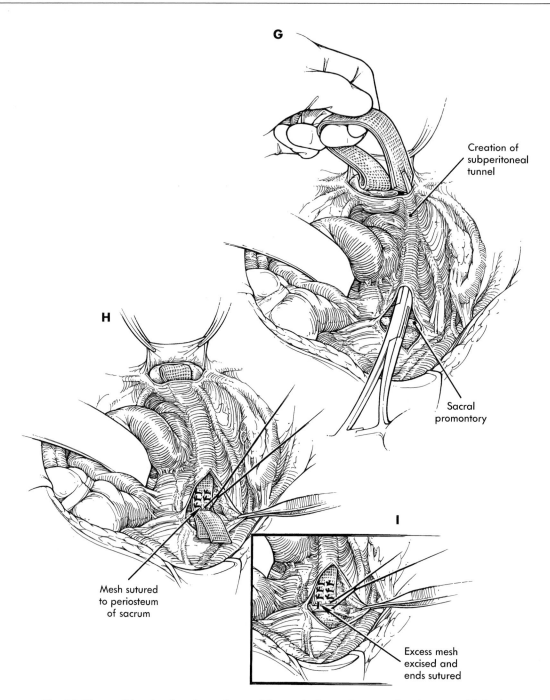

G

Creation of
subperitoneal
tunnel

Sacral
promontory

H

Mesh sutured
to periosteum
of sacrum

I

Excess mesh
excised and
ends sutured

Fig. 26-39, cont'd A subperitoneal tunnel beneath the peritoneum has been established, and a long Kelly forceps is introduced to grasp the free ends of the polyester or fascia **(G),** which is drawn through the tunnel and sewn to the presacral fascia and periosteum **(H). I,** The excess mesh is excised.

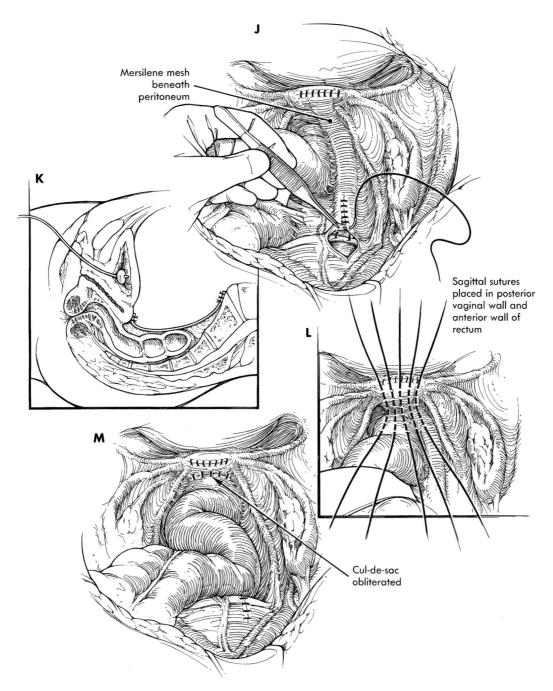

Mersilene mesh
beneath
peritoneum

Sagittal sutures
placed in posterior
vaginal wall and
anterior wall of
rectum

Cul-de-sac
obliterated

Fig. 26-39, cont'd   J, The peritoneum is closed. **K,** Sagittal view shows the end result of the sacral colpopexy. The surfaces of the cul-de-sac of Douglas are approximated by sagitally placed sutures **(L)** and have thus been obliterated **(M),** and the abdomen is closed.

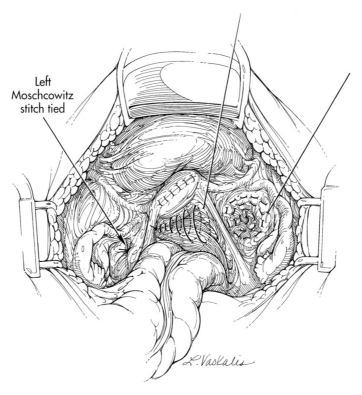

Fig. 26-40   Bilateral Moschcowitz obliteration of cul-de-sac. The closed vaginal vault is noted in the center of the illustration. A circumferential spiral obliteration has been performed on the left, and the suture tied. A similar closure has been placed on the right and awaits tying. A separate suture is closing the central portion of the cul-de-sac between the uterosacral ligaments. Alternatively, if the uterosacral ligaments were surgically weak, this central spot would be the site for a sacral colpopexy.

vault—through the full subepithelial fibromuscular thickness of the vaginal wall but not into the vaginal lumen. The midpoint of a 2 to 8 inch piece of polyester (Mersilene) mesh folded longitudinally (alternatively, a large strip of fascia) is brought to the vaginal apex; the braided plastic sutures are threaded through it and tied securely.

Using a long, curved intestinal clamp or kidney stone forceps for dissection, the operator can establish a tunnel that extends from the inferior edge of the incision over the sacral promontory, beneath the peritoneum across the posterolateral aspect of the right side of the cul-de-sac, to the cut edge of the peritoneum overlying the vaginal apex (see Fig. 26-39, *G* and *I*). (Alternatively, the operator may incise the peritoneum of the cul-de-sac longitudinally and reflect it.) With the curved clamp running through the subperitoneal tunnel, the operator grasps the free end of the mesh (or fascia) now attached to the apex of the vagina and by withdrawing the clamp draws it to the promontory of the sacrum.

Using a strong, but small, half-circle needle with a trochar point, the operator places three pairs of the same 2-0 braided nonabsorbable sutures in the presacral ligament and periosteum and fixes them to the plastic or fascial bridge. A little slack is left in the strip, and the sutures are tied. Excess ends of the bridge are excised, the peritoneum is closed with fine absorbable suture, and the cul-de-sac obliterated (Figs. 26-39, *J* to *M,* and 26-40). Unless an anterior col-

porrhaphy has been planned, a suprapubic pin-up of the urethrovesical junction may be appropriate to reduce the risk of postoperative urinary stress incontinence, and the vagina is distended overnight with a splinting iodoform or plain gauze pack. The patient is permitted out of bed on the first postoperative day, and the urinary catheter is removed at the same time as the vaginal packing.

Complications of Sacral Colpopexy. Addison et al.[1] have observed an occasional patient after abdominal sacral colpopexy with re-recurrent vaginal vault eversion and believe that the complication can be avoided by attaching permanent material to a wide area of the vagina with multiple sutures and a performing a meticulous culdoplasty using permanent sutures brought through the suspensory mesh.

Hemorrhage from laceration of a vessel entering one of the sacral foramina can be brisk and massive. Suture or coagulation of the torn vessel rarely controls the bleeding, nor does the local application of packing or hemostatic agents, because the edge of the injured vein will have retracted into the ostium. Success in quickly controlling such hemorrhage has been reported from placement of a sterile stainless steel thumbtack into the sacrum.* Pressure with the tip of a long Kelly hemostat is applied to the center of the head of the tack. A lag screw can be used similarly if a larger opening

---

*References 23, 37, 39, 50, 51, 56.

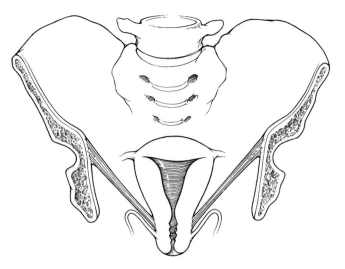

Fig. 26-41 Prolapse of the uterus, with marked elongation of the paracolpium.

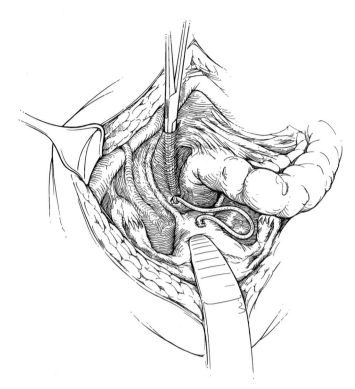

Fig. 26-42 Construction of a sacrocervical ligament. Any marked elongation of the cervix has been amputated transvaginally, and the abdomen opened. A strip of fascia lata has been sewn to the posterior cervix and lower uterine segment, and a tunnel has been established beneath the presacral peritoneum.

is encountered (it must, of course, be screwed into place). For a consultant in pelvic surgery or one who performs a good number of transabdominal sacral colpopexy operations or in a clinic where a number of these operations are performed, it may be prudent to have on hand a small sterile supply of such tacks or screws. The occasion to use them will be infrequent, but lifesaving. Sacral osteomyelitis has been reported[62] as a rare complication of sacral colpopexy.

Construction of a Sacrocervical Ligament. A patient with symptomatic genital prolapse who wishes to retain her fertility (Fig. 26-41) has several options from which to choose. A ring pessary combined with a program of vigorous perineal resistive exercises may be used to support the internal genitalia until childbearing is completed, after which the patient may elect a permanent reconstruction such as vaginal hysterectomy with repair. Strong functional pubococcygei are necessary to aid in pessary retention. If there is cervical elongation and preservation of the uterine corpus is desired, a Manchester-type procedure may be performed, with the knowledge that menses will continue as usual. However, subsequent pregnancy may be complicated by cervical stenosis, and should there be cervical incompetence, the risk of premature labor and delivery must be considered.[40] Suspension of the prolapsed uterus by transvaginal sacrospinous cervicopexy can be performed, but coincident colporrhaphy is not recommended because this may create a soft tissue obstruction that may impede future vaginal delivery. Subsequent pregnancy, labor, and delivery appear unaffected.

Another option to correct the uterine prolapse while conserving the uterus for reproduction is transabdominal construction of a sacrocervical ligament.[30,49] This relieves the symptoms of uterine prolapse and permits subsequent labor and vaginal delivery. This operation relieves the symptoms of uterine prolapse while making pregnancy, labor, and delivery possible, but does not preclude eventual progression of the other manifestations of prolapse, which might require a future reoperation. The operation is shown in Figs. 26-42 and 26-43.

Strips of fascia lata may be used as suture, particularly when fixing fascia lata to the posterior cervix.[16] The Gallie large-eyed needle is useful, and the fixation of the fascia-suture is ensured by the use of a slip-knot arrangement in which the easily frayed ends of the suture are tied with permanent ligatures (Fig. 26-44). The suture, having been passed through the point of anchorage, is now passed through its own body, as shown, and the slack is taken up.

CONCLUSION

Vaginal hysterectomy and repair, although usually successful, cannot serve all patients with massive eversion of the vagina equally well. The various causes, tissue strengths, and damages must be identified and correlated with a choice of different corrective surgical procedures. For those patients with vaginal vault prolapse but without surgically useful uterosacral–cardinal ligament support, the surgeon must add supplemental techniques for support of the vault. The ultimate goals are to relieve symptoms, restore the natural depth and position of the vagina, and effectively treat any coexistent pelvic disease, including cystocele, enterocele, and rectocele. This can be accomplished by using techniques that restore or preserve coital function.

It is usually unnecessary and often a distinct disservice to an active patient with prolapse to leave her with a short

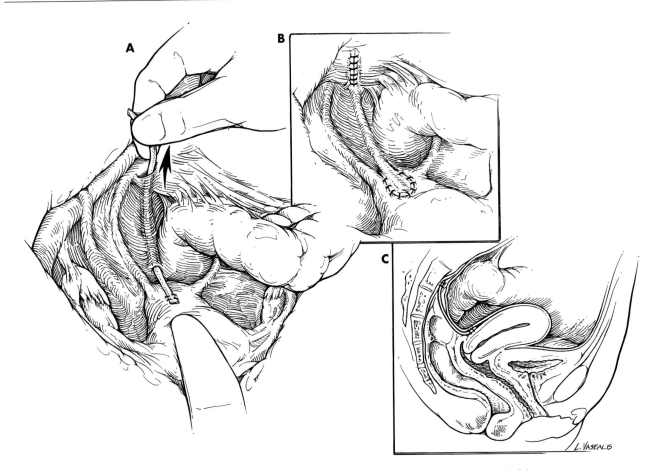

Fig. 26-43   A long forceps is introduced through this tunnel to grasp the free end of the strip. This is drawn through the tunnel **(A)** and sewn to the presacral fascia and periosteum **(B). C,** The final result. The uterus is once again within the pelvis, and there is a horizontal axis to the vagina.

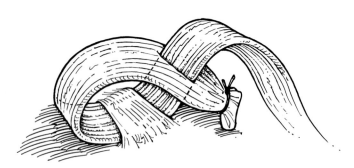

Fig. 26-44   When these strips of fascia lata are to be fixed to another surface, a slip-knot type of arrangement is useful. This can be placed as shown, often using a Gallie needle, which has a very wide eye through which the strip of fascia can be threaded.

vagina or to perform a partial or total colpectomy. When colpectomy is performed, however, the results are better if any coexistent enterocele has been identified and the sac has been excised. Accurate clinical perception and thoughtful and careful employment of an adequate remedial surgical procedure cannot help but improve the long-term result of the surgery employed.

REFERENCES

1. Addison WA, Timmons MC, Wall LL, Livengood CH III: Failed abdominal sacral colpopexy: observations and recommendations, *Obstet Gynecol* 74:480, 1989.
2. Alevizon SJ, Finan MA: Sacrospinous colpopexy: management of postoperative pudendal nerve entrapment, *Obstet Gynecol* 88:713, 1996.
3. Amreich J: Aëtiologie ünd Operation des Scheidenstumpf prolapses, *Wien Klin Wochenschr* 63:74, 1951.
4. Arthur HGE, Savage D: Uterine prolapse and prolapse of the vaginal vault treated by sacral hysteropexy, *J Obstet Gynecol Br Emp* 64:355, 1957.
5. Baden WF, Walker T: *Surgical repair of vaginal defects*, Philadelphia, 1992, JB Lippincott.
6. Barnhill D, Hoskins W, Heller P, et al: Repair of vaginal prolapse and perineal hernia after pelvic exenteration, *Obstet Gynecol* 65:764, 1985.
7. Bergamini V, Bouche M, Pecorari D: Isterocervicosuspensione laparoscopica: technica operatoria e risultati preliminari, *Giorn It Ost Gin* 17:114, 1995.
8. Burch JC: Urethrovaginal fixation to Cooper's ligament for stress incontinence, *Am J Obstet Gynecol* 81:2, 1961.
9. Cox OC: Hystero-colpectomy, *Sibley Mem Hosp Alumni Assoc Bull* 1:9, 1958.
10. Cruikshank SH: Sacrospinous fixation—should this be performed at the time of vaginal hysterectomy? *Am J Obstet Gynecol* 164:1072, 1991.

11. DeLancey JOL: Anatomic aspects of vaginal eversion after hysterectomy, *Am J Obstet Gynecol* 166:1717, 1992.
12. DeLancey JOL, Morley GW: Total colpocleisis for vaginal eversion, *Am J Obstet Gynecol* 176:1228, 1997.
13. Elkins TE, et al: Initial report of anatomic and clinical comparison of the sacrospinous ligament fixation to the high McCall culdeplasty for vaginal cuff fixation at hysterectomy for uterine prolapse, *J Pelv Surg* 1:12, 1995.
14. Falk HC: Uterine prolapse and prolapse of the vaginal vault treated by sacropexy, *Obstet Gynecol* 18:113, 1961.
15. Farrell SA, Scotti RJ, Ostergard DR, Bent AE: Massive evisceration: a complication following sacrospinous vaginal vault fixation, *Obstet Gynecol* 78:560, 1991.
16. Gallie WE, LeMesurier AB: A clinical and experimental study of the free transplantation of fascia and tendon, *J Bone Joint Surg* 4:600, 1922.
17. Hirsch HA, Käser O, Iklé FA: *Atlas of gynecologic surgery,* ed 3, Stuttgart, 1997, Thieme.
18. Holley RL, Varner RE, Gleason BP, et al: Recurrent pelvic support defects after sacrospinous ligament fixation for vaginal vault prolapse, *J Am Coll Surg* 180:444, 1995.
19. Holley RL, Varner RE, Gleason BP, et al: Sexual function after sacrospinous ligament fixation for vaginal vault prolapse, *J Reprod Med* 41:355, 1996.
20. Inman WB: Pelvic relaxation and repair including prolapse of vagina following hysterectomy, *South Med* 56:577, 1963.
21. Inmon WB, Bledsoe JW: Surgical repair of genital prolapse after hemipelvectomy, *Am J Obstet Gynecol* 123:766, 1975.
22. Jones HW Jr: Personal communication, 1990.
23. Khan FA, Fang OT, Nivatvongs S: Management of presacral bleeding during rectal resection, *Surg Gynecol Obstet* 165:272, 1987.
24. Kovac SR, Cruikshank SH: Successful pregnancies and vaginal deliveries after sacrospinous uterosacral fixation in five of nineteen patients, *Am J Obstet Gynecol* 168:1778, 1993.
25. Lind LR, Choe J, Bhatia, NN: An in-line suturing device to simplify sacrospinous vaginal vault suspension, *Obstet Gynecol* 89:129, 1997.
26. Marshall VF, Marchetti AA, Krantz KE: The correction of stress incontinence by simple vesicourethral suspension, *Surg Gynecol Obstet* 88:509, 1949.
27. Miyazaki FS: Miya hook ligature carrier for sacrospinous ligament fixation, *Obstet Gynecol* 70:286, 1987.
28. Morley GW, DeLancey JOL: Sacrospinous ligament fixation for eversion of the vagina, *Am J Obstet Gynecol* 158:872, 1988.
29. Nichols DH: Sacrospinous fixation for massive eversion of the vagina, *Am J Obstet Gynecol* 142:901, 1982.
30. Nichols DH: Fertility retention in the patient with genital prolapse, *Am J Obstet Gynecol* 164:1155, 1991.
31. Nichols DH, Milley PS, Randall CL: Significance of restoration of normal vaginal depth and axis, *Obstet Gynecol* 36:241, 1970.
32. Nichols DH, Randall CL: *Vaginal surgery,* ed 4, Baltimore, 1996, Williams & Wilkins.
33. Nichols DH: Transvaginal sacrospinous colpopexy, *J Pelv Surg* 2:87, 1996.
34. Papasakelariou C, Baker B: Simplifying sacrospinous ligament fixation, *Contemp Obstet Gynecol* April 1996, p 144.
35. Paraiso MF, Ballard LA, Walters MD, et al: Pelvic support defects and visceral and sexual function in women treated with sacrospinous ligament suspension and pelvic reconstruction, *Obstet Gynecol* 75:1423, 1996.
36. Parsons L, Ulfelder H: *An atlas of pelvic operations,* ed 2, Philadelphia, 1968, WB Saunders.
37. Patsner B, Orr JW Jr: Intractable venous sacral hemorrhage: use of stainless steel thumbtacks to obtain hemostasis, *Am J Obstet Gynecol* 162:452, 1990.
38. Percy NM, Perl JI: Total colpectomy, *Surg Gynecol Obstet* 113:174, 1961.
39. Qinyao W, Shi WJ, Zhao YR, et al: New concepts in severe presacral hemorrhage during proctectomy, *Arch Surg* 120:1013, 1985.
40. Richardson DA, Scotti RJ, Ostergard DR: Surgical management of uterine prolapse in young women, *J Reprod Med* 34:388, 1989.
41. Richter K: Die operative Behandlung des prolabierten Scheidengrundes nach Uterusextirpation, *Geburtshilfe Frauenheilkd* 27:941, 1967.
42. Richter K, Albrich W: Long-term results following fixation of the vagina on the sacrospinal ligament by the vaginal route (vaginaefixatio sacrospinalis vaginalis), *Am J Obstet Gynecol* 141:811, 1981.
43. Schlesinger RE: Vaginal sacrospinous ligament fixation with the autosuture endostitch device, *Am J Obstet Gynecol* 176:1358, 1997.
44. Sederl J: Zur Operation des Prolapses der blind endigenden Scheide, *Geburtshilfe Frauenheilkd* 18:824, 1958.
45. Sharp TR: Sacrospinous suspension made easy, *Obstet Gynecol* 82:873, 1993.
46. Shull BL, Capen CV, Riggs MW, Kuehl TJ: Preoperative and postoperative analysis of site-specific pelvic support defects in 81 women treated with sacrospinous ligament suspension and pelvic reconstruction, *Am J Obstet Gynecol* 166:1764, 1992.
47. Shull BL, Capen CV, Riggs MW, Kuehl TJ: Bilateral attachment of the vaginal cuff to iliococcygeus fascia: an effective method of cuff suspension, *Am J Obstet Gynecol* 168:1669, 1993.
48. Stoddard FJ, Myers RE: Connective tissue disorders in obstetrics and gynecology, *Am J Obstet Gynecol* 102:136, 1968.
49. Stoesser FG: Construction of a sacrocervical ligament for uterine suspension, *Surg Gynecol Obstet* 101:638, 1955.
50. Sutton GP: Thumbtacks, *Am J Obstet Gynecol* 164:931, 1991(letter).
51. Sutton GP, Addison WA, Livengood CH III, Hammond CB: Life-threatening hemorrhage complicating sacral colpopexy, *Am J Obstet Gynecol* 140:836, 1981.
52. Symmonds RE, Williams TJ, Lee RA, Webb MJ: Posthysterectomy enterocele and vaginal vault prolapse, *Am J Obstet Gynecol* 140:852, 1981.
53. Sze EH, Miklos JR, Partoll L, et al: Sacrospinous ligament fixation with transvaginal needle suspension for advanced pelvic organ prolapse and stress incontinence, *Obstet Gynecol* 89:94, 1997.
54. Tancer ML, Fleischer M, Berkowitz BJ: Simultaneous colporectosacropexy, *Obstet Gynecol* 70:951, 1987.
55. Thompson HG, Murphy CJ, Picot H: Hystero-colpectomy for treatment of uterine procidentia, *Am J Obstet Gynecol* 82:743, 1961.
56. Timmons MC, Kohler MF, Addison WA: Thumbtack use for control of presacral bleeding, with description of an instrument for thumbtack application, *Obstet Gynecol* 78:313, 1991.
57. Veronikis DK, Nichols DH: Ligature carrier specifically designed for transvaginal sacrospinous colpopexy, *Obstet Gynecol* 89:478, 1997.
58. Veronikis DK, Nichols DH, Wakamatsu MM: The incidence of low-pressure urethra as a function of prolapse-reducing technique in patients with massive pelvic organ prolapse (maximum descent at all vaginal sites), *Am J Obstet Gynecol* 177:1305, 1997.
59. Watson JD: Sacrospinous ligament colpopexy: new instrumentation applied to a standard gynecologic procedure, *Obstet Gynecol* 88:883, 1996.
60. Weber AM, Walters MD: Anterior vaginal prolapse: review of anatomy and techniques of surgical repair, *Obstet Gynecol* 89:311, 1997.
61. Weidner AC, et al: Sacral osteomyelitis: an unusual complication of abdominal sacral colpopexy, *Obstet Gynecol* 90:689, 1997.
62. White GR: Cystocele: a radical cure by suturing lateral sulci of vagina to the white line of pelvic fascia, *JAMA* 53:1707, 1909.
63. Zweifel P: *Vorlesungen über klinische gynäkologie,* Berlin, 1892, Hirschwald.

27 The Paravaginal Defect

DIONYSIOS K. VERONIKIS

Genital prolapse, and especially that of the anterior vaginal segment, remains one of the most challenging aspects of reconstructive pelvic surgery. Anterior segment prolapse, cystocele, results from inadequate support or insufficient stabilization at rest or during increases in intraabdominal pressure. Paravaginal defects are disturbances in the attachment of the anterior sulcus of the vagina to a connective tissue "bridge" that attaches the anterior sulcus to the arcus tendineus fascia pelvis. The paravaginal defect clinically presents as a cystocele resulting from a lateral separation of the vaginal wall attachments from the lateral pelvic sidewall(s). According to Baden and Walker, such a detachment should be suspected when the anterior vaginal wall is relaxed. If the anterior vaginal wall does not elevate when the patient squeezes the pelvic musculature, the connective tissue and vascular supports of the anterior vaginal wall may have been detached from the arcus tendineus fascia pelvis. The lateral vaginal wall is not attached directly to the arcus tendineus fascia pelvis, instead the anterior vaginal sulcus is attached to the arcus tendineus fascia pelvis by a meshwork of intervening connective tissue, a connective tissue "bridge." This intervening connective tissue may be subject to various strains and stretching, partial or complete avulsion. This type of strain is more common in parous patients as a result of trauma during labor and delivery and perhaps also can be attenuated, stretched, or avulsed with pull of massive genital prolapse, even in the nullipara.

In 1905, Ernest W. Hey Groves published a paper entitled "A new operation for the cure of vaginal cystocele." He stated in this manuscript that "If we regard the cystocele as a hernia, whose radical cure we have to undertake, it is not surprising that methods which depend for their success upon the fixation of so distensible a structure as the vaginal wall should lead to failure." He explained that "Vaginal cystocele exists under two conditions, that in which it only forms part of a uterine descent . . . and that in which it forms a distinct hernia or pouch, pushing the vagina before it, but leaving the uterus in a normal position." He further described the levator ani muscle complex, the "white line" of the pelvis fascia and its insertion. Although the description of his operative repair is not completely clear, he described the following: "A transverse incision is made from one labium majus to the other, about 3 cm behind the urethral orifice. The incision divides the whole thickness of the vagina. . . . The margins of the levatores ani muscles are then sought for and defined in either angle of the wound. It

will be found that they can easily be brought into apposition with little or no tension."

The first description of lateral cystocele repair incorporating the arcus tendineus fascia pelvis into the cystocele repair was by George R. White in 1909. White performed this repair on 19 patients over a 3-year period and, as he stated, always in connection with some other plastic operation.

White's classic paper described a surgical procedure that was designed to correct cystocele, a radical cure, by attaching the lateral vaginal sulci to the arcus tendineus fascia pelvis. One has to wonder what is meant by the term *radical cystocele* because it could conceivably include as much a displacement cystocele from lateral detachment as well as a displacement cystocele from an apical prolapse as well. White's 1909 paper did not receive much attention, and he again reported his views in 1912. Based on cadaver dissections, White wrote, "The easiest and simplest way to accomplish this is to incise the peritoneum at the side of the bladder, push the bladder aside until the white line comes into view, and then by the aid of an assistant's finger in the vagina, suture the anterior lateral side of the vagina to the white line of the pelvic fascia." Almost 50 years later, in 1961, John Christopher Burch, in performing a Marshall-Marchetti-Krantz operation, was unable to secure the sutures to the periosteum and concomitantly noticed the intravaginal finger elevating the vaginal wall to the "white line," the arcus tendineus fascia pelvis. After seven successful procedures, he believed that Cooper's ligament was a stronger attachment point. The paravaginal defect and its repair as it is known today was redescribed by Richardson through an abdominal retropubic exposure instead of the original transvaginal approach used by White.

CYSTOCELE AND THE PARAVAGINAL DEFECT

Cystocele results from trauma or damage to the vagina; either to the apical vaginal supports, to the lateral vaginal attachments, or to the vaginal wall itself. In examining and evaluating the anterior vaginal wall, one must have in mind that several distinct types of cystoceles exist and each may contribute partially or totally to anterior segment defects. All of the existing combinations must be recognized and corrected if surgical treatment is to be effective and durable.

Cystocele has been described according to whether it is anterior to the interureteric ridge (anterior cystocele) or posterior to it (posterior cystocele). Anterior cystocele is synonymous with urethrocele, in which straining or Valsalva efforts results in downward bulging or rotational descent of the urethra with or without a demonstrable tendency of the bladder to "herniate" behind the vesicourethral junction. The distal third of the vaginal wall and attachments underlies and supports the urethra. This rotational descent of the vesicourethral junction may be of varying degrees and is often associated with urinary incontinence. Pathologic dilation of the midurethra or distal urethra (true urethrocele) is uncommon. A true cystocele therefore does not include the distal vagina. Similarly, in patients with an intact cervix and uterus, the cervix occupies the upper third or so of the anterior vaginal wall. The length of the anterior vaginal wall plus the length of the cervix roughly equals the length of the posterior vaginal wall. Thus a distention cystocele is between the bladder neck and cervix. A distention cystocele is almost without exception the result of an overstretching of the vaginal wall beyond its ability to recover/involute after vaginal delivery, or it is the consequence of the atrophic changes of aging on the intrinsic structural components of the vaginal wall with or without earlier damage. Rugal folds once visible on the anterior vaginal epithelium are diminished with aging and may disappear as the physiologic and pathologic changes that occur behind the squamous epithelium and within the vaginal wall deep to the squamous epithelium continue. These processes allow the anterior vagina and bladder to "bulge" into the vaginal lumen. In a true distention cystocele the lateral attachments of the vagina are well supported. The transverse topographic length from vaginal sidewall to vaginal sidewall is increased. Therefore, almost without exception, the true distention cystocele is the result of attenuation of the anterior vaginal wall. The vagina, as an organ, responds to physiologic forces as well as to pathologic forces with the same response—stretching.

Lateral displacement cystocele is the result of pathologic elongation or detachment of the lateral vaginal attachments and support of the vagina. Etiologically, this is quite different from distention cystocele caused by connective tissue damage to the normal vaginal wall. The anterior vaginal segment also has superior attachments to the cervix. Thus the tissues supporting both the vagina and cervix are component parts of the cardinal ligaments and function as an anatomic unit. Displacement of one component is often followed by similar displacement of the other. Posthysterectomy eversion or prolapse of the upper vagina may also present as displacement cystocele by creating a "telescoping effect." If the upper vaginal segment does not descend, a telescoping effect and an apical displacement cystocele cannot occur. In its pure form, displacement cystocele represents an eversion of the vagina with relatively well-preserved rugal folds. The loss of support of the lateral vaginal attachments can be unilateral or bilateral.

Preserved rugae with descent of the anterior vaginal wall suggests a defect of the connective tissue structures that support the vagina and urethra bilaterally at the lateral pelvic wall along the arcus tendineus fascia pelvis. This type of anterior segment defect is a displacement cystocele, as is a cystocele from an upper vaginal vault prolapse. Descent of the upper vagina halfway between the ischial spines and hymen may easily be corrected by a surgical procedure directed only at the vaginal apex. Clinically, when the sulci disappear partially or completely, a paravaginal defect exists. When the anterior segment is evaluated, it must be determined whether the vaginal vault is partially or completely prolapsed, adding to the magnitude of a displacement cystocele. In addition, with the vaginal vault replaced, one must consider the extent of distention cystocele as well as the extent "imitating" displacement cystocele by the vault prolapse. Any coexistent paravaginal defects are then and only then evaluated. Repositioning the vaginal vault to the ischial spines with a ring forceps and labeling it a pure lateral displacement cystocele is an error in diagnosis. Yet, how often do residents, referring colleagues, and patients call a posthysterectomy vault prolapse a "dropped bladder"—cystocele! Hence, the biggest imitator of a cystocele in a posthysterectomy patient is an apical vaginal segment prolapse.

The surgical gynecologist contemplating surgical repair of anterior segment defects must consider that "pure" forms of individual anterior segment defects rarely occur. In general, one should anticipate a combination, "mixed cystocele," of the above types of defects.

DIFFERENTIAL DIAGNOSIS OF ANTERIOR SEGMENT DEFECTS

Examination of the patient with genital prolapse is facilitated by forceful Valsalva maneuver, especially in the standing position, to delineate defective vaginal sites that manifest themselves better under stress and to determine the extent and magnitude of all defects. However, paravaginal defects are best evaluated with the patient in the lithotomy position, initially at rest and then with forceful Valsalva maneuver to fully visualize descent of the anterior vaginal wall (Fig. 27-1). Subsequent evaluation must analyze the site or sites of defects with repositioning of the sulci (Fig. 27-2), as well as all other pelvic support defects if durable, long-term support of the anterior segment is to be obtained.

The importance of the damage caused by each component of the anterior vaginal segment may be noticeable at different levels within the anterior vaginal depth. Therefore, where are paravaginal defects along the vaginal depth? If the anterior vaginal segment is topographically divided into thirds, the paravaginal defects are in the middle third of the vagina. To study the relationship of vaginal support to uterine support, and vaginal support after hysterectomy, DeLancey examined vaginal support in cadavers that had previously undergone hysterectomy as well as cadavers with the uterus in place. The structures that supported the vagina were divided into three levels corresponding to different areas of support: levels I, II, and III. Although these three levels of vaginal support are continuous, surgically each of these three areas are repaired with different operations. Therefore a surgical procedure can be selected and directed to one of these three levels (I, II, or III).

One approach in evaluating patients with genital pro-

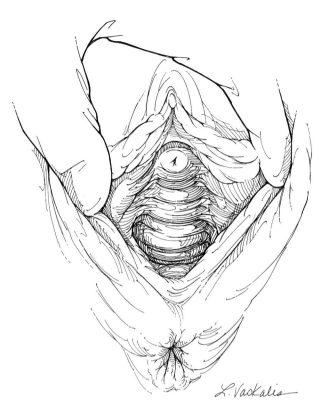

Fig. 27-1   Vaginal view of bilateral paravaginal defects. Displacement of the anterior vaginal wall is caused by lateral defects; the vaginal apex is well supported.

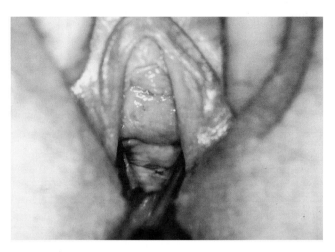

Fig. 27-2   Vaginal view of bilateral paravaginal defects repositioned with the Baden defect analyzer. A midline displacement cystocele, urethrocele, and altered urethral axis are also evident.

lapse is for the initial assessment to focus on the apical supports of the vagina. Descent of the vaginal apex or cervix suggests loss of connective tissue support between the vagina and the parametria, a level I defect. An undiagnosed partial vault prolapse may be spuriously treated surgically as a cystocele as a result of the telescoping effect of the anterior vaginal segment (from loss of apical support) in patients who have undergone hysterectomy. This apical defect is often associated with a midline defect of the vaginal wall (distention cystocele).

The literature in reconstructive pelvic surgery has not clearly stated the incidence and coassociation of paravaginal defects in patients with primary and recurrent prolapse. Richardson reported that about 85% of the cystoceles with descent of the anterior vaginal segment in his patients and more than 95% of the cystourethroceles with stress incontinence were caused by a paravaginal defect. Therefore 95% of his patients were treated with paravaginal defect repair.

Topographically dividing the anterior vagina into thirds permits evaluation of four distinct areas. This provides a useful paradigm that focuses on the defects and the surgical treatment that can be applied to their repair. As stated by DeLancey, these three levels of vaginal support are continuous with one another and therefore interdependent. The midvagina, level II, relies on a well-supported upper vagina (level I) to prevent an apical displacement cystocele that is caused by a telescoping effect of the anterior vaginal wall. As long as support of the upper vagina (level I) is intact, a "cystocele" or anterior segment defect is a support defect at

level II. Surgical correction of level I may be performed vaginally by unilateral or bilateral sacrospinous colpopexy, the Mayo-McCall culdeplasty, or an abdominal sacrocolpopexy. On the other hand, level III corresponds to the region of the vagina that extends 2 cm from the introitus to 3 cm above the hymenal ring and is fused with the surrounding structures. This is the area of the bladder neck, the urethrocele. In patients with total prolapse of the anterior vaginal wall and apex, urinary continence may be achieved by a "kinking" effect of the urethra. Reducing the cystocele and restoring the anatomic relationships of the anterior vaginal segment unmasks urinary incontinence. Depending on the type of incontinence and surgical approach, the urinary incontinence could be corrected by a vesicourethral sling or Burch urethropexy.

Thus the midportion of the anterior vaginal segment, level II, requires careful clinical evaluation because this is the site of both the midline distention cystocele and the lateral displacement cystocele (paravaginal defect). Therefore a true cystocele develops because of midline damage to the anterior vaginal wall or to the lateral connective tissue supports of the bladder, arcus tendineus fascia pelvis. Attenuation and breaks in the connective tissue and/or the muscularis of the anterior vaginal wall within level II results in descent of the anterior vaginal wall into the vaginal canal as a space-occupying mass, the cystocele. Because the distance from the left arcus tendineus fascia pelvis to the right arcus tendineus fascia pelvis is a fixed distance, any increase in the transverse anterior vaginal wall dimension along the length of level II will cause the anterior vaginal wall to bulge into the vaginal canal. Hence, an analogy can be drawn with respect to two fixed points such as clothesline poles and the clothesline between them.

Therefore the diagnosis of a paravaginal defect requires the vaginal apex, level I, to be repositioned in its normal anatomic position or at the site where reconstructive surgery will place it, then and only then should level II be evaluated. Preoperatively repositioning the vaginal apex in patients

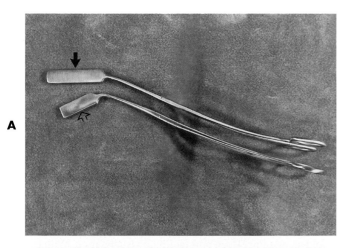

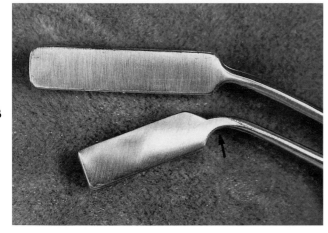

Fig. 27-3 **A,** Lateral view of the Baden vaginal defect analyzer (Zinnanti Surgical Instruments, Inc., Chatsworth, Calif.) *(solid arrow)* and modified Baden vaginal defect analyzer *(open arrow).* **B,** Shorter paddles on the modified Baden vaginal defect analyzer (Marina Medical, Hollywood, Calif.) reposition the lateral vaginal walls 1 cm from the ischial spine to 1 cm from the bladder neck. The distal bend *(arrow)* redirects the orientation of the body of the instrument and avoids periurethral pressure while facilitating replacement of the lateral vaginal wall along the trajectory of the arcus tendineus fascia pelvis without obscuring visualization.

with significant vault prolapse will avoid spuriously diagnosing an apical prolapse as a cystocele or as a paravaginal defect. Repositioning the vaginal apex is the initial step in correctly identifying the cause of level II defects and the complex nature of the pelvic floor defects. Huddleston evaluated patients with magnetic resonance imaging (MRI) preoperatively and then 4 to 30 days postoperatively after surgically correcting the paravaginal defects. This study effectively identified the paravaginal defects preoperatively and the persistent uncorrected vault prolapse, level I defects, postoperatively. The identification of the level I defects in the immediate postoperative MRI scans underscores the need to evaluate level II defects after level I has been repositioned, and if a level I defect exists it ought to be repaired.

Let us consider preoperative evaluation of a patient with an unreduced posthysterectomy vault prolapse to the level of the hymenal ring. The Baden defect analyzer (Fig. 27-3,

A and *B*) or a ring forceps may be used to reposition the sulci and elevate the vagina to the ischial spines. The vault prolapse and possible paravaginal defect are reduced and disappear as the most dependent portion of the vaginal apex is taken to the level of the ischial spines by the tip of the defect analyzer and as the sulci are elevated in the midvagina to the lateral pelvic sidewall, respectively. These findings may spuriously be diagnosed as a complete bilateral paravaginal defect. Alternatively, if the same patient was evaluated by initially reducing the apex of the prolapse with a disarticulated speculum, sponge stick, or preferably a scopette (rectal swab), this would immediately identify the vault prolapse as a level I defect. Then, with the vaginal apex repositioned, a lateral defect at level II may be evaluated by repositioning the sulci with the Baden vaginal defect analyzer or a curved ring forceps at rest and during Valsalva. When the vaginal apex is restored, the displacement cystocele from the apical prolapse is also noted; any remaining cystocele is the result of a midline defect. In clinical practice the magnitude of pelvic floor genital prolapse will undoubtedly yield variations in the severity of anterior segment defects, cystoceles. Multiple anterior segment site defects, "mixed cystocele," with midline distention, paravaginal defect, and apical descent components requires meticulous preoperative evaluation.

SURGICAL APPROACH TO PARAVAGINAL REPAIR

Pelvic floor defects can be repaired abdominally, vaginally, and laparoscopically. There is no right way, wrong way, or better method—only alternatives. These alternatives should be based on surgical indications, medical and surgical considerations such as coexistent abdominal pathologic conditions and other pelvic floor defects, and surgeon preference and training. As stated by David H. Nichols, "The operation should be made to fit the patient, not the patient the operation." Therefore, given the same set of clinical circumstances for a given patient and various surgeons, some alternatives are better for some patients and some alternatives are better for some surgeons. Ideally, the pelvic reconstructive surgeon ought to be able to operate with the same efficiency abdominally, vaginally, and laparoscopically depending on the pathologic condition, the surgical indications, and the patient's needs. Inherent to each approach are advantages and disadvantages. The advantages of an abdominal approach are (1) the arcus tendineus fascia pelvis is better visualized, (2) partial paravaginal defects can be repaired, (3) it is technically easier to perform, and (4) it may be combined with a Burch urethropexy. The laparoscopic approach offers the same advantages as the abdominal approach and is less traumatic to the anterior abdominal wall. However, the laparoscopic approach requires the surgeon to complete the "abdominal" operative procedure without direct retropubic palpation and requires advanced laparoscopic surgical skills and techniques. If a reconstructive surgeon performs a laparoscopic paravaginal repair in an identical manner as to the open abdominal repair, theoretically the complications and long-term results as they relate to the procedure should be the same.

Advantages of the transvaginal approach through a midline vaginal incision permit concomitant repair of distention cystocele and placement of a vesicourethral sling. In addition, repair of vault prolapse and enterocele as well as rectocele repair and reconstruction of the perineum may be performed through the same surgical exposure. The transvaginal approach can also be performed through two lateral incisions along the sulci of the anterior vaginal wall as originally described by White in 1909. This approach is indicated in patients with pure displacement cystoceles caused by isolated lateral paravaginal defects. Perhaps a possible disadvantage of the vaginal approach is the need to open the entire paravaginal space during repair for exposure to the lateral pelvic sidewall. A complete paravaginal repair will then be required, even if a partial defect was present.

Abdominal Retropubic Technique

If hysterectomy is indicated, the paravaginal defect repair is performed after completion of the hysterectomy and reconstruction of level I with a culdeplasty. If a laparoscopic assisted hysterectomy and laparoscopic Burch urethropexy with paravaginal defect repair is the indicated surgical treatment, the hysterectomy and culdeplasty should be completed before any reconstructive surgery is done. This will ensure mobility of the anterior segment and facilitate the vaginal portion of the hysterectomy without undue difficulty and unforeseen complications.

Proper patient positioning is critical; it will facilitate the operation by enhancing exposure, decreasing frustration between the repeated retropubic and vaginal manipulations, and decreasing the likelihood of nerve injury and compartment syndrome. Adjustable Allen stirrups, especially the PAL stirrups with featherlift (Allen Medical Systems, Cleveland, Ohio) enable easy intraoperative adjustment and provide excellent access to the lower abdomen and retropubic space by permitting the patient to be in a comfortable modified lithotomy position with access to the introitus and vaginal canal.

If an abdominal hysterectomy is to be performed, the placement of the incision should favor the exposure required for the hysterectomy with consideration that the retropubic space will need to be dissected. A high Pfannenstiel incision will compromise exposure to the retropubic space by creating an "awning" effect from the anterior abdominal wall as an anatomic obstacle that will require constant retraction as well as impede the reflection of light into the retropubic space in addition to creating shadowing.

In the absence of an abdominal hysterectomy, the low transverse incision is placed 2 fingerbreadths from the peak of the pubic symphysis and not from the most cephalad point of the pubic symphysis. This position will place the surgical exposure directly above the space of Retzius, minimize the amount of lateral retraction that will be required, avoid an awning effect, and facilitate visualization. With experience the length of the incision can be reduced to 3 inches. Use of a headlight provides shadow-free lighting in front of the surgeon, eliminating the frequent overhead light adjustments because the surgeon or assistant is blocking the light. If not already in place, the bladder is drained with a 14-Fr silicone coated catheter before reconstructive surgery is performed. The catheter is not connected to gravity drainage; if previously connected to gravity, it is disconnected from the Foley bag and clamped with a Kelly clamp. This allows easier manipulation of the Foley bulb in identifying the bladder neck and avoids the catheter from being pulled down in front of the introitus. The 5-ml Foley bulb is filled with 10 ml of saline.

The incision is then carried through the skin and subcutaneous fat to the fascia of the rectus abdominis, which is incised in the midline and extended laterally. The rectus muscles are sharply divided in the midline and gently reflected laterally with a medium-sized Richardson retractor. The goal of developing the retropubic space is gentle dissection because any bleeding will decrease exposure, obscure anatomic landmarks, and require frequent evacuation of the blood, further decreasing exposure as retractors are exchanged between surgeon and assistants.

Once the rectus muscle is reflected laterally the space of Retzius is developed by following the undersurface of the rectus muscle to the superior ramus of the pubic bone

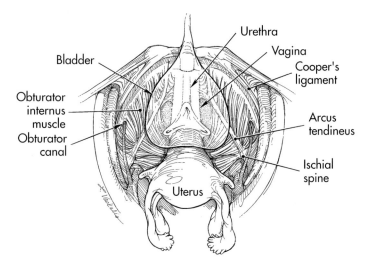

Fig. 27-4 Abdominal retropubic view of normal anatomic relationships. The ischial spine is distal to the obturator foramen. The trajectory of the arcus tendineus is from the ischial spine to the pubic symphysis. The obturator internus muscle is lateral to the arcus tendineus fascia pelvis.

(Fig. 27-4). Cooper's ligament is identified and noted. The loose areolar tissue can then gently be dissected from the pubic symphysis below and Cooper's ligament in a lateral to medial direction with blunt tissue forceps such as Singley. Initially, a narrow, malleable retractor is used to retract the bladder medially, and as dissection continues, a medium malleable retractor greatly facilitates exposure to the entire paravaginal space and provides bladder retraction. A mild curve in the narrow malleable retractor provides a smooth surface for an open sponge to be gently advanced between the malleable and the lateral pelvic sidewall. The malleable is then placed over the sponge and the process is repeated, usually two more times. The narrow malleable is exchanged for the medium malleable when the paravaginal space is fully dissected. The three sponges are left in place, and the same is performed on the contralateral paravaginal space. This sponge-malleable interchange effectively retracts the bladder medially with minimal abrasion as well as facilitates gentle dissection of the paravaginal space. One approach is to develop the left paravaginal space and leave the three sponges is position, then develop the right paravaginal space and maintain the exposure for suture placement and repair.

Before suture placement, the paravaginal defect as well as the arcus tendineus fascia pelvis should be visualized. The arcus tendineus fascia pelvis may be completely or partially visible on the lateral pelvic sidewall, or it may not be visible. If completely visible on the pelvic sidewall, from the back of the pubic symphysis to the ischial spine, the vaginal wall attachments have torn away from the arcus tendineus fascia pelvis. If partially visible, a portion of the arcus tendineus fascia pelvis may be on the vaginal wall and a portion on the pelvic sidewall. If the arcus tendineus fascia

pelvis is not visible on the lateral pelvic sidewall, it has remained with the vaginal wall attachments during detachment. The reconstructive intent is to reestablish fusion between the lateral pelvic sidewall and the vaginal wall. In those circumstances in which the arcus tendineus fascia pelvis is visible on the pelvic sidewall, the sutures will attach the vaginal wall to the arcus tendineus fascia pelvis (Fig. 27-5). In partial or complete avulsion of the arcus tendineus fascia pelvis from the pelvic sidewall, the attachment of the vaginal wall will be to the obturator internus fascia. In the latter situations a trajectory of the arcus tendineus fascia pelvis from the pubic symphysis to the ischial spine must be carefully plotted (Fig. 27-6). Although the back of the pubic symphysis is easily seen, the ischial spine is difficult to visualize from the retropubic space. However, from within the retropubic and paravaginal spaces, the position of the ischial spine can be identified with precision, 6 to 8 cm directly inferior to the obturator foramen. The surgeon's nondominant hand placed in the vagina can easily palpate the ischial spine at any time during the dissection as well as identify the bladder neck and elevate the vagina for countertraction during dissection (Fig. 27-7). In addition, manipulation of the vaginal wall by the vaginal hand can help identify the site of suture placement on the vaginal side by placing and replacing the vagina to the site of its intended postoperative lateral position. The vaginal hand also elevates the vagina up and away from vessels and bladder as well as provides tactile sensation of needle depth during suturing. The reconstructive goal is for the avulsed lateral vaginal wall to be sutured to the arcus tendineus fascia pelvis or along a trajectory on the fascia of the obturator internus muscle that runs from the ischial spine to the lower margin of the symphysis.

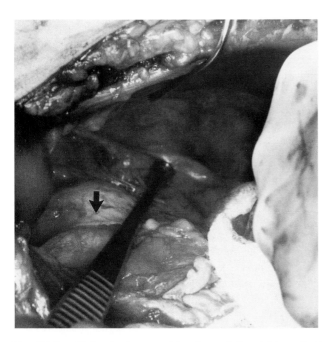

Fig. 27-5 Abdominal retropubic view of the right vaginal wall detached from the arcus tendineus fascia pelvis. Singley forceps show the arcus tendineus fascia pelvis. *Solid arrow* shows the bladder.

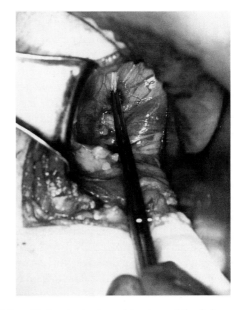

Fig. 27-6 Abdominal retropubic view of the left arcus tendineus fascia pelvis completely detached from the pelvic sidewall. Singley forceps are used to grasp the obturator internus muscle.

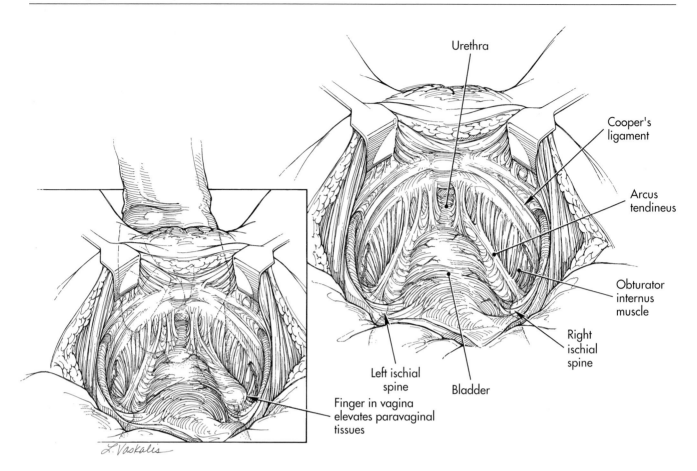

Fig. 27-7   Abdominal retropubic view of bilateral paravaginal defects. Complete avulsion of the lateral attachments between the vaginal wall and the arcus tendineus fascia pelvis *(inset)*. The surgeon's finger elevates the detached vaginal wall to the site of the arcus tendineus fascia pelvis at the level of the ischial spine.

After dissection of both paravaginal spaces, the defects are sutured with permanent braided suture material (Fig. 27-8) such as 2-0 Ethibond (Ethicon, Somerville, NJ). A long needle driver will permit suturing without the driving hand obscuring needle placement/rotation and visualization. As the vaginal finger presses the vagina toward the arcus tendineus fascia pelvis, the site of suture placement is selected and placed through the full-thickness vaginal wall, excluding the squamous epithelium. Because the most dependent portion of the operative field is at the ischial spine, blood collection in this area is inevitable. Therefore initiating suture placement near the ischial spine has the advantage of repairing this area before bleeding from needle passing and suturing further obscures the operative field. After the suture is recovered from the vaginal wall, the suture is passed through the arcus tendineus fascia pelvis and/or the fascia of the obturator internus muscle. The most cephalad suture should be placed approximately 1 to 2 cm from the ischial spine and additional sutures at 1- to 1.5-cm intervals (Fig. 27-9). It is generally easier to suture toward one's self. Therefore, on the patient's right, to further avoid inadvertently causing bleeding, the suture is initially passed through the arcus tendineus fascia pelvis and/or the fascia of the obturator internus muscle and then through the vaginal wall.

On the patient's left, the suture is passed through the vaginal wall first and then through the arcus tendineus fascia pelvis and/or the fascia of the obturator internus. Each suture may tagged with a numbered clamp until all sutures on both sides have been placed; usually 4 to 6 sutures will be required on each side to correct the paravaginal defect. An alternate approach to avoid suture entanglement is the use of McIntosh suture holding forceps (V. Mueller, Baxter Healthcare Corporation, Deerfield, Ill.). The McIntosh is a suture loom transversely placed on a nonpenetrating towel clamp that allows each suture to be secured within a groove.

If a Burch retropubic suspension will also be performed for genuine stress urinary incontinence, cystoscopic evaluation and indigo carmine evaluation for ureteral patency are performed after placement of the sutures through Cooper's ligament. The most cephalad paravaginal suture at the ischial spine is tied first, then the remaining ipsilateral paravaginal sutures, followed by the contralateral paravaginal sutures before any of the Burch sutures (Figs. 27-10 and 27-11).

Meticulous hemostasis is required not only with the dissection but also during suturing to ensure adequate repair because the needle will invariably exacerbate bleeding. Electrocautery, surgical clips, and 3-0 chromic sutures can

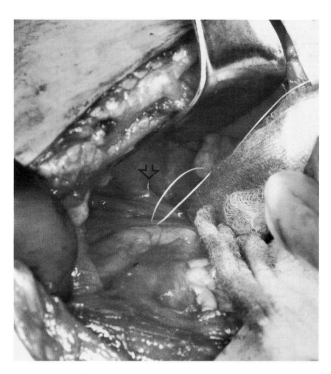

Fig. 27-8 Abdominal retropubic view. Initial suturing of a paravaginal defect. *Open arrow* shows the needle tip. The needle path has included the arcus tendineus fascia pelvis and the obturator internus.

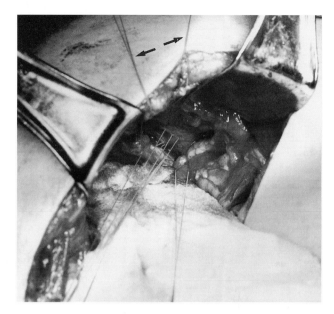

Fig. 27-9 Abdominal retropubic view. Sutures to correct a paravaginal defect have been placed and held. Note the defect between the suture pass. Sutures also placed through Coopers' ligament for Burch urethropexy *(solid arrows).*

be used for the sometimes very large veins coursing laterally around the bladder. Adequate lighting is essential; a headlight yields shadow-free focused lighting. Needle trauma to a vessel during suturing within the vaginal wall will usually stop bleeding with tying.

Vaginal Paravaginal Defect Repair

The transvaginal paravaginal defect repair is an alternative approach to repair the lateral defects causing anterior segment prolapse. The intent of the repair and the tissues to be repaired are the same as for the abdominal retropubic approach. A thorough understanding of the anatomy, the use of appropriate retractors designed for deep retraction, and the ability to mentally "visualize" the retropubic space and maintain a constant mental image of the final surgical repair are essential.

Patient positioning is once again given great detail to prevent injury and provide maximum exposure. The adjustable Allen stirrups, PAL stirrups with featherlift (Allen Medical Systems, Cleveland, Ohio) are also very useful for transvaginal surgery because leg elevation and hip rotation are not restricted to stirrup preselected positions. Intraoperative examination reconfirms the preoperative defects; if new defects are diagnosed, they must be repaired and the operative procedure is adjusted accordingly. If vaginal hysterectomy is indicated, it is performed first. A 14-Fr transurethral Foley is used to drain the bladder, 10 ml are placed in the bulb, and the end is clamped with a Kelly clamp. Marking sutures may be used to mark the most cephalad and

distal ends of the lateral sulcus so that as distortion during and from dissection occurs a reference point for suture placement may be maintained. One approach to selecting the marking suture reference point is to replace the vagina to the level of the ischial spine on both sides. Sutures are then placed approximately 1 cm from the ischial spine, at the level of the bladder neck and the midpoint between the two marking sutures. Dissection of the anterior vaginal segment is initiated by placing two Allis clamps on the anterior vaginal wall at the most dependent point. The vaginal incision is made with Noble-Mayo scissors directly into the vesicovaginal space. The incision is extended for the full length of the anterior vaginal segment, from the vaginal apex to 1 cm from the urethral meatus. Care is taken to maintain the dissection within the vesicovaginal space and to avoid splitting the anterior vaginal wall. Only sharp dissection is used with the Noble-Mayo scissors for the entire dissection. Dissection is maintained within the vesicovaginal space and is carried cephalad, caudad, and laterally to the full lateral limits of the vesicovaginal space. If the patient has undergone previous retropubic surgery, instilling 60 ml of infant milk formula into the bladder will identify any inadvertent bladder trauma. Dissection is then carried through the lateral limits of the vesicovaginal space and a fenestration between the vesicovaginal space and the paravaginal space is enlarged to the space of Retzius and the pelvic sidewall. A long Briesky-Navratil retractor is inserted into the paravaginal space, and the bladder is mobilized medially. Dissection is further facilitated by gently pushing open sponges against the

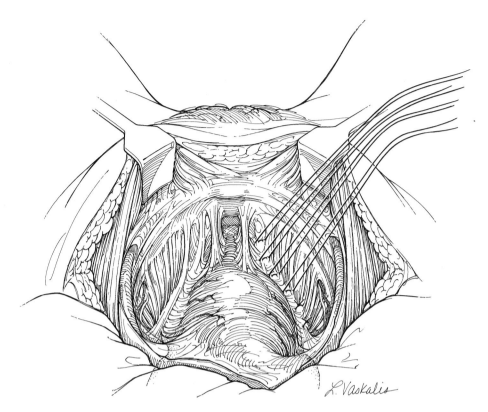

L. Vaskalis

Fig. 27-10   Abdominal retropubic view of a reconstructed right paravaginal defect.

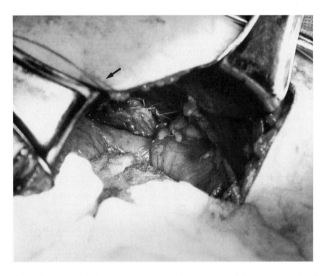

Fig. 27-11   Abdominal retropubic view. Right paravaginal sutures have been tied, approximating the lateral vaginal wall and the arcus tendineus fascia pelvis. *Solid arrow* shows the untied Burch urethropexy sutures.

Briesky-Navratil retractor and the pelvic sidewall. The Briesky-Navratil retractor is then placed over the sponge to decrease retractor slippage and to further retract the bladder and urethra medially. A total of three sponges are packed in this manner. In developing the paravaginal space, the surgeon must perform a full-length paravaginal repair. The ureters at this point are retracted medially and out of harm's way. Illumination is critical in visualizing the pelvic side-

wall, the obturator fascia, and the arcus tendineus pelvis, which are fully exposed. A headlight provides hands-free directed lighting but requires the surgeon to be comfortable in wearing a headlight. Alternatively, a lighted retractor of even the free laparoscopic fiberoptic cord directed into the paravaginal space will be of great help. Bleeding from small vessels may and should be controlled with electrocautery or with the use of a laparoscopic clip applicator because bleeding will decrease exposure. In contrast to the abdominal approach, after dissection of each paravaginal space, the sutures are placed through the arcus tendineus fascia pelvis and/or the obturator internus fascia. A Deschamps ligature carrier may be used and in certain clinical situations is preferred to a suture with a swedged-on needle. The disadvantage of the Deschamps ligature carrier is the need for passing all suture ends through a Mayo needle. The advantage of the Deschamps ligature carrier is the ability to pass a suture deep in the pelvis. I have found that with the correct retractors and focused assistants a doubly armed swedged-on needle placed with a long Haney needle driver is very efficient. The doubly armed 2-0 Ethibond braided suture on an SH needle (Ethicon, Somerville, NJ) allows both ends of the suture to be passed the respective tissues without the use of a Mayo needle. Suture twisting and entanglement may become a problem because all sutures ends will exit transvaginally and are affected by gravity. This time-consuming and frustrating portion of the operation can be effectively reduced by two simple maneuvers. The first is the use of two different color sutures: a green braided and a white braided Ethibond, which are alternatively placed. One

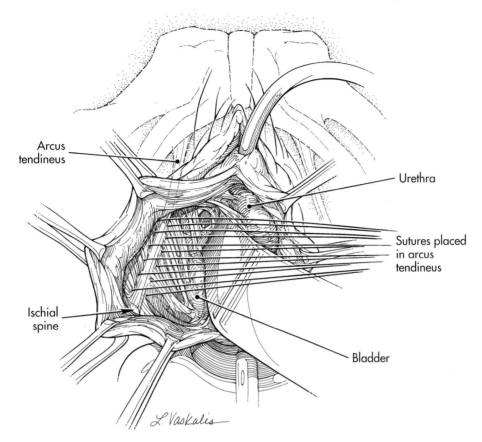

Arcus
tendineus

Urethra

Sutures placed
in arcus
tendineus

Ischial
spine

Bladder

L. Vaskalis

Fig. 27-12 Vaginal view showing initial placement of sutures through the arcus tendineus fascia pelvis. The full-thickness vaginal wall is held laterally, and the bladder is retracted medially.

approach is to place the green braided closest to the ischial spine and follow with the white braided and so on; generally four sutures will be required. The second is to hold the sutures in numbered clamps, but because gravity is unrelenting, this may still entangle the sutures. The use of a McIntosh suture holding forceps (V. Mueller, Baxter Healthcare Corporation, Deerfield, Ill.) further eliminates this problem. The McIntosh is a suture loom transversely placed on a nonpenetrating towel clamp, which is clamped onto the drapes cephalad or laterally. As each suture pass is completed, the suture ends are secured within a groove in the McIntosh suture loom.

The four sutures are placed through the arcus tendineus fascia pelvis and/or the obturator internus fascia from the ischial spine toward the symphysis pubis. Palpation of the ischial spine, the obturator foramen, and the back of the pubic symphysis is easily achieved transvaginally. Even if the arcus tendineus fascia pelvis has and can be seen as well as palpated, it is helpful for the surgeon to conceptualize a trajectory of the arcus tendineus fascia pelvis as suturing is initiated and focus is continually turned from the paravaginal space to the vaginal wall and vaginal lumen. Placing the first suture 1 to 2 cm from the ischial spine allows the surgeon to suture toward himself or herself and avoids entangling the distal sutures with the proximal needles and su-

tures during suturing while traversing the paravaginal space (Fig. 27-12). Each additional suture is placed at approximately 1-cm intervals (Fig. 27-13, *A* and *B*). If a vesicourethral sling will also be placed, the most distal suture should not be placed at the bladder neck because once this suture is tied it may negate the preferential action of the sling on the bladder neck by decreasing lift. Once all the lateral pelvic sidewall sutures are placed in the position required for each individual patient, the vaginal vault is placed in the proper desired postoperative position. If marking sutures were not used or were lost during dissection, the use of a ring forceps intraoperatively is very helpful and does not obscure the lateral vaginal sulci, as would the paddles from the Baden defect analyzer. With the ring forceps, the surgeon should open the fold where the dissected anterior vaginal wall crosses the edge of the forceps. The descending needle is then passed through the full thickness of the fibromuscular layer of the anterior vaginal wall. The remaining sutures are passed at the same distance on the anterior vaginal wall as they were on the lateral pelvic sidewall (Fig. 27-14). All of the sutures have a two-point penetration: the lateral pelvic sidewall (the arcus tendineus fascia pelvis and/or the obturator internus fascia) and the full-thickness anterior vaginal wall, excluding the squamous epithelium. Trauma to the bladder, urethra, or ureter is unlikely because all of these

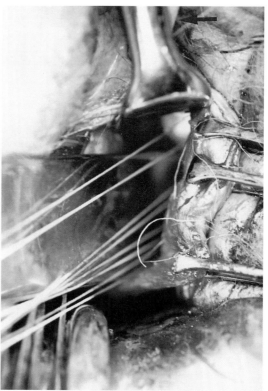
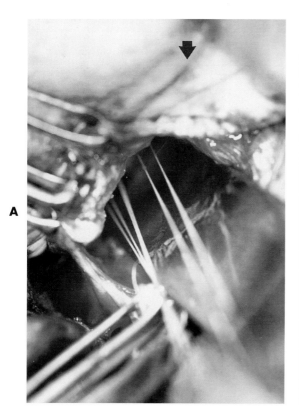

Fig. 27-13   **A,** Vaginal view. *Solid arrow* depicts approximate position of the pubic symphysis. The bladder is being retracted medially, the right paravaginal space is completely developed, and permanent sutures have been placed through the arcus tendineus fascia pelvis. **B,** Vaginal view. *Solid arrow* shows Foley catheter behind retractor. Permanent sutures placed through the left arcus tendineus fascia pelvis.

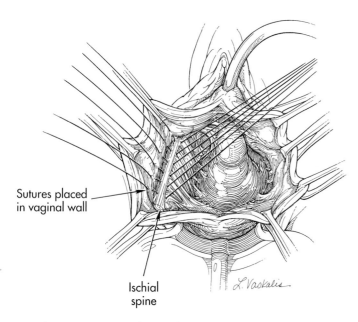

Sutures placed in vaginal wall

Ischial spine

Fig. 27-14   Vaginal view showing suture placement through the arcus tendineus fascia pelvis and the anterior vaginal wall, excluding the squamous epithelium.

structures are retracted medially and not involved directly in the suturing. However, a technical word of caution is required. The surgeon must attempt to estimate the amount of lateral paravaginal defect (displacement cystocele) and the extent of distention cystocele that will require midline plication. Care must be taken not to overcorrect the paravaginal defect because this may preclude midline reapproximation. Overcorrection may be achieved by placing the sutures too far medial on the anterior vaginal wall, above the arcus tendineus fascia pelvis, or a chosen trajectory on the obturator internus fascia or a combination of the aforementioned. The most significant of these is the extent of medial suture placement on the vaginal wall. It can almost be said that the sutures can not be placed too far laterally on the vaginal wall and strategic placement on the vaginal wall can compensate for less than ideal lateral wall placement. The sutures are not tied at this time, and the same sequence of steps is performed on the contralateral side (see Fig. 27-13, *A* and *B*). If a vesicourethral sling is to be placed, it is done at this time, in addition to the placement of any Kelly stitches to repair funneling. If a midline distention cystocele also needs repair, it is performed before sling placement, with one or more layers of 2-0 polyglycolic acid sutures. Alternatively, suburethral plication of the pubourethrovaginal ligament portion is of the urogenital diaphragm is performed with polydioxanone suture (Ethicon, Somerville, NJ).

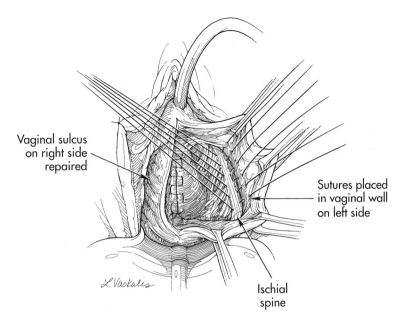

Vaginal sulcus
on right side
repaired

Sutures placed
in vaginal wall
on left side

Ischial
spine

L. Vackalis

Fig. 27-15 Vaginal view of a repaired midline distention cystocele, a right paravaginal defect, and a reconstructed sulcus. Sutures in the left arcus tendineus fascia pelvis and the vaginal wall remain to be tied. Trimming of the anterior vaginal wall and midline closure complete the reconstruction.

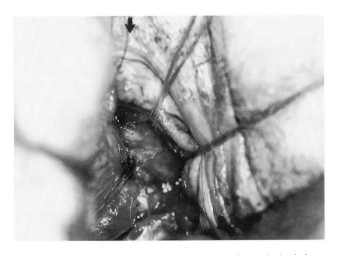

Fig. 27-16 Vaginal view of sutures placed through the left arcus tendineus fascia pelvis and the vaginal wall before they are tied. *Solid arrow* depicts approximate position of the pubic symphysis. The midline cystocele has been repaired, and the right paravaginal sutures have been tied. Note the thickness of the unsplit anterior vaginal wall.

If sacrospinous colpopexy or another apical support procedure has also been performed, those sutures are tied first. Then the lateral paravaginal sutures are tied in the order in which they were placed, first on one side and then on the other (Figs. 27-15 and 27-16). The midline cut edges of the vagina are brought together, trimming the excess as necessary to effect the desired midline result (Fig. 27-17, *A* and *B*). The anterior full-thickness vaginal wall is closed with a running subcuticular suture, or if a vesicourethral sling has been placed, the anterior vaginal wall is closed in two lay-

ers. Any additional posterior segment defects are repaired, and the vagina is lightly packed overnight if desired.

Laparoscopic Approach to Paravaginal Defect Repair

Laparoscopy is only a means of obtaining surgical exposure to organs, tissues, and structures. The surgical principles that apply to open surgery such as hemostasis, dissection, traction and countertraction, suturing, and gentle handling of tissues are also important in laparoscopic surgery. Similarly, the principles that have guided the development of a surgical procedure must be maintained with laparoscopic exposure; otherwise, the operations are not the same. All too often we bend these principles as a result of our own inadequacies, trying to think "open" while operating laparoscopically or just not being able to perform the "open" version of the operation laparoscopically. In general, what is performed open should be performed through the laparoscope, making the procedures identical in technique.

Laparoscopic surgery has the advantage of smaller abdominal incisions with perhaps respectively less abdominal pain and shortened recovery time. Disadvantages are the increased operative time, increased cost, and a steep learning curve in advanced laparoscopic surgery. Operative time and cost may decrease as experience is gained with laparoscopic surgery. It would make sense that before attempting to perform a laparoscopic retropubic procedure, the surgeon should have adequate experience in performing the same procedure through an open surgical exposure.

Patient positioning and preparation are the same as for the abdominal retropubic technique. Entry into the space or Retzius can be accomplished by a transperitoneal or an ex-

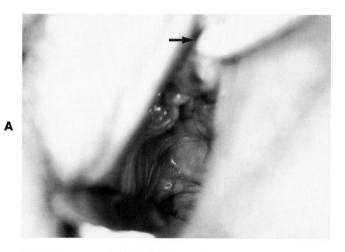

A

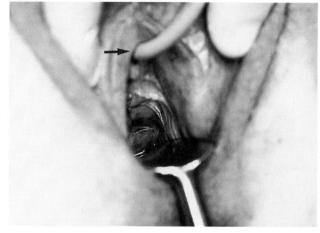

B

Fig. 27-17 **A,** Vaginal view of a repaired right paravaginal defect and a reconstructed right sulcus. *Solid arrow* shows Foley catheter. **B,** Vaginal view of a repaired left paravaginal defect and a reconstructed left sulcus. *Solid arrow* shows Foley catheter and correction of urethral axis.

traperitoneal approach. The choice will be based on surgeon's preference and other surgical indications that require transperitoneal surgery. A contraindication to the extraperitoneal approach using a preperitoneal distention balloon (Origin, Menlo Park, Calif.) is previous retropubic surgery. Also, with the extraperitoneal approach the balloon performs most of the dissection; however, the lack of intraperitoneal exposure significantly restricts surgical working space with instruments and especially suturing. The transperitoneal approach allows the surgeon to evaluate intraabdominal anatomy, permits a significantly larger working area for suturing, and allows concomitant culdeplasty. A disadvantage is that the peritoneal incision must be closed to avoid the small bowel from residing in the space of Retzius. This may be a significant concern if a future sling procedure is ever indicated.

The bladder is catheterized and emptied with a 14-Fr Foley, 10 ml are placed in the Foley bulb, and the end of the Foley is held with a Kelly clamp. The transperitoneal approach begins with creating a pneumoperitoneum, followed by inserting a 10-mm trocar at or below the umbilicus. After

the position of inferior epigastric vessels is evaluated, two additional lateral trocars are placed under direct laparoscopic guidance. Although the choice of trocar diameter is made on the basis of surgeon preference, a 10-mm trocar allows easy passage of the needle thorough the trocar sleeve, translating to efficient surgery and a time savings in the operating room. Essential to avoiding the creation of a cystotomy is the delineation of the bladder under the peritoneum. The bladder is retrograde filled with 300 ml of saline through the Foley. The upper bladder margin is clearly delineated, and using sharp dissection, a transverse incision is made 2 to 3 cm above the bladder reflection between the medial umbilical folds. Dissection with a blunt probe in the same manner as used in the abdominal procedure is performed. After the space of Retzius is developed and the lateral margins of the bladder are delineated, the weight of the full bladder facilitates dissection for a very short period. After this point the Kelly clamp should be released and the bladder emptied. Once the dissection has delineated the pubic symphysis, Cooper's ligament, the obturator internus muscle, the arcus tendineus fascia pelvis, the obturator foramen, and the ischial spine, a vaginal hand is inserted and any further dissection is completed. The ischial spine is palpated, and its position is noted. Bipolar cautery and laparoscopic clip applicators are useful for controlling any bleeding. Suturing is initiated near the ischial spine with 2-0 braided nonabsorbable suture, Ethibond on an SH needle (Ethicon, Somerville, NJ) identical to that used in the abdominal approach. A laparoscopic needle holder and an extracorporeal knot pusher are essential. Once all the sutures are tied extracorporeally, irrigation is performed, and if a Burch urethropexy is not performed, the space of Retzius is closed with interrupted sutures or staples.

The extraperitoneal approach requires a dissecting balloon (Preperitoneal Distention Balloon System, Origin, Menlo Park, Calif.) dissector. An infraumbilical incision is made to expose the subcutaneous tissues and the anterior rectus sheath. A 1.5-cm transverse incision is made in the rectus sheath just lateral to the midline, and the rectus muscle is retracted, exposing the posterior rectus sheath. The lubricated trocar and balloon assembly are inserted between the rectus muscle and the posterior rectus sheath. This is advanced in the midline inferiorly to the pubic symphysis. Under direct endoscopic visualization, the balloon is inflated and the retropubic space is dissected. The balloon and trocar are removed and replaced with a structural sealing balloon (Structural Balloon Trocar, Origin, Menlo Park, Calif.) designed with inflatable balloons on the sleeve to decrease carbon dioxide loss. The retropubic anatomy is further developed, and two additional trocar ports are placed under direct vision lateral to the inferior epigastric vessels. The operating surgeon places a finger in the vagina and elevates the vaginal wall to facilitate suturing. The principles of the laparoscopic repair are the same as those for the abdominal and vaginal approaches. The laparoscopic method is the same as that for the abdominal retropubic paravaginal defect repair. Suture entanglement is at times frustrating if the sutures are held and not tied immediately after placement. The transperitoneal approach allows the sutures to be placed over the bowel, and alternating between green and white sutures decreases confusion.

SUMMARY

There are several approaches to repairing lateral defects. One must keep in mind that paravaginal defects are only a portion of the entire reconstructive procedure. For the patient to have a durable and long-term result, all of the defects must be repaired. Until data on preoperative and postoperative urodynamic testing are available, the best indication for paravaginal defect repair is for the correction of lateral vaginal detachment.

SUGGESTED READINGS

Baden WF, Walker T: Evaluation of uterovaginal support. In Baden WF, Walker T, editors: *Surgical repair of vaginal defects,* Philadelphia, 1992, JB Lippincott.

Bonney V: On diurnal incontinence of urine in women, *J Obstet Gynaecol Br Emp* 30:358, 1923.

Burch JC: Urethrovaginal fixation to Cooper's ligament for correction of stress incontinence, cystocele, and prolapse, *Am J Obstet Gynecol* 81:281, 1961.

DeLancey JOL: Corrective study of paraurethral anatomy, *Obstet Gynecol* 68:91, 1986.

DeLancey JOL: Anatomic aspects of vaginal eversion after hysterectomy, *Am J Obstet Gynecol* 166:1717, 1992.

DeLancey JOL: Structural support of the urethra as it relates to stress urinary incontinence: the hammock hypothesis, *Am J Obstet Gynecol* 170:1713, 1994.

Kelly HA: Incontinence of urine in women, *Urol Cut Rev* 17:291, 1913.

Groves WHE: A new operation for the cure of vaginal cystocele, *Lons Obstet Soc Trans* 17:65, 1905.

Reiffenstuhl G: The clinical significance of the connective tissue planes and spaces, *Clin Obstet Gynecol* 25:811, 1982.

Richardson AC: How to correct prolapse paravaginally, *Contemp OB/GYN* 35:100, 1990.

Richardson AC, Edmonds PB, Williams NL: Treatment of stress urinary incontinence due to paravaginal fascial defect, *Obstet Gynecol* 57:357, 1981.

Richardson AC, Lyon JB, Williams NL: A new look at pelvic relaxation, *Am J Obstet Gynecol* 126:568, 1976.

Shull BL: How I do abdominal paravaginal repair, *J Pelvic Surg* 1:43, 1995.

Shull BL, Baden WF: A six-year experience with paravaginal defect repair for stress urinary incontinence, *Am J Obstet Gynecol* 160:1432, 1989.

Shull BL, Benn SJ, Kuehl TJ: Surgical management of prolapse of the anterior vaginal segment: an analysis of support defects, operative morbidity, and anatomic outcome, *Am J Obstet Gynecol* 171:1429, 1994.

Shull BL, et al: Preoperative and postoperative analysis of site-specific pelvic support defects in 81 women treated with sacrospinous ligament suspension and pelvic reconstruction, *Am J Obstet Gynecol* 166:1764, 1992.

Von Peham H, Amreich J: *Operative gynecology,* Philadelphia, 1934, JB Lippincott (Translated by LK Ferguson).

White GR: Cystocele: a radical cure by suturing lateral sulci of vagina to white line of the pelvic fascia, *JAMA* 53:1707, 1909.

White GR: An anatomic operation for the cure of cystocele, *Am J Obstet Dis Wom Child* 65:286, 1912.

28 Repair of Rectal Fistula and of Old Complete Perineal Laceration

DAVID H. NICHOLS

RECTAL FISTULA

Although occasionally congenital in origin,[41] the rectovaginal fistula seen in the developed countries of the world usually is the aftermath of trauma—either unrecognized or unrepaired, or inadequately and unsuccessfully repaired. Other causes of a rectovaginal fistula include the following:

Suture penetration of the rectal mucosa during episiotomy repair or perineorrhaphy

Crohn's disease

Infection and necrosis of a vaginal hematoma from hysterectomy, perineorrhaphy, or posterior colporrhaphy

Pelvic irradiation, particularly after trauma to the vagina in the presence of endarteritis obliterans

Growth of residual or recurrent cancer

A rectovaginal fistula may occur at any level within the vagina, but it occurs most commonly in the lower third, generally at the apex of an improperly healed repair of a fourth-degree perineal laceration caused by obstetric trauma. Difficulty expelling the fecal bolus with the first bowel movement after the repair may have caused the patient to strain excessively, thus compromising the repair at its weakest spot. Even though the surgeon may have approximated the tissue properly, such strain may result in a breakdown of the initial repair cranial to the perineal body, often between the fifth and tenth day after surgery. The liberal use of stool softeners and a low-residue diet for a few weeks postoperatively may prevent this complication.[17,33] Hauth et al.[17] have recommended early re-repair of rectal mucosal and anal sphincter dehiscence after an unsuccessful repair, but their patients all required a minimum of 10 days of hospitalization postoperatively, during which they were maintained on an initial "diet" of nothing by mouth followed by a no-residue diet for an additional week.

Fistulas may be single or multiple. Moreover, a single fistula may have several connecting tracts that communicate with one another within the subepithelial tissues, occasionally originating from several openings into the rectal lumen. Less commonly, a single opening in the rectal mucosa may communicate with several fistulous openings in the vagina and perineal skin. The relationship of a fistulous tract or tracts to the external anal sphincter is of paramount importance in planning surgical repair.

Observing the following principles in the management of rectovaginal fistula ensures the probability of successful surgical treatment:

1. At the time of fistula repair, granulation tissue, infection, and edema should be minimal.

2. The repair must interrupt the continuity of the fistula.

3. The repair need not involve levator plication, with its associated risk of dyspareunia, but the operator should interpose a layer of fresh tissue with an independent blood supply between the layers of repair, if possible, particularly with postirradiation fistulas.

4. The epithelialized fistulous tract should be excised, and the edges should be inverted into the lumen when possible.

5. Closure of the tissues of each organ using two suture layers, usually in a transverse axis, is advisable, because a second layer removes much of the tension from the suture line of the first layer.

6. The vaginal side of the fistula may be left open for drainage. When a rubber drain is used, it should be left in place for 2 to 7 days. The appropriate time for removal depends on how large the fistula was, how much drainage there is likely to be, and whether an abscess was encountered during the procedure.

Before repair, a relative degree of constipation provides reasonable fecal continence, but the patient usually is unable to control flatus. It is, in fact, the inability to prevent the involuntary loss of flatus that may first make the patient aware of the fistula and often accounts for her decision to seek surgical repair. While awaiting surgery, patients can use several simple techniques to reduce the quantity of flatus, much of which is related to unabsorbed nitrogen ingested with swallowed air. For example, not talking when having a mouthful of food, chewing food well, eating slowly without gulping, and finishing and swallowing one mouthful before taking another often reduce considerably the amount of air swallowed and thus the amount of gas that is likely to be expelled.

Diagnosis of Rectovaginal Fistula

Although some rectovaginal fistulas are asymptomatic, most are not. Incontinence of rectal gas or of liquid or solid stool when the perineum is intact and the external anal sphincter is functional suggests the presence of a fistula. When contaminants pass through the vagina, the bacterial concentration may precipitate chronic or recurrent vaginitis. The patient may experience dyspareunia when infection and fibrosis are present.

If the patient passes liquid stool through the fistula while passing solid stool through the rectum, a gastrointestinal-vaginal fistula in the upper vagina may have arisen from small bowel. The surgeon also should consider such a pos-

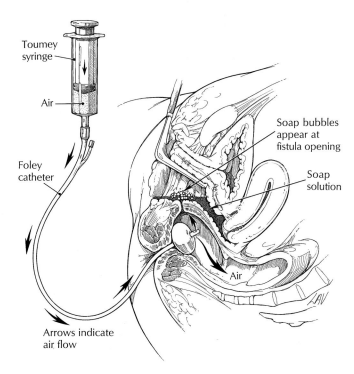

Fig. 28-1   Air bubble test for small rectovaginal fistula. The examining table is placed in the Trendelenburg position and a Foley catheter inserted into the rectum. The vagina is filled with mildly soapy water, and air is injected into the catheter. The appearance of soap bubbles in the vagina indicates the presence of a small rectovaginal fistula. (From Nichols DH, Randall CL: *Vaginal surgery,* ed 4, Baltimore, 1996, Williams & Wilkins.)

sibility if the vagina and vulva are excoriated, as may result from contact of the skin with digestive enzymes of the small intestine.

Diverticulosis. Intestinal diverticulosis may be suspected from the patient's history. Perforation of a diverticular abscess into the uterus may give rise to a ureterocolic fistula, or into the vagina, a colovaginal fistula. These are generally found at the vaginal vault. The diagnosis is confirmed by barium enema and sigmoidoscopy or colonoscopy or by retrograde vaginal fistulogram using water-soluble dye[49] infused under gravity pressure through a transrectal Foley catheter, the bulb inflated with air instead of liquid to improve radiovisibility. Surgery is generally by transabdominal route, with dissection of colon from vagina and primary fistulectomy with closure; however, if inflammation and abscess are noted, primary bowel resection and anastomosis are performed.[15]

Finding a Pinhole-Sized Fistula. When it is difficult to demonstrate a suspected pinhole-sized rectovaginal fistula, its specific site may be determined by filling the vagina of the recumbent patient with warm water or soapy water sufficient to cover the expected site of the fistula, placing a Foley catheter with a 10-ml bulb into the rectum, and instilling air through the catheter. A stream of air bubbles coming through the vaginal water pool indicates the site of the fistula through which a blunt probe can be placed (Fig. 28-1). If the vagina will not contain

the soapy water, the site of the fistula can be determined by instilling milk or a concentrated solution containing methylene blue or indigo carmine into the rectal Foley catheter and watching where it appears on the posterior vaginal wall. In seeking radiographic demonstration of the tract of a small rectovaginal fistula, one can inject a mixture of barium, mashed potato mix, and water into the rectum using a caulking gun. A lateral radiograph is taken while the patient bears down.

Surgical repair should be considered when a fistula has caused troublesome symptoms and when local edema and inflammation have subsided (usually coincident with relief of pain).

Preparation for Surgery

Because the standard antibiotic erythromycin-neomycin bowel preparation (1 g of each by mouth at 1:00, 2:00, and 11:00 PM the day before the operation)[34] is associated with a high incidence of troublesome gastrointestinal side effects, an alternative is to administer cefoxitin sodium (Mefoxin). An initial 2-g dose of cefoxitin should be given intravenously when the patient is on call to the operating room; another 2-g dose should be given 2 hours later, during surgery or in the recovery room if surgery is completed in less than 2 hours from the initial dose; and a third 2-g dose may be given 6 to 8 hours later. As Menaker[28] has stated, however, "systemic antibiotics administered preoperatively and for a

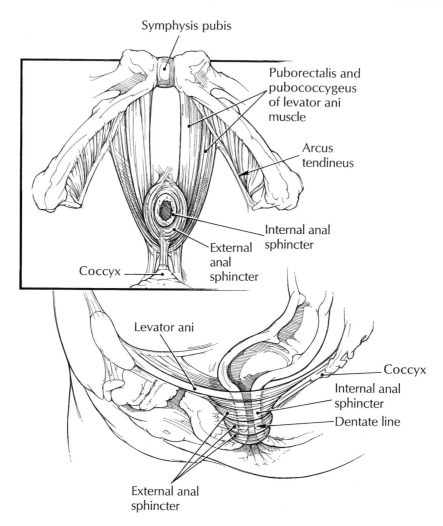

Fig. 28-2 Phantom drawings showing the anatomy of the puborectalis, pubococcygeus, and anal sphincter muscles. The relationships of the muscles to the rectum are shown in both frontal and sagittal views. The internal sphincter is a caudal continuation of the smooth muscle of the rectum and may be repaired by freshening and reuniting the torn rectal wall. (From Nichols DH, Randall CL: *Vaginal surgery,* ed 4, Baltimore, 1996, Williams & Wilkins.)

short perioperative interval . . . have little effect on intestinal colonization . . . antibiotics are not indicated merely to cover breaks in the operative technique." But Hibbard[18] has reported increased surgical success when antibiotic coverage is provided.

The patient should take only clear liquids by mouth for 2 days before admission to the hospital.

As part of the bowel preparation for surgery, drinking 3 or 4 L of chilled polyethylene glycol (PEG) 3350 electrolyte solution (NuLYTELY, GoLYTELY, Colyte)[3] the morning of the day before surgery, followed by two bisacodyl (Dulcolax) tablets to eliminate retained excess water in the bowel, usually is a more effective cleanser than preoperative enemas, because the incontinent patient usually cannot retain the latter. As an alternative, a half bottle of citrate of magnesia or two bisacodyl tablets are given the afternoon before admission. Two packaged (Fleet) enemas should be administered an hour apart the day before surgery; on the morning

of surgery, plain water or saline enemas should be administered until the return is clear.

Surgical Procedure

The gynecologic surgeon must consider several factors in choosing the most appropriate surgical procedure for a patient with a rectovaginal fistula. Foremost among these is the location of the fistula (lower, middle, or upper third of the vagina). Second is the cause of the fistula (trauma, postirradiation, postsurgery, postepisiotomy, Crohn's disease, active malignant disease). Additional considerations are the patient's age, the need for preserving or restoring coital function of the vagina, the presence or absence of a perineal body, and the integrity of the exterior anal sphincter.[42] As for all reconstructive surgery, the goals are to relieve the symptoms and to restore the anatomy and function to normal. The anatomy of the perineal muscles is shown in Fig. 28-2 and the functional anatomy in Fig. 28-3.

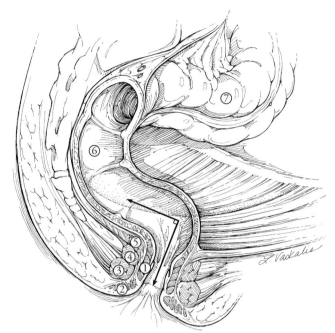

Structure	Function
1. Internal Anal Sphincter	*Tonic contraction (passive barrier)*
2. Subcutaneous Portion of External Anal Sphincter	*Active contraction (active barrier)*
3. Superficial Portion of External Anal Sphincter	
4. Deep Portion of External Anal Sphincter	
5. Puborectalis Portion of Levator Ani	*Maintains anorectal angle and active contraction (active barrier)*
6. Rectum	*Compliant reservoir*
7. Sigmoid	*Delays stool progression via contraction*

Fig. 28-3 Functional anatomy of anorectal canal.

The surgeon should be familiar with eight basic operative procedures involving repair of rectovaginal fistula:

1. Closure in layers without disrupting the perineum
2. Closure in layers after episioproctotomy
3. Transperineal mucosal flap transplant dorsal to an intact external sphincter
4. Transperineal mucosal layers and closure ventral to an intact external sphincter
5. Transrectal anterior rectal mucosal flap transplant
6. Noble-Mengert-Fish[29,35] anterior rectal flap operation
7. Transabdominal procedures for a fistula in the vault of an immobile vagina, which, when following radiation, may include temporary transverse colostomy
8. Colpocleisis or colpectomy

The gynecologic surgeon should be capable of performing all these procedures so that a technique or combination of techniques for the surgical treatment of a rectovaginal fistula can be chosen on the basis of what the individual patient needs. An effective surgical combination must be thoughtfully planned and carefully executed for each patient.

The gynecologic surgeon should perform a fistula repair only when there is no abscess, because an infection seriously impedes the quality of wound healing. When an abscess is unexpectedly encountered during surgery in the tissues between the rectum and the vagina, the operator must modify the intended procedure and perform a simple unroofing operation in which the full thickness of the vaginal wall overlying the abscess is widely excised. This permits immediate and adequate drainage. Such a wound granulates in from the bottom up; in some instances, the granulation of the base of the wound closes the communication with the rectum, and no further surgery is necessary.

When it is necessary to repair coexistent rectovaginal and vesicovaginal fistulas, the vesicovaginal fistula should be repaired first, or else postoperative scarring from the rectovaginal fistula repair may compromise the operative exposure. If the vesicorectovaginal fistula followed pelvic irradiation, usually the surgeon should perform a preliminary diverting transverse colostomy, followed in 2 or 3 months by repair of the vesicovaginal fistula in the usual manner, then repair of the rectovaginal fistula 2 months later, which may at times involve a colpocleisis, followed after 2 or 3 additional months by closure of the colostomy.

Rectovaginal fistulas resulting from an earlier obstetric trauma may be closed at the time of a subsequent delivery by episioproctorrhaphy. The excellent blood supply and laxity of the perineal muscles during pregnancy encourage healing. The operator makes a fresh incision to perform an episioproctotomy, "recreating" a fourth-degree laceration, excises the fistulous tract and scar tissue, and repairs the wound as if it were a new injury. In a nonpregnant patient, however, episioproctorrhaphy in the treatment of rectovaginal fistula may lead to postoperative infection with abscess formation that can destroy the integrity of the perineal body and external anal sphincter. Even without tissue destruction in abscess formation, infection in this area may initiate chronic painful inflammation, edema, and spasm of the pubococcygeal portion of the levator ani muscle, giving rise to the "levator syndrome" of levator spasm pain and tenderness that is so resistant to effective treatment.

In most cases, proctoscopy should precede rectovaginal or rectoperineal fistula repair. Occasionally it is difficult to demonstrate the rectal opening of the fistula, except by gentle probing while the patient is under anesthesia. When the fistula is not demonstrable with certainty, traction with an Allis clamp applied to the external secondary opening, as described by Bacon and Ross,[2] usually produces dimpling at the primary opening, which is often in an anal crypt. If visualization is still unclear, the surgeon may inject the fistulous tract with methylene blue, using a no. 18, 19, or 20 needle that has been cut off approximately 1 cm from its hub. Through an anoscope, the surgeon then looks for the blue dye as it comes through the rectum, as well as for branches of the fistula.[40]

As Corman[8] noted, genital fistulas have a high-pressure side and a low-pressure side. In the presence of a symptomatic fistula, the flow of material from a hollow viscus is always from the high-pressure side to the low-pressure side. With a rectovaginal fistula, the rectum is the high-pressure side and the vagina is the low-pressure side. Material flows from the rectum into the vagina, not from the vagina into the rectum. Primary attention must be given to secure and effective closure of the high-pressure side. Even if unattended, the low-pressure side (the vagina) generally closes spontaneously once the continuity of the fistula has been interrupted and the high-pressure side has been closed. Excising the epithelium that lines the vaginal fistulous opening and loosely approximating the sides of the vaginal defect (with the stitches far enough apart to permit postoperative drainage, if any) strengthens and hastens restoration of vaginal continuity over the rectum, however.

Because of the high vascularity of the pelvis, meticulous hemostasis in the area of fistula repair is essential to improve wound healing and reduce the chances of hematoma and abscess formation. Infiltration of up to 50 ml of a "liquid tourniquet" (e.g., 0.5 % lidocaine in 1:200,000 epinephrine solution) is helpful, although the surgeon may substitute phenylephrine hydrochloride (Neo-Synephrine), vasopressin (Pitressin), or saline solution in patients who have severe hypertension or coronary heart disease.

Effect of Location

Lower Third of the Vagina. Because of the almost complete absence of levator muscle anterior to the rectum and the proximity of an infected anterior anal crypt, the anterior anorectal canal is especially vulnerable to injury.[43] Stern et al.[46] have demonstrated that rectovaginal fistulas low in the vagina can be repaired using either a transvaginal or transanal approach. An endorectal approach permits simultaneous correction of coincident anorectal pathology, and, by leaving the vaginal defect open for drainage, postoperative infection is minimized, as is painful subvaginal scarring.

For the patient with an intact perineum, an intact external anal sphincter, and a fistula in the lower third of the vagina, the transperineal rectal flap sliding operation is appropriate. It does not disturb the perineal body, but does permit plication of an intact, although lax, external anal sphincter, if desired.

Episioproctotomy. Episioproctotomy permits excision of the entire fistulous tract followed by repair similar to that of a fresh fourth-degree perineal laceration (Fig. 28-4). The technique is generally simple to perform, but because it re-

quires transection and reunification of the three divisions of the external anal sphincter and of the lower part of the internal sphincter, there is a risk of recurrence as well as anal incontinence should healing be imperfect, compounding the original problem and requiring more sophisticated future reoperation.

Transperineal Rectal Flap Sliding Technique. A sliding rectal flap procedure, such as that described with the Noble-Mengert-Fish operation,[29,35] permits the mobilization and the excision of the portion of the anterior rectal wall that includes the fistula. If the external anal sphincter has been lacerated, its severed ends can be reunified and a perineal body constructed (Fig. 28-5).

Middle Third of the Vagina

Layered Closure. When the fistula is in the midvagina and the external anal sphincter and perineal body are intact, a layered closure is useful. The operator incises the full thickness of the vaginal wall (Fig. 28-6, *A*, p. 528) entering the rectovaginal space, and carefully separates the rectum from the vagina. Transecting the fistulous tract (see Fig. 28-6, *B*, p. 528), the operator excises the rectal tract in its entirety (see Fig. 28-6, *C*, p. 528). Two layers of submucosal interrupted size 3-0 polyglycolic acid–type mattress sutures, placed 2 or 3 mm apart in the rectal wall, are used to close the rectal wall (see Fig. 28-6, *D*, p. 529). These may be placed transversely or, if there is no risk of compromising the rectal lumen (see Fig. 28-6, *E*, p. 529), longitudinally in the muscular wall of the rectum,[25] depending on available exposure. A second layer not only reinforces the first, but also takes some of the tension from the first layer of closure.

The operator excises the epithelialized tract through the wall of the vagina and loosely approximates the opening in a longitudinal direction by interrupted sutures of polyglycolic acid (see Fig. 28-6, *F*, p. 529) placed at least 1 cm apart to allow for adequate postoperative drainage.

Alternatively, after irrigating the wound, the operator may split the posterior vaginal vault (Fig. 28-7, p. 530) and interpose a layer of rectovaginal septum from side to side; the edges of the vaginal incision are freshened and made symmetric, and the vagina is closed with interrupted sutures. When the operator has decided to use a layered closure after the excision of the epithelialized fistulous tract has created a fresh third-degree laceration and little other tissue is available for this use, the interposition of some "levator" stitches between the rectum and vagina, placed without palpable ridges, increases the thickness of the perineum and insulates the site of the fistula repair on the rectal side from that on the vaginal side.

Transverse Transperineal Repair. When the fistula is in the midvagina and the perineal body and external anal sphincter are intact, the transverse transperineal repair, which involves a transverse perineal incision, is also useful.[14,44] A failed Noble-Mengert-Fish operation can be an indication for the Thompson rectoperineoplasty[33,40] because this will avoid repeated and excessive stretching of the anterior rectal wall, which might compromise not only its

Text continued on p. 533

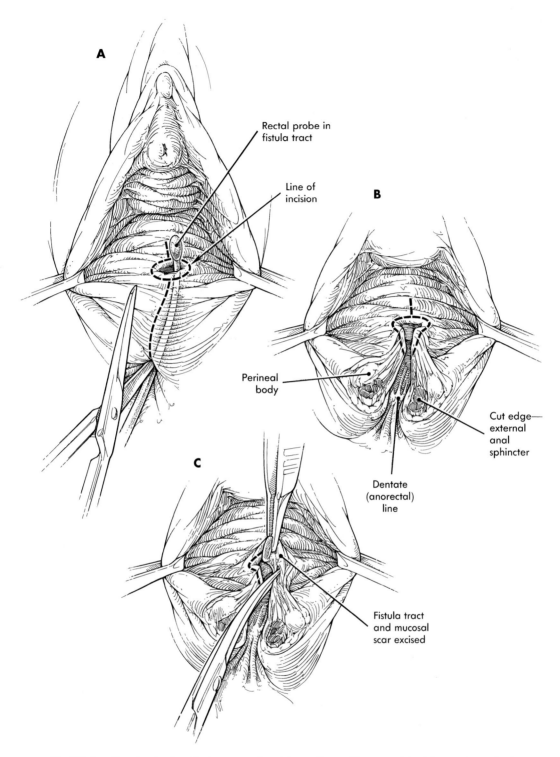

**Rectal probe in
fistula tract**

**Line of
incision**

A

B

**Perineal
body**

**Cut edge—
external
anal
sphincter**

**Dentate
(anorectal)
line**

C

**Fistula tract
and mucosal
scar excised**

Fig. 28-4   Repair of a fourth-degree perineal laceration with a coexistent low rectovaginal fistula. **A,** A malleable probe is inserted through the fistula tract. **B,** An incision along this probe exposes the tissue. **B** and **C,** The fistula tract is excised along the site of the *dashed line.*

Continued

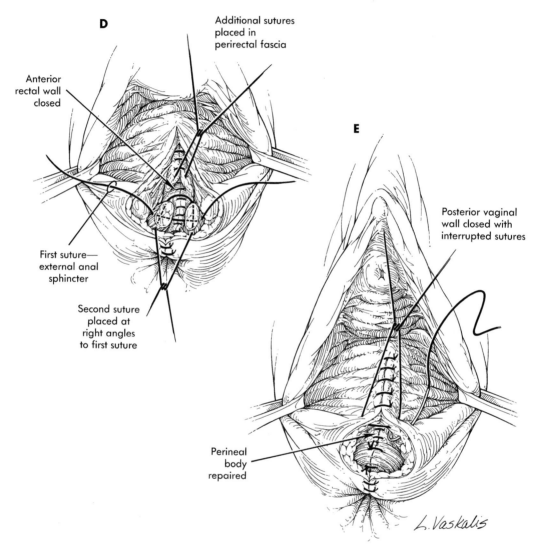

Fig. 28-4, cont'd   D, The submucosa and muscularis of the anterior rectal wall are closed with interrupted sutures, and this is inverted by an additional layer of sutures placed in the perirectal fascia. The edges of the external anal sphincter are dissected out and the scar tissue around their severed ends is reapproximated with two interrupted sutures placed at right angles to one another. **E,** The full thickness of the posterior vaginal wall is closed with interrupted sutures, and the perineal body is restored by a few interrupted stitches.

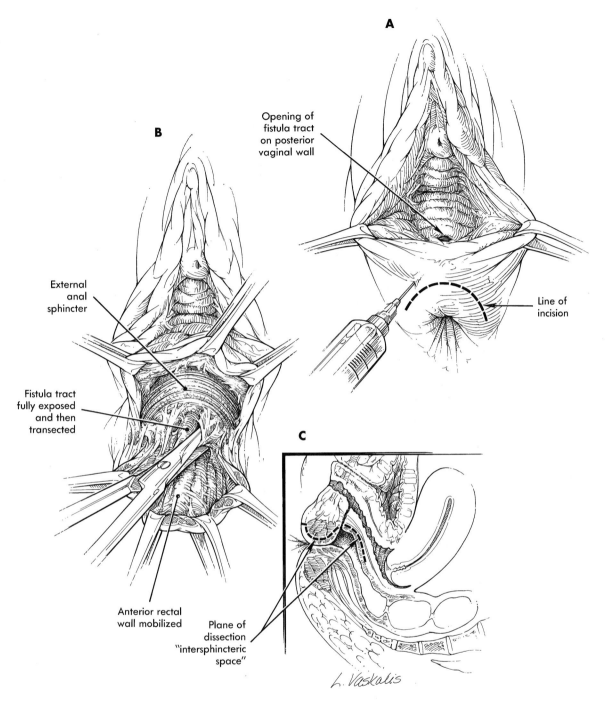

Fig. 28-5 Transperineal flap sliding technique for repair of rectovaginal fistula. **A,** The site of the fistula is shown, and the perineum and perineal body are thoroughly infiltrated by 1:200,000 epinephrine in 0.5% lidocaine. A semilunar incision is made around the anus, posterior to the external anal sphincter along the course of the *dashed line.* **B,** Allis clamps grasp the edges of the incision, and by gentle traction to those placed on the anterior portion of anus, the dissection proceeds beneath the capsule of the external anal sphincter into the intersphincteric space. The fistula tract is fully exposed as the anterior rectal wall is mobilized, and the tract is then transected. **C,** The path of dissection beneath the external anal sphincter and into the intersphincteric space. Traction to the anterior rectal wall and dissection.

Continued

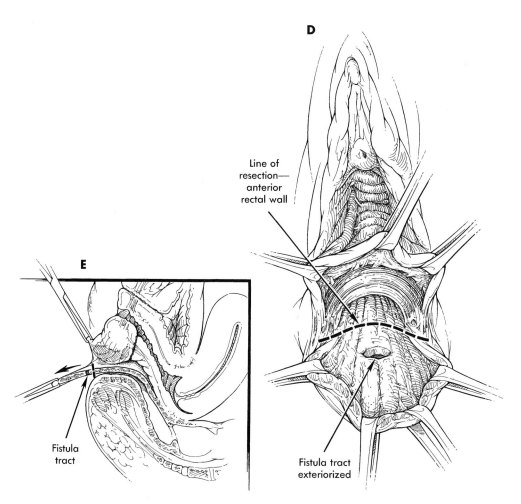

D

Line of
resection—
anterior
rectal wall

Fistula tract
exteriorized

E

Fistula
tract

Fig. 28-5, cont'd   D, Continued opening and dissection of the rectovaginal space, and gentle
traction to the anterior rectal wall exteriorizes the fistula. **E,** The anterior rectal wall including
the fistula is excised along the path of the *dashed line.*

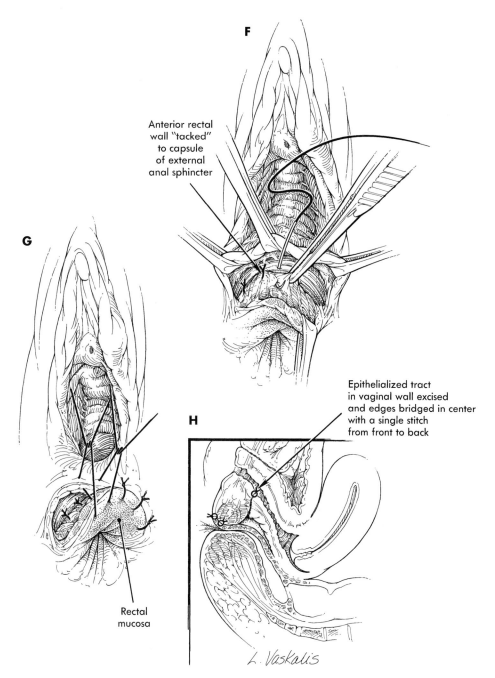

F

Anterior rectal
wall "tacked"
to capsule
of external
anal sphincter

G

Epithelialized tract
in vaginal wall excised
and edges bridged in center
with a single stitch
from front to back

H

Rectal
mucosa

L. Vaskalis

Fig. 28-5, cont'd   F, The anterior rectal wall is "tacked" to the capsule of the external anal sphincter. **G,** A second layer of interrupted PGA suture fixes the cut margin of the anterior rectal wall to the skin of the perineum. **H,** Sagittal section of the placement of these sutures; the epithelialized tract in the posterior vaginal wall is excised and the edges bridged in the center of the opening with a single stitch placed front to back.

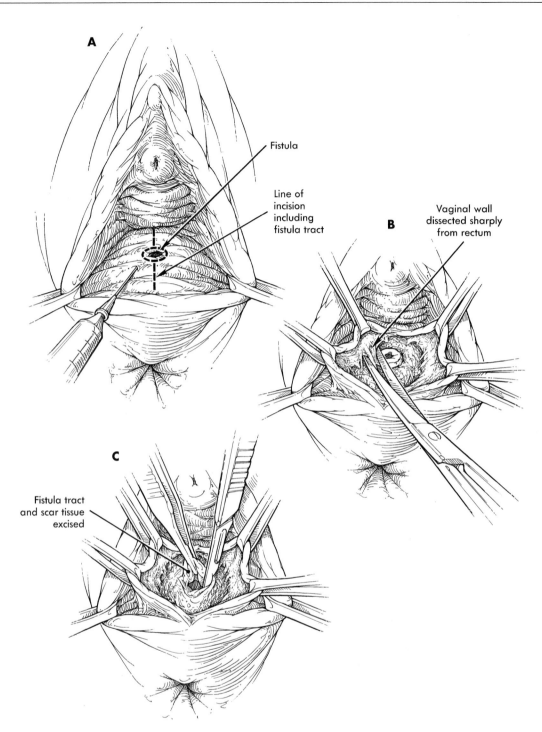

Fig. 28-6   Layered closure of a midvaginal rectovaginal fistula. **A,** The tissues around the site of the fistula are thoroughly infiltrated by 1:200,000 epinephrine in 0.5% lidocaine, and an incision is made along the path indicated by the *dashed line.* This incision circumscribes the tract of the fistula. **B,** The cut edges of the vagina are grasped by Allis clamps and sharply dissected from the anterior rectal wall. **C,** The fistula tract in its entirety is excised along with its surrounding scar tissue.

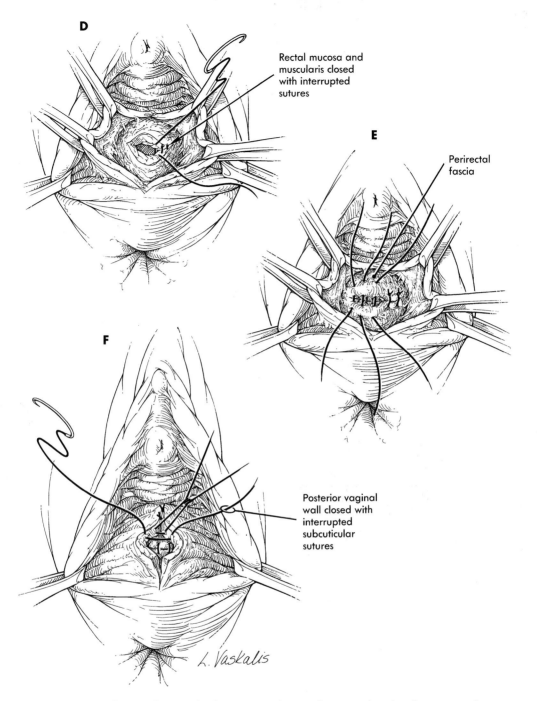

Rectal mucosa and
muscularis closed
with interrupted
sutures

Perirectal
fascia

Posterior vaginal
wall closed with
interrupted
subcuticular
sutures

L. Vaskalis

Fig. 28-6, cont'd   D, The rectal submucosa and muscularis are closed with interrupted sutures. **E,** The suture line is buried by a second layer of interrupted sutures in the muscularis and perirectal fascia. **F,** The wound may be thoroughly irrigated with sterile saline solution, and the posterior vaginal wall closed longitudinally and at right angles to the repair in the rectal wall using interrupted subcuticular sutures in the fibromuscular wall of the vagina.

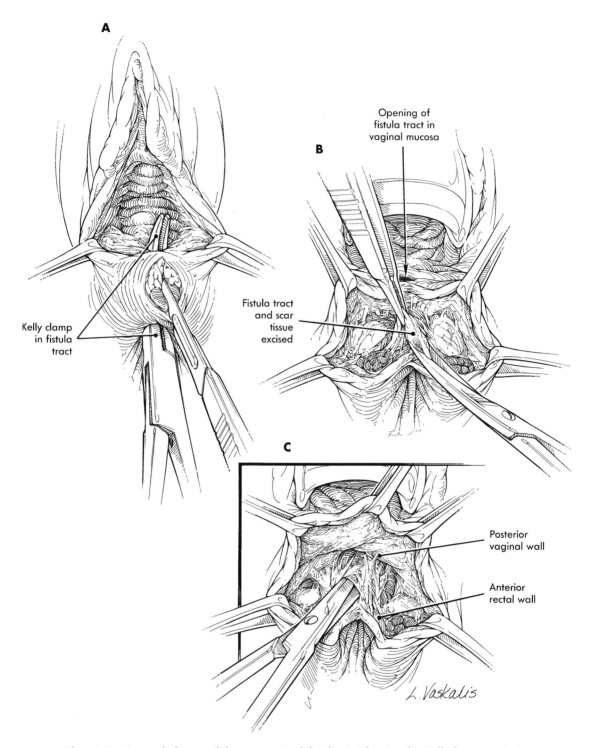

A

B

Opening of
fistula tract in
vaginal mucosa

Fistula tract
and scar
tissue
excised

Kelly clamp
in fistula
tract

C

Posterior
vaginal wall

Anterior
rectal wall

L. Vaskalis

Fig. 28-7   Layered closure of the rectovaginal fistula. **A,** The tip of a Kelly hemostat is inserted through the fistula tract and an incision made through the perineal body and internal sphincter. **B,** The entire fistula tract and scar tissue are excised. **C,** The anterior rectal wall is separated from the under surface of the posterior vaginal wall by sharp dissection.

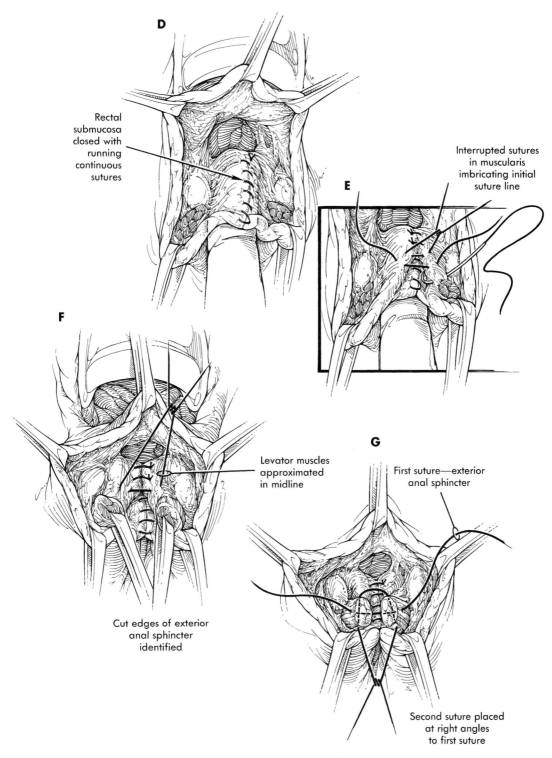

Rectal submucosa closed with running continuous sutures

Interrupted sutures in muscularis imbricating initial suture line

Levator muscles approximated in midline

First suture—exterior anal sphincter

Cut edges of exterior anal sphincter identified

Second suture placed at right angles to first suture

Fig. 28-7, cont'd   D, The freshened edges of the rectal submucosa are brought together with running continuous sutures placed in the submucosa. **E,** This is covered by a second layer of interrupted sutures in the muscularis of the rectum (internal anal sphincter), imbricating the initial suture line. **F,** The medial surfaces of the levator ani are approximated with interrupted sutures, and the cut edges of the external anal sphincter are identified and grasped with Allis clamps. **G,** The superficial external anal sphincter muscle is reapproximated with two interrupted sutures placed at right angles to each other.   *Continued*

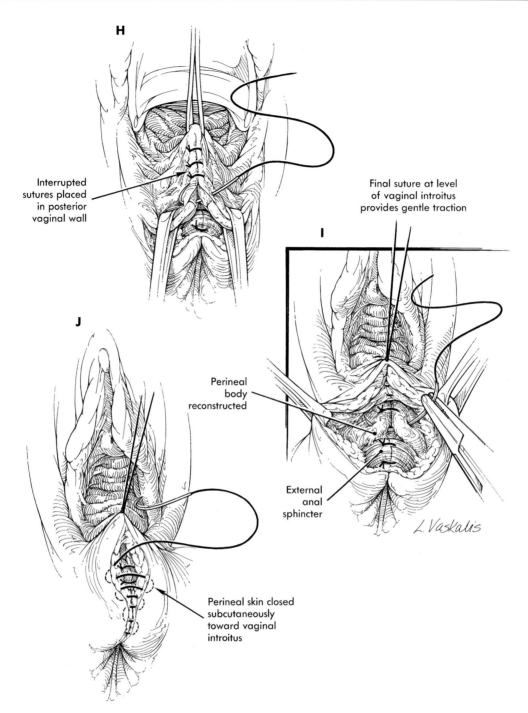

Fig. 28-7, cont'd   H, The freshened edges of the posterior vaginal wall are approximated by interrupted sutures. **I,** Upward traction to the lowermost of these sutures in the vaginal wall exposes the tissues from which the perineal body will be constructed; these are approximated with interrupted sutures. This takes much of the tension from the stitches placed within the external anal sphincter. **J,** The wound may be thoroughly irrigated with saline solution, and the perineal skin closed subcutaneously.

healing but also its effective function. In this procedure (Fig. 28-8), the operator injects the perineum, makes a transverse perineal incision, and then dissects beneath the posterior vaginal wall ventral or anterior to the external anal sphincter and enters the rectovaginal space. The passage of a malleable probe facilitates the identification of the fistula during dissection of the vaginal wall. After separating the rectum from the vagina, first laterally, then cranially to the fistula, the operator transects the fistula at its central portion. The transected fistula and the epithelialized tract are excised from both the rectal and vaginal walls.

The operator closes the rectal defect transversely with

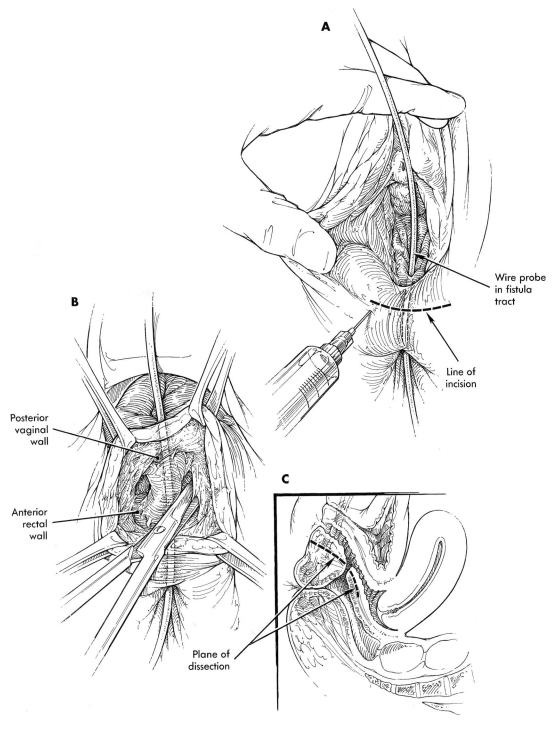

Fig. 28-8   Transperineal sphincter-sparing repair of rectovaginal fistula. **A,** A malleable probe has been inserted through the tract of the fistula, and the area to be dissected is thoroughly infiltrated by a solution of 1:200,000 epinephrine in 0.5% lidocaine. The perineum is incised transversely as shown. **B,** The dissection separates the vagina from the perineal body, and by sharp dissection, starting laterally, the entire tract of the fistula is exposed. **C,** The path of dissection.

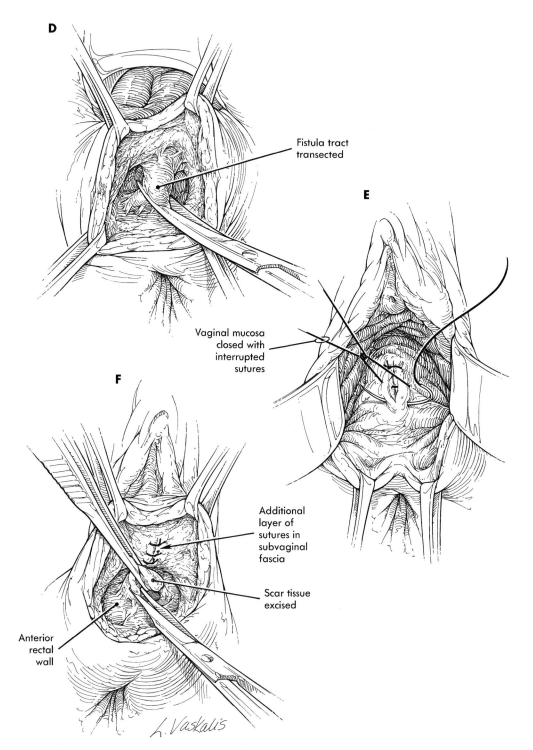

L. Vaskalis

Fig. 28-8, cont'd   D, After the tract has been isolated from the surrounding tissue, it is transected. The Allis clamps attached to the vagina are brought posteriorly, exposing the vaginal surface of the posterior vaginal wall. **E,** After the epithelized tract of the vaginal side of the fistula has been excised, the defect is closed with a few interrupted stitches of polyglycolic acid suture. **F,** The vaginal wall is again retracted anteriorly, and an additional layer of suture is placed in the fibromuscular layer of the vagina on the underside of the posterior vaginal wall. The fistulous tract in the rectum and its surrounding scar tissue are excised. A retractor is inserted into the rectovaginal space to better expose the anterior rectal wall.

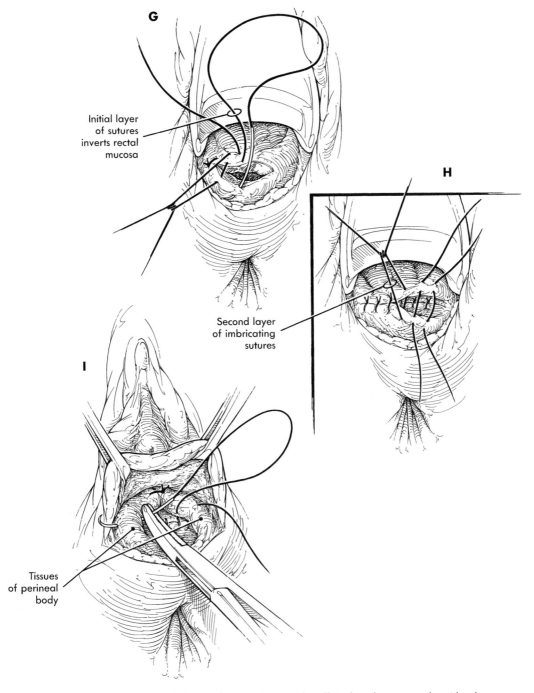

Fig. 28-8, cont'd   G, The defect in the anterior rectal wall is closed transversely with a layer of interrupted PGA sutures that inverts the rectal mucosa. **H,** A second layer of imbricating sutures is placed. **I,** The perirectal tissues and tissues of the perineal body are brought together in the midline by an additional layer of sutures.   *Continued*

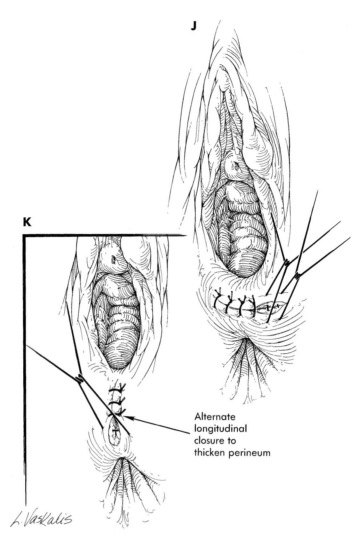

Alternate
longitudinal
closure to
thicken perineum

L. Vaskalis

Fig. 28-8, cont'd   **J,** The edges of the original excision in the perineal skin are brought together by a series of interrupted sutures. **K,** The perineal body can be thickened by closing the
incision from side to side, if desired. .

two layers, one of interrupted submucosal and the other of
intramural sutures, and then closes the vaginal wall longitudinally. A single layer of interrupted sutures may be placed
in the vagina, rather widely apart to permit possible postoperative drainage. The perineal skin may be closed transversely, but the skin and subcutaneous tissue may be approximated in the midline if the perineal body needs to be
lengthened (see Fig. 28-7, *K*).

Transrectal Mucosal Flap Transplant Technique.
When there is considerable fibrosis of the perineum and
transvaginal repair would so reduce the caliber of the vagina
and the size of the perineum that dyspareunia would be certain to follow surgery, an alternative surgical technique is
necessary to preserve the vaginal diameter and the integrity
of the external anal sphincter. One such operation is the
transrectal sliding mucosal flap operation.[12,19,21,33]

In this procedure, the patient is face down in a jackknife
position with small sandbags elevating the hips. The fistula
may be evident, and the operator may explore it from the
rectal side (Fig. 28-9) using a small malleable blunt probe

until the probe is palpable within the vagina. With a Smith
self-retaining retractor and a Sims retractor to provide exposure in the vagina, the rectal circumference of the fistula
may be infiltrated with dilute vasopressin (Pitressin) 0.5 ml
(10 pressor units) in 30 ml of normal saline or 0.5% lidocaine (Xylocaine) in 1:200,000 epinephrine (Adrenalin) solution. The rectal ostium is circumscribed by an incision
placed 0.5 to 1 cm from the margins of the tract (see Fig.
28-9). The operator extends this incision distally onto the
perineum and removes an inverted V-shaped wedge of skin
and subcutaneous tissue to expose the anal sphincter. Deepening the incision to permit the identification of both the internal and external anal sphincters, the operator may partially divide them to remove any tendency toward a ridge or
shelflike effect. The operator identifies the rectovaginal septum close to the posterior wall of the vagina, develops the
rectovaginal space, and mobilizes the anterior rectal wall for
approximately 3 cm above the site of the fistula. At this
point in the procedure, the operator places a figure-of-eight
suture through the rectal opening of the fistula and ties it to

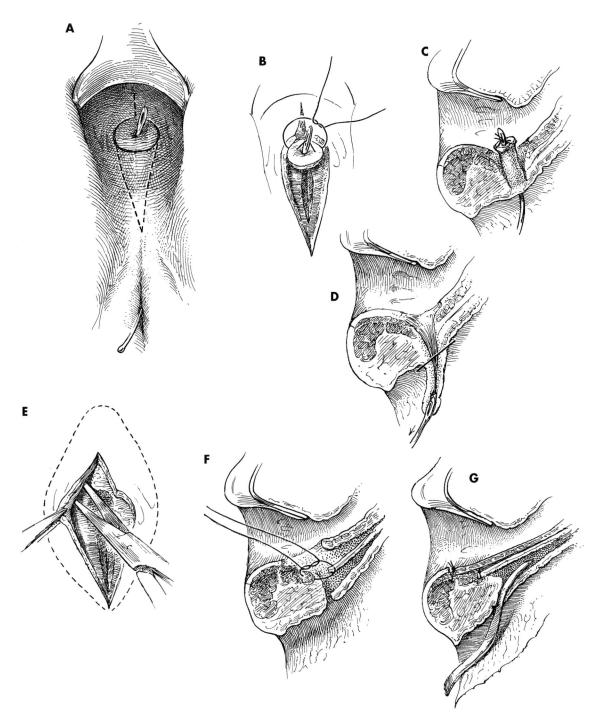

Fig. 28-9 The transrectal mucosal flap transplant. **A,** With the patient face down and in a jackknife position, the posterior metal wall is displaced by a retractor, and the fistula is explored from the rectal side by a small malleable probe. The rectal circumference of the fistula is infiltrated by 0.5% lidocaine in 1:200,000 epinephrine solution and the opening circumscribed by an incision placed 1 cm from the margin. This incision is extended distally onto the perineum, and a **V**-shaped wedge of epithelium is excised as indicated by the *dashed line.* **B,** Sufficient superficial fibers of the rectal side of the anal sphincter are incised to remove this as a postoperative obstruction to the passage of stool and gas, and the mobilized rectal opening of the fistula is sewn to the eye of the malleable probe. This is shown in sagittal section in **C. D,** Traction on the vaginal end of the probe is applied, inverting the fistulous tract into the vagina, where it is excised as indicated by the *dashed line.* **E,** The anterior rectal wall is separated from the vagina for about 2 cm. **F,** A series of interrupted sutures fixes the rectal wall to the internal anal sphincter. **G,** Another layer of sutures sews the mucosal edge of the anterior rectal wall to the posterior surface of the external sphincter. A small drain may be placed through the vaginal opening at the site of the previous fistula and fixed in place with a single absorbable stitch. (Modified from Nichols DH, Randall CL: *Vaginal surgery,* ed 4, Baltimore, 1996, Williams & Wilkins.)

the needle eye of the blunt probe. Traction on the probe from the vaginal side inverts the fistulous tract into the vagina, where the operator cuts it off flush with the vaginal skin. A series of interrupted 2-0 absorbable polyglycolic sutures is used to fix the rectal muscularis to the cranial edge of the external anal sphincter, and another layer of sutures is used to fix the mucosal edge of the anterior rectal wall to the posterior surface of the external anal sphincter. A small Malecot or Penrose drain may be placed through the vaginal opening at the site of the previous fistulous tract, sewn in place with a single absorbable suture, and the anal canal is lightly packed with a plug of petroleum jelly gauze. An indwelling Foley catheter is inserted into the bladder.

For primary repair of rectovaginal fistulas, Hibbard[18] has recommended proctotomy. However, for secondary repair of a layered closure and for a fistula high in the vagina or for a larger fistula, Hibbard[14] has recommended bringing in a separate and fresh blood supply to this area by performing a bulbocavernosus fat pad transplant (Martius graft).[18,20,44]

Upper Third of the Vagina. Fresh and unepithelialized fistulas in the upper third of the vagina, which usually are the result of postoperative pelvic abscess after hysterectomy, may close spontaneously if the patient follows a no-residue, elemental diet with clear liquids for several weeks to inactivate the lower bowel. Several weeks of local estrogen therapy are beneficial to wound healing, even preoperatively, if the patient is postmenopausal. Of the vault fistulas that do not close spontaneously, the small ones may be closed transvaginally by a Latzko partial colpocleisis. Laparotomy may be necessary to close larger fistulas, however.

After bowel preparation, the operator separates the rectum and the upper vagina by sharp dissection. After excision of the epithelialized margins, the rectal opening is closed transversely in two layers; the vaginal opening is closed longitudinally in one layer. The operator covers the site of each closure with a layer of mobilized peritoneum. Temporary colostomy usually is not necessary unless the patient has previously undergone therapeutic pelvic irradiation.

Effect of Etiology. When fistulas appear after therapeutic pelvic irradiation, usually years later as a result of the reduced blood flow associated with endarteritis obliterans, the gynecologist should first perform a biopsy of viable tissue from the fistula margin to rule out active malignant disease. If there is no evidence of malignancy, the gynecologist prescribes the nightly application of intravaginal estrogen cream to improve the local blood supply and thicken the genital epithelium. Repair should be delayed for approximately 1 year after the fistula is first noticed to permit adequate stabilization of the blood supply and further confirmation that there is no malignancy in the area. If repaired prematurely (before restabilization or arrest of the vascular obliteration), this type of fistula is likely to recur; furthermore, the recurrent fistula may be larger and more difficult to repair than the original.

Boronow's operation of partial colpocleisis of the upper vagina is frequently effective in the repair of a radiation-induced rectovaginal fistula.[7] The operator exposes the

somewhat fibrotic vaginal vault fistula by means of Schuchardt's incision (see Chapter 20) and carefully dissects the vagina from the anterior rectal wall for 1 to 2 cm in all directions at the site of the fistula. Hemostasis must be meticulous to prevent postoperative hematoma formation. The defect in the anterior rectal wall, the high-pressure side of the fistula, is closed transversely without tension by a two-layered interrupted fine polyglycolic acid suture technique. A bulbocavernosus fat pad on one or both sides is mobilized, swung beneath the anterior vaginal wall, and sewn in place to cover the site of the fistula repair, and the vagina is closed.

In general, the gynecologic surgeon performs colpocleisis only for a large fistula that is sometimes seen after irradiation, when the viability of the adjacent tissue is so poor that good wound healing is unlikely. It, of course, destroys the function of most or all of the vagina, and the patient must understand and accept this before the surgery takes place.

Sigmoid-vaginal fistula usually results from perforation of a sigmoid diverticulum coincident with abscess formation from diverticulitis. It generally occurs in an older patient with diverticulosis. A transabdominal operation, often combined with partial colectomy, is the proper surgical approach for this type of fistula.

Transabdominal closure generally is reserved for those rectovaginal fistulas that are relatively inaccessible from below and that are awkward to visualize, making repair of the bowel more difficult once the two organs have been separated. This situation usually is associated with a long-standing epithelialized fistula that developed after hysterectomy and pelvic abscess that may have limited vaginal mobility. When it follows pelvic irradiation, successful closure may require a temporary transverse colostomy and an interposing layer of fresh tissue with an independent blood supply (e.g., the omentum or the bulbocavernosus fat pad), since postirradiation fibrosis has obliterated local blood vessels and has led to endarteritis obliterans, which effectively reduces the blood supply to the irradiated tissues.

Other Types of Rectal Fistula

The appropriate treatment for anoperineal fistula that does not communicate with the anal sphincter is simple excision of a wide area of surrounding skin, at least 1 cm lateral to each side of the fistula (Fig. 28-10). The operator places a probe into the fistulous tract, incises through the full thickness of the overlying skin and subcutaneous tissue, and widely excises the surrounding skin margin, removing the fistulous tract. Any bleeding vessels are tied, and the wound is packed open to granulate in from the bottom. The skin margins should be the last portion of the wound to close. Although healing requires a 4- to 6-week period, the patient remains surprisingly comfortable and has little disability.

Rectovaginal Fistula from Crohn's Disease. Because standard surgical techniques do not generally resolve fistulas resulting from Crohn's disease, it is essential to recognize this disorder before recommending surgical repair of a fistula. The gynecologist should suspect Crohn's disease

VAGINORECTOPERINEAL FISTULA

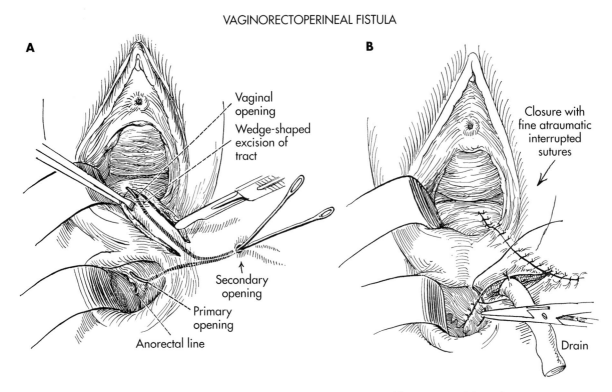

A

Vaginal opening

Wedge-shaped excision of tract

Secondary opening

Primary opening

Anorectal line

B

Closure with fine atraumatic interrupted sutures

Drain

Fig. 28-10   A, Probes are used to follow the tract and, if possible, are passed through its entire length. The injection of dye in the tract is seldom of any help and obscures the field of operation. If probes can be inserted, a wedge-shaped excision of the tract is carried out. All the infected tissue between the primary and secondary openings is removed. The excision of the tract going from the vagina to the perineum is shown. Subsequently the entire tract from the primary opening near the anorectal line to the skin of the perineum is excised. **B,** The anterior tract, after thorough and adequate excision from the vagina to the perineum, is closed with atraumatic interrupted sutures. After excision of the fistula-in-ano, several sutures are used to close the skin of the anoderm and invert it into the anal canal. Remnants of the rectal sphincter that can be approximated without tension are brought together with 2-0 PGA suture on atraumatic needles. A drain was inserted in the most dependent portion of the skin just lateral to the rectal sphincter. (From Ball TL: *Gynecologic surgery and urology,* ed 2, St Louis, 1963, Mosby.)

when there has been no mechanical trauma that would explain the origin of the fistula and the patient reports weight loss and frequent loose bowel movements, often accompanied by internal cramping. The fistula is invariably quite painful to touch (especially during the active phases of the disease), even when it has been present for a considerable length of time. Its edge has the roughened red appearance of granulation tissue. Biopsy, endoscopy, and study of the films of both upper and lower gastrointestinal radiography confirm the presence of Crohn's disease. The surgeon may consider repairing a Crohn's disease–induced rectovaginal fistula in the lower vagina during a temporary remission of the disease; the use of a sliding rectal flap operation permits the excision of the bowel wall that contains the fistula. The patient must be informed of the high risk of surgical failure or of exacerbation of the disease, however. Preoperative preparation may include the administration of metronidazole (Flagyl), 1000 mg daily along with 20 mg of prednisone daily, for 1 month.[5]

Because the prednisone may inhibit the usual rate of wound healing, a long-lasting monofilament synthetic suture such as polydioxanone (PDS) is useful in the deeper layers of repair and polyglycolic acid suture for the more superficial layers. Kodner[23] has emphasized the need for effective preliminary drainage of any associated abscess cavity by a small mushroom catheter (never a Malecot) sewn in place in a perirectal external opening to the abscess. The site should be inspected 2 weeks after the catheter has been placed and the catheter probably removed 1 week later. Although superficial fistula tracts occasionally may be managed by fistulotomy, sphincterotomy should be avoided, particularly if Crohn's disease is active.

When rectovaginal or anovaginal fistulas are caused by Crohn's disease, success may be achieved with surgical closure provided that the surgery is timed during a clearly inactive phase of the disease.[31] A rectal flap sliding technique is the preference of the author, providing that the fistula is low within the vagina and otherwise uncomplicated by stenosis or other fistula. Although Beecham[4] recommended coincident colostomy, we have not found this to be necessary in most instances.

Rectouterine Fistula and Diverticulosis. Unless associated with an invasive neoplasm, rectouterine fistulas are almost invariably the result of coexistent diverticulosis, in which diverticula became adherent to the posterior wall of the uterus and air abscesses formed, ultimately eroding into the uterine cavity. The condition produces a profuse, cloudy, watery discharge from the cervix in an amount that usually makes it necessary for the patient to wear a sanitary pad. Early in its course, the discharge may be intermittent, coinciding with flare-ups of activity within the abscess cavity, and the patient may be relatively comfortable between spells of watery leukorrhea. A barium enema and sigmoidoscopy readily confirm the diagnosis. Treatment is surgical, sometimes requiring a preliminary colostomy, a bowel resection and hysterectomy 2 or 3 months later, and closure of the colostomy as a tertiary procedure 2 or 3 months after the hysterectomy.

Vesicorectal Fistula. This fistula is a rare late complication of hysterectomy. Because of its location high within the vault of the vagina, successful repair usually requires a transabdominal approach with dissection followed by separate repair of each organ system. Depending on the size of the fistula and any previous irradiation, a preliminary diverting colostomy may be desirable.

POSTOPERATIVE CARE AFTER FISTULA REPAIR

Antibiotics that were administered preoperatively can be continued postoperatively for a short time unless significant diarrhea develops, in which case the antibiotic should be promptly discontinued and the diarrhea brought under control. The patient should have a clear liquid diet for 3 days; when she is passing gas, she is gradually changed to a low-roughage or bland diet for 3 weeks. Stool softeners should be given, and, if there has been no bowel movement by the seventh day, a gentle laxative should be added. Small doses of GoLYTELY are preferable to an enema at this time.

The vaginal drain should be removed between the fifth and seventh postoperative days, depending on the amount of drainage and the stability of the patient's temperature. Sitz baths given twice daily after the drain has been removed may make the patient more comfortable. Coitus is not permitted until the end of the third postoperative month.

Stool softeners such as docusate sodium (Colace) should be given for 5 weeks. Tincture of opium, 10 drops in water three times a day for the first 5 days, is often helpful if cramps are troublesome. When a partial colpocleisis has been performed, intravaginal estrogen cream should be instilled nightly for many weeks until healing, followed by long-term weekly use.

Late recurrence of rectovaginal fistula, even 10 or 15 years after the original repair, occasionally occurs, so periodic follow-up examinations are desirable.

REPAIR OF OLD COMPLETE PERINEAL LACERATION

Kelly once noted that genital prolapse was only rarely observed in patients with a complete and unrepaired perineal laceration.[22] Because the principal effectiveness of the pubococcygei and levator ani in supporting the birth canal is exerted *posterior* to the rectum where their fusion forms the levator plate, a laceration through the anterior rectum, perineal body, and posterior vagina is not likely to be the result of forces simultaneously exerted in a way that overstretches the major sources of the uterine support. Although such a laceration disrupts the anal sphincter, many of these patients, by vigorously exercising the pubococcygeus over a long period, develop a hypertrophy in this muscle that permits a side-to-side sphincterlike action that helps hold the sides of the fistula in opposition and accomplishes a semblance of anal continence. This mechanism does not restore control of flatus, but it may result in continence of the stool, particularly if the patient is careful to maintain a helpful degree of constipation. To test for fecal incontinence, a packaged enema may be given to the patient in the office to see if she can retain it voluntarily.

According to Miller and Brown,[30] the successful repair of an old laceration of the perineum has three essential requirements: (1) evidence of a good blood supply, (2) absence of infection in the tissues involved, and (3) closure of the repair with no tension on the sutures that reapproximate the tissues. It is equally important to excise all scar tissue to ensure that the tissues being reapproximated are similar to those of a fresh fourth-degree laceration. Layer-by-layer reconstruction of the rectal wall perirectal connective tissue, anal sphincter, and rectovaginal septum before closure of the overlying vaginal floor should be accomplished by means of terraced rows of fine absorbable suture, although such a repair occasionally breaks down, leaving a rectovaginal fistula. This discouraging result is particularly likely in a postmenopausal patient with atrophic tissues and a reduced blood supply.

Age reduces intestinal peristalsis, especially in the postmenopausal years. Nicotine withdrawal indirectly reduces peristalsis in those who have just stopped smoking before hospitalization, tending to invite postoperative constipation.

The results are best when an obstetric laceration is properly repaired immediately after delivery, when the vascularity of the perineum and perivaginal tissues favors rapid healing. Patients may seek a repair of a complete perineal laceration at any time, however, even years after the original injury. In these patients, scar tissue is appreciable, wound healing is poorer, and the fistula is more likely to recur. When the laceration to be repaired is an old one, it is important for the surgeon to choose an operation that provides the optimal chance of success involving only one repair procedure.

Partial or total denervation of the external anal sphincter, the internal sphincter, and of the levator ani can result from a combination of many factors.[16,45,47,48] Occult damage can be measured even after uncomplicated vaginal delivery, although it generally heals rapidly. Straining at stool may contribute to further damage, as may damage to the motor nerve roots of S3 and S4 from coincidental disc disease or spinal canal stenosis from osteoarthritis. Manning and Pratt[27] described their surgical results as best following the first repair; they noted difficulty in finding the frayed ends of the external anal sphincter when they were buried in scar tissue. They thought the symptomatic improvement after surgery to restore anal incontinence was less when the patient has been clinically diagnosed as having an irritable bowel syndrome. Pezim et al.[39] from the same institution concluded from examination of their own data that because 48% of their incontinent patients had been labeled as having irritable bowel before presentation, a much higher percentage than one would find among the normal population, in most cases the diagnosis was unwarranted. Their postsurgical results were equally satisfactory in this group, and they concluded that surgical repair should be offered to such patients with assurance of equal success. Although Fang et al.,[10] following on the work of Blaisdell,[6] reported better results with overlapping sphincteroplasty, acceptance of this conclusion is by no means universal. Not only may it be surgically difficult to dissect the external anal sphincter from surrounding scar tissue, but excessive dissection may compromise both the blood and the nerve supplies of the sphincter. Classic descriptions of the transected external anal sphincter characterize it as a narrow bundle to be sought just beneath the perianal skin and distinctly caudal to the internal sphincter.[19,37] More recent studies using MRI come to quite a different conclusion. Aronson et al.[1] have observed from their MRI studies that the external sphincter normally is a strong ellipsoidal cylinder complex that surrounds the distal portion of the internal anal sphincter in an adult for 3 to 4 cm and is thicker anteriorly and posteriorly than laterally. They submit that surgical reapproximation of this *entire muscular cylinder* should be followed by a more effective restoration of sphincter function than that following reapproximation of just the superficial subcutaneous portion of the external anal sphincter. This author agrees and no longer makes a decisive effort to dissect the external anal sphincter medially from its surrounding tissues. The free but scarred ends of the lacerated external sphincter should be sought and grasped so that they may be sewn together as a part of the perineal reconstruction, but combining this with full perineal reconstruction will produce the best anatomic and functional result. Fecal continence is the result of effective interaction and support between not only the external and internal anal sphincters,[16] but also the whole of the pelvic diaphragm including its puborectalis portion.[26]

Anal Endosonography

Pudendal nerve terminal motor latency combined with anal ultrasonography provides critical diagnostic data concerning both neuropathic and anatomic sphincter damage.[11,13]

EXTERNAL ANAL SPHINCTERPLASTY

It is well known from repair of a Maylard incision (see Chapter 13) that sutures placed directly in the cut margins of the striated muscle do not convey much strength to the re-

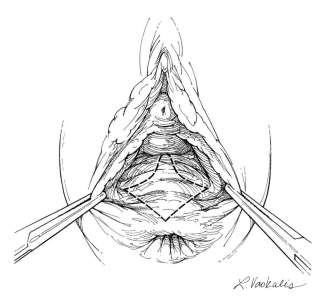

Fig. 28-11   Exterior anal sphincteroplasty. The perineal and vaginal incision to expose the underlying remnants of the exterior anal sphincter is identified by the *dashed line*.

union. Rather, it is the reunion of the capsule or fascial sheath surrounding the muscles that permits a strong bridge of scar tissue to develop between the ends of the transected muscle fibers. This observation can be applied safely to the perineum when external anal sphincter reconstruction is desired, reestablishing circular continuity of the external anal sphincter mechanism. In most instances after an appropriate perineal incision (Fig. 28-11) it is sufficient to mobilize extensively the scar surrounding the severed or damaged ends of the full length of the entire external sphincter by sharp dissection of the rectum from the overlying vagina. The medial portions of scar tissue of the three named portions of external anal sphincter are grasped bilaterally in Allis clamps and traction applied to identify them, the dissection often having been carried out with the gloved index finger of the operator's opposite hand inserted into the rectum so that the full-thickness of the rectal wall can be palpated. Once these scars have been identified and grasped by three or four Allis clamps on each side of the canal (Fig. 28-12), an incision is made on each side lateral to this grasped condensation of scar tissue, freeing the scar from any direct attachment to the pelvic diaphragm (Fig. 28-13) and permitting these two condensations, one from each side, to be united in the midline by a relatively tension-free series of interrupted polyglycolic acid–type sutures (Fig. 28-14). This permits a midline union of the scar tissue from each side to which the anal sphincter fibers are attached at each side, reestablishing the physiologic continuity of the sphincter circle and therefore restoring its function (Fig. 28-15). A perineorrhaphy or perineoplasty reestablishes the integrity of the perineal body and completes the reconstruction.

Layered Closure

Rectum and vagina are separated by dissection through the dense scar tissue between them. The separation is carried

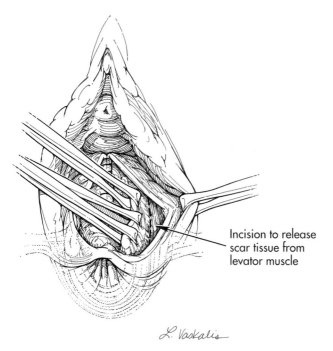

Fig. 28-12   Scar tissue containing the remnants of the subcutaneous, superficial, and deep portions of the external anal sphincter have been grasped by Allis clamps and an incision made along their lateral margins to free this tissue from the levator muscle.

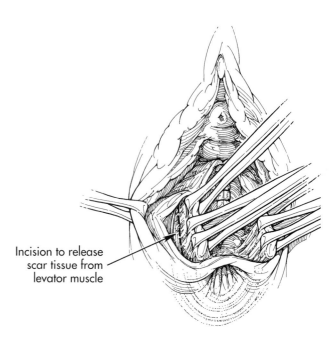

Fig. 28-13   A similar dissection is accomplished on the opposite side of the pelvis.

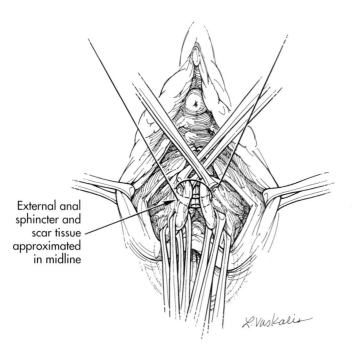

Fig. 28-14   The tissue grasped by matching Allis clamps is approximated by a series of polyglycolic acid mattress sutures.

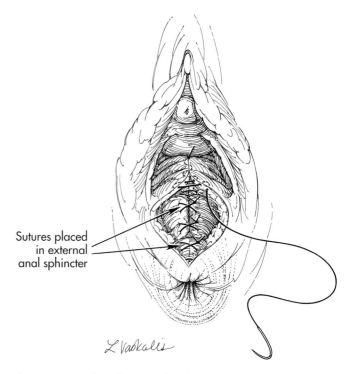

Fig. 28-15   When these stitches have been tied just enough to approximate the sides, but not enough to induce strangulation, the vaginal and perineal skin is closed by running subcuticular suture.

into the rectovaginal space (Fig. 28-16). The scarred ends of the external anal sphincter are identified and grasped in Kocher or Allis clamps or by a towel clip and held for later reapproximation. The submucosal rectal wall and anoderm are closed (see Fig. 28-16, *D*). A second layer approximates the perirectal fascia and muscularis, and the ends of the external anal sphincter are brought together. The perineal body

should be restored by a few buried interrupted stitches, and the skin of the posterior vaginal wall and perineum closed with interrupted sutures.

The Noble-Mengert-Fish anterior rectal flap operation often has been recommended for the repair of an old perineal laceration.[29,33,35] Primary healing with restoration of function usually follows the Warren-Miller-Brown vaginal

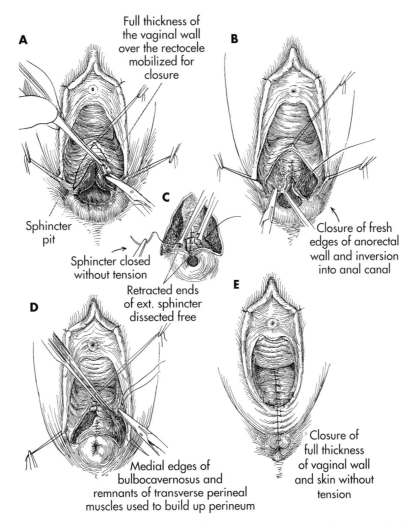

Fig. 28-16 Traction sutures are placed, outlining a triangular area to be denuded. The apex of this triangle is above any scar tissue in the vagina, while the angles of the base are over the sphincter pits **(A)**. The incision is carried high enough so that the full thickness of the vaginal wall over a rectocele or lateral vaginal wall relaxation can be mobilized to aid in the closure. The dissection is continued until the full thickness of the vagina is mobilized and separated from the rectal wall and mucosa. The scar tissue in the vaginal and rectal walls is excised so that fresh edges are approximated, and the rectal and anorectal walls are inverted into the canal by interrupted sutures of 2-0 PGA on atraumatic needles **(B)**. These sutures extend just to the submucosa and precisely approximate the tissues. The retracted ends of the external sphincter are located and mobilized sufficiently for approximation in the midline without tension **(C)**. They are sutured together with interrupted sutures of 2-0 PGA on atraumatic needles. The medial edges of the bulbocavernosi and remnants of the transverse perineal muscles are used to build up the perineal body over and above the reunited external sphincter **(D)**. The anterior edges of the levators are approximated in the midline to give additional support. The full thickness of the vaginal wall and the skin of the perineum are closed by interrupted sutures **(E)**. They are approximated without tension and inspected again so that scar tissue is not incorporated into the wound. (From Ball TL, *Gynecologic surgery and urology,* ed 2, St Louis, 1963, Mosby.)

flap operation as well.[9,30,50] The surgeon often chooses between the two operations on the basis of the size of the vagina. The rectal flap operation does not remove vaginal membrane and can be used in a patient with a smaller vagina, whereas the vaginal flap operation makes the vagina measurably smaller and therefore is appropriate when this is desired.

Rectal Flap Operation

In principle and usefulness, the rectal flap operation (Noble-Mengert-Fish procedure[29,33,35]) is not unlike the mucosal flap operations for rectovaginal fistula, but the rectal flap operation is a procedure of choice when the integrity of the external anal sphincter has been disturbed. The rectal flap operation is especially useful if an old fourth-degree laceration extends no more than 3 or 4 cm into the anal canal. By freeing up and pulling down the anterior rectal wall and suturing the undersurface of the mobilized segment of anterior rectal mucosa to the anal sphincter and the cut edge of the rectal wall to the perineal skin outside of the former anal canal, the surgeon can cover the area where the sutures not protected by such a flap are often disrupted postoperatively.

Brief electrical stimulation with an electrosurgical needle electrode not only aids hemostasis, but also can help identify striated muscle. An occasional buried stitch should include a superficial bite of the anal sphincter. The lower edge of the remaining flap of the anterior rectal wall is fixed to the skin of the perineum by several interrupted 2-0 absorbable polyglycolic acid–type sutures placed not more than 1 to 2 cm apart.

Vaginal (Warren) Flap Operation

The bowel is cleansed by an electrolyte purgative,[3] such as NuLYTELY or Colyte or by enemas until the return is clear, in preparation for the vaginal flap operation. To begin the procedure, the surgeon makes an inverted V-shaped incision in the posterior vaginal wall. The incision should be wide enough to leave the introitus with the desired caliber when the sides of the vagina are subsequently united[30,50] (Fig. 28-17). The base of this vaginal flap is continuous with the margin of the anterior rectal wall.

By sharp dissection through any scar tissue, the surgeon develops the avascular space between the rectum and vagina for several inches, mobilizing the anterior rectal wall. Stretching the rectal wall by traction to the free end of the vaginal flap will bring it and the V-shaped vaginal flap to beneath the site of the external anal sphincter. Then, grasping the buried ends of the sphincter, the surgeon places synthetic 2-0 mattress sutures, long-lasting but absorbable, but without tying them just yet.

The perineal body is reconstituted by several side-to-side sutures that are tied. After this, the anal sphincter stitches can be tied, and the perineal skin can be closed from side to side. The undersurface of the vaginal flap is sewn to the external anal sphincter and perineal skin, and the excess tissue in the flap is trimmed and removed.

The anal sphincter fibers will retract and shorten. Therefore the reconstructed anal canal should admit one fingerbreadth comfortably at the time of the surgery; if not, the operator should make a paradoxic sphincter incision as described by Miller and Brown.[9,30] Such an incision should be made between the 4-o'clock and 5-o'clock positions, cleanly through the perineal skin and anal sphincter and perpendicular to the muscle fibers of the sphincter. The sphincter remains relaxed, and the patient may not be completely continent until the formation of scar tissue reunites the sphincter ends and restores a degree of functional competence. This healing requires between 8 and 12 weeks, and the patient should be so informed.

Restoration of Continence by Repair of a Lacerated Anal Sphincter

Anal sphincter incompetence is almost invariably the result of an obstetric laceration that interrupted the integrity of the sphincter, generally in the midline near the 12-o'clock position. The anterior wall of the rectum may or may not have been torn as well. If the repair of the fresh injury does not heal properly, various situations may develop. For example, the rectal tear may have healed, but not the sphincter or perineal body; when this occurs, sphincter incontinence results. The perineal body and skin may have healed, but not the rectal laceration. The sphincter repair or some part thereof may or may not have healed. A rectovaginal fistula may form, sometimes, but not always, leading to sphincter incontinence. When the healing process has stabilized after the injury or previous repair and any raw areas have become epithelialized, the defective area should be reconstructed, provided, of course, that the patient is symptomatic and desires a restoration.

Symptoms and Etiology. Symptoms of anal sphincter insufficiency are those of rectal incontinence (i.e., inability to control rectal gas or feces, especially when liquid). At times, soiling may precipitate a troublesome vaginitis.

Damage to the nerves, often involving the pudendal nerve, which essentially denervates the pelvic diaphragm and the external anal sphincter, may cause anorectal incontinence.[37] This can be suspected during the preoperative pelvic examination if the patient cannot voluntarily contract her pubococcygeal muscles and her external anal sphincter. The diagnosis can be confirmed by electromyography. Acquired nerve damage usually results from straining at stool or from a difficult or prolonged labor. Myoplasty can tighten a loose external sphincter system, but if the muscles have been denervated, the prognosis for functional improvement is guarded. The prognosis for postsurgical function is better in a patient who has unilateral or partial residual innervation. A good internal (involuntary) sphincter system aids rectal continence.

Other, less common causes of anal sphincter incompetence include peripheral neuropathy (e.g., caused by diabetes), diseases of the central nervous system, spinal cord, or cauda equina, and postsurgical trauma (e.g., after laminectomy). The condition may be associated with the perineal

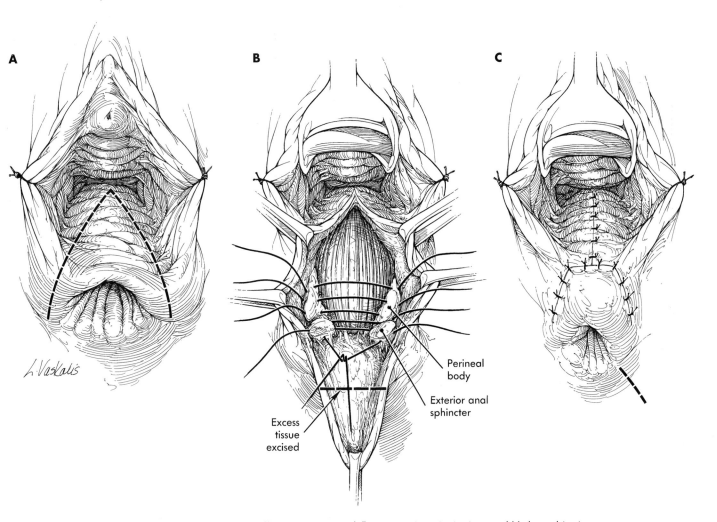

Fig. 28-17   The Warren-Miller-Brown vaginal flap operation. **A,** An inverted V-shaped incision is made through the full thickness of the vagina and skin of the perineum, opening into the rectovaginal space. Traction is applied to the vaginal skin overlying the rectum at the site noted by the asterisk. This is freed laterally from the surrounding scar tissue, exposing the site of the perineal body and the ends of the anal sphincter. **B,** These are united from side to side with a series of interrupted stitches of absorbable polyglycolic acid–type sutures. When the perineal body has been restored and the sphincter ends approximated, the flap is trimmed as shown and turned up to cover the sphincter repair. The posterior vaginal wall and skin of the perineum are closed by a series of interrupted stitches. If the reconstructed anal canal does not readily admit 1 fingerbreadth, the paradoxic sphincter incision of Miller and Brown can be performed (see text). The site is shown by the *dashed line* at the bottom right of **C.** (Modified from Nichols DH, Randall CL: *Vaginal surgery,* ed 4, Baltimore, 1996, Williams & Wilkins.)

descent syndrome or with rectal prolapse. Some patients who have chronic diarrhea may really harbor an undiagnosed sphincter incompetence secondary to not only sphincter laceration, but also sphincter denervation. A sphincter plication usually is ineffective in a patient whose rectal sphincter weakness is not the result of a previous sphincter laceration. Medical treatment, including the administration of loperamide hydrochloride (Imodium), may be helpful.

Novak's Operation for Restoration of Anal Sphincter Competence.   Novak described an operation to restore sphincter integrity and anal continence in a patient who had lost continence as a result of laceration.[36] Often, the opera-

tion is necessary because of the postoperative breakdown of an earlier repair of a fourth-degree obstetric laceration and, occasionally, of the perineum. The operation provides good exposure to the critical areas, particularly the ends of the lacerated anal sphincter and the tissue from which the perineum will be reconstructed. An essential step is the placement of the stitches so that they reinforce or restore the integrity of the perineal body and take much of the tension from the ends of the recently approximated external anal sphincter, splinting or bracing this repair and aiding in the integrity of its healing. If this tissue has been adequately identified and mobilized, it is not necessary to bring the medial borders of the pubococcygeal muscles together in front of the rectum, thus reducing the risk that painful ridges will form in the newly approximated tissue and cause subsequent dyspareunia. Polyglycolic acid–type 1-0 or 2-0 suture is used. When the perineum has "disappeared," it must be mobilized and reconstructed as an integral part of the repair, which effectively decreases the strain on the sphincter repair during its healing phase.

As in the rectal flap and vaginal flap operations, before surgery to restore anal sphincter competence the bowel should be cleansed by a mechanical bowel preparation, either with electrolyte or enemas, until clear. Traction stitches are placed. The damaged tissues must be mobilized carefully, and scar tissue must be freed by sharp dissection. None of the tissue needs to be discarded. The torn ends of the sphincter will be buried in scar tissue, but they can be identified by the subcutaneous dimples. An incision resembling the letter W is made with the knife through the skin margin between the vagina and rectum and extended upward *lateral* to the cut ends of the sphincter. After the rectovaginal space has been entered, the vagina is carefully separated front the anterior wall of the rectum up to the site of the previously placed traction suture.

When the cut edge of the vagina has been grasped with Allis forceps, the surgeon frees the scar tissue by both sharp and blunt dissection with wide mobilization of the vagina from the rectum. This procedure clearly exposes the caudal portion of the rectovaginal space and the site of the perineum. A traction stitch is placed in the muscularis of the anterior rectal wall. The application of upward tension to this latter suture makes the dimpling that identifies the scar of the torn edges of the external anal sphincter more noticeable, and the edges are grasped with Allis clamps or Kocher forceps. The scarred ends of the sphincter may be excised from the surrounding scar tissue by sharp dissection, and polydioxanone or polyglycolic acid–type sutures are placed in the retracted scarred ends of the sphincter. If the freed sphincter is long enough, the ends can be overlapped. For recurrent cases, a suture of a permanent monofilament, Prolene, Novofil, or Surgilene, can be used, provided that it can be effectively buried.

If the anterior anal wall has a V-shaped defect, it is approximated by interrupted submucosal polyglycolic acid–type sutures, and a second reinforcing layer is placed to reduce the tension on the first layer.

The perineal body is reinforced or reconstructed by a series of horizontally placed interrupted sutures, the stitch in the anal sphincter is tied, a second and perhaps third reinforcing mattress suture is placed in the muscle itself and tied, and the perineal skin is closed vertically.

Anal Incontinence after Sphincter Repair

For those patients complaining of persistent anal incontinence 3 to 12 months after sphincteroplasty, a retrorectal levatorplasty or post anal repair should be considered[38] (see Chapter 29). Persistent, substantial, and socially disabling anal incontinence after medical, surgical, or biofeedback

therapy is an indication for permanent colostomy—the site in a location visible to the patient, off the belt line, and away from abdominal scars and deformities[26] (see Chapter 51).

Postoperative Care

Postoperative care after all these procedures is similar. A clear liquid and nonresidue diet should be followed for 5 days, and constipation should be encouraged during this period. A rectal tube may be used for short intervals, however, to overcome any difficulty in expelling flatus. Stool softeners are administered and a gentle laxative is given on the fourth day, at which time a gradual return to the house diet should begin. An initial bowel movement usually is desirable by the seventh postoperative day. Stool softeners are given for a month postoperatively.

REFERENCES

1. Aronson MP, Lee RA, Berquist TH: Anatomy of anal sphincters and related structures in continent women studied with magnetic resonance imaging, *Obstet Gynecol* 76:846, 1990.
2. Bacon HE, Ross ST: *Atlas of operative technique: anus, rectum, and colon,* St Louis, 1954, Mosby.
3. Beck DE, Harford FJ, DiPalma JA: Comparison of cleansing methods in preparation for colonic surgery, *Dis Colon Rectum* 28:491, 1985.
4. Beecham CT: Recurring rectovaginal fistulas, *Obstet Gynecol* 40:323, 1972.
5. Bernstein LH, Frank MS, Brandt LJ, Boley SJ: Healing of perineal Crohn's disease with metronidazole, *Gastroenterology* 79:357, 1980.
6. Blaisdell PC: Repair of the incontinent sphincter ani, *Surg Gynecol Obstet* 70:692, 1940.
7. Boronow RC: Management of radiation-induced vaginal fistulas, *Am J Obstet Gynecol* 1:1, 1971.
8. Corman ML: *Colon and rectal surgery,* Philadelphia, 1984, JB Lippincott.
9. Crossen HS, Crossen PJ: *Operative gynecology,* ed 6, St Louis, 1948, Mosby.
10. Fang DT, Nivatvongs S, Vermeulen FD, et al: Overlapping sphincteroplasty for acquired anal incontinence, *Dis Colon Rectum* 27:720, 1984.
11. Felt-Bersma RJ, Cuesta MA, Koorevaar M, et al: Anal endosonography: relationship with anal manometry and neurophysiologic tests, *Dis Colon Rectum* 35:944, 1992.
12. Gallagher DM, Scarborough RA: Repair of low rectovaginal fistula, *Dis Colon Rectum* 5:193, 1962.
13. Genadry RR, Nichols DH: Recurrent anal incontinence. In Nichols DH, editor: *Reoperative gynecologic and obstetric surgery,* St Louis, 1997, Mosby.
14. Goligher JC: *Surgery of the anus, rectum, and colon,* ed 3, London, 1975, Bailliere Tindall.
15. Grissom R, Snyder TE: Colovaginal fistula secondary to diverticular disease, *Dis Colon Rectum* 34:1043, 1991.
16. Haadem K, Dahlstrom JA, Ling L, Ohrlander S: Anal sphincter function after delivery rupture, *Obstet Gynecol* 70:53, 1987.
17. Hauth JC, Gilstrap LC III, Ward SC, Hankins GD: Early repair of an external sphincter ani muscle and rectal mucosal dehiscence, *Obstet Gynecol* 67:806, 1986.
18. Hibbard LT: Surgical management of rectovaginal fistulas and complete perineal tears, *J Obstet Gynecol* 130:139, 1977.
19. Hirschman LJ: *Synopsis of ano-rectal diseases,* ed 2, St Louis, 1942, Mosby.
20. Hodgkinson CP: Correcting failed rectovaginal fistula repair. In Sanz LE, editor: *Gynecologic surgery,* Oradell, NJ, 1988, Medical Economics Books.
21. Jackman RJ: Rectovaginal and anovaginal fistulas: a surgical procedure for treatment of certain types, *J Iowa State Med Soc* 42:435, 1952.

22. Kelly HA: *Operative gynecology,* vol I, New York, 1898, D Appleton.

23. Kodner IJ: Anal procedure. In Wilmore DW et al, editors: *Care of the surgical patient,* New York, 1997, Scientific American.

24. Laird DR: Procedures used in the treatment of complicated fistulas, *Am J Surg* 76:701, 1948.

25. Leacher TC, Pratt JH: Vaginal repair of the simple rectovaginal fistula, *Surg Gynecol Obstet* 124:1317, 1967.

26. Madoff RD, Williams JG, Caushaj PF: Fecal incontinence, *N Engl J Med* 326:1102, 1992.

27. Manning PC, Pratt JH: Fecal incontinence caused by lacerations of the perineum, *Arch Surg* 88:569, 1964.

28. Menaker GH: The use of antibiotics in surgical treatment of the colon, *Surg Gynecol Obstet* 164:581, 1987.

29. Mengert WF, Fish SA: Anterior rectal wall advancement, *Obstet Gynecol* 5:262, 1955.

30. Miller NF, Brown W: The surgical treatment of complete perineal tears in the female, *Am J Obstet Gynecol* 34:196, 1937.

31. Morrison JG, Gathright JB Jr, Ray JE, et al: Results of operation for rectovaginal fistula in Crohn's disease, *Dis Colon Rectum* 32:497, 1989.

32. Nichols DH, editor: *Reoperative gynecologic and obstetric surgery,* St Louis, 1997, Mosby.

33. Nichols DH, Randall CL: *Vaginal surgery,* ed 4, Baltimore, 1989, Williams & Wilkins.

34. Nichols RL: Bowel preparation: perioperative care. In Wilmore DW et al, editors: *Care of the surgical patient,* New York, 1998, Scientific American.

35. Noble GH: A new operation to complete laceration of the perineum designed for the purpose of eliminating danger of infection from the rectum, *Trans Am Gynecol Soc* 7:357, 1902.

36. Novak F: *Surgical gynecologic techniques,* New York, 1978, John Wiley & Sons.

37. Oh C, Kark AE: Anatomy of the external anal sphincter, *Br J Surg* 59:717, 1972.

38. Penninckx F: Fecal incontinence: indications for repairing the anal sphincter, *World J Surg* 16:820, 1992.

39. Pezim ME, Spencer RJ, Stanhope CR, et al: Sphincter repair for fecal incontinence after obstetrical or iatrogenic injury, *Dis Colon Rectum* 30:521, 1987.

40. Rock JA, Thompson JD: *Te Linde's operative gynecology,* ed 8, Philadelphia, 1992, JB Lippincott.

41. Rock JA, Woodruff JD: Surgical correction of a rectovaginal fistula, *Int J Gynaecol Obstet* 20:413, 1982.

42. Rosenshein NB, Genadry RR, Woodruff JD: An anatomic classification of rectovaginal septal defects, *Am J Obstet Gynecol* 137:439, 1980.

43. Russell TR, Gallagher DM: Low rectovaginal fistulas, *Am J Surg* 134:13, 1977.

44. Sanz LE, Blank K: The Martius graft technique for rectovaginal fistulas. In Sanz LE, editor: *Gynecologic surgery,* Oradell, NJ, 1988, Medical Economics Books.

45. Snooks SJ, Henry MM: Fecal incontinence due to external anal sphincter division in childbirth is associated with damage to the innervation at the pelvic floor musculature: a double pathology, *Br J Obstet Gynecol* 92:824, 1985.

46. Stern H, Gamliel Z, Ross T, Dreznik Z: Rectovaginal fistula: initial experience, *Can J Surg* 31:359, 1988.

47. Swash M: New concepts in incontinence, *Br Med J* 290:4, 1985.

48. Swash M, Henry MM: Unifying concept of pelvic floor disorders and incontinence, *J R Soc Med* 78:906, 1985.

49. Tancer ML, Veridiano NP: Genital fistulas caused by diverticular disease of the sigmoid colon, *Am J Obstet Gynecol* 174:1547, 1996.

50. Warren JC: A new method of operation for the relief of rupture of the perineum through the sphincter and rectum, *Trans Am Gynecol Soc* 7:322, 1882.

29 Perineal Descent, Retrorectal Levatorplasty, and Rectal Prolapse

DAVID H. NICHOLS

PERINEAL DESCENT SYNDROME

The levator plate, formed by the fusion of the bellies of the pubococcygeal muscles, for the most part posterior to the rectum, extends to the insertion of these muscles on the coccyx and lower portion of the sacrum.[8,33] When the plate is intact, it is more or less horizontal; when markedly attenuated, however, it becomes a loose hammock. As the plate sags, it tips (Fig. 29-1) and, with any increases in intraabdominal pressure, may permit those structures that lie on it to slide downward (Fig. 29-2). These structures, principally the vagina and the rectum, not only may descend, but also may occasionally telescope when intraabdominal pressure increases along their axes.

In a rare patient, the pelvic diaphragm and the levator plate may sag to such a degree that the patient actually sits on her anus (Fig. 29-3). She may describe an unusual bearing-down sensation and difficulty with evacuation. The harder she strains in attempting evacuation, however, the greater the levator funneling, the smaller the subsequent diameters of the anus and the stool, and thus the more difficult evacuation becomes. As a result, the condition may be associated with chronic constipation, obstipation so severe that digital manipulation is necessary for evacuation, or the deliberate abuse of laxatives to achieve an almost chronic state of diarrhea. Some patients may evacuate by sitting on a board with a 3-inch hole, the edges of which exert counterpressure around the sides of the anus.[14]

A pelvic examination with the patient in the lithotomy position reveals a pathologic and almost vertical vaginal and rectal axis and a short, tipped levator plate posterior to the rectum, but it is easiest to demonstrate this condition while the patient is sitting on the examination table. After placing a hand beneath the anus, the examiner can feel the anus descend still further as the patient strains. This descent or prolapse of both the anus and perineum must be clearly differentiated from rectal prolapse, which is an actual intussusception of the bowel through the anal sphincter and anus. Any maneuver that raises intraabdominal pressure (e.g., straining, coughing) causes the weakened pelvic floor to descend, from which rapid recovery may not take place even after the fecal bolus has been passed. Reduction in the anorectal angle may encourage redundant mucosa to plug the anal canal, obstructing defecation and producing a sensation of incomplete emptying that further encourages straining. At times, the condition produces not only its characteristic symptom complex, but also a feeling of pelvic and rectal pressure or falling out when standing. The patient occasionally may find it very difficult to sit comfortably.

Prolapse of the anus and perineum may result from a variety of causes, including trauma, obstetric damage, defective innervation,[19,21,34,36] aging, and chronically increased intraabdominal pressure. There appear to be three kinds of perineal prolapse. One is the result of traumatic stretching of the pelvic diaphragm in multiple pregnancies and is associated with constipation or obstipation. Another, more common type is neuropathically induced, probably by stretching of the pudendal nerve during labor or consequent to long-standing constipation and straining at stool.[21,35,43] More common in a parous than in a nonparous patient, this neuropathy may lead to degeneration of the muscular cells of the levator ani that is histologically demonstrable and more or less irreversible. Urinary stress incontinence may accompany this neuropathic condition.[21] Although neuromuscular activity can be measured electromyographically,[18,20,21,46,50] it can be estimated to some degree by the patient's ability or inability to contract her pubococcygei and external anal sphincter voluntarily. The third type is a combination of the other two.

Constipation may be an early symptom of perineal descent. Anal incontinence is not associated as long as anal sphincter pressure remains normal.[7] The loss of the integrity of an intact pelvic diaphragm may make voluntary bearing-down efforts more necessary, more frequent, and more intense. These efforts may stretch the pudendal nerve,[19,21] damaging the innervation of both the pelvic diaphragm and the external anal sphincter, leading to partial paralysis and atrophy of these muscles. If the protective internal sphincter mechanism becomes overburdened, perineal prolapse occasionally results, with subsequent obstipation and later rectal incontinence. When perineal prolapse correlates with a decreased perception of rectal fullness, some of the neuromuscular receptors within the levator ani may degenerate, making the success of anatomic surgical reconstruction less likely.

Provided that the conduct of any labor has been proper, it is quite possible to prevent perineal prolapse through good bowel habits, even including the use of a mild laxative or suppository, if necessary, and increased bulk in the diet. A greater intake of water (because some degree of systemic dehydration may accompany the diminution of thirst that takes place with aging) and regular pubococcygeal isometric resistive exercises also are helpful.

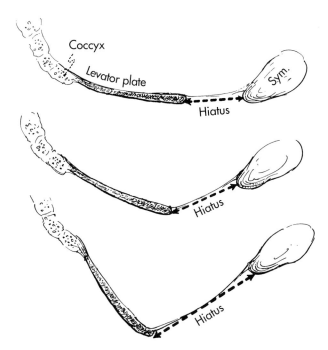

Fig. 29-1 As the levator plate sags, the genital hiatus becomes larger. In addition, the pull of gravity and the forces of intraabdominal pressure accentuate the strain on the pelvic suspensory system. *Sym,* Symphysis pubis. (Modified from Berglas B, Rubin IC: *Surg Gynecol Obstet* 97:672, 1953.)

RETRORECTAL LEVATORPLASTY (SURGICAL REPAIR)

Reconstruction of a damaged levator muscle produces a functionally more favorable result when the nerve supply is intact than when the nerve supply is significantly defective, whatever the cause. Severe pudendal neuropathy may render even biofeedback training ineffective. Biofeedback is most likely to be beneficial to a patient who still has some degree of rectal sensation and some ability to voluntarily contract the external anal sphincter.[29,39] When descent of the anus and rectum and sagging of the normally horizontal levator plate are associated with long-standing severe constipation and marked decrease in the diameter of the stool while straining, retrorectal levatorplasty with colporrhaphy may be curative. The coexistence of rectal incontinence and perineal prolapse suggests severe neuropathology, and the postsurgical prognosis is less favorable. However, retrorectal levatorplasty with colporrhaphy or the less extensive Parks postanal repair[35] may re-create a useful anal valve that may help these patients.

The Parks postanal repair[35] is a technique designed to restore a defective anorectal angle in patients with fecal incontinence secondary to denervation of the pelvic musculature. Parks attributed its success in such cases primarily to re-creation of an effective anorectal flap-valve mechanism, and secondarily to mechanical improvement of the function of puborectalis muscle fibers resulting from their plication. In this operation, an incision is made between the anus and

coccyx and carried into the intersphincteric "space" between the external and internal anal sphincters. The puborectalis portions of the levatores ani are sewn together *behind* the rectum, re-creating an anorectal angle. Yoshioka and Keighley[54] have been less optimistic about the rate of success and quality of continence following the Parks repair.

Uniting the medial portions of the pubococcygei between the vagina and rectum and anterior to the latter thickens the tissues of the perineum by interposing a muscular layer not initially well developed in this area and helps restore an anorectal angle, but it does not shorten the muscles, restore the defective axis of the plate, or correct the pathologic descent of the anus and rectum. The literature on techniques that have been used to achieve their goals is sparse, although there have been reports of lengthening the levator plate by the transperineal approach of Lange[25] and by the transabdominal approach used in various modifications of the operation of Graham.[13,15,17] Barrett[6] suggested a transperineal approach by incision and dissection between the anus and vagina, "posteriorly to the rectum in properly selected cases and the separated levator reunited with attachment of the rectal wall to this muscle," but apparently did not document any effort to pursue his idea. It is possible to plicate the pubococcygeal muscles posterior to the rectum by means of a transabdominal approach; however, it is difficult to obtain adequate exposure deep within the pelvis by means of this technique, and the operator cannot satisfactorily approach pathologic vaginal displacements with associated cystocele and rectocele through the same operative exposure.

Clinical experience with the Kraske or sacral transperineal approach to some surgical lesions of the rectum has reaffirmed the safety of this route,* and this approach has been used to correct levator deficiencies.[30,31] This transperineal retrorectal approach allows the operator to shorten the pubococcygei and puborectalis as necessary, as well as to unite the medial bellies of these muscles in the midline posterior to the rectum, thus lengthening the levator plate and advancing the genital hiatus anteriorly. By attaching the posterior rectal wall to the internal periosteum of the lower sacrum with a series of interrupted sutures, then sewing together the bellies of the pubococcygei *behind* the rectum, and shortening them as necessary, the operator can also establish a relatively horizontal axis to the rectum and to the vagina overlying it. This procedure makes it possible to suspend the elongated rectum[11,23,44] and, by performing appropriate supplemental anterior and posterior colporrhaphy,[41,47] to correct any coexistent cystocele and rectocele. Any enterocele should be excised.[53]

A preventive antibiotic, usually one dose of a cephalosporin, is given 1 hour preoperatively. An electrolyte bowel preparation and a liquid diet are given the day before surgery, or alternatively a mechanical bowel preparation may be given the night before.

For the procedure, the patient usually is placed in the Kraske jackknife position (Fig. 29-4), although the standard

*References 9, 10, 17, 22-24, 26, 28, 32, 51.

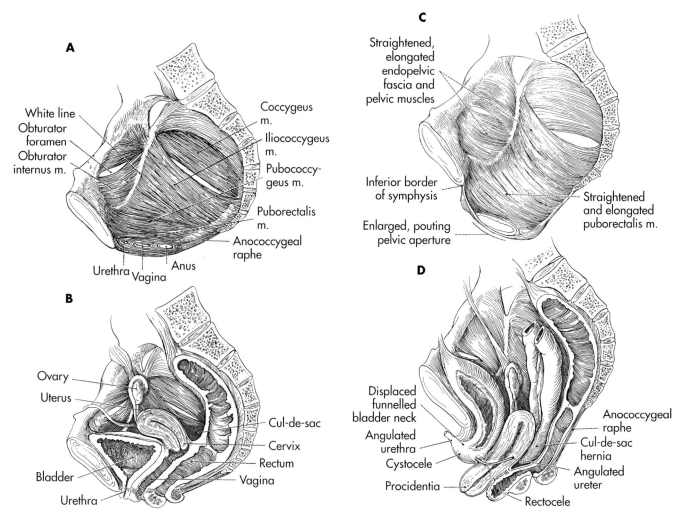

Fig. 29-2   **A,** The musculature of the side wall of the pelvis. Notice the almost horizontal inclination of the anococcygeal raphe and the dependent portion of the pubococcygeal muscle just above it, which is called the *levator plate*. **B,** A side view of the pelvic organs in their normal position. Notice that the vagina rests on the rectum, which in turn lies on the almost horizontal levator plate. **C,** Side view of the pelvis in which the muscles and their fasciae have become attenuated and are sagging. The pelvic basin is now funneled, and the levator plate is tipped. **D,** As a consequence of the soft tissue attenuation, a genital prolapse has developed. Notice the protruding bladder, uterus, and vagina, as well as a rectocele and an enterocele. The levator plate is tipped, and the organs above it are literally sliding downhill in their descent. (From Ball TL: *Gynecologic surgery and urology,* ed 2, St Louis, 1963, Mosby.)

Fig. 29-3   Sagittal section of the pelvis shows elongation and sagging of the levator plate. The usual angle between the anal canal and the rectum has been lost, as has the horizontal axis of the rectum and the upper vagina. (From Nichols DH, Randall CL: *Vaginal surgery,* ed 4, Baltimore, 1996, Williams & Wilkins.)

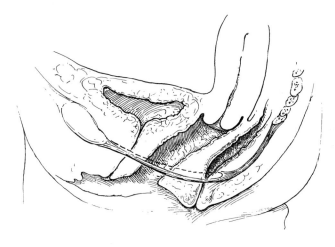

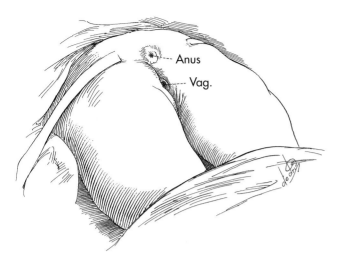

Fig. 29-4 "Jackknife" position. A sandbag has been placed beneath the hips, and the gluteal muscles are pulled apart by wide strips of adhesive tape fastened to the edges of the operating table. (From Nichols DH, Randall CL: *Vaginal surgery,* ed 4, Baltimore, 1996, Williams & Wilkins.)

lithotomy position may be used in those patients with plenty of room in the pelvis and for whom colporrhaphy is also planned. The operator makes a midline incision from the sacrum to the site of the external anal sphincter. After identifying the anococcygeal raphe (which varies significantly in strength and length among individuals), the operator separates it from the coccyx. The latter is grasped in a towel clip for traction but is not removed. Fat is displaced, and the undersurfaces of the pubococcygei and the levator plate are identified. The operator incises the levator plate in the midline, separating the right muscle belly from the left. The rectum is identified and separated from the levator muscles and plate. The rectococcygeal muscle (of Treitz) or ligament is identified and, if present, transected. (Like the anococcygeal raphe, this structure also varies in length and strength.) The retrorectal (or presacral) space is explored. Then the undersurface of the sacrum is cleansed of fat and loose connective tissue, exposing the periosteum.

The operator places three plication stitches in the posterior rectal wall 1 cm apart and ties but does not cut them (Fig. 29-5, *A*). Using an overglove, the operator performs a rectal examination to determine whether any sutures have penetrated the rectal mucosa; if so, they must be replaced because of the risk of abscess or fistula. These sutures are sewn to the presacral fascia (see Fig. 29-5, *B*). Polyglycolic acid–type sutures (Dexon or Vicryl) or longer-lasting polyglactin-type (PDS or Maxon) are used throughout the procedure. For patients who have chronic respiratory disease and therefore likely to have chronically increased intraabdominal pressure, a synthetic *nonabsorbable* monofilament suture may be used to provide firmer future resistance to recurrent herniation. A large dental mirror and a fiberoptic headlight help the operator visualize the placement of these stitches. After placing all stitches, the operator ties them, beginning with the most cranial suture. The coccyx is

not generally removed, and the middle sacral artery is ligated only if required to improve the exposure.

At this point, this operator uses a series of interrupted sutures (see Fig. 29-5, *C*) to sew together the medial borders of the levators (pubococcygei and puborectalis) in the midline *posterior* to the rectum; this procedure restores the integrity and length of the levator plate and displaces the rectum forward. The operator then shortens the undersurface of both right and left limbs of each pubococcygeal muscle (part of the anterior portion of the pelvic diaphragm) with Z-type sutures (see Fig. 29-5, *C*) and reattaches the lower rectum to the medial surfaces of the pubococcygei, suspending the rectum higher within the pelvis than it had been suspended preoperatively. The anococcygeal raphe is shortened by resection of the now excess length as necessary and reattached to either the coccygeal periosteum or to the gluteal fascia. A drain is not used. The subcutaneous tissue and the skin are closed with interrupted sutures.

If coincident anterior and posterior colporrhaphy, vaginal hysterectomy, or excision of any enterocele is necessary and has not yet been performed, the patient is repositioned in the conventional lithotomy position. If the perineal body has been separated from the connective tissue of the external anal sphincter, it should be reattached by a figure-of-eight stitch, which further stabilizes both the perineum and the anus (see Chapter 22). Fig. 29-6 illustrates the preoperative findings and postoperative results.

RECTAL PROLAPSE

When the patient complains of "hemorrhoids," although none is found at the time of examination, gynecologists must consider a previously undiagnosed intermittent (present only with straining) prolapse of the rectum or a mucosal prolapse. The patient, after the bowel has been given a preliminary mechanical preparation, should be asked to squat and to bear down heavily, as by a Valsalva maneuver. The surgeon carefully inspects the anus and confirms either hemorrhoids, mucosal prolapse, or rectal prolapse.

Hemorrhoids are lobular, with a visible sulcus between the masses of tissue. Prolapsing mucous membrane, being a single layer, is thinner to palpation than is the thickness of a true rectal prolapse with its multiple layers. The mucosal folds of a mucosal prolapse are radial in their direction, in contrast to those of rectal prolapse, which are arranged concentrically.[45]

To the patient so afflicted, rectal prolapse is of overwhelming clinical importance. Fortunately, genital prolapse is not often coincident with rectal prolapse[4] because it has a different etiology (Fig. 29-7). Rectal prolapse is probably the result of a rectorectal intussusception, rather than a sliding hernia.[45] A distended, freely mobile segment of rectal wall may virtually intussuscept into the previously normal caliber of the anal canal. Forcing defecation may be a contributing factor. The anatomic abnormalities noted in conjunction with rectal prolapse are probably the result, not the cause, of the prolapse.

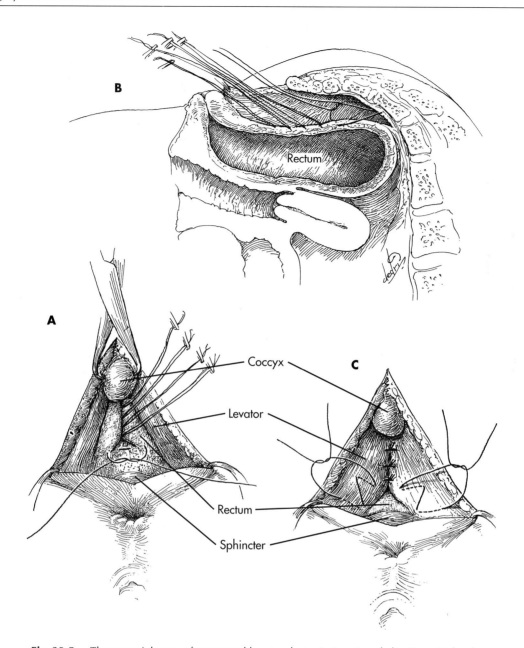

Fig. 29-5 The essential steps of retrorectal levatorplasty. **A,** A series of plication stitches have been placed 1 cm apart in the posterior wall of the rectum, tied, and left long. **B,** These are anchored individually to the anterior periosteum of the sacrum. **C,** The levator plate is restored and lengthened by bringing the pubococcygei of each side together in the midline between the coccyx and rectum. The bellies of the pubococcygei may be shortened by a **Z** stitch placed as shown in **C.** (From Nichols DH: *Surg Gynecol Obstet* 154:251, 1982.)

Rectal prolapse occurs predominantly in women who are thin and elderly; aging may have helped to diminish the tone of the pelvic muscles in these patients. Women with rectal prolapse are more likely to be nulliparous than multiparous, may suffer from chronic constipation, with chronic straining at stool, and may have abused laxatives. There is sometimes a coincident uterine prolapse.[4,25] Because the pelvic diaphragm and levator plate are tipped, the pelvic basin acts as a funnel, and as it becomes longer, the outlet opening becomes smaller, resulting in almost ribbonlike stools that become increasingly narrowed as the patient strains harder.

The symptoms of rectal prolapse are primarily rectal protrusion with straining or lifting, incomplete bowel movements, and rectal incontinence. As the condition progresses and the prolapsed rectum remains outside a greater portion of the time, bleeding develops. The physical findings are often clear enough to indicate the diagnosis, but the protrusion of the bowel when the patient strains (e.g., during a Valsalva maneuver) provides confirmation. The walls of the protruded rectum are thick, especially anteriorly, and an enterocele sac that contains small bowel may be present. The anus is usually patulous, up to 3 or 4 fingerbreadths in diameter, and the condition is surprisingly painless.[26]

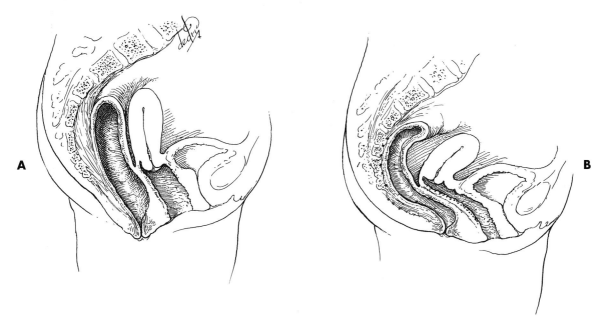

Fig. 29-6   A, Preoperative prolapse of the anus and perineum with tipping of the levator plate and elongation of the attachment of the rectum to the anterior surface of the sacrum. **B,** The result of surgery. The rectum has been approximated to the anterior periosteum of the sacrum, and the levator plate has been lengthened posterior to the rectum and the pubococcygei shortened as necessary. The axis of the lower rectum and upper vagina are more or less horizontal. An anorectal angulation is again present, and the anus is no longer the most dependent portion of the perineum. (From Nichols DH: *Surg Gynecol Obstet* 154:251,1982)

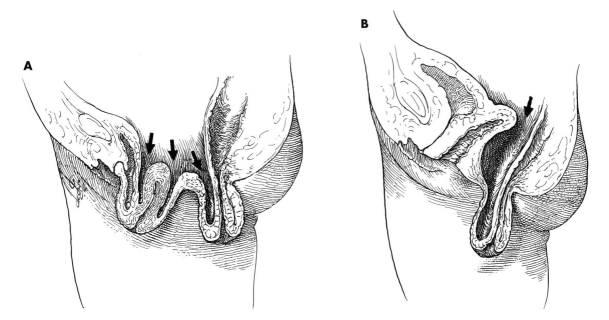

Fig. 29-7   **Rectal prolapse associated with enterocele. **A, Rectal prolapse is coincident with genital procidentia. **B,** The rectal prolapse is posterior to the vagina, which is not involved. (From Nichols DH: *Obstet Gynecol* 40:257, 1972.)

Most successful treatments for rectal prolapse in an otherwise healthy patient have been transabdominal,[30] although some surgeons have used the transperineal approach especially in elderly and debilitated patients, occasionally with coincident postanal levator repair,[16,38,40] and combinations of the transabdominal and transperineal approaches. Simple obliteration of the cul-de-sac on the rationale that the rectal prolapse is a sliding hernia (Moschcowitz) has not been consistently effective; the recurrence rate has been about 63%.[37] Intraabdominal and transperineal plication of the levator muscles has been employed, but lasting success has been obtained by transabdominal rectal and sigmoid suspension operations with or without the use of foreign materials.[4,42,49]

Retrorectal levatorplasty may be effective for some early stages of rectal prolapse. Perineal anal encirclement (for example, by the Thiersch technique) has been recommended with hesitation for elderly or poor-risk patients, although this technique requires the insertion of a foreign body around the anus, which decreases the anal diameter and risks fecal impaction as well as ulceration of the epithelium, requiring removal of the implant.[52] Unless the surgeon has special training and experience in rectal surgery, he or she should enlist the cooperation of an appropriate surgical consultant when planning and performing the necessary reconstruction.

Because prolapse of the rectum often is associated with rectal incontinence, especially in the presence of coincident anal sphincter damage, both internal and external sphincters, but especially the former, successful treatment of rectal prolapse requires some appreciation of the normal mechanisms of lower bowel function and a knowledge of the possible causes of any pathologic alterations.

Normal Lower Bowel Function

To a great extent, bowel function is the product of habit. The contents of the sigmoid colon are evacuated by first voluntarily relaxing the pelvic diaphragm (unlocking the colic valve) and relaxing the external anal sphincter. When the return is full, the internal sphincter opens. Modest increases in intraabdominal pressure obtained, for example, by bearing down, force the stool content downward. The gastrocolic reflex pattern regularly assists in this process by promoting intestinal peristalsis. A disorder that affects any of these steps predisposes a person to or causes constipation.

The levator ani and the external anal sphincter differ from the other striated muscles of the body in that they maintain a constant state of tone that is inversely proportional to the quantity of the rectal content. Neuromuscular pressure receptors within the levator ani are responsible for mediating its tone and apparently communicate with the central nervous system by way of the pudendal nerve on each side of the body, which generally arises from S3 and S4. Because intestinal peristalsis continues around the clock, although at apparently various degrees of intensity, this tone is responsible for rectal continence.

The contraction of the levator ani and puborectalis muscles pulls the genital hiatus toward the pubis, placing the rectum at an angle that allows it to function effectively as a valve, according to the observations of Parks.[33-35,48] There is a reflex reciprocity with the tone of the external anal sphincter. These muscles are innervated by the pudendal nerve and its accessory branches, and they function in synergism. The innervation of the puborectalis is less certain, although it may come from a sacral plexus component.

Pathologic Dysfunction of the Lower Bowel

Constipation may appear as an early symptom of perineal descent. A rectocele does *not* commonly cause constipation, however, although both may occur simultaneously. The primary symptoms of a rectocele are aching after a bowel movement and an inability to empty the bowel completely so that manual expression is often necessary for full evacuation. Posterior colporrhaphy should relieve these primary symptoms, but it will not necessarily relieve constipation other than that produced when stool is caught in a pocket of the rectal wall, precluding complete emptying of the bowel. Many women with a rectocele are not constipated, and many more women without a rectocele are constipated.

Either congenital or acquired pathologic conditions of the pudendal nerve can alter its efficiency and thus affect the ability of the neuromuscular receptors within the levator ani to influence pressure and maintain the responsive muscular tone of the levator ani.[27] Acquired damage may result from the trauma of the stretching of the pelvic floor during childbirth and quite possibly from chronic excessive straining at stool. Regular and excessive bearing down during defecation may stretch the pudendal nerves, destroying anatomic integrity, consequently weakening the muscles that they innervate, and occasionally resulting in a permanent loss of muscle tone in the denervated pelvic diaphragm and external anal sphincter. The neuropathic loss of the tone of the anal sphincter permits it to relax at inopportune times, resulting in rectal incontinence that may be most difficult to remedy surgically. The Parks group has suggested that this loss of voluntary muscle tone within the pelvic diaphragm may be coincident with urinary stress incontinence.[21]

Henry[19] described the relationship between rectal prolapse and rectal incontinence as follows:

> I think the primary pathology is one of neuropathy affecting the pelvic floor—in many patients a consequence of damage to the pudendal nerve, damage inflicted by traumatic childbirth. Incontinence may not develop initially if the internal anal sphincter is functioning normally. Pelvic floor denervation initiates rectal prolapse because of disruption of the anorectal flap valve. The prolapse starts with descent of the anterior rectal wall and at a later stage a circumferential complete prolapse intussuscepts through the anus. The dilatation of the internal anal sphincter caused by the prolapsing rectum then destroys the only mechanism protecting anorectal continence and a major functional problem results. Because the internal sphincter recovers, many patients recover a reasonable degree of control after successful repair of the prolapse. If continence is not recovered within six months, we will offer the patient a transperineal post-anal repair (of the puborectalis and the pelvic diaphragm).

Types and Combinations of Anorectal Prolapse

When a rectal prolapse and massive genital prolapse coexist (see Fig. 29-7, *A*), they should be treated simultaneously if possible. The cause and treatment of each are entirely different from one another. Often the rectal prolapse involves a pathologically long sigmoid colon and coincident enterocele. After appropriate diagnostic workup, including sigmoidoscopy, barium enema, and other studies depending on the presence of coexistent rectal incontinence, this can be treated surgically by large bowel resection with low anastomosis and rectopexy attaching the rectal "stalk" to the periosteum of the sacrum or even sacrospinous rectopexy (see Chapter 26). This is followed by appropriate treatment of the genital prolapse. If the latter is associated with poor cardinal-uterosacral ligament strength and colpopexy to a nongynecologic strong structure is planned, a transvaginal sacrospinous colpopexy with colporrhaphy may be done. If the surgeon and patient prefer a transabdominal route for treatment, an abdominal sacrocolpopexy with Halban-type stitches sagittally obliterating the cul-de-sac (see Chapter 23) should be done at the same operation and, if possible, immediately after the treatment of the bowel prolapse. Because the vagina is anterior to the rectum, the sacrocolpopexy must be performed anterior to the rectopexy. This surgical program is not to be taken lightly; however, use of the circular stapler improves the case and speed of large intestinal low anastomosis. Overall, there appears to be a small (1%) but significant risk of anastomotic leakage with subsequent peritonitis and all of its problems.[52] If not overly elongated a rectopexy may be considered, in which the peritoneal coat of the mobilized rectum and rectosigmoid are sewn to the "ligament" established between the vaginal vault and sacrum, fixing them in the sacral hollow.[4] Such colporrhaphy as might be necessary should be accomplished by a separate transvaginal route.

For older patients with massive eversion of the vagina including large cystocele and rectocele and a simultaneous but shorter (less than 5 cm) prolapse of the rectum, the surgeon may elect a transperineal approach to each. Transvaginal excision of any enterocele, sacrospinous colpopexy, and colporrhaphy are followed by resection of the prolapsed rectal mucosa and longitudinal accordion pleating of the muscularis followed by reunification of the mucosa and replacement of the resultant "doughnut" back within the anal canal, essentially the Delorme operation.[29,49]

For younger patients, transperineal, full-thickness resection of the type recommended by Altemeier[1-3] for rectal prolapse may be chosen in anticipation of the patient's longer life span and postoperative perception of discomfort.

Some Surgical Treatments for Rectal Prolapse

Delorme-Type Mucosal Stripping Operation.[5,12,29]

The combined prolapse is noted in Fig. 29-8, *A*.[5] It is replaced within the pelvis, and the colpopexy and colporrhaphy are accomplished. The rectal procidentia is gently pulled back into the operative field, and an incision is made just distal to the pectinate line down to the superficial layers

of the muscularis (see Fig. 29-8, *B*). This is the first of two techniques of reducing the rectal procidentia. First is the accordion type of plication. Because the peritoneal sac from the cul-de-sac has already been reduced and retracted upward during the reduction of the hernia vaginally, it is not necessary to locate and deal with the hernial sac, as it would be were this an isolated operation for rectal procidentia alone.

The surgeon encounters a general ooze of blood from the operative area during this dissection. Distinct bleeding points are clamped and ligated. Final hemostasis is obtained when the longitudinal plication sutures are tied.

Fig. 29-8, *C,* shows a method of denuding the mucosa and underlying muscularis mucosa from the rectal procidentia. Four or five longitudinal segments are selected, and, as the mucosa is separated by sharp dissection, it is rolled on a Halstead clamp. Specific arterial bleeding points are ligated during this denudation. As the denudation is continued distally, the terminal end of the intussusception is reached. This dissection is continued until a small edge of mucosa at the distal end of the prolapse is left for anastomosis (see Fig. 29-8, *D*). Fig. 29-8, *E,* shows the denudation of the mucosa from the posterior aspect. The blood loss during this dissection is carefully estimated, and one or more units may be needed for replacement.

Accordion pleating sutures are placed longitudinally about 2 cm apart. These should penetrate the muscular coats of the rectal wall but preferably not pass through the full thickness of the rectum (see Fig. 29-8, *F*). The preferred material is 0 polyglycolic acid–type suture on a fine Ferguson needle. After all the pleating sutures have been placed, they are tied by the operator while the assistants gradually draw up on the untied sutures and reduce the prolapse (see Fig. 29-8, *G*).

The mucosal edges should approximate each other without tension. A few additional sutures in the muscularis may be needed to permit approximation. Sutures of 2-0 polyglycolic acid on chromic catgut are used to close the mucosa (see Fig. 29-8, *H*).

The doughnut formed by the accordion method of pleating is replaced in the pelvis through the dilated rectal sphincter (see Fig. 29-8, *I*). Attention is directed to further support of the rectum by the transvaginal approach.

Altemeier-Type Full-Thickness Resection.[1-3,5,40] As

an alternative method, the rectal prolapse may be amputated. This is preferred in younger patients for whom the doughnut resulting from the plication technique may impinge on the posterior vaginal wall and cause a constriction. This is unimportant when the vagina need not be a functional organ. Fig. 29-9, *A* (p. 559), shows angle sutures placed just above the white line (distal to the white line as seen with the rectum inverted). These should be placed through all layers to prevent retraction when the procidentia is amputated.

Fig. 29-9, *B* (p. 559), shows the layers in midsagittal section. The layers to be approximated are shown because the intussuscipiens (outer layers) and intussusceptum

Text continued on p. 560

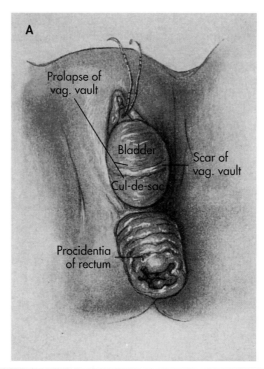

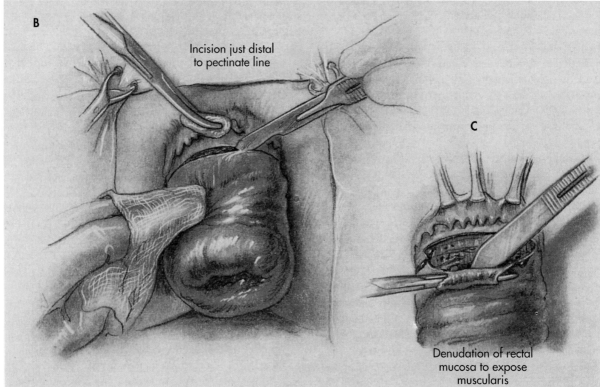

Fig. 29-8   Delorme-type mucosal stripping operation. **A,** A combined genital posthysterectomy prolapse and rectal prolapse. **B,** A circumferential incision is made to remove the protruding rectal mucosa. **C,** The prolapsed rectal mucosa is dissected from the underlying muscularis. (From Ball TL: *Gynecologic surgery and urology,* ed 2, St Louis, 1963, Mosby.)

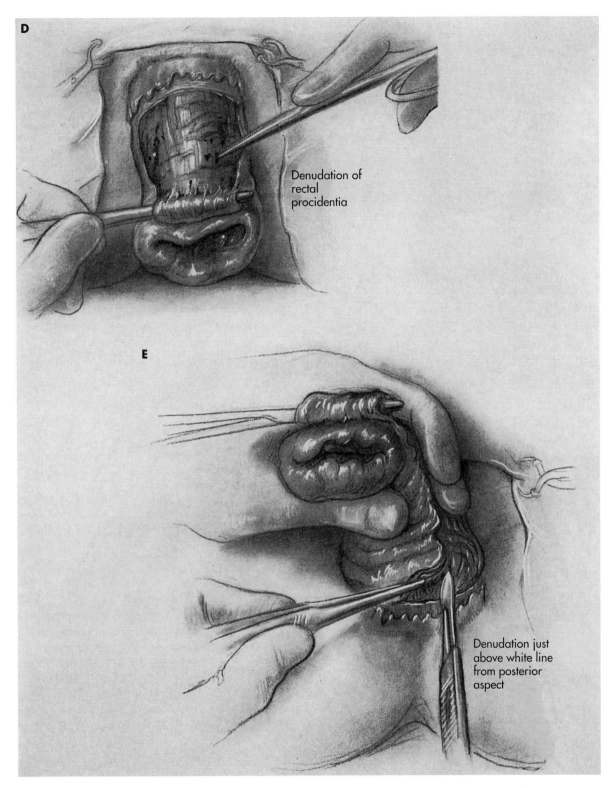

Fig. 29-8, cont'd   D, Mucosa denudation continues. **E,** Denudation progresses posteriorly to a limit just above the white or dentate line.   *Continued*

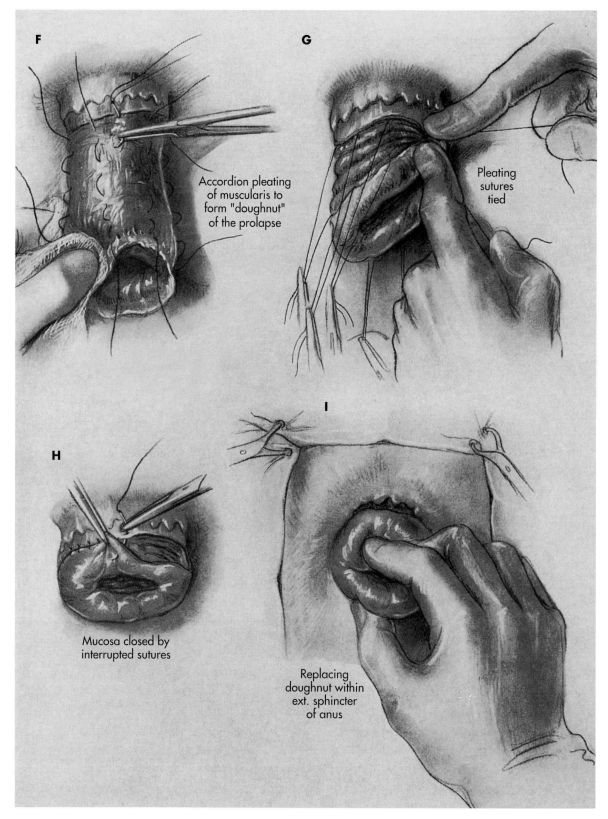

Fig. 29-8, cont'd   F, A series of longitudinally placed pleating stitches is placed in the muscularis. **G,** When all pleating sutures have been placed, they are tied in sequence. **H,** The mucosal edges are closed by interrupted sutures. **I,** The "doughnut" is gently replaced within the anal canal. (From Ball TL: *Gynecologic surgery and urology*, ed 2, St Louis, 1963, Mosby.)

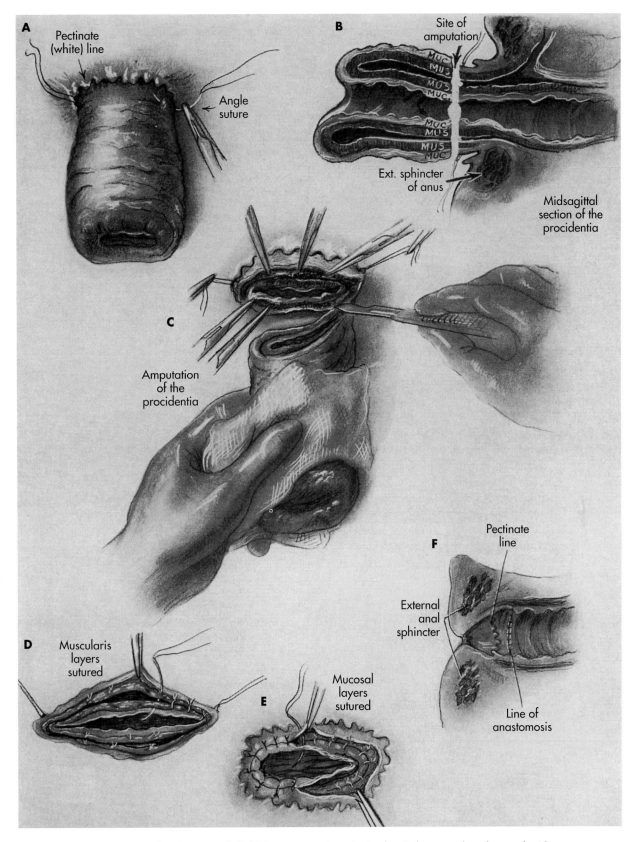

A

Pectinate
(white) line

Angle
suture

B

Site of
amputation

MUC
MUS
MUC
MUS
MUC
MUS
MUS
MUC

Ext. sphincter
of anus

Midsagittal
section of the
procidentia

C

Amputation
of the
procidentia

D

Muscularis
layers
sutured

E

Mucosal
layers
sutured

F

Pectinate
line

External
anal
sphincter

Line of
anastomosis

Fig. 29-9 Altemeier-type full-thickness resection. **A,** Angle stitches are placed to each side of the prolapsed rectum. **B,** Sagittal section through the prolapse shows the site of amputation. **C,** Procidentia is amputated. **D,** Muscularis layers are sewn together by interrupted sutures. **E,** Mucosal layers are sutured with interrupted sutures. **F,** Sagittal drawing shows the site of the bowel reanastomosis at the completion of the operation. A petroleum jelly gauze plug is placed in the rectum, and the vagina is packed with gauze.

(inner layers) are best delineated in midsagittal section. The hernial sac of peritoneum that would prolapse between the two anterior layers is missing because it was dissected out and reduced during the mobilization of the cul-de-sac hernia transvaginally.

The prolapsed rectum is then amputated (see Fig. 29-9, *C*). The bleeding points are clamped and tied. If the mucosa of the bowel tends to retract, it can be grasped with Allis clamps. The muscularis of the rectum is anastomosed with interrupted sutures of 2-0 polyglycolic acid–type suture (see Fig. 29-9, *D*). A clamp technique, continuous sutures, or the use of other suture materials may be elected according to the preference of the surgeon. The angle sutures are removed if they distort the approximation of either the mucosal or muscular layers during the anastomosis.

Fig. 29-9, *E,* shows the approximation of the muscularis of the bowel. This is done with 2-0 polyglycolic acid–type suture. The line of anastomosis is inverted behind the external sphincter of the anus. Its position, in midsagittal section, is shown in Fig. 29-9, *F.* The "doughnut" is replaced inside the anal canal, and the vagina is packed with plain or iodoform gauze. A Foley catheter is placed into the bladder. Removal of the dilating rectal wedge should soon help to narrow the widened levator hiatus.

Postoperative Care

The vaginal pack and petroleum jelly gauze plug in the rectum are removed in 24 hours. The patient's diet is modified, depending on whether the rectal procidentia was accordion-pleated or resected. With a bowel resection, even though retroperitoneal, the patient is maintained on intravenous fluids for the first 2 days. Vitamins and milliequivalents of potassium as indicated are added to the infusions. Blood chemistry studies to include serum potassium and chlorides are made for the first few days. The diet is progressed to clear liquids, then a soft diet as tolerated, and finally to a regular diet by the eighth day or sooner. This is modified, depending on the postoperative course of the patient. If the rectal procidentia is accordion-pleated, the patient can proceed to a regular diet much sooner. Intubation is seldom necessary, but the usual indications may necessitate this occasionally.

With a thorough bowel preparation before surgery and the preceding dietary routine, a warm mineral oil enema of 240 ml can be administered about the sixth postoperative day. If the patient is not uncomfortable, a tap water enema can be deferred until the eighth or ninth day. All this must be adapted to the individual patient and situation.

The patient is progressively ambulated, beginning by getting out of bed the day after the operation. Urinary antiseptics are administered. Because of the extent of the operation, some surgeons prefer to give combined therapy consisting of one sulfonamide preparation and one wide-spectrum antibiotic. The selection of drugs may be guided by the cultures and sensitivity tests if a bacteriuria was found. The catheter is removed on the fifth postoperative day, and residuals are measured.

REFERENCES

1. Altemeier WA, Culbertson WR: Technique for perineal repair of rectal prolapse, *Surgery* 58:758, 1965.
2. Altemeier WA, Culbertson WR, Schowengerdt C, Hunt J: Nineteen years' experience with the one-stage perineal repair of rectal prolapse, *Ann Surg* 173:993, 1971.
3. Altemeier WA, Giuseffi J, Hoxworth P: Treatment of extensive prolapse of the rectum in aged or debilitated patients, *Arch Surg* 65:72, 1952.
4. Amico JC, Marino AW Jr: Prolapse of the vagina in association with rectal procidentia, *Dis Colon Rectum* 11:115, 1968.
5. Ball TL: *Gynecologic surgery and urology,* ed 2, St Louis, 1963, Mosby.
6. Barrett CW: Hernias through the pelvic floor, *Am J Obstet Dis Women* 59:553, 1909.
7. Bartolo DC, Read NW, Jarratt JA, et al: Differences in anal sphincter function and clinical presentation in patients with pelvic floor descent, *Gastroenterology* 85:68, 1983.
8. Berglas B, Rubin IC: Study of the supportive structures of the uterus by levator myography, *Surg Gynecol Obstet* 97:672, 1953.
9. Bevan AD: Carcinoma of rectum—treatment by local excision, *Surg Clin* 1:1233, 1917.
10. Crowley RT, Davis DA: A procedure for total biopsy of doubtful polypoid growths of the lowest bowel segment, *Surg Gynecol Obstet* 93:23, 1951.
11. Davidian UA, Thomas CG: Transsacral repair of rectal prolapse, *Am J Surg* 123:231, 1972.
12. Delorme R: Sur le traitement des prolapsus du rectum totaux part l'excision de la muquese rectale au rectal-colique, *Bull Soc Chir Paris* 26:498, 1900.
13. Efron G: A simple method of posterior rectopexy for rectal procidentia, *Surg Gynecol Obstet* 145:75, 1977.
14. Gallagher DM: Personal communication.
15. Goligher JC: The treatment of complete prolapse of the rectum by the Roscoe Graham operation, *Br J Surg* 46:323, 1958.
16. Gopal KA, Amshel AL, Shonberg IL, Eftaiha M: Rectal procidentia in elderly and debilitated patients, *Dis Colon Rectum* 27:376, 1984.
17. Graham R: Operative repair of massive rectal prolapse, *Ann Surg* 115:1007, l942.
18. Haskell B, Rovner H: Electromyography in the management of the incompetent anal sphincter. Proceedings of the American Proctologic Society, Cleveland, June 1966.
19. Henry MM: Personal communication, Sept 2, 1987.
20. Henry MM, Swash M: Assessment of pelvic floor disorders and incontinence by electrophysiological recording of the anal reflex, *Lancet* 17:1290, 1978.
21. Henry MM, Swash M, editors: *Coloproctology and the pelvic floor,* ed 2, London, 1992, Butterworths.
22. Jenkins SG, Thomas CG: An operation for the repair of rectal prolapse, *Surg Gynecol Obstet* 114:381, 1962.
23. Klingensmith W, Dickinson WE, Hays RS: Posterior resection of selected rectal tumors, *Arch Surg* 110:647, 1975.
24. Kraske P: Zur Extirpation Hochsitzender Mastdarmkrebse, *Vehr Dtsch Ges Chir* 14:464, 1885.
25. Lange F: *Intestinal and anal surgery.* Quoted in Hadra BE, editor: *Lesions of the vagina and pelvic floor,* Philadelphia, 1888, McMullin.
26. Lockhart-Mummery JP: Rectal prolapse, *Br Med J* 1:345, 1939.
27. Madoff RD, Williams JG, Caushaj PF: Fecal incontinence, *N Engl J Med* 326:1002, 1992.
28. Mason AY: Trans-sphincteric surgery of the rectum, *Prog Surg* 13:66, 1974.
29. McCaffrey JF: Delorme repair for prolapse of the rectum following "failed" Ripstein operation, *Am J Proctol Gastroenterol Colon Rectal Surg* 34:5, 1983.
30. Nichols DH: Retrorectal levatorplasty for anal and perineal prolapse, *Surg Gynecol Obstet* 154:251, 1982.
31. Nichols DH: Retrorectal levatorplasty with colporrhaphy, *Clin Obstet Gynecol* 25:939, 1982.

32. O'Brien PH: Kraske's posterior approach to the rectum, *Surg Gynecol Obstet* 142:412, 1976.

33. Parks AG: Modern concepts of the anatomy of the anorectal region, *Postgrad Med J* 34:360, 1958.

34. Parks AG: Anorectal incontinence, *Proc R Soc Med* 68:681, 1975.

35. Parks AG, Porter NH, Hardcastle J: The syndrome of the descending perineum, *Proc R Soc Med* 59:477, 1966.

36. Parks AG, Swash M, Urich H: Sphincter denervation in anorectal incontinence and rectal prolapse, *J Br Soc Gastroenterol* 18:656, 1977.

37. Pemberton J de J, Stalker LK: Surgical treatment of complete metal prolapse, *Am Surg* 109:799, 1939.

38. Prasad ML, Pearl RK, Abcarian H, et al: Perineal proctectomy, posterior rectopexy, and postanal levator repair for the treatment of rectal prolapse, *Dis Colon Rectum* 29:547, 1986.

39. Ramanujam PS, Venkatesh KS: Perineal excision of rectal prolapse with posterior levator ani repair in elderly high-risk patients, *Dis Colon Rectum* 31:704, 1988.

40. Ramanujam PS, Venkatesh KS, Fietz MJ: Perineal excision of rectal procidentia in elderly high-risk patients, *Dis Colon Rectum* 37:1027, 1994.

41. Redding MD: The relaxed perineum and anorectal disease, *Dis Colon Rectum* 8:279, 1965.

42. Ripstein CB, Lanter B: Etiology and surgical therapy of massive prolapse of the rectum, *Ann Surg* 157:259, 1963.

43. Roig JV, Villoslada C, Lledo S, et al: Prevalence of pudendal neuropathy in fecal incontinence, *Dis Colon Rectum* 38:952, 1995.

44. Romer-Torres R: Sacrofixation with Marlex mesh in massive prolapse of the rectum, *Surg Gynecol Obstet* 149:709, 1979.

45. Schoetz DJ Jr, Veidenheimer MC: Rectal prolapse—pathogenesis and clinical features, In Henry MM, Swash M, editors: *Coloproctology and the pelvic floor,* ed 2, London, 1992, Butterworths.

46. Sharf B et al: Electromyogram of pelvic floor muscles in genital prolapse, *Int J Gynaecol Obstet* 14:2, 1976.

47. Sullivan ES et al: Transrectal perineal repair: an adjunct to improved function after anorectal surgery. Proceedings of the American Proctologic Society, New Orleans, April 1967.

48. Swash M, Snooks SJ, Henry MM: Unifying concept of pelvic floor disorders and incontinence, *J R Soc Med* 78:906, 1985.

49. Tancer ML, Fleischer M, Berkowitz BJ: Simultaneous colporectosacropexy, *Obstet Gynecol* 70:951, 1987.

50. Taverner D, Smiddy FG: An electromyographic study of the normal function of the external anal sphincter and pelvic diaphragm, *Dis Colon Rectum* 2:153, 1959.

51. Turner GG: Ideals and the art of surgery, *Surg Gynecol Obstet* 52:273, 1931.

52. Watts JD, Rothenberger DA, Goldberg SM: Rectal prolapse—treatment. In Henry MM, Swash M, editors: *Coloproctology and the pelvic floor,* ed 2, London, 1992, Butterworths.

53. Wiersema JS: Treatment of complete prolapse of the rectum by the vaginal approach, *Arch Chir Neerl* 28:25, 1976.

54. Yoshioka K, Keighley MPB: Critical assessment of the quality of continence after postanal repair for faecal incontinence, *Br J Surg* 78:1054, 1989 [Erratum *Br J Surg* 79:356, 1990].

30 Abdominal Hysterectomy

DANIEL L. CLARKE-PEARSON

Hysterectomy is the second most commonly performed operation in the United States, exceeded only by cesarean section. However, the number of hysterectomies has declined over the past two decades from approximately 649,000 in 1980[7] to approximately 556,000 in 1994.[9] Of the entire U.S. population, 18.5 million women have undergone a hysterectomy, and 37% of American women will undergo a hysterectomy by age 60.[16] It is estimated that the total cost for hysterectomies in 1994 was $5 billion.[9] Of all hysterectomies, 63% are performed in women between the ages of 15 and 44 years (median age 40.9 years).[16] Over the past two decades, there has been a significant decline in the length of stay for in-hospital recovery after hysterectomy, which in 1978 was approximately 8 days. Vaginal hysterectomy is now often done as an outpatient procedure,[19] and most patients who undergo an abdominal hysterectomy have only a 2- to 3-day postoperative hospital stay.

INDICATIONS

There are many indications for performing hysterectomies, and approximately 75% are performed through an abdominal incision. In addition, there are large regional variations in the number of hysterectomies performed and the frequency of abdominal and vaginal approaches.[1] The most common indications for abdominal hysterectomy are removal of symptomatic fibroid tumors, treatment of symptoms caused by endometriosis, correction of uterine descensus (prolapse), and cancer or endometrial hyperplasia. When symptoms are considered, 90% of hysterectomies are performed for the relief of bleeding, pain, or both.[6]

Removal of symptomatic uterine fibroids is the most common indication for performing a hysterectomy, accounting for approximately 39.5% of all hysterectomies.[13] Reasons most commonly reported include uncontrolled uterine bleeding, pelvic or abdominal pain and pressure, gastrointestinal symptoms (e.g., rectal pressure), and genitourinary symptoms (e.g., hydronephrosis or urinary frequency). Also noted as a reason is rapid expansion of fibroids. In past decades, a uterine size of greater than 12 weeks' gestation was considered an indication for hysterectomy, although this indication has undergone reevaluation in recent years, and

many authors now believe that hysterectomy for asymptomatic uterine fibroids is unnecessary.[17] Hysterectomy for uterine fibroids appears to be more commonly performed in African-American women than in white women.[21] On the other hand, rates for hysterectomies for treatment of endometriosis, prolapse, and cancer are higher in white women.[21] The selection of a vaginal or an abdominal hysterectomy for treatment of uterine fibroids is most often based on the size of the fibroids and the surgeon's estimation whether the surgery can be performed successfully through the vaginal route. Certainly techniques of morselization and laparoscopy have allowed the vaginal removal of a myomatous uterus of up to 14 to 16 weeks' gestational size in many women (see Chapters 19 and 20). Furthermore, the preoperative use of gonadotropin-releasing hormone (GnRH) agonists often results in a reduction in uterine size and the conversion from an abdominal to a vaginal approach in a significant number of women in whom initial uterine size is approximately 14 to 18 weeks' gestation.[18] Stovall et al.[18] note that GnRH agonists are of little help in converting the approach from abdominal to vaginal in women with uterine size greater than 18 weeks' gestation and that the use of GnRH agonists is not cost effective in an excessively large uterus.[2]

Endometriosis is the second most common indication for performing a hysterectomy and is most often associated with the symptom of chronic pelvic pain. The frequency of hysterectomy for the treatment of a diagnosis of endometriosis has been increasing over the past few decades, although the reason for this increase is not entirely clear. It may be that treatment of symptomatic endometriosis is more common because of delay in childbearing in American women, that endometriosis is diagnosed more accurately by American gynecologists (predominantly by use of the laparoscope for diagnosis), or that American gynecologists have liberalized their indications for performing hysterectomy for the treatment of symptomatic endometriosis. Over the past two decades, there have also been significant advances in the medical management of endometriosis with pharmacologic agents such as Provera (medroxyprogesterone), danazol, and GnRH agonists. Furthermore, there have been substantial advances in pain management, with a number of nonsteroidal antiinflammatory agents currently available.

Symptomatic uterine relaxation and prolapse are usually managed by a vaginal hysterectomy, which is often combined with additional surgical procedures to repair pelvic floor defects (see Chapters 19, 21, 22, 23, 26, 27, and 29). It is reasonable to perform an abdominal hysterectomy in patients with prolapse, in whom other intraabdominal procedures (e.g., sacral colpopexy) are also to be performed.

Chronic pelvic inflammatory disease may also be an indication for abdominal hysterectomy. In most patients, the hysterectomy is performed to treat chronic pelvic pain. The primary disease process often involves the adnexa (tubal ovarian abscesses and adhesions), although the uterus is commonly removed at the same time. However, the patient's opinion about whether hysterectomy should be performed must be clearly understood during the preoperative discussion because some patients, given the option for new reproductive technologies, might wish to preserve the uterus and achieve pregnancy through the use of donor oocytes and in vitro fertilization.

Chronic bleeding, unresponsive to medical management, is another common indication for hysterectomy. Bleeding may be caused by a number of gynecologic conditions, including uterine polyps, endometrial hyperplasia, fibroids, adenomyosis, disordered endometrial proliferation, coagulopathies, and cervical or uterine malignancy. Patients should be evaluated with endometrial biopsy, hysteroscopy, or dilation and curettage (D&C). For most patients, a hysterectomy should be considered only if management with hormones failed.

Emergency hysterectomies are most often performed in the postpartum setting to treat hemorrhage, uterine rupture, uterine atony, or endometritis unresponsive to antibiotic therapy. Septic, spontaneous, therapeutic, or criminal abortion may be associated with myonecrosis requiring hysterectomy, and a ruptured cornual ectopic pregnancy may require management by hysterectomy, although often conservative surgery can be performed, thus preserving the uterus.

Two decades ago, cervical intraepithelial neoplasia was a common primary indication for abdominal hysterectomy. Today, conservative management, as outlined in Chapter 17, has such a high success rate (with much decreased cost and morbidity) that hysterectomy is rarely recommended. On the other hand, endometrial carcinoma, endometrial carcinosarcoma, leiomyosarcoma, stromal sarcoma, ovarian carcinoma, fallopian tube carcinoma, and early invasive cervical carcinoma (stage IA1) are appropriate indications for abdominal hysterectomy. On rare occasions, abdominal hysterectomy is recommended for the treatment of apparent chemotherapy resistance, gestational trophoblastic disease invading the myometrium, or rectal carcinoma arising adjacent to or involving the uterine fundus.

Hysterectomy is also often performed in association with the treatment of benign adnexal disease. This is most commonly recommended in menopausal women or in premenopausal women, who will have both ovaries removed. However, in the treatment of adnexal pathologic conditions,

abdominal hysterectomy is not mandatory (unless the patient has cancer). This particular circumstance should be discussed preoperatively and a decision made by the patient about whether she wishes to have a hysterectomy performed. In evaluating this issue, Grover et al.[8] have found that women who had an elective hysterectomy at the time of adnexal surgery had a slight increase in short-term morbidity, which was counterbalanced by a slight increase in average life expectancy among perimenopausal women who had a hysterectomy performed. Furthermore, Grover et al. found that performing a hysterectomy at the time of adnexal resection resulted in slight cost savings. It was estimated that 10% of patients who had an elective hysterectomy under these circumstances would not need a second procedure at a later point to remove the uterus because of development of other benign or malignant gynecologic disease. However, it is more difficult to assess the full benefit that might be realized by women who may avoid the use of progestins while taking estrogen replacement therapy, those who may avoid future gynecologic symptoms, and those who would avoid minor surgical procedures such as endometrial biopsy, D&C, or colposcopy. Overall, the analysis of Grover et al. supports the selected use of concurrent hysterectomy at the time of bilateral salpingo-oophorectomy in patients who desire uterine removal and who are willing to take the risk of increased short-term morbidity and the possibility of unknown long-term complications.

ALTERNATIVE MANAGEMENT

Alternative management of gynecologic conditions, which might avoid the need for hysterectomy, is becoming more common and will likely result in the need for fewer abdominal hysterectomies in the future. As noted previously, endometriosis may also be managed by the use of medications such as progestins, danazol, and Lupron (leuprolide). Furthermore, conservative surgery with fulguration, laser vaporization, or conservative resection of endometriosis and endometriomas often can avoid the need for hysterectomy. The evaluation of "dysfunctional" uterine bleeding and management with hormonal manipulation based on findings of endometrial biopsy or D&C commonly will control bleeding, which in past decades required treatment by hysterectomy. With advances in hysteroscopic surgery (see Chapter 41), a symptomatic polyp or submucous myoma can often be removed, thereby preserving the uterus and avoiding hysterectomy. Intractable bleeding may also be managed alternatively by hysteroscopic resection or ablation of the endometrium. Finally, pain, which was a common indication for a hysterectomy in the past, has been managed in many patients with the early use of appropriate antibiotics for pelvic inflammatory disease, with antiinflammatory medications, and with thorough psychiatric evaluation. The outcomes of nonsurgical management of leiomyomas, abnormal bleeding, and chronic pelvic pain were studied by Carlson et al.,[4] who found that approximately 25% of patients initially treated nonsurgically subsequently underwent hysterectomy. In patients who did not require immediate hysterectomy, approximately 25% with abnormal bleeding and 50% with chronic pelvic pain reported continued symptoms after 1 year of follow-up. In the group with chronic pelvic pain, only 30% reported improvement in the pain after 12 months of treatment. Furthermore, patients with leiomyomas who were managed nonsurgically had no significant change in their symptoms or quality of life for over 1 year. Although medical management is certainly reasonable and should be considered, many patients in this study did not achieve resolution of symptoms or improvement in quality of life until they had undergone a hysterectomy.

Having outlined the most common indications for abdominal hysterectomy, it must be noted that a number of less morbid surgical alternative management options are available that should be considered by the gynecologist. The use of GnRH agonists for the management of fibroids,[18] for example, might shrink the fibroids to a size that would be appropriate for vaginal surgery. Myomectomy might be considered, especially when pregnancy or the preservation of fertility is desired. Myomectomy compares favorably with hysterectomy, with similar amounts of blood loss and transfusion requirements when controlled for uterine size.[11] Visceral injuries (e.g., ureteral, bladder, or bowel injuries) were more commonly encountered in the hysterectomy group.[11]

PREOPERATIVE PREPARATION

Before undergoing a hysterectomy the patient should have had a complete gynecologic evaluation as well as an evaluation of her general health and potential for surgical complications. Furthermore, the patient should be prepared before surgery using strategies known to prevent postoperative complications such as infection or venous thromboembolus. This evaluation and management are outlined in detail in Chapter 5, but some significant reminders are reviewed in this section.

The gynecologic evaluation should include ascertainment that the Pap smear is normal and that there is no indication of associated malignancy of the cervix or endometrium. Abnormal uterine bleeding should have been evaluated by endometrial biopsy, hysteroscopy, or D&C. Furthermore, anemia associated with abnormal bleeding should have been corrected by the use of iron, folate, or recombinant erythropoietin. Uncorrected anemia should be further evaluated to rule out other sources of bleeding such as a gastrointestinal malignancy or active peptic ulcer disease. Attempts should be made to stop the uterine bleeding with the use of progestins, oral contraceptives, or GnRH agonists. Stovall et al.[18] found that the preoperative use of GnRH agonists resulted in a significant increase in hemoglobin level and decreased blood loss for women with uterine myomatas of 14 to 18 weeks' gestational size when they were given GnRH agonists for 2 months before a hysterectomy. If anemia is severe or bleeding cannot be controlled, preoperative red blood cell transfusion may be required.

Preoperative evaluation of patients undergoing hysterectomy should follow routine guidelines wherein healthy young women do not necessarily require studies such as chest x-ray studies or electrocardiograms. Certainly, in low-risk patients, preoperative coagulation testing is not cost effective,[14] and a preoperative intravenous pyelogram should be done only in specific patients in whom ureteral compromise might be anticipated based on associated pelvic pathologic conditions, prior pelvic surgery, or other mullerian anomalies that might be associated with urologic anomalies.[15] I believe strongly that mechanical bowel preparation should be part of the preoperative preparation, although oral antibiotic bowel preparation is rarely recommended unless concurrent colon surgery is anticipated.

The use of prophylactic antibiotics to reduce febrile morbidity and urinary tract and wound infections is controversial. Although the literature is clear that patients undergoing vaginal hysterectomy benefit substantially from the use of prophylactic antibiotics, it is less clear that those undergoing abdominal hysterectomy benefit from prophylactic antibiotics. However, most of the literature supports the use of prophylactic antibiotics; therefore I would generally recommend the perioperative use of a first-generation cephalosporin.

Prevention of deep venous thrombosis and pulmonary embolism is also an important preoperative consideration, and prophylaxis by the use of low-dose heparin, low-molecular-weight heparin, or pneumatic leg compression should be offered to patients at moderate to high risk of developing deep vein thrombosis or pulmonary embolism. In general, this includes all women undergoing hysterectomy who are older than age 40 and younger women with other risk factors (e.g., a history of deep vein thrombosis or pulmonary embolism, obesity, thrombophilic conditions, and cancer).

The need for preoperative type and cross-match of packed red blood cells for possible intraoperative transfusion during a hysterectomy should be carefully considered for cost effectiveness. In general, the risk of blood transfusion after a hysterectomy ranges from 1% to 25%.[12] Clearly, transfusions are not given often enough in most patients undergoing hysterectomy to warrant a type and cross-match of one to two units of blood preoperatively because most of this blood would be discarded, increasing the cost of health care. On the other hand, patients with a marginal preoperative hemoglobin level or those in whom excessive blood loss is anticipated (e.g., those with extensive endometriosis, a massively enlarged fibroid uterus, or advanced ovarian cancer) should have appropriate estimations of blood requirements and blood made available for transfusion. The use of autologous blood donation before elective hysterectomy was evaluated by Kanter,[12] who found that in those patients who had autologous blood donated, there was an associated increase in preoperative anemia and a more liberal blood transfusion policy, resulting in a significant increase in the incidence of transfusion with its associated risks. It was concluded that preoperative autologous donation before hysterectomy is unnecessary and would not significantly eliminate the need for allogenic blood transfusion.

As part of the preoperative planning process, other associated conditions should be recognized and addressed. Problems such as pelvic floor prolapse, enterocele, cystocele, or incontinence should be identified based on history and physical examination. Appropriate urodynamic workups should be done if necessary. Other associated surgical procedures necessary to correct these pelvic floor defects should be incorporated into the information the patient is given as well as into informed consent. In the past, elective ("incidental") appendectomy was often advised or undertaken routinely. It appears that for most adult women, this is not necessarily appropriate and due consideration should be given to the pros and cons of appendectomy when an otherwise normal appearing appendix is encountered. These issues are discussed in detail in Chapter 51.

An important issue is the question of preservation or removal of the ovaries at the time of hysterectomy. Wilcox et al.[21] have reported that approximately 37% of women between the ages of 15 and 44 years have a bilateral salpingo-oophorectomy performed at the time of hysterectomy, whereas 68% of women older than 45 years have a bilateral salpingo-oophorectomy. The proportion of patients undergoing bilateral salpingo-oophorectomy is approximately 6 of 10 of those who undergo abdominal hysterectomy and only 1 of 10 of those who have a vaginal hysterectomy. Although most would agree that removal of normal ovaries at the time of hysterectomy in a menopausal patient is appropriate, a more important question is whether to remove ovaries in premenopausal women. In premenopausal women, the physician needs to consider a balance between the benefits of preserving the ovaries, which include continued ovarian function and production of female hormones as well as androgens. Ovaries retained after hysterectomy continue to function nearly normally, although their life span may be slightly shortened. The continued production of hormones in the premenopausal patient clearly reduces the risk of osteoporosis, coronary artery disease, and vasomotor symptoms. The risks of retaining the ovaries include the possibilities of subsequent ovarian neoplasm (benign or malignant) and the development of residual ovary syndrome. Although the lifetime risk of developing epithelial ovarian cancer in American women is 1 in 70, it is clearly increased in women with a family history of ovarian and breast cancer. Therefore a careful family history should be obtained when assessing whether the patient might have a significantly increased risk of developing ovarian cancer. This information should sway the decision whether ovaries should be preserved or removed. The residual ovary syndrome, which is associated with pain and dyspareunia, can be a chronic disabling condition.

If ovaries are preserved, it is recommended that the blood supply be conserved as well and not be compromised or interrupted by performing a salpingectomy (unless the fallopian tube is diseased). Also, if the ovary is preserved, I would recommend that it be attached to the pelvic sidewall rather than allowed to fall into the cul-de-sac or possibly become adherent to the vaginal cuff. The risk of needing a second operation for new pathologic conditions of the ovary is estimated to be approximately 1% to 3%. In general, it is recommended that women who are premenopausal (younger than age 45) and who have normal ovaries and an average risk for ovarian cancer have their ovaries retained for the beneficial effects of their own hormone production. However, this is clearly an informed consent issue, which should be carefully discussed with the patient, and the patient's wishes should be followed after she understands the risks and benefits of these decisions.

Recent discussion has focused on the potential value of preserving the cervix when an abdominal hysterectomy is performed. Before the early 1950s, subtotal hysterectomies were commonly performed in the United States. Subsequently the trend has swung strongly toward total abdominal hysterectomy with complete removal of the uterus and cervix. More recently, some have advocated preservation of the cervix to allegedly improve sexual function or reduce vaginal prolapse and provide continued pelvic support. Those who believe that elective supracervical hysterectomy is appropriate have argued that there is better sexual function, improved libido, and improved orgasmic response if the cervix is left in place. These contentions are entirely unproven, and a careful review of the literature shows contradictory information as to the exact role of the cervix in any of these matters. Until more information is available, the clinician should allow the patient the choice if reasonable, and patients should be fully informed. Clearly, patients who have a history of abnormal Pap smears or other cervical pathologic conditions or have uterine malignancy should be counseled against preserving the cervix. There are, of course, times where supracervical hysterectomy is an appropriate procedure to prevent potential complications. This is especially true in patients who have significant scarring between the bladder and cervix or the cervix and rectum. This might occur after cesarean section, extensive endometriosis, pelvic inflammatory disease, or advanced ovarian carcinoma. Furthermore, in a patient whose condition is unstable (e.g., a woman with postpartum hemorrhage), complete removal of the cervix may be ill advised when a higher priority for the prudent surgeon is to complete the surgical procedure as quickly as possible.

Other issues that should be discussed during the preoperative preparation of the patient include basic matters dealing with surgery including the expected length of recovery in the hospital and at home, when the patient might return to work, and her limitations of activities in the weeks after surgery. Patients may also wish to have information about the location of the incision, which anesthetic would be appropriate, or which pain medications would be used in the postoperative period. The clinician should be aware that despite the fact that most patients achieve an improved sense of well-being after hysterectomy,[3,6] depression, the most common psychiatric complication after surgery, may occur. To minimize the risk for postoperative depression, the clinician should have a clear understanding preoperatively of the patient's psychological state, of the stability of her marital relationship, and of any history of depression. Also important are her views on further pregnancies and her understanding of the indications of surgery.

SURGICAL TECHNIQUE

The safe removal of the uterus through an abdominal incision has been described by many authors over the decades, each with particular emphasis on variations in technique that the particular surgeon believed would result in better or improved surgical outcome. In fact, there are probably about as many variations on technique as there are surgeons who perform this specific gynecologic procedure. Given that there are no randomized trials that compare the various surgical techniques, we may assume that in general, slight variations in technique result in minimal or no change in ultimate outcome. Key philosophical issues that must always be addressed include the following goals:

1. Minimizing surgical trauma
2. Protecting adjacent organs, including the bladder, pelvic vessels, ureter, and rectum
3. Minimizing blood loss
4. Minimizing surgical complications such as infection, hemorrhage, venous thromboembolus, and sexual dysfunction
5. Avoiding subsequent vaginal vault prolapse
6. Achieving an uncomplicated postoperative recovery

The abdomen should be opened through an incision allowing adequate exposure to perform the anticipated surgical procedure. Although a Pfannenstiel incision may be appropriate for most hysterectomies performed for benign gynecologic conditions, the surgeon must be aware of the possibility of the need for additional exposure (e.g., for a large pelvic mass or proper surgical staging of ovarian or endometrial carcinoma, or when a difficult dissection is anticipated).

After abdominal incision, the abdomen and pelvis should be explored to ascertain any coexisting problems that might need to be dealt with during this same surgical procedure. The pelvic organs should be explored and exposed using appropriate retraction and packs. A variety of self-retaining abdominal retractors are available, and most surgeons have their own preferences. Given the flexibility of exposure of many areas and the variety of depths of retractor blades, I routinely use a Bookwalter retractor for all abdominal hysterectomies.

After the pelvis and key anatomic landmarks are evaluated, the uterus is grasped with long Kelly clamps across the uterine cornu, incorporating the round ligament and fallopian tube. Care should be taken to avoid trauma and tearing of the uterine vessels or fallopian tube. Traction and countertraction are two key elements in the successful performance of a hysterectomy. With the uterus grasped, the assistant may retract it in any direction, allowing the surgeon optimal exposure. The round ligament is first divided. Tra-

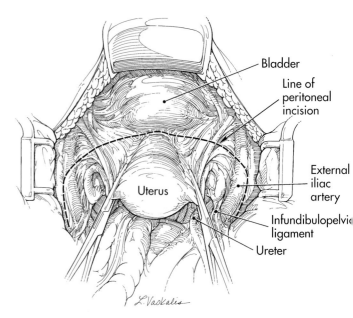

Fig. 30-1 Peritoneal incision. The uterus is grasped by two long Kelly clamps placed adjacent to the fundus and across the fallopian tube and round ligament. The pelvic peritoneum is incised by dividing the round ligament and extending the peritoneal incision cephalad just lateral to the external iliac artery overlying the psoas muscle. The incision is also carried along the anterior broad ligament and across the vesicouterine fold.

ditionally, the ligament has been suture ligated to incorporate the blood supply (Sampson's artery) in the base of the round ligament. Recently, I have found equal success using electrocautery to divide the round ligament, thus avoiding the expenditure of suture material and the time required to ligate and tie the round ligament.

It is my personal preference to identify the ureter both from a transperitoneal perspective (viewed through the peritoneum along the pelvic sidewall) and also from a retroperitoneal perspective. To identify the ureter in the retroperitoneum, the peritoneum lateral to the infundibulopelvic ligament is incised (Fig. 30-1). On the lateral aspect of the pelvis, the psoas muscle is identified. Moving medially, the external iliac artery and common iliac artery are identified. As the peritoneum on the medial aspect of the pelvis is mobilized, the infundibulopelvic ligament (ovarian vessels) is encountered (Fig. 30-2). Inferior to the ovarian vessels is the ureter. Anatomically, the ureter invariably crosses in the pelvis at the bifurcation of the common iliac artery into the internal and external iliac arteries. If the surgeon is unable to identify the ureter deeper in the pelvis, the dissection should be taken to the level of the common iliac bifurcation to ascertain the location of the ureter. With proper training and experience, the ureter can be identified in this manner in a matter of 30 seconds in most patients. Identification of the ureter early in the surgical procedure allows the surgeon to use this as a reference point and easily reidentify it later if the procedure becomes more difficult or complicated. In other words, it is optimal to have identified the ureter before a complication occurs rather than trying to identify it in the

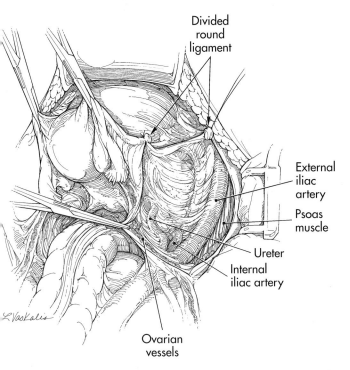

Divided
round
ligament

External
iliac
artery

Psoas
muscle

Ureter

Internal
iliac artery

Ovarian
vessels

Fig. 30-2 Identification of retroperitoneal structures. With the peritoneum incised, the dissection should proceed from lateral to medial, identifying the external iliac artery and vein, the internal iliac artery, the ovarian vessels, and the ureter. The ureter and the ovarian vessels will remain adherent to the medial leaf of the broad ligament and peritoneum. Invariably, the ureter crosses into the pelvis at the bifurcation of the common iliac artery.

midst of attempting to control bleeding or when distorted anatomy is encountered deeper in the pelvis.

If the fallopian tube and ovary are to be removed, the ovarian vessels should be isolated, clamped, divided, and ligated (Fig. 30-3, *A*). With the ureter clearly identified, I routinely pass a pointed clamp from lateral to medial, penetrating the peritoneum just beneath the ovarian vessels and above the ureter. The vascular pedicle is then clamped on the distal and proximal end and divided between these two clamps. The proximal vascular pedicle is free tied and suture ligated with the suture tied fore and aft distal to the free tie (see Fig. 30-3, *B*). The peritoneum on the posterior aspect of the broad ligament may be incised to allow mobilization of the adnexa. If exposure is adequate, I will usually free tie the distal ends of the ovarian vessels and then tie them to the Kelly clamps on the cornu of the uterus to hold them with the specimen so that they are not in the surgeon's way (Fig. 30-4). Alternatively, the adnexa may be transected next to the Kelly clamps and removed from the operative field.

If the tubes and ovaries are to be preserved, a window should be made in the posterior leaf of the broad ligament just lateral to the uterus. Using sharp dissection, the proximal round ligament stump should be pulled medially and the uteroovarian anastomosis and fallopian tube isolated as a pedicle. Again, good surgical technique dictates that this

pedicle be as small as possible and inclusion of extraneous tissue in it be avoided. The clamp on the distal portion of the fallopian tube should be placed as close to the Kelly clamp on the uterus as possible, thereby avoiding clamping of the ovary or compromising the ovarian blood supply (Fig. 30-5, *A*). The tube and uteroovarian vessels are free tied and suture ligated (Fig. 30-5, *B*).

The peritoneum on the anterior aspect of the broad ligament and overlying the vesicouterine junction must be incised. This incision should be carefully placed at the junction where the bladder reflects along the upper cervix or lower uterine segment (Fig. 30-6, p. 571). An incision placed too close to the uterus incises the uterine serosa, making development of the bladder flap more difficult because the initial dissection must be performed in dense attachment of uterine serosa to the myometrium. On the other hand, an incision of the peritoneum too close to the bladder may result in bladder injury. When anatomy is not distorted, the proper area of incision is easily identified by grasping the peritoneum with atraumatic forceps and identifying where it becomes pliable and loose just beneath its more dense attachment to the myometrium (uterine serosa). The incision of the broad ligament and vesicouterine peritoneum extends across the entire pelvis. With upward and posterior traction on the uterus and downward traction on the bladder (with smooth forceps), the plane between the bladder and cervix is opened using sharp and blunt dissection (Fig. 30-7, p. 571). I am against the idea of using a sponge stick to advance the "bladder flap." In my opinion, in uncomplicated procedures the bladder flap is easily mobilized with traction and blunt and sharp dissection and direct visualization. On the other hand, when the bladder flap is more adherent (e.g., after cesarean section), the use of a sponge stick is more likely to traumatize tissue and tear into an inappropriate plane, which is more likely to injure the bladder. If "blunt" pushing is to be performed in advancing the bladder flap, I would advise using the surgeon's forefinger or thumb. Using this "surgical tool" the surgeon at least has tactile sensation to determine when tissues are densely adherent and not pliable versus the "feel" of the proper plane (Fig. 30-8, p. 572).

After advancing the bladder from the cervix, I routinely palpate to be certain the bladder has been advanced past the lower aspect of the cervix. In advancing the bladder, sharp dissection is often needed to mobilize paravesical fat from the anterior lateral side of the lower uterus and cervix. Care must be taken to avoid injury to the uterine vessels or bladder pillar. Having advanced the bladder flap, I next skeletonize the uterine vessels, removing as much fat and peritoneum as is safe, to isolate a uterine vascular pedicle (Fig. 30-9, p. 572). I find it particularly helpful to pull the uterus forward (toward the bladder) and, by grasping the remaining posterior peritoneum along the broad ligament, incise that peritoneum to its junction on the cervix (see Fig. 30-9, *B*, p. 572). This step in the procedure avoids clamping a large pedicle of peritoneum, fat, and blood vessels, thereby minimizing the amount of tissue incorporated in the ligature. The

Text continued on p. 572

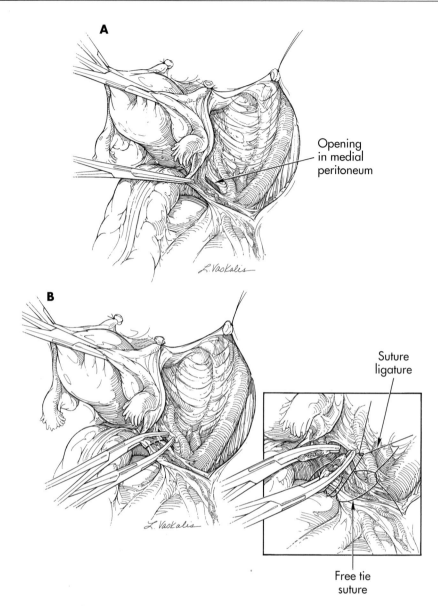

A

Opening
in medial
peritoneum

L. Vaskalis

B

Suture
ligature

L. Vaskalis

Free tie
suture

Fig. 30-3 **A,** Isolation of the ovarian vessels. When salpingo-oophorectomy is to be performed, the ovarian vessels should be isolated by developing a window beneath them (the infundibulopelvic ligament) through the pelvic peritoneum. Care should be taken to avoid injury
to the ureter. **B,** Clamping, dividing, and ligating the ovarian vessels. The ovarian vessels are
cross-clamped proximal to the ovary and fallopian tube. They are then ligated with a proximal
free tie and a distal fore and aft suture ligature.

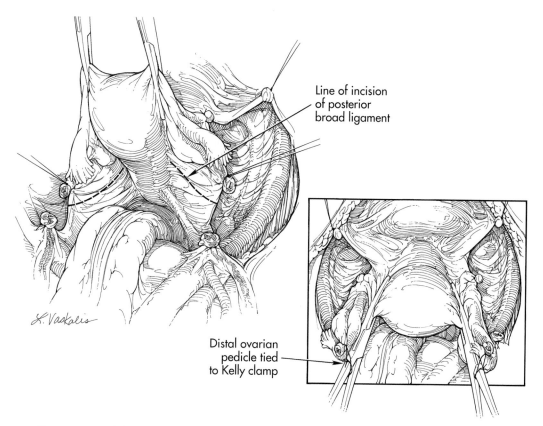

Line of incision
of posterior
broad ligament

Distal ovarian
pedicle tied
to Kelly clamp

L. Vaskalis

Fig. 30-4 Mobilization of the tube and ovary. The peritoneum on the posterior aspect of the broad ligament has been incised toward the uterus, thus mobilizing the tube and ovary. To isolate the tube and ovary from the operative field, the distal ovarian vessel pedicle is tied to the Kelly clamp, which has been placed across the uterine cornua.

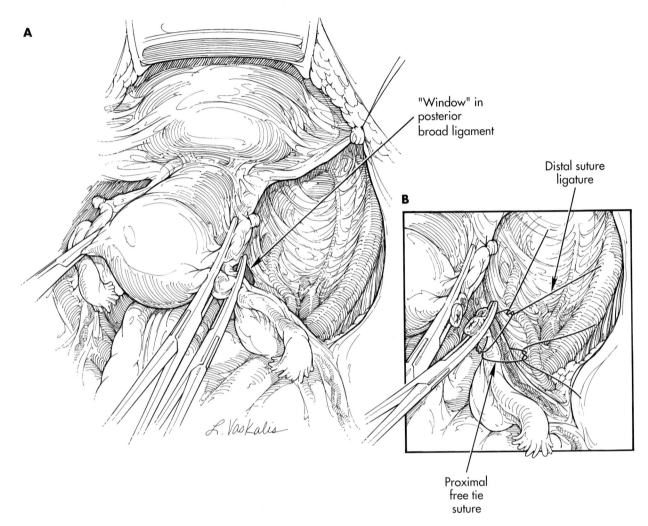

A

"Window" in
posterior
broad ligament

B

Distal suture
ligature

L. Vaskalis

Proximal
free tie
suture

Fig. 30-5   A, Preservation of the tube and ovary. When a hysterectomy is performed in which the tube and ovary are to be preserved, the fallopian tube and ovarian vessels are clamped and divided adjacent to the uterus. A "window" is made in the posterior aspect of the broad liga-ment adjacent to the uterus, and a pedicle is created, which is clamped incorporating the fal-lopian tube and ovarian vessels. Care should be taken to avoid clamping across a portion of the ovary or the round ligament. **B,** Dividing and ligating the tube and ovarian vessels. The clamp on the proximal fallopian tube and ovarian vessels is removed after the pedicle has been free-tied and sutured fore and aft.

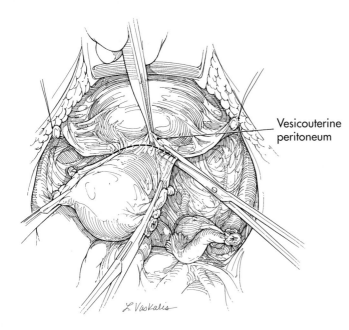

Vesicouterine
peritoneum

Fig. 30-6   Vesicouterine peritoneum. The peritoneum overlying the junction between the bladder and the cervix is incised immediately adjacent to the cervix where the peritoneum is easily tented up with forceps.

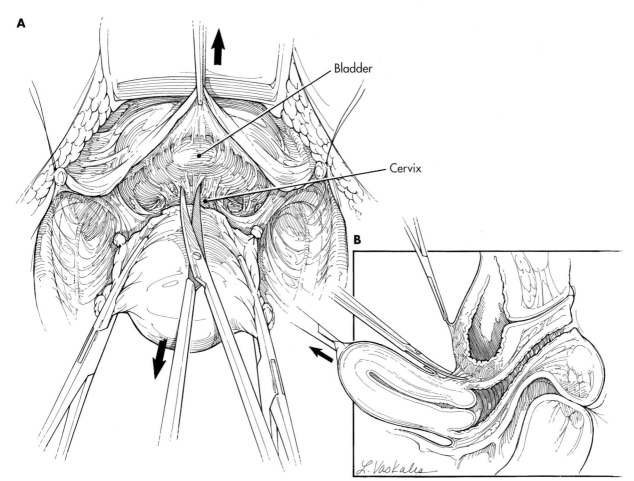

A

Bladder

Cervix

B

Fig. 30-7   A, Mobilization of the bladder. Using sharp and blunt dissection, the surgeon can mobilize the bladder from its attachment to the cervix and upper vagina using Metzenbaum scissors. Upward traction is provided by Kelly clamps across the uterine cornua, and inferior traction on the bladder is provided by smooth forceps. Care should be taken to avoid tearing or cutting vessels on the lateral aspects of the cervix and bladder pillars. **B,** Sharp dissection of bladder from the cervix and upper vagina. A sagittal view of similar dissection demonstrating the plane to be dissected between the cervix and bladder. The Metzenbaum scissors are placed immediately against the cervix, thereby using the firm cervix as a base for dissection.

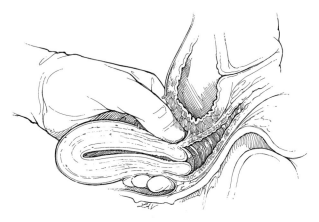

Fig. 30-8   Blunt dissection of the bladder from the cervix. The bladder may be further advanced using blunt dissection with the operator's thumb or forefinger grasping around the cervix. I do not recommend the use of a sponge stick in this situation because I believe that the surgeon's thumb has better tactile sense to determine when the dissection is going smoothly versus when there is an area of adherence that must be cut sharply.

uterine vessels are exposed and clamped. Most gynecologists use a curved Heaney-Ballentine clamp. My preference is to use the Parametrium clamp (Marina Medical, Hollywood, Fla.) because my perception is that this clamp has better holding power and also has a longer shank, thereby avoiding placement of the surgeon's hand in the surgical field. The uterine vessels are doubly clamped and divided between the two clamps (Fig. 30-10). The vessels in the distal clamp are suture ligated using a transfixion suture of 2-0 Vicryl. I prefer to use a smaller needle (CT 2) as big needles are sometimes difficult to manipulate in small areas of the pelvis. The upper parametrial clamp is left attached to the uterus to prevent "back bleeding," thus minimizing blood loss as well as keeping the surgical field as bloodless as possible.

After ligation of the primary uterine blood supply, a second clamp is placed just inferior to the uterine vessels and adjacent to the cardinal ligament (Fig. 30-11). Although some surgeons begin to use clamps with straight jaws at this point in the procedure, I have found that using the lower centimeter of the parametrial clamp works just as effectively and is more efficient in that the nurse does not have to pass different clamps from the instrument table. Having taken this additional pedicle of tissue, which is likewise suture ligated, the ureter begins to fall away from the side of the cervix.

At this point in the hysterectomy, I routinely open the rectovaginal septum. This is easily created by incising the serosa along the posterior aspect of the cervix at the level of the first cardinal ligament pedicle (Fig. 30-12, *A*). After this serosa is incised, the uterus should be pulled forward and the posterior peritoneum grasped with smooth pickups. Sharp dissection is required to mobilize the serosa off the distal cervix (see Fig. 30-12, *B*). Once this has been accomplished, the rectovaginal septum is easily developed using blunt dissection of a fingertip. To minimize bleeding, at this

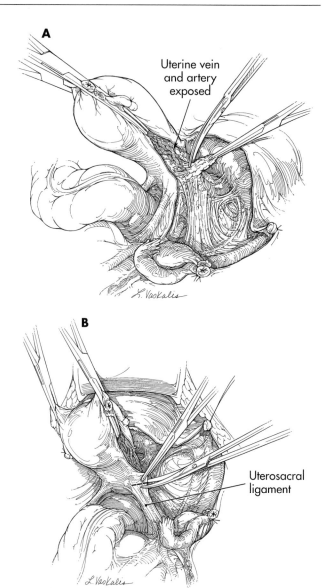

Fig. 30-9   Skeletonizing the uterine vessels. The fat and areolar tissue around the uterine vessels should be removed to expose the vessels more clearly and to obtain a vascular pedicle devoid of excess tissue. **A,** Sharp dissection of the areolar tissue surrounding the uterine vessels is performed using Metzenbaum scissors and smooth pickups. Do not "push" the tissue caudad because this will often tear fragile veins in the area. **B,** The peritoneum of the posterior aspect of the broad ligament is incised toward the uterosacral ligament to further skeletonize the uterine vessels and also to begin to create the rectovaginal septum.

step of the procedure the surgeon should focus on the central cervix and vagina between the uterosacral ligaments. Although this step is not always required, I find it an important skill to develop as it is paramount to protecting the rectum in patients with distorted pelvic anatomy. Furthermore, it is my feeling that by developing the rectovaginal septum, the uterosacral ligament and cardinal ligament complex are more easily identified and incorporated in the vaginal cuff closure later in the surgical procedure.

A

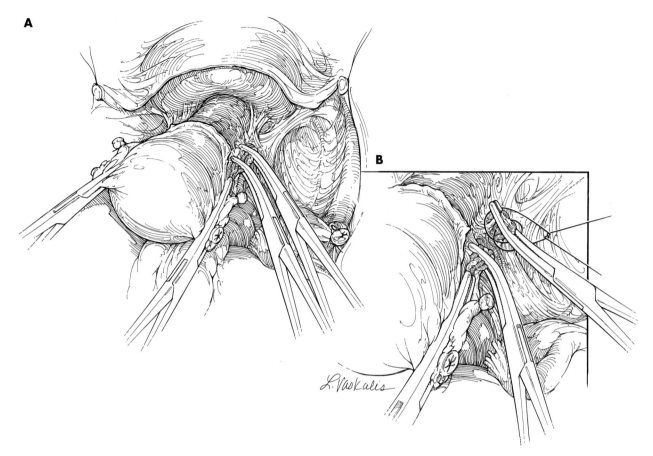

Fig. 30-10   Clamping of the uterine vessels. **A,** After isolation of the uterine vessels, two clamps are placed perpendicular to the axis of the uterine vessels as they ascend along the side of the lower uterine segment. **B,** Two parametrial clamps are placed, and the vessels are divided between the clamps. The distal vascular pedicle is transfixed using 2-0 Vicryl suture. There is no need to double-clamp or double-ligate the uterine vessels.

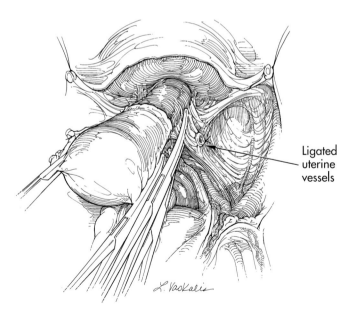

Ligated uterine vessels

Fig. 30-11   Clamping the paracervical tissues. The next clamp is placed immediately adjacent to and parallel to the cervix, incorporating the paracervical tissues. These clamps are placed medial and inferior to the previously ligated uterine vessels.

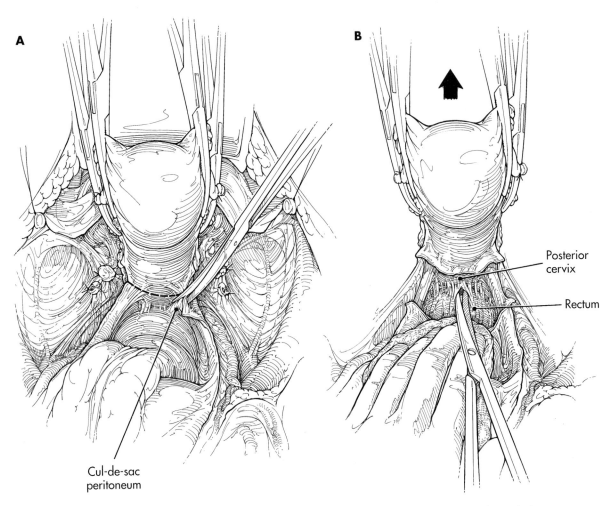

Fig. 30-12 **A,** Creation of the rectovaginal septum. After the cardinal ligament is ligated, the peritoneum over the posterior aspect of the cervix is incised between the uterosacral ligaments. **B,** Dissection of the rectovaginal septum. Using upward traction on the uterus and downward traction on the rectum, a plane is created with sharp dissection of Metzenbaum scissors between the posterior cervix and the rectum. At a position just beneath the cervix, the plane becomes loose and is easily dissected with blunt dissection of the finger.

The remainder of the cardinal ligament and paracervical tissues are clamped, divided, and suture ligated immediately adjacent to the cervix. At each step, the back blade of the clamp is placed within the rectovaginal septum, thus incorporating the upper, mid, and lower portions of the uterosacral ligament with the cardinal ligament (Fig. 30-13). Depending on the length of the cervix, the number of times the paracervical and cardinal ligaments are clamped and divided varies. I encourage surgeons to avoid large pedicles (which I disparagingly call "Gyn-Hog Bites"). Not only are large pedicles more likely to result in a larger amount of necrotic tissue, but they are also more likely to slip out of the clamp or have sutures that become loosened as the large pedicle liquefies.

When the vaginal attachment to the cervix is encountered, I cross-clamp the vaginal angles (incorporating the uterosacral ligaments) with parametrial clamps and incise the attachment of the vagina to the cervix (Fig. 30-14). There is only a rare occasion when an additional margin of

vaginal cuff should be removed. If additional vaginal cuff should be removed (e.g., to encompass a high-grade vaginal dysplasia adjacent to the cervix), it is my recommendation that this vaginal incision be made thorough a transvaginal approach at the beginning of the procedure to be certain that the entire lesion is incorporated with a clear margin. If additional vaginal cuff is required, the surgeon must be careful when placing the clamps lateral to the vagina in that the ureter becomes very close to this region. A modified radical hysterectomy, which will allow visualization and lateral retraction of the ureter, is highly recommended (see Chapter 37). The central portion of the vagina anteriorly and posteriorly is incised, and its connection to the cervix and the uterus and cervix is inspected to ensure that there is no remaining cervical tissue that has been transected.

The technique for closure of the vaginal cuff seems to inspire more clinical opinion and argument than any other portion of an abdominal hysterectomy. One of the primary debates is whether to close the vaginal cuff or leave it open.

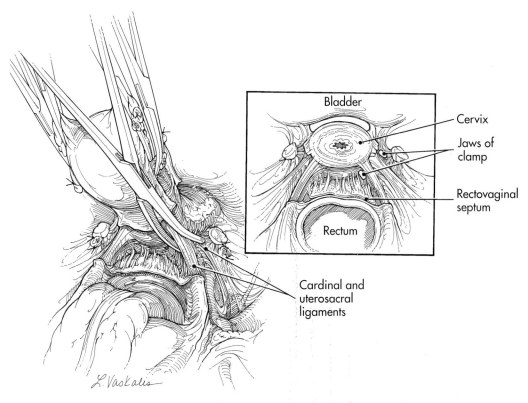

Fig. 30-13   Clamping of the cardinal and uterosacral ligament complex. After development of the rectovaginal septum and thereby isolation of the uterosacral ligament, clamps are now placed adjacent to the cervix, which incorporate both the cardinal and uterosacral ligament in the same bite. This will lend support to the upper vagina.

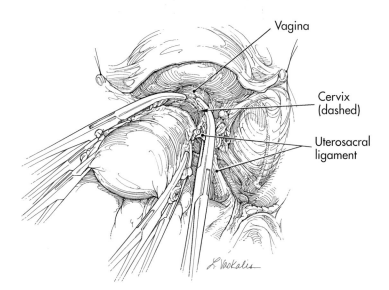

Fig. 30-14   Cross-clamping the upper vagina and uterosacral ligament complex. Once the cardinal and paracervical tissues have been divided, the vaginal angle is then cross-clamped. The posterior blade of the clamp incorporates the uterosacral ligament along with the vaginal angle.

Furthermore, the exact method by which to manage the vaginal angles seems to often cause debate and leads prominent surgeons to place their name on particular techniques used to close the vaginal cuff. Given that there is no evidence that leaving the vaginal cuff open in routine proce-

dures improves the patient's outcome, my opinion is that vaginal cuff closure results in less granulation tissue and less bleeding. Furthermore, I am unaware of any evidence that a particular suturing technique of the vaginal angle results in improved vaginal vault support. Therefore my technique is to transfix the vaginal angle, incorporating the first 1.5 cm of tissue along the lateral vaginal wall and uterosacral ligament (Fig. 30-15). Incorporating additional vaginal tissue, which might be contained in the vaginal cuff clamp, will result in shortening and narrowing of the upper vagina, which is undesirable. Having transfixed the vaginal angles, which should incorporate the vaginal artery, I hold these two sutures. If the remaining vaginal cuff is vascular, I will close

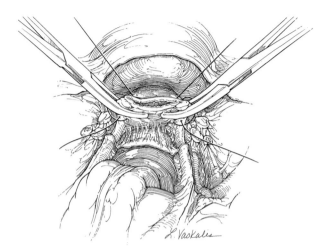

Fig. 30-15 Transfixion of the vaginal angle. Vaginal angles are transfixed using 0 Vicryl suture. Care should be taken not to incorporate an excessive amount of vaginal angle, thereby avoiding shortening or narrowing the upper vagina.

the central portion of the cuff with figure-of-eight sutures (Fig. 30-16, *A*). These sutures incorporate not only the anterior and posterior vaginal cuff but also the tissue in the rectovaginal septum and the posterior peritoneum. This is important to stop the slight vascular oozing from this surgical plane (rectovaginal septum), which has been developed. On the other hand, I do not routinely incorporate the peritoneum of the bladder flap with the vaginal cuff. For patients who seem to have minimal bleeding from the vaginal cuff, I will "run" the central portion of the vaginal cuff incorporating the anterior and posterior vagina with the rectovaginal septum peritoneum in a running locking closure from one angle to the other (see Fig. 30-16, *B*).

In concluding the hysterectomy, the pelvis is irrigated and inspected for hemostasis. If there is bleeding from pedicles, the bleeding points should be carefully identified and then managed with ligature, clips, or cautery, depending on the specific circumstance. I do not close the peritoneum along the lateral pelvic sidewall.

If the ovaries have been left in the pelvis, I routinely suture the uteroovarian ligament pedicle to the lateral pelvic peritoneum to keep the tube and ovary from falling into the deeper pelvis or becoming attached to the vaginal cuff, which might lead to dyspareunia (Fig. 30-17).

Depending on the patient's needs, other surgical procedures may have preceded or will follow the performance of the abdominal hysterectomy. These procedures are often related to pelvic floor relaxation or prolapse and are discussed

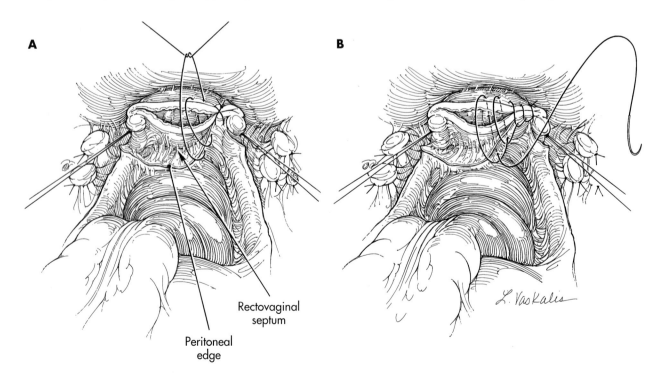

Rectovaginal septum

Peritoneal edge

Fig. 30-16 **A,** Closure of the vaginal cuff with interrupted figure-of-eight sutures. One method for closure of the vaginal cuff is to place figure-of-eight sutures. These sutures include the anterior and posterior vagina, the rectovaginal septum, and cul-de-sac peritoneum. When tied, the rectovaginal septum is obliterated and a small culdoplasty is created. **B,** Vaginal cuff closure using a continuous, locking suture. The cuff may be closed by a running, locking suture of 0 Vicryl. This suture extends from one vaginal angle to the other, incorporating the vagina, the rectovaginal septum, and posterior peritoneum of the cul-de-sac.

elsewhere in this book. Despite the lack of an apparent enterocele on preoperative evaluation, I find it common to identify a large cul-de-sac (pouch of Douglas). After completion of the abdominal hysterectomy, if the patient does have a large cul-de-sac, it is reasonable to obliterate this defect to prevent a subsequent symptomatic enterocele. This may be accomplished either with a Halban's culdeplasty or a Moschcowitz culdoplasty (see Chapter 23). Whichever culdeplasty is chosen, the surgeon must be particularly careful to avoid incorporating or causing significant deviation of the ureter.

The laparotomy pads and retractors are removed, and the abdominal wall is closed as is appropriate for the particular incision chosen. An intraperitoneal or vaginal cuff drain is not routinely left in the pelvis. The only time I drain the pelvis with a closed suction device (Jackson-Pratt drain or Blake drain) is if there is evidence of infection. If a drain is placed, it should be exited through a separate "stab" incision in the lower abdominal wall and should not exit through the abdominal incision itself.

STRATEGIES FOR MANAGING THE DIFFICULT ABDOMINAL HYSTERECTOMY
Preoperative Preparation

Because of disease and anatomic distortion, a hysterectomy may be one of the most challenging procedures that a pelvic surgeon encounters. Careful preoperative planning and excellence in surgical skill with the armamentarium of a variety of surgical strategies will result in the optimal outcome in these difficult procedures.

Preoperatively, the surgeon must be aware of potential difficulties. Although this may be obvious when dealing with a large pelvic mass or an obvious ovarian malignancy, less serious distortion may yet render a procedure difficult. For example, the "bladder flap" may be severely compromised and distorted in a patient who has had a previous cesarean section. Anatomy may be substantially distorted in patients who have had previous abdominal or pelvic surgery that appeared to have been uncomplicated. Disease processes such as endometriosis, fibroids, and pelvic inflammatory disease are commonly associated with anatomic distortion and difficulty in performing an abdominal hysterectomy. Having recognized these potential problems preoperatively, the surgeon should consider the following changes from his or her normal preoperative preparation:

1. Although informed consent should routinely incorporate discussion regarding the potential for injury to other pelvic viscera, this should be further emphasized and documented in the preoperative discussion with the patient whom the surgeon anticipates may have a distorted anatomy.
2. Mechanical bowel preparation must be complete in these patients and is reemphasized here despite the fact that I believe mechanical bowel preparation should be part of the routine preparation for even the simplest abdominal hysterectomy.
3. Although parenteral prophylactic antibiotics are of controversial benefit in patients undergoing abdominal hysterectomy, I would recommend them for patients who are anticipated to have difficult or prolonged procedures.
4. Planning the surgical procedure and anticipating needed equipment are critically important. I would recommend positioning the patient in Allen stirrups to allow for transvaginal, transrectal, and cystoscopic evaluation if necessary during the abdominal procedure. Placing the patient in a modified Whitmore position in Allen stirrups allows total flexibility, making it easy for the surgeon to perform proctoscopy or cystoscopy, for example. Positioning in Allen stirrups also allows for a second assistant to more closely visualize and assist with the surgical procedure.
5. The benefit of a skilled first assistant cannot be overestimated. The surgeon may wish to specifically request that a partner or other surgical technician who is skilled at assisting in difficult surgery be part of the surgical team from the beginning of the procedure.
6. The surgeon should book enough time on the surgical schedule so that he or she does not feel rushed and so that the procedure may be accomplished without others waiting past their expected "start time."

In the course of a difficult hysterectomy, exposure of the operative field is extremely important, and I would recommend the use of the Bookwalter retractor, which allows maximum flexibility in achieving exposure. Furthermore, the multiple retractor blades, which can be connected to the

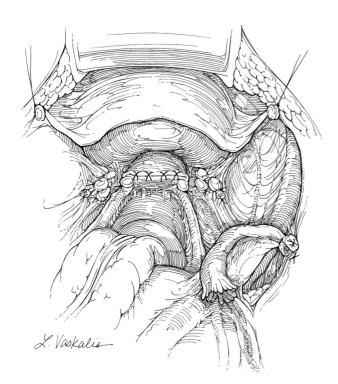

Fig. 30-17   Attaching the tube and ovary to the lateral peritoneum. To avoid the tube and ovary becoming adherent to the vaginal cuff or deep pelvis, the ovarian pedicle is sutured to the lateral pelvic peritoneum adjacent to the psoas muscle.

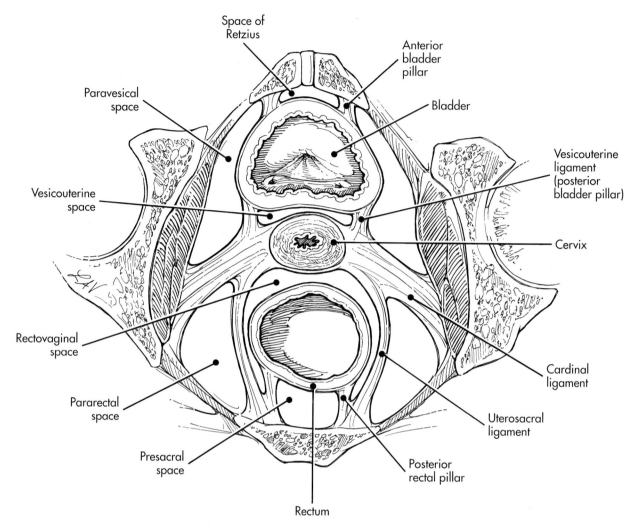

Fig. 30-18   Retroperitoneal spaces and ligaments of the pelvis. The retroperitoneal spaces (which are relatively avascular) may be used to the surgeon's advantage in difficult pelvic dissections.

stabilized ring, frees up the assistant's hands for more important duties than holding retractors.

Proper instrumentation is also extremely important for the successful outcome of a difficult hysterectomy. This might include a set of longer instruments, the availability of vascular clips, a Bovie tip extender, additional suction, or special lighting (e.g., a headlight or fiberoptic lighting system attached to the retractor or suction tip).

1. Although blood is not routinely typed and cross-matched in preparation for an abdominal hysterectomy, this might be considered for patients in whom the procedure is likely to be complicated.
2. Selection of the optimal abdominal incision is critical when a difficult hysterectomy is performed. Exposure to dissect distorted surgical planes and to control bleeding is also important and in general is best achieved by a midline incision. If a Pfannenstiel incision has been selected and more exposure is needed, conversion to a Cherney incision should be strongly considered as this usually allows excellent exposure to the pelvis (see Chapter 13).

One of the most important intraoperative skills necessary to perform a difficult hysterectomy is the ability to identify and establish normal anatomy. Key structures that must be protected in the course of a difficult abdominal hysterectomy include the bladder, rectum, ureters, and pelvic blood vessels. In nearly all gynecologic conditions requiring hysterectomy, the retroperitoneal spaces are essentially free of distortion and should therefore be used in the course of establishing normal anatomy. The gynecologist must have the skills to open carefully and identify the anatomy in the retroperitoneum. These steps become simplified as the gynecologist gains skill by repeatedly working in this area and is encouraged to develop these skills on "routine" procedures so that at the time when they are required for a difficult case, the surgeon has a comfort level and confidence in accomplishing the necessary tasks.

Surgical Technique

The key retroperitoneal spaces in the pelvis are shown in Fig. 30-18 and include the paravesical and pararectal spaces on the lateral pelvis and the rectovaginal septum and the

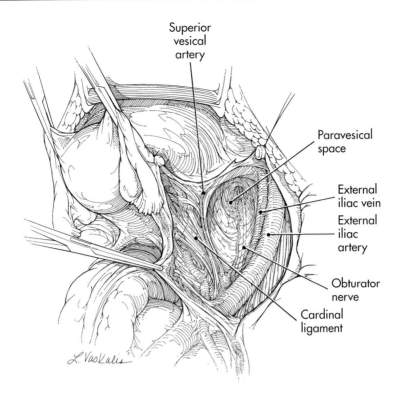

Superior
vesical
artery

Paravesical
space

External
iliac vein

External
iliac
artery

Obturator
nerve

Cardinal
ligament

L. VasKalis

Fig. 30-19   Developing of the paravesical space. After opening of the lateral pelvic peritoneum, the paravesical space is created by bluntly dividing the tissue between the external iliac
artery and vein and the bladder. In creating this space, the superior vesicle artery remains medially attached to the bladder. For orientation, the pararectal space is also shown, which was
created upon opening of the lateral pelvic sidewall (see Fig. 30-20). Between these two spaces
are the cardinal ligament, parametria, and uterine vessels.

vesicovaginal septum in the center of the pelvis. They also
include the space of Retzius (retropubic space) and the presacral space. In nearly all difficult hysterectomies, the lateral pelvic sidewall must be opened to protect the pelvic
blood vessels and the ureter. To open the pararectal and
paravesical spaces, the lateral pelvic peritoneum should be
incised over the psoas muscle (see Figs. 30-1 and 30-2).
Some surgeons recommend dividing the round ligament, but
this is not absolutely necessary; in fact, the round ligament
is sometimes obscured or obliterated by pelvic pathologic
conditions. Therefore dividing the peritoneum lateral to the
external iliac artery and opening the retroperitoneal space
are safely accomplished, and there are no vital structures at
this level of the pelvis. The retroperitoneal dissection should
then proceed medially, reflecting the medial peritoneum off
the retroperitoneal space. As the dissection proceeds medially, the genitofemoral nerve and external iliac artery are
first encountered. They are often encased in fat and lymphoid tissue, and palpation may be the first clue as to the location of the artery. Exposure of the artery allows anatomic
orientation. As the dissection proceeds further medially over
the external iliac artery, the external iliac vein will be next
encountered just inferior to the artery.

The dissection proceeds cephalad, and the bifurcation of
the common iliac artery into the external and internal iliac
arteries can be identified. At this location on the medial aspect of the peritoneum is the ureter (see Fig. 30-2). With the
ureter retracted medially and the hypogastric artery re-

tracted laterally, the perirectal space can be developed. This
is an avascular plane. The paravesical space is developed by
identifying the distal external iliac artery and vein. The
paravesical space is opened by retracting medially the adipose and areolar tissue which lies just medial to the external
iliac artery and vein (Fig. 30-19). On the medial aspect of
the paravesical space is the superior vesicle artery (obliterated umbilical artery). Having opened the pararectal and
paravesical spaces, the tissue between the two is the
"parametrium" or cardinal ligament, which contains not
only the lymphatic drainage from the cervix but also the
uterine artery and vein (Fig. 30-20). To specifically identify
the origin of the uterine artery, the dissection may proceed
along the anterior surface of the hypogastric artery until the
first main branch medial is identified (the uterine artery).
Alternatively, the dissection may proceed cephalad along
the superior vesicle artery until the origin of the uterine artery is identified (Fig. 30-21). Careful dissection on top of
the hypogastric and superior vesicle artery leaves little risk
of trauma to any vessels. On the other hand, if the dissection
proceeds medial to the hypogastric artery or the superior
vesicle artery, the surgeon is likely to tear into the uterine
vein or artery before it is completely identified. Identification of the uterine artery may be particularly helpful when a
modified radical (type II) hysterectomy is necessary. Furthermore, having identified the ureter on the medial aspect
of the pelvic peritoneum, the surgeon has the option to mobilize the ureter from the peritoneum and thus protect it

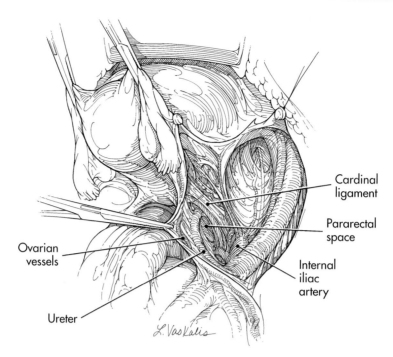

Fig. 30-20   Developing the pararectal space. The pararectal space is bounded by the external iliac artery and vein, hypogastric artery (internal iliac), and distal common iliac artery laterally and medially by the ureter and ovarian vessels.

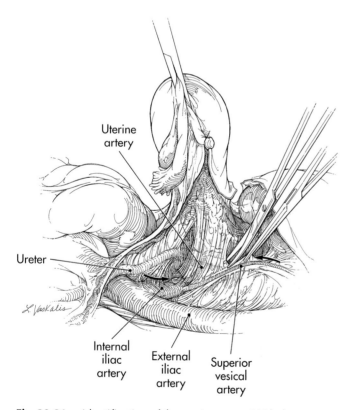

Fig. 30-21   Identification of the uterine artery. With the paravesical and pararectal spaces opened, the uterine artery may be found as it branches from the anterior division of the internal iliac artery by either dissection along the hypogastric artery caudad or along the superior vesicle artery cephalad. The dissection along the hypogastric artery and superior vesical artery should remain anterior to the artery. Dissection medially may injure the uterine veins.

from injury if the dissection is difficult on the lateral pelvic sidewall or in the posterior cul-de-sac or uterosacral ligament. In addition, with the ureter identified, it may be dissected from the paracervical tunnel in the course of more distal mobilization, required to manage disease in the parametria or an expanded lower uterine segment or cervix such as that found with a broad ligament or cervical myoma.

To protect the rectum, the surgeon must have the ability to develop the rectovaginal septum. Most vaginal surgeons use this relatively avascular plane when performing a posterior colporrhaphy transvaginally. To gain access to the rectovaginal septum from the abdominal approach, an incision is required along the junction between the cervix and vagina (see Fig. 30-12). However, in patients in whom the posterior cul-de-sac is obliterated by adhesive conditions such as endometriosis, pelvic inflammatory disease, or ovarian cancer, it may be impossible to identify the true cul-de-sac. Therefore, to develop the rectovaginal septum, the surgeon must make an incision higher on the cervix to create a plane between the cervical serosa and the cervical stroma (Fig. 30-22). With sharp dissection to free the serosa from the cervix, the rectovaginal septum will ultimately be encountered. Thereafter (unless there is disease extending into the rectovaginal septum such as with endometriosis), blunt dissection will mobilize the vagina away from its loose attachments to the rectum in the midline (see Fig. 30-12, *B*). The uterosacral ligaments lie on either side of this dissection. To connect between the uterosacral ligaments and the pararectal space, the ureter logically must be mobilized from its attachments to the medial peritoneum and retracted laterally. These are the same steps that the gynecologic oncologist uses in performing a radical hysterectomy

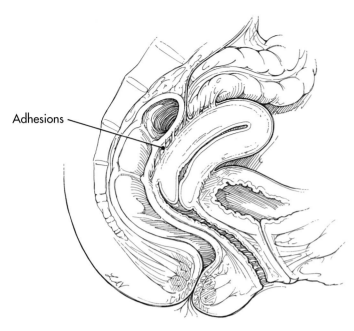

Adhesions

Fig. 30-22 Sigmoid colon densely adherent to the posterior uterus and cervix. This illustration shows the problem of a dense adherent rectosigmoid colon to the posterior aspect of the uterus and cervix, and obliterating the posterior cul-de-sac.

but are also skills necessary for performing difficult surgery on the posterior and lateral aspects of the uterus and cervix (Fig. 30-23, *A*).

Extensive dissection of the rectovaginal septum and rectosigmoid colon often results in a broad area of denuded rectosigmoid colon and rectovaginal septum. Hemostasis is usually best achieved by a series of sutures placed along the rectovaginal septum and denuded rectum in a Halban style closure. Tieing these sutures down invariably stops bleeding, which might otherwise be difficult to control with cautery, clips, and isolated sutures (see Fig. 30-23, *B*). This also results in the obliteration of the cul-de-sac and prevents enterocele formation.

The vesicovaginal septum may also be obliterated by adhesive disease that may occur after a cesarean section or endometriosis implants. Although developing the "bladder flap" is usually relatively simple in an uncomplicated procedure, it may be extremely difficult in patients with dense adhesions and scarring. In these patients, the bladder is at particular risk for injury. When it is difficult to establish the traditional bladder flap, I generally use four strategies, which assist in moving the bladder away from the lower uterus and cervix.

1. *The incision may be made higher on the uterus, incising the serosa (Fig. 30-24).* With sharp dissection (and often cautery to control oozing from the myometrium), the bladder and uterine serosa can be mobilized caudad, leaving the uterine serosa (and some myometrium and cervical stroma) attached to the bladder. This is a difficult dissection in that there is no anatomic plane in this region, and therefore the surgeon is essentially creating a "plane."

2. *The peritoneum overlying the bladder away from the diseased area may be incised (Fig. 30-25).* Using careful dissection, the peritoneum overlying the dome of the bladder can then be dissected toward the cervix, establishing a plane between the peritoneum and the bladder. In the most central portion of this attachment, the surgeon will be dissecting directly on bladder muscularis, and some bleeding may be encountered, which can usually be easily controlled with cautery. However, remaining in this plane will ultimately develop the bladder flap with ease. Most of the dissection should initially be placed in the center of the bladder, where it overlies the lower uterine segment and cervix. Because there may be distorted anatomy, the surgeon is advised to palpate the location of the cervix to remain oriented as to where the bladder is probably attached. Lateral attachments of the perivesical fat can likewise be freed with sharp and blunt dissection to more fully mobilize the bladder and also allow the ureter to be retracted laterally.

3. *The bladder dome may actually be opened, thereby allowing visualization and palpation of the bladder mucosa and muscularis (Fig. 30-26).* In creating an intentional cystotomy, the surgeon may palpate the cervix through the bladder wall and use this context clue to establish where the bladder is actually attached to the cervix and assist in mobilization. At the completion of the procedure, the bladder dome can be easily closed with little risk of fistulization. In my opinion it is much more desirous to open the dome of the bladder to identify anatomy rather than run the risk of causing cystotomy near the trigone in the course of developing the vesicovaginal plane.

4. *The paravesical space can often be used to help identify the cervix (Fig. 30-27).* Many times the difficulty in developing the vesicovaginal septum is caused by adhesions and scar tissue near the bladder flap, but not involving the lower cervix or upper vagina. Therefore, by approaching the cervix from the paravesical space, the lower cervix can initially be identified and an unscarred plane developed between the lower cervix and bladder. Having identified this plane and the cervical stroma, the surgeon can then proceed with dissection toward the fundus of the uterus, thereby releasing the more densely attached bladder from the cervix.

Other key techniques to performing a difficult abdominal hysterectomy include the issue of traction and countertraction to establish planes and to allow safe dissection. If possible, the uterus should be grasped at its cornu so that it can be manipulated and put on traction. If the uterus cannot be grasped, the medial portion of the divided round ligament should be grasped in a Kelly clamp. Grasping both round ligaments will allow traction and manipulation of the uterus, which has not been identified at this portion of the procedure (Fig. 30-28, p. 585). If only the upper portion of the uterine fundus is identifiable, this may be grasped for traction

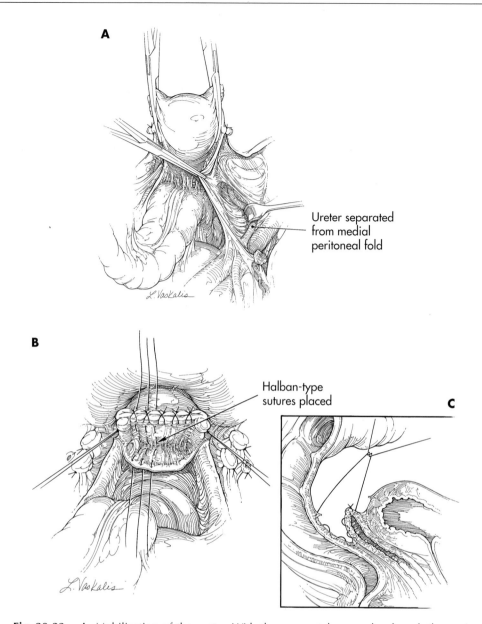

Fig. 30-23   **A,** Mobilization of the ureter. With the pararectal space developed, the ureter may be isolated from its loose attachments to the medial peritoneum. This is done with sharp and blunt dissection. By mobilizing the ureter and retracting it laterally, the uterosacral ligament and rectosigmoid colon, which is adherent to the posterior aspect of the uterus, may be dissected without fear of injury to the ureter. **B** and **C,** Closure of a large rectovaginal septum. After extensive dissection of the rectovaginal septum, especially when the colon has been adherent to the posterior cervix, a denuded portion of the colon may have some persistent oozing. This is usually easily controlled by placing Halban-type sutures, incorporating the vaginal cuff and rectal muscularis in a row of interrupted sutures, which when tied control bleeding and serve as a culdeplasty.

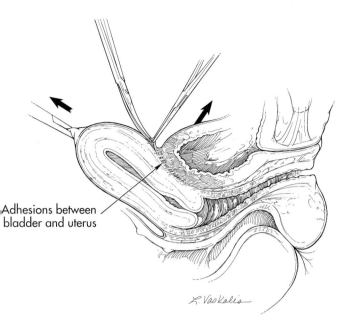

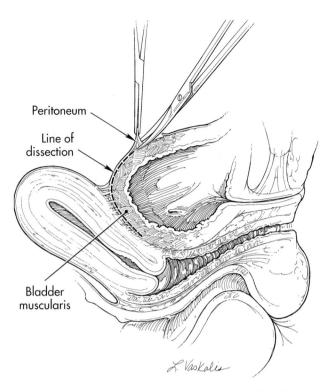

Fig. 30-24 The difficult bladder flap. In this illustration the bladder is densely inherent to the lower uterus. With traction on the uterus to pull it superiorly and traction to pull the bladder inferiorly, sharp dissection may then be performed in developing the space between the uterus and bladder. It is important to provide traction to facilitate this dissection.

Fig. 30-25 Alternative approach to an adherent bladder. The plane between the bladder and uterus may be approached by incising the peritoneum on the dome of the bladder. By lifting the peritoneal incision with forceps (or Allis clamps), sharp dissection will develop a plane between the peritoneum and the bladder muscularis. There are often small vessels in this plane, which can be controlled with electrocautery.

purposes in a Lahey tenaculum. Traction and countertraction are particularly important when the retroperitoneal spaces are developed. In this case, the medial peritoneum should be pulled medially by the assistant while the surgeon opens the spaces. Likewise the bladder or rectosigmoid colon may be put on traction by use of smooth pickups or a Babcock clamp to move it in the opposite direction of the uterus, thereby allowing dissection between the two organs.

Other techniques for successful completion of a difficult abdominal hysterectomy include the following:

1. The use of an intrafascial approach to the cervix will allow detachment of the uterus from the bladder (Fig. 30-29). When an intrafascial hysterectomy is performed, the fascia along the cervix is incised and clamps are placed within this fascial plane. Therefore some of the fascia of the cervix is left attached to the bladder.

2. When difficulty is encountered with either a scarred bladder flap or an obliterated posterior cul-de-sac, the surgeon should seriously consider the possibility of performing a supracervical or subtotal hysterectomy. Although this approach has been decried in the past, it should be considered to avoid complications of cystotomy or rectal injury and is especially appropriate in patients who do not have uterine or cervical malignancy or a history of high-grade cervical intraepithelial neoplasia. To perform a supracervical hysterectomy, the bladder flap must be advanced from the

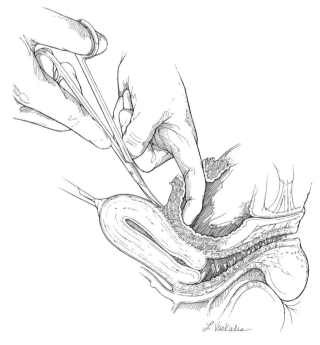

Fig. 30-26 Alternative approach to densely adherent bladder flap. If the bladder is so densely adherent to the uterus that a plane cannot be established easily, the dome of the bladder may be incised and the surgeon's finger used to palpate the bladder wall, thus protecting the bladder wall from a dissection that might go too deep into it.

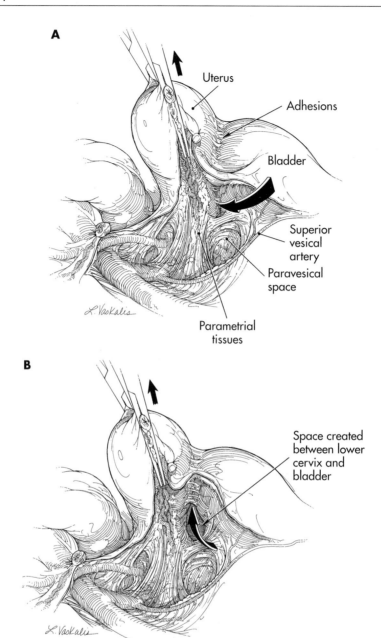

Fig. 30-27 **A,** Approaching the bladder from the paravesical space. With the paravesical space opened, the lower uterine segment and the cervix can be identified just superior to the superior vesicle artery. This area often is not adherent, and the bladder may be dissected off the lower cervix. **B,** Once the bladder has been mobilized from the lower cervix, the dissection can be carried cephalad between the bladder and the uterus, thereby protecting the bladder by more direct visualization of the appropriate plane. Anterior traction on the uterus provides additional exposure.

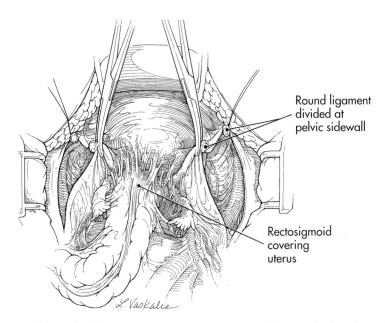

Fig. 30-28 Distorted pelvic anatomy; traction on the round ligaments. In patients in whom the pelvic anatomy is distorted and it is difficult to find the uterine fundus to provide traction, the round ligaments may be divided on the lateral pelvis and the medial round ligaments grasped with Kelly clamps, thereby allowing traction of the uterus. This often facilitates the dissection of the adhesions from the uterus, tubes, and ovaries and also facilitates opening the retroperitoneal spaces.

upper cervix and the rectum mobilized far enough away from the posterior cervix to identify the uterine blood supply. With the uterine vessels clamped, divided, and ligated, the cervix may then be transected and the uterine fundus removed from the operative field (Fig. 30-30). In some instances, removal of the uterine fundus by performing a supracervical hysterectomy will allow better exposure of the cervix and identification of the planes between the cervix and bladder and cervix and rectum, thereby allowing completion of the hysterectomy with more optimal exposure. I have found this technique particularly helpful in performing a total abdominal hysterectomy for patients who have large uterine fibroids. After removing the large uterine fundus, which is obscuring the view deeper in the pelvis, it is often easy then to remove the cervix as a separate specimen. If it is believed that removal of the cervix is too dangerous, the cervical stroma should be oversewn with figure-of-eight sutures of 0 Vicryl to achieve hemostasis. The advantage of ablating or resecting the endocervical canal is debatable in my opinion.

3. When it is difficult to free the rectosigmoid colon from the back of the cervix and uterus, a "reverse" hysterectomy may facilitate the dissection (Fig. 30-31). To perform this procedure, the bladder flap must be mobilized from the cervix and upper vagina. I prefer to also control the uterine blood supply. Before putting additional clamps along the paracervical or cardinal ligaments, the anterior vagina is incised and

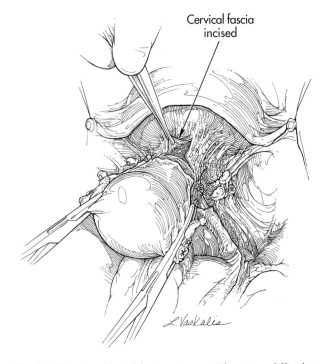

Fig. 30-29 Intrafascial hysterectomy. When it is difficult to mobilize the bladder from the cervix, the cervical fascia may be incised with a scalpel and mobilized from the cervix, leaving the fascia attached to the bladder. Clamps are then placed inside the fascia to complete the hysterectomy.

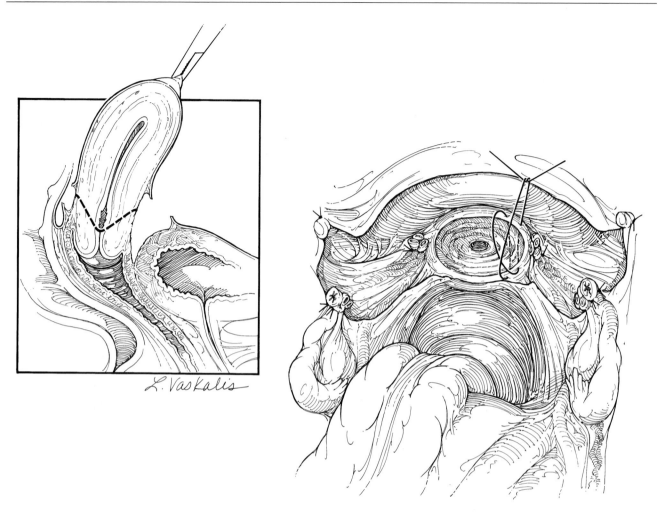

L. Vaskalis

Fig. 30-30 Supracervical hysterectomy. After the uterine vessels are controlled and ligated, the uterus is amputated from the cervix using a scalpel. The remaining cervix is then oversewn with figure-of-eight sutures of 0 Vicryl to achieve hemostatis.

a retractor is placed in the vagina to pull the bladder and anterior vagina caudad (see Fig. 30-31, *A* and *B*). A tenaculum is then placed on the anterior lip of the cervix, and it is lifted cephalad, thereby exposing the posterior vaginal wall. The posterior vaginal wall is then incised, and the upper portion is grasped with Alice clamps or long-toothed pickups (see Fig. 30-31, *C*). By staying in the midline of the posterior vagina, the surgeon can perform a sharp dissection, developing in a reverse manner the rectovaginal septum (see Fig. 30-31, *D*). Once this septum is started and the rectum is identified and separated from the vagina, the dissection can then be carried cephalad between and through the scar tissue obliterating the posterior cul-de-sac. Palpation from the intraperitoneal surface of the cul-de-sac as well as along the rectovaginal septum helps the surgeon identify and understand his or her location relevant to the vagina, cervix, and rectum. Once the rectovaginal septum is mobilized from the cervix, clamps may be placed at first along the paravaginal tissue and then moving cephalad toward the uterine vessels along the cardinal ligament and

paracervical tissues (see Fig. 30-31, *E*). This is essentially the sequence of removing the uterus during a vaginal hysterectomy. At all times, care must be taken to ensure that the clamps are placed adjacent to the cervix and not allowed to be located more laterally so as to avoid injury of the ureter. If necessary, the ureter should be mobilized from a portion of the paracervical tunnel by dividing the paracervical tunnel immediately superior to the ureter (type II hysterectomy) and then reflecting the ureter laterally.

After a difficult dissection, the surgeon must be fully cognizant of potential unrecognized injuries. It is critically important to identify injuries at the time of the surgical procedure rather than run the risk of an unrecognized injury until days or sometimes weeks postoperatively. Although these techniques are discussed in separate chapters of this text, it is worthwhile to reiterate them here so that the surgeon can recognize the armamentarium of possible methods of evaluation.

1. Potential injury to the ureter should be assessed to make certain that the ureter has not been ligated or transected. The most straightforward method of doing

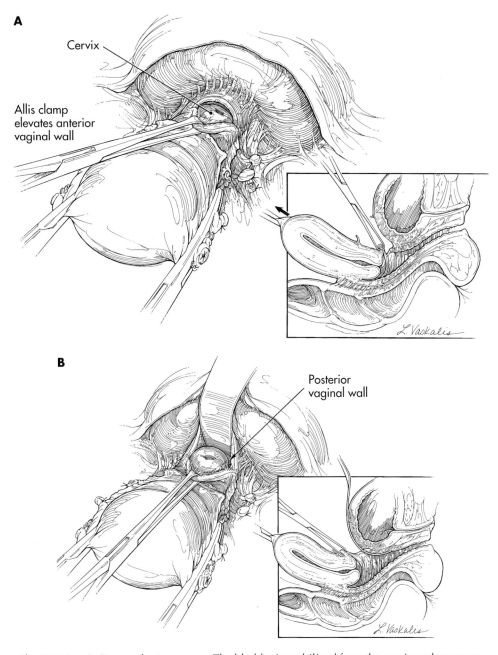

Fig. 30-31   **A,** Reverse hysterectomy. The bladder is mobilized from the cervix and upper vagina. The anterior vagina is opened just distal to the cervix. **B,** Exposure of the posterior vaginal wall. A narrow Deaver retractor is placed into the vagina, elevating it to gain better exposure to the posterior vaginal wall and the cervix.   *Continued*

this is to give intravenous indigo carmine (1 ampule; 5 ml). Inspection of the ureter and the pelvis is then carried out to be certain that no indigo carmine–colored urine leaks into the pelvis. Cystoscopy should then be performed to visualize indigo carmine being extruded from both ureteral orifices. If there is no evidence of dye coming from a ureteral orifice, retrograde stents should be passed to ascertain whether there is an area of obstruction, kinking, or ligation. If cystoscopy cannot be performed, the surgeon may consider performing telescopy (Fig. 30-32) or simply opening the bladder dome and visualizing the ureteral orifices. Retrograde stents may also be placed using either of these later techniques.

2. Potential rectal injury should be assessed by the "bubble test." Proctoscopy is performed to approximately 8 cm. The pelvis is filled with saline, and the surgeon compresses the sigmoid colon above the area of possible injury. The assistant manipulating the proctoscope then insufflates air into the rectum, and the rectum is observed for any bubbles coming through the saline. Identification of bubbles at this time indicates rectal injury, which should be repaired as discussed in Chapter 51.

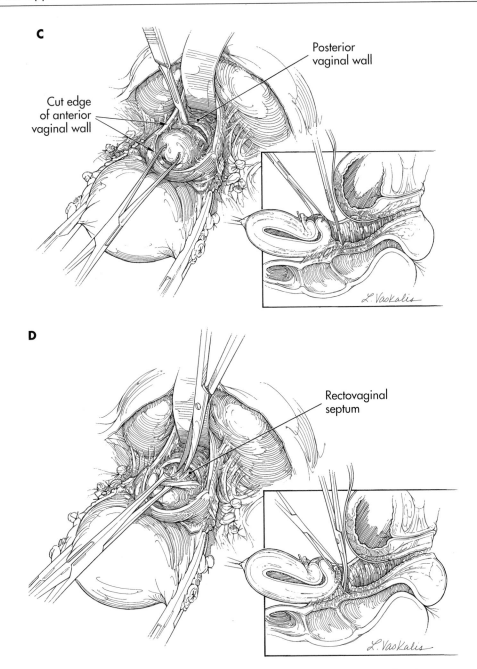

Fig. 30-31, cont'd C, Incision of the posterior vagina. The cervix is grasped with a tenaculum and pulled cephalad, thereby exposing the posterior vagina. The central portion of the posterior vagina is incised with a scalpel (15 blade on a long handle) and grasped. **D,** Creation of a rectovaginal lifted cephalad septum. An Allis clamp is placed on the posterior vagina. Using sharp dissection with Metzenbaum scissors, the rectovaginal septum is created dissecting cephalad.

3. Injury to the bladder is assessed initially by filling the bladder and ensuring there is no leak. I prefer to fill the bladder with 300 ml of sterile infant formula diluted with saline. The bladder dome and base must be carefully inspected to identify any leak of the white milk that has been instilled into the bladder. I prefer infant formula over a dye such as indigo carmine or methylene blue because these vital dyes tend to stain

tissues and therefore reassessment after repair of the cystotomy is somewhat compromised by the presence of stained bladder muscularis or mucosa.

COMPLICATIONS

The occurrence of acute complications associated with hysterectomy are reported in the literature to range between

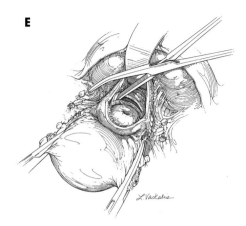

E

Fig. 30-31, cont'd   E, Once the rectovaginal septum has been developed, clamps may be placed from a caudad to a cephalad direction (similar to a vaginal hysterectomy). The first set of clamps is incorporated in the uterosacral ligaments and paracervical tissues. Throughout the dissection traction is placed on the cervix, helping to identify the plane between the cervix and rectum. All clamps must be immediately adjacent to the cervix and uterus to avoid ureteral injury.

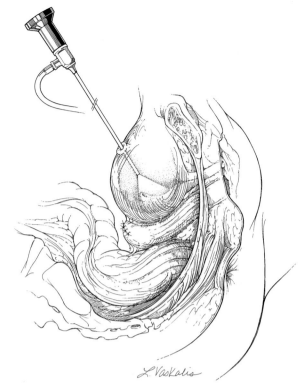

Fig. 30-32   Telescopy. A cystotomy is created in the dome of the bladder. A purse-string suture is placed around the cystotomy, and a cystoscope is inserted into the cystotomy. Using cystoscopic techniques, the bladder is filled and visualized to identify ureteral orifices and bladder anatomy.

25% and 50% of all patients.[7] Many of these complications are minor and have no long-term consequence. In the Maine Women's Health Study,[3] approximately 7% of patients had serious complications after hysterectomy. Factors found to increase the risk of complications included increasing age, urgent or emergency surgery, complicated and distorted anatomy, obesity, the lack of antibiotic or venous thromboembolism prophylaxis, inadequate bowel preparation, and the personal experience of the surgeon.

The most common complication after hysterectomy is febrile morbidity. This morbidity may be assigned to a number of causes, including urinary tract infection, pulmonary complications, pelvic surgical site infection, abdominal wound infection, and septic pelvic thrombophlebitis. The risks of febrile morbidity are increased in patients who have active or chronic pelvic inflammatory disease or who have the compounding factors listed previously. Although the literature is not in complete agreement, it appears that short-term single-agent first-generation cephalosporins administered before surgery can reduce the risk of febrile morbidity in most patients undergoing abdominal hysterectomy. The evaluation and management of patients with febrile complications after hysterectomy are outlined in Chapters 5 and 33.

The second most common complication associated with abdominal hysterectomy is intraoperative and postoperative hemorrhage. The risk of intraoperative bleeding is increased by extensive disease such as endometriosis or cancer or a large mass that obscures the operative field. If the uterus is enlarged to greater than 500 g, Hillis et al.[10] has demonstrated a substantially increased risk of intraoperative bleeding. This observation is confirmed by Stovall et al.[18] and leads to the recommendation that patients with 14 to 16 weeks' gestational size uterine fibroids be given 2 months of preoperative GnRH agonist treatment to reduce uterine size and thereby reduce intraoperative blood loss.

Urinary tract injury is a relatively uncommon yet serious complication of abdominal hysterectomy. It is estimated that injury to the ureter occurs in 0.2% to 0.5% of patients and injury to the bladder occurs in 0.3% to 0.8% of patients.[7] The risks of a urinary tract injury are increased when there is distorted anatomy, a large mass, extensive adhesions, or cancer. Careful identification of pelvic structures and recognition of the course of the ureter will likely prevent this complication. Immediate recognition of the complication and repair are critical to avoid a poor outcome and potential medicolegal implications.

An uncommon complication of abdominal hysterectomy is nerve injury, which most commonly involves the femoral nerve. This injury is not secondary to direct surgical trauma of the nerve but is almost always the result of improper positioning of the patient on the operating room table or improper placement of the self-retaining retractors, which compress the psoas muscle and femoral nerve. Most of these femoral nerve injuries are self-limited, and recovery should be expected within a few weeks to a few months. Physical therapy should be undertaken to assist the patient in adjusting to these neurologic deficits until recovery has occurred.

Postoperative death after hysterectomy is estimated to be 12 per 10,000 cases. A disproportionately higher incidence of postoperative mortality is seen when hysterectomy is associated with pregnancy (29.2 per 10,000) or cancer (37.8 per 10,000).[22] Deaths are most commonly caused by pulmonary embolism, infection, myocardial infarction, bowel obstruction, or cerebral vascular accident. Existing conditions that increase the risk of death include emergency surgery, postpartum hemorrhage, preexisting sepsis, and cancer.

Clarke et al.[6] and Carlson et al.[3] both have reported that after abdominal hysterectomy, 95% of patients have recognized resolution of their gynecologic symptoms and significant improvements in their quality of life. Compared with preoperative status, most patients indicate an increase in sexual desire and enjoyment despite the fact that the frequency of sexual activity is unchanged. Follow-up in excess of 1 year after surgery by Carlson et al.[3] has confirmed the continued resolution of symptoms, although they acknowledge the fact that there are short-term complications immediately after surgery that are likely to temporarily diminish the patient's quality of life. Because these minor complications are transient, they often are not discussed by the surgeon. It would seem prudent, however, for patients to be fully informed of short-term complications so that they do not have unrealistic expectations as to the rapidity of their recovery or the transient pain they may encounter.

Certainly there is a subgroup of patients who develop postoperative depression or decreased libido. This accounts for approximately 7% to 8% of patients as reported by Carlson et al.[5] Patients at increased risk of experiencing postoperative depression include those with a history of depression, those with a poor sense of well-being preoperatively, those with an unstable or unhappy marital relationship, those who desire pregnancy, and those who do not believe that there is an indication to have surgery performed. Furthermore, there are a multitude of views regarding female sexuality, menstruation, and childbearing that vary from one culture to another, and these should be evaluated preoperatively so that the physician's personal outlook does not overshadow the patient's own cultural perspective.

MEDICAL AND LEGAL ISSUES

Complications associated with hysterectomy are among the most common sources for medicolegal action after gynecologic surgery. Although this is discussed in Chapter 11, it is important to reiterate that the most common reasons for malpractice action include ureteral injury, the feeling that the patient underwent an unnecessary hysterectomy, and postoperative death.[20] Ureteral injury and prevention of fatal complications are discussed at length in other sections of this text and are not reiterated here. The issue of alleged unnecessary hysterectomy continues to be an important issue requiring the physician to clearly offer the patient informed consent and document this informed consent discussion. If alternative methods of management were not discussed or

tried, the patient has an increased likelihood of being angry postoperatively when symptoms do not fully resolve or the patient's expectations are not achieved.

REFERENCES

1. Bachman GA: Hysterectomy: a critical review, *J Reprod Med* 35:839, 1990.
2. Bradham DD, Stovall TG, Thompson CD: The use of GnRH agonists before hysterectomy: a cost simulation, *Obstet Gynecol* 85:401, 1995.
3. Carlson KJ, Miller BA, Fowler FJ: The Maine Women's Health Study. I. Outcomes of hysterectomy, *Obstet Gynecol* 83:556, 1994
4. Carlson KJ, Miller BA, Fowler FJ: The Maine Women's Health Study. II. Outcomes of nonsurgical management of leiomyomas, abnormal bleeding and chronic pelvic pain, *Obstet Gynecol* 83:566, 1994.
5. Carlson KJ, Nichols DH, Shiff I: Indications for hysterectomy, *N Engl J Med* 328:856, 1993.
6. Clarke A, Black N, Rowe P, et al: Indications for and outcome of total abdominal hysterectomy for benign disease: a prospective cohort study, *Br J Obstet Gynecol* 102:611,1995.
7. Easterday CL, Grimes DA, Riggs JA: Hysterectomy in the United States, *Obstet Gynecol* 62:203, 1983.
8. Grover CM, Kuppermann M, Kahn JG, et al: Concurrent hysterectomy at bilateral salpingo-oophorectomy: benefits, risks and costs, *Obstet Gynecol* 88:907, 1996.
9. Graves E, Gillum B: National hospital discharge survey: annual summary, 1994, *National Center for Health Statistics, Vital Health Statistics,* 13(126), 1997.
10. Hillis SD, Marchbanks PA, Peterson HB: Uterine size and risk of complications among women undergoing abdominal hysterectomy for leiomyomas, *Obstet Gynecol* 87:539, 1996.
11. Iverson RE, Chelmow D, Strohbehn K, et al: Relative morbidity of abdominal hysterectomy and myomectomy for management of uterine leiomyomas, *Obstet Gynecol* 88:415, 1996.
12. Kanter MH, van Maanen D, Anders KH, et al: Preoperative autologous blood donations before elective hysterectomy, *JAMA* 276:798, 1996.
13. Lepine LA, Hillis SD, Marchbanks PA: Hysterectomy surveillance: United States, 1980-1993. CDC Surveillance Summaries, August 8, 1997, *MMWR* 46:1-14, 1997.
14. Myers ER, Clarke-Pearson DL, Olt GJ, et al: Preoperative coagulation testing on a gynecologic oncology service, *Obstet Gynecol* 83:438, 1994.
15. Piscitelli JT, Simel DL, Addison WA: Who should have intravenous pyelograms before hysterectomy for benign disease? *Obstet Gynecol* 69:541, 1987.
16. Pokras R, Hufnagel VG: Hysterectomy in the United States, 1965-1984, *Am J Public Health* 78:852, 1988.
17. Reiter RC, Wagner PL, Gambone JC: Routine hysterectomy for large asymptomatic uterine leiomyomata: a reappraisal, *Obstet Gynecol* 79:481, 1992.
18. Stovall TG, Summitt RL, Washburn SA, et al: Gonadotropin-releasing hormone agonist use before hysterectomy *Am J Obstet Gynecol* 170:1744, 1994.
19. Summitt RL, Stovall TG, Lipscomb JH, et al: Outpatient hysterectomy: determinants of discharge and rehospitalization in 133 patients, *Am J Obstet Gynecol* 171:1480, 1994.
20. Whitelaw JM: Hysterectomy: a medical legal perspective, 1975-1985, *Am J Obstet Gynecol* 162:1451, 1990.
21. Wilcox LS, Koonin LM, Pokras R, et al: Hysterectomy in the United States, 1988-1990, *Obstet Gynecol* 83:549, 1994.
22. Wingo PA, Huezo CM, Rubin GL, et al: The mortality risk associated with hysterectomy, *Am J Obstet Gynecol* 152:803, 1985.

31 Myomectomy

SAMANTHA M. PFEIFER and CELSO-RAMÓN GARCÍA

Uterine myomas are among the most common tumors encountered in women. These tumors vary in appearance and specific distortions. Although derived from a single myometrial cell, their histologic composition can be quite varied, depending on how they have been influenced in their progressive development. These tumors may contain primarily smooth muscle but may have varying densities of fibrous elements derived from interstitial tissues. In addition, there may be varying degrees of degeneration, hemorrhage, and even calcification. The simple tumor is preferentially called a myoma but is often called fibroid, fibromyoma, leiomyoma, leiofibroma, fibroleiomyoma, and so forth, synonymously. Multiple myomas are particularly confusing because they can produce a variety of symptoms depending on the number, the size and location, and any associated pathologic condition that may accompany their presence. In light of the clinical variation in symptoms, each woman so afflicted will have different needs, the most important of which is the need to have her symptoms corrected without the loss of reproductive function.

Recent technologic advances applied to diagnose and manage this variable tumor entity have been hailed as useful, but at the same time, their application has clouded the issues. Never have we had the ability to assess the pelvic structures as well as we have at present. At the same time, never have we had so many various approaches to address the management of the problem from both a medical and surgical viewpoint. This variety exists despite the fact that myomectomy is basically a simple procedure. However, it does require dedication to a meticulous pursuit of excellence and mature experience in dealing with the anatomic variations of the myomas. In addition, it also requires the ability to address the specific needs of the woman. Therefore it is well to review the various factors that should be considered when deciding what to do and how to counsel each woman in light of her specific situation and considerations.

ANATOMIC CONSIDERATIONS

It is estimated that some 20% to 25% of women of reproductive age have myomas.[13,14] They are more common during or after the third decade and are rare before the age of 20 years. A threefold higher incidence in African-American than white women has been reported.[13,14,18] Myomas are found in various locations within and around the uterus. The subserous and intramural uterine locations are most common (Fig. 31-1). Pedunculated myomas can be seen arising from below the serosal surface but also from the submucosal myometrium. The submucosal myomas have an incidence of 5% to 10%.[6] They may be broad based or may arise on a narrow pedicle as a submucous pedunculated myoma. The latter can be extruded through the endocervix and can be associated with varying degrees of uterine inversion (Fig. 31-2).[45,82] Cervical and intraligamentous myomas (parauterine) are less common, with an incidence of 5% and 2.4%, respectively.[48] Parametrial and perisalpingeal locations are less common.[60] A parasitic myoma can arise from a pedunculated subserosal myoma that undergoes torsion, subsequently deriving its blood supply from another source with which it has interacted. Accordingly, they most commonly are found in the omentum.

Myomas can vary considerably in size from small seedlings (millimeters) to enormous, tumors, which have been reported to reach more than 100 lb.[51,89] Rates of myoma growth are unpredictably variable, and the explanation for this variability is equally vexing. Myomas are typically benign uterine tumors, occurring as multiple tumors, although less commonly, they may be solitary. Rapidly enlarging solitary tumors are more likely malignant than the multiple cohorts. Each myoma tends to be a discrete, elliptically spheroid pseudoencapsulated mass, often interlacing with another myoma in the myometrium, producing a lobulated shape of the uterine body. Cut sections disclose a whorl-like pattern of smooth muscle and fibrous connective tissue. The fibrous connective tissue forms a pseudocapsule around the myoma. Hemorrhage and degeneration, usually in the central aspect of the tumor, are seen when the myoma outgrows its blood supply. Necrosis of myomas can subsequently occur. Hyalinization, fibrosis, and calcification are late sequelae. Infection of a necrotizing myoma (pyomyoma) can also occur, usually after pregnancy, after instrumentation of the myomatous uterus, in association with an ascending infection, or by hematogenous spread.[42,97]

SYMPTOMATOLOGY

Symptomatic myomas have been reported in approximately 20% to 50% of patients. The severity of these parallels the degrees of pathologic findings, which are more notable during the latter years of reproductive potential. The wide array of symptoms includes abnormal uterine bleeding, which occurs in approximately 30% of patients and is seen more often with submucous myomas. Abdominal and pelvic pain, abdominal enlargement, and gastrointestinal pressure symp-

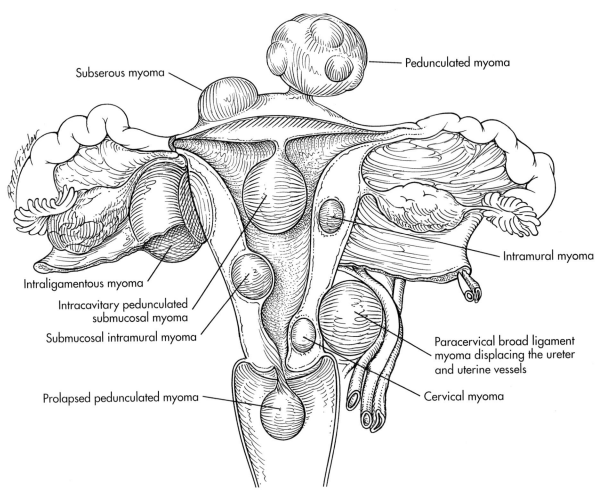

Subserous myoma

Pedunculated myoma

Intramural myoma

Intraligamentous myoma

Intracavitary pedunculated
submucosal myoma

Submucosal intramural myoma

Paracervical broad ligament
myoma displacing the ureter
and uterine vessels

Cervical myoma

Prolapsed pedunculated myoma

Fig. 31-1   A diagrammatic array of uterine myomata.

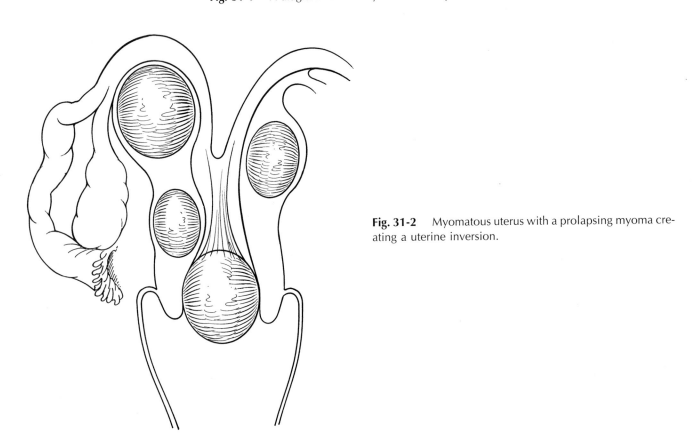

Fig. 31-2   Myomatous uterus with a prolapsing myoma creating a uterine inversion.

toms (backache and constipation) are related to the impingement of the tumor on the adjacent organs. These distortions of the anatomy can also elicit dysfunctions of the urinary bladder (urinary frequency and urinary retention) or, on rare occasions, even obstruction of the ureters. Pedunculated or enlarging myomas arising from the serosal surface can be attached by a thick stalk. Occasionally, they may be mistaken for an adnexal mass. Those with a thinner stalk may undergo torsion, giving rise to acute or recurrent abdominal pain. Pedunculated submucous myomas are often associated with heavy bleeding and have led to uterine inversion and sepsis when prolapsed through the cervix. Pain caused by necrosis of a myoma can be seen with rapidly growing myomas and during pregnancy.

Myomas may cause infertility through mechanisms such as compression of oviducts and distortion of the endometrial cavity or perhaps as an intrauterine device (IUD)-like effect seen especially with pedunculated submucous myomas.[18] Pregnancy loss has been attributed to myoma constraint on uterine cavity expansion. Pregnancy loss rates as high as 75% to 80% have been reported; the rate in women without myomas is 30%.[14]

ETIOLOGIC CONSIDERATIONS

Although the cause of myomas is unknown, several factors have been implicated. Evidence appears to support the fact that myomas, like many other benign tumors, are monoclonal.[80,94] Cytogenetic studies have found clonal chromosome arrangements in 50% to 60% of myomas studied. The most common abnormalities reported involve a translocation of chromosomes 12 and 14, specifically, t[12;14].[q14-15,q23-24].[26,59,80,94] The many different cytogenetic abnormalities described support the hypothesis that different genetic loci may be responsible for the development of myomas, and these differences may explain the heterogeneity seen in the clinical presentation. Recently, Brosens et al.[11] have described karyotyping in myomas, with submucous myomas having significantly fewer karyotype abnormalities than either intramural or subserosal myomas. Familial uterine myomas[52] have been reported; however, the actual incidence is unknown.

For years, estrogen has been causatively implicated in the pathophysiology of myomas. This theory is supported by the observation that myomas grow principally during the years of active ovarian function. Myomas are not seen before puberty; after menopause, they not only do not grow but are believed to decrease in size.

Nelson[65] was the first to demonstrate the association between estrogen and myomas by stimulating myomas to grow in guinea pigs after the administration of large doses of estrogens, which he thought to be a dose-related effect. Estrogen and progesterone receptors have been demonstrated in myoma tissue.[76,91,93,96] It is also of interest that the concentration of estrogen receptors is found to be greater in myoma tissue than in the myometrium.[18]

Epidermal growth factor has been demonstrated in myoma tissue as well as in the myometrium.[45,82] Its receptor is present in low concentrations, and no difference has been demonstrated among endometrium, myometrium, and myomas. However, the role of epidermal growth factor in myomas is unknown.

MANAGEMENT CONSIDERATIONS

Because the cause of myomas is not understood, preventing their occurrence is not feasible. Also, it should be recognized that no long-term medical therapies with proven safety are available for treatment of myomata. Thus treatment of myomas is usually surgical and should address the specific symptoms and needs of the woman. Conservational versus extirpative treatment must be individualized according to the woman's age, medical status, uterine size, and involvement of the myomatous uterus. This should address the importance of the uterus to the specific woman, including the desire for future reproduction. Selection of appropriate management for each woman is highly subjective and requires careful discussion and counseling on all the issues. Moreover, the surgeon's empathy, experience, and ability play a fundamental role. Careful consideration must be given to ensure appropriate individualized treatment.

When the myomas are asymptomatic and particularly if they are 3 months in gestational size or less, most concur that nothing need be done.[13] These patients should be followed by periodic evaluation, including pelvic examination and ultrasound evaluation, every 6 to 12 months to assess possible changes in the rate of growth. A rapid growth rate may suggest malignancy and requires more frequent evaluation with possible intervention. Women exhibiting only minimal changes in uterine mass and those who remain asymptomatic should be counseled about the need for careful, expectant follow-up, although medical or surgical intervention is not warranted.

The increased effort and experience required to perform myomectomy with limited risks lead many to conclude that there must be a justification for the need to preserve uterine function. Hysterectomy often is looked on as the definitive approach with which many surgeons feel most comfortable. Multiple myomectomy is most compelling when the aim is to improve fertility or to relieve a symptomatic myomatous distortion in the woman desirous of preserving her reproductive function. In general, the risks associated with myomectomy are prolonged operative time, blood loss, intestinal obstruction secondary to adhesions of bowel to the uterine operative sites, and the probability of myoma recurrence. These two latter complications of myomectomy, cited for their future potential for pelvic surgery, are often viewed as outweighing the potential benefit to be gained by myomectomy. Of course, hysterectomy is not without risks, and the importance of the uterus to the specific woman must not be underestimated. Sincere, careful counseling of the woman is key, and her desires must be weighed carefully. The woman should be counseled to seek another opinion when a consensus is not reached.

Infertile women with symptomatic myomas deserve every effort needed to preserve their uterine function. Successful pregnancies in women who have undergone myomectomy for intramural, subserosal, and submucosal myomas are reported to be in the range of 48% to 62%.[13,34,83] Pregnancy rates of 53% have been reported when submucosal myomas exceeding 5 cm in diameter were removed.[3,34,83] The fact that most of the pregnancies occur within the first year (75% to 80%) after myomectomy despite years of prior infertility supports the concept that myomectomy restores fertility. Nonetheless, no evidence supports the theory that the excision of small solitary myomas (less than 5 cm) significantly improves fertility.[8]

The feminist community argues for preservation of the reproductive organs and for myomectomy rather than hysterectomy at any age. This large group believes not only that hysterectomy is a reproductive loss but also that it contributes adversely to their sexual feelings through dyspareunia and the loss of deep orgasm. Moreover, they also point out that hysterectomy with and without oophorectomy is also associated with myocardial infarction related to estrogen deficiency secondary to premature ovarian failure. Several epidemiologic studies support this contention.[5,16,87] Significant disagreement still exists regarding the advisability of performing a myomectomy, especially in a woman older than age 40, in whom reproductive needs may be unrealistic and the distortion extensive. Although it may severely affect some women who perceive it as a loss of their femininity, it is important that the woman be counseled about the recurrence of myomas. There are those who raise concern regarding the appropriateness of myomectomy under these circumstances because subsequent myoma growth may lead to the need for reoperation. Myomas recur in at least 15% to 20% of women who have undergone myomectomy.

The difficulties associated with making the diagnosis of a leiomyosarcoma, although a rare occurrence, is another factor of concern. The clinical presentation is not reliable, and the diagnosis may not be made at the time of dilation and curettage (D&C). Radiographic studies, including magnetic resonance imaging (MRI), are not reliable in diagnosing early nonmetastatic uterine sarcomas. The malignant transformation of myomas is viewed with less concern because this is exceedingly rare, occurring in less than 0.1% of women with myomas.[13]

Increased size of myomas may be associated with greater risk in performing a myomectomy for some. Indeed, this need not be. Safe restorative surgery is facilitated by attention to meticulous hemostasis, careful appropriate dissection, rapid reconstruction, and so forth. However, the presence of coexisting pathologic conditions can make the surgery prolonged and tedious. In the more severe circumstances with the presence of myriad myomas and extensive adnexal disease, the "simpler" extirpative approach through hysterectomy might be preferable. For most whose situation may not be as severe, the goal probably should be the removal of all myomas with preservation of reproductive function. Proximity of the myomas to the oviducts and endometrial cavity is not a reason for leaving the myomas. Microsurgical dissection techniques may be needed to resect such myomas and repair the defects. Removal of all myomas to ensure the lowest risk of recurrence should be the aim.

Preoperative Evaluation and Patient Preparation

Before myomectomy, patients should have a complete history and physical examination, and all existing medical problems should be addressed. Preoperative screening should include a Pap smear to evaluate cervical cytologic findings and an endometrial biopsy or uterine curettage to diagnose possible chronic endometritis and/or malignancy. Hysterosalpingography is indicated to evaluate possible uterine cavity distortion and tubal distortion or compression by the myomas. Hysteroscopy can also evaluate the uterine cavity but not the oviducts. More recently, sonohysterography has gained acceptance as an alternative to evaluate the uterine cavity for submucosal and intracavitary pedunculated myomas and polyps. An abdominal ultrasound or an excretory urogram is helpful in identifying ureteral dilation, although it may not be routinely requested. Ultrasound and MRI have become useful adjuncts to define the location and size of the myomas and perhaps differentiate between an ovarian mass and a pedunculated myoma.[24,43] With good resolution, MRI scans not only may offer the advantage of distinguishing between myoma and adenomyosis but also may alert the surgeon to a leiomyosarcomatous appearance.[62] Laparoscopy is especially helpful in evaluating the size, location, and number of myomas as well as the presence of additional pelvic pathologic conditions that may influence the decision to proceed with the myomectomy (e.g., severe endometriosis, chronic pelvic adnexal inflammatory disease). Through such preoperative evaluation the extent of the myomas and the relation to the total clinical features can be assessed, and the physician can more accurately counsel the patient, who will feel better informed regarding her surgical options.

Anemia must be corrected before surgery. This can best be accomplished by a high-iron diet and with iron supplementation (e.g., ferrous sulfate, 325 mg four times daily after meals). In some patients, when menstrual blood loss has been severe, combinations of estrogen and progestagen or a gonadotropin-releasing hormone (GnRH) agonist have been used to stop vaginal bleeding to facilitate the correction of anemia *in conjunction with iron therapy*. The use of GnRH agonists has recently become popular, and they can be administered by daily subcutaneous injection (Lupron [leuprolide], 0.5 to 1.0 mg/day), by depot intramuscular form (Lupron, 3.75 mg or 7.5 mg every month), or by nasal spray (nafarelin [Synarel]), one to two puffs per nostril twice a day. The GnRH approaches have not had U.S. Food and Drug Administration (FDA) approval for the management of myomata. Bleeding can be stopped acutely with these regimens. Combinations of estrogens and progestogens, such as those used with high-dose oral contraceptives, have long been shown to be effective for the control of uterine bleeding. This was the initial approved indication for Enovid by the FDA. Three tablets of Estinyl (ethinyl estradiol), 0.05 mg (total of 0.15 mg), and Norlutin (norethindrone), 10 mg, is a dosage level of the estrogen-progestagen combination that halts dysfunctional uterine bleeding associated with submucous myomas. It can be used for 6 to 8 weeks together with hematinic therapy to correct anemia and allow the surgery to be scheduled. It should be used only as a short-term approach to stop bleeding and reverse anemia before surgery. Prolonged use results in subsequent uterine bleeding, requiring increases in dosage of this estrogen-progestogen combination, and also effects increases in uterine and myoma size. However, it does not contribute to an estrogen-deficient menopausal state as do the releasing hormone analogs with their skeletal and other implications.

In all patients planning to have a multiple myomectomy, autologous and directed donor blood donation should be discussed with the patient before surgery is scheduled. Presurgical autologous blood donation has been suggested as well as use of a directed donor. Some recommend that two units of autologous blood be available for surgery. However, this approach has not been proven to be sound in severely anemic women. Preoperative donation of blood can detract from the hemic buildup of an iron therapy if the blood was not donated. Moreover, two units of blood might be inadequate were there significant bleeding at surgery. Such a situation could warrant the need for four units or more from the blood bank, which is what the patient believes she is avoiding by autologous preoperative donations. Although autologous blood may be available, giving patients transfusions may not be as innocuous as some believe and can lead to cardiac overload and other risks associated with transfusions in general.[74] Blood from a directed donor can be collected before the procedure; however, this carries similar risks to the patient as blood from the blood bank pool. With greater awareness and careful screening, this risk has become small. The estimated risk of transmitting the human immunodeficiency virus (HIV) is about 1 in 450,000 to 1 in 660,000, but the probability estimate is now believed to have been lowered to 1 in 26 million as a result of improvement in screening and better sensitivity of enzyme-linked immunosorbent assays.[53,90] The risk of hepatitis still remains a concern. The careful surgeon who is aware of the need to use every technique to attain meticulous hemostasis can avoid excessive blood loss. With such care the need for transfusion can be virtually eliminated. However, the patient should be carefully counseled about these risks and the possible need for transfusion no matter how rare these occurrences may be.

MYOMECTOMY APPROACHES

Myomectomy is performed most commonly by the laparotomy route. Vaginal myomectomy, laparoscopic myomectomy, and myomectomy by hysteroscopic resection are performed under special circumstances. For the present, abdominal myomectomy must be viewed as the gold standard. More data are needed to ensure that these alternative approaches are superior in every way. Prolapsed myomas should be approached vaginally. Laparoscopic approaches can be vexing in the removal of the myomas from the abdominal cavity. Moreover, it may be impossible to locate all of the myomas. If the smaller ones are not removed, one can expect higher recurrence rates.

Abdominal Myomectomy—The Open Surgical Route

In carrying out the myomectomy, certain basic principles should be adhered to. Meticulous attention to hemostasis is essential. Most myomectomies can best be accomplished using a Pfannenstiel or a transverse incision in the abdomen, reserving a midline incision for much larger myomas (e.g., arising above the umbilicus). The midline incision is less time-consuming but is not as strong an incision as a transverse one. Moreover, it leaves the woman with a visible scar.

Good exposure, good assistance, and careful isolation of the tumor or tumors are essential to reduce blood loss. Moreover, meticulous hemostatic incision techniques help guard against insidious blood loss. The use of the Shaw heated scalpel is strongly recommended. The time it takes to master its use is justified because it does reduce the "insensible" blood loss incurred in opening the anterior abdominal wall. The dissection of the anterior sheath of the rectus abdominis muscle should be made in a curvilinear manner as in the creation of a significant U-shaped flap. This should start from the initial midline transverse fascial incision and extend laterally with a cephalad course on each side to a level approaching that of the umbilicus (Figs. 31-3 to 31-6). This U-shaped flap of the anterior sheath of the rectus affords excellent exposure to the abdominal cavity after the recti have been retracted laterally. The peritoneum is then opened vertically in the midline. Occasionally, the lower pole of the peritoneal incision may need to be extended in a lateral direction, avoiding the bladder.

Of significance is excellent retraction. This can best be achieved by the use of the Iron Intern or the Buckwalter retractor. It is ideally suited because it gives excellent exposure. It also has a gentle steady traction, which protects tissue from pressure points while also avoiding posterior pelvic compressions, which otherwise could lead to undesirable nerve and vessel trauma. The time taken to place these retractors is rewarded not only by excellent exposure but also by superior postoperative patient recovery. The retractor has a built-in safety clutch, which does not permit traumatic tissue pressures.

Hemostasis can be ensured with myometrial injection of vasoconstrictors such as dilute epinephrine, oxytocin (Pitocin), or vasopressin (Pitressin), as well as tourniquet application. Vasopressin should be injected into the myometrium as a dilute solution (20 U in 40 to 50 ml of normal saline). This can be used for small myomas or in conjunction with other techniques. Repeat use of dilute vasopressin may be needed. Although some report a histamine reaction, it has not been reported in many hundreds of myomectomies over 30 years.[34,78]

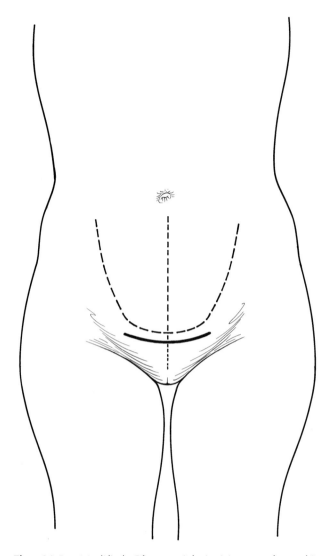

Fig. 31-3 Modified Pfannenstiel incision: a low skin incision.

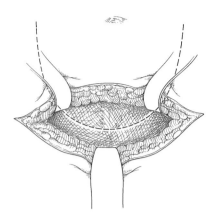

Fig. 31-4 Modified Pfannenstiel incision. Dissection exposing anterior sheath of the rectus. Tunneling of dissection at each angle follows dotted line.

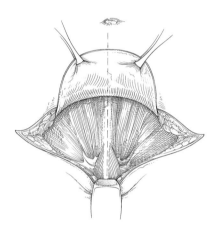

Fig. 31-5 Modified Pfannenstiel incision. Shows flap of anterior sheath of rectus muscle that has been dissected free from the muscle bellies.

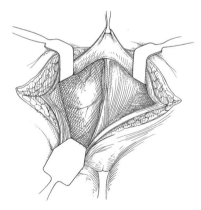

Fig. 31-6 Modified Pfannenstiel incision. Right rectus muscle belly retracted, exposing the peritoneum before the celomic cavity is opened.

The tourniquet technique is well suited to large myomatous uteri with multiple intramural and submucous myomas. Reducing the intraoperative blood loss can be ensured by placing the tourniquet around the uterine mass. The tourniquet should be low enough to compress the infundibulopelvic ligaments and cervix, as well as to include the adnexa, which should be above the tourniquet to avoid being compressed. In this way, the uterine blood supply to the uterus and the blood supply by way of the ovarian anastomosis from the infundibulopelvic vessels is contained. A simple piece of sterile rubber tubing or a catheter can serve as the tourniquet. The tourniquet is tightened in a stepwise fashion by alternately clamping with a Kelly clamp, pulling on the tourniquet, and again clamping with another Kelly clamp (Fig. 31-7). This repeated Kelly clamping and snugging of the tubing are continued until the compression is deemed adequate to constrict the blood flow. When vasopressin is injected into the myometrium before the application of the tourniquet, a vasoconstriction ensures reduction of the blood volume within the organ. As a result, there is less bleeding from the initial uterine incision because the vaso-

constriction has expressed the uterine blood into the peripheral circulation—a small autologous transfusion, as it were. This technique can be used for larger myomas as well as for smaller submucosal myomas. An alternative method of tourniquet application, suggested by Rubin[84] in the 1930s, re-

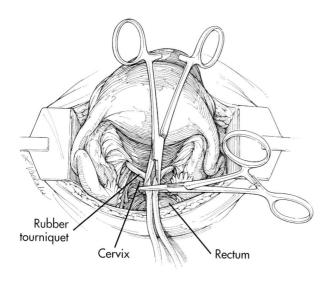

Rubber
tourniquet

Cervix   Rectum

Fig. 31-7 The rubber tourniquet is being applied to encompass the entire uterine mass. Note that the tourniquet application encompasses the adnexa and thus limits the flow of the uterine and the infundibulopelvic vessels. The rubber tourniquet is tightened in a stepwise application of Kelly clamps. Although the initial clamp crosses both segments of rubber tubing, it is strongly recommended that the subsequent clamps grasp the tubing so that the two arms of the tubing are opposed when the clamp is crossed as is depicted in the more proximal application. This ensures that the rubber tubing does not slip through the clamp. It is not necessary to open a passage in the broad ligament to exclude the infundibulopelvic vessels. Avoiding this dissection reduces the potential of postoperative periadnexal adhesions to these dissected areas. (From Pfeifer SM, Garcia CR: Myomectomy. In Nichols DH, editor: *Reoperative gynecologic and obstetric surgery,* ed 2, St Louis, 1997, Mosby.)

quires opening windows in the broad ligament through which the tourniquet is passed. This technique is particularly useful in patients with pelvic adhesions or broad ligament myomas for which application of the tourniquet across both the infundibulopelvic and uterine vessels is not feasible. Adequate hemostasis can be achieved with this application. This approach does not restrict the ovarian blood flow. It also has the disadvantage of creating broad ligament trauma. During the removal of multiple myomas, the tourniquet application may become loose. The surgeon should be continually aware of the possible need for application of a second tourniquet to ensure continued compression of the vessels and thorough hemostasis. Continual hemostasis can be maintained through appropriate compression, appropriate suture, and repeat injection of dilute vasopression as needed.

Anoxia to the follicles causes them to become atretic during the current cycle; however, in the next cycle, a new crop of follicles develops from the primordial germ cells, which are resistant to the anoxia. This regeneration of follicles in the subsequent cycles has been consistent over the years even when the tourniquet has been in place some 5 hours.

The Shaw scalpel, electrocautery, and laser[63,81] are use-

ful tools for removing small myomas. Moreover, traction and compression are also helpful in reducing blood loss and in the dissection of the myomas when tourniquets are not applied.

When the uterus is approached, the most important consideration is assessing the location and direction of the blood supply. A second consideration is to make as few incisions in the uterus as possible. The latter leads to a decreased chance of adhesion formation secondary to the effects of the uterine trauma. Posterior uterine wall incisions are of concern because of the potential for adhesions of bowel to these areas. Greater care in their repair is stressed.

Unless in the midline, the incision on the uterus should be made parallel with the course of the vascular bed of vessels. This is important when a more lateral uterine site is to be dissected. A vertical incision is preferable in the relatively avascular midline (Figs. 31-8 and 31-9). Once through the serosa, the incision should be carried down through the myometrium into the pseudocapsule of the myoma. After the myoma has been exposed, it may be grasped with a towel clamp, and traction can be applied. This traction reduces blood loss when a tourniquet has not been applied. The myoma is dissected free from the surrounding myometrium using a combination of sharp but principally blunt dissection (Fig. 31-10). The latter ensures remaining within the pseudocapsule. Strulli scissors and a periosteal elevator are particularly well suited to this purpose, as are the surgeon's fingertips. Constant traction on the myomas and a twisting motion are helpful. This dissection should not be difficult as long as the correct plane is maintained.

The dissection is carried down to the pedicle that contains the main blood supply to the myoma. The pedicle should be isolated, clamped, and ligated before the removal of the myoma as the first step in ensuring hemostasis (Figs. 31-11 and 31-12). Through the wall of the myometrial defect, other myomas are often detected and should also be dissected and excised. These surgically dissected uterine wall defects are repaired in a meticulous manner through the approximation of the tissues. This restores the anatomy previously distorted by the growing myomas. Several methods are suggested. The preferred approach uses a suture applied as a continuous concentric spiraling stitch, using vertically linear or radial bites. This closure is begun with a figure-of-eight stitch placed at the base of the operative defect. The important aspect of this stitch encompasses not only the anatomic reconstruction but also the securing of hemostasis. Both of these are achieved by closing all of the dead space (see Fig. 31-12). It is most important to ensure continuous traction by snugging the stitch after each bite and maintaining constant tension on the suture as these stitches are being placed. Closing the defect is best accomplished by use of fine absorbable suture such as 3-0 or 4-0 polyglactin (Vicryl). Catgut should be avoided because of its inherent reactivity and lower tensile strength. The serosa is closed using a baseball stitch that approximates the myometrium and inverts the serosa to minimize adhesion formation

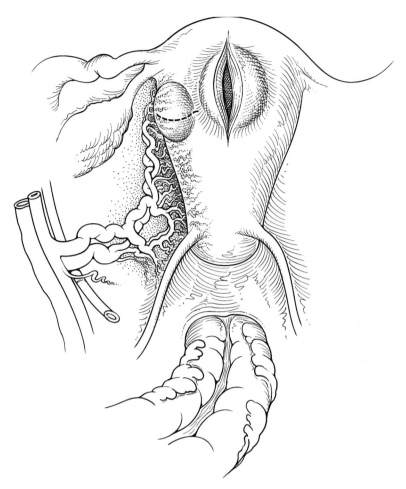

Fig. 31-8 Myomectomy incisions. The incisions should parallel the vasculature, except in the midline where the "avascularity" should be taken advantage of with a vertical or midline incision.

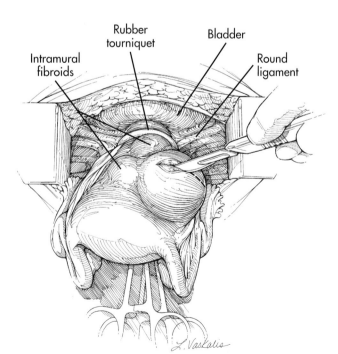

Intramural fibroids

Rubber tourniquet

Bladder

Round ligament

Fig. 31-9 The site of the anterior uterine wall incision is selected as the thinnest area over the myoma. Dissection after the removal of the first myoma allows access to the other myomas. A transverse incision of the uterine wall over the myoma parallels the lateral uterine vascular distribution. This limits the potential of bleeding better than a vertical incision made in this lateral location, which would cut across the vascular distribution. By contrast, in the midline the relative avascularity would allow a vertical incision. (From Pfeifer SM, Garcia CR: Myomectomy. In Nichols DH, editor: *Reoperative gynecologic and obstetric surgery,* ed 2, St Louis, 1997, Mosby.)

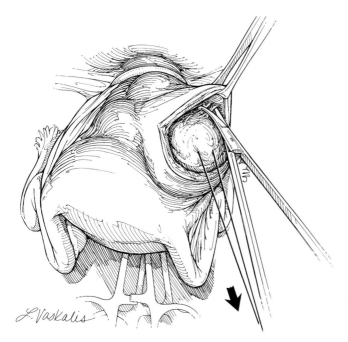

Fig. 31-10 Using a traction stitch or a towel clamp can elevate the tumor to facilitate the dissection through the layers of pseudocapsule. This dissection can be carried out with blunt and sharp dissection. A Kelly clamp, a periosteum elevator, and Strulli's scissors can be used for this dissection, but traction elevating the myoma is essential. (From Pfeifer SM, Garcia CR: Myomectomy. In Nichols DH, editor: *Reoperative gynecologic and obstetric surgery*, ed 2, St Louis, 1997, Mosby.)

(Fig. 31-13). For this approximation, 4-0 or 5-0 Vicryl sutures are used.

It is most important to identify all of the myomas. If small myomas remain, the risk of them developing into larger myomas increases. This appears to be related to the high recurrence rates sometimes observed. Position and presence of myomas are determined by palpating the uterine wall carefully through the incision(s) and defects. Some myomas may be identified only by palpation through the defect created by the removal of the prior excised myomas. When palpated, the myoma is preferably removed through this existing incision. Incision techniques that also offer hemostasis, such as the Shaw scalpel, laser, and bipolar cautery, should be used. The removal of the myoma is accomplished by incising the myometrium overlying the myoma and removing the tumor as described above. Several myomas can be removed through the same incision in this manner. In doing so, care must be taken to identify blood supply, ensuring hemostasis when all of the defects that have been created are closed. It is helpful to remove all myomas before closing defects to not confuse the digital palpation of sutured areas with remaining myomas.

With deep intramural or submucous myomas, the endometrial cavity may be exposed or entered. It is best to avoid entry into the endometrial cavity because this could lead to adhesion formation (Asherman's syndrome). If the cavity is entered, care should be exercised in the repair. The cavity

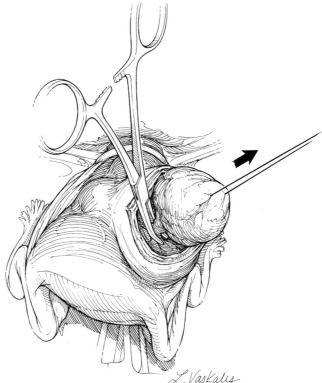

Fig. 31-11 As the base of the myoma is reached, the vascular pedicle is clamped, the myoma is extirpated, and the vascular pedicle is suture ligated. After the extirpation of the myoma shown in the figure, the remaining adjacent myomas can be reached by tunnelling dissection from the initial defect to avoid additional uteral incisions. The dead space from these distant myomectomies must be obliterated before the initial defect is closed, as depicted in Fig. 31-12. (From Pfeifer SM, Garcia CR: Myomectomy. In Nichols DH, editor: *Reoperative gynecologic and obstetric surgery*, ed 2, St Louis, 1997, Mosby.)

can be packed using ¼ inch Iodoform gauze packing (Fig. 31-14). The endometrial cavity must be approximated using a fine running stitch with 5-0 or 6-0 Vicryl, taking care to ensure that the suture is free from the packing. The pack can be removed vaginally some 72 hours postoperatively.

Special care must be taken when myomas impinge on the oviducts. The course of the oviduct may be distorted by the myoma. Unless care is exercised, the oviducts may be injured or occluded during removal and repair. The preoperative hysterosalpingography is useful in identifying variant anatomy. During surgery, a nylon stent of no. 1 monofilament nylon with a fine polished end may also be placed by way of the distal end of the tube to identify the oviduct by palpation during the resection. Microsurgical techniques are essential.

When a large myoma is removed, it is tempting to use the approach that Bonney described as the monk's cowl type of closure (Fig. 31-15). This approach should be reviewed as being of historical import. Such a repair is significantly anatomically unphysiologic in its context and should not be

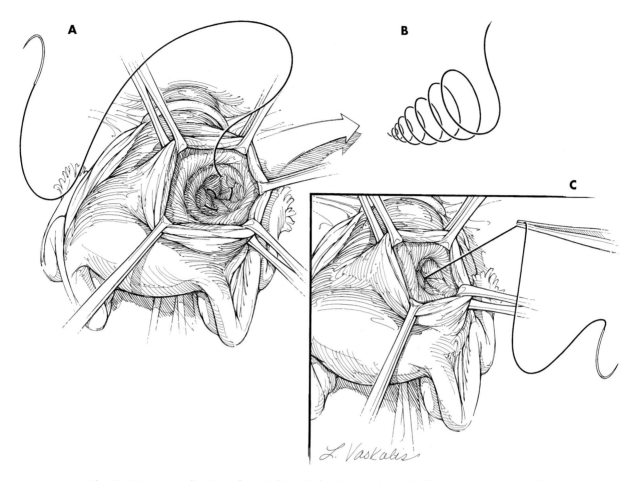

Fig. 31-12   **A,** Application of a spiraling stitch, shown schematically, closes the defect after the myoma has been removed. Initial placement of several deep spiraling stitches in layers. **B,** Schematic diagram of spiraling stitch. **C,** The spiraling stitch in the lower layer has been cinched with firm pressure with diamond-tip forceps. The spiraling stitch is then continued to successively obliterate the remaining defect. This spiraling stitch not only repairs the defect but also is hemostatic. (From Pfeifer SM, Garcia CR: Myomectomy. In Nichols DH, editor: *Reoperative gynecologic and obstetric surgery,* ed 2, St Louis, 1997, Mosby.)

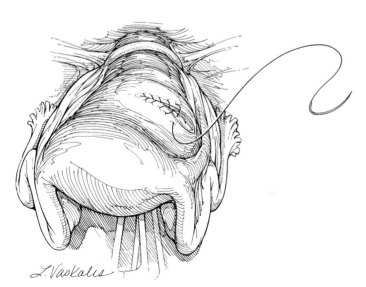

Fig. 31-13   The superficial closure of the myomectomy defect can be accomplished with a subserosal, a Lembert, or, as illustrated, a baseball stitch, using a 4-0 polyglactin suture. The baseball stitch allows for a smooth approximation of the wound edges and also is hemostatic. Antiadhesion coverings have not been necessary. (From Pfeifer SM, Garcia CR: Myomectomy. In Nichols DH, editor: *Reoperative gynecologic and obstetric surgery,* ed 2, St Louis, 1997, Mosby.)

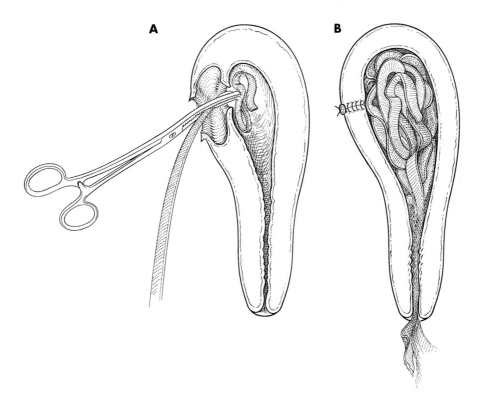

Fig. 31-14   **A-B,** Introduction of an intrauterine iodoform pack. This is done particularly when multiple entries to the cavity have occurred. Care must be exercised to prevent suturing the gauze in the closing of the defect.

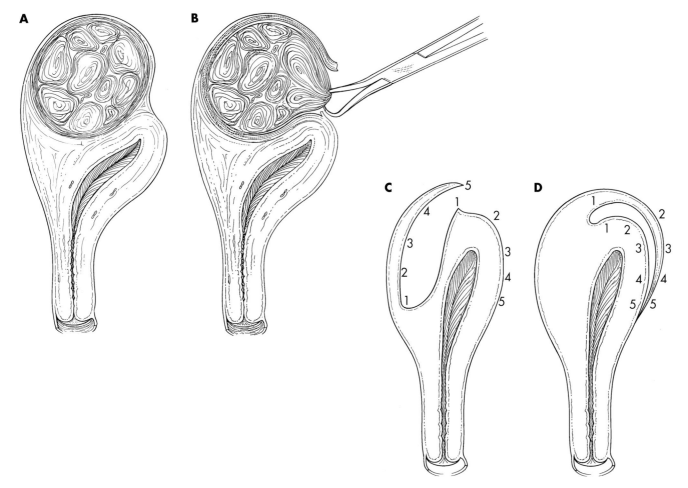

Fig. 31-15   **A-D,** Myomectomy. Repair of defect according to Bonney's monk's cowl technique.

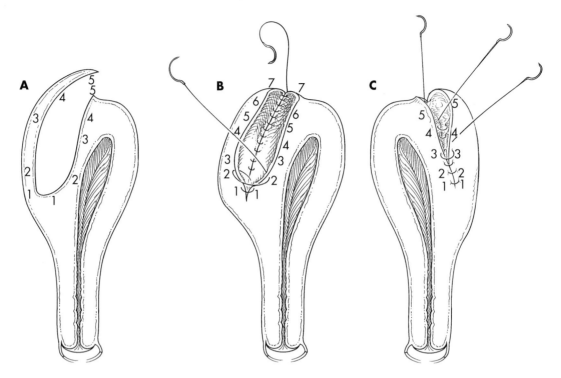

Fig. 31-16 **A-C,** Myomectomy cavity repair. Reconstruction of defect through repair approximating the anterior wall to the posterior wall in layers for a more anatomic reconstruction.

used. Reconstruction as outlined previously produces a more physiologic anatomic restoration (Fig. 31-16).

Myomas, even when multiple and of 10- to 14-cm diameter in size, do not, per se, dictate hysterectomy. Meticulous conservative uterine surgery allows extirpation and reconstruction of large myomas while preserving uterine function. With recurrent myomas, the technique of repeat myomectomy is similar to that described earlier when the myoma is initially dissected from the uterus.

Postoperatively, adhesion prophylaxis is recommended. Dexamethasone-promethazine solution, high-molecular-weight dextran solution, and Ringer's lactated solution have all, alone or in combination, been instilled in the abdominal cavity before closure as antiadhesion prophylaxis. Although Fayez and Schneider[27] have reported no significant difference among these techniques, the dexamethasone-promethazine regimen has the advantage of accelerating the patient's postoperative recovery period with few, if any, side effects when used in a short, low-dose protocol.* Early ambulation and resumption of perfunctory activities are associated with that approach.

Intercede and Gore-Tex have been advocated for prevention of adhesions. Much work has to be done before use of these materials can be recommended routinely. Adhesions can occur with Intercede unless meticulous hemostasis is at-

tained. A subsequent procedure is needed for removal of Gore-Tex. Prevention of adhesion formation or reformation is still best addressed by adhering to strict meticulous surgical principles. Constant irrigation using a dilute solution of heparinized saline (5000 U/L) is helpful to prevent clot formation, which potentially can be viewed as a step in adhesion formation.

Laparoscopic Myomectomy

Laparoscopic myomectomy is an appealing concept because major abdominal wall surgical trauma is avoided, which often permits the woman to resume her normal physical activities sooner—often 12 to 24 hours after the procedure. The laparoscopic approach may be well suited for small superficial or pedunculated myomas. However, limitations occur with larger myomas, especially in intramural locations. The larger the myoma, the more significant the problems that can be encountered with this technique. The integrity of the uterine scar is a significant concern. The laparoscopic suturing technique is crude when compared with the microsurgical technique of laparotomy. Accumulation of an intramural hematoma at the incision site and extensive use of thermal energy for hemostasis can lead to poor healing at the uterine incision site. Nezhat et al.[67] reported finding uterine indentation at all sites of laparoscopic removal of deep subserosal and intramural myomas. There is concern regarding the strength of the uterine wall for subsequent pregnancies. In fact, uterine rupture has been described during pregnancy after laparoscopic removal of deep and superficial subserosal myomas.[23,73] Laparoscopic suture to

---

*Low-dose protocol: 20 mg of dexamethasone and 25 mg of promethazine dissolved in 250 ml of normal saline instilled into the pelvis at the end of the procedure, followed by 12.5 mg of promethazine and 2 mg of dexamethasone every 4 hours for nine doses postoperatively.

close uterine defects is associated with significant adhesion formation.[67] Removing the myoma from the abdominal cavity after resection may require culdotomy or morselization techniques. Reported complications after laparoscopic myomectomy include extensive iatrogenic adenomyosis and uterine leiomyoma growing in an abdominal wall incision.[70,71] To overcome some of these difficulties Nezhat et al.[68] have proposed laparoscopically assisted myomectomy whereby myomas are identified and retracted to the abdominal wall where minilaparotomy is performed with closure of the uterus using conventional multilayer suturing.

Laparoscopic myomectomy offers many advantages but can be a difficult procedure with significant complications. The criteria for selecting women for this procedure have not been determined.

Laparoscopic myolysis has been advocated with the laparoscopic application of the neodymium:yttrium-aluminum-garnet (Nd:YAG) laser or the bipolar needle for coagulation of the blood supply of the myoma.[38,39] The intent is to cause atrophy and necrosis of the myoma by destroying its immediate blood supply. The most experienced advocate describes treating myomas up to 10 cm in diameter after GnRH pretreatment. The experience is based on 300 cases, but the complications are not fully detailed. The morbidity rate is said to be low. It is well known that necrosing myomas can and do produce pain, fever, and other symptoms and findings. Pyomyoma can also be expected, although it is rare.

Recently, cryomyolysis has been reported whereby myomas are frozen. The authors report a 10% mean volume decrease in the size of the fibroid after the procedure.[98] Further studies are warranted.

Vaginal Uterine Myomectomy and Hysteroscopic Approaches

Often, women with submucosal myomas have heavy vaginal bleeding (80% to 90%) and not necessarily an enlarging uterus. Previously, the abdominal approach was the only method available for removal of these myomas. Vaginal myomectomy was reserved only for pedunculated myomas protruding through the cervix. However, with the technical advances in hysteroscopy, selected submucous myomas are being resected vaginally.

Prolapsed submucous myomas are relatively rare, occurring in 2.5% of patients.[6] Patients have menorrhagia, anemia, and foul vaginal drainage. These myomas can be necrotic and infected, causing systemic signs of infection in up to 13% of patients.[6,40] On examination, they can often have the appearance of a malignancy. Rarely, the patient can have a complete uterine inversion caused by prolapsing of the myoma through the cervix.[45,82] The bladder and ureters are also exteriorized in this condition, and care is needed to avoid injury to these structures and to the uterine fundus during repair.[45] Vaginal myomectomy carries a lower morbidity rate than abdominal hysterectomy in these patients.[6,82] Prolapsed myomas are often attached to the cervical or endometrial cavity by a stalk. Removal of the tumors

involves ligating the stalk or twisting the stalk to remove the myoma. Alternatively, a tonsil snare can greatly facilitate removal.

Morselization, hysterectomy, vaginal hysterectomy, and Dührssen's incisions have been used for large myomas.[21] A less traumatic approach using laminaria to dilate the cervix has facilitated exposure and removal of the myoma.[40] Myomas ranging from 10 to 180 g have been removed using this technique. Success rates of 90% to 94% have been reported.[6,40] Unfortunately, early experiences with vaginal myomectomy have had some complications, including uterine perforation (1%), excessive bleeding requiring insertion of Foley catheter as a tamponade (0% to 5%), febrile morbidity (1% to 6%), and cervical laceration with subsequent cervical incompetence (5%). Prophylactic antibiotics should be used. It should be pointed out that the incidence of malignancy in these tumors is similar to that for other myomas and is reported to be as high as 2% to 3%.[40,82]

Hysteroscopic Resection of Intrauterine Myomas

Submucous myomas that are nonprolapsing, if small, can sometimes be removed by sharp curettage. However, hysteroscopic removal, first described by Norman et al. in 1957,[69] is now a preferable alternative to abdominal myomectomy for most submucous myomas. Hysteroscopic resection of myomas should be considered when there is definite evidence of submucous myomas proven by hysterosalpingogram, sonohysterography, hysteroscopy, or MRI. However, before resection endometrial assessment should be performed to rule out a neoplastic cause of bleeding. It is probably preferable to limit the use of hysteroscopic resection to myomas less than 4 cm, although larger myomas have been resected.[44] Sixty percent of the myoma should protrude into the endometrial cavity to allow safe resection with minimal bleeding and reduce the risk of uterine perforation. Resection of myomas at the same level on opposing walls should be avoided because the dissected areas can and do grow together, leading to intrauterine adhesions.

The technique with the operative hysteroscope or resectoscope involves shaving the protruding myoma to the level of the endometrium or, in the case of the laser, vaporizing out the myoma. Simultaneous laparoscopy has been advocated with removal of large myomas to avoid injury to the uterus. The fragments of myoma can be removed at the time of the operative hysteroscopy. Some leave the fragments within the cavity to be expelled with menses. More experience is needed to assess the various approaches. Complete resection of the myoma has not always been possible, and repeat hysteroscopic resection or definitive surgery has been required. The frequency with which this occurs has not always been reported. Some suggest the use of GnRH preoperatively with ablation of the endometrium and then resection of the submucous myomas. Neuwirth et al.[66] reported that, of 26 patients, 9 required further surgery after hysteroscopic resection of a myoma. Other small series have reported no need for further surgery. Although larger submucous myomas have been managed by repeated hysteroscopic resections on sequential procedures, not only is this approach fraught with risks but pregnancy rates and safety have yet to be assessed. Great care needs to be taken that appropriate counseling be given before a woman who desires to preserve reproductive function selects these approaches.

Hysteroscopic resection of submucosal myoma can be accomplished using the resectoscope at a power of 60 W cutting current.[88] The preference for laser applications has been the Nd:YAG laser at a power of 80 W.[22] The CO_2 laser can only be used with a CO_2 distending medium. Gas-cooled fiber tips should never be used because several deaths have been attributed to gas embolism.[2]

Maintenance of adequate uterine distention and clarity of view call for the use of a pump such as the electric Nezhat or the N_2 driven Davol disposable pump. When glycine is used as the distending medium, visualization of the cavity is good. However, hyponatremia has been reported with glycine.[95] Hyskon also allows a clear view of the uterine cavity because the pressure controls the bleeding that is present. However, high-molecular-weight dextran has been associated with pulmonary edema and disseminated intravascular coagulation defects. These side effects are related to the length of the procedure and the volume of the distention medium used.

Donnez et al.[22] described a technique for resection of myomas whose largest portion was located in the uterine wall.[32] They treated the patient preoperatively with GnRH agonist. An Nd:YAG laser was then used to resect the myoma hysteroscopically. The remaining portion of the myoma was drilled with the laser to destroy the vascularity. After an additional 8 weeks of GnRH analog therapy, repeat hysteroscopy revealed the residual portion of the myoma protruding, which could be readily resected. These authors reported 100% success and no complications. Most submucous resectionists advocate the preoperative use of GnRH agonist therapy for submucous myomas because the size of the myoma is reduced by an average of 38%.[22] Moreover, the uterine myometrium is made atrophic and the vascularity is also reduced. However, severe intractable hemorrhage has been reported when GnRH agonist therapy is used for submucous myomas.[32]

Endometrial ablation has also been used for treatment of hypermenorrhea and polymenorrhea.[7,46] This approach has been used in place of myomectomy or as an aid to reduce bleeding in the associated resection of myomas. Endometrial ablation is accomplished by using the rollerball[7] followed by the use of the resectoscope[20,49] or the laser.[19,41,57,58] Concerns about using the endometrial ablation procedure include burying a nidus of endometrium. Reports of hematometra have been described after endometrial ablation[41] and support a concern about widespread use of endometrial ablation without stringent indications. Longer-term follow-up is needed. We still do not know the extent of the problem secondary to burying endometrial nidi.

Uterine Artery Embolization

Several studies have evaluated the success of bilateral uterine artery embolization predominantly for treatment of menometrorrhagia or mass syndrome attributed to fibroids.[10,77] In the largest study by Ravina et al.,[78] 80 patients were available for analysis. The treatment of 9 patients failed. Menstrual periods returned to normal in 60 of 67 (89%) patients with menorrhagia. Pelvic pain requiring analgesia was observed, lasting 12 to 18 hours. The effect of this procedure on subsequent pregnancy has yet to be investigated, and therefore it should not be recommended for patients who desire preservation of childbearing potential.

MYOMECTOMY AND PREGNANCY

The incidence of myomas during pregnancy has been cited by Phelan[75] to range from 0.09% to 3.9%. Until recently, myomas during pregnancy were believed to enlarge secondary to endogenous hormonal tropism. More recently this has been challenged* because some 80% of uterine myomas followed by ultrasonography during pregnancy were unaltered or decreased in size.

The impact of myomas during pregnancy depends on the location and extent of the myoma. Complications of myomas arising during pregnancy include pain as a result of degeneration of the myoma or torsion of a pedunculated myoma. Other problems include pregnancy loss, premature labor, abruption, growth restriction, malpresentation, and sepsis. Myomas in the lower uterine segment increase the likelihood of malpresentation, cesarean section, and postpartum hemorrhage. In early pregnancy compression can be related to urinary retention. Other complications are radiculopathy and fetal deformities.

Degeneration of myomas during pregnancy occurs rarely—in 5% to 8% of patients. The cause is unclear, but such myomas can be symptomatic. Indeed, in some instances they can be severely painful and tender with leukocytosis, and they can initiate premature labor requiring tocolytic therapy. The use of ultrasonography[56] and/or MRI[17] of these painful myomas discloses characteristic cystic spaces in these tumors and decreases the need for diagnostic exploratory surgery in these women. Medical management with analgesics, such as acetaminophen, nonsteroidal antiinflammatory medication (before 34 weeks' gestation) and narcotics, as well as bed rest and tocolytic therapy, is usually successful.

Myomectomy has been advocated by some for the relief of pain in those women who do not respond to supportive medical management. The surgery is not without risk. Indeed, when at all possible it is probably better to treat the compelling complication medically. The problematic myoma(s) can then be addressed more reasonably after the pregnancy as an interim procedure before another pregnancy. There are a few, albeit small, studies reporting on myomectomy during pregnancy. Although Glavind et al.[36] describe no surgical complications, they did indicate that in 2 of 11 women, pregnancies were terminated as abortions after myomectomy. Burton et al.[12] reported 6 antepartum myomectomies. All of the myomas were of the pedunculated va-

---

*References 1, 35, 56, 64, 67, 76.

riety with stalk size of 2 to 5 cm. All pregnancies progressed to term. Exacoustos and Rosari[25] performed 13 myomectomies before 26 weeks' gestation for subserous or pedunculated myomas. Five of these women delivered prematurely between 32 weeks and term. No neonatal deaths occurred. Pelosi et al.[72] reported on a laparoscopic myomectomy performed in the second trimester of pregnancy for a symptomatic pedunculated 1500-g fibroid.

Although the complications reported appear minimal, selection of patients is paramount. There are no controlled studies to evaluate antepartum myomectomy. It is generally held that myomectomy during pregnancy should be limited to symptomatic pedunculated myomas with stalks of less than 5 cm.

Concerns have been raised regarding the advisability of myomectomy at the time of cesarean section. As with resection of myoma during pregnancy, resection at cesarean section often leads to severe bleeding, which may not easily be controlled and may lead to hysterectomy. Obviously, a small myoma in the incisional area may need to be resected with care to ensure hemostasis. Burton et al.[12] reported on 13 women who had incidental removal of myomas from submucosal, intramural, or subserosal locations. In 9 of these women the myomas were asymptomatic, but 1 of the cases was complicated by hemorrhage.

Myomectomy Complications

Blood Loss. Anemia is the most common complication after myomectomy. Strict adherence to a meticulous hemostatic technique as described previously is essential to avoid this. Preoperative fluid loading helps increase intravascular volume and promote hemodilution. Preoperatively, iron replacement and diet can be used to maximize hemoglobin for an anemic patient. *Transfusions should be used only when the need is urgent.* Transfusions should not be given to the patient merely because she stored her own blood. This should be made clear to the patient before donation.

Hematoma Formation. Seroma and hematoma formation can occur postoperatively. Meticulous closure of the defects in the myometrium avoids this. Patients may develop pain or fever when seromas or hematomas occur. MRI and ultrasound are useful in making the diagnosis. Management involves conservative and supportive therapy and antibiotics. Surgical intervention is rarely necessary and preferably avoided.

Hysteroscopic Complications. Complications of a hysteroscopic resection include hemorrhage and uterine perforation. The true incidence is not available because there are no well-controlled studies and complications with these clinical experiences occur sporadically. Concomitant use of laparoscopy is advocated to minimize the risk of uterine perforation. It is apparent that the incidence decreases with experience but is lowest with those who are cautious. Hyponatremia and other electrolyte problems require careful vigilance with time and volume control.

Myoma Recurrence after Myomectomy. The recurrence rate of myomas after myomectomy is reported to be 5% to 30%.[14] Fedele et al.[28] found a 27% cumulative 10-year recurrence among 622 patients who underwent myomectomy between 1970 and 1984 at the University of Milan. More recently Fedele et al.[29] reported a 50% recurrence of myoma within 5 years after myomectomy with ultrasound monitoring. García reported a 15% recurrence rate in 200 patients (unpublished data presented at the October, 1988, meeting of the International Federation of Gynecology and Obstetrics). The recurrence rate reported depends on the skill and care of the surgeon in removing all of the myomas detected at the time of the initial surgery. As discussed later in this chapter, the recurrence rate is higher in patients treated preoperatively with GnRH agonists. If these small, seemingly insignificant myomas are ignored, they may develop into significant myomas.

Leiomyosarcoma

Leiomyosarcoma has been found in 0.1% to 0.7% of uterine myomas.[13,54] Occasionally, this diagnosis can be made preoperatively by D&C.[67] However, most leiomyosarcomas may not be diagnosed until the intraoperative or postoperative period. Leiomyosarcoma is found more often in solitary myomas and in tumors showing rapid growth, necrosis, hemorrhagic areas, and poor demarcation. The diagnosis is confirmed only after microscopic evaluation of the tissue sections reveals more than 10 mitoses per 10 high-powered field.[94]

Malignant transformation similar to leiomyosarcoma occurs in 0.1% to 0.7% of patients undergoing myomectomy.[13,54] This is most often associated with increased age of the patient, abnormal uterine bleeding, rapid growth, and especially with solitary tumors.

Pregnancy after Myomectomy

Appropriately performed myomectomy should improve the probability of pregnancy in those who would otherwise be fertile. Nonetheless, myomas can occasionally be resected from areas that may contribute to difficulties in either gamete tubal transport or implantation. With the techniques detailed previously, fertility appears enhanced or restored.

Generally speaking, there is less need for delay of attempted conception because the risk of potential immediate pregnancy is less after myomectomy than after other infertility procedures. By the time the earliest pregnancy occurs, which is no sooner than 2 to 3 months after surgery and more often 6 months to 1 year, these patients experience no difficulty in safely bringing the pregnancy to term.

The mode of obstetric delivery is important. Cesarean section is advocated especially when intramural, submucosal, and large subserosal myomas have been removed. Small subserosal and some hysteroscopically removed submucosal myomas are not thought to present a contraindication to the trial of labor.

CONTROVERSIAL ISSUES

Despite the lack of approval by the FDA for the use of GnRH analogs in the management of myomas, they have been used extensively for this purpose. These medications are synthetic peptide analogs of GnRH. Their effect is to downregulate the pituitary gland, thereby creating a hypoestrogenic or menopausal state. Although the effects are believed to be reversed after discontinuing the medication, this is not universally the case.

Treatment with the GnRH agonists for 6 months has resulted in a shrinkage of the volume of myomas by 20% and shrinkage of total uterine volume in the range of 35% to 50%.[61,85,86] Initially, this was thought to be a significant advantage of this approach. However, several observations have been reported that may temper the initial enthusiasm for this therapy. First, the reduction in uterine volume has been shown to be greater than the reduction in myoma volume, 42.7% versus 30.4%, respectively, after 6 months of treatments.[85] This difference is explained by the fact that the GnRH agonist causes shrinkage of myometrial cells but not fibrous or interstitial elements, which can make up a significant proportion of the myoma. Response of myomas to GnRH agonist therapy may also vary with the karyotype, with myomas exhibiting an abnormal karyotype being less responsive to GnRH agonists than those with normal karyotype.[11] Second, the reduction in size is transient. Myomas and uteri have been shown to return to pretreatment size within 4 months of completing the medication. Third, the return of ovarian function may be delayed.

Furthermore, the volume reduction observed can be misleading. Because the formula for calculating volume of a sphere or of a spheroid involves the cube of the radius, the reduction in volume in large myomas represents proportionately only a small reduction in the diameter. The volume reduction of 4% in a 10-cm myoma represents a 1.7-cm reduction in diameter. However, a similar percentage reduction in volume of a small myoma represents a greater proportionate reduction in diameter. Thus the effect of the GnRH agonist ovarian suppression on small seedlings is more significant because they may be reduced to an undetectable size, thereby making removal at time of myomectomy impossible. This has been proposed as the reason for the higher recurrence rates seen in postmyomectomy patients pretreated with GnRH agonists compared with those who had no treatment. Fedele et al.,[28] in a careful prospective well-designed study, reported a 63% recurrence rate in patients treated preoperatively with GnRH agonists versus 13% recurrence rate in those not treated. Meticulous resection of all myomas without a menopausal state of estrogen suppression should provide a better long-term cure rate. Another advantage ascribed to the use of GnRH agonists has been a reported decrease in intraoperative myomectomy blood loss.[31] However, more recent reports have not supported this conclusion.[28]

The most significant problem with the use of GnRH agonists has been their side effects. A 2% to 6% decrease in bone mineral density has been observed after the 6-month course.[50] The mean values approach normal in most patients 6 months after treatment. There is concern for those women who do not have a return to normal bone mineral content levels. It has been advocated that the addition of estrogen

and progestin as add-back therapy to the GnRH agonist can prevent the bone mineral content loss.[33] However, at the clinical seminar and workshop on the use of bisphosphonates presented during the 1995 Annual Meeting of the American Society of Reproductive Medicine, Dr. Charles H. Chestnut and Uwe Ultich reported that even at 3 months of GnRH agonist therapy, despite concomitant add-back therapy, biopsies of cancellous bone disclosed microfractures on scanning electron microscopy. Such degenerative changes are not reversible. The use of alendronate therapy, which appears to be protective, along with calcium was suggested. Other effects include hot flashes (70% to 100%), vaginal dryness (30% to 60%), and effects on lipids.[35,37,55,61,85] Because of these effects, those who use GnRH agonists should limit the course to a maximum of 6 months. The use of repeated courses of GnRH agonists for reduction of uterine volume is not an acceptable approach. "Add-on" progesterone therapies may or may not be acceptable and need more careful evaluation of efficacy and safety.

For these reasons, preoperative treatment with GnRH agonists has become a less favored alternative. However, pretreatment with GnRH agonists appears to have a significant benefit in facilitating vaginal hysterectomy in those patients who would otherwise have required abdominal hysterectomy. Myomatous uteri the size of 14 to 18 weeks' gestation have been successfully removed vaginally after pretreatment with GnRH agonists.[18] Of course, morselization could be used in those cases in which previously GnRH agonists had been used and the potential problems of GnRH therapy can be avoided.

In a woman who had previously undergone myomectomy and has a recurrent symptomatic myomatous uterus, the decision must be made to proceed with repeat myomectomy versus hysterectomy. The chance of successfully achieving pregnancy may be less favorable than with primary myomectomy. Although complications of myomectomy are uncommon, the overall risk is probably greater than that for hysterectomy. However, the effect of hysterectomy on the specific woman is difficult to quantify. Using a nondirective approach, one can usually guide the 40- to 45-year-old woman away from myomectomy. Supracervical hysterectomy is a reasonable alternative especially because preservation of the cervix is an acceptable alternative in those who feel strongly about preserving their organs from a sexuality standpoint. Pap smear and colposcopy have allowed for preservation of the healthy cervix with reasonable risk.

CONCLUSIONS

Myomectomy can be a difficult and often time-consuming procedure. However, with meticulous attention to technique, the procedure can be accomplished safely and effectively with relatively assured hemostasis. Myomectomy affords the option of preserving the uterus for patients with symptomatic uterine myomas who desire to preserve their reproductive organs. However, careful assessment of the patient and counseling are essential. At this time, it is difficult to compare the advantages of the various approaches to the management of uterine myoma. Assessment of the management by the alternative approaches through minimally invasive techniques still leaves many questions about the risks and true advantages of the so-called day surgery approaches. Reports of the degree of incapacitation of the patient after the procedures are biased because they do not consider the competence of the surgeon. Patients having abdominal surgery, when appropriately screened, can and have gone home in 48 hours or less. The advantages claimed by the use of minimally invasive approaches are indeed very attractive. However, information about the selection of subjects, the problems encountered, and the complications, as well as the assessment of not only the short-term but also the long-term outcomes, still is not easily assessible. The attractiveness of minimally invasive approaches, as presented by their enthusiasts, is so beguiling, when they are uncomplicated, that this euphoric aura tends to override the serious concerns that have been raised. Until better comparisons, preferably randomized studies and under strict oversight conditions, are available, surgeons will continue to assume the responsibility for selecting the therapeutic modality for their patients based on their own clinical appraisal of which approach is best suited for the level of the patient's pathologic condition and the surgeon's own assessment of personal competence.

Since cure without deformity or loss of function must ever be surgery's highest ideal, the general proposition that myomectomy is a greater surgical achievement than hysterectomy is incontestable.[8]

Victor Bonney

REFERENCES

1. Aharoni A, et al: Patterns of growth of uterine leiomyomas during pregnancy: a longitudinal study, *Br J Obstet Gynaecol,* 95:510, 1988.
2. Baggish MS, Daniell JF: Catastrophic injury secondary to the use of coaxial gas-cooled fibers and artificial sapphire tips for intrauterine surgery: a report of five cases, *Lasers Surg Med* 9:581, 1989.
3. Bakaknia A, Rock JA, Jones HW Jr: Pregnancy success following abdominal myomectomy for infertility, *Fertil Steril* 30:644, 1978.
4. Barter JF, Izpak C, Creasman WT: Uterine leiomyomas with retroperitoneal lymph node involvement, *South Med J* 80:1320, 1987.
5. Beamis ELG, et al: Ovarian functions after hysterectomy with conservation of the ovaries in premenopausal women, *J Obstet Gynecol Br Commonw* 76:969, 1969.
6. Ben-Baruch G, et al: Immediate and late outcome of vaginal myomectomy for prolapsed pedunculated submucous myoma, *Obstet Gynecol* 72:858, 1988.
7. Bent AE, Ostergaard DR: Endometrial ablation with the neodymium:YAG laser, *Obstet Gynecol* 75:923, 1990.
8. Bonney V: The technique and result of myomectomy, *Lancet* Jan 24, 1931, p 171.
9. Bonney V: *A textbook of gynaecological surgery,* ed 6, New York, 1953, Hoebel.
10. Bradley EA, et al: Transcatheter uterine artery immobilization to treat large uterine fibroids, *Br J Obstet Gynecol* 105:235, 1998.
11. Brosens I, et al: Clinical significance of cytogenetic abnormalities in uterine myomas, *Fertil Steril* 69:232, 1998.
12. Burton CA, et al: Surgical management of leiomyomata during pregnancy, *Obstet Gynecol* 74:707, 1989.
13. Buttram VC Jr: Uterine leiomyomata—etiology, symptomatology and management. In *Gonadotropin down-regulation in gynecological practice,* New York, 1986, Alan R Liss.
14. Buttram VC Jr, Reiter RC: Uterine leiomyomata: etiology, symptomatology and management, *Fertil Steril* 36:433, 1981.
15. Candiani GB, et al: Risk of recurrence after myomectomy, *Br J Obstet Gynecol* 98:385, 1991.
16. Centerwall BS: Premenopausal hysterectomy and cardiovascular disease, *Am J Obstet Gynecol* 139:58, 1981.
17. Curtis M, et al: Magnetic resonance imaging to avoid laparotomy in pregnancy, *Obstet Gynecol* 82:833, 1993.
18. Damewood MD, Rock JA: Reproductive uterine surgery, *Obstet Gynecol Clin North Am* 14:1049, 1987.
19. Davis JA: Hysteroscopic endometrial ablation with the neodymium YAG laser, *Br J Obstet Gynaecol* 96:928, 1989.
20. DeCherney AH, et al: Endometrial ablation for intractable uterine bleeding: hysteroscopic resection, *Obstet Gynecol* 70:668, 1987.
21. Dicker D, et al: The management of prolapsed submucous fibroids, *Aust NZ J Obstet Gynaecol* 26:308, 1986.
22. Donnez J, et al: Neodymium:YAG laser hysteroscopy in large submucous fibroids, *Fertil Steril* 54:999, 1990.
23. Dubuisson JB, et al: Uterine rupture during pregnancy after laparoscopic myomectomy, *Human Reprod* 10:1475, 1995.
24. Dudiak CM, et al: Uterine leiomyomas in the infertile patient: preoperative localization with MR imaging versus US and hysterosalpingography, *Radiology* 167:627, 1988.
25. Exacoustos C, Rosati P: Ultrasound diagnosis of uterine myomas and complications in pregnancy, *Obstet Gynecol* 82:197, 1993.
26. Fan SX, et al: Cytogenetic findings in nine leiomyomas of the uterus, *Cancer Genet Cytogenet* 47:179, 1990.
27. Fayez JA, Schneider PJ: Prevention of pelvic adhesions formation by different modalities of treatment, *Am J Obstet Gynecol* 157:1184, 1987.
28. Fedele L, et al: Treatment of GnRH agonists before myomectomy and the risk of short-term myoma recurrence, *Br J Obstet Gynecol* 97:393, 1990.
29. Fedele L, et al: Risk of recurrence after myomectomy, *Br J Obstet Gynaecol* 95:385, 1991.
30. Ford JM, et al: Metastasizing leiomyoma of the uterus, *Aust NZ J Obstet Gynaecol* 28:154, 1988.
31. Friedman AJ, et al: A randomized placebo-controlled, double-blind study evaluating the efficacy of leuprolide acetate depot in the treatment of uterine leiomyomata, *Fertil Steril* 51:251, 1989.
32. Friedman AJ: Vaginal hemorrhage associated with degenerating submucous leiomyomata during leuprolide acetate treatment, *Fertil Steril* 52:152, 1989.
33. Friedman AJ, et al: Treatment of leiomyomata uteri with leuprolide acetate depot in a double-blind placebo controlled multicentered study: The Leuprolide Study Group, *Obstet Gynecol* 77:720, 1991.
34. García C-R, Tureck RW: Submucosal leiomyomas and infertility, *Fertil Steril* 42:16, 1984.
35. George M, et al: Long-term use of LH-RH agonist in the management of uterine leiomyomas: a study of 17 cases, *Int J Fertil* 34:19, 1989.
36. Glavind K, et al: Uterine myoma in pregnancy, *Acta Obstet Gynecol Scand* 69:617, 1990.
37. Golan A, et al: D-Trp-6 luteinizing hormone-releasing hormone microcapsules in the treatment of uterine leiomyomas, *Fertil Steril* 52:406, 1989.
38. Goldfarb HA: Bipolar laparoscopic needles for myoma coagulation, *J Am Assoc Gynecol Laparoscopists* 2:175, 1995.
39. Goldfarb HA: Laparoscopic coagulation of myoma (myolysis), *Obstet Gynecol Clin North Am* 22(4):807, 1995.
40. Goldrath MH: Vaginal removal of the pedunculated submucous myoma: historical observations and development of a new procedure, *J Reprod Med* 35:921, 1990.
41. Goldrath MH, Fuller TGA, Segal S: Laser photovaporization of endometrium for the treatment of menorrhagia, *Am J Obstet Gynecol* 140:14, 1981.

42. Greenspoon JS, et al: Pyomyoma associated with polymicrobial bacteremia and fatal septic shock: case report and review of the literature, *Obstet Gynecol Surv* 45:563, 1990.

43. Gross BH, Silver TM, Jaffe MH: Sonographic features of uterine leiomyomas: analysis of 41 proven cases, *J Ultrasound Med* 2:401, 1983.

44. Hallez JP, Perino A: Endoscopic intrauterine resection: principles and technique, *Acta Eur Fertil* 19:17, 1988.

45. Henderson PR: A large submucous fibroid polyp causing inversion of the uterus, *Aust NZ J Obstet Gynaecol* 20:251, 1980.

46. Hill D, Maher P: Treatment of menorrhagia by endometrial ablation, *Med J Aust* 152:564, 1990.

47. Hofmann GE, et al: Binding sites for epidermal growth factor in human uterine tissues and leiomyomas, *J Clin Endocrinol Metab* 58:880, 1984.

48. Honore LH: Parauterine leiomyomas in women: a clinicopathologic study of 22 cases, *Eur J Obstet Gynecol Reprod Biol* 11:273, 1981.

49. Indman PD, Sodentrom RM: Depth of endometrial coagulation with the urologic resectoscope, *J Reprod Med* 35:633, 1990.

50. Johanse JS, et al: The effect of a gonadotropin-releasing hormone agonist analog (Nafarelin) on bone metabolism, *J Clin Endocrinol Metab* 67:701, 1988.

51. Jonas HS, Masterson BJ: Giant uterine tumor: case report and review of the literature, *Obstet Gynecol* 50(suppl):2S, 1977.

52. Kulenthran A, Sivanesaratnam V: Recurrent uterine myomata in three sisters—an uncommon occurrence, *Int J Gynecol Obstet* 27:289, 1988.

53. Lackritz EM, et al: Estimated risk of transmission of the immunodeficiency virus by screened blood in the United States, *N Engl J Med* 333:1721, 1995.

54. Leibsohn S, et al: Leiomyosarcoma in a series of hysterectomies performed for presumed uterine leiomyomas, *Am J Obstet Gynecol* 4:968, 1990.

55. Letterie GS, et al: Efficacy of a gonadotropin-releasing hormone agonist in the treatment of uterine leiomyomata: long-term follow-up, *Fertil Steril* 51:951, 1989.

56. Lev-Toaff AS, et al: Leiomyomas in pregnancy: sonographic study, *Radiology* 164:375, 1987.

57. Loffler FD: Laser ablation of the endometrium, *Obstet Gynecol Clin North Am* 15:77, 1988.

58. Lomano JM: Dragging technique versus blanching technique for endometrial ablation with the Nd:YAG laser in the treatment of chronic menorrhagia, *Am J Obstet Gynecol* 159:152, 1988.

59. Mark J, et al: Cytogenetical observations in human benign leiomyomas, *Anticancer Res* 8:621, 1988.

60. Matamala MF, et al: Leiomyomas of the ovary, *Int J Gynecol Pathol* 7:190, 1988.

61. Matta WHM, Shaw RW, Nye M: Long-term follow-up of patients with uterine fibroids after treatment with the LHRH agonist buserelin, *Br J Obstet Gynecol* 96:200, 1989.

62. Mayer DP, Shiplov V: Ultrasonography and magnetic resonance imaging, *Obstet Gynecol Clin North Am* 22:667, 1995.

63. McLaughlin DS: Metroplasty and myomectomy with the CO_2 laser for maximizing the preservation of normal tissue and minimizing bone loss, *J Reprod Med* 30:1, 1985.

64. Muram D, et al: Myomas of the uterus in pregnancy: ultrasonographic follow-up, *Am J Obstet Gynecol* 138:16, 1980.

65. Nelson WO: Endometrial and myometrial changes, including fibromyomatous nodules, induced in the uterus of the guinea pig by the prolonged administration of oestrogenic hormone, *Anat Rec* 68:99, 1937.

66. Neuwirth RS: Hysteroscopic management of symptomatic submucous fibroids, *Obstet Gynecol* 62:509, 1983.

67. Nezhat C, et al: Laparoscopic myomectomy, *Int J Fertil* 36:175, 1991.

68. Nezhat C, et al: Laparoscopically assisted myomectomy, a report of a new technique in 57 cases, *Int J Fertil* 39:39, 1994.

69. Norman WB, et al: Hysteroscopy, *Surg Clin North Am* 37:1377, 1957.

70. Ostrzenshi A: Uterine leiomyoma particle growing in an abdominal wall incision after laparoscopic retrieval, *Obstet Gynecol* 89:853, 1997.

71. Ostrzenshi A: Extensive iatrogenic adenomyosis after laparoscopic myomectomy, *Fertil Steril* 69:143, 1998.

72. Pelosi MA, et al: Laparoscopic removal of a 1500-g symptomatic myoma during the second trimester of pregnancy, *J Am Assoc Gynec Laparosc* 2:457, 1995.

73. Pelosi MA, et al: Spontaneous uterine rupture at thirty-three weeks subsequent to previous superficial laparoscopic myomectomy, *Am J Obstet Gynecol* 177:1547, 1997.

74. Penner M, et al: Benefits and risks of autologous blood donation, *Infusionther Transfus Med* 21:64, 1994.

75. Phelan JP: Myomas and pregnancy, *Obstet Gynecol Clin North Am* 22:801, 1995.

76. Puukka MJ, et al: Oestrogen receptors in human myoma tissue, *Mol Cell Endocrinol* 6:35, 1976.

77. Ravina JH, et al: Arterial embolization to treat uterine myomata, *Lancet* 346:671, 1995.

78. Ravina JH, et al: Recourse to particular arterial embolization in the treatment of some uterine leiomyoma (in French), *Bull Acad Nat Med* 181:233, 1997.

79. Reich H: Laparoscopic myomectomy, *Obstet Gynecol Clin North Am* 22:757, 1995.

80. Rein MS, et al: Cytogenetic abnormalities in uterine leiomyomata, *Obstet Gynecol* 77:923, 1991.

81. Reyniak JV, Corenthal L: Microsurgical laser technique for abdominal myomectomy, *Microsurgery* 8:92, 1987.

82. Riley P: Treatment of prolapsed submucous fibroids, *South Am Med J* 62:22, 1982.

83. Rosenfeld DL: Abdominal myomectomy for otherwise unexplained infertility, *Fertil Steril* 46:328, 1986.

84. Rubin I: Progress in myomectomy: surgical measures and diagnostic aids favoring lower morbidity and mortality, *Am J Obstet Gynecol* 44:196, 1942.

85. Schlaff WD, et al: A placebo-controlled list of a depot gonadotropin-releasing hormone analogue (leuprolide) in the treatment of uterine leiomyomata, *Obstet Gynecol* 74:856, 1989.

86. Shaw RW: Mechanism of LHRH analogue action in uterine fibroids, *Horm Res* 32(suppl 1):150, 1989.

87. Siddle N, Sarrel P, Whitehead M: The effect of hysterectomy on the age of ovarian failure, *Fertil Steril* 47:94, 1987.

88. Siegler AM: Therapeutic hysteroscopy, *Acta Eur Fertil* 17:467, 1986.

89. Singhabhandhu B, et al: Giant leiomyoma of the uterus: report of a case and review of the literature, *Am Surg* 39:391, 1973.

90. Sloand EM, et al: Safety of the blood supply, *JAMA* 274:1368, 1995.

91. Soules KMR, McCarty KS Jr: Leiomyomas: steroid receptor content: variation within normal menstrual cycles, *Am J Obstet Gynecol* 143:6, 1982.

92. Stovall TG, et al: A randomized trial evaluating leuprolide acetate before hysterectomy as treatment for leiomyomas, *Am J Obstet Gynecol* 164:1420.

93. Tamaya T, Fujimoto J, Okada H: Comparison of cellular levels in steroid receptors in uterine leiomyoma and myometrium, *Acta Obstet Gynecol Scand* 64:307, 1985.

94. Townsend DE, et al: Unicellular histogenesis of uterine leiomyomas as determined by electrophoresis of glucose-6-phosphate dehydrogenase, *Am J Obstet Gynecol* 107:1168, 1970.

95. Van Bove MJ, et al: Dilutional hyponatremia associated with intrauterine endoscopic laser surgery, *Anesthesiology* 71:449, 1989.

96. Wilson EA, Yang F, Rees ED: Estradiol and progesterone binding in uterine leiomyomata and in normal uterine tissues, *Obstet Gynecol* 55:20, 1980.

97. Wong TC, Bard DS, Pearce LW: Unusual case of IUD-associated post-abortal sepsis complicated by an infected necrotic leiomyoma, suppurative pelvic thrombophlebitis, ovarian vein thrombosis, hematoperitoneum and drug fever, *J Ark Med Soc* 83:138, 1986.

98. Zreik TG, et al: Cryomyolysis, a new procedure for the conservative treatment of uterine fibroids, *J Am Assoc Gynecol Laparosc* 5:33, 1998.

32 Presacral Neurectomy

JOHN F. STEEGE

Central pelvic pain that is associated with intercourse, worsens during menstruation, and is present during other times of the menstrual month is caused most often by endometriosis. Although medical therapies such as non-steroidal antiinflammatory drugs (NSAIDs), oral contraceptives, progestational agents, and gonadotropin-releasing hormone analogs control pain in most patients, approximately 20% of patients do not obtain sufficient relief or else have substantial side effects. Hysterectomy, usually with removal of both ovaries, relieves the pain in these cases, but alternatives are needed when preservation of the uterus is desired. Several types of neuroablative procedures have been designed for this situation, the most commonly performed of which is presacral neurectomy.

INDICATIONS

The most common indication for presacral neurectomy is central pelvic endometriosis refractory to medical therapy.[24] On occasion, presacral neurectomy also may be used to treat primary dysmenorrhea that does not respond to intensive medical treatment. Neuroanatomical relationships suggest that sources of pain treated by this procedure are limited to the uterus and the immediately adjacent uterosacral ligaments, posterior and anterior cul-de-sacs, and proximal fallopian tubes and round ligaments.

CONTRAINDICATIONS

Physical instability of the patient should preclude the performance of this elective procedure. Perhaps more important, unrealistic expectations for relief of adjacent but perhaps unrelated complaints should be a major concern for the clinician. Since presacral neurectomy may impair the motility of the colon and the bladder,[4,23] patients with severe refractory constipation or any past history of urinary retention should be carefully evaluated and counseled. In patients with chronic pelvic pain, the clinician should consider the potentially addictive, anticholinergic effects of antidepressants commonly used to treat chronic pain.

Although most patients who are candidates for this procedure can be approached laparoscopically, those with extensive prior abdominal surgery (especially involving massive adhesions or bowel obstruction) and patients who are obese are more likely to require laparotomy.

HISTORY OF PRESACRAL NEURECTOMY

Presacral neurectomy was first introduced by Jaboulay[19] and Ruggi[30] in 1899 but was received with significant skepticism. Cotte[7] began performing the procedure in the early 1920s and over the next 15 years performed over 1500 procedures. He reported a greater than 98% success rate in relieving the pain of dysmenorrhea and did not report any significant complications with bladder, bowel, or sexual function.

Other authors such as Pfanneuf and Meigs[23] used the procedure less frequently, performing about three to eight procedures per year in their extensive referral practices. These authors observed problems of constipation and urinary retention in some patients but again did not apparently rigorously inquire about sexual changes.

Black[2] in 1964 reported the results of his own personal series as well as the results of approximately 10,000 procedures queried by questionnaire from practitioners around the United States. This report and others[10] consisted of open clinical trials predominantly involving women with dysmenorrhea, as well as some with pelvic endometriosis. The approach fell out of favor after the introduction of oral contraceptives in the mid-1960s and NSAIDs in the early 1970s. These agents appeared to control severe dysmenorrhea in many women who previously would have been considered candidates for neuroablative procedures.

The introduction of more aggressive techniques for treating endometriosis in the 1970s (e.g., Danocrine) and the introduction of gonadotropin-releasing oral agonists in the 1980s have relegated neuroablative procedures to a smaller group of patients.

Further open uncontrolled trials[16,22,27] suggested that the inclusion of presacral neurectomy with conservative resection procedures for endometriosis provided additional pain relief. This hypothesis was finally subjected to controlled trials in the late 1980s.[4,33]

EFFICACY

With the exception of Cotte's unusually optimistic report,[8] the majority of the literature suggests that primary dysmenorrhea can be relieved in approximately 85% of cases, with secondary dysmenorrhea relieved in 67% to 75%.[2] Two controlled trials compared the additive benefit of presacral neurectomy with that achieved by conservative resection of endometriosis in women with stage III and stage IV disease. Tjaden[33] randomized eight women to conservative resection by laparotomy, with or without the addition of presacral neurectomy. Of this initial group, the four women who were treated with presacral neurectomy obtained good pain relief, whereas the four who were treated only with conservative resection received no pain relief. At this point as statistical significance was reached, the study was terminated by the Institutional Review Board. The authors went on to perform the procedure in 17 patients, achieving success in 15. Of some concern is that the failure to relieve pain in any of the four women treated with conservative resection alone diverges substantially from the bulk of the prior literature.[27] A larger, similarly structured trial[4] of 71 women demonstrated that the addition of presacral neurectomy relieved the exacerbation of central pelvic pain associated with menstruation but did not significantly improve central pelvic pain at other times of the month, lateral pelvic pain, or dyspareunia.

For obvious clinical and ethical reasons, no trials have evaluated the effect of using only presacral neurectomy to treat central pelvic pain. One study[5] reported that presacral neurectomy was more effective than laparoscopic uterosacral nerve ablation for the treatment of refractory primary dysmenorrhea.

Regeneration of peripheral nerves occurs at a steady pace, allowing sensation to emerge about 12 to 18 months after neurolysis. Autonomic (e.g., sympathetic) nerves also may regenerate but may take longer to do so.[18] For this reason, follow-up of presacral neurectomy and other pelvic neuroablative procedures should probably be carried out for at least 2 to 3 years before final appraisal of efficacy.

PELVIC DENERVATION

The reasons for the variable results in the clinical reports reviewed above are multiple and include patient selection, the presence of nociceptive signals emanating from other organs, and simultaneous or subsequent treatment of endometriosis using nonsurgical therapies. In addition, anatomic variation in the nerve supply to the pelvic viscera is often held responsible for the variable results in neuroablative procedures.[13]

It would appear that enervation of the pelvic floor and viscera is redundant. Nociceptive signals may leave the pelvis by a variety of routes.[29] Sympathetic afferents arising from the central pelvic viscera traverse the inferior hypogastric plexus en route to the sympathetic chain through the superior hypogastric plexus. However, additional afferents may travel through the nervi erigentes to the sacral routes, and some sympathetic fibers may ascend through pathways more laterally placed than usual. These collateral supplies may account for failure of presacral neurectomy in the immediate postoperative period and for those failures during the course of longer observation.

Understanding this neurologic redundancy raises fascinating and challenging questions for investigators and clinicians. Does the state of being in chronic pain alter the balance of nociceptive signals originating in these various pathways? Does individual variation in neural transmission

pathways alone account for variable outcomes after presacral neurectomy? Can diagnostic blocks or laparoscopic pain-mapping procedures inform the clinician and the patient about the potential outcome of a presacral neurectomy or other neuroablative procedure?

Anesthetic blockade of the superior hypogastric plexus was introduced in 1990.[26] To date, this has been done almost universally under fluoroscopic control, using a posterior approach with the patient prone. Using a posterolateral approach adjacent to the L5 vertebral body, 7-inch, 22-gauge needles are passed on each side. Contrast is injected to document accurate retroperitoneal placement in the presacral space. Anesthetic is then injected, and pain relief assessed. The procedure is highly technical and costly, taking approximately 1 hour in the fluoroscopy suite. Potential complications include retroperitoneal bleeding from adjacent great vessels, although long-lasting or life-threatening complications have not been reported.

More recently, a similar block has been accomplished during microlaparoscopy under conscious sedation techniques.[32] Direct passage of a needle into the retroperitoneal space via laparoscopy is more difficult in an obese patient, because the presacral area is obscured by bowel and omental fat. Assuming these hurdles can be overcome, it may possible to intraoperatively assess the potential benefit of adding a presacral neurectomy to a planned laparoscopic procedure for endometriosis.

TECHNIQUE

Preoperative preparation should include thorough counseling of the patient concerning the risks of potential bleeding or visceral injury. A thorough mechanical bowel preparation is indicated especially with a laparoscopic approach, and the patient should expect laparotomy in the event of substantial bleeding.

The anatomic approach and results should be essentially similar whether approached by laparoscopy or by laparotomy. In the case of laparotomy, the large colon is packed away to expose the presacral area, and the small bowels are similarly eliminated from the field by a combination of Trendelenburg positioning and bowel packing. Laparoscopically, a greater degree of Trendelenburg position, in combination with a left lower quadrant probe used for large bowel retraction, usually accomplishes adequate exposure of the presacral area.

The presacral peritoneum may then be incised along the axis of the spine from approximately the lower margin of S1, continuing the incision cephalad to the level of the bifurcation of the aorta. Alternatively, as is often done when performing this procedure laparoscopically, the peritoneum can simply be transversely incised at or slightly caudad to the sacral promontory. Performed in this manner, the peritoneum seems to retract itself adequately to allow a thorough retroperitoneal approach (Fig. 32-1).

Gentle blunt dissection exposes glistening periosteum over the L5 and S1 vertebral bodies. It is perhaps useful to start on either side of the midline, thus avoiding the middle sacral artery and vein (Fig. 32-2). Although these vessels generally do present in the midline, their anatomic location is somewhat variable. Dissection is most readily carried out with cotton pledgets when done by laparotomy or with the laparoscopic equivalent. The author finds that dissecting gently with two instruments in a transverse direction provokes less bleeding, in contrast to axial dissection parallel to the direction of the middle sacral artery and vein. Once the periosteum is adequately viewed, the dissection can be car-

ried out to the medial aspect of the right ureter and to the base of the mesosigmoid on the left side. Fibroadipose tissue containing nerve fibers can be divided by creating pedicles and then transecting and suture ligating them. Laparoscopically, the pedicles are often simply coagulated with bipolar forceps or clipped and divided at several levels. The midline portion of the presacral retroperitoneal tissue can then be approached. Ideally, the middle sacral artery and vein can be gently dissected away from surrounding structures and left alone. If this is not possible, then a suture ligature can be placed cephalad and caudad about 3 to 4 cm apart and the intervening segment removed along with adjacent neural fibers. When performed laparoscopically, such sutures require placement with exquisite care, as these vessels often have fibrous attachments to the periosteum itself and the vein may tear upon retraction. When the middle sacral vessels are of substantial size, they will exceed the upper limits of size for vessels that can be adequately controlled by bipolar electrocoagulation.

The major complication of this procedure is bleeding from either the middle sacral artery and vein or from presacral veins that are increasingly prevalent the further one operates caudad to the inferior margin of S1. For this reason, it is prudent to stay cephalad to the S1-S2 interspace. Many methods have been used to control bleeding in this area, with perhaps the most successful being placement of stainless steel thumbtacks directly into the periosteum and bone.[25]

The particular risks associated with the laparoscopic approach make it appropriate only for surgeons who have substantial experience with laparoscopy. Perhaps the even

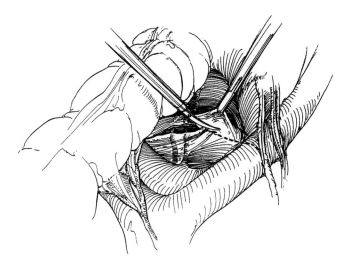

Fig. 32-1 Landmarks for performing a presacral neurectomy as viewed from a laparoscope inserted into the umbilical trocar.

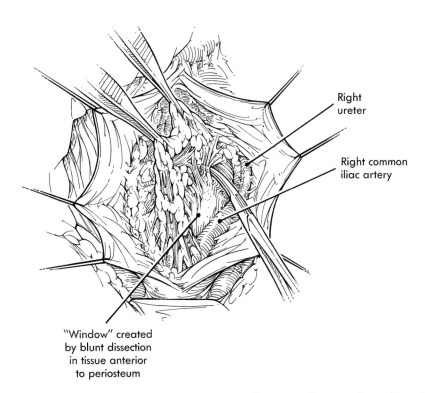

Right ureter

Right common iliac artery

"Window" created by blunt dissection in tissue anterior to periosteum

Fig. 32-2 A window is created in the retroperitoneal tissues as they are elevated anterior to the sacral promontory. Blunt dissection is begun medial to the right ureter.

greater hazard is that, since presacral neurectomy can be performed laparoscopically, both the patient and physician may underestimate the risks, with resultant overuse of the procedure. In addition, given the challenging nature of the procedure, the laparoscopist may have a tendency to err on the side of caution and do a less than complete denervation procedure. This may leave the patient with an inadequate degree of pain relief and with the mistaken impression that everything possible has been done in terms of neuroablative procedures. Once the presacral space has been operated on, repeat procedures can be quite difficult because of postoperative scarring.

COMPLICATIONS

As described above, bleeding is the major risk of the procedure.[20,25] Three deaths due to hemorrhage have been reported.[9,15] Less dramatic complications include short-term urinary retention,[1,2] long-term urinary urgency,[14,23] constipation in up to one third of patients,[2,4,5,20] and painless labor.[2,4] Vaginal dryness may occur during the first 6 months after surgery,[28] and small bowel obstruction may occur.[2]

It is noteworthy that reports of alterations of sexual function are entirely absent from the literature. This author suspects that alterations must occur, but in most cases they are subtle. Enthusiasm for returning to supracervical hysterectomy is growing, with the potential benefits of improved pelvic support and better retention of cervical sensitivity in sexual function offered as rationales. It would seem to this author that if the cervix does indeed provide an important sensory input to sexual response, then presacral neurectomy should eliminate this component. Further careful clinical observation would be desirable.

OTHER DENERVATION PROCEDURES

Doyle[12] in the 1950s designed a procedure in which the uterosacral ligaments on each side were transected and then reapproximated in a side-by-side fashion with an intervening layer of intact peritoneum between their severed ends. He accomplished this procedure either transvaginally or by laparotomy and reported improvement in the discomfort from dysmenorrhea to approximately the same degree as that seen following presacral neurectomy. The laparoscopic equivalent of this procedure has not been reported in the literature, although it would seem feasible. Beginning in the 1970s, laparoscopic uterosacral nerve ablation was reported, with techniques varying from partial to complete transection of the uterosacral ligaments. Clinical surveys reported 60% to 70% of patients having substantially reduced dysmenorrhea.[6] A subsequent controlled trial reported persistent relief of primary dysmenorrhea in only 45% of 11 subjects at 1-year follow-up.[21] Complications of this procedure include potential ureteral injury and altered pelvic support. Four cases of pelvic relaxation following this procedure have been reported to date.[11,17]

Denervation of the sympathetic supply of the ovary also has been attempted to relieve pain around the ovary during menstruation. Fleigner[14] described resolution of "ovarian dysmenorrhea" following division of the infundibulopelvic ligament in a few cases. Browne[3] reported 21 cases treated in a similar manner, with 16 cured and 1 patient receiving partial relief of her pain. Given the potential effect of this procedure on ovarian circulation, with the potential of postoperative chronic cyst formation,[3] it may prove prudent to exhaust all medical means of management first and to further document the ovarian source of pain by microlaparoscopic pain mapping and selective anesthetic blockade.

CONCLUSION

Presacral neurectomy and other neuroablative procedures seem to be again increasing in popularity. Among the reasons for this phenomenon is the ready ability to accomplish the procedure laparoscopically. Nevertheless, the existing evidence suggests that the benefit of presacral neurectomy is uncertain at best and is limited to partial relief of central menstrually associated pelvic pain. Further randomized trials of this treatment are needed and should be performed in well-defined populations studied with valid psychometric techniques. Follow-up should be lengthy, as reenervation may occur over several years. The relatively new techniques of pain mapping with microlaparoscopy may prove of additional diagnostic value and hence assist with patient selection.[31]

REFERENCES

1. Black WT: Presacral sympathectomy for dysmenorrhea and pelvic pain, *Am Surg* 103:903, 1936.
2. Black WT: Use of presacral sympathectomy in the treatment of dysmenorrhea, *Am J Obstet Gynecol* 89:16, 1964.
3. Browne OD: Survey of 113 cases of primary dysmenorrhea treated by neurectomy, *Am J Obstet Gynecol* 57:1053, 1949.
4. Candiani GB, Fedele L, Vercellini P, et al: Presacral neurectomy for the treatment of pelvic pain associated with endometriosis: a controlled study, *Am J Obstet Gynecol* 167:100, 1992.
5. Chen FP, Chang SD, Chu KK, Soong YK: Comparison of laparoscopic presacral neurectomy and laparoscopic uterine nerve ablation for primary dysmenorrhea, *J Reprod Med* 41:463, 1996.
6. Corson SL, Unger M, Kwa D, et al: Laparoscopic laser treatment of endometriosis with the Nd:YAG sapphire probe, *Am J Obstet Gynecol* 160:718, 1989.
7. Cotte G: La sympathectomie hypogastrique a-t-ella sa place dana la therapeutique gynecologique? *Presse Med* 33,98, 1925.
8. Cotte MG: Resection of the presacral nerve in the treatment of dysmenorrhea, *Am J Obstet Gynecol* 33:1030, 1937.
9. Cotte MG: Technique of presacral neurectomy, *Am J Surg* 78:50, 1949.
10. Counseller VS, Winchell McKS: The treatment of dysmenorrhea by resection of the presacral sympathetic nerves: evaluation and end results, *Am J Obstet Gynecol* 28:61, 1934.
11. Davis GD: Uterine prolapse after laparoscopic uterosacral transection in nulliparous airborne trainees: a report of three cases, *J Reprod Med* 41:279, 1996.
12. Doyle EB: Paracervical uterine denervation by transection of the cervical plexus for the relief of dysmenorrhea, *Am J Obstet Gynecol* 11:70, 1955.

13. Elant L: Surgical anatomy of the so-called presacral nerve, *Surg Gynecol Obstet* 57:51, 1933.

14. Fleigner JRH, Umstad MP: Presacral neurectomy—a reappraisal, *Aust N Z J Obstet Gynecol* 31:76, 1931.

15. Fontaine R, Herrmann LG: Clinical and experimental basis for surgery of pelvic sympathetic nerves in gynecology, *Surg Gynecol Obstet* 133:54, 1932.

16. Garcia CR, David SS: Pelvic endometriosis: infertility and pelvic pain, *Am J Obstet Gynecol* 129:740, 1977.

17. Good MC, Copas PR, Doody MC: Uterine prolapse after laparoscopic uterosacral transection, *J Reprod Med* 72:995, 1993.

18. Hannington-Kiff JG: Sympathetic nerve blocks in painful limb disorders. In PD Wall, R Melzack, editors: *Textbook of pain,* London, 1994, Churchill Livingstone.

19. Jaboulay M: Le traitment del la nevralgie pelviene par la paralysie due sympathique sacre, *Lyon Med* 90:102, 1899.

20. Lee RB, Stone K, Magelssen D, et al: Presacral neurectomy for chronic pelvic pain, *Obstet Gynecol* 68:517, 1986.

21. Lichten EM, Bombard J: Surgical treatment of primary dysmenorrhea with laparoscopic uterine nerve ablation, *J Reprod Med* 32:37, 1987.

22. Mahfoud HK, Hewitt SR: A place for presacral neurectomy, *Ir Med J* 74:198, 1981.

23. Meigs JV: Excision of the superior hypogastric (presacral nerve) for primary dysmenorrhea, *Surg Gynecol Obstet* 68:723, 1939.

24. Metzger DA: Nerve cutting procedures for pelvic pain. In Steege JF, Metzger DA, Levy BS, editors: *Chronic pelvic pain: an integrated approach,* Philadelphia, 1997, WB Saunders.

25. Patsner B, Ozz WJ: Intractable venous sacral hemorrhage: use of stainless steel thumbtacks to obtain hemostasis, *Am J Obstet Gynecol* 162:452, 1990.

26. Plancarte R, Amescua C, Patt RB, Aldrete JA: Superior hypogastric plexus block for pelvic cancer pain, *Anesthesiology* 73:236, 1990.

27. Polan ML, DeCherney A: Presacral neurectomy for pelvic pain in infertility, *Fertil Steril* 34:557, 1980.

28. Rock J, Jones H: *Reparative and reconstructive surgery of the female generative tract,* Baltimore, 1983, Williams & Wilkins.

29. Rogers R: Pelvic neuroanatomy. In Steege JF, Metzger DA, Levy B, editors: *Chronic pelvic pain: an integrated approach,* Philadelphia, 1977, WB Saunders.

30. Ruggi G: La Simpathectomia abdominale utero-ovarica come mezzo di cura di alcune lesioni interne degli organi genitali della donna, Bologna, Zanichelli, 1899.

31. Steege, JF: Microlaparoscopy. In Steege JF, Metzger DA, Levy B, editors: *Chronic pelvic pain: an integrated approach,* Philadelphia, WB Saunders, 1977.

32. Steege JF: Superior hypogastric block during microlaparoscopic pain mapping, *J Am Assoc Gynecol Laparoscopists* 5:265, 1998.

33. Tjaden B, Schlaff WD, Kimball A, Rock JA: The efficacy of presacral neurectomy for the relief of dysmenorrhea, *Obstet Gynecol* 76:89, 1990.

33 Pelvic Infection

SEBASTIAN FARO

Pelvic infections can be divided anatomically into those of the lower and upper genital tracts. Lower genital tract infections can be subdivided into those involving the vulva, the vestibule, and the vagina. Infections of the vulva usually are caused by bacteria that inhabit the skin and cause diseases such as furunculosis, carbunculosis, pyodermatitis, erysipelas, and impetigo. These infections tend to be unimicrobial, most commonly caused by *Staphylococcus aureus* and *Streptococcus pyogenes.* Skin infections not associated with an advancing cellulitis are most frequently treated with topical antibiotics. If an advancing cellulitis is present or the infection appears to have penetrated the deeper tissues, systemic antibiotic therapy should be started (i.e., first-generation cephalosporins or, if penicillinase-producing staphylococci are suspected, a penicillin such as nafcillin). Occasionally these infections form abscesses, requiring incision and drainage. In contrast, hidradenitis suppurativa is a complex infection that may be polymicrobial and often does not respond to antimicrobial treatment. Hidradenitis typically begins as an inflammatory process in which infection is secondary. The infectious process should be thought of as an abscess, and the reduced blood flow to the infected area is the likely reason that antibiotic therapy usually is unsuccessful.

Infections of the upper genital tract (i.e., the uterus and fallopian tubes) usually are more serious and often require the patient to be hospitalized. These infections are treated with systemic antibiotics administered orally or parenterally. Upper genital tract infections can lead to infertility and damaged fallopian tubes, resulting in ectopic pregnancy, or abscess formation (e.g., pyosalpinx or tuboovarian abscess). Surgical intervention often is necessary to treat abscesses.

Infections of the genital tract have a microbial cause that is derived either from the patient's own vaginal ecosystem or an exogenous source. The majority of infections originating from an exogenous source are caused by sexually transmitted organisms (i.e., sexually transmitted disease, or STD). These organisms can cause a local infection but also may cause systemic disease, disrupt pregnancy, and cause significant postoperative morbidity. The most common sexually transmitted organisms that can cause postoperative morbidity are *Neisseria gonorrhoeae, Chlamydia trachomatis, Trichomonas vaginalis,* and the human immunodeficiency virus (HIV). Although STD may play a role in postoperative infection, infections caused by a patient's own endogenous vaginal bacteria are more likely to cause significant and more frequent postoperative infection. There-fore an understanding of the vaginal ecosystem is most helpful in treating patients with a pelvic infection.

VAGINAL MICROFLORA

The bacterial microflora of the lower genital tract resembles the fecal flora except that the vagina is not as densely populated and usually does not contain abscessogenic bacteria (e.g., *Bacteroides fragilis* and the *B. fragilis* group). The endogenous vaginal bacterial population consists of gram-positive and gram-negative aerobic, facultative, and obligate anaerobes. In the healthy state the microflora of the vagina is dominated by commensal bacteria, which suppress or act antagonistically toward the growth of potentially pathogenic bacteria. A delicate balance exists between these two populations of bacteria (commensal versus pathogenic), which in turn must interact with environmental factors originating from the host and the exogenous environment. This dynamic but delicate equilibrium is tightly linked to the metabolic and hormonal activities of the host.[26,49] One crucial factor is the hydrogen ion concentration, which depends on the metabolic activity of the bacterial community and the host. The normal hydrogen ion concentration of the vagina is between 3.8 and 4.2. The predominant bacteria at this hydrogen ion concentration are the commensals on the following list, *Lactobacillus* being the dominant genus:

Lactobacillus spp.
Diphtheroids
Bacillus spp.
Nonhemolytic streptococci

Lactobacillus acidophilus is the dominant bacterium in the healthy vagina and is thought to suppress the growth of other bacteria, especially the pathogenic organisms, by production of lactic acid and hydrogen peroxide. The production of lactic acid aids in maintaining the pH between 3.8 and 4.2, which is unfavorable to the growth of many gram-positive and gram-negative bacteria. Hydrogen peroxide is toxic to the anaerobic bacteria.[18,28,29]

Many environmental factors, both exogenous and endogenous, can disturb the delicate equilibrium that exists in the healthy vagina. Once the pH is altered and the hydrogen ion concentration decreases, the pH rises, becoming more alkaline. A pH greater than 4.5 is more favorable to the growth of noncommensal, or pathogenic, endogenous bacteria. These co-inhabitants of the healthy vagina usually are present in concentrations of less than 1000 organisms per milliliter of vaginal fluid, but when the acidity of the vagina decreases they begin to reproduce more vigorously, exceeding 10,000 to 100,000 organisms per milliliter of vaginal fluid. Eventually these potentially pathogenic bacteria dominate and essentially become the microflora of the vagina (see the box below).

Numerous studies have attempted to define the vaginal flora in healthy and unhealthy states. Undoubtedly the hydrogen ion concentration is a key factor in maintaining the vaginal ecosystem in a state of equilibrium that allows the commensal bacteria to dominate. The hydrogen ion concentration can influence the growth of all the various members of the endogenous microflora. When vaginal equilibrium is disrupted, at least three distinct bacteriologic conditions may exist: (1) bacterial vaginitis, typified by the growth of various bacteria such as *Enterococcus faecalis, Streptococcus agalactiae,* and *Escherichia coli*[15]; (2) *Gardnerella vaginalis* vaginitis, characterized microscopically by the presence of clue cells (i.e., epithelial cells with adherent gram-negative rods that obscure the cytoplasmic membrane), aggregates or clumps of floating bacteria in the vaginal discharge, and the noticeable absence of white blood cells[17]; and (3) bacterial vaginosis, defined as an overgrowth of anaerobic bacteria and a decrease in lactobacilli, characterized microscopically by numerous individual free-floating bacteria, a noticeable absence of white blood cells, and the presence of clue cells.

Patients with abnormal vaginal bacterial flora typically have an altered hydrogen ion concentration (pH greater than 4.5). Bacterial vaginitis usually is not characterized by a large number of anaerobes, which typically produce amines that give the vaginal fluid a fishy odor and therefore a negative KOH or amine test. Microscopically, clue cells are not present, as is commonplace in the vaginal discharge of patients with *G. vaginalis* vaginitis and bacterial vaginosis, and the flora is dominated by anaerobic or facultative anaerobic bacteria. Patients with bacterial vaginitis usually have an increased amount of vaginal discharge, which may be clear, dirty gray, greenish, or yellow, typically do not have a foul odor, and may report some vaginal discomfort.[15]

Individuals with *G. vaginalis* vaginitis have a homogenous liquid discharge, often foul-smelling, and may have a burning sensation. The pH is usually greater than 4.5, and the KOH test is positive. Microscopic examination reveals the presence of clue cells and clumps of free-floating bacteria in the vaginal discharge. Typically the microflora is dominated by large numbers of *G. vaginalis* and the number of other bacteria is much smaller (e.g., greater than 100,000 versus 1000).[8] Bacterial vaginosis, in contrast to *G. vaginitis,* is characterized by an overgrowth of anaerobic bacteria and a decrease in lactobacilli, and *G. vaginalis* may or may not be present. The discharge is homogenous, dirty gray, runny, and usually has an amine odor when mixed with concentrated potassium hydroxide (KOH test). Microscopically there are large numbers of bacteria, which are free floating and contain both gram-positive and gram-negative bacteria. Typically white blood cells are not present to any large degree in the vaginal discharge of patients with bacterial vaginosis, hence the suffix *-osis* to indicate the absence of an inflammatory reaction.[21,22,45,46] *G. vaginalis* is a common inhabitant of the vaginal flora in patients with bacterial vaginosis. *G. vaginalis* may be isolated from the vaginas of up to 40% of women with a healthy vaginal ecosystem. It may be that *G. vaginalis* vaginitis is a precursor to bacterial vaginosis.

Endogenous bacterial vaginal flora apparently plays a role in infections of the female genital tract as well as in vaginitis, cervicitis, endometritis, salpingitis, postpartum endometritis, and perhaps even pelvic abscesses, all of which may be considered as stages in pelvic inflammatory disease. This is an important complex of infections, since the end result may place the patient at risk for ectopic pregnancy, infertility, or perhaps castration.

LOWER GENITAL TRACT INFECTIONS
Hidradenitis Suppurativa

Hidradenitis suppurativa originates in the apocrine sweat glands and is initiated by closure of the duct or pore, which prevents egress of the gland contents. The gland also becomes colonized with bacteria that inhabit the skin and perhaps bacteria that are derived from the normal vaginal flora. The skin overlying the groin and labia is exposed to the vaginal discharge, which contains numerous gram-positive and gram-negative bacteria, both aerobic and anaerobic. Therefore hidradenitis of the vulva and groin has the potential to be a complex polymicrobial infection.[30,35,36] Closure of the duct or pore probably is initiated by bacteria colonizing the gland, inducing an inflammatory reaction in the cell's lining and surrounding the duct and resulting in swelling and closure of the duct. The gland becomes distended as it fills with mucus and bacteria, thus forming an abscess. Eventually the abscessed gland may rupture at the skin surface, resulting in the drainage of a foul-smelling purulent material that is characteristic of hidradenitis suppurativa. The abscessed gland also may rupture below the skin surface, infecting the surrounding tissue. Fistulas may form to

---

ENDOGENOUS MICROFLORA OF THE LOWER GENITAL TRACT

GRAM-POSITIVE	GRAM-NEGATIVE
Streptococcus agalactiae	*Escherichia coli*
Stapylococcus aureus	*Enterobacter agglomerans*
Staphylococcus epidermidis	*Enterobacter aerogenes*
Enterococcus faecalis	*Enterobacter cloacae*
	Klebsiella pneumoniae

ANAEROBES	
Peptostreptococcus	*Proteus mirabilis*
Bacteroides	*Proteus vulgatus*
Fusobacterium	
Prevotella	

other apocrine glands, which eventually become infected, resulting in a chronic infection as these glands abscess and rupture and lead to infection of other apocrine glands. Typically, as the apocrine gland infection progresses to an abscess, nodules form on the skin surface. The area surrounding the infected gland becomes erythematous, swollen, and tender. The nodules suppurate and drain a thick, purulent, foul-smelling exudate. The recurrent formation of inflamed nodules that suppurate is a characteristic feature of this infection. Following rupture of an abscessed apocrine gland, fibrosis and hypertrophic scaring occur in the tissue overlying skin.

Hidradenitis suppurativa characteristically occurs in the axilla, groin, external genitalia, and perianal area. The recurrences or exacerbations typically occur during menses, which coincides with an increase in gland activity. No antibiotic treatment currently available can effectively cure this infection. Although antibiotic studies have not been conducted because it is difficult to obtain a significant number of patients, antibiotic regimens providing activity against anaerobes and facultative anaerobes appear to be most effective. The regimen should possess activity against bacteria such as *Propionibacterium, Peptostreptococcus, Staphylococcus,* and *Escherichia coli.* Two factors may be responsible for the inability to treat this infection successfully with antibiotics: (1) limited understanding of the microbiological makeup and (2) an inability to achieve adequate levels of antibiotics in the inflamed and infected tissue. The fibrosis that accompanies the infection may cause decreased vascular supply to the area, thereby preventing adequate levels of antibiotic in the tissue.

When antibiotic therapy fails, surgery is the only recourse. Basically one of two operative approaches can be chosen. The first consists of excision of the infected tissue, including a margin of noninfected tissue and the underlying subcutaneous tissue but not the fascia. The incision can be closed primarily or allowed to heal by secondary intention. The second approach consists of a skinning procedure and skin graft. The skinning procedure is preferred if large areas are involved, which, if excised, would create large defects and leave behind unsightly scars. Whichever procedure is chosen, it is extremely important that all infected tissue be removed. If infected tissue remains, the process resumes within 12 months or less.

Vulvovaginitis

Other microorganisms, such as viruses, play an important role in causing infections of the lower genital tract (e.g., molluscum contagiosum, condyloma acuminata, and herpes).[1,6,11] *Candida* is the most common fungus that causes lower genital tract infections and usually involves both the external genitalia and the vagina.[27] Vaginitis is the most common disease of the lower genital tract due to fungi, bacteria, viruses, parasites, and protozoans. These infections rarely lead to upper genital tract infections; however, they often can be responsible for chronic infections. Patients who have recurrent vaginal infections should be examined for the presence of yeast in the oral cavity. Any

symptoms that reflect possible infection of the gastrointestinal tract should be thoroughly investigated. Consideration should be given to screening the patient for HIV antibody because esophageal candidiasis is often an indication of HIV infection.

Epidemiology

Patients make approximately 1,000,000 outpatient visits to gynecologists per year for complaints of vaginitis. This probably represents a portion of the number of actual cases. Vaginitis obviously accounts for a significant amount of money spent on health care. In some cases the physician is unable to treat the individual's problem and may inform the patient that her condition is psychosomatic. Thus patients with recalcitrant vaginitis, be it yeast or bacterial, often avoid or alter their sexual activity because of embarrassment, making this condition both a health and a social problem.

Attempts have been made to link bacterial vaginitis or vaginosis with more severe infections such as premature rupture of amniotic membranes, premature labor, postpartum endomyometritis, pelvic inflammatory disease, and postoperative pelvic cellulitis. The connection between bacterial vaginosis and upper genital tract infection is gaining strength and is founded on the hypothesis that most of these infections are polymicrobial. The bacterial isolates from such sites as amniotic fluid, the endometrium, and the vaginal cuff in patients with pelvic cellulitis resemble the bacteriology of the lower genital tract. However, it must be emphasized that the bacterial isolates are often obtained not from the site of actual infection but from an area in close proximity, so this conclusion is based on an extrapolation from the available data.

UPPER GENITAL TRACT INFECTIONS

Upper genital tract infections include cervicitis, endometritis, salpingitis, and tuboovarian abscess. Other common infections that may occur in the pelvis, although not related to the female organs, are appendicitis and diverticulitis. Both of these infections are important because they are frequently confused with pelvic inflammatory disease and can damage the fallopian tubes, especially in patients 35 years of age or older. Subsequently the patient may be infertile or, if pregnancy can be achieved, it may be ectopic. The infections of the upper genital tract tend to be more serious and may give rise to systemic infection resulting in bacteremia, sepsis, and septic shock.

Crucial to the successful treatment of any pelvic infection is an understanding of the microorganisms responsible for the disease. Pelvic infections in women generally are caused by bacteria either introduced from the environment (most commonly STD) or by endogenous vaginal microflora. Although the specific role of endogenous microflora in the production or development of upper genital tract infection has not been delineated, an association appears to exist between their presence in the lower genital tract and upper genital tract infection.

PELVIC INFLAMMATORY DISEASE

Epidemiology

Pelvic inflammatory disease (PID) occurs predominantly among sexually promiscuous women between the ages of 15 and 44 years old, with the incidence peaking in women between 18 and 25 years of age.[51,52] Acute pelvic inflammatory disease may occur in 1% of sexually active women and in approximately 1.5% to 2% of sexually active teenagers between 15 and 19 years of age.

The relevance of these numbers of patients is manifested in the cost of treating PID and its sequelae. Approximately 1,000,000 patient visits per year can be attributed to PID. These generate between 200,000 and 300,000 hospitalizations per year, which in turn result in 110,000 operative procedures yearly. Several investigators have attempted to project the economic impact of this disease based on best estimates of the incidence of hospitalization and ambulatory patient visits to physicians. In the United States the estimated cost of treating PID and its sequelae ranges from $300 million to $3 billion a year.[39,41,51] The sequelae may be not only physically traumatic but also psychologically devastating. Approximately 25% of women who have had PID will be left with chronic pelvic pain, infertility, or at risk for ectopic pregnancy.[19,50,54]

Individuals at risk for contracting PID are primarily those with multiple sex partners or with a partner who has multiple sex partners. Patients exposed to gonorrhea are at risk for developing upper genital tract infection. Approximately 20% of women who contract cervical gonococcal infection, if left untreated or treated inappropriately, will develop pelvic inflammatory disease (i.e., endometritis or salpingitis).[44,54] Several factors have been found to be associated with the development of PID:

1. Unmarried and sexually active
2. Sexually promiscuous
3. History of exposure to a sexually transmitted disease
4. Presence of an intrauterine device
5. Use of oral contraceptives
6. Adolescence

The patient who is known to have more than one sexual contact, directly or indirectly and regardless of age should be evaluated for the presence of a sexually transmitted disease. If a sexually transmitted organism is found (e.g., *Trichomonas vaginalis, Herpes simplex, Neisseria gonorrhoeae, Chlamydia trachomatis,* human papillomavirus), specimens should be obtained for the detection of other sexually transmitted organisms.

Microbiology

The microbiologic makeup of PID has not been completely elucidated. There is controversy over which organism—*N. gonorrhoeae* or *C. trachomatis*—is most frequently responsible. The microbial causes of PID are as follows:

1. *N. gonorrhoeae*
2. *C. trachomatis*
3. Polymicrobial, nongonococcal, and nonchlamydial bacteria, ascending from the lower genital tract

4. Iatrogenic placement of bacteria during a diagnostic or therapeutic procedure

N. gonorrhoeae continues to be a leading isolate from patients diagnosed as having acute PID. In studies conducted on the Baylor gynecologic service at the Ben Taub Hospital, which renders care for an indigent population, *N. gonorrhoeae* was recovered from 50% to 60% of the patients and *C. trachomatis* from 16% to 20% of the patients with acute PID.[13,15,24] This is consistent with isolation rates reported by other investigators[12,23,48,53] (e.g., 10% to 81% for *N. gonorrhoeae* and 5% to 20% for *C. trachomatis*). Sweet et al.[48] reported a recovery rate of 48% for *N. gonorrhoeae* and 23% for *C. trachomatis* from patients with PID. Sweet et al., in studying chlamydial and gonococcal colonization rates during the menstrual cycle, recovered *N. gonorrhoeae* from 40% of the patients and *Chlamydia* from 27%. Judson and Tavelli[23] reported in 1986 that *N. gonorrhoeae* was recovered from 27% of patients attending a sexually transmitted disease clinic, whereas 18% harbored *C. trachomatis,* and 16% had both organisms. Neither organism was found in 39% of the patients with symptoms suggestive of acute PID. However, the experience in Sweden has been different. *C. trachomatis* has been isolated from 40% to 50% of the patients, and *N. gonorrhoeae* has been recovered from 10% to 15% of individuals with PID.[20,25,32,33] Kristensen et al. reported a 13% isolation rate for *N. gonorrhoeae* and 24% for *C. trachomatis.*[30,46]

Although U.S. data differ from the Scandinavian, empiric management of patients with acute salpingitis should include treatment for both organisms until definitive microbiologic data become available. Coinfections with *N. gonorrhoeae* and *C. trachomatis* have been reported to occur in 25% to 60% of women with gonorrhea who also have *Chlamydia.*[54,55]

Diagnosis

The initial infection begins with cervicitis, which usually is asymptomatic and all too often goes unnoticed. Signs of cervicitis are as follows:

1. Endocervical purulent discharge
2. Cervical bleeding with minor trauma
3. Cervical pain with intercourse

It is uncommon for a patient to recognize a cervical infection, since it is usually asymptomatic. This is the primary reason for the delay in diagnosis. However, the patient may relate that she has spotting after or pain during sexual intercourse. Frequently the physician notes the presence of endocervical pus when obtaining a Pap smear or, perhaps more commonly, notes that the cervix bleeds easily while obtaining endocervical cells for a Pap smear with a cotton-tipped applicator. The physician also may note that the endocervical epithelium is hypertrophic. Any of these observations during the pelvic examination should lead the physician to ask questions relating to frequency of sexual intercourse, number of sexual partners, and, if the patient has only one partner, whether she knows or suspects that other individuals may be involved with her partner and whether her consort has any symptoms that might suggest a genital tract infection. The patient's endocervix should be cultured for *N. gonorrhoeae,* and *C. trachomatis.* The urethra should be cultured for *N. gonorrhoeae, C. trachomatis, Ureaplasma,* and *Mycoplasma. The* vaginal discharge should be examined for *T. vaginalis.*

If gram reagents are readily available, then a gram stain of the endocervical specimen should be performed. If gram-negative intracellular diplococci are found, this can be taken as presumptive evidence for the presence of *N. gonorrhoeae.* The patient should be treated with a single dose of cefotaxime 125 mg intramuscularly. If no bacteria are seen on the Gram stain, and squamous epithelial cells are rarely seen, but white blood cells are present (5/hpf) and no detectable pathogen is observed (e.g., *T. vaginalis* or *Candida*), then it is reasonable to suspect the presence of *C. trachomatis.* The patient should be treated with doxycycline

---

ANTIBIOTIC CHOICES FOR THE TREATMENT OF *N. GONORRHOEAE* AND *C. TRACHOMATIS* CERVICITIS

FIRST CHOICE FOR TREATMENT OF *CHLAMYDIA TRACHOMATIS*

Oral Regimens
Doxycycline 100 mg bid for 7 days
Azithromycin 1 g in a single dose

ALTERNATIVE CHOICES

Oral Regimens
Ofloxacin 300 mg bid for 7 days
Erythromycin base 500 mg qid for 7 days
Sulfisoxazole 500 mg qid for 10 days

FIRST CHOICE FOR TREATMENT OF *NEISSERIA GONORRHOEAE*

Single Dose
Ceftriaxone 125 mg intramuscularly
Cefixime 400 mg orally
Ciprofloxacin 500 mg orally
Ofloxacin 400 mg orally

ALTERNATIVE CHOICES

Intramuscularly—Single Dose
Spectinomycin 2 g
Ceftizoxime 500 mg
Cefotaxime 500 mg
Cefotetan 1 g
Cefoxitin 2 g

Oral—Single Dose
Cefuroxime axetil 1 g
Cefpodoxime proxetil 200 mg
Enoxacin 400 mg
Lomefloxacin 400 mg
Norfloxacin 800 mg

Centers for Disease Control and Prevention: *MMWR* 42:51, 1993.

(100 mg twice daily for 7 days) or another suitable antibiotic (see the box below, left). Regimens used to treat *N. gonorrhoeae* in a single dose are not effective for treating *C. trachomatis.*

Most antibiotic regimens currently available for the treatment of *C. trachomatis* require 7 days, with the exception of azithromycin, which has been approved for use in a 1 g single dose. Ofloxacin is the only quinolone that has been approved by the FDA for the treatment of chlamydial infections. This is important because the other quinolones have activity against *N. gonorrhoeae* but not *C. trachomatis.* Therefore if any of these quinolones are used to treat cervicitis suspected of being caused by *N. gonorrhoeae,* an anti-*Chlamydia* must be included in the treatment regimen. Another point of consideration when treating cervical infections due to either *N. gonorrhoeae, C. trachomatis,* or both is that the infection may have ascended to the upper genital tract. Therefore it is highly probable that the patient would derive more benefit from a long versus a short treatment regimen (7 days versus 1). This concept is important because the goals of treatment are twofold: eradication of the infection organism(s) and prevention of damage to fallopian tubes.

Although the progression from cervicitis to endometritis may be perceived as asymptomatic, in fact the symptoms are typically subtle. The most common symptoms of gonococcal or chlamydial endometritis are listed in the box below.

Patients who have an intrauterine device, have multiple sexual partners, or are having sex with an individual who has multiple sexual partners are at risk for upper genital tract infection. These patients are likely to experience rapid progression to salpingitis, which may be asymptomatic. Thus patients suspected of having endometritis should be evaluated as follows:

1. Cleanse the cervix with Betadine.
2. Allow the Betadine to dry.
3. Insert a Pipelle into the uterine cavity and obtain a biopsy specimen.
4. Divide the specimen into two parts: place one part of the specimen in an anaerobic transport tube and save the other portion for histologic evaluation.

The specimen for culture should be processed for *N. gonorrhoeae, C. trachomatis, Mycoplasma hominis, Ureaplasma urealyticum,* and aerobic, facultative, and obligate anaerobic bacteria. If an intrauterine device is present it should be removed because it serves as a nidus for infection.

SUBTLE SIGNS OF GONOCOCCAL OR CHLAMYDIAL ENDOMETRITIS

1. Vague lower abdominal pain
2. Breakthrough bleeding on oral contraceptive pills
3. Irregular uterine bleeding; no irregular bleeding on OCPs
4. Uterine tenderness to palpation

The device should be cultured for *Actinomyces,* and the laboratory should be alerted to the possible existence of this bacteria. *Actinomyces* when present with an anaerobe can develop into a synergistic infection that can be quite destructive. Penicillin needs to be included in the treatment regimens of patients with endometritis in which *Actinomyces* is present. Treatment regimens for endometritis are listed in the box below.

Trovafloxacin is a quinolone that has recently been released. This is a broad-spectrum fluoroquinolone that can be administered parenterally or orally. Although levofloxacin has anaerobic activity, it does not have the broad spectrum of activity of trovafloxacin. Levofloxacin has been approved for treatment of pelvic inflammatory disease.

All patients treated for PID, regardless of the stage, should be reevaluated within 72 hours to determine if improvement has occurred. If there is no improvement, then the patient should be reevaluated to determine if the initial diagnosis was correct. If the initial diagnosis is correct, then administration of parenteral antibiotics should be considered.

Treatment of PID previously focused on the administration of intravenous antibiotics because of their broad spectrum of antibacterial activity. However, the newer antibiotics, which are available for oral administration, also have a broad spectrum of antibacterial activity. In selected cases this permits the treatment of PID in an outpatient setting. However, not all patients are suitable for outpatient treatment. Criteria for outpatient treatment are as follows. First, the antibiotic agent selected must be active against *N. gonorrhoeae, C. trachomatis,* aerobic bacteria, and facultative and obligate anaerobic bacteria.

Second, the patient must be able to tolerate oral antibiotic therapy. Third, the patient's disease must be uncomplicated; that is, there must be no evidence of peritonitis or a tuboovarian abscess.

Before deciding to institute outpatient therapy for PID, the physician must rule out appendicitis, ectopic pregnancy, ruptured hemorrhagic ovary, and so forth. Additionally, there should not be any suggestion of a pelvic abscess, nor any nausea and vomiting. Patients must be able to return for a follow-up examination within 72 hours of commencing therapy.

Adolescents, because they tend not to be compliant, and individuals who are HIV positive or pregnant should not be treated with oral antibiotics. Patients who are being treated with oral antibiotics and have not demonstrated improvement 48 to 72 hours after beginning therapy should be hospitalized. Specimens for the culture of *N. gonorrhoeae, C. trachomatis,* and aerobic, facultative, and obligate anaerobic bacteria should be obtained. Patients who have failed outpatient therapy or who show no improvement within 48 to 72 hours of receiving intravenous therapy should undergo laparoscopic examination of the pelvis, specifically the fallopian tubes, ovaries, cul-de-sac, appendix, and surface of the liver. Laparoscopic examination enables the physician to establish a correct diagnosis and institute appropriate treatment. If the diagnosis of PID is established, the patient should be treated with intravenous antibiotics.

Patients hospitalized for the treatment of endometritis or salpingitis should receive antibiotics until all signs and symptoms of infection have resolved (see the box on the left). Therapy should be continued for a minimum of 48 hours before changing to an oral regimen of comparable antibiotics. It is imperative that the oral regimen continue to provide broad antibacterial coverage including *N. gonorrhoeae* and *C. trachomatis.* The patient should be reevaluated within 72 hours after discharge from the hospital and again within 2 to 10 days. Individuals initially found to have positive cultures for either *N. gonorrhoeae, C. trachomatis,* or both should be recultured within 7 to 10 days after release from the hospital. A negative test for *N. gonorrhoeae* and *C. trachomatis* after treatment indicates the success of antibiotic therapy. Therefore patients must be educated regarding transmission and prevention of reinfection of STD if treatment is to be effective.

Critical to the management of PID are early institution of antibiotic therapy, early surgical intervention if warranted, and early follow-up after the patient has been discharged from the hospital. The emphasis on early treatment is to prevent damage to the fallopian tubes, which, if damaged, can result in ectopic pregnancy, infertility, pyosalpinx, hydrosalpinx, and tuboovarian abscess. The tragedy of this disease is that it primarily affects young women of reproductive age. Prevention of salpingitis depends on the recognition of the early signs of PID.

Furthermore, identification of patients with cervicitis or endometritis represents the initial opportunity to prevent salpingitis in individuals who are at risk for upper genital

---

ANTIBIOTIC TREATMENT REGIMENS FOR ENDOMETRITIS

1. Amoxicillin/clavulanic acid
   N. gonorrhoeae
   C. trachomatis
   Actinomyces
   Aerobic bacteria
   Facultative and obligate anaerobic bacteria
2. Clindamycin + ofloxacin
   Chlamydia
   N. gonorrhoeae
   C. trachomatis
   Gram-positive aerobes
   Aerobic bacteria
   Facultative and obligate anaerobic bacteria
3. Metronidazole + ofloxacin
   Obligate anaerobic bacteria
4. Trovafloxacin
   N. gonorrhoeae
   C. trachomatis
   Aerobic bacteria
   Facultative and obligate anaerobic bacteria

ANTIBIOTIC REGIMENS FOR THE TREATMENT OF PELVIC INFLAMMATORY DISEASE

AMBULATORY PATIENTS

1. Ceftriaxone 250 mg intramuscularly in a single dose, or cefoxitin 2 g intramuscularly plus probenecid 1 g orally in a single dose, plus doxycycline 100 mg orally bid for 14 days*
2. Amoxicillin 500 mg orally tid for 10 days*
3. Trovafloxacin 200 mg qd for 10 days
4. Clindamycin 450 mg orally qid, or metronidazole 500 mg orally bid for 14 days, plus ofloxacin 400 mg bid for 14 days*

HOSPITALIZED PATIENTS

1. Cefotetan 2 g q12h, or ceftizoxime 1 g q8h, or cefoxitin 2 g q8h administered intravenously, plus doxycycline 100 mg orally bid for 7 days*
2. Clindamycin 900 mg q8h plus gentamicin 2 mg/kg of body weight followed by a maintenance dose of 1.5 mg/kg q8h administered intravenously*
3. Ampicillin/sulbactam 3 g intravenously q6h,* or piperacillin/tazobactam 3.375 g intravenously q6h,* or levofloxacin 200 mg q12h intravenously

*Centers for Disease Control: *MMWR* 42:75, 1993.

DIFFERENTIAL DIAGNOSIS FOR ACUTE SALPINGITIS

1. Ectopic pregnancy
2. Appendicitis
3. Ruptured appendix
4. Endometriosis
5. Torsion of an adnexa
6. Diverticulitis
7. Infection of Meckel's diverticulum
8. Abscess of Meckel's diverticulum

---

tract infection. Once salpingitis has occurred, patients may experience the sequelae of this tragic infection. An individual who has a single episode of salpingitis has a 13% chance of being infertile; if a second episode of salpingitis occurs the risk is approximately 33%, and if three episodes have occurred the risk is 75%. Thus it is extremely important that the treatment for both *C. trachomatis* and *N. gonorrhoeae* be complete.

ACUTE SALPINGITIS

Acute salpingitis is a difficult diagnosis to establish. No laboratory or physical findings are pathonomic of PID or acute salpingitis. Individuals who have fever, lower abdominal pain, purulent cervical discharge, tenderness or pain on motion of the cervix and uterus, and tenderness on gentle palpation of the adnexa most likely have acute salpingitis. However, these signs of infection are not always present. The accepted criteria for making a clinical diagnosis are as follows: (1) fever, (2) lower abdominal pain, and (3) cervical motion and adnexal tenderness. In addition, the patient may have one or more of the following: an elevated white blood cell count, nausea and vomiting, evidence of pelvic peritonitis, a pelvic mass, and a purulent cervical discharge. The diagnosis must be differentiated from those clinical conditions that can easily mimic acute salpingitis (see the box above, right).

Patients with acute salpingitis should have specimens obtained from the endocervix for the isolation and identification of *N. gonorrhoeae* and *C. trachomatis*. Obtaining an endocervical specimen for the isolation and identification of aerobic and anaerobic bacteria is of no value.

The cervical specimens only reflect the vaginal flora. An endometrial biopsy should be obtained, preferably with a Pipelle. The tissue can easily be divided into two major portions, one for histologic evaluation and for the isolation of *N. gonorrhoeae, C. trachomatis, Mycoplasma, Ureaplasma,* and aerobic and anaerobic bacteria. The isolated aerobes and anaerobes should be identified, and antibiotic sensitivities should be performed. Although almost all patients with acute salpingitis respond to one of the recommended regimens of antibiotic therapy (see the box above, left), it is the patient who fails or who progresses to advanced PID that is of concern.

C. trachomatis is truly a unique organism not only because of its biphasic life cycle, but also because of its ability to cause persistent infection. Cell culture systems have demonstrated that this organism can assume a morphological state of arrested growth and persist intracellularly.[16,37,38] Persistent infection is significant because *C. trachomatis* may establish a long-term residence within the host cell, remain viable but inactive, and will likely be cultured negative. The abnormal persistent forms also have a differential expression of key chlamydial antigens and continued synthesis of heat shocked protein 60 (hsp 60), which is an immunopathologic protein (antigen) and reduced synthesis is of major outer membrane protein (MOMP).[34,47,57]

Chlamydia induces the production of cytokines, in particular, gamma interferon (IFN-γ). Gamma interferon activates mononuclear phagocytes, fibroblasts, epithelial cells, and restricts replication of chlamydia.[9,10,42] Gamma interferon has been shown to serve as a macrophage activating factor that induces microbial products of oxygen metabolism. IFN-γ inhibits growth of both *C. psittaci* and *C. trachomatis* by inducing the nonconstitutive enzyme indoleamine 2,3-dioxygenase, which is responsible for the degradation of tryptophan.[10] Gamma interferon restricts replication of *C. trachomatis* at high concentrations, whereas in low concentrations it causes the formation of morphologically aberrant forms.[43] The persistent aberrant forms do express key antigens (e.g., hsp 60 and reduced synthesis of MOMP, reduction in 60-CD envelope protein, and lipopolysaccharide).[4] Removal of IFN-γ results in recovery of normal forms and infectivity.

The aberrant forms seen with exposure to IFN-γ are similar to those seen when the organism is exposed to penicillin. Penicillin-exposed chlamydial cells release h5p60.[5] The effect of penicillin on *Chlamydia* may have a significant effect on treatment of patients with a penicillin. However, in a study in which patients with culture-positive chlamydial involvement who were treated with amoxicillin/clavulanic acid (Augmentin) and cultured after treatment at 1, 3, and 6 weeks, *Chlamydia* was not recovered.[31] More long-term studies of penicillin need to be conducted to determine if penicillins and short-term treatments are truly effective. This is especially needed because the aberrant persistent forms appear to be immunologically active.

Complications

Pelvic inflammatory disease evolves into a complex infection when the large and small bowel become adherent to the adnexa, simulating an abscess. The bowel becomes inflamed, edematous, and densely adherent to the inflamed adnexa. The mucosal lining of the bowel becomes injured and develops microscopic breaks or leaks, permitting the transmigration of bacteria that are endogenous to the large bowel. These bacteria, many of which are abscessogenic and may interact synergistically with organisms already present in the infected tissue, form an abscess. Synergy can occur between bacteria such as *E. coli* and *B. fragilis,* and perhaps between *E. faecalis* and *B. bivivus.* The patient with acute, uncomplicated salpingitis, that is, one who does not have a pelvic complex or mass, should respond to antibiotic therapy within 48 to 72 hours. The patient should become afebrile, and the white blood cell count should decrease. If signs of peritonitis were present on admission, these should be abating, the patient's appetite should be returning, and a general sense of well-being should be present. However, if the patient continues to have spiking temperatures (101° F), a persistent or elevated white blood cell count, and no change in the physical findings, it is imperative that a pelvic examination be repeated.

If a mass is detected, an ultrasonogram should be obtained, which may provide information concerning the number of masses, their size, whether they are unilocular or multilocular, and their location with respect to the uterus and bowel. The thickness of the wall of the mass can also be evaluated. This information may have a bearing on the treatment plan. A thick-walled multilocular mass is probably less likely to respond to antibiotic therapy than is a thin-walled, unilocular mass. The thick rind that is commonly found encasing a tuboovarian abscess is usually associated with thrombosed vessels that supply the abscess. This implies that blood flow is minimal at best, and the tissue may be necrotic. Antibiotics cannot be carried to the infected sites in sufficient quantities, nor can they penetrate the thick wall of the abscess. Thus the effectiveness of the antibiotic will be limited to preventing bacteremia, and it will not eradicate the abscess. In addition, ultrasonography may assist in fa-

cilitating percutaneous drainage of the abscess. Specimens obtained should be cultured for the organisms mentioned thus far.

If a pelvic mass is present, a computed tomography (CT) scan will detail its location with respect to other structures, identify whether it is solid or cystic, and provide information about the nature of the fluid it contains (e.g., blood, pus, serous fluid). The CT scan is also of assistance in detecting and locating intraabdominal abscesses, including interloop bowel and subhepatic and subdiaphragmatic abscesses. The location of the abscess is important because it will determine whether percutaneous drainage can be attempted or whether laparotomy is needed. The presence of gas in the abscess cavity indicates that anaerobic organisms are present. Gas in the tissue planes of the abscess suggests that a necrotizing infection is present (e.g., a clostridial or bacterial synergistic infection making surgical intervention imperative).

There are no specific clinical findings or laboratory tests that establish the presence of PID. Ideally laparoscopy should be performed to examine the pelvic cavity, but if this is not possible culdocentesis may prove helpful.

Before performing culdocentesis, a digital vaginal-rectal examination should be done to determine whether the cul-de-sac is clear. Combining this examination with ultrasonography will help make the culdocentesis successful. The fluid aspirated via culdocentesis can provide important clues for diagnostic evaluation and patient management. The presence of purulent fluid is suggestive of acute salpingitis. A ruptured tuboovarian abscess or pyosalpinx is unlikely unless the patient has signs of peritonitis or a mass on examination. Aspiration of nonclotting blood suggests an ectopic pregnancy, hemorrhagic corpus luteum, or retrograde menstruation. Aspiration of blood that clots suggests that the bleeding is recent or that a vessel has been injured. If serous fluid is aspirated, it should be gram stained and the fluid also tested for amylase. If numerous white blood cells are found, the patient may be suffering from acute salpingitis or another acute inflammatory process, such as appendicitis or pancreatitis.

Laparoscopy enables a more definitive examination of the fallopian tubes, ovaries, uterus, and cul-de-sac. Fluid from the cul-de-sac should be aspirated via the laparoscope and cultured for aerobic and anaerobic bacteria associated with salpingitis. If a tissue biopsy is obtained from the fallopian tube or adhesive tissue is removed, it should also be cultured as directed earlier. If an abscess is found at the time of laparoscopy, it should be drained and a catheter left in place to allow continued drainage and permit lavaging of the abscess cavity. If the pelvic organs cannot be seen and evaluated, or the patient is believed to have right-sided salpingitis and the appendix cannot be examined, laparotomy should be performed.

An exploratory laparotomy is also indicated in patients with a surgical abdomen who are suspected of having a ruptured or leaking tuboovarian abscess. If the tubes are inflamed but not occluded, the pelvis and abdomen should be irrigated copiously with saline. If pyosalpinx is present unilaterally or bilaterally, salpingostomies should be performed. Fluid obtained should be gram stained and cultured. If tuboovarian abscesses are present, a bilateral salpingo-oophorectomy is indicated. In those infrequent instances in which only one adnexum is abscessed and the contralateral adnexum is normal, the involved adnexum should be removed.

Operative management of the tuboovarian abscess begins with thorough counseling of the patient. It is imperative that the patient understand that removal of her reproductive organs will place her in a postmenopausal state. She will require hormone replacement, which may not be entirely successful in relieving the vasomotor symptoms, and she may note a decrease in her desire for sexual activity. Injury to the bowel may necessitate a colostomy, and there is the risk that one or both ureters may be damaged.

Another approach to the operative management of tuboovarian abscess is incision and drainage. This approach is especially important to consider in the young nulliparous patient. The procedure may be accomplished via a percutaneous approach using ultrasonography, CT scan, laparoscopy, or laparotomy. Regardless of which method is used, a catheter should be left in place to allow for drainage and lavage with an antibiotic solution.

Time may not be sufficient to allow for preoperative bowel preparation, but high-dose antibiotics should be administered before commencing the operative procedure. Intravenous fluid should be administered, and the patient should be stable, in electrolyte balance, and euglycemic if possible. A ruptured tuboovarian abscess is to be considered life-threatening, and such patients are at risk for gram-negative sepsis. If aggressive management is not undertaken, they are likely to progress rapidly from sepsis to septic shock to adult respiratory distress syndrome. Therefore operative intervention should not be delayed.

The operative procedure begins with a generous vertical incision. The subdiaphragmatic, subhepatic, and subpelvic areas should also be thoroughly explored for abscesses. The appendix should be examined to determine whether it is ruptured. The appendix may be densely adherent to the tuboovarian abscess, making it difficult to determine its degree of involvement; in such a case, the appendix will have to be removed. Once the pelvic organs have been identified and isolated, a decision must be made as to whether they should be removed or drainage attempted.

If the patient is nulliparous or desires to retain her reproductive organs, drainage may be attempted but may be unsuccessful; she should be apprised of this and also of the possibility that her condition may fail to improve or may deteriorate, necessitating a total hysterectomy with bilateral salpingo-oophorectomy. If drainage is to be undertaken, the abscesses should be opened and all loculations disrupted. If necrotic or gangrenous tissue is present, the adnexa should be removed. Drains, preferably Jackson-Pratt or of similar large bore, should be placed into the cavities created and attached to a closed suction apparatus. The drains also

can be used to lavage the cavities with antibiotic solution. Tetracycline antibiotics (including doxycycline) can cause significant adhesion formation and therefore should not be used.

A diagnosis of diverticulitis should be entertained in patients who are over 35 years of age and have PID and a pelvic mass, especially in the left lower quadrant. Diverticulitis is a likely cause, especially in those patients with a unilateral adnexal mass. Patients with diverticulitis are at risk for having an inflamed diverticulum become adherent to the fallopian tube or ovary. Pressure necrosis may occur at the point of attachment, thus providing a conduit for the passage of infected material from the colon (diverticulum) into the adnexa. Infection is likely to occur, which can develop into an abscess. These patients have pain and localized peritonitis. If the abscess should leak, then generalized peritonitis may occur. A CT scan with contrast can outline the diverticulum and the adnexal mass.

Patients should have a bowel preparation performed before undergoing surgery, since the area of bowel involved in this process is often indurated, inflamed, and infected. A colostomy may be necessary, particularly if a primary anastomosis cannot be performed. A broad-spectrum antibiotic regimen should be initiated for these patients (see the box below).

Management

The most difficult decision regards whether a hysterectomy is necessary when the fallopian tubes and ovaries are abscessed (a tuboovarian abscess). If it is a unilateral condition, a unilateral salpingo-oophorectomy can be performed with preservation of the contralateral adnexa. Often a pyosalpinx is present and the ovary is not involved. However, adhesions that involve the ovary usually are present, which often necessitates a salpingo-oophorectomy. If the ovary appears normal and the capsule of the ovary has not been violated, the ovary does not need to be removed. Leaving one or both ovaries in place allows the patient the opportunity of in vitro fertilization and an endogenous supply of estrogen, progesterone, and androgens. If both tubes and ovaries are abscessed, the decision becomes more difficult. Currently it is more common to perform a total hysterectomy with a bilateral salpingo-oophorectomy. However, consideration should be given to preserving the uterus, since it is not affected by the disease process. This permits the patient to consider embryo transfer as a possibility for bearing children. Whatever the extent of the surgery, the procedure

---

ANTIBIOTIC REGIMENS FOR POLYMICROBIC INFECTIONS

1. Piperacillin/tazobactam
2. Clindamycin + ampicillin + gentamicin
3. Metronidazole + ampicillin + gentamicin

along with its possible complications should be explained in detail before the operation. The following complications are possible: damage to the bladder, ureters, and bowel; the possibility of a colostomy, hemorrhage, recurrent infection, or pulmonary embolus; and the possibility of additional operative procedures.

If the abdomen and pelvis contain free pus at the time of laparotomy, regardless of the amount, and the pelvic organs are inflamed but no abscess is found, then no tissue or organ need be removed. Often the tube appears to be markedly edematous if the fimbriae are not completely agglutinated and the tube is patent, but nothing need be done surgically. The edema and inflammation will resolve, and healing may occur with little residual scarring. The pelvis and abdomen should be irrigated with copious amounts of saline (3 to 6 L), and all fluid should be removed. Some individuals prefer to use an antibiotic-containing solution. The author has not found this necessary or advantageous. When the abdomen is opened and subjected to the atmosphere, the oxygen present is toxic to the anaerobes, and the number of aerobic and facultative bacteria is reduced to unimportant concentrations by the washing, leaving an inoculum too small to induce infection. Couple this with the fact that antibiotic serum and tissue levels will be maintained during as well as after the operative procedure, and continuation of the infection is unlikely. The remaining inoculum size will be too small to effectively reproduce in the presence of adequate antibiotic concentrations. If an inoculum is left behind in an area not adequately served by antibiotics, then a reinfection is likely, but since the bowel has not been injured, bacteria will not leak into the pelvic cavity, so infection is not likely to occur. If purulent fluid is found upon entering the abdomen, an aliquot should be aspirated, placed in an anaerobic transport vial, and immediately taken to the laboratory. The specimen should be gram stained and processed for the isolation of aerobic, facultative, obligate, gram-positive, and gram-negative bacteria. The grain stain can be of great value in modifying antibiotic therapy. The patient is most likely taking a cephalosporin (e.g., cefotetan, cefoxitin, ceftizoxime) or clindamycin plus gentamicin, since these are the most commonly used antibiotics for the treatment of PID. Doxycycline may or may not be given at this time. If the gram stain reveals the presence of gram-positive cocci, streptococci or enterococci may be present. All but the latter organism are covered by any of the antibiotic regimens given above. Ampicillin should be added to the currently administered antibiotic regimen if enterococcus is suspected. A great deal of concern has been voiced over the significance of *Chlamydia;* whether it is isolated or not, it is recommended that the patient receive antibiotic therapy that is effective in eradicating this organism. We have not frequently found *C. trachomatis* in the presence of advanced pelvic inflammatory disease. However, the patient receiving clindamycin plus gentamicin should be well covered. Clindamycin has been shown to have activity against *C. trachomatis.* The combination of clindamycin plus gentamicin has recently been shown to be synergistic in vitro against *C. trachomatis.*[40]

Once the patient's abdomen and pelvis have been completely and thoroughly washed, the bowel should be completely inspected, and if adhesions are found between loops of bowel, they should be taken down carefully. This may be done easily by sharp dissection. If blunt dissection is employed and resistance is encountered in attempting lysis of adhesions between loops of bowel, bowel and peritoneum, or bowel and another organ, this technique should be abandoned and sharp dissection used. It is important not to damage the serosa of the bowel, since this causes the formation of dense adhesions and may result in bowel obstruction. Since the bowel may be edematous, vigorous lysis of adhesions may result in evulsion of large amounts of serosa, thus exposing the subserosal surface. If the bowel is further traumatized or becomes greatly distended, spontaneous breaks in the mucosa can occur. This can result in leakage of bowel contents, carrying bacteria into the peritoneal cavity. Peritonitis and intraperitoneal abscesses can develop. This necessitates a second exploratory laparotomy, which increases the risk for intraoperative complications, as well as for infection.

If the patient is found to have a pyosalpinx, unilaterally or bilaterally, and the ovaries are not involved in the infectious process, a neosalpingostomy is acceptable. The fallopian tubes should be copiously irrigated with sterile saline. A single stitch of permanent monofilament suture 40 gauge should be used to fix the ends of the incised fimbriae to the tubal serosa. The patient must be informed that this procedure was performed and that she is now at risk for ectopic pregnancy. If possible, a small tubal specimen from the end of the tube that was opened should be excised and cultured, especially for *N. gonorrhoeae* and *C. trachomatis.*

Parenteral antibiotic therapy should be continued until the patient has been afebrile for 48 hours, is tolerating oral liquids and solid nourishment, and pulse and white blood cell count is normal. A pelvic examination should be performed to determine if the pelvic organs are normal. The patient requires antibiotic therapy for at least an additional 7 days. The choice should depend on whether *Chlamydia* was present. If the organism was isolated, then the patient should receive doxycycline; if it was absent and the infection was polymicrobial, then perhaps amoxicillin/clavulanic acid (Augmentin) (500 mg orally three times a day for 10 days) (Table 33-1).

Table 33-1 Oral Antibiotic Regimens for Posthospital Treatment of PID

Antibiotic	Dosage	Duration (days)
Augmentin (Ampicillin/clavulanic acid)	500 mg tid	10
Metronidazole + oxfloxacin	500 mg bid	10
	300 mg bid	10
Clindamycin + oxfloxacin	450 mg tid	10
	300 mg tid	10
Trovafloxacin	300 mg qd	10

Ideally the patient should be reexamined within 72 hours of being discharged from the hospital to determine whether an exacerbation of the infection is occurring, whether the medication is being taken appropriately, and to emphasize the serious nature of the infection. This education process is necessary and can be accomplished only by informing the patient that her infection could yet result in serious sequelae. The patient also should be given oral contraceptive pills to prevent pregnancy and possible abscess formation if the infection has not been eradicated. Her sex partner should be examined, and if she was found to harbor the gonococcus or *Chlamydia,* he also should be treated. It would be advisable for her to have complete pelvic rest for at least 3 to 6 weeks after discharge from the hospital. Patients who have undergone an exploratory laparotomy but have not had a hysterectomy should have a laparoscopic examination 6 weeks after they have recovered from their initial infection. This is necessary to assess the residual damage from the infection and surgery. At this time patency of the fallopian tubes can be assessed, lysis of adhesions can be performed, and a determination of the result of the initial infection can be established. A more definitive prognosis can be afforded the patient then, as well as guidelines to follow if she desires pregnancy.

REFERENCES

1. Adam E, Kaufman RH, Adler-Storthz K, et al: A prospective study of association of herpes simplex virus and human papillomavirus infection with cervical neoplasia in women exposed to diethylstilbestrol in utero, *Int J Cancer* 35:19, 1985.
2. Aly R, Britz MB, Marbach HI: Quantitative microbiology of human vulva, *Br J Dermatol* 101:445, 1979.
3. Amsel R, Totten PA, Spiegel CA, et al: Nonspecific vaginitis: diagnostic criteria and microbial and epidemiologic association, *Am J Med* 74:14, 1983.
4. Beatty WL, Byrne GI, Morrison RP: Morphological and antigenic characterization of interferon-l-mediated persistent *Chlamydia trachomatis* infection in vitro, *Proc Natl Acad Sci USA* 90:3998, 1993.
5. Beatty WL, Morrison RP, Byrne GI: Characterization of long-term chlamydial persistence and recovery of infectivity in cell culture, abstract D-151, Washington, DC, 1993 American Society of Microbiology.
6. Becker TM, Blount JH, Douglas J, Judson FN: Trends of molluscum contagiosum in the United States 1966-83, *Sex Transm Dis* 13:88, 1986.
7. Bhatia NN, Bergman A, Broen TM: Advanced hidradenitis suppurativa of the vulva: a report of three cases, *J Reprod Med* 29:436, 1984.
8. Brown D Jr, Kaufman RH, Gardner HL: Gardnerella vaginalis vaginitis: the current opinion, *J Reprod Med* 29:300, 1984.
9. Byrne GI, Krueger DA: Lymphokine-mediated inhibition of *Chlamydia psittaci* replication in mouse fibroblasts in neutralized by anti-gamma interferon immunoglobulin, *Infect Immun* 42:1152, 1986.
10. Byrne GI, Lehemann LK, Landry GJ: Induction of tryptophan catabolism is the mechanism for gamma-interferon-mediated inhibition of intracellular *Chlamydia psittaci* replication in T24 cells, *Infect Immunol* 53:347, 1986.
11. Corey L, Holmes KK: Genital herpes simplex virus infection: current concepts in diagnosis, therapy, and prevention, *Ann Intern Med* 98:973, 1983.
12. Crombleholme WR, Ohm-Smith M, Robbie MO, et al: Ampicillin/sulbactam versus metronidazole-gentamicin in the treatment of soft tissue pelvic infections, *Am J Obstet Gynecol* 156:507, 1987.
13. Dodson MR, Fare S: The polymicrobial etiology of acute pelvic inflammatory disease and treatment regimens, *Rev Infect Dis* 7:696, 1985.
14. Faro S, Phillips LE: Nonspecific vaginitis or vaginitis of undetermined etiology, *Int J Tissue React* 9(2):173, 1987.
15. Faro S et al: Ceftizoxime versus cefotaxime in the treatment of hospitalized patients with pelvic inflammatory disease, *Curr Ther Res* 43:349, 1985.
16. Galasso GJ, Manire GP: Effect of antiserums and antibiotics on persistent infection of HeLa cells with meningopneumonitis virus. *J Immunol* 86:382-385, 1961.
17. Gardner HC, Dukes CD: Haemophilus vaginalis vaginitis: a newly defined specific infection previously classified "nonspecific" vaginitis, *Am J Obstet Gynecol* 69:962, 1955.
18. Hammann R, Kronibus A, Lang N, Werner H: Quantitative studies on the vaginal flora of asymptomatic women and patients with vaginitis and vaginosis, *Zentralbl Bakteriol Mikrobiol Hyg* 265:451, 1987.
19. Hartford SL, Silva PD, diZerega GS, Yonekura ML: Serologic evidence of prior chlamydial infection in patients with tubal ectopic pregnancy and contralateral tubal disease, *Fertil Steril* 47:118, 1987.
20. Henry-Suchet J, Utzmann C, De Brux J, et al: Microbiologic study of chronic inflammation associated with robot factor infertility: role of *Chlamydia trachomatis, Fertil Steril* 47:274, 1987.
21. Hill LVH: Anaerobes and *Gardnerella vaginalis* in nonspecific vaginitis, *Genitourin Med* 61:114, 1985.
22. Holst E, Wathne B, Hovelius B, Mardh PA: Bacterial vaginosis: microbiological and clinical findings, *Eur J Clin Microbiol* 6:536, 1987.
23. Judson FN, Tavelli BG: Comparison of clinical and epidemiological characteristics of pelvic inflammatory disease classified by endocervical cultures of *N. gonorrhoeae* and *Chlamydia trachomatis, Genitourin Med* 62:230, 1986.
24. Kirshon B, Faro S, Phillips LE, Pruett K: Correlation of ultrasonography and bacteriology of the endocervix and posterior cul-de-sac of patients with severe pelvic inflammatory disease, *Sex Transm Dis* 15:103, 1988.
25. Kristensen GB, Bollerup AC, Lind K, et al: Infections with *Neisseria gonorrhoeae* and *Chlamydia trachomatis* in women with acute salpingitis, *Genitourin Med* 61:179, 1985.
26. Larsen B, Galask RP: Vaginal microbial flora: composition and influences of host physiology, *Ann Intern Med* 96:926, 1982.
27. Leegaard M: The incidence of *Candida albicans* in the vagina of healthy young women, *Acta Obstet Gynecol Scand* 63:85, 1984.
28. Lidbeck A, Gustafsson JA, Nord CE: Impact of *Lactobacillus acidophilus* supplement on human oropharyngeal and intestinal microflots, *Scand J Infect Dis* 19:531, 1987.
29. Lidbeck A, Edlund C, Gustafsson JA, et al: Impact of *Lactobacillus acidophilus* on the normal intestinal microflora after the administration of two antimicrobial agents, *Antimicrob Agents Inf* 16:329, 1988.
30. Lycke E, Lowhagen GB, Hallhagen G, et al: The risk of transmission of genital *Chlamydia trachomatis* infection is less than that of genital *Neisseria gonorrhoeae* infection, *Sex Transm Dis* 7:6, 1980.
31. Mann MS et al: Treatment of cervical chlamydial infection with amoxicillin/clavulanate potassium, *Infect Dis Obstet Gynecol* 1:104, 1993.
32. Mardh PA, Lind I, Svensson L, et al: Antibodies to *Chlamydia trachomatis, Mycoplasma hominis and Neisseria gonorrhoeae* in sera from patients with acute salpingitis, *Br J Vener Dis* 57:125, 1981.
33. Moller BR, Mardh PA, Ahrons S, Nussler E: Infection with *Chlamydia trachomatis, Mycoplasma hominis, and Neisseria gonorrhoeae* in patients with acute pelvic inflammatory disease, *Sex Transm Dis* 8:198, 1981.
34. Morrison RP, Lyng K, Caldwell HD: Chlamydial disease pathogenesis: ocular hypersensitivity elicited by a genus-specific 57-kD protein, *J Exp Med* 169:663-667, 1989.
35. Mortimer PS: Mediation of hidradenitis suppurative by androgens, *Br Med J* 292:245, 1986.

36. Mortimer PS, Dawber RP, Gales MA, Moore RA: A double-blind controlled cross-over trial of cyproterone acetate in females with hidradenitis suppurativa, *Br J Dermatol* 115:263, 1986.

37. Moulder JW: The psittacosis group as bacteria. *CIBA lectures in microbial biochemistry,* New York, 1964, John Wiley & Sons.

38. Moulder JW, Levy NJ, Schulman RP: Persistent infection of mouse fibroblast (L-cells) with *Chlamydia psittaci:* evidence for a cryptic chlamydial form, *Infect Immunol* 30:874, 1980.

39. Nettleman MD, Jones RB: Cost-effectiveness of screening women at moderate risk for genital infections caused by *Chlamydia trachomatis, JAMA* 260:207, 1988.

40. Pearlman MD, Faro S, Riddle GD, Tortolero G: In vitro synergy of clindamycin and aminoglycosides against *Chlamydia trachomati, Antimicrob Agents Chemother* 34:1399, 1990.

41. Rice DP, Hodgson TA, Kopstein AN: The economic costs of illness: a replication and update, *Health Care Fin Rev* 7:61, 1985.

42. Rothermel CD, Rubin BY, Murray HW: l-interferon in the factor in lymphokine that activates human macrophages to inhibit intracellular *Chlamydia psittaci* replications, *J Immunol* 131:2542, 1983.

43. Shemer Y, Sarov I: Inhibition of growth of *Chlamydia trachomatis* growth, *Curr Microbiol* 16:9, 1987.

44. Spence MR: Epidemiology of sexually transmitted disease, *Obstet Gynecol Clin North Am* 16:453, 1989.

45. Spiegel CA, Amsel R, Holmes KK: Diagnosis of bacterial vaginosis by direct gram-stain of vaginal fluid, *J Clin Microbiol* 18:170, 1983.

46. Stamm WE, Guinan ME, Johnson C, et al: Effect of treatment regimens for *Neisseria gonorrhoeae* on simultaneous infection with *Chlamydia trachomatis, N Engl J Med* 310:545, 1984.

47. Su H, Watkins NG, Zhang YX, Caldwell HD: *Chlamydia trachomatis*–host cell interactions: role of the chlamydial outer membrane protein as an adhesin, *Infect Immunol* 58:1017, 1990.

48. Sweet RL, Blankfort-Doyle M, Robbie MO, Schacter J: The occurrence of chlamydial and gonococcal salpingitis during the menstrual cycle, *JAMA* 255:2062, 1986.

49. Tsai CC, Semmens JP, Semmens EC, et al: Vaginal physiology in the postmenopausal woman: pH value, transvaginal electropotentiated difference and estimated blood flow, *South Med J* 80:987, 1987.

50. Walters MD, Eddy CA, Gibbs RS, et al: Antibodies to *Chlamydia trachomatis* and risk for tubal pregnancy, *Am J Obstet Gynecol* 159:942, 1988.

51. Washington AE, Arno PS, Brooks MA: Economic cost of pelvic inflammatory disease, *JAMA* 255:1735, 1986.

52. Washington AE, Johnson RE, Sanders LL: *Chlamydia trachomatis* infection in the United States: what are they costing us? *JAMA* 257:2070, 1987.

53. Westergaard L, Phillipsen T, Scheibel J: Significance of *Chlamydia trachomatis* infection in postabortal pelvic inflammatory disease, *Obstet Gynecol* 60:322, 1980.

54. Westrom L: Effect of acute pelvic inflammatory disease, *Obstet Gynecol* 60:322, 1980.

55. Westrom L: Pelvic inflammatory disease: bacteriology and sequelae, *Contraception* 36:111, 1987.

56. Westrom L et al: Taxonomy of vaginosis: bacterial vaginosisa definition, *Scand J Urol Nephrol* 86:259, 1984.

57. Zhang YX, Stewart S, Joseph T, et al: Protective monoclonal antibodies recognize epitopes located on major outer membrane protein of *Chlamydia trachomatis, J Immunol* 138:575, 1987.

34 Methods of Female Sterilization

JAROSLAV F. HULKA

Female sterilization is a popular method of family planning in the United States. It is the leading method among married women over the age of 30, which also is the average age at which a woman in the United States undergoes sterilization. About 500,000 such operations are performed every year, about half of these at the time of delivery (postpartum sterilization) and about half in a nonpregnant state (interval). This chapter reviews the techniques available and appropriate for these procedures.

GENERAL CONSIDERATIONS

Voluntary sterilization is legal in the United States and is funded by the federal government through Medicaid. Certain selection criteria should be kept in mind when offering sterilization to appropriate patients. The patient should be *mature,* with her decision based on solid emotional grounds. She should be *informed,* aware of the contraception alternatives and of the risks of sterilization. Finally, she should be *unpressured,* not making this permanent decision under stress (e.g., during separation or divorce, at the time of delivery or abortion). Younger women (under 30) appear to have a greater risk for regret and a greater tendency to request reversal[28]; for these women, a more reversible technique should be offered.

Involuntary sterilization for mentally retarded patients is an option in many states. North Carolina has model legislation for this process, involving presentation and documentation of the patient's condition by parents or guardians to a judge while the clerk of court acts on behalf of the patient. When the judge is convinced that sterilization is in the patient's and society's best interest, a court order is issued directing the surgeon to sterilize the patient.

STERILIZATION AT CESAREAN SECTION
Pomeroy Technique

The Pomeroy technique is probably the one most commonly performed sterilization methods worldwide and serves as the gold standard against which other techniques are measured. Pomeroy's associates published his technique in 1930.[4] A loop of tube is elevated by forceps or Babcock, an absorbable no. 1 plain catgut suture creates a loop of the tube, and the loop is excised for documentation by the pathology laboratory. Fig. 34-1 illustrates this classic method.

Irving Technique

In 1924, Irving[17] described a method that does not destroy the tube and achieves high success. The isthmus is divided, and the proximal stump is buried in myometrium, with the distal stump buried in the leaves of the broad ligament (Fig. 34-2). This technique has had no known failures but is associated with more morbidity than simple tubal ligation. Because no tube is destroyed, reversibility of this technique is high.

Fimbriectomy

It is easy to grasp the distal end of the tube, ligate, and excise the fimbria. This results in permanent sterilization, since reversal is seldom successful. Failures in this technique have come from disregarding the fimbria ovarica, a strand of fimbria connecting the tube to the ovary. This structure maintains patency and allows pregnancy if it is not identified and separately divided (Fig. 34-3).

POSTPARTUM STERILIZATION

After vaginal delivery, sterilization can be accomplished with ease through a minilaparotomy incision just below the umbilicus, where the uterus and its tubes lie postpartum. The tubal ligation is best delayed until it is certain that the newborn is healthy. Postpartum sterilization often is deferred until 6 weeks after delivery. If the child is obviously robust and healthy, a comfortable plan is to have the delivery accomplished with a epidural catheter, leaving the catheter indwelling until the operating room or labor room is available for this elective procedure.

Minilaparotomy provides limited access to the tube, so the Irving technique or a fimbriectomy may not be feasible. The Pomeroy technique is the one most universally used in this situation. Care must be taken to ensure that the tube, not the round ligament, is operated on.

The Uchida technique[36] involves injection of saline-epinephrine solution into the tubal musculature to separate serosa from muscle layer. The edematous tube is incised, and the inner circular muscle of the tube can be identified and excised. The proximal stump is then buried beneath this edematous serosa, and the distal stump ligated outside the serosa (Fig. 34-4, p. 630). The reversibility of this technique depends entirely on how much of the inner circular tubal lumen is excised for the pathology specimen.

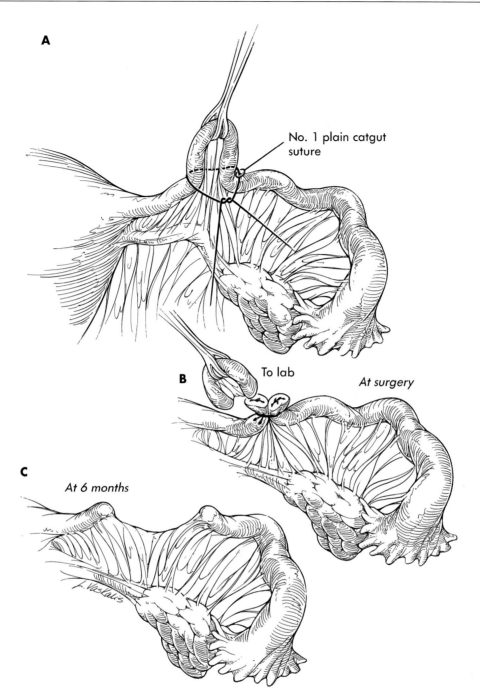

A

No. 1 plain catgut suture

B

To lab

At surgery

C

At 6 months

Fig. 34-1 Pomeroy technique. **A,** A Babcock clamp, scissors, and a length of no. 1 plain catgut are all the equipment necessary. **B,** A specimen confirms that tube and not round ligament was divided. **C,** Six months after division, the stumps have separated to about 3 cm apart. Elegantly simple and effective, this is the gold standard against which all other methods are compared.

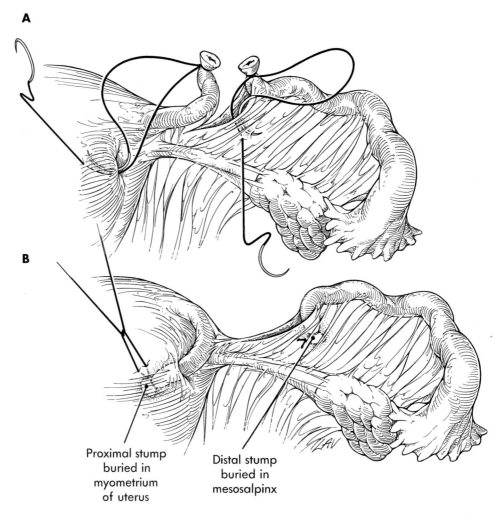

Proximal stump
buried in
myometrium
of uterus

Distal stump
buried in
mesosalpinx

Fig. 34-2   Irving technique. **A,** The divided isthmic stumps are drawn underneath peritoneum to ensure occlusion. **B,** The proximal stump is drawn under uterine, the distal stump under mesosalpingeal peritoneum. No failures with this method have been reported.

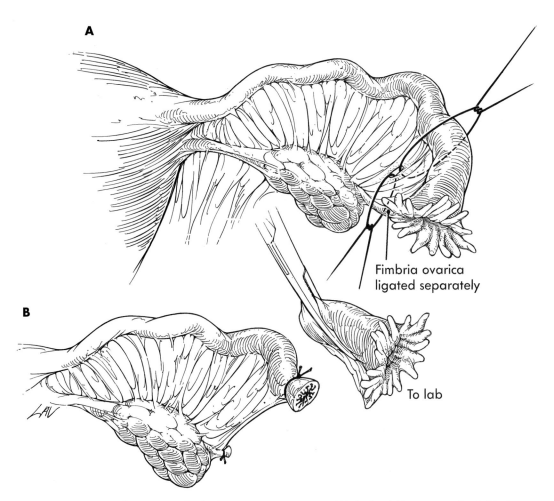

A

B

Fimbria ovarica
ligated separately

To lab

Fig. 34-3   Fimbriectomy. If a fimbria ovarica is present **(A)**, it should be separately divided to free the tubal fimbria for complete excision **(B).** This method is rarely reversed successfully.

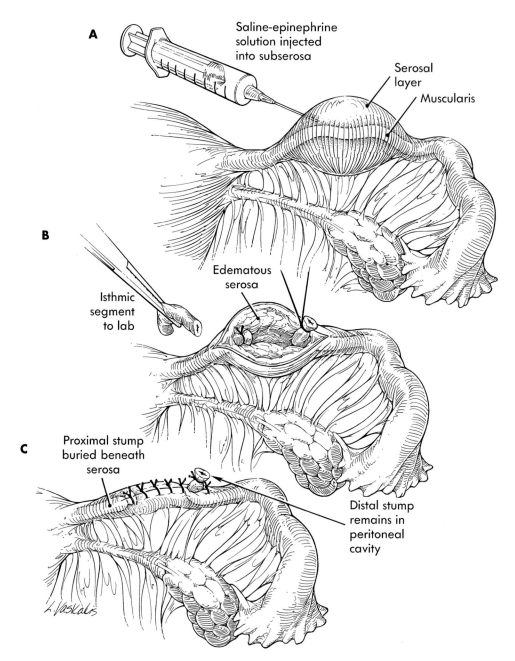

Fig. 34-4   Uchida technique. **A,** Saline-epinephrine solution dissects the loose longitudinal musculature from the hard inner circular muscle of the isthmus. **B,** Uchida recommends stripping and excising this inner segment to minimize failures. **C,** This distal stump is drawn and tied outside the mesosalpinx.

Clip Application

Although tantalum hemostatic clips do not work for tubal occlusion,[13] spring-loaded clips designed for laparoscopy can be placed by hand onto the postpartum tube.[19] The isthmus of the tube is held stretched between two Babcock clamps as the thumb and third finger close the jaws and the index finger pushes the spring into locked position (Fig. 34-5). Clips appear to cause lower morbidity compared to the Pomeroy technique, facilitating the mother's earlier recovery to full activity.

INTERVAL (NONPREGNANT) STERILIZATION

The introduction of laparoscopy in the 1970s was a major contributor to women's acceptance of sterilization as a method of family planning. The original unipolar electrocoagulation technique by Steptoe,[31] described in his textbook of laparoscopy, paved the way for worldwide use of the laparoscope and development of simpler and safer techniques.

Sterilization as an elective procedure not associated with pregnancy was infrequent before the acceptance of laparos-

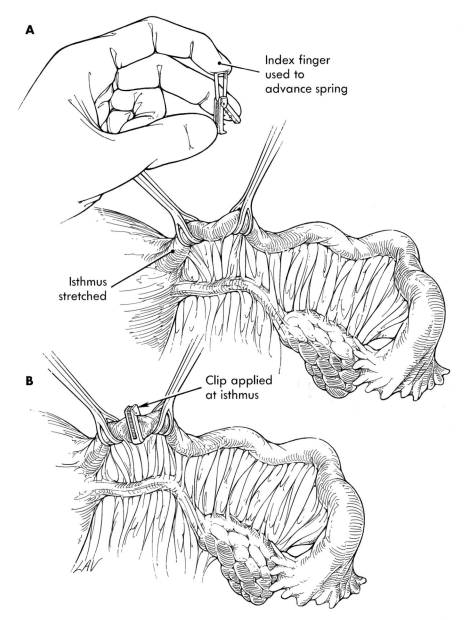

A

Index finger
used to
advance spring

Isthmus
stretched

B

Clip applied
at isthmus

Fig. 34-5   Clip at laparotomy. Two Babcocks, one close to the uterus, put a segment of isthmus on the stretch. **A,** A spring clip is held between thumb and third finger and placed on the stretched segment like a clothespin on a clothesline. **B,** The index finger pushes the metal spring over the plastic jaws to lock the clip on the isthmus.

copy. Many vaginal surgeons were performing a vaginal fimbriectomy as described by Kroener (see Fig. 34-3).[18] Other vaginal approaches incorporated the use of tantalum clips. However, compared with laparoscopic approaches, vaginal methods have been associated with a higher morbidity from postoperative infection, as well as higher pregnancy rates as a result of incomplete removal of the fimbria. Although a few good surgeons still recommend vaginal sterilization, this is no longer the trend in the United States.

Similarly, minilaparotomy has been introduced in developing countries as a means of avoiding the expensive equipment necessary for laparoscopy. In trained hands and with the patient under general anesthesia, minilaparotomy

is an effective and comfortable method of sterilization using the simple Pomeroy technique. However, with the patient under local anesthesia, abdominal entry usually is sufficiently uncomfortable to make this procedure less acceptable by patients, particularly if laparoscopy is available as an alternative. For this reason, minilaparotomy also has been abandoned in the United States except by a few skilled practitioners.

Unipolar Coagulation and Division

Unipolar coagulation and division was the first technique used by gynecologists learning both laparoscopy and electrocoagulation techniques. The tube is grasped, and current

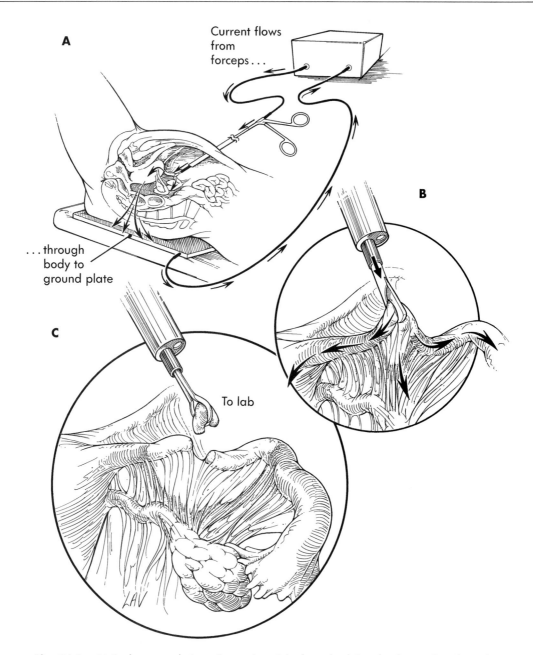

Fig. 34-6   Unipolar coagulation. Steptoe's original method involved grasping the tube **(A)**, elevating it **(B)**, and passing coagulating current through it until blanching occurred **(C).** Division with scissors sometimes resulted in bleeding from incompletely sealed mesosalpingeal vessels. Current running through the body caused skin and bowel burns.

is passed through the tube (and body) to a base plate (Fig. 34-6). This produces considerable destruction of the tube but is associated with hemorrhage from incompletely coagulated vessels severed at the time of tubal division. Deaths were associated with unipolar coagulation,[21] perhaps as much because of complications of trocar entry as electrocoagulation of bowel. This method was abandoned by most laparoscopists in favor of the less destructive techniques described below.

Bipolar Coagulation

Bipolar coagulation was developed independently in the early 1970s by Rioux in Canada, Kleppinger in the United

States, and Hirsch in Germany. The Kleppinger technique emerged as the most popular method of laparoscopic sterilization in the United States. The bipolar technique is the simplest to perform technically and is the most common method of laparoscopic sterilization today. The poles of the forceps conduct electricity between them, with no current flow beyond the forceps, so the patient is not part of the circuit (Fig. 34-7). Failures after bipolar coagulation have resulted from incomplete coagulation, sometimes because of inappropriate generators.[30] The end point of successful coagulation is indicated by a current flow meter on the appropriate or matched generator. When the flow diminishes and ceases, the tubal tissue has been desiccated to the point that

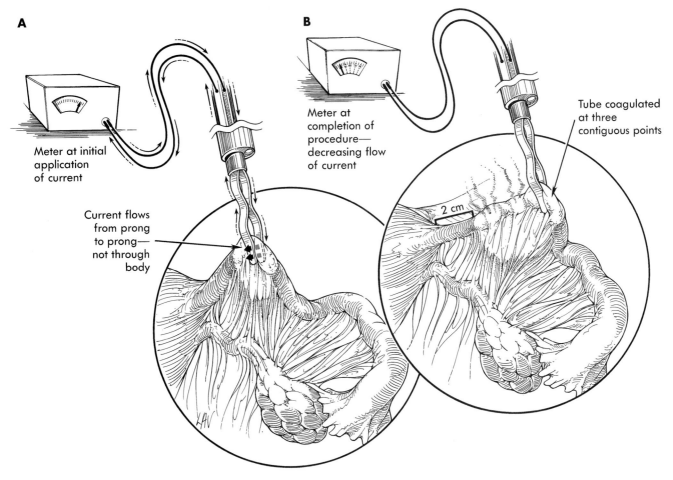

A

Meter at initial application of current

Current flows from prong to prong— not through body

B

Meter at completion of procedure— decreasing flow of current

Tube coagulated at three contiguous points

2 cm

Fig. 34-7   Bipolar coagulation. **A,** Current passes only through the tube from prong to prong of the forceps. **B,** Three contiguous burns are needed to prevent spontaneous recanalization. The end point for coagulation is tissue desiccation, at which point current ceases to flow through the dry, nonconducting tube. A meter on the generator to monitor current flow is thus necessary.

it no longer conducts electricity and the forceps can be moved to the next area for coagulation. Kleppinger stresses coagulation of three contiguous areas. This results in at least 3 cm of tube being destroyed and prevents spontaneous recanalization, occurring as a result of the healing process bringing the two stumps closely together.[9] Recent reports have noted a high incidence of ectopic pregnancy after bipolar coagulation,[20] which may be the result of fistula formation between the uterus and peritoneum when the tube is destroyed too close to the uterus.[32] Sperm can travel through these uteroperitoneal fistulas, reach the egg in the distal tubal segment, and cause an ectopic pregnancy (Fig. 34-8). This has led to the recommendation that the tube be grasped at least 2 to 3 cm away from the uterocornual junction at the time of sterilization so that a stump of isthmus remains to absorb the intrauterine fluid under pressure and minimize fistula formation.

Silastic Band Application

The Silastic band for sterilization was developed simultaneously by In Bae Yoon and Coy Lay in the early 1970s.

Widely distributed by the U.S. Agency for International Development, the band was offered as a nonelectric (and therefore safer) method of tubal occlusion. The fallopian tube is drawn 1.5 cm into a 0.5 cm diameter metal cylinder, destroying 3 cm of tube. A Silastic ring stretched on the outside of the cylinder is released to form an occlusion at the base of this knuckle (Fig. 34-9). Over time, about 3 cm of constricted tube undergoes necrosis and the tubes separate. Similar to the Pomeroy technique in theory, the laparoscopic application of band is associated with a 2.5% incidence of hemorrhage from stretching the vessels underneath the tube or tearing the tube itself. For this reason, Yoon et al.[40] have recommended that bipolar coagulation be available to manage this complication. Postoperatively, patients have pain from hypoxic necrosis of the tube in the band. This subsides in 48 to 96 hours and can be diminished somewhat by topical application of anesthesia at the time of band application.

Spring Clip Application

Devised in the 1970s as a mechanical alternative to electrocoagulation, the spring clip occludes the isthmus of the tube

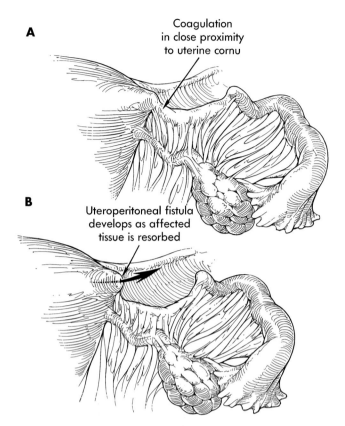

A

Coagulation in close proximity to uterine cornu

B

Uteroperitoneal fistula develops as affected tissue is resorbed

Fig. 34-8 Fistula formation. Destroying the isthmus too close to the uterus (**A**) may allow a uteroperitoneal fistula (**B**) to develop, through which sperm can reach the distal stump through the peritoneum. A fertilized ovum lodges as an ectopic pregnancy, a late serious complication of bipolar coagulation. Leaving a stump of isthmus should minimize this risk.

by two plastic jaws, compressing the tube by a stainless steel spring, pressing the jaws together.[14] Spring clip application by laparoscopy requires careful surgical technique to ensure that the clip is completely across the isthmus of the tube (Fig. 34-10). The Centers for Disease Control and Prevention (CDC) has recently published its findings of a 10-year follow-up study of several sterilization methods. High failure rates were reported the first 3 years after clip applications were made, presumably because of inadequate training leading to improper applications.[34,35] However, after the third year, annual clip pregnancy rates were similar to all other methods studied.

The spring clip is the most reversible of the techniques[28] because less than 5 mm of tube is destroyed between the jaws of the clip. For this reason, it should be considered for a woman under 30.

Cautery Techniques

True cautery is the direct application of heat to tissue, in contrast to electrocoagulation and desiccation, in which electrical energy flows through tissue and heats it. In the United States, the Waters technique involves drawing the tube into a 10-mm insulated sheath with an electrode hook

and applying current to the hook until the wire heats, cauterizes, and divides the tube in the sheath. The need for another 10-mm abdominal puncture has limited the appeal of this method. In Germany, the Semm Endotherm forceps is placed across the tube, and one prong of the forceps is heated to 100° C, cauterizing the tube. The time (30 to 60 seconds) required for each cautery has limited the popularity of this method.

TECHNIQUES UNDER INVESTIGATION

The laser has been tried for tubal division at laparoscopy but offers no advantage over standard techniques. Burying the fimbria in a pouch of broad ligament peritoneum and burying the ovary in an artificial plastic pouch have been evaluated in animals but have not been used with humans because of the increased morbidity compared to standard techniques. Various other clips have been devised (Bleier clip, Filshie clip). The Bleier clip has been discontinued because of a high pregnancy rate due to the tube's slipping into spaces within the jaws of the clip. The Filshie clip, a combination of tantalum and silicone, has recently been approved by the FDA for distribution in the United States, but there are few published articles concerning comparative efficacy of this method with others, or the extent to which this silicone implant is associated with systemic reaction.

A number of hysteroscopic approaches have reached the human trial stage only to prove less cost effective than standard laparoscopic techniques. In Europe, plastic tubal plugs developed by Steptoe in England and Hamou in France were abandoned after ectopic pregnancies developed. In the United States, the Silastic plug[8] was extensively evaluated[11] and found to be efficacious in about 85% to 90% of candidates, but technical failures persisted despite two or three hysteroscopic reapplications. The technique was intended to be reversible, but reversibility has not been demonstrated. Other hysteroscopic approaches have included destroying the endometrium by freezing or coagulation, but these approaches have been abandoned or are still in preclinical evaluation stages. Similarly, the introduction of methylcyanoacrylate (Crazy Glue) into the tube has been clinically tested overseas but is not ready for clinical use. Chinese researchers have experimented with formalin injection into the tube, but reports of the efficacy and safety of this approach are incomplete. Although there are still active research projects concerning alternative sterilization techniques, the existing laparoscopic approaches of mechanical or electrocoagulation tubal occlusion remain the standard against which these alternatives must be measured in terms of cost, efficacy, and safety.

STERILIZATION FAILURES

To study the pregnancy rate following sterilization techniques, a large number of patients (more than 1000) must be followed for a 2- to 3-year period with a high rate (over 85%) of follow-up. This enormously difficult task has been

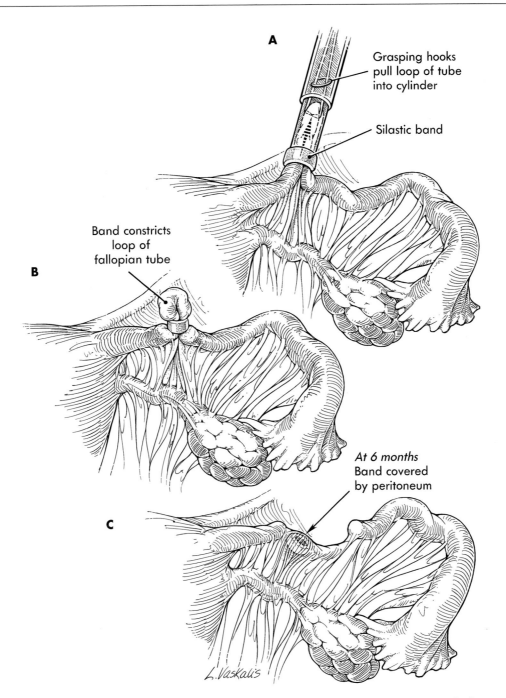

A, Grasping hooks pull loop of tube into cylinder

Silastic band

B, Band constricts loop of fallopian tube

At 6 months Band covered by peritoneum

L.Vaskalis

Fig. 34-9   Silastic band. **A,** About 3 cm of tube is drawn into a 5-mm cylinder over which a Silastic band has been stretched. **B,** Releasing the band constricts the knuckle of tube with eventual necrosis. **C,** As with the Pomeroy, 6 months later the stumps are about 3 cm apart.

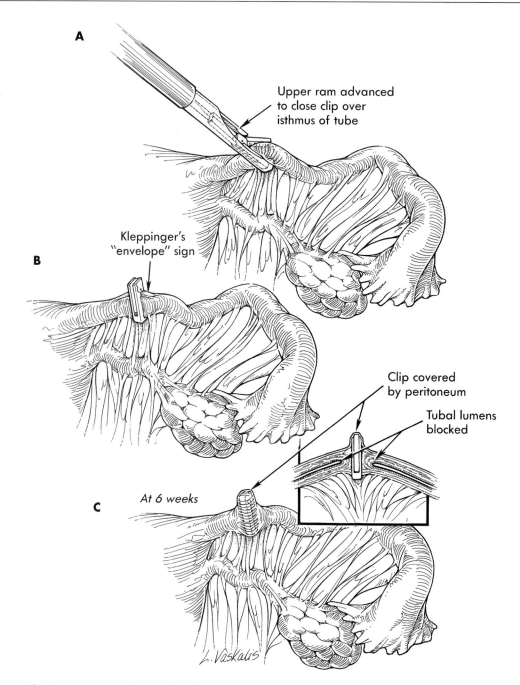

A

Upper ram advanced
to close clip over
isthmus of tube

B

Kleppinger's
"envelope" sign

Clip covered
by peritoneum

Tubal lumens
blocked

At 6 weeks

C

L. Vaskalis

Fig. 34-10 Spring clip. **A,** The isthmic portion (first 2 to 3 cm of tube) is maneuvered into the open jaws of the clip until it is snug against the hinge. **B,** Closing the clip will create the "Kleppinger envelope sign" **(C),** a fold of tubal peritoneum in the hinge of the clip. Failure to get the clip completely across the isthmus results in pregnancy. Some routinely use two clips close together on each tube.

accomplished very few times: by Johns Hopkins University in the early days of electrocoagulation and by the University of North Carolina in the development of the spring clip. The CREST study of the Centers for Disease Control and Prevention has revealed a much higher 10-year pregnancy rate than was first appreciated for all methods.[23] The latest ACOG technical bulletin on sterilization[1] found that the cumulative risk of pregnancy was highest among women sterilized at a young age with bipolar coagulation (54.3 per 1000) and spring-loaded clip application (52.1 per 1000). However, it is important to note that in another study of sterilization failures, all spring-loaded clip failures were attributed to misapplication.[33] The overall 10-year cumulative pregnancy rates for all methods was 18.5 (per 1000), with 24.8 for bipolar, 7.5 for unipolar, 17.7 for silicone rubber, 36.5 for spring clip, 20.1 for interval partial salpingectomy, and 7.5 for postpartum partial salpingectomy. Thus postpartum "Pomeroy" emerges as a far more effective sterilization method than had previously been thought.

Ectopic pregnancy is a rare but life-threatening form of pregnancy failure requiring early intervention for safe management. The most recent CDC study,[22] a 10-year follow-up study, found that 65% of all pregnancies following bipolar coagulation were ectopic, compared to 43% for interval "Pomeroy," 29% for band, 20% for postpartum "Pomeroy," 17% for unipolar coagulation, and 15% for spring clip.

For this reason, to minimize the risks of fistula formation we strongly recommend that a segment of isthmic tube next to the uterus be left when bipolar coagulation is used. Women with less tissue damage (from Pomeroy, band, and spring clip sterilization) have relatively less risk of ectopic pregnancy.

COMPLICATIONS
Morbidity and Mortality

With widespread teaching of laparoscopic sterilization, major complication rates, defined as those requiring laparotomy for repair, have remained below 2 : 1000 for the past decade. Mortality has not been reported since 1982.[16] This makes the one-time risk of sterilization comparable to the annual risk of morbidity from oral contraceptives and probably explains why this method is so popular among U.S. women whose families are complete.

Posttubal Syndrome

Approximately 6 million women in the United States have now undergone tubal sterilization. Many of these women's presenting symptoms are menometrorrhagia and pain, leading to the impression of a "posttubal syndrome" as a justification for hysterectomy. In an intensive analysis of this possibility, two prospective studies have recently been performed. Shain et al.[27] reported more initial menorrhagia, menstrual irregularity, and dysmenorrhea among women undergoing bipolar coagulation or Pomeroy ligation than among women undergoing mechanical tubal occlusion. Rulin et al.[26] reported a larger study showing only an increase in dysmenorrhea among sterilized women.

Endocrine Changes

In a related issue, sterilization altering ovarian function has been observed independently by Radwanska et al.[25] and Donnez et al.[7] In these studies, women who had undergone Pomeroy or coagulation sterilization had lower luteal progesterone levels (9 to 10 ng/ml) than normal controls or patients who had undergone clip sterilization (15 to 18 ng/ml). The authors postulated that extensive destruction of the vasculature with Pomeroy or coagulation interfered with luteal function. However, other studies in both humans[3] and animals have failed to confirm these studies. After salpingectomy and hysterectomy, monkeys failed to reveal significant alterations in ovarian endocrine secretion.[5] The conclusion to be drawn at the moment is that neither endocrine nor symptomatic changes after sterilization have been consistently reported and that the posttubal syndrome remains to be documented.

Regret and Reversibility

The permanent suspension of the reproductive function is not met with universal relief. Between 5% and 15% of women experience some form of regret over losing this function, but only 1% to 2% of sterilized women actually undergo reversal.[28] Because the average age of women requesting sterilization is 30, half of the requests are from women below this age. Recently, data from the United States[37] confirmed earlier findings that British[38] and Canadian[10] women under age 30 were more likely to request reversal later, usually after divorce and remarriage. The obstetrician-gynecologist thus faces a dilemma of whether to deny sterilization to hundreds of younger women who would benefit from the freedom from contraceptives and their risks in order to protect the reproductive ability of the few who may change their minds.

Recent experience with reversal has led to the insight, first proposed by Silber and Cohen,[29] that success of reversal sterilization is directly related to the length of tubal tissue remaining after sterilization. This was indirectly reported by Winston,[39] who found that anastomosis of isthmus to isthmus (after the least tubal damage) resulted in the highest success rates. A survey of microsurgeons who had performed reversal of clip sterilization[15] found an 87% intrauterine pregnancy rate. A review of the literature[28] revealed that unipolar coagulation, the most destructive method, had the lowest reversal rate, and the clip (least destructive) the highest. Fig. 34-11 presents the nature of the repair necessary after different sterilization techniques.

Selection of the sterilization technique appropriate to a young patient should include preserving the option of reversal by choosing a minimally destructive method. It is important to stress that all sterilization procedures are *permanent*, requiring microsurgical procedures for reversal. In this context, if women are contemplating more pregnancies later in life, sterilization is not appropriate. However, patients and doctors make honest mistakes, and the younger patient is at greater risk for requesting reversal after divorce and remar-

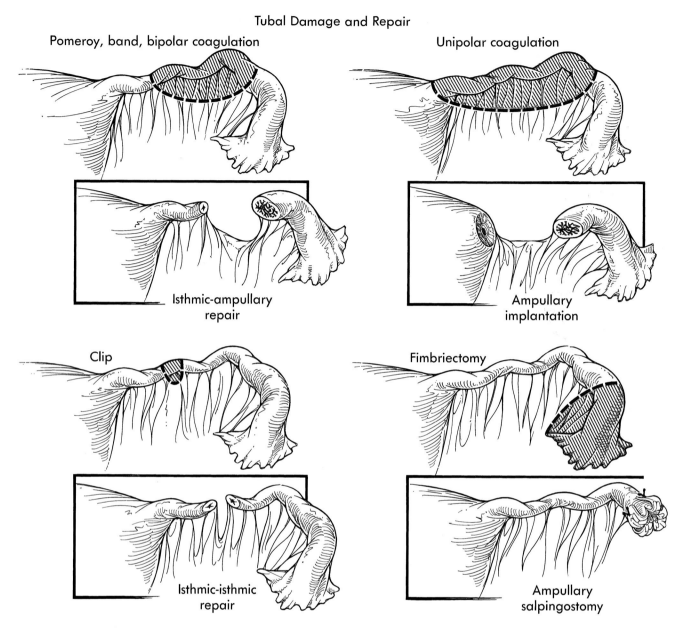

Tubal Damage and Repair

Pomeroy, band, bipolar coagulation

Isthmic-ampullary repair

Unipolar coagulation

Ampullary implantation

Clip

Isthmic-isthmic repair

Fimbriectomy

Ampullary salpingostomy

Fig. 34-11 Reversibility. Destroying a large portion of tube, particularly the junction of isthmus and ampulla, markedly diminishes the chance for a successful intrauterine pregnancy. (Adapted from Hulka JF: *Textbook of laparoscopy,* Philadelphia, 1985, Grune & Stratton.)

riage. This is the single area in which the spring clip appears to offer a clear advantage over other methods.

COMPARISON OF TECHNIQUES

The trend in laparoscopic sterilization in the United States has been away from unipolar coagulation in favor of bipolar coagulation, band, and clip. Fig. 34-12 presents the latest data, based on surveys of AAGL members.[16] A review of the literature concerning pregnancy failures and their management[12] revealed that no pregnancies were reported following the Irving procedure. Interestingly, cornual resection (a sterilization technique no longer recommended) had a

higher subsequent pregnancy rate than the Pomeroy technique, and these pregnancies were interstitial or ectopic.

All laparoscopic sterilizations have a method failure of between 2 and 5 pregnancies per 1000 procedures *per year,* with a 10-year cumulative rate ranging from 7.5/1000 to 54.3/1000. Failures appear to depend more on the age of the patient (young women are more fertile and more likely to be fertile again) and training of the physician than on the technique used.

The *bipolar* method is the simplest to perform and the most popular method in the United States today but requires proper matched equipment (forceps and generator). Failures continue for years after the procedure and often consist

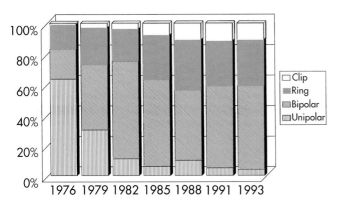

Fig. 34-12 Changing techniques in laparoscopic sterilization. Unipolar electrocoagulation has been displaced by bipolar coagulation as the leading method in the United States. (From American Association of Gynecologic Laparoscopists 1993 Membership Survey: *J Am Assoc Gynecol Laparosocp* 2:137, 1993.)

Table 34-1 Safety and Efficacy: Comparison of Sterilization Methods

	Coagulation	Band	Clip
Safety			
Days of readmissioin for complications	10.5	5.5	2.1
Late ectopic rate (%)	44	15	4
Reversibility			
Term pregnancies following reversal (%)	41	72	84
Efficacy			
1-year method failure range (rate per 1000)	1.9-2.6	3.3-4.7	1.8-5.9

Data from Chi IC et al,[6] Phillips JM et al,[24] and Siegler AM et al.[28]

of ectopic pregnancies, as recently reported from Scandinavia.[20] The cumulative bipolar failure rate in 6 years was 1.18%, all extrauterine. These authors urged the preservation of a 2 cm proximal isthmic stump to decrease the chance of subsequent fistula formation and ectopic pregnancy.

The *band* method is a widely used and good nonelectric method, although backup bipolar coagulation is recommended for occasional bleeding. Postoperative pain from the constricted tube is most severe with this technique.

The *clip* requires careful surgical technique to ensure proper placement across the isthmus of the tube. Nonetheless, it is the least destructive and therefore the most reversible technique and should be offered to women below age 30 seeking sterilization. Pregnancies after clip applications appear to occur mostly within the first 3 years, with long-term follow up studies showing few pregnancies afterward. Thus the long-term cumulative pregnancy rates with bipolar sterilization and the clip are similar.

Unipolar coagulation still has advocates among skilled practitioners, in whose hands patients will be well served, but this technique is not recommended for a younger patient who may later desire sterilization reversal.

Complication rates have been measured[6] for coagulation, band, and clip. All techniques had a similar rate of readmission for complications, but coagulation required a 10.5-day average stay (to rule out or manage bowel perforation); the band, 5.5 days (to rule out or manage pelvic infection); and the clip, 2.1 days, a statistically significant difference.

The comparative data available for safety and efficacy of different sterilization methods are summarized in Table 34-1.

I have consistently recommended that physicians choose the technique with which they are most comfortable and continue to provide this service to their patients until surgical misadventure or compelling reasons in the literature motivate a change of techniques.

REFERENCES

1. American College of Obstetricians and Gynecologists, Committee on Technical Bulletins with Pollack AE: Sterilization, ACOG Technical Bulletin 222, 1996.
2. American College of Obstetricians and Gynecologists: Sterilization for women and men, APO 11, April 1991.
3. Bhiwandiwala PP, Mumford SD, Feldblum PJ: A comparison of different laparoscopic sterilization occlusion techniques in 24,439 procedures, *Am J Obstet Gynecol* 144:319, 1982.
4. Bishop E, Nelms WF: A simple method of tubal sterilization, *N Y State J Med* 30:214, 1930.
5. Castracane VD, Moore GT, Shaikh AA: Ovarian function in hysterectomized Macaca fascicularis, *Biol Reprod* 20:462, 1979.
6. Chi IC, Potts M, Wilkens L: Rare events associated with tubal sterilizations: an international experience, *Obstet Gynecol Surv* 41:7, 1986.
7. Donnez J, Wauters M, Thomas K: Luteal function after tubal sterilization, *Obstet Gynecol* 57:65, 1981.
8. Erb RA, Reed TP: Hysteroscopic oviductal blocking with formed-in-place silicone rubber plugs: method and apparatus, *J Reprod Med* 23:65, 1979.
9. Fishburne JI Jr, Hulka JF: Tubal healing following laparoscopic electrocoagulation, *J Reprod Med* 16:129, 1976.
10. Gomel V: Profile of women requesting reversal of sterilization, *Fertil Steril* 30:39, 1978.
11. Houck RM et al: Hysteroscopic tubal occlusion with formed-in-place silicone plugs: a clinical review, *Obstet Gynecol* 62:587, 1983.
12. Hulka JF, Mitchell L: Resterilization after tubal sterilization failure. In Nichols DH, editor: *Reoperative gynecologic surgery,* St Louis, 1991, Mosby.
13. Hulka JF, Omran Kr: Comparative tubal occlusion: rigid and spring-loaded clips, *Fertil Steril* 23:633, 1972.
14. Hulka JF, Mercer JP, Fishburne JI, et al: Spring clip sterilization: 1-year follow-up of 1079 cases, *Am J Obstet Gynecol* 125:1039, 1976.
15. Hulka JF, Noble AD, Letchworth AT, et al: Reversibility of clip sterilizations, *Lancet* 2:927, 1982.
16. Hulka JF, Peterson HB, Phillips JM: American Association of Gynecologic Laparoscopists 1988 Membership Survey on Laparoscopic Sterilization, *J Reprod Med* 35:584, 1990.
17. Irving FC: A new method of insuring sterility following cesarean section, *Am J Obstet Gynecol* 8:335, 1924.
18. Kroener WF Jr: Surgical sterilization by fimbriectomy, *Am J Obstet Gynecol* 104:247, 1969.
19. Lee SH, Jones JS: Postpartum tubal sterilization: a comparative study of Hulka clip application and the modified Pomeroy technique, *J Reprod Med* 36:703, 1991.

20. Makar AP, Vanderheyden JS, Schatteman EA, et al: Female sterilization failure after bipolar electrocoagulation: a 6-year retrospective study, *Eur J Obstet Gynecol Reprod Biol* 37:237, 1990.

21. Peterson HB, DeStefano F, Rubin GL, et al: Deaths attributable to tubal sterilization in the United States, 1977 to 1981, *Am J Obstet Gynecol* 146:131, 1983.

22. Peterson HB, Xia Z, Hughes JM, et al: The risk of ectopic pregnancy after tubal sterilization: US Collaborative Review of Sterilization Working Group, *N Engl J Med* 336:762, 1997.

23. Peterson HB, Xia Z, Hughes JM, et al: The risk of pregnancy after tubal sterilization: findings from the US Collaborative Review of Sterilization, *Am J Obstet Gynecol* 174:1161, 1996.

24. Phillips JM, Hulka JF, Hulka B, Corson SL: American Association of Gynecologic Laparoscopists 1979 membership survey, *J Reprod Med* 26:529, 1981.

25. Radwanska E, Berger GS, Hammond J: Luteal deficiency among women with normal menstrual cycles, requesting reversal of tubal sterilization, *Obstet Gynecol* 54:189. 1979,

26. Rulin MC, Davidson AR, Philliber SG, et al: Changes in menstrual symptoms among sterilized and comparison women: a prospective study, *Obstet Gynecol* 74:149, 1989.

27. Shain RN, Miller WB, Mitchell GW, et al: Menstrual pattern change 1 year after sterilization: results of a controlled, prospective study, *Fertil Steril* 52:192, 1989.

28. Siegler AM, Hulka J, Peretz A: Reversibility of female sterilization, *Fertil Steril* 43:499, 1985.

29. Silber SJ, Cohen R: Microsurgical reversal of female sterilization: the role of tubal length, *Fertil Steril* 33:598, 1980.

30. Soderstrom RM, Levy BS, Engel T: Reducing bipolar sterilization failures, *Obstet Gynecol* 74:60, 1989.

31. Steptoe PC: *Laparoscopy in gynaecology,* Edinburgh, 1967, Livingstone.

32. Stock RJ: Histopathologic changes in tubal pregnancy, *J Reprod Med* 30:923, 1985.

33. Stovall TG, Ling FW, O'Kelley KR, Coleman SA: Gross and histologic examination of tubal ligation failures in a residency training program, *Obstet Gynecol* 76:461, 1990.

34. Stovall TG, Ling FW, Henry GM, Ryan GM Jr: Method failures of laparoscopic tubal sterilization in a residency training program: a comparison of the tubal ring and spring-loaded clip, *J Reprod Med* 36:283, 1991.

35. Stovall TG, Ling FW, Lipscomb GH, et al: A model for resident surgical training in laparoscopic sterilization, *Obstet Gynecol* 83:470, 1994.

36. Uchida H: Uchida tubal sterilization, *Am J Obstet Gynecol* 121:153, 1975.

37. Wilcox LS, Chu SY, Eaker ED, et al: Risk factors for regret after tubal sterilization: 5 years of follow-up in a prospective study, *Fertil Steril* 55:927, 1991.

38. Winston RML: Why 103 women asked for reversal of sterilisation, *Br Med J* 2:305, 1977.

39. Winston RML: Microsurgery of the fallopian tube: from fantasy to reality, *Fertil Steril* 34:521, 1980.

40. Yoon IB, King TM, Parmley TH: A 2-year experience with the Falope ring sterilization procedure, *Am J Obstet Gynecol* 127:109, 1977.

35 Adnexal Surgery for Benign Disease

DAN C. MARTIN

Laparoscopic techniques are replacing many laparotomy techniques for adnexal surgery. Some of the emphasis on laparoscopy is because of physicians' perceived need to admit patients who have had a laparotomy. However, laparotomy performed as an outpatient can be as cost effective and useful to patients as laparoscopy for many operations.[6] Laparoscopy is excellent for visualization. Palpation and handling are enhanced at laparotomy. Techniques for both approaches are covered in this chapter.

OVARIAN CYSTS

The chance of opening and spilling an ovarian cancer is a major concern that is balanced against a patient's need to preserve an ovary. This risk applies to both laparoscopy and laparotomy. If an ovarian cystectomy is to be performed, then preparation for any spill of tumor is necessary. Preoperative assessment by ultrasonography, magnetic resonance imaging, or tumor markers such as CA125, alpha-feta protein, and chorionic gonadotropin may be useful. These concepts are covered in Chapter 39 on malignant ovarian tumors.

Staging of ovarian cancer is necessary. Incomplete staging and treatment occurs not only at laparoscopy[64] but also at laparotomy.[109] Various protocols of staging include dilation and curettage, total hysterectomy with bilateral salpingo-oophorectomy if the patient does not wish to preserve fertility, cytologic washings of the pelvic cavity, washings from the pericolic gutters, washings from the subdiaphragmatic area, manual exploration of the upper abdomen, documentation of ascites, biopsy or resection of any adhesions adjacent to the primary tumor, examination for and biopsy of surface excrescences, examination for and biopsy of any solid areas, visualization and palpation of serosal surfaces of the large bowel, removal of the infracolic omentum if abnormal, aortic lymph node sampling, pelvic lymph node sampling, random biopsies of peritoneal sites including the pericolic gutters and hemidiaphragm, and wedge resection of the contralateral ovary if saved.[98,99,109]

Delay in treatment after inadvertent opening of an ovarian cancer may have significant implications.[64] The ill effects of spill of ovarian cancer at laparoscopy have been documented.[18,40,52,64] Implantation of cancer[19,33,52] has occurred at the trocar sites. Of note, only 7.4% of stage I ovarian cancer was removed using an endobag in one study.[52] Progression was noted in 53% of patients after this type of treatment. Implantation and metastasis have been microscopically visible as early as 8 days after surgery.[52] This occurs with both small and large incisions.[40,48,64] The CO_2 environment of laparoscopy may accentuate this problem.[112] Rupture may increase the stage of the patient's malignancy and mandate the use of chemotherapy in patients otherwise treated with surgery alone.[98]

If the ovary is to be removed intact at laparoscopy, bagging is used. The neck or entire bag is exteriorized through a small incision before opening the cyst. Since endometriosis and ovary can be transplanted into any incision,[17] bagging may be useful with endometriosis and dermoids in addition to malignancy.[17,65] Bagging also can decrease the operating time.[16] This can be accomplished even with large cysts with the bag placed and retrieved through a minilaparotomy, which can be extended if necessary. Allis clamps or temporary sutures maintain an air seal while the cyst is moved into the bag.

Drilling of cysts for diagnosis generally gives no additional histologic information. Because the therapeutic value of drilling is low and the potential for spill is high, aspiration of ovarian cysts should be abandoned.[46]

Teratomas

If ovarian cystectomy is to be performed, adequate control is needed to avoid rupture and spill. Laparotomy is used when control cannot be maintained at laparoscopy. Oophorectomy may sometimes be more reasonable than ovarian cystectomy for teratomas.

If a teratoma is spilled while doing a cystectomy with a head-down tilt, the patient and table must be reversed to put the head in an up position in order to keep the fluid in the pelvis. The pelvic volume is approximately 20 to 80 ml, and spill into the upper abdomen can occur rapidly with irrigation. Two (2.1%) episodes of peritonitis were reported among 97 patients who underwent puncture of a teratoma.[17]

Chocolate Cysts of the Ovary

Chocolate cysts of the ovary can be an endometrioma, residual of a hemorrhagic corpus luteum, or nonspecific. When these are opened and examined, the general appearance of an endometrioma is a mottled lining with red or brown areas on a white fibrotic base. Corpora lutea tend to have a smoother, more uniformly brown or yellow-brown lining. Biopsy specimens for confirmation of endometriosis are best taken from the red streaks of tissue coming off the base. Specimens taken from the brown areas frequently show hemosiderin for either old corpora lutea or endo-

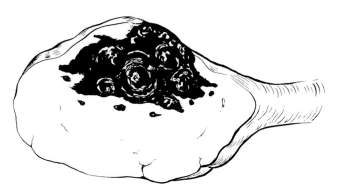

Fig. 35-1   Small ovarian endometriomas of up to 20 mm may be irregular in their infiltration and frequently have little or no fibrotic reaction.

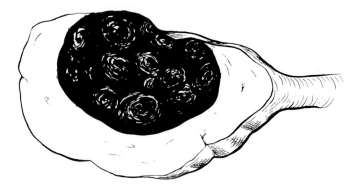

Fig. 35-2   As endometriomas exceed 2 cm, they are more likely to be flattened and have a regular round configuration. The interior content of these consists of blood and debris. A thin lining at the inner wall may have glands and stroma, a nonspecific hemosiderin containing lining, or a nonspecific flat lining. When these are greater than 2 cm, the glands and stroma have not infiltrated more than 1.5 mm into the fibrotic capsule. On the outside of the fibrotic capsule is a rim of healthy ovary that is removed in the process of stripping the ovaries.

metriomas. The chance that a biopsy will miss a cancer is small,* but the consequences are significant.[54,64] Stripping techniques can be used that remove the entire capsule for complete histologic analysis. However, these techniques are more difficult and may not be more effective for endometriosis than biopsy followed by coagulation. In addition, stripping removes not only the pseudocapsule but also a thin rim of healthy ovary immediately adjacent to the capsule. With large endometriomas, this small rim may have adequate volume to compromise the overall function of the ovary. Preoperative sonography and serologic markers may aid in clinical decisions regarding specific patients.

The chance that an unexpected ovarian cancer will be opened in treating endometriosis is small.[17,75,86] A larger concern may be identification.[43] The French experience with 629 masses showed 12 tumors with low malignant potential and 7 ovarian cancers.[17] The worry is that these more common cancers would be opened in the process of taking care of what is thought to be endometriosis. Biopsy of any peritoneal component needs to be performed for histology, especially with those of subtle appearance.[70,71] Morselization and extraction at laparoscopy should be avoided, since this can implant either cancer and endometriosis into the incision. When endometriomas are removed at laparoscopy, bagging with exteriorization of the bag before opening the bag is necessary to decrease spill and to decrease implantation into the incision.

Chocolate cysts less than 5 mm have little or no fibrotic reaction and tend to be irregular in their infiltration (Fig. 35-1). These are generally biopsied and then coagulated or vaporized. Various techniques are used for cysts between 5 to 20 mm and are chosen on the basis of the appearance as the procedure progresses. For cysts greater than 2 cm, the fibrotic reaction is prominent, and stripping of the pseudocapsule is accomplished in a slow but deliberate fashion. Stripping also may remove a rim of healthy ovary (Fig. 35-2). At laparotomy, Metzenbaum scissors can be used to spread through this area by progressively moving them into dissection plane. At laparoscopy, two grasping forceps are

usually all that are needed. However, as the cysts exceed 4 cm, a third grasping forceps or a transabdominal suture to hold the tissue to the anterior abdominal wall frequently increases visualization. In addition, a dissection technique using high-pressure water also may be useful in developing this tissue plane.[16,82]

As the stripping approaches the hilum, special attention and care are used to avoid the hilar vessels. When stripping is difficult in this area, generally the capsule is amputated above the hilar vessels and the remnant base coagulated. When these cysts have been greater than 5 cm, laparoscopies have taken up to 5 hours. Treating these large chocolate cysts by biopsy and coagulation followed by examinations and sonograms may help to preserve healthy ovarian tissue. However, this increases the risk of missing an ovarian cancer.[18]

In the management of these chocolate cysts, an incision is made at the most dependent portion so that the walls tend to collapse back together at the end of the procedure. Sutures are generally avoided, since suturing techniques have been shown to increase adhesions in both peritoneum[29,30,84] and in ovaries.[2,12,13,23,90] Furthermore, the highest pregnancy rates reported with ovarian cystectomy at laparoscopy was the 92% by Reich[93] when no other factors were present. This is similar to Martin's report of an 80% pregnancy rate following treatment of severe endometriosis using laser and no sutures.[67] When ovarian suturing is needed, laparotomy with true intracapsular closure is preferred. The use of fibrin glue has been suggested to avoid the ischemic sequelae of suturing.[1,27] This commercial glue is not yet available in the United States. Furthermore, results and complications of glues have mixed reports.

The risk of endometrioid ovarian cancer increases with age. Approximately 57% of patients with endometrioid carcinoma were postmenopausal. Ovarian endometriosis was

*References 17, 74, 75, 86, 89, 106.

coexistent in 26% of this group.[24] Hysterectomy decreases the general risk of ovarian cancer by half[88] and can be considered in any female. This may be relevant in patients with ovarian endometriosis.[24] Although hormone replacement therapy is of particular concern in endometriosis patients, 88% of exogenous endometrioid adenocarcinomas occur with no estrogen supplementation.[11]

An additional concern is the 20% overall increase in cancers noted in one study. An increased incidence of breast cancer was found in 63 patients, ovarian cancer in 14 patients, and non-Hodgkin's lymphoma in 13 patients in this group of 20,686 patients.[10] Since hysterectomy decreases the general risk of ovarian cancer by half,[88] this should be considered in patients with ovarian endometriosis.[24]

PROPHYLACTIC OOPHORECTOMY

The frequency of the routine use of prophylactic oophorectomy is variable. Fong[31] noted that 22% of English physicians routinely remove ovaries by age 49 as opposed to 81% of American physicians; 15% of English and 5% of American physicians do not routinely remove ovaries at any age. Several papers have recommended hysterectomy by age 40 and others at age 45.

There are several considerations regarding prophylactic oophorectomy at the time of hysterectomy. These includes the risk of cancer, the chance of reoperation for cysts, the chance of reoperation for endometriosis, the chance of reoperation for pain, increasing difficulty of ovarian removal when anatomy is distorted by previous surgery, the problems associated with surgical menopause, and the side effects and risks of hormone replacement therapy when used.*

Prophylactic oophorectomy seems reasonable in almost all cases involving a family history of ovarian cancer to decrease the risk of subsequent cancer. However, in low-risk patients, if the ovaries are normal at the time of hysterectomy, the chance of cancer in the future appears to be around 0.25%.[31]

There is also a 5% chance of reoperation with subsequent adnexal disease when the ovaries are saved. Most of these are cysts. In patients with pelvic pain, the reoperation rate had been reported to be as high as 47% in patients with endometriosis. Furthermore, surgical technical difficulty can be greater at a second surgery if the ovaries are removed in the presence of distorted anatomy.

Hormone replacement therapy is covered later in this chapter.

ADHESIONS
Needle and Trocar Insertion

In the treatment of patients with known pelvic or abdominal adhesions, insertion techniques are more important than usual.[37,47,53] Increased preparation of the patient for the possibility of bowel damage includes obtaining informed

---

*References 8, 20, 28, 35, 58, 81.

consent and performing bowel preparation. Although mini-laparotomy, open trocar insertion, and safety trocars have proponents who state a decreased chance of complications, this has not been the general observation in clinical use. Veress needle, direct insertion of reusable trocars, and direct insertion of disposable trocars revealed 22%, 6%, and 0% minor complications and no major complications.[85] There is no one technique that is universally accepted.[97]

Techniques of insertion include percussion of the gas in the stomach with use of nasogastric tubes for decompression when needed and percussion of liver dullness, using intraabdominal negative pressure to pull saline through the hub and injecting 10 ml of saline through the needle, followed by aspiration to check for contents.

Before surgery, informed consent and preoperative preparation for patients with histories of pelvic and abdominal adhesions and previous abdominal surgery need to include the possibility of laparotomy for bowel repair. Different general surgeons consider bowel preparation to be anything from helpful to essential in these patients.

Adhesion Prevention

Laparoscopic techniques result in fewer new adhesions than laparotomy techniques.[26,61,62] In addition, many studies have both suggested and denied that multiple agents help in adhesion prevention. Of the agents suggested, three are FDA approved—Interceed (TC7) (Johnson & Johnson Medical Division, Arlington, Tex.),[25,44] Gore-Tex (W. L. Gore and Associates, Inc., Flagstaff, Ariz.),[9] and Seprafilm (Genzyme, Cambridge, Mass.). The advantage of Interceed is that it can be cut into small pieces and laid into the pelvis through a laparoscope. At this time, Gore-Tex still requires suturing, is not absorbable, and, when used in infertility patients, needs a second operation for removal in order to allow egg transit. Seprafilm is approved for laparotomy but is very difficult to use at laparoscopy.

Lysis of Adhesions

Filmy adhesions (Fig. 35-3) can be lysed using several techniques. Although blunt dissection and lysis has been abdicated, the abraded surfaces, with their oozing and biochemical activity, may adhere more readily than surfaces that are cleanly cut and hemostatic. Data in the past suggest that adhesions are more common with ischemic tissue than dead tissue.[29,30,84]

Scissors and coagulation are very useful for making upper abdominal incisions from the omentum and epiploic fat to the anterior abdominal wall. These are progressively cut, and coagulation is used when bleeding occurs. Many of these adhesions are avascular. A significant area of concern is that the adhesions seen through the laparoscope can sometimes hide bowel on the other side. Care is taken to identify both sides of the adhesions when possible, and this sometimes includes placing the laparoscope through a lower port to obtain a view from the other side. Furthermore, in the attempt to avoid bowel, dissections have been kept so far anterior that the bladder has been entered. This has re-

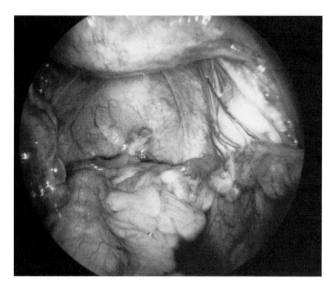

Fig. 35-3 Filmy adhesions are easy to lyse with any equipment. Blunt lysis is avoided, because this increases bleeding and petechial hemorrhage.

quired minilaparotomy, repair of the bladder, and indwelling catheterization.

Lasers and electrosurgery can be used to cut the adhesions under direct visualization. The electrosurgical knife and fiber-equipped lasers disperse rapidly in space and need no backstop. On the other hand, a CO_2 laser will continue in space until tissue is hit. This can be dangerous or it can be used to advantage by using the adherent tissue as its own backstop. A pulsed CO_2 laser technique is sometimes helpful in controlling this possibility.

Dense adhesions are more difficult to control with scissors and coagulation, and there is an increased chance that bowel is hidden in these. Slow dissection with electrosurgical knife or with lasers is generally performed.[21,83,104]

TUBAL SURGERY
Infertility Surgery

Tubal microsurgical anastomosis generally has been performed at laparotomy and can be carried out on an outpatient basis with significant savings.[6] This has been performed as an outpatient in Memphis since 1987 following correspondence with Robert Hunt.[42] The total cost for the surgeon, anesthesiologist, and surgery center is less than $4800 and averages about 2 hours. However, others have tried tubal anastomosis at laparoscopy. Although a few authors have had success,[56,117] others have reported lower success rates in the range of 35% to 40%.[49,96] These low success rates are more compatible with reports at meetings. In many gynecologists' hands, laparoscopic tubal anastomosis is less successful than open anastomosis. In addition, laparoscopic cases can be prolonged. Koh averaged 6 hours for his first five cases and 3 hours for the next five.[56] This can be compared with an average of less than 2 hours for outpatient laparotomy. At a development level, adding robotic control has potential in precision, but adds to time and expense.[66]

Laser preparation of the tubal segments before microsurgical anastomosis has been used at laparotomy.[4,5] This reportedly improved hemostasis and enhanced preservation of the normal tissue. However, high power density was needed because low power density is associated with low success[55] and with tubal stenosis.[107] Few gynecologists use these techniques today.

Other tubal surgery that may be reasonable at laparoscopy includes adhesiolysis, cuff salpingostomy for hydrosalpinx (Fig. 35-4), and salpingotomy for tubal gestation.[110] Laparoscopic results often have been compatible with microsurgical results. However, these have not been corrected for stage for adequate comparison.

Using standard microsurgery at laparotomy for hydrosalpinges, Boer-Miesel noted significant differences in term and ectopic pregnancy rates depending on the tubal stage. She reported a 59% term rate, 18% abortion rate, and 4% ectopic rate in the 25% of patients with class I tubes as opposed to a 3% term pregnancy rate and 16% tubal pregnancy rate in the 34% of patients with class III tubes. The largest group in her series (41%) was class II tubes, with a 17% term pregnancy rate, a 5% abortion rate, and a 27% tubal pregnancy rate.[7] Using adhesion, tubal fibrosis, and mucosal appearance on HSG as screening criteria, Hull separated patients into two groups. The first had a favorable 2-year chance of pregnancy at around 50%, whereas the second had less than a 12% pregnancy rate.[77] If tubal surgery is to be cost effective, screening[7,41,51,80] is needed.

Laparoscopic salpingostomy techniques have included the use of scissors to open up the tube followed by coagulation of any bleeders.[34] Some other surgeons use a Bruhat or modified Bruhat procedure.[69] This includes opening the tube along radial scarred lines in the tube. A probe inside the tube helps in both the identification of the folds and can serve as a backstop for the CO_2 laser when used. The tube is opened using high power density laser or electrosurgical techniques. This is then turned back using a defocused technique of the laser with low power density or by using a coagulator as a heat source. This can be accomplished by coagulating saline in the jaws and keeping those near the serosa of the tube. However, direct application of electrical current to the serosa of the tube can coagulate the deep vasculature and destroy the tube. If electrosurgery is used, care is taken to avoid excess tubal damage.

Procedures such as salpingectomy circumvent the passage of hydrosalpinx fluid into the uterine cavity and may benefit the developing environment for embryos.[77] In vitro fertilization pregnancy rates increase with salpingectomy for hydrosalpinges.[79,80,113] Salpingectomy for a hydrosalpinx has other potential advantages. Anecdotally, pelvic pain decreases in some patients, although recurrent vaginitis and discharge decrease in others. The discharge or infection fluid may be related to the passage of hydrosalpinx fluid mentioned by Mukherjee.[77]

Cancer is a concern in infertility patients having tubal surgery. In those undergoing tubal microsurgery, 1.1% of patients between 18 to 37 years of age had ovarian malignancy. This was compared to 0.02% at appendectomy or

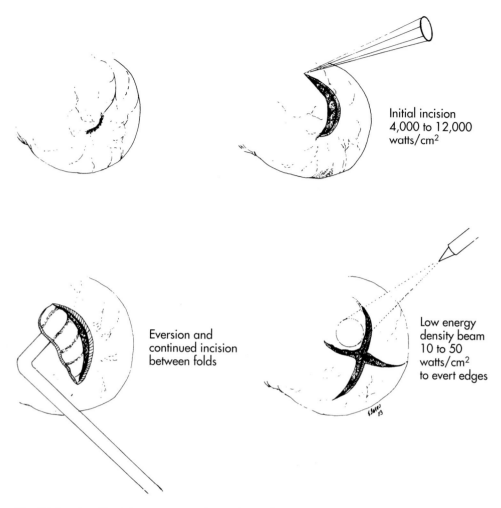

Initial incision
4,000 to 12,000
watts/cm²

Eversion and
continued incision
between folds

Low energy
density beam
10 to 50
watts/cm²
to evert edges

Fig. 35-4 A cuff salpingostomy can be performed with several types of equipment. The Bruhat technique using a carbon dioxide laser is performed by making an incision into the tube at high power density (greater than 4000 watts/cm²) and then coagulating the serosal surface to turn back the tube using low power density beam of less than 50 watts/cm².

cholecystectomy in this same group.[59] The degree of risk is similar to that reported by a collaborative ovarian cancer study that showed risks of 0.03% in women with three or more term pregnancies or four or more years of oral contraceptive use as opposed to 1.6% in women with no pregnancies and no oral contraceptive use by age 65.[36] Although there has been concern that clomiphene increases this risk,[115] the risk associated with resistance to clomiphene is not necessarily a result of using clomiphene. Infertility due to ovarian and peritoneal factors may be associated with cancer and with the use of clomiphene as independent factors. In addition, infertility and tubal surgery have relationships to psammoma bodies, endosalpingiosis, and chlamydia IgG titers.[70-72] Any suspicious lesion should be biopsied. Suspicious lesions may not be seen unless all adhesions are lysed.[42,109,110]

Ectopic Pregnancy

Yao and Tulandi of McGill University[116] and Jain et al.[45] published reports on the history of development of ectopic pregnancy and on the clinical techniques for its treatment, as

well as provided a review of the literature on this topic. These two references may be of interest to anyone studying tubal pregnancies. Laparoscopy has by and large replaced laparotomy as the primary surgical approach to the treatment of tubal pregnancy.[45,116] Laparotomy is still used when it is a quicker procedure in unstable patients and in the middle of the night when laparoscopy teams are not available.

Ectopic pregnancies are treated at laparoscopy just as they are treated at laparotomy. Linear salpingostomy (Fig. 35-5) is used in patients desiring to preserve fertility. The injection of vasopressin (Pitressin) along the antimesenteric border of the tube can be used to aid in hemostasis. A diluted solution of 1 mU vasopressin (0.1 ml of a 10-mU ampule) is used in 50 ml of normal saline and is injected using a spinal needle placed directly through the abdominal wall. After the antimesenteric incision is made, the products of conception are removed from the tube. Frequently these spontaneously extrude but more often require general teasing of the trophoblastic tissue from the bed. When multiple clots are in the tube, the distal and proximal margins of the incision are

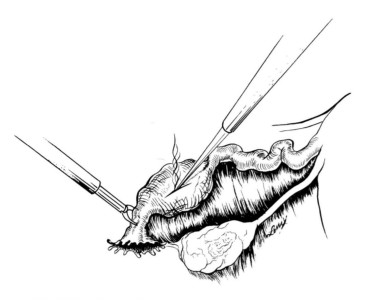

Fig. 35-5 Linear salpingotomy for an ectopic pregnancy can be performed with a laser, unipolar cautery, or scissors. Pitressin injection is used to decrease bleeding, and bipolar coagulation may be helpful in obtaining hemostasis.

closely observed to be sure that the trophoblastic tissue is not at the margin and hidden by the clots. Sutures do not appear to be beneficial.[111] Persistent ectopic pregnancy has been a problem in 5% of patients treated by this technique.[91] All patients having conservative surgery should undergo follow-up HCG titers to ensure these are declining. Depending on the speed of decline, these titers can be measured anywhere from every 3 days to every 2 weeks. It is not uncommon for titers to be positive for up to 24 days and uncommonly longer than that.

Salpingectomy is a technically easier procedure and is useful in patients who not desire to preserve fertility and in patients who have significant tubal damage from rupture. This technique can be performed using bipolar coagulation for hemostasis and scissors for the excision, loops for hemostasis followed by excision, or other devices such as the GIA. In all these techniques, the tube is removed intact through a minilaparotomy or colpotomy incision. Morselizing the tube may spread the ectopic and result in persistence.[63,94]

Laparoscopic techniques also have been adequate for the care of both unruptured[39] and ruptured[95] interstitial pregnancies. With experience, indications for laparoscopic surgery increase and the contraindications are few and resolve around the hemodynamic and medical status of the patient and the surgical history. Patients who are hemodynamically unstable, those with a history of diaphragmatic hernia, and patients who have known extensive pelvic adhesions appear to be best treated at laparotomy. Laparotomy also is used when laparoscopic equipment and a laparoscopic team are not available.

In addition to laparoscopic treatment, systemic and local injection of methotrexate have been used.[62] Furthermore, some authors suggest use of methotrexate after surgery.[100]

In general, the success rates after systemic injection are more predictable than those after local injection.[116] Although some studies report excellent results with local laparoscopic injection of methotrexate, others have reported much more variable results.[76,101]

STEIN-LEVENTHAL SYNDROME

Although wedge resection of the ovary was of major significance before clomiphene and gonadotrophin therapy,[50,108,114] adhesions could decrease fertility.[13,14,73,90] Several alternative techniques have been tried at laparoscopy. The treatment at laparoscopy has consisted of microcyst puncture, biopsy of the multiple microcystic areas, furrowing of the ovary, and true wedge resection.* The changes in hormones after wedge and laparoscopic techniques show a decrease in testosterone and luteinizing hormone.[2,103] Pregnancy rates after laparoscopic treatment have been reported to range from 52% to 57%.[2,22,103]

UTERINE SUSPENSION

Although indications for uterine suspension are difficult to define, this can be performed in patients who appear to have symptomatic retroversion or in patients in whom there is extensive posterior dissection and the surgeon wishes to attempt to keep the uterine fundus out of the posterior pelvis during healing. This can be a simple triplication of the round ligament or a Gilliam-type suspension at laparotomy. The Gilliam suspension suspends the round ligament to the rectus fascia. For this, a Kelly clamp is placed through the fascia above the round ligament. The ligament is grasped about one third to one half the length of the round ligament and then pulled through the peritoneum and back to the fascia. This is performed on both sides before suturing to ensure that no excess tension is distorting the tube. Two Tevdek sutures are used to anchor this to the external oblique fascia.

A technique similar to the Gilliam suspension can be performed at laparoscopy. Lateral incisions are made and the external oblique fascia identified. Pressure is placed to be sure that the site is above the insertion of the round ligament. An Allis clamp is placed through the fascia at this level and worked retroperitoneally down the round ligament under direct visualization through the laparoscope. This is taken one third to one half the length of the round ligament and then pushed through the peritoneum into the peritoneal cavity. The round ligament is grasped at this point and pulled back on itself to the fascia. Two Tevdek sutures are used to anchor this to the external oblique fascia. This is performed on both sides, and the incision is closed. In that these are outpatient surgeries, a Marcaine and morphine block of this area is generally performed. (Marcaine and morphine blocks are covered in the section on techniques.) Simple techniques include placing a loop ligature or a Falope ring around the round ligament in order to shorten this.

---

*References 2, 22, 32, 34, 57, 78.

Other surgeons have pulled the round ligament directly anterior and tacked this to the fascia. This technique can produce open areas lateral to the suspension and the possibility of internal herniation.

HORMONE REPLACEMENT THERAPY

When adnexal surgery results in castration, hormone replacement therapy (HRT) is generally indicated. There appear to be fewer deaths from ischemic heart disease and from osteoporotic fractures; however, there may be more breast cancer, endometrial cancer deaths, and deaths from gallbladder disease. In one estimate, for every 5813 lives saved, 252 are lost.[47,111] In that estrogen replacement therapy is associated with a significant increase in overall health[111] and is protective against cancers such as colon,[112] estrogen replacement therapy should not be withheld in light of the minimal risk it appears to represent.

There are specific concerns in patients treated for endometriosis. The addition of progesterone in patients with residual endometriosis after "radical" surgery appears appropriate.[45] The use of "definitive" surgery for endometriosis[21,113,114] decreases the chance that estrogen treatment is needed. There may be no compelling reason to delay HRT in women with endometriosis.[115]

Although HRT is initially started in 39% to 89% of patients, this decreases to 13% to 51% over time.[44] The amount of estrogen may be minimized by using a comprehensive hormonal approach,[48] which uses not only estrogen but also progesterone, testosterone, and DHEA. In addition to hormone treatment, many other alternatives can be chosen, including weight-bearing exercise, aspirin use, moderate alcohol intake, smoking cessation, vitamin D and calcium supplementation, and regular sexual activity.[116,117]

Laparoscopic techniques are replacing many laparotomy techniques for adnexal surgery, partly because of the perception that inpatient admission is needed after laparotomy. However, laparotomy may be as cost effective and useful to patients as laparoscopy if performed on an outpatient basis. Although laparoscopy is excellent for visualization, palpation and handling are enhanced at laparotomy. This appears to be particularly true for tubal anastomosis, for which time and cost are decreased and success rates higher using outpatient laparotomy in most hands. In all but the most obvious cases of benign adnexal tumor, preparations for staging of ovarian cancer need to be discussed preoperatively. In young patients and those who desire to preserve fertility, waiting for permanent sections may be a better answer than proceeding on the basis of frozen section. However, delay in definitive treatment must be avoided, since this increases the chance of dissemination.

REFERENCES

1. Adamyan LV, Myinbayev OA, Kulakov VI: Use of fibrin glue in obstetrics and gynecology: a review of the literature, *Int J Fertil* 36:76, 1991.
2. Armar NA, McGarrigle HHG, Honour J, et al: Laparoscopic ovarian diathermy in the management of anovulatory infertility in women with polycystic ovaries: endocrine changes and clinical outcome, *Fertil Steril* 53:45, 1990.
3. Ballweg ML: Coping with painful sex. In Ballweg ML, editor: *Endometriosis sourcebook,* Chicago, 1995, Contemporary Books.
4. Bellina JH: Lasers in gynecology, *World J Surg* 7:692, 1983.
5. Bellina JH: Microsurgery of the fallopian tube with the carbon dioxide laser: analysis of 230 cases with 2-year follow-up, *Lasers Surg Med* 3:255, 1983.
6. Berger GS: Outpatient pelvic laparotomy, *J Reprod Med* 39:569, 1994.
7. Boer-Meisel ME, te Velde ER, Habbema JDF, Kardaun JWPF: Predicting the pregnancy outcome in patients treated for hydrosalpinx: a prospective study, *Fertil Steril* 45:23, 1986.
8. Bonnier P, Romain S, Giacalone PL, et al: Clinical and biologic prognostic factors in breast cancer diagnosed during postmenopausal hormone replacement therapy, *Obstet Gynecol* 85:11, 1995
9. Boyers SP, Diamond MP, DeCherney AH: Reduction of postoperative pelvic adhesions in the rabbit with Gore-Tex surgical membrane, *Fertil Steril* 49:1066, 1988.
10. Brinton LA, Gridley G, Persson I, et al: Cancer risk after a hospital discharge diagnosis of endometriosis, *Am J Obstet Gynecol* 176:572, 1997.
11. Brooks JJ: Malignancy arising in extragonadal endometriosis, *Cancer* 40:3065, 1977.
12. Brosens IA, Ballaer PV, Puttemans P, Deprest J: Reconstruction of the ovary containing large endometriomas by an extraovarian endosurgical technique, *Fertil Steril* 66:517, 1996.
13. Brumsted JR, Deaton J, Lavigne E, Riddick DH: Postoperative adhesion formation after ovarian wedge resection with and without ovarian reconstruction in the rabbit, *Fertil Steril* 53:723, 1990.
14. Buttram Jr VJ, Vaquero C: Post-ovarian wedge resection adhesive disease, *Fertil Steril* 26:874, 1975.
15. Calle EE, Miracle-McMahill HL, Thun MJ, Heath CW Jr: Estrogen replacement therapy and risk of fatal colon cancer in a prospective cohort of postmenopausal women, *J Natl Cancer Inst* 87:517, 1995.
16. Campo S, Garcea N: Laparoscopic conservative excision of ovarian dermoid cysts with and without an endobag, *J Am Assoc Gynecol Laparosc* 5:165, 1998.
17. Canis M, Mage G, Pouly JL, et al: Laparoscopic diagnosis of adnexal cystic masses: a 12-year experience with long-term follow-up, *Obstet Gynecol* 83:707, 1994.
18. Canis M, Pouly JL, Wattiez A, et al: Laparoscopic management of adnexal masses suspicious at ultrasound, *Obstet Gynecol* 89:679, 1997.
19. Childers JM, Aqua KA, Surwit EA, et al: Abdominal-wall tumor implantation after laparoscopy for malignant conditions, *Obstet Gynecol* 84:765, 1994.
20. Col NF, Eckman MH, Kaeas RH, et al: Patient-specific decisions about hormone replacement therapy in postmenopausal women, *JAMA* 277:1140, 1997.
21. Daniell JF: Laparoscopic enterolysis for chronic abdominal pain, *J Gynecol Surg* 5:61, 1989.
22. Daniell JF, Miller W: Polycystic ovaries treated by laparoscopic laser vaporization, *Fertil Steril* 51:232, 1989.
23. De Leon FD, Edwards M, Heine MW: A comparison of microsurgery and laser surgery for ovarian wedge resections, *Int J Fertil* 35:177, 1990.
24. DePriest PD, Banks ER, Powell DE, et al: Endometrioid carcinoma of the ovary and endometriosis: the association in postmenopausal women, *Gynecol Oncol* 47:71, 1992.
25. Diamond MP, Cunningham T, Linsky CB, DeCherney AH: Laparoscopic application of Interceed (TC7) in the pig, *J Gynecol Surg* 5:45, 1989.
26. Diamond MP, Operative LSG, Daniell JF, et al: Postoperative adhesion development after operative laparoscopy: evaluation at early second-look procedures, *Fertil Steril* 55:700, 1991.

27. Donnez J, Nisolle M, Karaman Y, et al: CO_2 laser laparoscopy in peritoneal endometriosis and in ovarian endometrial cyst, *J Gynecol Surg* 5:361, 1989.

28. Duun S, Roed-Petersen K, Michelsen JW: Endometrioid carcinoma arising from endometriosis of the sigmoid colon during estrogenic treatment, *Acta Obstet Gynecol Scand* 72:676, 1993.

29. Ellis H: The cause and prevention of postoperative intraperitoneal adhesions, *Surg Gynecol Obstet* 133:497, 1971.

30. Ellis H: Internal overhealing: the problem of intraperitoneal adhesions, *World J Surg* 4:303, 1980.

31. Fong YF, Lim FK, Arulkumaran S: Prophylactic oophorectomy: a continuing controversy, *Obstet Gynecol Surv* 53:493, 1998.

32. Gadir AA, Mowafi RS, Alnaser HMI, et al: Ovarian electrocautery versus human menopausal gonadotrophins and pure follicle-stimulating hormone therapy in the treatment of patients with polycystic ovarian disease, *Clin Endocrinol* 33:585, 1990.

33. Gleeson NC, Nicosia SV, Mark JE, et al: Abdominal wall metastases from ovarian cancer after laparoscopy, *Am J Obstet Gynecol* 169:522, 1993.

34. Gomel V: Operative laparoscopy: time for acceptance, *Fertil Steril* 52:1, 1989.

35. Hargrove JT, Osteen KG: Alternative method of hormone replacement therapy using the natural sex steroids, *Infertil Reprod Med Clin North Am* 6:653, 1995.

36. Hartge P, Whittemore AS, et al, The Collaborative Ovarian Cancer Group: Rates and risks of ovarian cancer in subgroups of white women in the United States, *Obstet Gynecol* 84:760, 1994.

37. Hasson HM: Open techniques for equipment insertion. In Martin DC, editor: *Manual of endoscopy,* Santa Fe Springs, NM, 1990, AAGL.

38. Hickman TN, Namnoum AB, Hinton E, et al: Timing of estrogen replacement therapy following hysterectomy with oophorectomy for endometriosis, *Obstet Gynecol* 91:673, 1998.

39. Hill GA, Segars JH, Herbert CM: Laparoscopic management of interstitial pregnancy, *J Gynecol Surg* 5:209, 1989.

40. Hsiu J, Given F, Kemp G: Tumor implantation after diagnostic laparoscopy biopsy of serous ovarian tumors of low malignant potential, *Obstet Gynecol* 68:905, 1986.

41. Hull M, Fleming CF: Tubal surgery versus assisted reproduction: assessing their role in infertility therapy, *Curr Opin Obstet Gynecol* 7:160, 1995.

42. Hunt R: Personal communications on outpatient laparotomy for microsurgical anastomosis, 1987.

43. Hunt RB: Laparoscopic management of adnexal masses. Paper presented at Gynecologic Surgery for Clinicians, Chicago, May 14, 1997.

44. Interceed TABSG: Prevention of postsurgical adhesions by Interceed (TC7), an absorbable adhesion barrier: a prospective, randomized multicenter clinical study, *Fertil Steril* 51:933, 1989.

45. Jain A, Solima E, Luciano AA: Ectopic pregnancy, *J Am Assoc Gynecol Laparosc* 4:515, 1997.

46. Jansen FW, Tanahatoe S, Veselic M, Trimbos B: Laparoscopic aspiration of ovarian cysts: an unreliable technique in primary diagnosis of (sonographically) benign ovarian lesions, *Gynaecol Endosc* 6:363, 1997.

47. Jarrett JC: Laparoscopy: Direct trocar insertion without pneumoperitoneum, *Obstet Gynecol* 75:725, 1990.

48. Kadar N: Laparoscopic management of gynaecological malignancies: time to quit? I. *Gynaecol Endosc* 6:135, 1997.

49. Katz E, Donesky BW: Laparoscopic tubal anastomosis: a pilot study, *J Reprod Med* 39:497, 1994.

50. Katz M, Carr PJ, Cohen BM, Millar RP: Hormonal effects of wedge resection of polycystic ovaries, *Obstet Gynecol* 51:437, 1978.

51. Khare VK, Consonni R, Martin DC, Winfield AC: Use of algorithmic pathways to develop quality, cost-effective clinical care, *J Am Assoc Gynecol Laparosc* 2:169, 1995.

52. Kindermann G, Maassen V, Kuhn W: Laparoscopic management of ovarian tumors subsequently diagnosed as malignant, *J Pelvic Surg* 2:245, 1996.

53. Kleppinger RK: Closed techniques for equipment insertion. In Martin DC, editor: *Manual of endoscopy,* Santa Fe Springs, NM, 1990, AAGL.

54. Kline RC, Wharton JT, Atkinson EN, Burke TW, Gershenson DM, Edwards CL: Endometrioid carcinoma of the ovary: retrospective review of 145 cases, *Gynecol Oncol* 39:337, 1990.

55. Klink F, Großpietzsch R, Von Kitzing L, et al: Animal in vivo studies and in vitro experiments with human tubes for end-to-end anastomotic operations by a CO_2-laser technique, *Fertil Steril* 30:100, 1978.

56. Koh C, Janik GM: Laparoscopic microsurgical tubal anastomosis. In Adamson G, Martin D, editors: *Endoscopic management of gynecologic disease,* New York, 1996, Raven.

57. Kojima E, Yanagibori A, Otaka K, Hirakawa S: Ovarian wedge resection with contact Nd:YAG laser irradiation used laparoscopically, *J Reprod Med* 34:444, 1989.

58. Kritz-Silverstein D, Wingard DL, Barrett-Connor E, Morton DJ: Hysterectomy, oophorectomy, and depression in older women, *J Women's Health* 3:255, 1994.

59. Lais CW, Williams TJ, Gaffey TA: Prevalence of ovarian cancer found at the time of infertility microsurgery, *Fertil Steril* 49:551, 1988.

60. Lobo R: Benefits and risks of estrogen replacement therapy, *Am J Obstet Gynecol* 173:982, 1957.

61. Luciano AA, Whitman G, Maier DB, et al: A comparison of thermal injury, healing patterns, and postoperative adhesion formation following CO_2 laser and electromicrosurgery, *Fertil Steril* 48:1025, 1987.

62. Lundorff P, Halin M, Kallfelt B, et al: Adhesion formation after laparoscopic surgery in tubal pregnancy: a randomized trial versus laparotomy, *Fertil Steril* 55:911, 1991.

63. Lundorf P, Hahlin M, Sjoblom P, Linblom B: Persistent trophoblast after conservative treatment of tubal pregnancy: prediction and detection, *Obstet Gynecol* 77:129, 1991.

64. Maiman M, Seltzer V, Boyce J: Laparoscopic excision of ovarian neoplasms subsequently found to be malignant, *Obstet Gynecol* 77:563, 1991.

65. Marconi G, Quintana R, Rueda-Leverone NG, Vighi S: Accidental ovarian autograft after a laparoscopic surgery: case report, *Fertil Steril* 68:364, 1997.

66. Margossian H, Garcia-Tuiz A, Flacone T, et al: Robotically assisted laparoscopic tubal anastomosis in a porcine model: a pilot study, *J Laparosc Endosc Adv Surg Tech* 8:69, 1998.

67. Martin DC: CO_2 laser laparoscopy for endometriosis associated with infertility, *J Reprod Med* 31:1089, 1986.

68. Martin DC: Surgical treatment of endometriosis, *Clin Consul Obstet Gynecol* 7:190, 1995.

69. Martin DC, Diamond MP: Operative laparoscopy: comparison of lasers with other techniques, *Curr Probl Obstet Gynecol Fertil* 9:563, 1986.

70. Martin DC, Khare VK, Miller BE: Association of *Chlamydia trachomatis* immunoglobulin gamma titers with dystrophic peritoneal calcification, psammoma bodies, adhesions, and hydrosalpinges, *Fertil Steril* 63:39, 1995.

71. Martin D, Khare V, Parker L: Clear and opaque vesicles: endometriosis, psammoma bodies, endosalpingiosis, or cancer. In Coutinho EM, Spinola P, de Moura LH, editors: *Progress in the management of endometriosis,* New York, 1994, Parthenon.

72. Martin DC, Khare VK, Miller BE, Batzer FR: Association of positive *Chlamydia trachomatis* and *Chlamydia pneumoniae* immunoglobulin gamma titers with increasing age, *J Am Assoc Gynecol Laparosc* 4:583, 1997.

73. McLaughlin DS: Evaluation of adhesion reformation by early second-look laparoscopy following microlaser ovarian wedge resection, *Fertil Steril* 42:531, 1984.

74. Molpus KL: Pathophysiology and management of endometriosis in menopause, *Infertil Reprod Med Clin North Am* 6:805, 1995.

75. Mostoufizadeh M, Scully RE: Malignant tumors arising in endometriosis, *Clin Obstet Gynecol* 23:951, 1980.

76. Mottla G, Rulin M, Guzick D: Lack of resolution of ectopic pregnancy by intratubal injection of methotrexate, *Fertil Steril* 57:685, 1992.

77. Mukherjee T, Copperman AB, McCaffrey C, et al: Hydrosalpinx fluid has embryotoxic effects on murine embryogenesis: a case for prophylactic salpingectomy, *Fertil Steril* 66:851, 1996.

78. Murphy AA: Operative laparoscopy, *Fertil Steril* 47:1, 1987.

79. Murray DL, Sagoskin AW, Widra EA, Levy ML: The adverse effect of hydrosalpinges on in vitro fertilization pregnancy rates and the benefit of surgical correction, *Fertil Steril* 69:41, 1998.

80. Nackley AC, Muasher SJ: The significance of hydrosalpinx in in vitro fertilization, *Fertil Steril* 69:373, 1998.

81. Namnoum AB, Hickman TN, Goodman SB, et al: Incidence of symptom recurrence after hysterectomy for endometriosis, *Fertil Steril* 64:898, 1995.

82. Nezhat F, Nezhat C: Operative laparoscopy for the treatment of ovarian remnant syndrome, *Fertil Steril* 57:1003, 1992.

83. Nezhat C, Winer W, Cooper JD, et al: Endoscopic infertility surgery, *J Reprod Med* 34:127, 1989.

84. Nezhat CR, Nezhat FR, Metzger DA, Luciano AA: Adhesion reformation after reproductive surgery by videolaseroscopy, *Fertil Steril* 53:1008, 1990.

85. Nezhat FR, Silfen SL, Evans D, Nezhat C: Comparison of direct insertion of disposable and standard reusable laparoscopic trocars and previous pneumoperitoneum with Veress needle, *Obstet Gynecol* 78:148, 1991.

86. Nezhat F, Nezhat C, Allan CJ, et al: Clinical and histologic classification of endometriomas: implications for a mechanism of pathogenesis, *J Reprod Med* 37:771, 1992.

87. Norwitz E: Managing the menopause without estrogen, *The Female Patient* 22:42, 1997.

88. Parazzini F, Negri E, La Vecchia C, et al: Hysterectomy, oophorectomy, and subsequent ovarian cancer risk, *Obstet Gynecol* 81:363, 1993.

89. Parker WH, Berek JS: Management of selected cystic adnexal masses in postmenopausal women by operative laparoscopy: a pilot study, *Am J Obstet Gynecol* 163:1574, 1990.

90. Portuondo JA, Melchor JC, Neyro JL, Alegre A: Periovarian adhesions following ovarian wedge resection or laparoscopic biopsy, *Endoscopy* 16:143, 1984.

91. Pouly JL, Mahnes H, Mage G, et al: Conservative laparoscopic treatment of 321 ectopic pregnancies, *Fertil Steril* 46:1093, 1986.

92. Redwine DB: Endometriosis persisting after castration: clinical characteristics and results of surgical management, *Obstet Gynecol* 83:405, 1994.

93. Reich H, McGlynn F: Treatment of ovarian endometriomas using laparoscopic surgical techniques, *J Reprod Med* 31:577, 1986.

94. Reich H, DeCaprio J, McGlynn F, et al: Peritoneal trophoblastic tissue implants after laparoscopic treatment of tubal ectopic pregnancy, *Fertil Steril* 52:337, 1989.

95. Reich H, McGlynn F, Budin R, et al: Laparoscopic treatment of ruptured interstitial pregnancy, *J Gynecol Surg* 6:135, 1990.

96. Reich H, McGlynn F, Parente C, et al: Laparoscopic tubal anastomosis, *J Am Assoc Gynecol Laparosc* 1:16, 1993.

97. Rosen DMB, Lam AM, Chapman MC, Cario GM: Methods of creating pneumoperitoneum: a review of techniques and complications, *Obstet Gynecol Surv* 53:167, 1998.

98. Rubin SC, Lewis JL: Surgery for cancer of the ovary. In Nichols DH, editor: *Gynecologic and obstetric surgery,* St Louis, 1993, Mosby.

99. Rutledge FN: Surgical treatment of ovarian cancer. In Te Linde RW, editor: *Operative gynecology,* Philadelphia, 1992, JB Lippincott.

100. Seifer D: Persistent ectopic pregnancy: an argument for heightened vigilance and patient compliance, *Fertil Steril* 68:402, 1997.

101. Shalev E, Peleg D, Bustan M, et al: Limited role for intratubal methotrexate treatment of ectopic pregnancy, *Fertil Steril* 63:20, 1995.

102. Stovall TG, Ling FW, Gray LA: Single-dose methotrexate for treatment of ectopic pregnancy, *Obstet Gynecol* 77:754, 1991.

103. Sumioki H, Utsunomyiya T, Matsuoka K, et al: The effect of laparoscopic multiple punch resection of the ovary on hypothalamopituitary axis in polycystic ovary syndrome, *Fertil Steril* 50:567, 1988.

104. Sutton C, Macdonald R: Laser laparoscopic adhesiolysis, *J Gynecol Surg* 6:155, 1990.

105. Sutton CJ, Ewen SP, Jacobs SA, Whitelaw NL: Laser laparoscopic surgery in the treatment of ovarian endometriomas, *J Am Assoc Gynecol Laparosc* 4:319, 1997.

106. Taylor PJ: The Canadian Consensus Conference on Endometriosis, *J Soc Obstet Gynaecol Can* 15:1, 1993.

107. Taylor MV, Martin DC, Poston W, et al: Effect of power density and carbonization on residual tissue coagulation using the continuous wave carbon dioxide laser, *Colposc Gynecol Laser Surg* 2:169, 1986.

108. Toaff R, Toaff ME, Peyser MR: Infertility following wedge resection of the ovaries, *Am J Obstet Gynecol* 124:92, 1975.

109. Trimbos JG, Schueler JA, van Lent M, et al: Reasons for incomplete surgical staging in early ovarian carcinoma, *Gynecol Oncol* 37:374, 1990.

110. Tulandi T: Reconstructive tubal surgery by laparoscopy, *Obstet Gynecol Surv* 42:193, 1987.

111. Tulandi T, Guralnick M: Treatment of tubal ectopic pregnancy by salpingotomy with or without tubal suturing and salpingectomy, *Fertil Steril* 55:53, 1991.

112. Volz J, Koster S, Schaeff B, Paolucci V: Laparoscopic surgery: the effects of insufflation gas on tumor-induced lethality in nude mice, *Am J Obstet Gynecol* 178:793, 1998.

113. Wainer R, Camus E, Camier B, et al: Does hydrosalpinx reduce the pregnancy rate after in vitro fertilization, *Fertil Steril* 68:1022, 1997.

114. Weinstein D, Polishuk WS: The role of wedge resection of the ovary as a cause for mechanical sterility, *Surg Gynecol Obstet* 141:417, 1975.

115. Whittemore AS, Harris R, Itnyre J, The Collaborative Ovarian Cancer Group: Characteristics relating to ovarian cancer risk: collaborative analysis of 12 US case-control studies, *Am J Epidemiol* 136:1184, 1992.

116. Yao M, Tulandi T: Current status of surgical and nonsurgical management of ectopic pregnancy, *Fertil Steril* 67:421, 1997.

117. Yoon TK, Sung HR, Cha SH, et al: Fertility outcome after laparoscopic microsurgical tubal anastomosis, *Fertil Steril* 67:18, 1997.

36 Surgery for Vulvar Cancer

GEORGE W. MORLEY and R. KEVIN REYNOLDS

Cancer of the vulva is one of the less frequently encountered malignancies of the female genital tract with a reported incidence of 4% among all gynecologic tumors. Vulvar malignancy usually affects women of advanced years; more than two thirds of the cases occur in women between 60 and 80 years of age. Invasive carcinoma of the vulva is seen in about 2 per 100,000 women per year.

The etiology of squamous cell carcinoma of the vulva can be divided into two groups based on the age of the patient. Younger women appear to be at a higher risk for basaloid and warty types of squamous vulvar carcinoma, whereas older women are more likely to develop keratinizing squamous cell carcinoma. Human papillomavirus (HPV) is detectable in 86% of basaloid and warty squamous cancers. Risk factors for this type of cancer include multiple sexual partners, early age at coitarche, and smoking. In comparison, only 6% of keratinizing squamous cell vulvar cancers are associated with HPV. These cancers are associated with lichen sclerosis and hyperplastic dystrophy in 19% and 33% of patients, respectively. Smoking and sexual history appear to have less effect on the risk of developing a keratinizing squamous cell vulvar cancer. Women with no history of HPV exposure may have other risk factors associated with the development of vulvar squamous cell carcinoma, including occupational exposure to carcinogens, caffeine consumption, and chronic granulomatous infections.[25]

The incidence of VIN has increased dramatically in the last three decades (Fig. 36-1). Between 1961 and 1992, the age at the time of diagnosis of VIN decreased from a mean of 52.7 years to 35.8 years. Untreated VIN may progress to invasive cancer in up to 88% of cases, whereas treated VIN progresses to invasion in only 4% of cases.[14]

Many advances have been made in the treatment of carcinoma of the vulva over the past 25 years. Previously, basically three forms of therapy were used to treat this malignant lesion: a total vulvectomy was considered the treatment of choice for preinvasive disease; radical vulvectomy and regional lymphadenectomy were the treatment for invasive disease; and palliative vulvectomy was reserved for treatment of the unresectable or incurable condition. In a comparative study from the University of Michigan Medical Center covering a 40-year period from 1935 to 1975, researchers reported a 20% incidence of lesions too extensive

to be treated therapeutically as a curative procedure.[18] In a more recent series reported from the University of Michigan, the incidence of palliative vulvectomy had decreased to approximately 5%.[12]

CLASSIFICATION OF VULVAR CANCER

The 1995 revision of the International Federation of Gynecology and Obstetrics (FIGO) definitions for surgical staging of vulvar carcinoma is presented in the box on p. 651.[6] These rules do not apply to the staging of malignant melanoma of the vulva.

Following is the TNM classification of carcinoma of the vulva (FIGO).

T	Primary Tumor
T_{is}	Preinvasive carcinoma
T_1	Tumor confined to the vulva and/or perineum, ≤ 2 cm in largest diameter
T_{1a}	Tumor invades ≤ 1 mm
T_{1b}	Tumor invades > 1 mm
T_2	Tumor confined to vulva and/or perineum, > 2 cm in largest diameter
T_3	Tumor of any size with adjacent spread to urethra, vagina, and/or anus
T_4	Tumor of any size infiltrating bladder and/or rectal mucosa, and/or fixed to bone
N	**Regional Lymph Nodes**
N_0	No lymph node metastasis
N_1	Unilateral regional node metastases
N_2	Bilateral regional node metastases
M	**Distant Metastasis**
M_0	No clinical metastases
M_1	Spread to pelvic nodes or distant metastasis
Stage	**Carcinoma in situ Microinvasion**
Stage 0	T_{is}
Stage Ia	$T_{1a} N_0 M_0$
Stage Ib	$T_{1b} N_0 M_0$
Stage II	$T_2 N_0 M_0$
Stage III	$T_3 N_0 M_0$, $T_3 N_1 M_0$, $T_1 N_1 M_0$, $T_2 N_1 M_0$
Stage IVa	$T_1 N_2 M_0$, $T_2 N_2 M_0$, $T_3 N_2 M_0$, $T_4 N_0 M_0$, $T_4 N_1 M_0$, $T_4 N_2 M_0$
Stage IVb	$T(any) N(any) M_1$

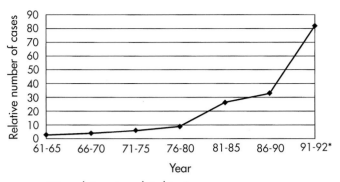

*Year data extrapolated to 4 years

Fig. 36-1   Changing incidence of VIN.

ASSESSMENT OF REGIONAL LYMPH NODES

Early in the second half of this century, pelvic lymphadenectomy began to be used selectively rather than routinely along with the bilateral groin lymphadenectomy in the treatment of invasive carcinoma of the vulva. Once its routine use was discontinued, it was then thought to be indicated only in the treatment of carcinoma of the clitoris or Bartholin's gland, in the presence of positive groin lymph nodes, in vulvar melanomas, or for urethral or vaginal involvement. It is now known that the chance of direct involvement of the pelvic lymph nodes in any of these conditions is virtually nonexistent without the initial involvement of the groin lymph nodes. Therefore pelvic lymphadenectomy essentially has been eliminated from the initial surgical approach to the treatment of invasive carcinoma of the vulva. A randomized gynecologic oncology study demonstrated that pelvic radiation therapy was significantly more effective than pelvic lymphadenectomy for treatment of patients who had groin lymph node metastases. The 2-year survival was 68% in the radiated group compared with 54% in the lymphadenectomy group.[10]

Other significant modifications of the therapy for carcinoma of the vulva have been made in the past 15 to 20 years, especially involving the treatment of regional lymph nodes, and have been made without any compromise in survival rates. Currently, if a patient has a *unilateral* vulvar lesion that does not involve either the clitoral-paraclitoral tissue or the perineal body, then initial treatment consists of an *ipsilateral* groin (inguinal and femoral) lymph node dissection, which is considered a well-accepted treatment of this lesion. If there is proven nodal involvement on the ipsilateral side, however, then a contralateral groin dissection is required. Lesions involving clitoral or perineal tissues are still treated with bilateral groin lymph node dissections along with the radical vulvectomy, since bilateral lymphatic drainage can occur from either of these sites.

ALTERATIONS IN THE VULVAR PHASE

The philosophy of "it is better to overtreat than to undertreat" continues to be an appropriate approach to treat-

---

INTERNATIONAL FEDERATION OF GYNECOLOGY AND OBSTETRICS (FIGO) SURGICAL STAGING OF VULVAR CARCINOMA

STAGE 0

T_{is} — Carcinoma in situ, intraepithelial carcinoma

STAGE I

$T_1 N_0 M_0$ — Tumor confined to the vulva and/or perineum—2 cm or less in greatest dimension, nodes not palpable

T_{1a} — Tumor invades ≤ 1 mm

T_{1b} — Tumor invades >1 mm

STAGE II

$T_2 N_0 M_0$ — Tumor confined to the vulva and/or perineum—more than 2 cm in greatest dimension, nodes not palpable

STAGE III

$T_3 N_0 M_0$
$T_3 N_1 M_0$ — Tumor of any size with:
(1) adjacent spread to the lower urethra and/or the vagina, or the anus and/or
(2) unilateral regional (groin) lymph node metastasis

$T_1 N_1 M_0$
$T_2 N_1 M_0$

STAGE IVa

$T_1 N_2 M_0$
$T_2 N_2 M_0$ — Tumor invades any of the following: upper urethra, bladder mucosa, rectal mucosa, pelvic bone, and/or bilateral regional (groin) lymph node metastasis

$T_3 N_2 M_0$
T_4 any N M_0

STAGE IVb

Any T, any N, M_1 — Any distant metastasis including pelvic lymph nodes

---

ment of invasive genital malignancies. However, during the past 15 years gynecologic oncologists have been able to modify the vulvar phase of treatment simply because of their increased understanding of the disease process regarding both diagnosis and treatment, as well as because of earlier seeking of medical attention by patients when a sore or growth appears in the vulvar area. No longer is a total radical vulvectomy always considered the treatment of choice for invasive vulvar cancers. In fact, in the presence of a unilaterally localized vulvar lesion, a subtotal or hemiradical vulvectomy can be performed. The surgical limits of the vulvar phase of this treatment are modified further when an anterior or posterior malignant lesion is encountered.[5]

SURGICAL APPROACHES TO TREATMENT

By tradition, surgery has been the mainstay of therapy for all carcinoma of the vulva. Once the patient has undergone a complete physical and medical evaluation with appropriate corrective measures undertaken and has understood the details of the surgery along with the inherent risks involved, she is then prepared for the surgical treatment. Almost all patients are treated with prophylactic heparin or sequential compression devices (SCD), and antibiotics are used liberally as a preventive measure.

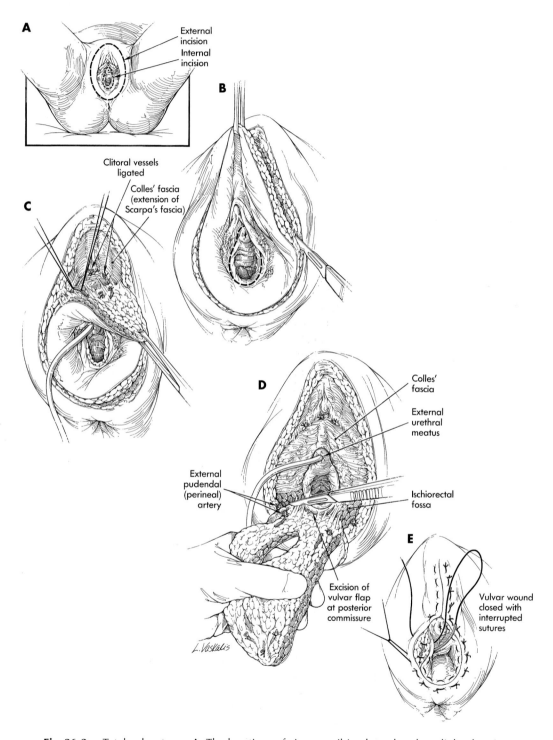

Fig. 36-2   Total vulvectomy. **A,** The locations of circumscribing lateral and medial vulvar incisions. The medial incision is at the hymenal ring. **B,** Skin and subcutaneous tissues are excised using a knife (as shown) or electrocautery technique. **C,** Dissection is carried down to Colles' fascia with excision of all subcutaneous tissue superficial to it. **D,** Posterior dissection involves excision of an appropriate portion of ischiorectal fat. **E,** Vulvar wound is then closed in a manner reflecting the preference of the operating surgeon.

Treatment of Preinvasive Carcinoma of the Vulva

Once surgical excision is considered the treatment of choice for preinvasive disease of the vulva, then several options are available for care, including wide local excision with satisfactory margins, laser photoablation, subtotal or total vulvectomy, or skinning vulvectomy with or without a skin grafting. However, the size of the lesion and the age and health status of the patient must be taken into consideration in making the final therapeutic choice. No longer is only one form of therapy the treatment of choice. The recurrence rate is essentially the same when results from wide local excision versus total vulvectomy are compared.

Most of these lesions, which are usually quite localized, can be satisfactorily controlled with a wide local excision and negative margins. However, often a multifocal lesion is present, and this may require a subtotal or total vulvectomy followed by primary closure of the defect with easy approximation of the skin edges (Fig. 36-2). This treatment requires the removal of the skin lesion with 1 to 2 cm of clinically clear margins and enough subcutaneous tissue for the pathologist to determine the limits of the offending lesion accurately. This dissection extends down to the level of Colles' fascia, which is the perineal extension of Scarpa's fascia, that is present in the abdominal wall. Throughout the dissection, one must keep in mind the end result and attempt to avoid a deformity or sexual dysfunction, although control of the disease is the primary goal.

More than 30 years ago, Rutledge and Sinclair[23] introduced the skinning vulvectomy and split-thickness skin graft vulvoplasty as treatment of the more diffuse or advanced, yet still preinvasive, lesion. In the skinning vulvectomy, only the epidermis and dermis are excised (Fig. 36-3). The split-thickness skin graft is taken from either the buttocks or some aspect of the upper thigh. Meticulous hemostasis of the recipient site and careful application of the donor skin are all that is required in obtaining a satisfactory "take" of the graft. Preservation of the subcutaneous tissue in this way provides the patient with an excellent cosmetic and functional result. It must be remembered that a skinning vulvectomy *without* the need for a skin graft vulvoplasty also is a perfectly reasonable way to treat many of these patients, since the paravulvar tissues and distal vaginal mucosa can be easily mobilized and approximated in the usual fashion.

Extramammary Paget's disease of the vulva, however, must *not* be managed with a skinning vulvectomy, but rather by a wide subtotal or total vulvectomy to include some of the subcutaneous tissue, since three characteristic features are unique to this condition. First, the lesion grows horizontally or laterally within the basal epidermis, and histologically this horizontal spread is greater than that seen clinically on initial inspection. For this reason, wide margins of resection should be obtained. Intraoperative frozen section examination may be helpful in reducing subsequent recurrence. A more concentrated solution of acetic acid on a sponge placed up against the margins for 1 to 2 minutes also may help to better outline the intraepithelial extension. Second, whereas most intraepithelial lesions of the vulva have a regular, uniform, and constant basement membrane, in Paget's disease the basement membrane is highly irregular

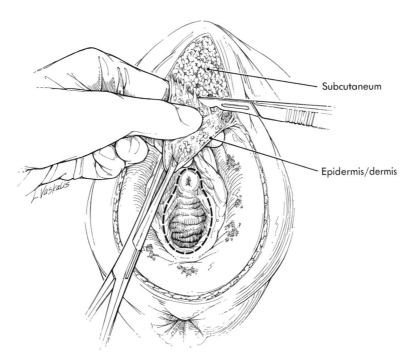

Subcutaneum

Epidermis/dermis

Fig. 36-3   Skinning vulvectomy. Skin incisions are essentially the same as in total vulvectomy. The epidermal/dermal layer of skin is dissected free of underlying subcutaneous tissue. The defect is covered by a split-thickness skin graft; more commonly the wound can be closed per primum.

and its rete pegs push into the dermis to varying depths. A skinning vulvectomy in this situation would more than likely cut across some of these rete pegs, leading to incomplete resection of the lesion and thus the likelihood of recurrence. Last, approximately one fourth to one third of all patients with extramammary Paget's disease of the vulva have invasive adenocarcinoma of either the underlying apocrine gland structures, or more distantly, to include Bartholin glands, as well as endometrial, ovarian, or colorectal tissues.

In view of these characteristic features, Paget's disease of the vulva should be treated by a more traditional type of hemi-, subtotal, or total vulvectomy. This includes the epidermis, dermis, and underlying subcutaneous fat tissue.

Alternative methods of treatment of preinvasive disease of the vulva include topical 5-fluorouracil (Efudex) and carbon dioxide laser therapy, the latter having almost universally replaced cryosurgery in popularity. The disadvantage of 5-fluorouracil is that painful ulcerations arise in the treated area, and only short-term remissions have been reported in most instances. Although laser therapy is used by many gynecologists in the treatment of this condition and these areas heal well cosmetically, the main disadvantages include (1) prolonged healing, (2) no tissue available for the pathologist to determine the depth of disease and presence or absence of margin involvement, (3) hazards to health care personnel from vaporization inhalation, and (4) pain.

Treatment of Microinvasive Lesions of the Vulva

A microinvasive lesion of the vulva is defined as 2 cm or less in diameter and 1 mm or less in depth measuring from the dermal-epidermal junction. This diagnosis can be applied only to an excisional biopsy specimen. These lesions can be satisfactorily treated with a wide local excision or some lesser form of vulvectomy. A groin lymphadenectomy need not be performed, and the 5-year survival rate approximates 100%.

A number of gynecologic oncologists define a superficially invasive carcinoma of the vulva as a 2 cm or less primary lesion with a 1 to 3 mm depth of stromal invasion. These individuals recommend that either an ipsilateral or bilateral (when indicated) superficial groin lymph node dissection and an adequate wide local excision or a partial radical vulvectomy be considered initially as adequate therapy. A superficial dissection of the groin nodes requires that all inguinal lymph nodes lying superficial to the fascia lata be removed. If any of the superficial groin lymph nodes are positive for metastatic disease, however, then an ipsilateral deep groin lymph node dissection must be performed. The deep groin lymph nodes are located in the femoral triangle and lie medial to and parallel to the femoral vein.

Parenthetically, verrucous and basal cell carcinomas are special cases in that these malignancies rarely spread to regional lymph nodes, and wide local excision usually is considered adequate therapy.

Treatment of Invasive Carcinoma of the Vulva

In choosing the appropriate treatment for invasive vulvar carcinoma, the histologic type of lesion, as well as its size and location, must be considered. Squamous cell carcinoma accounts for almost 90% of all vulvar cancers, whereas melanoma is present in 6% to 10%. Other rarer types of vulvar neoplasms include Bartholin's gland adenocarcinoma, adenoid cystic carcinoma, basal cell carcinoma, and various types of sarcoma.

The traditional treatment of choice for invasive carcinoma of the vulva is radical vulvectomy and bilateral groin lymph node dissection with both the inguinal and femoral lymph nodes being excised.

This operation is accomplished through one of the two types of incisions most frequently used today: (1) the trapezoid, or "butterfly," incision (Fig. 36-4, A), used primarily for larger, more involved lesions as an en bloc procedure and for some lesions involving the clitoral and paraclitoral area, and (2) the "three-in-one" incision (see Fig. 36-4, B), which employs separate incisions for the radical vulvectomy and the two groin lymph node dissections. Both techniques have been used selectively and the results are equally satisfactory. Use of the three separate incisions lessens the incidence of wound infection and tissue necrosis, but the classic "butterfly" incision must not be totally abandoned, since clitoral and paraclitoral lesions have a threefold increased incidence of groin lymph node involvement.

Smaller lesions can be treated with further modifications of the three-in-one incision (see Fig. 36-4, C). For example, a radical partial or hemivulvectomy allows for conservation of unaffected vulvar tissues, especially in the region of the clitoris when these areas are uninvolved. Currently a unilateral radical vulvectomy accompanied by an ipsilateral groin lymph node dissection is considered the treatment of choice for a single unilateral lesion that does not encroach on the clitoris or perineal body. Under the latter two circumstances, a bilateral groin lymph node dissection is required. If positive lymph nodes are encountered on the ipsilateral groin side when treating a unilateral lesion, then a contralateral groin lymphadenectomy is indicated. If a margin of normal-appearing vulvar epithelium of at least 1 cm in width can be obtained on all sides of a T1 lesion, the likelihood of a local recurrence is significantly reduced. Heaps et al. noted no local recurrence when 1 cm margins were obtainable, and almost a 50% chance of recurrence if the margin was less than 1 cm. The distance a lesion must be located from the midline before it may be considered a lateral lesion remains undefined, with different authors advocating various definitions. Finally, the vulvar incisions are still further modified when treating an anterior or posterior malignant lesion (see Fig. 36-4, D and E). The final decision on which incision is to be used depends totally on the knowledge and experience of the operating surgeon.

The radical vulvectomy usually is performed after the groin lymph node dissections have been completed, irrespective of the type of incision used to perform the combined procedure. The groin lymph node dissection in

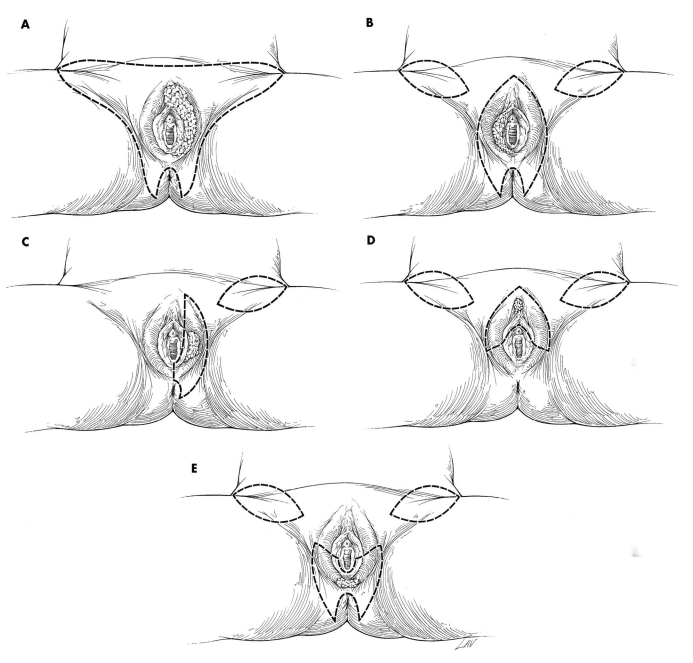

Fig. 36-4   Incisions. **A,** Trapezoid, or "butterfly," incision, commonly used for advanced lesions or when the lesion involves the clitoral-paraclitoral area. **B,** "Three-in-one" incision, used for excision of lesser, more localized invasive lesions or lesions involving the perineal body. **C,** Hemivulvar incision and ipsilateral groin incision (if lymph nodes are negative), used for unilateral invasive lesions of labial tissues. **D,** Anterior vulvar incision and bilateral groin incisions, used to begin dissections for small anterior vulvar lesions. **E,** Posterior vulvar and perineal incision and bilateral groin incisions, used to begin dissections for perineal lesions.

the three-in-one incision usually is a full-thickness dissection using elliptical incisions measuring approximately 12 to 15 cm in length and 5 to 8 cm in width at its widest point. The development of skin flaps with undermining dissection is another technique used by other surgeons. Most important, one must not compromise the length, depth, or width of this dissection, since a permanent cure of this disease is our primary goal. These full-thickness wounds often heal per primum, and even if with wound disruption, the final result is a linear scar at the end of the healing period. If the trapezoid, or butterfly, incision is used as an en bloc approach to the primary lesion and its regional lymph nodes, the full-thickness principle is still of paramount importance, since the elliptical groin masses are removed in continuity with the vulvar tissue to be excised subsequently.

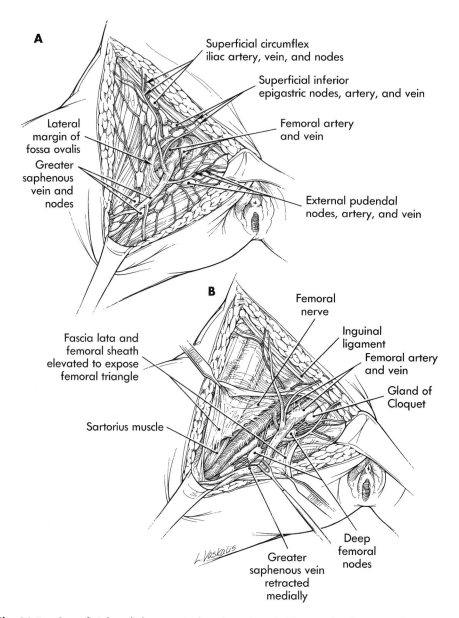

Fig. 36-5 Superficial and deep groin lymph nodes. **A,** The randomly situated superficial groin lymph nodes are located superficial to the fascia lata and alongside superficial arteries and veins in this compartment. **B,** The deep groin lymph nodes lying deep to the fascia lata and femoral sheath are located in a more orderly manner, lying medial and parallel to the femoral vein. The most cephalad lymph node in this chain is the gland of Cloquet (or Rosenmuller's node).

Since the main indication for the groin dissection is not only to interrupt the lymphatic drainage of the vulva but also to excise all the lymph nodes in this area, the surgeon must have an in-depth knowledge of the anatomic structures in this region. The groin lymph nodal tissue is divided into two compartments, referred to as either the inguinal and femoral lymph nodes or the superficial and deep groin lymph nodes, respectively (Fig. 36-5). These compartments are separated by the fascia lata and femoral sheath, which is the portion of the fascia lata that overlies the femoral triangle. The lymph node bearing tissue in the superficial groin or inguinal compartment lies alongside the various veins

draining the specific areas, that is, the saphenous, external pudendal, superficial circumflex iliac, and superficial inferior epigastric vessels. Both blunt and sharp dissection are used in developing an en bloc specimen from these areas. Either 2-0 chromic catgut or synthetic absorbable suture material is used to accomplish hemostasis and ligation of lymphatic channels. A 6 to 7 cm segment of saphenous vein is frequently excised, and all of this tissue is included in the specimen. Many gynecologic oncologists now believe that resection of the saphenous vein is not necessary, however, and when preserved it may help to lessen the incidence of the dependent edema otherwise so commonly seen in the postoperative period. If a portion of the saphenous vein is excised, then the remaining stumps are ligated with 3-0 transfixing silk suture.

The femoral sheath and cribriform fascia cover the femoral canal, which also is referred to as the *femoral triangle.* The lymphatic channels from the superficial groin lymph nodes perforate the cribriform fascia as they drain into the underlying deep groin lymph nodes, and the saphenous vein drains directly into the femoral vein in the region of the fossa ovalis. The deep groin or femoral lymph nodes are located in a more orderly fashion just medial and parallel to the femoral vein. The femoral sheath divides this area into three compartments by septa that are attached to the underlying muscular tissue. The lateral compartment contains the femoral artery; the middle compartment, the femoral vein; and the inner compartment, the femoral lymph nodes. The femoral nerve lies lateral to and *outside* the femoral sheath. Exposure of this nerve at the time of dissection is not only unnecessary but contraindicated.

Classically, inguinal lymphadenectomy involves removal of both the superficial and deep inguinal nodes. Superficial inguinal nodes are the nodes above the fascia lata and cribriform fascia, and the deep inguinal nodes are those beneath the cribriform fascia and within the femoral triangle. A number of studies have demonstrated that deep inguinal nodes are likely to be positive for metastatic disease if the superficial nodes are negative. Nevertheless, ipsilateral recurrence following negative superficial lymphadenectomy occurs in 5% to 8% of patients, presumably from metastases that bypassed the superficial nodes, according to Hacker.[8] Lymphatic mapping with isosulfan blue dye has demonstrated lymph drainage from the vulva directly into the deep inguinal nodes, bypassing the superficial nodes in 8% of patients.[15]

The gland of Cloquet, or Rosenmuller's node, is the uppermost lymph node in the femoral chain. It is located in the upper part of the femoral canal, high in the fossa ovalis, and is often referred to as the *sentinel node.* This node is included in the groin lymph node en bloc dissection. Approximately seven or eight of the remaining lymph nodes in this chain lie distal to the fossa ovalis and underneath the femoral sheath. They are accessed through a longitudinal incision in the overlying femoral sheath. Once these nodes have been excised, the edges of the femoral sheath are reapproximated using absorbable sutures. After further pathologic research, if the gland of Cloquet is negative for metastatic disease, it is suspected by the senior author that the lesser nodes in this chain will be consistently negative and may not have to be excised. This implies that the removal of the lymph nodes in the fossa ovalis, to include the gland of Cloquet, can be easily added to the superficial groin lymph node dissection as a satisfactory groin dissection if the gland of Cloquet is negative for metastatic disease.

On the infrequent occasion when the femoral canal cannot be covered as indicated above, the sartorius muscle is transplanted from its lateral insertion along the inguinal ligament and reattached to the medial portion of the ingui-

nal ligament using absorbable sutures. This acts as a protective covering to the femoral vessels when the femoral sheath in this area has been sacrificed during the dissection.

If an indication for a pelvic lymph node dissection should exist, a linear incision is made through the external oblique aponeurosis and the internal oblique and transverse muscles in the lower abdominal wall, above and parallel to the inguinal ligament. The deep inferior epigastric vessels are clamped, divided, and ligated to aid in this exposure. The dissection is continued down through these flank muscles until the retroperitoneal area is entered. With the peritoneum and its attached ureter reflected medially and superiorly, the pelvic lymph nodes are exposed and excised through this retroperitoneal approach, again using both blunt and sharp dissection. Once hemostasis is obtained, the groin wounds are closed in the usual fashion with interrupted absorbable suture. The use of Jackson-Pratt drains is strictly a reflection of the surgeon's preference. In our experience at the University of Michigan, drains do not have a significant effect on wound complications.

Knowledge of the boundaries of the dissection is important in performing radical vulvectomy. The lateral circumferential incision is along the labiocrural crease bilaterally (Fig. 36-6, *A*). These incisions are connected to each other anteriorly either by en bloc dissection of the groin lymph nodes or by an elliptical incision above the base of the clitoris if separate incisions are used. Posteriorly, a crescent-shaped incision anterior to the anal verge connects the lateral labiocrural incisions. The medial circumferential incision begins anterior to the external urethral meatus and courses down and posteriorly around the introitus at the level of the hymenal ring. For more advanced lesions, the boundaries of dissection must obviously be individualized to give satisfactory wide margins of safety. These incisions and subsequent dissections can be performed with either the scalpel or the electrocautery knife—again depending on the preference and familiarity of the surgeon. Most important, this dissection must move along with dispatch, temporarily having the assistant apply pressure with hemostatic packs until the specimen is removed rather than stopping to tie off the minor bleeders as one goes along. This dissection is continued down to the inferior fascia of the urogenital diaphragm anteriorly and into the ischiorectal fossa posteriorly (see Fig. 36-6, *B* and *C*). The inferior fascia of the urogenital diaphragm is an extension of the rectus abdominis fascia from the abdominal wall down onto the perineum. Care must be taken to isolate and ligate the clitoral and pudendal vessels that supply this area. A major portion of the bulbocavernosus, ischiocavernosus, and superficial transverse perineal muscles is included in this en bloc dissection. The internal pudendal arteries and veins are located at the 4- and 8-o'clock positions as one faces the perineum (see Fig. 36-6, *D*).

Once the specimen is removed, bleeding from the venous plexus, located in the bulbocavernosus muscle, which also contains the vestibular bulb, is best controlled using an all-inclusive, continuous absorbable suture as a "whip stitch" around the introital opening of the vagina (see Fig. 36-6, *E*

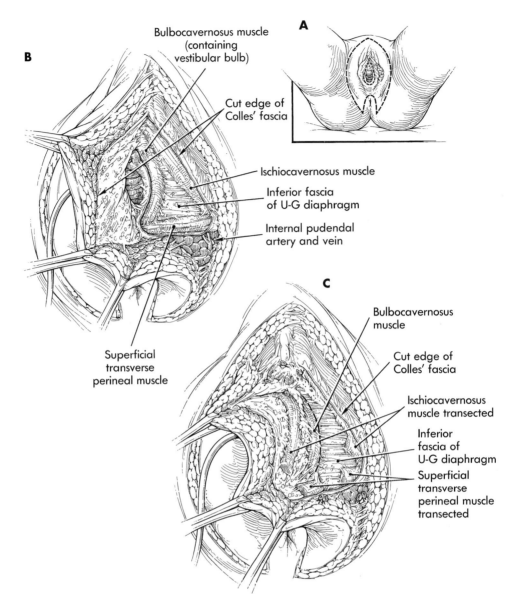

Fig. 36-6 Radical vulvectomy. **A,** Lateral skin incision is located along labiocrural crease with appropriate distances from lesion. Anteriorly it extends up over the mons pubis and posteriorly it is completed with a crescent-shaped incision anterior to the rectum. Medial incision usually is satisfactorily located along the hymenal ring and anterior to the external urethral meatus. **B,** Colles' fascia is dissected and retracted off underlying muscle bundles as a "cutaway" to show location of bulbocavernosus, ischiocavernosus, and superficial transverse perineal muscles. **C,** En bloc dissection performed in radical vulvectomy is extended down to the inferior fascia of the urogenital diaphragm. This en bloc specimen contains the muscle bundles referred to in **B.**

and *F*). Once hemostasis has been obtained, wound closure is performed in a preferential manner. *Remember, mapping and identification of margins are required before sending the specimen to the pathologist.*

POSTOPERATIVE CARE AND COMPLICATIONS

Once the immediate postoperative and postanesthetic periods have passed, patients undergoing this type of surgery usually have a progressively satisfactory course. Most of these patients continue with prophylactic anticoagulant and antibiotic therapy for a reasonable period, and they remain strictly confined to bed for approximately 48 hours assuming a modified semi-Fowler's position to avoid tension on the wound edges. Conservative measures such as logrolling and intermittent movement of the lower extremities are permissible during this period as methods of improving circulation. Sequential compression devices applied to the lower extremities may be used in place of anticoagulation therapy. Subsequently patients are allowed progressive ambulation,

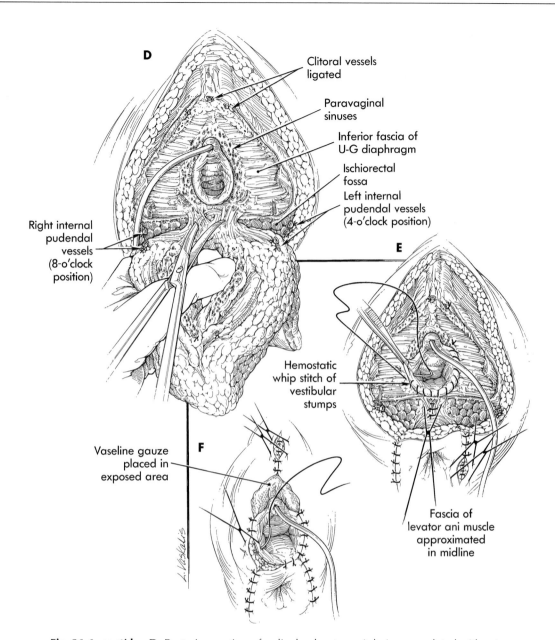

Clitoral vessels ligated

Paravaginal sinuses

Inferior fascia of U-G diaphragm

Ischiorectal fossa

Left internal pudendal vessels (4-o'clock position)

Right internal pudendal vessels (8-o'clock position)

Hemostatic whip stitch of vestibular stumps

Vaseline gauze placed in exposed area

Fascia of levator ani muscle approximated in midline

Fig. 36-6, cont'd **D,** Posterior portion of radical vulvectomy is being completed with extensive resection in the chiorectal fossa. Note that internal pudendal vessels are located in 4- and 8-o'clock positions. **E,** Continuous running "whip stitch" to include vestibular venous stumps and the distal edge of the vaginal mucosa is used as a hemostatic absorbable stitch. This venous plexus was part of the vestibular bulb contained within the bulbocavernosus muscles. **F,** Most vulvar incisions can be approximated primarily. A Foley catheter is inserted into the bladder, and dressings are applied to the wound. Vaseline gauze is placed over the exposed area, which ultimately heals as a linear scar.

and the indwelling catheter is removed on the fourth or fifth postoperative day.

The most common postoperative complications seen in these patients are wound cellulitis and wound disruption, which occur to some degree in approximately 30% to 40% of patients. Usually these separations are not great and are treated conservatively with debridement and open packing. An attempt to reapproximate the wound edges at a later date

is considered unwise because these wounds heal secondarily with a normal-appearing linear scar as their end point.

One must be aware that hemorrhage, although occurring infrequently, can be the result of anticoagulants prescribed prophylactically or of frequent, long-term self-administration of salicylates and similar drugs, as used by many elderly people. Pulmonary embolization itself is rarely reported as a complication of this procedure.

Not infrequently a lymphocyst appears in the groin region. This complication occurs in less than 10% of the cases, and its incidence can be further reduced by careful attention to ligation of the lymphatic vessels in both the superficial and deep groin compartments. Lymphocysts require frequent aspiration followed by local compression to the area. Only on rare occasions does the causative lymphatic vessel need to be surgically isolated and ligated. The usual postoperative complications, which are unrelated to the procedure itself, must also be kept in mind by the attending surgical team throughout the remainder of the hospitalization.

Late complications are of a more permanent nature and primarily are related to alterations of the vaginal introitus, the urinary tract system, and the lower extremities. Introital stenosis of the vagina may give rise to dyspareunia; however, this can easily be corrected using relaxing incisions at the introitus or by performing a reversed perineorrhaphy. Fissuring or "cracking" of the perineum is not uncommon, and a vitamin A and D ointment or other nonmedicated skin softener applied one or two times daily often softens up this inelastic tissue.

Now that less advanced malignant lesions of the vulva are being seen, postsurgical disfigurement is less frequently encountered, even though the local anatomy and appearance of the operative site are obviously altered. Infrequently, a far advanced lesion may require extensive therapeutic surgical intervention, which may necessitate reconstructive vulvoplasty. A number of techniques have been described, which include the classic Z-plasty approach, the myocutaneous gracilis flap technique, and the rhomboid skin flap mobilization.[2,21,27] Again, these procedures are seldom indicated. Finally, if sexual function is satisfactory following primary healing and only local appearance is of concern, patients should probably receive sexual counseling rather than undergo surgical correction of these changes.

A number of patients complain of misdirection of the urinary stream during micturition. The patient can avoid this embarrassment by repositioning herself on the toilet seat or by attaching a plastic deflector to the commode. This annoyance can be prevented at the time of surgery by repositioning the external urethral meatus more proximally on the anterior vaginal wall 1 to 2 cm in from the introitus. If an external urethral stenosis is encountered as a late complication, an external urethral meatotomy may be the only corrective step required.

Not uncommonly, pelvic relaxation with the appearance of a cystocele or rectocele or symptoms of stress urinary incontinence are reported during a follow-up examination. These changes may or may not be related to the radical surgery itself but are easily corrected through well-known nonsurgical or surgical approaches.

Probably the most annoying late complication for the patient and the most frustrating complication for the physician is swelling of the lower extremities, much of which can be avoided if the patient is instructed to use elastic stockings prophylactically for the first 6 months after surgery. In spite of this preventive measure, leg edema develops in a number of patients and must then be treated therapeutically with compression stockings worn almost continuously when ambulatory. To date, surgical intervention has not been successful. Preservation of the saphenous vein at the time of groin lymph node dissection may help to reduce this complication without any compromise of survival. The overall mortality reported of 1% to 2% following radical pelvic surgery for carcinoma of the vulva seems reasonable given that this is a disease of the elderly.

MALIGNANT MELANOMA

Melanoma of the vulva is the second most common type of vulvar malignancy, accounting for about 10% of diagnoses. Three types of melanoma occur on the vulva—superficial spreading malignant melanoma, nodular melanoma, and acral lentiginous melanoma. Most melanoma lesions are pigmented, but amelanotic lesions are not rare. The FIGO anatomic staging system used for squamous cell carcinoma of the vulva is not used for staging vulvar melanoma. The following micro-staging using lesion thickness, described by Breslow, is the best predictor of a prognosis.[20,25]

Breslow's Level	Thickness of Lesion
I	<0.76 mm
II	0.76-1.5 mm
III	1.51-3.0 mm%
IV	>3.0 mm

The Breslow system has been incorporated into the American Joint Commission on Cancer (AJCC) staging system for melanoma, which was adopted in 1992.

In the past, treatment of melanoma of the vulva involved radical vulvectomy and bilateral groin lymphadenectomy. A number of authors have demonstrated that more conservative resection is possible without compromising survival.[16,20,26] Lesion thickness should be taken into account when planning the margin of resection. For lesions less than 1 mm in thickness, a 1 cm margin of resection is adequate. All other lesions should have a 2 cm or greater margin of resection depending on its thickness. The deep margin of resection for vulvar melanoma should extend to the underlying fascia. Inguinal lymphadenectomy for patients with no palpable lymphadenopathy is controversial and has not been shown to improve survival. Palpable nodes should be studied either by fine needle aspiration or biopsy. Patients with lesions less than 1.5 mm in thickness are unlikely to have lymphatic metastases. Some authors advocate elective lymphadenectomy when the lesion is greater than 1.5 mm. Survival following treatment for melanoma is closely correlated with lesion thickness.

RESULTS

The results of collective experience over a 50-year period (1935 to 1990) at the University of Michigan Medical Center are similar to those reported in the literature.[12,17] During this time, almost 500 patients with invasive carcinoma of the vulva were treated with some type of radical vulvar surgery in this institution.

From a review of a collected series over a 20-year literature search,[1,7,17,24] there is a 35% incidence of groin lymph node involvement when all stages of the disease are analyzed—the nodes being involved in 12% to 15% of the cases with stage I disease and in 90% with stage IV disease. The overall 5-year survival rate for all stages approximates 60%, with almost 85% survival in patients with stage I disease. Only a 12% to 15% survival is to be expected in stage IV disease. Given that the regional lymph nodes are negative for metastases, an overall 5-year survival rate of 85% for all stages can be anticipated. The absolute 5-year survival rate for patients with stage I disease and negative lymph nodes approximates 95%. If the regional lymph nodes are positive for metastatic disease, the overall 5-year survival rate drops to around 40%. Again, the lymph node status significantly influences survival; however, it has been shown that the survival rates for patients having only one groin node involvement is essentially equal to the survival of patients with no regional lymph node involvement.

Patients with advanced vulvar cancer are still seen in our clinics, and they present a unique and difficult problem. A surgical approach to advanced vulvar cancer usually involves some type of pelvic exenteration, especially when the primary lesion is geographically located in close proximity to the bladder anteriorly or to the bowel posteriorly. Often these patients respond quite satisfactorily to this radical pelvic surgery, and although the series at Michigan[19] is small, the overall survival approximates 60%. Recently, Boronow and others[3,22] have reported on preoperative irradiation for patients with an advanced lesion. They found that lesser surgery could be anticipated following preoperative irradiation, thus satisfying the goal of preservation of the visceral organs. Boronow reported a 72% 5-year survival rate using this type of combination therapy in patients with stages III and IV carcinoma of the vulva.[4] Radiation therapy alone and postoperative pelvic irradiation are other options still being considered.[10,13] An alternative approach using combined chemo-radiation followed by limited resection has been reported to be effective for these patients.

Approximately 10% of patients have a recurrence of the vulvar malignancy at the primary site.[9,11] The mainstay of therapy for this recurrent disease is wide local excision with or without radiation therapy depending on the surgical margins and the presence or absence of metastatic disease to the regional lymph nodes. Again, the status of the lymph nodes is a significant prognostic factor. When the recurrences remain localized to the vulva, surgical resection of the involved area with wide and deep margins can provide an excellent survival rate for these patients.

Medicine has always been in transition, and it will continue to be so. Results of the treatment of invasive carcinoma of the vulva in the next several years should reflect the current knowledge gleaned from a variety of facts that include (1) a 25% to 35% inaccurate clinical assessment of groin lymph nodes, (2) a threefold increase in groin lymph node involvement in clitoral/perineal lesions, (3) an essentially equal 5-year survival rate for patients with negative groin lymph nodes versus patients with one positive groin lymph node, (4) a 5-year survival rate for all patients in all stages dropping approximately 50% when groin lymph nodes are positive, (5) an ipsilateral groin lymph node dissection only in a unilateral lesion if the lymph nodes are negative, (6) a preservation of body image and sexual response through conservation of normal tissue through a partial or hemiradical vulvectomy when feasible, and (7) a frequently satisfactory survival rate when recurrences are usually treated with radical local excision and supplemental regional lymph node dissection when required.

In closing, it was Mr. Stanley Way of Newcastle-on-Tyne, England, a noted gynecologic oncologist, who once said, "Surgery will one day become obsolete in the treatment of cancer of the vulva." It is hoped that through a better understanding of the biology of the disease and through continued advances in radiation therapy, chemotherapy, and immunotherapy or their combinations, we may be able to provide a new and better direction in the treatment of invasive carcinoma of the vulva in the future.

REFERENCES

1. Annual Report: International Federation of Gynecology and Obstetrics, vol 18, 1988.
2. Barnhill DR, Hoskins WJ, Metz P: Use of the rhomboid flap after partial vulvectomy, *Obstet Gynecol* 62:444, 1983.
3. Boronow RC: Therapeutic alternative to primary exenteration for advanced vulvovaginal cancer, *Cancer* 1:233, 1973.
4. Boronow RC, Hickman BT, Reagan MT, et al: Combined therapy as an alternative to exenteration for locally advanced vulvovaginal cancer. II. Results, complications, and dosimetric and surgical considerations, *Am J Clin Oncol* 10:171, 1987.
5. Burrell MO, Franklin EW III, Campion MJ, et al: The modified radical vulvectomy with groin dissection: an eight-year experience, *Am J Obstet Gynecol* 159:715, 1988.
6. Creasman WT: New gynecologic cancer staging, *Gynecol Oncol* 58:157, 1995 (editorial).
7. Hacker NF, Berek JS, Lagasse LD, et al: Individualization of treatment for stage I squamous cell vulvar carcinoma, *Obstet Gynecol* 63:155, 1984.
8. Hacker NF: Current treatment of small vulvar cancers, *Oncology* 4:21, 1990.
9. Heaps JM, Fu YS, Montz FJ, et al: Surgical-pathologic variables predictive of local recurrence in squamous cell carcinoma of the vulva, *Gynecol Oncol* 38:309, 1990.
10. Homesley HD, Bundy BN, Sedlis A, Adcock L: Radiation therapy versus pelvic node resection for carcinoma of the vulva with positive groin nodes, *Obstet Gynecol* 68:733, 1986.
11. Hopkins MP, Reid GC, Morley GW: The surgical management of recurrent squamous cell carcinoma of the vulva, *Obstet Gynecol* 75:1001, 1990.
12. Hopkins MP, Reid GC, Vettrano I, Morley GW: Squamous cell carcinoma of the vulva: prognostic factors influencing survival, *Gynecol Oncol* 43:113, 1991.
13. Jafari K, Magdotti M: Radiation therapy in carcinoma of the vulva, *Cancer* 47:686, 1981.
14. Jones RW, Rowan DM: Vulvar intraepithelial neoplasia. III. A clinical study of the outcome in 113 cases with relation to the later development of invasive vulvar carcinoma, *Obstet Gynecol* 84:741, 1994.

15. Levenback C, Burke TW, Gershenson DM, et al: Intraoperative lymphatic mapping for vulvar cancer, *Obstet Gynecol* 84:164, 1994.

16. Look KY, Roth LM, Sutton GP: Vulvar melanoma reconsidered, *Cancer* 72:143, 1993.

17. Malfetano J, Piver MS, Tsukada Y: Stage III and IV squamous cell carcinoma of the vulva, *Gynecol Oncol* 23:192, 1986.

18. Morley GW: Infiltrative carcinoma of the vulva: results of surgical management, *Am J Obstet Gynecol* 124:874, 1976.

19. Morley GW, Hopkins MP, Lindenauer SM, Roberts JA: Pelvic exenteration, University of Michigan: 100 patients at 5 years, *Obstet Gynecol* 74:934, 1989.

20. Podratz KC, Gaffey TA, Symmonds RE, et al: Melanoma of the vulva: an update, *Gynecol Oncol* 16:153, 1983.

21. Rankin R, Pinkney JR: The use of Z-plasty in gynecologic operations, *Am J Obstet Gynecol* 117:231, 1973.

22. Rotmensch J, Rubin SJ, Sutton HG, et al: Preoperative radiotherapy followed by radical vulvectomy with inguinal lymphadenectomy for advanced vulvar carcinomas, *Gynecol Oncol* 36:181, 1990.

23. Rutledge F, Sinclair M: Treatment of intraepithelial carcinoma of the vulva by skin excision and graft, *Am J Obstet Gynecol* 102:806, 1968.

24. Trelford JD, Deer DA, Ordorica E, et al: Ten-year prospective study in a management change of vulvar carcinoma, *Am J Obstet Gynecol* 150:288, 1984.

25. Trimble EL, Lewis JL Jr, Williams LL, et al: Management of vulvar melanoma, *Gynecol Oncol* 45:254, 1992.

26. Trimble EL et al: Heterogeneous etiology of squamous carcinoma of the vulva, *Obstet Gynecol* 87:59, 1996.

27. Wheeless CR Jr, McGibbon B, Dorsey JH, Maxwell GP: Gracilis myocutaneous flap in reconstruction of the vulva and female perineum, *Obstet Gynecol* 54:97, 1979.

37 Surgical Staging of Cervical Cancer and Radical Abdominal Hysterectomy and Pelvic Lymphadenectomy

KUNIO MIYAZAWA

HISTORICAL PERSPECTIVE

It was on Christmas day in 1809 in Danville, Kentucky, that Dr. Ephraim McDowell performed the first successful exploratory laparotomy and oophorectomy in the history of pelvic surgery. The operation took only 25 minutes.[17,22,47,53] Subsequent successful removal of the ovary in the hands of a few skillful surgeons led others to attempt the removal of not only a large uterine fundus but also the entire uterus. Laparohysterectomy was first performed by Clay of Manchester, England, in 1843, although Heath in the same district was said to have attempted removal of an adnexal mass that was found to be an enlarged uterus at the time of exploration and subjected to subtotal hysterectomy.[4,39] After these pioneer procedures, hysterectomy was performed several hundred times in Europe but was not well recognized in the United States. After much dissection of many cadavers, Wilhelm Alexander Freund[20] of Breslau (now Wroclow), Poland, introduced the most refined technique of abdominal hysterectomy on January 30, 1878, on a patient with cancer of the uterus. Although there was great interest in this procedure, most surgeons preferred the vaginal hysterectomy for the treatment of cancer of the cervix because of very high mortality due to peritonitis subsequent to abdominal hysterectomy. As time passed it became clear that at best only 17% of patients were free of cervical cancer 2 years after vaginal hysterectomy.[9] In the early nineteenth century an attempt was made without success to treat cervical cancer by simple cervical amputation. The use of simple abdominal hysterectomy was not successful either.

The modern surgical treatment of cervical carcinoma may be traced to John Clark at Johns Hopkins Hospital who undertook a radical abdominal operation for the treatment of invasive cervical cancer in 1895.[27] In 1907 Wertheim of Vienna first described 500 patients with cervical cancer treated by a radical surgical procedure, which was popularized mainly in Europe.[61] In 1921 Okabayashi[38] introduced his technique of removing the widest parametrium and the cancer-infiltrated area according to Takayama, who developed and described his method at the Japanese Gynecological Association Meeting 10 years previously. In May 1934 Bonney[6] of London presented his operative technique of Wertheim's operation at the annual meeting of the American Gynecological Society. Taussig of St. Louis, Missouri, in 1934 published his iliac lymphadenectomy technique for irradiated patients.[54-56] In 1944 Meigs[28] of Boston

published his radical surgical procedure. He called this operation the Wertheim-Clark plus Taussig operation by which he proved that the procedure could be carried out with a mortality rate of 1% by a specially trained gynecologist.[28-31] In 1952 Yagi[62] reported on his 333 patients treated by Okabayashi's radical hysterectomy and pelvic lymphadenectomy. Since then, various modifications have been introduced by pelvic surgeons to reduce operative morbidity and mortality and to bring about a better quality of life.

Over the past 30 to 40 years, much advancement and improvement have been made in anesthesia, intensive care, antibiotics, and blood component therapy, as well as surgical techniques, resulting in better operability and improved complication and survival rates. At the same time, the incidence of invasive cervical carcinoma in the United States has declined to the third most common of the female genital tract cancers, whereas 30 years ago it was the most common invasive cancer. As a result of increased understanding of the natural history of cervical cancer, the surgical approach to early invasive cervical carcinoma has been changing gradually from a radical approach to a conservative procedure resulting in decreased mortality and morbidity, as well as a better quality of life.[2]

Surgical staging has become a popular method to define the exact extent of the disease. Laparoscopy has been receiving attention as a cost-effective procedure for lymph node evaluation in determining the extent of the cancer accurately through definitive tissue diagnosis, thus establishing a proper treatment plan.

PREOPERATIVE CONSIDERATIONS
Indications

Given that early cervical carcinoma may be managed by either surgery or radiation therapy with similar outcomes, the following are the most common indications for radical surgical management of early invasive cervical carcinoma:

1. A young patient who needs preservation of ovarian function
2. Any patient who desires preservation of sexual vaginal function
3. Any patient for whom radiation treatment is contraindicated (such as a history of severe pelvic inflammatory disease or inflammatory bowel disease)
4. Any patient who desires a short treatment time

Contraindications

The following are considered contraindications of radical surgical management of early invasive cervical carcinoma:

1. Serious medical condition
2. Metastasis to paraaortic nodes
3. Metastasis to multiple pelvic nodes
4. Carcinoma involving parametrial region or vesico-uterine space
5. Massive obesity
6. Old age (However, Lawton and Hacker[24] suggest that chronologic age is a poor determinant of surgical risk and elderly patients can go through radical surgery almost as well as their younger counterparts.)
7. Barrel-shaped lesion of the cervix (should be treated by radiotherapy and extrafascial hysterectomy, especially when the lesion is larger than 5 cm)

The most important decision a pelvic surgeon must make before a surgical procedure consists of how to individualize therapy and whether to use radiation therapy or radical hysterectomy. The benefits and risks (both short-term and long-term effects) of both treatments should be fully explained to the patient so that she may make an informed decision.

Preparation

History and Physical Examination. A careful history is a sine qua non for preoperative evaluation. Particular attention should be paid to the patient's current general physical status, history of medical illnesses, and unusual problems such as ease of bruising and bleeding. Recent ingestion of aspirin-containing drugs should be ruled out. Review of each organ system should be carefully carried out. Existing iron deficiency anemia should be corrected in advance with oral iron and multivitamins. Smoking should be stopped to prevent postoperative atelectasis. The degree of cardiovascular tolerance to exercise is a good indication of her physical stress reserve.

Laboratory Studies. In addition to the routine preoperative evaluation of blood count, platelet and differential, and urinalysis, a renal and hepatic profile should be obtained. Chest x-ray film and electrocardiogram are to be ordered. Patients who smoke, are obese, or have an existing lung disorder should undergo an arterial blood gas analysis and pulmonary function tests, which assist the patient postoperatively. An intravenous pyelogram (or CT scan) is commonly obtained for metastatic workup.

Preoperative Orders. Adequate blood should be available, although for cost effectiveness, blood from most patients needs only to be typed and screened. A review of one series reported a mean blood loss of 1400 ml from radical hysterectomy.[34] The patient should have a thorough mechanical and antibiotic bowel preparation. Use of 4 L of GoLYTELY 1 day before the surgery provides a good bowel preparation. The patient should be taught pulmonary toilet with an incentive spirometer. The patient should walk as much as possible on the ward and should be advised to resume this as soon as possible after surgery. Prophylaxis of venous thromboembolism should be initiated perioperatively.

STAGING CONSIDERATIONS

When we discuss "staging of cervical cancer" it is extremely important to define which staging system we are talking about. There are two approaches: clinical staging and surgical staging. Obviously it is crucial that clinicians understand the differences between these systems so that everyone is of the same mind when discussing the stage of cervical cancer.

Clinical FIGO Staging

FIGO (Federation International Obstetrics and Gynecology) established a clinical staging system with clear rules to follow for each clinical case. Adequate staging requires cervical biopsy, cystoscopy, proctosigmoidoscopy, chest x-ray study, and an intravenous pyelogram (or CT scan). FIGO clinical staging is based on a careful clinical examination that must be performed before any therapy is undertaken. Optimal clinical staging usually is conducted under general anesthesia when cystoscopy and sigmoidoscopy are planned jointly by a team of experienced examiners such as a gynecologic oncologist and a radiation oncologist. Clinical staging cannot be changed once assigned. Presently available modern diagnostic tools such as CT and MRI study are being used more frequently than examinations such as lymphangiography. Although these examinations provide valuable information to clinicians, the established clinical staging should not be changed. Adherence to the established rules will assist in overall improved communication among clinicians all over the world and yield more reliable statistical data in the comparison of various treatment methods.

In 1994 the International Federation of Gynecology and Obstetrics updated and revised the staging of cervical cancer[52] (see the box on the next page). However, clinical staging is often deficient for overall evaluation and follow-up of cervical cancer patients. This is primarily because the FIGO clinical staging system is based on the belief that cervical cancer is mainly a local disease in the female pelvis and that lack of extensive surgical evaluation makes it impossible for developing countries to participate in a surgical staging system. This reality must be appreciated, since invasive cervical cancer is still the major cause of death from cancer of women in developing countries. The lack of adequate Pap smear screening programs results in a delay in diagnosis and treatment of cervical intraepithelial neoplasia, resulting in about 450,000 new cases annually of invasive cervical cancer.

Surgical Staging System

The surgical staging system was born when Nelson reported staging laparotomy for 13 patients with stages IIB and III carcinoma of the cervix at the annual clinical meeting of the Society of Gynecologic Oncology in January 1970. Nelson commented that the impetus for his work was the case of a young woman with stage IIA cervical carcinoma who underwent laparotomy with the surgical intention of radical hysterectomy and pelvic lymphadenectomy, but a large single paraaortic node was infiltrated with metastatic epidermoid carcinoma. In his initial report 7 of 13 patients were found to have histologically proven metastatic disease

1995 FIGO STAGING (MONTREAL) FOR CARCINOMA OF THE CERVIX UTERI

STAGE I

The carcinoma is strictly confined to the cervix (extension to the corpus should be disregarded).

Stage IA

Invasive cancer identified only microscopically.

All gross lesions even with superficial invasion are stage IB cancers.

Invasion is limited to measured stromal invasion with maximum depth of 5.0 mm and maximum width of 7.0 mm.

Stage IA1

Measured invasion of stroma no deeper than 3.0 mm and no wider than 7.0 mm.

Stage IA2

Measured invasion of stroma deeper than 3.0 mm and no greater than 5.0 mm and no wider than 7.0 mm.

The depth of invasion should not be more 5.0 mm taken from the base of the epithelium, either surface or glandular, from which it originates. Preformed space involvement (vascular or lymphatic) should not alter the staging but should be specifically recorded to determine its effect on future treatment decisions.

Stage IB

Clinical lesions confined to the cervix or preclinical lesions greater than stage IA.

Stage IBl

Clinical lesions no greater than 4.0 cm.

Stage IB2

Clinical lesions greater than 4.0 cm.

STAGE II

The carcinoma extends beyond the cervix but has not extended to the pelvic wall. The carcinoma involves the vagina but not as far as the lower third.

Stage IIA

No obvious parametrial involvement.

Stage IIB

Obvious parametrial involvement.

STAGE III

The carcinoma has extended to the pelvic wall. On rectal examination, there is no cancer-free space between the tumor and the pelvic wall. The tumor involves the lower third of the vagina. All cases with a hydronephrosis or nonfunctioning kidney are included unless they are known to be due to other causes.

Stage IIIA

No extension to the pelvic wall.

Stage IIIB

Extension to the pelvic wall and/or hydronephrosis or nonfunctioning kidney.

STAGE IV

Extension beyond the true pelvis or clinical involvement of the mucosa of the bladder or rectum.

A bullous edema as such does not permit a case to be allotted to stage IV.

Stage IVA

Spread to adjacent organs.

Stage IVB

Spread to distant organs.

From The Society of Gynecologic Oncologists: *Clinical practice guidelines: management of gynecologic cancers,* Oct 1996.

in the paraaortic nodes above the bifurcation of the aorta. Nelson's work at the New York Downstate Medical Center was confirmed by other independent studies.[35] The technique has evolved into a retroperitoneal approach to the lymph nodes, thereby avoiding adhesions and a subsequent increase in bowel complications from radiation.

Surgical staging can provide crucial information to guide surgical or radiotherapy management. Furthermore, data obtained from various management strategies eventually lead to the most effective care of cancer patients for better survival and prognostic indicator analysis. Various attempts are being made to determine lymph node status through minimally invasive technology such as fine needle aspiration, which is guided under CT scanning or MRI. The most important thing to remember is that the purpose surgical staging is to establish the extent of the disease accurately before deciding on treatment. When surgical staging is considered together with histopathological evaluation of the primary lesion, prognostic factors may be more accurately assessed. For example, Patsner et al.[40] reported that 2 of 125 patients with FIGO stage IB invasive cervical cancer carcinoma had

metastases to the paraaortic nodes at exploration for radical hysterectomy. Both patients with microscopic paraaortic nodal metastases had grossly positive pelvic node involvement. This led the authors to conclude that paraaortic node sampling can be limited to patients with suspicious pelvic or paraaortic nodes when the clinical stage IB cervical carcinoma is 3 cm or less in diameter. It is hoped that a new staging system based on clinical and surgical evaluation together with histopathological analysis will be entertained worldwide. This will result in improved staging and better care of cancer patients.

Surgical staging by laparoscopy is a newly and rapidly developing technology for evaluating lymph node status for cervical carcinoma and other gynecologic malignancies. There is a surge of interest among gynecologic oncologists in applying this surgical technology to the evaluation of lymph node status before definitive treatment is initiated in the management of cervical carcinoma. Querleu et al.[42] reported their experience with laparoscopic pelvic lymphadenectomy in the staging of 39 patients with early carcinoma of the cervix. They concluded that it is possible to remove the first line of regional lymph nodes (obturator, external iliac, and hypogastric lymph nodes) with minimal surgical trauma. They believed the risk of missing a positive node is low, as a skip metastasis is rare in early cervical carcinoma. The average number of lymph nodes removed ranged from 3 to 22, with a mean of 8.7.

Occult metastasis to the paraaortic lymph node accounts for a significant number of treatment failures in patients with advanced cervical carcinoma who are treated by radiation alone. We know that routine paraaortic node sampling of cervical cancer patients yields valuable information for treatment planning. The experience of Childers et al.[7] with laparoscopic pelvic and paraaortic lymphadenectomy shows that the number of nodes removed averaged 31.4, and subsequently an average of 2.8 additional nodes were removed at the time of radical hysterectomy. They report no significant complication, with discharge on the first postoperative day if no additional surgery is performed. In their preliminary data Fowler et al.[18] reported no lymph nodes missed by laparoscopic lymphadenectomy among 12 patients who underwent laparoscopic pelvic and paraaortic lymphadenectomy for cervical cancer. Similar data were reported by Recio et al.[43] of 12 patients with stage IB2 cervical carcinoma (lesion 5 cm or more) who underwent pretreatment transperitoneal laparoscopic staging pelvic and paraaortic lymphadenectomy. An average of 25 lymph nodes were obtained (18 pelvic and 7 paraaortic). Pelvic nodal metastasis was found in 3 patients, all of whom had a negative CT scan. They emphasized the feasibility of this method, as well as its association with minimal morbidity, short hospital stay, and minimal delay before radiation therapy. The technique has been used in Europe and the United States and also has begun to be used in countries where cervical cancer still remains a common disease. Chu et al.[8] in Taiwan reported their preliminary experience using laparoscopic pelvic or paraaortic lymphadenectomy for surgical staging procedure in the pretreatment evaluation of cervical carcinoma in 67 patients. They found an average of 14.2 nodes from the right side and 12.5 nodes from the left in pelvic lymphadenectomy and 8 nodes from both sides in paraaortic lymphadenectomy. They concluded that this is an efficient and feasible surgical staging technique.

TECHNICAL ASPECT
Radical Abdominal Hysterectomy and Pelvic Lymphadenectomy

Review of Meig's Operative Technique. Professor E. Wertheim's paper, "The Extended Abdominal Operation for Carcinoma Uteri," was translated into English and appeared in August 1912.[61] Since this original work, many modifications have appeared. The procedure that became popular in the United States is that of Dr. Joe V. Meigs in Boston, with his first publication in 1944.[28] Various modifications have followed. For details of modifications of this procedure, the reader can refer to various textbooks on pelvic surgery. Major points are presented here briefly for review purposes.[31,32]

This procedure could be accomplished in the following manner. After a Foley drainage system is placed into the patient's bladder, careful pelvic and rectal examinations are performed to determine the extent of the tumor and its mobility. The vagina and cervix are painted with Schiller's solution, and any unstained area is identified. After the extent of the tumor is determined, the abdominal portion of surgery begins. The operating surgeon usually stands on the left side of the patient while the patient is kept in a Trendelenburg position. A midline incision is made from the mons pubis to the umbilicus. The pyramidalis muscle at the lower end is preserved. If necessary for better exposure the incision could be extended to the right side of the umbilicus. To provide an extra space for pelvic dissection, the fascial incision proceeds down to the symphysis. Exploration of the abdominal cavity and contents is carried out, with special attention given to the paraaortic area. If an enlarged node above the bifurcation is detected, it must be dissected for frozen section diagnosis. The abdomen is packed in a systematic manner, a self-retaining retractor is placed, and the uterus is grasped with a double hook or tenaculum. With adequate upward tension on the uterus, the pelvic cavity and organs are inspected and palpated for any sign of tumor extension.

The peritoneal reflection on the lower uterine region is entered by a small superficial incision and extended laterally with the aid of the index finger and scissors. The peritoneal edge is pulled to reflect the median raphe. Fine fibers between the bladder and vagina are incised. The round ligament and infundibulopelvic ligament are ligated and dissected if ovarian preservation is not applicable. Then the same procedure is carried out on the opposite side. Next, the paravesical space and pararectal space are explored bilaterally. Care should be exercised so as not to injure the internal vein in exploration of the pararectal space because this causes tremendous unnecessary bleeding between the ureter and hypogastric vessels. The cardinal ligament (Web) is now palpated for any evidence of tumor invasion. It usually is soft bilaterally when free from tumor. Bilateral pelvic lymph nodes are palpated in the entire chain; if any enlarged node is present, it should be removed for frozen section diagnosis. With the uterus pulled to the opposite side, the ureter is identified on the medial flap of the peritoneum and the uterine vessels are noted arising from the hypogastric vessels. The uterine artery is ligated and dissected at the origin bilaterally. It is important to spare the superficial vesical artery at this point. The ureter is separated gently from the underlying medial leaf of the peritoneum without damaging the ureteral sheath in which there is a longitudinal arterial blood supply to the ureter. Further dissection is made, separating the bladder from the lower end of the cervix and the anterior vaginal wall. The posterior peritoneum in the rectovaginal space is widely incised transversely, and the rectovaginal space is entered ensuring that the rectum is away from the cervix and vagina. With the bladder well advanced and the rectum separated, the ureter is dissected away from the tissues that lie above and beneath it. With the ureter under light traction, it is untunneled, and the tissue overlying the ureter is divided without causing any trauma to the ureter. The ureter is freed from all attachments until it enters the bladder. The most lateral aspect of the bladder is dissected free from the underlying tissue. The same procedure is applied to the opposite side. The deep uterosacral ligament is severed closer to the rectum, and the cardinal ligament is incised as laterally as possible. The same is applied to paracervical and paravaginal tissues. The vagina is removed, including the upper 3 to 4 cm portion, depending on tumor extension and Schiller's staining. The cuff is closed by interlocking suture.

With the uterus removed and pelvic dissection completed, dissection of the regional lymph nodes follows, beginning lateral to the external iliac vessels along the psoas muscle. With retraction of the external iliac vessels, the obturator space becomes accessible. The genitofemoral nerve is preserved. All lymph node–bearing tissue is removed from the pelvic wall down to the obturator nerves. Dissection moves upward to the common iliac vessels, and the distal and proximal ends are ligated to prevent lymphocyst formation. All lymphatic and surrounding fat is removed from the external iliac vessels distally to the deep circumflex iliac vein. For the nodes of the obturator space, the external iliac artery and vein are retracted and the block of tissue is removed. The lateral tissue along the external iliac vessels is removed. Extreme care should be taken to remove the tissue from the hypogastric vessels and presacral area without injury to the vein.

Complete hemostasis is obtained from the operating site. The ureters and bladder are inspected, and rectal injuries are ruled out. The peritoneum is closed, placing the ureters in the retroperitoneal space, and a Hemovac drain is placed in both retroperitoneal cavities. The abdomen is closed in three layers.

Introduction of Uchida's Technique of Radical Hysterectomy and Pelvic Lymphadenectomy.[57,58] It is my greatest privilege to present Uchida's technique here for the surgical management of cervical cancer, with narrative and illustrations provided to make it clear and simple. His technique was born as a result of more than 4500 radical hysterectomies he performed over the past 45 to 50 years. His technique has been mastered by many Asian gynecologic oncologists. It originated with Okabayashi's technique, which was later modified by Yagi and others.[34,38,62] The most impressive point of his technique is an average operating time of 75 minutes with minimal blood loss, yet resulting in an excellent 5-year survival rate. Few differences exist between his technique and a standard radical hysterectomy, which the author would like to point out as the text progresses.

After the patient is properly prepared and draped, a low abdominal longitudinal incision is made. After the abdomen is explored, a self-retaining retractor is used to expose the pelvis widely. Two pairs of Uchida's uterine clamps are applied to the sides of the uterus, including the round and uteroovarian ligaments. Because of the catches on the clamp

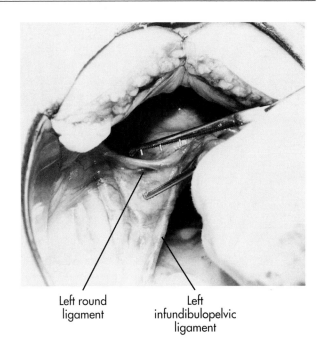

Left round   Left
ligament   infundibulopelvic
                    ligament

Fig. 37-1 Uchida's uterine clamp with its special catches avoids slippage during uterine manipulation.

it is easy to manipulate the uterus during the operative procedure (Fig. 37-1).

The round and infundibulopelvic ligaments are ligated and severed. The broad ligament is now widely separated between two sheets (Fig. 37-2). The uterine artery is isolated, ligated, and severed at its origin (Fig. 37-3). The ureter is separated in one scissors stroke from the posterior leaf of the broad ligament (Fig. 37-4). The same procedure is carried out on the opposite side of the pelvis.

Lymphadenectomy starts with the paraaortic region. Along the common iliac and external iliac vessels, lymph nodes and fatty tissue are removed by the "peeling off" technique. The very fine space between the blood vessel and the lymphatic system is detected by peeling off the lymphatic tissue (Fig. 37-5). Lymph tissue should be removed from the external iliac vessels in one block, including the hypogastric chain. It should be noted that the clamp is used to peel off the lymphatic tissue. The obturator space is next explored, and the obturator nerve and vessels are identified. The same technique is used to clear the lymphatic system in this area. The obturator nerve is easily visible, naked and white (Fig. 37-6, *A*). The obturator nodes are removed as an entire block. The same procedure is applied to the opposite side of the lymphatic chain.

Now, the rectovaginal space is opened widely, creating a large rectovaginal sac (Fig. 37-6, *B*). The pararectal space and paravesical space are opened bilaterally. The cardinal ligament is completely isolated now. The lymphatic system and blood vessels around the root of the ligament are squeezed and pushed upward to the uterine side. The cardinal ligament is now narrow and thin with remaining naked, thick vessels (Fig. 37-7). This is clamped near the sidewall, cut, and ligated. The deep uterosacral ligament is clamped

Text continued on p. 674

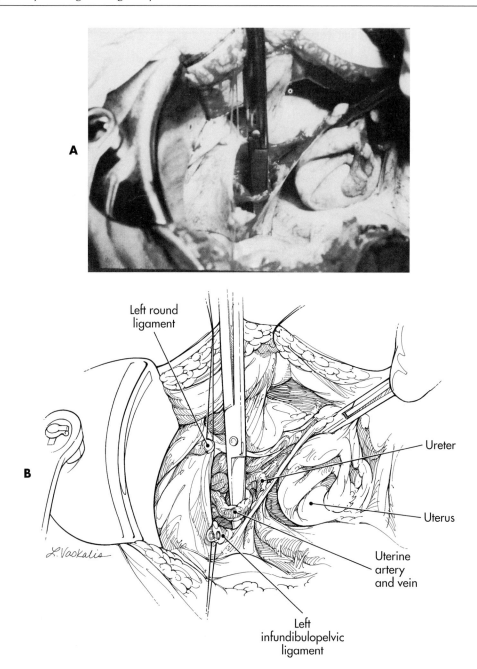

Fig. 37-2 **A,** The round and infundibulopelvic ligaments are ligated and severed. The retroperitoneal space is entered by separating between two sheets of broad ligaments and the uterine vessels are identified. **B,** Schematic of **A.**

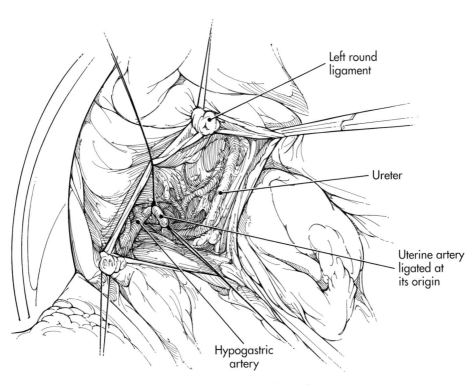

Left round
ligament

Ureter

Uterine artery
ligated at
its origin

Hypogastric
artery

Fig. 37-3   The uterine artery is ligated at its origin.

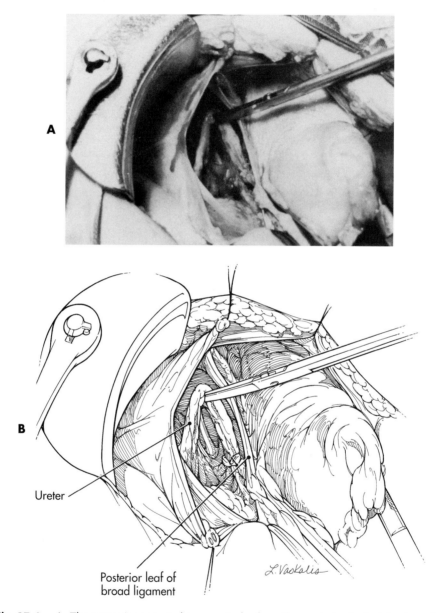

Ureter

Posterior leaf of
broad ligament

Fig. 37-4   **A,** The ureter is separated in one stroke from the posterior leaf of the broad ligament. **B,** Schematic of **A.**

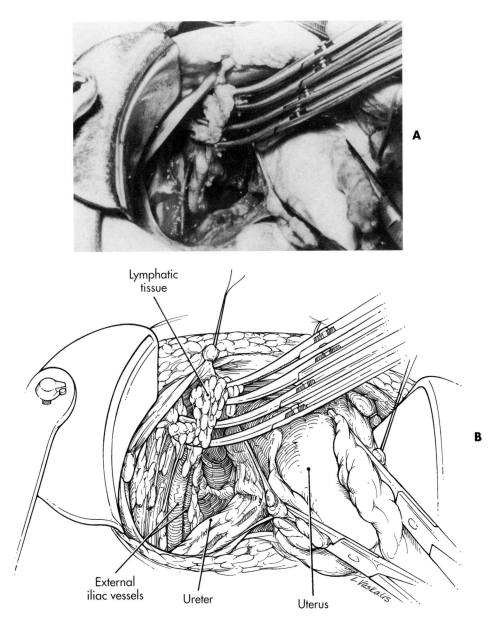

Fig. 37-5   **A,** Lymph nodes and fatty tissue are removed by peeling off lymphatic tissue.
B, Schematic of **A.**

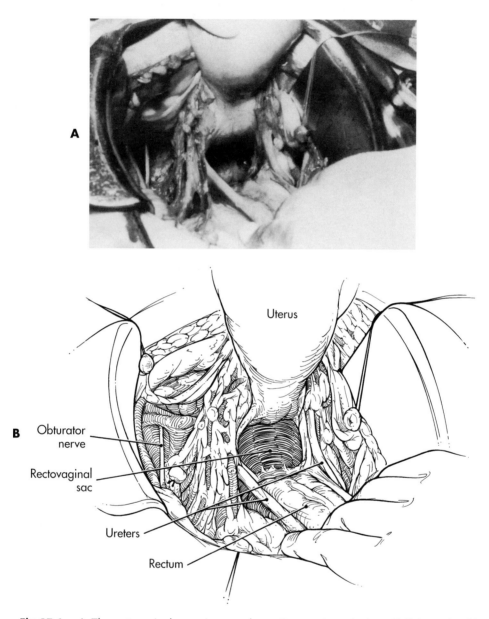

A

B   Obturator
nerve

Rectovaginal
sac

Ureters

Rectum

Uterus

Fig. 37-6   **A,** The rectovaginal space is opened, creating a rectovaginal sac. **B,** Schematic of **A.**

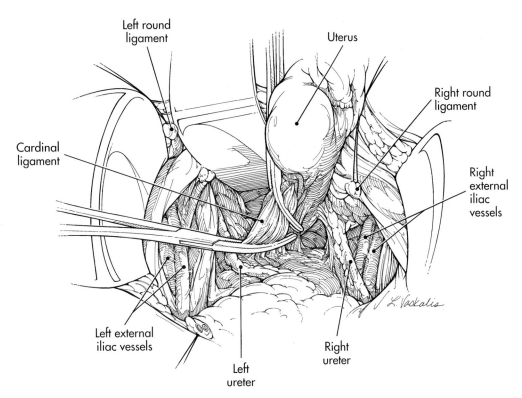

Fig. 37-7 The cardinal ligament is doubly clamped before it is resected from the left pelvic sidewall. Each uterosacral ligament is then clamped, cut, and sutured.

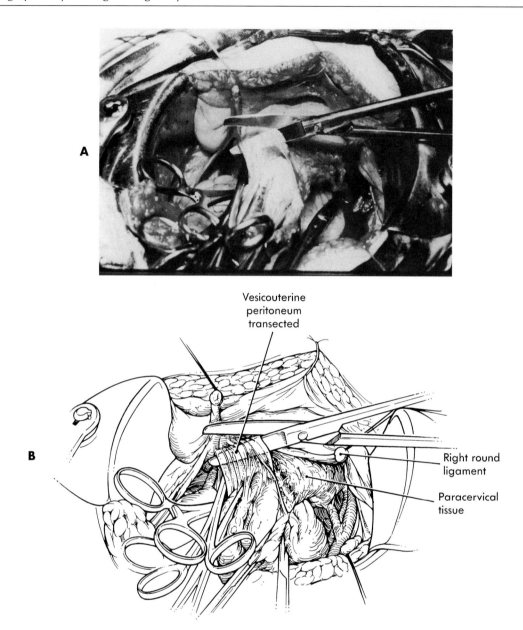

Vesicouterine
peritoneum
transected

Right round
ligament

Paracervical
tissue

Fig. 37-8 **A,** The vesicouterine peritoneum is incised transversely after a tentlike space is created. **B,** Schematic of **A.**

near the rectum, cut, and sutured. Next, vesicovaginal exposure is begun by placing and pushing a scissors between the vesicouterine peritoneum and the cervix. Use of the scissors is important to create a tentlike space. The peritoneum is cut transversely (Fig. 37-8). It is crucial to confirm that there is no bleeding when the medial portion of the bladder is separated from the vagina. The lateral margin of the vesicouterine ligament should not be touched because it bleeds excessively. To separate the ureter from this area, a special instrument is used—Uchida's ureter scoop, which has grooves on both edges. By suspending with two pairs of forceps the portion where the ureter goes into the bladder pillar, a triangular space is produced (Fig. 37-9). The ureter scoop is pushed through the fine space between the anterior portion of the vesicouterine ligament and the ureter, and two

pairs of long and thin forceps are inserted just above the ureter (Fig. 37-10). The anterior portion of the vesicouterine ligament is incised along the two long thin forceps on the uterine side. When the two pairs of forceps are turned over, the ureter appears under the scoop. The forceps are placed away from the bladder (Fig. 37-11). When the two pairs of the forceps are further turned aside, departing further from the ureter, a space can be noticed beside the ureter and between the cervix and the bladder. Uchida found no bleeding to occur even if the tissue adjacent to the uterus is not clamped. To separate the ureter from the uterus, this space is pushed through and opened (Fig. 37-12). Fig. 37-12, *B,* illustrates how the bladder pillar and the ureter can be manipulated. Through this space two pairs of slim forceps are inserted and an incision is made between the forceps to

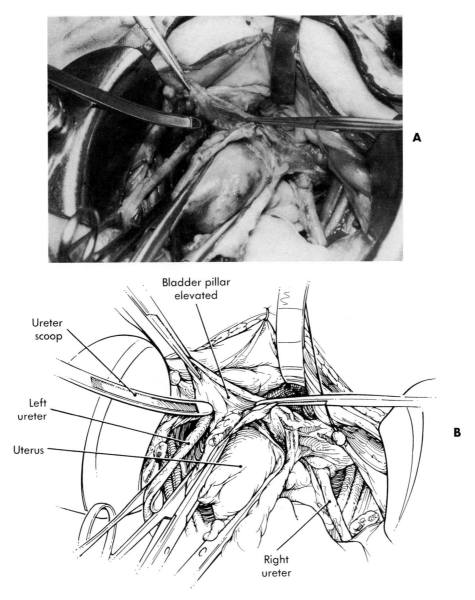

Fig. 37-9 **A,** Using Uchida's ureter scoop and two pairs of forceps, the bladder pillar is elevated and a triangular space is produced. **B,** Schematic of **A.**

separate the ureter from the cervix. The posterior layer is separated and incised. Both layers are ligated with fine suture. The ureter can be noted (Fig. 37-13).

Uchida's paracolpium clamps are used to separate the connecting tissue around the vagina. This clamp has catches on the tip. Two pair of clamps are placed in the paravaginal tissue (Fig. 37-14). Paravaginal tissue is cut between two clamps. The catches are very effective for grasping the soft paracolpium tightly without any slippage. The paravaginal tissue is excised between the clamps and ligated. The vagina is amputated, and the uterine specimen is removed (Fig. 37-15). The entire vagina should be inspected before closure of the cuff (Fig. 37-16). The vaginal cuff is closed by running interlocking sutures to provide and retain enough length of vagina and facilitate good postoperative drainage. Two drains are inserted into the pelvic cavity through the vagina

and fixed to the vaginal wall with very fine catgut. The edge of the bladder flap is sutured to the vaginal cuff and the rectal peritoneal edge to the cuff with chromic catgut. The ureters are placed in the abdominal cavity by closing the retroperitoneum. This replacement of the ureters in the abdominal cavity can maintain ureters straight to the bladder through the abdominal peritoneal cavity. Uchida believes that such placement of the ureters prevents formation of a ureteral fistula and pyelitis. The abdominal cavity receives 100 ml of antibiotic solution, the peritoneum and fascia are closed with continuous catgut, and the skin incision is reapproximated with clips.

Uchida states that before he achieved success with this operation, he had to overcome innumerable difficulties. Some characteristics of Uchida's technique are summarized here. No suction apparatus is used during the procedure,

Text continued on p. 681

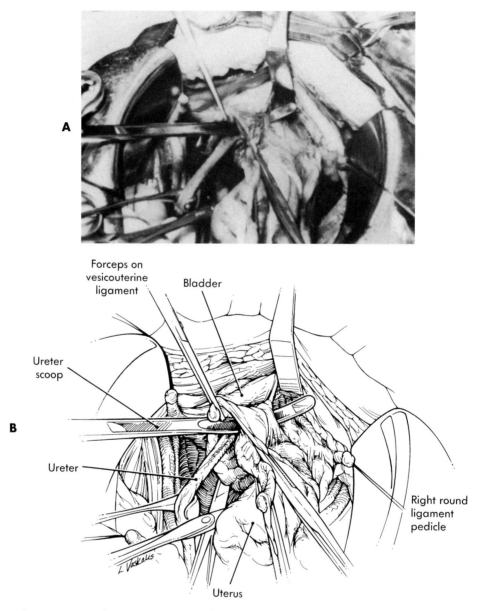

Fig. 37-10   A, The ureter scoop is pushed through the space between the anterior portion of vesicouterine ligament and ureter, and forceps are inserted above the ureter. **B,** Schematic of **A.**

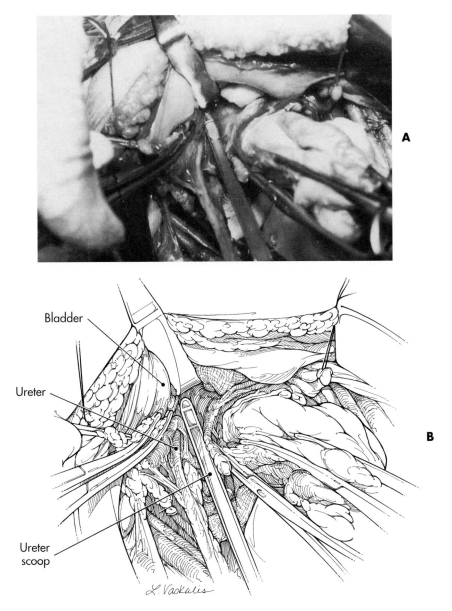

Fig. 37-11   **A,** When two pairs of forceps are turned over, away from bladder, the ureter appears under the scoop. **B,** Schematic of **A.**

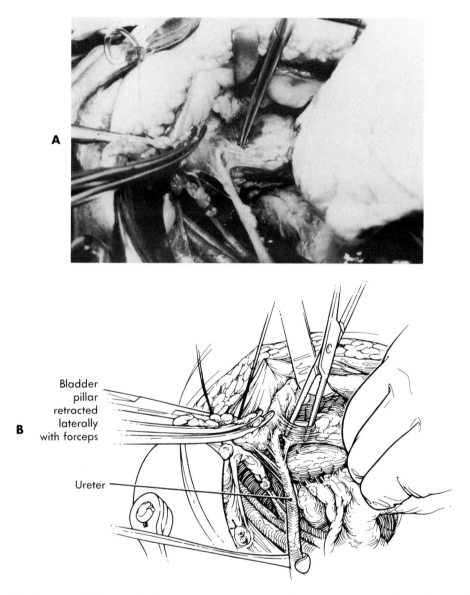

Fig. 37-12 **A,** To separate the ureter from the uterine side, forceps are used to push through and are then opened. **B,** Manipulation of bladder pillar and ureter.

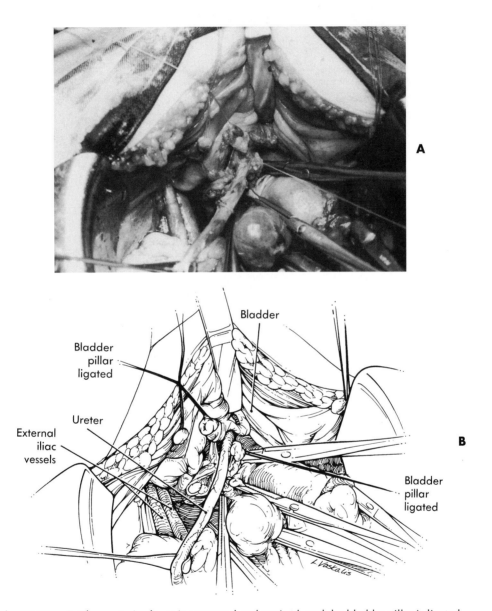

Fig. 37-13 **A,** The posterior layer is separated and excised, and the bladder pillar is ligated.
B, Schematic of **A**.

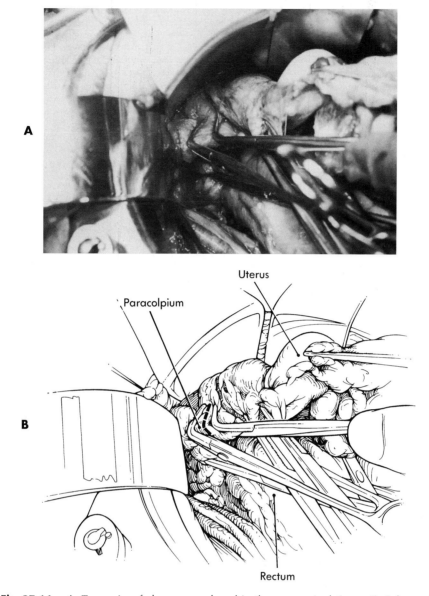

Fig. 37-14   **A,** Two pairs of clamps are placed in the paravaginal tissue. **B,** Schematic of **A.**

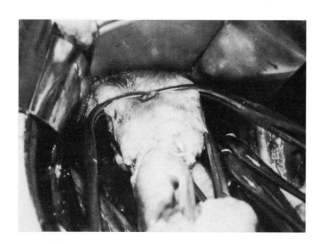

Fig. 37-15   The vagina is clamped bilaterally to include adequate vaginal cuff below the cervix.

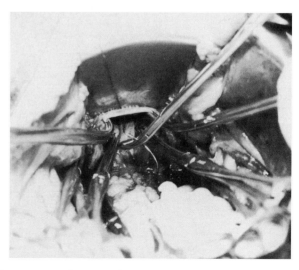

Fig. 37-16   The vaginal cuff is sutured with one continuous running stitch.

because very little bleeding occurs. Only gauze is used for pressing bleeding tissue. During dissection, anatomic avascular fine spaces between tissues or organs are used for the procedure. He emphasizes detection of anatomic fine avascular spaces between tissues or organs and expanding these spaces rather than making frequent incisions and amputations. This technique reduces blood loss greatly during this operative procedure. Successful surgery depends on special instruments, in particular, a uterine clamp with catches at the tip that can hold up the uterus during the procedure, a Paracolpium clamp with catches at the tip that can grasp the paravaginal tissue firmly (preventing slipping), and a ureteral scoop that is used for separating the ureter from the vesicouterine ligaments. Other unique techniques include separating the ureter from the posterior leaf of the broad ligament in one stroke, peeling off lymph nodes and tissue from the arteries and veins in one entire block for lymphadenectomy, as if a snake's skin were being shed, squeezing the cardinal ligament toward the uterus to make it narrow and thin and incising as close as possible to the pelvic sidewall, and separating the ureter by Uchida's ureteral scoop through the small space between the anterior portion of the vesicouterine ligament and the ureter.

As a result of practicing these principles of radical hysterectomy and lymphadenectomy, it is Uchida's experience that no blood transfusion has become necessary in most cases. A complete resection of the lesion most often brings a favorable result and plays a principal role in treatment, even if the treatment is supplemented by chemotherapy, radiation treatment, and immune therapy. The following points should be stressed to bring about a successful radical hysterectomy.

1. *Do not waste time.* Start the easy dissection first rather than spending a lot of time struggling to dissect the difficult area. Traditionally, closure of peritoneum has been considered necessary after radical hysterectomy, but Franchi et al.[19] have shown in their randomized study that nonclosure of pelvic and parietal peritoneum at radical abdominal hysterectomy and node dissection are not associated with increased postoperative morbidity. Likewise, abdominal closure can be easily accomplished without closing the peritoneum. The recent report by Colombo et al.[14] showed that in a randomized comparison of continuous versus interrupted mass closure of midline incisions in patients with gynecologic cancer, the continuous closure is faster and cost effective and that the interrupted closure was not found superior to the continuous closure as far as short- and long-term wound healing and security among 632 patients randomly compared.

2. *Use fingers properly.* This example is observed when fingers are being directed toward the posterior cul-de-sac. The peritoneal defect of the posterior cul-de-sac can be enlarged easily and safely without causing bleeding by placing three fingers (index, middle, and fourth fingers) and by a dorsal sweep in the avascular space, thus separating between rectum and vagina adequately before the uterosacral ligaments are incised as shown in Fig. 37-17.

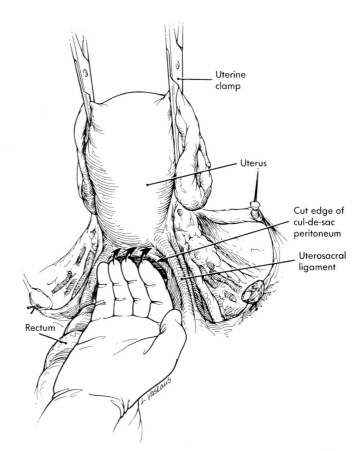

Fig. 37-17   Three fingers (index, middle, fourth) are placed, and by a dorsal sweep the space between rectum and vagina is expanded.

3. *Maintain uterine traction.* Uterine traction together with countertraction produces better visualization not only of the pelvic cavity but also of the clear living anatomy of pelvic structures. With proper uterine traction and countertraction, separation of the uterus from adjacent structures becomes easy. This principle is stressed in Fig. 37-18. The operating team should apply this principle always, since repeated practice brings about a smoother and easier surgical procedure for everyone involved.

4. *Enter the avascular spaces.* This principle is applicable to any pelvic surgical procedure but more so when performing radical hysterectomy and pelvic node dissection and paraaortic node exploration. It is bloodless when in these spaces. Gentle entry and manipulation result in a faster and problem-free pelvic surgical procedure.

5. *Master living anatomy.* Standard textbook and cadaver anatomy is different from that found in living patients. Full recognition of the anatomic variety and an appreciation for individualization not only prevents unnecessary damage to crucial neighboring organs and vascular structure but also minimizes surgical complications.

6. *Use a simple set of operative instruments.* Most operating room tray tables have multiple instruments. It is

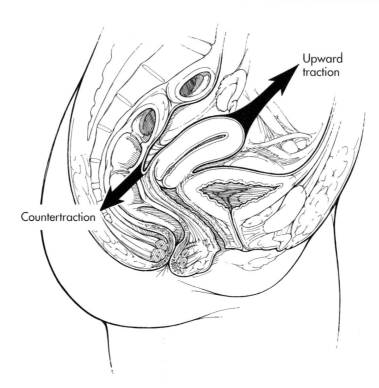

Fig. 37-18   Upward uterine traction with downward countertraction.

obvious that 80% of the sterilized instruments are not used by the operating team, and this is especially true with radical hysterectomy and pelvic node dissection. A pelvic surgeon should become familiar with surgical instruments that are used in most procedures and become very good at using a limited number of instruments.

7. *Use imagery technique.* Life is full of unexpected events, and so is pelvic surgery, especially extensive procedures such as radical hysterectomy and lymphadenectomy. To some pelvic surgeons this undoubtedly becomes an exciting challenge, but to others a fearful expectation of poor surgical result and complication. It is crucial that a pelvic surgeon always think positively about the result of the procedure. Conversation or self-talk by the operating pelvic surgeon such as, "This is a wonderful case. All is working well and she is doing fine," is a first step toward establishing the rapid recovery of the patient. A positive attitude and thinking, together with entertaining this type of imagery, does a great deal to help the operating health care team, including the chief pelvic surgeon. Dare not think such an idea as "something will go wrong this morning" even if such a thought arises inside. Change it to a positive, wonderful image immediately.

Modified Radical Abdominal Hysterectomy

Piver et al.[41] reported five classes of extended hysterectomy for women with cervical cancer in 1974. Class I represents extrafascial hysterectomy, ensuring removal of all cervical tissue. The goal of class II is to remove more paracervical tissue without disturbing the blood supply to the distal ureters and bladder. Uterine vessels are ligated just medial to the ureters. The medial half of the cardinal ligament is removed, and uterosacral ligaments are resected midway between uterus and their sacral attachments. The upper one third of the vagina is removed. The aim of class III is to remove the parametrial and paravaginal tissues widely together with pelvic lymph nodes. The uterine vessels are ligated at the origin from the hypogastric vessels. A small lateral portion of the pubovesical ligament between the lower end of the ureter and the superior vesical artery is preserved. The uterosacral ligaments are resected at the sacral attachments and the cardinal ligaments at the pelvic side wall. One half of the vagina is removed. Class IV removes all periureteral tissue with extensive excision of the perivaginal tissues. This procedure is different from class III in that the ureters are completely resected from the pubovesical ligament, the superior vesical artery is not spared, and three fourths of the vagina is excised. The procedure is for anteriorly involved central recurrence with the goal of preserving the bladder. Class V removes centrally recurrent cancer involving portions of the distal ureter or bladder with removal of distal ureter or bladder and ureteroileoneocystotomy.

When carcinoma of the cervix has been diagnosed to be at an earlier stage, less radical procedures have been used more often.[2] Whereas radical hysterectomy with pelvic lymphadenectomy removes the entire cardinal ligament and all lymph nodes in the pelvis (type III hysterectomy), the modified hysterectomy removes only the medial portion of

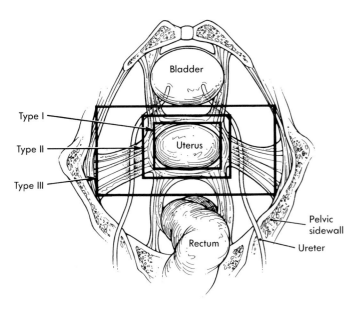

Fig. 37-19 Different types of abdominal hysterectomy: type I, simple hysterectomy; type II, modified radical hysterectomy; and type III, radical hysterectomy.

the cardinal ligament and no lymph nodes, as shown in Fig. 37-19 (type II hysterectomy).[44] The major difference is that the ureter has not been freed from the posterior attachment as in a radical procedure. The ureters are moved laterally, but the blood supply to the ureters is conserved, as the uterine vessels are ligated medial to the ureters.

The procedure may be most commonly used for surgical treatment of microinvasive carcinoma of the cervix. Figs. 37-20 to 37-22 illustrate the differences between the uterine specimen and adjacent tissue removed by simple hysterectomy, modified radical hysterectomy, and radical hysterectomy with pelvic lymphadenectomy. Understanding the principle of this procedure can be used to perform hysterectomy for cervical myoma or bulky endocervical barrel-shaped tumors that require hysterectomy after pelvic irradiation treatment. Whereas the radical hysterectomy removes the entire cardinal ligament, this procedure removes the medial half of the cardinal ligament, thus decreasing the exposure of the ureter to operative trauma.

The round ligament is transected and ligated at the lateral border to expose wider retroperitoneal space. When ovarian conservation is not needed, the infundibulopelvic ligament also is transected and ligated. Posterior parietal peritoneum is incised along the external iliac artery from the infundibulopelvic ligament to the round ligament. The retroperitoneal space is exposed through avascular space dissection with the fingers while applying gentle tension to the medial edge of the incised peritoneum. Ureteral peristalsis is fully visible. The ureter is not dissected from the peritoneal attachment. The bladder peritoneum is incised widely, and the bladder is sharply dissected from the uterine and cervical attachment. Blunt dissection is gently carried toward the origin of the uterine artery from the hypogastric artery. The uterine vessels are dissected, clamped, cut, and ligated just

medial to the ureter (Fig. 37-23). The surgeon's index finger is gently placed in the paracervical tunnel anteriorly and medially to the ureter for dissection, and the vesicouterine ligament is incised with the ureter being unroofed (Fig. 37-24). At this point the ureter is displaced laterally, and the uterosacral ligament is incised, as well as part of the medial portion of the cardinal ligament (Fig. 37-25). The technique shown in Fig. 37-17 provides safe separation of the vagina from the rectum. The paravaginal tissue is clamped and ligated. The same is applied to the opposite side. The tip of the cervix is palpated by the surgeon's thumb and index finger. The upper vaginal cuff is removed 2 to 3 cm below the cervix by placing the right-angle clamp across the upper vagina bilaterally and transecting below the clamp. During this process attention is given to not injuring the bladder by applying traction and countertraction, demonstrated in Fig. 37-18. Here, the technique of modified radical hysterectomy is described briefly after Uchida's method.[59]

Uchida's Subradical Abdominal Hysterectomy with Regressive Ureteral Separation. After the abdomen is opened through a low mid-subumbilical incision, careful abdominal and pelvic exploration is performed. The uterus is grasped with Uchida's uterine clamps and lifted. The right round ligament is ligated and cut, and the incision is extended to open the broad ligament widely. The uterine vessels are identified, ligated medial to the ureter, and cut. If ovarian preservation is not required, the right infundibulopelvic ligament is clamped, cut, and ligated. The ureter is mobilized laterally in one stroke by using the back portion of Metzenbaum scissors. The same procedure is applied to the opposite side. The peritoneum of the posterior cul-de-sac is opened transversely, and the rectovaginal space is deeply opened. The uterosacral ligament is clamped, cut, and ligated deeply on the both sides. The uterovesical peritoneum is incised transversely, and the vesicouterine space is pushed distally to expose paravaginal tissue anteriorly. The vesicouterine ligament of the lateral attachment is identified. A thin clamp is inserted medially along the ureter toward the pelvis from the bladder side opposite to the direction of the flow of urine, and it is widely opened, two fine clamps are placed, and the tissue is cut in the middle and ligated. The ureter is replaced laterally now, and parametrial, paracervical, and paravaginal tissue is clamped, cut, and ligated. Each vaginal angle is clamped, and the vagina is amputated. Each vaginal angle is ligated and the vaginal cuff is closed by a running interlocking suture. The retroperitoneum is closed by continuous suture. The specimen usually includes 2 to 3 cm of vaginal cuff with partial parametrium, with paracervical and paravaginal tissue attached. The abdomen is closed in three layers. Uchida stated that his subradical abdominal hysterectomy takes 15 to 20 minutes longer than a simple hysterectomy, which usually takes him 20 to 25 minutes.

Extraperitoneal Lymphadenectomy

The staging classification for carcinoma of the cervix is established by the International Federation of Gynecology and

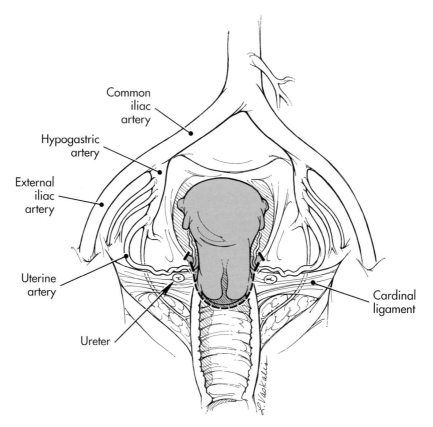

Common iliac artery

Hypogastric artery

External iliac artery

Uterine artery

Ureter

Cardinal ligament

Fig. 37-20 The shaded area represents a specimen removed by simple abdominal hysterectomy.

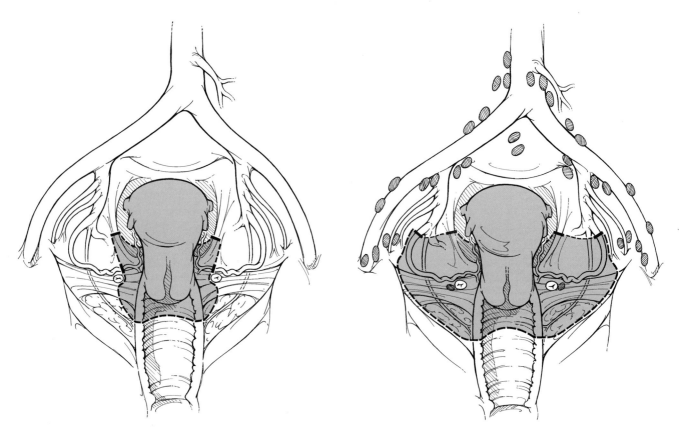

Fig. 37-21 The shaded area represents a specimen removed by modified radical abdominal hysterectomy.

Fig. 37-22 The shaded area represents a specimen removed by radical abdominal hysterectomy.

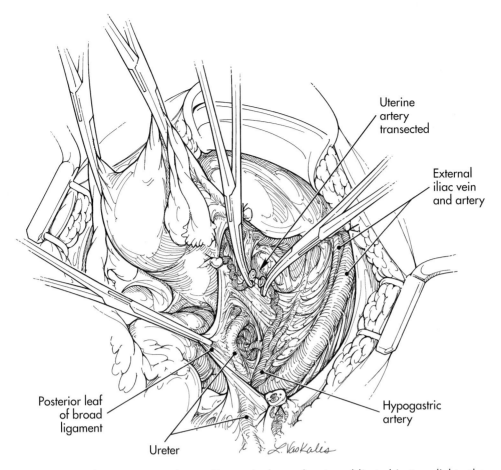

Fig. 37-23 The uterine vessels are dissected, clamped, cut, and ligated just medial to the ureter.

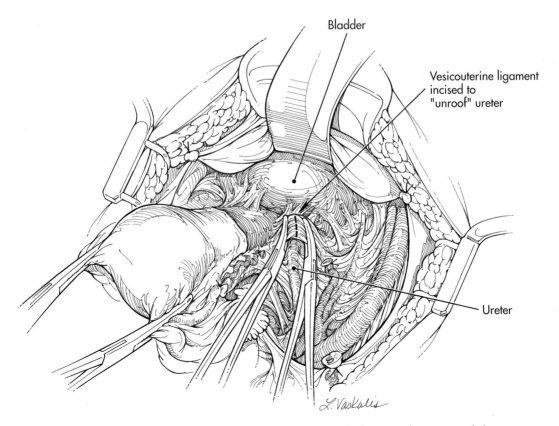

Fig. 37-24 The vesicouterine ligament is incised with the ureter being unroofed.

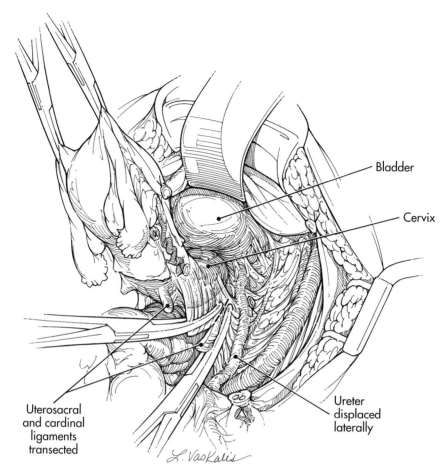

Bladder

Cervix

Uterosacral
and cardinal
ligaments
transected

Ureter
displaced
laterally

L. VasKalis

Fig. 37-25 The ureter is displaced laterally, and the uterosacral ligament, as well as a part of the medial portion of the cardinal ligament, is incised.

Obstetrics (FIGO) and includes clinical and some radiographic evaluation for assessment of tumor extension. Cystoscopy, sigmoidoscopy, chest x-ray study, intravenous pyelography, and barium enema are included when indicated. However, this staging system does not quite adequately reflect the true status of a patient's pelvic and paraaortic lymph nodes.[1] Noninvasive methods for assessing nodal metastasis such as lymphangiography or CT scanning are not always reliable.[23] Because lymph node metastasis of cervical cancer adversely affects patient survival, accurate evaluation is essential in modifying a treatment plan. Historically, transperitoneal pelvic and paraaortic node dissection has been associated with increased intestinal complications when followed by conventional or extended field radiation therapy.[3,60] On the other hand, Berman et al.[5] reported a very low morbidity after performing pelvic and paraaortic lymphadenectomy extraperitoneally through a lateral J-shaped vertical incision in the left abdominal wall. Downey et al.[16] reported a similar extraperitoneal approach through a low mid-subumbilical incision. In general, the abdominal incision may be made through a lateral J-shaped vertical incision, a low mid-subumbilical incision, or a paramedian incision (Fig. 37-26). This could be adjusted according to the site and extent of tumor involvement. The fascia

is cut in the same direction as the skin incision. The peritoneum is rolled medially until the psoas muscle is visible. The round ligament and inferior epigastric vessels can be ligated and cut for a better exposure to the opposite side of the pelvis. With the help of wide, large retractors the left ureter is identified on the peritoneum, and this is pushed medially to expose the vessels (Fig. 37-27). Left paraaortic node dissection begins from the region of the second lumbar spine down to the bifurcation of the aorta. This is followed by dissection of the common iliac, external iliac, hypogastric, and obturator lymph node chain on the left side (Fig. 37-28). For right-sided dissection, care should be taken to remove the peritoneum very gently from the underlying great vessels, especially the inferior vena cava. It also is important to identify the right ureter and the inferior mesenteric artery when exposing the vessels of the right side. The same lymphadenectomy is carried out. The separate specimen is sent for each chain. Many surgical staging protocols call for a small peritoneal opening, peritoneal washing, and gentle exploration and determination of gross tumor extension. Any gross lesion should be biopsied if found. A suction drain is placed in the retroperitoneal cavity, and the wound is closed. For paraaortic node sampling, such structures as the bifurcation of the aorta, inferior vena cava, ovarian ves-

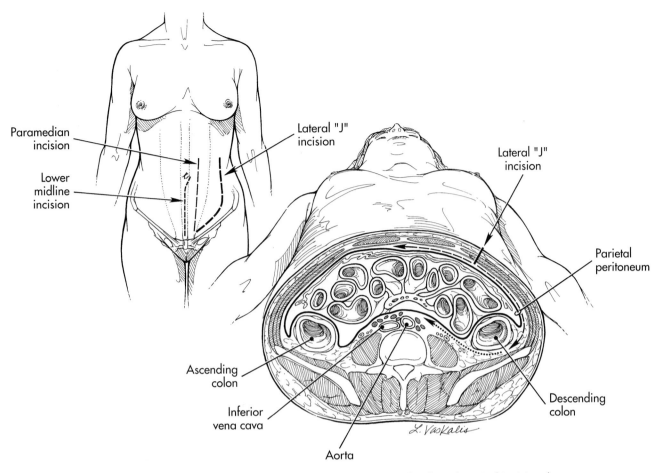

Fig. 37-26   The abdominal incision is made through a lateral J-shaped vertical incision, low mid-subumbilical incision, or paramedian incision.

sels, the inferior mesenteric artery, the ureters, as well as a portion of the duodenum must be identified. Any enlarged or suspicious nodes are excised or biopsied if not resectable.

This technique is used to evaluate lymph node status and tumor extent of invasive cervical carcinoma before radiation therapy at various medical centers. Pelvic surgeons who perform this procedure must have the proper training and experience to handle any associated vascular, intestinal, and genitourinary complications that might occur during the procedure. The position of the patient on the operating table also assists an operating team by tilting either side of the table to obtain better exposure of the deeper vessels and nodes. It appears that this technique will be used less frequently in the future because laparoscopic pelvic and paraaortic lymphadenectomy have been popularized, as mentioned previously in the surgical staging section.

POSTOPERATIVE CONSIDERATIONS
Prevention and Management of Complications

Vascular and Pulmonary Complications. Although rare, massive pulmonary embolism remains the most common cause of death postoperatively.[48]

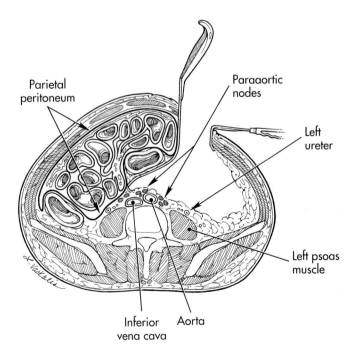

Fig. 37-27   The retroperitoneal space is reached without entering the peritoneal cavity.

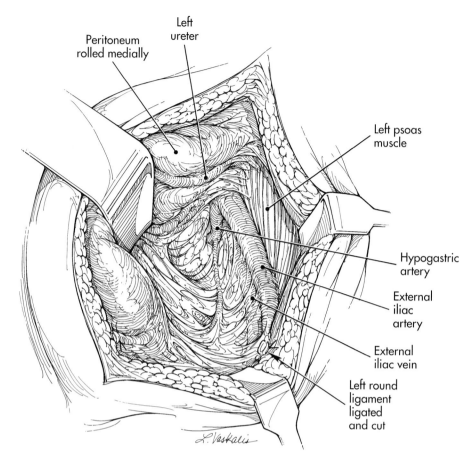

Peritoneum
rolled medially

Left
ureter

Left psoas
muscle

Hypogastric
artery

External
iliac
artery

External
iliac vein

Left round
ligament
ligated
and cut

L. Vaskalis

Fig. 37-28   Large retractors are used to expose the pelvic vessels for lymphadenectomy.

The incidence of pulmonary embolism is reported to vary from 0.3% to 3.0%. Because a massive pulmonary embolism usually is fatal, its prevention becomes crucial. Venous thrombosis is asymptomatic in 50% of cases. Malignancy is known to be associated with a hypercoagulable state. Postoperative immobility and multiple traumas to the pelvic vessels create a favorable source for development of silent thrombosis and subsequent sudden thromboembolic phenomena. Classical use of minidose heparin introduced by Kakkar[10] in 1975 has been challenged by the use of intermittent pneumatic cuff compression and prolonged preoperative use of minidose heparin.[12] Clarke-Pearson et al.[10] reported effective prevention of thrombosis with no bleeding problem with the use of 5000 units of heparin preoperatively every 8 hours for 2 to 9 doses given subcutaneously and continuously postoperatively for 7 days. It is important to monitor activated thromboplastin times and platelet counts preoperatively and postoperatively. Randomized trials of low-dose heparin and intermittent pneumatic calf compression for prevention of deep venous thrombosis after gynecologic cancer surgery by Clarke-Pearson et al.[11] showed that both provided similar reduction in the incidence of postoperative venous thrombosis, but postoperative bleeding complications were more frequent in the low-dose heparin group.

Pulmonary complications are considered to be the most common cause of morbidity and mortality after major surgery. The most common pulmonary complication, atelectasis, results in hypoxia due to partial or complete collapse of the alveolar spaces. Prevention should start before surgery by instructing patients on the use of inspirometer, deep breathing, and early ambulation. The most sensitive test for early detection of microatelectasis is arterial blood gas, which usually reveals lowered Po_2 and O_2 saturation with normal Pco_2.[27] Chest physiotherapy should be provided early for the patient. She should receive adequate pain medication frequently, stay in a sitting position often, with frequent deep inspiration to avoid other serious pulmonary complications such as pneumonia, hypoventilation, acute ventilatory failure, and adult respiratory distress syndrome.

Urinary Complications.   Temporary paralysis of the bladder is the most common complication of radical hysterectomy. Interruption of parasympathetic and sympathetic nerve fibers contained in the pelvic nerve plexus produces temporary and prolonged bladder dysfunction. The degree of bladder dysfunction appears to be directly related to dissection of the inferolateral aspect of the cardinal ligament and the deep uterosacral ligament. Sasaki et al.[46] reported on a surgical technique to preserve the posterior portion of the cardinal ligament, by which they have shown a beneficial effect on bladder function. Use of prolonged bladder drainage by a Foley catheter or a suprapubic catheter assists in preventing overdistention of the bladder. Shingleton et al.[50] reported an advantage of suprapubic drainage over transurethral catheters and encountered very few long-term bladder complications without intermittent self-catheterization.

Vesicovaginal fistula is rare even when the bladder is extensively dissected from the anterior cervix and vagina. To detect bladder injury, a bladder irrigation set should be employed before the procedure and the bladder distended with sterile water and methylene blue dye before reperitonealization. This assists the pelvic surgeon in finding an unexpected bladder injury. Immediate repair of the rent on the operating table is the best way to manage this complication. If found a few days postoperatively, ureteral damage also should be ruled out by injecting 5 ml of 0.8% indigo carmine into a vein. A tampon placed into the vagina should demonstrate the presence of a ureterovaginal fistula. Intravenous pyelography assists in localizing the ureteral fistula. Ureterovaginal fistula, which previously was a very common problem, is found in less than 1% of contemporary radical hysterectomies.[25,50] Suction drainage has made a significant contribution in reducing this complication.[36,50] It is manifested about 1 or 2 weeks postoperatively with a watery vaginal discharge. The history reveals the presence of vague elevated temperature and/or pelvic discomfort during the postoperative period. A retrograde cystoscopic procedure can identify a fistula and an attempt should be made to insert a catheter to the involved renal pelvis through a damaged ureter in order to bring a communication which could be established in 2 to 3 weeks. A retrograde catheterization can be attempted again later if reduction of tissue edema is expected. Surgical repair is best performed with ureteroneocystostomy if the fistula is in the lower pelvis. End-to-end ureteral anastomosis is indicated for the fistula located 5 cm or more above the ureterovesical junction.[37]

Infectious Complications. Febrile morbidity develops in an estimated 25% to 30% of patients after radical hysterectomy.[50] Significant causes include urinary tract infection, pelvic cellulitis and abscess, wound infection, and pulmonary atelectasis. Prophylactic antibiotics, suction drainage, perioperative care, and surgical technique resulted in a remarkably low incidence of serious infectious complications.[48] Because of prolonged catheterization, urinary tract infection can be seen after radical hysterectomy in up to 10% of patients despite use of prophylactic antibiotics. For a high-risk patient, urinary antiseptics are encouraged as long as she is using a urinary catheter.

Sevin et al.[49] advised closure of the vaginal cuff to reduce pelvic infection by avoiding an ascending infection through the vagina; however, others have reported a few infectious problems with the open vaginal cuff technique. Randomized trials of an open versus closed vaginal vault in preventing postoperative morbidity after abdominal hysterectomy have been conducted by Colombo et al.[13] and failed to show any advantage to either of the two methods. Ac-

cording to Mattingly,[27] prophylactic broad-spectrum antibiotics reduce the incidence of pelvic cellulitis to less than 5% of all radical hysterectomies. The use of antibiotic irrigation at the time of the procedure seems associated with a significantly lower incidence of pelvic and wound infection.[33] Pelvic infection, if it occurs, should be treated aggressively with antibiotics and drainage. The author concludes that careful surgical technique and prophylaxis remain the most important factors in preventing postoperative morbidity.

Wound care is an important aspect in preventing a serious wound problem such as dehiscence and evisceration. Skin preparation stands as the first line of defense. Applying an agent such as aqueous solution of povidone-iodine and air drying is most effective in preparing a patient for surgery.[26] Fascial closure with an absorbable monofilament synthetic suture such as polydioxanone (PDS) and polyglyconate (Maxon) provides retention of about 50% strength at 4 weeks.[45] Their tensile strength is greater than that of Dexon and Vicryl. Fascial suture should be placed loosely for single layer "mass" closure, no closer than 1 cm from the edge and 1 cm between bites. Any surgical patient with fever should receive immediate attention to the wound, especially in the early postoperative phase. Early wound infection, usually caused by group A beta-hemolytic streptococcus, requires immediate antibiotic therapy and excision of necrotic tissue. Gallup et al.[21] evaluated the effect of subcutaneous closed drainage systems and prophylactic antibiotics on the wound breakdown rate in 197 obese patients undergoing gynecologic surgery. They found subcutaneous drains plus prophylactic antibiotics decrease postoperative morbidity. It appears that the thickness of subcutaneous tissue is the most significant risk factor associated with abdominal wound infection after abdominal hysterectomy.[52]

Lymphatic Complications. In modern medical practice lymphocyst formation has become a very infrequent complication of radical hysterectomy. Most series reveal an incidence of up to 3%.[35] This low incidence is the result of the effectiveness of suction drainage of the pelvis. Shingleton et al.[50] report that this complication is very rare even without routine ligation of lymphatics. Although most lymphocysts are not symptomatic, serial ultrasound study may detect a silent progressive lymphocele that could be corrected by percutaneous catheter drainage on an outpatient basis.[15] Lymphedema of the lower extremities is sometimes seen after radical hysterectomy, especially in those patients with radiation treatment combined with the procedure.

Follow-Up

Because most recurrences of early cervical cancer are observed within the first 24 months after initial therapy, the patient should be seen every 3 months during this period. If there is no recurrence, then she is seen every 6 months for an additional 3 years. At each visit a thorough careful history should be taken regarding her general health. Physical examination includes her weight and careful examination for supraclavicular and groin nodes, abdominal masses, and hepatomegaly. The vaginal cuff should be inspected, as well as the lower vagina and suburethral legion. A Pap smear is taken. Rectovaginal examination is performed to evaluate for any sign of recurrence. A chest x-ray film is taken every year, and a CT scan may be ordered for any questionable case of recurrence.

The key to successful pelvic surgery is to find the avascular spaces and dissect each swiftly. Because this usually is not detailed in textbooks, it must be learned through experience. Living anatomy of the pelvic structure is available to any pelvic surgeon through various pelvic surgeries, especially in procedures such as radical hysterectomy and pelvic lymphadenectomy. We must appreciate the three-dimensional pelvic structure each time we operate. Concentration balanced with delicate fingers appears to guide where we should be and how to obtain avascular spaces based on each precious experience. Time efficiency is essential for a prolonged pelvic surgical procedure. Each minute the patient spends on the operating table should be used efficiently. Our goal should be clear. When we encounter an unexpected difficulty we can seek an easier area in which to work to increase the safety of our patients. As long as our goal is clear and focused we should be able to find a plane to dissect. Although in some cases it seems almost impossible to continue our planned procedure because of various adhesions or dense fibrosis, we should remember that by recalling the living anatomy and seeking a hidden avascular plane we can find an easy path to dissect. It has always been better when we ask for divine guidance and intercession. We are trying to save and improve the life of our patient who is seeking more time to live on this earth.

ACKNOWLEDGMENT

The author gives his thanks to Dr. Hajime Uchida for providing the photographs relating to his radical hysterectomy technique.

REFERENCES

1. Averette HE, Dudan RC, Ford JH Jr: Exploratory celiotomy for surgical staging of cervical cancer, *Am J Obstet Gynecol* 113:1090, 1972.
2. Averette HE, et al: How radical should surgery be for cervical cancer? *Contemp Obstet Gynecol* July 1990, p 91.
3. Ballon SC, Berman ML, Lagasse LD, et al: Survival after extraperitoneal pelvic and paraaortic lymphadenectomy and radiation therapy in cervical carcinoma, *Obstet Gynecol* 57:90, 1981.
4. Benrubi GI: History of hysterectomy, *J Fla Med Assoc* 75:533, 1988.
5. Berman ML, Lagasse LD, Watring WG, et al: The operative evaluation of patients with cervical carcinoma by an extraperitoneal approach, *Obstet Gynecol* 50:658, 1977.
6. Bonney MS: The treatment of carcinoma of the cervix by Wertheim's operation, *Am J Obstet Gynecol* 30:815, 1935.
7. Childers JM, Hatch K, Surwit EA: The role of laparoscopic lymphadenectomy in the management of cervical carcinoma, *Gynecol Oncol* 47:38, 1992.
8. Chu KK, Chang SD, Chen FP, Soong YK: Laparoscopic surgical staging in cervical cancer—preliminary experience among Chinese, *Gynecol Oncol* 64:49, 1997.
9. Clark JG. In Kelly HA, Noble CP, editors: *Gynecology and abdominal surgery*, Philadelphia, 1907, WB Saunders.
10. Clarke-Pearson DL, DeLong E, Synan IS, et al: A controlled trial of two low dose heparin regimens for the prevention of postoperative deep vein thrombosis, *Obstet Gynecol* 75:684, 1990.
11. Clarke-Pearson DL, Synan IS, Dodge R, et al: A randomized trial of low-dose heparin and intermittent pneumatic calf compression for the prevention of deep venous thrombosis after gynecologic oncology surgery, *Am J Obstet Gynecol* 168:1146, 1993.
12. Clarke-Pearson DL, Synan IS, Hinshaw WM, et al: Prevention of postoperative venous thromboembolism by external pneumatic calf compression in patients with gynecologic malignancy, *Obstet Gynecol* 63:92, 1984.
13. Colombo M, Maggioni A, Zanini A, et al: A randomized trial of open versus closed vaginal vault in the prevention of postoperative morbidity after abdominal hysterectomy, *Am J Obstet Gynecol* 173:1807, 1995.
14. Colombo M, Maggioni A, Parma G, et al: A randomized comparison of continuous versus interrupted mass closure of midline incisions in patients with gynecologic cancer, *Obstet Gynecol* 89:684, 1997.
15. Conte M, Panici PB, Guariglia L, et al: Pelvic lymphocele following radical paraaortic and pelvic lymphadenectomy for cervical carcinoma: incidence rate and percutaneous management, *Obstet Gynecol* 76:268, 1990.
16. Downey GO, Potish RA, Adcock LL, et al: Pretreatment surgical staging in cervical carcinoma: therapeutic efficacy of pelvic lymph node resection, *Am J Obstet Gynecol* 160:1055, 1989.
17. Ellis H: *Famous operations,* Media, Pa, 1984, Harwal.
18. Fowler JM, Carter JR, Carlson JW, et al: Lymph node yield from laparoscopic lymphadenectomy in cervical cancer: a comparative study, *Gynecol Oncol* 51:187, 1993.
19. Franchi M, Ghezzi F, Zanaboni F, et al: Nonclosure of peritoneum at radical abdominal hysterectomy and pelvic node dissection: a randomized study, *Obstet Gynecol* 90:622, 1997.
20. Freund WA: Extirpation of the entire uterus by a new method, *Am J Obstet* 11:648, 1878.
21. Gallup DC, Gallup DG, Nolan TE, et al: Use of a subcutaneous closed drainage system and antibiotics in obese gynecologic patients, *Am J Obstet Gynecol* 175:358, 1996.
22. Gray L Sr: *The life and times of Ephraim McDowell,* 1987, VG Reed and Sons.
23. Hann LE, Crivello MS: Imaging techniques in the staging of gynecologic malignancy, *Clin Obstet Gynecol* 29:715, 1986.
24. Lawton FG, Hacker NF: Surgery for invasive gynecologic cancer in the elderly female population, *Obstet Gynecol* 76:287, 1990.
25. Lee YN, Wang KL, Lin MH, et al: Radical hysterectomy with pelvic node dissection for treatment of cervical cancer: a clinical review of 954 cases, *Gynecol Oncol* 32:135, 1989.
26. Masterson BJ: Skin preparation, *Clin Obstet Gynecol* 31:736, 1988.
27. Mattingly RF, Thompson JD: *Te Linde's operative gynecology,* ed 6, Philadelphia, 1985, JB Lippincott.
28. Meigs JV: Carcinoma of the cervix—The Wertheim operation, *Surg Gynecol Obstet* 78:195, 1944.
29. Meigs VJ: Gynecology: carcinoma of the cervix, *N Engl J Med* 230:577, 1944.
30. Meigs JV: The Wertheim operation for carcinoma of the cervix, *Am J Obstet Gynecol* 49:542, 1945.
31. Meigs JV: Radical hysterectomy with bilateral pelvic lymph node dissections: a report of 100 patients operated on 5 or more years ago, *Am J Obstet Gynecol* 62:854, 1951.
32. Meigs JV: *Surgical treatment of cancer of the cervix,* New York, 1954, Grune & Stratton.
33. Miyazawa K, Hernandez E, Dillon MB: Prophylactic topical cefamandole in radical hysterectomy, *Int J Gynecol Obstet* 25:133, 1987.
34. Nakano R: Abdominal radical hysterectomy and bilateral pelvic lymph node dissection for cancer of the cervix, *Gynecol Obstet Invest* 12:281, 1981.
35. Nelson JF: Surgical staging of cervical cancer. In Nichols DH, editor: *Gynecologic and obstetric surgery,* St Louis, 1993, Mosby.

36. Newton M, Newton ER: *Complications of gynecologic and obstetric management,* Philadelphia, 1988, WB Saunders.

37. Nichols DH: *Clinical problems, injuries, and complications of gynecologic surgery,* ed 2, Baltimore, 1988, Williams & Wilkins.

38. Okabayashi H: Radical abdominal hysterectomy for cancer of the cervix uteri, *Surg Gynecol Obstet* 33:335, 1921.

39. Palmer CD: Laparotomy and lapro-hysterectomy: their indications and statistics for fibroid tumors of the uterus, *Trans Am Gynecol Soc* 5:361, 1880.

40. Patsner B, Sedlacek TV, Lovecchio JL: Para-aortic node sampling in small (3 cm or less) stage IB invasive cervical cancer, *Gynecol Oncol* 44:53, 1992.

41. Piver MS, Rutledge F, Smith JP: Five classes of extended hysterectomy for women with cervical cancer, *Obstet Gynecol* 44:265, 1974.

42. Querleu D, Leblanc E, Castelain B: Laparoscopic pelvic lymphadenectomy in the staging of early carcinoma of the cervix, *Am J Obstet Gynecol* 164:579, 1991.

43. Recio FO, Piver MS, Hempling RE: Pretreatment transperitoneal laparoscopic staging pelvic and paraaortic lymphadenectomy in large (5 cm) stage IB2 cervical carcinoma: report of a pilot study, *Gynecol Oncol* 63:333, 1996.

44. Ridley JH: *Gynecologic surgery, errors, safeguards, salvage,* ed 2, Baltimore, 1981, Williams & Wilkins.

45. Sanz LE: Wound management—matching materials and methods for best results, *Contemp Obstet Gynecol* Nov 1987, p 86.

46. Sasaki H, Yoshida T, Noda K: Urethral pressure profiles following radical hysterectomy, *Obstet Gynecol* 59:101, 1982.

47. Schachner A: *Ephraim McDowell, "Father of ovariotomy and founder of abdominal surgery,"* Philadelphia, 1921, JB Lippincott.

48. Schaffer G, Graber EA, editors: *Complications in obstetrics and gynecologic surgery,* Hagerstown, Md, 1981, Harper & Row.

49. Sevin BU, Ramos R, Lichtinger M, et al: Antibiotic prevention of infections complicating radical abdominal hysterectomy, *Obstet Gynecol* 64:539, 1984.

50. Shingleton HM, Orr JW: *Cancer of the cervix,* Philadelphia, 1995, JB Lippincott.

51. Soper DE, Bump RC, Hurt WG: Wound infection after abdominal hysterectomy: effect of the depth of subcutaneous tissue, *Am J Obstet Gynecol* 173:465, 1995.

52. Society of Gynecologic Oncologists Medical Practice and Ethics Committee: Clinical practice guidelines 1:19, 1996.

53. Sparkman RS: Presidential address: The woman in the case, *Ann Surg* 189:529, 1979.

54. Taussig FJ: Iliac lymphadenectomy with irradiation in the treatment of cancer of the cervix, *Am J Obstet Gynecol* 28:650, 1934.

55. Taussig FJ: The removal of lymph nodes in cancer of the cervix, *Am J Roentgenol Radium Therapy* 34:354, 1935.

56. Taussig FJ: Iliac lymphadenectomy for group II cancer of the cervix, *Am J Obstet Gynecol* 45:733, 1943.

57. Uchida H: Radical operation for cancer of the cervix. Presented by film at the Seventh Asian Congress of Obstetrics and Gynecology, Bangkok, Nov 1977.

58. Uchida H: Radical operation for cancer of the cervix. Presented by film at the Tenth World Congress of Gynecology and Obstetrics, San Francisco, Oct 1982.

59. Uchida H: Subradical hysterectomy with regressive ureter separation, *Obstet Gynecol Therapy* 59:44, 1989.

60. Weiser EB, Bundy BN, Hoskins WJ, et al: Extraperitoneal versus transperitoneal selective paraaortic lymphadenectomy in the pretreatment surgical staging of advanced cervical carcinoma (A Gynecologic Oncology Group study), *Gynecol Oncol* 33:283, 1989.

61. Wertheim E: The extended abdominal operation for carcinoma uteri (based on 500 operative cases), *Am J Obstet* 66:169, 1912.

62. Yagi H: Treatment of carcinoma of the cervix uteri, *Surg Gynecol Obstet* 95:552, 1952.

38 Transperitoneal Laparoscopic Lymphadenectomy

JOEL M. CHILDERS

THE EVOLUTION

The laparoscopic extraperitoneal lymph node sampling of Daniel Dargent ushered modern operative laparoscopy into the world of gynecologic oncology and is described in Chapter 66. The technique described here is a transperitoneal approach to both pelvic and paraaortic lymph nodes that Dr. Earl Surwit and I developed beginning in 1990. The first transperitoneal pelvic lymphadenectomies were reported in 1991 by Querleu et al.[6] Reports on low laparoscopic paraaortic lymphadenectomy in patients with cervical, endometrial, and ovarian cancer soon followed.[1-4,7] The final phase of development of laparoscopic lymphadenectomy came with the ability to perform high paraaortic or infrarenal lymphadenectomies, which is necessary for cancer staging in patients with ovarian and fallopian tube cancer.[2,3,5]

Lymph nodes found from the abdominal aorta to the pelvic floor can be the primary sites of metastases in cervical, vaginal, endometrial, ovarian, and fallopian tube carcinomas. Most gynecologic malignancies are either staged surgically or managed surgically. Lymphadenectomy is the foundation of surgical staging for gynecologic malignancies. Most gynecologic oncologists perform a selective lymphadenectomy or a lymph node sampling for gynecologic malignancies with the exception of early carcinoma of the cervix, in which a complete or therapeutic lymphadenectomy is performed. Most of the regional lymph nodes are removed during a lymph node sampling procedure. However, emphasis is not placed on skeletonizing the vessels, as is done in a therapeutic, or complete, lymphadenectomy.

INDICATIONS

Currently, vulvar, endometrial, and ovarian carcinomas are surgically staged. Part of the surgical staging of malignancies involving these sites includes evaluation of the regional lymph nodes. Laparoscopic lymphadenectomy could potentially be used in the surgical staging of cancer in patients with endometrial and ovarian carcinomas. Although cervical cancer is a clinically staged malignancy, the laparoscopic lymphadenectomy can be incorporated into the surgical management of this disease.

CERVICAL CANCER

Laparoscopic lymphadenectomy may be used in two categories of patients with cervical cancer. The first category consists of patients with early cervical cancer who are considered candidates for radical hysterectomy. A "therapeutic" pelvic lymphadenectomy is performed laparoscopically, and the radical hysterectomy can be accomplished laparoscopically or vaginally.

The second category of patients includes those with early or late cervical cancer whose primary treatment will be radiotherapy. Because these patients are to receive standard whole-pelvis radiotherapy, they require only sampling of the lymph nodes high (cephalad) in the radiation field and just outside the radiation field. This includes the proximal common and low paraaortic lymph nodes bilaterally. A thorough inspection for intraperitoneal disease should be carried out in these patients as well. Albeit a rare phenomenon, the presence of intraperitoneal disease would certainly change their treatment plans. This laparoscopic approach in patients scheduled for radiotherapy is controversial because of the higher incidence of postirradiation regional enteric complications associated with extended-field radiotherapy in patients who undergo transperitoneal paraaortic lymphadenectomy. The alternative, extraperitoneal lymphadenectomy, is described in Chapter 37.

OVARIAN CARCINOMA

Laparoscopic lymphadenectomy can be used in two categories of patients with ovarian carcinoma in two situations. The first category includes patients with presumed early (stage I or II) ovarian carcinoma who require surgical staging. In these patients, unilateral or bilateral lymphadenectomy is required from the renal vessels to the pelvis. This includes sampling the obturator lymph nodes, the external, internal, and common iliac lymph nodes, and the paraaortic nodes both above and below the inferior mesenteric artery.

The second category of patients eligible for laparoscopic lymphadenectomy includes those with advanced ovarian carcinoma who have undergone surgical debulking and platinum-based chemotherapy and have no evidence of disease after treatment. A thorough evaluation of the entire intraperitoneal cavity and sites of disease remaining after the surgical debulking should be done first, and the lymphadenectomy should be the final step of a laparoscopic second-look procedure and performed only if no other evidence of disease is found.

ENDOMETRIAL CARCINOMA

Patients with clinical stage I adenocarcinoma of the endometrium may be managed with a combined laparoscopic and vaginal surgery approach. If a laparoscopically assisted surgical staging procedure is to be performed, a thorough inspection of the intraperitoneal cavity, procurement of intraperitoneal washings, and a lymphadenectomy should be performed in addition to the vaginal hysterectomy. Laparoscopically assisted surgical staging can also be used in the patient whose cancer was not surgically staged at the time of hysterectomy. When endometrial cancer is staged, it is particularly important to sample the pelvic lymph nodes, including the obturator, external, internal, and common iliac lymph nodes. Removal of the paraaortic lymph nodes is left to the discretion of the individual surgeon but, when performed, includes only the lymph nodes below the inferior mesenteric artery.

The operative technique described in this chapter is radically different from that of most gynecologic operative laparoscopic procedures. This procedure requires solid knowledge of the retroperitoneal anatomy and a high level of comfort with retroperitoneal operative techniques. It also requires the surgeon to change his or her way of operating.

This operative shift is required for both traditional laparoscopists and laparotomists. The laparotomist will no longer be able to use retractors in the retroperitoneal space and will no longer need multiple clips. The laparoscopist will not need standard laparoscopic instruments or techniques. Bipolar electricity is rarely used, aquadissection is never used, lasers are of no benefit, and irrigation may be performed only at the end of the procedure, if at all.

This technique relies heavily on proven surgical principles: traction and countertraction, use of proper surgical planes, sharp and blunt dissection, and use of both hands by the surgeon. It also requires the surgeon to become a virtuoso with the oldest, least expensive, most common energy source available: monopolar electricity. Horror stories about laparoscopic use of monopolar electricity outdate us all. Experts in electrical physics shun its use, based on theory. However, with this procedure, monopolar electricity is safe and efficient if certain principles are understood and important anatomic structures are kept out of harm's way.

If the operative laparoscopist performs the lymph node dissection outlined in this chapter, only two instruments will be used (scissors and graspers), only one instrument will be removed from its port during the entire procedure (a grasper to extract nodes as they are dissected), the surgeon will operate with both hands, and the assistant will provide exposure and visualization. A 30-minute operation quickly becomes a 2-hour operation if traditional laparoscopic techniques are used.

Once the gynecologist has mastered the technique of laparoscopic lymphadenectomy, a whole new world opens up. Most early gynecologic malignancies and some advanced carcinomas can now be surgically managed laparoscopically. As the surgeon's vaginal and laparoscopic operative skills improve, many laparotomies may be avoided.

This shift is already taking place in many practices, and it is safe to say that the gynecologic oncologist of the early twenty-first century will be an operative laparoscopist.

SURGICAL TECHNIQUES
Preoperative Considerations

Bowel Preparation. Having the large and small bowel evacuated facilitates the laparoscopic approach to the paraaortic nodes. This is easily accomplished by having the patient on a liquid diet for 2 days before the procedure and administering one bottle (240 ml) of magnesium citrate 1 and 2 days before the procedure. An enema on the morning of admission will aid in the evacuation of the lower bowel.

Anesthesia Considerations

General anesthesia is used. An endotracheal tube is placed, and end-tidal carbon dioxide is monitored. A nasogastric or oral gastric tube is inserted to empty the stomach contents before placement of the primary trocar or Veress needle. A pulse oximeter is used, and a Foley catheter is placed. The patient's arms are tucked to the sides with consideration for padding of the ulnar nerve. Sequential compression stockings are currently used.

Operating Room Considerations and Instrumentation

In general, the procedure can be accomplished with a few simple laparoscopic instruments. It is necessary to have (1) sharp scissors with monopolar electrocautery capabilities (these should have Metzenbaum-like tips), (2) grasping forceps with tips large enough to grab large nodal bundles and extract them through a 12-mm laparoscopic sleeve, and (3) an irrigation-suction apparatus. I prefer disposable scissors because they are always sharp. A 10-mm laparoscopic telescope with a 0-degree lens is preferable for most cases. On occasion, the laparoscopic clip-applier may be needed. This is most commonly used for perforating veins over the vena cava.

Operative Technique

Port Placement. Four laparoscopic ports are needed to perform this procedure (Fig. 38-1). The primary port is placed in the umbilicus and should be at least 10 mm in size for use with a 10-mm telescope and camera. I believe it is important to place the umbilical port in the base of the umbilicus at a 90-degree angle to the abdominal wall, as opposed to a subumbilical insertion at a 45-degree angle. The latter method of subumbilical port placement can lead to a large amount of abdominal tissue between the site of insertion on the skin and the site of entrance into the intraperitoneal cavity. This large fulcrum of skin makes it difficult to direct the laparoscopic camera to the upper abdomen or to the paraaortic area. With placement through the base of the umbilicus, the umbilical port can easily be directed to the pelvis or the upper abdomen. Furthermore, with a skin incision made in the base of the umbilicus by a no. 11 blade

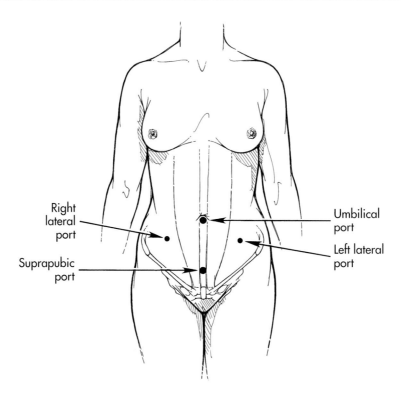

Fig. 38-1   The location of the four laparoscopic port sites. A 10- to 12-mm port is needed in the umbilicus and a 12-mm port is needed suprapubically. The two lateral ports should be 5 mm in size and are lateral to the inferior epigastric vessels.

scalpel and with upward traction on the anterior abdominal wall by towel clips, the peritoneal cavity is, in most instances, entered. When this is done, the umbilical sleeve can be placed into the intraperitoneal cavity without a trocar. This is safer than direct trocar insertion and quicker than open laparoscopy. The three ancillary ports are placed under direct laparoscopic visualization. Two 5-mm trocars and sleeves are placed lateral to the inferior epigastric vessels and the rectus muscle bilaterally. The third ancillary port is placed in the midline above the symphysis and should be 12 mm in size to allow removal of the nodal tissue, which at times can contain sizable specimens.

Inspection of the Intraperitoneal Cavity. After the laparoscopic ports are in place and before the patient is placed in Trendelenburg position, it is important to explore the entire intraperitoneal cavity. This should be done in a systematic fashion and should specifically include areas to which gynecologic malignancies metastasize. If pelvic washings are to be taken, they should be obtained before any operative procedures are undertaken.

Laparoscopic Pelvic Lymphadenectomy. Laparoscopic lymphadenectomy, like lymphadenectomy performed at laparotomy, can be accomplished in a number of ways. In general, however, it is easier if the surgeon stands on the side opposite that of the nodes to be dissected (Fig. 38-2). The telescope is placed through the umbilical port and is held by the assistant. The assistant also uses a grasper, placed through the ipsilateral lateral port. The surgeon uses a grasper through the lower midline port and scissors with monopolar cautery capability through the ipsilateral lateral port.

The peritoneum is picked up and incised over the psoas muscle near the external iliac artery, between the round and infundibulopelvic ligaments. These ligaments can be left intact, but greater exposure is offered if they are transected. The broad ligament is opened, and the obliterated umbilical artery is identified (Fig. 38-3). This built-in retractor is retracted medially, opening the paravesical and obturator spaces. The obliterated umbilical artery can easily be identified in the pelvis of thin patients adjacent to the external iliac vein. In patients with more adipose tissue the umbilical artery can be identified in the pelvis by pushing on it at the anterior abdominal wall and watching for its movement in the pelvis. The avascular plane between the obliterated umbilical artery and external iliac vein is easily opened, exposing the obturator space very nicely.

It is advisable to perform the obturator lymphadenectomy first because blood, lymph fluid, or irrigation fluid can accumulate in this dependent area and may obscure visualization somewhat if these nodes are not removed first. The obturator nerve is identified, and the nodal tissue on the anterior surface of the nerve is dissected off bluntly. The nodal tissue along the medial aspect of the external iliac vein is then dissected off along the length of the vein. When this dissection is performed, care should be taken not to damage any aberrant or accessory veins emptying into the external iliac vein. The proper plane between the nodal tissue and the vein can be easily identified by seizing nodal tissue with the

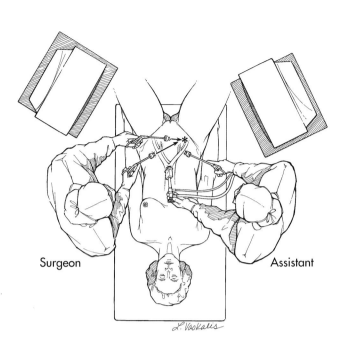

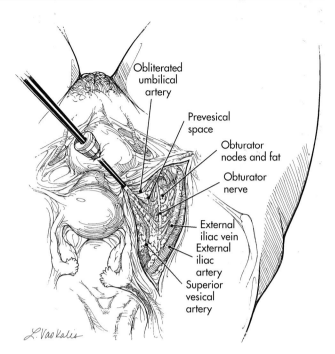

Fig. 38-2 The surgeon, standing on the patient's left side, removes the right-side pelvic lymph nodes, using scissors through the left lateral port and graspers through the suprapubic port. The assistant, on the patient's right side, holds the laparoscope placed through the umbilicus and offers exposure using an instrument placed through the right lateral port.

Fig. 38-3 A grasper placed through the suprapubic port is used to retract the obliterated umbilical artery medially, exposing the obturator and paravesical space.

grasper and retracting it medially. The scissor tips can be placed into the space and opened, and the remaining tissue can be easily separated bluntly.

It is my preference to then follow the nodal bundle distally to the pelvic wall and transect the nodal package at the pelvic wall with monopolar electrocautery. I use a fulgurating technique in which the scissor tips are held adjacent to the nodal tissue to be transected, and the spark is allowed to jump to the nodal tissue. Traction on the nodal bundle is mandatory. Once this is completed, the only remaining attachment of the obturator nodal package is at the junction of the hypogastric and external iliac arteries. This is usually the most difficult part of removing the obturator nodes. Adequate visualization can be difficult to obtain because the nodal bundle starts to course laterally. Furthermore, the ureter crosses the iliac vessels in this area, making injury to the ureter more likely during this portion of the dissection. The safest way to extract the cephalad extent of this bundle is by blunt traction, pulling the node away from the vein and underlying obturator nerve. The nodal bundle is removed intact through the lower 10 to 12 mm port using the large forceps.

Removal of the external lymph nodes is performed in a fashion similar to that of laparotomy. The assistant retracts the distal transected round ligament, offering exposure to the distal external iliac vessels, and the surgeon substitutes monopolar electricity for surgical clips. This dissection is accomplished by creating a plane in the adventitia of the external iliac artery and dissecting it up to the circumflex iliac

artery. Effort should be made to avoid damaging the genitofemoral nerve laterally. The dissection can be extended proximally to the point where the ovarian vessels and/or the ureter crosses the iliac vessels. Here, the assistant must retract the ureter in a cephalad and medial direction (Fig. 38-4). The nodal dissection can then be continued up the distal common iliac artery.

When the left pelvic lymph nodes are removed, it is necessary to take down the rectosigmoid colon from the left pelvic sidewall. This can be accomplished by incising the peritoneum in this area along the white line of Toldt, which will give access to the retroperitoneal space. If mobilization of the rectosigmoid colon is not required, the same incision, as previously described, is made between the round ligament and the ovarian vessels. The surgeon stands on the right side of the patient and operates through the midline port with graspers and the lateral port with scissors.

At the end of the procedure, the operative site can be irrigated and inspected to ensure that hemostasis is adequate. The peritoneum is left open, and no drains are used.

Laparoscopic Paraaortic Lymphadenectomy. Sampling of the paraaortic lymph nodes cannot be accomplished without adequate exposure, which requires placement of the omentum, transverse colon, and small bowel into the upper abdomen. The laparoscope can be placed temporarily through the suprapubic port to obtain a more panoramic view. The omentum can be flipped on its pedicle and placed atop the liver. The stomach should be adequately decompressed. Next, the small bowel should be flipped on its mesenteric pedicle in a cephalad direction and splayed out across the upper abdomen. Trendelenburg position, good

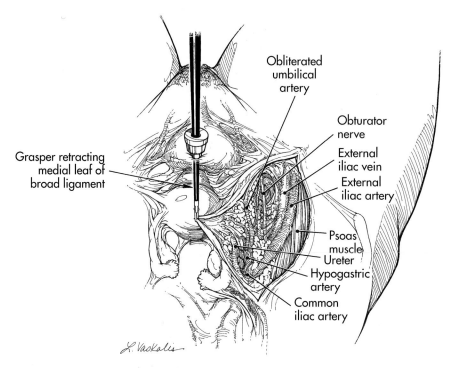

Fig. 38-4   Right retroperitoneal pelvic anatomy. A grasper placed through the suprapubic port is retracting the medial leaf of the broad ligament, pulling the ureter medially away from the bifurcation of the common iliac vessels.

bowel preparation, and occasionally, lateral tilt of the operating table assist in keeping the bowel in the upper abdomen. It is during this process that the small bowel can be inspected for metastatic disease. This "packing" of the bowel is extremely important, and time should be taken to accomplish this correctly, lest time be lost later. Occasionally, the use of additional 5-mm left or right upper quadrant ports to keep the bowel in the upper abdomen may be required to accomplish a paraaortic lymphadenectomy, especially in heavier patients. Depending on the patient's anatomy, the transverse duodenum can often be visualized as it crosses the vena cava and aorta. Lifting the mesentery of the small bowel as it crosses the aorta aids in visualizing the third portion of the duodenum. Sometimes the peritoneum over the aorta and proximal right common iliac artery will need to be incised and mobilized before the transverse duodenum can be visualized. The aorta, right common iliac artery, and ureter as it crosses the right iliac vessels are landmarks that should be identified before beginning the dissection.

Right-Sided Paraaortic Lymphadenectomy. There are a number of ways to sample the paraaortic lymph nodes laparoscopically. The surgeon can stand on the side of the patient or between the patient's legs (Figs. 38-5 and 38-6). The telescope can be placed through the umbilical or suprapubic port. The technique described here mimics that of the procedure performed at laparotomy and is therefore easy to learn.

The surgeon, on the left side of the patient, performs the procedure with graspers in the lower midline port and scissors in the left lateral port, identical to that of the pelvic dissection (see Fig. 38-6). The assistant holds the camera in the

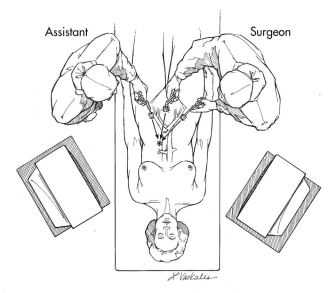

Fig. 38-5   The surgeon stands on the patient's right side to perform the left paraaortic lymph node procedure. Scissors are placed through the left lateral port, and graspers are placed through the suprapubic port. The monitor is moved up toward the patient's head for the comfort and orientation of the surgeon. It is easy to see how the surgeon could stand between the patient's legs as well.

umbilical port and uses graspers in the right lateral port. It is helpful to rotate the camera so that the aorta and vena cava are horizontal on the color monitor, with the patient's head to the right of the monitor. It is also helpful to move the monitors from the foot of the operating table to the side of

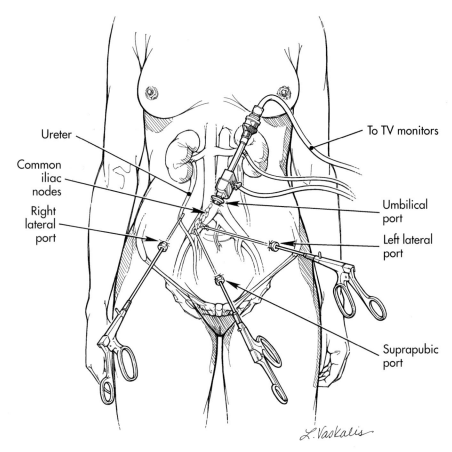

Fig. 38-6   With scissors placed through the left lateral port and graspers placed through the suprapubic port, a surgeon standing on the patient's left side can remove the right-sided paraaortic nodes. The grasper placed through the right lateral port is used to retract the ureter and ovarian vessels laterally.

the patient, either near the umbilicus or near the patient's head. In this situation, two monitors may be necessary.

An incision is made in the peritoneum over the aorta. This incision is extended down the right common iliac artery to where the ureter crosses the iliac vessels and up the aorta to the mesentery of the small bowel or the transverse duodenum. The peritoneum is lifted with graspers, and blunt dissection is performed laterally toward the right psoas muscle. The right ureter is identified and lifted away from the underlying psoas muscle (Fig. 38-7). The grasper in the midline port then is used to elevate the ureter anteriorly and laterally. The right psoas muscle and tendon of the psoas should be easily seen.

The assistant then places his or her grasper (in the right lateral port) beneath the ureter to retract it anteriorly and laterally out of the operative field. This also creates a small "tent," which helps prevent small bowel from falling into the operative field.

The surgeon then dissects the nodal and fatty tissue off the aorta by first sharply developing the adventitial plane of the aorta. This arterial dissection is continued in a cephalad and caudad direction, up the aorta and down the common iliac artery, using the scissors and electrocautery as needed. Lateral dissection is then performed toward the psoas muscle so that the nodal bundle is separated from the underlying vena cava.

Care should be taken to avoid lacerating perforating vessels when unroofing the vena cava. It is uncommon to encounter a perforator from the vena cava that cannot be controlled with monopolar electricity. Only through experience will the surgeon gain an appreciation for which perforating vessels should be clipped. If any doubt exists, the clip applicator should be used, but, as stated, with experience this is an uncommon event. Dissection is continued up and down the vena cava. Small vessels and lymphatic channels are easily coagulated with monopolar electricity.

One end of the nodal bundle is then transected. This can be easily and quickly performed, using short bursts of monopolar electrocautery in a fulgurating fashion. Once the nodal package is transected at one end, it is easy to peel the bundle off the vena cava toward the opposite end. Transection of the remaining end is again accomplished by monopolar electrocautery. When the cephalad end of this bundle is transected, care should be taken not to injure the transverse duodenum, and when the caudad end of the bundle is transected, care should be taken not to injure the right ureter. The nodal tissue is extracted using the large forceps through the lower midline port. The operative field is irrigated, and hemostasis is secured.

If the nodal tissue over the right common iliac artery is to be removed as well, this can be accomplished through the

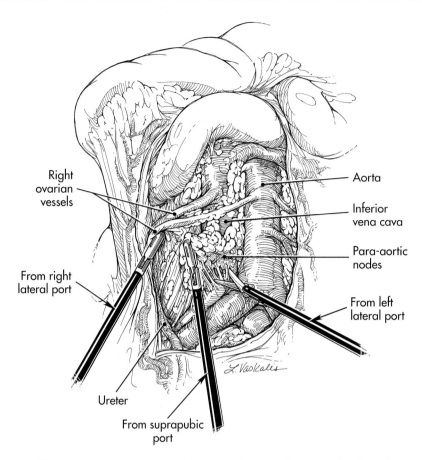

Right
ovarian
vessels

Aorta

Inferior
vena cava

Para-aortic
nodes

From right
lateral port

From left
lateral port

Ureter

From suprapubic
port

L. Vaskalis

Fig. 38-7 The right ureter can be retracted in a caudad direction, exposing the right common iliac artery and its bifurcation. An incision is made in the peritoneum medial to the ureter to perform this maneuver.

same peritoneal incision. The assistant uses his or her grasper to retract the ureter atraumatically in a caudad direction. This will provide exposure to the nodal tissue over this artery and beyond its bifurcation (Figs. 38-6 to 38-8). The nodal dissection is then continued down the common iliac to the proximal internal and external iliac vessels.

Left-Sided Paraaortic Lymphadenectomy. The surgeon, on the right side of the patient or between the patient's legs, performs this procedure using a grasper placed through the lower midline and scissors through the right lateral port (Figs. 38-5 and 38-9). The assistant holds the telescope and camera through the umbilical port. The camera is rotated so that the surgeon is comfortably oriented.

If the peritoneal incision has not already been made, an incision is made similar to that used for the right-sided paraaortic lymphadenectomy. This incision over the aorta is extended in the cephalad direction as far as possible. The mesentery of the small bowel or the third portion of the duodenum will limit the cephalad extent. The incision is extended in a caudad direction over the proximal left common iliac artery.

The surgeon first dissects in the adventitial plane of the aorta in a cephalad and caudad direction. It is important to extend this adventitial dissection as far as possible in both directions to allow ample room to perform the lymphade-

nectomy safely. On the left side, the cephalad extent will be limited by the inferior mesenteric artery. Care should be taken to avoid injuring this artery because its origin on the abdominal aorta is often difficult to identify. The more the aorta and left common iliac are "cleaned off," the more space and visibility the surgeon will have.

Only *after* the adventitia over the aorta has been adequately dissected free should lateral dissection toward the left psoas muscle be carried out. I believe this greatly assists in the identification of the proper surgical plane for lateral dissection. The surgeon can safely dissect beneath the left ureter and mesentery of the rectosigmoid using this plane. This differs from the right-sided paraaortic lymphadenectomy, in which lateral dissection is carried out after making the peritoneal incision but before dissecting the aortic adventitia. Identification of the proper plane is critical. If the surgeon dissects laterally anterior to the proper plane, which is easy to do, the left lumbar veins, ureter, or inferior mesenteric artery may be left posterior and subsequently injured during extraction of the nodes.

Lateral dissection is performed until the psoas muscle and its tendon are identified. The assistant now places the grasper (left lateral port) into the dissected space beneath the mesentery of the rectosigmoid colon and the left ureter (Fig. 38-10). This retraction is paramount for adequate ex-

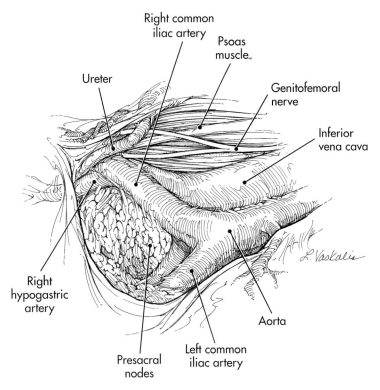

Fig. 38-8   The surgeon, standing on the patient's right side, has access to the left paraaortic nodes. Scissors are placed through the right lateral port and graspers are placed through the suprapubic port.

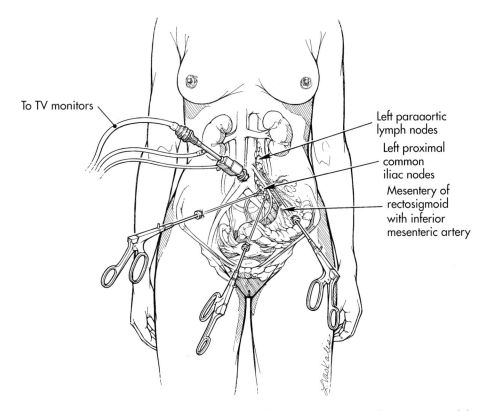

Fig. 38-9   The instrument placed through the left lateral port retracts the mesentery of the rectosigmoid colon with the inferior mesenteric artery as well as the left ureter and left ovarian vessels.

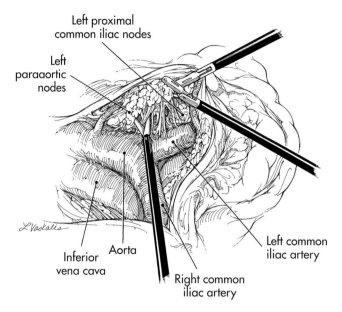

Fig. 38-10 The surgeon removes the lower left paraaortic lymph node bundle. With the mesentery of the rectosigmoid colon and the left ureter retracted laterally by the assistant, the surgeon grasps the left paraaortic nodal bundle with the graspers and elevates the nodal bundle away from the aorta and left common iliac artery, allowing the scissors to sharply dissect the nodal chain.

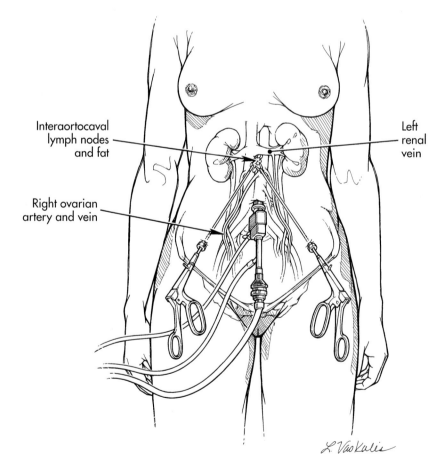

Fig. 38-11 The high paraaortic nodes can be accessed by standing on either the left or right side of the patient or between the patient's legs. Monitors must be placed at the head of the table for the surgeon and assistant to be completely oriented.

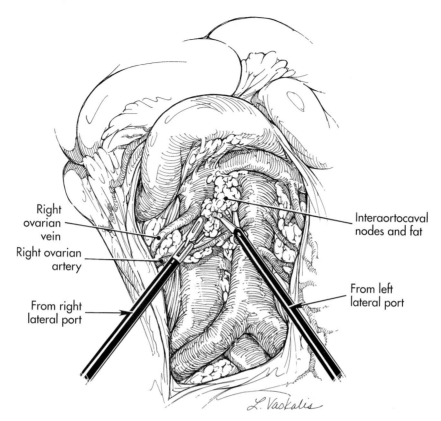

Fig. 38-12   If necessary, nodal tissue between the aorta and the vena cava can easily be sampled.

posure, which is mandatory because the left-sided paraaortic lymph nodes in this area are lateral to the aorta.

Once adequate exposure has been created, the surgeon grasps the nodal bundle adjacent to either the aorta or the proximal common iliac artery and lifts anteriorly while simultaneously slightly pushing down on the aorta with the scissors. This frees the loose attachments between these two structures and assists in dissecting beneath the nodal chain. A window is created beneath the nodal chain at its caudad end by this blunt dissection. Transection of the nodal chain is easily accomplished with scissors and electrocautery. The dissection is then extended in a cephalad direction using blunt and sharp dissection and electrocautery with the scissors as needed. The nodal chain is then transected at the cephalad end near the inferior mesenteric artery. The specimen is removed through the lower midline 12-mm port, and the operative field is irrigated and inspected for hemostasis.

Infrarenal Paraaortic Lymphadenectomy. To sample the paraaortic lymph nodes above the inferior mesenteric artery, the avascular plane between the transverse duodenum and the vena cava and the aorta is opened by blunt and sharp dissection. This dissection is continued in a cephalad and *lateral* direction. The assistant provides exposure by maintaining upward retraction on the transverse duodenum. These higher nodes can be removed with the surgeon standing on either the left or right side of the patient or between the patient's legs (Fig. 38-11).

After adequate cephalad exposure is obtained, the nodal dissection is begun. On the right, this is simply a matter of continuing the previously performed lymphadenectomy up to the origin of the ovarian vein, which may enter the vena cava distal to or very near the left renal vein (Figs. 38-7 and 38-12). On the left, the surgeon is faced with the lateral location of the nodal chain and working around the inferior mesenteric artery. The left renal and ovarian veins must be identified as soon as possible (Fig. 38-13). They are often disguised in the endoabdominal fascia and could be easily damaged. Once these vessels are located, dissection in the adventitia of the aorta should be carried out. With generous use of monopolar electricity, annoying small bleeding vessels will be minimized. The ovarian artery may need to be sacrificed; this can be done with clips or bipolar or monopolar electricity. The nodal bundle is transected near the left renal vein. This entire dissection can be performed with scissors and monopolar electricity.

A WORD OF WARNING

If performed properly, laparoscopic lymphadenectomy is a two-person, four-port operation. Once the operation begins, the only instrument to be removed from a port is the grasper, through the suprapubic port site, and this is done only to remove lymph nodes as they are dissected.

Like most operations, laparoscopic lymphadenectomy can be accomplished in a number of ways. However, one of

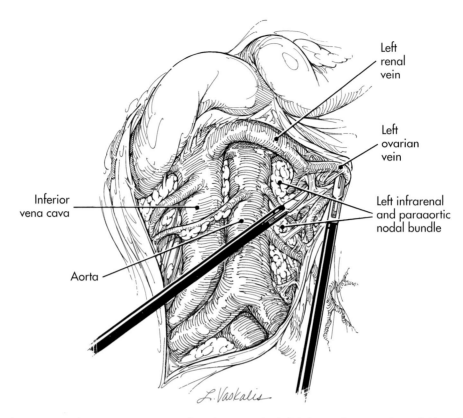

Fig. 38-13   The surgeon creates a plane between the left infrarenal paraaortic nodal bundle and the left ovarian vein. Creation of this natural surgical plane allows better identification of the left infrarenal nodes. Often, lumbar veins draining into the ovarian vein will be encountered.

the biggest pitfalls is using traditional laparoscopic surgical techniques for this procedure. This usually results in irrigating and aspirating too frequently and overuse of clip applicators and bipolar electrocautery forceps. For this operation, these steps are time-consuming and generally unnecessary. This constant changing of laparoscopic instruments only slows the process.

Another common pitfall is the inappropriate use of monopolar electricity. The greatest mistake is using another instrument to accomplish what monopolar electricity can accomplish. This results only in loss of valuable time and possibly an increase in the cost of the operation (e.g., disposable clip applicators). In my experience, bipolar energy and clip applicators are virtually never needed for pelvic lymphadenectomies and only rarely for low paraaortic lymphadenectomies. Another mistake with monopolar electricity is its misuse. When it is used appropriately, only short bursts of electrical energy are required. In most instances the fulgurating technique is all that is needed. Occasionally, large vessels will need to be coapted. In these instances the vessel is grasped, and the scissors apply "cutting" current to the grasper.

As the surgeon becomes adept at this process, the lymph node bundles removed will be virtually intact. Some of these bundles, like the obturator nodal bundle, can be large, and therefore use of a 12-mm suprapubic port is strongly

recommended. Large lateral ports are not necessary and only increase the incidence of postoperative pain and the likelihood of postoperative bowel herniation.

If the surgeon is not careful with hemostasis, the retroperitoneal tissue is readily blood stained, which absorbs light, and even with excellent cameras visualization is decreased. Preoperative bowel preparation is mandatory.

In the pelvis the most common complications will be injury to the genitofemoral nerve and injury to an aberrant or accessory obturator vein. Experience and attention to detail will minimize the frequency of these complications. Injury to the left pelvic ureter near the bifurcation of the common iliac vessels can be prevented by a good assistant who retracts the ureter medially without causing trauma while the surgeon is operating in this area.

Proper identification of the appropriate surgical planes is mandatory. In the pelvis, the key is in learning to quickly identify the obliterated umbilical artery. This key landmark is the door to the avascular plane that opens the obturator space. In the right paraaortic area, the crucial plane is between the right ureter and the right ovarian vessels anteriorly and the vena cava nodal pad and psoas muscle posteriorly. The right ureter must be separated from the psoas muscle to avoid injury. In the left paraaortic area, the crucial plane is beneath the inferior mesenteric artery, the left ureter, and the left ovarian vessels. This plane is more posterior than one may think. If the adventitial plane over the aorta and left common iliac artery are not cleaned off first, it is easy for the surgeon to dissect laterally toward the psoas muscle in the wrong plane. It is here where the left lumbar veins, ureter, and inferior mesenteric artery can easily be damaged during lymph node dissection. When the infrarenal lymph nodes are removed, it is mandatory that enough blunt and sharp dissection be performed to allow identification of the left renal vein as it crosses the aorta and the left ovarian vein as it empties into the left renal vein, before the lymphadenectomy is performed. If the lymph nodes are attacked, before these landmarks are properly identified, disastrous results may ensue.

CONCLUSIONS

Laparoscopic lymphadenectomy is in its infancy. The role that this technique will play in the management of patients with pelvic malignancies is yet to be determined. Initial reports indicate that laparoscopic lymphadenectomy, both pelvic and paraaortic, is feasible, adequate, and safe. Use of this technique will avoid an abdominal incision when surgical management of patients with early endometrial, ovarian, and cervical malignancies is undertaken.

It is imperative that the survival of patients with pelvic malignancies not be compromised by use of laparoscopic lymphadenectomy. Currently, survival data for patients with pelvic malignancies who have been managed with laparo-

scopy are lacking. The learning curve associated with this surgical procedure is significant and is unlikely to be overcome by the surgeon with no experience in abdominal pelvic and paraaortic lymphadenectomy or by the experienced oncologic surgeon who performs this laparoscopic procedure only occasionally. Only the experienced, committed oncologic surgeon will master laparoscopic pelvic and paraaortic lymphadenectomy. Future clinical trials with experienced surgeons and long-term survival data will help determine the role of laparoscopic lymphadenectomy in oncology.

REFERENCES

1. Childers J, Hatch K, Surwit E: The role of laparoscopic lymphadenectomy in the management of cervical cancer, *Gynecol Oncol* 47:38, 1992.
2. Childers JM, Hatch KD, Surwit EA: Laparoscopic para-aortic lymphadenectomy in gynecologic malignancies, *Obstet Gynecol* 82:741, 1993.
3. Childers J, et al: Laparoscopic surgical staging of ovarian cancer, *Gynecol Oncol* 59:25, 1995.
4. Querleu D: Laparoscopic para-aortic node sampling in gynecologic oncology: a preliminary experience, *Gynecol Oncol* 49:24, 1993.
5. Querleu D, LeBlanc E: Laparoscopic infrarenal para-aortic node dissection in the restaging of carcinomas of the ovary and fallopian tube, *Cancer* 73:1467, 1994.
6. Querleu D, LeBlanc E, Castelain B: Laparoscopic pelvic lymphadenectomy in the staging of early carcinoma of the cervix, *Am J Obstet Gynecol* 164:579, 1991.
7. Spirtos N, et al: Laparoscopic bilateral pelvic and para-aortic lymph node sampling: an evolving technique, *Am J Obstet Gynecol* 173:105, 1995.

39 Surgery for Cancer of the Ovary

STEPHEN C. RUBIN and IVOR BENJAMIN

Ovarian cancer is the leading cause of death in women with gynecologic malignancies. Although it accounts for only approximately 27% of new gynecologic cancer cases each year in the United States, this disease kills more U.S. women each year than all the other gynecologic malignancies combined. In 1998, the Surveillance Research Program of the American Cancer Society estimated that there would be 25,400 new cases and 14,500 deaths from ovarian cancer in that year.[59] As with many cancers, survival for patients with ovarian cancer is directly related to stage of disease at the time of diagnosis. It is unfortunate that most patients remain asymptomatic until their disease has progressed to advanced stages. Furthermore, no effective screening modalities are available, making early diagnosis uncommon and generally serendipitous. Therefore it is not surprising that according to the 1991 International Federation of Gynecology and Obstetrics (FIGO) report including data on nearly 10,912 patients with ovarian cancer, only 23% of patients had stage I disease at presentation.[104] The major advances that have been made in the chemotherapy of ovarian cancer over the last 15 years have tended to overshadow our enhanced understanding of the role of the gynecologic cancer surgeon in the management of this disease. Surgery remains the cornerstone of the treatment of ovarian cancer, playing a critical part in diagnosis and staging, removal of tumor, assessment of response to chemotherapy, and palliation of symptoms, including intestinal obstruction. The role of surgery in the management of ovarian cancer can be considered in three categories:

1. Primary
   a. Establish diagnosis, histology, and grade of the cancer
   b. Define extent of the disease (staging)
   c. Resect tumor (primary cytoreduction)
   d. Resect tumor at interval (cytoreduction performed midway through a planned course of combination chemotherapy)
2. Secondary
   a. Assess response to therapy (second-look laparotomy)
   b. Resect tumor (secondary cytoreduction after completion of a course of chemotherapy)
3. Supportive and palliative
   a. Relieve intestinal obstruction
   b. Alleviate pleural effusion or ascites
   c. Establish intravenous access
   d. Establish intraperitoneal access

Despite the importance of surgery in the management of this disease, in all patients with disease beyond stage IA,

surgery alone is inadequate treatment for ovarian cancer. Without adjunctive chemotherapy, progression of the disease is inevitable. At the same time, the success of both chemotherapy and radiotherapy depends heavily on appropriate surgery. This true synergy among the therapeutic modalities highlights the fact that ovarian cancer requires an interdisciplinary approach to treatment. This approach brings together the gynecologic surgeon, the medical and radiation oncologists, the pathologist, the nurse oncologist, and a number of supporting professionals including psychiatrists, nutritionists, geneticists, and social workers. Although this chapter deals only with the surgical management of ovarian cancer, such surgery should be part of a comprehensive multimodality program for the management of the disease.

HISTOGENETIC CLASSIFICATION OF OVARIAN TUMORS

The ovary can give rise to a remarkable variety of neoplasms, both benign and malignant. A comprehensive classification of these tumors, adopted by the World Health Organization (WHO) in 1973[138] and more recently described by Scully et al. in 1994[137] is based on currently accepted concepts of their histogenesis. Tumors may arise from any of the three main types of cells that make up the ovary: (1) the coelomic surface epithelium (actually mesothelium) that covers the ovary, (2) the cortical mesenchymal stroma and sex cords, and (3) the germ cells. The WHO classification for the common epithelial tumors is given in the box on p. 705. Epithelial tumors comprise approximately 60% of all ovarian tumors and about 90% of malignant ovarian tumors. Although this chapter does not deal specifically with the surgical management of the less common stromal and germ cell malignancies of the ovary, for the most part the same principles and techniques apply. Epithelial ovarian tumors are subdivided according to the predominant pattern of differentiation of the coelomic epithelial cell. These patterns tend to resemble the normally differentiated epithelium of the various areas of the female genital tract. The most common epithelial tumors are those of serous differentiation. The epithelium of these tumors contains a mixture of ciliated, goblet, and intercalated cells resembling those of the fallopian tube.

Mucinous tumors contain endocervical type epithelium with tall columnar mucin-producing cells or intestinal type epithelium with goblet cells. Other tumors, designated endometrioid, produce epithelium resembling that found in the

WORLD HEALTH ORGANIZATION HISTOLOGIC CLASSIFICATION OF EPITHELIAL OVARIAN TUMORS

I. Common epithelial tumors
  A. Serous tumors
    1. Benign
      a. Cystadenoma and papillary cystadenoma
      b. Surface papilloma
      c. Adenofibroma and cystadenofibroma
    2. Of borderline malignancy (carcinoma of low malignant potential)
      a. Cystadenoma and papillary cystadenoma
      b. Surface papilloma
      c. Adenofibroma and cystadenofibroma
    3. Malignant
      a. Adenocarcinoma, papillary adenocarcinoma, and papillary cystadenocarcinoma
      b. Surface papillary carcinoma
      c. Malignant adenofibroma and cystadenofibroma
  B. Mucinous tumors
    1. Benign
      a. Cystadenoma
      b. Adenofibroma and cystadenofibroma
    2. Of borderline malignancy (carcinoma of low malignant potential)
      a. Cystadenoma
      b. Adenofibroma and cystadenofibroma
    3. Malignant
      a. Adenocarcinoma and cystadenocarcinoma
      b. Malignant adenofibroma and cystadenofibroma
  C. Endometrioid tumors
    1. Benign
      a. Adenoma and cystadenoma
      b. Adenofibroma and cystadenofibroma
    2. Of borderline malignancy (carcinoma of low malignant potential)
      a. Adenoma and cystadenoma
      b. Adenofibroma and cystadenofibroma
    3. Malignant
      a. Carcinoma
        (1) Adenoacarcinoma
        (2) Adenocanthoma
        (3) Malignant adenofibroma
      b. Endometrioid stromal sarcomas
      c. Mesodermal (müllerian) mixed tumors, homologous, and heterologous
  D. Clear cell (mesonephroid) tumors
    1. Benign: adenofibroma
    2. Of borderline malignancy (carcinoma of low malignant potential)
    3. Malignant: carcinoma and adenocarcinoma
  E. Brenner tumors
    1. Benign
    2. Of borderline malignancy (proliferating)
    3. Malignant
  F. Mixed epithelial tumors
    1. Benign
    2. Of borderline malignancy
    3. Malignant
  G. Undifferentiated carcinoma
  H. Unclassified epithelial tumors

From Serov S, Scully R, Sobin L: Histological typing of ovarian tumors. In *International histological classification of tumors,* No. 9, pp. 17-18. Geneva, 1973, World Health Organization.

endometrium. Related to the endometrioid group are the clear cell tumors, formerly misclassified as mesonephric. The so-called Brenner tumors produce epithelium resembling the transitional cells lining the urinary tract. Many ovarian tumors contain mixtures of the various types of epithelium, and some are so undifferentiated that they cannot be classified by this schema. Table 39-1 shows this classification of differentiated epithelial tumors of the ovary.

EPIDEMIOLOGY OF EPITHELIAL OVARIAN CANCER

Epithelial cancers of the ovary most commonly occur in women in the early postmenopausal age range, the average age at diagnosis being about 54 years. Fig. 39-1, based on data from more than 8000 patients from the FIGO 1988 Annual Report,[103] shows the distribution of cases by age. Epithelial ovarian cancer is rare in women younger than age 20, with a yearly incidence rate of less than 1 in 100,000 in this age group. This rate rises to about 33 per 100,000 at age 55. Although it is not generally appreciated, the incidence rate

continues to rise thereafter, peaking at 52 cases per 100,000 women per year at age 78.[139]

Although the cause of epithelial ovarian cancer remains unknown and risk factors are poorly defined, some generalizations can be made. The epidemiologic observation that incidence rates are highest in industrialized countries suggests that some as yet undefined environmental factors play a role in the cause of the disease. A major exception to this observation is Japan, where recorded rates of developing ovarian cancer are among the lowest in the world. The risk of ovarian cancer is related to several aspects of reproductive and hormonal status. Young age at first pregnancy is recognized as protective,[60] whereas the risk is higher for women who have no or few children. Early menarche and late menopause have been associated with an increased risk.[40] The effect of obesity on the risk of developing ovarian cancer is controversial. In a large prospective study, Lew and Garfinkel[155] found that women who were 40% or more overweight had an increased risk of dying of ovarian cancer compared with women who were of average weight.[64] Other studies have shown no relationship between body weight and risk.

Table 39-1 Histogenetic Classification of Epithelial Ovarian Tumors

Differentiation	Benign Tumor	Borderline Tumor	Malignant Tumor
Tubal	Serous cystadenoma	Borderline serous tumor	Serous carcinoma
Endocervical	Mucinous cystadenoma	Borderline mucinous tumor	Mucinous carcinoma
Endometrial	Endometrioid adenofibroma*	Borderline endometrioid tumor*	Endometrioid carcinoma
Clear cell	Clear cell adenofibroma*	Borderline clear cell tumor*	Clear cell carcinoma
Urothelial	Brenner tumor	Proliferating Brenner tumor*	Malignant Brenner tumor*

Modified from Gompel C, Silverberg S, Zaloudek C: The ovary. In Silverberg S, Zaloudek C, editors: *Pathology in gynecology and obstetrics,* Philadelphia, 1985, JB Lippincott.
*Rare.

A number of studies have reported that the use of oral contraceptives decreases the risk of epithelial ovarian cancer. In a large case-control study published in 1987, the Centers for Disease Control and Prevention reported that women who had used oral contraceptives had a risk of epithelial ovarian cancer of 0.6 compared with those who had never used them.[4,63] This protective effect was noted in women who had used oral contraceptives for as little as 3 to 6 months and persisted for 15 years. This effect was independent of the specific type of oral contraceptive used. This observation was confirmed by a case-control study reported by Rosenberg et al.,[124] which compared 441 women with recently diagnosed invasive ovarian cancer to 2065 control women. The inverse association of risk with 3 years of use or more was consistently present across categories of age, parity, interview year, and geographic area. It was apparent for as long as 15 to 19 years after cessation of the oral contraceptive. A similar result (0.7 relative risk reduction) was noted in an Italian case-control study reported by Parazzini et al.[101]

Several reports have suggested a relationship between high ovarian cancer mortality and high total intake of dietary fat, especially fats of animal origin.[31,120,123] A case-control study by Risch et al.[120] showed that saturated fat consumption was associated with increasing risk of ovarian cancer (odds ratio 1.20 for each 10 g/day of intake; 95% confidence interval 1.03 to 1.40; one-sided $p = .0082$). No relationship was seen with intake of unsaturated fats. Egg consumption also appeared related to increased risk (odds ratio 1.42 for each 100 mg of egg cholesterol per day; 95% confidence interval 1.18 to 1.72; two-sided $p = .0002$).[123]

The known association of environmental carcinogens, specifically asbestos, with mesotheliomas, has led some to suggest a similar cause for cancers of the ovarian epithelium, which shares a common embryologic origin with the peritoneal mesothelium. In a case-control study of ovarian cancer, Cramer et al.[29] noted that women with ovarian cancer were significantly more likely to report the regular use of talc as a dusting powder on the perineum or sanitary napkins, providing a possible route of direct ovarian exposure.

Some reports have suggested an association between viral infections and the development of ovarian cancer. McGowan et al.[83] found that patients with ovarian cancer had had rubella in their teens more often than a control

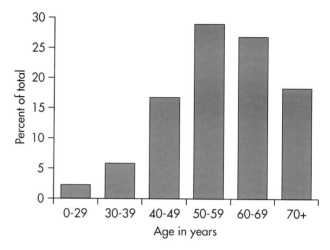

Fig. 39-1 Age distribution of patients with epithelial ovarian cancer. Based on data from the International Federation of Gynecology and Obstetrical (FIGO) 1988 Annual Report.[39]

group. A history of mumps has been suggested to increase the risk of ovarian cancer,[30] although others have suggested a protective effect.

Although most cases of ovarian cancer are considered sporadic, with no discernible familial tendency, there is now growing evidence that a subset of ovarian cancers do have a heritable genetic basis. Lynch and others described early observations regarding familial associated ovarian cancer in the 1970s and 1980s.[72,73,110] These cancers tend to occur at an earlier age than the sporadic variety and are generally of the serous or undifferentiated cell types. Classically, Lynch et al.[71] described three variants of familial ovarian cancer: (1) site-specific ovarian cancer, (2) ovarian cancer associated with colon and endometrial cancers, and (3) ovarian cancer associated with breast cancer. In 1994, the first breast-ovarian cancer gene (BRCA1) was cloned.[86] In 1995, BRCA2 was cloned.[152] The clinical course of patients harboring germline mutations of BRCA1 or BRCA2 is still being elucidated. Rubin et al.[26] reported on clinical and pathologic features of ovarian cancer in 53 women with germline mutations of BRCA1. They reported that the actuarial median survival for the 43 patients with advanced-stage disease was 77 months, compared with 29 months for the matched control subjects ($p < .001$). These data suggest that

BRCA1-associated epithelial ovarian cancer may occur at an earlier age and be more indolent than sporadically occurring cancers. In a similar series from Japan, Aida et al.[2] also reported an increased survival for women harboring a germline mutation in BRCA1 (115 versus 53 months).

Management of women from families with a clear history of familial ovarian cancer or a known germline mutation in BRCA1 or BRCA2 is controversial. As yet, no clear evidence shows that surveillance of such women with serum markers, sonography, laparoscopy, or frequent pelvic examinations is of any benefit, although some form of intensified surveillance and early intervention for adnexal enlargement or pelvic symptoms seems appropriate. Many would recommend prophylactic excision of the ovaries after age 35 if the woman has completed childbearing, recognizing that there have been reports of peritoneal carcinomatosis developing in women who previously had undergone prophylactic bilateral oophorectomy at which time normal ovaries were removed.[145] However, it is important that women considering prophylactic surgery receive adequate preoperative counseling. Multidisciplinary services have been established, facilitating an informed decision.[15,51] At a minimum, this evaluation should include a pedigree analysis and possible deoxyribonucleic acid (DNA) testing for germline mutations in affected individuals from selected families. More difficult yet is the problem of women with a history of one or more first-degree relatives (mother, sister, or daughter) with ovarian and/or breast cancer when none of the affected family members has undergone genetic testing.

NATURAL HISTORY AND PATTERNS OF SPREAD

Epithelial cancers of the ovary generally begin as cystic intraovarian growths, probably developing in invaginations of the normal ovarian surface epithelium. The tumors grow within the substance of the ovary for some time before dissemination begins by one of several routes. The rate of growth of early tumors and the length of time they remain confined to the ovary before spread are unknown. When spread does occur, two main routes are involved: exfoliation of cells into the peritoneal cavity and spread by lymphatic dissemination. Occasionally, bloodborne spread to distant organs may be seen, but in general, ovarian cancer remains confined to the peritoneal cavity and retroperitoneal lymphatics for most, if not all, of its natural history. In the past, spread of ovarian cancer by way of the lymphatics received little attention. Over the past 15 years, it has become clear that lymphatic spread is common in patients with advanced intraperitoneal ovarian cancer and that even when the disease appears grossly confined to the ovaries, lymph nodes may already be involved.

The primary lymphatic drainage of the ovary follows the blood vessels in the infundibulopelvic ligament to terminate in aortic lymph nodes at approximately the level of the renal hilus.[111] Secondary channels traverse the broad ligament and terminate in the iliac lymph nodes. Spread may also occur by way of uterine cornual and tubal lymphatics along the path of the round ligament to terminate in the inguinal lymph nodes. Although the clinical significance of lymphatic spread is uncertain in women with advanced intraperitoneal disease, in cases in which the tumor appears grossly to be confined to the ovary, the detection of such spread is of critical importance.

The intraperitoneal spread of ovarian cancer has appropriately received much greater attention than spread by way of the lymphatics. After growing for some time within the ovary itself, ovarian tumors eventually breach the capsule of the ovary where they may involve adjacent organs by direct extension or exfoliation. In its earliest form, intraperitoneal spread is clinically occult and must be actively searched for by the operating surgeon, or the patient's cancer may be staged inappropriately and then undertreated. In advanced cases, an amorphous mass of tumor may engulf the pelvic organs and obscure anatomic landmarks. Intraperitoneal spread by exfoliation of malignant cells from the surface of the ovary leads to viable tumor cells being carried throughout the peritoneal cavity by the normal clockwise circulation of the peritoneal fluid. Typically, tumor cells implant and grow as nodules on the parietal and visceral peritoneal surfaces, including the intestinal serosa, omentum, paracolic gutters, and undersurfaces of the diaphragm, particularly on the right. This initially produces the characteristic picture of miliary carcinomatosis so common in women with advanced ovarian cancer. Such metastatic implants can also become large. The specific surgical management of both occult and advanced intraperitoneal spread is discussed in subsequent sections.

Relatively late in the natural history of the disease, ovarian cancer can also spread beyond the peritoneal cavity to involve distant organs. Tumor cells may traverse the diaphragmatic lymphatics to involve the pleural space, producing malignant pleural effusions and pleural metastases. In one autopsy series of ovarian cancer patients, 36% had pleural metastases.[17] The disease may also spread by hematogenous dissemination to involve a variety of organs, most commonly the liver.

STAGING OF CANCER OF THE OVARY

The stage of a malignant tumor is determined by the extent of disease at the time of diagnosis. Once properly assigned, the stage does not change if the disease progresses or recurs. Unlike the staging systems for many malignancies, the staging system used for cancer of the ovary is based on a surgical determination of the extent of disease. Because the stage of a patient's ovarian cancer correlates strongly with prognosis and is the basis for the selection of appropriate therapy, proper surgical staging is a critical element in the management of these patients. In 1985, the FIGO Cancer Committee[39] revised the surgical staging system for ovarian cancer to reflect not only the results of a thorough exploration of the areas at risk of spread but also a more precise determination of the extent of such spread. This system is

FIGO STAGING SYSTEM FOR OVARIAN CANCER

Stage I: Growth limited to the ovaries
  IA: Growth limited to one ovary; no ascites; no tumor on the external surfaces; capsule intact
  Ib: Growth limited to both ovaries; no ascites; no tumor on the external surfaces; capsule intact
  Ic: Tumor either stage Ia or stage Ib but with tumor on the surface of one or both ovaries; or with capsule ruptured; or with ascites present containing malignant cells or with positive peritoneal washings
Stage II: Growth involving one or both ovaries with pelvic extension
  IIa: Extension and/or metastases to the uterus and/or tubes
  IIb: Extension to other pelvic tissues
  IIc: Tumor either stage IIa or IIb but with tumor on the surface of one or both ovaries; or with capsule(s) ruptured; or with ascites present containing malignant cells or with positive peritoneal washings

Stage III: Tumor involving one or both ovaries with peritoneal implants outside the pelvis and/or positive retroperitoneal or inguinal nodes; superficial liver metastases equals stage III; tumor is limited to the true pelvis but with histologically verified malignant extension to small bowel or omentum
  IIIa: Tumor grossly limited to the true pelvis with negative nodes but with histologically confirmed microscopic seeding of abdominal peritoneal surfaces
  IIIb: Tumor of one or both ovaries; histologically confirmed implants of abdominal peritoneal surfaces, none exceeding 2 cm in diameter; nodes negative
  IIIc: Abdominal implants greater than 2 cm in diameter and/or positive retroperitoneal or inguinal nodes
Stage IV: Growth involving one or both ovaries with distant metastases; if pleural effusion is present, there must be positive cytologic test results to allot a case to stage IV; parenchymal liver metastases equals stage IV

From Cancer Committee of FIGO: *Gynecol Oncol* 25:383, 1986.

Table 39-2 Distribution by Stage of Ovarian Cancer Patients

Stage	Patients	
	No.	%
I	2230	26.1
II	1313	15.4
III	3339	39.1
IV	1391	16.3
Unstaged	268	3.1
TOTAL	8451	100.0

Data summarized from 1988 FIGO Annual Report.

shown in the box above. Generally, early ovarian tumors are completely asymptomatic, although they occasionally may produce pain associated with rupture or torsion. Once the tumor has grown to considerable size, patients may complain of symptoms relating to pressure on the bladder or rectum such as urinary frequency, constipation, or tenesmus. With the development of ascites, they may notice abdominal bloating and an increase in the size of their waistline despite a loss of appetite. Because of the lack of specific symptoms early in the course of the disease, in most patients, cancer of the ovary is not diagnosed until the malignancy has spread beyond the ovary. Table 39-2, taken from the FIGO 1988 Annual Report, shows the distribution by stage of more than 8000 patients with epithelial cancers of the ovary reported to FIGO from 95 participating institutions around the world.[103] In only about one quarter of these patients was ovarian cancer diagnosed in stage I, and in more than 50%, it was not diagnosed until stage III or IV disease was present.

PRIMARY SURGICAL MANAGEMENT OF APPARENT EARLY OVARIAN CANCER

Early ovarian cancers are most often detected at the time of exploration in a patient with an adnexal mass. Because the preoperative diagnosis of early ovarian cancer cannot be made definitively, nor the possibility excluded, the surgeon faced with a patient with an adnexal mass is well advised to form an opinion about the likelihood of malignancy and to base the preoperative evaluation, discussion with the patient, and operative approach on this assessment.

With the ready availability of techniques such as sonography, computed tomography (CT), and magnetic resonance imaging (MRI), most patients with a persistent adnexal mass have some form of imaging of the mass performed preoperatively. Apart from confirming the presence of the mass, such tests may provide information about the precise size, composition, location, and origin of masses that may aid the clinician in refining the differential diagnosis. However, such techniques are not accurate in distinguishing benign from malignant masses because there is broad overlap in the imaging characteristics of each. Transvaginal color flow sonographic imaging to detect tumor neovascularization appears promising as a means of distinguishing benign from malignant ovarian tumors, but its clinical utility is still unclear.[16] Often, measurement of serum markers such as CA 125 is performed. If levels are elevated, suspicion should be increased, although CA 125 may be elevated in a variety of benign conditions including endometriosis and pelvic inflammatory disease[48,75] and may, in fact, be normal in many patients with early ovarian cancers.[102] However, the likelihood of malignancy increases with increasing age, increased levels of CA 125, and increasing size and complexity of the mass on transvaginal sonography.[6,38] Most women older than age 50 with a CA 125 greater than 100 units/ml and a complex pelvic mass larger than 5 cm will have ovarian cancer. The presence of ascites also greatly increases the likelihood that a pelvic mass is caused by an ovarian malignancy.

The role of laparoscopy in the primary management of ovarian cancer is in evolution. Small case series have reported the use of laparoscopy for staging and/or debulking of ovarian cancer.[3,95,115] In a large series from Austria, Wenzl et al.[150] presented data on 16,601 laparoscopic surgeries for adnexal masses. In 108 cases, malignant ovarian tumors were found. Of these 108 patients, 20 were treated with laparoscopy alone. In 22 patients, laparoscopy was followed by immediate laparotomy. A delayed laparotomy (3 to 1415 days) was performed in 54 patients. Staging revealed FIGO classifications from stages IA to IV. Others have described their experience with nodal dissection as a potential alternative to restaging laparotomy.[25,116,117]

Laparoscopy may prove useful in selected patients with adnexal masses. Chi et al.[24] reported a series of 34 patients with a history of nongynecologic malignancies who presented with adnexal masses. In six patients, metastatic non-gynecologic malignancies were confirmed, thereby sparing the patient the morbidity of an exploratory laparotomy. All six of these patients had preoperative imaging studies that showed solid and/or complex adnexal masses, and five of six had elevated preoperative CA 125 levels. Two primary ovarian cancers were identified by frozen section. These patients underwent immediate laparotomy.

Before surgery for an adnexal mass, the experienced clinician forms an opinion as to the likelihood of malignancy based on the patient's age, the size and characteristics of the mass, and other factors. In all but the most clear-cut cases of benign disease, the physician should discuss the possibility of malignancy with the patient, review the surgical options if cancer is found, and ascertain the patient's wishes regarding these options. If the physician is uncomfortable with this type of discussion or if the suspicion of malignancy is high, consultation with a gynecologic oncologist should be obtained. In addition to the traditionally available references available for physicians and patients, the Internet is becoming an increasingly valuable resource for cancer information.

In the operating room, pelvic examination should be performed after the induction of anesthesia to allow a final assessment of the pelvic findings before exploration. If the adnexal mass is suspicious or other indications for evaluation of the endometrium exist, dilation and curettage (D&C) should be performed. The information obtained from this may aid in the decision-making process if an apparent early ovarian malignancy is found in a young woman who wishes to preserve fertility, because one is more comfortable leaving the uterus if the endometrium and uterine serosa are apparently free of disease. The choice of incision is determined by the surgeon's level of suspicion regarding malignancy. A low transverse incision, which does not allow surgical exposure of the upper abdomen necessary for a proper ovarian cancer operation, should be avoided in favor

of a vertical incision if there is a significant risk of cancer being found. If the patient insists on this as the initial incision, the possibility of her needing a second upper abdominal incision if a malignancy is found should be discussed.

When the abdomen is entered, cytologic washings should be taken from the pelvic cavity by saline lavage. If the ovaries are suspicious, washings should also be taken from both paracolic gutters and subdiaphragmatic areas before surgery in the pelvis. Manual exploration of the upper abdominal structures should be performed to identify any obvious abnormalities. The pelvic organs should be inspected, and the pathologic condition of the ovaries should be identified. As the operation progresses, the surgeon constantly should be refining the estimate of the risk of malignancy based on inspection and palpation of the ovarian mass. The presence of ascites, bilateral ovarian involvement, surface excrescences, adherence to surrounding structures, or obvious solid areas in the ovarian tumor increase the chance of malignancy. The importance of such assessment lies in its effect on the operative management. In younger women with nonsuspicious masses, the surgeon may consider cystectomy with preservation of the remaining portion of the ovary. To the extent that cystectomy increases the risk of intraoperative rupture of an ovarian tumor, it should be avoided if that tumor might be malignant. Intraoperative rupture of a cystic ovarian cancer limited to the ovaries with resultant spillage of viable tumor cells into the peritoneal cavity worsens prognosis, as reflected in the official staging system.

After removal of the tumor, a frozen section should be studied. If malignancy is identified and there is no evidence of obvious metastatic disease, the role of further surgery is primarily diagnostic. Based on an understanding of the patterns of spread of ovarian cancer and of the patient's wishes for future fertility as determined in the preoperative discussion, a complete cancer staging operation should now be performed. This procedure should include a meticulous abdominal exploration, with special attention given to visualization and palpation of the serosal surfaces of the small and large intestine. The infracolic omentum is removed (Fig. 39-2) by serially clamping, transecting, and ligating the omental attachments to the transverse colon. Most gynecologic oncologists do not remove the gastrocolic portion of the omentum if it is grossly normal because this adds little to the diagnostic accuracy of the omentectomy and increases the risk of damage to adjacent structures, including the mesentery of the transverse colon and the vessels along the greater curvature of the stomach.

Aortic lymph nodes should be sampled, as should pelvic lymph nodes on the side of the primary tumor. The aortic lymph nodes can be approached by several routes. Either the ascending or the descending colon can be detached from its lateral peritoneal attachments and reflected medially to allow exposure of the aorta and vena cava. A somewhat simpler technique that usually provides adequate exposure for these purposes involves direct incision of the posterior parietal peritoneum overlying the right common iliac artery and the lower aorta. The small bowel must be packed above

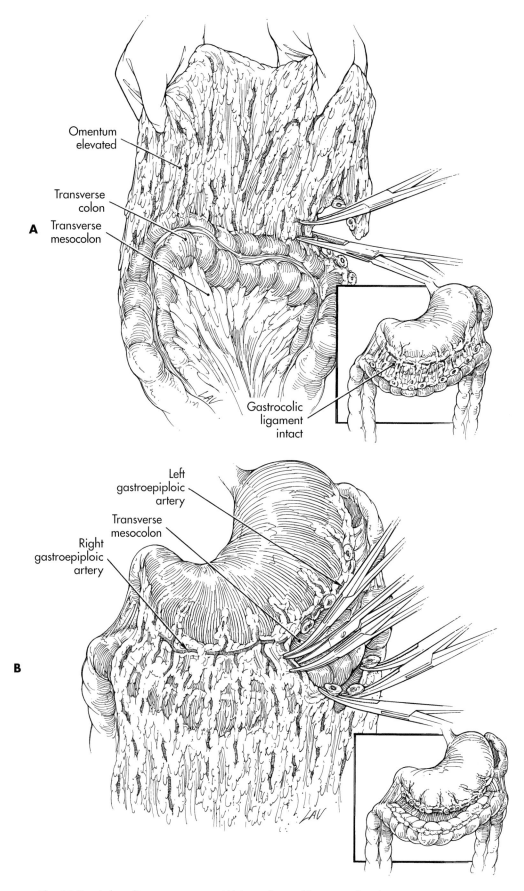

Fig. 39-2 Infracolic omentectomy **(A)** is performed by removing the omentum near its attachments to the transverse colon. If there is gross involvement of the gastrocolic omentum this can also be resected **(B).**

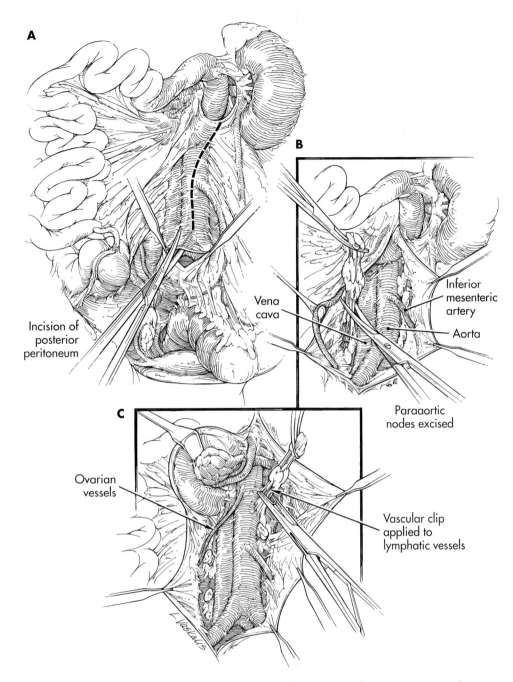

Fig. 39-3   Paraaortic node dissection for staging of apparent early ovarian cancer. The posterior parietal peritoneum overlying the aorta is incised (**A**), and the nodal tissue stripped from the vena cava (**B**) and the aorta (**C**) to the level of the left renal hilus.

the operative field or displaced from the abdominal cavity. The retroperitoneal fat overlying the common iliac artery and the lower aorta is incised to expose the wall of the vessel and identify the proper plane of dissection. The right ureter should be carefully identified and retracted laterally. This procedure provides access to the fatty node-bearing tissue overlying the aorta and the vena cava, which is then carefully stripped from the vessels by blunt and sharp dissection, using stainless steel or titanium clips for hemostasis (Fig. 39-3). The dissection can be carried upward to approximately the level of the renal hilus. Through the same

posterior parietal incision, the retroperitoneal space can be developed toward the left, elevating and mobilizing the mesentery of the descending colon and the inferior mesenteric artery and vein and retracting them laterally to allow dissection of the nodes along the left common iliac artery and the left side of the aorta. This is particularly important if the primary tumor developed in the left ovary.

Pelvic lymph nodes on the same side as the primary tumor can be sampled by incising the peritoneum overlying the external iliac artery as far as the inguinal ligament. The ureter should be identified and retracted medially. The nodal tissue can be stripped from the external iliac artery and vein, with care taken to avoid injury to the genitofemoral nerve, which lies along the psoas muscle just lateral to the vessels. If desired, nodal tissue can also be removed from the obturator fossa beneath the vessels. Although the yield is low, many gynecologic oncologists recommend taking random peritoneal biopsies from multiple sites in the pelvis, from the lateral paracolic gutters, and from the undersurfaces of both hemidiaphragms.

If the patient is not concerned about future childbearing, total hysterectomy and bilateral salpingo-oophorectomy should be completed if malignancy is found. In younger women who wish to preserve fertility and who have no anatomic or functional barrier to successful pregnancy, it may be possible to preserve the uterus and the uninvolved tube and ovary. For this to be safe requires that there be no evidence of spread beyond the primary tumor as determined by complete surgical staging, including a generous wedge biopsy of the contralateral ovary. The results of the preexploration D&C become important to rule out endometrial involvement. If the tumor is stage IA and well differentiated histologically, surgery alone should be curative in more than 90% of patients. Women with stage I moderately or poorly differentiated tumors have a good likelihood of cure after adjuvant treatment with chemotherapy and may be able to retain fertility if the opposite ovary and uterus are left in place. Obviously, these issues must have been discussed with the patient preoperatively if the appropriate intraoperative decision is to be made. If they have not, it is generally best to perform the most conservative operative procedure possible and to subject the patient to reoperation if necessary. The same would apply if the frozen section diagnosis of malignancy is uncertain. The surgical approach to apparent early ovarian cancer is summarized as follows:

1. Vertical incision
2. Multiple cytologic washings
3. Intact tumor removal
4. Complete abdominal exploration
5. Removal of remaining ovary, uterus, tubes (may be preserved in selected patients)
6. Omentectomy
7. Lymph node sampling
8. Random peritoneal biopsies, including diaphragm

The importance of a careful staging operation lies in the fact that a significant proportion of patients with ovarian cancers that appear grossly to be confined to a single ovary actually have microscopic spread detected by surgical staging. Table 39-3 shows the incidence of subclinical metastases in a relatively large group of women undergoing surgical staging for what appeared to be stage I ovarian cancer. Identification of these women with microscopic metastases will define more accurately their prognosis and allow them to receive potentially curative chemotherapy.

Unfortunately, incomplete surgical staging of ovarian cancer continues to be a major problem in the United States. A 1997 report by Munoz et al.,[91] using data from the National Cancer Institute's Surveillance, Epidemiology, and

Table 39-3 Subclinical Metastases in Apparent Early Ovarian Cancer

Site	Patients	Involvement (%)
Peritoneal washings	79	33
Aortic nodes	58	10
Diaphragm	44	11
Omentum	27	3

From Piver MS, Barlow JJ, Lele SB: *Obstet Gynecol* 52:100, 1978.

End Results (SEER) program, found that only 10% of women with presumptive stage I and II ovarian cancer received the recommended staging and treatment. Furthermore, it has been shown by McGowan et al.[84] that complete surgical staging is much more likely to be performed appropriately by fellowship trained gynecologic oncologists when compared with general obstetrician-gynecologists and general surgeons. A review of 291 procedures performed at several community and university-based hospitals showed differences in the likelihood of complete surgical staging being performed by specialists. Accurate staging was performed 97% of the time by gynecologic oncologists in patients for whom they were the primary surgeon. In only 52% of procedures performed by general obstetrician-gynecologists and in only 35% of those performed by general surgeons was the cancer adequately staged. In 1993, The Commission on Cancer of the American College of Surgeons reported that in only 21% of patients with newly diagnosed ovarian cancer was a gynecologic oncologist the primary surgeon.[97] Most staging procedures were performed by general obstetrician-gynecologists (45%) or general surgeons (21%). From this same data set, it was shown that gynecologic oncologists performed more hysterectomies, oophorectomies, omentectomies, and lymph node and peritoneal biopsies than did other specialists.

PRIMARY SURGICAL MANAGEMENT OF ADVANCED OVARIAN CANCER

Unfortunately, the typical ovarian cancer patient has advanced, rather than early, disease at presentation. Such patients may have obvious ascites and large pelvic and upper abdominal masses indicative of widespread malignancy. In such patients, the goal of the surgery is primarily one of "debulking," or cytoreductive surgery. Unlike the experience with many other human solid tumors for which aggressive surgery is indicated only if all tumor can be resected, for ovarian cancer, there is substantial theoretical and clinical evidence that debulking short of complete tumor removal is of benefit to the patient. Removal of bulky tumor masses with a resultant decrease in the formation of ascites may contribute to the patient's comfort and improve her ability to maintain adequate nutrition. In addition, removal of large, poorly vascularized tumor masses with relatively low growth fractions may directly improve the response of remaining areas of tumor to chemotherapy by allowing more tumor cells to enter the active phase of the cell cycle, in which sensitivity to cytotoxic chemotherapy is greatest.[140] Because a given dose of chemotherapy will kill a constant fraction of the cancer cells present, regardless of the initial cell population,[141] cytoreduction should decrease the number of cycles of chemotherapy necessary, thus decreasing host toxicity and the development of spontaneous chemotherapy-resistant tumor cell populations.[44] Although mechanisms of acquired chemoresistance in ovarian cancer patients have not been clearly determined,[131] it is reasonable to assume that this might also be decreased by cytoreduction, which allows a decreased duration of exposure to chemotherapy.

Clinical studies supporting the concept of debulking in advanced ovarian cancer go back more than two decades.[37,90] Griffiths, in 1975,[45] was able to quantify residual disease accurately after surgery in ovarian cancer patients and showed a tripling of median survival time to 39 months in patients with no residual tumor who received melphalan. More recently, reports of prospective clinical trials involving both non–platinum-based and platinum-based combination chemotherapy regimens in ovarian cancer have supported the concept of primary cytoreductive surgery.[99,156] In general, studies examining the effect of cytoreductive surgery have reported an increase in the likelihood of a surgically documented complete response to chemotherapy (negative second-look),[125] an increase in median survival,[52] and a decrease in the risk of recurrence after a negative second-look[132] for patients undergoing optimal primary cytoreduction. The definition of "optimal" primary cytoreduction has varied among reports and is generally defined as removal of all tumor masses greater than a certain maximum diameter in size, often 2 cm. This implies a "threshold" effect, in which cytoreduction of large tumor masses does not improve outcome unless they are reduced below a certain critical size. Therefore most gynecologic oncologists believe that, unless optimal cytoreduction can be accomplished, aggressive surgery is unwarranted. For example, it would be inappropriate to perform a major colon resection to debulk a pelvic tumor mass if there was a large volume of unresectable disease in the upper abdomen. However, in a reanalysis of Gynecologic Oncology Group (GOG) Protocol 97, Hoskins et al.[54] examined the potential prognostic value of the maximal diameter of disease after primary cytoreductive surgery in a group of patients with suboptimally cytoreduced (residual diameter greater than 1 cm) stage III epithelial ovarian cancer. This protocol also included adjuvant treatment with platinum-based chemotherapy. In this group of patients, no relationship between survival and the size of the tumor at the time of initial exploration was appreciated. This analysis demonstrated a difference in survival based on the diameter of the largest residual tumor mass before the initiation of chemotherapy. Patients with suboptimal disease who were able to have their tumor cytoreduced to less than 2 cm had a significantly improved survival compared with those patients left with greater than 2 cm residual disease. This analysis further supports the

benefits of primary cytoreduction even when "optimal" residual disease cannot be achieved.

The preoperative evaluation of the patient with suspected advanced ovarian cancer must be tailored to the clinical situation. Imaging studies such as CT, sonography, or MRI may be performed to confirm the presence of a mass and to look for ascites and evidence of metastatic disease. However, more than one of these studies is usually redundant. A barium enema should be considered to ascertain the extent of colonic involvement and to rule out a colonic primary tumor with metastases to the ovary. The preoperative discussion with the patient and her family should include a thorough review of the differential diagnosis, the risk of malignancy, and the surgical options that might be used depending on the operative findings, including intestinal resection and possible colostomy. We generally use a 2-day outpatient regimen of cathartics and enemas to cleanse the large intestine in case intestinal surgery is needed. In addition, postoperative recovery of bowel function may be improved if the colon is evacuated preoperatively. We also routinely use perioperative intravenous antibiotics and prophylaxis for deep venous thrombosis (either sequential compression stockings or low-dose subcutaneous heparin). During the bowel preparation, patients are encouraged to drink copious quantities of clear liquids in order to compensate for the dehydration associated with cathartics and ascites formation.

In the operating room, cystoscopy and proctoscopy may be performed under anesthesia to evaluate the bladder and lower colon. The abdomen should be entered through a vertical incision extending from the pubic symphysis into the upper abdomen. When the abdomen is entered, ascites, if present, should be collected for cytologic evaluation. If none is present, saline washings can be taken, although in the presence of obvious intraperitoneal metastases, this may contribute little useful information.[126] A general exploration of the entire peritoneal cavity should be performed to assess the extent and resectability of both the pelvic and upper abdominal disease and to identify any other pathologic conditions present. The aortic and pelvic lymph nodes should be palpated because these are often involved in advanced ovarian cancer.[154] Often, patients with advanced ovarian cancer have extensive pelvic and upper abdominal disease and widespread abdominal carcinomatosis. Such situations can test the judgment of even the most experienced gynecologic cancer surgeon, who will have to determine the feasibility of optimal cytoreduction and weigh the benefits of such a procedure against the operative risks.

The surgical approach to the debulking of an extensive pelvic tumor is a retroperitoneal one. Even when the intraperitoneal pelvic anatomy is obliterated by massive tumor involvement, the retroperitoneal tissue planes are generally preserved and can be developed with relative ease. The infundibulopelvic ligament should be identified at the pelvic brim, and the parietal peritoneum lateral to it should be incised (Fig 39-4). Retracting the infundibulopelvic ligament medially, the retroperitoneal space can be developed medi-

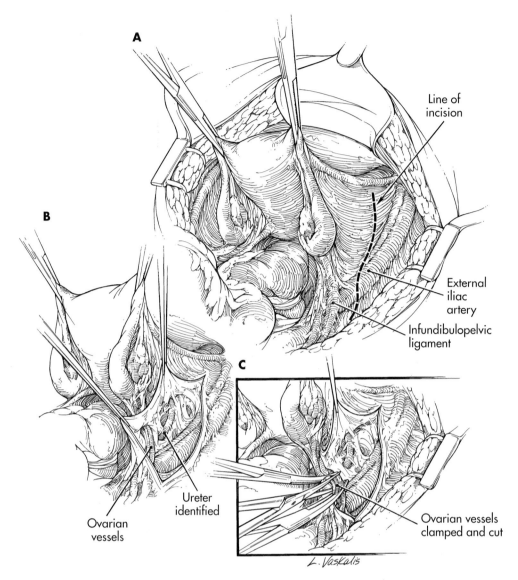

L. Vaskalis

Fig. 39-4 The retroperitoneal approach to the pelvis. The peritoneum in incised lateral to the infundibulopelvic ligament (**A**). Blunt development of the retroperitoneal space allows visualization of the ureter (**B**) before ligation of the ovarian vessels at the pelvic sidewall (**C**).

ally to identify the ureter and isolate the ovarian supply, which is then ligated and transacted. By controlling the ovarian blood supply before any manipulation of the tumor, blood loss can be reduced. With the ureter under direct vision, a combination of blunt and sharp dissection can be used to free the tumor from the pelvic sidewall and cul-de-sac, stripping the peritoneum from these areas if necessary. The uterus should be removed in most patients. Tumor nodules lateral or posterior to the uterus can often be removed in continuity with the uterine specimen by performing the type of dissection used in a modified radical hysterectomy, unroofing the ureter as it passes through the base of the broad ligament, and ligating the uterine vessels at this point. If removing the uterus will not contribute significantly to debulking of the pelvic tumor or if hysterectomy cannot be accomplished easily because of tumor encasement, the clinician may decide to leave the uterus in place or perform a supracervical hysterectomy. In extreme cases in which a bulky ovarian cancer involves the rectosigmoid colon, this can be resected together with the uterus by performing a procedure similar to posterior exenteration. The introduction of intestinal stapling devices has extended the ability to restore intestinal continuity in these patients by performing low colonic anastomoses. If this cannot be accomplished, colostomy is necessary. If a low colonic anastomosis is considered to be a possibility based on the preoperative findings, the patient's position on the operating table should allow direct access to the perineum to allow use of the stapling device through the anus. This can be accomplished by supporting the patient's legs in stirrups in a modified lithotomy position.

In the upper abdomen, omentectomy can be performed by dividing the omentum from its attachments to the transverse colon (see Fig. 39-2). If the gastrocolic omentum is involved, the dissection can be continued upward to the greater curvature of the stomach (see Fig. 39-2). In most patients the omental tumor can be removed completely from the colon without intestinal resection. If it cannot, resection of the transverse colon should be performed if it contributes to an optimal debulking procedure. Occasionally, extensive omental tumor may extend upward along the left side of the omentum to involve the spleen, necessitating splenectomy.[89] Primary reanastomosis of the transverse colon can usually be accomplished after mobilization of the splenic or hepatic flexures. Bulky tumor involvement may require resection of other areas of the intestine, most commonly the terminal ileum, cecum, and ascending colon. Such aggressive cytoreductive procedures are justified only if they result in optimal tumor reduction or if there is evidence of obstruction.

The role of lymph node resection in advanced ovarian cancer remains unclear. Most patients with advanced ovarian cancer have involvement of retroperitoneal lymph nodes.[20,153] In a retrospective series, Burghardt et al.[19] reported improved survival in patients with advanced ovarian cancer undergoing lymphadenectomy compared with historical control subjects. This same group also reported that the incidence of lymph node metastases after chemotherapy was approximately the same as that seen in patients with newly diagnosed ovarian cancer, implying that chemotherapy may not be effective against retroperitoneal disease. Although these data are interesting, they await confirmation. Lymphadenectomy is not considered a standard part of the surgical management of advanced ovarian cancer.

Patients with ovarian cancer often have clinical features that increase the risk of incisional complications, including advanced age, obesity, medical conditions, vomiting as a result of postoperative chemotherapy, and perhaps most important, an advanced intraabdominal malignancy. In the past, surgeons often used retention suture closures in such patients. Closure techniques similar to that commonly known as the Smead-Jones closure, first described in 1941,[56] have been used with great success to avoid fascial dehiscence. These techniques, essentially internal retention sutures, incorporate large bites of fascia, rectus muscle, and peritoneum in a bulk closure that is extremely resistant to disruption. Several authors have reported good results using a bulk closure with a continuous monofilament nonabsorbable polypropylene or delayed absorbable suture.[4,41,58]

SECOND-LOOK LAPAROTOMY

With regard to ovarian cancer, the term *second-look laparotomy* has been used with a variety of meanings. It has been used to describe all secondary operations, including those performed for resection of known residual, progressive, or recurrent cancer; operations done for relief of symptoms such as intestinal obstruction; and operations performed to evaluate the response of tumor to treatment. In current use, the term most commonly designates an exploratory operation performed in a patient who has completed a planned program of chemotherapy and has no clinical evidence of cancer. The primary goal of such an operation is to determine whether ovarian cancer is still present. A secondary goal may be to resect residual disease, if detected.

Second-look laparotomy has become a common part of the management of ovarian cancer for a number of reasons. Because ovarian cancer is a disease that generally remains confined to the peritoneal cavity and retroperitoneal lymph nodes for most or all of its natural history, it lends itself to reassessment by laparotomy. With the use of aggressive primary cytoreductive surgery and platinum-based combination chemotherapy, a large proportion of patients with ovarian cancer have no clinically detectable tumor at the completion of their chemotherapy. No noninvasive method of reassessment of these patients that approaches the accuracy of surgical reexploration is available.

Laparoscopy has been investigated as a less invasive alternative to second-look laparotomy. Berek et al.,[11] reporting on 119 laparoscopic examinations performed in patients with ovarian cancer, observed a 14% incidence of major complications requiring laparotomy, most involving intestinal perforation. Ozols et al.[100] have reported a false-negative rate of more than 50% in ovarian cancer patients undergoing reassessment laparoscopy. Although recent reports have been more favorable,[1] in view of the high false-negative rate, the significant risk of complications, and the inability to resect residual disease by laparoscopy, this technique has not gained much acceptance in the reassessment of patients with ovarian cancer.

A number of authors have reported their results using imaging techniques such as CT, sonography, and MRI for detection of residual ovarian cancer after chemotherapy. Although these techniques may be useful in detecting large tumor masses, they are poor at detecting intraperitoneal tumor masses in the clinically important size range of less than 2 cm.[57,70,92] In one series, CT failed to detect large omental tumor cakes and abdominal and pelvic masses up to 3 cm in size.[18] Such techniques in no way approach the accuracy of surgical exploration in detecting residual disease.

Cytologic analysis of peritoneal fluid obtained by culdocentesis has been suggested as a means of detecting persistent cancer after treatment.[82] However, it has been demonstrated that most women with biopsy-proven residual ovarian cancer in the peritoneal cavity have cytologically negative peritoneal washings. Rubin et al.[126] reported on 96 women undergoing reexploration for ovarian cancer at Memorial Sloan-Kettering who had washings taken with the abdomen open at the time of laparotomy. Only 34% of patients with biopsy-proven gross intraperitoneal disease had positive washings.

The serial measurement of serum levels of CA 125 has been a significant advance in the management of ovarian cancer.[10] Such measurements correlate well with tumor response or nonresponse during chemotherapy. However, serum levels are often normal in patients with small amounts of tumor, and multiple studies have confirmed that many patients with normal CA 125 levels have tumor found on exploration. Rubin et al.[130] reported on CA 125 levels and surgical findings in 96 patients undergoing secondary operations for ovarian cancer. More than half the patients who had normal CA 125 levels had cancer documented at surgery. Similar findings have been reported by other authors.[14,85,98] Although an elevated CA 125 level appears to be a reliable predictor of persistent tumor, it has been our practice to perform second-look laparotomy on patients with elevated values to document the extent and location of tumor and attempt secondary cytoreduction[53] before the initiation of second-line chemotherapy protocols. To a large extent, the benefits of second-look laparotomy are related to the efficacy of second-line therapy for ovarian cancer. Given the encouraging results reported with second-line intraperitoneal chemotherapy in patients with small-volume disease,[77,119] second-look laparotomy is likely to continue to play an important role in the management of ovarian cancer.

The surgical procedure is similar to that performed for the initial staging of apparently early-stage ovarian cancer. The details of the patient's initial operation for ovarian cancer should be reviewed by the surgeon performing the second-look procedure, particularly with regard to the location and extent of areas of tumor left at the end of the initial surgery. The abdomen should be entered through a vertical incision adequate to allow full evaluation of the upper abdomen. If obvious tumor is identified, frozen section confirmation should be obtained, and involved areas should be resected if optimal cytoreduction appears possible. When no tumor is evident after initial exploration, the operation may actually become more difficult because the surgeon must undertake a careful and thorough evaluation of the entire peritoneal cavity and selected retroperitoneal structures to detect areas of occult tumor. Washings for cytologic analysis should be obtained from multiple sites within the peritoneal cavity. Although these are not particularly sensitive in detecting residual disease, they may occasionally be the only positive finding. The upper abdomen should be carefully explored, including the undersurfaces of both hemidiaphragms. Some surgeons use a sterile proctoscope or laparoscope to aid in visualization of the diaphragm. Suspicious areas should be biopsied. If no suspicious areas are seen, random biopsies or scrapings for cytologic examination should be obtained. Any remaining omentum should be removed. The intestines should be carefully examined. All adhesions should be lysed, and portions should be submitted for pathologic analysis. Biopsy samples are taken from both paracolic gutters. In the pelvis, biopsy samples should be taken from the peritoneal surfaces of the bladder, rectum, and pouch of Douglas. The surgical pedicles from the initial operation, particularly the stumps of the infundibulopelvic ligaments, should be identified and a biopsy performed. Any remaining internal reproductive organs are generally removed. A thorough sampling of the paraaortic and pelvic lymph nodes should be performed. If no tumor is identified, a carefully performed second-look operation may take several hours and produce in excess of 20 individual histologic specimens.

Table 39-4 Clinical Correlates of Second-Look Laparotomy

Feature	Percent Negative
Stage	
I	82
II	71
III	34
IV	33
Residual tumor after primary cytoreduction	
None	76
Optimal	46
Suboptimal	23
Histologic grade	
1	56
2	60
3	41

Many reports on second-look laparotomy have appeared in the literature. We have compiled data from 27 reports comprising more than 2000 patients.* Overall, about 55% of patients undergoing second-look laparotomy had cancer detected. The likelihood of finding residual cancer at second-look laparotomy can be related to several clinical and histologic factors, including stage, the amount of residual tumor left after the initial ovarian cancer operation, and perhaps the histologic grade of the tumor. Table 39-4 shows information compiled from the above cited references that relates these features to the probability of having no tumor found at the time of second-look laparotomy. Among the strongest predictors of findings at second-look laparotomy is the amount of tumor remaining after the initial operation for ovarian cancer, once again suggesting a benefit for aggressive primary cytoreduction.

The amount of tumor detected at second-look laparotomy has a clear effect on prognosis. In some reports, most patients with gross tumor detected died within 3 years.[113,136] More recent reports of salvage regimens for such patients portray a somewhat brighter picture, particularly in patients who are able to undergo optimal secondary cytoreduction, discussed as follows. Patients who have no visible disease found at second-look laparotomy but who have histologic or cytologic evidence of microscopic disease have a better outlook. Copeland et al.[28] reported a survival of 96% and 71% at 2 and 5 years, respectively, in a group of 50 patients with only microscopic disease found at second-look laparotomy. Treatment of such patients with intraperitoneal chemotherapy regimens may improve survival.

Patients with no tumor detected at the time of second-look laparotomy have generally been thought to have a good prognosis, with recurrence rates reported in the range of 20% to 30%. A review by Rubin and Lewis[125] of second-look laparotomy identified 12 studies published be-

---

*References 7, 9, 13, 21-23, 27, 32, 33, 36, 42, 43, 49, 65, 69, 81, 87, 88, 107, 112, 114, 121, 122, 142, 144, 148, 149.

tween 1980 and 1986 that provided information about recurrences after a negative exploration. In these combined series, the overall recurrence rate was 18%, with 26% of patients with stage III or IV disease having recurrence. All of these reports included patients treated with non–platinum-containing chemotherapy. Subsequent studies by Rubin et al.[127,132] have demonstrated that the risk of recurrence in patients achieving a negative second-look laparotomy after platinum-based chemotherapy approximates 50%, with essentially all recurrences taking place within the first 5 years after second-look laparotomy.[134] Multivariate analysis showed that stage, histologic grade, and the amount of tumor remaining after primary cytoreduction were significant predictors of recurrence after negative second-look laparotomy. In a phase II trial of three courses of intraperitoneal cisplatin and etoposide as consolidation therapy after pathologically negative second-look surgical reassessment for stage IIC-IV epithelial ovarian cancer, Barakat et al.[8] noted a significant increase in disease-free survival (DFS) compared with nonprotocol patients treated concurrently who underwent observation alone. With a median follow-up of 36 months, 14 of 36 (39%) in the protocol group had recurrences, compared with 25 of 46 (54%) of those undergoing observation alone. Median DFS for the patients observed is 28.5 months and had not been reached in the consolidation group at the time of the report.

SECONDARY CYTOREDUCTION

Although the benefits of primary cytoreduction in ovarian cancer are well established, the role of debulking surgery later in the course of the disease is considerably less clear. Because more than half of patients undergoing second-look laparotomy have tumor detected and most have gross disease, many patients are potential candidates for secondary cytoreductive operations. Patients who experience tumor recurrence after a negative second-look operation and patients who undergo reexploration after several cycles of chemotherapy to resect previously unresectable tumor (interval debulking) are examples of other situations in which secondary cytoreduction may be applied. The surgical principles and technical considerations are essentially the same as in primary debulking, except that the operation is likely to be more difficult because of prior surgery and the effects of treatment, particularly intraperitoneal therapy, on the condition of the abdominal contents. The reported rates of successful secondary cytoreduction vary from about 25% to 84%,* depending on the patient population, the surgeon's skill and aggressiveness, and the definition of "success" used. Whether secondary cytoreduction conveys a survival benefit is controversial. In a relatively small series reported by Chambers et al.[23] and Luesley et al.,[68] no survival benefit was associated with secondary cytoreduction. In a report from the Mayo Clinic, Podratz et al.[114] described 116 patients with positive second-look laparotomy and found

4-year survival to be substantially greater in those with microscopic residual tumor compared with those with larger tumors. Hoskins et al.[53] found that patients whose tumors were reduced to microscopic residual tumors at the time of a positive second-look procedure had a 5-year survival of 51%, compared with less than 10% of patients left with gross disease. Other authors have also reported an improved survival after optimal cytoreduction at the time of second-look laparotomy.[65] It seems likely that the value of secondary cytoreduction depends strongly on what therapy is used after surgery. Promising second-line therapies based on increasing the exposure of tumor cells to cytoxic agents, such as intraperitoneal therapy or intensive intravenous therapy with autologous bone marrow support or colony-stimulating factors, will probably be most effective in patients with small-volume residual disease.[79,80]

An interval debulking procedure is becoming more popular in the management of advanced-stage ovarian cancer. Interval debulking applies when at the conclusion of primary cytoreductive surgery, bulky intraperitoneal tumor deposits remain, and a short program of chemotherapy is given before a planned second attempt at surgical cytoreduction. It has been shown both retrospectively[61] and in a prospective study by Ng et al.[96] that a high proportion of such patients can have optimal cytoreduction at the secondary procedure. Whether this will result in an improved outcome remains to be demonstrated and probably depends in part on the type of therapy used after the second operation. In one report, patients who underwent interval cytoreduction and then continued intravenous chemotherapy had no survival advantage over those who did not have interval cytoreduction.[94] On the other hand, Hakes et al.,[47] reporting on a subset of patients described by Ng et al.,[96] found that 47% of patients who underwent optimal interval cytoreduction followed by four courses of intraperitoneal platinum had a subsequent negative reexploration, a rate of complete pathologic response almost twice that usually reported for advanced ovarian cancer.

There is increasing evidence that interval cytoreductive surgery may provide a survival advantage for patients with advanced epithelial ovarian cancer. Several reports have demonstrated the feasibility for achieving optimal cytoreduction during an interval debulking procedure.[61,62,96,151] However, the most compelling evidence that interval debulking procedures are beneficial comes from the Gynecological Cancer Cooperative Group of the European Organization for Research and Treatment of Cancer (EORTC), which reported the results of a large, prospective, randomized trial of interval debulking surgery in patients with stages IIb through IV epithelial ovarian cancer.[147] In the EORTC trial, patients with ovarian cancer who underwent primary cytoreductive surgery with suboptimal residual were evaluated after three cycles of cisplatin (75 mg/m^2) and cyclophosphamide (750 mg/m^2) chemotherapy given every 3 weeks. Patients with a complete response, partial response or stable disease were assigned randomly ($N = 319$) to either undergo an exploratory laparotomy for

---

*References 12, 46, 68, 74, 118, 145.

interval debulking surgery ($N = 140$) or not undergo surgery ($N = 138$) before receiving three additional cycles of cisplatin and cyclophosphamide.

A survival advantage for patients who underwent the interval debulking surgery was observed in this trial. The results were stratified on the basis of the residual disease at interval cytoreductive surgery. Patients who were found to have small-volume (less than 1 cm) disease upon secondary laparotomy (median survival 41.6 months) and those who were found to have large-volume disease but were able to achieve optimal status (less than 1 cm) (median survival 26.6 months) as a result of the interval cytoreductive surgery. This group survived significantly longer than patients with bulky disease (median survival 19.4 months) or those in the no interval surgery arm (median survival 20.0 months).

Presently, it is difficult to recommend interval debulking surgery as a routine clinical practice for a variety of reasons. Interpretation of the data from the EORTC study is limited in that no patients were treated with paclitaxel. Because paclitaxel is now considered a component of standard induction chemotherapy for epithelial ovarian cancer, its influence on the efficacy of interval cytoreductive procedures is unknown. In addition, first-line treatment plans that incorporate an interval debulking procedure would mandate at least two major operations in the primary treatment of advanced ovarian cancer, unless a neoadjuvant chemotherapy approach, which is currently unproven, is taken. Therefore, although the results of the EORTC study are encouraging, interval debulking is not a component of standard care. Last, how a second-look operation would fit into an interval debulking approach is unknown. A second-look operation at the completion of an interval debulking regimen would require a third laparotomy.

To address the role of paclitaxel as a component of front-line therapy that includes interval cytoreductive surgery, the GOG developed Protocol 152. This phase III randomized study, which compares six cycles of cisplatin and paclitaxel versus three cycles of cisplatin followed by secondary cytoreductive surgery and three additional cycles of chemotherapy, has recently completed accrual. However, it will take several years to gather adequate follow-up data on this group of patients to draw meaningful conclusions regarding the impact of interval cytoreductive surgery.

PALLIATIVE OPERATIONS

Despite the advances in our understanding of ovarian cancer that have accrued in the last decade, early diagnosis is still unusual, and most women with disease diagnosed in the advanced stages die of the disease within 2 to 4 years. Because of the tendency of the disease to remain confined largely to the peritoneal cavity, many of these women eventually develop intestinal obstruction. In general, these patients are fully alert, are in little or no pain, and might otherwise enjoy a reasonable quality of life, albeit for a limited time, were it not for the intestinal obstruction that necessitates gastric drainage and intravenous hydration. Although percutaneous

endoscopic gastrostomy[50,76] and home intravenous therapy have been helpful in the management of intestinal obstruction, the question often arises about whether an attempt to surgically relieve the obstruction would be appropriate. The physician making such a decision must weigh a number of factors, including the patient's overall medical condition, the extent of her cancer, prior therapeutic interventions, and the likelihood of a response to further cancer treatment. In addressing this issue, several authors have attempted to define factors that would predict a favorable outcome after exploration for intestinal obstruction in patients with advanced ovarian cancer. According to Krebs and Goplerud,[58] advanced age, poor nutritional status, palpable tumor masses, ascites, and prior irradiation are factors associated with a poor outcome. Clarke-Pearson et al.[26] reported that nutritional status and the amount of cancer remaining at the completion of the operation for intestinal obstruction were related to the duration of postoperative survival. On the other hand, Rubin et al.[129] found no clinical features that were predictive of operability or duration of survival after surgery. We do not believe it is possible to define firm criteria for deciding on surgery. Such decisions must be made on an individual basis after a frank discussion with the patient and her family.

If the patient is deemed to be a candidate for operation, consideration should be given to the use of preoperative total parenteral nutrition because these patients are often in poor condition nutritionally and therefore at increased risk for perioperative complications. A barium enema should be performed to determine whether the obstruction involves the colon. In a report of 54 operations performed for intestinal obstruction on ovarian cancer patients, Rubin et al.[129] found that the site of obstruction was in the small intestine alone in 44%, the large intestine alone in 33%, and involved both small and large intestine in 22%. At the time of surgery, a definitive procedure for relief of obstruction was performed in 79% of the patients in this series. The obstruction was not correctable in the remaining patients at the time of exploration. Of the patients undergoing a definitive procedure, about 80% were discharged from the hospital eating a regular or low-residue diet. Their mean postoperative survival was 6.8 months. Other authors have reported similar findings.[58,109,146] Although survival is short, surgery may allow patients with intestinal obstruction to regain intestinal function and significantly improve the quality of their remaining months of life.

SURGICAL CONSIDERATIONS OF INTRAPERITONEAL THERAPY

Intraperitoneal therapy is one of a number of methods used to intensify the exposure of ovarian cancer cells to cytotoxic agents. The pharmacologic basis for intraperitoneal therapy has been well described by Dedrick et al. from the National Cancer Institute.[35] Multiple studies have documented the efficacy of this approach in selected patients with ovarian cancer,[67,78] and some have documented responses in tumors that had been resistant to intravenous chemotherapy.[119]

The delivery of drugs into the peritoneal cavity has been accomplished using a variety of catheter systems.* Catheters that exit the skin (transcutaneous) require more maintenance and appear to have a substantially higher rate of infection than systems using a totally implanted port and catheter. The implanted systems consist of a stainless steel or titanium port with a Silastic septum. The port is attached with a locking collar to a Silastic tube with multiple side holes that is tunneled subcutaneously along the abdominal wall before entering the peritoneal cavity in the midabdomen. The technique of placement of the port and catheter has been well described by Pfeifle et al.[106] The port should be placed in a subcutaneous pocket and anchored to the fascia with permanent suture. Implantation of the port over the lower rib cage provides it with a firm support, which facilitates percutaneous puncture of the Silastic septum. These systems require no maintenance between uses.

The largest experience with totally implanted subcutaneous port and catheter systems has been reported by Rubin et al.[128] and Davidson et al.[34] In the latter report, the authors described their experience with 227 patients receiving catheters for the first time for treatment in a variety of prospective intraperitoneal chemotherapy trials, most lasting from 5 to 6 months. These patients received a total of 1331 courses of chemotherapy during the study period. There were a total of 40 (17.6%) catheter-related complications noted, including an 8.8% rate of catheter blockage, generally caused by the formation of a fibrous sheath around the intraperitoneal portion of the catheter. An additional 8.8% of patients experienced catheter-associated infections. Included among these were eight patients with late erosion of the catheter into the intestinal lumen. The occurrence of profuse diarrhea shortly after chemotherapy infusion should alert the clinician to this possibility. Although the authors could not demonstrate a statistically significant increase in the rate of infection, they recommend against inserting catheters at the time of surgery on the large intestine.

The major technical problem associated with intraperitoneal chemotherapy is the formation of adhesions that limit the free distribution of the infusate within the peritoneal cavity, thus abrogating much of the advantage of direct drug delivery. These adhesions form as a result of the multiple insults suffered by the peritoneal contents: surgery, cancer, and the intraperitoneal treatment itself. There is no effective means of preventing the formation of adhesions or of eliminating them once formed. If blockage of the catheter occurs, radiographic contrast studies should be used to determine whether the blockage is caused by formation of a fibrous sheath around the catheter itself or by development of extensive adhesions within the peritoneal cavity. Repeat laparotomy for removal of a fibrous sheath may allow continued intraperitoneal chemotherapy. If the cause of catheter blockage is extensive intraperitoneal adhesions, repeat laparotomy with extensive lysis of adhesions usually does not result in long-term reestablishment of catheter patency.

*References 17, 55, 93, 105, 106, 108, 135.

REFERENCES

1. Abu-Rustum NR, Barakat RR, Siegel PL, et al: Second-look operation for epithelial ovarian cancer: laparoscopy or laparotomy? *Obstet Gynecol* 88:549, 1996.
2. Aida H, Takakuwa K, Nagata H, et al: Clinical features of ovarian cancer in Japanese women with germ-line mutations of BRCA1, *Clin Cancer Res* 4:235, 1998.
3. Amara DP, Nezhat C, et al: Operative laparoscopy in the management of ovarian cancer, *Surg Laparosc Endosc* 6:38, 1996.
4. Anonymous: The reduction in risk of ovarian cancer associated with oral-contraceptive use: The Cancer and Steroid Hormone Study of the Centers for Disease Control and the National Institute of Child Health and Human Development, *N Engl J Med* 316:650, 1987.
5. Archie J, Feldtman R: Primary abdominal wound closure with permanent, continuous running monofilament sutures, *Surg Gynecol Obstet* 153:721, 1981.
6. Bailey CL, Ueland FR, Land GL, et al: The malignant potential of small cystic ovarian tumors in women over 50 years of age, *Gynecol Oncol* 69:3, 1998 (comments).
7. Ballon SC, Portnuff JC, Sikic BI, et al: Second-look laparotomy in epithelial ovarian carcinoma: precise definition, sensitivity, and specificity of the operative procedure, *Gynecol Oncol* 17:154, 1984.
8. Barakat RR, Almadrones L, Venkatraman ES, et al: A phase II trial of intraperitoneal cisplatin and etoposide as consolidation therapy in patients with stage II-IV epithelial ovarian cancer following negative surgical assessment, *Gynecol Oncol* 69:17, 1998.
9. Barnhill DR, Hoskins WJ, Heller PB, et al: The second-look surgical reassessment for epithelial ovarian carcinoma, *Gynecol Oncol* 19:148, 1984.
10. Bast RC Jr, Klug TL, St John E, et al: A radioimmunoassay using a monoclonal antibody to monitor the course of epithelial ovarian cancer, *N Engl J Med* 309:883, 1983.
11. Berek JS, Griffiths CT, Leventhal JM: Laparoscopy for second-look evaluation in ovarian cancer, *Obstet Gynecol* 58:192, 1981.
12. Berek JS, Hacker NF, Lagasse LD, et al: Survival of patients following secondary cytoreductive surgery in ovarian cancer, *Obstet Gynecol* 61:189, 1983.
13. Berek JS, Hacker NF, Lagasse LD, et al: Second-look laparotomy in stage III epithelial ovarian cancer: clinical variables associated with disease status, *Obstet Gynecol* 64:207, 1984.
14. Berek JS, Knapp RC, Malkasian GD, et al: CA 125 serum levels correlated with second-look operations among ovarian cancer patients, *Obstet Gynecol* 67:685, 1986.
15. Biesecker, BB., Boehnke M, Calzone K, et al: Genetic counseling for families with inherited susceptibility to breast and ovarian cancer, *JAMA* 269:1970, 1993. (Published erratum appears in *JAMA* 270:832, 1993.).
16. Bourne T, Campbell S, Steer C, et al: Transvaginal colour flow imaging: a possible new screening technique for ovarian cancer, *Br Med J* 299:1367, 1989 (comments).
17. Braly P, Doroshow J, Hoff S: Technical aspects of intraperitoneal chemotherapy in abdominal carcinomatosis, *Gynecol Oncol* 25:319, 1986.
18. Brenner DE, Shaff MI, Jones HW, et al: Abdominopelvic computed tomography: evaluation in patients undergoing second-look laparotomy for ovarian carcinoma, *Obstet Gynecol* 65:715, 1985.
19. Burghardt E, Lahousen M, Stettner H: The significance of pelvic and para-aortic lymphadenectomy in the operative treatment of ovarian cancer, *Baillieres Clin Obstet Gynaecol* 3:157, 1989.
20. Burghardt E, Pickel H, Lahousen M, et al: Pelvic lymphadenectomy in operative treatment of ovarian cancer, *Am J Obstet Gynecol* 155:315, 1986.
21. Cain JM, Saigo PE, Pierce VK, et al: A review of second-look laparotomy for ovarian cancer, *Gynecol Oncol* 23:14, 1986.
22. Carmichael JA, Shelley WE, Brown LB, et al: A predictive index of cure versus no cure in advanced ovarian carcinoma patients—replacement of second-look laparotomy as a diagnostic test, *Gynecol Oncol* 27:269, 1987.

23. Chambers SK, Chambers JT, Kohorn EI, et al: Evaluation of the role of second-look surgery in ovarian cancer, *Obstet Gynecol* 72:404, 1988.

24. Chi DS, Curtin JP, Barakat RR: Laparoscopic management of adnexal masses in women with a history of nongynecologic malignancy, *Obstet Gynecol* 86:964, 1995.

25. Childers JM, Surwit EA: Current status of operative laparoscopy in gynecologic oncology, *Oncology (Huntingt)* 7(11):47-51, 1993 (discussion 7[11]:53-54, 57).

26. Clarke-Pearson DL, DeLong ER, et al: Intestinal obstruction in patients with ovarian cancer: variables associated with surgical complications and survival, *Arch Surg* 123:42, 1988.

27. Cohen CJ, Bruckner HW, Goldberg JD, et al: Improved therapy with cisplatin regimens for patients with ovarian carcinoma (FIGO III and IV) as measured by surgical end-staging (second-look surgery)—the Mount Sinai experience, *Clin Obstet Gynaecol* 10:307, 1983.

28. Copeland LJ, Gershenson DM, Wharton JT, et al: Microscopic disease at second-look laparotomy in advanced ovarian cancer, *Cancer* 55:472, 1985.

29. Cramer DW, Welch WR, Scully RE, et al: Ovarian cancer and talc: a case-control study, *Cancer* 50:372, 1982.

30. Cramer DW, Welch WR, Cassells S, et al: Mumps, menarche, menopause, and ovarian cancer, *Am J Obstet Gynecol* 147:1, 1983.

31. Cramer DW, Welch WR, Hutchison GB, et al: Dietary animal fat in relation to ovarian cancer risk, *Obstet Gynecol* 63:833, 1984.

32. Curry SL, Zembo MM, Nahhas WA, et al: Second-look laparotomy for ovarian cancer, *Gynecol Oncol* 11:114, 1981.

33. Dauplat J, Ferriere JP, Gorbinet M, et al: Second-look laparotomy in managing epithelial ovarian carcinoma, *Cancer* 57:1627, 1986.

34. Davidson SA, Rubin SC, Markman M, et al: Intraperitoneal chemotherapy: analysis of complications with an implanted subcutaneous port and catheter system, *Gynecol Oncol* 41:101, 1991.

35. Dedrick RL, Myers CE, Bungay PM, et al: Pharmacokinetic rationale for peritoneal drug administration in the treatment of ovarian cancer, *Cancer Treat Rep* 62:1, 1978.

36. de Gramont A, Drolet Y, Varette C, et al: Survival after second-look laparotomy in advanced ovarian epithelial cancer: study of 86 patients, *Eur J Cancer Clin Oncol* 25:451, 1989.

37. Delclos L, Quinlan E: Malignant tumors of the ovary managed with post operative megavoltage irradiation, *Radiology* 93:659, 1969.

38. DePriest PD, Gallion HH, Pavlik EJ, et al: Transvaginal sonography as a screening method for the detection of early ovarian cancer, *Gynecol Oncol* 65:408, 1997.

39. FIGO Cancer Committee: Staging announcement, *Gynecol Oncol* 25:383, 1986.

40. Franceschi S, La Vecchia C, Helmrich SP, et al: Risk factors for epithelial ovarian cancer in Italy, *Am J Epidemiol* 115:714, 1982.

41. Gallup DG, Nolan TE, Smith RP: Primary mass closure of midline incisions with a continuous polyglyconate monofilament absorbable suture, *Obstet Gynecol* 76:872, 1990.

42. Gallup DG, Talledo OE, Dudzinski MR, et al: Another look at the second-assessment procedure for ovarian epithelial carcinoma, *Am J Obstet Gynecol* 157:590, 1987.

43. Gershenson DM, Copeland LJ, Wharton JT, et al: Prognosis of surgically determined complete responders in advanced ovarian cancer, *Cancer* 55:1129, 1985.

44. Goldie JH, Coldman, AJ: A mathematic model for relating the drug sensitivity of tumors to their spontaneous mutation rate, *Cancer Treat Rep* 63:1727, 1979.

45. Griffiths CT: Surgical resection of tumor bulk in the primary treatment of ovarian carcinoma, *Natl Cancer Inst Monogr* 42:101, 1975.

46. Griffiths CT, Parker LM, Fuller AF Jr: Role of cytoreductive surgical treatment in the management of advanced ovarian cancer, *Cancer Treat Rep* 63:235, 1979.

47. Hakes, EA: High intensity intravenous cyclophosphamide/cisplatin and intraperitoneal cisplatin for advanced ovarian: a preliminary report, *Proc ASCO* 8: 152, 1989.

48. Halila H, Stenman UH, Seppala M: Ovarian cancer antigen CA 125 levels in pelvic inflammatory disease and pregnancy, *Cancer* 57:1327, 1986.

49. Ho AG, Beller U, Speyer JL, et al: A reassessment of the role of second-look laparotomy in advanced ovarian cancer, *J Clin Oncol* 5:1316, 1987.

50. Hopkins MP, Roberts JA, Morley GW: Outpatient management of small bowel obstruction in terminal ovarian cancer, *J Reprod Med* 32:827, 1987.

51. Hoskins KF, Stopfer JE, Calzone KA, et al: Assessment and counseling for women with a family history of breast cancer: a guide for clinicians, *JAMA* 273:577, 1995.

52. Hoskins WJ: The influence of cytoreductive surgery on progression-free interval and survival in epithelial ovarian cancer, *Baillieres Clin Obstet Gynaecol* 3:59, 1989.

53. Hoskins WJ, Rubin SC, Dulaney E, et al: Influence of secondary cytoreduction at the time of second-look laparotomy on the survival of patients with epithelial ovarian carcinoma, *Gynecol Oncol* 34:365, 1989.

54. Hoskins WJ, McGuire WP, Brady MF, et al: The effect of diameter of largest residual disease on survival after primary cytoreductive surgery in patients with suboptimal residual epithelial ovarian carcinoma, *Am J Obstet Gynecol* 170:974, 1994 (discussion 170:979).

55. Jenkins J, Sugarbaker PH, Gianola FJ, et al: Technical considerations in the use of intraperitoneal chemotherapy administered by Tenckhoff catheter, *Surg Gynecol Obstet* 154:858, 1982.

56. Jones T, Newell E, Brubaker R: The use of alloy steel wire in the closure of abdominal wounds, *Surg Gynecol Oncol* 72:1056, 1941.

57. Khan O, Cosgrove DO, Fried AM, et al: Ovarian carcinoma follow-up: US versus laparotomy, *Radiology* 159:111, 1986.

58. Krebs HB, Goplerud DR: Surgical management of bowel obstruction in advanced ovarian carcinoma, *Obstet Gynecol* 61:327, 1983.

59. Landis SH, Murray T, Bolden S, et al: Cancer statistics, 1998, *CA Cancer J Clin* 48:6, 1998.

60. La Vecchia C, Decarli A, Franceschi S, et al: Age at first birth and the risk of epithelial ovarian cancer, *J Natl Cancer Inst* 73:663, 1984.

61. Lawton FG, Redman CW, Luesley DM, et al: Neoadjuvant (cytoreductive) chemotherapy combined with intervention debulking surgery in advanced, unresected epithelial ovarian cancer, *Obstet Gynecol* 73:61, 1989.

62. Lawton F, Luesley D, Redman C, et al: Feasibility and outcome of complete secondary tumor resection for patients with advanced ovarian cancer, *J Surg Oncol* 45:14, 1990.

63. Lee N: The reduction in risk of ovarian cancer associated with oral-contraceptive use: The Cancer and Steroid Hormone Study of the Centers for Disease Control and the National Institute of Child Health and Human Development, *N Engl J Med* 316:650, 1987.

64. Lew EA, Garfinkel L: Variations in mortality by weight among 750,000 men and women, *J Chronic Dis* 32:563, 1979.

65. Lippman SM, Alberts DS, Slymen DJ, et al: Second-look laparotomy in epithelial ovarian carcinoma: prognostic factors associated with survival duration, *Cancer* 61:2571, 1988.

66. Reference deleted in proofs.

67. Lucas WE, Markman M, Howell SB: Intraperitoneal chemotherapy for advanced ovarian cancer, Am J Obstet Gynecol 152 (4), 474-478, 1985.

68. Luesley DM, Chan KK, Fielding JW, et al: Second-look laparotomy in the management of epithelial ovarian carcinoma: an evaluation of fifty cases, *Obstet Gynecol* 64:421, 1984.

69. Lund B, Williamson P: Prognostic factors for outcome of and survival after second-look laparotomy in patients with advanced ovarian carcinoma, *Obstet Gynecol* 76:617, 1990.

70. Lund B, Jacobsen K, Rasch L: Correlation of abdominal ultrasound and computed tomography scans with second- or third-look laparotomy in patients with ovarian carcinoma, *Gynecol Oncol* 37:279, 1990.

71. Lynch HT, Bewtra C, Lynch JF: Familial ovarian carcinoma: clinical nuances, *Am J Med* 81:1073, 1986.

72. Lynch HT, Guirgis HA, Albert S, et al: Familial association of carcinoma of the breast and ovary, *Surg Gynecol Obstet* 138:717, 1974.

73. Lynch HT, Albano W, Black L, et al: Familial excess of cancer of the ovary and other anatomic sites, *JAMA* 245:261, 1981.

74. Maggino T, Tredese F, Valente S, et al: Role of second look laparotomy in multidisciplinary treatment and in the follow up of advanced ovarian cancer, *Eur J Gynaecol Oncol* 4:26, 1983.

75. Malkasian GD Jr, Podratz KC, Stanhope CR, et al: CA 125 in gynecologic practice, *Am J Obstet Gynecol* 155:515, 1986.

76. Malone JM Jr, Koonce T, Larson DM, et al: Palliation of small bowel obstruction by percutaneous gastrostomy in patients with progressive ovarian carcinoma, *Obstet Gynecol* 68:431, 1986.

77. Markman M, Reichman B, Hakes T, et al: Intraperitoneal chemotherapy as treatment for ovarian carcinoma and gastrointestinal malignancies: the Memorial Sloan-Kettering Cancer Center experience, *Acta Med Aust* 16:65, 1989.

78. Markman M, Hakes T, Reichman B, et al: Intraperitoneal therapy in the management of ovarian carcinoma, *Yale J Biol Med* 62:393, 1989.

79. Markman M, Reichman B, Hakes T, et al: Responses to second-line cisplatin-based intraperitoneal therapy in ovarian cancer: influence of a prior response to intravenous cisplatin, *J Clin Oncol* 9:1801, 1991.

80. Markman M, Rothman R, Hakes T, et al: Second-line platinum therapy in patients with ovarian cancer previously treated with cisplatin, *J Clin Oncol* 9:389, 1991.

81. McCusker MC, Hoffman JS, Curry SL, et al: The role of second-look laparotomy in treatment of epithelial ovarian cancer, *Gynecol Oncol* 28:83, 1987.

82. McGowan L, Bunnag B: The evaluation of therapy for ovarian cancer, *Gynecol Oncol* 4:375, 1976.

83. McGowan L, Parent L, Lednar W, et al: The woman at risk for developing ovarian cancer, *Gynecol Oncol* 7:325, 1979.

84. McGowan L, Lesher LP, Norris HJ, et al: Misstaging of ovarian cancer, *Obstet Gynecol* 65:568, 1985.

85. Meier W, Stieber P, Eiermann W, et al: Serum levels of CA 125 and histological findings at second-look laparotomy in ovarian carcinoma, *Gynecol Oncol* 35:446, 1989.

86. Miki Y, Swensen J, Shattuck-Eidens D, et al: A strong candidate for the breast and ovarian cancer susceptibility gene BRCA1, *Science* 266:66, 1994.

87. Miller DS, Ballon SC, Teng NN, et al: A critical reassessment of second-look laparotomy in epithelial ovarian carcinoma, *Cancer* 57:530, 1986.

88. Milsted R, Sangster G, Kaye S, et al: Treatment of advanced ovarian cancer with combination chemotherapy using cyclophosphamide, Adriamycin and cis-platinum, *Br J Obstet Gynaecol* 91:927, 1984.

89. Morris M, Gershenson DM, Burke TW, et al: Splenectomy in gynecologic oncology: indications, complications, and technique, *Gynecol Oncol* 43:118, 1991.

90. Munnell EW: The changing prognosis and treatment in cancer of the ovary: a report of 235 patients with primary ovarian carcinoma 1952-1961, *Am J Obstet Gynecol* 100:790, 1968.

91. Munoz KA, Harlan LC, Trimble EL: Patterns of care for women with ovarian cancer in the United States, *J Clin Oncol* 15:3408, 1997.

92. Murolo C, Costantini S, Foglia G, et al: Ultrasound examination in ovarian cancer patients: a comparison with second look laparotomy, *J Ultrasound Med* 8:441, 1989.

93. Myers CE, Collins JM: Pharmacology of intraperitoneal chemotherapy, *Cancer Invest* 1:395, 1983.

94. Neijt JP, ten Bokkel Huinink WW, van der Burg ME, et al: Randomized trial comparing two combination chemotherapy regimens (CHAP-5 v CP) in advanced ovarian carcinoma, *J Clin Oncol* 5:1157, 1987.

95. Nezhat CR, Amara P, Teng N, et al: Management of ovarian cancer by operative laparoscopy, *J Am Assoc Gynecol Laparosc* 2(suppl):S35, 1995.

96. Ng LW, Rubin SC, Hoskins WJ, et al: Aggressive chemosurgical debulking in patients with advanced ovarian cancer, *Gynecol Oncol* 38:358, 1990.

97. Nguyen HN, Averette HE, Hoskins W, et al: National survey of ovarian carcinoma. VI. Critical assessment of current International Federation of Gynecology and Obstetrics staging system, *Cancer* 72:3007, 1993.

98. Niloff JM, Bast RC Jr, Schaetzl EM, et al: Predictive value of CA 125 antigen levels in second-look procedures for ovarian cancer, *Am J Obstet Gynecol* 151:981, 1985.

99. Omura GA, Bundy BN, Berek JS, et al: Randomized trial of cyclophosphamide plus cisplatin with or without doxorubicin in ovarian carcinoma: a Gynecologic Oncology Group Study, *J Clin Oncol* 7:457, 1989.

100. Ozols RF, Fisher RI, Anderson T, et al: Peritoneoscopy in the management of ovarian cancer, *Am J Obstet Gynecol* 140:611, 1981.

101. Parazzini F, La Vecchia C, Negri E, et al: Oral contraceptive use and the risk of ovarian cancer: an Italian case-control study, *Eur J Cancer* 27:594, 1991.

102. Patsner B, Mann WJ: The value of preoperative serum CA 125 levels in patients with a pelvic mass, *Am J Obstet Gynecol* 159:873, 1988 (comments).

103. Pettersson F: *Annual report of the results of treatment in gynecological cancer,* Stockholm, 1988, International Federation of Gynecology and Obstetrics.

104. Pettersson F: *International Federation of Gynecology and Obstetrics Report,* Stockholm, 1991, International Federation of Gynecology and Obstetrics.

105. Pfeiffer P, Asmussen L, Kvist-Poulsen H, et al: Intraperitoneal chemotherapy: introduction of a new "single use" delivery system—a preliminary report, *Gynecol Oncol* 35:47, 1989.

106. Pfeifle CE, Howell SB, Markman M, et al: Totally implantable system for peritoneal access, *J Clin Oncol* 2:1277, 1984.

107. Phibbs GD, Smith JP, Stanhope CR: Analysis of sites of persistent cancer at "second-look" laparotomy in patients with ovarian cancer, *Am J Obstet Gynecol* 147:611, 1983.

108. Piccart MJ, Speyer JL, Markman M, et al: Intraperitoneal chemotherapy: technical experience at five institutions, *Semin Oncol* 12(suppl 4):90, 1985.

109. Piver MS, Barlow JJ, Lele SB, et al: Survival after ovarian cancer induced intestinal obstruction, *Gynecol Oncol* 13:44, 1982.

110. Piver MS, Mettlin CJ, Tsukada Y, et al: Familial Ovarian Cancer Registry, *Obstet Gynecol* 64:195, 1984.

111. Plentyl A, Friedman E: *Lymphatic system of the female genitalia,* Philadelphia, 1971, WB Saunders.

112. Podczaski ES, Stevens CW Jr, Manetta A, et al: Use of second-look laparotomy in the management of patients with ovarian epithelial malignancies, *Gynecol Oncol* 28:205, 1987.

113. Podratz KC, Malkasian GD Jr, Hilton JF, et al: Second-look laparotomy in ovarian cancer: evaluation of pathologic variables, *Am J Obstet Gynecol* 152:230, 1985.

114. Podratz KC, Schray MF, Wieand HS, et al: Evaluation of treatment and survival after positive second-look laparotomy, *Gynecol Oncol* 31:9, 1988.

115. Pomel C, Provencher D, Dauplat J, Gauthier P, et al: Laparoscopic staging of early ovarian cancer, *Gynecol Oncol* 58:301, 1995.

116. Querleu D: Laparoscopic paraaortic node sampling in gynecologic oncology: a preliminary experience, *Gynecol Oncol* 49:24, 1993.

117. Querleu D, LeBlanc E: Laparoscopic infrarenal paraaortic lymph node dissection for restaging of carcinoma of the ovary or fallopian tube, *Cancer* 73:1467, 1994.

118. Raju KS, McKinna JA, Barker GH, et al: Second-look operations in the planned management of advanced ovarian carcinoma, *Am J Obstet Gynecol* 144:50, 1982.

119. Reichman B, Markman M, Hakes T, et al: Intraperitoneal cisplatin and etoposide in the treatment of refractory/recurrent ovarian carcinoma, *J Clin Oncol* 7:1327, 1989.

120. Risch HA, Jain M, Marrett LD, et al: Dietary fat intake and risk of epithelial ovarian cancer, *J Natl Cancer Inst* 86:1409, 1994.

121. Roberts WS, Hodel K, Rich WM, et al: Second-look laparotomy in the management of gynecologic malignancy, *Gynecol Oncol* 13:345, 1982.

122. Rocereto TF, Mangan CE, Giuntoli RL, et al: The second-look celiotomy in ovarian cancer, *Gynecol Oncol* 19:34, 1984.

123. Rose DP, Boyar AP, Wynder EL: International comparisons of mortality rates for cancer of the breast, ovary, prostate, and colon, and per capita food consumption, *Cancer* 58:2363, 1986.

124. Rosenberg L, Palmer JR, Zauber AG, et al: A case-control study of oral contraceptive use and invasive epithelial ovarian cancer, *Am J Epidemiol* 139:654, 1994.

125. Rubin SC, Lewis JL Jr: Second-look surgery in ovarian carcinoma, *Crit Rev Oncol Hematol* 8:75, 1988.

126. Rubin SC, Dulaney ED, Markman M, et al: Peritoneal cytology as an indicator of disease in patients with residual ovarian carcinoma, *Obstet Gynecol* 71(6 Pt 1):851, 1988 (comments).

127. Rubin SC, Hoskins WJ, Hakes TB, et al: Recurrence after negative second-look laparotomy for ovarian cancer: analysis of risk factors, *Am J Obstet Gynecol* 159:1094, 1988.

128. Rubin SC, Hoskins WJ, Markman M, et al: Long-term access to the peritoneal cavity in ovarian cancer patients, *Gynecol Oncol* 33:46, 1989.

129. Rubin SC, Hoskins WJ, Benjamin I, et al: Palliative surgery for intestinal obstruction in advanced ovarian cancer, *Gynecol Oncol* 34:16, 1989.

130. Rubin SC, Hoskins WJ, Hakes TB, et al: Serum CA 125 levels and surgical findings in patients undergoing secondary operations for epithelial ovarian cancer, *Am J Obstet Gynecol* 160:667, 1989.

131. Rubin SC, Finstad CL, Hoskins WJ, et al: Expression of P-glycoprotein in epithelial ovarian cancer: evaluation as a marker of multidrug resistance, *Am J Obstet Gynecol* 163(1 part 1):69, 1990.

132. Rubin SC, Hoskins WJ, Saigo PE, et al: Prognostic factors for recurrence following negative second-look laparotomy in ovarian cancer patients treated with platinum-based chemotherapy, *Gynecol Oncol* 42:137, 1991.

133. Rubin SC, Benjamin I, Behbakht K, et al: Clinical and pathological features of ovarian cancer in women with germ-line mutations of BRCA1, *N Engl J Med* 335:1413, 1996 (comments).

134. Rubin SC, Randall T, Armstrong K, et al: Ten year follow-up of ovarian cancer patients having negative second-look laparotomy, *Obstet Gynecol* 93:21, 1999.

135. Runowicz CD, Dottino PR, Shafir MK, et al: Catheter complications associated with intraperitoneal chemotherapy, *Gynecol Oncol* 24:41, 1986.

136. Schwartz PE, Smith JP: Second-look operations in ovarian cancer, *Am J Obstet Gynecol* 138:1124, 1980.

137. Scully RE, Bonfiglio TA, Kuman RJ, et al: *Histological typing of female genital tract tumors (International Histological Classification of Tumors)*, ed 2, Springer-Verlag, 1994, New York.

138. Serov S, Scully R, Sobin L: Histological typing of ovarian tumors. In: *International histological classification of tumors*, Geneva, 1973, World Health Organization.

139. Silverberg E: *Statistical and epidemiological information on gynecological cancer*, New York, 1996, American Cancer Society.

140. Skipper HE: Thoughts on cancer chemotherapy and combination modality therapy (1974), *JAMA* 230:1033, 1974.

141. Skipper H, Schabel EJ, Wilcox V: Experimental evaluation of potential anticancer agents. XII. On the criteria and kinetics associated with "curability" of experimental leukemia, *Cancer Chemother Rep* 35:1, 1964.

142. Smirz LR, Stehman FB, Ulbright TM, et al: Second-look laparotomy after chemotherapy in the management of ovarian malignancy, *Am J Obstet Gynecol* 152 (6 part 1):661, 1985.

143. Smith JP, Delgado G, Rutledge F Second-look operation in ovarian carcinoma: postchemotherapy, *Cancer* 38:1438, 1976.

144. Sonnendecker EW: Is routine second-look laparotomy for ovarian cancer justified? *Gynecol Oncol* 31:249, 1988.

145. Tobacman JK, Greene MH, Tucker MA, et al: Intra-abdominal carcinomatosis after prophylactic oophorectomy in ovarian-cancer-prone families, *Lancet* 2:795, 1982.

146. Tunca JC, Buchler DA, Mack EA, et al: The management of ovarian-cancer-caused bowel obstruction, *Gynecol Oncol* 12(2 part 1):186, 1981.

147. van der Burg ME, van Lent M, Buyse M, et al: The effect of debulking surgery after induction chemotherapy on the prognosis in advanced epithelial ovarian cancer: Gynecological Cancer Cooperative Group of the European Organization for Research and Treatment of Cancer, *N Engl J Med* 332:29, 1995 (comments).

148. Webb MJ, Snyder JA Jr, Williams TJ, et al: Second-look laparotomy in ovarian cancer, *Gynecol Oncol* 14:285, 1982.

149. Webster KD, Ballard LA Jr: Ovarian carcinoma; second-look laparotomy postchemotherapy: preliminary report, *Cleve Clin Q* 48:365, 1981.

150. Wenzl R, Lehner R, Husslein P, et al: Laparoscopic surgery in cases of ovarian malignancies: an Austria-wide survey, *Gynecol Oncol* 63:57, 1996.

151. Wils J, Blijham G, Naus A, et al: Primary or delayed debulking surgery and chemotherapy consisting of cisplatin, doxorubicin, and cyclophosphamide in stage III-IV epithelial ovarian carcinoma, *J Clin Oncol* 4:1068, 1986.

152. Wooster R, Bignell G, Lancaster J, et al: Identification of the breast cancer susceptibility gene BRCA2, *Nature* 378:789, 1995 (comments). (Published erratum appears in *Nature* 379:749, 1996.)

153. Wu PC, Qu JY, Lang JH, et al: Lymph node metastasis of ovarian cancer: a preliminary survey of 74 cases of lymphadenectomy, *Am J Obstet Gynecol* 155:1103, 1986.

154. Wu PC, Lang JH, Huang RL, et al: Lymph node metastasis and retroperitoneal lymphadenectomy in ovarian cancer, *Baillieres Clin Obstet Gynaecol* 3:143, 1989.

155. Wynder EL, Dodo H, Barber HR: Epidemiology of cancer of the ovary, *Cancer* 23:352, 1969.

156. Young RC, Chabner BA, Hubbard SP, et al: Advanced ovarian adenocarcinoma: a prospective clinical trial of melphalan (L-PAM) versus combination chemotherapy, *N Engl J Med* 299:1261, 1978.

40 Pelvic Exenteration and Pelvic Reconstruction

JOHN T. SOPER

BACKGROUND

In 1948, Brunschwig reported the first series of patients treated with a single stage operation consisting of en bloc resection of the gynecologic organs, bladder, and rectum for the treatment of pelvic malignancy.[6] In early series of patients treated with pelvic exenteration, the operative morbidity and mortality rates were extremely high, approaching 70%.[6,11] The past 50 years have seen steady improvements in the operative morbidity and mortality of this procedure.[11] Although no single advance in medical or surgical technology has resulted in these improvements, they can be attributed in part to better patient selection, improved surgical instrumentation and techniques, advanced anesthetic techniques, and improved intensive care unit and general postoperative support. Additional factors include modern blood banking methods, broad-spectrum antibiotics, total parenteral nutritional support, and improved radiologic techniques.

Experience led to improved selection of patients, with the operation usually performed on those with central pelvic malignancy, most commonly after failure of curative attempts with radiotherapy.[11] A variety of malignancies can be treated with this ultraradical procedure, most often including squamous malignancies of the cervix, vagina, and vulva. Some patients with adenocarcinoma of the cervix, uterus, colon, or rectum and rare patients with ovarian epithelial adenocarcinomas are treated with exenteration. Because of the protean nature of the operation, exenteration is not a suitable procedure for patients whose malignancies are unlikely to be cured with this operation because of tumor biology or location.

Pelvic exenteration comprises three basic operations (Fig. 40-1) with several variations, depending on the location of disease and amount of reconstruction that is performed.[11] Total pelvic exenteration (see Fig. 40-1, *A*) consists of an en bloc removal of the bladder, gynecologic organs, and rectosigmoid colon. Anterior exenteration (see Fig. 40-1, *B*) is a combination of radical hysterectomy-vaginectomy with cystectomy, and posterior exenteration (see Fig. 40-1, *C*) is a combination of radical hysterectomy-vaginectomy with rectosigmoid resection. Infralevator exenterations include removal of the structures below the pelvic diaphragm. In performing supralevator exenterations, the pelvic viscera are resected at the level of the levator plate/pelvic diaphragm, leaving the introitus intact. In selected patients the bladder and vagina are resected below the pelvic diaphragm, and the anus and distal rectum are preserved. Pelvic exenteration is occasionally combined with radical resections of the vulva.

With the development of surgical stapling devices and advanced sophistication of plastic surgery reconstruction techniques, increasing numbers of women are undergoing simultaneous attempts to reconstruct the pelvis, restore bowel continuity, and create continent urinary conduits.[11,27,33] In addition to being beneficial to the patient's body self-image, attempts to reconstruct the pelvis appeared to decrease complications by filling the empty pelvis with vascularized tissue, resulting in a decrease in pelvic infectious complications and fistulas of the gastrointestinal or genitourinary tract.

A survey of surgical results with exenteration indicates survival ranging between 30% and 60% in most recent series generated over the past 15 years and operative mortality decreasing to less than 10%.* Most series report a decreasing incidence of operative mortality during the later years of their study interval.

PATIENT SELECTION

Because a pelvic exenteration is an ultraradical operation with the potential for extreme effects on body self-image and complications, patient selection is of utmost importance. The patient have not only must have a malignancy that can potentially be cured with this procedure, but also also must be medically and psychologically able to withstand the procedure. Furthermore, the psychological effects of an "aborted" exenteration on the patient and her family must be considered when discussing this treatment option for patients who have only a small possibility of being candidates for this procedure.

The preoperative evaluation includes a careful consideration of the type of malignancy and prior therapy. In general, women with squamous malignancies of the female genital tract that spread by local invasion of adjacent structures and with a relatively orderly progression of lymphatic metastasis are potential candidates. In contrast, adenocarcinomas more often metastasize via intraperitoneal dissemination. Sarcomas and melanomas of the female genital tract also have a tendency for hematogenous dissemination, but occasionally, patients in these categories are suitable candidates for exenteration.

Patients who have been treated with a previous radical hysterectomy, even if followed by radiation therapy, are

---

*References 1, 7, 9, 20, 25, 26, 28.

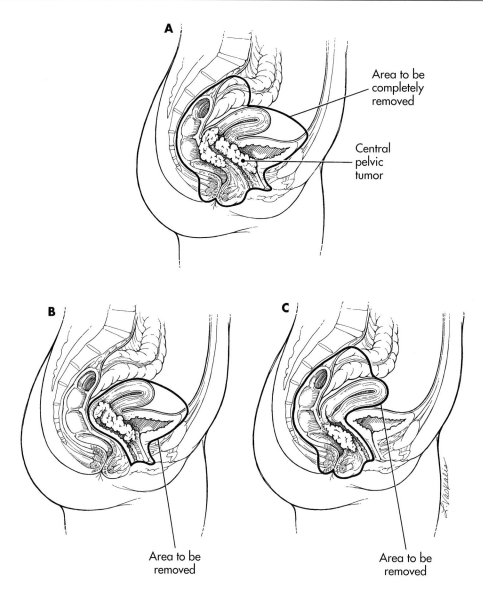

Fig. 40-1 Schematic representations of total **(A)**, anterior **(B)**, and posterior **(C)** exenteration with perineal phase (infralevator exenteration). The extent of the operation is dictated by tumor anatomy and prior therapy (see text).

rarely candidates for exenteration. In addition to having prior extensive pelvic dissections, which leads to increased difficulty in performing the procedure, some series have demonstrated the patterns of recurrence in these patients are rarely suitable for exenteration and that patients who have isolated central recurrences after radical hysterectomy often have recurrences outside of the pelvis after exenteration.[11] Furthermore, patients who have persistent or rapidly recurring central gynecologic malignancies are at an increased risk for recurrence after pelvic exenteration, even when disease is centrally localized. Several series have documented recurrence rates in excess of 80% among patients undergoing exenteration within 2 years of their primary therapy.[11]

On physical examination, a biopsy should be performed for any sites suspicious for distant lymphatic metastasis. Pelvic examination should be used to carefully evaluate the location, size, and mobility of the tumor. The patient with a bulky, poorly mobile tumor that clinically extends beyond the medial parametrium is unlikely to have disease that can be cured with exenteration.

Before sophisticated radiographic techniques were developed, patients with centrally recurrent pelvic malignancies who had a "triad of trouble" were considered to have inoperable disease.[11] This included the presence of ureteral obstruction on intravenous pyelogram, suggesting nodal disease or tumor involvement of the pelvic sidewall. Pain in a sciatic nerve distribution is an indication of perineural invasion of the posterior pelvic sidewall. Lower extremity edema is often associated with lymphatic obstruction. Even today, the simultaneous occurrence of these three findings indicates a patient who is unlikely to have disease that would be appropriate for treatment with pelvic exenteration.

Radiographic evaluation of a potential candidate for exenteration should include chest x-ray film or a computed tomography (CT) scan of the lungs and CT scan of the abdomen and pelvis. Biopsy should be performed on any suspicious extrapelvic lesions by using the CT-directed fine-needle aspirate technique, which has a high sensitivity and specificity for metastatic disease, particularly involving the retroperitoneal lymph nodes. A pelvic magnetic resonance imaging (MRI) scan may be helpful in determining whether pelvic induration is caused by radiation change or active malignancy, particularly if more than 12 months have elapsed since completion of radiotherapy. Patients who have evidence of extrapelvic or lateral pelvic sidewall disease by these radiographic techniques are not suitable candidates for exenteration.

In many patients, examination under anesthesia is helpful for determining resectability of central pelvic disease. A Tru-Cut biopsy can be obtained from indurated or thickened parametrium. The presence of malignant cells in the lateral parametrial tissues is an indication of unresectability. On other occasions, questionable findings on a clinical pelvic examination can be resolved, with a better determination of the mobility of the central pelvic structures while the patient is under anesthesia. Biopsies on samples obtained from the distal vagina may also aid in making a decision regarding the extent of vaginal resection necessary to encompass disease.

Each patient must be evaluated carefully before undergoing exploration for exenteration to determine whether there are factors that might increase the morbidity or mortality of the procedure, including general medical condition and nutritional status, obesity, and age. Appropriate consultation should be obtained to aid in the perioperative management of those who have significant medical comorbidities. Although there is a general increase in medical comorbidities among older women, many series have included patients older than 70 years who have successfully undergone exenteration and adapted postoperatively.[28] Advanced age by itself is not a contraindication of the procedure. Likewise, obesity may increase the difficulty of the procedure and increase perioperative complications, but it is not a contraindication to exenteration by itself.

Finally, the patient's general psychological status and support systems must be evaluated. Each patient must be mentally able to accept and deal with the changes in body self-image that accompany this procedure. Even if a partial (anterior or posterior) exenteration is contemplated, the patient must be aware of the possibility of an undesired stoma. Furthermore, it is imperative that each patient have the family and social support to aid during the recovery period from this operation.

Despite the considerations just discussed, exploratory laparotomy to determine resectability is the final determinant as to whether the patient is a suitable candidate for this procedure. During exploration, the upper abdomen is carefully assessed for any sign of metastatic disease and the retroperitoneal spaces are explored to exclude lymph node metastases and to determine resectability of the pelvic tumor. Several absolute contraindications for performance of exenteration exist. Peritoneal carcinomatosis and even transperi-

toneal penetration of tumor portend rapid recurrence, often before the patient has recovered from surgery.[30] Likewise, bulky paraaortic and pelvic or microscopic paraaortic metastatic disease indicates a poor prognosis, even if all lymph nodes are resected.[30] Tumor involvement of the pelvic sidewall or bone has traditionally been accepted as an absolute contraindication to performance of exenteration. However, patients occasionally have been treated with ultraradical resections of the symphysis or hemipelvis, with some long-term survivors. In addition, placement of afterloading catheters for the purpose of delivering postoperative brachytherapy has been advocated as deliberate treatment for pelvic sidewall recurrences of cervical cancer by some investigators. However, the results of these extended techniques are too limited to recommend universally.

Microscopic involvement of pelvic lymph nodes as a contraindication for pelvic exenteration is a controversial topic. In some series, no patients with microscopic pelvic lymph node metastases survived, although other series have demonstrated 5-year survival of up to 23%.[30] Therefore the decision to proceed with an exenteration in the face of microscopic pelvic lymph node metastases should be carried out with an appreciation for the extent of pelvic lymph node involvement, the interval from treatment to recurrence, and especially the age and desires of the patient.

Occasionally, a concurrent surgical complication that would seriously increase the morbidity of an exenteration, such as pelvic abscess, occult fistula, or severe intraoperative hemorrhage, is encountered. The decision to abort the exenteration should not be made lightly in these circumstances because most often exenteration provides the patient with her only chance for cure.

Preoperative Preparation of the Patient

It is important that every patient be fully informed about the nature and extent of exenteration. Although I do not routinely obtain a formal psychiatric consultation, this should be obtained if the clinician has concerns regarding the patient's ability to adapt to the postoperative state.

Patients undergo counseling by a stomal therapist so that they can anticipate the bodily function changes that accompany urostomy or colostomy. It is often helpful to recruit a previous patient who is surviving after exenteration to help in the preoperative counseling of patients. The patient's home environment should be assessed so that appropriate support can be arranged during the postoperative recovery after discharge from the hospital.

Before surgery, each patient undergoes a mechanical bowel preparation consisting of at least 2 days of clear liquids and cathartics (GoLYTELY, Fleets Phospho Soda, or magnesium citrate) followed by enemas on the night before surgery. If necessary, patients are admitted preoperatively for hydration. Each patient receives preoperative prophylactic antibiotics that include coverage for anaerobic bacteria (e.g., cefoxitin). Thromboembolic prophylaxis consisting of either intermittent compression boots or intermediate-dose subcutaneous heparin (5000 U every 8 hours) or low-dose low-molecular-weight heparin is initiated in the operating room. Clipping or shaving of the abdomen and mons is performed in the operating room.

The patient is positioned in the modified lithotomy ("ski jump") position using Allen stirrups. The sterile field extends from the nipples to the knees, allowing access to the upper abdomen and inner thigh to maximize the options for pelvic reconstruction with rectus or gracilis myocutaneous flaps. A Bookwalter retractor and headlight are helpful in obtaining exposure during the procedure. A cell saver may be used during the initial phases of an exenteration but should not be used after the bowel or vagina has been entered because of bacterial contamination.

Intraoperative Exploration

A vertical incision is usually used to explore patients for exenteration. Although a muscle-cutting Maylard transverse incision offers good exposure to the pelvis, it limits the options for vaginal reconstruction because rectus flaps are not available for use after this incision.[27] The upper abdomen is carefully explored, and frozen section samples are taken from any suspicious lesions for biopsy. The presence of abdominal metastases is an absolute contraindication to performance of exenteration.

The peritoneum overlying the right common iliac artery (Fig. 40-2) is elevated and incised parallel to the aorta, cephalad and medially to the ureter inferiorly. The lym-

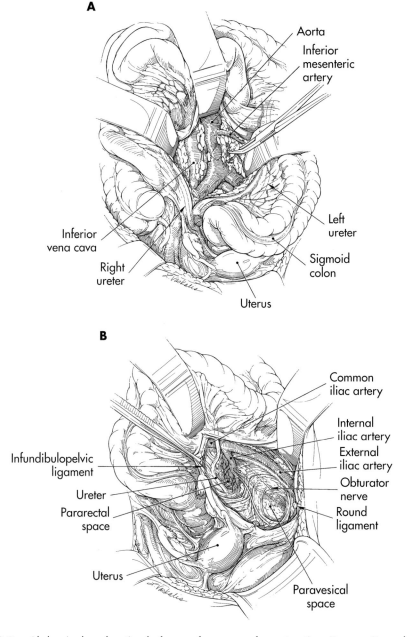

Fig. 40-2 Abdominal exploration before performance of exenteration. Transperitoneal sampling of paraaortic lymph nodes (**A**) and pelvic lymph nodes (**B**) is performed to exclude metastases outside of the ureteral pelvis.

phatic fat pad overlying the vena cava and right side of the distal aorta is removed, using sharp and blunt dissection and hemoclips for hemostasis. Lymph nodes overlying and lateral to the right common iliac artery are likewise removed, and both specimens are submitted for frozen section. During this transperitoneal dissection, the right ureter is mobilized laterally and carefully preserved. The retroperitoneal dissection is then extended to the left (see Fig. 40-2, *A*), across the midline under the inferior mesenteric artery and anterior to the aorta and sacral promontory to expose the left common iliac artery and distal left side of the aorta. The left ureter is retracted along with the sigmoid colon anteriorly and laterally. Lymph nodes overlying and lateral to the distal aorta and left common iliac artery are removed and submitted for frozen section analysis.

While awaiting frozen section results, the surgeon can develop the pelvic retroperitoneal spaces using sharp and blunt dissection (see Fig. 40-2, *B*). The ureters are preserved, and dissection should be performed carefully to avoid hemorrhage at this early stage of the procedure. Frozen sections are obtained from pelvic lymph nodes and any suspicious lesions at or near the anticipated resection margins (e.g., lateral cardinal ligament adjacent to the pelvic sidewall). Nothing irreversible has been done at this portion of the operation, so the exenteration can be aborted if frozen sections indicate that the malignancy is not resectable.

OPERATIVE TECHNIQUE

When it has been determined that the patient is a suitable candidate for exenteration, the surgeon should individualize the resection based on the patient's prior surgery and location of tumor. Although it is reasonable to attempt to be conservative by performing a partial exenteration to preserve bodily function, this should be tempered by the need to obtain surgical margins clear of disease. Furthermore, extensive dissection of a rectovaginal or vesicovaginal plane in the face of extensive central radiation results in a high risk of fistula formation.

Several possible combinations exist for pelvic exenteration. In addition to total, anterior, and posterior exenteration, a supralevator exenteration removes tissue only above the levator plate and pelvic diaphragm, whereas an infralevator exenteration removes tissues below the pelvic diaphragm to the vaginal introitus. The operative technique is also influenced by the extent of reconstruction that is performed after exenteration.

Total Pelvic Exenteration

The presacral, pararectal, paravesical, and prepubic (space of Retzius) spaces are developed by using sharp and blunt dissection (Fig. 40-3) to the level of the levator plate (Fig. 40-4). The infundibulopelvic ligaments are divided. The upper cardinal ligaments are developed into pedicles that are clamped, divided, and suture ligated with absorbable suture (Vicryl) at the pelvic sidewalls. Depending on tumor anatomy, the anterior division of the hypogastric artery can be isolated and ligated on each side. This reduces the pulse

pressure to the central pelvis and may reduce operative blood loss. However, when the hypogastric artery has been ligated, the secondary blood supply to the gracilis muscle is sacrificed, and this must be considered if a gracilis flap is used for vaginal reconstruction.[29] Alternatively, the uterine arteries can be separately isolated and ligated at their origin. If the patient has undergone prior pelvic lymph node dissection combined with radiation, the pararectal space may be obliterated; rather than running the risk of increased complications from hemorrhage by attempting to dissect these spaces, it is sometimes preferable to develop the presacral space and space of Retzius, leaving a broad plane of fibrosis and cardinal ligament laterally, which must be taken in several pedicles during the exenteration.

A mesenteric window is created adjacent to the midsigmoid colon, and the serosa of the bowel is cleared of fat using sharp and blunt dissection and electrocautery for hemostasis. The GIA stapler is used to transect and staple the colon. The mesentery is then developed in the pedicles that are cross-clamped, divided, and suture ligated. The sigmoid colon is then reflected anteriorly and the presacral space developed further, with division and ligation of the remaining uterosacral ligaments, to the level of the levator plate (Fig. 40-5, *A*). Any attachments of the bladder to the pubis are controlled hemostatically and divided (see Fig. 40-5, *A*).

Dissection of the presacral space should be directed toward the sigmoid colon so that the presacral veins are avoided. Disruption of the presacral veins can result in catastrophic blood loss. The ureters are mobilized off of the medial leaf of the broad ligament and divided at or below the pelvic brim to obtain the greatest length of ureter without devascularizing the ureter by "digging it out" of dense radiation fibrosis. Ligating the ureters at this time is helpful (see Fig. 40-5, *A*) because it allows ureteral dilation to occur during the remainder of the case leading to creation of the urinary conduit.

The cardinal ligaments are developed into pedicles that are clamped, divided, and suture ligated adjacent to the pelvic sidewall (see Fig. 40-5, *B*). The upper portions of the cardinal ligaments are often developed during dissection of the presacral space. The lower portions of the cardinal ligaments are usually the last pelvic ligaments to be divided. They must be controlled to the level of the levator plate before the specimen is removed (see Fig. 40-5, *B*).

If a supralevator exenteration is performed, the specimen is amputated at the level of the levator plate. A perineal phase is required if an infralevator exenteration is to be performed (see Fig. 40-5, *B*). Often, a second team of surgeons will perform this phase of the operation and assist during pelvic reconstruction, which expedites performance of the procedure. The vagina, urethra, and anus are circumscribed with a scalpel. Blunt dissection is used to develop the lateral paravaginal and perineal body pedicles, which are divided, and to continue the dissection to the pelvic diaphragm. The levator plate is then circumscribed, and the specimen is removed. Additional hemostasis is achieved in the pelvis. This often requires interrupted figure-of-eight sutures along the edges of the levator plate. If the anus has been removed, sigmoidos-

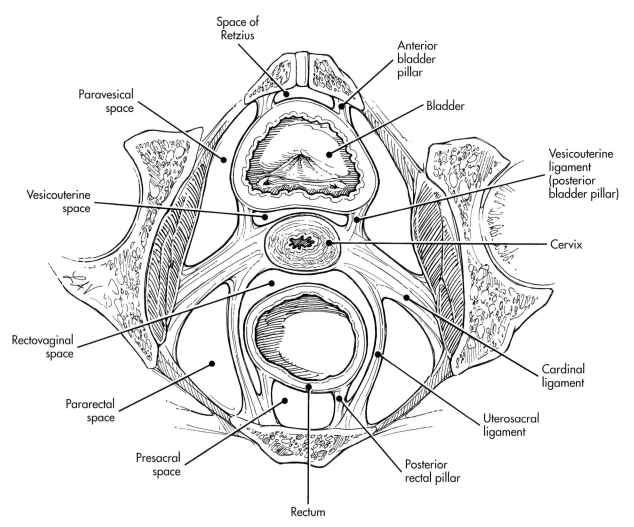

Fig. 40-3 Schematic cross-section of the pelvis illustrating relationships of the pelvic viscera, pelvic ligaments, and the avascular spaces that are developed during exenteration (see text).

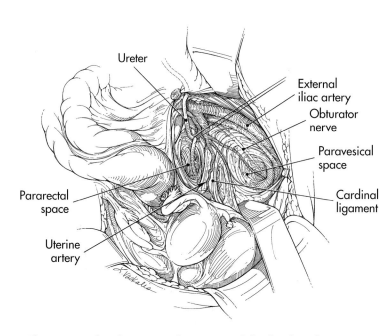

Fig. 40-4 The pararectal and paravesical spaces are fully developed. Any suspicious areas adjacent to the pelvic sidewalls are sampled for frozen section analysis.

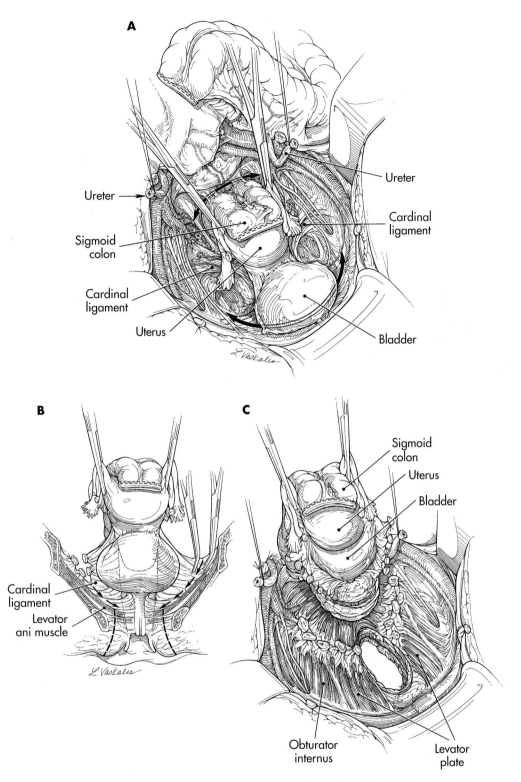

Fig. 40-5   Total pelvic exenteration. **A,** The ureters are ligated and divided. The sigmoid colon has been divided with a GIA stapler and the mesenteric pedicles, including the superior hemorrhoidal artery, have been controlled. The hypogastric or uterine arteries are usually individually ligated. The colon is mobilized anteriorly from the presacral space by dividing the posterior rectal pillars, and the bladder is fully mobilized. Dissection in the direction of the arrows produces broad cardinal ligaments laterally on each side of the central pelvis. **B,** The cardinal ligaments and lateral fibrovascular pedicles are sequentially clamped and divided to the levator plate. **C,** Simultaneous perineal dissection allows en bloc removal of the specimen or the specimen can be transected from above at the level of the levator plate.

tomy and colostomy are performed and matured after closure of the abdominal wall, as described in Chapter 50.

If rectosigmoid reanastomosis is to be performed and the anus is preserved, the posterior vagina is dissected off of the anus beginning at the level of the introitus to the appropriate level for division of the rectum. Using upward traction, the isolated rectum can then be cross-clamped or stapled by transabdominal or transvaginal route, allowing amputation of the specimen.

Anterior Exenteration

An anterior exenteration basically consists of a radical hysterectomy-vaginectomy in conjunction with cystectomy. The pararectal, perivesical, and anterior spaces are developed. The rectovaginal septum is developed by using sharp and blunt dissection. The uterine arteries are isolated at their origin, divided, and ligated and the lateral cardinal ligaments are developed in the pedicles that are cross-clamped, divided, and suture ligated. The infundibulopelvic ligaments are divided and suture ligated. The distal ureters are mobilized from the medial leaf of the broad ligament, divided, and ligated. The uterosacral ligaments are isolated, clamped, and divided adjacent to the rectum. Similar to total pelvic exenteration, the procedure continues until the levator plate is reached, when a decision is made whether an infralevator or supralevator exenteration is to be performed.

Posterior Exenteration

In general, posterior exenteration with extensive removal of the anterior vaginal wall is inappropriate if the patient has received extensive radiation to the base of the bladder. In these situations, it is preferable to perform a total pelvic exenteration or, if appropriate, to preserve a portion of the anterior vaginal mucosa. This would reduce the potential risk of inducing a urinary fistula.

A posterior exenteration is essentially a radical hysterectomy-vaginectomy performed in conjunction with rectosigmoid resection. The upper cardinal ligaments and uterine artery are controlled as previously noted. The ureter is completely immobilized off of the medial leaf of the broad ligament to its insertion into the ureteric tunnel. The presacral space and posterior uterosacral ligaments are managed similarly to a total pelvic exenteration. After division of the sigmoid colon and its mesentery, the posterior dissection is continued to allow anterior mobility of the specimen. The bladder is mobilized off of the vagina using sharp dissection. Similar to performance of a radical hysterectomy, the ureteric tunnel is unroofed by developing the anterior vesicouterine ligaments that are cross-clamped, divided, and suture ligated. The base of the bladder and distal ureters are further mobilized, and the posterior vesicouterine ligaments are developed into pedicles. If the anterior vagina is to be preserved, it is entered and the lateral vaginal walls are incised at approximately 10 and 2 o'clock. The remainder of the procedure is completed, similar to a total pelvic exenteration.

PELVIC AND VAGINAL RECONSTRUCTION

After completion of exenteration, it is important to ensure pelvic hemostasis before proceeding to pelvic reconstruction. "Empty pelvis syndrome" was commonly observed after pelvic exenteration in the early experience with this operation, before surgeons made an attempt to reconstruct the pelvis and vagina.[14,19] This consisted of massive loss of fluid and electrolytes from the denuded and radiated pelvic tissues. These patients were prone to postoperative infections, bowel obstructions, and fistula formation. The purpose of pelvic and vaginal reconstruction is to obturate the pelvic cavity with tissue bulk and bring in a new blood supply to irradiated tissues.[27] A secondary goal is to restore function of bowel and vagina, which may be beneficial to the patient's body image. In general, efforts to reconstruct the pelvis and vagina should proceed from the posterior pelvis to the anterior pelvis, as this facilitates exposure.

Low Pelvic Rectosigmoid Reanastomosis

In appropriate patients the anus and distal rectum can be preserved, allowing the potential for normal bowel function. Performance of a low pelvic reanastomosis of the colon has been made easier by the introduction of automatic end-to-end (EEA) stapling devices, which provide a reliable full-thickness anastomosis deep in the pelvis as illustrated in Chapter 51.

In general, the largest diameter device should be used to avoid stenosis. A full-thickness purse-string suture of 2-0 monofilament is placed around the distal end of the sigmoid colon. The rectal stump can also be controlled with a purse-string suture, but the stapler can be used to anastomose through a prior staple line. The stapler is advanced through the rectal stump, and the anvil is placed on the central pole. The purse-string suture in the distal sigmoid colon is tied down around the central pole, the device is tightened, and anastomosis performed. The stapler is withdrawn and should be inspected to make sure that there are two full tissue donuts around the central post. A "bubble test" is performed by immersing the anastomosis in water, inflating air through a sigmoidoscope, and inspecting the staple line for leakage of air. The staple line is reinforced with interrupted sutures of 3-0 silk or Vicryl. In radiated patients, it is prudent to perform a diverting colostomy.

If less than 4 to 6 cm of rectal stump is preserved, a J-pouch may decrease the incidence of fecal incontinence, tenesmus, and diarrhea.[33] It also allows an increase in the size of the EEA device used for anastomosis. Approximately a 10-cm length of distal sigmoid is doubled back on itself and anchored with a serosal suture. Colotomy is made at the outside apex of the curve. Serial applications of the GIA stapler are used to detubularize the intestine, allowing approximately 8 cm of communication between the proximal and distal limbs of the J-pouch. Before each firing of the GIA stapler, appendix epiploicae and fat should be cleared from the serosa of the bowel so that they do not compromise the staple line. The internal aspect of the J-pouch is inspected for hemostasis along the staple line. A purse-string suture of 2-0 monofilament is used around the colotomy, and anastomosis is performed with the EEA stapler as described previously.

Vaginal Reconstruction Techniques

A variety of techniques have been used in an attempt to create a functional vagina after pelvic exenteration.[14,27] The earliest attempts consisted of suturing omentum or peritoneum over a pelvic pack to allow epithelialization to occur gradually. Split-thickness skin grafting techniques have been applied to omentum and peritoneal flap, providing an epithelialized neovagina.[14,27] The bulbocavernosus myocutaneous flap can be used to provide a partial neovaginal reconstruction and brings vascularized, nonradiated tissue into the vagina but is generally insufficient for complete vaginal reconstruction.[10] I most commonly use gracilis myocutaneous or rectus myocutaneous flaps for vaginal reconstruction because these provide vascularized, nonradiated tissue, in addition to tissue bulk to obturate the pelvic cavity. Both of these techniques can be used for partial or complete vaginal reconstructions.

Gracilis Flap Neovagina

Myocutaneous flaps based on the gracilis muscle of the medial thigh have become widely used for neovaginal reconstruction since the first report by McCraw et al.[17] This thin straplike muscle is the most medial adductor of the thigh but can be sacrificed without loss of function. The gracilis originates from the pubic tubercle and runs posterior to the adductor longus, inserting into the medial tibial plateau. The major blood supply is derived from a vascular pedicle originating from branches of the medial femoral circumflex artery, and this supports a large territory of skin extending along the proximal two thirds of the medial thigh, posterior to the adductor longus. The dominant vascular pedicle enters the deep gracilis muscle with paired venae comitantes and nerve approximately 6 to 8 cm distal to the pubic tubercle after passing between the adductor longus and brevis muscles. An accessory blood supply is derived from anastomotic terminal branches of the obturator and pudendal vessels entering within the proximal 1 to 3 cm of the muscle. Although these accessory vessels are not as well defined as the dominant vascular pedicle, they have been used to support short gracilis flap that can be successfully used for vulvovaginal reconstructions.[8,29]

Fig. 40-6 illustrates the use of a gracilis flap for neovaginal formation during pelvic exenteration. The guideline is drawn on the medial thigh from the pubic tubercle to the medial tibial plateau along the margin of the adductor longus muscle. The skin island supplied by the gracilis will be located posterior to this line. If a long flap is to be used, an ellipsoid skin island 10 to 20 cm long and 6 to 10 cm wide will be developed with a proximal margin 4 to 6 cm distal to the crural fold (see Fig. 40-6, A). Skin islands up to 25 cm in length can be developed, but the distal third of the skin in the medial thigh is supplied via the sartorius muscle with a variable watershed of blood supply beyond the midthigh.

An ellipsoid 10 to 14 cm long and 5 to 8 cm wide with the proximal margin at the crural fold is used for the short flap (see Fig. 40-6, A).[8,29]

A full-thickness skin incision is made along the anterior and distal margin of the skin island through the fascia lata (see Fig. 40-6, B). The skin is loosely anchored to the fascia with temporary interrupted sutures to prevent shearing of the fat and skin away from the underlying fascia during manipulation. The belly of the gracilis muscle is identified at the distal tip of the flap, posterior to the adductor longus. It is isolated and divided with electrocautery. The remainder of the full-thickness incision from skin to fascia is completed around the margin of the skin island.

The gracilis is mobilized from its bed with sharp and blunt dissection working, from the distal tip of the flap toward the origin so that the dominant vascular pedicle can be identified (see Fig. 40-6, B). With its paired venae comitantes, the dominant vascular pedicle is easily distinguished from the loose areolar tissue between the muscles.[16,17,27] The nerve usually enters with, or just proximal to, the dominant vascular pedicle. If a classic long flap is used, the pedicle is mobilized (see Fig. 40-6, B). If a short flap is used, the pedicle is cross-clamped, divided, and ligated (see Fig. 40-6, B).[8,29] The nerve can usually be spared to provide muscular innervation and sensation of the skin island, but it may be sacrificed. The remainder of the gracilis flap is mobilized to its origin. If a short flap is used, the 2 to 3 cm of proximal gracilis muscle should not be aggressively skeletonized so that the small accessory vessels are not stripped away.

A subfascial tunnel is constructed to the vaginal introitus with sharp and blunt dissection. The fascia should allow passage of the gracilis flap freely without pressure. The flaps are rotated posteriorly through the tunnels and are allowed to hang freely between the patient's legs (see Fig. 40-6, C). The neovaginal tube is constructed by approximating the skin edges with interrupted absorbable suture, beginning at the distal tips of the flap (see Fig. 40-6, C). The temporary sutures anchoring skin to fascia are cut, and the proximal skin margins are left open to form the introitus. The neovaginal tube is then rotated posteriorly into the pelvis and anchored to the levator plate and symphysis or sacral hollow with interrupted sutures (see Fig. 40-6, D). The redundant skin is trimmed, and the proximal skin of the flap is sutured to the introitus. If gracilis flaps are used to create a neovagina during an exenteration, the neovagina can be constructed by a second team without interruption of the abdominal procedure, resulting in minimal prolongation of operative time and no added blood loss.[7,13,17,29] The thigh incisions are irrigated and closed in layers over closed suction drains. Patients are allowed to ambulate within 24 to 48 hours of surgery.

Complications specific to the gracilis flap are often encountered but are rarely life-threatening. Major flap loss is encountered in 10% to 15% of patients and does not appear to be increased in patients receiving the short gracilis flap.[2,7,13,17,29] Minor loss of skin from the margins of the flap is commonly encountered. Other complications include

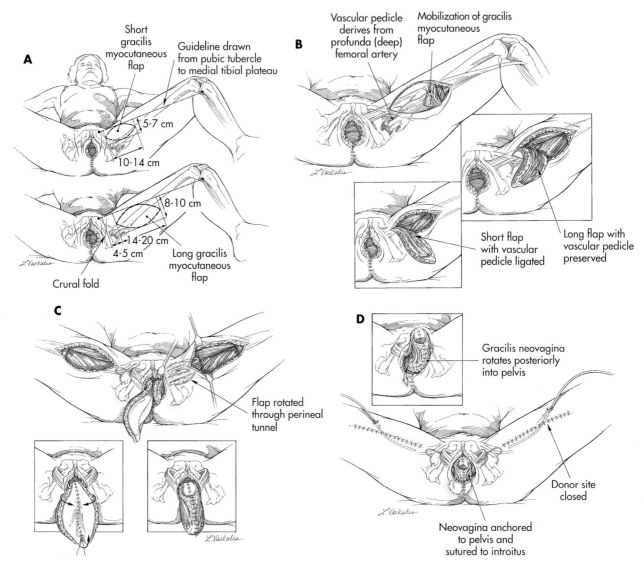

Fig. 40-6 Gracilis myocutaneous flap for neovaginal reconstruction. **A,** Relative size and location of the short and long gracilis flap. **B,** Mobilization of the gracilis myocutaneous flap and identification of the primary vascular pedicle. Dissection proceeds from the distal muscle toward the pubis. The primary vascular pedicle is identified along the anterior margin of the muscle, approximately 6 to 8 cm distal to the pubic tubercle. The vascular pedicle is preserved if a long flap is used, but can be deliberately sacrificed if a short gracilis flap is developed *(insets)*. **C,** Formation of the neovagina. The flaps are rotated through the perineal tunnel into the pelvic defect. The neovagina is intubated by approximating the skin edges *(inset)*. The distal tips of the flap become the vaginal apex. **D,** The neovagina rotates posteriorly into the pelvic defect *(inset)* to fill the cavity. The neovagina is anchored to adjacent tissues to prevent prolapse and sutured to the introitus. The donor site is closed over suction drains.

donor site hematoma or abscess, introital stenosis, and vaginal vault prolapse. Prolapse of the neovagina can be prevented by meticulously anchoring the neovagina to adjacent structures with permanent sutures.

Inferior Rectus Abdominis Flap

The inferior rectus abdominis flap, based on the inferior epigastric artery pedicle, can support a variety of transverse or vertical skin islands.[31] The deep inferior epigastric artery originates from the distal external iliac artery, coursing up-

ward and medially to the lateral border of the rectus abdominis muscles. The artery travels with paired venae comitantes, entering the rectus sheath at approximately the level of the arcuate line, ascending along the deep belly of the muscle. It divides into several branches below the level of the umbilicus and travels within the belly of the muscle to anastomose with branches of the superior epigastric system above the level of the umbilicus.[31] Branches are given to the peritoneum, muscle, and skin, extending off all portions of the inferior epigastric system, usually radiating away from the umbilical region. These anastomose liberally with branches of the superior epigastric artery, intercostal and lumbar arteries, and superficial and deep vessels from the groin and across the midline with branches of the contralateral deep inferior epigastric system. The entire rectus muscle and overlying abdominal skin can be supported by the deep inferior epigastric system, even if the superior epigastric artery and secondary vessels are divided. This richly anastomotic blood supply of the anterior abdominal wall allows support of both vertical and transverse skin islands that can extend far beyond the level of the underlying strip of anterior rectus fascia.[13] Transverse or vertical skin islands are usually mobilized above the level of arcuate line so that the posterior sheath can provide additional support to the abdominal wall after closure of the donor site.

Principles for development of inferior rectus abdominis flaps are similarly used for vertical or transverse islands. The skin island is defined and incised along the superior border through the anterior rectus sheath (Fig. 40-7, *A*). The belly of the rectus muscle is mobilized with blunt dissection, proceeding from the rectus diastasis off the posterior sheath to define the lateral margin of the muscle, and the anterior fascial incision is extended to this point. The muscle is divided and anastomotic vessels connecting to this superior epigastric system are ligated. The remaining borders of the skin are incised to the level of the anterior fascia, and the subcutaneous fat is mobilized back to the lateral and medial margins of the rectus muscle. After the anterior rectus fascia is incised along the lateral borders, the muscle and fascia are elevated. The inferior margin of the fascial strip is incised. It is important to retain the fascia over at least one to two segments of the rectus muscle so that several perforating vessels will supply the skin island.

The rectus muscle inferior to the skin island is mobilized from both the posterior and anterior fascial sheaths using sharp and blunt dissection (see Fig. 40-7, *B*). If a flap is being raised in conjunction with the midline incision, this can be performed very rapidly, working from the medial to lateral aspect of the muscle. The lateral tendinous insertions and segmental nerve vascular bundles of the muscle are isolated and divided. The deep inferior epigastric pedicle is dissected free, if necessary, and can be isolated to the external iliac vessels to facilitate mobilization of the rectus muscle.

Usually a 12- to 14-cm by 4- to 6-cm skin island will provide a sufficient neovagina. The neovaginal tube is formed by approximating the skin edges with absorbable sutures (see Fig. 40-7, *B*). The neovagina is rotated into the pelvis, suturing the open end of the neovagina to the introitus (see Fig. 40-7, *C*). During rotation of the flap, the vascular pedicle should be observed to determine that there is no twisting or tension on the vessels. In morbidly obese patients with bulky subcutaneous tissues, a bulky myocutaneous flap might produce enough pressure to cause venous congestion and skin slough of the flap. In these patients, use of a myoperitoneal flap or myosubcutaneous flap with a split-thickness skin graft might be preferable to a myocutaneous flap.[27]

Because the vascular pedicle is extremely predictable and the anterior abdominal wall has an excellent blood supply, very satisfactory results have been reported for most series of patients with inferior rectus abdominis flap pelvic reconstructions, with close to 100% flap viability.[18,24,32] In patients with severe atherosclerosis of the lower extremities, preoperative angiography should be used to ensure patency of the inferior epigastric arteries before developing this flap because anecdotal reports have documented loss of an extremity in patients who had severe occlusion of the vessels to the lower leg and derived perfusion from retrograde flow through the inferior epigastric system.[24] The anterior fascial defect should be closed using either primary closure or synthetic mesh in an attempt to prevent hernia (see Fig. 40-7, *C*). Usually, the anterior rectus fascial defect can be closed primarily. A minor disadvantage for use of this flap for neovaginal reconstruction during exenteration is interruption of the operative "flow" of the exenteration while the flap is being raised.[27] Unlike the gracilis flap, construction of a rectus flap adds extra time to the operation because flap construction takes place within the abdominal operative field.

Both of these techniques for vaginal reconstruction provide adequate tissue bulk to obturate the denuded pelvis and provide neovascularization to the radiated pelvis. Both techniques provide a neovagina that is satisfactory for coitus and is not prone to stenosis. In my experience, approximately 45% of patients who undergo neovaginal reconstruction resume sexual activity after exenteration.

Omental Lid

The omentum is often used to revascularize the pelvis and provide a buffer between the intestines and raw pelvic surfaces.[28] The omentum is mobilized off the transverse colon, and, beginning at the hepatic flexure, vascular pedicles are divided and ligated (Fig. 40-8). The vascular pedicles in the region of the splenic flexure are retained so that the omental flap is perfused from branches of the left gastroepiploic vessels. The resulting flap is rotated into the pelvis along the left gutter and loosely sutured to the pelvic structures to form a "carpet" without attempting to form a sling (see Fig. 40-8).[28] This reduces the chances of development of an internal hernia. Closed suction drains are usually placed into the pelvis under the omental carpet.

URINARY CONDUIT

Since Brunswick's initial reports of pelvic exenteration with cutaneous ureterostomy or wet colostomy,[6] a variety of urinary conduits have been devised that provide satisfactory urinary drainage with separation of the urine and fecal streams. An isolated ileal conduit was first used by Bricker[5] and has been widely adopted for pelvic exenteration. Unfortunately, the terminal ileum often receives significant radiation with the potential for increased incidence of complications at the site of intestinal anastomosis and complications related to the conduit.[4,21,28] Jejunal conduits are associated with a high rate of metabolic complications because of elec-

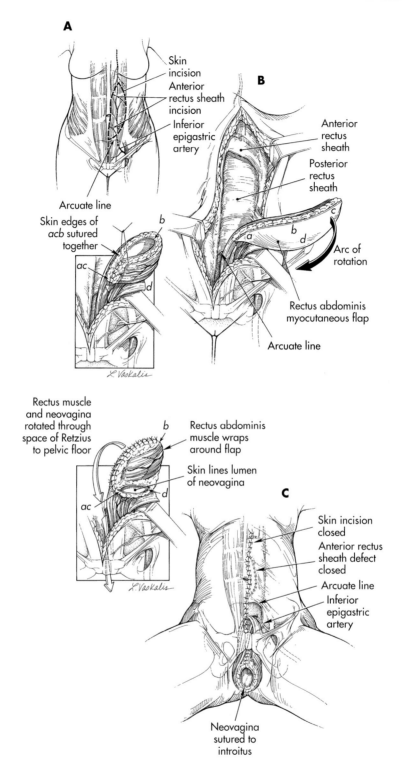

Fig. 40-7 Vertical inferior rectus abdominis flap for neovaginal reconstruction. **A,** Development of the myocutaneous flap. Because of the rich blood supply, the flap can extend several centimeters beyond the underlying anterior rectus fascia. **B,** Development of the neovaginal tube. The rectus muscle is divided distally and mobilized off the anterior and posterior rectus sheath. The inferior epigastric vessels are preserved. The flap is intubated by approximating the skin edges *(inset).* **C,** Completion of the rectus abdominis neovagina. The flap is rotated into the pelvis below the arcuate line and sutured to the introitus *(inset).* The inferior epigastric vessels must not be kinked to ensure good perfusion and venous drainage of the flap. The anterior rectus sheath defect should be repaired with primary closure, if possible.

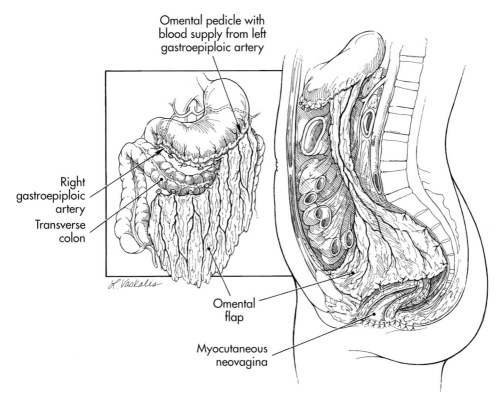

Omental pedicle with blood supply from left gastroepiploic artery

Right gastroepiploic artery

Transverse colon

Omental flap

Myocutaneous neovagina

Fig. 40-8   Use of omental flap as a carpet to cover the pelvic defect after exenteration. The omentum is mobilized off the transverse colon. The vascular supply from the left gastroepiploic artery is preserved. The omentum is sutured into the pelvis as a carpet. It may serve as a recipient site for split-thickness skin graft.

trolytes from the urine. In general, use of the nonirradiated transverse colon is associated with fewer complications than ileal conduits.[28] Techniques for construction of various urinary conduits are detailed in Chapter 46.

More recently, continent conduits have been developed in an attempt to eliminate the incontinent urinary stoma. Although the Kock pouch has gained wide acceptance among urologists, this requires detubularization of a large segment of ileum,[12] which is often unsuitable because of adhesions and previous radiation therapy. The Miami or Indiana continent conduit uses detubularized ascending and transverse colon as a urinary reservoir.[15,23] The continence mechanism consists of tapered distal ileum reinforced with purse-string sutures at the ileocecal valve.

Before the continent conduit is performed, the hepatic flexure is divided and the ascending colon is mobilized off the retroperitoneal structures (Fig. 40-9, *A*). The omentum is mobilized off the transverse colon. Appendectomy is performed. A 10- to 14-cm segment of distal ileum is divided with staplers, and the mesentery is developed into pedicles (see Fig. 40-9, *A*). The ileocecal branch of the superior mesenteric artery must be preserved because it provides the blood supply to the colonic reservoir. The midtransverse colon is divided with staplers, and the mesentery is developed into pedicles. Usually, either the entire middle colic artery or at least the right branch of the middle colic artery is pre-

served (see Fig. 40-9, *A*) to provide additional perfusion of the reservoir.[15,23]

The colonic segment is detubularized by opening the colon along the anterior tinea (see Fig. 40-9, *B*). Direct mucosa-to-mucosa ureteral anastomosis is performed in the posterior wall over ureteral stents. The colonic defect is closed using a two-layer technique with absorbable sutures or stapled with absorbable staplers (see Fig. 40-9, *B*), folding the tip of the transverse colon to the cecum. The terminal ileum is tapered over a 12-Fr catheter (see Fig. 40-9, *B*), using serial applications of GIA staplers or suture to narrow the antimesenteric portion of the ileum.[15,23]

A double or triple purse-string suture of 2-0 silk is used to reinforce the ileocecal valve and provide continence (see Fig. 40-9, *C*).[15,23] The ureteral stents are brought out through a stab incision in the anterior colonic reservoir. The urinary conduit is brought to the skin through a full-thickness incision in the right lower quadrant or umbilicus. The ileocecal valve should be snug against the anterior abdominal wall, without twisting. Excess terminal ileum is trimmed and full-thickness sutures are used to anchor the conduit to the skin, without a formal rosebud stoma.

The ureteral stents and catheter are removed approximately 3 weeks after surgery, after radiographic studies have documented no leak or ureteral obstruction. The patient is instructed about intermittent catheterization and frequent

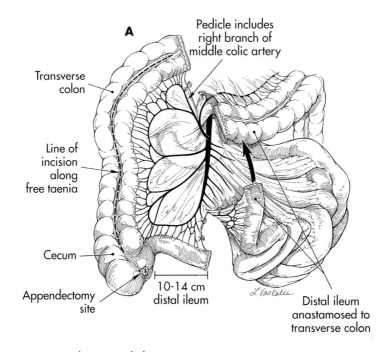

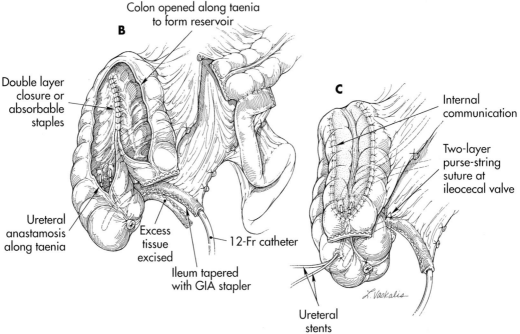

Fig. 40-9   Formation of a right colonic continent conduit. **A,** The distal ileum and right colon are isolated and mobilized. The terminal ileum and mid-transverse colon are divided with staplers. Appendectomy is performed. Either the entire middle colic artery or the main right branch of the middle colic artery (shown) is preserved. **B,** The colon is opened along the anterior tinea and detubularized using a double-layer closure or absorbable staples to approximate the bowel wall. The terminal ileum is tapered over a 12-Fr catheter with serial applications of the GIA stapler. **C,** Before the anterior wall of the reservoir is closed, the ureters are anastomosed along a tinea, and ureteral stents are brought out through the anterior wall. The ileocecal valve is reinforced with purse-string sutures to provide continence.

flushing of the conduit. Short-term results indicate no significant increase in complications related to use of this continent conduit, even in previously irradiated patients.[15,23]

COMPLICATIONS OF EXENTERATION

It is not surprising that serious morbidity occurs in approximately half of all patients undergoing pelvic exenteration.* Complications relating to comorbid medical conditions and more commonly performed gynecologic procedures are covered elsewhere in this text. Intraoperative complications are usually related to hemorrhage and problems related to the mechanics of the reconstructive phase of exenteration. Blood loss in excess of 2000 ml is not unusual. Management of intraoperative hemorrhage is discussed in Chapter 15. Surgery involving irradiated bowel and genitourinary tissues has a high incidence of obstruction or fistula formation, related to fibrostenosis of these tissues. Approximately one third of patients undergoing exenteration will develop a life-threatening surgical complication in the immediate or delayed postoperative period.[25,28] Usually reexploration and surgical correction during the immediate postoperative period are associated with a very high surgical mortality rate; therefore urologic or gastrointestinal complications are often managed conservatively.[4,28]

SUMMARY

Although pelvic exenteration remains a treatment of last resort and is associated with a high morbidity rate, current techniques are associated with survival of approximately half of all patients who undergo this operation. In most of these women, previous attempts to cure the malignancy have failed. Because of advances in surgical and supportive techniques, the operative mortality has decreased to between 5% and 10% and most patients who survive the malignancy are able to adapt to the changes in body image that are imposed by these procedures. Advances in reconstructive techniques have helped diminish the frequency and severity of surgical complications of exenteration. Increased application of rectosigmoid reanastomosis and performance of continent urinary conduits has increased the number of patients who are able to undergo this procedure without requiring a permanent colostomy or incontinent urostomy.

REFERENCES

1. Averette HA, et al: Pelvic exenteration: a 15 year experience in a general metropolitan hospital, *Am J Obstet Gynecol* 150:179, 1984.
2. Becker DW Jr, et al: Musculocutaneous flaps in reconstructive pelvic surgery, *Obstet Gynecol* 54:178, 1979.
3. Becker JS, et al: Vaginal reconstruction performed simultaneously with pelvic exenteration, *Obstet Gynecol* 63:318, 1984.
4. Bladou F, et al: Incidence and management of major urinary complications after pelvic exenteration for gynecologic malignancies, *J Surg Oncol* 58:91, 1995.
5. Bricker EM: Bladder substitution after pelvic evisceration, *Surg Clin North Am* 30:1511, 1950.
6. Brunschwig A: Complete excision of the pelvic viscera for advanced carcinoma, *Cancer* 1:177, 1948.
7. Cain JM, et al: The morbidity and benefits of concurrent gracilis myocutaneous graft with pelvic exenteration, *Obstet Gynecol* 74:185, 1989.
8. Copeland CJ, et al: Gracilis myocutaneous vaginal reconstruction concurrent with total pelvic exenteration, *Am J Obstet Gynecol* 160:1095, 1989.
9. Curry SL, et al: Pelvic exenteration: a 7-year experience, *Gynecol Oncol* 11:119, 1981.
10. Hatch KD: Construction of a neovagina after exenteration using the vulvobulbocavernosus myocutaneous graft, *Obstet Gynecol* 63:110, 1984.
11. Hatch KD, Mann WJ Jr: Exenterative surgery of the female pelvis. In Mann WJ Jr, Stovall TG, editors: *Gynecologic surgery*, New York, 1996, Churchill Livingstone, p 535.
12. Kock ND, et al: Urinary diversion via a continent ileal reservoir: clinical results in 12 patients, *J Urol* 128:469, 1982.
13. Lacy CG, et al: Vaginal reconstruction after exenteration with use of gracilis myocutaneous flaps: The University of California, San Francisco experience, *Am J Obstet Gynecol* 158:1278, 1988.
14. Magrina JF, et al: Vaginal reconstruction in gynecologic oncology: a review of techniques, *Obstet Gynecol Surg* 36:1, 1981.
15. Manuel RS, et al: Indiana pouch continent urinary reservoir in patients with previous pelvic irradiation, *Obstet Gynecol* 75:891, 1990.
16. McCraw JB, Arnold PJ, editors: *McCraw and Arnold's atlas of muscle and musculocutaneous flaps,* Norfolk, VA, 1986, Hampton Press.
17. McCraw JB, et al: Vaginal reconstruction with gracilis myocutaneous flaps, *Plast Reconstr Surg* 58:176, 1976.
18. McCraw JB, et al: Correction of high pelvic defects with the inferiorly based rectus abdominis myocutaneous flap, *Clin Plast Surg* 7:123, 1980.
19. Morley GW, et al: Vaginal reconstruction following pelvic exenteration: surgical and psychological considerations, *Am J Obstet Gynecol* 116:996, 1973.
20. Morley GW, et al: Pelvic exenteration, University of Michigan: 100 patients at 5 years, *Obstet Gynecol* 74:934, 1989.
21. Orr JW Jr, et al: Urinary diversion in patients undergoing pelvic exenteration, *Am J Obstet Gynecol* 142:883, 1982.
22. Orr JW Jr, et al: Gastrointestinal complications associated with pelvic exenteration, *Am J Obstet Gynecol* 145:325, 1983.
23. Penalver MA, et al: Continent urinary diversion in gynecologic oncology, *Gynecol Oncol* 34:274, 1989.
24. Pursell SH, et al: Distally-based rectus abdominis flap for reconstruction in radical gynecologic procedures, *Gynecol Oncol* 37:234, 1990.
25. Roberts WS, et al: Major morbidity after pelvic exenteration: a seven year experience, *Obstet Gynecol* 69:617, 1987.
26. Rutledge FN, et al: Pelvic exenteration: analysis of 296 patients, *Am J Obstet Gynecol* 129:881, 1977.
27. Soper JT: Grafts and flaps in gynecologic surgery. In Mann WJ Jr, Stovall TG, editors: *Gynecologic surgery,* New York, 1996, Churchill Livingstone.
28. Soper JT, et al: Pelvic exenteration: factors associated with major surgical morbidity, *Gynecol Oncol* 35:93, 1989.
29. Soper JT, et al: Short gracilis myocutaneous flaps for vulvovaginal reconstruction after radical pelvic surgery, *Obstet Gynecol* 74:823, 1989.
30. Stanhope CR, et al: Palliative exenteration what, when and why? *Am J Obstet Gynecol* 152:12, 1985.
31. Taylor GI, et al The versatile deep inferior epigastric (inferior rectus abdominis) flap, *Br J Plast Surg* 37:330, 1984.
32. Tobin GR, et al: Vaginal and pelvic reconstruction with distally based rectus abdominis myocutaneous flaps, *Plast Reconstr Surg* 81:62, 1988.
33. Wheeless CR Jr: *Atlas of pelvic surgery*, ed 2, Philadelphia, 1988, Lea & Febiger, 1988.

*References 4, 7, 21, 22, 25, 28.

41 Hysteroscopy

CHARLES M. MARCH

The exact incidence of infertility and pregnancy wastage caused by structural uterine abnormalities is unknown. However, such pathologic conditions have been identified in 5% to 10% of infertile couples and in up to one third of women with recurrent pregnancy loss. Although intrauterine defects have been found in 13% of asymptomatic women undergoing surgical sterilization, up to 62% of patients who are infertile have been reported to have lesions.[11,84] Losses in the second trimester and early in the third trimester are likely to be caused by congenital anomalies and submucosal myomas.

Before the advent of hysteroscopy, gynecologists could investigate the uterine cavity only indirectly. Although members of other surgical specialties such as orthopedics and urology have considered endoscopy to be one of their indispensable diagnostic and therapeutic tools, gynecologists have not embraced hysteroscopy with the same enthusiasm. Table 41-1 demonstrates the differences between the urinary bladder and the uterus with respect to endoscopy and highlights the limitations that uterine anatomy places on gynecologists. Thus, for many decades, we used only hysterosalpingography, ultrasound, curettage, and the limited palpatory sensations afforded by the tip of a uterine sound to detect intrauterine pathologic conditions. Although the deficiencies of these different approaches have been known, difficulties with adequate illumination and the lack of suitable uterine distending media hindered acceptance of hysteroscopy, a procedure described in 1869 by Pantaleoni.[64]

Cold-light fiberoptics solved the problem with illumination. However, only after Edström and Fernström[22] demonstrated the feasibility of using a highly viscous dextran solution to provide both uterine distention and a clear view even in the presence of blood and cellular debris did hysteroscopy emerge as a valuable procedure with many applications.

Hysteroscopy not only permits the nature of a lesion suggested by ultrasound or hysterography to be confirmed but also allows the surgeon to plan therapy and to assess the defect's proximity to tubal ostia or the internal cervical os. All of these benefits accrue without exposure to radiation. A comparison of hysterosalpingography (HSG) and hysteroscopy is shown in Table 41-2. These two studies should be considered complementary rather than competing or mutually exclusive. The advantages of hysteroscopy make it the first choice for patients who are likely to have uterine pathologic conditions. However, as a screening procedure, HSG is preferred for those physicians who do not have office hysteroscopy available. In addition, for infertile patients the additional information about the fallopian tubes that can only be obtained by HSG makes this procedure invaluable.

INDICATIONS
Sterilization

The first widespread application of hysteroscopy was transcervical sterilization under direct visualization (see the box on p. 739). Although this application remains investigational and therefore is outside the scope of this chapter, a brief summary is warranted. Fulguration of the tubal ostia was adopted as a rapid, simple method of achieving tubal closure.[66] However, this technique has a high failure rate and is associated with many ectopic pregnancies, especially intramural pregnancies.[15] Excessive thermal damage to the intramural portion of the tube has been postulated as the cause of this complication.[50] A variety of plugs, implants, and sclerosing agents have had an unacceptably low rate of success.[24,75] Formed-in-place silicone plugs have been approved in some European countries, but adequate data were never available to permit approval in the United States.[48,69]

Reproductive Failure

Unexplained infertility and recurrent abortion continue to frustrate gynecologists and their patients. Although it was believed that direct inspection of the uterine cavity in women with normal hysterograms would provide important information about the preimplantation phase of the endometrium and thus provide clues to diagnosis and treatment, this hope has not been realized. Although the correlation between the presumptive diagnosis of a uterine abnormality detected by HSG and the definitive diagnosis established by hysteroscopy is excellent, discrepancies do occur.[76,79] If the properly performed hysterogram is normal and if no new symptoms have developed nor intrauterine surgery performed since the last HSG had been obtained, hysteroscopy

Table 41-1 Endoscopy of the Uterus and Urinary Bladder

Uterus	Urinary Bladder
Virtual cavity, thick muscle	Thin muscle
Distended by high pressure	Distended by gavity only
Fragile lining, bleeds easily	Resistant epithelium
Cyclic epithelial changes	None
Communicates with peritoneal cavity	No communication

Table 41-2 Comparison of Hysterosalpingography and Hysteroscopy

Hysterosalpingography	Hysteroscopy
Outlined by contrast	Direct view of cavity
Presumptive diagnosis	Definitive diagnosis
Localization difficult	Lesion location mapped
No surgery possible	Surgery possible
Tubal study also	Uterine evaluation only
Low cost	Moderate cost
Minimal radiation	No radiation

is unnecessary.[26] However, if any of the necessary elements of that radiographic study are absent (long axis of the uterus parallel to the film plate, view of endocervical canal, view of the uterus during the early filling phase, or absence of uterine contractions that obscure the upper fundus) or if a cavity defect is present, hysteroscopy is a mandatory step in the evaluation of the infertile woman, all those with recurrent abortion, and the patient with only one second trimester loss. Obviously, the iodine contrast media for hysterography should not be introduced via a balloon catheter, which would obscure the lower uterine segment and endocervical canal.

Intrauterine Pathologic Conditions

Hysteroscopy is used to establish the presence of the following intrauterine pathologic conditions.

1. Intrauterine adhesions can be diagnosed definitively and their extent classified. Synechiae can be lysed completely and safely under direct vision. The success of treatment can be evaluated by repeat hysteroscopy (or HSG) at a later date.
2. The nature and extent of congenital uterine anomalies can be defined if hysteroscopy is combined with laparoscopy. A treatment plan can then be formulated. The septate uterus can be unified and the results assessed by a follow-up hysteroscopy or HSG.
3. Embedded intrauterine devices (IUDs) can be visualized and removed under direct vision, thereby minimizing endometrial trauma.
4. Endometrial polyps can be differentiated from submucous leiomyomas, which is not always possible by HSG. The polyps should be excised under direct vision and then their bases should be curetted or fulgurated to reduce the risk of recurrence.

INDICATIONS FOR HYSTEROSCOPY

I. Sterilization
II. Reproductive failure
   A. Unexplained infertility
   B. Recurrent abortion
III. Intrauterine pathologic conditions
   A. Confirm abnormal HSG
   B. Intrauterine adhesions
   C. Congenital anomalies
   D. Embedded intrauterine devices (IUDs)
   E. Abnormal bleeding
      1. Polyps
      2. Myomas
      3. Carcinoma
      4. Endometrial ablation/resection
   F. Proximal tubal obstruction
   G. Assisted reproductive technologies

---

5. Submucous leiomyomas can be differentiated from polyps, their extent can be evaluated, and biopsy or resection can be performed. If pedunculated, the lesion can be excised completely.
6. In cases of abnormal bleeding, structural abnormalities of the uterine cavity can be detected and classified so that appropriate medical or surgical treatment can be used. Malignancies occasionally missed by curettage can be diagnosed. Endometrial carcinoma can be staged more accurately than by fractional curettage. Endometrial ablation and/or resection can be performed.
7. In some patients with proximal tubal obstruction, only a small portion of the intramural segment of tube is occluded, and the placement of a series of wires and catheters in a coaxial fashion under hysteroscopic and laparoscopic guidance may achieve patency. As an extension of hysteroscopy, falloposcopy has been recommended as a method of evaluating the endosalpinx before surgery or gamete intrafallopian transfer (GIFT). This technique appears very promising.

INSTRUMENTATION
Hysteroscopes

Hysteroscopes are of three types: rigid panoramic, rigid contact, and "flexible" panoramic. Most panoramic hysteroscopes are modified cystoscopes. The telescope may have an outer diameter of 2.7 to 4.0 mm. The telescope may have a 0-degree viewing angle and thus provide a straight-on view or may have a Foroblique lens that is offset from the horizontal by 12, 15, 25, or 30 degrees. Some telescopes have a focusing knob that allows them to be used as a contact device. Others allow magnification. The sheaths for panoramic hysteroscopes may be 3.3 to 4.5 mm in diameter and are only for diagnostic use. These are ideally suited for office work without anesthesia or after a paracervical block has been introduced. For operative hysteroscopy, 5.0- to 8-mm sheaths are available to permit the placement of one or two accessory instruments. One hysteroscope (Fig. 41-1) has two accessory channels. In its sheath the four channels (telescope, medium, and two accessory) are completely isolated from one another; this is one of a number of panoramic hysteroscopes that can provide true continuous flow. Some sheaths have a modification at their distal end, the Albarran bridge, which allows the accessory instrument to be deflected toward a lesion. This modification is especially valuable for patients whose tubal ostia are eccentrically placed and who wish to have transcervical tubal surgery—sterilization or relief of proximal tubal obstruction. Another operating panoramic hysteroscope has an offset eyepiece and accepts rigid accessory instruments.

Two hysteroscopes can be considered "mini" or "micro" hysteroscopes. Both are 0-degree fiberoptic telescopes. One is 1.2 mm and has a 2.5-mm diagnostic sheath. This telescope may also be used with a 3.7-mm operating sheath, which accepts 4-Fr instruments or 5-mm continuous flow inner-outer sheath combination. The flexible fiberoptic hysteroscope from Imagyn is 1.6 mm, is enclosed in a disposable sheath, and uses a low viscosity liquid medium for uterine distention.

The microcolpohysteroscope provides a magnified view of the endocervix and uterine cavity and may be useful in evaluating patients with cervical intraepithelial neoplasia lesions that extend into the canal.[35] If the full extent of the lesion can be seen, directed biopsy may reduce the need for conization.

The contact hysteroscope (Fig. 41-2) is an office instrument that is valuable for diagnosing all types of intrauterine pathologic conditions, but not for therapy.[2] The hallmark of contact hysteroscopy is simplicity. Neither a light source nor distending medium is necessary. Two instruments are available: one with a 6-mm diameter and one of 8 mm. The former is favored because it requires less cervical dilation. Biopsy/grasping forceps that fit over the 6-mm endoscope can be used to remove embedded IUDs. A focusing device

that increases the depth of field is a mandatory attachment. Because the contact hysteroscope does not provide a panoramic view of the cavity, most physicians find it more difficult to master than the panoramic hysteroscope. Achieving complete inspection of the cavity requires discipline and patience. However, its simplicity of use and maintenance makes the contact hysteroscope a valuable and convenient diagnostic tool. It may also be used as a cystoscope, an amnioscope, and a vaginoscope.

"Flexible" hysteroscopes (Fig. 41-3) are not truly flexible but rather steerable.[45] The outer diameter varies between 3.5 and 4.8 mm, and the distal end can be deflected over an arc of 130 to 160 degrees. Rotating the entire instrument makes it possible to view the entire cavity. The 1-mm media channel can be used to deliver either carbon dioxide (CO_2) or 5% glucose in water. The larger flexible hysteroscope can be used for surgery and has a 2-mm operating channel for biopsy forceps and microscissors. The view afforded by flexible hysteroscopes that are composed of multiple fibers rather than a single rod-lens system is somewhat inferior to that obtained by a rigid telescope, but because the leading edge can be maneuvered around lesions and because it can provide a parallel view of even the most eccentrically placed tubal ostium, this instrument can help cannulate tubes and deliver a balloon to relieve obstruction or a plug or chemical to cause sterilization.

The choice of hysteroscope depends on the goals of the user and the needs of the patient. All instruments have a role, and the "complete" hysteroscopist will be able to use all types well.

Ancillary Equipment

The ancillary equipment available includes an aspirating cannula, biopsy forceps, scissors, alligator-jaw grasping forceps, and monopolar or bipolar electrodes. The aspirating cannula and electrodes are both flexible and are 5 to 7 Fr. The aspirating cannula is really an essential instrument rather than an accessory one. Because blood and cellular debris may be present before the hysteroscopy is begun or as a

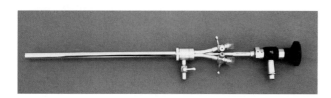

Fig. 41-1 Double channel hysteroscope.

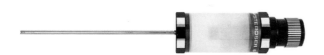

Fig. 41-2 Contact hysteroscope.

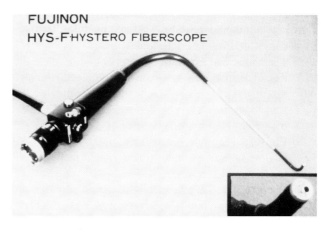

Fig. 41-3 "Flexible" hysteroscope.

consequence of intrauterine surgery, a method of maintaining a clear field of view is important. Even though dextran media are not miscible with blood and continuous-flow instruments permit thorough rinsing of the cavity, an aspirating catheter permits pinpoint clearing of certain regions, especially the cornual recesses and tubal ostia.

Scissors can be used to incise a septum, to lyse adhesions, or to excise a polyp or pedunculated submucosal myoma. Biopsy forceps should be used to document the histology of any lesion that is not resected. Alligator-jaw grasping forceps can retrieve retained IUDs or other foreign bodies. All of these instruments can be flexible, semirigid, or rigid, depending on the sheath used. Rigid instruments are the most durable. They can be used with an offset eyepiece hysteroscope or can be an integral part of the sheath. The latter instruments are called optical hysteroscopes. The forceps or scissors remain a fixed distance in front of the telescope and cannot be moved. Because depth of field is poor with monocular instruments, this class of instrument may be associated with an increased risk of uterine perforation and a relative inability to approach eccentrically placed lesions.

Coagulation can be obtained via flexible electrodes or a fiber to deliver laser energy from an argon or neodymium:yttrium-argon-garnet (Nd:YAG) source. The latter can use a bare 600-mm fiber or one with a sapphire tip. If the latter is used, the tip *cannot* be cooled with gas. Electrodes may be unipolar or bipolar. A bipolar electrode can be used in an electrolyte-containing solution and can be used for control of bleeding and for resection of myomas or polyps. This electrode may also be suitable for endometrial ablation.

A four-pronged "cervical-sealing" tenaculum, which reduces the leakage of medium through a patulous cervix, is well designed and permits the telescope to be passed through its prongs.[29] At the base of each prong is a broad ball, which limits the depth of penetration of the prong and exerts pressure against any vessel that may have been punctured. A simple bivalve speculum with only one attachment between both blades permits it to be removed easily after insertion of the telescope, thereby reducing patient discomfort.

Resectoscope

The urologic resectoscope has been modified for use by the gynecologist (Fig. 41-4). This instrument has inner and outer sheaths to provide continuous flow of the low-viscosity medium. Although this instrument can be used with only the inner sheath, which has an insulated tip, most gynecologic surgeons prefer the continuous-flow instrument because of its ability to clear the operative field of blood and cellular debris. Commercially available resectoscopes have outer sheath sizes between 22 and 27 Fr. The medium is instilled via the inner sheath into the uterus and then flows out via perforations in the outer sheath. Either gravity or suction can be used to withdraw the medium. Most instrument companies have modified the outflow sheath by placing outflow holes around the entire sheath.

The FemRx disposable resectoscope sheath can be adapted to most manufacturers' telescopes. This unit permits continuous aspiration of tissue fragments, which are morselized within the fluid return path. Saline can be used as the distending medium, and the electrode can cut or ablate tissue.

The Working Element. The electrodes extend a maximum of 4 cm beyond the end of the outer sheath. Two types of working elements are available to extend and retract the electrodes over that distance—two-handed and one-handed mechanisms. The two-handed mechanism, exemplified by the Stern-McCarty unit, works on a rack and pinion lever. Two types of one-handed models are the Baumrucker and Iglesias mechanisms, both of which use a spring mechanism.

The most common electrodes used in gynecologic surgery are the roller ball and the cutting loop. A number of variations of the roller ball with a bar or cylinder configuration are available, ranging in diameter from 2 mm upward. The cutting loops available are generally between 5 and 8 mm in outer diameter. One modified roller bar electrode has deep grooves, which permit very high-energy contact points, allowing myomas to be vaporized (Fig. 41-5). If this electrode is used, a representative sample should be obtained so that the pathologist can verify that the tumor is benign. Another electrode with application in gynecology is the knife, useful in cutting septa and synechiae. The bipolar Versapoint electrode permits electrosurgery to be performed with an electrolyte-containing medium such as normal saline or lactated Ringer's solution, thereby eliminating the risk of electrolyte imbalance, a potentially lethal complication of low-viscosity media. This electrode is used with a continuous-flow hysteroscope, not a resectoscope.

Conversion to Operating Hysteroscope. The Circon/ACMI resectoscope allows the outflow sheath mechanism to be converted to use as an operating hysteroscope by use of a bridge. This bridge allows the surgeon to use a 7-Fr operating channel for insertion of semirigid instruments or a laser fiber.

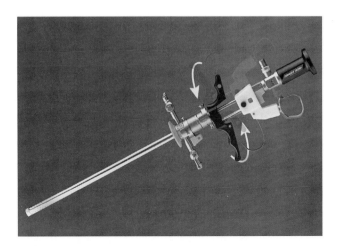

Fig. 41-4 Continuous-flow gynecologic resectoscope.

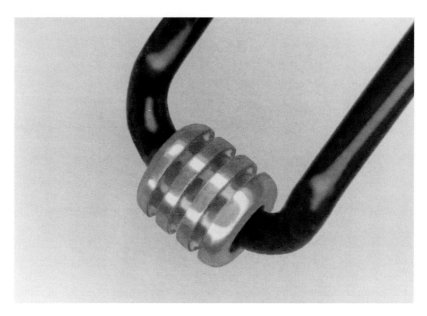

Fig. 41-5   Electrode for vaporizing myomas.

TECHNIQUE

Hysteroscopy may be performed at any time during the menstrual cycle except during menses. However, visualization is best within 2 to 3 days after the cessation of menstrual flow. The endometrium is thin early in the cycle, but later the tubal ostia may become obscured by endometrial growth. In addition, the endometrium is less friable in the early proliferative phase. If hysteroscopy is performed during the secretary phase, the couple must use adequate contraception.

Hysteroscopy may be performed in the office. For both patients and physicians, office hysteroscopy is invaluable (Table 41-3). The ability to provide a diagnosis almost instantaneously reduces patient anxiety, allows a treatment plan to be formulated quickly, and is easily accommodated into even the busiest patient and physician schedules. Minor procedures can be performed, thereby freeing up the operating room for more difficult procedures. Cost is reduced, and patient safety is maintained. No special preoperative instructions or tests are necessary. For patients with a history of pelvic infection, a cervical culture should be obtained before surgery. Pelvic tenderness should be considered possible evidence of infection and may dictate postponing the procedure. For most patients, prophylactic antibiotics are unnecessary. For brief procedures, premedication with 600 mg of ibuprofen is sufficient. If a longer or more difficult hysteroscopy is anticipated, intravenous (IV) meperidine, midazolam, propofol, or diazepam should be given for sedation. Concurrence with conscious sedation protocols will assure patient safety. The use of these drugs mandates that the patient leave the office in the care of another. If general or regional anesthesia is necessary, an outpatient surgical unit provides an adequate setting and the patient may be discharged in a few hours.

Table 41-3   Advantages of Office Hysteroscopy

For the Patient	For the Physician
More convenient	Less paperwork
More rapid diagnosis	Easily accommodated
Less preoperative evaluation	Greater productivity
Less frightening	No extra preoperative or postoperative visits
Equal safety	Minor surgery possible
Faster recovery	Simplifies operating schedule

Before application of the cervical tenaculum and introduction of the paracervical block, the cervix is sprayed with 20% benzocaine. After introduction of a paracervical block with 5 ml of 1% chloroprocaine without epinephrine into each uterosacral ligament, the uterine cavity is sounded. If necessary, the cervix is then dilated to between 2 and 8 mm, and the hysteroscope is engaged in the external os and advanced into the uterine cavity only if the view is clear. A 2.5-mm sheath is used if the procedure is to be diagnostic only, and a 5- to 8-mm sheath is used for operative procedures. Because the anterior and posterior uterine walls are in apposition, the cavity must be distended by one of three different types of media (described in the following section) to ensure proper visualization. After inspection of the endocervical canal and lower uterine segment, the hysteroscope is advanced into the cavity, and the lateral walls, upper fundus, both cornual recesses, and both tubal ostia are inspected in a systematic fashion. If necessary, scissors may be introduced through the operating channel of the hysteroscope for lysis of minimal synechiae. In addition, polyps may be excised, a biopsy may be performed on an area of atypical endometrium, and embedded IUDs may be removed. Resection of myomas or lysis of moderate or severe adhesions requires general or regional anesthesia. If a uterine division is found, simultaneous laparoscopy is necessary to differentiate the bicornuate from the septate anomaly. If the anomaly proves to be septate, the laparoscopist will guide the hysteroscopist in treating the defect and preventing uterine perforation.

MEDIA
Low Viscosity

An inexpensive medium is 5% glucose in water. It is introduced via an IV infusion bag. The rate of flow is controlled by gravity or by increasing the infusion pressure by a hand pump or a pressure cuff. The high-volume, high-flow-rate system of delivery increases uterine cramping and thus hinders the use of this medium for office procedures. Another disadvantage of this type of medium is that it mixes with blood, thus obscuring vision. Normal saline, Ringer's lactate, 3.3% sorbitol, or 1.5% glycine may also be used for hysteroscopy and have the same attributes and limitations as glucose in water.[36] Electrolyte-containing media cannot be used if an electrosurgical procedure is planned unless a bipolar electrode is used. A laser fiber can also be used in a medium that contains electrolytes.

Carbon Dioxide

A special insufflator is required (the CO_2 insufflator used to create the pneumoperitoneum for laparoscopy *must not* be used).[47] CO_2 is instilled at a flow rate of 25 to 100 ml/min at a maximum pressure of 200 mm Hg. Because the refractile index of CO_2 is 1.00, the appearance of the tissue is more "true to life" than with other media.[46] There is less magnification than with other media because of the lower index of refraction of CO_2. A patulous cervix limits the ability to maintain adequate uterine distention. During prolonged procedures, up to 500 ml of CO_2 may be needed to compensate for both absorption and spill into the peritoneal cavity. Intraperitoneal CO_2 will cause shoulder pain when the patient resumes an erect position. This medium is perfectly suited for office diagnostic procedures.

High Viscosity

Dextran, being immiscible with blood, provides excellent visualization. It is instilled via a 50-ml syringe attached to large-diameter (5-mm) infusion tubing. Wide-bore tubing facilitates the introduction of this viscous medium. Intermittent delivery of 5- to 10-ml volumes to enhance visualization results in less uterine cramping. This medium is very difficult to remove from instruments; thus instruments *must* be rinsed immediately after the procedure with copious amounts of hot water. Two forms of dextran have been used for hysteroscopy. The first, Rheomacrodex, is a 10% dextran solution with a molecular weight of 40,000 Da in 5% glucose in water. The second, Hyskon Hysteroscopy Fluid, is a 32% dextran solution with a molecular weight of 70,000 Da in 10% glucose in water. This medium was developed specifically for use in hysteroscopy.[22] The excellent clarity and

Table 41-4 Classification of Intrauterine Adhesions by Hysteroscopic Findings

Class	Findings
Severe	More than three fourths of uterine cavity involved; agglutination of walls or thick bands; ostial areas and upper cavity occluded
Moderate	One fourth to three fourths of uterine cavity involved; no agglutination of walls, adhesions only; ostial areas and upper fundus only partially occluded
Minimal	Less than one fourth of uterine cavity involved; thin or filmy adhesions; ostial areas and upper fundus minimally involved or clear

From March CM, Israel R, March AD: *Am J Obstet Gynecol* 130:653, 1978.

minimal equipment needed make Hyskon the medium of choice for operative hysteroscopy. Almost all examinations can be completed with one 100-ml bottle. For difficult operative procedures, much larger volumes may be necessary, but the total amount absorbed should not exceed 250 ml.

CONTRAINDICATIONS

The absolute contraindications to hysteroscopy are acute pelvic infection, invasive cervical cancer, and inadequate equipment or training. Active uterine bleeding, pregnancy, a recent uterine perforation, and uterine cancer are relative contraindications. If Hyskon is used to distend the uterine cavity, a satisfactory examination can usually be accomplished even if the patient is bleeding heavily. If the low-viscosity media are used in a continuous-flow system, similar results can be obtained because the blood and cellular debris will be flushed from the cavity. The contact hysteroscope may also be used in patients with a recent uterine perforation. Although hysteroscopy may be used to diagnose and stage cancer, the potential for tumor dissemination has prevented its widespread use. This theoretical objection does not apply if contact hysteroscopy is performed and is of lesser concern if CO_2 is used for panoramic hysteroscopy. CO_2 has been shown to lead to reflux of endometrial cells much less often compared with a liquid medium.[4,67]

SPECIFIC PROCEDURES
Intrauterine Adhesions

Lysis of adhesions under direct vision is safer and more complete than blind curettage or hysterotomy. Before adhesiolysis is begun, the extent of the disease is classified (Table 41-4 and Fig. 41-6).[1,54] Under hysteroscopic guidance, it is possible to cut only scar tissue, thereby sparing adjacent normal endometrium and permitting it to be a source for endometrial regrowth over the freshly dissected surfaces. Each adhesive band is identified and divided with miniature scissors (Fig. 41-7). Restoration of normal uterine architecture can be achieved even in women with complete

THE AMERICAN FERTILITY SOCIETY CLASSIFICATION OF INTRAUTERINE ADHESIONS

Patient's Name _____ Date _____ Chart # _____

Age _____ G _____ P _____ Sp Ab _____ VTP _____ Ectopic _____ Infertile Yes _____ No _____

Other Signficant History (i.e. surgery, infection, etc.) _____

_____

HSG _____ Sonography _____ Photography _____ Laparoscopy _____ Laparotomy _____

Extent of Cavity Involved	<1/3	1/3 -2/3	>2/3
	1	2	4
Type of Adhesions	Filmy	Filmy & Dense	Dense
	1	2	4
Menstrual Pattern	Normal	Hypomenorrhea	Amenorrhea
	0	2	4

Prognostic Classification   HSG*   Hysteroscopy   Additional Findings: _____
                             Score   Score

Stage I   (Mild)   1-4   _____   _____   _____
Stage II   (Moderate) 5-8   _____   _____   _____
Stage III (Severe)   9-12   _____   _____   _____
*All adhesions should be considered dense

Treatment (Surgical Procedures): _____

_____

_____

_____

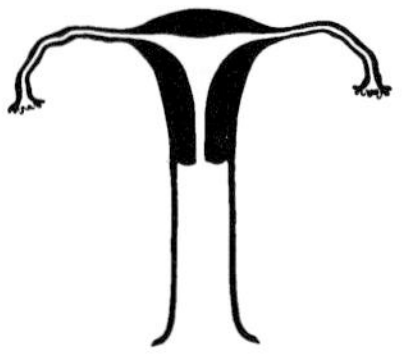

Prognosis for Conception & Subsequent Viable Infant*
_____ Excellent (> 75%)
_____ Good   (50% - 75%)
_____ Fair   (25% - 50%)
_____ Poor   (< 25%)
*Physician's judgment based upon tubal patency.

Recommended Followup Treatment: _____

_____

_____

Property of
The American Fertility Society

Drawing

HSG Findings

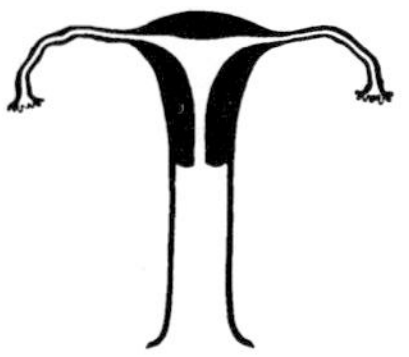

Hysteroscopy Findings

For additional supply write to:
The American Fertility Society
2140 11th Avenue, South
Suite 200
Birmingham, Alabama 35205

Fig. 41-6   AFS Classification of intrauterine adhesions. (From American Fertility Society: The American Fertility Society classification of adnexal adhesions, distal tubal occlusion, tubal occlusion secondary to tubal ligation, tubal pregnancies, müllerian anomalies and intrauterine adhesions, *Fertil Steril* 49:944, 1988.)

uterine obliteration. However, patients who have very extensive disease should undergo simultaneous laparoscopy. The laparoscopist will guide the hysteroscopist to reduce the risk of uterine perforation. If the intensity of the light source for the laparoscope is reduced greatly, the laparoscopist will more readily detect dissection into the myometrium because the light of the hysteroscope will begin to shine brightly through the uterine serosa at a single point. In contrast, after the cavity's configuration has been restored, the uterus will have a uniform glow. After adhesiolysis, an inflatable splint (Fig. 41-8) is placed in the cavity and retained for 5 to 7 days. During this time period, a broad-spectrum antibiotic is prescribed. Postoperative use of a splint may reduce the chances that the raw dissected surfaces will readhere.[51] This

same splint may also be used to tamponade bleeding points if some degree of myometrial dissection has occurred.

Rock et al.[73] described a technique of simultaneous laparoscopy and hysteroscopy for the treatment of patients with extensive lower uterine segment and midfundal adhesions who have a small normal upper fundal "pocket." Under laparoscopic guidance, methylene blue is introduced into that pocket via a needle. The hysteroscopist then searches for and dissects toward the trail of blue dye to reach the upper cavity.

Conjugated equine estrogens (2.5 to 5 mg/day) are given to all patients for 30 to 60 days, and medroxyprogesterone acetate (10 mg) is added during the last 5 days of estrogen therapy.[51] The dosage and duration of the estrogen therapy

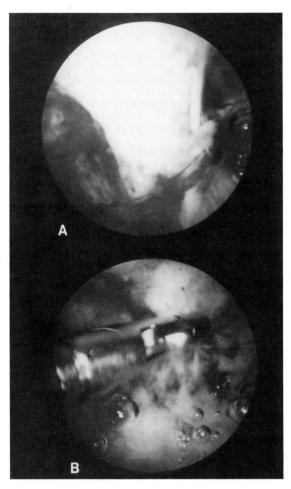

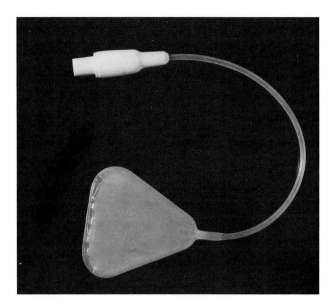

Fig. 41-8 Inflatable intrauterine splint used to maintain separation of uterine walls after adhesiolysis.

Fig. 41-7 **A,** Intrauterine scar as seen through the hysteroscope. **B,** Division of scar using miniature scissors. (From March CM: Hysteroscopy and the uterine factor in infertility. In Lobo RA, Mishell DR Jr, Paulson RJ, et al, editors: *Mishell's textbook of infertility, contraception and reproductive endocrinology,* ed 4, Cambridge, MA, 1997, Blackwell Scientific.)

Table 41-5 Results of Lysis of Intrauterine Adhesions Using Hysteroscopy

Before		After	
Findings	**No. of Patients**	**Findings**	**No. of Patients**
Amenorrhea	183	Normal menses	168
		Hypomenorrhea	6
		Amenorrhea	9
Hypomenorrhea	50	Normal menses	48
Infertile	119	Conceived	90

Table 41-6 Principles of Treating Intrauterine Adhesions

Goal	Method
Restore normal uterine architecture	Hysteroscopic lysis
Prevent readherence	Splint
Promote endometrial overgrowth	High-dose estrogen
Verify uterine normalcy	Follow-up hysteroscopy or hysterosalpingography

are adjusted depending on the extent of adhesion formation. High-dose sequential estrogen-progestin therapy maximally stimulates the endometrium so that the previously scarred surfaces are reepithelialized. The adequacy of therapy should be assessed accurately by repeat hysteroscopy or by HSG after the steroid-induced withdrawal bleeding. If the HSG is normal, complete resolution may be presumed. However, an abnormal HSG does not definitively indicate persistent adhesions and the hysteroscopy should be repeated.

The results of this approach to the first 275 patients with intrauterine adhesions (IUAs) are summarized in Table 41-5. Of the 183 patients who originally had symptoms of secondary amenorrhea, 168 have cyclic, spontaneous, painless menses of normal flow and duration; 6 have hypomenorrhea; and 9 have remained amenorrheic. Of the 50 who had hypomenorrhea before therapy, 48 have normal menses. After one hysteroscopic treatment, 90% of our patients have had a normal follow-up hysteroscopy or HSG. Although most of the others have needed a second procedure only to

restore normal uterine architecture, a few women have needed three to six operations. Therefore our approach to patients with IUAs is four pronged (Table 41-6). The importance of a postoperative study to verify normalcy of the cavity before permitting conception cannot be overemphasized. Severe obstetric complications have been reported in patients who conceived before postoperative studies were performed to document complete resolution of the adhe-

Table 41-7   Gestational Outcome after Treatment for Intrauterine Adhesions*

Method	No. of Pregnancies	First or Second Trimester Losses No. (%)	Term No. (%)
Traditional*	369	104 (28)	147 (40)
Hysteroscopic	99	14 (14)	85 (86)

From Jewelwicz R, et al: *Obstet Gynecol* 47:701, 1976. Reprinted with permission from The American College of Obstetricians and Gynecologists.

*Includes blind disruption of adhesions; data gathered from the literature. Hysteroscopic data are from the author's series.

Table 41-8   Successful Pregnancy Rates after Lysis of Adhesions in Patients with Prior Poor Outcome

Reference	Pretreatment	Posttreatment
52	14/84 (16.7%)	33/38 (86.8%)
86	8/266 (3.0%)	85/95 (89.5%)
42	189/484 (39.0%)	77/113 (68.1%)
10	40/122 (32.8%)	28/33 (84.8%)
63	9/57 (15.8%)	14/20 (70.0%)
Total	260/1013 (25.7%)	237/299 (79.3%)

sions.[27] It is likely that these women had persistent disease, causing the subsequent obstetric problems.

The pregnancy results with the approach are excellent and surpass those with other types of therapy[40,52] (Table 41-7). Of these 275 patients, 119 wished to conceive and had no other known infertility factors. Of the 119, 90 (75%) conceived 99 times, and 85 (86%) of the 99 pregnancies went to term. Placental complications were mild and unusual. Two patients had placenta previa, and two required manual removal of the placenta. A fifth patient had retained placental fragments, which were detected when a curettage was performed to stop hemorrhage 3 weeks after delivery. After hysteroscopic adhesiolysis, her follow-up HSG had been abnormal but she conceived before another hysteroscopic procedure could be performed. The results of this management plan are superior to those achieved by outdated treatment modalities such as blind disruption of adhesions by a sound or curette.

Among patients with prior poor obstetric outcomes and in whom the diagnosis of IUAs was made, hysteroscopic therapy has improved the prognosis dramatically (Table 41-8). The data from this medical center include only those who had a complete evaluation for recurrent abortion and in whom no factor other than IUA was found. Among this group, 86.8% of pregnancies resulted in an infant who survived compared to 16.7% before therapy.

Congenital Anomalies

Uterine anomalies are found in 1% to 2% of all women, in 4% of infertile women, and in 10% to 15% of women with recurrent spontaneous pregnancy loss before 20 weeks.[6]

Congenital uterine anomalies may be classified as follows:

1. Unicornuate: complete developmental arrest of one müllerian duct.
2. Didelphic: a complete lack of fusion, with duplication of corpus and cervix. The duplication may extend into the vagina. This anomaly is associated with premature delivery and abnormal presentations.
3. Bicornuate: partial lack of fusion and associated with a single or septate cervix. The defect is manifested externally and internally. This is the most common anomaly and is associated with malpresentations and premature delivery.
4. Septate: a partial lack of resorption of the midline septum. In some, the upper cavity is normal.[80] This defect is manifested internally only. It may be associated with a septate cervix. This is the anomaly most often associated with recurrent first trimester abortions.[72]
5. Arcuate: a very mild, asymptomatic form of septate uterus. It is a hysterographic or hysteroscopic diagnosis only and has no reproductive consequences.
6. Rudimentary horn: incomplete development of one horn. The horn may be either communicating or noncommunicating. The latter is more common. Rudimentary horns may or may not have functioning endometrium.

Abortion and obstetric problems such as premature labor and abnormal fetal presentations are the most common symptoms in patients with uterine anomalies.[77] Uterine defects have not been proven to cause primary infertility. Although two thirds of pregnancies in women with uterine duplications progress to term, abortion has been reported to occur in as many as 30% of pregnancies in women with septate uteri.[37] If the endometrium present in a noncommunicating rudimentary horn is functional, recurrent abdominal pain, hematometra, and even rupture simulating an ectopic pregnancy may occur. Longitudinal vaginal septa, which are usually asymptomatic, may be found alone or combined with other müllerian anomalies, especially uterus didelphys. Some patients with a septate vagina have one side obstructed; thus the outflow of one uterus is restricted to a variable degree, and a mass forms as a result of hydrocolpos and/or hematocolpos.

HSG and hysteroscopy (Fig. 41-9) can be used to delineate uterine defects and serve as a baseline before treatment. The HSG also provides information regarding tubal patency. Before metroplasty, a complete investigation is mandatory so that other infertility factors and other causes of recurrent abortion can be ruled out.

Only the anomalies related to in utero diethylstilbestrol (DES) exposure and the septate uterus are definitely associated with early reproductive failure. A uterine septum is not usually an indication for surgery in infertile patients because

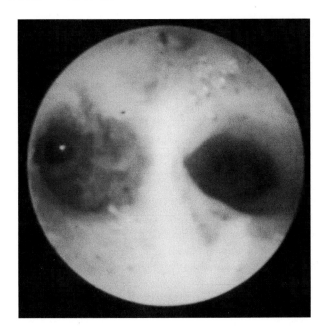

Fig. 41-9 Hysteroscopic view of uterine septum. (From March CM: Hysteroscopy and the uterine factor in infertility. In Lobo RA, Mishell DR Jr, Paulson RJ, et al, editors: *Mishell's textbook of infertility, contraception and reproductive endocrinology,* ed 4, Cambridge, MA, 1997, Blackwell Scientific.)

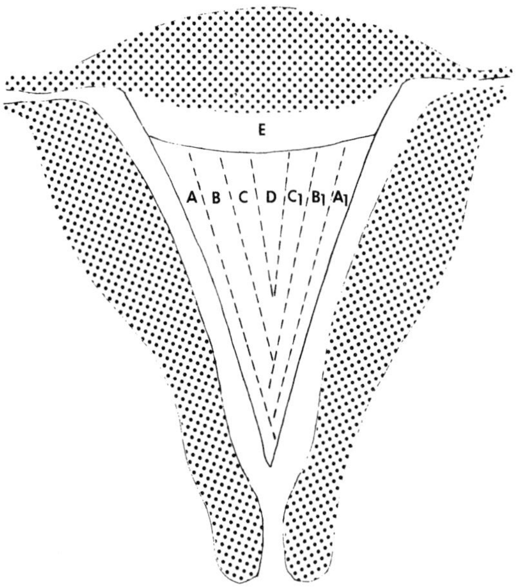

Fig. 41-10 Diagram of surgical approach to wide uterine septum. Sequential incisions are made through all of area A, then A_1, B, B_1, C, C_1, and D. Finally, the residual notch E is incised. (From March CM, Israel R: *Am J Obstet Gynecol* 156:834, 1987.)

this defect has not been reported to cause infertility. Laparotomy with uterine unification and incision or excision of the septum was formerly the procedure of choice for women with this anomaly and a history of recurrent abortion. The procedures advocated by Tompkins and by Rock and Jones[71] were the most popular. Hysteroscopic treatment of septa has relegated these procedures to antiquity.

Hysteroscopy is used not only to assess the size and extent of the septum but also to treat the anomaly.[14] Simultaneous laparoscopy is needed to verify that the uterus is unified externally and also to provide guidance for the hysteroscopist. Flexible scissors are passed through the operating channel of the hysteroscope, and the central portion of the anteroposterior column of the septum is incised. If the width of the septum is 3 cm or less at the top of the fundus, the incision is carried cephalad from the most inferior point of the septum and directed laterally as the most superior aspect of the uterus is approached. The fibroelastic band of tissue retracts immediately and does not bleed. The dissection is continued until the septum is incised completely, and the uterine architecture is normalized.[38,53] Broader septa are treated differently. The incision is begun at the most inferior portion of the septum, and the scissors are directed superiorly along one lateral margin of the septum up to 0.5 cm from the junction with normal myometrium (Fig. 41-10). Next, the other lateral margin is incised up to the same level, and subsequently each new lateral aspect is incised alternatively until only a short broad notch (see Fig. 41-10, *E*) between the tubal ostia remains. Finally, this notch is incised beginning from one cornual recess and progressing to the

other. This approach is used because minimal bleeding usually occurs at the interface between myometrium and septum, and if treatment of this portion is delayed until the end of the procedure, blood loss is minimized and excellent visualization is ensured throughout the duration of the surgery. The dissection is complete when both tubal ostia can be visualized simultaneously even when the hysteroscope is high in the cavity, when the hysteroscope can move freely from one cornual recess to another, and/or when the laparoscopist observes that the entire uterus glows uniformly, even when the distal end of the hysteroscope is located in one cornual recess.

If the cervix is septate also, it is not incised because this area is very vascular, because cervical incompetence may ensue, and because the cervical portion of the septum will not hinder labor. The hysteroscope is placed in one horn and a uterine sound in the other. The sound is used to deflect the septum toward the hysteroscope and the scissors that incise it just above the internal os. After a small communication has been made between the two horns, the remaining upper portion of the septum is treated as described previously.

Some have used a laser (Nd:YAG, KTP, or argon) or even a resectoscope to incise the septum. These instruments offer no advantage over scissor incision and cause more tissue damage.[8] In addition, anatomic results are worse when a resectoscope is used.[20] There is no need to place an intrauterine splint.

The patient may be discharged from the surgery unit a few hours after the procedure is finished. To epithelialize the area over the incised septum, conjugated estrogens

(1.25 mg/day) are prescribed for 25 days. Medroxyprogesterone acetate (10 mg/day) is given during the last 5 days of the estrogen treatment. Office hysteroscopy or HSG should be performed after the withdrawal menses. If normal, the patient may attempt to conceive immediately thereafter.

Preoperative and postoperative HSGs of a patient treated by hysteroscopic incision are shown in Fig. 41-11. Outcomes have been excellent in four series of hysteroscopic treatment of patients with uterine septa and histories of recurrent abortion.[13,20,53,65] The rates of abortion were reduced from 95% (pretreatment) to less than 15% (posttreatment) (Table 41-9).[53] These results equal those of abdominal metroplasty.[74] A comparison of transfundal and transcervical techniques for incision of the septate uterus is shown in Table 41-10. These differences were demonstrated most clearly in a report by a single surgeon who compared his personal results.[25] The multiple advantages of hysteroscopic therapy make it the method of choice for treating uterine septa. In fact, because this method of treatment is so easy and safe, it may permit us to expand the indications for treating patients with uterine septa. For example, it should be used before in vitro fertilization or GIFT and may be used before complex therapy such as ovulation induction with gonadotropins or even for patients with unexplained infertility. The value of hysteroscopic treatment of uterine septa for these expanded indications remains uncertain.

However, its value for those with reproductive failure is unquestioned. This operation has made abdominal metroplasty for the septate uterus obsolete.

Currently, the most common müllerian anomaly is that which follows in utero exposure to DES. Typical radiographic findings include a T shape with cornual constriction bands and pretubal bulges, lower uterine segment dilation, and small cavities with irregular borders resembling intrauterine adhesions. These findings occur in more than 80% of women who have typical DES changes in the cervix or vagina. These anomalies may be confirmed by hysteroscopy. Although most investigators believe that hysteroscopy is not of therapeutic value, Nagel and Malo[58] reported an improved gestational outcome in a small number of patients with recurrent pregnancy loss after hysteroscopic incision of the lateral uterine walls.

Excessive Bleeding

Curettage and hysterectomy are often used as methods of controlling abnormal bleeding. A dilation and curettage (D&C) is usually required if the patient has evidence of endometrial hyperplasia or if the biopsy cannot exclude malignancy and in patients who have profuse bleeding, hypovolemia, or recurrent bleeding or in whom medical therapy has failed. Curettage has no place in the long-term management of dysfunctional uterine bleeding (DUB). More than 68% of patients with DUB treated by curettage alone have recurrences of excessive bleeding. If the patient is anovulatory, intermittent progestational therapy will prevent recurrences

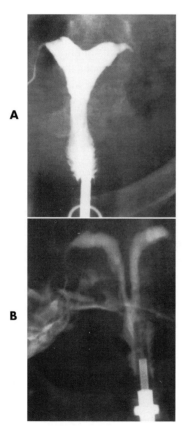

Fig. 41-11 Preoperative **(A)** and postoperative **(B)** hysterogram of patient with septate uterus who underwent hysteroscopic treatment.

Table 41-9 Reproductive Outcome before and after Hysteroscopy Metroplasty (*N* = Number of Pregnancies)*

	Preoperatively (*N* = 240)	Postoperatively (*N* = 63)
Term, survived	7	51
Premature, survived	5	4
Premature, neonatal death or stillbirth	16	—
Spontaneous abortion	212	8
Successful	12(5%)	55(87%)

*Data from March CM, Israel R: *Am J Obstet Gynecol* 156:834, 1987.

Table 41-10 Comparison of Hysteroscopic and Abdominal Metroplasty

Hysteroscopic	Abdominal
Minor surgery	Major surgery
Outpatient	Inpatient
½-hour operating time	2-hour operating time
Contraception for 1 month	Contraception for 3 months
Vaginal delivery	Cesarean section needed
Postoperative hysteroscopy or hysterosalpingography	Postoperative hysteroscopy or hysterosalpingography

in most patients. In one study of those with ovulatory menorrhagia, menstrual blood loss was unchanged 2 months or more after D&C.[61] Hysteroscopic examination of the endometrial cavity at the time of D&C helps rule out the presence of polyps or submucosal myomas. Among 113 patients who had abnormal bleeding that was investigated by both curettage and hysteroscopy, either a polyp or a submucosal myoma was found in 58 (85%) of the 68 whose excessive bleeding persisted for 6 months or more; 26 (84%) of the 31 women who had secretary endometrium had a cavity defect; of the 78 whose abnormal bleeding recurred despite having had one or two curettages in the previous 6 months, 58 (78%) had a polyp and 18 (23%) had a myoma; and of the 33 with minimal uterine enlargement, 24 (73%) had a submucosal myoma.

Comparisons between office hysteroscopy and pelvic ultrasound via an endovaginal transducer with or without fluid enhancement have been reported by many investigators. Towbin et al.[81] reported that in patients with abnormal uterine bleeding, hysteroscopy had sensitivity and specificity of 79% and 93%, respectively. In contrast, the sensitivity and specificity of ultrasound were 54% and 90%. Preliminary studies comparing hysteroscopy and saline infusion sonography at this institution have continued to demonstrate the superiority of hysteroscopy in the diagnosis of intracavity causes of abnormal uterine bleeding. Obviously, the instant availability of directed biopsy would also favor hysteroscopy in the evaluation of these patients, especially if a small caliber endoscope is used. However, depending on the physician's experience and the equipment available, he or she may prefer to use ultrasound as a screening test.

Among 342 patients who underwent both hysteroscopy and curettage, uterine inspection and directed biopsy were six times more likely to demonstrate more advanced pathologic conditions than did curettage in the group of 71 women whose histologic findings were not in agreement.[30] If the patient is bleeding heavily, a clear view can be obtained if patience is combined with a high-viscosity medium such as Hyskon or one of the low-viscosity media together with a continuous-flow instrument.

Endometrial Carcinoma

Although the standard method of differentiating stage I endometrial carcinoma from stage II disease is fractional curettage, errors in staging occur 10% to 15% of the time. For physicians who treat all women in both stages with primary surgery of the same type and who use intraoperative findings or the final pathology report as a guide to selection for further surgery or adjunctive therapy, this distinction is not critical. However, contact hysteroscopy or panoramic hysteroscopy with CO_2 is a safe and accurate method of differentiating between these two stages and of providing important information about the progression of the disease.[78]

Endometrial Polyps

Endometrial polyps (Fig. 41-12) are often a cause of menometrorrhagia and often cannot be removed completely with polyp forceps and/or a curette.[5] However, hysteroscopic excision by means of scissors or a loop electrode is an easy procedure. If scissors are used to excise the polyp, its base should be fulgurated or curetted to reduce the risk of recurrence. If curettage rather than excision under hysteroscopic control is used for removal, the hysteroscope must be reinserted to verify that no polyps or fragments thereof remain.

Leiomyomata Uteri

Leiomyomas of the uterus are the most common solid pelvic tumor and occur in 20% of women 35 years of age or older.[56] Despite their frequency, their cause and pathophysiology remain unclear, although they appear to be unicellular in origin.[83] Myomas arise most often during the third and fourth decades and therefore have an important impact upon reproductive performance. Because first pregnancies are delayed beyond age 35 more commonly today, the relative incidence of myomas in women attempting to conceive is rising. Myomas tend to be multiple and to grow slowly. Most patients are asymptomatic but have firm nodular masses that distort the uterine contour. Infertility, abortion (during either the first or second trimester), premature labor, and abnormal presentations have all been associated with the presence of submucous myomas.[7]

Intramural and submucous myomas have the greatest impact on reproductive capability. Submucous myomas may hinder endometrial nutrition and afford a poor implantation

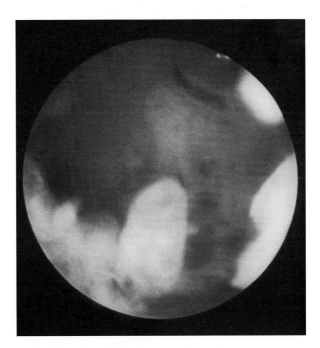

Fig. 41-12 Hysteroscopic view of an endometrial polyp. A feathery appearance and transillumination distinguish a polyp from a myoma. (From March CM: Hysteroscopy and the uterine factor in infertility. In Lobo RA, Mishell DR Jr, Paulson RJ, et al, editors: *Mishell's textbook of infertility, contraception and reproductive endocrinology,* ed 4, Cambridge, MA, 1997, Blackwell Scientific.)

site (resulting in abortion or infertility). Large intramural myomas may cause enlargement of the endometrial cavity (possibly resulting in poor sperm transport) and may occasionally occlude the intramural portion of the tube(s). Both types, but particularly the submucous variety, may not allow normal uterine enlargement during pregnancy and thus lead to abortion and premature labor.

The diagnosis of intramural myomas is usually made at the time of bimanual examination. The presence of submucous tumors may be suspected during curettage, but HSG or hysteroscopy is necessary for confirmation. Smooth, circular, or crescent-shaped defects persisting after the entire cavity is filled suggest submucous myomas (Fig. 41-13). Occasionally, it is impossible to differentiate the defect caused by a myoma from that of an endometrial polyp or a gestational sac. HSG also gives prognostic information because significant tubal disease would contraindicate conservative surgery unless the patient is interested in in vitro fertilization. HSG may also demonstrate the filling of multiple channels in the tumor mass that communicate with the endometrial cavity, and thus the diagnosis of adenomyosis can be made (Fig. 41-14).

The definitive diagnosis of a submucosal myoma is made by hysteroscopy. Direct visualization can establish the nature of the defect(s) more accurately and pinpoint the location, size, and relation to the tubal ostia and internal os (Fig. 41-15).

Because myomas develop and enlarge during the reproductive years and especially during pregnancy but tend to involute after delivery and after menopause, all medical methods of treatment have been directed toward inducing estrogen deficiency. The response to progestins has been variable, but high-dose medrogestone acetate has been shown to induce significant degeneration, fibrosis, and hya-

linization.[32] The response to danazol has been variable.[18] Recently, a significant reduction in myomas has been demonstrated with gestrinone, an antiestrogen antiprogesterone, when administered orally or vaginally[12] and with RU 486.[57] Preoperative treatment with a potent gonadotropin-releasing

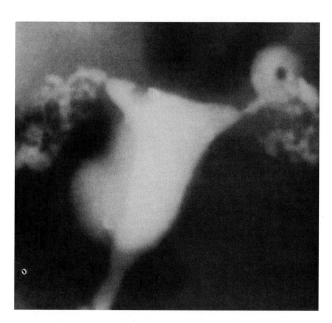

Fig. 41-14 Adenomyosis. (From March CM: Hysteroscopy and the uterine factor in infertility. In Mishell DR Jr, Davajan V, Lobo RA, editors: *Infertility, contraception and reproductive endocrinology,* ed 3, Cambridge, MA, 1991, Blackwell Scientific.)

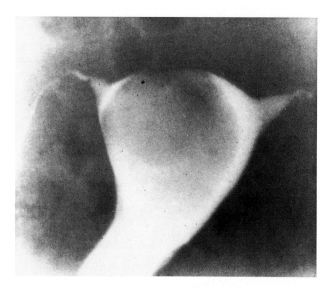

Fig. 41-13 Hysterogram of patient with submucous myoma. (From March CM: Hysteroscopy and the uterine factor in infertility. In Lobo RA, Mishell DR Jr, Paulson RJ, et al, editors: *Mishell's textbook of infertility, contraception and reproductive endocrinology,* ed 4, Cambridge, MA, 1997, Blackwell Scientific.)

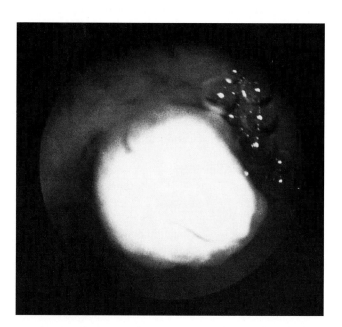

Fig. 41-15 Pedunculated submucous leiomyoma visualized with the hysteroscope. Myomas appear white and glistening. (From March CM: Hysteroscopy and the uterine factor in infertility. In Lobo RA, Mishell DR Jr, Paulson RJ, et al, editors: *Mishell's Textbook of infertility, contraception and reproductive endocrinology,* ed 4, Cambridge, MA, 1997, Blackwell Scientific.)

hormone (GnRH) agonist such as nafarelin or leuprolide causes cellular myomas to shrink markedly and thus facilitates surgery.[44] Maximal tumor shrinkage occurs after 3 months of therapy.[28] Before surgery, anemic patients should be treated with a GnRH agonist and iron until their iron stores have been replenished. The medical management of myomas cannot replace surgery for the symptomatic infertile woman or one with recurrent abortion because ovarian function is restored promptly after the agonist is discontinued and myomas usually return to their original size within 3 months. Calcified myomas and those that are fibrous and avascular do not respond to medical treatment.

Indications for myomectomy are (1) to conserve the uterus in a woman with large or symptomatic myomas and (2) to improve reproductive potential. Before performing a myomectomy to improve reproductive potential, a complete infertility investigation must be carried out to place the role of the myoma(s) in proper perspective. Additional infertility factor(s) should be corrected, if possible, before surgery. Subsequent pregnancy rates are reduced if myomectomy is performed in patients with multifactorial infertility. Smaller myomas (less than 7 cm) may be resected or, if pedunculated, may be excised under hysteroscopic control.

Three types of instruments have been used. A standard operating hysteroscope with scissors has been used to resect submucosal myomas. The line of resection follows that of the adjacent normal endometrial surface. This technique is most suitable for myomas in the center of the endometrial cavity and has been used to resect solitary or multiple myomas of up to 5 cm in diameter. After resection, the mass must be morselized to permit removal via the cervical os.

Another approach involves using a resectoscope (see Fig. 41-4) and "shaving" the myoma gradually to a point even with the normal endometrial surface[34,60] (see the box below). This technique may be used for larger myomas and for those more eccentrically placed (Fig. 41-16). If multiple submucosal myomas are present and if these myomas occupy most of the endometrial surface and/or oppose one another, endoscopic resection is not advised. Much of the endometrial surface will be damaged by resection, and the risk of synechiae formation is high. An alternative for moderate-sized opposing wall myomas is a two-stage procedure, that is, resecting the myomas at 2-month intervals so that only one uterine surface is raw at one time.

After the induction of anesthesia and a pelvic examination, the uterine cavity is sounded and the cervix is dilated to 9 mm. The resectoscope and all tubing are filled with medium, the instrument is introduced into the endocervical canal, and systematic inspection of the cavity is performed (see the box below). The technique of resecting a myoma involves the systematic shaving of the intracavitary portion of the tumor. If the depth of myometrial involvement is thought to be great, preoperative magnetic resonance imaging (MRI) should be performed. This study will identify myomas that have an intramural component so large that transuterine resection would be of little value if only the intracavitary component were excised or dangerous if the resection were carried far into the uterine wall. Any large surface vessels are coagulated before the resection is begun. The resection is carried out, beginning with the portion of the myoma that bulges most into the uterine cavity. The electrosurgical unit is set initially at 50 W, but more power is often needed, especially for tumors that are more fibrous. Cutting current only is used. The resecting loop is passed superior to the myoma and withdrawn back toward the insulated sheath. As the loop passes the tumor, it is activated and a piece of the myoma is excised. The loop should be activated only when it is completely in view and not in contact with adjacent normal endometrium or a tubal ostium. As fragments are resected, they should be pushed superior to the myoma to maintain a clear view. If the view becomes obscured, the fragments should be rinsed out of the cavity or retrieved with polyp forceps. All of the resected tumors should be sent to the laboratory for examination (see Fig. 41-15).

As the resection progresses, some of the tumor that had been intramural is commonly extruded into the cavity and becomes available to the resecting electrode. The resection may be continued to a point even with the normal adjacent endometrium or even to just below this level but no further.

STEPS IN HYSTEROSCOPIC MYOMECTOMY

Inspection of cavity
Coagulation of surface vessels
Resection of myoma(s)
Coagulation of cut vessels
Evacuation of chips
Reinspection
Conjugated equine estrogens (CEEs) (1.25 mg/day for 21 days)
Medroxyprogesterone acetate (10 mg/day, days 16 to 21 of CEEs)

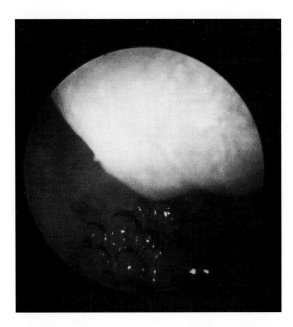

Fig. 41-16   Large myoma via hysteroscope.

If the resection is continued into the underlying muscle, significant hemorrhage may occur and the risk of uterine perforation is a real one. Moreover, deep dissection is usually unnecessary. If a small intramural component is left in situ, uterine contractions over the ensuing weeks often cause that fragment to be extruded into the uterine cavity and subsequently aborted.

This mechanism probably explains the high rate of success even if a portion of the myoma remains. One technique that increases the likelihood that the residual component will be expelled is to coagulate the intramural component with an electrode or laser fiber, thereby causing necrosis. Myomas that are located on the most superior aspect of the uterus are more difficult to resect because access to them is limited. Newer loops and other cautery elements are being designed to permit excision of these masses. At present, the easiest access to these myomas is with a quartz fiber transmitting energy from an Nd:YAG laser or a bipolar electrode delivered via a panoramic hysteroscope.

Operator caution is critical to endoscopic resection of submucosal myomas. Tumors that are attached to the region of the internal cervical os are more vascular, and injury to large vessels may occur. Abdominal removal should be considered. Myomas that have a large intramural component (more than half of the uterine wall) may be resected, but these tend to cause recurrent symptoms shortly after surgery. If the MRI scan demonstrates that the submucosal myoma extends close to the uterine serosa, an abdominal approach should be used. The same approach is needed in patients who have bothersome symptoms related to other myomas that are intramural or subserosal. A combined approach of resection of myomas and endometrial ablation may be used in women with multiple or solitary submucosal myomas who do not wish to conserve fertility. Pretreatment with a GnRH agonist, danazol, or a progestin should be used before ablation to induce endometrial atrophy.

Since Neuwirth[60] reported resecting of submucosal myomata with a resectoscope, the value of this technique has been proven by other investigators. The largest published experience is that of Hallez et al.[33] Of my patients, 90% have had no recurrence of bleeding over 2½ to 12 years of follow-up (Table 41-11). Similar results have been reported by others.[85] Recently, Hallez et al.[33] reported a single-stage hysteroscopic myomectomy for tumors that had a significant intramural component. After the intracavitary component has been excised, manual abdominal pressure is used to force the intramural component into the cavity, and this portion is then resected.

Recently, the Nd:YAG laser has been used to resect a submucosal myoma.[21] Most investigators were experienced hysteroscopists before undertaking resection of submucosal myomas via a resectoscope or laser. A thorough preoperative investigation and correction of anemia will reduce the risk of complications. Although simultaneous laparoscopy has not been used at the University of Southern California (USC) center, it may be helpful, especially during a surgeon's early experience with this valuable approach to the symptomatic submucosal leiomyoma. In contrast to abdominal myomectomy, patients may attempt to conceive 1 month after surgery and may deliver vaginally. If a GnRH agonist is used before myomectomy, estrogen therapy should be used immediately after surgery to reduce the risk of adhesion formation. HSG or repeat hysteroscopy should be performed before conception.

Endometrial Ablation

Laser photovaporization of the endometrium has been investigated for treatment of menorrhagia.[31] An Nd:YAG laser was used under hysteroscopic visualization. Before the procedure, all patients were given danazol (800 mg/day) for 2 to 3 weeks. An additional 2 weeks of danazol treatment followed the laser procedure. This regimen cured 203 of 210 patients, including many with organic lesions such as submucosal myomas. Similar results have been reported by Loffer,[49] using a "nontouch" technique to destroy the endometrium. Photovaporization causes varying degrees of uterine contraction, scarring, and adhesion formation, as follow-up HSGs and hysteroscopy showed. DeCherney et al.,[19] Townsend et al.,[82] and Vancaille[87] have used a standard urologic resectoscope or a modified one that permits continuous flow of the distending medium (and therefore reduced fluid absorption) to destroy the endometrium with cautery. The instruments used are different but the techniques of endometrial destruction are similar. Preoperative endometrial sampling is mandatory to rule out the presence of any endometrial atypicalities. If the patient has more than minimal uterine enlargement or other symptoms related to leiomyomata, this procedure will not relieve all of her complaints. The use of a drug to cause endometrial atrophy before surgery will facilitate ablation and increase efficacy. At USC leuprolide acetate is used for 2 months before surgery.

Surgery is performed on an outpatient basis under general or regional anesthesia. The results of endometrial ablation are similar irrespective of whether a resectoscope or a laser is used. I prefer to use the former: the instrument is readily available and less costly, and the procedure can be performed more rapidly. A 2.5-mm roller electrode is used to coagulate the endometrium. The electrosurgical unit is set at 80 W, but occasionally 100 W or more are needed. The end point is a series of overlapping dark brown or black furrows. The thermal injury must be conducted down to the basalis so that the endometrium will not regenerate. Although a loop electrode may be used to resect the endo-

Table 41-11   Results of Hysteroscopic Resection of Myomas

Number	60
Follow-up	2½-12 yr
Largest	
Pedunculated	8 cm
Sessile	6 by 4 cm
Recurrence (6)	
Abdominal myomectomy	3
Hysterectomy	2
Repeat resection	1

metrium, the depth of resection is more difficult to control and therefore damage to uterine muscle may occur with resultant hemorrhage and increased absorption of medium. A continuous-flow resectoscope is used. Sorbitol, glycine, and Hyskon all provide a clear view. The ablation is begun in the cornual regions and carried inferiorly to just above the level of the internal os. Ablation below this point increases the risk of damage to large blood vessels. Medroxyprogesterone acetate (150 mg) is given intramuscularly on the day of the procedure to maintain hypoestrogenism and therefore facilitate adhesion formation. Two months after surgery the uterine cavity is sounded to disrupt adhesions in the lower segment so that the process of endometrial obliteration proceeds from above downward. Thereby the chance of development of hematometra is reduced.

Endometrial ablation is an alternative to hysterectomy when other modalities have failed, are contraindicated, or are undesirable. The goal of endometrial ablation is relief of hypermenorrhea, and thus hypomenorrhea or normal menses should be considered successful outcomes. Only about two thirds of patients develop amenorrhea. The rest have hypomenorrhea, and the failure rate is 5% to 10%. Therefore any patient who demands amenorrhea might be served better by hysterectomy. However, the avoidance of major surgery, the faster return to normal activity, reduced hospitalization and cost make ablation attractive to many women even if the risk of failure is significant.[59]

All patients must be willing to accept sterilization as a consequence of the surgery, and although the risk of subsequent pregnancy is small, some have advocated simultaneous tubal sterilization. If the patient is at risk for pregnancy, a barrier method should be used until long-term amenorrhea has been documented. When postmenopausal hormone replacement therapy is given to these patients, a progestin should be added to the estrogen to protect any remaining islands of endometrium from unopposed estrogen stimulation.

Tubal Obstruction

The cause of proximal tubal obstruction remains obscure. In many cases the presumptive diagnosis, made by HSG, is proven incorrect when laparoscopy with transcervical hydrochromoperturbation is performed. Most of these patients have spasm at the proximal uterotubal junction during HSG.

Others have anatomic damage at both the proximal and distal tubal regions or at only the proximal segments. Those with bipolar disease should probably undergo in vitro fertilization because the results of microsurgery remain poor. Those with salpingitis isthmica nodosa usually have a poor prognosis because the disease tends to be extensive and progressive and produces a predisposition to ectopic pregnancy. Until recently, tubal reimplantation or microsurgical tubocornual anastomosis was the only method of treating patients who had occlusion of the proximal fallopian tube. Although transcervical balloon tuboplasty (TBT) under fluoroscopic control is probably efficacious, treatment via hysteroscopy offers advantages.[51] Most TBT protocols require that patients have normal distal tubes. Therefore laparoscopy is usually a prerequisite to TBT. During that laparoscopy, coaxial dilation of the proximal fallopian tube under hysteroscopic guidance is a convenient alternative to TBT because treatment is carried out at the same time, thereby speeding management and reducing cost and discomfort.

Novy, Deaton, and Kerin and their respective coauthors[17,41,62] described hysteroscopic cannulation. Novy et al.[62] described transcervical cannulation of the proximal oviduct with a 3-Fr Teflon catheter and flexible guidewire, 0.043 cm in diameter. Deaton et al.[17] used a 0.97-mm urologic stainless-steel guidewire with a flexible tip that is introduced into the operating channel of the 7-mm operating hysteroscope. The tip of the guidewire is placed at the tubal ostium and pressure is applied. Often, the end of the hysteroscope must be placed within 2 mm of the ostium to provide extra stability for the guidewire. After the tip of the guidewire enters the tubal ostium, its position is documented by laparoscopy, the guidewire is withdrawn, and patency is confirmed by use of either dextran or indigo carmine. The technique of Kerin et al. uses guidewire cannulation (a no. 32 guidewire) and direct balloon tuboplasty under hysteroscopic, falloposcopic, and laparoscopic control.[41]

Transcervical tubal cannulation and balloon tuboplasty, either radiographically, hysteroscopically, or in the future ultrasonographically, offer important new advances in the diagnosis and treatment of fallopian tube disease (Table 41-12).[70] There are numerous causes for proximal fallopian tube obstruction. Some of these, such as spasm, filmy adhesions, and various types of mucous plugs or debris, are

Table 41-12 Treatment of Proximal Tubal Obstruction

Author	N	Patients			
		Tubal Patency		IUP	ECT
		Immediate	6 Mo		
Capitanio	108	81	35	23	—
Thurmond	100	86	75	39	6
Confino	77	92	82	35	5
Lisse	41	84	57	31	—
Platia	21	76	75	38	13

Modified from Risquez F, Confino E: *Fertil Steril* 60:211, 1993.

IUP, Intrauterine pregnancy; *ECT,* ectopic pregnancy.

probably effectively treated by tubal cannulation or balloon tuboplasty. More significant lesions, such as those produced by salpingitis isthmica nodosa, severe fibrosis, endosalpingiosis, or previous reconstructive surgery, have a much lower chance of being corrected by the transcervical approach.

Recently, Das et al.[16] and Rausan and Garcia[68] reported equal results with hysteroscopic tubal catheterization and microsurgical tubocornual resection and reanastomosis. If HSG indicates proximal tubal occlusion, it is reasonable to proceed with laparoscopy with hydrotubation. Then if bilateral patency is confirmed, no further procedures need to be done unless the patient requires hysteroscopy. When either or both fallopian tubes are blocked proximally, diagnostic hysteroscopy with selective tubal hydrotubation is indicated. If this does not result in documented patency of the fallopian tube, transcervical tubal cannulation can be performed. If this is unsuccessful, the patient can undergo laparotomy for repair during that operation or at a later date, depending on her wishes. Alternatively, given the overall nature of the patient's fertility status, in vitro fertilization might be the ideal recommendation.

As an adjunct to salpingography and to assess the tubal surface anatomy after relief of proximal obstruction and/or before salpingostomy, falloposcopy has emerged as a tool of the future. Although falloposcopy has been performed from the peritoneal side, more recently the falloposcope has been passed into the tube after being guided up to the tubal ostium via a flexible hysteroscope.[41]

Foreign Bodies

The combination of ultrasound and alligator-jaw grasping forceps can remove most "lost" or embedded IUDs. This approach is safer than the use of an IUD hook. Rather than subjecting all patients to hysteroscopy, USC uses a simple flow chart (Fig. 41-17). The first step is to provide a second method of contraception as soon as the possibility of an expelled or extrauterine device is encountered. After the next menstrual period, an attempt is made to retrieve the filaments from the endocervical canal. If they are not detected, an ultrasound is performed. If the device is judged to be in or near the uterus, the cavity is sounded to "palpate" the de-

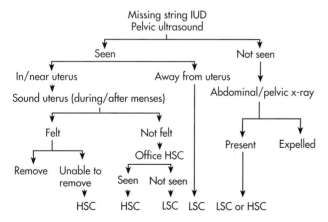

Fig. 41-17 Algorithm for locating and removing an intrauterine device whose filaments cannot be identified.

vice. If the device is felt, it is retrieved via an alligator-jaw grasping forceps or hysteroscopy. If it cannot be felt, hysteroscopy is used to confirm its location. If the IUD cannot be detected by ultrasound, one or more imaging procedures should be used to localize the device, which is then removed by the appropriate surgical procedure. However, for those who have the capability of office hysteroscopy, it can readily be performed before the imaging studies outlined on the right side of Fig. 41-16. If an embedded device is partially intracavitary, the base is grasped with forceps and the device, forceps, and hysteroscope are withdrawn as a single unit. If only a small portion of the device is visible, it may be partially extrauterine and may have involved the bowel. In these instances simultaneous laparoscopy is advised.

POSTOPERATIVE CARE

Little care is needed after hysteroscopy. Those who have had only local anesthesia may leave the office after a brief rest period. If a parenteral narcotic or tranquilizer has been administered, the patient may leave in the care of another after 1 hour. If general anesthesia has been used, standard guidelines of the hospital or day surgery unit are followed. Bleeding, usually light, should be expected for a few to 10 days. Mild cramping should persist for less than 1 day. Coitus may be resumed in 1 week, and if the patient wishes to conceive, she may attempt to do so after 1 month provided that all adjunctive therapy has been completed and that any necessary postoperative inspection of the cavity proves it to be normal.

COMPLICATIONS AND MANAGEMENT

Complications have been uncommon, and most have been mild in the more than 8000 hysteroscopies performed at USC. The frequency of complications can be reduced if strict guidelines are followed:

1. Prior training and proctoring
2. Careful history and physical examination
3. Operation during follicular phase
4. Advancement of the telescope only in a clear field
5. No overdilation of the cervix
6. Media volume monitoring
7. Use of electrosurgery and laser with care
8. Liberal use of simultaneous laparoscopy

Pain is usually mild to moderate during hysteroscopy. Most brief hysteroscopies can be performed on an outpatient basis using paracervical block anesthesia. Meperidine, midazolam, diazepam, propofol, or a prostaglandin synthetase inhibitor may be used to supplement the paracervical block. Cramps increase substantially if the operating time exceeds 20 to 30 minutes. After hysteroscopy, mild cramping may persist for a few hours and is easily controlled with a mild analgesic.

Bleeding

In the USC series of more than 8000 procedures, bleeding has occurred in 12 patients, usually secondary to a laceration at the site of tenaculum placement. In 2 women, a branch of the uterine artery was severed, and tamponade using an intrauterine balloon successfully arrested the bleeding. In another patient, heavy bleeding necessitating transfusion occurred after IUD placement after incision of a uterine septum (splints are no longer used after hysteroplasty). Bleeding may also occur after extensive dissection of synechiae or resection of polyps or a submucous myoma. Almost all bleeding is caused by myometrial injury, not incision of a septum, scar, polyp, or myoma.

Infection

Only three of the USC patients have developed pelvic infection after hysteroscopy. Two had histories of salpingitis, and one was found to have a cervical culture positive for *Neisseria gonorrhoeae* when she was admitted for IV antibiotic therapy. Broad-spectrum antibiotic therapy, including an agent effective against anaerobic organisms, such as clindamycin or chloramphenicol, should be instituted immediately if symptoms of infection develop.

Prophylactic antibiotic therapy for hysteroscopy is unnecessary.

Uterine Perforation

Uterine perforation is a rare complication of hysteroscopy and usually occurs only in patients with the most severe IUAs. If the dissection proves to be extremely difficult, general anesthesia should be administered and laparoscopy performed simultaneously to reduce the chance of uterine perforation. Central perforations may be managed by observation only. Antibiotics are not used, and hospitalization is unnecessary.

The use of electrocautery and lasers inside the uterus increases the potential sequelae of uterine perforation because bowel or bladder injury or damage to large blood vessels may occur. The surgeon can only activate the electrosurgical electrode or fire the laser when the view is clear and all of the electrode or laser fiber can be seen. If a resectoscope is used, the electrode should only be activated when it is being withdrawn toward the sheath, never going away. For patients undergoing endometrial ablation, the endocervical canal and internal os should not be treated because of the risk of damage to large blood vessels.

Endometrial Dislocation

The subsequent development of endometriosis is probably only a theoretical complication. Avoidance of hysteroscopy during menses further reduces the risk.

Anesthetic Accidents

The rare anesthetic complications are related to the agents used rather than to the hysteroscopic procedure itself.

Complications Related to the Medium

Allergic reactions to dextran occur rarely. If a large amount of dextran enters the venous circulation, circulatory overload is possible.[43,89] A symptom complex consisting of acute noncardiogenic pulmonary edema and disseminated intravascular coagulation has occurred in 12 of the USC patients.[39] All received large volumes (600 to 800 ml) of Hyskon and had extensive dissection of their endometrial surfaces. To avoid this serious complication, it is advisable to limit the total amount of Hyskon used to 250 ml or less, even if this means that the procedure must be terminated prematurely and completed at a later date. Hyskon enters the vascular system and can draw almost 9 ml of fluid from the extravascular space for each 1 ml of Hyskon absorbed. After approximately 200 ml of Hyskon is absorbed, platelet dysfunction will result.[55]

Acute fluid overload has also been reported when large volumes of glucose in water, glycine, saline, or sorbitol have been used.[88] If large volumes of glucose in water have been absorbed, hyperglycemia and hyponatremia may develop.[9] Electrolyte imbalance can occur if large amounts of sorbitol or glycine are absorbed. Prolonged operating time and deep myometrial dissection predispose to greater amounts of fluid being absorbed.[23] If low-viscosity media are used, intake and output must be recorded accurately at 15-minute intervals. Only rarely should fluid absorption exceed 3000 ml. Two recent advances in technology should make the use of low-viscosity fluid safer. One is the introduction of a bipolar electrode and a modified loop electrode so that electrolyte-containing solutions can be used for electrosurgical procedures. The second is the development of infusion pumps that deliver low-viscosity fluids under pressure and that measure inflow and outflow continuously during surgery and provide real-time measurement of the fluid deficit. These monitoring devices reduce nursing time and physician anxiety and improve patient safety. Their use will probably become widespread in the immediate future. In some patients, potent diuretics have been used prophylactically. If fluid overload or pulmonary edema occurs, treatment is identical to that used when these events are not preceded by intrauterine surgery. The use of warm low-viscosity media will reduce the occurrence of hypothermia.

CO_2 acidosis and arrhythmias are probably only theoretical complications if the proper insulator is used. However, deaths have occurred when the sheathed fiber used to deliver Nd:YAG energy had a sapphire tip that was cooled by gas delivered at a high rate of flow.[3] These tips should be cooled by the liquid medium being used to distend the cavity. If CO_2 is used as the uterine distending medium, a bare fiber should deliver the laser energy.

LEARNING HYSTEROSCOPY

Although hysteroscopy is easier to learn than laparoscopy, a disciplined approach and patience are necessary. Books, postgraduate courses, and a preceptorship serve to get the novice ready to perform diagnostic hysteroscopy, first under supervision and then independently. After the physician becomes adept at recognizing normal and abnormal structures, excision of polyps and small pedunculated myomas and lysis of minimal adhesions may be undertaken. Incision of septa and more extensive adhesions and the management of larger myomas are procedures of moderate difficulty and risk. If the entire cavity is obliterated by scar tissue or if a laser or resectoscope is to be used inside the uterus, an accomplished hysteroscopist should be in charge of the procedure.

REFERENCES

1. American Fertility Society: The American Fertility Society classification of adnexal adhesions, distal tubal occlusion, tubal occlusion secondary to tubal ligation, tubal pregnancies, müllerian anomalies and intrauterine adhesions, *Fertil Steril* 49:944, 1988.
2. Baggish MS: Contact hysteroscopy: a new technique to explore the uterine cavity, *Obstet Gynecol* 59:350, 1979.
3. Baggish MS, Daniell MS: Death caused by air embolism associated with neodymium: yttrium-aluminum-garnet laser surgery and artificial sapphire tips, *Am J Obstet Gynecol* 161:877, 1989.
4. Bartosik D, Jacobs SL, Kelly LJ: Endometrial tissue in peritoneal fluid, *Fertil Steril* 46:796, 1986.
5. Burnett JE: Hysteroscopy-controlled curettage for endometrial polyps, *Obstet Gynecol* 24:621, 1964.
6. Buttram VC Jr, Gibbons WE: Mullerian anomalies: a proposed classification (an analysis of 144 cases), *Fertil Steril* 32:40, 1979.
7. Buttram VC Jr., Reiter RC: Uterine leiomyomata: etiology, symptomatology and management, *Fertil Steril* 36:433, 1981.
8. Candiani GB, et al: Argon laser versus microscissors for hysteroscopic incision of uterine septa, *Am J Obstet Gynecol* 164:87, 1991.
9. Carson SA, et al: Hyperglycemia and hyponatremia during operative hysteroscopy with 5% dextrose in water distention, *Fertil Steril* 51:341, 1989.
10. Caspi E, Peripinial S: Reproductive performance after treatment of intrauterine adhesion, *Int J Fertil* 20:249, 1975.
11. Cooper JM, Houck RM, Rigberg HS: The incidence of intrauterine abnormalities found at hysteroscopy in patients undergoing elective hysteroscopic sterilization, *J Reprod Med* 10:659, 1983.
12. Coutinho EM, Goncalves MT: Long-term treatment of leiomyoma with gestrinone, *Fertil Steril* 51:939, 1989.
13. Daly DC, Maier D, Soto-Albors C: Hysteroscopic metroplasty: six years experience, *Obstet Gynecol* 73:201, 1989.
14. Daly DC, Walters RA, Soto-Albors CE, et al: Hysteroscopic metroplasty: surgical technique and obstetric outcome, *Fertil Steril* 39:623, 1983.
15. Darabi KF, Roy K, Richart RM: Collaborative study on hysteroscopic sterilization procedures: final report. In Sciarra JJ, Zatuchni GL, Speidel JJ, editors: *Risks, benefits and controversies in fertility control,* Hagerstown, MD, 1978, Harper & Row.
16. Das K, Nagel TC, Malo JLS: Hysteroscopic cannulation for proximal tubal obstruction: a change for the better, *Fertil Steril* 63:1009, 1995.
17. Deaton JL, Gibson M, Riddick DH, et al: Diagnosis and treatment of cornual obstruction using a flexible tip guidewire, *Fertil Steril* 53:232-236, 1990.
18. DeCherney AH, Maheux R, Polan ML: A medical treatment for myomata uteri, *Fertil Steril* 39:429, 1983.
19. DeCherney AH, Diamond MP, Lang G, Polan ML: Endometrial ablation for intractable uterine bleeding: hysteroscopic resection, *Obstet Gynecol* 70:668, 1977.
20. DeCherney AH, Russell JB, Graebe RA, et al: Resectoscopic management of mullerian fusion defects, *Fertil Steril* 45:726, 1986.
21. Donnez J, Sandow J, Schrurs B, et al: Treatment of uterine fibroids with implants of gonadotropin-releasing hormone agonist: assessment by hysterography, *Fertil Steril* 51:947, 1989.
22. Edström K, Fernström I: The diagnostic possibilities of a modified hysteroscopic technique, *Acta Obstet Gynecol Scand* 49:327, 1970.
23. Emmanuel MH, Hart A, Wamsteker K, et al: An analysis of fluid loss during transcervical resection of submucous myomas, *Fertil Steril* 68:881, 1997.
24. Falb RD, Lower BR, Crowley JP, Powell TR: Transcervical fallopian tube blockage with gelatin-resorcinol-formaldehyde (GRF). In Sciarra JJ, Droegemuller W, Speidel JJ, editors: *Advances in female sterilization techniques,* Hagerstown, MD, 1976, Harper & Row.
25. Fayez JA: Comparison between abdominal and hysteroscopic metroplasty, *Obstet Gynecol* 68:399, 1986.
26. Fayez JA, Mutie G, Schneider PJ: The diagnostic value of hysterosalpingography and hysteroscopy in infertility investigation, *Am J Obstet Gynecol* 156:558, 1987.
27. Friedman A, DeFazio S, DeCherney A: Severe obstetric complications after aggressive treatment of Asherman syndrome, *Obstet Gynecol* 67:864, 1986.
28. Friedman AJ, Rein MS, Harrison-Atlas D, et al: A randomized, placebo-controlled, double-blind study evaluating the efficacy of leuprolide acetate depot in the treatment of uterine leiomyomata, *Fertil Steril* 51:251, 1989.
29. Gimpelson RJ: Preventing cervical reflux of the distention medium during panoramic hysteroscopy, *J Reprod Med* 31:592, 1986.
30. Gimpleson RJ, Rappold HO: A comparative study between panoramic hysteroscopy with directed biopsies and dilatation and curettage, *Am J Obstet Gynecol* 158:489, 1988.
31. Goldrath MH, Fuller TA, Segal S: Laser photovaporization of endometrium for the treatment of menorrhagia, *Am J Obstet Gynecol* 140:14, 1981.
32. Goldzieher JW, et al: Induction of degenerative changes in uterine myomas by high-dose progestin therapy, *Am J Obstet Gynecol* 96:1078, 1966.
33. Hallez JP, Netter A, Cartier R: Methodical intrauterine resection, *Am J Obstet Gynecol* 156:1080, 1987.
34. Hallez JP: Single-stage total hysteroscopic myomectomy; indications, techniques, and results, *Fertil Steril* 65:703-708, 1995.
35. Hamou J: Microhysteroscopy, *J Reprod Med* 26:375, 1981.
36. Haning RV Jr, Harkins PG, Uehling DT: Preservation of fertility by transcervical resection of a benign mesodermal uterine tumor with a resectoscope and glycine distending medium, *Fertil Steril* 33:209, 1980.
37. Heinonen PK, Saarikoski S, Pystynen P: Reproductive performance of women with uterine anomalies, *Acta Obstet Gynecol Scand* 61:157, 1982.
38. Israel R, March CM: Hysteroscopic incision of the septate uterus, *Am J Obstet Gynecol* 149:66, 1984.
39. Jederkin R, Olsfanger D, Kessler I: Disseminated intravascular coagulopathy and adult respiratory distress syndrome: life threatening complications of hysteroscopy, *Am J Obstet Gynecol* 162:44, 1990.
40. Jewelwicz R, Khalaf S, Neuwirth RS, et al: Obstetric complications after treatment of intrauterine synechiae (Asherman's syndrome), *Obstet Gynecol* 47:701, 1976.
41. Kerin J, Daykhovsky L, Segalowitz J, et al: Falloposcopy: a microendoscopic technique for visual exploration of the human fallopian tube from the uterotubal ostia to the fimbria using a transvaginal approach, *Fertil Steril* 54:390-400, 1990.
42. Lancet M, Kessler I: A review of Asherman's syndrome, and results of modern treatment, *Int J Fertil* 33:14, 1988.
43. Leake JF, Murphy AA, Zacur HA: Noncardiogenic pulmonary edema: a complication of operative hysteroscopy, *Fertil Steril* 48:497, 1987.
44. Letterie GS, Shawker TH, Coddington CC, et al: Efficacy of a gonadotropin-releasing hormone agonist in the treatment of uterine leiomyomata: long-term follow-up, *Fertil Steril* 51:951, 1989.
45. Lin BL, et al: Flexible hysterofibroscope: the development of a new flexible hysterofiberscope and its clinical application, *Acta Obstet Gynecol Jpn* 39:649, 1987.
46. Lindemann H-J: The use of CO_2 in the uterine cavity for hysteroscopy, *Int J Fertil* 17:221, 1972.
47. Lindemann H-J, Siegler AM, Mohr J: The hysteroflator 1000s, *J Reprod Med* 16:145, 1976.
48. Loffer FD: Hysteroscopic sterilization with the use of formed-in-place silicone plugs, *Am J Obstet Gynecol* 149:261, 1984.
49. Loffer FD: Hysteroscopic endometrial ablation with the Nd:YAG laser using a nontouch technique, *Obstet Gynecol* 69:679, 1987.
50. March CM, Israel R: A critical appraisal of hysteroscopic tubal fulguration for sterilization, *Contraception* 11:261, 1975.

51. March CM, Israel R: Intrauterine adhesions secondary to elective hysteroscopic diagnosis and management, *Obstet Gynecol* 48:422, 1976.

52. March CM, Israel R: Gestational outcome following hysteroscopic lysis of adhesions, *Fertil Steril* 36:455, 1981.

53. March CM, Israel R: Hysteroscopic management of recurrent abortion caused by septate uterus, *Am J Obstet Gynecol* 156:834, 1987.

54. March CM, Israel R, March AD: Hysteroscopic management of intrauterine adhesions, *Am J Obstet Gynecol* 130:653, 1978.

55. McLucas B: Hyskon complications in hysteroscopic surgery, *Obstet Gynecol Surv* 46:196, 1991.

56. Miller NF, Ludovici PP. On the origin and development of uterine fibroids, *Am J Obstet Gynecol* 70:720, 1955.

57. Murphy AA, Kettel LM, Morales AJ, et al: Regression of uterine leiomyomata in response to the antiprogesterone RU486, *J Clin Endocrinol Metab* 76:513, 1993.

58. Nagel TC, Malo J W: Hysteroscopic metroplasty in the diethylstilbestrol-exposed uterus and similar nonfusion anomalies; effects on subsequent reproductive performance, a preliminary report, *Fertil Steril* 59:502, 1993.

59. Nagale F, Rubinger T, Magos A: Why do women choose endometrial ablation rather than hysterectomy, *Fertil Steril* 69:1063, 1998.

60. Neuwirth RS: A new technique for and additional experience with hysteroscopic resection of submucous fibroids, *Am J Obstet Gynecol* 131:91, 1978.

61. Nilsson L, Rybo G: Treatment of menorrhagia, *Am J Obstet Gynecol* 110:713, 1971.

62. Novy MJ, Thurmond AS, Patton P, et al: Diagnosis of cornual obstruction by transcervical fallopian tube cannulation, *Fertil Steril* 50:434, 1988.

63. Oelsner G, David A, Insler V, et al: Outcome of pregnancy after treatment of intrauterine adhesions, *Obstet Gynecol* 44:341, 1974.

64. Pantaleoni DC: On endoscopic examination of the cavity of the womb, *Med Press Circ* 8:26, 1869.

65. Perino A, Mencaglia L, Hamou J, et al: Hysteroscopy for incision of uterine septa: report of 24 cases, *Fertil Steril* 48:321, 1987.

66. Quiñones RG, Aznar RR, Duran HA: Tubal electrocauterization under hysteroscopic control, *Contraception* 7:195, 1973.

67. Ranta H, Risto A, Oksanen H, Heinonen PK: Dissemination of endometrial cells during carbon dioxide hysteroscopy and chromotubation among infertility patients, *Fertil Steril* 53:751, 1990.

68. Rauson MX, Garcia AJ: Surgical management of cornual-isthmic tubal obstruction, *Fertil Steril* 68:887, 1997.

69. Reed TP III, Erb R: Hysteroscopic tubal occlusion with silicone rubber, *Obstet Gynecol* 61:388, 1983.

70. Risquez F, Confino E: Transcervical tubal cannulation, past, present, and future, *Fertil Steril* 60:211-226, 1993.

71. Rock JA, Jones HW Jr: The clinical management of the double uterus, *Fertil Steril* 28:798, 1977.

72. Rock JA, Schlaff WD: The obstetrical consequences of utero-vaginal anomalies, *Fertil Steril* 43:681, 1985.

73. Rock JA, Singh M, Murphy AA: A modification of technique for hysteroscopic lysis of severe uterine adhesions, *J Gynecol Surg* 9:191, 1993.

74. Rock JA, Zacur HA: The clinical management of repeated early pregnancy wastage, *Fertil Steril* 39:123, 1983.

75. Sciarra JJ: Hysteroscopic approaches for tubal closure. In Zatuchni GL, Lablock MH, Sciarra JJ, editors: *Research frontiers in fertility regulation,* Hagerstown, MD, 1980, Harper & Row.

76. Siegler AM: Hysterography and hysteroscopy in the infertile patient, *J Reprod Med* 18:143, 1977.

77. Stein AL, March CM: The outcome of pregnancy in women with müllerian duct anomalies, *J Reprod Med* 35:411, 1990.

78. Sugimoto O: Hysteroscopic diagnosis of endometrial carcinoma, *Am J Obstet Gynecol* 121:105, 1975.

79. Taylor PJ: Correlations in infertility: symptomatology, hysterosalpingography, laparoscopy and hysteroscopy, *J Reprod Med* 18:339, 1977.

80. Toaff ME, Lew-Toaff AS, Toaff R: Communicating uteri: review and classification with introduction of two previously unreported types, *Fertil Steril* 41:661, 1984.

81. Towbin NA, Gviazda IM, March CM: Office hysteroscopy versus transvaginal ultrasonography in the evaluation of patients with excessive uterine bleeding, *Am J Obstet Gynecol* 174:1678, 1996.

82. Townsend DE, Richart RM, Paskowitz RA, et al: "Rollerball" coagulation of the endometrium, *Obstet Gynecol* 76:310, 1990.

83. Townsend DE, Sparks RS, Baluda MC, et al: Unicellular histogenesis of uterine leiomyomas as determined by electrophoresis of glucose-6-phosphate dehydrogenase, *Am J Obstet Gynecol* 107:1168, 1970.

84. Valle RF: Hysteroscopy in the evaluation of female infertility, *Am J Obstet Gynecol* 137:425, 1980.

85. Valle RF: Hysteroscopic removal of submucous leiomyomas, *J Gynecol Surg* 6:89, 1990.

86. Valle RF, Sciarra JJ: Intrauterine adhesions: hysteroscopic diagnosis, classification, treatment, and reproductive outcome, *Am J Obstet Gynecol* 158:1459, 1988.

87. Vancaille T: Electrocoagulation of the endometrium with the ball-end resectoscope, *Obstet Gynecol* 74:425, 1989.

88. Witz CA, Silverberg KM, Burns WN, et al: Complications associated with the absorption of hysteroscopic fluid media, *Fertil Steril* 60:745, 1993.

89. Zbella EA, Moise J, Carson SA: Noncardiogenic pulmonary edema secondary to intrauterine instillation of 32% dextran 70, *Fertil Steril* 43:479, 1985.

42 Restoration of Tubal Patency

ROBERT B. HUNT

Recently, I spoke with a gentleman just completing his reproductive endocrinology fellowship in Boston. To my amazement, he disclosed that he had not yet performed a tubal anastomosis. As evidenced by the paucity of articles relating to tubal reconstructive surgery in peer review journals over the past 10 years, I am concerned that this proven and valuable technology is being relegated to the shelves of gynecologic history. If one does not perform these technically challenging procedures often, one quickly loses the skills needed to accomplish superior surgery. In my view, reconstructive surgery remains a valuable option for many couples with tubal factor infertility. Viable pregnancy rates after expert correction of many tubal conditions compare favorably with those achieved with assisted-reproductive technologies (ART) and should be offered to the applicable couple as an alternative to ART or when ART has failed or is unavailable. This chapter addresses operations performed by laparotomy. The reader is referred to Chapter 7, which addresses laparoscopic approaches to tubal surgery.

PREOPERATIVE EVALUATION
Fertility Testing

Which tests to perform preoperatively on an infertile couple with tubal factor infertility vary from couple to couple. The following should be considered: status of sperm, usually determined by either semen analysis or postcoital test; *Chlamydia* antibody or appropriate cervical cultures for sexually transmitted disease; complete blood count and sedimentation rate test to rule out active pelvic inflammation; midluteal phase serum progesterone to assess ovulation; and sometimes a day 3 serum follicle-stimulating hormone level to determine oocyte reserve. In an older woman, I often perform a clomiphene challenge test. Usually, evaluation of fallopian tubes by laparoscopy or hysterosalpingogram (HSG) would have already been done. If available, I review HSG films, pertinent operative and pathology reports, and operative photographs.

Counseling

The couple should be informed of other options of management, such as ART. Adequate information concerning details of the proposed operation and postoperative recovery should be discussed. Risks of the operation and realistic expectation of outcome, including ectopic pregnancy, should be a part of the informed consent process. I find it best to go through these details with the couple at the time that I recommend tubal surgery. I then send a letter reviewing these same details to the couple with a copy to the referring provider. My written informed consent is also given to the couple to be read, signed, witnessed, dated, and returned to the office before surgery. This stepwise informed consent process is an excellent policy because the couple is then well versed, and information imparted to the couple is documented. This makes good medical and legal sense.

I am often confronted with a woman 40 years or older who is a candidate for reproductive surgery. If her oocyte reserve appears adequate and other fertility factors are satisfactory, I proceed with surgery, provided the woman's age does not exceed 44 years.[8,33]

GENERAL CONSIDERATIONS FOR SURGERY
Magnification

I find the operating microscope of great value for tubal anastomosis, whereas ×2.5 operating loupes are perfectly adequate for adhesiolysis, fimbrioplasty, or salpingostomy.* The headlamp is of enormous help when using operating loupes or when operating with no magnification.

Anesthesia

General, epidural, or spinal anesthesia is satisfactory for pelvic operations if no assessment laparoscopy is done; otherwise, I prefer general anesthesia.

Incision

If a woman has had previous lower abdominal surgery, I generally use the same incision; otherwise, I open the skin and subcutaneous tissue transversely and fascia and peritoneum vertically.[17] This lessens the chance of injury to ilioinguinal nerves, provides excellent pelvic exposure, and causes less postoperative pain than the Pfannenstiel incision. The incision is made just large enough to allow pelvic surgery to be accomplished expertly.

Microsutures

Synthetic absorbable and nonabsorbable sutures for microsurgery have been compared.[12,19,20,24,30] Some minor histologic differences among them have been demonstrated in animal studies but not enough to affect patency or pregnancy rates. I do not recommend the use of catgut because catgut produces considerable tissue reaction. I choose microsuture by needle design, color contrast, tensile strength, and suture memory. My preferred needle design is a taper

---

*References 4, 9, 13, 23, 26, 28, 37.

needle with a cutting tip and suture materials are nylon and polybutester.

Antibiotics

I administer antibiotics immediately before beginning the operation and order one or two doses postoperatively; however, prophylactic antibiotics have not been shown to improve pregnancy rates. My preferred antibiotic is doxycycline, 100 mg, dissolved in intravenous fluids. I also add 10 ml of 4.2% sodium bicarbonate (Neut, Abbott Laboratories, Chicago, IL) to intravenous fluids containing doxycycline to neutralize the acidity caused by doxycycline. This may lessen the risk of superficial phlebitis.

Pelvic Preparation

After the woman has been anesthetized, I perform a pelvic examination to determine the orientation of the uterus and to rule out adnexal masses. I then insert an intrauterine catheter connected to a syringe and tubing filled with dilute indigo carmine. Kerlix gauze soaked in Ringer's lactate solution is inserted into the posterior vaginal fornix to prevent the catheter from being expelled and to elevate the uterus. The ure-thra is irrigated, and a Foley catheter is inserted for continuous bladder drainage. After the patient has been draped for laparotomy, the syringe and tubing connected to the intrauterine catheter is removed. A sterile syringe and tubing on the sterile field, filled with dilute indigo carmine, is connected by the circulating nurse to the tubing joined to the intrauterine catheter. This allows me to control tubal lavage from the surgical field.

An orogastric tube is inserted into the stomach, and the stomach is decompressed. The orogastric tube is removed at the conclusion of the operation.

Once the abdomen has been opened and general abdominal exploration completed, the woman is placed in the Trendelenburg position. A Kirschner retractor is positioned over a wound protector, the bowel is displaced cephalad with three folded and saturated abdominal packs, and the posterior cul-de-sac is packed with a single Kerlix gauze sponge saturated with Ringer's lactate and placed over a sump drain. The drain is connected to continuous suction to remove excess fluid. A silicone mat may be placed over the Kerlix gauze pad to provide a background unencumbered by packing (Fig. 42-1).

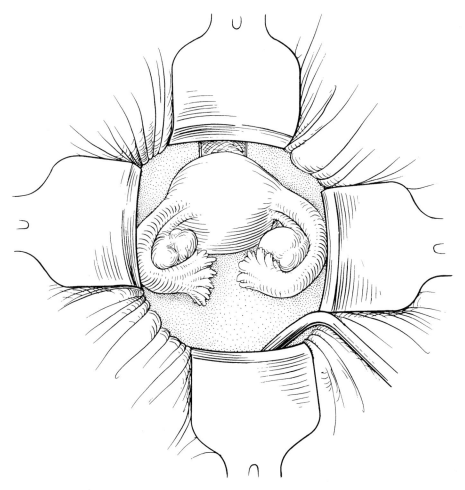

Fig. 42-1   Placement of the Kirschner retractor and exposure of pelvic structures are accomplished. (From Hunt RB: Pelvic preparation and choice of incision for laparotomy. In Hunt RB, editor: *Atlas of female infertility surgery,* ed 3, St Louis, 1999, Mosby.)

Irrigant

Animal studies have revealed that balanced salt solutions do not cause fimbrial edema, whereas saline does.[2] Therefore I favor Ringer's lactate for hydroflotation, that is, fluid left in the abdomen at the conclusion of the operation. For irrigation, I use 1.5% glycine because this electrolyte-free fluid allows an open vessel to be identified and coagulated while irrigant is being directed to the site.

TUBAL ANASTOMOSIS

Tubal anastomosis is applicable for repair of localized tubal obstruction caused by conditions such as salpingitis isthmica nodosa, endometriosis, or previous tubal sterilization. The same principles exist for each anastomosis: excise diseased tissue; achieve meticulous hemostasis, yet preserve blood supply; and accomplish a precise, tension-free anastomosis.

Techniques described here are a distillate of those developed by my colleagues and me and are applicable to most tubal obstructions for which anastomosis is indicated.

Cornual Anastomosis

When confronted with a woman with cornual obstruction, I initially attempt to relieve the obstruction by cannulation, guided by either the hysteroscope or fluoroscope.[29] If this is unsuccessful and the woman is deemed a good candidate for tubal anastomosis, I proceed. I believe it is advisable to wait for at least one menstrual cycle before performing definitive surgery.

The rationale for cornual anastomosis was established by Ehrler.[6] He noted that the intramural tube was preserved in most patients with proximal tubal disease. Based on this observation, he offered tubal anastomosis as an alternative to tubal implantation. Although clinical results were unsuccessful, he paved the way for others to refine the operation.

The four most common histologic abnormalities associated with cornual occlusion were obliterative fibrosis (38.1%), salpingitis isthmica nodosa (23.8%), chronic tubal inflammation (21.4%), and endometriosis (14.3%).[7] To remove diseased tissue, I usually resect a portion of the intramural tube and often most of the isthmus.

After pelvic preparation has been completed and the abdomen opened, approximately 1 to 2 U of dilute vasopressin (20 U in 100 ml of Ringer's lactate) is injected into the uterine fundus near the cornu to reduce small vessel bleeding (Fig. 42-2). Because vasopressin has been associated with significant hypertension, the anesthesiologist should be alerted about its use.

Dissection begins at midisthmus and is conducted under a continual stream of irrigant. Bipolar coagulation with microbipolar forceps is used judiciously. The peritoneal incision is made over the tube (Fig. 42-3). A dissecting rod and forceps are of enormous help in rotating the tube to improve exposure.

The tube is transected with iris scissors (Fig. 42-4). Great care must be taken to avoid damage to nutrient vessels located immediately beneath the tube. It is often best to obtain hemostasis superiorly first because this strategy prevents

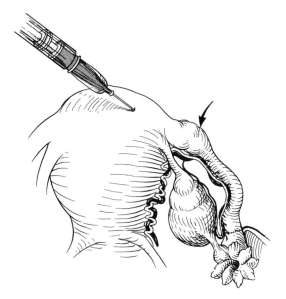

Fig. 42-2   Typical cornual thickening *(arrow)* seen in salpingitis isthmica nodosa. The myometrium is injected with 1 to 2 U of vasopressin. (From Hunt RB: Tubal anastomosis by laparotomy. In Hunt RB, editor: *Atlas of female infertility surgery*, ed 3, St Louis, 1999, Mosby.)

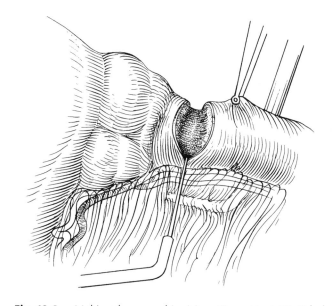

Fig. 42-3   Making the serosal incision. (From Hunt RB: Tubal anastomosis by laparotomy. In Hunt RB, editor: *Atlas of female infertility surgery*, ed 3, St Louis, 1999, Mosby.)

blood from running over inferior vessels that need to be controlled (Fig. 42-5). Tiny vessels and those located very close to the mucosa should not be coagulated because they generally stop bleeding on their own. If bleeding is brisk, gentle pressure may be applied to facilitate identification and control.

The proximal tube is grasped with heavy toothed forceps, and the tube is lifted superiorly (Fig. 42-6). The tube is dissected from the mesosalpinx by incising the peritoneum on either side and releasing underlying connective tissue. Dissection is continued until the uterus is reached.

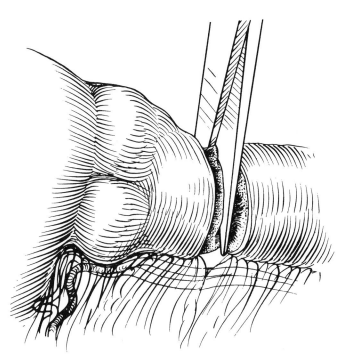

Fig. 42-4 A perpendicular cut is made in the tube. (From Hunt RB: Tubal anastomosis by laparotomy. In Hunt RB, editor: *Atlas of female infertility surgery,* ed 3, St Louis, 1999, Mosby.)

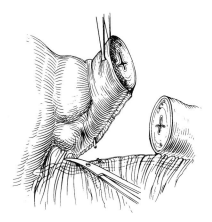

Fig. 42-6 The proximal tube is lifted superiorly and released from the mesosalpinx. Care is taken to spare nutrient vessels. (From Hunt RB: Tubal anastomosis by laparotomy. In Hunt RB, editor: *Atlas of female infertility surgery,* ed 3, St Louis, 1999, Mosby.)

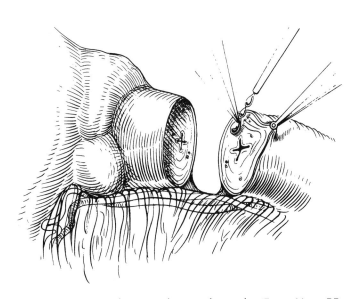

Fig. 42-5 Bipolar coagulation of vessels. (From Hunt RB: Tubal anastomosis by laparotomy. In Hunt RB, editor: *Atlas of female infertility surgery,* ed 3, St Louis, 1999, Mosby.)

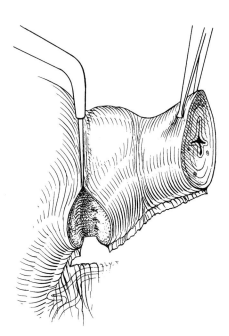

Fig. 42-7 A serosal incision is made over the cornu. (From Hunt RB: Tubal anastomosis by laparotomy. In Hunt RB, editor: *Atlas of female infertility surgery,* ed 3, St Louis, 1999, Mosby.)

With traction applied to the proximal tube, a peritoneal incision is made over the cornu (Fig. 42-7). Keeping in mind that nutrient vessels curve inferiorly to become part of the uterine arterial and venous complex, the tube is transected with a single cut with iris scissors (Fig. 42-8). Occasionally, an open venous sinus is encountered. To prevent excessive tissue damage from coagulation, a 6-0 or 8-0 suture is used to close the sinus.

Normal tissue is seldom found at the initial site of transection. To facilitate deeper dissection, a 6-0 suture is placed through the tubal lumen (Fig. 42-9). Gentle traction is applied, and dissection is continued with microscissors or a microelectrode just outside circular muscle. Each time a 2-mm segment is freed, it is excised with a 15-degree ophthalmic scalpel, and the proximal tube is checked for patency and normalcy (Figs. 42-10 and 42-11). If the intramural tube is difficult to visualize, crescents of myometrium overlying the intramural tube are excised.

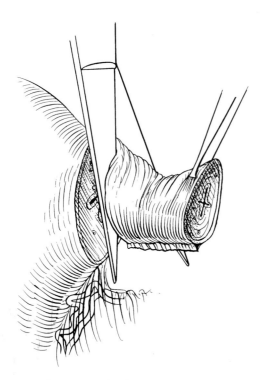

Fig. 42-8 The proximal tube is excised. (From Hunt RB: Tubal anastomosis by laparotomy. In Hunt RB, editor: *Atlas of female infertility surgery,* ed 3, St Louis, 1999, Mosby.)

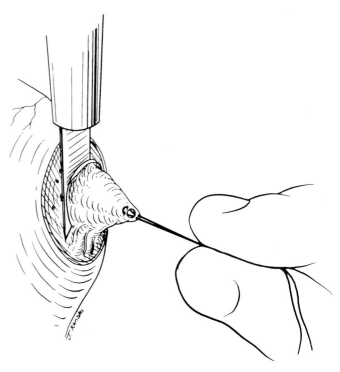

Fig. 42-10 A segment of the intramural tube is excised with a disposable ophthalmic scalpel. (From Hunt RB: Tubal anastomosis by laparotomy. In Hunt RB, editor: *Atlas of female infertility surgery,* ed 3, St Louis, 1999, Mosby.)

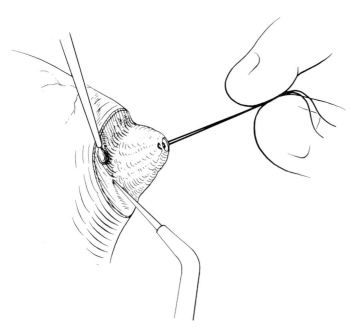

Fig. 42-9 A suture of 6-0 material has been placed through the intramural tube for traction, and dissection is continued. (From Hunt RB: Tubal anastomosis by laparotomy. In Hunt RB, editor: *Atlas of female infertility surgery,* ed 3, St Louis, 1999, Mosby.)

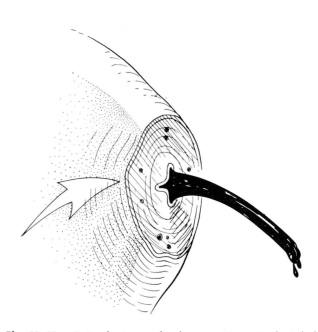

Fig. 42-11 A steady steam of indigo carmine exits the tubal lumen. (From Hunt RB: Tubal anastomosis by laparotomy. In Hunt RB, editor: *Atlas of female infertility surgery,* ed 3, St Louis, 1999, Mosby.)

A healthy proximal fallopian tube should have the following characteristics:

1. When lavaged, indigo carmine should flow uninterrupted. If not, a no. 0 or no. 1 monofilament suture is threaded through the tubal lumen into the uterine cavity and removed. This strategy may dislodge particulate matter, such as displaced endometrial tissue. It may also relieve obstruction caused by polyps or intratubal adhesions.
2. The tubal mucosa should appear velvety when lightly stained with indigo carmine.
3. The tubal musculature should be well perfused.

4. The myometrium should be devoid of fibrosis or pathologic conditions.

Once preparation of the proximal segment has been completed, attention is turned to the lateral segment. Retrograde lavage is carried out. If the isthmus is obstructed at the site of transection or appears abnormal, additional tube is excised. The medial extreme of the lateral segment is grasped with heavy toothed forceps, the peritoneum is incised on either side and connective tissue beneath the tube released, and the tube is dissected away from nutrient vessels until normal tube has been reached (Fig. 42-12). After the peritoneum investing the tube is incised, the tube is transected with iris scissors (Figs. 42-13 and 42-14). Hemostasis is achieved and patency documented (Fig. 42-15). Often, the healthy tube is first encountered at the ampullary-isthmic junction. This is fortuitous because anastomosis can be effected without having to correct a large luminal disparity.

Stay sutures of 6-0 material on tapered needles are placed, and sutures are held with fine hemostats (Fig. 42-16). Great care must be taken to avoid misaligning the tubal lumina because the purpose of stay sutures is to relieve tension at anastomosis sites and to maintain alignment.

If tension exists when tubal segments are brought together, additional steps must be taken to relieve it. The following strategies are useful: incise the peritoneum widely on either side of the mesosalpinx; position moist sponges lateral to the uterus on the contralateral side and lateral to the adnexa on the ipsilateral side; consider removing some vaginal packing to bring the proximal tube to the level of the distal tube.

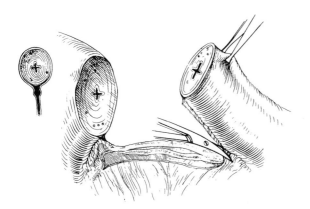

Fig. 42-12 The distal tube is dissected from the underlying mesosalpinx. (From Hunt RB: Tubal anastomosis by laparotomy. In Hunt RB, editor: *Atlas of female infertility surgery,* ed 3, St Louis, 1999, Mosby.)

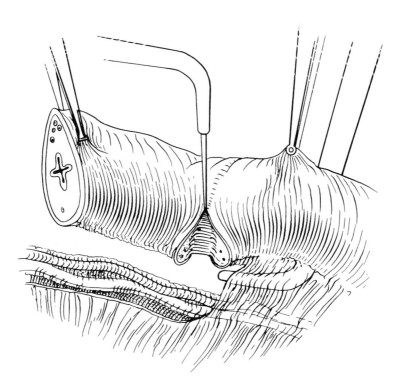

Fig. 42-13 A serosal incision is made over the isthmus. (From Hunt RB: Tubal anastomosis by laparotomy. In Hunt RB, editor: *Atlas of female infertility surgery,* ed 3, St Louis, 1999, Mosby.)

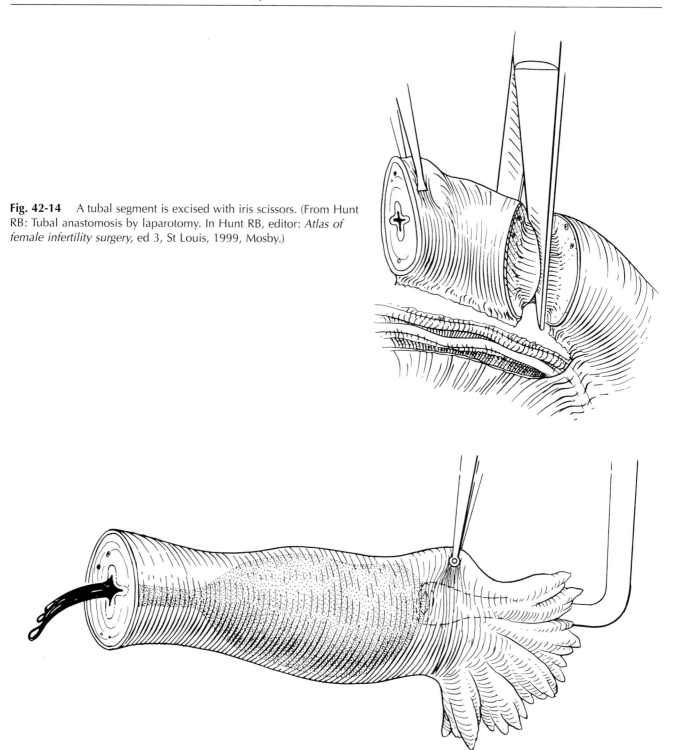

Fig. 42-14 A tubal segment is excised with iris scissors. (From Hunt RB: Tubal anastomosis by laparotomy. In Hunt RB, editor: *Atlas of female infertility surgery*, ed 3, St Louis, 1999, Mosby.)

Fig. 42-15 Retrograde lavage confirms tubal patency. (From Hunt RB: Tubal anastomosis by laparotomy. In Hunt RB, editor: *Atlas of female infertility surgery*, ed 3, St Louis, 1999, Mosby.)

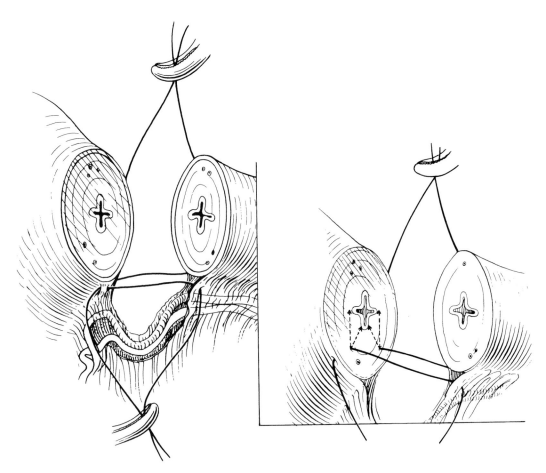

Fig. 42-16   Stay sutures have been placed to align the tubal segments and ultimately to relieve tension at the anastomosis site. (From Hunt RB: Tubal anastomosis by laparotomy. In Hunt RB, editor: *Atlas of female infertility surgery,* ed 3, St Louis, 1999, Mosby.)

With the operating microscope properly adjusted and centered, anastomosis begins. An 8-0 or 9-0 suture is placed extramucosally at the 6 o'clock position so that the knot will be outside the tubal lumen (Fig. 42-17). If the medial portion of the distal segment is ampulla, I incorporate a tiny bit of mucosa in the suture because ampullary muscle is thin; however, I include only muscularis in isthmic and intramural segments. The knot is tied and cut. Stay sutures may be tied at this time or later (Fig. 42-18).

The first of two lateral sutures is placed but left untied. The remaining lateral suture is placed. The 12 o'clock suture is positioned, and all sutures are tied (Figs. 42-19 through 42-22). Patency is tested by transuterine lavage. If the myometrial defect is large, it is partially diminished (Fig. 42-23). The serosa is approximated (Fig. 42-24). Additional sutures of 6-0 material may be required to close the anterior mesosalpinx. The overall tubal length is determined and recorded. The completed anastomosis is shown in Fig. 42-25.

Leakage at the anastomosis site often occurs and is acceptable, provided no tissue tension exists at the site and the flow of indigo carmine through the fimbriated end is adequate. What is not acceptable is for indigo carmine to leak at the site of anastomosis but not appear at the fimbriated end. If the proximal tube does not fill with dye, yet the uterus expands when dye is injected, one may massage the uterus manually in the vicinity of the cornu. This sometimes relieves the apparent obstruction. If the uterus does not expand at the time of lavage, the intrauterine catheter should be removed by the circulating nurse. An 18-gauge needle connected to a 20-ml syringe and tubing filled with indigo carmine is inserted through the top of the uterine fundus and advanced into the uterine cavity transabdominally. The lower uterine segment is occluded either manually or with a specially designed clamp (Shirodkar, Buxton, or Mulligan), and tubal lavage is effected. If these maneuvers are unsuccessful and proximal patency was documented at the time of anastomosis and a precise anastomosis was performed, the anastomosis need not be redone.

Tubotubal Anastomosis

Most women being considered for tubotubal anastomosis on my service have undergone tubal sterilization.[38] Techniques shown in this chapter are applicable whether the obstruction was caused by sterilization, endometriosis, fibrosis, or partial salpingectomy.

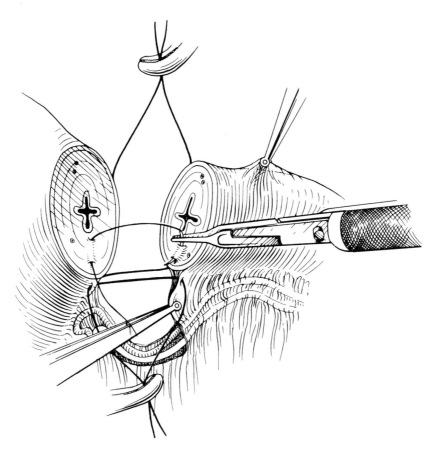

Fig. 42-17 An 8-0 or 9-0 suture is placed at the 6 o'clock position. (From Hunt RB: Tubal anastomosis by laparotomy. In Hunt RB, editor: *Atlas of female infertility surgery,* ed 3, St Louis, 1999, Mosby.)

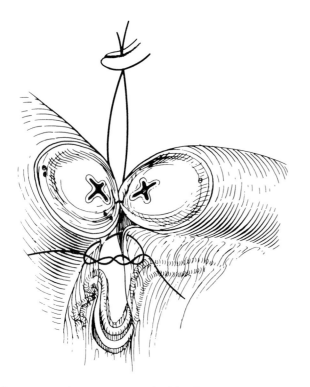

Fig. 42-18 The suture at 6 o'clock has been tied. Stay sutures may be tied now or later. (From Hunt RB: Tubal anastomosis by laparotomy. In Hunt RB, editor: *Atlas of female infertility surgery,* ed 3, St Louis, 1999, Mosby.)

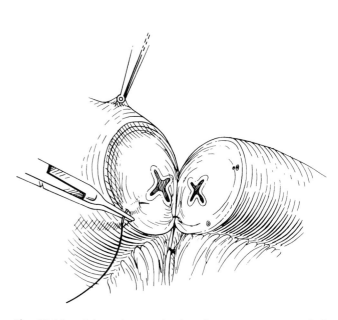

Fig. 42-19 A lateral suture is placed. (From Hunt RB: Tubal anastomosis by laparotomy. In Hunt RB, editor: *Atlas of female infertility surgery,* ed 3, St Louis, 1999, Mosby.)

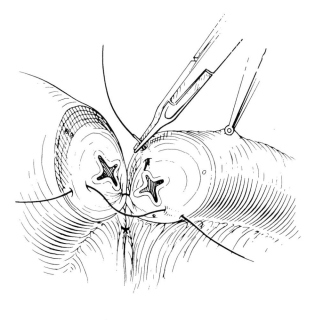

Fig. 42-20   The remaining lateral suture is placed. Both lateral sutures may be tied now or later. (From Hunt RB: Tubal anastomosis by laparotomy. In Hunt RB, editor: *Atlas of female infertility surgery*, ed 3, St Louis, 1999, Mosby.)

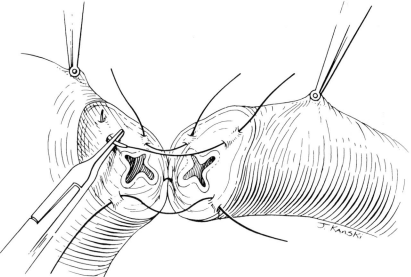

Fig. 42-21   The inner layer of sutures is completed with placement of the 12 o'clock suture. (From Hunt RB: Tubal anastomosis by laparotomy. In Hunt RB, editor: *Atlas of female infertility surgery*, ed 3, St Louis, 1999, Mosby.)

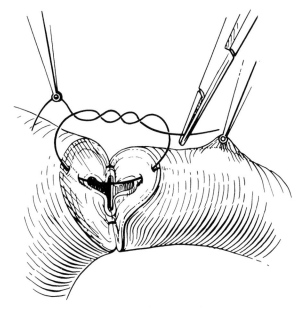

Fig. 42-22   All sutures comprising the inner layer are tied. (From Hunt RB: Tubal anastomosis by laparotomy. In Hunt RB, editor: *Atlas of female infertility surgery*, ed 3, St Louis, 1999, Mosby.)

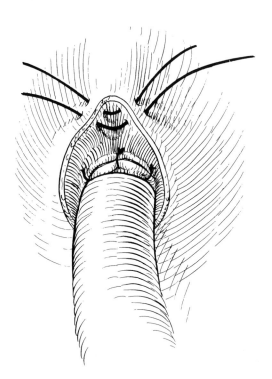

Fig. 42-23 The superior defect is narrowed with transverse sutures of 6-0 or 8-0 material. (From Hunt RB: Tubal anastomosis by laparotomy. In Hunt RB, editor: *Atlas of female infertility surgery,* ed 3, St Louis, 1999, Mosby.)

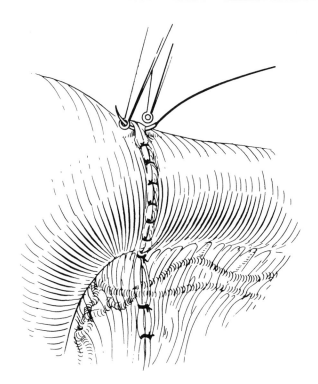

Fig. 42-24 Serosal sutures are placed and tied. Note the technique to facilitate grasping the needle with ring forceps. (From Hunt RB: Tubal anastomosis by laparotomy. In Hunt RB, editor: *Atlas of female infertility surgery,* ed 3, St Louis, 1999, Mosby.)

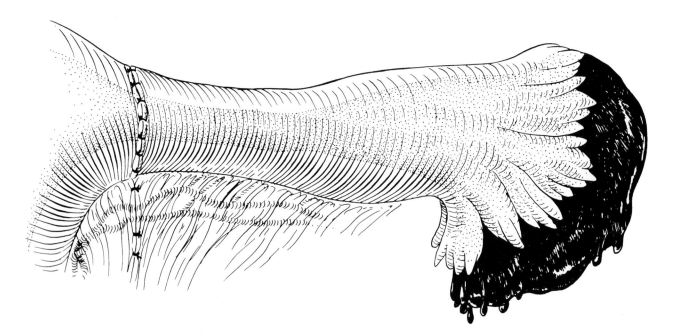

Fig. 42-25 Indigo carmine exits the fallopian tube at completion of the anastomosis. (From Hunt RB: Tubal anastomosis by laparotomy. In Hunt RB, editor: *Atlas of female infertility surgery,* ed 3, St Louis, 1999, Mosby.)

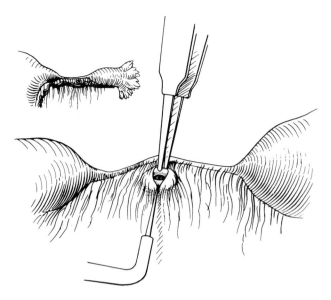

Fig. 42-26 Fallopian tube appearance after Falope ring sterilization. (From Hunt RB: Tubal anastomosis by laparotomy. In Hunt RB, editor: *Atlas of female infertility surgery,* ed 3, St Louis, 1999, Mosby.)

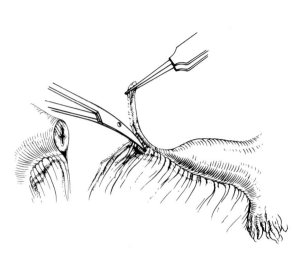

Fig. 42-28 The fibrous band is dissected toward the distal tubal segment. (From Hunt RB: Tubal anastomosis by laparotomy. In Hunt RB, editor: *Atlas of female infertility surgery,* ed 3, St Louis, 1999, Mosby.)

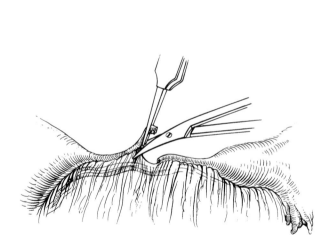

Fig. 42-27 The fibrous band joining tubal segments is divided and dissected toward the proximal tubal segment. (From Hunt RB: Tubal anastomosis by laparotomy. In Hunt RB, editor: *Atlas of female infertility surgery,* ed 3, St Louis, 1999, Mosby.)

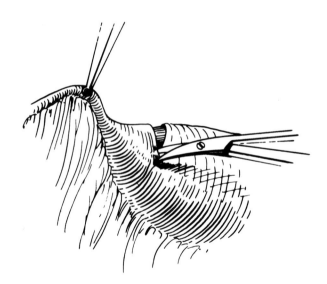

Fig. 42-29 The serosal cap is excised with microscissors. (From Hunt RB: Tubal anastomosis by laparotomy. In Hunt RB, editor: *Atlas of female infertility surgery,* ed 3, St Louis, 1999, Mosby.)

Fig. 42-26 represents typical findings after tubal sterilization by Falope ring. The ring is grasped with heavy toothed forceps and excised. A bundle of fibrous tissue connects proximal and distal tubal segments. This bundle is grasped, lifted superiorly, and dissected until the proximal segment is reached (Fig. 42-27). The proximal segment is prepared for anastomosis. Approximately 0.5 to 1.0 cm of tube is excised because this portion is usually diseased.[5,27,32,34] The proximal tube may be transected at up to a 30-degree angle to provide a slightly larger tubal lumen.

The lateral segment is next addressed. The fibrous bundle is dissected to its termination at the medial portion of the lateral segment, in this case the ampulla (Fig. 42-28). A small cap of serosa is excised, taking care not to damage the underlying mucosa (Fig. 42-29). Thermal energy is avoided because of the thinness of ampullary wall. Tubal distention by retrograde lavage will define the most medial extent of the lateral segment. This site is grasped with ring forceps and a tiny bit is excised, thus creating a small tubal opening (Fig. 42-30). Patency may be checked by retrograde lavage,

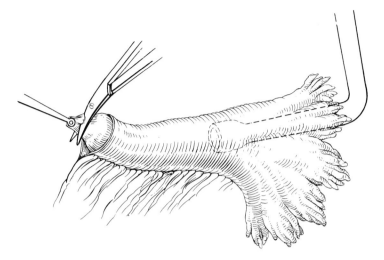

Fig. 42-30   The medial extreme of the lateral segment is opened with microscissors. (From Hunt RB: Tubal anastomosis by laparotomy. In Hunt RB, editor: *Atlas of female infertility surgery,* ed 3, St Louis, 1999, Mosby.)

but this must be done very gently or ampullary mucosa will spill out, making anastomosis much more difficult. Stay sutures of 6-0 material are placed and held (Fig. 42-31). Typically four 8-0 or 9-0 sutures are placed in the inner layer, and all sutures are tied (Fig. 42-32). After patency is confirmed, serosal 8-0 sutures are placed and tied. Additional 6-0 sutures are placed in the anterior mesosalpinx as necessary for closure.

Occasionally, visibility is hampered by abundant ampullary mucosa draping over the proposed site of suture placement. The mucosa may be brushed back with the needle tip or ring forceps as each suture is placed. Another strategy is to lift the lateral sutures superiorly and replace the ampullary mucosa with ring forceps or irrigation.

Occasionally, a large luminal disparity exists, even after the proximal tube is cut at a 30-degree angle. A larger opening, usually ampullary, may be narrowed with 8-0 or 9-0 sutures placed transversely (Figs. 42-33 through 42-35). Alternatively, anastomosis may be performed in the standard manner but by fashioning the larger opening to the smaller one. Often, five or six sutures are required to accomplish this. Because the ampulla so readily conforms to the smaller isthmic opening, I generally prefer the latter strategy.

Obstruction sometimes occurs in the ampulla. The technique is the same as that for ampullary-isthmic anastomosis described previously. Because luminal disparity is generally not a problem, the proximal and lateral segments are cut at right angles and standard anastomosis is effected. Usually five or six 8-0 or 9-0 sutures are required because of the relatively large lumina (Figs. 42-36 through 42-41).

If at least 2 cm of distal ampulla with healthy fimbriae is present and the proximal ampulla is deciliated, I often resect a portion of the proximal ampulla, being careful not to create too large a luminal disparity.

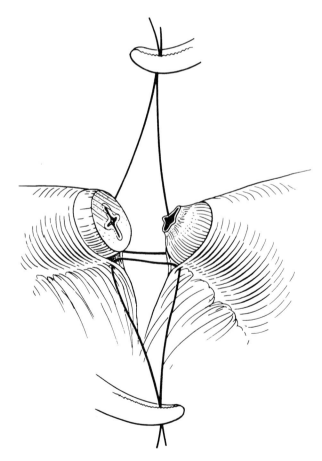

Fig. 42-31   The proximal tube has been cut at a 30-degree angle to compensate for luminal disparity. (From Hunt RB: Tubal anastomosis by laparotomy. In Hunt RB, editor: *Atlas of female infertility surgery,* ed 3, St Louis, 1999, Mosby.)

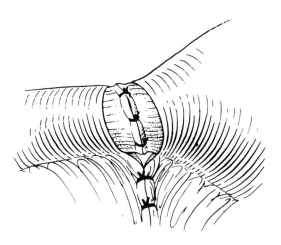

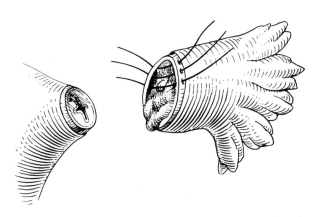

Fig. 42-32   The inner layer of sutures 8-0 or 9-0 have been placed and tied. Note closure of mesosalpinx with 6-0 or 8-0 sutures. This will be followed by placement of serosal 8-0 sutures to complete the anastomosis. (From Hunt RB: Tubal anastomosis by laparotomy. In Hunt RB, editor: *Atlas of female infertility surgery,* ed 3, St Louis, 1999, Mosby.)

Fig. 42-33   Transverse 8-0 or 9-0 sutures have been placed to correct luminal disparity. (From Hunt RB: Tubal anastomosis by laparotomy. In Hunt RB, editor: *Atlas of female infertility surgery,* ed 3, St Louis, 1999, Mosby.)

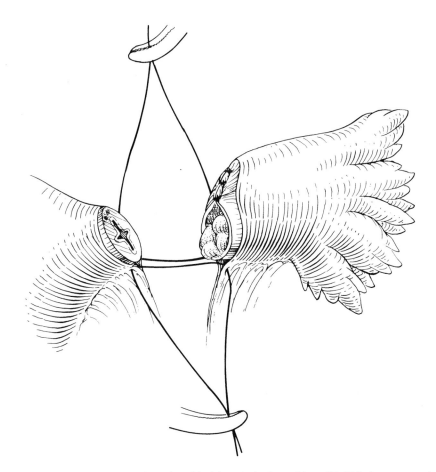

Fig. 42-34   Stay sutures are placed and held or tied. (From Hunt RB: Tubal anastomosis by laparotomy. In Hunt RB, editor: *Atlas of female infertility surgery,* ed 3, St Louis, 1999, Mosby.)

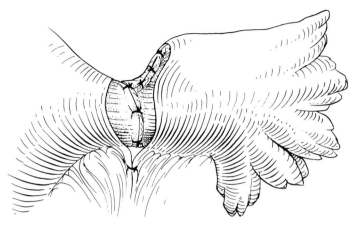

Fig. 42-35   Inner layer of sutures are placed and tied. Serosa will be approximated next, thus completing anastomosis. (From Hunt RB: Tubal anastomosis by laparotomy. In Hunt RB, editor: *Atlas of female infertility surgery,* ed 3, St Louis, 1999, Mosby.)

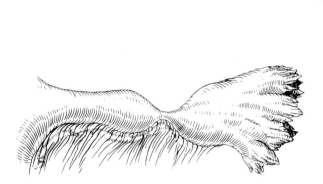

Fig. 42-36   Ampullary obstruction. (From Hunt RB: Tubal anastomosis by laparotomy. In Hunt RB, editor: *Atlas of female infertility surgery,* ed 3, St Louis, 1999, Mosby.)

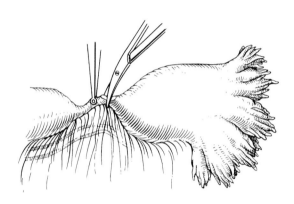

Fig. 42-37   The fibrous band joining the two segments is divided. (From Hunt RB: Tubal anastomosis by laparotomy. In Hunt RB, editor: *Atlas of female infertility surgery,* ed 3, St Louis, 1999, Mosby.)

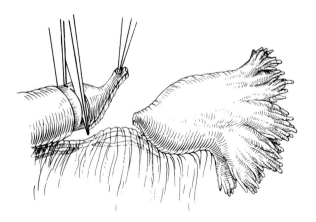

Fig. 42-38   The proximal segment is cut vertically. (From Hunt RB: Tubal anastomosis by laparotomy. In Hunt RB, editor: *Atlas of female infertility surgery,* ed 3, St Louis, 1999, Mosby.)

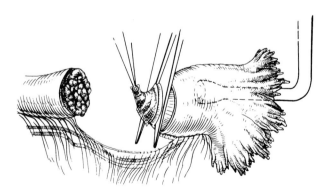

Fig. 42-39   The distal segment is prepared similarly. (From Hunt RB: Tubal anastomosis by laparotomy. In Hunt RB, editor: *Atlas of female infertility surgery,* ed 3, St Louis, 1999, Mosby.)

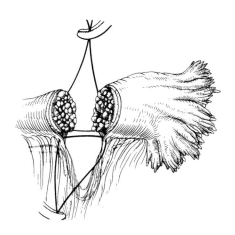

Fig. 42-40 Stay sutures are placed and tied. (From Hunt RB: Tubal anastomosis by laparotomy. In Hunt RB, editor: *Atlas of female infertility surgery,* ed 3, St Louis, 1999, Mosby.)

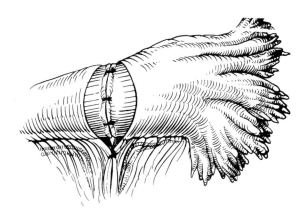

Fig. 42-41 The inner layer of 8-0 or 9-0 sutures are placed and tied. The serosa will be approximated next with 8-0 sutures. (From Hunt RB: Tubal anastomosis by laparotomy. In Hunt RB, editor: *Atlas of female infertility surgery,* ed 3, St Louis, 1999, Mosby.)

SALPINGOSTOMY

After adhesiolysis, attention is focused on the distal tube, which is released from the underlying ovary and a normal anatomic relationship is achieved (Figs. 42-42 through 42-44).

I prefer the technique advanced by Kosasa and Hale.[18] The distal tube is stabilized with a Babcock forceps and distended with indigo carmine injected transcervically. The distal tube is opened with a microelectrode, microscissors, or a laser, and the opening is enlarged with a fine hemostat (Figs. 42-45 and 42-46). The cut edges are grasped with fine hemostats, which are rotated outwardly, providing significant mucosal eversion (Fig. 42-47). Mucosal bridges and fibrous bands are divided. The mucosa is fixed with 6-0 sutures (Fig. 42-48). The process is continued until the mucosa has been everted and fixed circumferentially (Figs. 42-49 through 42-51). Tubal and ovarian defects are repaired (Fig. 42-52). After salpingostomy has been completed, the ampullary mucosa may be inspected with a standard hysteroscope (tuboscopy or falloposcopy) inserted transabdominally through the distal end of the tube and advanced to the ampullary-isthmic junction. The ampulla is distended with Ringer's lactate, and the hysteroscope is slowly withdrawn. An excellent view of the ampullary mucosa is usually obtained, allowing one to determine prognosis.[14]

To avoid adherence of the tube and ovary to the lateral pelvic sidewall, peritoneal platforms may be developed (Fig. 42-53, p. 777). This is accomplished by placing a 3-0 suture just beneath ovary, beginning at the lateral one third of the ovary. Several passes are made through the peritoneum, advancing toward the uterus. The suture is anchored just inferior to insertion of uteroovarian ligament and tied. The ureter must not be distorted by the suture. To avoid culde-sac adhesion reformation, one may triplicate round ligaments, using no. 0 absorbable or nonabsorbable synthetic materials (Fig. 42-54, p. 777).

POSTOPERATIVE FOLLOW-UP

Careful monitoring of these patients is important. They are seen 3 to 4 weeks after surgery. The couple may attempt pregnancy after the postoperative visit. At the time of the visit, the woman is again cautioned about the possibility of an ectopic pregnancy and is instructed to contact her responsible provider as soon as pregnancy is suspected. HSG is usually recommended after 4 months of unsuccessful attempts at conception. The couple is followed approximately every 2 months to review the fertility evaluation and to plan the next step. This practice keeps the couple involved in the process, which at times can be discouraging. I often obtain consultation with colleagues involved in ART for assistance in ovulation enhancement.

PREGNANCY RESULTS
Cornual Anastomosis

Cornual anastomosis has yielded excellent results. Of 43 women undergoing the procedure to reverse sterilization, 26 (61%) achieved pregnancy with only 1 (2.3%) ectopic pregnancy (EP). Of 28 patients, 18 (64.3%) experienced term pregnancy after cornual anastomosis for several indications.[3]

Results after anastomosis for correction of pathologic cornual occlusion have also been excellent. One series reported that 27 of 48 (56.2%) women had a term pregnancy and 6.2% had an EP.[10] Of 27 patients undergoing anastomosis, 53.2% consummated a viable pregnancy, but 11% developed an EP.[25] Term pregnancy rates in two additional series were 15 of 26 (57.7%)[22] and 36 of 82 (44%)[4] women. EP rates were 15.4% and 7%, respectively. Collected series of 506 women undergoing cornual anastomosis for proximal occlusion revealed 274 (54%) with intrauterine pregnancy and 18 (3.6%) with EP.[31]

Text continued on p. 778

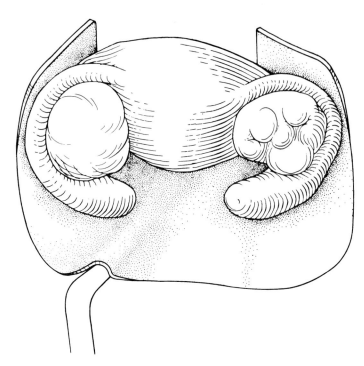

Fig. 42-42 Adhesiolysis is complete and exposure obtained. (From Hunt RB, Verhoeven HC, Schlosser HLS: Adhesiolysis, fimbrioplasty, and salpingostomy. In Hunt RB, editor: *Atlas of female infertility surgery*, ed 3, St Louis, 1999, Mosby.)

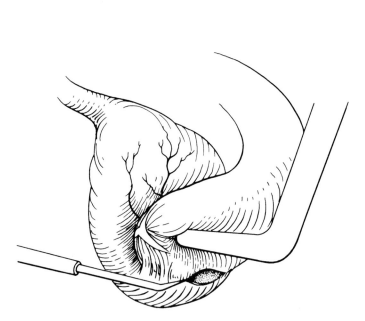

Fig. 42-43 The distal tube is mobilized from ovary. (From Hunt RB, Verhoeven HC, Schlosser HLS: Adhesiolysis, fimbrioplasty, and salpingostomy. In Hunt RB, editor: *Atlas of female infertility surgery,* ed 3, St Louis, 1999, Mosby.)

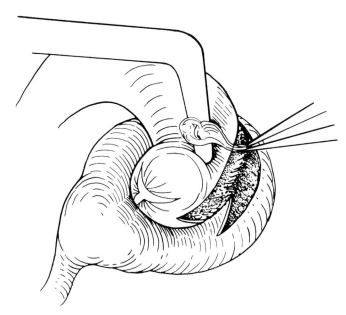

Fig. 42-44 Hemostasis is obtained with bipolar coagulation. (From Hunt RB, Verhoeven HC, Schlosser HLS: Adhesiolysis, fimbrioplasty, and salpingostomy. In Hunt RB, editor: *Atlas of female infertility surgery,* ed 3, St Louis, 1999, Mosby.)

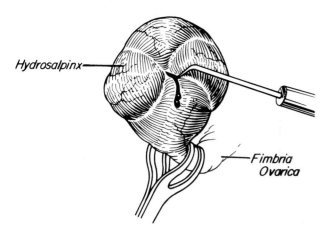

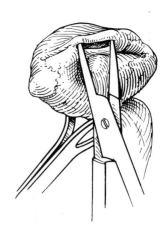

Fig. 42-45 The fimbria ovarica is stabilized with Babcock forceps and the distended distal tube is opened with a microelectrode. (From Hunt RB, Verhoeven HC, Schlosser HLS: Adhesiolysis, fimbrioplasty, and salpingostomy. In Hunt RB, editor: *Atlas of female infertility surgery*, ed 3, St Louis, 1999, Mosby.)

Fig. 42-46 The tubal opening is enlarged with a fine hemostat. (From Hunt RB, Verhoeven HC, Schlosser HLS: Adhesiolysis, fimbrioplasty, and salpingostomy. In Hunt RB, editor: *Atlas of female infertility surgery*, ed 3, St Louis, 1999, Mosby.)

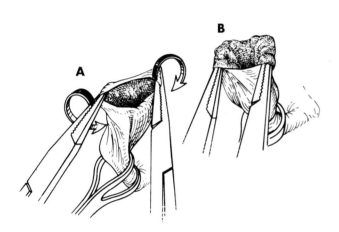

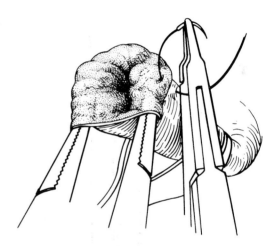

Fig. 42-47 The mucosa is grasped with fine hemostats **(A)** and everted by outward rotation **(B).** (From Hunt RB, Verhoeven HC, Schlosser HLS: Adhesiolysis, fimbrioplasty, and salpingostomy. In Hunt RB, editor: *Atlas of female infertility surgery*, ed 3, St Louis, 1999, Mosby.)

Fig. 42-48 The mucosa is fixed to the serosa by 6-0 sutures, either synthetic absorbable or nonabsorbable. (From Hunt RB, Verhoeven HC, Schlosser HLS: Adhesiolysis, fimbrioplasty, and salpingostomy. In Hunt RB, editor: *Atlas of female infertility surgery*, ed 3, St Louis, 1999, Mosby.)

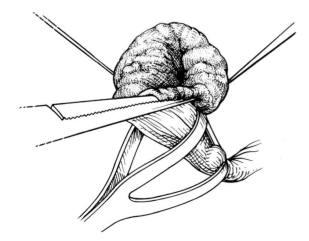

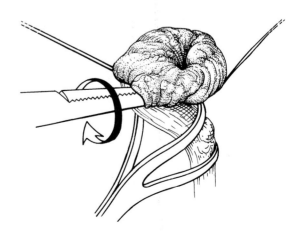

Fig. 42-49 The inferior edge of the mucosa is grasped and everted. (From Hunt RB, Verhoeven HC, Schlosser HLS: Adhesiolysis, fimbrioplasty, and salpingostomy. In Hunt RB, editor: *Atlas of female infertility surgery*, ed 3, St Louis, 1999, Mosby.)

Fig. 42-50 Rotation is continued. (From Hunt RB, Verhoeven HC, Schlosser HLS: Adhesiolysis, fimbrioplasty, and salpingostomy. In Hunt RB, editor: *Atlas of female infertility surgery*, ed 3, St Louis, 1999, Mosby.)

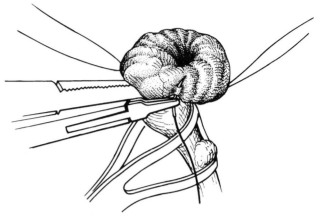

Fig. 42-51 The process is continued until all mucosa is everted and fixed with sutures. (From Hunt RB, Verhoeven HC, Schlosser HLS: Adhesiolysis, fimbrioplasty, and salpingostomy. In Hunt RB, editor: *Atlas of female infertility surgery,* ed 3, St Louis, 1999, Mosby.)

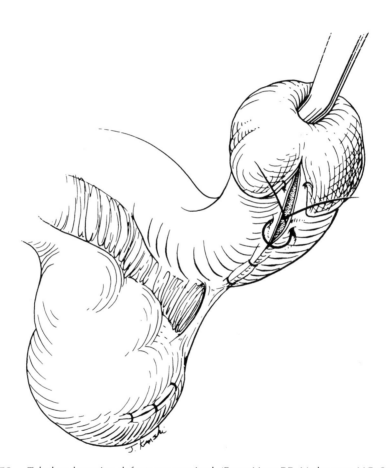

Fig. 42-52 Tubal and ovarian defects are repaired. (From Hunt RB, Verhoeven HC, Schlosser HLS: Adhesiolysis, fimbrioplasty, and salpingostomy. In Hunt RB, editor: *Atlas of female infertility surgery,* ed 3, St Louis, 1999, Mosby.)

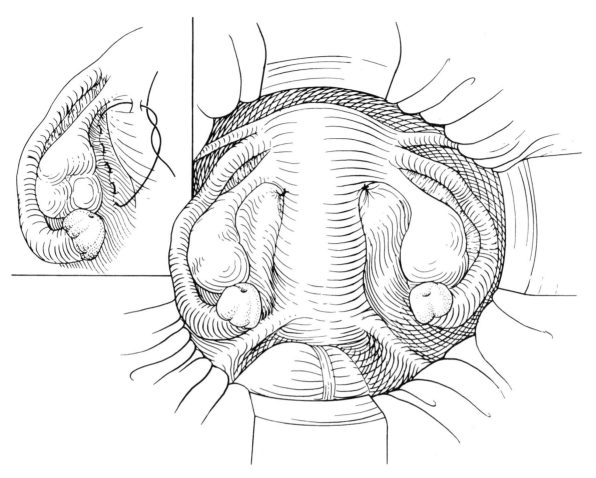

Fig. 42-53   Peritoneal platforms are developed *(inset)*. (From Hunt RB, Verhoeven HC, Schlosser HLS: Adhesiolysis, fimbrioplasty, and salpingostomy. In Hunt RB, editor: *Atlas of female infertility surgery,* ed 3, St Louis, 1999, Mosby.)

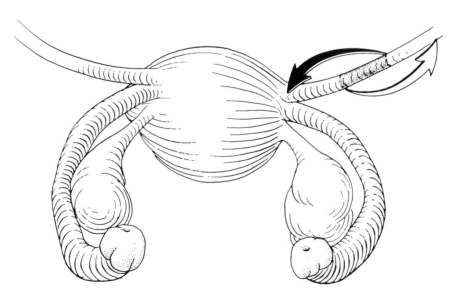

Fig. 42-54   Graphic representation of round ligament triplication. (From Hunt RB, Verhoeven HC, Schlosser HLS: Adhesiolysis, fimbrioplasty, and salpingostomy. In Hunt RB, editor: *Atlas of female infertility surgery,* ed 3, St Louis, 1999, Mosby.)

Tubotubal Anastomosis

Most reported results are based on reversal of tubal sterilization, and these have been excellent. Of 118 women undergoing tubotubal anastomosis, 93 (78.8%) achieved term pregnancy and 2 (1.7%) experienced EP.[11] Collected series of 1803 women after anastomosis revealed that 1149 (63.7%) had an intrauterine pregnancy and 68 (3.8%) had an EP.[31]

One investigator reported a 61.1% pregnancy rate after anastomosis for reversal of sterilization if the longer oviduct was 4 cm or less.[37] The mean time to conceive in this subgroup of women was 19.1 months. Another report found different results. When the longer tube was 7 cm or greater, 75% of women conceived successfully, whereas only 16% conceived successfully when the longer tube was less than 7 cm.[16] Another report found much better outcomes if the longer fallopian tube was at least 4 cm in length.[27] Although the minimal length of fallopian tube required for conception in the human has not been determined, I take a very positive view. If at least 2 cm of healthy ampulla with normal fimbriae is present in the longer tube, I proceed with anastomosis.

Salpingostomy

To determine pregnancy outcomes in women having undergone salpingostomy, one needs to follow them for at least 5 years.

Outcomes for 143 women undergoing distal salpingostomy in one clinic were as follows: 19.6% term pregnancy, 4.2% abortion, and 2.1% EP.[35] Collected series of 692 women from seven centers revealed term pregnancy rates to vary between 18% and 31% (median 24%) and EP rates between 0% and 18% (median 10%).[1]

Collected series from 14 centers consisted of 1275 women with the following results: 21% term pregnancy and 8% EP. Women found to have favorable prognosis had a term pregnancy rate of 59% and an EP rate of 4% compared with a term pregnancy rate of 4% and an EP rate of 16% among those thought to have a poor prognosis.[21]

The Mayo Clinic reported a 29% term pregnancy rate among 71 women who underwent salpingostomy.[36] For women found to have moderate adhesions the rate of success was 39% compared with 27% among those with severe adhesions. These findings are consistent with the report of direct correlation between the extent and type of adhesions and pregnancy outcomes after salpingostomy.[15]

What about repeat salpingostomy? In collected series of 135 women undergoing repeat salpingostomy from five centers, the reported term pregnancy rates ranged from 8.4% to 33% (median 10%).[1]

CONCLUSION

The physician should be in a position to offer the infertile couple afflicted with tubal factor infertility the very best in ART and microsurgical skills. The method of treatment can then be matched to the woman, and not the woman to the method of treatment. The patient will be most appreciative, and the physician will experience the joy of having offered the best therapy for the couple.

REFERENCES

1. Bateman BG, Nunley WC Jr, Kitchin JD III: Surgical management of distal tubal obstruction—are we making progress? *Fertil Steril* 48:523, 1987.
2. Blandau RJ: Comparative aspects of tubal anatomy and physiology as they relate to reconstructive procedures, *J Reprod Med* 21:7, 1978.
3. Diamond E: A comparison of gross and microsurgical techniques for repair of cornual occlusion in infertility: a retrospective study, 1968-1978, *Fertil Steril* 32:370, 1979.
4. Donnez J, Casanas-Roux F: Prognostic factors influencing the pregnancy rate after microsurgical cornual anastomosis, *Fertil Steril* 46:1089, 1986.
5. Donnez J, et al: Tubal polyps, epithelial inclusions, and endometriosis after tubal sterilization, *Fertil Steril* 41:564, 1984.
6. Ehrler P: Anastomose intramurale de la tromp, *Bull Fed Soc Gynecol Obstet* 17:866, 1965.
7. Fortier KJ, Haney AF: Pathologic spectrum of uterotubal junction obstruction, *Obstet Gynecol* 65:93, 1985.
8. Glock JL, et al: Reproductive outcome after tubal reversal in women 40 years of age or older, *Fertil Steril* 65:863, 1996.
9. Gomel V: Microsurgical reversal of female sterilization: a reappraisal, *Fertil Steril* 33:587, 1980.
10. Gomel V: An odyssey through the oviduct, *Fertil Steril* 39:144, 1983.
11. Gomel V: *Microsurgery in female infertility,* Boston, 1983, Little, Brown.
12. Gomel V, McComb P, Boer-Meisel M: Histologic reaction to polyglactin-910, polyethylene, and nylon microsuture, *J Reprod Med* 25:56, 1980.
13. Hedon B, Wineman M, Winston RML: Loupes or microscope for tubal anastomosis? An experimental study, *Fertil Steril* 34:264, 1980.
14. Henry-Suchet J, et al: Prognostic value of tuboscopy vs hysterosalpingography before tuboplasty, *J Reprod Med* 29:609, 1984.
15. Hulka JF: Adnexal adhesions: a prognostic staging and classification system based on a five-year survey of fertility surgery results at Chapel Hill, North Carolina, *Am J Obstet Gynecol* 144:141, 1982.
16. Hulka JF, Halme J: Sterilization reversal: results of 101 attempts, *Am J Obstet Gynecol* 159:769, 1988.
17. Hunt RB, Acuna HA: Pelvic preparation and choice of incision. In Hunt RB, editor: *Atlas of female infertility surgery,* Chicago, 1986, Mosby.
18. Kosasa TS, Hale RW: Treatment of hydrosalpinx using a single incision eversion procedure, *Int J Fertil* 33:319, 1988.
19. Laufer N, et al: Macroscopic and histologic tissue reaction to polydioxanone, a new, synthetic, monofilament microsuture, *J Reprod Med* 29:307, 1984.
20. Leader A, et al: Histologic reaction to a new microsurgical suture in rabbit reproductive tissue, *Fertil Steril* 40:815, 1983.
21. Marana R, Quagliarello J: Distal tubal occlusion: microsurgery versus in vitro fertilization: a review, *Int J Fertil* 33:107, 1988.
22. McComb P: Microsurgical tubocornual anastomosis for occlusive cornual disease: reproducible results without the need for tubouterine implantation, *Fertil Steril* 46:571, 1986.
23. McCormick WG, Torres J: A method of Pomeroy tubal ligation reanastomosis, *Obstet Gynecol* 47:623, 1976.
24. Neff MR, Holtz GL, Betsill WL Jr: Adhesion formation and histologic reaction with polydioxanone and polyglactin suture, *Am J Obstet Gynecol* 151:20, 1985.
25. Patton PE, Williams TJ, Coulam CB: Microsurgical reconstruction of the proximal oviduct, *Fertil Steril* 47:35, 1987.
26. Pauerstein CJ: Why has not man a microscopic eye? *Fertil Steril* 34:289, 1980.
27. Rock JA, et al: Tubal anastomosis following unipolar cautery, *Fertil Steril* 37:613, 1982.

28. Rock JA, et al: Comparison of the operating microscope and loupe for microsurgical tubal anastomosis: a randomized clinical trial, *Fertil Steril* 41:229, 1984.

29. Rosch J, et al: Selective transcervical fallopian tube catheterization: technique update, *Radiology* 168:1, 1988.

30. Sojo D, Pardo JD, Nistal M: Histology and fertility after microsurgical anastomosis of the rabbit fallopian tube with nylon and polyglactin sutures, *Fertil Steril* 39:707, 1983.

31. Sotrel G: *Tubal reconstructive surgery,* Philadelphia, 1990, Lea & Febiger.

32. Stock RJ: Postsalpingectomy endometriosis: a reassessment, *Obstet Gynecol* 60:560, 1982.

33. Trimbos-Kemper TCM: Reversal of sterilization in women over 40 years of age: a multicenter study in the Netherlands, *Fertil Steril* 53:575, 1990.

34. Vasquez G, et al: Tubal lesions subsequent to sterilization and their relation to fertility after attempts at reversal, *Am J Obstet Gynecol* 138:86, 1980.

35. Verhoeven HC, et al: Surgical treatment for distal tubal occlusion, *J Reprod Med* 28:293, 1983.

36. Williams TJ: Surgical procedures for inflammatory tubal disease, *Obstet Gynecol Clin North Am* 14:1037, 1987.

37. Winston RML: The future of microsurgery in infertility, *Clin Obstet Gynecol* 5:607, 1978.

38. Winston RML: Reversal of tubal sterilization, *Clin Obstet Gynecol* 23:1261, 1980.

43 Surgery to Repair Disorders of Development

JOHN A. ROCK and RONY A. ADAM

EMBRYOLOGY

The reproductive organs in the female (and also in the male) consist of external genitalia, gonads, and an internal duct system between the two. These three components originate embryologically from different primordia and in close association with the urinary system and hindgut (Figs. 43-1 and 43-2). Even in the 3.5- to 4-mm embryo, the bilateral thickenings of the coelomic epithelium known as the gonadal ridges medial to the mesonephros (primitive kidney) in the dorsum of the coelomic cavity can be recognized. At about the sixth week of gestation, in the 17- to 20-mm embryo, the gonad can be distinguished as either a testis or an ovary.

In the female, the labia minora and majora develop from the labioscrotal folds, which are ectodermal in origin. The phallic portion of the urogenital sinus gives rise to the urethra. The müllerian (paramesonephric) duct system is stimulated to develop preferentially over the wolffian (mesonephric) duct system, which regresses in early female fetal life. The cranial parts of the wolffian ducts can persist as the epoöphoron of the ovarian hilum; the caudal parts can persist as Gartner's ducts. The müllerian ducts persist and attain complete development to form the fallopian tubes, the uterine corpus and cervix, and a portion of the vagina.

Origins of the Müllerian Ducts

About 37 days after fertilization, the müllerian ducts first appear lateral to each wolffian duct as invaginations of the dorsal coelomic epithelium. The site of origin of the invaginations remains open and ultimately forms the fimbriated ends of the fallopian tubes. At their point of origin, each of the müllerian ducts forms a solid bud. Each bud penetrates the mesenchyme lateral and parallel to each wolffian duct. As the solid buds elongate, a lumen appears in the cranial part, beginning at each coelomic opening. The lumina extend gradually to the caudal growing tips of the ducts.

Eventually, the caudal end of each müllerian duct crosses the ventral aspect of the wolffian duct. The paired müllerian ducts continue to grow in a medial and caudal direction until they eventually meet in the midline and become fused together in the urogenital septum. The septum between the two müllerian ducts gradually disappears, leaving a single uterovaginal canal lined with cuboidal epithelium. The most cranial parts of the müllerian ducts remain separate and form the fallopian tubes. The caudal segments of the müllerian ducts fuse to form the uterus and part of the vagina. The cranial point of fusion is the site of the future fundus of the uterus.

Development of the Vagina

The vagina is formed from the lower end of the uterovaginal canal, which developed from the müllerian ducts and the urogenital sinus (see Fig. 43-2). The point of contact between the two is the müllerian tubercle. A solid vaginal cord results from proliferation of the cells at the caudal tip of the fused müllerian ducts. The cord gradually elongates to meet the bilateral endodermal evaginations (sinovaginal bulbs) from the posterior aspect of the urogenital sinus below. These sinovaginal bulbs extend cranially to fuse with the caudal end of the vaginal cord, forming the vaginal plate. Subsequent canalization of the vaginal cord occurs, followed by epithelialization with cells derived mostly from endoderm of the urogenital sinus. Recent proposals hold that only the upper one third of the vagina is formed from the müllerian ducts and that the lower vagina develops from the vaginal plate of the urogenital sinus. Recent studies also suggest that the vaginal canal is actually open and connected to a patent uterus and tubes, even in early embryonic life, and that the vagina develops under the influence of the müllerian ducts and estrogenic stimulation. There is general agreement that the vagina is a composite formed partly from the müllerian ducts and partly from the urogenital sinus.[134]

At about the twentieth week, the cervix takes form as a result of condensation of stromal cells at a specific site around the fused müllerian ducts. The mesenchyme surrounding the müllerian ducts becomes condensed early in embryonic development and eventually forms the musculature of the female genital tract. The hymen is the embryologic septum between the sinovaginal bulbs above and the urogenital sinus proper below. It is lined by an internal layer of vaginal epithelium and an external layer of epithelium derived from the urogenital sinus (both of endodermal origin), with mesoderm between the two. It is not derived from the müllerian ducts.

CLASSIFICATION OF UTEROVAGINAL ANOMALIES

Classifications of uterovaginal anomalies were originally organized on the basis of clinical findings. Our improved understanding of the developmental biology underlying uterovaginal anomalies has enabled categorization on the basis of embryology.[3] Our discussion follows a suggested modification of the American Fertility Society (AFS) classification of uterovaginal anomalies (see the box on p. 783).

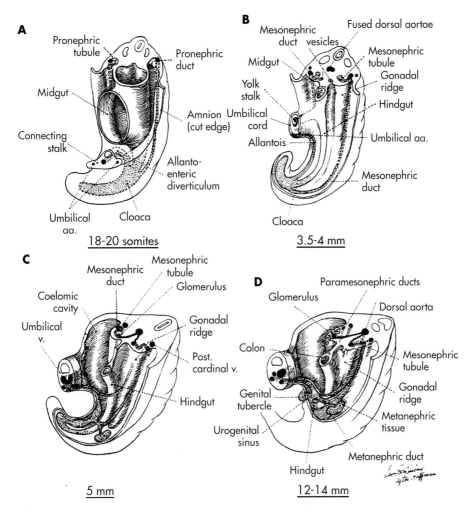

Fig. 43-1   Diagrammatic representation of the development of the female reproductive organs and structures in early embryogenesis. **A,** At the 18- to 20-somite stage (fourth week), the gonadal ridges have not yet begun to form. **B,** In the 3.5- to 4-mm embryo (fifth week), the gonadal ridges can be recognized as thickenings of the coelomic cavity just medial to the mesonephric tubules. (Gonadal differentiation into either testis or ovary does not occur until the sixth week of development.) The allantoenteric diverticulum is joined caudally to the dilated cloaca. **C** and **D,** The genital tubercle and labial folds form in the region just anterior to the cloaca. The cloaca later divides into the ventral urogenital sinus and the dorsal rectum. The development of the urinary system closely parallels that of the reproductive system. The nonfunctioning pronephric tubules shown in **A** develop to form the mesonephric ducts shown in **B** and **C.** The permanent kidneys eventually develop from the metanephric tissue, and the urinary collecting system develops from the metanephric ducts. The paramesonephric (müllerian) ducts are apparent by the 12- to 14-mm stage (**D**) (their subsequent development is illustrated in Fig. 43-2). (From Rock JA, Thompson JD: *TeLinde's operative gynecology,* ed 8, Philadelphia, 1997, Lippincott-Raven.)

This classification of four groups is based on recognizable embryologic aberrations.

Class I: Dysgenesis of the Müllerian Ducts

Dysgenesis of the müllerian ducts, also called agenesis of the uterus and vagina (the Mayer-Rokitansky-Küster-Hauser syndrome), is an impairment of the reproductive system characterized by no reproductive potential other than that achieved by in vitro fertilization in a host uterus.

Class II: Disorders of Vertical Fusion of the Müllerian Ducts

Disorders of vertical fusion can be considered to represent faults in the junction between the down-growing müllerian ducts (müllerian tubercle) and the up-growing derivative of the urogenital sinus. Typically, these disorders are characterized by an atretic portion of vagina that can be quite thick, extending through more than half the distance of the vagina, or it can be quite thin and limited to a small obstructing membrane.

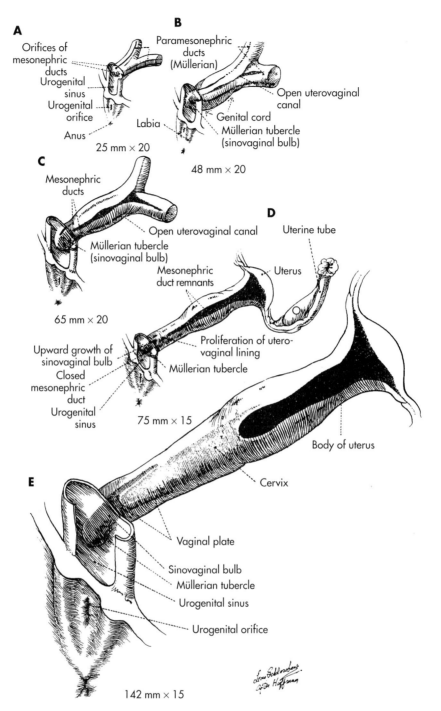

Fig. 43-2 Further development of the paramesonephric (müllerian) ducts and the urogenital sinus. **A,** Early development of the paramesonephric ducts. The cranial ends of the paramesonephric ducts develop first. These ends remain open to form the fimbriated ends of the fallopian tubes. The paramesonephric ducts grow caudally, cross the mesonephric ducts ventrally, and **(B)** eventually fuse together to form the uterovaginal canal. **C,** Further caudal development brings this structure into contact with the wall of the urogenital sinus, producing the müllerian tubercle. The caudal ends of the fused paramesonephric ducts form the uterine corpus and cervix. Together with the urogenital sinus, they also form the vagina. The cranial point of fusion of the paramesonephric ducts marks the location of the future uterine fundus. The fallopian tubes form from the unfused cranial parts of the paramesonephric (müllerian) ducts. The proliferation of the lining of the uterovaginal canal above the upward growth of the sinovaginal bulb from below **(D)** forms the vaginal plate **(E),** which later becomes canalized to leave an open vaginal canal. Thus the vagina is of composite origin. The mesonephric ducts in the female degenerate but can persist into adult life as Gartner's ducts. (From Rock JA, Thompson JD: *TeLinde's operative gynecology,* ed 8, Philadelphia, 1997, Lippincott-Raven.)

A transverse vaginal septum can develop at any location in the vagina but is more common in the upper vagina at the point of junction between the vaginal plate and the caudal end of the fused müllerian ducts. This defect presumably is caused by failure of absorption of the tissue that separates the two or by failure of complete fusion of the two embryologic components of the vagina. A large segment of vagina can be atretic. In past reviews, this has been termed partial vaginal agenesis with a uterus present. Elucidation of the cause of a high transverse vaginal septum is more difficult. A local abnormality of the vaginal mesoderm or failure of canalization of the epithelial vaginal plate can provide the answer, but why the abnormality should occur at this particular site is not evident. The proportion of the vagina originating from the urogenital sinus can at times be considerably more than one fifth, and a high transverse vaginal septum thus may represent the junction of an abnormally long urogenital sinus contribution and a short müllerian portion.

Regardless of the length of the septum, a disorder of vertical fusion should be regarded as a transverse vaginal septum and classified as either obstructed or unobstructed. The so-called partial vaginal agenesis with uterus and cervix present is probably a misnomer for a large segment of atretic vagina. Cervical agenesis or dysgenesis is also included in the group of disorders of vertical fusion.

Class III: Disorders of Lateral Fusion of the Müllerian Ducts

Disorders of lateral fusion of the two müllerian ducts can be symmetric-unobstructed, as with the double vagina, or asymmetric-obstructed, as with unilateral vaginal obstruction. Obstructions associated with disorders of lateral fusion are particularly noteworthy because they are observed clinically only as unilateral obstructions that almost invariably are associated with absence of the ipsilateral kidney. Bilateral obstruction is thought to be associated with bilateral agenesis and subsequent nonviability of the developing embryo.

The three varieties of asymmetric obstruction with ipsilateral renal agenesis are as follows:

1. Unicornuate uterus with a noncommunicating horn that contains menstruating endometrium
2. Unilateral obstruction of a cavity of a double uterus
3. Unilateral vaginal obstruction

The five groups of symmetric-unobstructed disorders of lateral fusion are as follows:

1. The didelphic uterus
2. The septate uterus
3. The bicornuate uterus
4. The T-shaped uterine cavity, which may be hypoplastic and irregular and which is associated with diethylstilbestrol (DES) exposure in utero
5. The unicornuate uterus with or without a rudimentary horn

The first three groups are types of double uteri; differentiation between a septate uterus (second group) and a bicor-

---

AMERICAN FERTILITY SOCIETY CLASSIFICATION OF UTEROVAGINAL ANOMALIES

Class I. Dysgenesis of the müllerian ducts
Class II. Disorders of vertical fusion of the müllerian ducts
    A. Transverse vaginal septum
        1. Obstructed
        2. Unobstructed
    B. Cervical agenesis or dysgenesis
Class III. Disorders of lateral fusion of the müllerian ducts
    A. Asymmetric-obstructed disorder of uterus or vagina usually associated with ipsilateral renal agenesis
        1. Unicornuate uterus with a noncommunicating rudimentary anlage or horn
        2. Unilateral obstruction of a cavity of a double uterus
        3. Unilateral vaginal obstruction associated with double uterus
    B. Symmetric-unobstructed
        1. Didelphic uterus
            a. Complete longitudinal vaginal septum
            b. Partial longitudinal vaginal septum
            c. No longitudinal vaginal septum
        2. Septate uterus
            a. Complete
                (1) Complete longitudinal vaginal septum
                (2) Partial longitudinal vaginal septum
                (3) No longitudinal vaginal septum
            b. Partial
                (1) Complete longitudinal vaginal septum
                (2) Partial longitudinal vaginal septum
                (3) No longitudinal vaginal septum
        3. Bicornuate uterus
            a. Complete
                (1) Complete longitudinal vaginal septum
                (2) Partial longitudinal vaginal septum
                (3) No longitudinal vaginal septum
            b. Partial
                (1) Complete longitudinal vaginal septum
                (2) Partial longitudinal vaginal septum
                (3) No longitudinal vaginal septum
        4. T-shaped uterine cavity (diethylstilbestrol related)
        5. Unicornuate uterus
            a. With a rudimentary horn
                (1) With endometrial cavity
                    (a) Communicating
                    (b) Noncommunicating
                (2) Without endometrial cavity
            b. Without a rudimentary horn
Class IV. Unusual configurations of vertical-lateral fusion defects

Modified from the American Fertility Society classification of müllerian anomalies, *Fertil Steril* 49:952, 1988.

nuate uterus (third group) requires visualization of the fundus. The septum within the septate uterus is complete or partial. When the septum is complete, there inevitably are two cervices with a longitudinal vaginal septum that can extend to the introitus or partially down the vagina. The bicornuate uterus also can have a partial or almost complete separation of the uterine cavities. The term *arcuate* uterus is used primarily by radiologists to refer to a slight septum in the uterine fundus that forms no clear separation of the uterine cavities. This type of uterus is usually included in the category of partial septate uterus.

The unicornuate uterus may have an attached horn with a cavity that communicates with the unicornuate uterus, or there may be no uterine horn or a uterine horn with no cavity. Some debate has focused on whether the unicornuate uterus with a communicating horn can represent a hypoplastic side of a bicornuate uterus.

Class IV: Unusual Configurations of Vertical-Lateral Fusion Defects

This final category, unusual configurations of vertical-lateral fusion defects, includes combinations of uterovaginal anomalies and other disorders. Unusual uterovaginal configurations have been described that do not fit a particular category, and vertical and lateral fusion disorders can coexist.

Unusual configurations of vertical-lateral fusion defects can be seen with abnormalities of the lower urinary tract. Singh et al.[126] have described a patient who was noted to have a persistent hymen and a longitudinal vaginal septum with a didelphic uterus. The patient was noted also to have a double urethra and bladder and left renal agenesis.

Obstructive lesions require immediate attention to relieve retrograde flow of trapped mucus and menstrual blood and increasing pressure on surrounding organs and structures. When no obstruction is present, attention may not be required immediately, but it will always be required eventually to establish or improve reproductive or coital function.

DYSGENESIS OF THE MÜLLERIAN DUCTS
Overview

The disorders of müllerian agenesis include congenital absence of the vagina and uterus. Often referred to in the literature simply as congenital absence of the vagina (vaginal agenesis), this condition is more accurately labeled aplasia (or dysplasia) of the müllerian ducts because the lower vagina generally is normal but the middle and upper two thirds are missing. Despite the absence of the uterus, rudimentary uterine primordia are found that are comparable to each other in size and appearance. Tubes and ovaries in patients with congenital absence of the müllerian ducts generally are normal. The syndrome, usually called the Mayer-Rokitansky-Küster-Hauser syndrome, is associated with a heterogeneous group of disorders that have a variety of genetic, endocrine, and metabolic manifestations and associated anomalies of other body systems (Fig. 43-3).[52,53] The incidence of the syndrome is estimated at approximately 1 per 10,000 female births.[34]

Individuals with classic Mayer-Rokitansky-Küster-Hauser syndrome usually are first seen by a gynecologist at age 14 to 15 years with primary amenorrhea. Such young women have a normal complement of chromosomes (46,XX) and usually have normal ovaries and secondary sex characteristics, including external genitalia. Menstruation does not appear at the usual age because the uterus is absent, but ovulation occurs regularly. However, polycystic ovaries or gonadal dysgenesis occasionally occurs in patients with müllerian agenesis.

Many patients with müllerian agenesis have associated anomalies of the upper müllerian duct system along with associated anomalies of other organ systems. By gentle rectal examination, the physician can feel an absence of the midline müllerian structure that should represent the uterus. The physician will instead feel a smooth band (possibly a remnant of the uterosacral ligaments) that extends from one side of the pelvis to the other. In classic Mayer-Rokitansky-Küster-Hauser syndrome, the uterus is represented by bilateral rudimentary uterine bulbs that vary in size, are not usually palpable, are connected to small fallopian tubes, and are located on the lateral pelvic side wall adjacent to normal ovaries.[98] Depending on their size, these rudimentary uterine bulbs may or may not contain a cavity lined by endometrial tissue (Fig. 43-4). If present, the endometrial tissue can appear immature or, rarely, can show evidence of cyclic response to ovarian hormones. The endometrial cavity does not communicate often with the peritoneal cavity because the tube may not be patent at the point of junction between the tube and the rudimentary uterine bulb. In rare instances, however, active endometrium can exist within the uterine anlagen and the endometrial cavity, enabling communication with the peritoneal cavity through patent fallopian tubes. Reports have described several patients with functioning endometrial tissue in one or both rudimentary uterine bulbs (see Fig 43-4, *B*). The patient can develop a large hematometra as a result of cyclic accumulation of trapped blood. Cyclic abdominal pain is relieved by excision of the active uterine anlagen.[110] A patient with Mayer-Rokitansky-Küster-Hauser syndrome was reported who had a 4-cm endometrioma removed from the left ovary by laparotomy at the time of operation to create a vagina. Myomas have been known to form in the muscular wall, and mild dysmenorrhea has been attributed to their presence.

Chakravarty[16] and Singh and Devi[125] have demonstrated that the rudimentary bulbs have the potential for function. These authors used these rudimentary uterine bulbs to reconstruct a midline uterus. The reconstructed uterus was then connected to a newly constructed vagina. A surprising number of patients who have undergone this procedure have experienced cyclic menstruation, although recurrent stenosis and obstruction of the rudimentary horns are the most common results of such efforts. The authors have had no experience with this technique and question its usefulness.

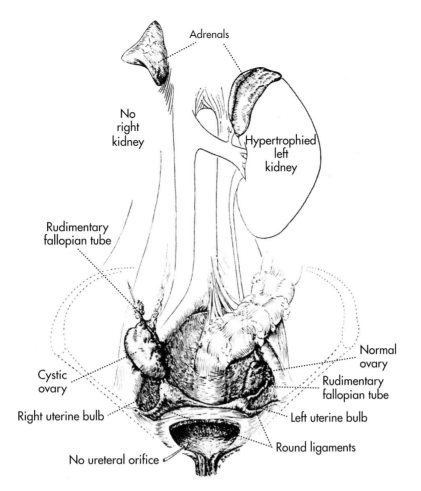

Fig. 43-3 Typical findings in a patient with Mayer-Rokitansky-Küster-Hauser syndrome. Note the absence of the right kidney and right ureteral orifice. The uterus is represented by bilateral rudimentary uterine bulbs joined by a band behind the bladder. The ovaries appear normal although there is malposition of the right ovary. (From Rock JA, Thompson JD: *TeLinde's operative gynecology,* ed 8, Philadelphia, 1997, Lippincott-Raven.)

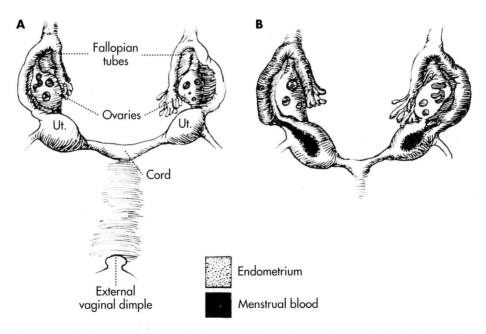

Fig. 43-4 Patients with congenital absence of the vagina can show variation in the development of the upper müllerian ducts. **A,** Bilateral rudimentary uterine bulbs without endometrium. **B,** Bilateral rudimentary uterine bulbs containing a cavity lined with functioning endometrial tissue. Cross-sectional view shows presence of menstrual blood. (From Rock JA, Thompson JD: *TeLinde's operative gynecology,* ed 8, Philadelphia, 1997, Lippincott-Raven.)

However, these rudimentary uterine bulbs usually are insignificant structures that cause no problems.

Depending on the timing of the teratogenic influence, kidneys may be absent or fused or in unusual locations in the pelvis. Ureters can be duplicated or can open in unusual places such as the vagina or uterus. Jones and Rock[74] have pointed out that failure of lateral fusion of the müllerian ducts with unilateral obstruction is associated consistently with absence of the kidney on the side with obstruction. Bilateral obstruction has not been observed clinically, presumably because it would be associated with bilateral renal agenesis, a condition that would not allow the embryo to develop. According to Thompson and Lynn,[133] 40% of female patients with congenital absence of the kidneys are found to have associated genital anomalies. Fore et al.[43] reported that 47% of patients in whom evaluation of the urinary tract was performed had associated urologic anomalies. In other studies, approximately one third of patients with complete vaginal agenesis were found to have significant urinary anomalies, including unilateral renal agenesis, unilateral or bilateral pelvic kidney, horseshoe kidney, hydronephrosis, hydroureter, and a variety of patterns of ureteral duplication. A significant number of patients with partial vaginal agenesis also have associated urinary tract anomalies.

Associated skeletal anomalies have been recognized since congenital absence of the vagina was first described. In a review of 574 reported cases, Griffin et al.[50] found a 12% incidence of skeletal abnormalities. Most of these abnormalities involve the spine (e.g., wedge vertebrae, fusions), but the limbs and ribs can also be involved. Other anomalies include syndactyly, absence of a digit, congenital heart disease, and inguinal hernias, although the latter are more often present in patients with androgen insensitivity syndrome than in patients with Mayer-Rokitansky-Küster-Hauser syndrome.

Clinical Evaluation

The evaluation of a young teenager with primary amenorrhea begins with a careful history, especially eliciting complaints of cyclic pelvic pain. Obtaining a basal body temperature chart may help differentiate such pain as being ovulatory or dysmenorrhea originating from well developed rudimentary uterine bulbs. Careful pelvic and rectal examinations are crucial to determine whether the vagina and uterus are present. Note should be made regarding secondary sexual characteristics (breast development, pubic hair pattern, and external genitalia).

The congenital absence of the vagina must be differentiated from an imperforate hymen with cryptomenorrhea. The diagnosis is facilitated by placing a metal catheter or similar instrument in the urethra and a finger in the rectum. If the metal instrument in the urethra is easily felt through the anterior rectal wall, the vagina is most likely absent. On the other hand, an intervening mass felt between the rectal finger and the instrument in the urethra may represent hematocolpos accumulated behind an imperforate hymen.

Additional diagnostic testing includes a buccal smear to determine presence or absence of the chromatin body. If the chromatin body is absent or if gonadal dysgenesis, androgen insensitivity syndrome, or a variant of the classic Mayer-Rokitansky-Küster-Hauser syndrome is suspected, a complete chromosomal analysis should be performed. An intravenous pyelogram should be done to evaluate the urinary tract and survey for spine anomalies. If a pelvic mass is present, additional special studies, including ultrasonography, should be performed to differentiate between hematometra, hematocolpos, endometrial and other cysts, and pelvic kidney. Evaluation with magnetic resonance imaging (MRI) has been suggested for the evaluation of primary amenorrhea. Overall, high levels of correlation have been noted between MRI diagnosis and subsequent findings. Laparoscopy is rarely necessary to complete the evaluation of patients suspected for müllerian agenesis.

Psychological Preparation of the Patient

Insufficient attention has been given to the psychological aspects of this problem. The patient with congenital absence of the vagina cannot be made into a whole person simply by creating a perineal pouch for intercourse. Establishment of sexual function is only one concern and may be the easiest problem to correct. Evans[33] reported that 15% of his patients have real psychiatric difficulty. Evans et al.[34] and David et al.[26] suggest that psychiatric help should be initiated before any surgery is undertaken.

Learning about this anomaly, especially at a young age, is a shock and is accompanied by diminished self-esteem. Such patients can be encouraged by having their gynecologist offer appropriate surgery to establish coital function. The gynecologist can point out that, functionally, the patient will be like thousands of young women who have had a hysterectomy because of serious pelvic disease and who have satisfied their desire to be a parent through adoption. Another reproductive option may be in vitro fertilization and implantation into a donor uterus.

METHODS OF CREATING A VAGINA

Techniques for creating a vagina may be classified as nonsurgical or surgical, with no consensus as to the best approach (see the box on p. 787). Regardless of the technique used, the patient must understand her crucial role in successfully maintaining a patent vagina until regular intercourse is taking place. The single most important factor in determining the success of vaginoplasty is the psychosocial adjustment of the patient to her congenital vaginal anomaly. The usual timing of surgery for vaginal agenesis is at 17 to 20 years of age and when the patient is emotionally mature and intellectually reliable enough to manage the vaginal form used to maintain the neovaginal space.

Nonsurgical Methods

In 1938, Frank[44] described a method of creating an artificial vagina without operation. In 1940, he reported remarkably

CLASSIFICATION OF METHODS TO FORM A NEW VAGINA

NONSURGICAL (INTERMITTENT PRESSURE ON THE PERINEUM)
Active dilation
Passive dilation
Vecchietti procedure

SURGICAL
Without use of abdominal contents
Without cavity dissection
   Vulvovaginoplasty
   Constant pressure
No attempt to line cavity (now unacceptable)
Lining cavity with artificial material (oxidized regenerated cellulose)
Lining cavity with grafts
   Split-thickness skin grafts (McIndoe operation)
   Dermis grafts
   Amnion homografts
Lining cavity with flaps
   Musculocutaneous flaps
   Fasciocutaneous flaps
   Subcutaneous pedicled skin flaps
   Labial skin flaps (can be created with tissue expander)
   Penoplasty (transsexualism)
With use of abdominal contents (cavity lining with)
   Peritoneum
   Free intestinal graft
   Pedicled intestine

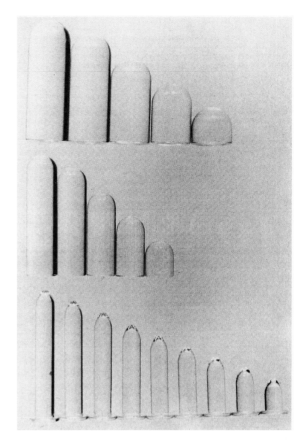

Fig. 43-5 Vaginal dilators for use in Ingram passive dilation technique to create a new vagina. The set consists of 19 dilators of increasing length and width. (Courtesy of Faulkner Plastics, Tampa, FL. From Rock JA, Thompson JD: *TeLinde's operative gynecology,* ed 8, Philadelphia, 1997, Lippincott-Raven.)

satisfactory results in eight patients treated by this method.[45] His follow-up study showed that a vagina formed in this manner remained permanent in depth and caliber, even in patients who neglected dilation for more than 1 year. It has been emphasized that the pelvic floor itself is embryologically deficient in some patients. Indeed, the ease with which some patients are able to create a vagina with intercourse alone or with other intermittent pressure techniques can be explained on this basis.

Rock et al.[116] at the Johns Hopkins Hospital reported that an initial trial of vaginal dilation was successful in 9 of 21 patients.

Prompted by the rewarding results of Broadbent and Woolf,[11] Ingram[62] has described a passive dilation technique of creating a new vagina. Instructing his patients in the insertion of dilators (Fig. 43-5) specially designed for use with a bicycle seat stool, Ingram was able to produce satisfactory vaginal depth and coital function in 10 of 12 patients with vaginal agenesis and 32 of 40 patients with various types of stenosis.

The Ingram technique for passive dilation has several advantages. The patient is not required to press the dilator against the vaginal pouch. A series of graduated Lucite dilators slowly and evenly dilate the neovaginal space. The patient should be carefully instructed in the use of dilators, as recommended by Ingram, beginning with the smallest dilator. The patient is instructed with the use of a mirror how to place a dilator against the introital dimple. The dilator may be held in place with a light girdle and regular clothing worn over this.

The patient sits on a racing type bicycle seat that is placed on a stool 24 inches above the floor. She is instructed to sit leaning slightly forward with the dilator in place for at least 2 hours/day at 15- to 30-minute intervals. The patient is usually followed at monthly intervals and can be expected to graduate to the next size larger dilator about every month. Sexual intercourse may be attempted after the use of the largest dilator for 1 or 2 months. Continued dilation is recommended if intercourse is infrequent. In our experience, functional success rates approach 80% (personal communication, J. A. Rock). Thus passive dilation should be suggested as an initial therapy for vaginal creation. If dilation is unsuccessful, operative vaginoplasty is indicated.

Surgical Methods

Intermediate between surgical and nonsurgical methods, the Vecchietti operation[136] involves surgically placing an olive-shaped acrylic dilator on the perineum. The olive is connected by suture, which is passed subperitoneally to a traction device placed on the lower abdomen. Postoperatively, progressive, constant traction is placed on the olive, which creates a neovagina by invagination within 6 to 9 days. The original Vecchietti operation is an abdominal procedure, which recently has been adapted to a laparoscopic technique.[138]

During the past three decades, experience has proved the Abbe-Wharton-McIndoe procedure (more popularly called the McIndoe operation) to be generally superior to others for dealing with the complete absence of a vagina. In special circumstances, either the Williams method of creating a vulvovaginal pouch or the sigmoid transplant of Pratt may be indicated.

Historical Development of Surgical Procedures

In 1907, Baldwin[7] used a double loop of ileum to line a space dissected between the rectum and bladder, leaving the mesentery connected to the bowel. The continuity of the intestinal tract was reestablished by an end-to-end anastomosis. He reported that the new vagina was absolutely normal in every way. In 1910, Popaw[107] constructed a vagina using a portion of the rectum that was moved anteriorly. This operation was modified by Schubert in 1911. The rectum was severed above the anal sphincter and moved anteriorly to serve as the vagina. The sigmoid colon was sutured to the anus to reestablish the continuity of the intestinal tract. Both operations had soberingly high morbidity and mortality, and their popularity declined. Today, segments of sigmoid are used most often to create a vaginal pouch or extend vaginal length in patients who have lost vaginal function as a result of extensive surgery or irradiation for pelvic malignancy.

Less formidable procedures involving dissection of a space between the bladder and rectum and lining of this space with flaps of skin from the labia or inner thighs also were tried. Significant scarring resulted, and hair usually grew into the vagina. Extensive plastic procedures to construct a vagina are no longer necessary or desirable unless there is the problem of maintaining a vaginal canal after an extensive exenterative operation for pelvic malignancy. In this case, the physician may want to consider using the gracilis myocutaneous flap technique described by McCraw et al. in 1976.[89]

The Abbe-Wharton-McIndoe Operation

Overview. The operation most popular today for creating a new vagina began with simple surgical attempts to create a space between the bladder and the rectum.[1] These early attempts were often made in patients with cryptomenorrhea. However, such a space usually would constrict because the surgeon would fail to recognize the importance of prolonged continuous dilation until the constrictive phase of healing was complete.

At the Johns Hopkins Hospital in 1938, Wharton[140] combined adequate dissection of the vaginal space with continuous dilation by a balsa form that was covered with a thin rubber sheath and was left in the space. He did not use a split-thickness skin graft. Instead, he based his operation on the principle that the vaginal epithelium has remarkable powers of proliferation and in a relatively short time will cover the raw surface. Recalling that a similar procedure occurs in the fetus when the epithelium of the sinovaginal bulbs and the urogenital sinus form the vaginal canal, Wharton[141,142] merely applied this same principle in the adult. This simple procedure is entirely satisfactory as long as the space is kept dilated long enough to allow the epithelium to grow in. However, even after several years, the vault of the vagina occasionally remains without epithelial covering. Coital bleeding and leukorrhea result from the persistent granulation tissue, and the vaginas constructed by this method tend to be constricted by scarring in the upper portion. In Counseller's 1948 report from the Mayo Clinic[19] of 100 operations to construct a new vagina, 14 were performed by Wharton's method, with excellent results in all 14 patients. It was stated that the disadvantages of persistent granulation tissue with bleeding and leukorrhea were of no consequence. This has not been our experience.

When inlay skin grafts were first used to construct a new vagina, the results were poor because the necessity for dilation of the new vagina again was not recognized. Severe contraction, uncontrolled by continuous or intermittent dilation, almost invariably spoiled the results. Although Heppner, Abbe, and others preceded him by many years in using a skin-covered prosthesis in neovaginal construction,[1] it was Sir Archibald McIndoe, at the Queen Victoria Hospital in England, who popularized the method and gave it substantial clinical trial.[91,92] He emphasized the three important principles used today in successful operations for vaginal agenesis:

1. Dissection of an adequate space between the rectum and bladder
2. Inlay split-thickness skin grafting
3. The cardinal principle of continuous and prolonged dilation during the contractile phase of healing

Other tissues, such as amnion and peritoneum, have been used to line the new vaginal space, but they have not had substantial success. However, Tancer et al.[132] reported good results with human amnion. Karjalainen et al.[79] stated that a more physiologic result was achieved with an amnion graft than with a skin graft. Nevertheless, concerns about the transmission of human immunodeficiency virus with human amnion now limit this option. More recent small series report satisfactory short-term results using regenerated oxidized cellulose (Interceed) as the vaginal lining.[65,123] The limited experience with this technique renders it a less attractive option at this time.

Technique of the Abbe-Wharton-McIndoe Operation

Taking the Graft. After a careful pelvic examination is performed under anesthesia to verify previous findings, the patient is positioned for taking a skin graft from the buttocks. For cosmetic reasons, the graft should not be taken from the thigh or hip unless for some reason it cannot be obtained from the buttocks. Patients may be asked to sunbathe in a brief bathing suit before coming to the hospital so that its outline can be seen; an attempt should be made to take the graft from both buttocks within these borders. The quality of the graft determines to a great extent the success of the operation. We have found the Padgett electrodermatome to be the most satisfactory instrument for taking the graft. With relatively little experience and practice, the gynecologic surgeon can successfully cut a graft of controlled width and thickness (Fig. 43-6). The instrument is set and checked for taking a graft approximately 0.018 inch thick and 8 to 9 cm wide. The total graft length should be 16 to 20 cm. If the entire graft cannot be taken from one buttock, a graft 8 to 10 cm long will be needed from each buttock.

The skin of the donor site is prepared with an antiseptic solution (povidone-iodine), which is then thoroughly washed away. The skin is lubricated with mineral oil as assistants steady and stretch the skin tight. Considerable pressure should be applied uniformly across the dermatome blade. The thickness of the graft must have minimum variation. A graft that is a little too thick is better than one that is a little too thin. There should be no breaks in the continuity of the graft. The graft is placed between two layers of moist gauze, and the donor sites are dressed. The donor site is soaked with a dilute solution of epinephrine for hemostasis, and a sterile dressing is applied. A pressure dressing placed over the site can be removed on the seventh postoperative

day. The sterile dressing will dry in place over the donor site and ultimately will fall off by itself. Moistened areas on the dressing can be dried with cool air. If there is separation and evidence of superficial infection, merbromin (Mercurochrome) can be applied to these areas.

Creating the Neovaginal Space. The patient is placed in the lithotomy position and a transverse incision is made through the mucosa of the vaginal vestibule (Fig. 43-7, *A*). The space between the urethra and bladder anteriorly and the rectum posteriorly is dissected until the undersurface of the peritoneum is reached. This step may be safer with a catheter in the urethra and sometimes a finger in the rectum to guide the dissection in the proper plane. After incising the mucosa of the vaginal vestibule transversely, the physician often is able to create a channel on each side of a median raphe (see Fig. 43-7, *B*), starting with blunt dissection and then dilating each channel with Hegar dilators or with finger dissection. In some instances it may be necessary to develop the neovaginal space by dissecting laterally and bringing the fingers toward the midline. The median raphe is then divided, thus joining the two channels. This maneuver is helpful in dissecting an adequate space without causing injury to surrounding structures.

To avoid subsequent narrowing of the vagina at the level of the urogenital diaphragm, it may be helpful to incise the margin of the puborectalis muscles bilaterally along the midportion of the medial margin (see Fig. 43-7, *C*). Although useful in all circumstances, incision of the puborectalis muscle is more important in patients with androgen insensitivity syndrome with android pelves, in which the levator muscles are more taut against the pelvic diaphragm, than in patients with gynecoid pelves. Incision of the puborectalis muscle causes no difficulty with fecal incontinence, significantly improves the ease with which the vaginal form can be inserted into the canal in the postoperative period, and has eliminated the problem of contracture of the upper vagina caused by a poorly applied form. The dissection should be carried as high as possible without entering the peritoneal cavity and without cleaning away all tissue beneath the peritoneum. A split-thickness skin graft will not take well when applied against a base of thin peritoneum. All bleeding vessels should be ligated by clamping and tying them with very fine sutures. It is essential that the vaginal cavity be dry to prevent bleeding beneath the graft. Bleeding will cause the graft to separate from its bed, resulting in the inevitable failure of the graft to implant in that area and in local graft necrosis.

Preparing the Vaginal Form. Early skin grafts were formed over balsa, which has the advantages of being an inexpensive, easily available, light wood that can be sterilized without difficulty. It also can be whittled easily in the operating room to a proper shape to fit the new vaginal space. However, uneven pressure from the form can cause a skin graft to slough in places, and pressure spots also are associated with an increased risk of fistula formation. The Counseller-Flor (1957) modification[20,21] of the McIndoe tech-

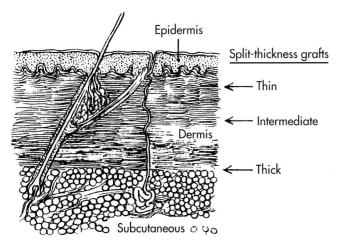

Fig. 43-6 Section of split-thickness skin grafts. Grafts should be uniform in thickness. The Padgett electrodermatome is set to take a graft approximately 0.018 inch thick. A graft that is slightly thick is better than a thin graft. (From Rock JA, Thompson JD: *TeLinde's operative gynecology,* ed 8, Philadelphia, 1997, Lippincott-Raven.)

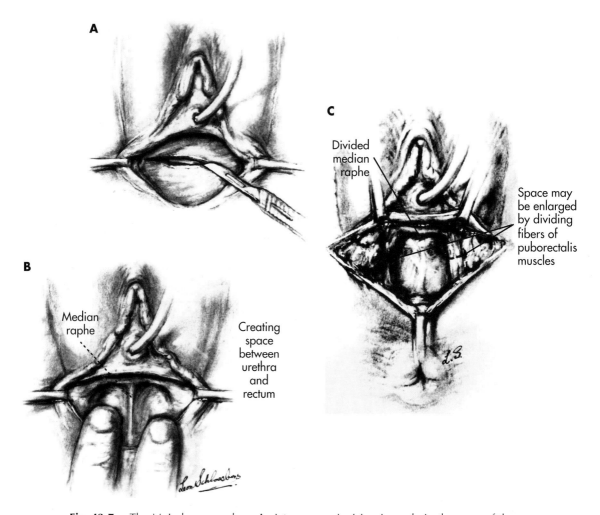

Fig. 43-7 The McIndoe procedure. **A,** A transverse incision is made in the apex of the vaginal dimple. **B,** A channel can usually be dissected on each side of the median raphe. The median raphe is then divided. Careful dissection prevents injury to the bladder and rectum. **C,** A space between the urethra and bladder anteriorly and the rectum posteriorly is dissected until the undersurface of the peritoneum is reached. Incision of the medial margin of the puborectalis muscles will enlarge the vagina laterally. (From Rock JA, Thompson JD: *TeLinde's operative gynecology,* ed 8, Philadelphia, 1997, Lippincott-Raven.)

nique uses, instead of the rigid balsa form, a foam rubber mold shaped for the vaginal cavity from a foam rubber block and covered with a condom. The foam rubber is gas sterilized in blocks measuring approximately 10 by 10 by 20 cm. The block is shaped with scissors to approximately twice the desired size, compressed into a condom, and placed into the neovagina (Fig. 43-8, *A* through *C*). The form is left in place for 20 to 30 seconds with the condom open to allow the foam rubber to expand and conform to the neovaginal space (see Fig. 43-8, *D*). The condom is then closed, and the form is withdrawn. The external end is tied with 2-0 silk, and an additional condom is placed over the form and tied securely (see Fig. 43-8, *E* and *F*).

Sewing the Graft over the Vaginal Form. The skin graft is then placed over the form and its undersurface is exteriorized and sewn over the form with interrupted vertical mattress 5-0 nonreactive sutures (see Fig. 43-8, *G* and *H*).

Where the graft is approximated, the undersurfaces of the sutured edges are also exteriorized.

The graft should not be "meshed" to make it stretch farther, and the edges of the graft should be approximated meticulously around the form without gaps. Granulation tissue develops at any place where the form is not covered with skin. Contraction usually occurs where granulation tissue forms. After the form has been placed in the neovaginal space, the edges of the graft are sutured to the skin edge with 5-0 nonreactive absorbable sutures, with sufficient space left between sutures for drainage to occur. The physician must be careful not to have the form so large that it causes undue pressure on the urethra or rectum. A balsa form should have a groove to accommodate the urethra. With a foam rubber form, this is unnecessary. A suprapubic silicone catheter is placed in the bladder for drainage. If the labia are of sufficient length, then the form can be held in

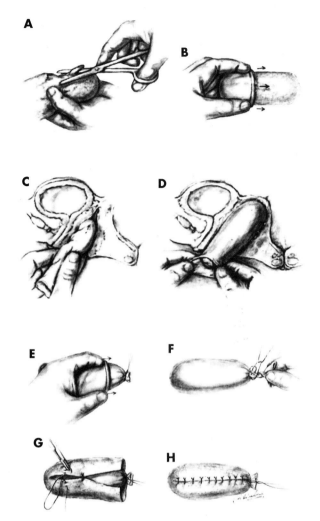

Fig. 43-8 Counsellor-Flor modification of the McIndoe technique. **A,** A form is cut from a foam rubber block. **B,** A condom is placed over the form. **C,** The form is compressed and placed into the vagina. **D,** Air is allowed to expand the foam rubber, which accommodates to the neovaginal space. The condom is closed and the form removed. **E,** A second condom is placed over the form and (**F**) tied securely. **G,** The graft is then sewn over the form with interrupted 5-0 nonreactive sutures. **H,** The undersurfaces of the sutured edges of the graft are exteriorized. The vaginal form is ready for insertion into the neovagina. (From Rock JA, Thompson JD: *TeLinde's operative gynecology,* ed 8, Philadelphia, 1997, Lippincott-Raven.)

place by suturing the labia together with two or three nonreactive sutures.

Replacing with a New Form. After 7 to 10 days, the form is removed and the vaginal cavity is irrigated with warm saline solution and inspected. This is usually performed with mild sedation and without an anesthetic. The cavity should be inspected carefully to determine whether the graft has taken satisfactorily in all areas of the new vagina. Any undue pressure by the form should be noted and corrected. It is especially important that there not be too much pressure superiorly against the peritoneum of the cul-de-sac. Such a constant upward pressure could result in

weakness with subsequent enterocele formation. The new vaginal cavity must be inspected frequently to detect and to prevent pressure necrosis of the skin graft.

The patient is given instructions on daily removal and reinsertion of the form and is taught how to administer a low-pressure douche of clean warm water. She is advised to remove the form at the time of urination and defecation, but otherwise to wear it continuously for 6 weeks. A neoprene form, which is much easier to remove and keep clean than a foam rubber form, is substituted for the original form in 6 weeks. A new form is molded with a sterile sheath cover (condom) to fit the size of the vaginal canal. The patient is instructed to use the form during the night for the following 12 months. If the caliber of the vagina has not changed by that time, it is unlikely to occur later and insertion of the form at night can be done intermittently until coitus is a frequent occurrence.[114] However, if there is the slightest difficulty in inserting the form, the patient should be advised to use the form continuously again. Most patients are able to maintain the form in place simply by wearing a panty girdle and perineal pad. Douches are advisable while there is residual vaginal healing and discharge.

Results and Complications. Results with the McIndoe operation have improved over the years. Recently reported percentages of satisfactory results have ranged from 80% to 100%. The serious complications formerly associated with the McIndoe operation have been significantly reduced by improvements in technique and greater experience. Serious complications do still occur, however, including a 4% postoperative fistula rate (urethrovaginal, vesicovaginal, and rectovaginal), postoperative infection, and intraoperative and postoperative hemorrhage. Graft failure is also still reported as an occasional complication and often leads to the development of granulation tissue, which might require another operation, curettage of the granulation tissue down to a healthy base, and even regrafting. Minor granulation can be treated with silver nitrate application. The functional result is more important than the anatomic result in evaluating the success of this operation. Although a vaginal depth of only 4 cm is adequate for some couples, in most instances a vagina smaller than 4 cm causes major problems.

The postoperative results have improved significantly since the balsa vaginal form was replaced by the foam rubber form. Between 1950 and 1989, the McIndoe operation was performed on 94 patients at the Johns Hopkins Hospital. During these 39 years, 83% of the 94 patients had complete taking of the graft; in only 3 patients was there a significant area over which the graft failed. Alessandrescu et al.[2] recently reported on 201 patients undergoing vaginoplasty. Complications consisted of two rectal perforations (1%), one intraoperative and one 10 days postoperatively; eight graft infections (4%); and 11 infections of the graft site (5.5%).

Urethrovaginal fistula has occurred rarely since the introduction of the suprapubic catheter and the foam rubber form. The catheter is removed when the patient is voiding well and has no residual urine. In general, the patient is able to void without difficulty within the first few days of the procedure. Prophylactic broad-spectrum antibiotics, started within 12 hours of surgery and continued for 7 days, have definite value in reducing the incidence of graft failures from infection in the operative site.

Because of the excellent results obtained after a modified McIndoe vaginoplasty, this operation is recommended as the preferred procedure for women unable or unwilling to obtain a neovagina with dilation methods. Women with a flat perineum with no dimple or pouch have no alternative other than the McIndoe vaginoplasty to obtain a neovagina for comfortable sexual relations.

It is important that a McIndoe operation be performed correctly the first time. If the vagina becomes constricted because of granulation tissue formation, injury to adjacent structures, or failure to use the form properly, subsequent attempts to create a satisfactory vagina will be more difficult. The first operation has the best chance of success.

Development of Malignancies. At least 10 case reports exist of malignant disease developing in a vagina created by various techniques; these reports were reviewed by Gallup et al.[46] The authors reported a patient who was initially treated for intraepithelial malignancy by total vaginectomy combined with a split-thickness skin graft vaginoplasty to reconstruct a functional vagina. The authors noted a lesion in her vaginal apex 7 years later. These findings suggest that epithelium transplanted to the vagina can assume the oncogenic potential of the lower reproductive tract. It is therefore important that patients have long-term follow-up examinations after split-thickness skin graft vaginoplasty.

The Williams Vulvovaginoplasty

Construction of a perineal bridge to help contain the vaginal mold was a routine part of the operation described by McIndoe, but it was not adopted subsequently by others. However, Williams described a similar vulvovaginoplasty procedure in 1964[143] and advised that it could be used to create a vaginal canal.[144] In 1976, he reported that the procedure was unsuccessful in only 1 of 52 patients.[145] Feroze et al.[42] reported that the anatomic results were good in 22 of 26 patients. According to these authors, the advantages of the Williams operation are its technical simplicity, its absence of serious local complications even when performed as a repeat procedure, the ease of postoperative care, the absence of postoperative pain, the speed of recovery, the possible elimination of dilators and consequent applicability to patients who do not intend to have regular intercourse in the near future, and the higher success rates of primary and repeat procedures. The technique is not applicable to patients with poorly developed labia. It also results in an unusual angle of the vaginal canal, which is reported to straighten to a more normal direction with intercourse. If a very high perineum is created, urine can momentarily collect in the pouch after urination, giving the impression of postvoid incontinence. Failure of the suture line to heal by primary intention will

result in a large area of granulation tissue and most likely an unsatisfactory result.

Williams believes that if the urethral meatus is patulous, a vulvovaginoplasty should not be performed because the urethra might be stretched further by coitus. He suggests that varying deficiencies in muscular and fascial tissue can explain why some patients with uterovaginal agenesis are able to develop a satisfactory vaginal canal with simple intermittent pressure with coitus, whereas others are prone to develop enteroceles.

The technique of vulvovaginoplasty described by Williams is as follows (Fig. 43-9). A horseshoe-shaped incision is made in the vulva to extend across the perineum and up the medial side of the labia to the level of the external urethral meatus. The success of the operation depends on the appropriation of sufficient skin to line the new vagina. Therefore the initial mucosal incisions are made as close to the hairline as possible and approximately 4 cm from the midline. After complete mobilization, the inner skin margins are sutured together with knots tied inside the vaginal lumen. A second layer of sutures approximates subcutaneous fat and perineal muscles for support. Finally, the external skin margins are approximated with interrupted sutures. If the procedure is performed properly, it should be possible to insert two fingers into the pouch to a depth of 3 cm. An indwelling bladder catheter is used. The patient is confined to bed for 1 week in an effort to avoid tension on the suture line. Examinations are avoided for 6 weeks, at which time the patient is instructed in the use of dilators. Capraro and Gallego[15] have advised a modification of the Williams technique. They make the U-shaped incision in the skin of the labia majora at the level of the urethra or even lower, claiming that this modification results in a vulva more normal to sight and touch and still satisfactory for intercourse and that it will avoid trapping of stagnant urine in the vaginal pouch. Other modifications have been made by Feroze et al.[42] and by Creatsas.[22]

The Williams vulvovaginoplasty is a useful operation and should certainly be considered the operation of choice for patients needing a follow-up to an unsatisfactory McIndoe operation or a supplement to a small vagina resulting from extensive surgery or radiation therapy. Rarely will a patient with a solitary kidney low in the pelvis not have room for dissection of an adequate vaginal space.

Acquired Vaginal Insufficiency

Unusual types of infection and atrophy rarely can cause closure of part of the vagina, but acquired vaginal inadequacy most often is the result of treatment of various gynecologic malignancies with surgery or radiation or a combination of both. Restoration and maintenance of vaginal function are important elements of the treatment plan for such malignancies, especially when the patient is young and otherwise healthy. The techniques of vaginal reconstruction in gynecologic oncology have been reviewed by Magrina and Masterson,[85] by Pratt,[108] and by McCraw et al.[89]

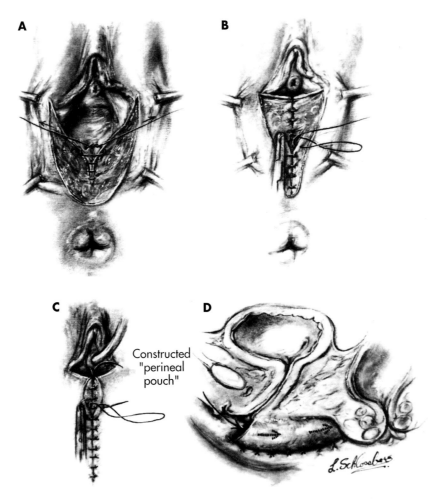

Constructed "perineal pouch"

Fig. 43-9   The Williams vulvovaginoplasty. **A** through **C,** A 3-0 polyglycolic acid sutures can be used throughout to close both inner and outer skin margins and the tissue between. **D,** The entrance to the pouch should not cover the external urethral meatus. (From Rock JA, Thompson JD: *TeLinde's operative gynecology,* ed 8, Philadelphia, 1997, Lippincott-Raven.)

DISORDERS OF VERTICAL FUSION

The problems associated with vertical fusion include transverse vaginal septum with or without obstruction. Although imperforate hymen is a vertical fusion problem, the hymen is not a derivative of the müllerian ducts; therefore this condition is discussed later in this chapter.

Transverse Vaginal Septum

No reliable epidemiologic data exist regarding the incidence of transverse vaginal septum. Reported incidences vary from 1 in 2100 to 1 in 72,000. It is probably less common than congenital absence of the vagina and uterus. It has been diagnosed in newborns, infants, and older adolescent girls. Its cause is unknown, although McKusick et al.[93] have suggested that some and perhaps most cases result from a female sex-limited autosomal-recessive transmission. There is a developmental defect in vaginal embryogenesis that leads to an incomplete fusion between the müllerian duct component and the urogenital sinus component of the vagina. The incomplete vertical fusion results in a transverse vaginal septum (AFS IIA) that varies in thickness and can be lo-

cated at almost any level in the vagina (Fig. 43-10). Lodi[82] has reported that 46% occur in the upper vagina, 40% in the midvagina, and 14% in the lower vagina.[82] Rock et al.[121] have noted septa in the upper, middle, and lower thirds of the vagina in 46%, 35%, and 19% of patients, respectively. In general, the thicker septum is noted to be more common closer to the uterine cervix. In contrast to congenital absence of the müllerian ducts, the transverse vaginal septum is associated with few urologic or other anomalies. Imperforate anus and bicornuate uterus can be found, as reported by Mandell et al.[87] The lower surface of the transverse septum is always covered by squamous epithelium. The upper surface can be covered by glandular epithelium, which is likely to be transformed into squamous epithelium by a metaplastic process after correction of the obstruction.

In neonates and young infants, imperforate transvaginal septum with obstruction can lead to serious life-threatening problems caused by the compression of surrounding organs by fluid that has collected above the septum. The fluid undoubtedly comes from endocervical glands and müllerian glandular epithelium in the upper vagina that have been

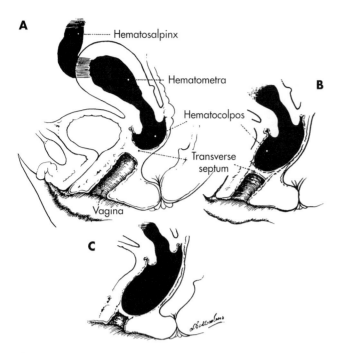

Fig. 43-10   Positions of septum responsible for complete vaginal obstruction. High **(A)**, mid **(B)**, and low **(C)** transverse vaginal septa. Note the position of the hematocolpos. Lower vaginal septa allow more blood to accumulate in the upper vagina. The vaginal mass shown in **C** is more accessible through rectovaginal examination. (From Rock JA, Thompson JD: *TeLinde's operative gynecology,* ed 8, Philadelphia, 1997, Lippincott-Raven.)

stimulated by the placental transfer of maternal estrogen. Continued fluid collection in infants, even after the first year, has been reported; thus the possibility of a fistula between the upper vagina and the urinary tract should be considered. The distended upper vagina creates a large pelvic and lower abdominal mass that can displace the bladder anteriorly, displace the ureters laterally with hydroureters and hydronephrosis, compress the rectum with associated obstipation and even intestinal obstruction, and limit diaphragmatic excursion to indirectly compress the vena cava and produce cardiorespiratory failure. Fatalities have been reported. The hydrocolpos develops along the axis of the upper vagina and therefore may not necessarily cause the outlet or perineum to bulge when there is compression of the mass from above. After careful preoperative radiologic and endoscopic investigations of the infant, the septum should be removed through a perineal approach. Bilateral Schuchardt incisions may be required to ensure that the septum has been removed. Because of the subsequent tendency for vaginal stenosis and reaccumulation of the fluid in the upper vagina, follow-up studies to assess the recurrence of urinary obstruction are important. Vaginal reconstruction may be required in later years to allow satisfactory menstruation and coitus.

A hematocolpos may not develop until puberty. Symptoms include cyclic lower abdominal pain, no visible menstrual discharge, and gradual development of a central lower

abdominal and pelvic mass. Sometimes, a small tract will open in the septum, some menstrual blood will escape periodically, and symptoms will be variable. A septum large enough to allow pregnancy to occur can still cause dystocia during labor. Cyclic hematuria may be present if a communication between the bladder and upper vagina exists. The pelvic organs of a woman with a transverse vaginal septum are shown in Fig. 43-11. The woman developed severe cyclic pain at the time of onset of menstruation but had no external bleeding until menstrual blood finally began to flow through the small sinus. Pelvic examination per rectum revealed a cervix and a normal-sized corpus. The ovaries were palpable but adherent, probably because of organized blood from hematosalpinx and hematoperitoneum. Remarkably, the woman had little dysmenorrhea after beginning to menstruate externally. Coitus was fairly satisfactory before surgical correction, but the shortness of the vagina was something of a handicap. The obstructing membrane was excised and an anastomosis of the upper and lower vagina was performed.

The findings of 26 patients with complete transverse vaginal septum reported from the Johns Hopkins Hospital by Rock et al.[121] have shown that associated congenital anomalies include urinary tract anomalies, coarctation of the aorta, atrial septal defect, and malformations of the lumbar spine. Vaginal patency and coital function were successfully established in all patients, and 7 of 19 patients attempting pregnancy eventually had children. The incidence of endometriosis and spontaneous abortion was high. A lower pregnancy rate and more extensive endometriosis were present when the transverse septum was located high in the vagina, suggesting that retrograde flow through the uterus and fallopian tubes occurs earlier in these patients. More extensive dissection between the bladder and rectum was required to identify the upper vagina when the septum was thick and high. Exploratory laparotomy was necessary in 5 patients to guide a probe through the uterine fundus and cervix and to assist in locating a high hematocolpos.

Surgical Technique

A transverse incision is made through the vault of the short vagina (see Fig. 43-11, *A*). A probe is introduced through the septum after a portion of the barrier has been separated by sharp and blunt dissection. The physician usually finds some areolar tissue in dissecting the space between the vagina and the rectum. Palpation of a urethral catheter anteriorly and insertion of a double-gloved finger along the anterior wall of the rectum posteriorly will provide the proper surgical guidelines so that the bladder and rectum can be avoided during this blind procedure. After the dissection is continued for a short distance, the cervix can usually be palpated and continuity can be established with the upper segment of the vagina (see Fig. 43-11, *B* and *C*). The lateral margins of the excised septum are extended widely by sharp knife dissection to avoid postoperative stricture formation. The edges of the upper and the lower vaginal mucosa are undermined and mobilized enough to permit anastomosis with the

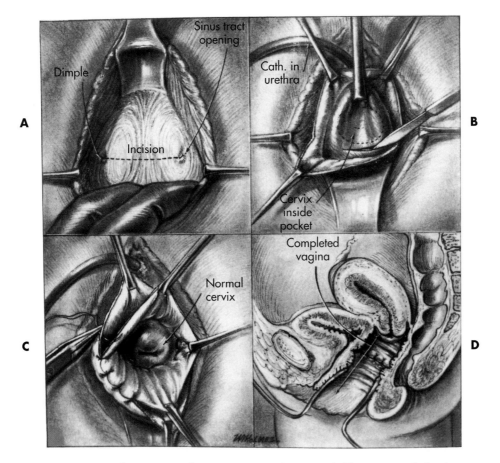

Fig. 43-11   Surgical correction of transverse vaginal septum. **A,** The upper end of a short vagina. The small sinus tract opening, through which the patient menstruated, is shown. The line of incision is drawn through the mucous membrane between the vaginal dimple and the sinus. **B,** Areolar tissue is dissected through to the pocket of mucosa that covered the cervix. The mucosa is incised. **C,** An anastomosis is made between the lower vagina and the upper vagina. **D,** Completed vagina. It is slightly shorter than normal but of normal caliber. (From Rock JA, Thompson JD: *TeLinde's operative gynecology,* ed 8, Philadelphia, 1997, Lippincott-Raven.)

use of interrupted delayed-absorbable sutures (see Fig. 43-11, *C*). Fig. 43-11, *D,* shows the completed anastomosis with a vagina that is of normal caliber but has a length slightly shorter than average. A soft foam rubber vaginal form covered with a sterile latex sheath can be placed in the vagina and removed in 10 days for evaluation of the healing process. The form can be worn for 4 to 6 weeks until complete healing has occurred. After this, coitus is permitted. If the patient is not sexually active, vaginal dilation may be necessary to maintain established patency. Alternatively, a silicone elastomer (Silastic) vaginal form can be inserted at night until the constrictive phase of healing is complete.

If the length of the obstructing transverse septum is such that reanastomosis of the upper and lower septum is impossible, as is the case with a high transverse vaginal septum, in which a significant portion of vagina is atretic, a space is created between the rectum and bladder to permit identification of the obstructed vagina (Fig. 43-12). The mass that has resulted from accumulated menstrual blood must be distinguished from the bladder anteriorly and the rectum posteriorly, a process that is facilitated by the mass itself. When differentiation is impossible, however, exploratory laparotomy can be performed. During this procedure, a probe is passed through the fundus of the uterus to tent out the vaginal septum and enable the surgeon to excise it from below and resect it safely.

In most surgical procedures to remove the high transverse vaginal septum, the obstructing membrane can be readily identified (Fig. 43-13), after which the operator can probe the mass with an aspirating needle to identify old menstrual blood. The upper vagina is then opened and the septum excised. Because the distance between the septum and the upper vagina is too great to permit an anastomosis, an indwelling acrylic resin (Lucite) form, consisting of a bulbous end and a channel through which menstrual blood can drain, is placed into the vagina and anchored with a retaining harness. The bulbous end of the form will in most instances be retained in the upper vagina and should be left in place for 4 to 6 months while epithelialization is accomplished. After its removal, vaginal dilation should be practiced daily for 2 to 4 months to prevent contracture of the space. It is essential to the success of the operation that the

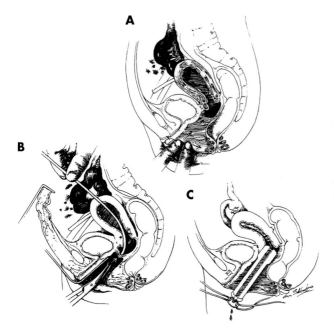

Fig. 43-12 Correction of an atretic vagina. **A,** A large portion of atretic vagina is palpated with two fingers. Once the vaginal space is developed, it may be necessary to open the abdomen via laparotomy and pass a probe through to the uterine fundus **(B)** to tent out the septum, which may then be safely excised. **C,** An acrylic resin (Lucite) form is then placed into the vagina and secured with rubber straps. (From Rock JA, Thompson JD: *TeLinde's operative gynecology,* ed 8, Philadelphia, 1997, Lippincott-Raven.)

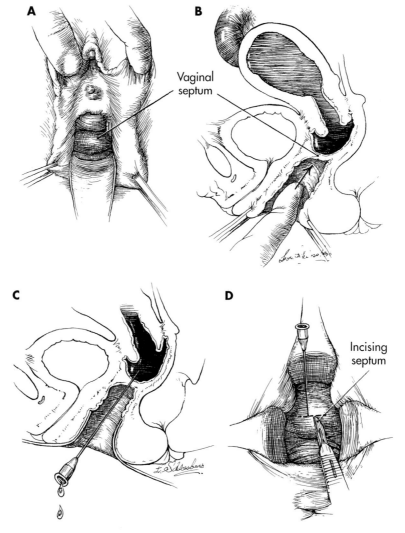

Vaginal septum

Incising septum

Fig. 43-13 A high transverse vaginal septum. **A,** The neovaginal space is dissected, revealing a high obstructing vaginal membrane. **B,** This can be palpated with the middle finger. **C,** A needle is then placed into the mass. **D,** The incision is made with a sharp knife, and considerable bleeding can occur. (From Rock J: *Semin Reprod Endocrinol* 4:24, 1986.)

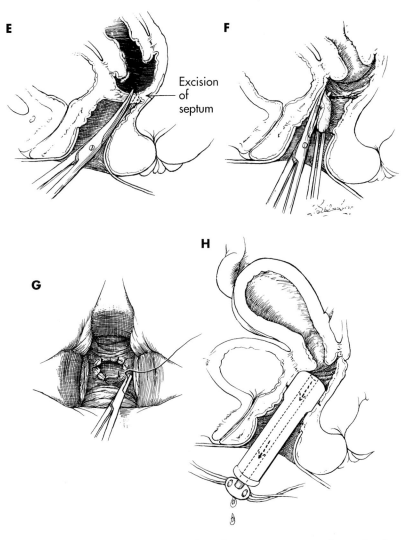

Fig. 43-13, cont'd   E, The septum is excised. **F,** The septum is removed. **G,** After the septum is removed, the wall of the septum is oversewn with interrupted sutures of 2-0 chromic catgut. **H,** Because the distance between the septum and the upper vagina is too great to allow anastomosis, an acrylic resin (Lucite) form is placed in the vagina so that epithelialization can occur over the form while vaginal patency is maintained. The form, in place, is fitted with a plastic retainer. Rubber straps can be placed through the retainer and attached to a waist belt to allow constant upper pressure so that the form is retained in the upper vagina. Modification of this method includes a small adapter to allow drainage through the acrylic resin (Lucite) form, preventing the accumulation of old blood and mucus in the upper vagina.

new space not become constricted; to avoid constriction, the form must be worn for many months during the constrictive phase of healing. As an alternative to the Lucite form, the physician can consider using a split-thickness graft to bridge the gap. The graft is usually sutured in situ in the vagina rather than sutured to a form. An ingenious but rather complicated Z-plasty method of bridging the gap has been described by Garcia[47] and by Musset.[100] A simpler flap method was described by Brenner et al.[10]

A transverse vaginal septum diagnosed after the onset of puberty presents numerous problems. Often, a large segment of the vagina is absent, making anastomosis of the upper and lower segments difficult. Furthermore, postoperative vaginal dilation is necessary to prevent stenosis at the anastomosis site. Poor compliance with dilation in a poorly motivated pubertal patient is always a concern. However, rarely is the surgeon able to delay vaginoplasty until the patient is more mature because the cyclic abdominal pain caused by the hematocolpos increasingly becomes more severe. Thus a difficult vaginoplasty can have less than optimal results.

Hurst and Rock[61] have described an alternative approach to maximize surgical resection and anastomosis in women with a high transverse vaginal septum. Aspiration of the hematocolpos under ultrasound guidance was necessary to relieve the acute pain and delay surgery. Continuous oral contraceptives were used to delay recurrence of hematocolpos. Most important, vaginal dilation was used to lengthen the

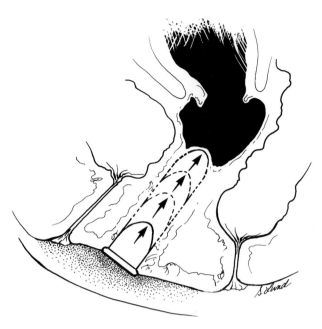

Fig. 43-14 High transverse vaginal septum **(A)**, demonstrating a small hematocolpos and hematometra. Upper to lower vaginal anastomosis at this stage can result in stenosis at the anastomosed site. **B,** Vaginal depth is increased with passive dilation using progressively larger dilators. **C,** A primary upper to lower vaginal anastomosis can be performed easily after dilation. (From Rock JA, Thompson JD: *TeLinde's operative gynecology,* ed 8, Philadelphia, 1997, Lippincott-Raven.)

lower vaginal segment to facilitate resection and reanastomosis (Fig. 43-14). The approach proved to be successful in all three patients.

CONGENITAL ABSENCE OR DYSGENESIS OF THE CERVIX

Agenesis or atresia of the cervix (AFS class IIB) is a relatively uncommon müllerian anomaly. When this anomaly does occur, it is often in association with the absence of a portion of or all of the vagina. In many patients with cervical agenesis or atresia, retention of menstrual blood initiates symptoms of cyclic lower abdominal pain without menstrual flow, causing the patient to seek gynecologic evaluation and care. In the past, diagnosis was suspected on the basis of a history and physical findings but was not proved until the time of surgery. Today, diagnosis of cervical agenesis or atresia is still usually difficult before operation, but the possibility of making a correct diagnosis before surgery does exist, with the help of modern diagnostic tools. Early diagnosis offers significant advantages in patient care, the most important of which is effective presurgical planning and preparation.

Diagnosis

Patients with congenital absence of the cervix present a diagnostic challenge. Patients with cervical aplasia with a functioning midline uterine corpus have aplasia of the lower

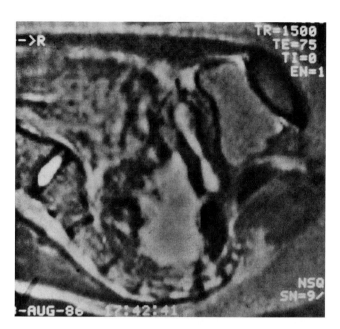

Fig. 43-15 Magnetic resonance imaging T1 image showing atretic segment of distal cervix. The tip of an atretic cervix is shown. No vagina is noted. (From Rock JA, Thompson JD: *TeLinde's operative gynecology,* ed 8, Philadelphia, 1997, Lippincott-Raven.)

two thirds of the vagina with an upper vaginal pouch. Similarly, some patients will have a considerable atretic segment of vagina and an upper vaginal pouch with a properly developed uterine cervix and corpus above. Differentiation of these two müllerian anomalies is essential. Ultrasonography may be helpful. Valdes et al.[135] have reported the use of preoperative ultrasonography in the evaluation of two patients with atresia of the vagina and cervix. MRI has been found to be helpful in confirming this diagnosis, as reported by Markham et al.[88] The lower uterine segment and cervical tissue can be carefully examined (Fig. 43-15). With cervical dysgenesis there is no vaginal dilation with the accumulation of blood, as seen with high transverse vaginal septum. Both ultrasonography and MRI are most helpful when they are correlated with the findings of a careful pelvic examination under anesthesia.

Anatomic Variations of Congenital Cervical Anomalies

Two basic categories of cervical anomalies have been observed in several configurations. Patients exhibiting the first type, cervical aplasia, lack a uterine cervix (Fig. 43-16, *A*), and the lower uterine segment narrows to terminate in a peritoneal sleeve at a point well above the normal communication with the vaginal apex. The second type, cervical dysgenesis, can be described as four subtypes:

1. Cervical body consisting of a fibrous band of variable length and diameter (endocervical glands may be noted on pathologic examination) (see Fig. 43-16, *B*)
2. Intact cervical body with obstruction of the cervical os (the cervix is usually well formed, but a

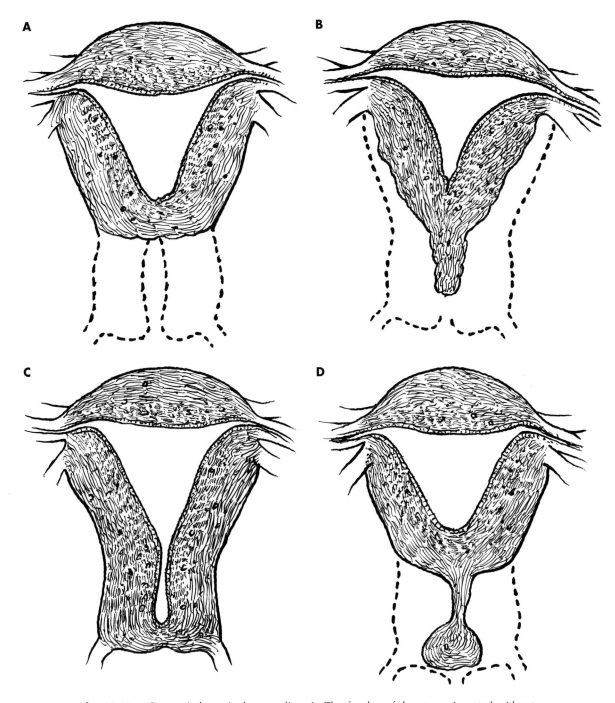

Fig. 43-16   Congenital cervical anomalies. **A,** The fundus of the uterus is noted without a cervix. **B,** The cervical body consists of a fibrous band of variable length and diameter that can contain endocervical glands. **C,** The cervical body is intact with obstruction of the cervical os. Variable portions of the cervical lumen are obliterated. **D,** Stricture of the midportion of the cervix, which is hypoplastic with a bulbous tip. No cervical lumen is identified. (From Rock JA, Thompson JD: *TeLinde's operative gynecology,* ed 8, Philadelphia, 1997, Lippincott-Raven.)   *Continued*

portion of the endocervical lumen is obliterated) (see Fig. 43-16, *C*)

3. Stricture of the midportion of the cervix (which is hypoplastic with a bulbous tip and no identifiable cervical lumen) (see Fig. 43-16, *D*)

4. Fragmentation of the cervix (with portions that can be palpated below the fundus and that are not connected to the lower uterine segment) (see Fig. 43-16, *E*)

Associated anomalies of the urinary tract are rare but can occur. Variable portions of the vagina can be atretic. Cervi-

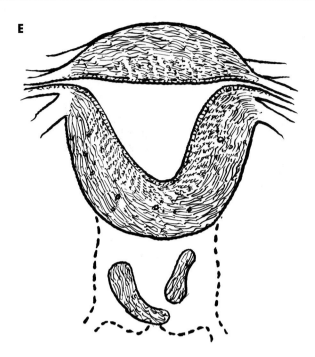

Fig. 43-16, cont'd   E, Cervical fragmentation in which portions of the cervix are noted with no connection to the uterine body. Hypoplasia of the uterine cavity can be associated with cervical cord fragmentation. (From Rock JA, Thompson JD: *TeLinde's operative gynecology,* ed 8, Philadelphia, 1997, Lippincott-Raven.)

cal obstruction is most often associated with a vagina of normal length.

Treatment

When both the vagina and cervix are absent and a functioning uterine corpus is present, it is difficult to obtain a satisfactory fistulous tract through which menstruation can occur. Many methods have been tried, most of them involving creation of a passage through the dense fibrous tissue between the uterine cavity and the vagina and placement of a stent to keep the tract open.[66] Occasional successes in maintaining an open passageway and normal cyclic menstruation have been reported, but endocervical glands do not develop and there is no way to compensate for the absence of the cervical mucus, which plays an important role in sperm transport. Even though cyclic ovulatory periods can be achieved in a few patients, pregnancy is unlikely. Eventually the uterovaginal tract closes from constriction by fibrous tissue. Endometriosis can develop along the tract. Endometriosis also can develop in ovaries and other pelvic sites because of retrograde menstruation.[103] Recurrent and severe pelvic infection is common and may require total hysterectomy and removal of both ovaries. As in vitro fertilization procedures began to offer the possibility for a host uterus to carry a pregnancy to term, procedures to establish a fistulous tract were abandoned. Nevertheless, Cukier et al.[23] in 1986 reported treating a patient with congenital absence of the cervix by construction of a splint that extended into the neocervical canal such that a split-thickness skin

graft could actually be placed within the endocervical canal. This patient has continued to menstruate without difficulty, although pregnancy has not been accomplished.

Many authors have recommended hysterectomy as an initial procedure for a patient with a functioning uterine corpus and congenital absence of the cervix and vagina. A hysterectomy will eliminate much needless suffering from associated problems such as cryptomenorrhea, sepsis, endometriosis, and multiple operations.[111] If the hysterectomy is performed soon enough, before the problems become great, it may be possible to conserve the ovaries and their useful functions. There are recommendations to the contrary, in articles by Farber and Marchant[35] and by Farber and Mitchell,[36-38] but most agree with authors Geary and Weed,[49] Maciulla et al.,[84] Dillon et al.,[31] Niver et al.,[102] and Jones and Rock[74] that a recommendation for a hysterectomy as the initial primary therapy is realistic in these patients, with few exceptions. The reconstructive surgeon should be prepared to perform a vaginoplasty with use of a split-thickness graft if hysterectomy is performed, particularly if there has been a vaginal dissection.[119] If the neovaginal space is allowed to close and scar, future operations to develop an adequate neovagina are associated with increased risks of graft failure and fistula formation.

Despite the overall poor results from reconstruction for congenital absence of both the cervix and the vagina, clinical experience suggests that cannulization procedures can be worthwhile for a few carefully selected patients with adequate stroma to allow a cervicovaginal anastomosis. If a long segment of cervix is fibrous cord, a cervical grafting technique may be required. If a fragmented cervix is noted, hysterectomy is usually warranted. Those few patients who have achieved a pregnancy after cervical reconstruction have had a well-formed cervical body.

DISORDERS OF LATERAL FUSION

Failures of lateral fusion of the two müllerian ducts cause vaginal anomalies that are grouped as obstructed or unobstructed.

Unobstructed Double Uterus (Bicornuate, Septate, or Didelphic Uterus)

Overview. Complete failure of medial fusion of the two müllerian ducts can result in complete duplication of the vagina, cervix, and uterus. Partial failure of fusion can result in a single vagina with a single or duplicate cervix and complete or partial duplication of the uterine corpus. A failure of absorption of the uterine septum between the two fused müllerian ducts causes the septum to persist inside the uterus to a variable extent, but the external appearance remains that of a single uterus. The septum can be so complete that it divides both the uterine cavity and endocervical canal into two equal or unequal components. More often, incomplete disappearance of the septum will leave only the upper uterine cavities divided. Each of these and a variety of other forms of double uteri will have their own individual features of clinical significance. When no obstruction is present, surgical reconstruction is performed primarily because of difficulties with reproduction.

Some aspects of lateral fusion disorders remain controversial because information is still inaccurate or incomplete. Many reports are based on small samples of selected patients, patients in whom one anomaly or another has been diagnosed on the basis of incomplete data, and patients who have received unification operations without preliminary studies to rule out other causes of reproductive difficulty. A comparison of results from one series to the next is difficult because authors have used different classifications based on a variety of embryologic, anatomic, physiologic, functional, and radiologic considerations. Unknown numbers of uterine anomalies may have escaped detection because reproductive performance is generally acceptable and gynecologic difficulties do not necessarily occur.

Historical Development of Surgical Procedures. In 1882, Ruge first reported on the excision of a uterine septum in a woman who had miscarried twice. The woman subsequently carried a pregnancy to term. Paul Strassmann of Berlin and later Erwin Strassmann, his son, were strong advocates of uterine unification operations.[129-131] The studies of Jones and Jones[72] have contributed greatly to our understanding of the management of uterine anomalies. Their studies began with a report in 1953 of a series that was started in 1936. Updates have been published from time to time. Wheeless, Rock, Andrews, and others have joined in these reports.[4,74,75]

Diagnosis of Uterine Anomalies. If a uterine anomaly is associated with obstruction of menstrual flow, it will cause symptoms that will come to the attention of the gynecologist shortly after menarche. Unobstructed uterine anomalies are diagnosed later in a variety of circumstances. Young girls may notice difficulty in using tampons or later difficulty in coitus if a longitudinal vaginal septum is present. This can lead to the diagnosis of an associated uterine anomaly. A patient with an anomalous upper urinary tract on intravenous pyelogram may be found to have a uterine anomaly on gynecologic evaluation. A uterine anomaly is occasionally found when a patient complains of dysmenorrhea or menorrhagia or when a dilation and curettage (D&C) is performed for abortion or some other indication. A palpable mass may be a uterine anomaly but should be confirmed as such by ultrasonography, hysterography, or laparoscopy. Semmens[124] has pointed out that the diagnosis of a uterine anomaly can also be made from astute observation of an abnormal uterine contour during pregnancy, either in the antepartum period or at the time of abdominal or vaginal delivery. The abnormal contour is caused by a combination of fetal malpresentation and an anomalous uterus. An anomalous uterus can also be diagnosed when a pregnancy occurs despite the presence of an intrauterine contraceptive device. Persistent postmenopausal bleeding despite recent D&C can lead to diagnosis of an anomalous uterus. Sometimes, the diagnosis is made as an incidental finding at laparotomy. However, most uterine anomalies are diagnosed

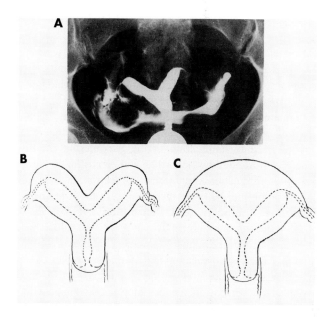

Fig. 43-17   A, A hysterogram of a double uterus. A bicornuate uterus (**B**) and a septate uterus (**C**) are types of double uteri. Visualization of the fundus is required to determine the type of uterus. (From Rock JA, Thompson JD: *TeLinde's operative gynecology,* ed 8, Philadelphia, 1997, Lippincott-Raven.)

after hysterosalpingography to evaluate infertility or reproductive loss, usually from repeated spontaneous abortion.

Proper technique during the performance of hysterosalpingography to diagnose uterine anomalies is important. The hysterogram must be taken at right angles to the axis of the uterus for a true assessment of the deformity to be made. The study is best done under fluoroscopy. A septate uterus cannot be distinguished from a bicornuate uterus by hysterogram alone (Fig. 43-17). The external uterine configuration also cannot usually be determined by pelvic examination alone, but some idea of the configuration can be obtained by ultrasonography. McDonough and Tho[90] have suggested the use of double-contour pelvic pneumoperitoneum-hysterographic studies for precise identification of müllerian malformations. Transvaginal hysterosonography has been recently described in the preoperative diagnosis of uterine malformations, especially septae, with good correlation with hysteroscopic findings.[32,122] Three-dimensional ultrasound has been reported to allow differentiation between arcuate and bicornuate uteri.[78] Of course, laparoscopy has greater sensitivity. If the uterine corpus has not been previously visualized, the physician must be prepared to correct either anomaly (i.e., obstructed or unobstructed), depending on the findings at laparotomy.

A complete investigation should also include an assessment of tubal patency and an intravenous pyelogram. A variety of upper urinary tract anomalies are seen, including absence of one kidney, horseshoe kidney, pelvic kidney, duplication of the collecting system, and ectopically located ureteral orifices. The lower urinary tract (bladder and urethra) is much less often anomalous.

Uterine Anomalies and Menstrual Difficulties. Dysmenorrhea and abnormal and heavy menstrual bleeding have been reported to be a common occurrence with any form of double uterus and to be relieved after unification operations. Capraro et al.[14] reported on several patients in whom dysmenorrhea was cured by metroplasty. Erwin Strassmann[129,130] also believed that all cases of dysmenorrhea and menorrhagia associated with uterine anomalies were relieved by unification of the two uterine cavities. Generally, however, dysmenorrhea and menorrhagia are inappropriate indications for uterine unification, and the operation should not be performed solely for these reasons.

Uterine Anomalies and Reproductive History. Although some uterine anomalies can cause infertility, most patients with uterine anomalies are able to conceive without difficulty. There is no question that uterine anomalies can be associated with perfectly normal reproductive performance. Overall, however, the incidences of spontaneous abortion, premature birth, fetal loss, malpresentation, and cesarean section are clearly increased when a uterine anomaly is present. Unfortunately, it is impossible to predict which patients with uterine anomalies will have these problems.

The cause of reproductive failure in patients with uterine anomalies remains unclear. Mahgoub[86] believes that the presence of a uterine septum can lead to abortion because of diminished intrauterine space for fetal growth caused by implantation of the placenta on a poorly vascularized septum. Mizuno et al.[95] have attached importance to the inadequacy of vascularization of the uterine septum. Associated cervical incompetence, luteal phase insufficiency, and distortion of the uterine milieu have all been implicated in the cause of increased reproductive loss. However, it is as yet unexplained why some patients with a uterine anomaly have normal reproductive function, whereas others abort early in pregnancy. Interestingly, it has been reported that the chance for a liveborn child increases with each pregnancy loss. It is unknown whether this apparent "conditioning" of the uterus is the result of better vascularization, better myometrial stretching and accommodation, or some other factor.

A medical history of three or more episodes of spontaneous abortion or premature labor merits hysterosalpingography to determine whether structural abnormalities of the uterus are present. An abnormality will be found in about 10% of such patients. Among patients who repeatedly abort early in the second trimester, the incidence may be higher. The cause of spontaneous abortion is complex, and a complete workup should be done even when an anomalous uterus has been found.[120] A careful history should include a detailed discussion of each previous pregnancy loss and inquiry into DES exposure or other drug or chemical toxicity, specific medical illnesses, and exposure to contagious diseases. A family history should emphasize reproductive failures among family members of both the patient and the husband. Specific medical diseases such as thyroid disease, diabetes mellitus, renal disease, and systemic lupus erythematosus should be ruled out. The possibility of infection by such agents as *Neisseria gonorrhoeae*, *Chlamydia*, *Myco-*

plasma, *Toxoplasma*, and *Listeria* should be considered. Chromosome analyses should be done. Abnormalities in aborted tissue are found in more than 50% of spontaneous abortions, and abnormalities appear in up to one fourth of couples with a history of habitual abortion. Identifying such couples makes it possible to offer genetic counseling for subsequent pregnancies. Uterine leiomyomas, especially lower uterine segment and submucous leiomyomas, can cause spontaneous abortion. Basal body temperature charts, serum progesterone determinations, and endometrial biopsies timed in the luteal phase will help determine the presence of luteal phase deficiency. The cervix should be studied for incompetence.

Couples with multiple causes for reproductive loss should have all other problems corrected before metroplasty is considered. Indeed, correcting other factors first may correct the problem of reproductive loss without metroplasty. In 1977, Rock and Jones[112] reported on seven patients who had anomalous uterine development and extrauterine factors in the etiology of their reproductive loss. These patients had already had 16 pregnancies, 5 (31%) of which resulted in a liveborn child. After therapy to correct the extrauterine factor, the success rate increased to 71%. Stoot and Mastboom[128] reported an impressive increase in reproductive performance among patients with uterine anomalies by simple improvement of abnormal carbohydrate metabolism.

The Double Uterus and Obstetric Outcome. The percentage of term pregnancies in an unselected series of women with various types of double uteri who have not been operated on is unknown. For all types combined, it is probably approximately 25%. In patients selected for operation, it probably increases from approximately 5% to 10% to approximately 80% to 90%. Because patients with uterine anomalies who have relatively normal obstetric histories cannot be identified, there is confusion in the literature about which anomalies are more often associated with obstetric difficulties and which are relatively benign in their effect.[117] Special diagnostic procedures to detect uterine anomalies are not usually performed before reproductive performance is tested. A didelphic uterus is the exception. This anomaly can be diagnosed easily on routine pelvic examination by identification of two complete cervices and perhaps also a longitudinal vaginal septum. A study by Heinonen and Pystynen[55] in Finland of 182 women with uterine anomalies indicated that pregnancies in the septate uterus had a better fetal survival rate (86%) than they did in the complete bicornuate uterus (50%) or in the unicornuate uterus (40%). These findings differ from prevailing opinions that the septate uterus is associated with the highest reproductive loss, as proposed by Jones and Jones.[72,76]

In 1968, Capraro et al.[14] reported on 85 patients with uterine anomalies seen between 1962 and 1966. One uterine anomaly was seen for every 645 admissions (0.145%). Metroplasty was considered necessary in only 14 (16%) of these 85 patients. According to Jones and Jones, only one third of patients with a double uterus have important reproductive problems. In most instances the presence of a double uterus is not in itself an indication for metroplasty.

In 1980, Jewelewicz et al.[68] estimated the spontaneous abortion rate to be 33.8% in women with a bicornuate uterus, 22.2% in those with a septate uterus, and 34.6% in those with a unicornuate uterus.[68] More recently, Ludmir et al.[83] reported that high-risk obstetric intervention did not significantly increase the fetal survival rate for uncorrected uterine anomalies. Capraro et al.[14] found a preoperative fetal salvage rate of 33.3% for the septate uterus, 10% for the bicornuate uterus, and 0% for the didelphic uterus. Postoperatively, the fetal salvage rate was 100% for the bicornuate uterus, 80% for the septate uterus, and 66% for the didelphic uterus. The report gives the improved salvage figures, compared with several previous studies, after abdominal metroplasty.

Anomalies and Infertility. Opinions differ considerably in terms of whether infertility is a proper indication for metroplasty. Erwin Strassmann[129,130] stated that primary infertility could be cured in 60% of patients with uterine anomaly if all other causes of infertility were excluded. Strassmann reported eight metroplasties for primary sterility that yielded nine pregnancies and seven liveborn children, although the number of patients who conceived was not given. Similar reports of small numbers of patients can be found throughout the literature. Heinonen and Pystynen[55] indicated that uterine anomalies are rarely the reason for infertility. Nonuterine causes of infertility must be ruled out before metroplasty, as a last resort, is considered.

Certainly, a full infertility investigation to rule out other causes should be completed before the anomalous uterus is blamed. Even when no other cause for infertility is found, except for a septate or bicornuate uterus, metroplasty may not be indicated. This question of when to perform metroplasty simply has not yet been answered. The decision is difficult and becomes even more difficult when the opportunity for metroplasty presents itself because a septate or bicornuate uterus requires laparotomy for some other reason, such as endometriosis or tubal occlusion.

The Didelphic Uterus. A didelphic uterus with two hemicorpora is easily diagnosed because all patients will be found to have two hemicervices visible on speculum examination, and most, if not all, will have a longitudinal sagittal vaginal septum. In the series reported by Heinonen et al.,[56] all 21 patients with a didelphic uterus had a vaginal septum. Conversely, a patient with a longitudinal vaginal septum will usually be found to have a didelphic uterus.[54] This indication for uterine unification is related to the role of this anomaly as a causative factor in reproductive loss. Of all the uterine anomalies (except an arcuate uterus), the didelphic uterus is associated with the best possibility of a successful pregnancy. However, there is still some increase in perinatal mortality, premature birth, breech presentation, and cesarean section for delivery. Heinonen et al.[56] reported a fetal survival rate of 64% without metroplasty. Musich and Behrman[99] stated that the didelphic uterus offers the best chance for a successful pregnancy (57%) and should not be considered an appropriate indication for metroplasty. However,

Jones[77] considered the didelphic uterus to give the worst obstetric outcome. In our opinion, a unification operation for a didelphic uterus is not often indicated, and the results may be disappointing, especially when an attempt is made to unify the cervix. This procedure not only is technically difficult in a patient with a complete didelphic anomaly, but also can result in cervical incompetence or cervical stenosis.

The Septate Uterus. Most patients evaluated for repeated abortion and found to have a uterine anomaly will have a septate uterus. A few will have other anomalies, mostly the bicornuate uterus. In our experience, fetal survival rates are higher after septate uterus repair than after other repairs. In 1977, Rock and Jones[112] reported on 43 patients with septate uteri selected for Jones metroplasty at the Johns Hopkins Hospital. Of these 43 patients, 95% became pregnant postoperatively, 73% carried to term, and 77% delivered a liveborn child. Similar results have been reported after hysteroscopic or resectoscopic incision of the uterine septum. Recently, the histologic features of the septum in this abnormal uterus have been described. Dabirashrafi et al.[24] noted less connective tissue in uterine septa. Poor decidualization and placentation were suggested as a cause.[24]

Finally, the AFS class VA uterus (a double cervix and uterine cavity with a single fundus) can result from a rotation abnormality during the descent of the müllerian ducts. If the dextrorotating müllerian ducts overrotate, Rock theorizes (personal observations, J. A. Rock, 1991) that the septum fails to absorb after fusion of the ducts. In virtually every patient with a complete septate uterus, the left cervix is higher than the right. In one patient, one cervix has been noted above the other (Fig. 43-18). This rotation abnormal-

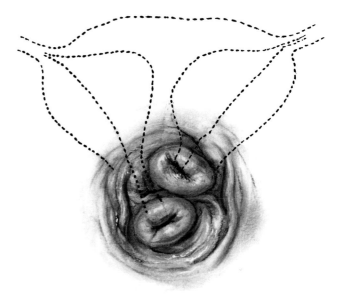

Fig. 43-18 A double uterus with two cervices and a single fundus (class V). Note that the left cervix is positioned over the right cervix. This rotation abnormality may be a factor associated with a lack of absorption of the uterine septum. (From Rock JA, Thompson JD: *TeLinde's operative gynecology*, ed 8, Philadelphia, 1997, Lippincott-Raven.)

ity may be a factor associated with lack of absorption of the uterine septum in these patients.

Surgical Techniques for Uterine Unification

Traditionally, the septate uterus has been unified with either the Jones or the Tompkins procedure. Clinical reports by Chervenak and Neuwirth,[17] Daly et al.,[25] DeCherney et al.,[28] and Israel and March[63] have favorably compared hysteroscopic or resectoscopic incision of a uterine septum with the more traditional transabdominal approach. Term pregnancy rates after these procedures have approached 80% to 85%. Several attempts may be necessary to incise a wide septum, although the septum usually can be incised completely at the first operation.

Transcervical incision of a uterine septum for patients with a septate uterus has obvious advantages. Morbidity is decreased after the procedure and delivery can be vaginal. Term pregnancy rates are comparable to those after abdominal metroplasty for repeated pregnancy wastage.[39]

Most of the septa associated with a septate uterus can be cut through the cervix by way of the hysteroscope or the resectoscope. Nevertheless, cases of broad uterine septum can benefit from the wedge metroplasty, and reconstructive surgeons should be knowledgeable in its performance.

Transcervical Lysis of the Uterine Septum. Abdominal metroplasty for transfundal incision or for excision of the septum associated with the septate uterus generally has been abandoned. With hysteroscopic scissors, the procedure can be tedious, especially with a large, broad septum. Although the hysteroscope and scissors are still used for cutting the septum, the resectoscope has been found to be comparable. The optics are excellent, and the septum can be electrosurgically incised with little difficulty.

Before transcervical lysis of a uterine septum, a regimen of danazol or a gonadotropin-releasing hormone agonist for 2 months should be started to reduce the amount of endometrium that can obscure the surgeon's view during the procedure.[27] Transcervical lysis is usually performed in conjunction with laparoscopy under general endotracheal anesthesia. The uterine cavity is distended with dextran 70 (Hyskon) by way of the resectoscope, which is inserted into the cervix. The septum is then electrosurgically incised by advancing the cutting loupe, using the trigger mechanism of the resectoscope or with microscissors. The uterine septum is incised until the tubal ostia are visualized, and there is no appreciable evidence of the septum. The procedure is performed under simultaneous laparoscopy to limit the risks of uterine perforation. The laparoscopic light can be turned off so that the light from the hysteroscope can be clearly visualized through the fundus. Most patients can be discharged within 4 hours of the procedure. Antibiotic therapy is begun before the procedure, and the medication is continued for 5 days after surgery to limit the risks of infection. No intrauterine devices are used. If excessive bleeding occurs after the procedure, a Foley catheter should be placed in the uterine cavity for tamponade and removed in 4 to 6 hours.

Transcervical lysis also can be performed to repair a complete septate uterus (i.e., a single fundus with two cavities and two cervices). In this instance, a no. 8 Foley catheter is inserted into one cervix and indigo carmine is injected into the cavity. The other cavity is distended with dextran 70 (Hyskon) by way of the resectoscope. The septum is electrosurgically incised at a point above the internal cervical os until the Foley catheter is visualized. The septum is then incised in a superior direction until the tubal ostium is visualized, and there is no appreciable septum (Fig. 43-19). More recent reports suggest beginning the operation with Metzenbaum scissor incision of the cervical septum.[137]

After transcervical lysis of a uterine septum, a 2-month delay before attempting pregnancy is suggested to allow complete reabsorption of the septum. Delivery may be vaginal. The Jones procedure is used to repair a septate uterus when a particularly broad septum cannot be easily incised with the resectoscope. The Strassmann procedure is used for unification of a bicornuate uterus.

The Modified Jones Metroplasty. The technique of modified Jones metroplasty is a compromise between the classic Jones metroplasty and the Tompkins metroplasty. In the Jones operation the entire septum is removed. In the Tompkins operation a single median incision divides the uterine corpus and septum in half. The incision is carried inferiorly until the endometrial cavity is reached. Each lateral septal half is then incised to within 1 cm of the tubes. No septal tissue is removed. The myometrium is reapproximated, taking care not to place sutures too close to the interstitial portion of the tubes. Proponents of the Tompkins technique suggest that it is simpler than the classic Jones procedure, that it conserves all myometrial tissue and leaves the uterotubal junction in a more normal and lateral position, and that it provides better results than the Jones metroplasty. Good results with the Tompkins technique have been reported by McShane et al.[94]

In the modified Jones unification operation (Fig. 43-20), the abdomen is generally opened through a transverse incision. If only the unification operation is planned, a Pfannenstiel incision is permissible. The pelvic viscera are inspected. The septate uterus may demonstrate a median raphe across the fundus, but it is surprising how often the corpus looks normal. To facilitate manipulation, a traction suture of heavy silk is placed through the top of the septum. This suture will be removed from the site when the septum is excised.

No attempt is made to stain the uterine cavity with methylene blue. Normal unstained endometrial tissue can be easily differentiated from the myometrium.

Essentially two methods are used to control bleeding during this procedure. In the first, a tourniquet is applied at the junction of the lower uterine segment and cervix by inserting a 0.5-inch Penrose drain through an avascular space in the broad ligaments just lateral to the uterine vessels on each side. The tourniquet is placed around the lower uterine segment and is tied anterior to the uterus. Because the uterine

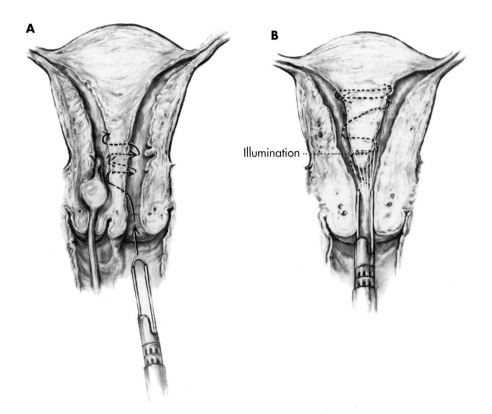

Fig. 43-19   Resectoscopic metroplasty. **A,** A Foley catheter is placed in one cavity of a complete septate uterus (AFS class VA uterus). The resectoscope is inserted in the opposite cavity, and the septum is incised until the catheter is visualized. The septum can be easily incised with the resectoscope until both internal os are visible. **B,** A septate uterus with a single cervix. The septum can be incised with the straight loupe of the resectoscope. (From Rock JA, Thompson JD: *TeLinde's operative gynecology,* ed 8, Philadelphia, 1997, Lippincott-Raven.)

corpus receives a significant blood supply through the ovarian arteries, tourniquets should also be tied around the infundibulopelvic ligaments of each side, using the same hole in the broad ligament. All tourniquets must be tied tightly enough to occlude both the arterial supply to and the venous drainage from the uterus. If only the venous drainage is occluded, the corpus will become engorged and congested and bleeding will be increased. If the arterial supply is occluded, the uterus will blanch and the bleeding will be minimal. A sterile Doptone can be used to establish disappearance of uterine artery pulsations. Hypotensive anesthetic techniques used in conjunction with the tourniquets will allow a uterine unification operation to be accomplished with negligible blood loss.

The alternative method for hemostasis uses up to 20 U of vasopressin that is diluted in 20 ml of saline and injected into the anterior and posterior walls of the uterus before the incision is made.

The uterine septum should be surgically excised as a wedge (see Fig. 43-20, *D*). The incisions begin at the fundus of the uterus. The approach to the endometrial cavity should be handled carefully so that it is not transected (see Fig. 43-20, *E*). The original incisions at the top of the fundus are usually within 1 cm, and sometimes even less, of the insertion of the fallopian tubes. If the incision is directed toward

the apex of the wedge, however, there seems to be little danger of transecting the tube across its interstitial transit in the myometrium.

After the wedge has been removed, the uterus is closed in three layers with interrupted stitches; 2-0 nonreactive suture on an atraumatic tapered needle is convenient. Two sizes of needles are needed—a ½-inch needle for the inner and intermediate layers and a large needle (¾ half-round) for the outer muscular layer. The inner layer of stitches must include about one third of the thickness of the myometrium because the endometrium alone is too delicate to hold a suture and it will be cut through. The inner sutures should be placed through the endometrium and the myometrium in such a way that the knot is tied within the endometrial cavity (see Fig. 43-20, *G* and *H*). While the suture is being tied, the two lateral halves of the uterus should be pressed together both manually and with guy sutures to relieve tension on the suture line and to reduce the possibility of cutting through. These sutures are placed alternately, first anterior and then posterior. After the first few stitches are placed and before the first layer is completed, the second layer can be started to reduce tension.

As the operation proceeds, the third layer of stitches is begun in the serosa both anteriorly and posteriorly (see Fig. 43-20, *I* through *K*). Finer, nonreactive suture material can

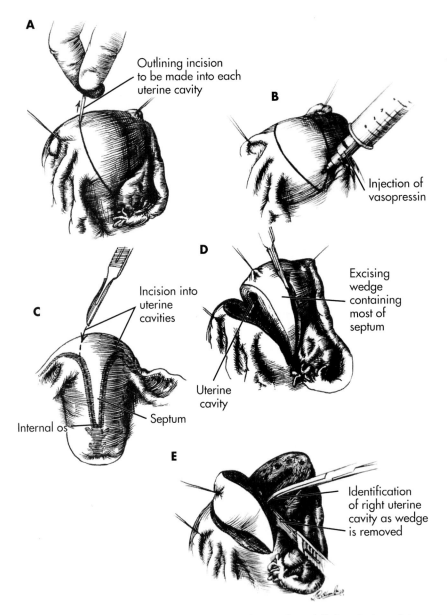

Fig. 43-20 The modified Jones metroplasty. See the text for a full description of the various steps in the operative repair of a septate uterus by excision of a wedge. (From Rock JA, Thompson JD: *TeLinde's operative gynecology,* ed 8, Philadelphia, 1997, Lippincott-Raven.)

be used to approximate the serosal edges of the uterus more precisely to prevent adhesion formation to the suture line (see Fig. 43-20, *K* and *L*). By the conclusion of the operation, the uterus appears near normal in configuration. The striking feature is usually the proximity of the insertions of the fallopian tubes. Special care must be exercised not to obstruct the interstitial portions of the fallopian tubes while placing the fundal myometrial and serosal sutures.

The final size of the uterine cavity seems to be relatively unimportant to reproductive capability; uterine symmetry appears to be a more important factor. The constructed cavity is often small compared with the normal uterus. Whether the surgeon removes the septum with the Jones procedure or lyses the septum transcervically, postoperative hysterogram

films often show small dog-ears that are leftover tags from the original bifid condition of the uterus. Such dog-ears do not seem to interfere with function, although a postoperative roentgenogram cannot be considered normal in the sense that it will not have the appearance of a normal endometrial cavity after such an operation. If a double cervix is present, the physician should not attempt to unify the cervix because an incompetent cervical os will be the result. To allow the uterine incision the best possible opportunity to heal, a delay of 4 to 6 months in attempting pregnancy is advised after abdominal metroplasty.

The Strassmann Metroplasty. The Strassmann procedure is not easily adapted to the septate uterus, but it is the procedure of choice for unification of the two endometrial

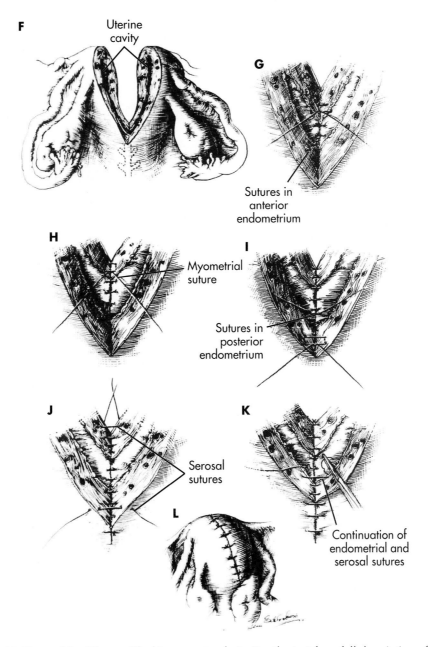

Fig. 43-20, cont'd The modified Jones metroplasty. See the text for a full description of the various steps in the operative repair of a septate uterus by excision of a wedge.

cavities of an externally divided uterus, both bicornuate and didelphic (Fig. 43-21). A bicornuate uterus cannot be repaired through transcervical lysis because perforation will result. When fusion of the two müllerian ducts has failed, inspection of the pelvic cavity often will reveal a broad peritoneal band that lies in the middle between the two lateral hemicorpora. This rectovesical ligament is attached anteriorly to the bladder, folds over and is attached between the uterine cornua, continues posteriorly in the cul-de-sac, and ends with its attachment to the anterior wall of the sigmoid colon and rectum. It is not invariably present, but when it is, its potential significance in the cause of the anomaly, possibly by preventing the two müllerian ducts from joining, must be considered. This rectovesical ligament must be re-

moved before a unification procedure can be performed (see Fig. 43-21, A).

For hemostasis, tourniquets are used in a manner similar to that described for the modified Jones procedure. The two uterine cornua are incised on their median sides in their longitudinal axes, deeply enough to expose the uterine cavities (see Fig. 43-21, B). Superiorly, the incision must not be too close to the interstitial portion of the fallopian tubes. Inferiorly, the incision is carried far enough to join the two sides into a single endocervical canal. If it appears that a deeper incision will compromise the competence of the cervix, a double cervical canal can be left. If the cervix is already duplex, it should not be joined. As the incision in the myometrium releases the internal stresses in the walls of the

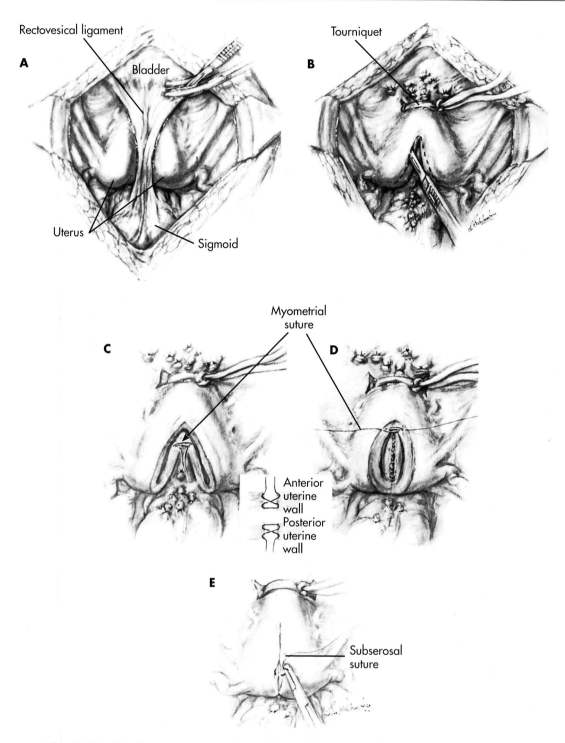

Fig. 43-21 The Strassmann metroplasty with modification. **A,** If a rectovesical ligament is found, it should be removed. **B,** An incision is made on the medial side of each hemicorpus and carried deep enough to enter the uterine cavity. The edges of the myometrium will evert to face the opposite side. **C** and **D,** The myometrium is approximated by use of interrupted vertical figure-of-eight 3-0 polyglycolic acid sutures. One should avoid placing sutures too close to the interstitial portion of the fallopian tubes. **E,** A continuous 5-0 polyglycolic acid subserosal suture is used as a final layer. Tourniquets are removed, and defects in the broad ligament are closed. (From Rock JA, Thompson JD: *TeLinde's operative gynecology,* ed 8, Philadelphia, 1997, Lippincott-Raven.)

hemicorpora, each one everts and is perfectly positioned for apposition, almost as if the original intention in embryologic development is finally to be realized. The suture technique for joining the two sides (see Fig. 43-21, C through E) is exactly the same as for the modified Jones procedure. The suture line in the uterine corpus should be observed for several minutes to determine the adequacy of hemostasis. Occasionally, one or two extra sutures need to be placed to control bleeding.

A uterine suspension can be performed as necessary. However, in the event of pregnancy, the shortened round ligaments can produce symptoms from an enlarging uterus. Presacral neurectomy in association with uterine unification should be considered only in patients with severe midline dysmenorrhea.

The cervix should be dilated to ensure proper drainage from the uterine cavity. This can be accomplished transvaginally after the abdominal procedure or from above by inserting a dilator through the cervical canal into the vagina, to be removed later.

The operative technique should always be consistent with the goal of maintaining or enhancing fertility and possibly achieving a successful pregnancy. Tissue surfaces should be kept moist throughout the procedure, and instruments should be selected and used in such a way that tissue damage is minimized. Abdominal packs should be placed in plastic bags to avoid adhesions, or no-lint laparotomy pads can be used. Talc should be carefully washed from gloves, and meticulous aseptic technique should be used. The appendix should not be removed. A solution of Ringer's lactate containing heparin and corticosteroid can be used for peritoneal lavage throughout the procedure.

Related Concerns

Cervical Incompetence Associated with a Double Uterus. When a patient with an anomalous uterus, with or without unification, becomes pregnant, she must be watched closely for evidence of cervical incompetence, especially if a history of previous reproductive loss suggests cervical incompetence. Heinonen et al.[56] were able to improve the fetal survival rate from 57% to 92% by cervical cerclage. Cerclage was used mostly in patients with a partial bicornuate uterus. In these patients the fetal salvage rate was improved from 53% before cerclage to 100% afterward. Prematurity also was decreased, from 53% to 3%. The authors stress that cervical incompetence, not the uterine anomaly, is the proper indication for cerclage in these patients. However, the frequency with which these problems are found together suggests the importance of doing a careful evaluation for both problems. Some reproductive losses from a uterine anomaly might be prevented by cerclage of an incompetent cervix during metroplasty. However, routine cerclage at the time of metroplasty is not recommended.

Attempts to unify a double cervix or a septate cervix also are not recommended because of the possibility of causing cervical incompetence. However, a double or septate cervix can adversely affect the outcome of delivery if vaginal delivery is attempted, and delivery should be by cesarean section if it appears that the cervix will cause dystocia.

Mode of Delivery after Metroplasty. The scar formed in the myometrium after unification is as strong as, if not stronger than, the scar formed after cesarean section. The biologic conditions under which healing occurs are entirely different in these two situations. Endomyometritis is a common complication after cesarean section but is not a complication of uterine unification. Of 71 known pregnancies in Strassmann's collected series reported in 1952,[130] 61 were delivered vaginally. There were no cases of uterine rupture during pregnancy or delivery. Despite evidence that the uterine scar heals securely after unification operations, our policy is to recommend delivery by elective cesarean section in all patients who have undergone abdominal metroplasty. Patients can deliver vaginally after a hysteroscopic or resectoscopic metroplasty.

Diethylstilbestrol-Related Uterine Anomalies. Exposure of the female fetus to DES can cause significant anomalous development of the uterus, as reported by Kaufman et al.[80] and by Haney et al.[51] The T-shaped uterus is the variant most commonly seen. It is associated with an increased rate of spontaneous abortions, preterm deliveries, and ectopic pregnancies.

Nagel and Malo[101] determined the feasibility of correcting the uterine malformations seen in DES-exposed women by incising constriction rings and septae. Their goal was to incise the irregular uterine walls until the cavity assumed a smooth, straight line from the lower uterine cavity to the uterine tubal ostium. Their results suggested that metroplasty can decrease pregnancy loss but does not enhance fertility. We suggest that in rare situations, a patient can benefit from a uterine reconstructive procedure but that most patients will not. Surgeons may never develop a large series to document the efficacy of surgical outcomes because patients with this anomaly will eventually age beyond reproductive years, and some latitude is required in patients who might possibly benefit from metroplasty.

DES-exposed patients must be monitored closely for evidence of dilation and effacement of the cervix early in pregnancy. Cervical cerclage may be indicated in some patients.

Unicornuate Uterus

Overview. A unicornuate uterus can be present alone or with a rudimentary horn or bulb on the opposite side. In a series reported by Heinonen et al.,[56] 11 of 13 patients with a unicornuate uterus had a rudimentary horn, and 2 did not. The rudimentary anlage (uterine muscle bundle or bulb) can communicate directly with the unicornuate uterus. In some instances there is no cavity within the anlage or there is no rudimentary horn. Most rudimentary horns are noncommunicating (90% according to O'Leary and O'Leary[104]). The two sides may be connected by a fibromuscular band, or there may be no connection and no communication between the two uterine cavities. In 1988, Fedele et al.[41] found that sonography was useful in determining the presence of not only a rudimentary horn but also a cavity within.

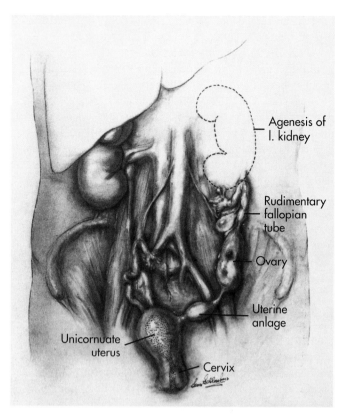

Fig. 43-22 A unicornuate uterus associated with ovarian malposition on the left. Note that the ovary and the tube are slightly above the pelvic brim. In this instance, the ovary measured 6 inches in length. (From Rock JA, Thompson JD: *TeLinde's operative gynecology,* ed 8, Philadelphia, 1997, Lippincott-Raven.)

Urinary tract anomalies are often associated with a unicornuate uterus. On the side opposite the unicornuate uterus, there may be a horseshoe or a pelvic kidney, or the kidney may be hypoplastic or absent. This is especially true if there is associated müllerian duct obstruction. In 1996, Fedele et al.[40] reported a 40% incidence of urinary tract anomalies in patients with a unicornuate uterus. When all müllerian duct derivatives and the kidney are absent on one side, this implies failure of development of the entire urogenital ridge, including the genital ridge where the ovary forms. In addition, the ovary may be malpositioned (Fig. 43-22). Rock et al.[115] reported a unilateral ovary located above the pelvic brim in patients with uterine anomalies. The orifice of the müllerian duct develops at about the level of the fourth thoracic vertebra (T4) in the embryo. The tip subsequently migrates along the course of the müllerian duct into the pelvis. The orifice of the duct or the fimbriated end of the tube comes to lie in the pelvis as a result of differential growth of the fetus. The subsequent differential growth is retarded so that the portion of the urogenital ridge that gives rise to both the gonad and tube does not displace into the pelvis. Malpositions of the ovary and tube are the result.

Reproductive Performance. According to Heinonen et al.,[56] the unicornuate uterus is associated with the poorest fetal survival (40%) of all uterine anomalies. In 1956, Jones

et al.[71] reported similar findings. The poor obstetric outcome may be explained by the abnormal shape, the insufficient muscular mass of the uterus, and the reduced uterine volume and inability to expand.

Moutos et al.[97] compared the reproductive performance of the unicornuate uterus with that of the didelphic uterus. Of 29 women with a unicornuate uterus, 20 produced a total of 40 pregnancies, whereas 13 women with a didelphic uterus produced a total of 28 pregnancies. The percentages of pregnancies resulting in preterm delivery, term delivery, and living children were similar in both groups. The authors concluded that reproductive performance of the unicornuate uterus was not different from that of the didelphic uterus, that it is uncommon for either malformation to be a primary cause of infertility, and that there is insufficient information to support recommendation of placement of a cervical cerclage in the absence of cervical incompetence. Thus there is no evidence that uterine reconstruction should be performed for patients with a unicornuate (or didelphic) uterus.

Because most patients with a unicornuate uterus will have a noncommunicating rudimentary uterine horn on the opposite side, there is danger of pregnancy in the rudimentary horn from transperitoneal migration of sperm or ovum from the opposite side. According to Holden and Hart,[60] some 350 instances of pregnancy in a rudimentary horn have been reported since the original case report by Mauriceau in 1669. O'Leary and O'Leary[104] found the corpus luteum on the side contralateral to the rudimentary horn containing a pregnancy in 8% of cases. Signs and symptoms of an ectopic pregnancy will develop with eventual rupture of the horn if the pregnancy is not detected early. Rupture through the wall of the vascular rudimentary horn is associated with sudden and severe intraperitoneal hemorrhage and shock. Death can occur in a few minutes. It is surprising that the current mortality rate has decreased to 5%.

Little, if anything, can be done to improve the reproductive performance of patients with a unicornuate uterus. The physician should observe these women closely for cervical incompetence and perform cerclage as indicated. Andrews and Jones[4] have suggested that removal of the rudimentary uterine horn may improve the chances of a successful pregnancy, but the experience is too small to support a definite recommendation. The asymmetric development of the unicornuate uterus with an opposing rudimentary uterine horn is not amenable to unification.

Longitudinal Vaginal Septum

Failure of fusion of the lower müllerian ducts that form the vagina can result in a vagina with a longitudinal septum. The septum can be partial or complete in any one of the symmetric unobstructed types of lateral fusion disorders. Young patients will have difficulty using tampons. In cases of didelphic uterus with a longitudinal vaginal septum, one uterine hemicorpus is usually better developed than the other. If intercourse consistently occurs on the vaginal side connected to the uterine hemicorpus that is less well developed, infertility or repeated abortion could result. For these reasons, the septum should be removed (when the patient is not pregnant) unless there is a contraindication. This can usually be accomplished easily with reasonable precautions against injury to the urethra, bladder, and rectum.

ASYMMETRIC OBSTRUCTION OF THE UTERUS OR VAGINA

Unicornuate Uterus and Noncommunicating Uterine Anlage Containing Functional Endometrium

If one müllerian duct develops normally and the opposite müllerian duct fails to develop or develops incompletely, a relatively normal unicornuate uterus is found on one side and the cervix, musculature, uterine cavity, endometrium, fallopian tube, blood supply, and ligamentous attachments are absent or hypoplastic to a varying degree on the other side. Obstruction to menstruation can also occur to varying degrees on the improperly developed side. For example, if a rudimentary uterine horn does not communicate externally but does have an endometrium-lined uterine cavity, clear symptoms of obstructed menstruation may begin soon after menarche and severe dysmenorrhea will be present. Unfortunately, cryptomenorrhea can be overlooked as the diagnosis because there will be cyclic menstruation from the opposite side. It is important to make the diagnosis as soon as possible, however, because if the lumen of the tube communicates with the endometrium cavity of the rudimentary uterus, retrograde menstruation and pelvic endometriosis will develop and reproductive potential can be destroyed. Occasionally, the fallopian tube connected to the rudimentary uterine horn may not be patent because of incomplete development (Fig. 43-23).

Unilateral Obstruction of a Cavity of a Double Uterus

Another example of a rare obstructed lateral fusion problem is the complete septum between two uterine cavities illustrated in Fig. 43-24. One cavity communicated with a cervix and the other did not. This could represent an example of unilateral failure of cervical development. The patient complained of incapacitating dysmenorrhea that appeared shortly after the menarche and lasted 5 days. A tense, cystic mass was palpable in the right half of the pelvis. The operation, described originally by Jones,[70] consisted of making an incision through the anterior wall of the cystic right portion of the uterus. It was found to contain old menstrual blood. The entire septum was excised, and the uterus was reconstructed by anastomosis of the two cavities. A continuous lockstitch was reinforced by interrupted myometrial sutures, and the plastic reconstruction of the uterus was completed by a third layer of interrupted sutures uniting myometrium and serosa.

Double Uterus with Obstructed Hemivagina and Ipsilateral Renal Agenesis

The unique clinical syndrome consisting of a double uterus, obstruction of the vagina (unilateral, partial, or complete), and ipsilateral renal agenesis is rare.[113] The renal agenesis

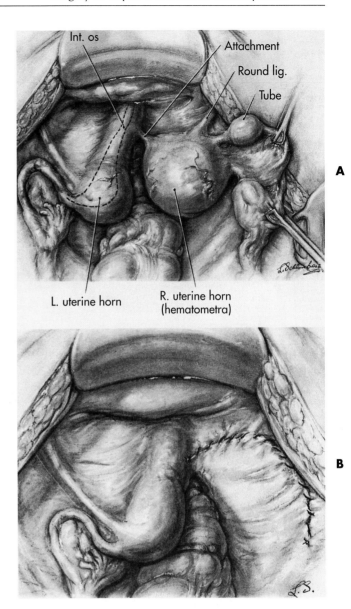

Fig. 43-23 **A,** A noncommunicating rudimentary horn with functional endometrium that contains menstrual blood under pressure. Note the congenital abnormality of the fallopian tube, which prevented retrograde menstruation. **B,** The same patient after excision of the rudimentary horn. (From Rock JA, Thompson JD: *TeLinde's operative gynecology,* ed 8, Philadelphia, 1997, Lippincott-Raven.)

(mesonephric involution) on the side of the obstructed vagina associated with a double uterus and double cervix suggests an embryologic arrest at 8 weeks of pregnancy that simultaneously affects the müllerian and metanephric ducts. The exact cause is unknown.

Diagnostic Groups. Clinical symptoms vary depending on the uterovaginal relations in individual patients, but the syndrome can be described generally in three groups. Group 1 patients have complete unilateral vaginal obstruction without uterine communication, resulting in a paravaginal mass and symptoms of severe dysmenorrhea and lower abdominal pain. Menses are regular. Group 2 patients have an incomplete unilateral vaginal obstruction without uterine

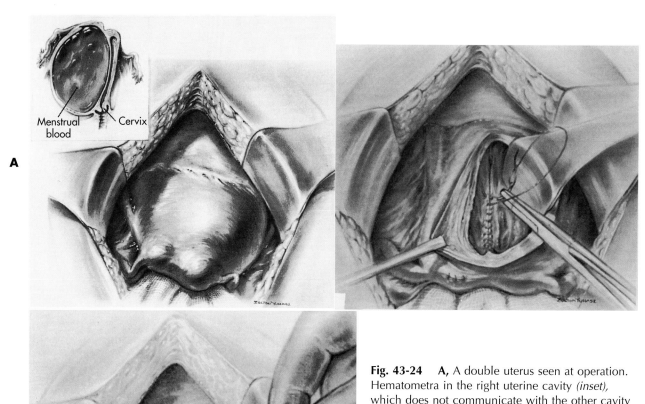

A

Menstrual blood   Cervix

B

C

Incision into left uterine cavity   Accessory osteum

Fig. 43-24   A, A double uterus seen at operation. Hematometra in the right uterine cavity *(inset),* which does not communicate with the other cavity or the cervical canal. **B,** The septum of the double uterus has been excised, and anastomosis is performed to unite the two cavities. **C,** Anastomosis is completed. The small incision in the left uterine cavity was made before the septum was removed for the purpose of orientation. (From Rock JA, Thompson JD: *TeLinde's operative gynecology,* ed 8, Philadelphia, 1997, Lippincott-Raven.)

communication. The presenting symptoms are lower abdominal pain, severe dysmenorrhea, excessive foul mucopurulent discharge, and in some instances, intermenstrual bleeding. Group 3 patients have complete vaginal obstruction with a laterally communicating double uterus. They have a paravaginal mass, lower abdominal pain, and dysmenorrhea. Menses are regular.

Because menses in patients with this syndrome are rarely irregular, the possibility of this syndrome as a diagnosis can easily be overlooked. A careful pelvic examination is necessary to make the correct diagnosis. MRI can identify the obstructed vagina, double uterus, and absence of a kidney on the side of the obstruction (Fig. 43-25), but it may not be helpful if there is incomplete vaginal obstruction or a uterine communication.

Complete unilateral vaginal obstruction (group 1) can go unrecognized for a number of years after the onset of menses. The vagina is distensible and can accommodate a large amount of accumulated blood in the obstructed side. There

is sufficient absorption of menstrual blood between periods, so each subsequent flow can add to the increments of accumulated blood without pain. Nevertheless, once retrograde menstruation occurs, endometriosis invariably is the result.

Surgical Treatment. Careful excision of the vaginal septum is the preferred treatment for a unilateral vaginal obstruction. Prophylactic antibiotics should be administered before surgery. After the vaginal pouch is opened, the surgeon should use suction and lavage to remove the pooled blood and mucus.

Because the obstructing septum is usually thick, removal can be difficult. Clamps should be used to isolate a generous vaginal pedicle while the suture is being tied in place to prevent slippage of tissue. Such pedicles generally retract during healing, and vaginal stenosis is thus avoided. In most instances, surgery is restricted to excision of the septum, and abdominal exploration is unnecessary. Uterine reconstruction is not indicated for cases of lateral communication of the uterine horns.

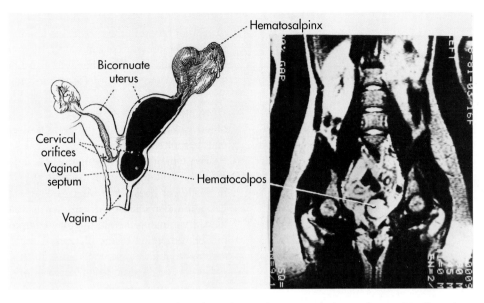

Fig. 43-25 A double uterus with unilateral complete vaginal obstruction and ipsilateral renal agenesis. Magnetic resonance imaging reveals the left hematocolpos, both uteri, and absence of the left kidney on the side of the vaginal obstruction. (From Rock JA, Thompson JD: *TeLinde's operative gynecology,* ed 8, Philadelphia, 1997, Lippincott-Raven.)

Reproductive performance for patients with this disorder is usually consistent with that of patients with a double uterus unless the delay in diagnosis and resection of the obstructing septum has been sufficient to destroy the tubal connection or to cause the development of endometriosis.

UNUSUAL CONFIGURATIONS OF VERTICAL-LATERAL FUSION DEFECTS

Müllerian duct anomalies can occur in association with a variety of other problems. For example, Stanton[127] reported that in a series of 70 patients with bladder exstrophy, 30 (43%) had reproductive tract abnormalities. He suggested that the true figures were actually higher. Müllerian abnormalities included absence of the vagina; septate vagina; unicornuate, bicornuate, and didelphic uterus; and absent uterus. Fewer müllerian anomalies are seen with epispadias. Jones[69] investigated anomalies of the external genitalia and vagina in 30 patients with bladder exstrophy seen at the Johns Hopkins Hospital and suggested operative techniques for correction of these anomalies. Techniques for the management of other gynecologic and obstetric problems (especially uterine prolapse) also have been discussed by Weed and McKee[139] and by Blakely and Mills.[9] A number of other rare combinations of congenital malformations of the vagina and perineum have been found in association with uterine anomalies. Their surgical correction, especially in children, is reported by Hendren and Donahoe[59] and by others.

Müllerian duct anomalies are seen with the McKusick-Kaufman syndrome, an autosomal-recessive disorder. Other clinical findings reported with this syndrome include hydrometrocolpos, postaxial polydactyly, syndactyly, congenital heart disease, intravaginal displacement of the urethral meatus, and anorectal anomalies. In 1982, Jabs et al.[64] also reported a case in the literature.

SURGICAL CONDITIONS OF THE EXTERNAL GENITALIA/VAGINA
Labial Adhesions

Labial agglutination in a young child is occasionally mistaken for congenital absence of the vagina. Labial anatomy will be distorted, whereas in vaginal agenesis external genitalia anatomy is normal. Daily local treatment with estrogen cream is all that may be required to treat this condition.

The Imperforate Hymen

The hymen, the junction of the sinovaginal bulbs with the urogenital sinus, is a thin mucous membrane, sometimes cribriform in urogenital sinus epithelium. The hymen is not derived from the müllerian ducts. The hymen usually is perforated during embryonic life to establish a connection between the lumen of the vaginal canal and the vaginal vestibule, and it usually is torn early in the prepubertal years. If there are no perforations through this membrane, the hymen is called imperforate (Fig. 43-26).

Although variations in hymen development occur, complete blockage by the hymen of the vaginal orifice is rare. In 1988, Pokorny and Kozinetz[106] described the various configurations and anatomic details of the prepubertal hymen. In a case series of 265 children with known genital problems, three main hymenal configurations were observed: fimbriated, circumferential, and posterior rim. Interestingly, bleeding without a history of trauma was associated with

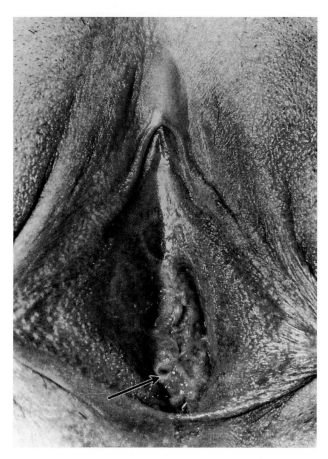

Fig. 43-26 Hymen that is almost imperforate. The pinhead-sized opening *(arrow)* was sufficient to permit pregnancy. (From Rock JA, Thompson JD: *TeLinde's operative gynecology*, ed 8, Philadelphia, 1997, Lippincott-Raven.)

hymenal bumps or breaks suggestive of trauma (31%) or with other hemorrhagic vulvar lesions (40%).

Clinical Presentation

If an imperforate hymen is noticed before puberty, the condition can be treated when it is entirely asymptomatic. When the hymen is incised, the vagina is found to contain mucoid fluid that is the result of accumulated cervical secretion.

Most patients first visit the gynecologist at 13 to 15 years of age, when symptoms begin to appear, but menstruation appears not to have begun. The symptoms after the onset of puberty result from the accumulation of menstrual blood. The blood of the first cycle period or two is collected in the vagina, which can hold a large volume of blood without undue stretching and with no other symptoms. This accumulated menstrual blood in the vagina is called hematocolpos. The patient may feel a slight fatigue and have cramping discomfort suggesting menstruation but will have no history of any passage of menstrual blood through the vaginal outlet.

As menstruation continues to occur, however, the vagina becomes greatly overdistended and the cervical canal also

will begin to dilate. *Hematometra,* the accumulation of menstrual blood in the uterine cavity, may occur. When the intrauterine pressure reaches a certain point, retrograde passage of blood into the tubes will cause hematosalpinx. Associated or other adhesion formation within or at the fimbriated ends of the tubes may seal them, so little or no blood will enter the peritoneal cavity. In some cases, however, blood passes freely into the peritoneal cavity, forming hematoperitoneum (Fig. 43-27).

The most common symptoms of vaginal overdistention are lower abdominal pain, discomfort in the pelvis, and pain in the lower back. Pain often is aggravated on defecation. Urination also can be difficult because pressure of the distended vagina on the urethra may compress the urethra and prevent emptying of the bladder. Cramplike pains recur in the suprapubic region, together with the common urologic symptoms of dysuria, frequency, and urgency; overflow incontinence may eventually develop.

A tender mass often is palpable suprapubically, the result of uterine enlargement and upward displacement, bladder distention, or both. If hematoperitoneum occurs, the irritation of the free blood may cause all the symptoms and signs of peritonitis. Protrusion of the hymen usually is visible. The protrusion sometimes is massive and dark in color because the occult blood shows through the stretched mucous membrane.

Between 1945 and 1981 at the Johns Hopkins Hospital, 22 patients with a mean age of 14.7 years were admitted for surgical correction of imperforate hymens. Associated anomalies, including urinary tract anomalies, were rare. Thirteen patients subsequently conceived, and 10 patients were observed to have living children as reported by Rock et al.[121] The great distensibility of the vagina probably protects the adolescent patient with an imperforate hymen from abnormal retrograde menstruation. Subsequent development of pelvic endometriosis with imperforate hymen as the cause is unlikely as long as the diagnosis is made reasonably early.

Surgical Treatment

When an imperforate hymen is discovered before puberty, the hymenal membrane can simply be incised, preferably at the 2-, 4-, 8-, and 10-o'clock positions. The quadrants of the hymen are then excised, and the mucosal margins are approximated with fine delayed-absorbable suture (Fig. 43-28). To prevent scarring and stenosis, which could result in dyspareunia, the hymenal tissue should not be excised too close to the vaginal mucosa. All unnecessary intrauterine instrumentation should be avoided because if hematocolpos has already developed (see Fig. 43-27), there is the risk of perforating the thin, overstretched uterine wall.

Generally, no further surgical intervention is needed. If the uterine mass does not regress within 2 to 3 weeks, however, inspection and dilation of the cervix should be performed to ensure that drainage from the uterus is satisfactory.

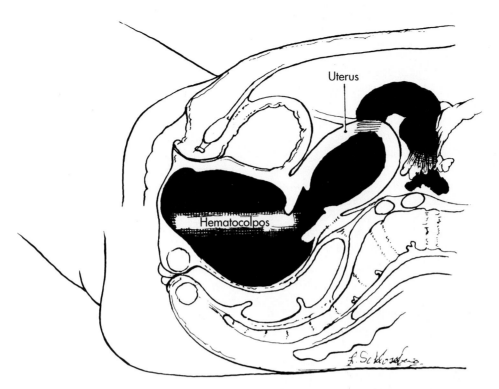

Fig. 43-27 Hematocolpos, hematometra, hematosalpinx, and hematoperitoneum consequent to an imperforate hymen. (From Rock JA, Thompson JD: *TeLinde's operative gynecology,* ed 8, Philadelphia, 1997, Lippincott-Raven.)

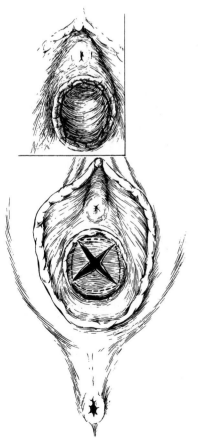

Fig. 43-28 Excision of imperforate hymen. Stellate incisions are made through the hymenal membrane at the 2-, 4-, 8-, and 10-o'clock positions. The individual quadrants are excised along the lateral wall of the vagina, avoiding excision of the vagina. Margins of vaginal mucosa are approximated with fine delayed-absorbable suture *(inset).* (From Rock JA, Thompson JD: *TeLinde's operative gynecology,* ed 8, Philadelphia, 1997, Lippincott-Raven.)

ANOMALIES OF THE EXTERNAL GENITALIA

When abnormal gonadal development is caused by ineffective suppression of the müllerian ducts, ambiguous external genitalia often will be accompanied by a small rudimentary uterus or a partially developed vagina. In addition, when there is a genetic loss of cytoplasmic receptor proteins within the androgenic target cells, such as with the androgen insensitivity syndromes (formerly called testicular feminization syndrome), the vagina will be incompletely developed because the existing male gonads suppress the development of the müllerian ducts. Because these genetically male patients are seen clinically as phenotypic XY females without a completely formed vagina, it is important that a vagina be surgically constructed so that these patients may have satisfactory sexual function in their female gender role.

Congenital rectovaginal fistula, imperforate (covered) anus, hypospadia, and other anatomic variants of cloacal dysgenesis also can occur. These anomalies can be associated with maldevelopment of the müllerian and mesonephric duct derivatives.

Sexually ambiguous external genitalia defects of the urogenital sinus are remarkably constant in appearance regardless of the cause of the anomaly. Such genitalia differ only in their degree of malformation and occupy a range of positions somewhere intermediate to the genitalia of a normal female and that of a normal male. These anomalies can be anatomically identical to each other whether their causative factor is congenital adrenal hyperplasia (CAH), male hermaphroditism, true hermaphroditism, or some other syndrome (see the box above). Furthermore, in the absence of a virilizing factor either from the normal embryonic testis or from an abnormal virilizing source such as the adrenal gland in CAH, the urogenital sinus invariably develops along female lines. In the presence of a virilizing influence, however, fusion of the scrotolabial folds may be sufficient to obscure or conceal the vagina from the outside or even to entirely suppress its formation, and a urethra will be formed for varying distances or along the entire length of the phallus. The essential elements of the operative procedure for reconstruction of ambiguous genitalia into female genitalia does not vary, regardless of the cause of intersexuality.

Construction of Female External Genitalia

Any reconstruction of the external genitalia with the objective of producing normal female appearance and function requires a full understanding of the surgical anatomy. It is especially important to accurately identify the site of communication of the vagina with the urogenital sinus. Briefly, the vaginal communication is almost always in relation to the caudal urogenital sinus derivatives. The vagina communicates with that portion of the urogenital sinus that in a male gives rise to the membranous portion of the male urethra and that in the female becomes the vaginal vestibule. The vagina almost never communicates with the portion of the urogenital sinus that becomes the prostatic urethra in the male or the entire urethra in the female. In 1989, Bargy et

ANOMALIES ASSOCIATED WITH HERMAPHRODITISM
Female hermaphroditism
Congenital adrenal hyperplasia
Nonadrenal androgenization
Maternal drug intake
Virilizing ovarian or adrenal tumors
Luteoma of pregnancy
Idiopathic
Male hermaphroditism
Central nervous system defects
Absence of gonadotropins
Abnormal gonadotropins
Deficiencies in enzymes involved in testosterone synthesis
Leydig cell agenesis
Gonadal dysgenesis
Partial androgen insensitivity (testicular feminization) syndrome
5α-Reductase deficiency
Y chromosome defect
True hermaphroditism

Adapted from Damario MA, Rock JA: Diagnostic approach to ambiguous genitalia. In Adashi EI, Rock JA, Rosenwaks Z, editors: *Productive endocrinology, surgery and technology,* Philadelphia, 1996, Lippincott-Raven.

al.[8] reviewed and confirmed these relations. If this usual relation is confirmed at surgery, the anomalously persistent urogenital sinus may be incised to the vaginal communication without fear of disturbing the urinary sphincter. Interestingly, hermaphrodites with anomalies of the external genitalia (Fig. 43-29) rarely have problems of urinary continence.

Hendren and Crawford[58] identified patients whose vagina entered the urogenital sinus in that portion from which the posterior urethra is derived. However, this unusual communication is seldom sufficiently posterior for urinary continence to be problematic.

One objective of the reconstruction procedure for external genitalia is to delay the procedure until the anomalous structures are of a size to permit easy identification of all structures, yet to complete the procedure before the anomalies may prove embarrassing or alarming to either the patient or the patient's family. Proceeding as early as possible may have many psychological advantages. As observed by Azziz et al.,[5] however, vaginal repair may be delayed until menarche, when maturity and the desire for sexual activity are usually well established.

Most hermaphrodites reared as girls have a vagina or vaginal pouch, although in some instances it is rudimentary. Only rarely is no vagina present, despite ambiguity of the external genitalia. The choice of operative procedure must conform to the observed anatomy. Thus these choices are considered in the context of several categories based on anatomic structure of the anomaly.

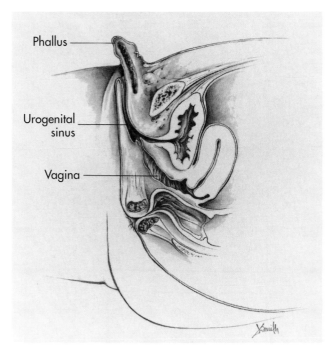

Fig. 43-29 Sagittal view of a patient with adrenogenital syndrome. Clitoromegaly and posterior fusion are present. (From Rock JA, Thompson JD: *TeLinde's operative gynecology,* ed 8, Philadelphia, 1997, Lippincott-Raven.)

Techniques Based on Specific Situations

When the Vagina Is Present. The basic operation is, in essence, a modification of one described at length by Young.[146] Neugebauer describes incision of the urogenital sinus in cases of hermaphroditism.

Patients with adrenal hyperplasia usually require reconstruction of the external genitalia exclusively. However, when exploratory laparotomy is necessary to remove contradictory sex structures in patients with other types of intersexuality or to establish the diagnosis, reconstruction of the genitalia may be accomplished at the same operation.

When the operation is performed at the ideal age, the structures are so small that it is impossible to introduce a finger into the urogenital sinus, and all tissues must be grasped throughout the operation with fine delicate tissue forceps. Operating loupes (2.5×) are of great benefit to the surgeon. Small bipolar forceps and microscissors are also useful. Fine, 5-0 or 6-0 synthetic absorbable suture material on an atraumatic needle is used throughout the procedure.

Initially, the urogenital sinus may be thoroughly investigated with a small McCarthy panendoscope to determine accurately the position and size of the vaginal communication. If a sound or catheter can be easily introduced into the meatus of the urogenital sinus and into the vagina, use of the endoscope may be omitted. Special care is needed not to introduce the sound into the urethra, which poses the danger of incising the distal urethral meatus. After the urogenital sinus is incised (to within 2 or 3 cm of the anus) the urethral orifice may be identified (Fig. 43-30, *A* and *B*). A small

Foley catheter may then be introduced through the urinary meatus for purposes of identification throughout the remainder of the operation (see Fig. 43-30, *C*). To attach the edges of the vagina to the skin, it is usually necessary to free the vagina posteriorly and laterally to secure sufficient mobilization to have these structures meet without tension. It is unnecessary to free the vagina anteriorly because this would require its separation from the urethra. Sufficient mobilization can ordinarily be obtained by lateral and posterior dissection. When sufficient freedom has been attained, the edges of the vagina may be secured to the skin with interrupted 5-0 sutures on an atraumatic reverse cutting needle. In the infant, four or five sutures around the edge of the vagina are usually sufficient. The edges of the incised sinus membrane may then be sutured to the skin anteriorly (see Fig. 43-30, *D* through *G*). A small sponge impregnated with Vaseline may be introduced into the vagina to try to maintain its patency during the healing process.

Attention is directed to the enlarged clitoris. Traditionally, the clitoris was simply amputated, and a nonfunctioning cosmetic clitoris was fashioned. Although several children so treated now have normal adult sexual function, the literature lacks follow-up data on large patient groups.

Alternatively, a newer technique has provided a somewhat better cosmetic result. This procedure attempts to preserve a shell of the glans on a pedicle flap. The shaft of the clitoris is subtotally resected, and the stumps are reanastomosed (Fig. 43-31). The nerve supply to the glans is severed during this procedure, with the result that sensation in the glans is diminished. However, sexual function seems to be satisfactory.

Rajfer et al.[109] have suggested a dorsal approach to the subtotal resection of the corpora (Fig. 43-32), which has the advantage of preserving the ventral nerve supply and which should preserve sensation in the glans. This approach is theoretically desirable and can be recommended for suitable patients. As mentioned previously, however, lack of clitoral sensation does not seem to significantly affect the later sexual behavior of patients treated by procedures that sever the dorsal nerves to the glans.

The indwelling catheter may be left in place for a few days until edema of the surrounding structures has subsided. An indwelling catheter is particularly useful in children with metabolic disorders that require accurate urine collection. A pressure dressing for 24 hours reduces the incidence of incisional hematoma.

When the Vaginal Orifice Is Obscured. As mentioned, preoperative identification and catheterization or sounding of the vaginal orifice are key to the performance of a successful one-stage procedure. When the vagina cannot be located by sounding, it sometimes can be seen by endoscopy. When sounding and vision both fail, an attempt before surgery to introduce a small (no. 4 or 5) ureteral catheter into the vagina by blindly probing through the endoscope along the posterior wall of the urogenital sinus may assist in the identification of the vagina. Sometimes this catheter will find the orifice. If so, it may be left within the vagina as a

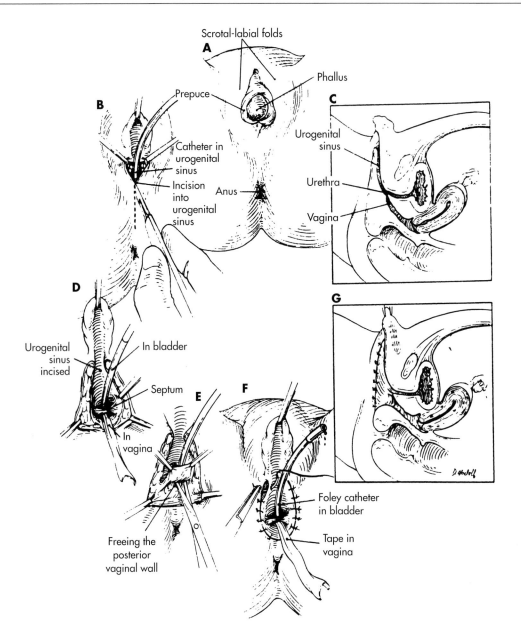

Fig. 43-30   **A,** The external genitalia of an 18-month-old patient with female hermaphrodit-ism caused by congenital adrenal hyperplasia. The operation is the same, regardless of the cause of the deformity. **B,** Beginning of the operation. Incision into the urogenital sinus. If the external meatus is large enough and the urogenital sinus will accommodate it, it is sometimes possible to introduce a catheter into the bladder through the urethra and introduce a sound into the vagina beside this. When the structures are large enough, this maneuver greatly facili-tates the operative procedure by ensuring their identification. **C,** Lateral view, which better shows the relations among the various structures. In this patient, in whom the anomaly was caused by congenital virilizing adrenal hyperplasia, the development of the müllerian ducts was entirely normal for a female. **D,** Situation after incision of the urogenital sinus. **E,** With the glass catheter in the bladder, the posterior vaginal wall is freed as far as necessary to make it possible to bring it to the skin edge without undue tension. **F,** The operative situation after the edges of the vagina are sutured to the skin and after the edges of the mucous membrane of the urogenital sinus are also sutured to the skin along the line of incision. **G,** Lateral view at the completion of the operation. (From Rock JA, Thompson JD: *TeLinde's operative gyne-cology,* ed 8, Philadelphia, 1997, Lippincott-Raven.)

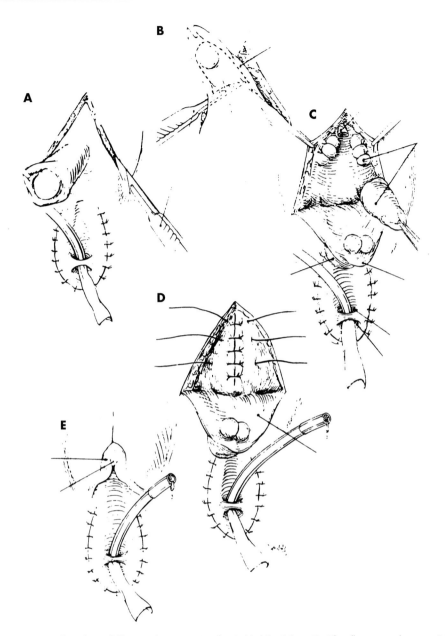

Fig. 43-31 The clitoral flap technique. **A,** The initial incision. **B,** The flap must be as wide as possible at the base to preserve the circulation for the glans. The glans cannot be preserved completely because the blood supply will be insufficient to maintain it. It must be as thin a shell of the glans as possible. **C,** The shaft of the phallus has been removed. **D,** There has been some closure of the space from which the corpora were removed. **E,** The flap has been sutured into place. (From Rock JA, Thompson JD: *TeLinde's operative gynecology,* ed 8, Philadelphia, 1997, Lippincott-Raven.)

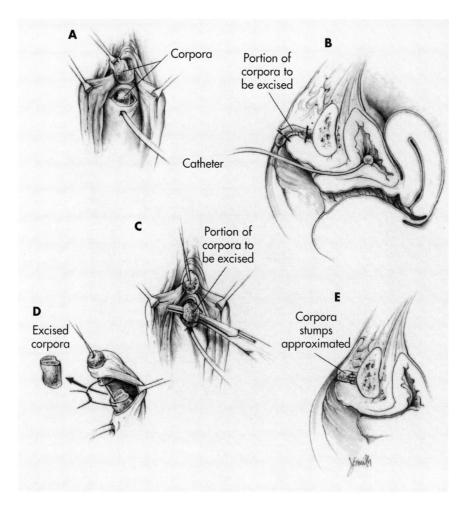

Fig. 43-32   Operation of Rajfer et al. **A** through **C,** Corpora are approached and removed through a posterior incision in the phallus. **D,** Diagram of the excised portion of the corpora. **E,** The corpora are removed and stumps approximated. (From Rock JA, Thompson JD: *TeLinde's operative gynecology,* ed 8, Philadelphia, 1997, Lippincott-Raven.)

guide during surgical exposure of the area (Fig. 43-33). In the event that the vaginal orifice cannot be located, a planned two-stage operation may be indicated. The objective of the first stage is to obtain cosmetically satisfactory female genitalia by removing the clitoris and partially excising the urogenital sinus without exteriorizing the vagina. The second stage, exteriorization of the vagina, may be postponed until a later date, when identification of the vaginal orifice by sounding becomes possible.

When the Vaginosinus Communication Is Blocked. Rarely does the vagina not communicate with the urogenital sinus. The vagina with the urogenital sinus is homologous with the hymenal area, and the hymen rarely is imperforate in an otherwise normal female. For such a circumstance, we have found it helpful to pass a sound downward from above to identify the vagina in the perineum. With such a guide, the edges of the vaginal epithelium can be located and sutured to the skin (Fig. 43-34). Until the uterus enlarges somewhat from its infantile state, the cavity is not large enough to accommodate even a uterine sound. Therefore, if such an operation is contemplated, it should not be done un-

til there is palpable enlargement of the uterus at the onset of puberty.

When the Vaginosinus Communication Is Deep. Hendren[57] has been especially interested in patients whose vaginosinus communication involves the proximal urethra. He has advocated an operation that disconnects the vagina from the urethra and repositions the vaginal orifice in the perineum. In his hands, this procedure seems to have been satisfactory for some patients. The procedure requires positioning the new vaginal orifice in the perineum (Fig. 43-35). Most patients with ambiguous external genitalia and a vagina have a vaginosinus communication well distal to the proximal urethra, and consideration of the procedure advocated by Hendren is not necessary.

Results of Revision of External Genitalia

Among 28 patients with adrenogenital syndrome and good follow-up treated at the Johns Hopkins Hospital, 22 (78.6%) needed further vaginal reconstructive surgery to achieve an adequate vaginal size to allow comfortable intercourse. Interestingly, of the 22 patients, 5 had undergone more than

Text continued on p. 826

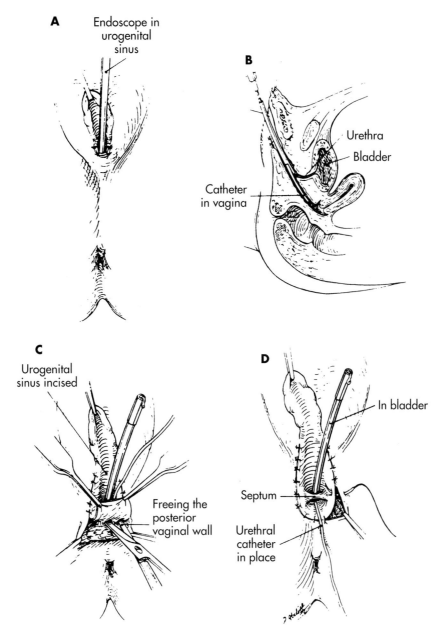

Fig. 43-33 Operative procedure when it is difficult to locate the vaginal orifice by sounding. An operative endoscope can be used to probe with a small ureteral catheter. **A,** The orifice is enlarged to accommodate the endoscope. **B,** The tip of the catheter has found the vaginal opening and entered the vagina. **C,** Freeing the posterior vaginal wall with the ureteral catheter in the vagina and a stiff catheter in the urethra. **D,** The vaginal portion of the operation is complete. (From Rock JA, Thompson JD: *TeLinde's operative gynecology,* ed 8, Philadelphia, 1997, Lippincott-Raven.)

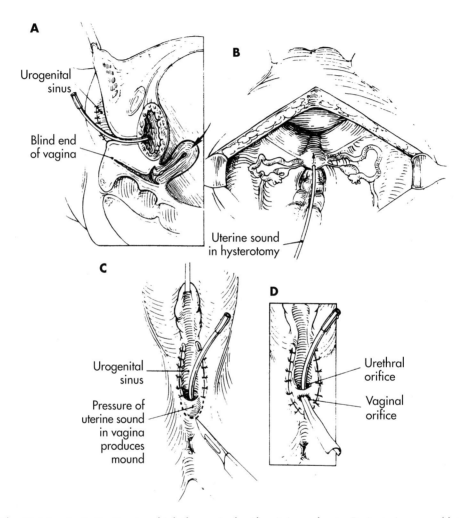

Fig. 43-34   **A,** A situation in which the vaginal orifice is imperforate. **B,** A uterine sound has been passed through the fundus into the vagina. **C,** The tip of the sound can be palpated in the perineum. **D,** The completed procedure. (From Rock JA, Thompson JD: *TeLinde's operative gynecology,* ed 8, Philadelphia, 1997, Lippincott-Raven.)

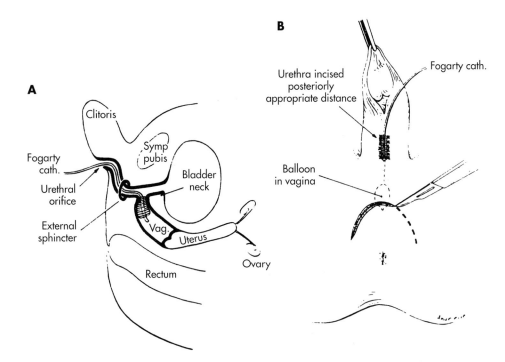

Fig. 43-35   A perineal pull-through vaginoplasty according to Hendren. **A,** Sagittal view in diagram of vaginal communication very high in the urogenital sinus. A small Foley catheter is placed in the vagina to aid in its manipulation and localization. **B,** The location of the initial incision in relation to the balloon in the vagina. A perineal pull-through vaginoplasty according to Hendren. (From Rock JA, Thompson JD: *TeLinde's operative gynecology,* ed 8, Philadelphia, 1997, Lippincott-Raven.)   *Continued*

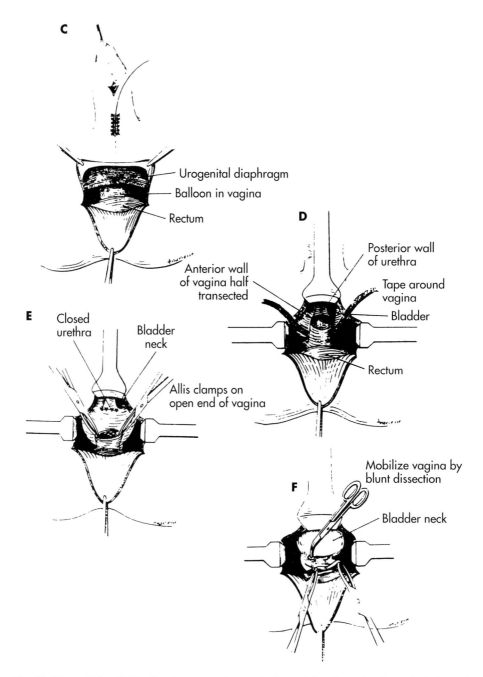

Fig. 43-35, cont'd   **C,** The flap is retracted posteriorly, and the dissection is carried along the anterior wall of the rectum until the vagina (as identified by the balloon) is approached. **D,** The vagina is identified by the Foley balloon catheter. The vagina is open. Care should be taken to pull a flap of vagina distal so that there will be no problem in closing the urethra. **E,** The urethra is closed. Clips are placed on the vagina to bring it down to the perineum. **F,** The vagina is further mobilized. A perineal pull-through vaginoplasty according to Hendren. (From Rock JA, Thompson JD: *TeLinde's operative gynecology,* ed 8, Philadelphia, 1997, Lippincott-Raven.)

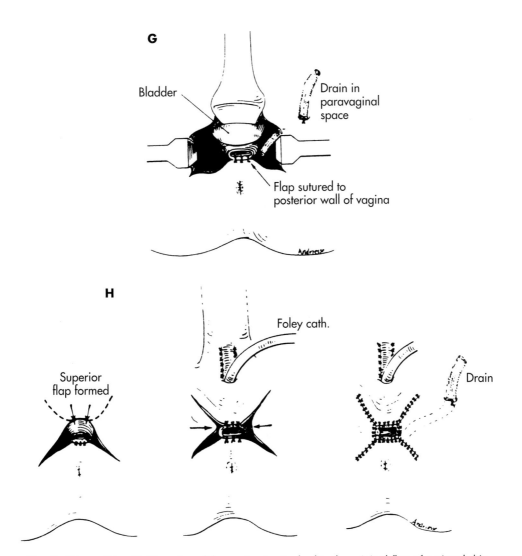

Fig. 43-35, cont'd   **G,** The edge of the vagina is attached to the original flap of perineal skin. **H,** Anterior and lateral flaps are attached. Note the use of a drain in the perivaginal space.

one surgical attempt at reconstruction. The mean age of patients undergoing repeat procedures was 7.1 years. The mean age at first surgery for the whole group was 23.6 months. Vaginal reconstructive surgery was performed on 18 of these patients and was successful in 13 (72%) of the procedures. It generally is recommended that exteriorization of the vagina be postponed until near puberty, when feminization occurs and the young woman is sufficiently mature to comply with a postoperative dilation program. The results of exteriorization performed during infancy must be followed carefully for evidence of narrowing, requiring regular dilation until puberty, to prevent vaginal stenosis.[6]

Interestingly, in a recent study of fertility and women with CAH, it was found that 36% of patients older than 16 years of age had never had heterosexual relations. Furthermore, there seemed to be a relatively high rate of homosexuality and consequent lack of vaginal coitus among female CAH patients.[59,96]

Secondary Operations

A secondary operation on the vaginal outlet may be required. This is generally the case if the basic operation is deliberately accomplished in two stages, whatever the reason. A secondary operation may be indicated, for example, when an infant's vaginal orifice is not readily identifiable, yet it seems desirable to construct cosmetically acceptable female genitalia at a very early age. In this circumstance the clitoroplasty can be done in the newborn, and the vagina may be exteriorized at puberty.

When the complete operation is attempted at an early age, the vagina is sometimes not satisfactorily exteriorized. Vaginal stenosis may require reconstruction at the time of puberty (Fig. 43-36). In this circumstance there usually has been a failure to carry the midline incision far enough posteriorly, and a second procedure will be required to complete the first one by continuing the midline incision far enough posteriorly.

In other cases, contraction at the vaginal outlet may occur even if the operation is adequately performed.[118] A minor revision of the vaginal orifice will be required to enlarge the vaginal orifice by making an incision in the midline and closing it at 90 degrees to the original axis of the original incision (Fig. 43-37). In some instances, flaps may need to be created to enlarge the vaginal orifice (Fig. 43-38). Labial tissue expanders have been advocated to reduce the risk of stenosis.[105]

BLADDER EXSTROPHY

Exstrophy of the bladder is a rare, congenital anomaly that occurs in 1:25,000 to 1:40,000 live births. There is a male predominance over females at a ratio of about 2:1. Classic bladder exstrophy is characterized by (1) absence of the lower anterior abdominal wall; (2) absence of the anterior wall of the bladder, leaving the posterior bladder wall and the ureteric orifices exposed; (3) a poorly defined bladder neck and urethra; and (4) wide separation of the pubic sym-

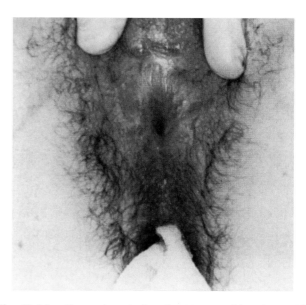

Fig. 43-36 External genitalia of a 15-year-old patient with vaginal stenosis. Revision of the external genitalia, including an exteriorization of the vagina, had been performed in infancy. (From Rock JA, Thompson JD: *TeLinde's operative gynecology,* ed 8, Philadelphia, 1997, Lippincott-Raven.)

physis. A genital abnormality typically present in females with bladder exstrophy is anterior displacement and narrowing of the vagina (Fig. 43-39) and separation of the clitoris into two distinct bodies[29] (Fig. 43-40).

Bladder exstrophy, cloacal exstrophy, and epispadias are variants of the exstrophy epispadias complex. These defects have been attributed to failure of the normal process of ingrowth of mesoderm and the consequent lack of reinforcement of the cloacal membrane. The normal cloacal membrane is bilaminar and occupies the caudal end of the germinal disc. An ingrowth of mesenchyme between the ectodermal and endodermal layers of the cloacal membrane forms the lower abdominal wall musculature and the pelvic bones. After mesenchymal ingrowth occurs, descent of the urorectal septum divides the cloacal membrane into the bladder anteriorly and the rectum posteriorly. The urorectal septum eventually meets with the posterior remnant of the cloacal membrane, which perforates to form the anal and urogenital sinus openings. The paired genital tubercles migrate medially and fuse in the midline anterior to the cloacal membrane before perforation. Without its normal support from mesenchymal derivatives, the cloacal membrane is subject to premature rupture. Depending on the extent of the intraumbilical defect and the stage of development when rupture occurs, bladder exstrophy, cloacal exstrophy, or epispadias will develop (Fig. 43-41).

Treatment

Our understanding of appropriate urologic management of bladder exstrophy has evolved greatly over the past few decades, and improved management has dramatically increased the life expectancy and quality of life of patients with this anomaly. Historical methods of treatment involved

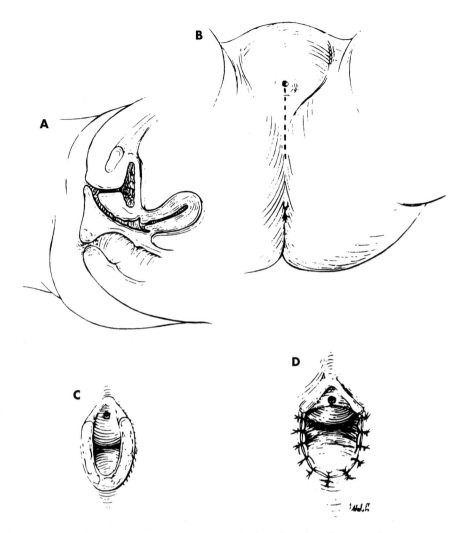

Fig. 43-37   **A,** Repeated operation on the vaginal outlet when the operation was not completed at the first procedure. **B,** The posterior incision. **C,** The vagina is exposed. **D,** The closure. (From Rock JA, Thompson JD: *TeLinde's operative gynecology,* ed 8, P hiladelphia, 1997, Lippincott-Raven.)

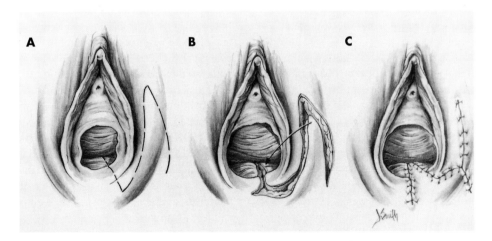

Fig. 43-38   Labial cutaneous flap. **A,** An incision is made through the labia skin and subcutaneous fat. **B,** The flap is rotated into the perineotomy incision and **(C)** is sutured in place by interrupted 3-0 delayed absorbable sutures. This may be repeated on the other side if required. (From Rock JA, Thompson JD: *TeLinde's operative gynecology,* ed 8, Philadelphia, 1997, Lippincott-Raven.)

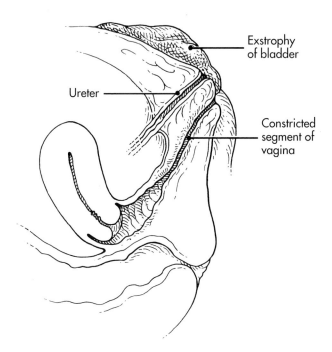

Fig. 43-39 Common gynecologic anomaly seen in females with bladder exstrophy. The vagina is rotated anteriorly and constricted over its distal portion. (From Rock JA, Thompson JD: *TeLinde's operative gynecology,* ed 8, Philadelphia, 1997, Lippincott-Raven.)

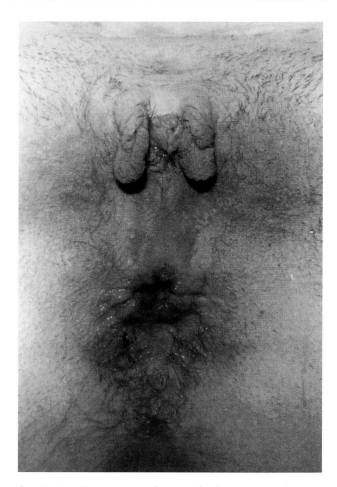

Fig. 43-40 Preoperative photograph of a patient undergoing reconstruction of the external genitalia. Note the bifid clitoris and small anterior vaginal orifice. (From Rock JA, Thompson JD: *TeLinde's operative gynecology,* ed 8, Philadelphia, 1997, Lippincott-Raven.)

bladder excision and a urinary diversion procedure such as ureterosigmoidostomy. These techniques are complicated by serious sequelae, including pyelonephritis, hyperchloremic acidosis, rectal incontinence, ureteral obstruction, and later development of malignancy.

Modern urologic management of bladder exstrophy relies on a staged approach to functional bladder closure. The initial procedure consists of primary bladder closure with or without iliac osteotomies to aid closure of the pelvic ring and growth and improvement of bladder capacity. The second-stage procedures usually involve bladder neck reconstruction to improve continence and bilateral ureteral reimplantations to prevent reflux.

The prognosis using modern-day procedures is good. Although deficiency of the pelvic floor and a predisposition for pelvic organ prolapse are not unusual with bladder exstrophy, the condition of bladder exstrophy itself can often be corrected and associated genital anomalies can be managed to allow comfortable sexual activity and possibly even pregnancy.

The adjunctive procedures that may be important with surgical correction of bladder exstrophy are those that address the correction of anterior displacement and narrowing of the vagina and separation of the clitoris into two distinct bodies that are so typically associated with bladder exstrophy.

The procedure for correcting the external genitalia has evolved from one that was first described by Jones in 1973.[69] Particular emphasis is placed on attainment of an adequate vaginal diameter without further predisposing to

subsequent prolapse. The first step is vertical incision into the posterior raphe of what resembles fused scrotolabial folds; next, Allis clamps are placed laterally for traction. Fine-needle point electrocautery is then used to further open the incision, with special care not to take this incision too far posteriorly. The lateral portions of the incision are secured with 3-0 nonreactive absorbable sutures for further traction. The posterior vaginal edges are undermined to allow their mobilization to the exterior. The vaginal mucosa is then approximated to the perineal surface with interrupted and figure-of-eight sutures, incorporating the superficial perineal muscles into the closure. In the more posterior portion of the closure, 2-0 nonreactive absorbable suture is used because this is the area of greatest tension. At completion, there is a significant increase in the diameter of the vagina, and the vaginal orifice usually will accommodate two fingers.

Postoperative active dilation therapy has recently been advocated. Experience with management of ambiguous genitalia has shown a decrease in the incidence of postoperative vaginal stenosis if dilation therapy is used during the constrictive phase (the first 6 weeks) of healing. Therefore,

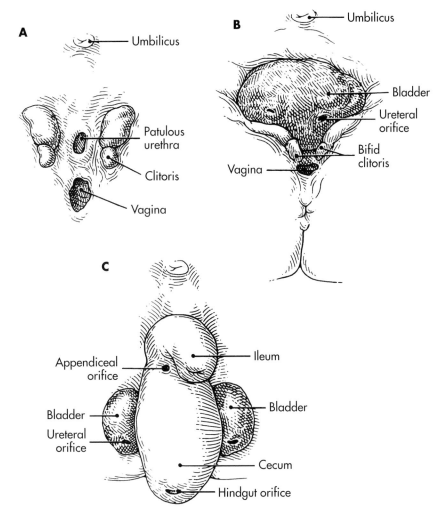

Fig. 43-41 Anatomic features of **(A)** epispadias, **(B)** classic bladder exstrophy, and **(C)** cloacal exstrophy in females. (From Rock JA, Thompson JD: *TeLinde's operative gynecology,* ed 8, Philadelphia, 1997, Lippincott-Raven.)

after reconstruction of the external genitalia and exteriorization of the vagina, appropriate-sized Lucite dilators are used once or twice a day for this 6-week period or until healing is complete.

Reapproximation of the bifid clitoris (Fig. 43-42) is primarily cosmetic and is not always performed. The technique involves excising a diamond-shaped area of skin and subcutaneous tissue between the clitoral bodies. The medial aspect of each side of the clitoris is then denuded and undermined to allow a central reapproximation with a side-to-side closure.

Adjunctive Treatments

Stanton[127] mentions that perineotomy was performed in six patients with bladder exstrophy in which the labia and clitoris are reapproximated by a Z-plasty technique. Still others have described rather extraordinary efforts to restore the mons pubis and female escutcheon with skin flaps of hair-bearing areas. However, these latter reports fail to mention correction of the vaginal anomaly.

Other series have described a wide range of both genital and extragenital abnormalities in association with bladder exstrophy. Stanton reviewed 70 patients with bladder exstrophy and observed an increased incidence of various müllerian anomalies. Eleven patients were also observed to have associated rectal prolapse. Blakely and Mills[9] observed various extragenital abnormalities in their series, including rectal prolapse, imperforate anus, exophthalmos, renal agenesis, and spina bifida.

Results

Jones[69] reviewed the records of all female patients in whom bladder exstrophy was diagnosed at Johns Hopkins Hospital over a 20-year time span. Of 18 patients with adequately described external genitalia, 13 had small, anteriorly displaced vaginal orifices, and the remaining 5 patients had vaginal orifices of normal size and location. Therefore, although demonstrating phenomena typical of bladder exstrophy, all female patients do not have the defect of narrowing of the vagina. Damario et al.[29] have recently updated

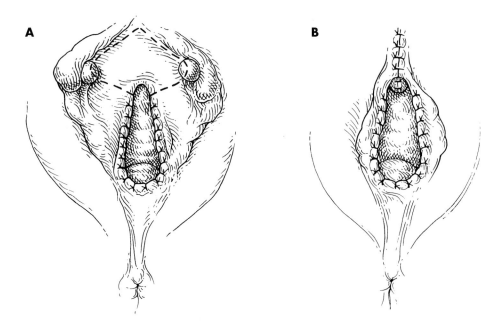

Fig. 43-42   Schematic depiction of procedure to reapproximate the clitoris. A vulvovagino-plasty has already been performed to exteriorize the vagina. **A,** A diamond-shaped piece of skin and subcutaneous tissue between the clitoral bodies is excised. **B,** The clitoral bodies are then undermined and mobilized to the center for a side-to-side reapproximation. (From Rock JA, Thompson JD: *TeLinde's operative gynecology,* ed 8, Philadelphia, 1997, Lippincott-Raven.)

the Hopkins series, documenting continued excellent long-term results.

Several series have reviewed subsequent pregnancy outcomes in patients with bladder exstrophy. Clemetson reviewed the literature extensively in 1958[18] and found 45 patients who had 64 pregnancies. A very high incidence of uterine prolapse was observed both before and after pregnancy. In addition, there was a higher incidence of premature labor and malpresentations (24%). Krisiloff et al.[81] also reported a high incidence of uterine prolapse related to pregnancy, which occurred in 6 of 7 women. Burbige et al.[12] reported on 14 pregnancies in patients with a history of bladder exstrophy. Uterine prolapse occurred in 7 of 11 patients, all of whom had undergone a previous urinary diversion procedure.

The mode of delivery in patients with prior urinary diversion procedures has primarily been spontaneous vaginal delivery. However, the increased incidence of premature labor and malpresentation has warranted an increased rate of cesarean sections for obstetric indications. In patients with a prior bladder reconstruction, most surgeons advocate an elective cesarean section to eliminate stress on the pelvic floor and to avoid trauma to the delicate urinary sphincter mechanism.

MANAGEMENT OF UTERINE PROLAPSE WITH BLADDER EXSTROPHY

Several mechanisms have been proposed to explain the high incidence of uterine prolapse in patients with bladder exstrophy. These mechanisms include (1) a deficiency of the

pelvic floor due to the wide separation of the pubic symphysis, (2) an inherent deficiency of the cardinal ligament complex, and (3) the normal axis and short length of the vagina.

Because wide separation of the pubic symphysis results in an enlarged genital hiatus and deficiency of the pelvic floor, it is possible that iliac osteotomy may be helpful in deterring pelvic organ prolapse by closer approximation of the levator ani and puborectal muscles. Although Gearhart and Jeffs[48] suggest that iliac osteotomies may not be necessary if primary bladder closure is performed in the first 72 hours of life, perhaps the procedure should be given increased consideration in female patients who present such a high risk for uterine prolapse later in life.

It appears important not to extend the midline perineal incision too far posteriorly in revision of the genitalia in these patients. As the incision proceeds posteriorly, the midline septum thickens to approximately 2 cm. At this point, the levator ani muscles may be severed, further enlarging the genital hiatus. Therefore it is prudent to be more conservative; postoperative dilator therapy may aid in achieving further vaginal diameter if needed.

The following case has illustrated this point. A 16-year-old nulliparous patient with bladder exstrophy and a history of staged bladder reconstruction underwent revision of the external genitalia. A large posterior incision into the perineal body had left a gaping introitus, and uterine prolapse had occurred several months after this procedure. The patient was referred to us at this point. Our initial approach was to reconstruct the perineal body to help contain the uterus and improve support to the pelvic floor. This reconstruction has been successful, without further prolapse 3 years after the procedure. A similar case was reported by Blakely and Mills,[9] who observed uterine prolapse occurring very soon after enlargement of the vaginal introitus.

Management of uterine prolapse associated with bladder exstrophy may be difficult. The patient often desires preservation of her childbearing capacity. Sacrospinous fixation of the cervix may be considered, although an abnormally short vagina may produce difficulty in obtaining the suspension without significant suture bridges. An abdominal sacrocervicopexy may also be considered. Dewhurst et al. described this approach in 1980.[30] They suspended the uterus to the sacrum using Ivalon sponge in a patient with procidentia after repair of bladder exstrophy.

The high historical incidence of uterine prolapse and the potential difficulties in managing this problem highlight the need for the reconstructive surgeon to give extra thought and care to revision of the external genitalia in females with bladder exstrophy. Inappropriate reconstruction may actually accelerate genital prolapse. In addition, elective cesarean section may be the most judicious mode of delivery for limiting traumatic insults to the pelvic floor that could further increase the propensity for prolapse.

REFERENCES

1. Abbe R: New method of creating a vagina in a case of congenital absence, *Med Rec* 54:836, 1898.
2. Alessandrescu D, et al: Neocolpopoiesis with split-thickness skin graft as a surgical treatment of vaginal agenesis: retrospective review of 210 cases, *Am J Obstet Gynecol* 175:131, 1996.
3. American Fertility Society: The American Fertility Society classification of adnexal adhesions, distal tubal occlusion, tubal occlusion secondary to tubal ligation, tubal pregnancies, müllerian anomalies and intrauterine adhesions, *Fertil Steril* 49:944, 1988.
4. Andrews MC, Jones HW: Impaired reproductive performance of the unicornuate uterus: intrauterine growth retardation, infertility, and recurrent abortion in five cases, *Am J Obstet Gynecol* 144:173, 1982.
5. Azziz R, et al: Congenital adrenal hyperplasia: long-term results following vaginal reconstruction, *Fertil Steril* 46:1011, 1986.
6. Bailez MM, et al: Vaginal reconstruction after initial construction of the external genitalia in girls with salt-wasting adrenal hyperplasia, *J Urol* 148:680, 1992.
7. Baldwin JF: The formation of an artificial vagina by intestinal transplantation, *Ann Surg* 40:398, 1984.
8. Bargy F, et al: The anatomy of intersexuality, *Surg Radiol Anat* 11:103, 1989.
9. Blakely CR, Mills WG: The obstetric and gynaecological complications of bladder exstrophy and epispadias, *Br J Obstet Gynaecol* 88:167, 1981.
10. Brenner P, Sedlis A, Cooperman H: Complete imperforate transverse vaginal septum, *Obstet Gynecol* 25:135, 1965.
11. Broadbent TR, Woolf RM: Congenital absence of the vagina: reconstruction without operation, *Br J Plast Surg* 30:118, 1977.
12. Burbige KA, et al: Pregnancy and sexual function in women with bladder exstrophy, *Urology* 28:120, 1986.
13. Reference deleted in proofs.
14. Capraro VJ, Chuang JT, Randall CL: Imported fetal salvage after metroplasty, *Obstet Gynecol* 31:97, 1968.
15. Capraro VJ, Gallego MB: Vaginal agenesis, *Am J Obstet Gynecol* 124:98, 1976.
16. Chakravarty BN: Congenital absence of the vagina and uterus—simultaneous vaginoplasty and hysteroplasty, *J Obstet Gynecol (India)* 27:627, 1977.
17. Chervenak FA, Neuwirth RS: Hysteroscopic resection of the uterine septum, *Am J Obstet Gynecol* 141:351, 1981.
18. Clemetson CAB: Ectopic vesicae and split pelvis: an account of pregnancy in women with treated ectopic vesicae and split pelvis, including a review of the literature, *J Obstet Gynecol Br Emp* 65:9730, 1958.
19. Counseller VS: Congenital absence of the vagina, *JAMA* 136:861, 1948.
20. Counseller VS, Davis CE: Atresia of the vagina, *Obstet Gynecol* 32:528, 1968.
21. Counseller VS, Flor FS: Congenital absence of the vagina, *Surg Clin North Am* 37:1107, 1957.
22. Creatsas GC: Creatsas modification of Williams vaginoplasty, *J Gynecol Surg* 7:219, 1991.
23. Cukier J, et al: Genital tract reconstruction in a patient with congenital absence of a vagina and hypoplasia of the cervix, *Obstet Gynecol* 68:325, 1986.
24. Dabirashrafi H, et al: Septate uterus: new idea on the histologic features of the septum in the abnormal uterus, *Am J Obstet Gynecol* 172:105, 1995.
25. Daly DC, et al: Hysteroscopic metroplasty: surgical technique and obstetrical outcome, *Fertil Steril* 39:623, 1983.
26. David A, et al: Congenital absence of the vagina: clinical and psychological aspects, *Obstet Gynecol* 46:407, 1975.
27. DeCherney A, Polan ML: Hysteroscopic management of intrauterine lesions and intractable uterine bleeding, *Obstet Gynecol* 61:392, 1983.
28. DeCherney AH, et al: Resectoscopic management of müllerian fusion defects, *Fertil Steril* 45:726, 1986.
29. Damario MA, et al: Reconstruction of the external genitalia in females with bladder exstrophy, *Int J Gynaecol Obstet* 44:245, 1994.
30. Dewhurst J, Topliss PH, Shepherd JH: Ivalon sponge hysterosacropexy for genital prolapse in patients with bladder exstrophy, *Br J Obstet Gynaecol* 87:67, 1980.
31. Dillon WP, Mudaliar NA, Wingate NB: Congenital atresia of the cervix, *Obstet Gynecol* 54:126, 1979.
32. DiNaro E, et al: The diagnosis of benign uterine pathology using endohysterosonography, *Clin Exp Obstet Gynecol* 23:103, 1996.
33. Evans TN: The artificial vagina, *Am J Obstet Gynecol* 99:944, 1967.
34. Evans TN, Poland ML, Boving RL: Vaginal malformations, *Am J Obstet Gynecol* 141:910, 1981.
35. Farber M, Marchant DJ: Reconstructive surgery for congenital atresia of the uterine cervix, *Fertil Steril* 27:1277, 1976.
36. Farber M, Mitchell GW: Bicornuate uterus and partial atresia of the fallopian tube, *Am J Obstet Gynecol* 134:881, 1979.
37. Farber M, Mitchell GW: Surgery for congenital anomalies of müllerian ducts, *Contemp Obstet Gynecol* 9:63, 1977.
38. Farber M, Mitchell GW: Surgery for congenital absence of the vagina, *Obstet Gynecol* 51:364, 1978.
39. Fayez JA: Comparison between abdominal and hysteroscopic metroplasty, *Obstet Gynecol* 68:399, 1986.
40. Fedele L, et al: Urinary tract anomalies associated with unicornuate uterus, *J Urol* 155:847, 1996.
41. Fedele L, et al: Ultrasound in the diagnosis of subclasses of unicornuate uterus, *Obstet Gynecol* 71:274, 1988.
42. Feroze RM, Dewhurst CJ, Welply G: Vaginoplasty at the Chelsea Hospital for women: a comparison of two techniques, *Br J Obstet Gynaecol* 82:536, 1975.
43. Fore SR, et al: Urologic and genital anomalies in patients with congenital absence of the vagina, *Obstet Gynecol* 46:410, 1975.
44. Frank RT: The formation of an artificial vagina without operation, *Am J Obstet Gynecol* 35:1053, 1938.
45. Frank RT: The formation of an artificial vaginal without operation, *NY State J Med* 40:1669, 1940.
46. Gallup DG, Castle CA, Stock RJ: Recurrent carcinoma in situ of the vagina following split thickness graft vaginoplasty, *Gynecol Oncol* 26:98, 1987.
47. Garcia RF: Z-plasty for correction of congenital transverse vaginal septum, *Am J Obstet Gynecol* 99:1164, 1967.

48. Gearhart JP, Jeffs RD: State of the art reconstructive surgery for bladder exstrophy at the Johns Hopkins Hospital, *Am J Dis Child* 143:1475, 1989.

49. Geary WL, Weed JC: Congenital atresia of the uterine cervix, *Obstet Gynecol* 42:213, 1973.

50. Griffin JE, et al: Congenital absence of the vagina, *Ann Intern Med* 85:224, 1976.

51. Haney AF, et al: Diethylstilbestrol-induced upper genital tract abnormalities, *Fertil Steril* 31:142, 1979.

52. Hauser GA, Keller M, Koller T: Das Mayer-Rokitansky-Küster-Hauser syndrom: uterus bipartitus solidus rudimetrarius cum vagina solida, *Gynecologia* 151:111, 1961.

53. Hauser GA, Schreiner WE: Das Mayer-Rokitansky-Küster-Hauser Syndrom, *Schweiz Med Wochenschr* 91:381, 1961.

54. Heinonen PK: Longitudinal vaginal septum, *Eur J Obstet Gynecol Reprod Biol* 13:253, 1982.

55. Heinonen PK, Pystynen PP: Primary infertility and uterine anomalies, *Fertil Steril* 40:311, 1983.

56. Heinonen PK, Saarikoski S, Pystynen P: Reproductive performance of women with uterine anomalies, *Acta Obstet Gynecol Scand* 61:157, 1982.

57. Hendren WH: Surgical management of urogenital sinus abnormalities, *J Pediatr Surg* 12:339, 1977.

58. Hendren WH, Crawford JD: Adrenogenital syndrome: the anatomy of the anomaly and its repair, *J Pediatr Surg* 4:49, 1969.

59. Hendren WH, Donahoe PK: Correction of congenital abnormalities of the vagina and perineum, *J Pediatr Surg* 15:751, 1980.

60. Holden R, Hart P: First-trimester rudimentary horn pregnancy: pre-rupture ultrasound diagnosis, *Obstet Gynecol* 61(suppl):56, 1983.

61. Hurst BS, Rock JA: Preoperative dilation to facilitate repair of high transverse vaginal septum, *Fertil Steril* 57:1351, 1992.

62. Ingram JM: The bicycle seat stool in the treatment of vaginal agenesis and stenosis: a preliminary report, *Am J Obstet Gynecol* 140:867, 1984.

63. Israel R, March CM: Hysteroscopic incision of the septate uterus, *Am J Obstet Gynecol* 149:66, 1984.

64. Jabs EW, Leonard CO, Phillips JA: New features of the McKusick-Kaufman syndrome, *Birth Defects* 18:161, 1982.

65. Jackson ND, Rosenblatt PL: Use of Interceed absorbable adhesion barrier for vaginoplasty, *Obstet Gynecol* 84:1048, 1994.

66. Jacob JH, Griffin WT: Surgical reconstruction of congenital atresia of the cervix, *Am J Obstet Gynecol* 82:923, 1961.

67. Reference deleted in proofs.

68. Jewelewicz R, Husami N, Wallach EE: When uterine factors cause infertility, *Contemp Obstet Gynecol* 16:95, 1980.

69. Jones HW: An anomaly of the external genitalia in female patients with exstrophy of the bladder, *Am J Obstet Gynecol* 177:748, 1973.

70. Jones HW: Reproductive impairment and the malformed uterus, *Fertil Steril* 36:137, 1981.

71. Jones HW, Delfs E, Jones GE: Reproductive difficulties in double uterus: the place of plastic reconstruction, *Am J Obstet Gynecol* 72:865, 1956.

72. Jones HW, Jones GE: Double uterus as an etiologic factor in repeated abortion: indications for surgical repair, *Am J Obstet Gynecol* 65:325, 1953.

73. Reference deleted in proofs.

74. Jones HW, Rock JA: *Reparative and constructive surgery of the female generative tract,* Baltimore, 1983, Williams & Wilkins.

75. Jones HW, Wheeless CR: Salvage of the reproductive potential of women with anomalous development of the müllerian ducts: 1868-1968-2068. *Am J Obstet Gynecol* 104:348, 1969.

76. Jones TB, et al: Sonographic characteristics of congenital uterine abnormalities and associated pregnancy, *J Clin Ultrasound* 8:435, 1980.

77. Jones WS: Obstetric significance of female genital anomalies, *Obstet Gynecol* 10:113, 1957.

78. Jurkovic D, et al: Three-dimensional ultrasound for the assessment of uterine anatomy and detection of congenital anomalies: a comparison with hysterosalpingography and two-dimensional sonography, *Ultrasound Obstet Gynecol* 5:233, 1995.

79. Karjalainen O, et al: Management of vaginal agenesis, *Ann Chir Gynaecol* 69:37, 1980.

80. Kaufman RK, et al: Upper genital tract changes associated with exposure in utero to diethylstilbestrol, *Am J Obstet Gynecol* 128:51, 1977.

81. Krisiloff M, et al: Pregnancy in women with bladder exstrophy, *J Urol* 119:478, 1978.

82. Lodi A: Contributo clinico statistico sulle malformazion della vagina osservate nella clinica Obstetrica e Ginecologica di Milano dal 1906 al 1950, *Ann Ostet Ginecol Med Perinat* 73:1246, 1951.

83. Ludmir J, et al: Pregnancy outcome of patients with uncorrected uterine anomalies managed in a high risk obstetric setting, *Obstet Gynecol* 75:907, 1990.

84. Maciulla GJ, Heine MW, Christian CD: Functional endometrial tissue with vaginal agenesis, *J Reprod Med* 21:373, 1978.

85. Magrina JF, Masterson BJ: Vaginal reconstruction in gynecological oncology: a review of techniques, *Obstet Gynecol Surv* 36:1, 1981.

86. Mahgoub SE: Unification of a septate uterus: Mahgoub's operation, *Int J Gynecol Obstet* 15:400, 1978.

87. Mandell J, Stevens PS, Lucey DT: Diagnosis and management of hydrometrocolpos in infancy, *J Urol* 120:262, 1978.

88. Markham SM, et al: Cervical agenesis combined with vaginal agenesis diagnosed by magnetic resonance imaging, *Fertil Steril* 48:143, 1987.

89. McCraw JB, et al: Vaginal reconstruction with gracilis myocutaneous flaps, *Plast Reconstr Surg* 58:175, 1976.

90. McDonough PG, Tho PT: Use of pelvic pneumoperitoneum: a critical assessment of 12 years experience, *South Med J* 67:517, 1947.

91. McIndoe AH: The treatment of congenital absence and obliterative conditions of the vagina, *Br J Plast Surg* 2:254, 1950.

92. McIndoe AH, Banister JB: An operation for the cure of congenital absence of the vagina, *J Obstet Gynaecol Br Emp* 45:490, 1938.

93. McKusick BA, Weilbaccher RG, Gragg GW: Recessive inheritance of a congenital malformation syndrome, *JAMA* 204:111, 1968.

94. McShane PM, Reilly RJ, Schiff I: Pregnancy outcomes following Tompkins metroplasty, *Fertil Steril* 40:190, 1983.

95. Mizuno K, et al: Significance of Jones-Jones operation on double uterus: vascularity and dating of endometrium in uterine septum, *Jpn J Fertil Steril* 23:9, 1978.

96. Money J, Schwartz M, Lewis VG: Adult erotosexual status and fetal hormonal masculinization and demasculinization: 46XX congenital virilizing adrenal hyperplasia and 46XY androgen-insensitivity syndrome compared, *Psychoneuroendocrinology* 9:405, 1984.

97. Moutos DM, et al: A comparison of the reproductive outcome between women with a unicornuate uterus and women with a didelphic uterus, *Fertil Steril* 58:88, 1992.

98. Murphy AA, Krall A, Rock JA: Bilateral functioning uterine anlagen with the Rokitansky-Mayer-Küster-Hauser syndrome, *Int J Fertil* 32:316, 1987.

99. Musich JR, Behrman SJ: Obstetric outcome before and after metroplasty in women with uterine anomalies, *Obstet Gynecol* 52:63, 1978.

100. Musset R: Traitement chirurgical des cloisans transcersales due vagin d'origine congenitale par la plastie en "Z" a l'Hospital Lariboisiere, *Gynec Obstet* 55:382, 1956.

101. Nagel TC, Malo JW: Hysteroscopic metroplasty in diethylstilbestrol-exposed uterus and similar fusion anomalies, *Fertil Steril* 59:502, 1993.

102. Niver DH, Barrette G, Jewelewicz R: Congenital atresia of the uterine cervix and vagina—three cases, *Fertil Steril* 33:25, 1980.

103. Nunley WC, Kitchin JD: Congenital atresia of the uterine cervix with pelvic endometriosis, *Arch Surg* 115:757, 1980.

104. O'Leary JL, O'Leary JA: Rudimentary horn pregnancy, *Obstet Gynecol* 22:371, 1963.

105. Patil V, Hixon FP: The role of tissue expanders in vaginoplasty for congenital malformations of the vagina, *Br J Urol* 70:554, 1992.

106. Pokorny SF, Kozinetz CA: Configuration and other anatomic details of the prepubertal hymen, *Adolesc Pediatr Gynecol* 1:97, 1988.

107. Popaw DD: Utilization of the rectum in construction of a functional vagina, *Russk Virach St Peter* 43:1512, 1910.

108. Pratt JH: Vaginal atresia corrected by use of small and large bowel, *Clin Obstet Gynecol* 15:639, 1972.

109. Rajfer J, Ehrlich RM, Goodwin WE: Reduction clitoroplasty via ventral approach, *J Urol* 128:341, 1982.

110. Rock JA, et al: A unilateral functioning uterine anlage with müllerian duct agenesis, *Int J Gynecol Obstet* 18:99, 1980.

111. Rock JA, et al: The clinical management of maldevelopment of the uterine cervix, *J Pelvic Surg* 1:129, 1995.

112. Rock JA, Jones HW: The clinical management of the double uterus, *Fertil Steril* 28:798, 1977.

113. Rock JA, Jones HW: The double uterus associated with an obstructed hemivagina and ipsilateral renal agenesis, *Am J Obstet Gynecol* 138:339, 1980.

114. Rock JA, Jones HW Jr: Vaginal forms for dilation and/or to maintain vaginal patency, *Fertil Steril* 42:187, 1984.

115. Rock JA, et al: Malposition of the ovary associated with uterine anomalies, *Fertil Steril* 45:561, 1986.

116. Rock JA, et al: Success following vaginal creation for müllerian agenesis, *Fertil Steril* 39:809, 1983.

117. Rock JA, Schlaff WD: The obstetrical consequences of uterovaginal anomalies, *Fertil Steril* 43:681, 1985.

118. Rock JA, Schlaff WD: Congenital adrenal hyperplasia: the surgical treatment of vaginal stenosis, *Int J Gynaecol Obstet* 24:417, 1986.

119. Rock JA, et al: The clinical management of congenital absence of the uterine cervix, *Int J Gynaecol Obstet* 22:231, 1984.

120. Rock JA, Zacur HA: The clinical management of repeated early pregnancy wastage, *Fertil Steril* 39:123, 1983.

121. Rock JA, et al: Pregnancy success following surgical correction of imperforate hymen and complete transverse septum, *Obstet Gynecol* 59:448, 1982.

122. Salle B, et al: Transvaginal hysterosonographic evaluation of septate uteri: a preliminary report, *Hum Reprod* 11:1004, 1996.

123. Sauer-Ramirez R, et al: Modification of the Abbe-Wharton-McIndoe technique using regenerated oxidized cellulose instead of a skin graft, *Ginecol Obstet Mex* 63:112, 1995.

124. Semmens JP: Abdominal contour in the third trimester: an aid to diagnosis of uterine anomalies, *Obstet Gynecol* 25:779, 1965.

125. Singh KJ, Devi L: Hysteroplasty and vaginoplasty for reconstruction of the uterus, *Int J Gynecol Obstet* 17:457, 1980.

126. Singh M, Gearhart JP, Rock JA: Double urethra, double bladder, left renal agenesis, persistent hymen, double vagina and uterus didelphys, *Adolesc Pediatr Gynecol* 6:99, 1993.

127. Stanton SL: Gynecologic complications of epispadias and bladder exstrophy, *Am J Obstet Gynecol* 119:749, 1974.

128. Stoot JE, Mastboom JL: Restriction on the indications for metroplasty, *Acta Eur Fertil* 8:79, 1977.

129. Strassmann EO: Plastic unification of double uterus, *Am J Obstet Gynecol* 64:25, 1952.

130. Strassmann EO: Operations for double uterus and endometrial atresia, *Clin Obstet Gynecol* 4:240, 1961.

131. Strassmann P: Die operative vereinigung eins deppelten uterus, *Zentralbl Gynakol* 31:1322, 1907.

132. Tancer ML, Katz M, Veridiano NP: Vaginal epithelialization with human amnion, *Obstet Gynecol* 54:345, 1979.

133. Thompson DP, Lynn HB: Genital anomalies associated with solitary kidney, *Mayo Clin Proc* 41:538, 1966.

134. Ulfelder H, Robboy SJ: The embryologic development of the human vagina, *Am J Obstet Gynecol* 126:769, 1976.

135. Valdes C, Malini S, Malinak L: Sonography in the surgical management of vaginal and cervical atresia, *Fertil Steril* 40:263, 1983.

136. Vecchietti G: Neovagina nella sindrome di Rokitansky Kuster Hauser, *Att Obstet Ginecol* 11:131, 1965.

137. Vercellini P, et al: Metroplasty for the complete septate uterus: does cervical sparing matter? *J Am Assoc Gynecol Laparosc* 3:509, 1996.

138. Veronikis DK, McClure GB, Nichols DH: The Vecchietti operation for constructing a neovagina: indications, instrumentation, and techniques, *Obstet Gynecol* 90:301, 1997.

139. Weed HC, McKee DM: Vulvoplasty in cases of exstrophy of the bladder, *Obstet Gynecol* 43:512, 1974.

140. Wharton LR: A simple method of constructing a vagina, *Ann Surg* 107:842, 1938.

141. Wharton LR: Further experiences in construction of the vagina, *Ann Surg* 111:1010, 1940.

142. Wharton LR: Congenital malformations associated with developmental defects of the female reproductive organs, *Am J Obstet Gynecol* 53:37, 1947.

143. Williams EA: Congenital absence of the vagina, a simple operation for its relief, *J Obstet Gynecol Br Commonw* 71:511, 1964.

144. Williams EA: Vulvo-vaginoplasty, *Proc R Soc Med* 63:40, 1970.

145. Williams EA: Uterovaginal agenesis, *Ann R Coll Surg Engl* 58:266, 1976.

146. Young HH: *Genital abnormalities, hermaphroditism and related adrenal diseases,* Baltimore, 1937, Williams & Wilkins.

44 The Repair of Urethral Injuries, Diverticula, and Fistula

RAYMOND A. LEE

The female urethra is well protected and rarely involved in injury except during childbirth or operation. Occasionally, usually as a result of a motor vehicle accident, a woman may experience an avulsion of the urethra, generally in the area of the bladder neck. Less commonly, women may experience a penetrating wound as a result of being impaled while fence climbing or being struck by farming tools; such injuries often result in hematoma of the vulva and laceration of the urethra. Occasionally, injuries to the vagina, rectum, and urethra result from a disproportion between the size of the penis and that of the vagina. These usually result in disruption of the posterior vaginal wall and the anal sphincter rather than trauma to the urethra and the base of the bladder.

Any injury to the urethra and anterior vaginal wall usually consists of a longitudinal laceration of the vaginal wall extending into the lateral vaginal fornix, but rarely is the urethra itself disrupted. I have seen several patients who were unaware that they had agenesis of the vagina and were attempting or experiencing intercourse in the urethra. Early in her experience, such a patient generally will have pain with few other symptoms. With sufficient time, the urethra dilates to accommodate a normal penis, and this process eventually results in significant urinary incontinence because of the stretched urethra and bladder neck but not because of laceration. Bleeding is not a frequent problem.

An appropriate diagnosis can generally be made on careful inspection of the area, but anesthesia may be required to ensure an accurate assessment of the urethra. This examination in combination with a cystourethroscopic examination assists in determining the integrity of the urethra, the bladder neck, and the base of the bladder. If they are found to be intact, depending on the degree of trauma, a urethral catheter may be required for a short time to ensure adequate drainage of the bladder during recovery. If a defect is noted in the urethra and the tissues can be assessed accurately, immediate operative repair may be accomplished by reconstructing the urethra, its supporting tissues, and the anterior vaginal wall with interrupted 4-0 delayed absorbable sutures.

Recently, complete disruption of the urethra at the bladder neck was found in a patient after forceps delivery. Cystoscopy revealed the bladder to be intact to the level of the bladder neck (Fig. 44-1). Immediate reconstruction was accomplished with the development of a tongue-shaped, inverted "U" flap of the anterior vaginal wall, superficial to the cervical pubic fascia (Fig. 44-2). Fig. 44-2 demonstrates a small curved forceps inserted through the external urethral meatus with its tips passing through the disrupted proximal portion of the urethra through an anterior vaginal wall laceration. Reconstruction is accomplished by placement of the first suture in the 12-o'clock position, approximating the bladder neck and proximal urethra (Fig. 44-3, A). After tying the first suture at 12 o'clock, all other sutures are placed, approximating essentially a full thickness of the urethra with each suture in an extramucosal position (see Fig. 44-3, B). All sutures are tied in the order they were placed. Careful reconstruction is accomplished around a no. 14 Foley catheter. The tongue of the anterior vaginal wall is then replaced in such a fashion that it avoids overlying suture lines. Fig. 44-4 shows the stippled area of urethral reconstruction under the flap of anterior vaginal wall.

URETHROVAGINAL FISTULA
Etiology

Prolonged labor continues to be a common cause of destruction of the urethra and base of the bladder in medically deprived countries,[6,13,16] whereas elective urethral and vaginal operation is the leading cause of these low-lying fistulas in the United States.[5,15] The excision of a friable, infected urethral diverticulum can be tedious and inexact.[10] Despite meticulous efforts to reconstruct the urethral floor accurately, infection and edema may lead to imperfect healing and fistula formation. In addition, overzealous plication of the urethra or the inadvertent intramural placement of a suture (vaginal or retropubic needle suspension) may produce a fistula of the urethra or, a greater calamity, actual slough of the entire floor and the bladder neck.[15]

Portions of this chapter were previously published in Lee RA: Surgical management of genitourinary fistulas. In WG Hurt, editor: *Urogynecological surgery,* Gaithersburg, MD, 1991, Aspen. By permission of the publisher.

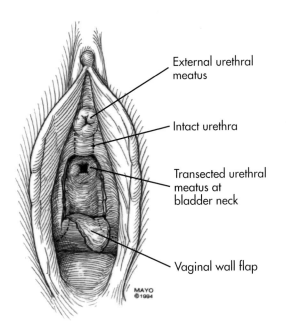

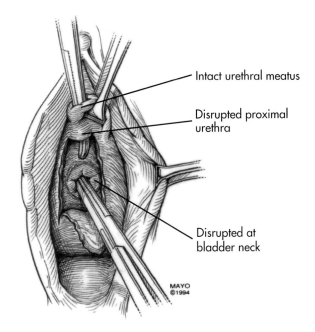

Fig. 44-1   External urethral meatus and distal urethra intact but totally separated from the proximal urethra entering the bladder. (By permission of Mayo Foundation.)

Fig. 44-2   Small curved forceps introduced through the external urethral meatus and intact distal urethra and a second forceps introduced through the proximal urethra in the bladder neck but separated from the distal urethral segment. (By permission of Mayo Foundation.)

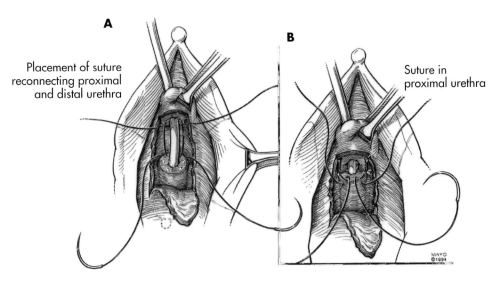

Fig. 44-3   **A,** Initial sutures placed in an extramucosal location in the 12-o'clock position. **B,** Working clockwise and counterclockwise, individual sutures approximate the disrupted segment with all sutures placed in an extramucosal location. (By permission of Mayo Foundation.)

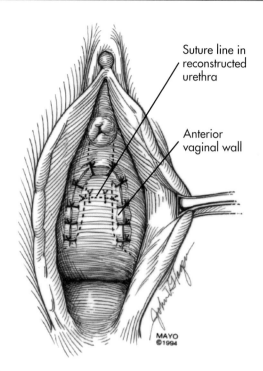

Suture line in
reconstructed
urethra

Anterior
vaginal wall

Fig. 44-4   Reconstructed urethra with replacement of the tongued, pedicled anterior vaginal wall flap. (By permission of Mayo Foundation.)

Clinical Symptoms

Patients who experience trauma to the urethra from forceps delivery or automobile accident have leakage immediately or within the first 24 hours after damage. If a urethral catheter is in place, either after delivery or trauma, removal of the catheter is generally followed promptly by leakage of urine. Patients who have undergone an operation generally have a catheter in place for 2 to 7 days. Some patients who have had an operation may have an unrecognized suture through the wall of the urethra; this generally results in necrosis of the tissue, possibly associated with hematoma formation or some degree of infection, the combination of which results in leakage of urine. The patient may initially be continent only to experience leakage 1 to 2 weeks postoperatively. Patients who have had irradiation generally note the leakage some time after the treatment, generally within 2 to 4 weeks after therapy.

Simple urethrovaginal fistula, depending on its location relative to the bladder neck, may not produce urinary incontinence and may not require operative repair. A fistula located near the bladder neck may be technically more difficult to repair, and urinary continence cannot be ensured. Even after what appears to be a successful repair, the patient may experience urinary stress incontinence due to fibrosis, fixation, and poor contractility of the urethral musculature. A more complex problem is presented by patients who have had a major slough resulting in a linear loss of the floor of the urethra and frequently involving the bladder neck and the base of the bladder.

Operative Repair

The basic phases of operative reconstruction consist of a linear incision, much like that for an anterior colporrhaphy, and mobilization of the vaginal mucosa laterally off the underlying cervicopubic fascia. This procedure must be accomplished in the proper bloodless tissue plane sufficiently lateral (to establish mobility) so that a tension-free closure of the urethra can be accomplished.

Once the fistula is completely mobilized and the scar tissue (fistula tract) is removed, the fistula is closed with fine 4-0 delayed absorbable sutures placed extramucosally, and the tissue edges are approximated free of tension and with excellent hemostasis. The presence of a small-caliber catheter within the urethra often assists in accurate placement of the sutures to close the fistulous tract. This initial suture line is imbricated with a second set of sutures, the most distal suture being just distal to the original suture line. Snug plication of the bladder neck by approximation, under the urethra, of the tissue (cervicopubic fascia) lateral to the urethra to create a tension-free second layer of sutures is mandatory for a successful repair. A tension-free closure of the vaginal wall as a third layer, or when necessary for the obliteration of dead space and actual replacement of the anterior vaginal wall with a pedicled-skin, fibrofatty labial graft, may be indicated.

A "second-stage" retropubic urethral vesical suspension for patients who have a good anatomic result with an apparently intact urethra but who nevertheless remain incontinent (intact urethra with stress incontinence) may be necessary at a later date. This result cannot be predicted at the time of closure of the urethral fistula.

Loss of the Floor of the Urethra

One of the most challenging forms of genitourinary fistula is the fistula that involves the loss of a major portion of the proximal urethra and bladder neck. Several operative techniques can correct the anatomic defect (urethrovaginal fistula), but urinary continence rather than the anatomic result is a far better criterion of a successful operation. Regardless of the operative technique selected, the surgeon cannot anticipate successful restoration of urinary continence in all patients who have loss of the urethra. Symmonds and Hill[15] reported on 50 Mayo Clinic patients with loss of the urethra. The causative factors are the same as those that result in simple urethrovaginal fistula—anterior colporrhaphy and repair of urethral diverticulum.

Operative Repair. A midline incision is made in the anterior vaginal wall and extended up and around the margins of the urethral defect (Fig. 44-5). The dissection is carried laterally to the descending pubic ramus much like that carried out for an anterior colporrhaphy (see Fig. 44-5). With appropriate traction on the edges of the urethral wall, the urethra is mobilized sufficiently that a tension-free closure can be constructed. All palpable bands of scar tissue that distort the urethra and the bladder neck must be dissected and released. In patients who have loss of a major portion of the proximal urethra and the bladder neck, it may be prefer-

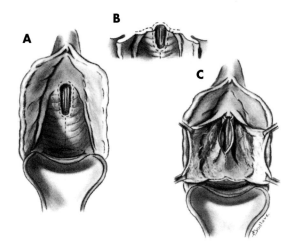

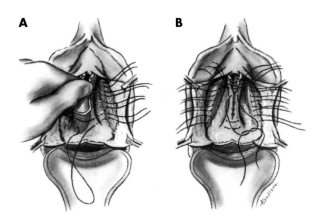

Fig. 44-5 Mobilization of tissue. **A,** Proposed midline incision about the defect. **B,** Proposed line of dissection about the urethra through the mucosa of the vagina. **C,** Wide mobilization of vaginal mucosa off the cervicopubic fascia. (From Symmonds RE: *Am J Obstet Gynecol* 103:665, 1969.)

Fig. 44-6 Closure of urethra. **A,** A finger through the bladder neck assists the placement of bladder neck and proximal urethral sutures. **B,** Reconstructed urethral tube with fine extramucosal sutures. (From Symmonds RE: *Am J Obstet Gynecol* 103:665, 1969.)

able to insert what will be the second row of interrupted sutures before reconstructing the urethra. If this procedure is done in this sequence, one can be assured that the suture is not within the lumen of the bladder or proximal urethra; thus the maximal amount of all available tissue can be used in attempting to reconstruct the urethra, and a satisfactory continence mechanism will result. A finger inserted through the defect (Fig. 44-6, *A*) into the bladder aids in identifying the bladder wall and the ureters (previously placed ureteral stents), and the suture can be accurately placed. This initial layer of sutures (2-0 delayed absorbable) is tagged and held laterally. The urethral reconstruction is accomplished over a small catheter (8 to 12 Fr) with the use of interrupted 3-0 delayed absorbable sutures. These sutures are placed in a manner that accurately inverts and approximates the epithelial edges without entering the urethra. On completion of the first layer (see Fig. 44-6, *B*), the sutures are tied in the order in which they were placed. The bladder can be tested by passing 200 ml of sterile evaporated milk solution or infant formula through the previously placed urethral catheter to ensure that the closure of the floor of the bladder, the proximal urethra, and the bladder neck is watertight.

After the urethral floor and the bladder neck have been constructed, the initially placed second row of sutures is tied to create a broad approximation of tissue that reinforces the initial suture line and the newly reconstructed urethra (Fig. 44-7). The sutures that act as plicating sutures to the bladder neck are tied and usually consist of 2-0 monofilament delayed absorbable sutures.

In this "much-operated" group of patients, occasionally a complete second layer of sutures cannot be obtained throughout the entire length of the urethra. In this circumstance, one needs to rely on the single set of sutures of the more distal portion of the urethra. Not infrequently, once the

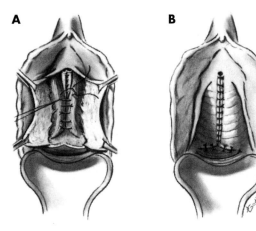

Fig. 44-7 Bladder neck and urethral plication and vaginal closure. **A,** Placement of the second layer; reconstruction sutures inverting the initial suture line of the newly reconstructed urethra. **B,** Tension-free closure of the anterior vaginal wall. (From Symmonds RE: *Am J Obstet Gynecol* 103:665, 1969.)

vaginal wall is incised and the dissection is performed, it is impossible to reapproximate the vaginal wall without undue tension. In this circumstance, I prefer to use a labial pad with an anterior pedicle (Fig. 44-8). The flap should be of sufficient width and length to replace the defect in the anterior vaginal wall. The flap is rotated into the vagina, filling the defect, where it is fixed with fine interrupted (4-0) delayed absorbable sutures in an accurate and meticulous fashion. The blood supply of the labial flaps has always proved to be adequate, regardless of whether the pedicle is based anteriorly or posteriorly. Once the repair is accomplished, a small vaginal pack is inserted to compress the pedicle and

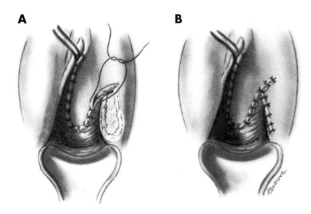

Fig. 44-8 **A,** Mobilization of the labial skin-fibrofatty flap. The placement of the pedicled fibrofatty labial flap replacing the defect in the anterior vaginal wall. **B,** Vaginal wall reconstruction. Individual sutures fixing the labial flap in place and closing the defect in the labia majora. (From Symmonds RE: *Am J Obstet Gynecol* 103:665, 1969.)

aid in obliterating any underlying dead space or venous oozing. The transurethral catheter is removed, and a suprapubic catheter is placed.

Postoperative Management. For patients in whom approximation of vaginal wall would result in tension on the suture line, I prefer to use a Martius-type (bulbocavernosus) muscle flap to obliterate the dead space and interpose a living tissue layer between the urethral and vaginal suture lines. When much of the lower anterior vaginal wall is absent or is the site of excessive scar, the wall should be completely replaced with a labial skin flap.

Postoperatively, the patient receives appropriate antibiotic coverage. The suprapubic catheter is clamped on the tenth postoperative day, when voiding may be undertaken. Almost always, the patient is voiding within the first week that the catheter is clamped, and only 1 of our last 25 patients has required suprapubic drainage for more than 20 days.

Despite adequate vesical neck plication and satisfactory elevation of the support of the urethra and even though an anatomically sound–appearing urethra has been obtained by the operation, some persistent urinary incontinence eventually may be noted. In this case, a second-stage retropubic suspension of the neourethra may be necessary at a later date. Obviously, the goal of surgical correction is to construct a urethra that provides sufficient resistance to ensure good urinary continence; regrettably, a neourethra that appears to be anatomically sound, perfectly supported, and in excellent position does not guarantee good urethral function and urinary control. A scarred, fixed, noncontractile urethra does not provide good urinary control regardless of the urethral angles or support.

In some instances, perhaps when there has been significant destruction of the proximal urethra and the smooth muscle of the bladder neck, a second-stage retropubic suspension may be necessary to increase urethral support and

resistance and provide better urinary control. Certainly, use of some type of labial flap to replace a deficient anterior vaginal wall or to reduce tension on the suture line frequently will improve the chance for successful repair. The type of vaginal closure required depends on the anatomic relationships noted after urethral bladder neck reconstruction. As our experience has increased, it has become apparent that approximately 70% of patients will not require a second-stage retropubic procedure.

Blaivas and Heritz[1] described 49 patients who underwent urethral or vesical neck reconstruction with vaginal flaps. A Martius labial pad flap was used in 47 patients, a gracilis flap in 1, and an anterior bladder tube in 1. In 41 patients an antiincontinence procedure consisted of a fascial pubovaginal sling placed over the labial fat pad flap without tension. Follow-up from 1 to 11 years showed that postoperative continence was obtained in 42 of 49 patients (86%). They concluded that a one-stage vaginal flap reconstruction and a pubovaginal sling procedure are effective in patients with extensive vesical neck or urethral damage.

I have been reluctant to perform a concomitant suspension because it might produce undesirable stress or pull on the suburethral suture line, promoting disruption of the urethral repair. The caliber of the new urethra is, of necessity, small. Although this was an initial concern of mine, urethral dilation is rarely required.

DIVERTICULUM OF THE URETHRA

Diverticulum of the female urethra causes untold misery in the patient and often is well disguised, resulting in a prolonged period of symptoms before diagnosis. Numerous investigative studies have been undertaken to clarify its cause and its clinical presentation. Various innovative techniques have been suggested to improve the accuracy of diagnosis of this elusive condition because surgical correction may be technically difficult and occasionally may result in serious complications. New operations and modifications of old procedures continue to be recommended.

Etiology

Several theories have been advanced to explain the pathogenesis of urethral diverticulum. Evidence for a congenital origin is based on case reports of children and neonates. The reports by Glassman et al.[4] of a diverticulum in a 6-hour-old female infant reinforced this concept. They suggested that the exact cause of their patient's diverticulum could be a collecting system duplication, now obliterated except for a tiny ectopic ureterocele. I have had no evidence to support the congenital origin of diverticulum of the urethra. Huffman[7] aptly likened the urethra to a tree from the base of which arise numerous stunted branches—the periurethral ducts and glands. In some patients they form a labyrinthine mass encircling the urethra on all sides with ducts opening into the lateral, dorsal, and a few ventral urethral walls. Most investigators agree with Routh,[12] who postulated that infection and obstruction of the periurethral glands result in the formation of retention cysts that when infected rupture into the lumen and give rise to a diverticulum. Urethral trauma from catheterization and childbirth has also been suggested as contributing to the formation of a diverticulum. Because 20% of my patients were nulliparous,[10] a finding also reported by Davis and TeLinde,[3] I do not support childbirth as an important causative factor. Rather, it appears that there are several different causative factors, any one of which may result in the formation of a diverticulum of the female urethra.

Clinical Presentation

Although the complaints of patients vary, most patients experience urgency, frequency, dysuria, and dyspareunia. A history of recurrent urinary tract infection is common; hematuria, dribbling after voiding, and urinary stress incontinence are rarely mentioned. A palpable, tender, suburethral mass is found in approximately 60% of patients; actual protrusion of a diverticulum from the vaginal introitus is rare.

Diagnosis

The diagnosis initially must be suspected but is customarily confirmed by cystourethroscopy or voiding cystourethrography. Double-balloon urethrography, although theoretically appealing, has not proved very efficacious in our experience. Vaginal ultrasonography has recently been proved to be an extremely effective diagnostic tool and may become the standard method.

Kim et al.[8] suggested that magnetic resonance imaging is accurate for showing urethral diverticula, but because of its high cost it should be considered only when urethroscopic or urethrographic findings are equivocal or when patients are unable to undergo these procedures and clinical findings strongly suggest a urethral diverticulum.

Huffman[7] found that most openings to the periurethral glands ended in the distal (external) third of the urethra; however, there is significant individual variation with openings extending throughout the entire length and involving the bladder neck. These findings correlate well with the site of origin of most diverticula of the urethra and further support a direct relationship between the periurethral ducts and the formation of diverticula.

Menville and Mitchell[11] reported that 85% of diverticula were located in the distal two thirds of the urethra. Cook and Pool[2] stated that the orifices were located more often in the middle of the urethra. In my experience, 65% of the diverticula are located in the proximal two thirds of the urethra and the bladder neck area, and an additional 20% of the diverticula have multiple sites of origin, most of which are in the midurethra with a second opening in the inner or outer segment. Only 15% are in the distal (external) third of the urethra. When cystourethroscopy is used in combination with urethrography, the size, ramifications, and number of diverticula usually can be determined. Occasionally, a saddlebag diverticulum or even multiple diverticula can be demonstrated with voiding cystourethrography when only a single orifice can be seen on urethroscopic examination.

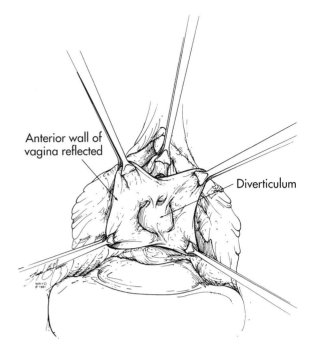

Fig. 44-9 Diverticulum exposed, with the vaginal lining and endopelvic fascia retracted. (From Lee RA: *Obstet Gynecol* 61:52, 1983. By permission of Mayo Foundation.)

Operative Technique

A vertical incision is made in the anterior vaginal wall, the underlying pubocervical fascia is exposed, and the lateral vaginal wall flaps are mobilized to the descending pubic ramus. A similar incision is made in the fascia, which is mobilized laterally to expose the underlying diverticulum (Fig. 44-9). The wall of the diverticulum is recognized as a smooth, shiny, thin-walled structure. The dissection must be sharp, accurate, and meticulous. Preoperative placement (coiling) of a ureteral catheter within the diverticulum to distend its walls when this can be accomplished may enhance the identification and dissection of the diverticulum (Fig. 44-10). Occasionally, the diverticulum is in immediate apposition or even perforating the pubocervical fascia, and it can be easily identified (perhaps even inadvertently entered) during the dissection. If the diverticulum is entered, the surgeon simply may introduce the tip of the left index finger into the diverticulum and, with appropriate traction with a broad Allis forceps on the edge of the diverticulum, further dissect it from the surrounding cervicopubic fascia (Fig. 44-11). Rarely, a linear incision is made through the full thickness of the urethra to expose the urethral floor and permit the passage of a probe through the ostium to aid in the identification of the diverticulum. Depending on the size of the diverticulum, it may present with loculations containing various amounts of urine, purulent material, necrotic debris, and even gravel; such loculations or septae should be incised. The use of Allis forceps on the rim of the diverticulum permits gentle traction on the wall of the diverticulum

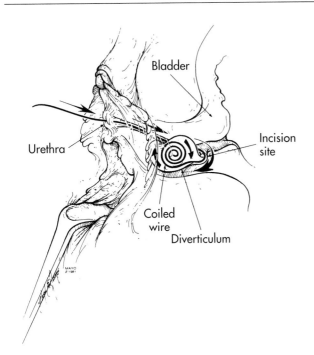

Fig. 44-10   Coiled ureteral catheter distends the diverticulum and aids in its identification and dissection. (From Lee RA: *Obstet Gynecol* 61:52, 1983. By permission of Mayo Foundation.)

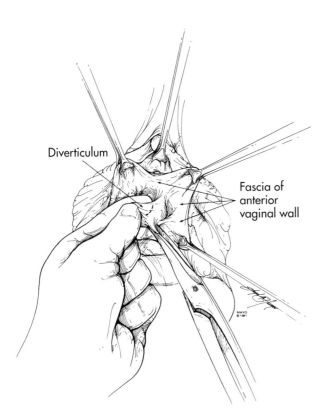

Fig. 44-11   A finger within the diverticulum permits traction, which aids in dissection and identification of the ostium. (From Lee RA: *Obstet Gynecol* 61:52, 1983. By permission of Mayo Foundation.)

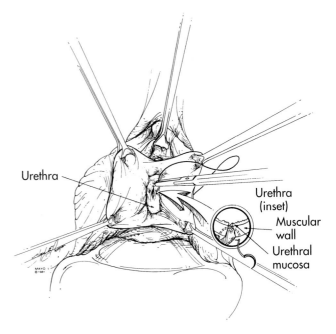

Fig. 44-12   After complete resection of the diverticulum, the urethra is closed with fine interrupted extramucosal chromic sutures. (From Lee RA: *Obstet Gynecol* 61:52, 1983. By permission of Mayo Foundation.)

and aids in the dissection with Metzenbaum scissors to ensure total excision.

Occasionally, the sac of the diverticulum extends laterally and upward around the urethra. Rarely, it may extend into the retropubic space, or the urethral orifice of the diverticulum may be located laterally or may even enter the roof of the diverticulum. In the latter instance the dissection is continued as far superiorly as possible, at which point the neck of the diverticulum is simply transected and permitted to retract; no attempt is made to close the defect in the urethra. In some patients, the diverticulum is saddle-shaped around the entire urethra or bladder neck; thus extensive dissection of the lower trigone or a major portion of the urethral floor is required.

The urethra is closed in a linear direction over a urethral catheter (the size varies depending on the size of the urethra and the size and shape of the defect in the urethra) with interrupted 4-0 delayed absorbable sutures (Fig. 44-12). Rarely, the tissues can be most appropriately approximated in a transverse direction to prevent tension on the suture line. After the urethral defect is repaired, the pubocervical fascia is imbricated in a side-to-side (vest-over-pants) fashion with 3-0 delayed absorbable sutures (Fig. 44-13). By providing two additional supporting layers and avoiding a superimposed suture line, this method appears to diminish the possibility of fistula formation. In addition, it provides good support for the proximal urethra and the bladder neck. Before closure of the vaginal wall, complete hemostasis must be accomplished with use of fine interrupted absorb-

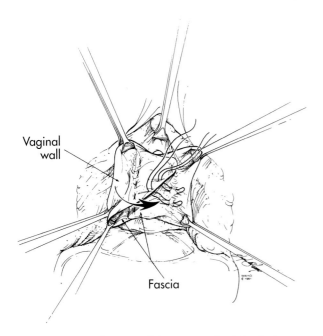

Fig. 44-13 Overlapping of the paraurethral fascia in a vest-over-pants fashion further supports repair and reduces the opportunity for formation of fistulas. (From Lee RA: *Obstet Gynecol* 61:52, 1983. By permission of The Mayo Foundation.)

able sutures and meticulous electrocoagulation; the vaginal wall is closed with 3-0 delayed absorbable suture material. A urethral retention catheter is inserted; generally, this remains in place until the sixth postoperative day. In individual cases, the complexity of the repair may require that the catheter be retained for a longer time.

Most repairs of diverticula are tedious and difficult and are associated with more loss of blood than one would expect from such a small incision. The potential for development of a serious complication depends on the size and the number of the diverticula, the degree of inflammation, and the friability of the tissues and the position of the ostium in relation to the floor of the urethra and the bladder neck. The resection of multiple, large, multiloculated or saddle-shaped diverticula can require extensive dissection about the floor of the urethra, the bladder neck, and the lower trigone. In these conditions the placement of ureteral catheters before the operation can facilitate identification of the ureters and actually reduce the risk of damage during the dissection. Actual or potential destruction or fixation of the smooth muscle of the urethra and the bladder neck produced by both the expanding inflammatory mass and the trauma associated with this excision can result in a urethral fistula or stress incontinence. Accurate reconstruction of the urethra and its supporting structures in combination with good hemostasis and routine antibiotic therapy for control of the infectious process significantly reduces the frequency of these potentially disabling complications.

Other surgical management applicable to individual situations should be considered. Lapides[9] reported a technique

of transurethral marsupialization or resection of the roof of the diverticulum by use of a transurethral knife electrode. This technique involves enlarging the orifice of the diverticulum by incising the roof linearly. The result is an internal marsupialization or saucerization of the diverticulum. This procedure, for certain complicated or recurrent diverticula depending on their size and the location of the urethra, deserves further consideration.

Another operative approach reported by Spence and Duckett[14] is applicable to patients with the ostium of the diverticulum distal (external) to the peak urethral closure pressure. The operative approach consists of a transvaginal marsupialization of the diverticulum with one blade of the scissors in the urethra and the other blade in the vagina. With the exception of lesions involving the distal third of the urethra, it is conceivable that with menopausal atrophy of pelvic supports and resulting loss of tone of the remaining smooth muscle, a significant incidence of urinary incontinence may result some years after what appeared to be a successful marsupialization procedure.

Complications and Results

Prompt, complete, and long-lasting relief of symptoms is usually obtained after successful diverticulectomy.[10] Urethroscopic examination demonstrates either a normal urethra or a shallow depression or a dimple at the operative site. We have seen no evidence of a urethral stricture in patients undergoing diverticulectomy. More than 80% of patients remain asymptomatic and have not required postoperative medical or surgical management. A small number of patients may have persistent pain, dyspareunia, or recurrent urinary tract infection. In this group, cystourethroscopy, cystourethrography, and appropriate cultures of the urine should be reevaluated. Rarely, there may be a recurrence of a diverticulum of the urethra, either in the same location or presumably a second diverticulum at another location. If it occurs in the same location, the original diverticulum may have been incompletely excised. Recurrence of a diverticulum elsewhere in the urethra may be a diverticulum that was overlooked during the original operation or may represent the development of a second diverticulum. Whatever the cause, the frequency of recurrent diverticular disease after diverticulectomy emphasizes the difficulties associated with the surgical treatment of this disease. Of 85 of our patients who underwent diverticulectomy, a urethrovaginal fistula developed in 1.[10] This followed the use of anticoagulant therapy necessary for the management of a myocardial infarction. A hematoma developed in the suture line, and a fistula developed later.

I continue to favor transvaginal excision of the diverticulum, even though it is a more complex and tedious operation. Resection of the diverticulum has provided a relatively good long-term rate of cure with an extremely low incidence of fistula and other serious complications.

Injury to the urethra, whether by trauma, childbirth, or operation, can result in disabling complications for the patient. The operative area is relatively small, the supporting tissues are of variable quality, and the wall of the urethra is thick. Given sufficient blood supply, laceration, fistula, loss of the floor, or diverticulum of the urethra can be reconstructed to form an intact tube. However, the functional result—a contractile, continent urethra—is more difficult to predict and cannot be ensured, even when the anatomic result appears satisfactory.

REFERENCES

1. Blaivas JG, Heritz DM: Vaginal flap reconstruction of the urethra and vesical neck in women: a report of 49 cases, *J Urol* 155:1014, 1996.
2. Cook EN, Pool TL: Urethral diverticulum in the female, *J Urol* 62:495, 1949.
3. Davis HJ, TeLinde RW: Urethral diverticula: an assay of 121 cases, *J Urol* 80:34, 1958.
4. Glassman TA, Weinerth JL, Glenn JF: Neonatal female urethral diverticulum, *Urology* 5:249, 1975.
5. Gray LA: Urethrovaginal fistulas, *Am J Obstet Gynecol* 101:28, 1968.
6. Hamlin RHJ, Nicholson EC: Reconstruction of urethra totally destroyed in labour, *Br Med J* 2:147, 1969.
7. Huffman JW: The detailed anatomy of the paraurethral ducts in the adult human female, *Am J Obstet Gynecol* 55:86, 1948.
8. Kim B, Hricak H, Tanagho EA: Diagnosis of urethral diverticula in women: value of MR imaging, *AJR Am J Roentgenol* 161:809, 1993.
9. Lapides J: Transurethral treatment of urethral diverticula in women, *Trans Am Assoc Genitourin Surg* 70:135, 1978.
10. Lee RA: Diverticulum of the female urethra: postoperative complications and results, *Obstet Gynecol* 61:52, 1983.
11. Menville JG, Mitchell JD Jr: Diverticulum of the female urethra, *J Urol* 51:411, 1944.
12. Routh A: Urethral diverticula, *Br Med J* 1:361, 1890.
13. Shigui F, Qinge S: Operative treatment of female urinary fistulas: report of 405 cases, *Chin Med J* 92:263, 1979.
14. Spence HM, Duckett JW Jr: Diverticulum of the female urethra: clinical aspects and presentation of a simple operative technique for cure, *J Urol* 104:432, 1970.
15. Symmonds RE, Hill LM: Loss of the urethra: a report on 50 patients, *Am J Obstet Gynecol* 130:130, 1978.
16. Vanderputte SR: Obstetric vesicovaginal fistulae: experience with 89 cases, *Ann Soc Belg Med Trop* 65:303, 1985.

45 Surgery for Urinary Stress Incontinence

DAVID H. NICHOLS and DIONYSIOS K. VERONIKIS

To effectively evaluate and treat urinary incontinence, the physician must have a thorough understanding of pelvic anatomy and lower urinary tract physiology. Based then on these concepts of normal anatomy and physiology, the cause and pathophysiology of stress urinary incontinence can be understood. More than 100 antiincontinence operations are described in the literature, and all of these operations use the same anatomy and affect the same physiology. However, as our comprehension of anatomy and physiology has evolved and scientific principles have been applied to surgical treatment as they relate to success, failure, and complications of these operations, the surgical treatments have been modified. Therefore, perhaps some of the principles that guided surgery for stress urinary incontinence in the past are no longer applicable. Instead, the choice of which antiincontinence operation to offer the patient should be guided by the indication(s) for surgery, which must include an accurate evaluation of contributing anatomic defects; the objective cause of the incontinence; concomitant alterations in physiology, including relevant neuropathy; and the patient's functional status. The goals that should underlie all surgical efforts in reconstructive pelvic surgery and urogynecology should be to restore anatomy, relieve symptoms, and restore function.[20]

The term *urinary incontinence* may refer equally to the patient's symptom, the physical sign of urine loss, or a specific urodynamic diagnosis. Urinary incontinence has been defined by the International Continence Society as a condition in which involuntary loss of urine is a social or hygienic problem that is objectively demonstrable. *Genuine stress urinary incontinence* is defined as involuntary loss of urine when, in the absence of a detrusor contraction, the intravesical pressure exceeds the maximum urethral pressure.[1] It is a urodynamic diagnosis and is not synonymous with the symptom or sign of stress urinary incontinence.

HISTORY AND PHYSICAL EXAMINATION

In general, patients with lower urinary tract dysfunction present with symptoms. The typical patient complaint (symptom) of stress urinary incontinence is the expulsion of urine with coughing, laughing, lifting, or sneezing. However, to a varying degree, symptoms have been shown to be misleading in all branches of medicine. If symptoms were reliable and diagnostic of specific diseases, further investigation would not be required before treatment. Chest pain is not diagnostic of myocardial infarction or compromised coronary blood flow requiring coronary artery bypass grafting. Lower urinary tract symptoms and patient history have been shown to correlate poorly with the objective urodynamic diagnosis of incontinence. Studies have shown that when patients are diagnosed by symptoms as having stress urinary incontinence and subsequently studied with urodynamics, only 40% to 60% of patients are objectively diagnosed with genuine stress urinary incontinence.[14,21,23]

All organ systems express dysfunction as an alteration in their physiology. The bladder and urethra have only two functions: storage and evacuation of urine. Therefore the bladder and urethra truly have a limited repertoire of expressing dysfunction. It is for this reason that the statement "the bladder is an unreliable witness" was made by Bates[3] in one of the early papers on urodynamics.

It is clear from careful objective analysis of bladder physiology correlated with symptoms that there is tremendous overlap of the presenting symptoms and objective urodynamic diagnoses. The diagnosis of genuine stress urinary incontinence must be unequivocally made before any surgical treatment is initiated. Diagnosis and surgical therapy based on symptoms have without doubt led to misdiagnosis and misapplication of surgical procedures.

The general medical history may be facilitated by providing the patient in advance with a questionnaire that addresses medical and surgical history, allergies, medications taken (with a special section on estrogen status), and social history. The focused urogynecologic history in patients with a complaint of urinary incontinence must include inquiries about obstetric, gynecologic, urologic, and neurologic conditions. The current urinary problem is reviewed in detail, including an estimate of severity, duration, and current and past treatments. Particular emphasis should focus on any previous antiincontinence and/or past pelvic surgery, and if prior surgery has been performed, a copy of the operative dictation is essential in determining the indications, execution, and details of the previous operation. In addition, if the procedure has failed, it is important to note when it failed, if the incontinence is the same or worse, and whether other symptoms are present. A focused urogynecologic physical examination should include observation for perineal irritation secondary to incontinence or from pad protection, evaluation of estrogen status, pelvic support/prolapse, loss of vaginal rugae, muscle tone, and neurologic assessment of S2-S4 nerve distribution. Stress incontinence is commonly associated with pelvic organ prolapse. Patients should be examined in both the dorsal lithotomy and standing posi-

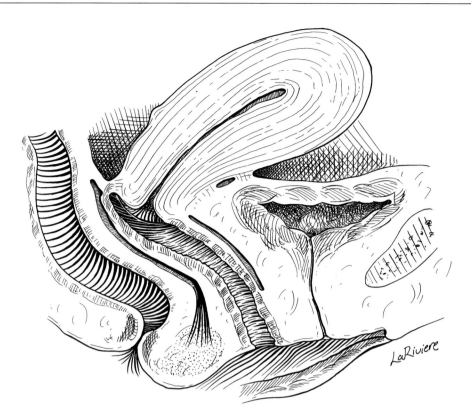

Fig. 45-1 Drawing of the female pelvis showing the usual location of the vesicourethral position at about the junction of the lower third with the upper two thirds of the back of the pubis.

tions to disclose any pelvic support defects. In addition, the patient should perform a Valsalva maneuver in both the lithotomy and standing positions. The presence of prolapse, just as the absence, reveals nothing about the cause or type of prolapse. A large cystocele and/or vault prolapse can prevent incontinence by causing urethral kinking.[25]

The assessment of urethral mobility can be performed by inspection and palpation or by the Q-tip test.[11] It cannot be overemphasized that urethral mobility does not diagnose stress urinary incontinence. Evaluation of urethral mobility is valuable because operative procedures are designed to stabilize the urethra and prevent rotational descent (Fig. 45-1). Inspection and palpation are usually reliable, especially in multiparous patients with significant hypermobility. However, care must be taken in patients with redundant periurethral vaginal tissue. With the patient in the dorsal lithotomy position, a Q-tip that is well lubricated with 2% lidocaine is gently introduced into the urethra and gently pulled back out of the bladder until some resistance is encountered placing the Q-tip at the urethrovesical junction. The resting angle form the horizontal is measured with an orthopedic goniometer. The patient is asked to cough and/or perform a Valsalva maneuver; the change in urethral axis is measured with the goniometer. A change in the angle of more than 30 degrees from the horizontal indicates poor anatomic support and urethral hypermobility[11,15] (Fig. 45-2). Continent women may have a positive Q-tip test, but it does not imply stress incontinence.[7,19] However, most

women with stress incontinence have a positive test.[6,15] The Q-tip test is unreliable in differentiating between the different types of urinary incontinence. Lack of hypermobility in patients with stress incontinence is associated with a 50% surgical failure rate.[7]

Urodynamics is a term used to describe a number of complementary tests performed individually or in combination. The principles and practice of urodynamics apply to the measurement of pressure within the bladder (P_{ves}) and urethra (P_{ura}) as well as within the vagina (P_{abd}) as a measure of abdominal pressure. A pressure transducer (microtip) is a device that converts a change in pressure into a change in electrical voltage. The change in electrical voltage can be amplified and recorded on a paper trace or can be digitized. Two microtip catheters record three direct positive pressures, P_{abd}, P_{ves}, and P_{ura}. The detrusor pressure ($P_{det} = P_{ves} - P_{abd}$) and the closure pressure ($P_{clo} = P_{ura} - P_{ves}$) can be calculated electronically by subtracting the direct channels among themselves.

Uroflowmetry is primarily used to determine whether the patient is voiding normally and to rule out bladder outlet obstruction. Cystometry is used to measure bladder pressure during filling and to diagnose detrusor instability, high compliant bladder, or noncompliant bladder, as well as genuine stress urinary incontinence and genuine stress urinary incontinence caused by intrinsic sphincteric deficiency. During cystometry, the bladder is filled through a small catheter (8 Fr) containing two pressure transducers 6 cm apart

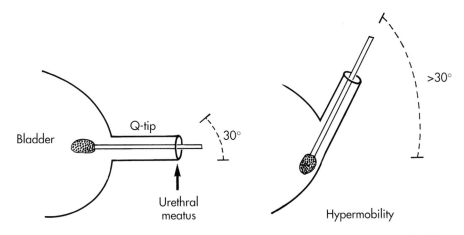

Fig. 45-2 Q-tip test. Resting angle on left and effect of Valsalva maneuver on urethral hypermobility on the right.

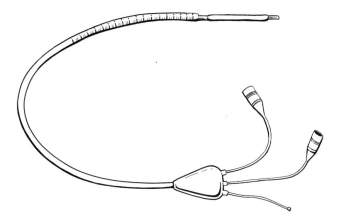

Fig. 45-3 Multichannel urethral/bladder pressure catheter.

(Fig. 45-3). The distal microtip transducer is P_{ves} and the proximal is P_{ura}. During cystometric testing, the distal transducer remains in the bladder and the proximal in the urethra. The diagnosis of genuine stress urinary incontinence is made during cystometry. Valsalva leakpoint evaluation is also performed during cystometry. During cystometry at a given volume (200 ml) and in the standing position, the patient is asked to perform the Valsalva maneuver. The lowest intravesical pressure (P_{ves}) that causes gross incontinence of urine is recorded as the Valsalva leakpoint pressure. A leakpoint of 60 cm H_2O has been correlated with intrinsic sphincteric deficiency.[17] Urethral profilometry is used to measure urethral pressure over the length of the urethra, functional urethral length, and closure pressure (Fig. 45-4). Urethral profilometry is the measurement of intraurethral pressure along the urethra by the proximal transducer (P_{ura}) drawn from the bladder neck to the external urethral meatus by a catheter puller, while the distal transducer (P_{ves}) continues to measure bladder pressure. Functional urethral length is that length of the urethra over which urethral pressure exceeds bladder pressure when measured concomi-

tantly. Total urethral length is the true anatomic urethral length. Closure pressure is the value calculated by subtracting bladder pressure from urethral pressure ($P_{clo} = P_{ura} - P_{ves}$). This reflects a positive urethral pressure that resists urine flow from the bladder. Low urethral pressure is closure pressure of less than 20 cm H_2O and is an indication of poor urethral function, which is associated with a significantly higher surgical failure rate than that of standard antiincontinence procedures.[8,24] A uroflow with the recording catheters in place is a pressure-flow and allows intraurethral pressure, intravesical pressure, intraabdominal pressure, detrusor pressure, closure pressure, and flow rate to be measured simultaneously. This allows the physician to determine voiding mechanism.

Urodynamics is essential to the comprehensive evaluation of the patient with urinary incontinence.

CHOICE OF PROCEDURE AND INDICATIONS

The selection of a particular surgical procedure should be individualized and based on (1) the underlying anatomic defects and physiologic abnormality responsible for incontinence; (2) the surgeon's preference, experience, and surgical skills; and (3) the patient's expectations. If the underlying pathophysiology is urethral hypermobility, the goal of surgery is to prevent rotational descent of the bladder neck. This goal may be accomplished by a number of methods. Short-term results of vaginal plications, needle suspensions, retropubic operations, and sling procedures all provide success rates of 85%.[4,5] However, longer-term results have shown that retropubic operations and sling procedures have higher success rates.[5] Patients with low urethral closure pressure have a significantly higher failure rate with retropubic operations.[8,24] Therefore, in patents with urethral hypermobility and low urethral closure pressure and/or intrinsic sphincteric deficiency, the most effective surgical treatment is sling urethropexy. In women, intrinsic sphincter deficiency is commonly associated with advanced genital

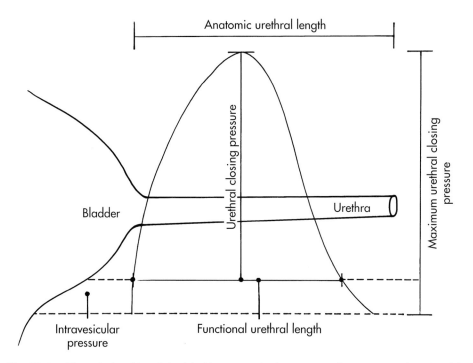

Fig. 45-4 The relationship of the bladder to urethral pressure. The anatomic length of the urethra is greater than the functional length. The closing pressure is greatest at the midpoint of the functional urethral length.

prolapse, multiple antiincontinence procedures, hypoestrogenism, aging, or a combination. The role of collagen injections as a bulking agent appears to be most indicated in the absence of hypermobility and intrinsic sphincteric deficiency.

Abdominal Retropubic Technique

In 1949, Marshall, Marchetti, and Krantz[16] (MMK) described a new operation for urinary incontinence by elevating and suturing the urethra and bladder neck to the pubic symphysis. In performing an MMK operation, Burch[9] found that the sutures often pulled out of the pubic periosteum. In his attempts to find alternative locations for suture attachment he initially tried the fascia overlying the obturator internus muscle.[9] However, he ultimately chose Cooper's ligament as the fixation point and in 1968 published his 9-year experience, reporting a 93% cure rate.[10] Burch also identified enterocele formation as a result of the procedure, presumably caused by a change in the vaginal axis.

Proper patient positioning is critical because it will facilitate the operation by enhancing exposure. Adjustable Allen stirrups, especially the PAL stirrups with featherlift (Allen Medical Systems, Cleveland, Ohio), enable easy intraoperative adjustment and provide excellent access to the lower abdomen and retropubic space.

If an abdominal hysterectomy is to be performed, the placement of the incision should favor the exposure required for the hysterectomy with consideration that the retropubic space will need to be dissected. A high Pfannenstiel incision will compromise exposure to the retropubic

space by creating an "awning" effect from the anterior abdominal wall as an anatomic obstacle that will require constant retraction as well as impede the reflection of light into the retropubic space in addition to creating shadowing.

In the absence of an abdominal hysterectomy, the low transverse incision is placed 2 fingerbreadths from the peak of the pubic symphysis and not from the most cephalad point of the pubic symphysis. This position will place the surgical exposure directly above the space of Retzius, minimize the amount of lateral retraction that will be required, avoid an awning effect, and facilitate visualization. Use of a headlight provides shadow-free lighting in front of the surgeon, eliminating the need to make frequent adjustments to overhead lights because the surgeon or assistant is blocking the light. If not already in place, the bladder is drained with a 14-Fr silicone-coated catheter before the reconstructive surgery is done. The catheter is not connected to gravity drainage; if previously connected to gravity, it is disconnected from the Foley bag and secured with a Kelly clamp. This allows easier manipulation of the distal end of the Foley in identifying the bladder neck and avoids the catheter from being pulled down in front of the introitus. The 5-ml Foley bulb is filled with 10 ml of saline.

The incision is then carried through the skin and subcutaneous fat to the fascia of the rectus abdominis, which is incised in the midline and extended laterally. The rectus muscles are sharply divided in the midline and gently reflected laterally with a medium-sized Richardson retractor. The goal of developing the retropubic space is gentle dissection because any bleeding will decrease exposure, ob-

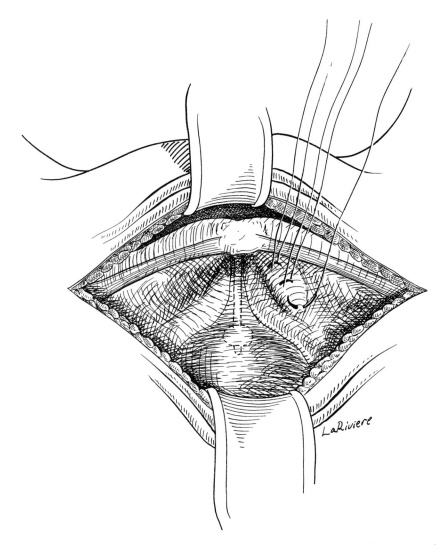

Fig. 45-5   Burch urethropexy. The retropubic space has been dissected, and the sutures have been placed through the fibromuscular wall of the vagina lateral to the urethra.

scure anatomic landmarks, and require frequent evacuation of the blood, further decreasing exposure as retractors are exchanged between the surgeon and assistants.

Once the rectus muscle is reflected laterally, the space of Retzius is developed by following the undersurface of the rectus muscle to the superior ramus of the pubic bone. Cooper's ligament is identified and noted. The loose areolar tissue can then gently be dissected from the pubic symphysis below and Cooper's ligament in a lateral to medial direction with blunt tissue forceps such a Singley. A narrow malleable retractor is used to retract the bladder medially.

The surgeon's nondominant hand may be placed in the vagina during retropubic dissection. The vaginal hand elevates the vagina up and away from vessels and bladder and provides tactile sensation of needle depth during suturing (Fig. 45-5).

After dissection of the space of Retzius, the vaginal wall is sutured with permanent braided suture material such as 2-0 Ethibond (Ethicon, Somerville, NJ). A long needle-driver will permit suturing without the driving hand obscuring needle placement/rotation and visualization. After the

suture is recovered from the vaginal wall, the suture is passed through Cooper's ligament (Fig. 45-6). Once all sutures are placed, usually four, cystoscopic evaluation and indigo carmine evaluation for ureteral patency are performed. After cystoscopic evaluation, the bladder is emptied, a Q-tip is placed in the urethra, and the operating room table is brought to a horizontal position. The sutures in the retropubic space are tied with enough tension to bring the Q-tip between 0 and −10 degrees. Under no instance should the vaginal wall be elevated to the Cooper's ligament.

Vesicourethral Sling

Hawksworth and Roux[13] long ago wrote that the most successful surgical means of supporting the vesicourethral junction are "sling" procedures of one type or another, whether the lateral walls of the vagina or urethra are plicated to the tissue that is normally found in that area, whether the vagina is attached to the back of the pubic symphysis, or whether the material is used as a transplantable sling to actually elevate the vesicourethral junction. The sling can be fashioned from abdominal fascia that has been

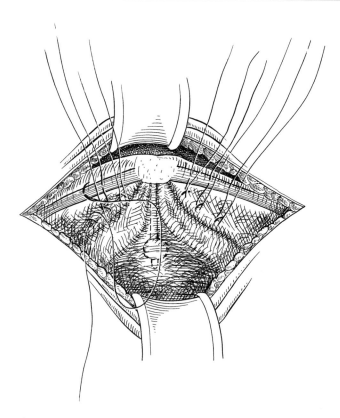

Fig. 45-6 Sutures have been passed through Cooper's ligament.

relocated, a harvested portion of fascia lata, or a synthetic material such as Mersilene mesh. The desired result is similar in all patients because the vesicourethral junction is elevated and supported to a point within the pelvis where the proximal urethra and bladder are simultaneously subject to increases in intraabdominal pressure.

The indications for use of a vesicourethral sling are recurrent urinary stress incontinence, low urethral pressure, or intrinsic sphincteric deficiency. Our choice for vesicourethral sling material is Mersilene mesh (not Mersilene tape). As an alternative, in patients with diabetes mellitus or severe asthma that requires steroid therapy, we prefer fascia lata. In these patient's an altered immune system may increase the incidence of infection. Mersilene mesh by its thinness and flexibility seems to be superior to other synthetic sling materials. When implanted suburethrally, it is virtually undetectable on physical examination. The use of synthetic materials also saves the patient the discomfort from obtaining a strip of fascia lata. The single-layered, porous Mersilene mesh has a predetermined length and width and can be cut to size intraoperatively or preoperatively. Mersilene mesh has a configuration that will allow stretch in one direction more than the other. This becomes critical in tailoring the sling in the direction of least stretch. The Mersilene mesh hammock or vesicourethral sling (available from Ethicon, Inc., Sommerville, NJ, catalog # RM43RRM54) measures no more than 2.5 cm maximum width at the center of its belly and tapers to 1.5 cm at each end of the hammock. It measures 32 cm in length. It is im-

portant that the maximum width of the mesh be no greater than 2.5 cm to aid in optimum positioning beneath the vesicourethral junction. A diameter any wider would bring the posterior margin of the sling too far into the posteroinferior surface of the bladder, and one with a narrower width may apply to much pressure and strangulate the urethra. Moir[18] has stressed the importance of cutting the sheet of gauze in the direction of least stretch. When there is risk of postoperative vaginal necrosis such as atrophic vagina, previous radiation, or extensive scarring from previous repair, the surgeon might want to select fascia lata as championed by Ridley as a modification of the Goebell-Frankenheim-Stoeckel procedure. The material is a homograft and not likely to be rejected or harbor any prolonged infection if deliberate exteriorization in the vagina is needed. Rectus fascia can also be obtained through a low transverse midline or Pfannenstiel incision. However, because the direction of fibers in this strip of tissue are oblique, the stress placed on this tissue will not be of maximum strength. To obtain a suitable long strip, an abdominal incision would require a crescent-shaped incision that would be cosmetically unattractive or that would require extensive dissection of the anterior abdominal wall through a low transverse incision. Theoretically, harvesting strips from the midline rectus fascia is associated with increased postoperative discomfort as well as the possibility of a postoperative wound hernia.

A strip of fascia lata is obtained by the technique suggested by Ridley.[22] Its overall width may be increased somewhat by increasing the distance between the parallel incisions when being harvested with a Masson stripper or a similar instrument. If the strip is too narrow, the suburethral pressure of the strap may be concentrated in too small an area, increasing the risk for pressure necrosis of the urethra. If the central belly of the sling is too narrow, it may be widened by central incisions. If there is evidence of funneling within the proximal urethra or low urethral closure pressure has been demonstrated preoperatively, the tissue surrounding the urethral wall at the vesicourethral junction may be strengthened and supported by imbrication with Kelly bladder neck plication sutures using polyglycolic-type sutures.

Technique of the Sling Operation. Careful patient positioning is required, and intraoperative adjustable Allen stirrups are of great benefit. The operation is begun suprapubically with a 2- to 5-cm incision through the skin overlying each groin, parallel to the inguinal canal, 2 cm cephalad and 2 cm lateral to the pubic symphysis. The length of the incision will be determined by factors such as distribution of subcutaneous adipose tissue. The incision is made medial to the pubic tubercle and extends laterally toward the anterior iliac spine. In patients with previous retropubic surgery such as an MMK procedure, these incisions are lateral to the site of retropubic scarring, which need not be disturbed. However, if the patient has previously undergone a Burch urethropexy to Cooper's ligament, a conventional Pfannenstiel incision through the skin and fascia should be considered and the stitches of the Burch procedure identified and cut. The vesicourethral junction is freed by sharp dissection from the back of the pubic symphysis and Cooper's ligament. Inadvertent cystotomy should be closed with two layers. An alternative method is to perform the dissection under direct cystoscopic visualization with a 70-degree scope. This is similar to laparoscopy, in which introduction of the 5-mm trocar is done under direct visualization. This will allow dissection within the space of Retzius while bladder integrity is visualized and maintained.

Each of the lateral incisions is taken down to the rectus sheath. The rectus sheath is opened by a 1- to 2-cm incision parallel to the skin incision. Each rectus muscle is penetrated by the tips of the curved Mayo scissors, with the curve directed toward the pubis. The closed scissor is advanced through the transversalis fascia into the space of Retzius. This can be done under direct cystoscopic visualization in patients who have had a Burch retropubic operation. If scissors are used, the tips are opened a small amount and withdrawn, enlarging the deeper incision. Digital confirmation and mild dissection can then be performed from the posterior surface of the obturator foramen across Cooper's ligament toward the pubic symphysis. A moist sponge is placed in each wound, and the procedure is then directed toward the vaginal portion. The intraoperative adjustable Allen stirrups being in a modified supine position can then be adjusted to a lithotomy position. This adjustment is very desirable because it affords great patient comfort and facilitates the operation.

A transurethral 14-Fr silicone-coated Foley catheter is inserted into the bladder, and the bladder is emptied of any contents. Experience will reveal that any trauma to the bladder from the suprapubic incisions can easily be recognized from the color of the urine. If any injury is suspected, cystoscopy should be performed at this point. If there is no evidence of injury, 50 ml of sterile infant formula is instilled in the bladder through the catheter to identify any unrecognized penetration of the bladder during the course of the vaginal dissection. Prompt appearance of the infant formula will be obvious and does not stain the surrounding tissues for the duration of the surgery, as would be true with the use of methylene blue and indigo carmine. The bulb on the Foley catheter is identified, and the vaginal wall is picked up between two Allis clamps placed at the 3- and 9-o'clock positions proximal to the position of the Foley bulb.

A longitudinal full-thickness vaginal incision is made between the clamps directly into the vesicovaginal space and carried through the anterior vaginal wall for the full extent of the cystocele using sharp dissection separating the vagina from the urethra to within 1 cm of the external urethral meatus (Fig. 45-7). The separation of bladder from vagina is carried posteriorly well beyond the bulb on the catheter (the full distance to the vault of the vagina if cystocele is to be repaired), and the dissection is carried laterally as far as required to fully repair the midline defect and/or into the paravaginal space if a paravaginal defect is also simultaneously being performed. Lateral dissection of the vaginal wall from

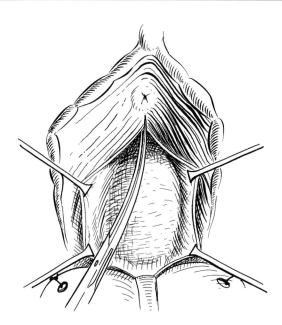

Fig. 45-7   Full-thickness anterior vaginal wall has been opened 1 cm from the urethral meatus.

the vesicourethral junction for patients who have previously undergone surgery may release troublesome scar tissue that may have been holding the internal urethral orifice open. The dissection is carried laterally at the level of the bladder neck and the vaginal retropubic portion of the tunnels are created (Fig. 45-8).

If there is evidence of urethral funneling within the proximal urethra, the tissues surrounding the urethral wall of the vesicourethral junction may be strengthened and supported with Kelly plication sutures using a 2-0 polyglycolic acid suture.

The position of the urethrovesical junction is carefully reconfirmed by palpating the site of the inflated Foley catheter bulb. The tissues of the urogenital diaphragm on each paraurethral side of the vesicourethral junction are perforated bluntly with the tips of the curved Mayo scissors. The scissors are directed upward and laterally away from the bladder toward the previously established retropubic inguinal tunnels into the space of Retzius. The scissors are opened 1 to 2 cm and withdrawn, enlarging the opening. It is important to stay close to the pubic rami but to avoid the periosteum. Some venous bleeding is occasionally seen and responds readily to tamponade. The sterile packs are removed from the abdominal incisions, and the surgeon inserts the tip of the left index finger through the abdominal incision into the patient's retropubic tunnel. The surgeon then introduces the tip of the uterine dressing forceps, convex side toward the operator, into the intravaginal tunnel through the urogenital diaphragm onto the patient until it meets the left index finger. The fascia lata strap or the precut Mersilene mesh is held in place transversely beneath the posterior urethra. The anterior margin of the sling belly is fixed to the undersurface of the lateral periurethral connective tissue by two interrupted 2-0 nonabsorbable synthetic

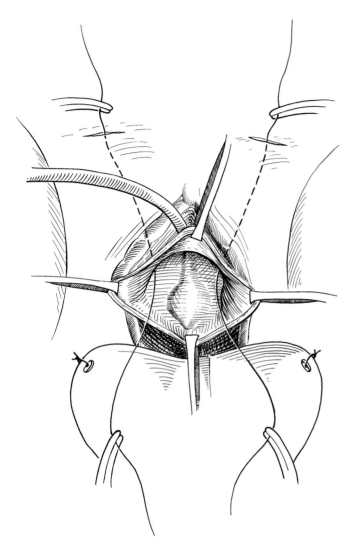

Fig. 45-8   Retropubic tunnels created, and pilot sutures passed through the tunnels.

sutures such as Ethibond (Fig. 45-9). The posterior edge of the belly is sewn to the bladder of the capsule with three additional interrupted sutures. Two sutures are placed lateral to the midline and one suture in the midline, fixing the sling to the bladder capsule. This stretches the sling anteroposteriorly without tension but with sufficient pull to remove wrinkles from the belly of the sling. Each pilot suture is then tied to the respective sling arm end, and the mesh is pulled through the retropubic tunnel, exiting through the abdominal incision.

If any cystocele repair or anterior colporrhaphy is to be accomplished, it is completed now. The edges of the anterior vaginal wall are trimmed only if necessary and are approximated in two layers. A deep or buried layer of interrupted 2-0 polyglycolic acid sutures is followed by a superficial layer of interrupted mattress sutures also with 2-0 polyglycolic acid sutures. After completing the anterior colporrhaphy, any posterior colporrhaphy and/or perineorrhaphy that may be indicated is performed. At this point, any cystoscopy that may be required is performed and the vagina is lightly packed

with 1-inch Iodoform gauze packing. The packing itself acts as a bolster supporting and elevating the vesicourethral junction. Once in place, the surgeon's attention is redirected to the abdomen and the sling is sewn to the point at which the sling arms cross the rectus aponeurosis, tightly enough only that any slack or wrinkles in the mesh are removed.

After the ends of the hammock have been securely anchored to the rectus fascia using nonabsorbable synthetic sutures, the excess tails are trimmed and removed from the operative field. Any remaining defects in the rectus fascial incision are closed with interrupted sutures of 2-0 Ethibond. The skin is closed with surgical clips or a subcuticular suture.

The wide belly of the sling distributes suburethral pressure over a wide area, and the sling neither constricts the urethra nor decreases its lumen (Fig. 45-10), although it appears to increase both urethral tone and intraurethral pressure by providing a firm support upon which the urethra may rest. In the rare event of unexpected bladder penetration during placement of the sling, any externally visible opening can be repaired. If good exposure is not available, the sling may be repositioned away from the penetration. The edges of the penetration are permitted to fall together. The catheter decompression of the bladder should be maintained for 5 to 7 days to permit the bladder to heal.

Postoperative Adjustments in Sling Tension. If the sling or other material has been placed to loosely to achieve an increase in intraurethral pressure sufficient to restore continence, this will become evident shortly after the Foley catheter has been removed, almost in the immediate postoperative period. Increasing the sling tension is easiest within the first 4 weeks after surgery, when fibrosis and scarring around the sling are still minimal. In situations requiring an increase in sling tension, the groin incisions are opened and the sling is released from its attachment to the abdominal aponeurosis and gentle traction on the sling arms should change the axis of the bladder neck. This is most noticeable with a Q-tip in the urethra. Preoperatively and intraoperatively, there should be a positive Q-tip angle, and with the Q-tip in position and both sling arms freed from the abdominal incisions, gentle traction is placed on the sling arms to a point that brings the bladder neck to 0 and no more than -10 degrees. Alternatively, the degree to which the sling may be tightened can be judged by simultaneous direct urethroscopy.

On the other hand, if there is postoperative urinary retention or incomplete bladder emptying, the sling may require adjustment. In the case of Mersilene mesh, if there is complete urinary retention within the first 2 weeks, the abdominal incisions may be opened, the sling arms may be released from the abdominal aponeurosis, and a urethral sound can be placed in the urethra with traction distally to free the sling arms. Resuturing of the sling arms to the fascia is not required. If the patient had surgery approximately 1 month prior or if there is complete urinary retention, the sling may be divided through a transvaginal incision. In release through the transvaginal route, the same procedure is

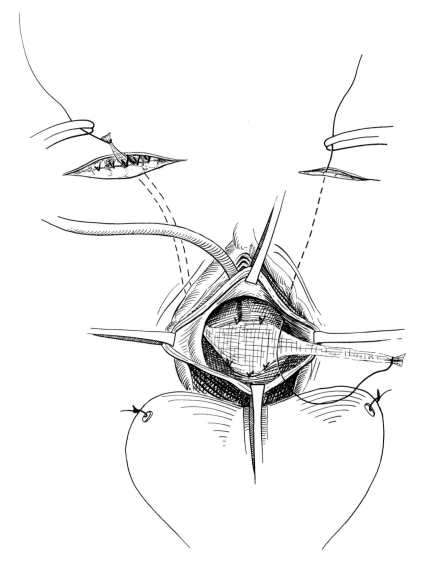

Fig. 45-9   The belly of the sling has been secured suburethrally. The right sling arm is shown sutured to the abdominal fascia.

followed by placing two Allis clamps on the anterior vaginal wall and making an incision directly into the vesicovaginal space. This space may be slightly obliterated because of postoperative inflammation. While the Foley is concomitantly being palpated, the bladder neck and bladder are "protected" by the sling. Therefore the dissection should be taken toward the sling material. In both situations in which the abdominal/fascia lata or Mersilene mesh was used, the sling can be readily identified with meticulous dissection. The sling can be divided in the middle, or the sling belly may be excised, depending on the amount of urinary retention or incomplete bladder emptying.

Periurethral Bulking Agents

Cross-linked collagen preparations (GAX) can be used to increase urethral coaptation in patients after previous incontinence operations have failed, particularly when the urethrovesical junction is otherwise well supported.[12] In addi-

tion, it may be used in patients with intrinsic sphincteric deficiency without a hypermobile urethra.[2]

Contigen is a sterile, nonpyrogenic material composed of highly purified bovine dermal collagen that is cross-linked with glutaraldehyde and dispersed in phosphate-buffered physiologic saline. It may be injected transurethrally or periurethrally in patients who are not sensitive to the collagen (this must be determined by preliminary intradermal inoculation 4 weeks before the treatment). In the periurethral method the urethra is anesthetized by 1% plain lidocaine injected at the 3- to 9-o'clock position. A 22-gauge spinal needle is inserted periurethrally at the 4-o'clock position, with the bevel directed medially, and is slowly advanced while its progress is followed through the 17-Fr sheath with a 0 - or 30-degree cystoscope until the needle tip is subepithelial and at the vesicourethral junction. The Contigen is injected until the bulge produced reaches the midline. The needle is removed, and the process is repeated at the

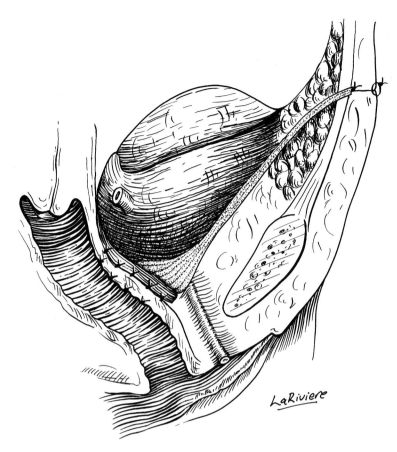

Fig. 45-10 Effect of sling in elevating the vesicourethral junction.

8-o'clock position on the opposite side. The injection is continued under direct cystoscopic visualization of the vesicourethral junction until the mucosal tissue of one side just touches that of the opposite side. Appell[2] has described considerable success and enthusiasm for the procedure in carefully selected patients.

The transurethral approach is facilitated by the Wolf aspiration-injection system (Richard Wolf Medical Instruments Corp., Vernon Hills, Ill.), which allows accurate submucosal injection. A 21-Fr urethroscope-cystoscope sheath allows visualization of the needle immediately as it emerges from the sheath, permitting direct visualization during needle placement and injection into the submucosal tissues. Patients with transient urinary retention empty their bladders by intermittent self-catheterization, which is taught preoperatively. An indwelling Foley catheter should not be placed because it will force the collagen around the Foley, disturbing the mucosal approximation.

Contigen, which is biodegradable, appears to be safe and efficacious, particularly in patients who do not manifest detrusor problems and have a urethrovesical junction that is fairly well stabilized in position. Contigen begins to degrade 12 weeks after injection. It stimulates and is replaced by the body's own collagen, retaining the effect of being a bulking agent. About a third of the patients will require a second injection of Contigen after 30 days if they are not dry,

and patients have then reported that they have remained dry for at least 12 months.[2] Follow-up, however, has been short.

SUMMARY

Surgery for stress urinary incontinence has many varied techniques and approaches. The surgeon's preferences and skills are of paramount importance in selecting the best surgical approach. The Burch urethropexy and the vesicourethral sling are the most effective and durable operations for stress urinary incontinence. Current expectations for long-term success on the part of the patient and surgeon almost mandates that the operations with the most durable results be selected for surgical treatment.

REFERENCES

1. Abrams P, Blaivas JG, Stanton SL, Andersen JT: The standardization of terminology of lower urinary tract function recommended by the International continence Society, *Int Urogynecol J* 1:45, 1990.
2. Appell RA: Injectables for urethral incompetence, *World J Urol* 8:208, 1990.
3. Bates CP, Whiteside CG, Turner Warwick R: Synchronous urine pressure flow cystourethrography with special reference to stress and urge incontinence, *Br J Urol* 42:714, 1970.
4. Bergman A, Ballard CA, Koonings P: Comparison of three surgical procedures for genuine stress incontinence: prospective randomized study, *Am J Obstet Gynecol* 160:1102, 1989.

5. Bergman A, Elia G: Three surgical procedures for genuine stress urinary incontinence: five-year follow-up of prospective randomized study, *Am J Obstet Gynecol* 173:66, 1995.

6. Bergman A, Koonings PP, Ballard CA: Negative Q-tip test as a risk factor for failed anti-incontinence surgery, *J Reprod Med* 34:157, 1989.

7. Bergman A, et al: Role of Q-tip test in evaluating stress urinary incontinence, *J Reprod Med* 32:273, 1987.

8. Bowen LW, et al: Unsuccessful Burch retropubic urethropexy: a case-controlled urodynamics study, *Am J Obstet Gynecol* 160:452, 1989.

9. Burch JC: Urethrovaginal fixation to Cooper's ligament for correction of stress incontinence, cystocele and prolapse, *Am J Obstet Gynecol* 81:281, 1961.

10. Burch JC: Cooper's ligament urethrovesical suspension for stress incontinence: 9 years' experience—results, complications, technique, *Am J Obstet Gynecol* 100:764, 1968.

11. Chrystle CD, Charme LS, Copeland WE: Q-tip test in stress urinary incontinence, *Obstet Gynecol* 38:313, 1971.

12. Eckford SD, Abrams P: Para-urethral collagen implantation for female stress incontinence, *Br J Urol* 68:586, 1991.

13. Hawksworth W, Roux JP: Vaginal hysterectomy, *J Obstet Gynaecol Br Commonw* 63:214, 1958.

14. Jarvis GJ, et al: An assessment of urodynamic examination in incontinence women, *Br J Obstet Gynaecol* 87:873, 1980.

15. Karram MM, Bhatia NN: The Q-tip test: standardization of the technique and its interpretation in women with urinary incontinence, *Obstet Gynecol* 71:807, 1988.

16. Marshall VF, Marchetti AA, Krantz KE: The correction of stress incontinence by simple vesicourethral suspension, *Surg Gynecol Obstet* 88:509, 1949.

17. McGuire EJ, et al: Clinical assessment of urethral function, *J Urol* 150:1452, 1993.

18. Moir JC: The gauze hammock operation, *J Obstet Gynaecol Br Commonw* 75:1, 1968.

19. Montz FJ, Stanton SL: Q-tip test in female urinary incontinence, *Obstet Gynecol* 67:258, 1986.

20. Nichols DH, Randall CL: *Vaginal surgery,* ed 4, Baltimore, 1996, Williams & Wilkins, p 384.

21. Powell PH, Shepherd AM, Lewis P, Feneley RCL: The accuracy of clinical diagnosis assessed urodynamically. In *Proceedings 10th meeting ICS Los Angeles,* 1980, p 3.

22. Ridley JH: Appraisal of the Goebell-Frangenheim-Stoeckel sling procedure, *Am J Obstet Gynecol* 33:680, 1969.

23. Sand PK, Hill RC, Ostergard DR: Incontinence history as a predictor of detrusor instability, *Obstet Gynecol* 71:257, 1988.

24. Sand PK, et al: The low pressure urethra as a factor in failed retropubic urethropexy, *Obstet Gynecol* 69:399, 1987.

25. Veronikis DK, Nichols DH, Wakamatsu MM: The incidence of low pressure urethra as a function of prolapse reducing technique in patients with massive pelvic organ prolapse (maximum descent at all vaginal sites), *Am J Obstet Gynecol* 177:1305, 1977.

46 Intraoperative Ureteral Injuries and Ureterovaginal Fistulas

W. GLENN HURT and EILEEN M. SEGRETI

The close anatomic relationship that exists between the lower urinary tract and the internal genitalia predisposes the distal ureter to involvement by gynecologic disorders and places it at risk for injury during pelvic surgery and radiation therapy. Intraoperative repair of ureteral injuries is successful in more than 90% of patients. Patients whose ureteral injuries are missed during the operation in which they occur are much more likely to have a poor result after a subsequent repair attempt.[8]

Unrecognized ureteral injuries or unsuccessful ureteral repairs may cause oliguria or anuria, fever, chills, and flank pain. If there is intraperitoneal or retroperitoneal leakage of urine, it may cause abdominal distention, ileus, and urinoma formation. Ultimately, a urinary fistula may develop or there may be ureteral obstruction with loss of renal function.

INCIDENCE OF URETERAL INJURY

Operative injuries to the ureter are most commonly associated with gynecologic or urologic surgery, rectosigmoid resections, and repeat surgical procedures within the pelvis and retroperitoneum. The surgical literature has historically attributed between 50% and 90% of all ureteral injuries to gynecologic procedures, but recent American publications report a significant increase in iatrogenic ureteral injuries that result from endourologic procedures.[1,25]

Although the true incidence of ureteral injuries at the time of major gynecologic surgery is unknown, studies suggest an incidence 0.4% to 2.5%.* Ureteral injury is much more likely to occur during an abdominal hysterectomy than during a vaginal hysterectomy.[29] There appears to be a increasing number of ureteral injuries associated with periaortic node dissections, obstetric procedures (e.g., cesarean sections and cesarean or postpartum hysterectomies), and operative laparoscopy.[1,23]

Pelvic surgery will never be free of ureteral injuries. However, it should be possible to minimize the risk of ureteral injury by identifying the course of the pelvic ureters and keeping them out of harm's way. Unfortunately, most surgical injuries to the ureter are not recognized at the time they occur. Therefore, to reduce the postoperative morbidity associated with ureteral injuries, it is important that whenever the ureter is jeopardized by a disease process or a surgical procedure, for the surgeon to demonstrate the integrity of the ureter by surgical dissection or intraoperative testing.

Some pelvic conditions that distort the anatomy, infiltrate the tissues, affect the blood supply, and predispose to ureteral injury are listed in the box on p. 855. Yet, Symmonds[29] reminds us that it is not the complicated surgical procedure that is responsible for most ureteral injuries; it is the "simple" abdominal hysterectomy performed for a benign indication (e.g., abnormal uterine bleeding, cervical intraepithelial neoplasia) that is most often associated with a ureteral injury. If this is true, it should be possible to prevent most ureteral injuries.

PREVENTION OF URETERAL INJURY

Preoperatively, the history and physical examination, urinalysis, urine culture, and blood chemistry measurements may give a clue to the condition of the urinary tract and its potential involvement by pathologic conditions. Preoperative intravenous urograms assist in detecting congenital anomalies of the urinary tract and in documenting involvement by pelvic tumors, pelvic inflammatory disease, or invasive processes such as endometriosis or cancer. Routine preoperative urograms have not been shown to lower the overall incidence of operative ureteral injuries.[21] Ultrasound examinations, computed tomography scans, magnetic resonance imaging, and radionucleotide scans can all document the preoperative integrity and function of the urinary tract, but they do not facilitate ureteral identification during pelvic surgery nor obviate the surgeon's obligation to identify the ureters.[3,15,29]

Preoperative placement of ureteral catheters to assist in the identification and the dissection of the ureters during surgery is not always practical or desirable. Ureteral catheterization cannot be expected to reduce the overall incidence of ureteral injuries, most of which occur in patients for whom there is no indication that their use is needed. When pelvic findings suggest the need for preoperative ureteral catheterization because of fixation of the tissues or malignancy, the catheters often are difficult to palpate within the ureter. It has been suggested that during dissection of a ureter, an unyielding ureteral catheter may, in fact, cause mucosal injury or predispose the ureter to devascularization or laceration.[29] If ureteral catheterization is needed during a difficult pelvic dissection, it can be easily performed by linear ureterotomy, suprapubic cystotomy, or cystoscopy. Most pelvic surgeons find this preferable to preoperative ureteral catheter placement.

Intraoperatively, the principles that contribute to the

*References 4, 6, 10, 17, 27, 29.

Large pelvic tumors
Cervical leiomyomas
Endometriosis
Ovarian remnants
Pelvic inflammatory disease
Pelvic malignancies
Pelvic hematomas and lymphocysts
Pelvic organ prolapse
Diverticulosis
Congenital anomalies
Pregnancy
Prior pelvic surgery
Prior radiation therapy

safety of all pelvic procedures include adequate exposure of the surgical field; adequate light within the surgical field; restoration of anatomic relationships; traction and countertraction to expose adjacent structures; dissection along tissue planes; appropriate dissection of extraperitoneal spaces; clamping, cutting, and suturing under direct vision; and the avoidance of mass ligation of tissues. These surgical principles help protect all vital organs. The most effective way to prevent ureteral injury during pelvic laparotomy is to identify the ureters as they enter the pelvis over the bifurcations of the common iliac arteries[15] and to trace the pelvic course of each ureter during dissection of the retroperitoneal spaces. In demonstrating the course of the ureter, its attachment to the pelvic peritoneum should be preserved. Every effort should be made to protect the blood supply to each ureter and the longitudinal network of the microvasculature within its adventitial sheath.

COMMON SITES OF URETERAL INJURY

Most ureteral injuries that result from gynecologic surgery occur in the lower third of the ureter. The three most common sites of ureteric injury at the time of hysterectomy are (1) at the pelvic brim where the ureters lie beneath the infundibulopelvic ligaments and over the bifurcations of the common iliac arteries, (2) lateral to the cervix where the ureters pass under the uterine arteries, and (3) lateral to the vaginal fornices where the ureters course adjacent to the cervix and upper vagina to enter the bladder.

Ureteral angulation, perforation, or ligation may occur during reperitonealization of the pelvis, posterior culdeplasty, or colporrhaphy or as a result of retropubic urethropexy/vaginopexy. Dissecting the ureter from within a pathologic process and "untunneling" the ureter near the bladder may result in devascularization or laceration.

In the obstetric patient, ureteral injury most often occurs as a result of extension of the uterine incision, suturing of the uterine incision, or an effort to control hemorrhage within one of the broad ligaments.[7] Cesarean and postpartum hysterectomies may be associated with ureteral injuries because of the increased vascularity of the pelvis, the distortion of the anatomy, the loss of tissue turgor that maintains the shape of the pelvic organs during traction and countertraction, and the effacement and dilatation of the cervix.

Ureteral injury as a result of pelvic radiation therapy for cervical cancer is uncommon (less than 0.5%). The immediate effect of radiation therapy is an inflammatory response; over time it causes devascularization and fibrosis of the tissues and places the ureter at risk for injury during subsequent surgical procedures.

DETECTION OF URETERAL INJURY

During surgery, if there is reason to suspect that ureteral injury has occurred, a number of procedures can be used to determine the location and extent of the injury. These include the following:

- *Ureteral dye injection:* Indigo carmine is injected through a 22-gauge needle into the ureter above the suspected site of injury. Resistance to the injection suggests ureteral obstruction, leakage of dye into the operative field below the injection site indicates ureteral injury, and excretion of dye in the urine suggests ureteral patency.
- *Intravenous dye injection:* Injection of intravenous indigo carmine (5 ml) should be followed in 5 to 10 minutes by the excretion of blue urine. Complete bilateral ureteral obstruction prevents urine from reaching the bladder. Unilateral ureteral obstruction cannot be detected by the intravenous administration of indigo carmine unless ureteral excretion is observed via cystotomy or cystoscopy (suprapubic or transurethral). Leakage of blue urine through an injured ureter into the operative site identifies an area of ureteral injury.
- *Intraoperative ureteral catheterization:* The ureter(s) may be catheterized during surgery by ureterostomy, cystotomy, or cystoscopy. A linear ureterotomy above the site of suspected injury permits catheter passage down the ureter and into the bladder. A cystotomy may be performed in the anterior wall of the bladder to visualize the ureteral orifices and to pass ureteral catheters. During an abdominal procedure, transurethral cystoscopy is a somewhat cumbersome method of ureteral catheter placement.
- *Intravenous excretory urography:* Constant infusion intraoperative intravenous urography may be performed during surgery to evaluate the integrity of the urinary tract.
- *Dissection of the ureter:* When there is concern about the integrity of a ureter, there is no substitute for dissecting the pararectal space and visualizing repetitive vermiculation of the ureter throughout its course.

SURGICAL ANATOMY OF THE URETER

The ureters are bilateral tubular structures, 25 to 30 cm in length, that serve as urinary conduits between the kidneys and bladder. The ureters originate rather indistinctly from the renal pelves lateral to the transverse processes of the first lumbar vertebra. They descend retroperitoneally, lateral to the transverse processes of the vertebrae, over the anterior surface of the psoas muscles to pass dorsal to the ovarian vessels and then cross the pelvic brim and enter the true pelvis. Within the pelvis they descend anterior to the bifurcations of the common iliac vessels, forming the posterior boundary of the ovarian fossae. They then pass under the uterine arteries and turn anteriorly, medial to the obturator vessels and nerve, to pass about the cervix and upper vagina to enter 1.5- to 2.0-cm intramural tunnels within the base of the bladder. The ureters open into the bladder on either end of the interureteral ridge (Mercier's bar) that forms the base of the trigone of the bladder.

In descent, the right ureter is crossed by the right colic and ileocolic vessels, and the left ureter is crossed by the left colic vessels. The ureters are slightly constricted and more firmly attached by their adventitial layer to adjacent structures at the ureteropelvic junction, as they cross anterior to the iliac vessels, and at the ureterovesical junction. The pelvic portion of the ureter is more intimately attached to the overlying parietal peritoneum than is the abdominal portion.

Congenital anomalies of the ureter are common. A bifid or Y-shaped ureter may connect anywhere between the ureteropelvic junction and the bladder. When there is ureteral duplication, the two ureters commonly cross within the retroperitoneal spaces and enter the bladder wall through the same ureteral tunnel but open into the bladder in a predictable relationship in which the upper ureteral orifice drains the lower pole and the lower ureteral orifice drains the upper pole of the kidney (Weigert-Meyer rule). The rare ectopic ureter may have its distal opening into the lower urinary tract anywhere between its normal location within the bladder and the external urethral meatus, or it may open into the vagina or vestibule.

The arterial supply to the ureter is unpredictable. The upper ureter usually receives a branch of the renal artery that descends within the adventitial sheath. The ureter may receive additional branches from the aorta and the ovarian, iliac, uterine, middle hemorrhoidal, superior vesical, and/or vaginal arteries. When no single artery runs the length of the ureter, there is usually a longitudinal anastomosis of branches of some or all of the arteries mentioned. In both cases, arteries within the adventitial layer of the ureter give off arterioles and capillaries that penetrate and supply its muscular and submucosal layers (Fig. 46-1).[12,13] The fact that the arterial blood supply to the ureter is unpredictable and may depend on only one or two vessels within the adventitial layer makes it important to handle the ureter with care and, when possible, to perform all dissection outside of the adventitial sheath.

The venous drainage of the ureter arises within its submucosal and muscular layers and forms a network within

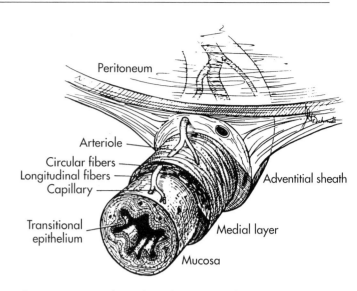

Fig. 46-1 Arterial supply and microvasculature of the ureter. (From Guerriero WG: *AUA update series*, vol II, lesson 22, p 1, Bellaire, TX, 1983, AUA Office of Education.)

the adventitial layer that closely parallels its arterial blood supply. The ureteral lymphatics arise in its muscular layer and drain from the upper ureter to the lumbar nodes along the aorta and inferior vena cava or from the lower ureter to the internal iliac nodes.

The nerve supply to the upper ureter comes from the celiac and aorticorenal plexus and that to the lower ureter from the superior and inferior hypogastric plexus. Its sympathetic supply arises in the T11, T12, and L1 spinal segments. The parasympathetic supply to the upper ureter arises from the celiac plexus and that to the lower ureter from S2, S3, and S4 sacral segments. The ureter receives primarily visceral sensory, not visceral motor, fibers. When the extrinsic nerve supply to the ureter is cut, ureteric pain is relieved and normal peristaltic activity is retained.

The wall of the ureter has three layers: an outer adventitial (Waldeyer's sheath) layer of connective tissue containing collagen, elastin, and nonmyelinated nerve fibers and blood vessels; a middle layer of smooth muscle fibers that interdigitate in a longitudinal, circular, and spiral fashion; and an inner mucosal layer of transitional epithelium resting on a basement membrane or lamina propria.

Animal experiments have shown that, after ureterotomy, mucosal healing is complete at 3 weeks, and smooth muscle bridging is complete at 6 weeks. Conduction of peristalsis across the anastomosis is not seen until 28 days after surgery. Ureters with extensive fibrosis, angulation, or poor smooth muscle regeneration may fail to regain their peristaltic activity. An oblique or spatulated end-to-end anastomosis heals faster and regains its peristaltic activity faster than a circular anastomosis.[24]

REPAIR OF URETERAL INJURY

Common types of ureteral injury are listed in the box on p. 857, left. Repairs are usually performed at the time of in-

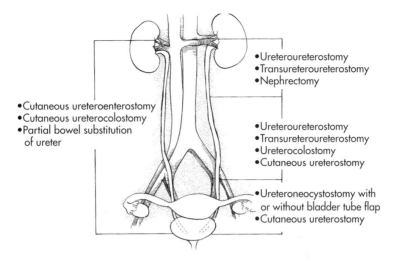

Fig. 46-2   Surgical procedures recommended for repair of ureteral injuries according to involved ureteral segment. (From Hurt WG, Dunn LJ: Complications of gynecologic surgery and trauma. In Greenfield LJ, editor: *Complications in surgery and trauma*, ed 2, Philadelphia, 1990, JB Lippincott.)

TYPES OF URETERAL INJURY

Angulation
Devascularization
Crushing
Ligation
Penetration
Laceration, partial or complete
Loss of segment

PRINCIPLES FOR SUCCESSFUL URETERAL REPAIR

1. Perform meticulous ureteral dissection using atraumatic instruments.
2. Preserve ureteral blood supply and microvasculature by leaving the peritoneal attachment and dissecting outside the adventitial sheath.
3. Perform a tension-free anastomosis.
4. Use the minimal amount of the smallest absorbable suture needed to obtain a watertight anastomosis.
5. Surround the anastomosis with retroperitoneal fat or omentum to assist healing.
6. Drain the retroperitoneal anastomotic site to prevent accumulation of urine, lymph, or blood.
7. Consider proximal urinary diversion, with or without stenting.

Modified from Schlossberg SM: *Semin Urol* 5:198, 1987.

jury or by subsequent laparotomy. A skilled vaginal surgeon might choose to repair a distal (last 3 cm) ureteric injury vaginally.[30] Whether the repair is performed abdominally or vaginally, the basic principles and techniques of ureteral repairs are similar.

Any significant angulation of the ureter should be released to prevent obstruction. Minor devascularization and crush injuries may not require additional treatment. Stenting the injured ureter may be beneficial.[26] A ligated ureter should have the suture removed and treated as if it were a crush injury. Partial lacerations of the ureter may be closed with several interrupted 4-0 absorbable sutures over a ureteral stent. The treatment of ureteral transection and the loss of a segment of ureter depends on the location of the injury. Fig. 46-2 shows treatment options for major ureteral injuries, and the box above, right, lists surgical principles for successful ureteral repair.

Unfortunately, most ureteral injuries that occur as a result of surgery are not recognized during the course of the surgical procedure. As a rule, when ureteral injuries that require definitive repair are recognized, it is best not to delay the repair,[31] unless it would be complicated by the presence of a pelvic infection or the patient's condition is too unstable for the operation to be completed.

URETERONEOCYSTOSTOMY

Ureteroneocystostomy, or ureteral reimplantation, is recommended for the repair of significant injuries to the lower 4 to 5 cm of either ureter. It is easier to perform and more likely to be successful than ureteroureterostomy. Most injuries that are the result of gynecologic surgery or pelvic radiation therapy involve this portion of the ureter and can be repaired by ureteroneocystostomy.[16]

The pelvic peritoneum is incised anterolateral to the ureter, where it crosses the bifurcation of the common iliac artery, and the peritoneal incision is continued caudally to the bladder. The distal ureter is meticulously dissected to prevent damage to its adventitial sheath and blood supply.

The ureter is ligated with permanent suture at the ureterovesical junction. Any damaged ureteral segment is excised. A 3-0 delayed absorbable tagging suture affixed to an atraumatic tapered needle is passed through the diameter of the distal ureter about 0.5 cm from its end. The needle is removed, and the ends of the untied suture are tagged with a small forceps.

An extraperitoneal cystotomy is performed in the dome of the bladder, and the ureteral orifices are identified. A finger is placed inside the fundus of the bladder, which is displaced toward the cut end of the ureter to determine the best site for a tension-free reimplantation. If direct reimplantation is to be performed, the entire thickness of the bladder wall is perforated with a right-angled forceps from within the bladder at the site of reimplantation. The tips of the forceps are opened about 1 cm to enlarge the hole in the bladder wall and to grasp the tagged end of the ureter, which is gently drawn through the bladder wall and into the bladder a distance of 1 cm. The end of the ureter is spatulated about 0.5 cm on opposite sides of its circumference, and the tagging suture is removed. Four 4-0 absorbable chromic sutures are placed to secure the distal ureteral flaps to the inside of the bladder wall (Fig. 46-3).

Several 3-0 delayed absorbable sutures are used to anchor the adventitial sheath of the ureter to the outside of the bladder wall. If a peritoneal flap was left attached to the ureter, it may be secured to the outside of the bladder wall with 3-0 or 4-0 delayed absorbable sutures.[11,29]

In adults with normal kidney function, no bladder outlet obstruction, and no history of significant urinary tract infections, direct reimplantation of the ureter is satisfactory. Hydrodynamically, the female bladder is a low-pressure organ, and because bladder outlet obstruction is uncommon, vesicoureteral reflux is a rare cause of upper urinary tract damage. However, if the upper urinary tract is compromised physiologically, a submucosal tunnel may be created within the wall of the bladder to prevent vesicoureteral reflux. A submucosal tunnel requires 2 cm of the length of the ureter. Therefore it is important to ensure that, as a result of the placement of 2 cm of the ureter in the tunnel, there will be no undue tension on the reimplantation site. The submucosal tunnel (e.g., modified Paquin,[20] Politano-Leadbetter[22]) may be created by passing closed Metzenbaum scissors or small tapered forceps (i.e., Adson tonsil forceps) obliquely through the outer visceral peritoneum and the muscular layer of the bladder. The distal three quarters or half of the tunnel should be submucosal before its final entry into a predetermined site for the new ureteral orifice within the bladder. The size of the tunnel may be increased by opening the scissors or forceps slightly as they are removed. An Adson tonsil forceps may be used to traverse the tunnel within the bladder wall to grasp the suture tag on the distal end of the ureter and to draw the tagging suture and distal ureter through the tunnel. The ureter may be fed into the tunnel as gentle traction is applied to the tagging suture. The distal ureter is secured to the mucosal and muscular layers of the bladder by several 4-0 absorbable sutures, and the tagging suture is removed. The adventitial sheath of the ureter may

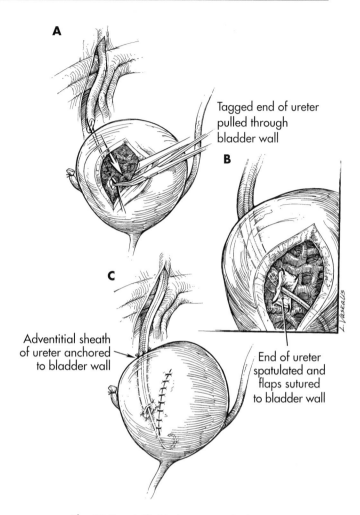

Fig. 46-3   A-C, Ureteroneocystostomy.

be anchored to the outer bladder wall by several 3-0 delayed absorbable sutures.

It is usually unnecessary to stent a ureter when an open, direct ureteroneocystostomy is performed. It is recommended that a ureteral stent (8-Fr double J ureteral catheter or polyethylene or polyurethane drainage tube) be placed if a submucosal tunnel is used.[26] Extraperitoneal drainage of the reimplantation site must be provided, preferably with a silicone closed suction drainage system. After placement of the drain, the opening in the peritoneum about the reimplanted ureter may be closed. A suprapubic or transurethral bladder drainage system is placed, and a two-layer closure of the cystotomy incision is performed using 3-0 absorbable or delayed absorbable suture. The bladder drainage system is usually discontinued after 7 to 10 days unless there is reason to keep the bladder drained longer. The drain from the reimplantation site is removed when there is no drainage or evidence of leaking urine.

URETEROURETEROSTOMY

Ureteroureterostomy is recommended for significant injuries above and just below the pelvic brim. It is often difficult

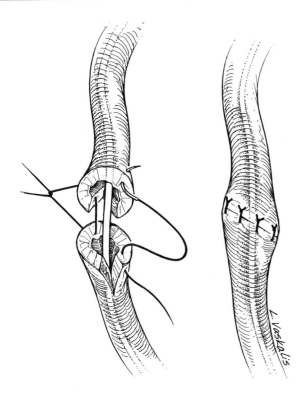

Fig. 46-4 Ureteroureterostomy.

to perform an end-to-end anastomosis on the lower 4 to 5 cm of either ureter; when it is attempted, it is likely to be unsuccessful.

The cut ends of a ureter may be joined when there will be no tension on the anastomosis. This is usually possible if less than 2 cm of ureteral length is lost. The damaged portion of the ureter is excised, and each end is dissected free of the peritoneum. One end of the ureter is spatulated anteriorly, and the opposite end is spatulated posteriorly to help prevent stenosis at the site of the anastomosis.[11] A vertical extraperitoneal cystotomy is performed in the dome of the bladder, and a ureteral catheter (8-Fr double J ureteral catheter or polyurethane or polyethylene drainage tube) is passed through the ureteral orifice up the distal ureteral segment and then up the proximal ureter into the renal pelvis as a stent for the anastomosis and to drain urine from the renal pelvis. The cut ends of the ureter are approximated with four or five interrupted 4-0 absorbable sutures that pass through the adventitial and muscular coats of the ureteral wall. The anastomosis should be watertight but not ischemic (Fig. 46-4). The distal end of the ureteral catheter may be brought out through the anterior bladder and abdominal wall and secured to the abdominal wall or to a suprapubic catheter or, alternatively, through the urethra and secured to a transurethral Foley catheter. An extraperitoneal suction drain should be placed adjacent to, but not touching, the ureteroureteral anastomosis. The catheters may usually be removed after 10 days. The suction drain is removed 24 hours later if there is no evidence of urinary leakage.

Laparoscopic ureteroureterostomy has been described[18];

however, a sufficient number of cases have not been reported to allow a comparison of outcome parameters with those of the traditional approach of open laparotomy.

BLADDER EXTENSION AND MOBILIZATION

When a ureteroneocystostomy or ureteroureterostomy is performed, the ureteral anastomosis *must* be tension free. This may require mobilization of the bladder by severance of the attachments to its anterior wall. A vesicopsoas hitch may be performed to elongate the bladder in the direction of the proposed anastomosis. Bladder flaps of the Boari-Ockerblad[2,19] or Demel[5] type have been recommended for further extension of the bladder fundus toward the site of a ureteral anastomosis, but they may be technically difficult to perform and may be a source of postoperative complications (e.g., flap necrosis, ureteral reflux, stenosis).

The upward mobility of the bladder may be increased to a moderate degree by dissecting the retropubic space (of Retzius) and freeing the dome of the bladder from its loose attachments to the retrosymphysis. This procedure often provides enough mobility of the bladder to relieve minor degrees of tension that may be placed on a ureteral anastomosis or reimplantation site. Downward displacement of the kidney may provide a tension-free anastomosis and bridge a large ureteral gap.

Vesicopsoas Hitch

If there is any question whether there will be tension on the reimplantation or anastomotic site after mobilization of the bladder, a vesicopsoas hitch may be performed to ensure that the reimplantation site is protected. The vesicopsoas hitch should be performed before reimplantation or reanastomosis of the ureter.

To perform a vesicopsoas hitch, one or two fingers are placed through an anterior vertical extraperitoneal cystotomy in the dome of the bladder, which is displaced toward the end of the ureter that is to be reimplanted. The leading point of the outer wall and muscular layer of the bladder are sutured to the psoas major fascia with several interrupted 2-0 or 1-0 delayed absorbable sutures. The bladder must be anchored to the psoas major fascia without undue tension to prevent pressure necrosis about the sutures and premature detachment of the bladder (Fig. 46-5).[11]

Boari-Ockerblad Bladder Flap

The bladder is fully mobilized by lysis of all attachments to its anterior wall. A vesicopsoas hitch is performed on the side of the reimplantation. A full-thickness, wide-based flap with adequate blood supply is cut out of the anterior bladder wall as shown in Fig. 46-6.[2,19] The distal ureter is reimplanted directly or by way of a submucosal tunnel into the upper end of the bladder flap with 4-0 interrupted absorbable or delayed absorbable sutures. The cut edges of the flap are approximated with one layer of interrupted 4-0 or 3-0 absorbable or delayed absorbable sutures.

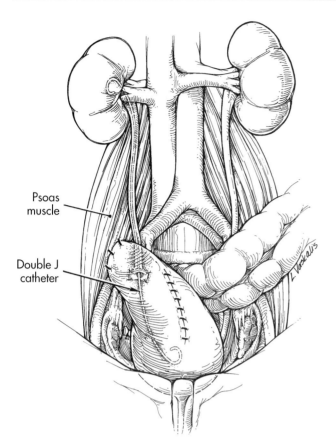

Psoas
muscle

Double J
catheter

Fig. 46-5 Vesicopsoas hitch.

Demel Bladder Flap

The bladder is fully mobilized by lysis of all attachments to its anterior wall. A vesicopsoas hitch is performed on the side of the reimplantation. A curved incision is made about the anterolateral wall of the bladder on the side of the ureteral reimplantation as shown in Fig. 46-7.[5] The distal end of the ureter is reimplanted directly or by way of a submucosal tunnel into the upper end of the bladder flap with 4-0 interrupted absorbable or delayed absorbable sutures. The incision in the bladder is closed with interrupted 4-0 or 3-0 absorbable or delayed absorbable sutures.

TRANSURETEROURETEROSTOMY

Transureteroureterostomy may be performed when there is loss of a significant portion of one of the lower ureters. This technique is technically easy and safe for palliating a difficult situation.[28] Its major disadvantage results from connecting the renal units proximal to the bladder where reflux and infection may damage both kidneys.

During the procedure, the distal end of the injured ureter is tied with a permanent suture at its ureterovesical junction. The proximal ureter is mobilized and carried retroperitoneally below the inferior mesenteric artery and in front of the great vessels to meet the opposite ureter. The recipient ureter is longitudinally incised, and an end-to-side anastomosis is performed using interrupted 4-0 absorbable sutures

placed through the adventitial and muscular layers of both ureters. The anastomosis should be watertight but not ischemic (Fig. 46-8).[11] The anastomotic site should be drained by an extraperitoneal suction drain. Stenting catheters are usually not necessary. The suction catheter is not removed until there is no drainage from the anastomotic site.

URETEROILEONEOCYSTOSTOMY

A segment of ileum can be interposed between a shortened ureter and the bladder. The advantage of this procedure over transureteroureterostomy is its isolation of the two renal units. Hence, infection of one ureterorenal unit does not directly jeopardize the other ureterorenal unit. The disadvantage of ureteroileoneocystostomy involves the creation of a bowel anastomosis.

In performing the procedure, a mobile segment of mid-ileum is selected to easily bridge the gap between the divided ureter and bladder. The mesentery is incised, and its blood vessels are appropriately ligated. Bowel clamps or the automatic gastrointestinal stapler is used to divide the ileum. A defect is created in the colonic mesentery through which the ileal segment is passed posteriorly. Small bowel continuity is then restored anterior to the planned ureteroileal anastomosis.

The ileal segment is irrigated, and the proximal end is sewn closed. The ureter is spatulated and brought through the antimesenteric side of the proximal portion of the ileal segment. An end-to-side mucosa-to-mucosa nontunneled anastomosis is created and secured with four to six interrupted absorbable 4-0 sutures. The anastomosis is performed without tension over a ureteral stent. A circular area of bladder is excised close to the trigone. The distal end of the ileal segment is sewn into the bladder with 3-0 absorbable suture using an end-to-side technique (Fig. 46-9). All anastomoses should be watertight and the surgical site drained. The stent and Foley catheter are left in place for 7 to 10 days.

CUTANEOUS URETEROSTOMY

Cutaneous ureterostomy is the least complicated and also the least permanent of all ureteral diversions. The distal end of the ureter is tied with permanent suture. The cut end of the ureter is brought out retroperitoneally, and a ureteral skin anastomosis is performed.[11] Stenting is usually unnecessary. Cutaneous ureterostomies, which are not considered permanent procedures, may be performed in patients whose chances of survival are expected to be limited or in cases in which the surgeon is not prepared to perform a definitive repair. A ureteral stent may be temporarily brought through the abdominal wall.

URETEROVAGINAL FISTULAS

Advances in endoscopic instrumentation have led to less invasive "endourologic" procedures for the treatment of

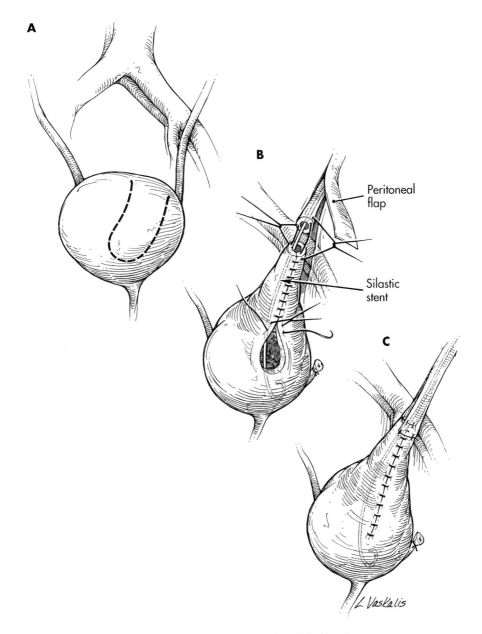

Fig. 46-6   A-C, Boari-Ockerblad bladder flap.

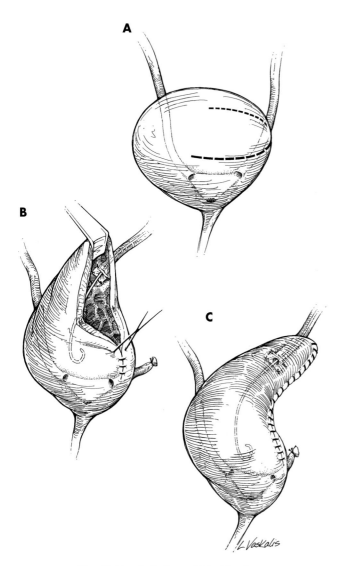

Fig. 46-7   A-C, Demel bladder flap.

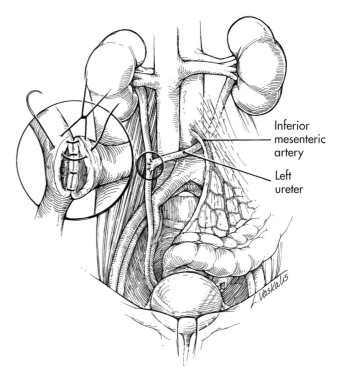

Fig. 46-8   Transureteroureterostomy.

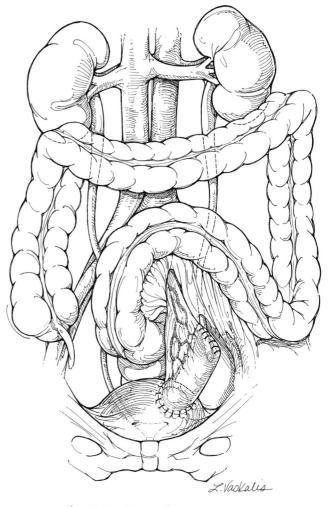

Fig. 46-9   Ureteroileoneocystostomy.

ureteric injuries that are recognized postoperatively. A recent report[9] compared 9 patients undergoing immediate open repair of ureterovaginal fistulas and strictures with 29 patients undergoing delayed open repair and with 25 patients undergoing primary endourologic treatment. The success rates were similar: 87%, 88%, and 90%, respectively. Only patients with unilateral ureteric injuries were treated endourologically.

Postoperative ureterovaginal fistulas are usually repaired transabdominally, either by ureteroneocystostomy or by a lower urinary tract reconstructive procedure. The operative procedure is selected according to the location and the extent of the ureteric injury (see Fig. 46-2). The surgical technique is the same as if the injury was repaired intraoperatively.

FOLLOW-UP OF URETERAL ANASTOMOSES

Prophylactic antibiotics (e.g., a cephalosporin) are recommended until all stents and drains are removed. The extravasation of urine into tissues often leads to infection, impaired healing, and fibrosis and can contribute to ureteral stenosis and loss of kidney function. Intravenous urography should be performed after the repair of ureteral injuries to detect ureteral stenosis and to evaluate kidney function.

REFERENCES

1. Assimos DG, Patterson LC, Taylor CL: Changing incidence and etiology of iatrogenic ureteral injuries, *J Urol* 152:2240, 1994.
2. Boari A: Contributo sperimentale alla plastica dell' uretere, *Atti Acad Sci Med Nat Ferrara* 68:149, 1894.
3. Cruikshank SH: Surgical method of identifying the ureters during total vaginal hysterectomy, *Obstet Gynecol* 67:277, 1986.
4. Daly JW, Higgins KA: Injury to the ureter during gynecologic surgical procedures, *Surg Gynecol Obstet* 167:19, 1988.
5. Demel R: Ersatz des Ureters durch eine Plastik aus der Harnblase (Vorlaufige Mitteilung), *Zentralbl Chir* 51:2008, 1924.
6. Dowling RA, Corriere JN Jr, Sandler CM: Iatrogenic ureteral injury, *J Urol* 135:912, 1986.
7. Eisenkop SM, et al: Urinary tract injury during cesarean section, *Obstet Gynecol* 60:591, 1982.
8. Fry DE, Milholen L, Harbrecht PJ: Iatrogenic ureteral injury, *Arch Surg* 118:454, 1983.
9. Giberti C, et al: Obstetric and gynaecological ureteric injuries: treatment and results, *Br J Urol* 77:21, 1996.
10. Goodno JA Jr, Powers TW, Harris VD: Ureteral injury in gynecologic surgery: a 10-year review in a community hospital, *Am J Obstet Gynecol* 172:1817, 1995.
11. Greenstein A, Koontz WW Jr, Smith MJV: Surgery of the ureter. In Walsh PC et al, editors: *Campbell's urology*, ed 6, Philadelphia, 1991, WB Saunders.
12. Guerriero WG: Ureteral trauma. In Guerriero WG, editor: *Management of acute and chronic urologic injury*, Norwalk, CT, 1984, Appleton-Century-Crofts.
13. Guerriero WG: Ureteral injury, *Urol Clin North Am* 16:237, 1989.
14. Reference deleted in proofs.
15. Manetta A: Surgical maneuver for the prevention of ureteral injuries, *J Gynecol Surg* 5:291, 1989.
16. Mann WJ, et al: Ureteral injuries in obstetrics and gynecology training program: etiology and management, *Obstet Gynecol* 72:82, 1988.
17. Miyazawa K: Urological injuries in gynecological surgery, *Hawaii Med J* 39:11, 1980.
18. Nezhat C, Nezhat F: Laparoscopic repair of ureter resected during operative laparoscopy, *Obstet Gynecol* 80:543, 1992.
19. Ockerblad NF: Reimplantation of the ureter into the bladder by a flap method, *J Urol* 57:845, 1947.
20. Paquin AJ Jr: Ureterovesical anastomosis: the description and evaluation of a technique, *J Urol* 82:573, 1959.
21. Piscitelli JT, Simel DL, Addison WA: Who should have intravenous pyelograms before hysterectomy for benign disease? *Obstet Gynecol* 69:541, 1987.
22. Politano VA, Leadbetter WF: An operative technique for correction of vesicoureteral reflux, *J Urol* 79:932, 1958.
23. Saidi MH, et al: Diagnosis and management of serious urinary complications after major operative laparoscopy, *Obstet Gynecol* 87:272, 1996.
24. Schlossberg SM: Ureteral healing, *Semin Urol* 5:197, 1987.
25. Selzman AA, Spirnak JP: Iatrogenic ureteral injuries: a 20-year experience in treating 165 injuries, *J Urol* 155:878, 1996.
26. Shore ND, Bragg KJ, Sosa RE: Indwelling ureteral stents, *Semin Urol* 5:200, 1987.
27. Solomons E, et al: A pyelographic study of injuries sustained during hysterectomy for benign conditions, *Surg Gynecol Obstet* 111:41, 1960.
28. Strup SE, Sindelar WF, Walther MM: The use of transureteroureterostomy in the management of complex ureteral problems, *J Urol* 155:1572, 1996.
29. Symmonds RE: Ureteral injuries associated with gynecologic surgery: prevention and management, *Clin Obstet Gynecol* 19:623, 1976.
30. Thompson JD, Benigno BB: Vaginal repair of ureteral injuries, *Am J Obstet Gynecol* 3:601, 1971.
31. Witters S, Cornelissen M, Vereecken R: Iatrogenic ureteral injury: aggressive or conservative treatment, *Am J Obstet Gynecol* 155:582, 1986.

47 Repair of Vesicovaginal Fistula

DAVID H. NICHOLS

SURGICAL PRINCIPLES IN BLADDER FISTULA SURGERY

The late Tom Ball[3] described the following surgical principles that are universally applicable to the successful closure of genitourinary fistulas.

1. Surfaces are to be opposed that will require all the factors concerned with the union of tissues to be as near normal as possible. Evaluate the patient's general health and nutrition. Postpone operation until any nutritional deficiencies are corrected by diet and supplementary therapy. Investigate the patient's blood chemistry with attention to plasma proteins, blood sugar, and electrolytes. Latent diabetes should be suspected and a sugar tolerance test performed in patients who have experienced multiple closure failures. The most skillful closure may fail when the essential conditions for proper wound healing are neglected.

2. Infection and the deposition of urinary salts about the edges of the fistula compromise healing. Upper urinary track disease should be eliminated by appropriate study and treatment and the bladder freed of infection by urinary antiseptics. An intravenous pyelogram, cystoscopy, and retrograde studies as indicated should precede the operation. Urine cultures and sensitivity tests—so you know you have one or more agents effective against any organism identified—guide your choice of antibiotics and other urinary antiseptics. The importance of confirming the presence of healthy edges by cystoscopic observation will be apparent to those who attempt a closure only to find themselves inverting tissue into an encrusted bladder mucosa. The preoperative preparation of the fistulous track requires attention to bladder irrigations and vaginal douches. The solutions should be mildly acidic because the deposition of urinary encrustations is most common in patients with alkaline urine. Water intake should be forced despite the discomfort that accompanies the increased output.

3. Study the accessibility of a fistula and the means by which the position on the operating table (lithotomy, Sims, knee-chest) may help bring it into the field. As Kelly said regarding accessibility, "Either the operator must go up to the fistula or the fistula must be brought down to the operator; or a combination of both may be necessary for success."

4. Regardless of how distant the track may seem from the vaginal aspect, it is not, with few exceptions, so far away as it is through a large abdominal panniculus, deep pelvis, and across the bladder through a suprapubic cystotomy. In short, everything favors the vaginal approach to all but a few fistulas. *From the abdomen you operate in the dark so far as the vaginal wall is concerned and at the bottom of a chasm on the bladder wall; from the vagina you see the vaginal wall directly, and the mucosa of the bladder can be visualized as often as necessary by the simplest of endoscopes!*

5. Remember that fistulas in the lateral sulci are accessible only with some risk of damage to the ureter unless this structure is positively identified. Place a catheter in the ureter, if possible, on the side of the fistula, and remove it only when all sutures in the fistula closure have been placed and tied. A small catheter can be left in place as a splint if the particular fistula involves the intramural ureter. If the catheter is removed, the ureteral orifice should be visualized with a simple observation endoscope to note the efflux of urine and whether it contains blood.

6. Schuchardt's incision, correctly performed, makes a high fistula readily accessible.

7. Vesicovaginal fistulas recognized during delivery are closed immediately only if the edges of the tear are clean, not edematous or necrotic, and the patient's condition is good. The frantic closure of a fistula after a long labor, edema and ischemia of the edges, and contamination of the tissue by repeated examinations and instrumentation will most surely result in complete breakdown of the wound and complicate future closure. Exercise restraint because the fistula may close spontaneously or closure may be a simple procedure in a few months.

8. Develop the patience to study, before and during a fistula repair, the direction, density, and firmness of the scar tissue adjacent to the fistula, not only in all directions, but also along its course directly to the bladder or through other structures. Master gynecologic surgeons—renowned for dexterity and speed—have the wisdom to proceed painstakingly and deliberately in performing a fistula repair. Remember that you can observe the pliability of the bladder wall through a cystoscope while manipulating the vaginal aspect of the fistulous track and add to your informa-

tion regarding the direction of forces that may disrupt your repair.

9. Midline vesicovaginal fistulas are best approached by a vertical (in axis of the vagina) incision that circumscribes the vaginal orifice of the fistula. After the separation and mobilization of the vaginal and bladder walls, the bladder is closed transversely and the vaginal wall vertically. By this method the ultimate strain on the suture lines is minimized, and the blood supply is left intact to both layers.

10. Lateral sulcus fistulas of small dimensions are best approached with a transverse vaginal incision because the blood supply to the vagina originates from that direction. A long vertical incision in the lateral vaginal wall, while leaving the lateral vaginal flap of the closure with an intact blood supply, may compromise the medial flap because it would have to receive vessels from above or across the midline.

11. Adequate mobilization of the bladder often requires a total hysterectomy, either vaginal or abdominal. This is necessary to remove a uterus to which the bladder adheres by dense scar tissue that would cause retraction of the edges of the fistula closure if left behind.

12. Fistulas often course through a cervical stump when they are the result of an emergency Porro section or other surgery to stem bleeding. Elimination of the entire fistula is best accomplished by excision of the cervical stump, which effects adequate mobilization of the bladder at the same time.

13. *Study the cause of a fistula and you will learn where to expect its edges to be scarred and retracted!* An example of this is a vault fistula after a total abdominal hysterectomy. The posterior edge of such a fistula is farthest from the introitus and coincides with the transverse scar of the vaginal vault. *This, then, is the segment of the opening that must be carefully mobilized!* In an obliteration type of procedure (Latzko), this must be recognized so that an adequate denudation is done posteriorly to cover the opening that anatomically lies in the anterior vaginal wall just as it is reflected anteriorly from the scar of the closed vaginal vault.

14. Recognize a situation in which the blood supply adjacent to the fistula is so impaired that it requires some type of transplant as an artificial means of providing nourishment to the flaps used in the closure. The gracilis muscle or a Martius graft (bulbocavernosus and vestibular bulb) is a source of a new blood supply.

15. Will the patient have gross urinary stress incontinence from an incompetent bladder neck after a successful fistula closure and thus be little better off than before? Studies of the position of the bladder neck before surgery by urethroscopy and urethrography may anticipate this complication, permitting the surgeon to incorporate some type of bladder neck

plication for restoration of the posterior urethrovesical angle and a competent bladder neck in his or her fistula repair.

16. The principles of bladder fistula surgery that permit approximation of the edges without strangulation or tension are put into effect the moment tissue is touched. Use traction sutures to gain exposure or fix tissues for dissection wherever possible.

17. Crushing instruments must not be used, and *all tissues are delicately handled and as little as possible.*

18. Aim for the approximation of broad, raw, healthy surfaces.

19. When a suture has to be tied under tension, the dissection has been inadequate, and this suture should be removed. It will only cause a sloughing of the immediate area and may doom the entire procedure to failure.

20. The availability of strong, small caliber, and atraumatic suture material has made the use of nonabsorbable material such as silkworm gut and silver or steel wire outmoded. Use small, round-body, atraumatic needles and interrupted sutures throughout. Purse-string, figure-of-eight, and other fancy variations are tissue stranglers and have no place in fistula surgery.

21. Characteristic of the anastomosis in most hollow structures (bowel, ureterovesical and ureterointestinal transplants, vascular surgery), the success of the closure, to a great extent, depends on the approximation of the internal lining of the structure. Strive to approximate mucosa to mucosa, with your sutures passing in the submucosa in the closure of a bladder fistula.

22. Close the bladder and vaginal walls in different planes so that as little as possible of one suture line is superimposed on the other. The exception to this principle is a situation in which such a closure would cause undue tension. The direction of retraction of the edges of the fistula may necessitate closure in the same plane to avoid tension, and this is more important than superimposition of the suture lines.

23. Do not neglect the use of the cystourethroscope during the course of an operation. It is invaluable in determining the proper eversion of healthy tissue and mucosa-to-mucosa approximation within the bladder.

24. A urethral catheter is satisfactory for fistulas in the base of the bladder, provided it does not lay on the suture line. A suprapubic cystotomy is used after an abdominal approach to some fistulas or a combined approach.

25. Postoperatively, the urinary track is kept free of infection by the use of an effective urinary antiseptic or a combination of drugs. The patient's nutrition is important, and appropriate electrolyte studies are done as indicated. Patients should be mobilized immediately and careful attention paid to the avoidance

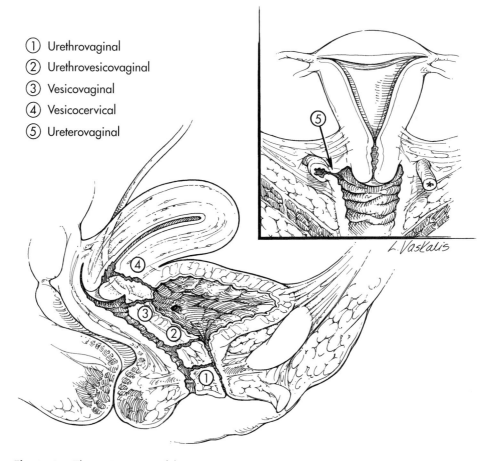

① Urethrovaginal
② Urethrovesicovaginal
③ Vesicovaginal
④ Vesicocervical
⑤ Ureterovaginal

L. Vaskalis

Fig. 47-1 The various sites of the more commonly seen urogenital fistulas are shown in sagittal section. A combination of fistulas is possible, and the tracks may course through several structures. Vesicouterine, vesicocervicovaginal, urethrovesicovaginal, and ureterovaginal fistulas are indicated. One or more fistulas may exist at the same time.

of straining to evacuate the bowel, coughing, or sneezing. Complete immobilization of the patient would seem to add little to the chance of successful closure because the patients still have to strain to evacuate their bowels.

In younger patients who have a history of urinary loss, particularly in those with evidence of congenital malformation of the genitalia, the surgeon must thoroughly inspect both the urinary track and the genital track. Intravenous pyelography may be the only way to determine whether the patient has an aberrant or third ureter opening into the vagina. It is equally important to confirm that the patient with a urinary fistula has two patent, normally placed ureters. If the patient has only a single kidney and ureter, the surgeon should certainly be aware of this fact before planning and undertaking repair of the fistula. The surgeon should also determine the relationship of the fistula to the ureteral orifices, bladder neck, and trigone by means of preoperative cystoscopy.

Trauma, necrosis secondary to invasion by neoplastic growth, or rarely the reaction to certain types of necrotizing inflammation, may lead to fistulas involving the female urinary track and genitalia. Genital track trauma is by far the most common cause.

Some possible locations of urinary fistulas are shown in Fig. 47-1. The cause, diagnosis, and treatment of each type of fistula is distinctive enough that the surgeon must be familiar with each one, bearing in mind that a patient may have more than one at a given time.

ACCIDENTAL INJURY TO ADJACENT STRUCTURES

Because unrecognized or unrepaired full-thickness trauma in the urinary or intestinal system usually results in the formation of a fistula, it is essential for the surgeon who is performing any gynecologic operation or obstetric procedure to recognize immediately any penetration of a neighboring viscus. The presence of a *small* amount of urine in the bladder is desirable at the time of *vaginal hysterectomy or anterior colporrhaphy* because its appearance in the operative field alerts the surgeon to a penetrating injury. Any suspicion of such an injury must be investigated thoroughly and an appropriate repair done without delay. Although the incidence of accidental penetration is small and becomes smaller as the experience of the surgeon increases, unexpected relationships may occasionally lead to accidental injuries no matter how often a surgeon operates.

Preoperatively, the surgeon should consider all sites of possible accidental trauma, such as an undesirable laceration, avulsion, or unwanted incision of nearby pelvic organs.

Any suspected injury must be evaluated and treated promptly. A problem that is neglected intraoperatively may eventually necessitate one or more secondary surgical procedures, which can be as damaging to the surgeon's reputation as to the patient's health. There is no room for procrastination in the hope that the suspected damage did not occur or will resolve itself. Therefore, as soon as any injury is recognized, the surgeon should mobilize the tissues sufficiently to accomplish the repair under direct vision. The remainder of the operation can then proceed as planned. The effective management of such problems requires candor, scientific objectivity, and confident surgical technique.

One indication of a possible bladder injury during the course of surgery is the escape of a recognizable urinelike fluid into the vagina. Therefore it is desirable that some urine remains in the bladder during vaginal surgery. Patients about to undergo vaginal surgery should be asked to void shortly before they come to the operating suite and then should be catheterized at the beginning of surgery only if bimanual examination reveals bladder overdistention.

It is best to repair a visceral injury with two or three layers of fine absorbable suture (e.g., 3-0 polydioxanone, polyg-lyconate, polyglycolic acid [PGA] type, or chromic catgut). In the repair of injuries to the bladder or ureter, however, knots should be extraluminal to reduce the risk of calculus formation at the site of the suture. Accurate approximation of the submucosal muscular layers must provide the primary support in these cases; although mucosal sutures are hemostatic, they supply minimal support. A layer of watertight running horizontal mattress sutures in the muscular layer inverts the previous stitches, and another layer of interrupted reinforcing mattress stitches may be added, if desired, to reduce the tension on the deeper layer (Fig. 47-2). The surgeon must always be careful to avoid tying mattress sutures so tightly as to strangulate the tissues involved.

After a recognized penetration in the bladder wall is repaired, the surgeon may test the repair for watertightness by instilling a methylene blue solution, an indigo carmine solution, or sterile milk (e.g., evaporated milk, canned condensed milk, infant formula milk from the nursery) and checking for leakage. (Sterile milk has the obvious advantage over dyes in that the leakage of milk does not cause prolonged staining of adjacent tissues.) If there is evidence of leakage at the initial repair, the surgeon should place additional reinforcing sutures and again test the repair for leakage. If the wall of the bladder is penetrated near its attachment to the cervix, the adjacent peritoneum can be mobilized and sewn over the site of the repair after the defect in the musculature has been repaired; such a peritoneal flap provides support and increases the blood supply to the area (see Fig. 47-2, *D*).

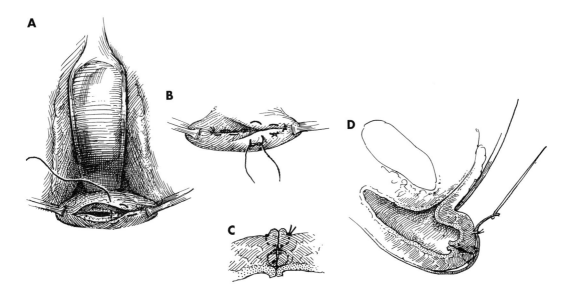

Fig. 47-2 Closure of accidental cystotomy is depicted. The defect has been identified and widely mobilized. A suture tagging the peritoneum is noted on the right side of **D.** If no mucosal stitch is used, a running mattress suture in the muscularis, starting and finishing lateral to the defect, may be placed as shown in **A.** This may be covered by a second layer of interrupted mattress sutures **(B),** establishing full-thickness reapproximation of the muscularis as seen in cross-section **(C).** An anterior peritoneal flap has been excised from the anterior surface of the uterus as shown **(D)** and tacked in place over the operative repair, providing the security of an additional fresh tissue layer. (From Nichols DH, Randall CL: *Vaginal surgery,* ed 4, Baltimore, 1996, Williams & Wilkins.)

If the ureteral orifices are near or part of an accidental laceration, the surgeon should insert ureteral catheters. Ureteroneocystostomy is advisable if the integrity of the ureters cannot be ensured.

If the ureter is transected, as may occur inadvertently when the patient has an undiagnosed duplication of the ureter on one or both sides, the severed ureter can be successfully reimplanted under direct vision. Postoperative splinting with both ureteral and urethral catheters is desirable for 2 weeks.

A fistula that follows an obstetric laceration should be repaired within 24 hours of the injury. However, if a fistula develops after hysterectomy or if the first attempt to repair a fistula fails the surgeon may allow 3 to 6 months to pass so that adequate lymphatic drainage can return to the tissue and the infection, swelling, and edema of surgery can subside. If necrosis and edema subside earlier, immediate repair should be considered.[24,27,28] If the fistula results from necrosis after irradiation, the vagina should be given local estrogen supplementation by transvaginal instillation of estrogen cream (1 to 2 g at bedtime, two or three times weekly) and the repair postponed for at least 1 year to permit progression of the causative endarteritis obliterans to cease.[29]

While awaiting the appropriate time for the repair of a fistula, the patient can obtain some temporary but welcome relief by wearing an intravaginal contraceptive diaphragm,[4,5,20,36] the center of which has been perforated by a 3-mm hole through which the tip of a Foley catheter has been inserted. The balloon is inflated with 5 to 10 ml of air and the base of the balloon cemented by a cyanoacrylate watertight glue or cement to the inside of the diaphragm to create a watertight seal. After the adhesive has dried for 15 minutes, the diaphragm can be inserted into the vagina and connected to a urinary leg bag. It has been recommended that an estrogen cream be applied to the edges of the diaphragm each time it is inserted to minimize trauma and that the diaphragm be removed for several hours every few days, either at night or during the day, to avoid vaginal ulceration. The resulting improvement makes it easier for the patient to wait until the condition of the tissues is optimal for surgical repair. Although some authorities recommend cortisone treatment to accelerate tissue preparation for surgery, it seems preferable to wait the length of time required for inflammation and edema to subside and not compromise wound healing by coincident steroid use, which may precipitate premature absorption of sutures.

Thompson and others[24,27,28] have described a technique of transvaginal repair of the distal ureter (i.e., along its lowest 3 cm). Ureteral catheters are inserted transurethrally, if possible. Palpation of the tip of this catheter identifies the area where operative exposure must be obtained. The proximal ureter is identified (if necessary, by the passage of urine made blue by an injection of intravenous indigo carmine) and dissected free. If the stump of a transected ureter is long enough to permit ureteroureteral anastomosis without tension, a series of four 4-0 PGA sutures are placed through the

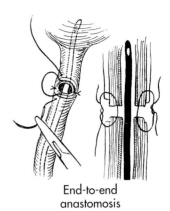

End-to-end
anastomosis

Fig. 47-3 Ureteroureterostomy. Damage may be treated by ureteroureterostomy if there are unmistakably viable segments above and below the injury, and the ureter can be anastomosed without tension. The ends are brought together with interrupted sutures of 4-0 PGA or chromic catgut on atraumatic needles. The sutures should not pass into the lumen and should accurately approximate mucosa to mucosa. The anastomosis may also be done side-to-side or end-to-side. An end-to-end anastomosis restores the normal course of the ureter—a surgical principle that is observed when possible. A small splinting catheter is left in place. (From Ball TL: *Gynecologic surgery and urology*, ed 2, St Louis, 1963, Mosby, p 542.)

muscularis (stent in place) (Fig. 47-3) and tied, establishing a ureteroureteral anastomosis. If the vesical stump of ureter is too short to be used safely, it is ligated and a ureteroneocystostomy is performed.

Technique of Transvaginal Ureteroneocystostomy

A small cystotomy is made that is large enough to permit retrieval of the vesical end of the ureteral catheter (or infant-sized plastic feeding tube as a substitute for the ureteral catheter), which has been introduced into the bladder through the urethra. The internal tip is brought out through the cystotomy wound and inserted into the lumen of the cut end of the proximal ureter. The stent is advanced along the ureteral lumen for several centimeters. The tip of the proximal ureter is spatulated or fish-mouthed for about 1 cm on each side, and a 3-0 or 4-0 PGA suture is placed through the full thickness of the ureteral wall (Fig. 47-4). Both ends of each suture are sewn through the full thickness of the bladder mucosa and muscularis, one set on each side of the cystotomy, and gentle traction is applied to them, drawing the spatulated end of the ureter into the bladder (Fig. 47-5). The transmural sutures are tied, fixing the ureter in place. Tension on the anastomosis is reduced by placing several circumferential interrupted PGA sutures that fix the external surface of the implanted ureter to the bladder muscularis. (A "psoas hitch" to the bladder to achieve this is not possible with this transvaginal operative exposure.) If the site of ureteral repair or anastomosis cannot be covered by the flap of anterior vaginal wall, a Martius graft (see Fig. 47-15) can be readily obtained and transposed into place.

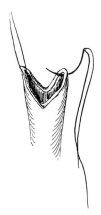

Fig. 47-4 Ureteroneocystostomy. A fish-mouth incision is made in the terminal ureter and traction sutures of 4-0 PGA or chromic catgut are placed in the edge of each flap. (From Ball TL: *Gynecologic surgery and urology*, ed 2, St Louis, 1963, Mosby, p 542.)

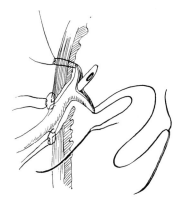

Fig. 47-5 The ureter is drawn into the bladder, and the traction sutures are threaded on fine needles and passed through the adjacent bladder wall to anchor the flaps. These are tied on the outside to just approximate the tissues without strangulation. A few sutures are used to anchor the ureter at the point of entrance into the bladder wall. They should be placed in the adventitia of the ureter and into the bladder wall without constricting the anastomosis. (From Ball TL: *Gynecologic surgery and urology*, ed 2, St Louis, 1963, Mosby, p 542.)

The vagina is packed, and the ureteral stent is taped to a transurethral Foley catheter. A postoperative intravenous pyelogram is obtained, and another is ordered on an outpatient basis 2 to 3 weeks after removal of the stent. The pyelogram may be repeated periodically for several years in an attempt to ensure the integrity of the anastomosis and absence of progressive hydroureter-hydronephrosis that would suggest ureteral stricture.

With an absorbent tampon in place within the vagina, 100 ml of dilute Congo red solution may be instilled into the bladder through a transurethral catheter. The catheter is removed, and the patient is instructed to stand and move around. After ½ hour, the vaginal tampon is removed and inspected. If the tip of the tampon is stained red, the dye will be presumed to have come from the Congo red, and the presence of a vesicovaginal fistula is likely. If the tampon is not stained, a fresh one is inserted into the vagina and the patient is given 5 ml of indigo carmine intravenously. The second tampon is removed after ½ hour and inspected. If the tip of the second tampon is stained blue, the dye will have come from the intravenous indigo carmine, and the presence of a vesicovaginal fistula should be suspected.

VESICOVAGINAL FISTULA

A history of low cervical cesarean section is a factor predisposing to the development of a vesicovaginal fistula after hysterectomy because cesarean section may alter tissue relationships between the bladder and the cervix, thus increasing the risk of inadvertent injury during hysterectomy. When a patient who has had a cesarean section must undergo hysterectomy, it is helpful to instill 60 ml of indigo carmine or methylene blue solution into the bladder preoperatively because it stains the mucosa. The violet-stained bladder mucosa can sometimes be seen *before* the bladder is opened, and violet-stained urine in the operative field is a priori evidence of unwanted penetration. Approximately 20% of the present generation of parous women who will require hysterectomy in the future will have a history of previous cesarean section.

When a vesicovaginal fistula develops after a hysterectomy, it is likely to be at the very apex of the vagina if the vaginal cuff was not closed or just anterior to the suture line if the vaginal cuff was closed. A vesicovaginal fistula in the lower vagina is more likely to occur after colporrhaphy.

A fistula first recognized after hysterectomy is usually the result of unrecognized penetration or laceration at the time of the primary operation, the result of trauma recognized but inadequately repaired, or sometimes the result of postoperative necrosis of a small area of bladder epithelium secondary to an infected hematoma or to devascularization by a suture placed into or immediately adjacent to the lumen of the bladder. Carelessly faced hemostatic mattress sutures in the bladder wall near the cut edge in the vagina may devitalize the spot of tissue in which they have been placed. In addition, incomplete surgical separation from the vaginal cuff during hysterectomy places the bladder at risk.

The presence of hematuria after the initial operative procedure should alert the surgeon to the possibility of a subsequent fistula, particularly if the bloody urine persists for longer than 48 hours after the operation. When this occurs, inspection by cystoscopy is advisable, and catheter drainage should usually continue for a number of days beyond the usual period until 48 hours from the time microscopic hematuria has disappeared. When a fistulous track, even a small one, is relatively short, the patient is usually incontinent. When the fistulous track is longer, especially if it is tortuous, the patient is likely to be incontinent only intermittently because the flow of urine through the track may be inversely proportional to the amount of urine within the bladder. If the fresh vesicovaginal fistula is tiny and urinary leakage ceases when a transurethral catheter is in place, it may heal spontaneously during 2 months of transurethral catheter drainage providing constant bladder decompression. Having the patient continuously wear a standard deeply placed intravaginal menstrual tampon will supply pressure from beneath the vaginal site of the fistula, helping keep it closed. If, on the other hand, the fistula leaks with the catheter in place and draining, spontaneous healing is unlikely and surgical repair should be promptly undertaken.[31] In addition, patients with this type of fistula are often prone to infection and calculus formation along the track. The presence of an intermittent spontaneous bloody urethral or urinary discharge is ominous, requiring evaluation and biopsy to rule out the presence of malignant disease, which may be coexisting with the fistulous track.

Miller[18] reports a useful method for diagnosing an obscure or very small vesicovaginal fistula: A Foley catheter with a 75-ml balloon is placed in the vagina, and the balloon is inflated to occlude the vaginal orifice. A cystoscope is inserted into the partly filled bladder, and a solution of methylene blue or indigo carmine is injected under pressure into the proximal vagina. A thin stream of dye will be seen, confirming and pinpointing the location of a small fistula, and its relationship to the trigone and ureteral orifices can be evaluated precisely.

Preoperative Considerations

The gynecologic surgeon must always consider the possibility of multiple fistulas when investigating a recognized fistula. Obviously, the surgical correction of the recognized fistula will not eliminate incontinence resulting from an unrecognized and thus unrepaired coexistent fistula. Both the surgeon and the patient may believe that the treatment failed when the apparent failure may be the result of the inadequacy of the preoperative study and appraisal. Careful review of the history and circumstances preceding the recognition of a fistula is essential.

Differentiation between a vesicovaginal and a ureterovaginal fistula is of primary importance. In making this distinction, many surgeons find that the tampon test is helpful.[10] A rather long menstrual tampon is inserted into the vagina, and 6 to 8 ounces of strongly colored methylene blue or indigo carmine solution is then injected into the bladder. The patient is instructed to walk around for 10 or 15 minutes, after which the tampon is examined. If only the lowest part is wet and blue, the patient presumably has urinary stress incontinence or detrusor instability; if the upper thirds are wet and blue, the patient probably has a vesicovaginal fistula; if the upper third is wet but not blue, the diagnosis is a damaged ureter.

General Principles of Repair

Several excellent techniques are available for the repair of a vesicovaginal fistula, and they are adaptable to a variety of clinical circumstances. There are also certain general principles that a surgeon should consistently adhere to in performing a urinary fistula repair, however. The surgeon should do the following:

1. Supplement or replace estrogen preoperatively and postoperatively if the patient is postmenopausal.
2. Postpone the repair until infection and inflammation have subsided, and healthy granulation tissue may be present.
3. Dissect, mobilize, and excise the epithelialized track and adjacent seat tissue until healthy, normal tissue is reached, thus converting the lesion to a fresh wound. As a rule, a fresh wound of bladder or rectum heals promptly and primarily if the initial repair is adequate and appropriate. It should be closed without tension.
4. Make lateral vaginal relaxing incisions if the repair has been closed under tension.
5. Try to interrupt the continuity of the fistulous track so that the orifice of repair in one viscus no longer overlies or underlies its counterpart in the other.
6. Approximate anatomically strong layers or flaps, and when available, interpose between the previous fistulous orifices a strong tissue layer that has an independent blood supply.
7. When infection or abscess formation is likely, provide adequate drainage of the low-pressure side of the previous track.
8. Catheterize the ureter at the time of the repair if it is adjacent to or incorporated in the fistula to avoid unintentional operative ureteral stricture. If the repair seems likely to compromise the ureter, a coincident ureteroneocystostomy may be desirable.
9. Decompress the bladder by catheter postoperatively. If the inflated bulb of a transurethral Foley catheter would touch the bladder side of the fistula, possibly interfering with the healing process, the catheter may be placed suprapubically (Fig. 47-6).

Techniques of Repair

Electrosurgical or chemical cautery of a very small fistulous opening may destroy the epithelial lining of the track and permit spontaneous healing in a small percentage of tiny fistulae.[7] Coagulation must be followed by immediate decompression of the bladder and constant drainage for 2 to 3 weeks. This technique is most likely to be effective when the fistula is only 1 or 2 mm in diameter, follows an oblique course, and has thick, healthy bladder wall around it, as may be seen after the inadvertent placement of a stitch through the bladder wall.

Most vesicovaginal fistulas seen in patients of the Western world occur after hysterectomy and are located in the vaginal vault just anterior to the scar representing the site where the cervix had been located. Most can be repaired by a transvaginal approach. Some complex and recurrent fistulas may be better treated by a transabdominal approach, and the O'Conor technique[21,22] (Fig. 47-7, *A* through *E*) is my procedure of choice. If there is any question during surgery about the integrity of the repair or its good blood supply, a

Text continued on p. 875

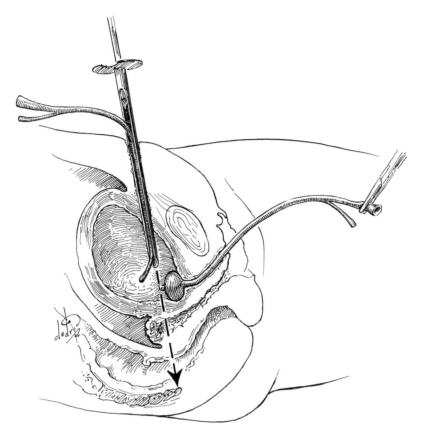

Fig. 47-6   Suprapubic cystostomy. The bladder has been distended by 400 ml of sterile saline solution instilled through a transurethral Foley catheter, shown in place and clamped. At a midline point 2 fingerbreadths above the superior border of the pubis, a no. 22 spinal needle was introduced through the anterior abdominal and bladder wall and pointed toward the coccyx. When a free flow of clear urine has been observed, the needle is immediately removed and a 1.5-cm transverse incision through the skin only is made using a no. 12 scalpel blade at the site of the needle puncture. The surgeon, having noted the approximate depth at which the spinal needle entered the bladder, bluntly introduces the Campbell trocar in the same direction until the characteristic "give" is noted. The sharply pointed obturator of the trocar is withdrawn about 1 inch, the blunt end of the sleeve is inserted an additional 1 to 2 inches, and the obturator is removed. There is prompt escape of urine and saline, and immediately a no. 16 Foley catheter is inserted through the trocar into the bladder as shown. The 5-ml bulb is inflated, the trocar is removed, and a brief tug on the catheter until resistance is encountered brings the now inflated bulb to the undersurface of the fresh cystostomy. (From Nichols DH, Milley PS: *Ob/Gyn Digest* 12:30, 1970.)

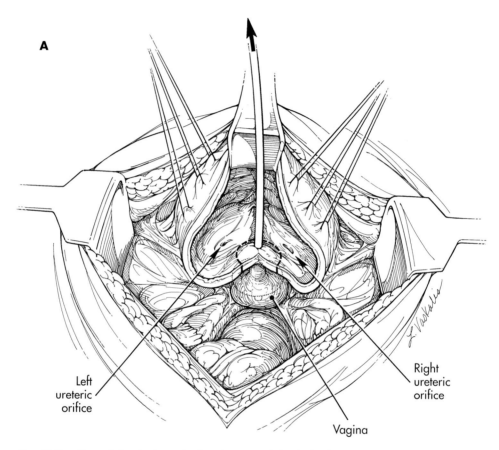

A

Left
ureteric
orifice

Right
ureteric
orifice

Vagina

Fig. 47-7   Transabdominal repair of vesicovaginal fistula by the O'Conor technique. **A,** The
abdomen has been opened and explored. Three guide sutures are placed in the bladder muscularis, as shown, and the bladder is opened by a generous midline incision providing adequate exposure of the trigone. The fistula has been identified, a Foley catheter is placed
through it from the bladder into the vagina as shown, and the bulb is inflated. The ureters may
be separately catheterized if desired. The fistulous track is circumcised by an incision indicated by the dashed line.

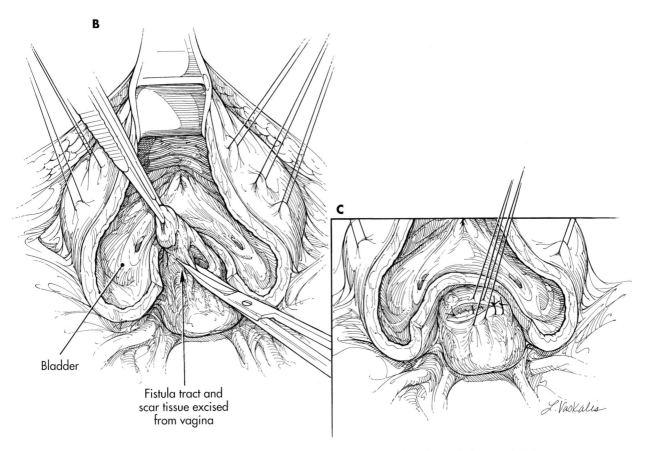

B

Bladder

Fistula tract and
scar tissue excised
from vagina

C

L. Vaskalis

Fig. 47-7, cont'd   **B,** A total excision of the fistulous track is performed after careful sharp dissection of the bladder from the underlying vagina. **C,** The vagina is closed separately by a series of interrupted sutures. If desired, a flap of omentum may be brought down and sewn in place between the vagina and bladder at the site of the previous fistula.

Continued

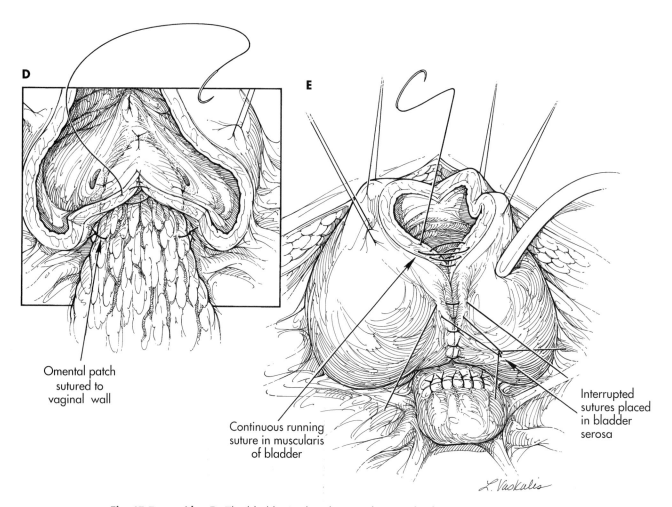

D

Omental patch
sutured to
vaginal wall

Continuous running
suture in muscularis
of bladder

E

Interrupted
sutures placed
in bladder
serosa

L. Vaskalis

Fig. 47-7, cont'd D, The bladder is closed in two layers. The first is a running stitch in the
muscularis. **E,** This is followed by a second layer of interrupted stitches at the "serosal surface,"
and a suprapubic cystostomy with placement of a Foley catheter is shown.

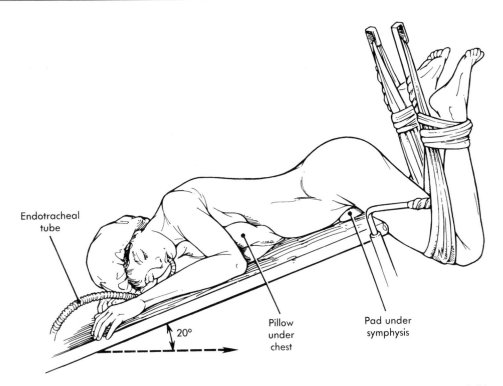

Fig. 47-8   Lawson's[15] prone position to improve the surgeon's view of the operative field when a vesicovaginal fistula is adherent to the pubic symphysis.

tip of omentum may be transposed and anchored in place between the bladder repair and that of the vagina.[29]

Most experienced gynecologic surgeons repair vesicovaginal fistulas by a transvaginal approach.[14,19,32] The transabdominal route is reserved for very unusual situations in which mobility is limited, the ureter is involved, earlier repeated attempts to repair the fistula have failed, or the fistula has developed in tissues previously irradiated.[19,24,25]

As Moir[19] has written, ". . . the vaginal operation is, from the patient's point of view, relatively simple; and, if need should arise, it can be repeated without much ado. This last argument can be epitomized by the cynical and doubtless exaggerated comments: 'The surgeon who chooses to operate on a vesicovaginal fistula through the abdominal wall is the surgeon who would remove a child's tonsils by dissecting through an incision in the side of the neck.' "

Rarely, after persistent or recurrent malignancy has been ruled out as a possible cause for the fistula, a transvaginal fistula repair will be chosen for a patient who had previously received radiation therapy. Generous and frequent applications of intravaginal estrogen cream should be given to such a patient for 1 month before surgery to thicken the vagina and for 1 month after surgery to promote healing. However, the surgeon generally will wish to insulate the fistula repair during the prolonged healing time by either a Martius bulbocavernosus fat pad transplant (if the patient has fleshy and thick labia majora)[6,17] or a gracilis muscle transplant as practiced by Ingelman-Sundberg[11] and described by Ball.[3]

A few special instruments can be very helpful for fistula repair, such as a pair of fine dissecting scissors, right-angled scissors, Sims hooks, and Sims or Breisky retractors. A small suction tip is desirable. A variety of scalpel blades and handles should also be available to the surgeon, particularly the no. 11- and no. 15-type blades and the no. 7-type scalpel handle. It is also extremely helpful to have a flexible operative schedule that allows the surgeon as much time as necessary for the particular reconstruction because the length of time required for an adequate operation is not always predictable.

Adequate exposure of the fistula is of paramount importance. If for any reason the exaggerated lithotomy position does not provide adequate exposure, as when the fistula is found to be fibrosed to the symphysis pubis, it may be necessary to use the knee-chest position or even the jackknife or Kraske position, in which the patient is face down with the hips well flexed, the table bent at this point, and extra padding supplied under the hips[15,23] (Fig. 47-8). This enables the surgeon to look down on the fistula. Adequate, well-focused lighting is equally important; at times the surgeon may find it advantageous to wear a forehead fiberoptic light to concentrate illumination and reduce annoying shadows.

The gynecologic surgeon should examine both sides of the fistulous track in choosing the appropriate procedure for the repair of a genital fistula. This examination will reveal the size of each aperture and will afford the surgeon a better opportunity to appraise scarring, fibrosis, and the possibility of multiple openings.

When biopsy of any suspicious area in the margin of the postirradiation fistula has excluded active malignancy, successful repair generally requires not only the delicate han-

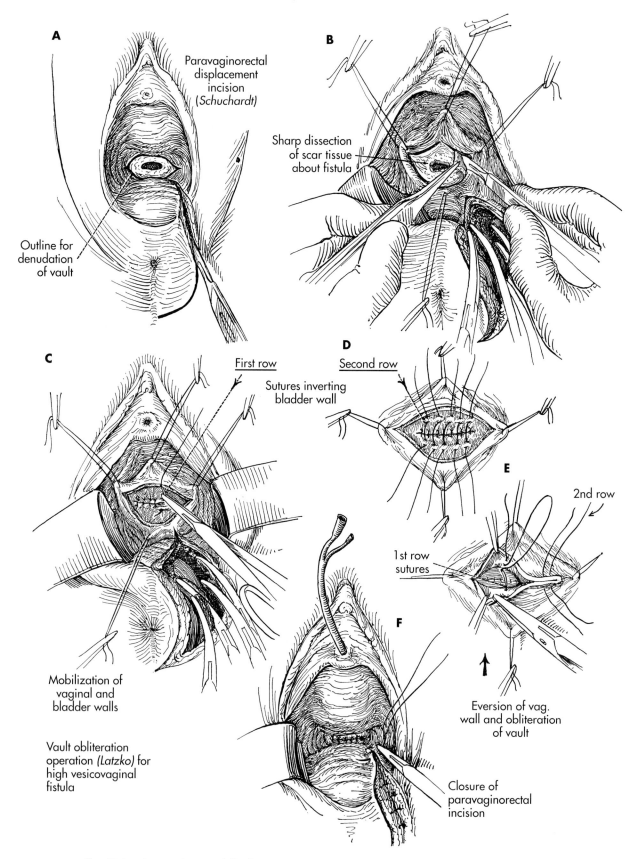

Fig. 47-9 Paravaginorectal displacement incision (Schuchardt) and Latzko closure of a vesicovaginal fistula. This technique of making the upper vagina accessible for fistula closure or radical surgery has been poorly understood. Many surgeons make a superficial cut in the perineum to permit the introduction of a larger retractor and describe this as the operation originally described by Schuchardt. Correctly performed, a paravaginorectal incision displaces the

vagina and rectum to the left (for right-handed surgeons) and changes the vagina from a tubular structure to a wide-open field of operation. This incision provides wide exposure of the operative field from the introitus to a point a few centimeters distal to the fistula. It extends posteriorly and laterally along the extensions of the obturator fascia on the levator ani. It is impossible not to cut some of the fibers of the levator muscles that pass posteriorly. The tissues to be incised may be infiltrated by no more than 50 ml of 0.5% lidocaine in 1 : 200,000 epinephrine—the "liquid tourniquet"—to reduce blood loss. Make an incision in the left lateral sulcus of the vagina about 6 cm above the introitus and carry it down through the full thickness of the vaginal wall. Continue this to the vulva, curving more laterally after the edge of the puborectalis is passed. At the mucocutaneous junction the incision is continued in a half circle about the anus to the midline posteriorly. It should clear the anus by at least 3 cm to avoid any fibers of the external sphincter ani muscle **(A)**. The incision is now carried deeper along the lateral wall of the rectum. Bleeding points from the inferior and middle hemorrhoidal vessels will be numerous and require ligation. The extension of the incision to the deeper layers in the perineum will cut the superficial and deep layers of the urogenital diaphragm, and the anal, deep, and superficial transverse perineal branches of the pudendal artery, vein, and nerve. Retractors are placed on either side to further expose the vaginal vault. The rectum and vagina tend to fall caudad from loss of support and in this way bring the vaginal vault closer to the surgeon **(C)**. The incision (after completion of the fistula repair) is closed in layers, using 2-0 chromic catgut **(F)**. Dead space is avoided particularly where the incision has opened up the ischiorectal fossa. Vault obliteration operation *(Latzko)*. **A,** Shows the outline for denudation of the vault about the area of the fistula. The scar tissue about the fistula is completely excised from both the vaginal and bladder walls. This excision should be carried a sufficient distance from the edges of the fistula to ensure removal of all the scar tissue even though it is anticipated that the vault will be shortened **(B)**. The vaginal and bladder walls are mobilized for some distance from the fistula. The bladder wall is then inverted toward the interior of the bladder by two rows of sutures of 4-0 PGA or chromic catgut on atraumatic needles **(C and D)**. The vaginal vault is partially obliterated by eversion of the vaginal wall toward the vaginal aspect. This is accomplished by two rows of sutures as shown in **E.** These sutures are placed so that broad, healthy surfaces oppose each other as the incision heals. The paravaginorectal incision is closed in layers **(F)**. (From Ball TL: *Gynecologic surgery and urology,* ed 2, St Louis, 1963, Mosby, p 232.)

---

dling and approximation of tissue but also the introduction of a new layer of tissue that will provide a new blood supply to the organs involved. If the labia are fleshy, it may be possible to obtain from them a bulbocavernosus fat pad for this new layer.[6] If the labial tissues are atrophic, a nonirradiated graft of omentum, with its blood supply intact, may be brought down and sutured in place to provide the new blood supply and the necessary insulation[29] (see Chapter 49).

Latzko Technique. If the patient has a deep vagina and a posthysterectomy fistula at the very apex of the vagina, the simplest and most effective operative repair is often the Latzko colpocleisis.[16,23,25] This technique is also useful for a small residual vault fistula that remains after the closure of a larger fistula. If there is any problem with exposure of the fistula, a preliminary episiotomy or Schuchardt-type incision (Fig. 47-9, *A*) is strongly recommended to improve accessibility and ensure visibility of the fistula.

It is not necessary or even desirable to excise the fistulous track into the bladder because the edges will be coapted in a linear fashion when the supporting tissues in the fibromuscular vaginal wall have been placed and tied. Furthermore, the location of this fistula after hysterectomy is such that it will be near the bladder trigone and not in the area of bladder that would expand and contract with normal bladder function. The ureters are not generally a part of the fistula, and the repair is in the fibromuscular wall of the vagina, well removed from the ureters, so ureteral catheterization is superfluous. By the same token, all vesicovaginal fistula repairs benefit from immediate postoperative inspection of this bladder by cystoscopy after injection of intravenous indigo carmine and waiting for it to appear at the ureteral orifice on each side, guaranteeing ureteral patency.

The insertion of a small or pediatric Foley catheter (no. 8) into the bladder through the fistula itself may facilitate the mobilization of a fistulous track. When the bulb on the catheter is inflated, the catheter not only serves as an identifying handle but also makes it possible to apply traction on the fistula in all directions.[12] If the fistulous opening is not big enough to permit the entry of a small Foley catheter, the surgeon can gently enlarge the opening by spreading the tips of a small hemostat or inserting a small Hegar dilator. Infiltration of the area with dilute epinephrine-lidocaine solution has a hemostatic effect; in addition, the local hemostatic effect of using small sponges (e.g., wisps, pushers, "peanuts") soaked in an epinephrine solution often improves visibility, especially when the surgeon is dissecting and mobilizing the healthy mucosal tissue. There may

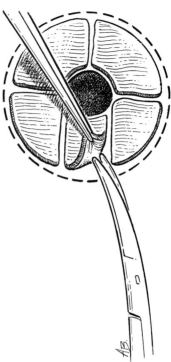

Fig. 47-10 Ueda's[30] alternative method of closing a large fistula.[15] The vaginal wall around the fistula is divided into five sections as shown. Four are removed, but the fifth, the width of the fistula, is developed as a flap. (From Nichols DH, Randall CL: *Vaginal surgery,* ed 4, Baltimore, 1996, Williams & Wilkins.)

be considerable oozing, but few vessels are large enough to require clamping and tying.

In this technique (see Fig. 47-9, *B*), the surgeon excises a 1.5- to 2-cm disk—*of only the superficial and middle layers of the vaginal epithelium*—from around the fistulous opening, which denudes but does not remove all the full thickness of the vaginal epithelium. (If the *full* thickness of both epithelium and fibromuscular layers of the vaginal wall were removed, the remaining soft muscular wall of the bladder muscle around the fistula might be too fragile to support the deeper layers of suture to be placed, and the repair might fail.) When approximated by suture, the disk effectively closes the area turned into the bladder lumen, where it will be subsequently covered by a process of vesical epithelialization. It is essential for the surgeon to excise outward from the line of the initial incision a disk of the more *superficial layers* of the vaginal membrane wide enough to ensure that the deeper fibromuscular tissue layer (i.e., vaginal wall denuded of superficial epithelium by excision of the epithelial disk) can be brought together as a thickened supporting layer beneath the segment of vaginal membrane that is being invaginated into the bladder lumen (see Fig. 47-9, *C*). Dissection of the bladder from the vagina at the vaginal vault may be difficult because usually there is no vesicovaginal space at this site—just one fused layer of vagina and bladder base. This is in contrast to the dissection in the midvagina where the two layers, bladder and vagina, can be identified and closed separately and independently. The excised disk of vaginal epithelium should be ovoid rather than round, usually with the long axis of the ovoid transverse across the vault so that the infolding of a portion of the vaginal wall does not constrict the vaginal caliber. When the depth of the vagina is likely to be more critical than the di-

ameter, the long axis and repair of the denuded ovoid of connective tissue that surrounds the invaginated segment of vaginal membrane can parallel the length rather than the width of the vagina.

The sutures of the first layer should be placed to bring together the narrow margins of preserved vaginal membrane around the fistula in what should effectively serve as a subcuticular closure of the denuded segment of vaginal wall, precluding a postoperative bladder diverticulum. Results are best if (1) mobilization is sufficient to permit approximation of the supporting connective tissue layer with no tension and with no irregular buckling of the surfaces as they are brought together, obliterating the angle at each side of the vault, and (2) no suture material goes into the lumen of the urinary track or through both bladder and vaginal walls into the lumen of the vagina.

If the bladder opening is too large to close from side to side without unusual tension, the surgeon may transpose a flap of vaginal wall to cover the defect (Figs. 47-10 and 47-11).[30] The instillation of sterile milk or infant formula into the bladder makes it possible to determine the watertightness of the repair because any presence of milk in the operative area indicates a leak; the surgeon must correct any leaks promptly. To avoid tangling the sutures that have been placed but not yet tied, the surgeon may clamp the free end pairs in small hemostats and then place each handle over the free tip of a long hemostat whose handle has been clamped to the drape by two towel clips.

The surgeon should place one or more additional layers of interrupted stitches (see Fig. 47-9, *D*), coapting the denuded vesical musculature, and should close the vaginal wall with interrupted sutures (see Fig. 47-9, *E* and *F*). If the closure is not watertight at the conclusion of the operation,

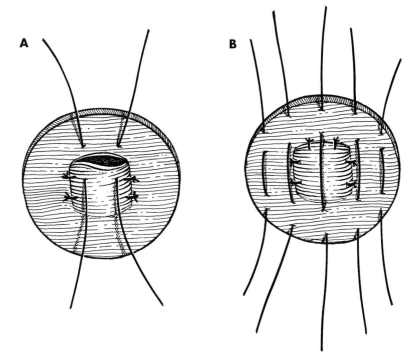

Fig. 47-11   **A,** The vaginal flap has been turned to cover the fistula and sewn in place by several interrupted sutures, sufficient to make closure watertight. **B,** A second layer of sutures approximates exposed tissues, and when these have been tied, the cut edges of the vagina are approximated by interrupted through-and-through sutures. (From Nichols DH, Randall CL: *Vaginal surgery,* ed 4, Baltimore, 1996, Williams & Wilkins.)

the surgeon should remove the stitches and reapproximate the wound as part of the same operation. When it is desirable not to overlap the vaginal closure over the vesical suture line, as in the repair of a recurrent fistula, the modification of Hurd[5] (Fig. 47-12) is effective. Because this requires undermining of the vaginal wall, however, it further shortens the vagina.

Bladder decompression by catheter drainage usually continues postoperatively for 10 to 14 days, but the patient should ambulate the day after surgery. The patient should take stool softeners to evacuate the bowel without straining. A 6% failure rate has been reported. If the repair fails (usually recognized promptly after surgery) and the patient wishes to attempt repair again, the surgeon can take the repair down and repeat the procedure 6 or 8 weeks later when epithelization is complete, paying special attention to dissecting and repairing the lateral tissues of the wound.

When used at the apex of the vagina, the Latzko technique may shorten the vagina by as much as 1 inch. If the shortened vagina causes a marital problem, the surgeon can create distal additional depth by using a Williams vulvovaginoplasty. As with any type of fistula repair, no coitus should be permitted for 2 months postoperatively.

Modified Latzko Technique of Repair. On occasion one will encounter a posthysterectomy vesicovaginal fistula in the very vault of a vagina that is already of shorter depth than one might wish. In this circumstance, after cystoscopy has clearly identified the site of the fistula and its freedom

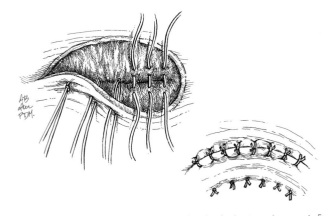

Fig. 47-12   Hurd's alternate method of closing the vault,[5] useful for a recurrent fistula. The posterior vaginal wall margin has been undermined for 1 1/2 cm, and ends of the final reinforcing layer of stitches approximating bladder wall have been tied, reinserted through all thickness of vaginal wall as shown, and tied again to avoid overlapping of bladder closure with that of vagina. The vaginal incision is closed by a separate layer. (From Nichols DH, Randall CL: *Vaginal surgery,* ed 4, Baltimore, 1996, Williams & Wilkins.)

from the ureteral orifices, a modified Latzko repair with minimal colpocleisis can be used.

Four guide sutures are placed in the vaginal vault surrounding the fistula, its track is probed, a no. 8 pediatric Foley catheter is inserted through the fistula, and the bulb is inflated. The vaginal skin of the tissues surrounding the site of the fistula is infiltrated with 1:200,000 epinephrine in 0.5% lidocaine, both for the temporary liquid tourniquet effect and to make the dissection easier.

A disk about 2.5 cm in diameter (Fig. 47-13, *A*) is demarcated around the periphery of the fistula, using traction on the catheter to improve exposure, and a smaller incision circumscribes the vaginal exit of the fistula. The disk is divided into two quadrants, and by sharp dissection into the vaginal wall, leaving only the deepest portion of vaginal skin still attached to the bladder, the disk is very carefully dissected free and removed. The cut edges of the vaginal incision are grasped by Allis clamps, and the thickest portion of the surrounding vaginal wall is undermined and sharply dissected

from its deeper layer for a circumferential distance of about 0.5 cm. A series of 4-0 PGA mattress stitches about 5 mm apart are placed in the raw area on the surface of the bladder and held, but not yet tied. When all are in place, the pediatric Foley bulb is deflated, the small catheter is removed from the fistula and a no. 16 transurethral Foley catheter is introduced into the bladder. The stitches are tied in the reverse order in which they had been placed (see Fig. 47-13, *B*), and 60 ml of sterile milk is instilled into the bladder to determine whether the first layer of repair is watertight. If any milk is seen in the operative wound, this spot is reinforced with additional stitches as necessary. The edges of the vaginal incision are then closed with interrupted 2-0 PGA mattress sutures placed about 0.5 cm apart in the same

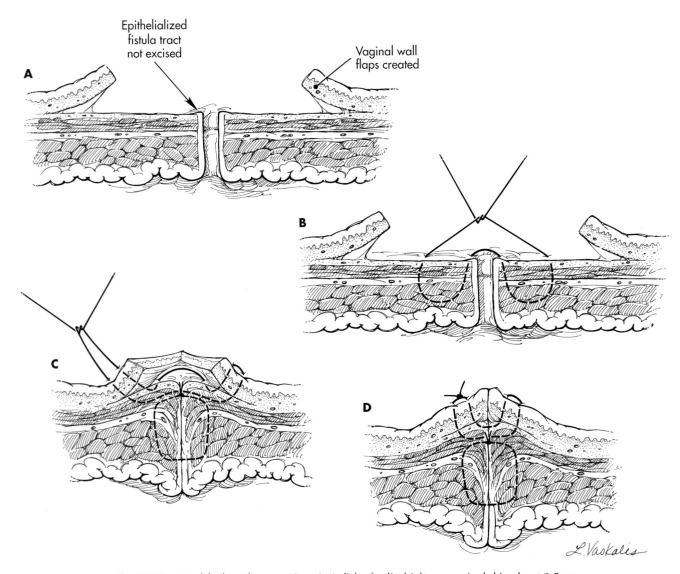

Fig. 47-13   Modified Latzko operation. **A,** A disk of split-thickness vaginal skin about 2.5 cm in diameter has been removed surrounding a vesicovaginal fistula. The deepest portion of vaginal skin is left on the bladder, as shown. **B,** Using 2-0 PGA suture a series of interrupted mattress stitches have been placed about 0.5 cm apart. When all are in place, they are tied and the repair is tested for watertightness. **C,** The vaginal skin is closed by a series of interrupted mattress stitches. **D,** Sagittal section of the final result after all stitches have been tied. Both entrance and exit of the fistula have been coapted.

axis as the underlying layer (see Fig. 47-13, *C* and *D*). No pack is used, and continuous bladder drainage is supplied.

Layered Closure Technique. Moir[19] reintroduced a modification of the standard Sims vaginal operation for the repair of vesicovaginal fistulas, particularly those distal to the vaginal apex. This operation, which has been popular for many years, does not shorten the vagina as does the Latzo "colpocleisis." Moir[19] went on to say:

> The treatment of vesicovaginal fistula has a fascination of its own. No branch of surgery calls for greater resource, never is patience so sorely tried, and never is success more dependent on the exercise of constant care both during operation and, even more perhaps, during the anxious days of convalescence. But never is reward greater. Nothing can equal the gratitude of the woman who, wearied from constant pain, depressed by an ever-growing sense of the humiliating nature of her infirmity, and desperate with the realization that her very presence is an offence to others, finds suddenly that she is restored to full health and able to resume a rightful place in the family—who finds, as it were, that life has been given anew and that she has again become a citizen of the world. To J. Marion Sims, more than to any man, is due the honour for this transformation. And if in these days a moment can be spared for sentimental reverie, look again, I beg, at the curious speculum and, gazing through the confused reflections from its bright curves, catch a fleeting glimpse of an old hut in Alabama and seven negro women who suffered, and endured, and had rich reward.

After obtaining suitable exposure, the surgeon injects or infiltrates the margins of the fistulous track, which are often quite vascular, with a few milliliters of 0.5% lidocaine in 1:200,000 epinephrine solution. A small Foley catheter may be inserted through the fistula (enlarged, if necessary, by the tip of a small hemostat) into the bladder, and the bulb is inflated. Traction on the catheter will stabilize the position of the fistula and bring it closer to the surgeon. Alternatively, guide sutures may be placed for traction (Fig. 47-14, *A*).

The surgeon circumscribes the circumference of the fistula with the point of the scalpel blade 0.5 cm from the edge of the fistula. After making a circular incision through the full thickness of the bladder wall (see Fig. 47-14, *B*), the surgeon removes the fistulous track. Any remaining fibrous tissue is carefully excised to a point where tissue vascularity is normal; it is desirable to remove as much scar and fibrous tissue as possible to convert the edges of the defect to a fresh operative wound. Then, with a no. 11 taper-pointed Bard-Parker blade, the surgeon makes a sagittal incision completely through the vaginal wall (but not into the bladder muscularis or cavity) for a distance of 1 cm superior and inferior to the fistula. The vaginal wall is undercut approximately 1 cm along each side of the fistulous track (see Fig. 47-14, *C*). Undercutting is continued until the bladder adjacent to the fistulous track is mobilized sufficiently to facilitate closure without tension.

If necessary for hemostasis, the surgeon may close the bladder mucosa with a layer of running 3-0 PGA or chromic suture, using a subcuticular stitch that inverts any exposed bladder mucosa into the lumen of the bladder. The bladder

muscularis is closed with interrupted sutures of 3-0 or 4-0 PGA suture (see Fig. 47-14, *D*).

As with the Latzko technique, the watertightness of the closure may be tested by examining the area for leakage after the instillation of sterile milk or infant formula into the bladder; additional sutures may be inserted as a second layer, if necessary. The bladder neck may be plicated prophylactically if desired (see Fig. 47-14, *E*). If there is any question about the viability of the tissues, either a Martius bulbocavernosus graft[6,17] (Fig. 47-15) or a gracilis muscle transplant can be used[3,11] (Figs. 47-16 and 47-17, pp. 884 and 886, respectively).

Gracilis Interposition Operation. The decision to use a new source of blood supply at the site of the fistula often will be determined at the time of operation. The surgeon will excise the fistulous track and then begin to mobilize layers to approximate viable tissue to viable tissue but finds that he or she is cutting through avascular scar tissue that cuts like plasterboard and bleeds little. The patient should have signed an informed operative permit because the leg incision to mobilize the gracilis is the length of the thigh. This should have been explained in detail. The patient should also be told that, if in the judgment of the surgeon the closure shows a good chance for success without a transplant, the muscle will not be used.

Surgical Anatomy of the Gracilis Muscle. The gracilis is a long, flat muscle that is the most medial of the adductors of the thigh. The fact that its upper portion is wide and flat, with an abundant blood supply, together with its proximity to the vagina makes it ideal for inclusion in plastic procedures for the cure of fistula. It arises from the medial margin of the body and ramus of the pubis by a thin, broad tendon about 6 cm in width. It becomes more round in the lower thigh and terminates in a round tendon, which passes behind the medial condyle of the femur, over the internal lateral ligament of the knee joint, and between the tendons of the semitendinosus and sartorius muscles, to be inserted into the proximal part of the medial aspect of the shaft of the tibia below the medial tuberosity. The long saphenous nerve passes between the tendons of the gracilis and sartorius. Loss of the gracilis as an adductor of the thigh and flexor of the knee is of no importance because the remaining muscles of the adductor group are more than adequate.

The general principles of fistula surgery—viable, fresh edges for approximation, liberal dissection to avoid tension of the suture lines, and the use of fine, atraumatic, catgut—apply here. Because the interposition of the muscle is done to supply blood to tissue with an inadequate supply, it is important to excise every fragment of scar tissue from the edges of the fistulous track. Excision of scar tissue may enlarge the opening, but if it removes scarred edges, the size of the fistula is unimportant.[3]

If the cut edge of the vaginal incision appears ragged, torn, or suspiciously thin, the surgeon may trim the edge. The full thickness of the vaginal membrane is closed from side to side with vertical mattress sutures of 2-0 PGA or polydioxanone (PDS) or polyglyconate (Maxon). These additional

Text continued on p. 887

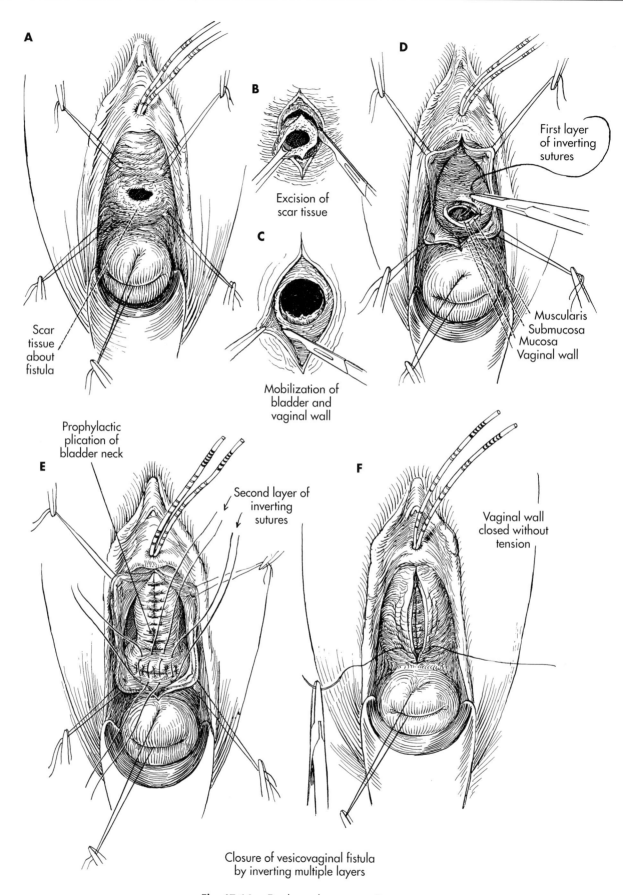

A

Scar
tissue
about
fistula

B

Excision of
scar tissue

C

Mobilization of
bladder and
vaginal wall

D

First layer
of inverting
sutures

Muscularis
Submucosa
Mucosa
Vaginal wall

E

Prophylactic
plication of
bladder neck

Second layer of
inverting
sutures

F

Vaginal wall
closed without
tension

Closure of vesicovaginal fistula
by inverting multiple layers

Fig. 47-14   For legend see opposite page.

Fig. 47-14, cont'd   Multiple-layer closure of a vesicovaginal fistula. **A,** Shows a vesicovaginal fistula in the bladder base that is readily accessible. The ureters may be catheterized to identify them in the event that the dissection is extended near the intramural ureter. Four traction sutures are placed about the fistulous track, and the tissue is grasped by instruments only when absolutely necessary. The scar tissue about the fistulous track is studied, and the direction of any retraction caused by this tissue is noted. The scar tissue about the fistula is completely excised **(B),** including that which has formed in the bladder musculature as well as the vaginal wall. By sharp dissection the plane of cleavage between the bladder and vaginal wall is located. Flaps, free of scar tissue, are mobilized for some distance from the fistula **(C).** The mobilization of healthy tissue extends far enough away from the fistulous track to ensure approximation without tension. The bladder mucosa is inverted toward the interior of the bladder by interrupted sutures of 4-0 PGA or chromic catgut on atraumatic needles **(D).** This suture passes through the muscularis of the bladder down to, but not including, the mucosa **(D).** In **E,** a second layer of inverting sutures has been placed in the bladder, and when sutures are tied, the bladder mucosa in the area of the former fistula will be precisely inverted toward the interior. If the fistula is in the bladder base and preoperative studies have indicated that the patient, after successful closure of the fistula, would have ordinary stress incontinence, a prophylactic plication of the bladder neck is done **(E).** The vaginal wall is closed with interrupted sutures in the opposite (longitudinal) direction to the closure of the bladder wall **(F).** The ureteral catheters are replaced by a silicone-coated 16-Fr transurethral Foley catheter. (From Ball TL: *Gynecologic surgery and urology,* ed 2, St Louis, 1963, Mosby, p 234.)

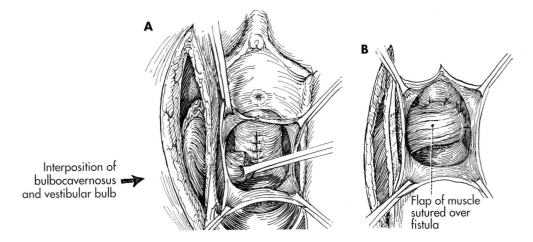

Interposition of bulbocavernosus and vestibular bulb →

Flap of muscle sutured over fistula

Fig. 47-15   Interposition of bulbocavernosus in a fistula repair. A lateral incision over the labia majora is made, and the bulbocavernosus and part of the vestibular bulb are mobilized, with care being exercised not to disturb the blood supply of the bulbocavernosus, which comes from the deep perineal branch of the external pudendal artery. This approaches the muscle near its point of origin, so care should be exercised not to disturb the major vessels. The vaginal wall is mobilized further on the lateral edge of the incision, and finally the anterolateral wall is dissected free along the upper portion of the descending pubic rami. A canal is formed behind the labia major and vaginal wall through which the bulbocavernosus can be drawn **(A).** The bulbocavernosus is detached anteriorly, and the free edge is observed for viability. The muscle is sutured across the area of the fistula or to the periosteum of the opposite pubic ramus **(B).** The full thickness of the vaginal wall is closed by interrupted sutures. The incision in the labia majora is likewise closed, and the skin edges are everted by interrupted sutures. (From Ball TL: *Gynecologic surgery and urology,* ed 2, St Louis, 1963, Mosby, p 234.)

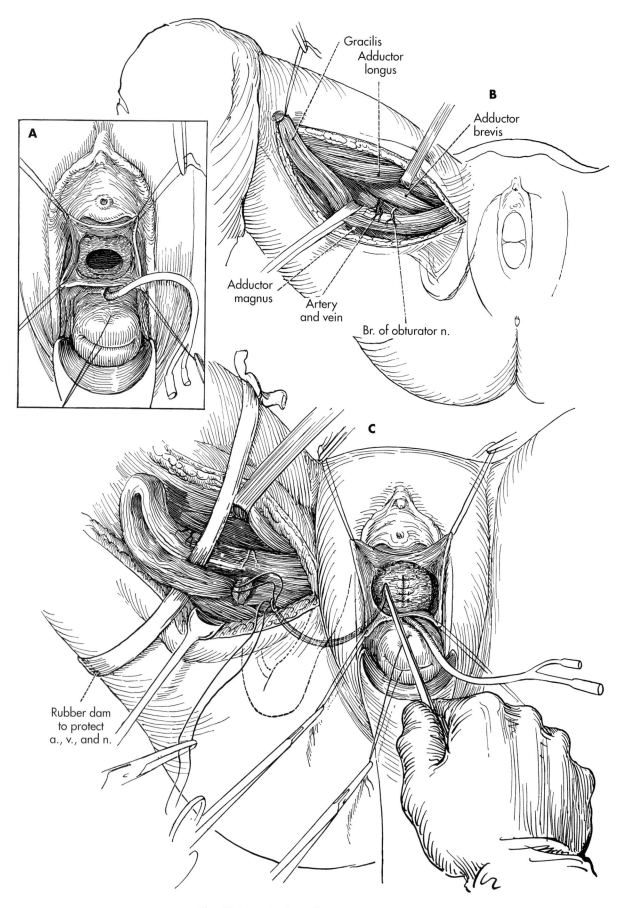

Fig. 47-16   For legend see opposite page.

Fig. 47-16, cont'd   Gracilis muscle interposition operation. The medial aspect of either the right or left leg is prepared and draped from the genitocrural fold to the region of the medial epicondyle of the knee. The vagina and vulva are prepared and draped. The preparation of the vaginal flaps about the fistula may be done in the knee-chest position, and the patient is turned around for the gracilis transplant. It is awkward to attempt to mobilize the gracilis with the patient in the knee-chest position. If exposure is adequate, the entire procedure is better done in the dorsal lithotomy position. The sketches accompanying this description were drawn with the patient in the dorsal lithotomy position, and the right gracilis was transplanted. The edges of the fistula are denuded of all scar tissue, and the natural line of cleavage between the bladder and anterior vaginal wall is entered when reasonably normal tissue is found some distance from the fistula. Continue the dissection farther until the bladder is freely mobilized and until the edges of the fistula will come together without tension. With large fistulas this may not be possible, and the transplanted muscle will be used to fill the gap. If the edges will come together, they are loosely approximated with interrupted sutures of 4-0 atraumatic chromic catgut. No attempt should be made to close the fistula in several layers, which adds a lot of suture material in the wound. The area of the fistula is then avoided and protected from trauma and pressure during the rest of the operation **(A).** If the fistula is at the bladder neck, trigone, or adjacent bladder base, it should be drained by a vaginal cystotomy as illustrated in **A.** A fistula in the bladder base may be drained by an indwelling catheter a long as it does not cause pressure on the edges of the wound or muscle transplant. A suprapubic cystotomy is preferable to an indwelling urethral catheter and can be done as a preliminary operation or at the time of the gracilis transplant procedure. The medial epicondyle of the femur is then palpated, and an incision is made through the skin and subcutaneous tela from here to a point on the descending ramus of the pubis and 2 cm below the inferior border of the symphysis **(B).** The fascia lata is then split along the course of the incision to within a few centimeters of the knee where it thickens and sends fibers into the joint capsule. The fascia lata is then dissected laterally and medially, exposing the gracilis, adductor longus, and, medial to the gracilis, the edge of the adductor magnus. The success of the transplant depends on the next maneuver. Retract the fascia lata laterally about 12 cm distal from the origin of the gracilis muscle. Gently lift up its lateral edge and look for the anterior branch of the obturator artery, vein, and nerve. It will be seen entering the lateral edge of the muscle together with some connective tissue extensions of the muscle sheath. In some patients the vessels are located by retracting the lateral edge of the gracilis medially. This is best done with a vein retractor, and once the bundle of vessels and nerve are located, the area must be carefully protected. To protect the blood and nerve supply, a rubber dam is sutured across the point of entrance of the vessels and attached to skin or adjacent muscle. During the ensuing phase of the operation, the blood and nerve supply can be compromised as the surgeon draws the muscle through the obturator foramen and under the bladder. The rubber dam serves as a landmark and prevents traction on the vessels **(C).** The gracilis is now dissected free from the other muscles of the adductor group to a point where its tendon is overlapped by the tendon of the sartorius. This portion of tendon is useful in passing the muscle through the obturator space but is later resected almost down to the belly of the muscle because the latter is the part that has an abundant blood supply. The distal portion of the muscle is bathed in wet gauze while the path for its transplantation between the bladder and vaginal wall is being prepared. The index finger is now inserted between the medial edge of the gracilis and the medial edge of the adductor magnus that lies behind and at a deeper level. Direct the dissecting finger posteriorly between the adductor magnus and the adductor brevis, which is anterior to the adductor magnus. This may avoid injuring the posterior branches of the obturator artery, vein, and nerve. The index finger of the other hand is then inserted between the bladder and vaginal wall and directed laterally until the most caudad edge of the obturator membrane is felt. The finger dissecting from the thigh then separates some of the fibers of the obturator externus to meet the finger in the vagina, with the obturator membrane interposed between them. The finger in the vagina will rupture some of the fibers of the levator ani and obturator internus in this dissection. A long, curved Kelly clamp is then passed along the index finger, dissecting from the thigh until the tip reaches the most caudad part of the obturator membrane. The clamp is then forced through the membrane and opened to make a passageway of sufficient size to admit the belly of the gracilis. It is important to make the opening adequate so the edges do not necrose the muscle or constrict its blood supply. A silk traction suture is inserted there in the tendon of the gracilis. A large curved clamp or large aneurysm needle is passed from the vaginal aspect, through the rent in the obturator membrane, and between the muscles, to emerge medial to the gracilis and a few centimeters from its origin. (From Ball TL: *Gynecologic surgery and urology,* ed 2, St Louis, 1963, Mosby, p 240.)

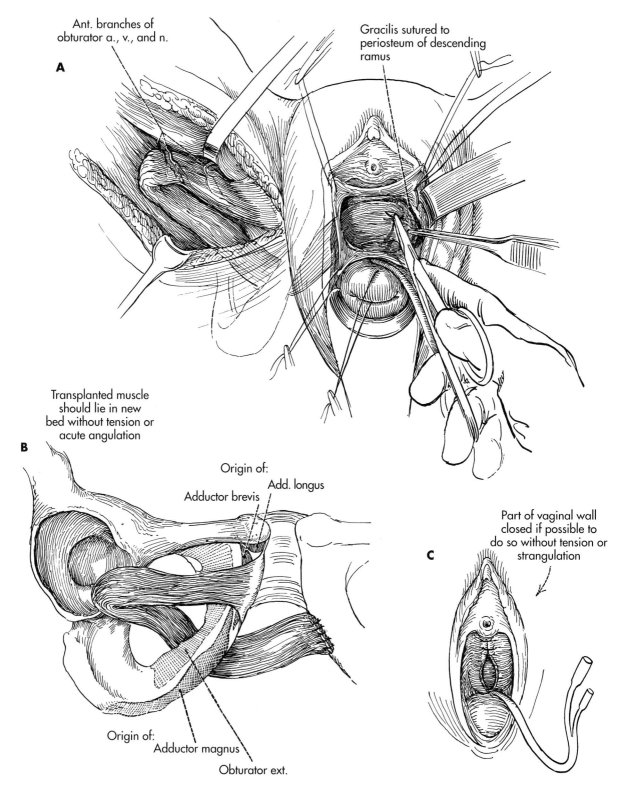

Ant. branches of
obturator a., v., and n.

Gracilis sutured to
periosteum of descending
ramus

A

Transplanted muscle
should lie in new
bed without tension or
acute angulation

B

Origin of:

Adductor brevis   Add. longus

Part of vaginal wall
closed if possible to
do so without tension or
strangulation

C

Origin of:
Adductor magnus

Obturator ext.

Fig. 47-17   The traction suture is drawn through this pathway and out the vagina. A clamp is used to grasp the tendon of the gracilis, and by a combination of pushing with the clamp and traction on the suture, the muscle is inserted through the obturator fossa and between the bladder and vaginal wall to the opposite descending ramus of the pubis **(A).** This must be accomplished without tension or angulation of the blood and nerve supply of the muscle **(B).** Because the detached distal end of the muscle retracts, it often seems that there is not enough muscle to reach across the vagina. This is not the case, and one finds ample length to span even the widest pubic arch. The viable ends of the muscle or tendon that have not been disturbed by traction suture or clamp are then sutured to the inner aspect of the opposite descending ramus of the pubis. These sutures pass through the remains of the attachment of the levator ani and the extensions of the obturator fascia that once formed the inferior layer of the urogenital diaphragm that in these patients has long since lost its identity. The muscle should now lie between the bladder and vaginal wall without tension and should cover the fistula. With large fistulas the muscle will present into the interior of the bladder and with a successful transplant soon become covered with bladder mucosa **(C)**. If the vaginal wall can be closed without tension, this is done with interrupted sutures of 2-0 PGA or chromic catgut, tied to provide approximation without strangulation. Should the anterior vaginal wall be so deficient that approximation is not feasible without tension, the edges should be sutured to the muscle graft in a few places to eliminate dead space, but again the sutures should be few and far between and not tied tightly **(C)**. The vagina should not be packed, nor should petroleum jelly, gauze, or other foreign bodies be placed against the suture lines to impede vascularization and healing. The leg incision is closed in layers with fine and medium silk sutures. There is no contraindication to early mobilization of the patient. (From Ball TL: *Gynecologic surgery and urology*, ed 2, St Louis, 1963, Mosby, p 240.)

---

layers of closure relieve much of the tension on the stitches of the first layer. The surgeon should place and hold all of these interrupted stitches before tying them; when the stitches are tied, the surgeon should be certain to incorporate a double turn on the first cast of each knot, followed by four additional casts of the suture, to prevent postoperative slipping. As Moir[19] correctly emphasized, these sutures should be only tight enough to approximate the tissue securely—not tight enough to strangulate the tissue. The ends of any *nonabsorbable* sutures should be left long to facilitate their removal on approximately the twenty-first postoperative day.

If necessary, the surgeon may make full-thickness lateral relaxing incisions in the vagina to relieve any tension on the suture line. The vagina should then be loosely packed with iodoform gauze for 24 hours and an indwelling catheter inserted to ensure bladder contraction for 10 days. If the patient is postmenopausal, both local and systemic estrogen should be administered through the postoperative period.

If the vaginal defect is too large to permit its edges to be coapted without tension, a *myocutaneous* bulbocavernosus transplant can be considered (Fig. 47-18).

Vaginal Lapping. For the larger vesicovaginal fistula, the dissection of the vaginal wall from the bladder wall *must* be sufficiently extensive to permit the mobilization and interposition of a large layer of subcutaneous tissue between the sutures that close the bladder and those that close the defect in the vagina. When the vaginal wall is suitably redundant, the vaginal lapping technique[1,13] may provide insulation and reinforcement for these suture layers.

The underlying fibromuscular layer of the right vaginal flap is split from the vaginal epithelium to the lateral margins of the vesicovaginal space (Fig. 47-19). Dissection along this line of cleavage should separate the musculoelastic layer of the vaginal wall from the overlying layer of vaginal epithelium. The vaginal flap of the left side is not similarly split, however; all connective tissue should remain attached to the epithelial layer of the left flap of the vagina to preserve as much of its blood supply as possible. Leaving

the vaginal muscularis attached to the epithelium on one side also effectively doubles the thickness of the connective tissue layer supporting the anterior vaginal wall.

Using a series of interrupted sutures of 2-0 PGA suture, the surgeon sews the medial edge of the right inner vaginal or fibromuscular flap to the undersurface of the unsplit full-thickness flap of the left vaginal wall, along the lateral extent of the vesicovaginal space. Each untied suture is held loosely until all have been placed; then all are tied (Fig. 47-20).

At this point, trimming an appropriate amount of the right epithelial covering layer of vaginal flap along the left lateral margin of the vesicovaginal space brings the edges of the vaginal membrane together again, making them roughly parallel over the now doubled fibromuscular tissue layers. Finally, the surgeon attaches the full thickness of the unsplit left vaginal flap to the cut edge of the right flap by a series of interrupted sutures of 2-0 PGA suture (Fig. 47-21). Any noticeable damage to or relaxation of the posterior vaginal wall and perineum could be repaired at this time.

Under rare circumstances, when the anterior vaginal wall is unusually thin and it is desirable to preserve the full vaginal depth and width, the Ocejo modification of the Watkins-Wertheim[8,33-35] interposition operation may be useful in patients who still have their uterus. In this modification, which Gallo[8] advocated, the surgeon amputates the cervix and excises the endometrium through a longitudinal incision in the anterior wall of the uterus, safely removing this potential source of future endometrial trouble or symptoms. The uterine fundus is interposed as a separate tissue layer between the bladder and the vagina and sewn into position as shown in Fig. 47-22 (p. 890).

Postoperative Care

Although the bladder of a patient who has been totally incontinent as a result of a vesicovaginal fistula is usually capable of physiologic regeneration and function within a few weeks, even when the incontinence has persisted for a number of years, the capacity of the bladder is likely to be rela-

Fig. 47-18   Myocutaneous bulbocavernosus transplant. When the defect in the vagina is of such size that its edges could not be approximated without tension and postoperative stenosis, a myocutaneous bulbocavernosus fat pad transplant can be accomplished as shown. A full-thickness labial skin incision has been made, circumscribing a piece of labial skin of a size sufficient to fill the defect in the anterior vaginal wall. The underlying fat pad and bulbocavernosus are carefully mobilized, and a tunnel is created by sharp and blunt dissection to unite the two incisions in the direction of the arrow and of a width sufficient to permit the myocutaneous flap to pass without compromising its blood supply. It has been sewn to the edges of the vaginal defect by a series of interrupted through-and-through sutures. (From Nichols DH, Randall CL: *Vaginal surgery,* ed 4, Baltimore, 1996, Williams & Wilkins.)

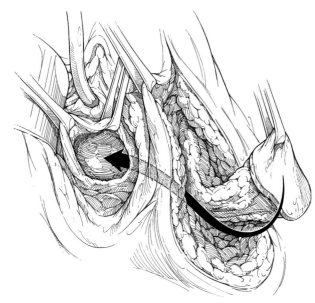

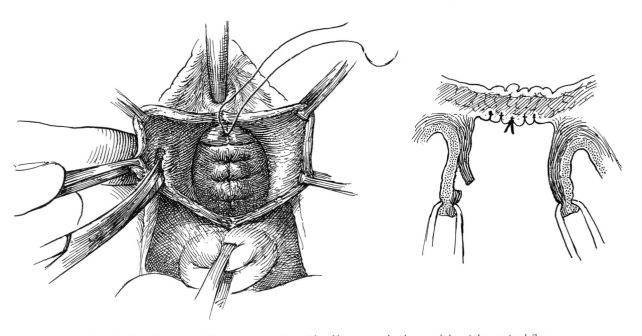

Fig. 47-19   The vaginal lapping operation. The fibromuscular layer of the right vaginal flap is dissected from superficial vaginal skin. (From Nichols DH, Randall CL: *Vaginal surgery,* ed 4, Baltimore, 1996, Williams & Wilkins.)

tively small immediately after the repair. The surgeon should warn the patient to expect a certain amount of urgency and should advise the patient of the need to empty her bladder frequently for the first few postoperative weeks, even during the night. It may be suggested that she set an alarm clock to arouse her for this purpose to avoid nocturnal distention. Because primary healing is so important, urinary antisepsis should be maintained for several weeks after the surgery. For postmenopausal patients, it is sometimes advisable to prescribe estrogen to improve vascularity and wound healing in these estrogen-sensitive tissues.

Any element of postoperative detrusor instability giving rise to precipitancy or incontinence must be sought and, if found, promptly treated, usually by a program of dietary caffeine restriction and bladder drill (voiding every 2 hours during the waking hours) supplemented by anticholinergic medication is necessary. "Closure of the fistula does not always mean success. Urinary continence must be restored."[32]

VESICOUTERINE AND VESICOCERVICAL FISTULA

If the escape of urine through the external cervical os is suspected but not identified, a standing lateral cystogram or hysterogram using a short-tipped cannula will supply the confirmation. "Menouria," which may consist of cyclic he-

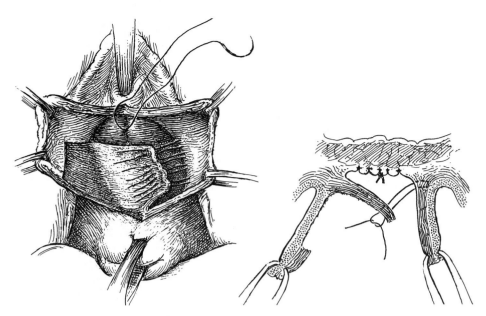

Fig. 47-20 The fibromuscular layer of the right vaginal flap is sewn to the undersurface of the unsplit left vaginal wall. The excess of the split right vaginal flap is trimmed. (From Nichols DH, Randall CL: *Vaginal surgery,* ed 4, Baltimore, 1996, Williams & Wilkins.)

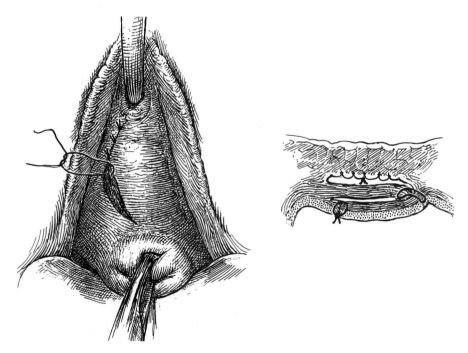

Fig. 47-21 The full thickness of the left flap is sewn to the right flap. (From Nichols DH, Randall CL: *Vaginal surgery,* ed 3, Baltimore, 1989, Williams & Wilkins.)

maturia, a vesicouterine fistula above the level of the internal cervical os, and apparent amenorrhea in the presence of a patent cervix but without coincident urinary incontinence has come to be known as Youssef's syndrome.[26,37] Urinary incontinence does not always occur with vesicocervical fistula; the sole symptom is sometimes menstrual hematuria, erroneously suggesting endometriosis of the bladder. In such instances, some valvelike structure has developed within a fistulous track, creating a flat effect that permits

fluid to pass from the uterus to the bladder but not in the reverse direction. Vesical endometriosis should have been excluded by careful cystoscopic examination.

Vesicocervical fistula has been reported after Shirodkar cervical cerclage.[9] A vesicouterine or vesicocervical fistula, with its accompanying incontinence, is almost invariably the result of a cesarean section during which a suture used in the repair of the uterine incision compromised the integrity of the bladder. Occasionally, such a fistula develops af-

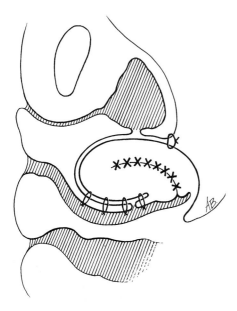

Fig. 47-22 The uterine corpus may be transposed between the bladder and vagina in certain patients with vesicovaginal fistula when blood supply is poor. In Ocejo's modification,[8] the endometrium has been removed by sharp dissection and the cavity obliterated by sutures as shown. An elongated cervix will have been amputated. (From Nichols DH, Randall CL: *Vaginal surgery*, ed 4, Baltimore, 1996, Williams & Wilkins.)

ter uterine rupture as a result of precipitate labor.[2] Surgery involves the anatomic dissection and separation of the bladder from the uterus at the site of the fistula, freshening of the edges, and separate repair of each organ with absorbable suture. Catheter decompression of the bladder for at least 10 days after surgery is desirable.

Such a fistula may be repaired either transvaginally or abdominally and the option of coincidental hysterectomy considered according to the patient's wishes for future reproduction. Normal subsequent pregnancy and delivery have been reported in patients in whom the uterus was retained.

URETEROVAGINAL FISTULA

Although freshly damaged or transected ureters may be transvaginally reimplanted into the bladder at the time of the initial injury—if the surgeon is familiar with the technique of repair[27,28]—the postoperative ureterovaginal fistula is most often approached through a transabdominal route, either for reconstruction or reimplantation.

Urinary Diversion

Permanent diversion of the patient's urine to a biologic reservoir appropriated from another system within the body may be required rarely. This subject is considered in Chapter 46.

REFERENCES

1. Aldridge AH: Modern treatment for vesicovaginal fistula, *J Obstet Gynecol Br Emp* 60:1, 1953.
2. Al-Juburi A, Aloosi I, Khundra S: Unusual vesicovaginal fistulas, *J Obstet Gynaecol* 4:264, 1984.
3. Ball TL: *Gynecologic surgery and urology*, ed 2, St Louis, 1963, Mosby.
4. Banfield PJ, Scott G, Roberts HR: A modified contraceptive diaphragm for relief of utero-vaginal fistula: a case report, *Br J Obstet Gynaecol* 98:101, 1991.
5. Dotters DJ, Droegemueller W: Diaphragm catheters for vesicovaginal fistula management, *Contemp Obstet-Gynecol Technol*, Special issue:45, 1992.
6. Elkins TE, De Lancey JOL, McGuire EJ: The use of modified Martius graft as an adjunctive technique in vesicovaginal and rectovaginal fistula repair, *Obstet Gynecol* 75:727, 1990.
7. Falk HC, Orkin LA: Nonsurgical closure of vesicovaginal fistulas, *Obstet Gynecol* 9:538, 1957.
8. Gallo D: *Ocejo modification of interposition operation*. In *Urologica Ginecologica*, Guadalajara, 1969, Gallo.
9. Golumb J, et al: Conservative treatment of vesicocervical fistula resulting from Shirodkar cervical cerclage, *J Urol* 149:833, 1993.
10. Hurd JK: *Vaginal repair of vesicovaginal fistula*. In Libertino JA, Zinman L, editors: *Reconstructive urologic surgery*, Baltimore, 1977, Williams & Wilkins.
11. Ingelman-Sundberg A: Repair of vesicovaginal and rectovaginal fistula following fulguration of recurrent cancer of the cervix after radiation. In Meigs JV, editor: *Surgical treatment of cancer of the cervix*, New York, 1954, Grune & Stratton.
12. Janisch H, Palmrich AH, Pecherstorfer M: *Selected urologic operations in gynecology*, Berlin, 1979, Walter de Gruyter.
13. Judd GE, Marshall JR: Repair of urethral diverticulum or vesicovaginal fistula by vaginal flap technique, *Obstet Gynecol* 47:627, 1976.
14. Keettel WC, et al: Surgical management of urethrovaginal and vesicovaginal fistulas, *Am J Obstet Gynecol* 131:425, 1978.
15. Lawson JB, Stewart DB: *Obstetrics and gynaecology in the tropics*, London, 1967, Arnold.
16. Latzko W: Postoperative vesicovaginal fistula, *Am J Surg* 58:211, 1942.
17. Margolis T, et al: Full thickness Martius grafts to preserve vaginal depth as an adjunct in the repair of large obstetric fistulas, *Obstet Gynecol* 84:148, 1994.
18. Miller BA: New diagnostic technics for an obscure vesicovaginal fistula, *Obstet Gynecol* 38:436, 1971.
19. Moir JC: *The vesicovaginal fistula*, London, 1967, Balliere, Tindall & Cassell.
20. Nichols DH, Randall CL: *Vaginal surgery*, ed 4, Baltimore, 1996, Williams & Wilkins, p 437.
21. O'Conor VJ Jr, et al: Suprapubic closure of vesicovaginal fistula, *J Urol* 109:51, 1973.
22. O'Conor VJ Jr: Repair of vesicovaginal fistula with associated urethral loss, *Surg Gynecol Obstet* 146:251, 1978.
23. Rock JA, Thompson JD, editors: *Te Linde's operative gynecology*, ed 8, Philadelphia, 1997, Lippincott-Raven.
24. Robertson JR: *Vesicovaginal fistulas*. In Slate WG, editor: *Disorders of the female urethra and urinary incontinence*, Baltimore, 1982, Williams & Wilkins.
25. Tancer L: Personal communication, 1985.
26. Tancer ML: Vesicouterine fistula—a review, *Obstet Gynecol Surv* 41:743, 1986.
27. Thompson JD: Transvaginal ureteral transection with vaginal hysterectomy and anterior colporrhaphy. In Nichols DH, editor: *Clinical problems, injuries and complication of gynecologic surgery*, ed 2, Baltimore, 1988, Williams & Wilkins.
28. Thompson JD, Benigno BB: Vaginal repair of ureteral injuries, *Am J Obstet Gynecol* 3:601, 1971.
29. Turner-Warwick R: The use of pedicle grafts in the repair of urinary track fistulae, *Br J Urol* 44:644, 1972.
30. Ueda T, et al: Closure of a vesicovaginal fistula using a vaginal flap, *J Urol* 119:742, 1978.
31. Wang Y, Hadley HR: Nondelayed transvaginal repair of high lying vesicovaginal fistula, *J Urol* 144:34, 1990.
32. Ward A: Personal communication, 1990.

33. Watkins TJ: The treatment of cystocele and uterine prolapse after the menopause, *Am Gynaecol Obstet J* 15:420, 1899.

34. Watkins TJ: Treatment of cases of extensive cystocele and uterine prolapse, *Surg Gynecol Obstet* 2:659, 1906.

35. Wertheim E: Zur plastichen Vermendung des Uterus bei Prolapsen, *Centralbl Gynäkol* 23:369, 1899.

36. Wolff HD, Gililand NA: Vaginal diaphragm catheters, *J Urol* 79:681, 1957.

37. Youssef AF: Menouria following lower segment cesarean section, *Am J Obstet Gynecol* 73:759, 1957.

48 Massive Vesicovaginal Fistula

E. CATHERINE HAMLIN and ROBERT F. ZACHARIN

The worldwide incidence of massive vesicovaginal fistula (Fig. 48-1) makes it the most common major gynecologic surgical problem existing today. Although it is rare in communities with access to expert medical help, in many countries such care is minimal or nonexistent and the problem is common. The tragedy, of course, is that such fistulas are entirely preventable.

CAUSES

Urinary fistula in the Western world usually results from pelvic surgery or pelvic malignancy and its treatment. Obstructed labor leading to fistula formation should not occur. In Third World countries there is a clear relationship between such fistulas and poor or absent obstetric care, associated with a wide range of contributing social conditions. The prime factor is unrelieved obstructed labor, leading to pressure necrosis. The duration of obstruction and the level at which descent of the presenting part is arrested determine the extent of tissue damage. Not only the bladder but commonly the urethra and ureters together with the rectum and cervix may be involved in the sloughing process. Associated medical factors include disproportion resulting from large babies or contracted pelvis, delay in diagnosis, and added difficulties of a traumatic delivery either by forceps, cesarean section, or a destructive procedure. Social factors with an important impact include poor diet and associated systemic diseases (e.g., malaria) that stunt growth, poor or absent medical care, obstruction to quick transport from villages to hospitals by distance or rugged terrain, and use of traditional remedies including deliberate genital tract injury and mutilation.

PATHOLOGIC FACTORS

Fistula site and extent are determined by the level of obstruction with the tissues passing through various phases from discoloration to eventual sloughing. The bladder wall is subjected to both mechanical pressure from the impacted presenting part and hydrostatic pressure from unrelieved retention of urine. The bladder neck and trigone area usually bear the brunt of the pressure, but often the urethra and ureters are included in the tissue loss. For some weeks after damage, necrotic debris continues to be discharged (Fig. 48-2), and healing follows by secondary intention. This process leads to gross scarring, adhesion to the ischiopubic rami, and cross-union between bladder and vaginal epithelial linings. Such a healing phase requires 10 to 12 weeks for completion. This healing process has several important clinical features to be appreciated when later surgical correction is being considered. Scar tissue is maximal at or near the fistula track but nevertheless extends, although diminished, into tissues well removed from the fistula. Scar tissue must be divided to allow access into the vagina and also to free the fistula from its attachment to pelvic bones. Only after satisfactory mobilization of the bladder and vagina will the true extent of the tissue deficit become apparent.

CLASSIFICATION

Site and size of the fistula determine what reparative measures will be necessary. There have been many proposals for classification, but most are too complex, attempting to consider every variant and failing to appreciate that there are no clear-cut divisions between these described varieties. In a clinical setting, important features are (1) the anatomic site of damage, (2) the size of the defect, and (3) the degree of associated scarring.

Fistula Site

The clinical grouping of fistulas involving the urinary bladder system is as follows:
1. Vesicovaginal fistula without urethral involvement
2. Vesicovaginal fistula with partial or complete urethral destruction
3. Vesicocervicovaginal fistula

Fistula Size

The following simplification into small, medium, and large is based on realities of surgical correction.

Small Fistula. Although small compared with other obstetric fistulas, it is not to be compared with a small posthysterectomy fistula. It lies in the anterior vaginal wall, does not involve the bladder neck or urethra, is not fixed to bone, and has minimal tissue deficit (Fig. 48-3).

Medium Fistula. A large area of the anterior vaginal wall and urethrovesical junction, including part of the proximal urethra, is lost. Bony adhesion is usual, and one or both ureteral orifices may be near the fistula edge and, on occasion, even outside (Fig. 48-4).

Large Fistula. A large amount of bladder floor, the urethrovesical junction, and often the whole urethra are affected, with the anterior vaginal wall replaced by massive scarring. The ureteral orifices are always displaced near to

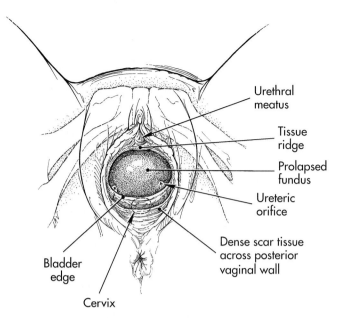

Fig. 48-1   Massive vesicovaginal fistula with bladder fundus prolapsing through the defect. Note the shortness of the urethra and the proximity of the ureteral orifices to the edge of the fistula. There is a dense band of scar tissue across the posterior vaginal wall. The uterine cervix can be palpated beyond the scar and the short vagina.

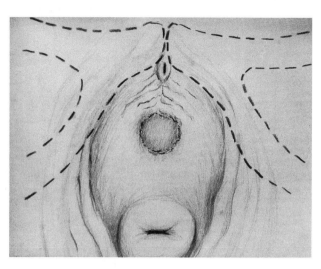

Fig. 48-3   Line drawing of a small fistula: central situation, minimal tissue deficit, and scarring without bony adhesion. (From Zacharin RF: *Obstetric fistula,* New York, 1988, Springer-Verlag.)

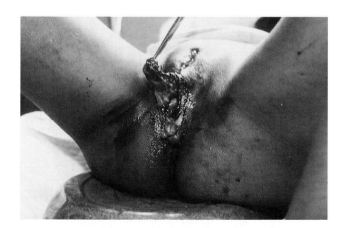

Fig. 48-2   Necrotic tissues discharged through the vulva some weeks after obstructed labor. (From Zacharin RF: *Obstetric fistula,* New York, 1988, Springer-Verlag.)

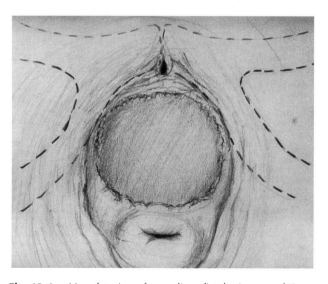

Fig. 48-4   Line drawing of a medium fistula: increased tissue deficit with scarring and the likelihood of ureteral involvement together with moderate bony adhesion. (From Zacharin RF: *Obstetric fistula,* New York, 1988, Springer-Verlag.)

the fistula margin or outside it. There are dense adhesions between the bladder remnant and pelvic bones (Fig. 48-5).

Fistula with Extensive Vaginal Scarring. The vagina is almost completely obliterated by scar tissue precluding insertion of even a fingertip. Preliminary "excavation" must take place before any anatomic characteristics of the fistula can be identified.

DIAGNOSIS AND INVESTIGATION

It is always wise to assume that there is something unusual about each patient and to conduct a thorough and thoughtful examination.[15] Accuracy in identification of physical signs is essential and usually straightforward, but suspicious granulating areas separate from the major defect must be investigated carefully with probe, dye, or vaginal swab test. A

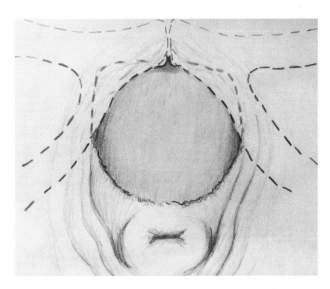

Fig. 48-5   Line drawing of a large fistula: massive tissue loss, scarring, and bony adhesion; the ureteral orifices may lie near to the fistula edge or even outside it. (From Zacharin RF: *Obstetric fistula,* New York, 1988, Springer-Verlag.)

ureterovaginal fistula, which may occur in association with a vesicovaginal fistula, must be excluded or confirmed by complete urologic assessment. An especially difficult diagnostic problem is a ureterovaginal fistula occurring at the lower end of the ureter, right against the bladder wall. The following are the important details in diagnosis.

Anatomic Facts

Significant anatomic facts include the following:
1. Site and size of the fistula into the vagina, its relation to cervix, bladder, urethrovesical junction, and urethra, cervix involvement, and identification of external os
2. Number of fistulas
3. Patency of the urethra
4. Relationship of ureteral orifices to the fistula and their proximity to the fistula edge (In larger fistulas, one or both orifices can lie outside the fistula edge, and this possibility must be clarified with certainty early on during reparative surgery.)

Pathologic Features

All of these features are compounded by previous attempts to correct the fistula surgically. The more attempts have been made, the more obvious are these changes.
1. Amount of tissue deficit.
2. Extent of scarring at the fistula edge and degree of associated vaginal fixity and stenosis.
3. Adhesion of the fistula to the ischiopubic rami and pubic bones.
4. Bladder inversion through the defect.
5. Presence of bladder calculi.
6. Progress of epithelial healing in the bladder and vagina as gauged by a return of normal epithelial appearance. After frequent surgical attempts to repair a fistula, return

to normal is much delayed. Assessment of normality is made by periodic vaginal inspections and cystoscopic examination of the bladder. Major indexes of normality are as follows:
   a. Loss of tissue edema and return of normal epithelial color.
   b. Softening and return of tissue mobility.
   c. Decrease in inflammatory reaction shown by results of the blanching test: compression of vaginal epithelium with the tip of a uterine sound produces significant blanching in inflamed tissues, which diminishes as healing progresses.

Additional Considerations

Finally, there must be an assessment of renal function, restoration of vulval and vaginal cleanliness before any surgery, and a general examination to exclude commonly associated problems, such as malaria, anemia, bilharziasis, and various parasitic infestations.

Consideration of all of these factors enables planning to begin, for both general and local preparation, and a decision to be made about an appropriate time for surgical intervention. General diseases, especially bilharziasis and malaria, must be treated and local vaginal cleanliness achieved by simple hygiene, especially mechanical scrubbing and washing and intravaginal douches. With long-standing fistulas, calculi must be sought and removed. Urinary tract infection is not a problem before surgery because of free urinary drainage but requires appropriate prophylaxis after fistula closure with the need for prolonged catheter drainage.

SURGICAL CORRECTION
Prophylaxis

Hamlin and Nicholson[8] succinctly described the causes of obstetric fistula as obstructed labor and obstructed transport. Therefore prophylaxis should be focused on these major problems. According to Lister[12]:

> The real answer as to what can be done in decreasing the incidence of fistula comes within the wide term of education of the patient, husband, relatives and influential people at the village level, and they should be made to realize that all women should be brought to hospital when undelivered after 24 hours, and also that certain women are high risk, i.e., short young girls, elderly primigravidae, grand multiparity, patients with still-births and those who have had operative deliveries in the past or a repaired vesicovaginal fistula. If all these women came to hospital early in labor or even attended an antenatal clinic, fistulae in many countries would become things of the past.

If bladder injury occurs during cesarean section, prompt recognition and careful management are needed to avoid cervicovesicovaginal fistula.

Difficulties Associated with Urinary Fistulas

Sir Reginald Watson-Jones, emphasizing the importance of controlled treatment of fractures, remarked, "Bones are filled not with red marrow; but with black in gratitude." Similar words might be used to underline the meticulous care necessary for successful fistula management.

The nature of the injury that caused the fistula and the type of fistula and its location are the main factors determining the result of attempted repair.[3] The two most important factors that can militate against a successful outcome are the amount of tissue deficit and dense fibrosis with adhesion to the rami and body of the pubic bones. The ability to mobilize grossly scarred tissues adequately without destroying blood supply and then to close them carefully in layers without tension is vital for successful repair. Associated vaginal stenosis can usually be overcome by adequate incision. Repair of a concurrent rectal defect should not be attempted until the bladder has been closed, although we have stated that our usual practice in Addis Ababa is to close both fistulas during one operation.[8] Scarring produced by repeated operations, particularly near the bladder neck, may result in a rigid patulous internal urinary meatus densely adherent to bone, further resulting in severe incontinence even if successful closure is achieved.

Methods Available for Surgical Correction

Vaginal Surgery. Hamlin and Nicholson[8] have performed all of their fistula operations with the patient in the lithotomy position. In their experience with 12,000 vaginal fistulas, they have never found it necessary to use the knee-chest position, the left lateral (Sims) position, or the abdominal approach. The vaginal approach embodies two techniques. The first, saucerization, was popularized by Sims but has been largely replaced by the alternative method of layered repair attributed to Mackenrodt. This second technique is also known as flap-splitting or dedoublement.

Ureteric Transplantation. Ureteric transplantation is usually unnecessary and in Third World countries with limited or absent medical care may in fact be lethal. Lawson[11] performed the procedure 30 times in 377 patients, but with increasing experience the technique was required much less often.

Principles of Vaginal Closure

Fistula surgery is difficult and demanding, and success will be gained only by meticulous attention to detail because the tissues are scarred and have a poor blood supply that leads to slow healing and tissue loss of greater or lesser degree. Accordingly, the best chance of surgical success is at the first attempt, so everything possible related to the surgery must be as right as conditions permit. The accepted time for all inflammatory changes and scar contraction to have subsided is 10 to 12 weeks, and surgical intervention during this time is considered unwise. Despite the increased risk of failure with early intervention, attempts to speed up healing using cortisone have been advocated. Similarly, selective intervention for surgically produced fistulas is suggested by some, believing the tissue reaction to be much less than that after obstetric trauma. Failure means a great emotional letdown and prolonged delay before a second attempt can be made, however. A more reliable result will follow thorough observance of the principles laid down long ago, but despite the best care, failures will still occur because the nature of the tissues precludes 100% success.

Immediate Preoperative Requirements

Intervention should be timed well away from the menstrual period, when the tissues become unduly vascular and engorged, making dissection more difficult. Similarly, the patient should stop taking oral contraceptives several weeks before surgery. Blood group and hemoglobin should be known, and blood should be available for replacement in patients requiring extensive surgery with gracilis muscle grafting. The following are additional considerations:

1. *Anesthesia:* Depending on availability, either low spinal or general anesthesia is suitable.
2. *Position on the operating table:* Throughout their experience over the past 33 years, Hamlin and Nicholson have used the exaggerated lithotomy position for every vaginal fistula operation.
3. *Lighting:* A properly focused, adequately bright theater light is essential.
4. *Vaginal access:* A variety of specula are necessary depending on the degree of stenosis. Access can be improved by episiotomy, but with gross degrees of scarring, a modified Schuchardt incision could be required.
5. *Suturing:* The labia are stitched with 2-0 silk. When feasible the fistula should be drawn toward the vaginal introitus using four guy sutures of 2-0 chromic catgut inserted about its periphery, but in many large obstetric fistulas, scarring and adhesion inhibit vaginal mobility to varying degrees.
6. *Proper instruments:* Essentials include a range of sharp-pointed scissors and fine-toothed dissecting forceps of adequate length so that the surgeon's hand does not obscure the field. A long-handled Bard-Parker scalpel with no. 11 blades, fine Allis forceps and skin hooks, a small neurosurgical sucker, and a range of fine needle-holders together with 2-0 chromic catgut and 2-0 nylon sutures on small curved strong needles are necessary.

Assessment under Anesthesia

All preoperative impressions should be confirmed and, if necessary, ureteral catheters passed.

Mobilization

The primary object of mobilization is to free the bladder from the vaginal wall, and flap-splitting is the standard procedure. First, the fistula is steadied, with guy sutures, Allis forceps, or transfixion with the point of the no. 11 scalpel blade. Next, the junctional zone between the bladder and vagina is incised, beginning where access is easiest (Fig. 48-6). The freed vaginal skin edge is held by Allis or long-toothed forceps, and incision of the junctional zone continues until the circular incision is complete. Then extensions of 1 to 2 cm are made anterior and posterior at the 6- and

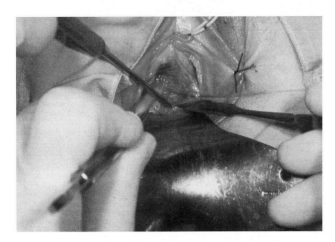

Fig. 48-6 Mobilization begins, using fine-toothed dissectors, a no. 11 blade, and a neurosurgical sucker. The traction suture can be seen on the right. (From Zacharin RF: *Obstetric fistula,* New York, 1988, Springer-Verlag.)

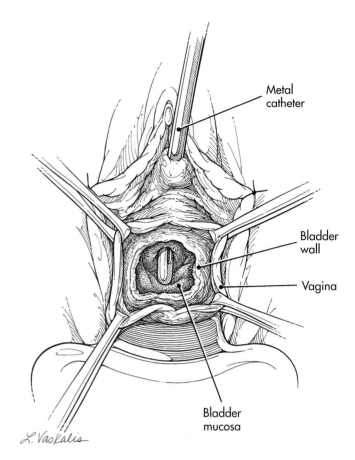

Fig. 48-7 Mobilization completed with a small fistula.

12-o'clock positions through the full thickness of the vaginal wall. Judicious use of suction enhances speed and accuracy, and progressive undercutting to free the bladder from the vagina is achieved using the no. 11 blade and sharp scissors. Ultimately, mobilization must be sufficient to allow bladder closure without tension, for tension means failure. Therefore the larger the defect, the more extensive the necessary mobilization (Fig. 48-7). Special attention must be directed to lateral extensions of the fistula, particularly bony adhesion to the ischiopubic rami. All such attachments must be freed using sharp scissors aided by palpation and finger pressure between bladder and vagina (Fig. 48-8). The finger detects ridges of scar tissue and areas of adhesion that need division so that the next tissue cut can be directed with accuracy.

Excision of Scar Tissue

Excision of scar tissue is a separate heading to emphasize the point that scar excision is never—*never*—necessary. This step, emphasized in many textbooks, has been copied, it would seem, from one publication to another but never by the pen of an experienced fistula surgeon. Excision of bladder scar tissue not only makes the tissue deficit present even greater, leading to a more difficult and more hazardous closure, but also creates unnecessary bleeding, which hinders closure and allows the bladder to fill with blood. One need only review the pathologic processes in the healing of a fistula to appreciate the fact that the bladder wall for some distance around is infiltrated heavily with scar tissue.

Care of the Ureters

With massive fistulas the likelihood of ureteral involvement at or near the fistula edge, or even outside it, must be presumed in each case until disproven. Early in dissection the orifices must be identified and catheterized so that mobilization proceeds superiorly, laterally, and centrally, carefully avoiding the lateral angles of the defect near the cervix (Fig. 48-9). It is important that the bladder be mobilized

centrally from the cervix. Pockets of freedom produced by this preliminary mobilization aid eventual ureteral orifice identification by freeing the bladder, but with larger fistulas, identification often can be made before any mobilization attempt begins.

Methods of Ureteral Orifice Identification

Methods to identify the ureteral orifice include the following:

1. After preliminary mobilization has been completed, the terminal ureter and orifice may be palpable. Eversion of the lateral angles of the fistula might enable the orifice to be seen, allowing the passage of a fine probe gently through the orifice, particularly if the probe lies flat on the bladder mucosa and is passed carefully in several areas in the anticipated line of the distal ureter (Fig. 48-10).
2. With a very large fistula, or when probing is unrewarded, 5 ml of 0.5% indigo carmine injected intravenously will produce telltale blue dye within 5 minutes and identify the orifices.
3. If dye investigation fails, a second indigo carmine injection or even a double dose together with 10 mg of intravenous furosemide (Lasix) will usually complete identification. When the ureters have been catheterized and the catheters drawn through the urethra by artery forceps, bladder mobilization can proceed and be safely completed (Fig. 48-11).

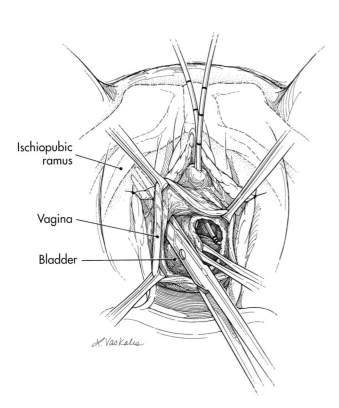

Fig. 48-8 Scissors free adhesions between the bladder and pubic ramus.

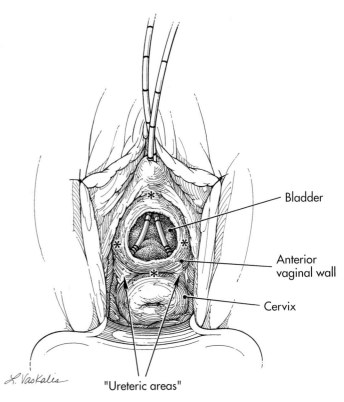

Fig. 48-9 Diagrammatic representation of areas to be mobilized at sites of asterisks and ureteral areas to be avoided until the ureters have been identified and catheterized.

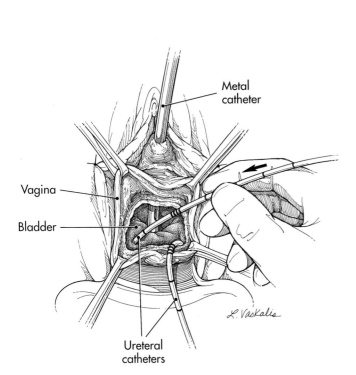

Fig. 48-10 Preliminary ureteral orifice identification, then passage of a ureteral catheter.

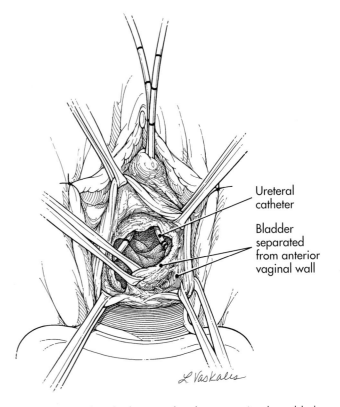

Fig. 48-11 When both ureteral catheters are in place, bladder mobilization can proceed.

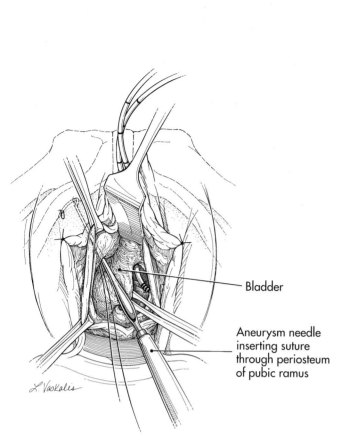

Fig. 48-12 Inserting a bladder stabilizing suture through the periosteum of the pubic ramus.

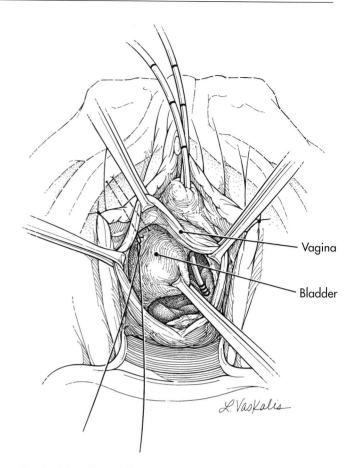

Fig. 48-13 The stabilizing suture is tied, anchoring the bladder to the pubic symphysis. (From Zacharin RF: *Obstetric fistula,* New York, 1988, Springer-Verlag.)

Bladder Wall Closure

Although there are no fixed rules to be followed, the bladder is usually closed with interrupted sutures of 2-0 chromic catgut (W565 Ethicon is recommended) while the surgeon observes the following principles:

1. The limits of the fistula are defined, and the bladder mucosa is inverted with interrupted sutures *passing through muscle and submucosal layers only, avoiding the bladder lumen.* Wide bites will prevent tearing out, and sutures should ensure apposition without strangulation. The surgeon should never forget that these tissues have been subjected to excessive trauma. Even though they appear nearly normal, they are far from it. Healing will be slow, for blood supply is much less then usual, and tight suturing is unnecessary and dangerous.

2. Before closure of larger fistulas is begun, the lateral edges of the bladder defect are identified on either side and the bladder wall immediately lateral to this is fixed to the periosteum of the ischiopubic ramus on that side (Fig. 48-12). Tying this suture is an important and key step that stabilizes the bladder against the rami, minimizing postoperative movements of the recent bladder suture line (Fig. 48-13).

3. Bladder wall closure begins laterally and moves centrally either in the natural transverse direction or in the anteroposterior direction should this seem more appropriate. Occasionally, a combination of transversely placed sutures laterally with centrally sited anteroposterior sutures can be the best method for closing a large defect (Fig. 48-14). The important principle to be remembered and reemphasized is that *there must never be any tension on this suture line.*

4. It is usually possible to insert a double layer of sutures with the outer overlapping the inner.

5. After fistula closure, the patency of the suture line must always be tested by injecting dye into the bladder through the catheter. Moderate pressure may be applied to the bladder, and any leaks detected will require extra sutures (Fig 48-15).

Grafting

In historical terms, the placing of a graft between the bladder and vagina is a relatively recent innovation, yet it ranks equally in importance with other principles of fistula closure. Some form of grafting should be used during the closure of every fistula because there is no point in saving this technique for future surgical attempts. Undoubtedly, a graft

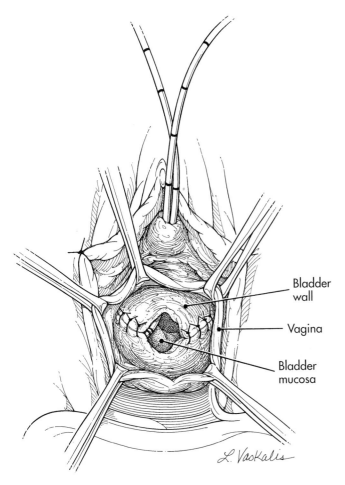

Fig. 48-14 A large fistula partly closed horizontally at the lateral extremities.

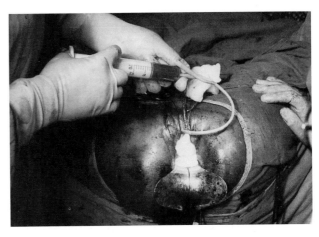

Fig. 48-15 Injecting methylene blue into the bladder to confirm a watertight closure. (From Zacharin RF: *Obstetric fistula,* New York, 1988, Springer-Verlag.)

enhances the quality of fistula closure and makes a successful outcome more likely. The two grafting techniques used are the Martius graft and the gracilis muscle graft.

Martius Graft. The Martius graft should be used with most fistulas, excluding very small and very large ones with urethral loss when it would be inadequate. Key points of the technique in taking this graft and placing it in position are that the fat pedicle must be mobilized back to the inferior margin of the ischiopubic ramus without disturbing the blood supply of the graft, and the tunnel for the graft must lie in close apposition to the inferior margin of the ramus to avoid undue bleeding. The tunnel should allow easy passage of the little finger to avoid strangulation, and the fat pedicle should be fixed in position over the closed fistula with anchor sutures, avoiding undue tension.

Gracilis Graft. Described originally by Garlock[5] and embellished by Ingelman-Sundberg,[9] the Gracilis graft was simplified by Hamlin and Nicholson,[7] making it similar in principle to a Martius graft in being transferred from the donor site subcutaneously into the vagina. It is required for correcting some large fistulas, especially those involving urethral reconstruction. The vaginal wound is closed with 2-0 monofilament nylon inserted as vertical mattress su-

tures, incorporating the underlying graft to help eliminate dead space. Just enough tension is applied to bring the skin edges into apposition without strangulation. Should there be a deficit of vaginal skin, a labial skin flap can be raised from the lesser labium of one or the other side and laid over the muscle or fat graft as a full-thickness skin graft.

Vaginal Pack

The vagina is packed gently but firmly with gauze soaked in paraffin. This pack remains for 48 hours, a step that encourages the various layers to adhere and minimizes dead space and hematoma formation.

Postoperative Management

Immediately after surgery, urine should be draining from all catheters. If not, intravenous furosemide (Lasix) will start a flushing action. Bladder washout should be avoided. Two important principles must be observed:

1. The bladder must be kept empty during the healing phase.
2. Antibiotics are required to prevent urinary tract infection as long as the catheter is required.

A nurse should be present until the patient fully recovers from the anesthesia, a precaution that minimizes any risk of interference with catheter drainage. Suction is never used because it has inherent problems. The patient is instructed to watch catheter drainage and to notify the nursing staff should there be any concern about adequacy of drainage. If any doubt exists, the catheter should be changed immediately without question. Depending on the size of the bladder defect, catheter drainage is required for a minimum of 10 days and up to 14 days for larger defects. Ureteral catheters remain in situ for 8 to 10 days to allow meatal edema to subside. After catheter removal, the patient usually has no difficulty voiding, but she must be observed carefully and catheterized at 4- to 6-hour intervals, depending on fluid intake, if she is unable to void. In practice, voiding usually occurs easily, and providing that volumes are 200 ml or

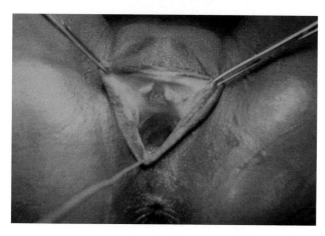

Fig. 48-16 The residual fistula after some months of healing without repair: "the urethra has vanished and the examiner looks straight into the bladder." (From Zacharin RF: *Obstetric fistula*, New York, 1988, Springer-Verlag.)

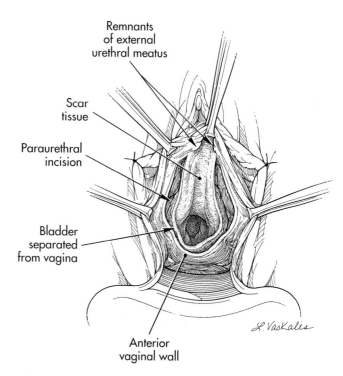

Fig. 48-17 Paraurethral incision outlining the new urethra.

more, no checks are necessary. The patient remains under supervision for a further 24 hours, a specimen of urine is checked for infection, and antibiotics are stopped. The sutures are removed just before discharge (about the sixteenth to twenty-fourth day). At discharge, the patient is instructed to avoid sexual intercourse for 3 months and to return if complications arise.

Complications

The addition of partial or complete urethral destruction to a vesicovaginal fistula has been regarded as a serious complicating factor that is difficult to correct. Many procedures have been designed to correct the situation. Hamlin and Nicholson,[7] drawing on extensive experience with difficult fistulas, have described their technique for reconstructing a urethra totally destroyed in labor, a detailed procedure that includes contributions from earlier publications by Martius, Chassar Moir, and Ingleman-Sundberg. The principles of repair are as follows:

1. Lithotomy with steep Trendelenburg tilt is the procedure to be used.
2. Posterolateral introital incision opens the stenosed vagina.
3. The vesical defect in these patients is such that usually ureteral orifices can be identified and catheterized. However, if not then, along with mobilization of tissues to be used in reconstructing the new urethra, bladder mobilization begins laterally and centrally, avoiding the ureteral areas. Then the ureters are identified and catheterized.
4. Remains of the external urethral meatus can be seen as two small epithelial elevations adherent anterior to the pubic bone, whereas the site of the absent urethra is marked by tough scar tissue joining urethral remnants to the ischiopubic rami and anterior edge of the bladder defect (Fig. 48-16).

5. Deep paraurethral incisions are made, demarcating tissue to be used in forming the new urethra. Extending the incisions deeply allows mobilization of this tissue, which is then rolled over a no. 12 Foley catheter to form the new urethra (Figs. 48-17 and 48-18).
6. The bladder is mobilized widely with special attention given to bony adhesion.
7. Before urethral closure is begun, the Foley and two ureteral catheters are held in place against the new urethral roof while the first inverting suture of 2-0 chromic catgut is placed. Then the urethral tube transmitting the three catheters is completed down to the bladder defect with a series of mattress sutures, not too many and not too tight (Fig. 48-19). During urethral reconstruction, the danger point at the urethrovesical junction is reinforced with extra sutures, drawing bladder muscle over this junctional zone to invert the join and minimize the risk of later stress incontinence.
8. The bladder is closed, rolling in the mucosa with the contained ureteral orifices and catheters. Often the bladder defect, because of its size, is closed transversely. It is important to insert anchor sutures to stabilize the bladder wall laterally against the ischiopubic rami. After closure, a dye test is performed.
9. The repair is reinforced with a gracilis muscle graft, and in some cases a Martius fat graft is also used.
10. The anterior vaginal wall is closed, if necessary, using a labial skin graft.

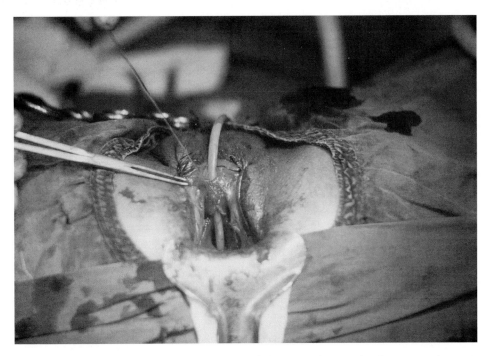

Fig. 48-18   Urethral reconstruction. (From Zacharin RF: *Obstetric fistula,* New York, 1988, Springer-Verlag.)

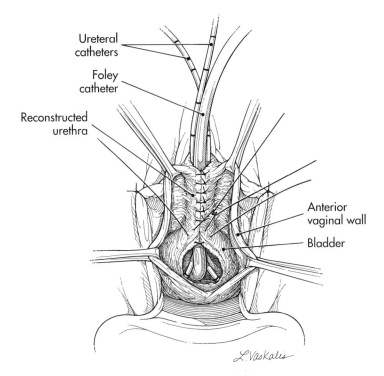

Fig. 48-19   Completion of urethral reconstruction.

REFERENCES

1. Bardescu N: Ein neues Verfahren fur die Operation der tiefen Blasen-Uterus-Scheidenfisteln, *Zentralbl Gynäkol* 24:170, 1900.

2. Blaikley JB: Colpocleisis for difficult vesicovaginal and rectovaginal fistulas, *Am J Obstet Gynecol* 91:589, 1965.

3. Carter B, et al: Vesicovaginal fistulas, *Am J Obstet Gynecol* 63:579, 1952.

4. Counsellor VS, Haigler FH: Management of urinary vaginal fistula in 253 cases, *Am J Obstet Gynecol* 72:367, 1956.

5. Garlock JH: The cure of an intractable vesicovaginal fistula by the use of a pedicled muscle graft, *Surg Gynecol Obstet* 47:255, 1928.

6. Greenslade NF: Vesico-vaginal fistula: a method of repair, *Aust NZ J Surg* 38:283, 1969.

7. Hamlin RHJ, Nicholson EC: Reconstruction of urethra totally destroyed in labour, *Br Med J* 2:147, 1969.

8. Hamlin RHJ, Nicholson EC: Personal communication, 1986.

9. Ingelman-Sundberg A: Pathogenesis and operative treatment of urinary fistula in irradiated tissue. In Youssef AF, editor: *Gynaecological urology,* Springfield, Ill, 1960, Charles C Thomas.

10. Kiricuta I, Goldstein AMB: The repair of extensive vesicovaginal fistulas with pedicled omentum: a review of 27 cases, *J Urol* 108:724, 1972.

11. Lawson SB: Vesico-vaginal fistula. In *Proceedings of the 1st International Conference of the Faculty of Gynaecology and Obstetrics,* Ibadan, Nigeria, 1977.

12. Lister U: Personal communication, 1986.

13. O'Conor VJ, et al: Suprapubic closure of vesico-vaginal fistula, *J Urol* 109:51, 1973.

14. Roen PR: Combined vaginal and transvesical approach in successful repair of vesicovaginal fistula, *Arch Surg* 80:6238, 1960.

15. Russell CS: The vesical fistula high in the vagina, *Proc R Soc Med* 59:1022, 1966.

16. Simon G: Fälle von Operation bei Urinfisteln am Weibe, Beobachtung einer Harnleiter-Scheidenfistel, 1856. Cited in Latzko W: Postoperative vesicovaginal fistulas: genesis and therapy, *Am J Surg* 58:211, 1942.

17. Su CT: A flap technique for repair of vesicovaginal fistula, *J Urol* 102:56, 1969.

18. von Dittel, 1893. Cited in Latzko W: Postoperative vesicovaginal fistulas: genesis and therapy, *Am J Surg* 58:211, 1942.

19. Weyrauch HM, Rous SN: Transvaginal-transvesical approach for surgical repair of vesicovaginal fistula, *Surg Gynecol Obstet* 123:121, 1966.

20. Zacharin RF: Grafting as a principle in the surgical management of vesicovaginal and rectovaginal fistulae, *Aust N Z Obstet Gynaecol* 20:10, 1980.

21. Zacharin RF: *Obstetric fistula,* New York, 1988, Springer-Verlag.

49 The Omental Flap in an Abdominal Repair of Complex Vesicovaginal Fistulas

RICHARD TURNER-WARWICK and CHRISTOPHER R. CHAPPLE

It is almost always possible to close urinary vaginal fistulas. Meticulous technique is naturally essential, but reliable success with the more complicated problems depends on the surgeon's ability to select the procedure best suited to the particular clinical situation and to vary it according to the findings in the course of the operation on the basis of wide personal experience.

Because urinary fistulas in women are commonly the result of gynecologic and obstetric complications, in addition to being an unpleasant inconvenience for the patient, they often present a medicolegal aspect. Therefore the essential goal of treatment is to resolve the situation without delay and without any complications. Failure should be a rare event.

The basic surgical option for the repair of a vesical fistula lies between a vaginal-approach procedure and an abdominal-approach procedure. Many surgeons have an instinctive personal preference for one of these, but this should not be the case. Although many simple vesicovaginal fistulas can be closed by a vaginal repair procedure, the access that this provides is relatively restricted, and any significant incidence of failure after this approach suggests that the abdominal approach is not being used enough. Similarly, a significant incidence of failure after a simple abdominal approach layer-closure can be resolved by a formal omental interposition procedure because in the absence of active tumor or infection, this procedure should be almost invariably successful.[2,13] Almost the only indication for urinary diversion after a fistula operation is urinary incontinence caused by irremediable sphincter damage.

Thus, ideally, the closure of even an apparently simple vesicovaginal fistula should be regarded as a procedure for a gynecourologic or urogynecologic specialist, and the surgeon who created the fistula is not always the best person to undertake its repair.

THE TIMING OF REPAIR

Even the smaller vesicovaginal fistulas rarely respond to conservative treatment by simple catheter drainage of the bladder. A definitive closure is almost invariably required.

Traditionally, a delayed repair has been advocated for the treatment of urinary fistulas to ensure that the local tissue reaction has settled. The major change in the management of postoperative vesical and ureteric fistulas in recent years has been an immediate repair procedure rather than a delayed one. However, this does not generally apply to ure-throvaginal fistulas because these are invariably associated with damage to the all-important intrinsic urethral sphincter mechanism on which continence depends. The appropriate procedure for these is usually a delayed definitive reconstructive sphincteroplasty.

When an omenta interposition procedure is used, the success of the closure is less dependent on the perfect healing of a simple layer-closure. Thus the timing of a repair must be carefully considered in each particular case.

FISTULOUS INJURIES
Gynecologic Injuries

The development of a simple vesicovaginal fistula is not invariably the direct result of a surgical misadventure. These fistulas are commonly large and located in the midline above the trigone. They often are not immediately identifiable, with the vaginal leakage starting a few days postoperatively. This type of fistula can result from a patch of ischemia that develops after the separation of a particularly thin-walled bladder from the anterior aspect of the uterus and cervix. Even the most experienced surgeons are not immune from this fortuitous complication.

The Surgical Significance of Infrequent Voiding

Patients who void infrequently have a characteristically thin-walled bladder, which predisposes them to the development of an ischemic supratrigonal vesicovaginal fistula. Thus carefully monitoring the postoperative voiding efficiency of patients with thin-walled bladders is generally advisable. A temporary prophylactic suprapubic catheter can be used to avoid overdistention or retention that can contribute to the development of necrosis of the ischemic patch and consequent fistulation.

Patients who void infrequently (at intervals of 4 to 6 hours or more) are prone to develop voiding difficulties after simple pelvic surgery and, incidentally, are also prone to late-onset urine infection.[3,4,10] Having identified this situation from the history preoperatively, it is wise to forewarn the patient that socially convenient infrequent voiding can be associated with a somewhat precarious degree of voiding dysfunction and cause voiding difficulties postoperatively. If, despite extra care, such a patient does develop a fistula, such a forewarning may help her understand that it was her particularly thin-walled bladder that was the underlying cause of the vesicovaginal fistula, not simply a surgical misadventure.

Principles of Transabdominal Layered Closure of a Fistula

The basic principles of the layered-closure of a fistula are well established, but many technical options are available.

After appropriate separation of the vagina and bladder, facilitated by a guiding finger in the vagina, the abnormal tissue at the margin of the fistula is resected. We always use polyglycolic acid (PGA) sutures—never catgut—and tie the knots on the lumen when possible. The technique of suturing and the duration of catheter drainage are discussed in the following section. The vagina is usually closed with a single layer of inverting interrupted sutures. If the tissue quality and the closure of the bladder are deemed sufficiently good for a simple layer-closure procedure, the bladder is closed with two layers of sutures. However, if any doubt exists about the success of this procedure, a single layer of carefully placed, interrupted, inverting sutures is used in combination with omental support.

Supporting the Closure of Complex Fistulas by Interposition Grafts

When the healing potential of the tissue around a fistula is compromised by fibrotic scar tissue resulting from infection, from the failure of previous repairs, or from irradiation, the reliability of a simple layer-closure procedure diminishes abruptly unless an additional well-vascularized transposition graft is interposed. The advisability of interposition support generally becomes obvious in the course of an operation, so surgeons generally should regard the recurrence of a fistula after a simple layer-closure procedure as an avoidable complication, even though it may be fortuitously inevitable at times.

A sizable flat of parapelvic peritoneum sometimes provides sufficient additional interposition support for a layer-closure, but this is generally inappropriate when it is also involved in the local pathologic conditions, especially irradiation. Pedicled muscle flaps, such as gracilis, can be used as a simple tissue-bulk interposition; however, skeletal muscle is ill-adapted to resist infection and to resolve inflammation, so it contributes little to the local healing reaction. Its vascular response potential is primarily related to exercise, and, ultimately, inactivity results in disuse atrophy and fibrosis.

Surgical Value of Omental Redeployment Support

The omentum is unique in that it is the only body tissue specifically developed for the purpose of resolving inflammation. This function is partly the result of its vascularization, which is capable of rapid augmentation in response to inflammation. However, the "magic" of the omentum fundamentally depends on its abundant lymphatic drainage, which is so good that it can rapidly reabsorb macromolecular inflammatory exudates, the accumulation of which can create purulent collections that compromise the healing of a repair. Thus the omentum acts as a physiologic drain that generally prevents the formation of pus in the peritoneal cavity except in locations it does not normally reach, such as the pelvis and the subdiaphragmatic areas.

Surgically, the omentum is invaluable for the support of more precarious urinary tract reconstructions.[12] Furthermore, unlike the retroperitoneal and retropubic fat, the omentum always regains its suppleness after an inflammatory response has subsided. Thus the omentum provides a unique urodynamic quality of support that is fundamentally important to the reliable success of functional reconstructions, especially sphincteroplasty, because it ensures the freedom of its subsequent functional movements.[2] Appropriately used, the omentum can virtually guarantee the closure of a vesicovaginal fistula (Fig. 49-1) or a complex vesicovaginorectal fistula (Fig. 49-2) provided an adequate bulk of it is appropriately mobilized and interposed between PGA-sutured closure lines of the vagina and the bladder/urethra.

The omentum should completely fill an interposition abdominoperineal tunnel that is properly developed laterally to admit three or four fingers so that a good tissue overlap is ensured. It should not be regarded simply as an "omental

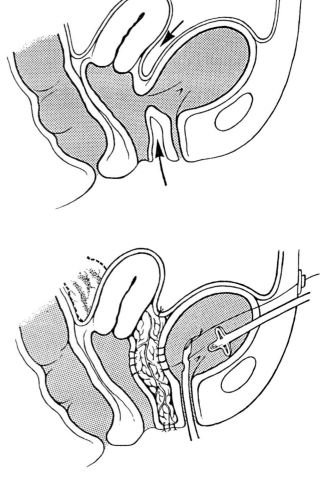

Fig. 49-1   Omental interposition for a recurrent vesicovaginal fistula after the creation of a wide intervening abdominoperineal tunnel. (© 1966, Institute of Urology.)

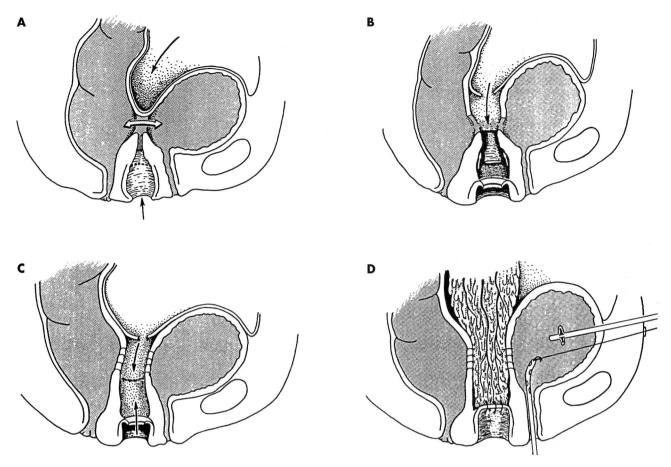

Fig. 49-2   A-D, The closure of a complex hysterectomy plus irradiation vesicovaginal fistula achieved by excising the stenotic vault of the irradiated vagina to create a wide abdomino-perineal tunnel for omental interpositioning. (© 1966, Institute of Urology.)

plug." The lower margin of the interposed omentum is anchored by including it in the perineal sutures used to close the vaginal wall opening, just proximal to the introitus, at the lower end of the abdominoperineal interposition tunnel.

Anatomic Basis of Omental Mobilization

The "magic" of the omentum depends on the "pulsating efficiency" of its vascularization, and this must be preserved during its mobilization. Preservation depends on an accurate knowledge of its anatomic features, which are detailed elsewhere.[2,6]

The blood supply of the omentum is derived from the right gastroepiploic branch of the gastroduodenal vessels and the left gastroepiploic branch of the splenic vessels (Fig. 49-3). The right gastroepiploic vascular pedicle is considerably larger than that on the left, and it directly supplies the major part of the omental apron. Within the omental apron, the collateral anastomoses between the vertical branches of the gastroepiploic arcade are relatively minor and somewhat unreliable.

In about 30% of patients, the omentum reaches the perineum without any mobilization of its vascular pedicles (see Fig. 49-3). Even so, when it is surgically redeployed to support reconstructive procedures in the pelvis, it is generally

advisable to separate its natural adhesion to the transverse colon and the mesocolon to avoid its distraction by gaseous distention of the bowel postoperatively.

Simple mobilization by division of its relatively minor left gastroepiploic vascular pedicle enables a further 30% of omental aprons to reach the perineum. Normally, this does not significantly reduce its blood supply.

In about 40% of patients (more in children whose apron is often relatively short), meticulous full-length mobilization of the right gastroepiploic vascular arcade from the stomach is required to enable it to be effectively redeployed in the pelvis. Because the bulk of a fully mobilized omentum is based on its slender vascular pedicle, this should be protected by mobilizing the right colon so that it can lie retroperitoneally behind this. Failure to do this can result in the division of the all-important pedicle during a subsequent laparotomy for obstruction, a complication we have seen during several retrievoplasty procedures. Thus, even when its apron is underdeveloped, as it often is in children, a normal omentum can always be redeployed into the pelvis.

Unfortunately, some surgical and gynecologic texts advocate basing the mobilization of the omentum on its relatively minor vascular pedicle on the left; others even elongate the apron by a simple horizontal incision that transects

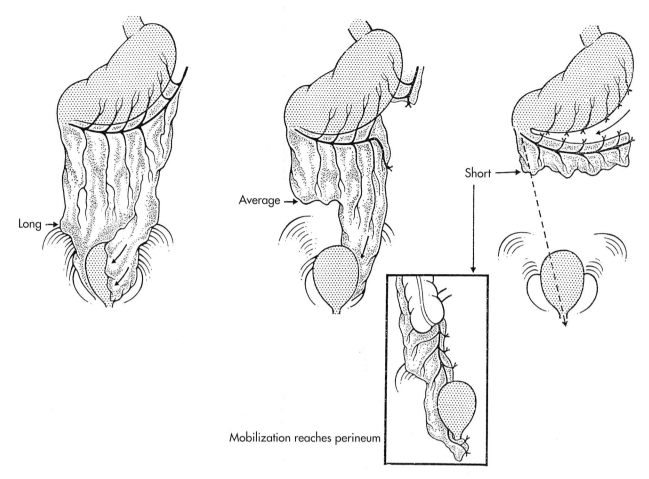

Fig. 49-3 In 30% of patients, the omental apron is long enough to reach the perineum after its simple separation from the transverse colon and mesocolon. In another 30%, an additional division of its left gastroepiploic pedicle is required. Formal mobilization of the whole length of its right gastroepiploic pedicle from the stomach is required in 40%. In such cases, the pedicle should be protected by positioning it behind the mobilized right colon, and a prophylactic appendicectomy is generally advisable. (© 1987, Institute of Urology.)

its vertical vessels, which inevitably reduces its pulsating efficiency. Furthermore, in about 10% of patients, there is no anastomotic junction between the right and the left gastroepiploic vessels that usually form a complete gastroepiploic arcade on the greater curvature of the stomach (Fig. 49-4).

Operative Procedure for Full-Length Mobilization of the Right Gastroepiploic Pedicle

A midline abdominal wall incision must always be used when reconstruction in the pelvis may require omental support; this is essential to enable the incision to be extended upward to provide appropriate surgical access to the stomach for the meticulous mobilization of its pedicle vessels. The need for an extended mobilization cannot be predicted preoperatively. It is fundamentally important to remember that there is only one omentum and that damage to its blood supply by inappropriate mobilization of its vascular pedicle

compromises not only the success of the procedure but also the success of a subsequent retrievoplasty.

The individual ligation of the 20 to 30 short gastric branches involves meticulous vascular technique to avoid damage to the main gastroepiploic pedicle vessels (Fig. 49-5); this takes time.

The operative procedure is as follows:

1. Bunch ligation of vessels foreshortens the pedicle and increases the risk that they may escape and bleed.
2. Absorbable ligatures should be used for mobilization of the omental pedicle vessels. Nonabsorbable sutures and Ligaclips can later lie exposed within a fistulous area and can result in stone formation.
3. The technique of the division of the short gastric vessels must be meticulous to avoid damage to the parent gastroepiploic vessels. The proximal end of these branches should be ligated in continuity, before division, not between hemostats. This is because their inadvertent escape can result in the immediate develop-

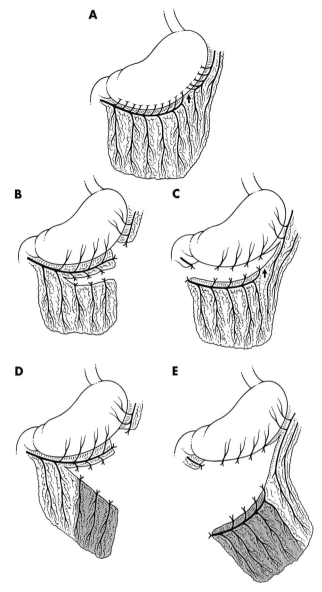

Fig. 49-4 **A,** In 10% of patients, the right and left gastroepiploic vessels do not anastomose to form an "arch." **B** and **C,** The omentum should not be mobilized by a horizontal incision across the apron below the gastroepiploic arch because this divides the vertical branches and the distal collateral communications between these are poor. **D** and **E,** The right gastroepiploic vessels vascularize more than two thirds of the omental apron. Mobilization of the omentum on the basis of the left gastroepiploic pedicle may result in ischemia if the gastroepiploic arch is incomplete. (© 1977, Institute of Urology.)

ture the last undivided branch or "window" the main pedicle vessel.

5. The slender pedicle vessels at the root of a fully mobilized right omental pedicle should be protected by relocating them behind the mobilized ascending colon. A prophylactic appendectomy avoids incidental surgical damage to the pedicle during a subsequent acute appendectomy immediately adjacent to it.

Avoidable Causes of Failure of Omental Interposition Repairs

Failure of an omental interposition repair can almost always be prevented by ensuring the following:

1. The size of the abdominoperineal interposition tunnel is adequate to provide a sufficient tissue overlap laterally. The tunnel should be 3 to 4 fingerbreadths wide.
2. A sufficient bulk of omentum is mobilized to fill the appropriately sized interposition tunnel.
3. Appropriate mobilization procedure and meticulous vascular technique are used to avoid impairment of the "pulsating efficiency" of the mobilized omentum.
4. The pedicle of a fully mobilized right gastroepiploic pedicle is relocated behind the mobilized ascending colon to protect it from subsequent surgery (see the previous section).

In our experience with secondary and tertiary repairs, the previous failure of an omental interposition procedure was almost always attributable to one or more of these. However, despite meticulous care, the occasional fortuitous loss of a fully mobilized omental flap is inevitable.

SOME PRINCIPLES OF RECONSTRUCTIVE SURGERY

The basic principles for the avoidance of postoperative complications are to anticipate them and to prevent them. The surgeon's inclination and ability to adapt a procedure according to the actual findings at the time of operation, many of which cannot be anticipated, however detailed the preoperative evaluation, are essential to success.[2,6,7]

Technique and Tissue Handling

Successful reconstructive surgery depends on technique and tissue handling. Almost all surgeons regard their surgical technique as "meticulous and immaculate"; however, some are more "tissue-sensitive" than others are. For instance, tissue forceps applied to tissue that will remain in situ should be used gently enough to apply to a fold of one's finger skin.

Sutures

Dexon and Vicryl sutures cause much less tissue reaction than catgut and are consequently much more suitable for urinary tract reconstruction. The author thankfully abandoned catgut for all urinary tract operations in 1970, when Davis and Geck pioneered the production of PGA sutures. Size for size, these are much stronger than catgut, enabling

ment of an interstitial hematoma in the omentum, and even greater care is then necessary to retrieve it for secure religation without damaging the main pedicle vessels. Hemostat ligation can be used for the gastric end because this is easy to retrieve if it slips off.

4. Once started, mobilization of the right gastroepiploic arch from the greater curvature of the stomach should be completed to its gastroduodenal origin; otherwise, there is a risk that traction on the pedicle might rup-

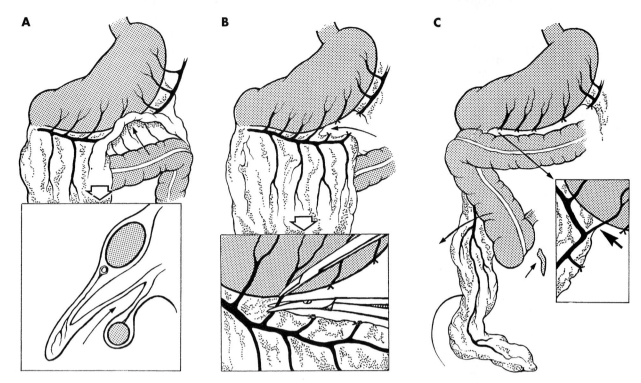

Fig. 49-5 Mobilization of the right gastroepiploic pedicle of the omentum requires meticulous vascular technique. **A,** Separation from the transverse mesocolon by development of the avascular plane is always advisable to prevent postoperative displacement of the redeployed omentum by gaseous bowel distention. **B,** Ligation-incontinuity reduces the risk of an interstitial hematoma developing. A risk of ligation between hemostats is vessel escape. Nonabsorbable ligature material should always be used. **C,** Once started, mobilization of the right gastroepiploic vessels from the stomach should be extended to their gastroduodenal origin; otherwise, tension on the pedicle at the point of the last undivided branch may rupture it. (© 1977, Institute of Urology.)

smaller sizes to be used, and they retain their tensile strength longer. The 30- to 40-day survival of the tensile strength of 3-0 and 4-0 PGA sutures is generally appropriate for urinary tract reconstruction. Catgut causes a severe tissue reaction, which is generally unacceptable for meticulous reconstructive surgery (except for certain special purposes when this excessive reaction is unimportant or even a particular advantage).

Interrupted sutures allow the best possible vascularization of the tissue intervening between the suture bites and are generally preferable when the vascularization is relatively precarious. If interrupted runs of a continuous suture are used, it is most important that they be snugged down lightly so they gently approximate the tissue without strangulating it. Consequently, assistants should be dissuaded from their natural instinct to use a continuous suture as an elevating retractor.

Postoperative Urine Drainage

Suprapubic catheter drainage of the urine is strongly advocated after all vesical fistula repairs; it is efficient, reliable, and less uncomfortable than a urethral catheter. Furthermore, at the conclusion of the drainage period, it is easy to

verify the restoration of voiding efficiency by clamping the suprapubic drainage and checking the postvoiding residual urine volumes before removing it. This compares favorably with the emotionally charged situation that can arise when only a urethral catheter is used, meaning that it has to be reinserted repeatedly for the management of a voiding difficulty—the "yo-yo catheter."[3,4,10]

An additional urethral catheter is insurance against early postoperative bladder distention that can occasionally arise as a result of obstruction of suprapubic catheter drainage. However, the use of a Foley balloon catheter is inadvisable because inadvertent traction on this can disastrously disrupt the bladder base closure; a urethral catheter is best retained by a sling suture, button-fixed on the abdominal surface.

Unobstructed catheter drainage is all that a fistula repair requires, hence the added safety of using an additional urethral catheter for the first week or so. Suction urinary drainage systems are unnecessary. Unfortunately, however, the caliber of the connecting tubes of many standard urologic drainage bag systems is so large that they have a tendency to retain air, and the consequent fluid levels in a hanging loop at the bedside can create a positive hydrostatic resistance to the flow or urine. If the internal diameter of the connecting tube does not much exceed the lumen of the catheter that it is draining, it remains bubble free so that, hanging by the bedside, it naturally creates a syphonic-suction negative pressure.

The duration of catheter drainage after a fistula repair should relate to the quality of the tissue healing of the particular patient; drainage should be maintained until it has served its intended function. This depends on the surgeon's judgment and, on the principle that there should be no brave surgeons, just brave patients, we maintain catheter drainage until we do not have to feel brave when deciding to discontinue it—in other words, at least 2 weeks after a simple fistula closure. Naturally, when the quality of tissue healing is relatively poor after infection, the failure of previous surgery or irradiation, a longer period is advisable, say 3 weeks, with a preliminary check on the watertightness of the suture line by suprapubic cystography.

Wound Drains and Antibiotics

The use of wound drains is a matter of the surgeon's personal preference. In general, the reliability of suture-line healing is enhanced when it is immediately surrounded by well-vascularized tissue; it is diminished by adjacent accumulations of inert hematoma and tissue fluid, especially if these become infected, as they tend to, in the pelvis. Consequently, we always use an appropriate wound drain for as long as we feel it is fulfilling its intended purpose. Suction drainage may be relatively inefficient when positioned within folds of omentum because this tends to get sucked into the fenestrations of the tubing and occlude them. A soft Penrose drain may be more efficient.

The use of prophylactic antibiotics is optional, but preferable. The problem is that a precarious suture line may occasionally separate as a result of infection before this is clinically identifiable. There is good evidence that the incidence of postoperative hip-prosthesis infection is significantly reduced by the use of prophylactic antibiotics.

Midline Abdominal Wall Incision and the "Suprapubic Cross Incision"

A midline incision in the abdominal wall is essential to provide access for the radical mobilization of the vascular pedicle of the omentum when necessary, the mobilization of which may be fundamental to the success of closure of a difficult fistula repair. The need for the mobilization of the pedicle of a short omental apron from the stomach cannot be predicted preoperatively, but in fact, a subumbilical midline abdominal wall incision is sufficient to achieve its effective transposition in more than half the patients in whom this is necessary.

The traditional transverse Pfannenstiel incision cannot be simply extended for an extensive mobilization of the omental pedicle. However, many patients with a vesicovaginal fistula have already had a Pfannenstiel-approach procedure, and the routine use of an additional vertical midline skin incision for a fistula repair results in a scar, which is a lasting

reminder of the complication and may contribute to the initiation of medicolegal proceedings.

The "suprapubic cross incision" was developed to enable most abdominal approach fistula repairs to be completed through the original Pfannenstiel skin incision (Fig. 49-6). After only a minor lateral extension of this horizontal skin incision, the upper and lower skin/subcutaneous tissue flaps are separated from the rectus fascia to enable a midline abdominal wall incision to be made up to the level of the umbilicus, leaving the original horizontal Pfannenstiel rectus sheath closure intact (with suture reinforcement if necessary).

In the event that upper abdominal access is required to mobilize the vascular pedicle of a short-apron omentum (30% to 40% of cases), this can be achieved by a relatively small additional midline epigastric skin incision and a supraumbilical extension of the midline incision in the abdominal wall under the wide skin bridge. Thus a secondary midline skin incision is avoided in most patients who require a postoperative fistula-repair procedure without compromising the option of a safeguarding omental interposition procedure in the event of need for this.

Increasing the Midline Incisional Access to the Retropubic Space

Simple application of surgical anatomy can greatly improve the midline incisional access to the retropubic space. Although traditional anatomic texts often describe a pubic attachment of the rectus abdominis aponeurosis to the pubic crest, in reality it spreads down, over the anterior surface of the pubis, to its inferior margin. After a distal prepubic extension of the midline incision into the prepubic aponeurosis, it can be reflected off the surface of the pubic bone by sharp dissection (Fig. 49-7).[8,12] This creates a remarkably effective exposure of the whole width of the upper border of the pubis.

COMPLEX VESICOVAGINAL FISTULAS

Fistula surgery that is "complex" because of impaired local tissue healing from infection, previous surgery, or irradiation may be further complicated by the additional involvement of the terminal ureter on one or both sides, by a urethral sphincter deficiency, by a coincident rectal fistula, by a vaginal abnormality, or by a "frozen pelvis" resulting from extensive radiation fibrosis. These naturally make an already difficult repair procedure even more difficult. However, almost all are nevertheless synchronously remediable by an appropriate variation of the available procedures.

Neovaginoplasty Fistulas

The creation of a neovagina involves the development of a neovaginal space between the bladder and the urethra anteriorly and the anorectum posteriorly. The development of this plane is relatively easy in simple congenital vaginal atresia. In gender-reassignment procedures, it is complicated by the dense adhesion of the male rectourethral liga-

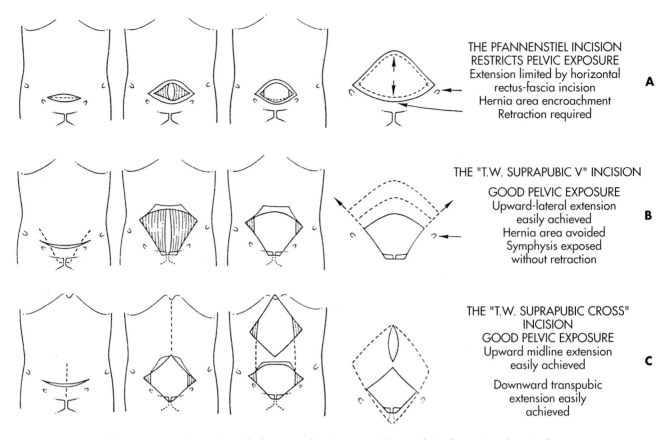

THE PFANNENSTIEL INCISION
RESTRICTS PELVIC EXPOSURE
Extension limited by horizontal
rectus-fascia incision
Hernia area encroachment
Retraction required

A

THE "T.W. SUPRAPUBIC V" INCISION

GOOD PELVIC EXPOSURE
Upward-lateral extension
easily achieved
Hernia area avoided
Symphysis exposed
without retraction

B

THE "T.W. SUPRAPUBIC CROSS"
INCISION
GOOD PELVIC EXPOSURE
Upward midline extension
easily achieved

Downward transpubic
extension easily
achieved

C

Fig. 49-6 **A,** The traditional Pfannenstiel incision provides a relatively restricted surgical access to the pelvis. The lateral extent of its horizontal incision in the rectus sheath is limited by the inguinal canal area, and the lower margin of the rectus sheath requires retraction. **B,** The Turner-Warwick suprapubic V incision uses the same horizontal skin incision, but the access to the pelvis and the lower abdomen is greatly improved by the V-shaped incision in the rectus sheath, which can be extended upward and laterally, if necessary, to provide a good exposure of the upper urinary tract without division of the rectus muscle. **C,** The Turner-Warwick suprapubic cross incision also uses the same horizontal skin incision, but its subumbilical midline incision in the abdominal wall can be extended upward to provide supraumbilical upper abdominal access for mobilization of the right gastroepiploic pedicle of the omentum from the stomach by using an additional vertical epigastric midline skin incision. (© 1974, Institute of Urology.)

ment. Postirradiation fistulas are naturally associated with extensive adhesions, which increase both the risk of injury and the difficulty of the reconstruction.

Various surgical options are available for the creation of a neovaginal lining. Split-skin and amnion can be satisfactory substitutes, but both have the disadvantage that the wall of the neovagina is very thin and its capacity is relatively small and tends to contract. Thus its size has to be maintained by regular intercourse or by the passage of dilators, which can occasionally result in neovaginal rupture and the development of a fistula into the rectum or the bladder. The resolution of neovaginal fistulas presents particular problems and an omentoneovaginoplasty can be a useful reconstructive procedure (see Fig. 49-7).

Postirradiation "Frozen Pelvis"

Inevitably, the effective treatment of carcinoma of the cervix by radiotherapy results in a degree of irradiation tissue

damage to the bladder and to the rectum. The extent or irradiation damage is not always directly related to the dose—there is considerable variation in the particular tissue response of the individual. Thus a given depth dose that causes a moderate reaction in one patient may cause extensive radiation fibrosis in another.

Severe radiation injury can result in incarceration of the rectum and ureters by radiation fibrosis and the development of a vesicovaginal fistula, occasionally associated with a radionecrotic cavity in the vaginal vault area. Traditionally, such a "frozen pelvis" has been treated by a urostomy and colostomy, but even this does not always relieve the unfortunate patient of an offensive purulent discharge from a radionecrotic cavity.

Although the fibrotic reaction in such patients is extensive, the anal canal, its sphincter mechanism, and the lower segment of the vagina are rarely severely damaged. Consequently, it is often possible to exenterate the fibrosis and to

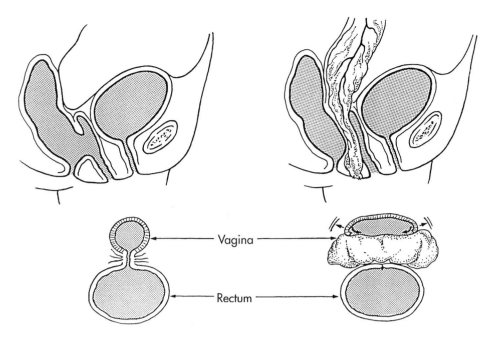

Fig. 49-7 A complex neovaginal-rectal fistula after a skin graft vaginoplasty for atresia, closed by separation and lateral fixation of the neovaginal skin strip. The surface of the interpositioned omentum opposed to the skin strip epithelializes, greatly increasing the vaginal capacity. (© 1973, Institute of Urology.)

restore bowel continuity by anastomosis of the mobilized unirradiated descending colon to the partially irradiated anal canal. Naturally, this anastomosis is potentially precarious, but if it is meticulous and it is wrapped with a well-vascularized omental flap, it is often successful.

The functional result of reconstructing a small-capacity irradiated bladder by a bowel-substitution cystoplasty depends primarily on whether the residual urethral sphincter mechanism is capable of maintaining continence. The cystoplasty/bladder-base anastomosis is potentially precarious, but again, this is generally successful if a good omental wrap can be achieved. The anastomosis of the unirradiated proximal ureters to the relatively unirradiated bowel cystoplasty rarely presents difficulties.

There is always a possibility of residual tumor cells in the fibrosis associated with an irradiation fistula, even when preoperative biopsy proves negative and even if the treatment was concluded 10 years or more previously. It is clearly inappropriate to attempt to close a fistula when the bulk of the pelvic induration associated with it is active, recurrent macroscopic tumor. However, when a patient develops a postirradiation vesicovaginal fistula and a representative preliminary biopsy shows only a few residual cells in extensive irradiation fibrosis, the local tumor may be relatively quiescent. Under these circumstances, because the prognosis is very poor, it is all the more important to resolve the incapacitating incontinence as swiftly and as efficiently as possible. Closure of such a fistula by omental interposition is a simpler procedure than a ureteroileal surface conduit, and it also offers the patient a good chance of normal voiding and urinary control for their few short remaining months.

CONCLUSION

It has long been recognized that the boundaries between some traditional areas of surgical specialization are inappropriate to the proper development and improvement of our care of patients. This is reflected in the evolution of a number of regional surgical specialities such as head and neck surgery, hand surgery, and so forth.

The proximity of the genital and the lower urinary tracts naturally results in a degree of structural and functional interdependence. Consequently, some incidence of urinary tract complications is inevitable during childbirth and gynecologic operations.

Within the traditional confines of gynecology and of urology, we have to recognize the need for cross-boundary training and subspecialization by the development of specialist interests in urogynecologic and in gynecourologic functional reconstruction. The natural progress of this must surely be the development of a small number of referral units with special expertise in a "horizontal specialty" of "pelvic surgery" to avoid the shortcoming of "committee surgery" in the pelvis for the treatment of complex congenital trauma, incontinence, and oncologic gynecourologic problems. Proper training in pelvic surgery should also involve an appropriate experience of reconstructive colorectal surgery.

Successful functional reconstruction should be primarily based on a particular aptitude for meticulous surgical minutiae and, furthermore, an instinctive inclination to adopt and to adapt procedures according to the findings at the time of operation. Thus, in addition to training in general gynecourology or urogynecology, a surgeon undertaking reconstructive procedures should have an additional period of training in plastic surgical techniques and tissue handling.

Because all parts of the urinary tract are specially developed to subserve a particular function, appropriate functional reconstruction requires not only an accurate understanding of the local anatomic structure but also personal hands-on experience of videourodynamic assessment, for which there is no substitute.

Finally, it is essential to appreciate that any operative procedure that fails, however well intentioned and well performed, inevitably complicates a subsequent retrievoplasty—"having a go" cannot be in the best interests of one's patients.

REFERENCES

1. Kirby RS, Turner-Warwick R: Reconstruction of the vagina by caecolo-vaginoplasty, *Surg Gynecol Obstet* 170:132, 1990.
2. Turner-Warwick R: The use of the omental pedicle graft in urinary tract reconstruction, *J Urol* 116:341, 1976.
3. Turner-Warwick R: Impaired voiding efficiency and retention in the female, *Clin Obstet Gynecol* 5:193, 1978.
4. Turner-Warwick R: Clinical urodynamics, *Urol Clin North Am* 6:13, 1979.
5. Turner-Warwick R: Female sphincter mechanisms and their relation to incontinence surgery. In Dubruyne FMJ, Van Karrenbrock PEUA, editors: *Practical aspects of urinary incontinence,* Dordrecht, 1986, Martinus Nijhoff.
6. Turner-Warwick R: Urinary fistula in the female. In *Campbell's urology,* Philadelphia, 1986, Saunders.
7. Turner-Warwick R: The Turner-Warwick bladder elongation psoas hitch BEPH procedure for substitution ureteroplasty. In Abrams P, Gingell JC, editors: *Controversies and innovations in urological surgery,* New York, 1988, Springer-Verlag.
8. Turner-Warwick R: Increasing surgical access to the retropubic space, *Br J Urol* 65:307, 1990.
9. Turner-Warwick R, Handley Ashken M: The functional results of cystoplasty with special reference to caecocystoplasty (and mention of caeco-vaginoplasty), *Br J Urol* 39:3, 1967.
10. Turner-Warwick R, Kirby RS: Urodynamic studies and their effect upon management. In Chisholm GD, Fair WR, editors: *Scientific foundations of urology,* ed 3, 1991, Heinemann.
11. Turner-Warwick R, Worth PHL: The psoas-hitch procedure for the replacement of the lower third of the urethra, *Br J Urol* 41:701, 1969.
12. Turner-Warwick R, Wynne EJC, Handley Ashken M: The use of the omentum in the repair and reconstruction of the urinary tract, *Br J Surg* 54:849, 1967.
13. Turner-Warwick R, et al: The 'supra-pubic V' incision, *Br J Urol* 46:39, 1974.

50 Surgery of the Small Intestine

DANIEL L. CLARKE-PEARSON

Surgery of the small intestine is a rarely planned procedure associated with surgery for benign gynecologic conditions. In most instances the gynecologist encounters an unexpected pathologic condition (e.g., Meckel's diverticulum, cancer, Crohn's disease) or finds that small intestinal surgery is necessary to correct an intraoperative injury.[3] The gynecologic oncologist, on the other hand, often anticipates performing resection of small intestine in the course of cytoreductive surgery for advanced ovarian cancer and in the management of obstruction or fistula associated with prior radiation therapy.[2] Although general surgical texts detail the technical procedures commonly used to correct small bowel injury and disease, this chapter offers an overview and an understanding of the principles used in small intestinal surgery as is relevant to the gynecologist.

ANATOMY

Successful surgery on the small intestine is predicated on a clear understanding of the anatomy of the small bowel and in establishing normal anatomy in surgical circumstances when it is initially distorted by disease.

The primary arterial blood supply to the stomach and small bowel derives from the celiac trunk and the superior mesenteric artery. The left gastric artery, arising from the celiac trunk, anastomoses with the right gastric branch of the hepatic artery. The gastric duodenal artery becomes the gastroepiploic artery, which runs along the greater curvature of the stomach. This is also the primary blood supply to the greater omentum. Other branches of the celiac trunk include the splenic artery, which passes posterior to the stomach, and the common hepatic artery. The lateral blood supply from the splenic artery includes the short gastric arteries, the left gastroepiploic arteries and blood supply to the pancreas (Fig. 50-1).

Distal to the celiac trunk and also arising from the abdominal aorta is the superior mesenteric artery, which supplies the jejunum and ileum as well as the right and transverse colon (Fig. 50-2). The ileal colic artery is an important branch that supplies the terminal ileum and cecum. Parallel to most of the arterial supply of the small intestine is a venous drainage system, which ultimately becomes the supe-

rior mesenteric vein that then joins the splenic vein, ultimately forming the portal vein.

The lymphatic drainage of the small intestine also parallels the arterial supply ultimately draining and passing to the root of the small intestine mesentery, which passes superiorly to the right of the aorta, terminating in the preaortic lymph nodes.

The small intestine is attached to the posterior abdominal cavity by a mesentery that crosses from the left to right; originally arising at the level of the second lumbar vertebra and passing obliquely to the right iliac fossa. The superior mesenteric vessels pass into the root of the mesentery in its upper portion. The adipose content of the mesentery progressively increases as it goes from the jejunum to the ileum. It will also be noted that the vascular arcades in the mesentery increase in number as one progresses distally along the small intestine. Usually, the first portion of the jejunum contains a single arcade, the second portion has two arcades, and the first part of the ileum has three arcades. The terminal ileum commonly has four arcades. This anatomic variation provides a rough indication of the portion of the small intestine being observed.

PREOPREATIVE EVALUATION AND PREPARATION

The preoperative evaluation of the patient for gynecologic surgery should also include an evaluation of the gastrointestinal tract when symptoms or signs warrant. Appropriate consultation with a gastroenterologist in a patient who has signs or symptoms of upper abdominal discomfort, pain, weight loss, or dyspepsia or who has guaiac-positive stools is critical to avoid the surprise finding of a gastrointestinal lesion at the time of surgery. For example, it should be recalled that approximately 10% of all ovarian malignancies are from metastatic sites, which include gastric carcinoma, colon cancer, pancreatic carcinoma, and breast cancer. Likewise, a "pelvic mass" could represent an inflammatory mass of small bowel and mesentery associated with Crohn's disease, a mucocele of the appendix, an appendiceal abscess, or a diverticular abscess. The value of a careful history and physical examination in selecting patients who would benefit from further gastrointestinal evaluation while at the

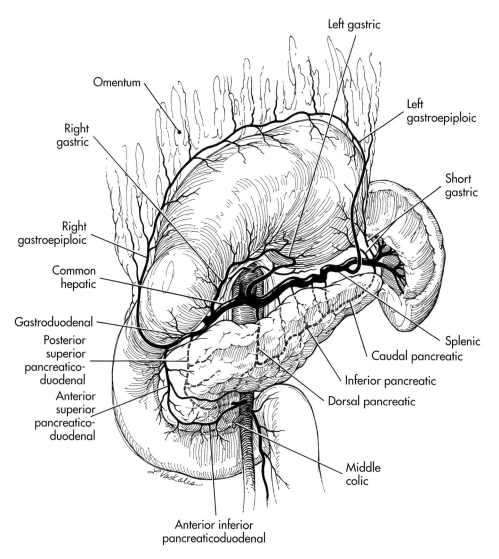

Fig. 50-1 Arterial supply arising from the celiac axis supplying the stomach, duodenum, spleen, and omentum. The stomach has been reflected superiorly and the posterior surface is exposed.

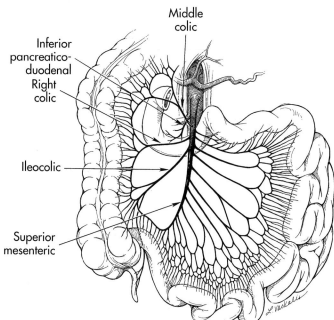

Fig. 50-2 Arterial blood supply arising from the superior mesenteric artery. Superior mesenteric artery supplies blood to the entire small intestine and ascending and transverse colon.

same time avoiding an expensive and extended workup in most patients who do not warrant it preoperatively cannot be underestimated.

Before any major abdominal and pelvic surgery, I would advise a mechanical bowel preparation in all patients. This would include a clear liquid diet for 24 hours and mechanical evacuation of the colon, using either magnesium citrate, GoLYTELY, or Phospho-Soda. Lower bowel preparation should be completed with an enema. Oral antibiotic bowel preparation (erythromycin and neomycin) should be instituted when colon surgery is anticipated or when the possibility of injury to the colon is a concern (e.g., in patients with a "fixed" pelvic mass, extensive endometriosis, or ovarian cancer, in patients undergoing cytoreductive surgery, and in patients undergoing pelvic surgery who have previously had pelvic radiation therapy). Because the unobstructed small intestine does not have a significant bacterial population, infection after small intestinal surgery is uncommon and the incidence is not significantly reduced by the use of oral preoperative antibiotics.

If, in the surgeon's opinion, the possibility exists that the patient might undergo intestinal surgery, this should be included in the informed consent discussion. The implications of this surgery, including the possibility of an ostomy, should be discussed, and if a stoma is anticipated, the patient should be referred to an enterostomal therapist preoperatively for counseling.

Finally, preoperative nutritional assessment should be done in women who appear to be malnourished. The sequelae of complications associated with a surgical patient who is malnourished can be substantial and can be significantly reversed by the judicious use of preoperative parenteral alimentation. (See Chapter 5 for more detailed discussion.)

PROBLEMS COMMONLY ENCOUNTERED BY THE GYNECOLOGIST

Intestinal Adhesions

With the large number of surgical techniques and procedures available to correct intraabdominal pathologic abnormalities, combined with the increased safety of anesthesia and postoperative recovery, many women have undergone at least one prior abdominal operation. Therefore intestinal adhesions are often encountered in the course of performing gynecologic surgery. Adhesions of the small bowel to the previous abdominal incision along the parietal peritoneum or into the pelvis or loop-to-loop adhesions between the small intestine and/or colon often must be freed before pelvic surgery is performed. On the other hand, the presence of adhesions per se does not constitute an indication for lysis. This is especially true if the adhesions are well formed and do not obstruct the surgeon's ability to carry out the gynecologic procedure planned. Indications for lysis of adhesions include the following:

1. The presence of adhesions between the small intestine and pelvic peritoneum or pelvic organs that interfere with dissection

2. Partial or complete intestinal obstruction manifest by dilation of the intestines proximally to the point of obstruction

3. The finding of adhesive "bands" or "banjo string" adhesions (This type of adhesion is a common cause of delayed small bowel obstruction.)

Adhesions should be lysed with sharp dissection rather than bluntly with the surgeon's fingers or sponge sticks. Keys to successful lysis of adhesions include excellent exposure of the operative field, good lighting, and traction and countertraction on the segment being dissected. When adhesions are so dense in one area that it is difficult to identify anatomy, the surgeon can often move to another or adjacent area, finding a more clearly demarcated plane in which to dissect; ultimately, this alternative approach frees up the more densely adherent region. In the course of adhesiolysis, the serosa or superficial muscle layer may be injured. These "denuded" areas should be oversewn with interrupted sutures perpendicular to the lumen of the small bowel (Fig. 50-3).

Enterotomy

Enterotomy is a common problem arising in the course of lysis of small bowel adhesions. Risk factors associated with enterotomies include dense adhesions fixed in the pelvis, endometriosis, pelvic inflammatory disease, and advanced gynecologic cancer. Intraoperative recognition of the enterotomy is extremely important, and the surgeon must carefully inspect all areas of small bowel that have been freed from adhesions. When an enterotomy is identified, repair should be accomplished only when there is adequate mobility of the bowel wall to ensure a tension-free repair. Further-

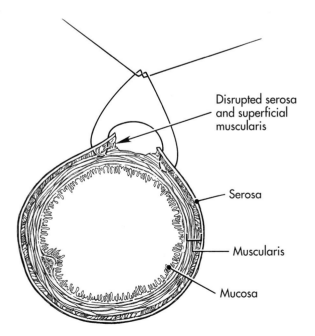

Fig. 50-3 Repair of seromuscular injury of the small bowel. Interrupted imbricating sutures used to reapproximate the injured seromuscular layer. If the extent of injury is such that the repair results in narrowing of the small bowel lumen, resection with reanastomosis should be performed.

more, adequate blood supply must be ensured. Finally, the caliber of the small bowel should not be compromised in this repair. If there are multiple areas of small bowel injury within a short segment, it is usually more prudent to resect the injured segment and make a single anastomosis rather than attempt repair of several enterotomies.

Although some surgeons rely on a single-layer closure for an enterotomy, I continue to close enterotomies in two layers. The line of closure should be created to make the enterotomy incision perpendicular to the axis of the small bowel, thereby avoiding narrowing the lumen. The first layer is an absorbable suture (2-0 or 3-0 Vicryl or chromic catgut) incorporating small bowel mucosa and muscularis.

The knot is tied into the lumen of the small bowel. The second layer is an imbricating layer of either a 2-0 or 3-0 silk or Vicryl. In this layer the knot is tied on the serosal surface rather than being buried in the muscularis (Fig. 50-4). Once the enterotomy is repaired, the bowel lumen should be palpated to ensure its patency and caliber.

Resection and Anastomosis

Small bowel resection and anastomosis may be required in the management of a segment of small bowel that has been injured, in the course of debulking ovarian carcinoma, or when correcting an intestinal obstruction caused by adhesions or radiation injury. Techniques of resection and anas-

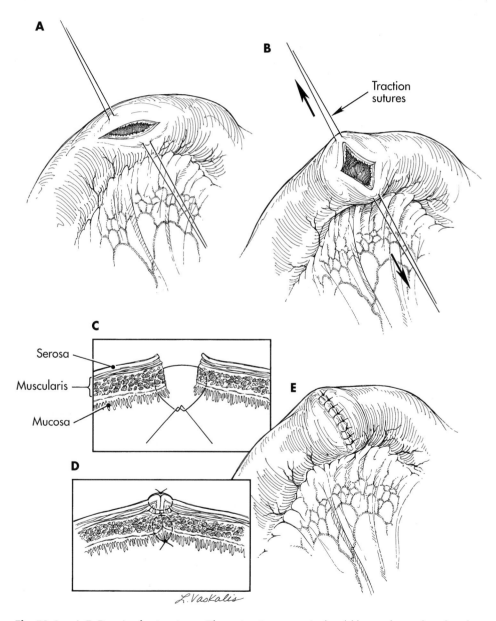

Fig. 50-4   A-E, Repair of enterotomy. The enterotomy repair should be performed so that the closure is perpendicular to the axis of the small bowel lumen. This will minimize the amount of narrowing of the small bowel. Traction sutures placed at what will ultimately be the apex of the enterotomy closure help align the bowel. Two-layer closure incorporating the mucosa and muscularis in the inner layer and the serosa and muscularis on the outer layer is recommended.

tomosis may be accomplished using hand-sewn methods or surgical staplers. There is no clear evidence that one technique is better than another as long as the following basic principles are followed:

1. The anastomosis should have adequate blood supply from either side.
2. The anastomosis should not be under tension.
3. The anastomosis should have an adequate lumen.

End-to-End Sutured Anastomosis. The small bowel segment to be resected should be identified, isolated, and mobilized from any adjacent adhesions. The mesentery beneath the area to be resected should be inspected to ensure that a dominant vascular pedicle is supplying the distal and proximal portions of the remaining small bowel. A defect is created between the small bowel serosa, and mesentery and atraumatic intestinal clamps are placed across the bowel. The bowel is then transected between the two clamps, avoiding spill of intestinal contents (Fig. 50-5, *A*). The remainder of the mesentery is divided by isolating vascular pedicles, which are clamped and suture ligated (see Fig. 50-5, *B*).

In creating the anastomosis, the surgeon moves the bowel clamps approximately 2 to 3 cm from the cut edge of the bowel and cleans the fat and mesentery off the bowel for approximately 5 mm from the anastomosis. Fresh, well-vascularized edges of small intestine should be ascertained, and if there is a question, additional bowel should be resected. The two sections of small bowel are brought together, and the seromuscular layer along the posterior wall is approximated using a Lembert imbricating stitch (Fig. 50-6, *A*). It should be noted that the knot to this interrupted suture is tied on the serosal side. A mucosal layer is then placed, beginning on the back wall of the bowel, but continuing until the entire bowel lumen is closed (see Fig. 50-6, *B*). In this case, the knots of the suture are placed in the bowel lumen. To complete the anastomosis, the seromuscular layer anteriorly is imbricated as well (see Fig. 50-6, *C*). I usually use 2-0 Vicryl for the mucosal layer and 2-0 or 3-0 silk for the serosa.

Where there is disparity between the lumen size of the two segments to be reanastomosed, a Cheatle incision may be created on the antimesenteric surface of the smaller lumen (Fig. 50-7, *A*). This will provide an increased diameter of lumen and will also allow a more even approximation of the two segments of the small bowel. Once the anastomosis is completed, the lumen should be palpated through the anastomotic ring to ensure adequate lumen caliber and patency. The suture line should be inspected carefully to ensure closure and hemostasis. Finally, the mesenteric defect should be closed so that an internal hernia does not result (see Fig. 50-7, *B*).

Side-to-Side (Functional End-to-End Stapled Anastomosis). Using gastrointestinal stapling devices, the surgeon can create a functional end-to-end anastomosis. Similar to the hand-sewn anastomosis, the segment to be resected is isolated from its mesenteric attachment, and a GIA stapler is placed across the bowel, closed, and fired, thus dividing and

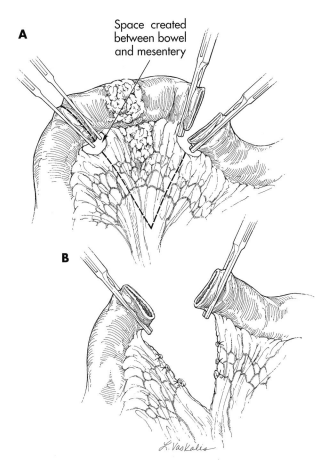

Fig. 50-5 Small bowel resection. **A,** Defects are created in the junction between the mesentery and serosa of the bowel so that two atraumatic intestinal clamps may be placed across the bowel lumen. **B,** After the bowel lumen is divided between the clamps, the mesentery of the bowel is likewise incised and the vascular arcades are clamped and ligated.

stapling both the proximal and distal lumen of that segment of bowel (Fig. 50-8, *A*). The small bowel mesentery blood supply is isolated, clamped, divided, and suture ligated (see Fig. 50-8, *B*). The edges of the distal and proximal segment of bowel are brought together and the antimesenteric portion of the staple line is transected (see Fig. 50-8, *C*). A GIA stapler is then placed into the lumen of both bowel segments, and the antimesenteric surfaces are approximated. The GIA stapler is closed and fired, thus creating a side-to-side anastomosis (see Fig. 50-8, *D*). To complete the anastomosis, the surgeon closes the remaining enterotomy with a TA55 stapler, making certain that the entire defect is brought into the staple line and that the prior GIA staple lines are overlapped by the TA55 stapler (see Fig. 50-8, *E*). The residual portion of bowel above the TA55 stapler is resected. Again, the bowel lumen should be palpated and patency and caliber reassured. Stapled anastomosis of this type usually results in a larger lumen than an end-to-end anastomosis. The mesentery of the small bowel is closed with interrupted sutures of 2-0 Vicryl, taking care to avoid suturing blood vessels in the mesentery (see Fig. 50-7, *B*).

Text continued on p. 922

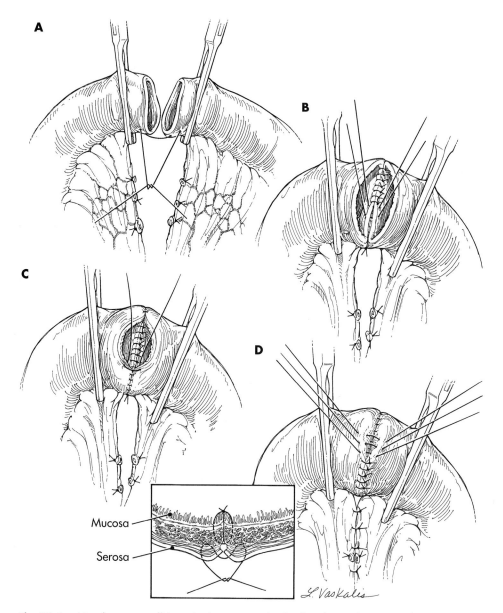

Fig. 50-6 Hand-sewn small intestinal anastomosis. **A,** The closure begins on the antimesentery surface approximating the seromuscular layer. **B,** The mucosal layer on the "back wall" is then closed. **C,** The mucosal layer closure continues onto the anterior wall, thus completing the mucosal closure circumferentially. **D,** Finally, the anterior seromuscular layer is closed using an imbricating suture. The mesenteric defect is likewise closed with care to avoid injury or hematoma of the mesenteric blood supply. *Inset,* The mucosa-muscularis closure with 2-0 Vicryl and knots tied in the bowel lumen is shown. The outer seromuscular layer embrocates the bowel wall with knots tied on the serosal surface.

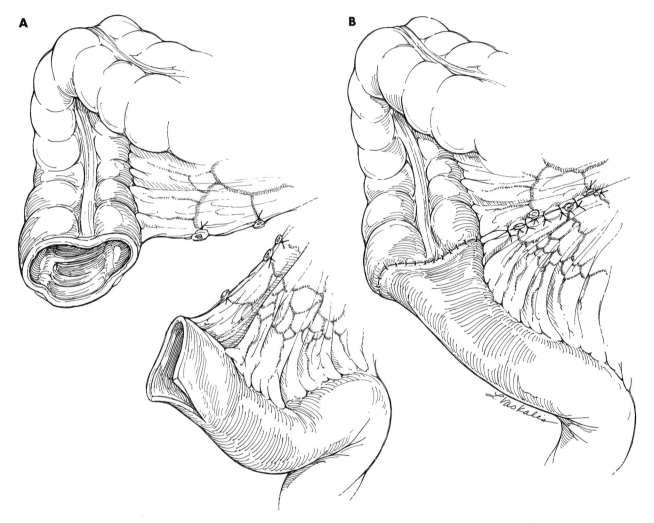

Fig. 50-7   A-B, Cheatle incision. To anastomose two bowel lumens of disparate sizes, an incision is made in the antimesenteric surface of the bowel with a smaller lumen, thereby enlarging the bowel lumen, which results in a tension-free anastomosis.

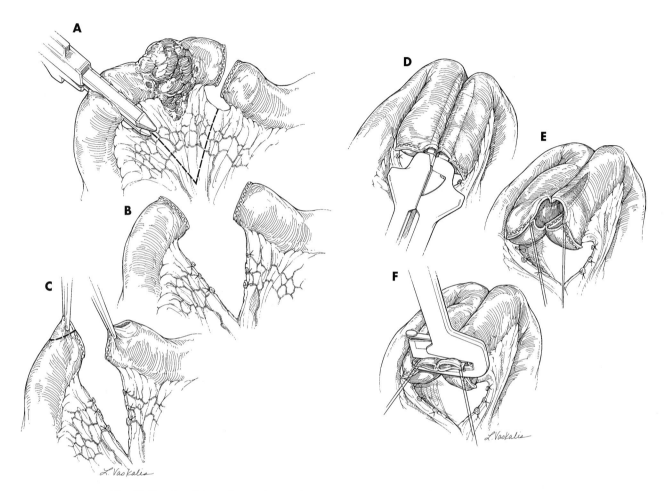

Fig. 50-8 Small bowel resection and reanastomosis using stapling devices. **A,** A mesenteric defect is made just beneath the bowel lumen, and the GIA stapler is introduced crossing the lumen. When the device is "fired," two rows of staples are applied, which are divided between a knife. **B,** After division of the small bowel lumen, the small bowel mesentery is divided, and the blood supply is ligated. **C,** The two portions of small bowel to be reanastomosed are approximated at their antimesenteric surfaces. The antimesenteric corners of the staple lines are transected. **D** and **E,** The GIA stapler is introduced with one "arm" in each lumen. The stapler is closed and fired, thereby creating an anastomosis between the two segments of small bowel. **F,** The remaining enterotomy is closed using a TA55 stapler with care to overlap the previous staple lines and to be certain that the full thickness of the small bowel enterotomy is incorporated in the staple line. The excess tissue above the stapler is excised.

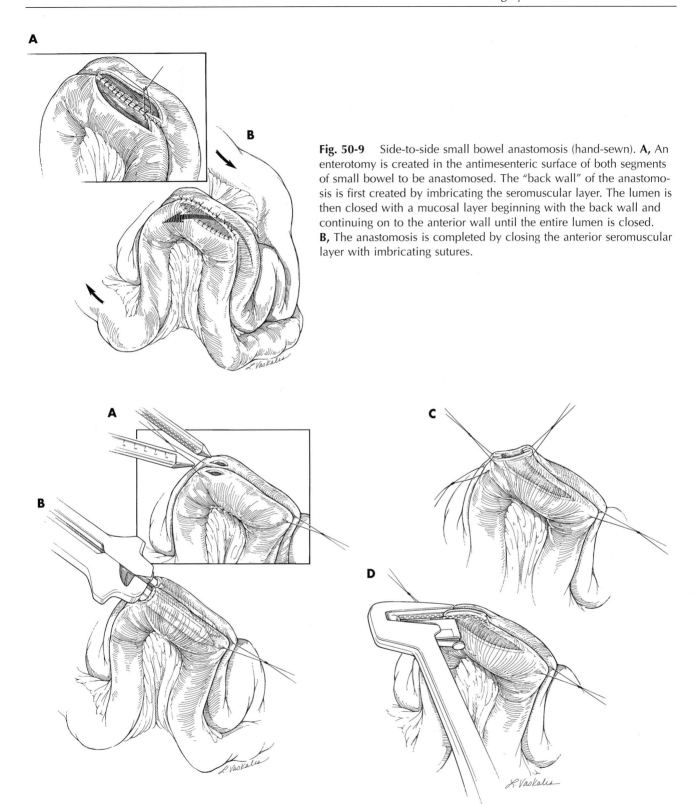

Fig. 50-9 Side-to-side small bowel anastomosis (hand-sewn). **A,** An enterotomy is created in the antimesenteric surface of both segments of small bowel to be anastomosed. The "back wall" of the anastomosis is first created by imbricating the seromuscular layer. The lumen is then closed with a mucosal layer beginning with the back wall and continuing on to the anterior wall until the entire lumen is closed. **B,** The anastomosis is completed by closing the anterior seromuscular layer with imbricating sutures.

Fig. 50-10 Side-to-side anastomosis created with a stapling device. **A,** The antimesenteric surfaces of both small bowel lumens are approximated, and a small incision is made in each antimesenteric surface to introduce the GIA stapling device. **B,** With the stapling device introduced into the lumen, it is fired, thereby creating the anastomosis. **C,** The remaining enterotomy is elevated with stay sutures. **D,** The enterotomy is then closed using the TA55 stapling device. The excess tissue above the stapling device is excised.

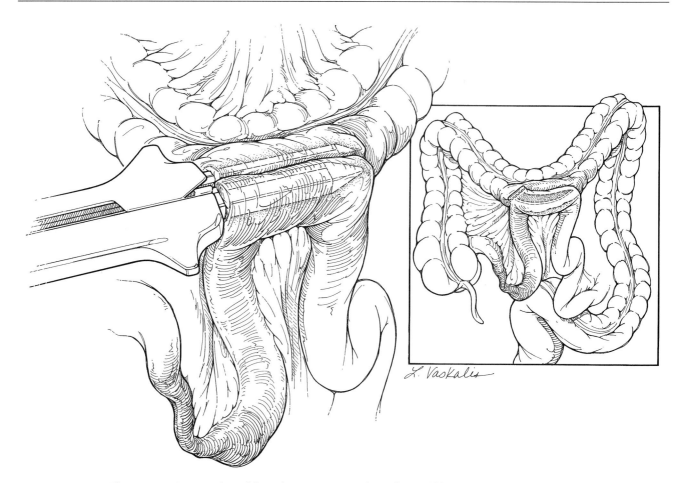

L. Vaskalis

Fig. 50-11 Bypass of small bowel to transverse colon. The small bowel may be bypassed to the ascending, transverse, or descending colon using a side-to-side stapling technique, observing the same principle as outlined in the legend to Fig. 50-10.

Side-to-Side Anastomosis. The technique of side-to-side anastomosis is usually performed to "bypass" a segment of obstructed bowel that cannot be resected. This may be most common in bypassing bowel that is obstructed and is densely adherent in the pelvis after radiation therapy. Small bowel that is extensively involved with ovarian carcinoma might also be "bypassed" rather than resected. Side-to-side anastomosis can be accomplished by either a hand-sewn technique (Fig. 50-9) or by using the GIA stapler (Fig. 50-10). Side-to-side bypass procedures may reanastomose small bowel to small bowel or small bowel to ascending or transverse colon (Fig. 50-11). Furthermore, the segment of small bowel, which is diseased, may be more completely isolated from the fecal stream by being transected and the distal lumen brought to the skin as a mucous fistula (Fig. 50-12).

POSTOPERATIVE CARE

Care of the patient after small bowel resection and anastomosis is focused on allowing the anastomosis to heal. Keys to promote healing include providing good nutrition, eliminating infection, and avoiding distention of the small bowel lumen. The patient should be given nothing by mouth (NPO) and have a nasogastric tube placed intraoperatively

to decompress the stomach and small bowel. Ileus may persist for several days postoperatively. If prolonged ileus is anticipated, nutritional assessment should be carried out to determine whether total parenteral nutrition should be instituted. Alternatively, an elemental diet may be administered through a jejunostomy tube or a Dubhoff catheter placed in the duodenum. Once a patient has good bowel sounds and passes flatus, an oral diet may be instituted promptly.

MECKEL'S DIVERTICULUM

Meckel's diverticulum may be encountered as an asymptomatic condition in the course of pelvic surgery in approximately 2% of patients. Meckel's diverticulum results from the failure of the closure of the intestinal end of the omphalomesenteric or vitelline duct, which was present in the first few weeks of fetal life as a portion of the primitive yolk sac. The diverticulum arises in the terminal ileum approximately 45 to 90 cm proximal to the ileal cecal valve on the antimesenteric border of the ileum. It may vary in length from 1 to 10 cm, although most are clinically obvious, measuring approximately 3 to 4 cm.[1] Meckel's diverticulum is commonly known to students and housestaff as the "disease of 2's": it occurs in 2% of the population, is twice as common

A

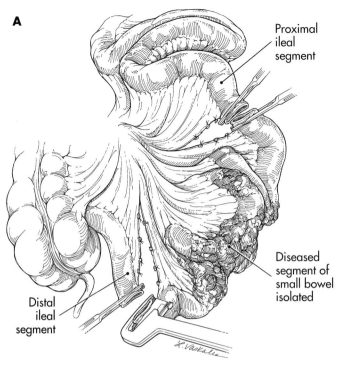

Proximal
ileal
segment

Diseased
segment of
small bowel
isolated

Distal
ileal
segment

Fig. 50-12   Small bowel resection with isolation of diseased segment and creation of a mucous fistula. Sometimes, the segment of diseased small bowel cannot safely be removed and therefore needs to be isolated. So that a "blind loop" is not created, a mucous fistula must be developed. **A,** The proximal and distal portions of the diseased small bowel are divided with either intestinal clamps or GIA stapling devices. **B,** The proximal and distal portions of small bowel to be reanastomosed are brought together and reanastomosed using either a hand-sewn or stapling technique. **C,** The diseased segment of small bowel that had been isolated is brought to the skin surface, and a mucous fistula stoma is created to allow drainage from the isolated segment.

B

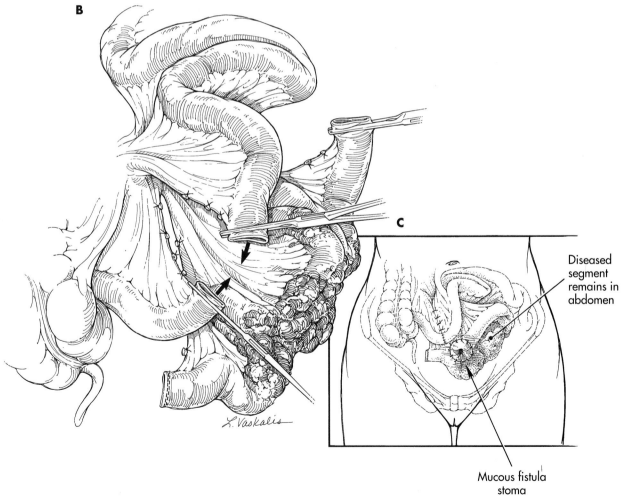

C

Diseased
segment
remains in
abdomen

Mucous fistula
stoma

in males as in females, and is usually found 2 feet from the ileocecal valve. In approximately 20% of patients, it may contain heterotopic gastric, colonic, or pancreatic mucosa.

Symptomatic Meckel's diverticulum is commonly encountered in the pediatric age group, although it can result in morbidity and mortality in the elderly as well. Serious complications and death from Meckel's diverticulum are almost always the result of a delay in diagnosis and therapy. Symptomatic Meckel's diverticulum may result from intussusception, diverticulitis within the diverticulum, volvulus of a segment of small bowel around a fibrous band connecting the diverticulum to the umbilicus, or a peptic ulcer arising in heterotopic gastric mucosa within the diverticulum. In gynecologic surgery, Meckel's diverticulum is nearly always encountered in an asymptomatic state, and one must question whether the diverticulum should be removed if found incidentally. Certainly, the diverticulum should be removed if there is any evidence of ectopic tissue (ectopic gastric mucosa), which may be suspected if there is a localized thickening of the diverticulum. In addition, the diverticulum should be removed if the orifice of the draining diverticulum appears to be narrow or if there is concern that the patient's symptoms are secondary to an abnormality of the diverticulum. Because it may be difficult intraoperatively to determine whether the diverticulum contains ectopic gastric mucosa, I routinely recommend resection of the diverticulum if encountered incidentally.

The basic surgical treatment of the Meckel's diverticulum requires the ligation of any separate blood supply arising from the mesentery of the ileum and crossing to the diverticulum. The diverticulum may then be clamped with intestinal clamps placed perpendicular to the axis of the lumen of the ileum, and the Meckel's diverticulum is resected. The small bowel lumen is then closed in two layers as outlined for a large enterotomy. Alternatively, using a GIA or TA55 stapler results in a rapid excision of Meckel's diverticulum (Fig. 50-13). The mortality and morbidity associated with resection of an uncomplicated Meckel's diverticulum should be negligible. Postoperative care should follow the guidelines for the care of a patient after a small bowel anastomosis.

Resection of a Meckel's diverticulum that may present as bleeding from the diverticulum, intussusception, or diverticulitis is more complicated. Surgical treatment should include segmental resection of the adjacent small bowel with primary reanastomosis of the ileum rather than a diverticulectomy, which might result in leaving ectopic gastric tissue behind or result in an anastomosis across an inflamed diverticular base.

SMALL INTESTINAL COMPLICATIONS OF LAPAROSCOPIC SURGERY

The ever-increasing use of the laparoscope to perform gynecologic procedures has resulted in an increased number of small intestinal injuries associated with laparoscopic surgery. Given the serious outcomes of unrecognized injury, the laparoscopic surgeon must be ever vigilant to prevent these complications and to identify them intraoperatively. Gastrointestinal injury occurs in approximately 1.6 per 1000 laparoscopic procedures, and it is reported that only 60% of these injuries are noted at the time of surgery.

Prevention of intestinal injury is key, and high-risk situations should be identified. Most intestinal injuries occur at the time of insertion of Veress needles or trocars. The incidence of these injuries is increased in patients who have had prior surgery, who have bowel adhesions, or who have intestinal distention. Patients who have had previous abdominal or pelvic surgery might best be operated on through an "open" technique. Alternatively, success with establishing a pneumoperitoneum by placing the Veress needle in the midclavicular line in the left upper quadrant (where adhesions from prior pelvic surgery are rare) has been reported.

Another key element in laparoscopic surgery, which should reduce the risk of intestinal complications, is the use of a sharp trocar. I often use spring-loaded "safety shield" trocars, but it must be acknowledged that this does not necessarily eliminate all possibility of intestinal injury. Adequate pneumoperitoneum should be achieved so that the second trocar can be inserted under direct visualization. Other techniques to confirm safe intraperitoneal entry as outlined in Chapter 7 should be followed.

Perforation of the bowel by the Veress needle is not usually a serious problem unless it has been torn by excessive lateral movement of the Veress needle or the mesenteric vessels have been injured. Injury by the Veress needle may be suspected if gastrointestinal contents are aspirated from the needle after it has been inserted or if a fecal smell is noted upon removal of the needle. Other signs of intraluminal entry of the needle include asymmetric abdominal distention, unexpected dilation of the small or large bowel, belching, or sudden passage of flatus.

Simple Veress needle penetrations of the small intestine or stomach usually will seal spontaneously without leakage of bowel contents. Administration of broad-spectrum antibiotics is suggested, and the patient should be observed for abdominal distention, tenderness, or other signs of peritonitis. Immediate laparotomy should be performed if any signs suggesting peritonitis are present. Injury by the Veress needle is more serious if a tear in the bowel has occurred. Therefore Veress needle injuries should be inspected carefully, and attention should be paid to ascertain whether there is a through-and-through penetration or whether the mesenteric vessels have been injured. Depending on the surgeon's skills, repair of a tear in the small bowel wall may be accomplished by either open or laparoscopic techniques.

The small intestine may also be injured by placement of either the primary or ancillary trocars or during the dissection of adhesions. Trocar injuries may result in bruising or penetration of one side of the small intestine, or result in a through-and-through perforation of the small bowel. Particularly dangerous injuries are those that go unrecognized.

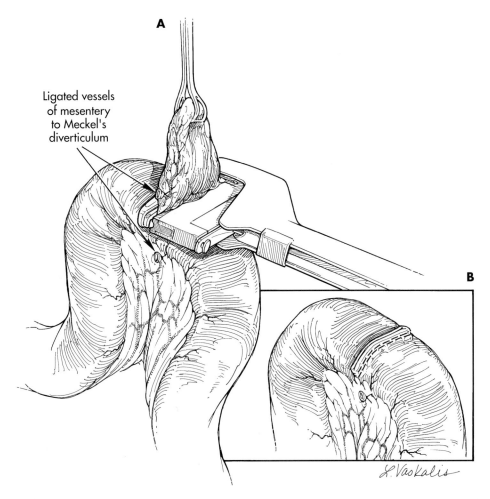

Ligated vessels
of mesentery
to Meckel's
diverticulum

A

B

L. Vaskalis

Fig. 50-13   Resection of Meckel's diverticulum may be performed using either intestinal clamps and a hand-sewn closure or the TA55 stapling device. **A,** The mesenteric blood supply of the Meckel's diverticulum is isolated, clamped, and ligated. The Meckel's diverticulum is then elevated, and the TA55 stapling device is applied across the base of the Meckel's diverticulum with an axis perpendicular to the small bowel lumen. After the device is fired, the Meckel's diverticulum is excised. **B,** The result of the stapled resection does not narrow the small bowel lumen. In patients with diverticulitis, extensive inflammation, or a question of ectopic tissue, which may not be entirely excised, segmental resection of the small bowel and Meckel's diverticulum is necessary.

Therefore it is recommended that the following precautions be taken:

1. Immediately upon placement of the primary trocar and sleeve, the laparoscope should be inserted and the area beneath the insertion site should be carefully inspected to determine whether there is any adjacent intestinal injury.

2. If it is strongly suspected that perforation has occurred but it is impossible to identify the perforation with the laparoscope, it is best to err on the side of caution and perform a laparotomy to examine the entire intestine and abdominal contents.

3. A through-and-through bowel injury, especially if it is adjacent to the anterior abdominal wall, may go entirely unrecognized (Fig. 50-14). Therefore a prudent surgeon will observe the withdrawal of the cannula through the laparoscope at the completion of the sur-

gical procedure. This may be the only opportunity to identify the lumen of the bowel that has been injured.

4. Insertion of secondary trocars should always be performed under direct visualization.

A small bowel perforation created by the insertion of trocar and cannula should be repaired using the same principles as those applied to closure of an enterotomy at an open procedure. In skilled hands, this may often be accomplished using laparoscopic suturing and knot-tying techniques. Laparotomy should be performed if the surgeon does not have sufficient skill to suture laparoscopically.

Unrecognized trocar and cannula injury to the intestine may result in serious and sometimes fatal peritonitis. The patient may initially do well but be seen 2 to 3 days postoperatively with increasing abdominal pain and signs of peritonitis, including abdominal distention, vomiting, rebound tenderness, and fever. Thermal damage injuries may not be-

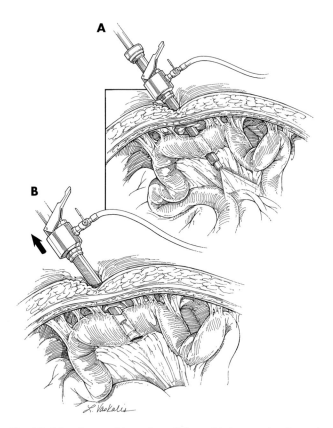

Fig. 50-14 Recognition of small bowel injury at the time of laparoscopy. **A,** Small bowel adherent to the anterior abdominal wall in the region of the initial port site has a high possibility of not being recognized. After introduction of the laparoscopic sheath and laparoscope, visualization of the pelvis may appear normal and the loop of bowel that has been crossed by the sheath and laparoscope may not be identified. **B,** To identify this occult injury, the laparoscope should be withdrawn into the lumen of the sheath and then the sheath should be observed as it is being withdrawn from the abdominal cavity. As the sheath exits through the loop of small bowel that has been injured, the injury may be recognized and immediately repaired.

come apparent for up to 10 days postoperatively. Because of the catastrophic consequences associated with delay in recognition and management of intestinal injuries, immediate laparotomy is strongly recommended in patients with suspected peritonitis. The advice that "the patient who has increasing postoperative pain following a laparoscopy has a bowel perforation until proven otherwise" should be a well-accepted motto of the laparoscopic surgeon.[6]

Electrical burns of the small intestine may range from superficial serosal blanching to full-thickness burns of the intestinal wall. Minor superficial burns may be watched expectantly. However, significant blanching of the bowel wall indicates a serious burn, which may undergo necrosis and delayed perforation. Obvious thermal injuries should be dealt with immediately. Because the spread of electrothermal damage is much greater than the area of obvious blanching, it is generally advised that a segment of bowel approximately 5 cm on either side of the margins of the

damaged site be excised and an anastomosis be performed.[6]

Incisional hernia from 10-mm and larger ports can result in yet another postoperative small bowel complication. The risks of incisional hernia increase in direct proportion to the size of the cannula inserted, and it is generally recommended that fascia be closed beneath ports that are 10 mm or larger. In such closure, it is recommended that the peritoneum also be approximated to avoid a Richter's hernia. A number of laparoscopic devices can be used to facilitate closure of the port site.

Signs of intestinal obstruction or pain at the port site may represent incarceration of small bowel or omentum. Management includes surgical exploration, release of the incarcerated tissue, and possible resection if infarction is recognized.

POSTOPERATIVE COMPLICATIONS
Ileus and Small Bowel Obstruction

After abdominal surgery, there is a reduction in the coordinated propulsion of the gastrointestinal tract, resulting in abdominal distention. This condition (ileus) varies among patients and is somewhat unpredictable. Furthermore, there is clear evidence that different portions of the gastrointestinal tract recover their function at different times. For example, the stomach remains atonic for approximately 18 to 24 hours postoperatively, whereas the small intestine regains its motility within a few hours of abdominal surgery. The colon, on the other hand, will not regain function until approximately 48 hours after abdominal surgery.

Despite this transient dysfunction of the intestinal tract, I usually instruct patients who have undergone uncomplicated abdominal or pelvic surgery within the first 12 hours of surgery to begin a liquid diet. In most patients, intestinal function returns promptly and the diet progresses to regular meals within 48 to 72 hours. Unfortunately, some patients develop an ileus, resulting in abdominal distention, nausea, and vomiting. A significant ileus may also result in respiratory compromise, wound dehiscence, or anastomotic leak. Treatment of an ileus includes bowel rest (NPO), replacement of intravascular volume and electrolytes, and nasogastric intubation and intestinal decompression.[5] It should be remembered that most of the air in the small intestine is swallowed, and even if a nasogastric tube is not removing large volumes of liquid gastrointestinal contents, it may still be preventing further introduction of air into the small bowel. Prolonged postoperative ileus (persisting for more than 4 days) should raise the concern that the patient may actually have a mechanical bowel obstruction. Throughout the conservative management of the ileus, the patient should be observed for signs of intestinal vascular compromise (ischemia or infarction), which would necessitate immediate laparotomy (e.g., rebound tenderness, fever, leukocytosis).

After abdominal surgery, intestinal obstruction may occur in 1% of 2% of patients. These obstructions are most commonly caused by adhesions of small bowel to the abdominal incision or to a pelvic operative site. Other postoperative small bowel obstructions might result from incarceration in an internal hernia caused by adhesions or a mesenteric defect or malrotation of the small bowel or volvulus. Initially, the patient may have signs and symptoms similar to those of an ileus, including abdominal distention and nausea or vomiting. Although surgical intervention may be necessary, conservative medical management most often results in the resolution of the obstruction. Management should include administration of intravenous fluids and electrolytes, nasogastric decompression, and complete bowel rest. During this course of medical management, the patient should be monitored carefully for any evidence of intestinal strangulation and intestinal vascular compromise or perforation. In particular, the patient should be monitored for leukocytosis, metabolic acidosis, fever, or worsening peritoneal signs. If the intestinal obstruction does not improve in 72 hours or if at any time there is evidence of bowel ischemia or perforation, the patient should be returned to the operating room immediately for laparotomy and correction of the obstruction.

Although abdominal x-ray films may be helpful in evaluating the patient with ileus or small bowel obstruction, the radiographic picture of small intestinal distention and air-fluid levels may be present in both conditions. It is therefore difficult to visibly differentiate between a simple ileus and an early or incomplete (partial) obstruction. Likewise, free air in the peritoneal cavity immediately after laparotomy may persist for several days and may not be a helpful sign in identifying viscus perforation versus the normal amount of free air seen in the abdomen postoperatively.

Nasogastric Tube Decompression

Postoperative use of the nasogastric tube after abdominal surgery has been advocated in patients in whom extended procedures might be associated with a higher risk of postoperative ileus developing. However, recent studies question the benefit of routine postoperative nasogastric decompression. In a randomized trial of patients undergoing major abdominal surgery for a gynecologic malignancy, there was clear evidence that postoperative nasogastric tube decompression did not reduce the incidence of gastrointestinal complications.[4] Postoperative nausea, vomiting, and abdominal distention occurred with equal frequency in the group who had nasogastric tubes and those who did not. Furthermore, it has been noted that the incidence of pulmonary complications, including atelectasis and pneumonia, was actually increased in patients who had nasogastric tubes for postoperative intestinal decompression. Therefore it is currently believed that postoperative nasogastric tube decompression in patients undergoing abdominal surgery does not provide any substantial benefit and does significantly increase the patient's discomfort. It remains the consensus that patients undergoing intestinal surgery or those who have had surgery for bowel obstruction may still benefit from nasogastric decompression. When nasogastric decompression is used, patients should be treated concurrently with cimetidine to reduce the risk of stress ulcers and gastritis developing.

REFERENCES

1. Ellis H: Meckel's diverticulum, diverticulosis of the small intestine, umbilical fistulae and tumors. In Schwartz SI, Ellis H, editors: *Maingot's abdominal operations,* East Norwalk, Conn, 1989, Appleton & Lange.
2. Krebs H, Goplerud DR: The role of intestinal intubation in obstruction of the small intestine due to carcinoma of the ovary, *Surg Gynecol Obstet* 158:467, 1984.
3. Krebs H, Goplerud DR: Mechanical intestinal obstruction in patients with gynecologic disease: a review of 368 patients, *Am J Obstet Gynecol* 157:577, 1987.
4. Pearl ML, et al: A randomized controlled trial of postoperative nasogastric tube decompression in gynecologic oncology patients undergoing intra-abdominal surgery, *J Obstet Gynecol* 88:399, 1996.
5. Petz DJ, Gamelli RL, Plicher DB: Intestinal intubation in acute mechanical small bowel obstruction, *Arch Surg* 117:334, 1982.
6. Soderstrom RM, Levinson C, Levy B: Complications of operative laparoscopy. In Soderstrom RM, editor: *Operative laparoscopy,* New York, 1993, Raven Press.

51   Surgery of the Colon and Appendix

DANIEL L. CLARKE-PEARSON and DAVID H. NICHOLS

The colon and some of its associated disease processes are commonly encountered by the gynecologist. Except for gynecologic oncologists, gynecologic surgeons rarely anticipate and perform their own colon surgeries. The exceptions to this statement include performing appendectomies and lysing adhesions from the sigmoid colon to other pelvic structures. On the other hand, an understanding of the common conditions of the colon and the common surgical procedures performed on the colon are indeed relevant to the gynecologic surgeon and will be discussed in this chapter.

ANATOMY

The colon occupies several anatomic locations throughout the abdomen and pelvis and alternates between a retroperitoneal and intraperitoneal structure. Because of the relative mobility of some segments and the fixation of other segments, somewhat different surgical approaches are required for different portions of the colon. The colon is easily distinguished from the small intestine by the presence of taeniae, sacculations (haustra coli), and fatty appendages (appendices epiploicae). Primary portions of the colon that "frame" the small intestine include the cecum, ascending colon, transverse colon, descending colon, sigmoid colon, and the rectum.

The blood supply to the colon arises from three primary sources: the superior mesenteric artery, the inferior mesenteric artery, and the middle and inferior hemorrhoidal branches, which arise from the internal iliac artery. Throughout most of the ascending, transverse, and descending colon is a rich collateral circulation supplied by the marginal artery (marginal artery of Drummond). As noted in Chapter 50, the superior mesenteric artery, which supplies all of the small intestine blood supply, also supplies the cecum, ascending colon, and the right side of the transverse colon. Predominant arteries include the ileocolic artery to the terminal ileum and cecum and the right and middle colic arteries. The inferior mesenteric artery supplies the left side of the transverse colon, the descending colon, and the sigmoid colon and upper rectum. Primary branches from the superior mesenteric artery include the left colic artery, the branches to the sigmoid colon, and the superior rectal artery. The rectum derives its blood supply from the internal iliac artery, which gives off branches including the middle and inferior rectal arteries (Fig. 51-1). The venous drainage of the colon ultimately feeds into the portal vein (Fig. 51-2). The right and transverse colon empty predominantly into the superior mes-

enteric vein, whereas the sigmoid and left colon drain into the inferior mesenteric vein, which drains into the splenic vein before entering the portal vein. Lymphatics of the colon largely follow the main arterial channels, which ultimately flow into the terminal nodes at the base of the main colic vessels and into the paraaortic nodes.

Detailed anatomy of the cecum and appendix is discussed in the appendectomy section later in this chapter.

Other important anatomic relationships to the colon may include the following.

Whereas the transverse colon is relatively mobile and may literally descend into the pelvis, the hepatic and splenic flexures are reasonably fixed in their location. It is especially important to recognize the relationship between the spleen and the splenic flexure of the colon. The most common cause of splenic injury intraoperatively is by too much downward traction on the descending or transverse colon, thereby tearing the spleen capsule, which is adjacent to the splenic flexure of the colon. From a gynecologist's point of view, this most commonly would happen in the course of performing an omentectomy. The splenic flexure needs to be mobilized by incising the paracolic gutter lateral to the left colon and by mobilizing the omentum and splenic flexure away from the spleen.

In the course of pelvic surgery, the surgeon needs to be aware of the relationship of the left ureter and ovarian vessels (in particular, the infundibulopelvic ligament). It is not uncommon to find that the sigmoid colon as it crosses the pelvic brim is immediately adjacent to these retroperitoneal structures and sometimes adhesions have made the sigmoid adherent to the left pelvic sidewall peritoneum. A retroperitoneal approach should be taken by incising the left paracolic gutter. Entering the retroperitoneum of the pelvis allows the surgeon to identify the ureter and ovarian vessels and thereby protect the ureter and control the ovarian vessels. Dissection in this region, especially when adhesions are present, increases the risk of injury to mesenteric arteries and veins of the sigmoid colon, which can bleed profusely.

The pelvic ureter lies lateral to the rectosigmoid colon. Given the usual approach to the retroperitoneum that most gynecologic surgeons take, the ureter is usually mobilized immediately because of the lateral approach to the retroperitoneum. On the other hand, the ureter may be allowed to remain in a lateral position if a more medial course of dissection on the colon is taken. However, in this course along the rectosigmoid colon, the surgeon must always bear in mind the location of the ureter.

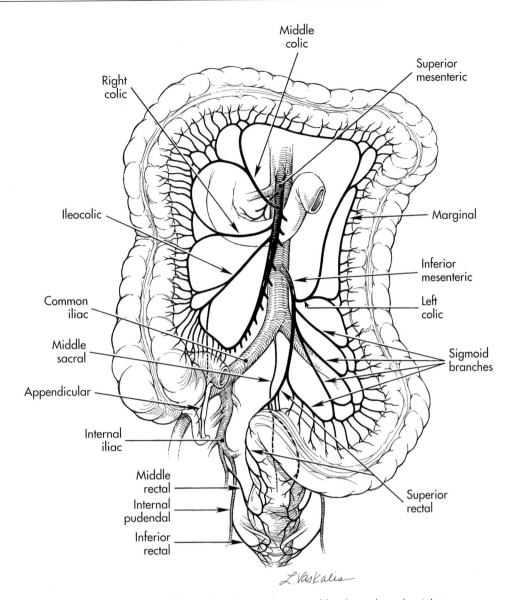

Fig. 51-1   Arterial supply of the colon. The predominant blood supply to the right transverse descending, and sigmoid colon comes from the superior mesenteric artery and the inferior mesenteric artery. There is rich anastomosis between these two dominant trunks especially supplied by the marginal artery. Blood supply to the distal sigmoid colon and rectum comes from distal branches of the inferior mesenteric artery and from the middle and inferior rectal arteries, which arise from the internal iliac artery.

The retroperitoneal portion of the rectum begins at the posterior cul-de-sac lying immediately behind the cervix and upper vagina. In its retroperitoneal course, the rectum is adjacent to the vagina, although there is an easily dissected plane (the rectovaginal septum) that may be entered from either a transperitoneal or transvaginal approach (as in the performance of a posterior colporrhaphy).

PREOPERATIVE PREPARATION

Patients who have symptoms related to the colon (e.g., worsening constipation, diarrhea, rectal bleeding, rectal pain, narrowing of the stool caliber) should receive appropriate gastrointestinal evaluation before pelvic surgery is undertaken. Studies that are particularly helpful include flexible proctosigmoidostomy, colonoscopy, and air-contrast barium enema. This evaluation is particularly important in planning the pelvic surgery approach for both benign conditions (e.g., extensive endometriosis) and cancer (especially ovarian cancer). Selective use of colonic evaluation as well as appropriate gastrointestinal medical consultation will allow the gynecologic surgeon to achieve the best outcome for the patient. However, this is not to say that every patient with a pelvic mass warrants a thorough colonic workup because the surgeon should select tests that are cost effective and perform them if the results will have some bearing on surgical outcome.

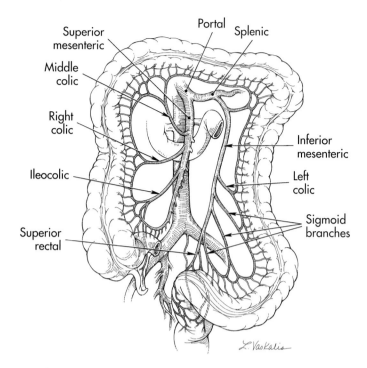

Fig. 51-2   The venous drainage of the colon ultimately feeds into the portal vein. The superior mesenteric vein drains directly into the portal vein, whereas the inferior mesenteric vein drains to the splenic vein.

Whether gastrointestinal surgery is anticipated or not, we feel strongly that mechanical bowel preparation should be part of the preoperative management of all patients having major pelvic surgery. This is especially important because most colon surgery and injury during gynecologic procedures is not anticipated. In patients who do not have adequate mechanical bowel preparation, the infection rate from the spill of colonic contents is substantially increased.[11] Although the colon and rectum cannot be thoroughly sterilized, the bacterial count can be sufficiently decreased by mechanical bowel preparation to reduce the incidence of infection. There are three commonly used bowel preparation techniques.

1. A clear liquid diet is begun 24 hours before the anticipated surgery. On the afternoon before surgery, the patient ingests 4 L of GoLYTELY at the rate of approximately 1 L/hr. The rectal effluent after this preparation should be clear. If it is not, the patient should drink more GoLYTELY. In patients who cannot tolerate the oral ingestion of this quantity of liquids, a small-gauge nasogastric tube may be placed and the GoLYTELY introduced at a steady rate.

2. Magnesium citrate may be used to cleanse the bowel, using its purgative effects. Again, the patient begins a clear liquid diet 24 hours before surgery and on the afternoon before surgery drinks 250 ml of magnesium citrate. Later that same evening we administer a Fleets enema to finally cleanse the distal colon.

3. The patient begins a clear liquid diet 24 hours before surgery and then ingests oral sodium phosphate (Fleets Phospho-Soda), 45 ml mixed in one glass of water at 4:00 PM followed by three glasses of water or clear fruit juice.

Each of these three bowel preparation regimens has its advocates, and it is not entirely clear which is preferable. In a study performed by Cohen et al.,[3] which in a blinded randomized fashion compared GoLYTELY with Fleets Phospho-Soda, it was found that endoscopists scored the bowel preparation as good-to-excellent in 90% of patients receiving Phospho-Soda compared with 70% of patients receiving GoLYTELY. Of the patients who received sodium phosphate preparation, 83% stated they would take the same preparation again compared with only 19% of the patients who received the GoLYTELY preparation. There were no clinically significant changes in weight or biochemical parameters in either group. Based on this one randomized trial evaluating bowel preparation at the time of colonoscopy, one can conclude that Fleets Phospho-Soda might be the most appropriate and best tolerated method for bowel preparation.

Complications of colon surgery are further reduced by the use of oral and intravenous antibiotics. For many years, colorectal surgeons believed that the preoperative use of oral antibiotic preparations such as neomycin and erythromycin reduced the risks of infectious complications. The usual regimen calls for administration of 1 g of neomycin and 1 g of erythromycin at 1, 2, and 11 PM on the day before surgery. For patients who will be having surgery late in the day, the timing of the administration of the erythromycin and neomycin should be delayed such that the last dose is given approximately 9 hours before surgery.

Parenteral antibiotics may also reduce the incidence of infectious and septic complications after colon surgery, although the results of randomized trials are somewhat variable and controversial. Today, most surgeons who anticipate performing colon surgery do not rely on parenteral antibiotics alone as their method of prophylaxis. In fact, most surgeons presently use both oral and parenteral antibiotics in addition to mechanical cleansing as preoperative preparation before elective colon resection in hopes of further reducing the postoperative infection rate. Whether the addition of a parenteral antibiotic to the oral antibiotic regimen actually improves outcome also remains controversial. In a large randomized study, there was no particular benefit shown with the addition of parenteral antibiotics.[4] In conclusion, we strongly believe that all patients undergoing major pelvic surgery should also have mechanical bowel preparation. Clearly, in patients for whom colon resection is anticipated (e.g., those with endometriosis, ovarian cancer invading the colon, or a constricting lesion), we would also add an oral neomycin-erythromycin preparation as outlined previously. In addition, we would suggest using oral antibiotics when there is an increased risk for colonic injury (e.g., patients with severe endometriosis, severe pelvic inflammatory disease, or a large pelvic mass).

Finally, preparation for surgery also includes consideration of positioning of the patient on the operating table. When even the most remote possibility of colonic injury or colon surgery exists, we place the patient in Allen stirrups in a modified lithotomy (Whitmore) position with her buttocks at the edge of the operating table. A sterile field is prepared for abdominal, vaginal, transperineal, and anal surgery. This will allow access to the vagina and rectum to perform proctoscopy, a "bubble test" (see the following section), or low rectal stapled anastomoses.

COMMON PROBLEMS ENCOUNTERED BY THE GYNECOLOGIC SURGEON
Rectal Injury

The most common unanticipated need for colon surgery in the course of performing a gynecologic operation is rectal injury. Rectal injury is most likely to occur during a difficult dissection where tissue planes and anatomy are distorted by severe adhesions, endometriosis, pelvic inflammatory disease, or cancer. Recognizing these high-risk situations, the gynecologic surgeon should have the patient prepared for potential colon surgery as outlined in the previous section.

Key to the prevention of rectal injury is a keen awareness of the anatomy and of surgical techniques to reestablish normal anatomy. The sigmoid colon adherent to the left pelvic sidewall should be mobilized by taking advantage of the left retroperitoneal space. By opening the left retroperitoneal space and thereby including the paravesical and pararectal spaces, the sigmoid colon may be mobilized medially. In addition, key vascular structures (common iliac, external iliac, and internal iliac arteries and veins) may be identified and protected and mobilized away from the colon. Furthermore, the surgeon must identify the ureter and, if necessary, mobilize it away from its attachments to the peritoneum, which may be adherent to the rectosigmoid mesentery (ureterolysis). Finally, the ovarian vessels should be identified as they course across the pelvic brim usually just superior to the ureter at this location. Further mobilization of the sigmoid colon can be achieved by opening the presacral space. The presacral space is an avascular plane lying behind the rectosigmoid colon and in front of the sacral vessels and left common iliac vein.

The other area of difficult dissection where rectal injury is likely to occur is in the region of the posterior cul-de-sac (pouch of Douglas). Again, with conditions that distort the anatomy in this region, the rectosigmoid colon may be densely adherent to the posterior uterus and cervix, and the posterior cul-de-sac may be entirely obliterated. In these situations, not only should lateral mobilization be achieved (as discussed previously) but the anatomy in the posterior pelvis needs to be restored by a sharp dissection. Blunt dissection and tearing through tissues with excessive traction most commonly results in denuding the muscularis of the colon and increases the risks of transrectal injury. If possible, the dissection should be performed adjacent to the posterior aspect of the uterus and on occasion must actually cross the uterine serosa. Because there is not an easily dissected plane, sharp dissection must ensue until the rectovaginal septum is encountered. Thereafter, in most situations, the rectovaginal septum is relatively avascular and

dissects easily with blunt dissection. Throughout the course of this dissection, traction and countertraction are extremely important, with traction being applied to pull the uterus forward, the adnexa laterally, and the colon posteriorly. Attempting to stay in the central portion of the uterus and the cervix also results in less chance of bleeding, injury to uterine vessels, or injury to the ureter. The ureter should be identified on either side of the pelvis in these difficult dissections because it is most likely to be injured adjacent to the uterosacral ligaments, where adhesive disease has obliterated the cul-de-sac and has caused the colon to be adherent to the uterosacral ligaments and pelvic peritoneum at this location. To protect the ureter, it must be dissected free from its peritoneal attachments and retracted laterally.

After completing a difficult dissection as already discussed, we routinely perform a "bubble test" to assess the rectosigmoid colon and to identify any occult injury that may have occurred (Fig. 51-3). The bubble test is performed easily, especially if the patient is positioned in Allen stirrups in a Whitmore position. A proctoscope is inserted into the rectum for a distance of approximately 8 cm. The pelvis is filled with saline, and the proximal sigmoid colon is grasped between the surgeon's hand and compressed, thereby keeping air from filling the ascending and transverse colon. The assistant with the proctoscope then insufflates air into the rectum, distending the rectosigmoid colon with air. Careful observation is made for any bubbles. If bubbles appear, the surgeon should aspirate the saline from the pelvis and follow the bubbles to the point where the rectum has been injured and then proceed with repair. Sometimes this is only a small "pinhole" injury that would not have been recognized without the bubble test. If there is no rectal injury, the proctoscope valve is opened, allowing the air to escape from the rectum, and the proctoscope is removed. Those using the proctoscope should change gown and gloves before resuming the abdominal and pelvic portion of the procedure.

When a rectal injury is recognized, the important steps of the repair include ensuring that there is an adequate blood supply to the tissues to be reapproximated, that the tissues edges are healthy, and that the reanastomosis or repair of the enterotomy is not under tension. Any damaged or poorly perfused tissue should be excised. In most cases, a simple two-layer enterotomy repair can be achieved. We usually close the mucosa and muscular layer with interrupted sutures of 2-0 Vicryl with a knot tied in the colon lumen. A second layer of seromuscular closure imbricates the mucosal layer (Fig. 51-4).

Patients who have received prior radiation therapy and who therefore have compromised blood supply in the rectosigmoid colon may benefit from the use of an omental J-flap to bring in additional blood supply to the region of the closure. In all patients, we copiously lavage the pelvis after the repair of the rectal injury and often will leave a Blake drain in the pelvis for several days postoperatively to remove serum and blood.

The question is often asked about the need for a diverting colostomy for patients who had inadequate or no mechanical bowel preparation preoperatively. Traditionally,

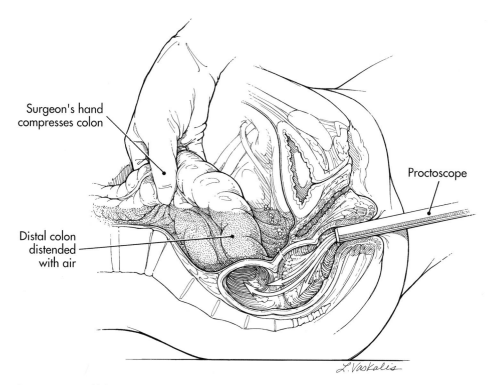

Fig. 51-3 "Bubble test." To evaluate the possibility of an occult rectal injury, the pelvis is filled with saline, and a proctoscope is introduced through the anus. The sigmoid colon at the pelvic brim is compressed between the surgeon's fingers and the rectosigmoid colon is insufflated with air. The appearance of bubbles coming from the rectum indicates rectal injury, which needs to be immediately repaired.

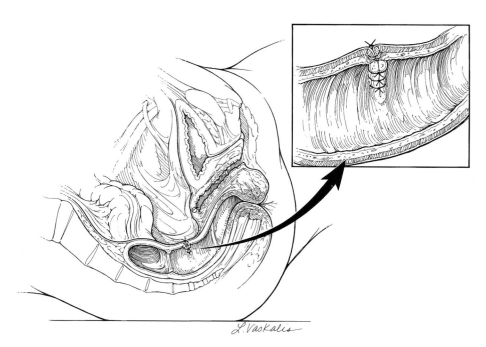

Fig. 51-4 After ensuring that all margins of the rectal injury (enterotomy) are healthy and have good vascular perfusion, the mucosal-muscular layer is closed with 2-0 Vicryl. The knots should be placed in the rectal lumen. A second layer imbricates the first layer, incorporating the serosa and muscularis. This suture line has its knots tied on the serosa.

performance of a diverting colostomy was seriously considered. However, this determination is now considered an issue of surgical judgment, and consultation with a colorectal surgeon is advised in most cases. In a randomized trial evaluating 114 patients with penetrating wounds to the colon who had not had mechanical bowel preparation, patients were assigned to either primary closure of the perforation or closure along with the diverting colostomy.[7] The authors found that complications related to sepsis occurred with equal frequency in both groups and that complication rates in the presence of significant fecal contamination, shock, and significant blood loss were all higher in the group undergoing diversion (colostomy). Therefore it is believed that even in patients with an unprepared bowel (e.g., in a trauma situation), primary repair of a penetrating colon injury is the management method of choice. Obviously, treatment with broad-spectrum antibiotics, which provide both gram-negative and anaerobic bacteria coverage should be instituted immediately in these situations, and we would again suggest closed suction drainage in this area. After closure of the rectum, a bubble test should be performed to assure that the closure is airtight.

Rectosigmoid Resection

The role of rectosigmoid resection in the debulking of ovarian cancer has been evaluated and elucidated over the past two decades. Because ovarian cancer remains an intraperitoneal lesion, the retroperitoneal spaces are relatively spared and may be easily opened in the pelvis, thereby "surrounding" the large pelvic tumor and at the same time protecting the important blood vessels and ureter. Furthermore, the distal involvement of the colon is usually down to but not extending past the peritoneal reflection, thereby preserving approximately 10 cm of distal rectum (the retroperitoneal portion of the rectum), which is free of cancer involvement. Having developed the retroperitoneal spaces, the surgeon can resect the rectosigmoid colon involved with the ovarian cancer and its mesentery with relative ease, often completely removing a large pelvic mass (Fig. 51-5). Use of these techniques obviously requires excellent surgical judgment, and they are not necessarily appropriate in every case of debulking surgery. However, there is evidence that by removing a large pelvic mass that invades the rectosigmoid colon, tumors may be optimally "debulked," and patients therefore have a better chance for prolonged disease-free survival. Furthermore, although more difficult to quantitate, resection of a large mass usually results in improved quality of life for the patient.

After resection of the rectosigmoid colon, the surgeon may either create a descending end colostomy with a Hartmann pouch (Fig. 51-6) or may proceed with low rectal anastomosis (Fig. 51-7). The use of circular stapling devices has substantially shortened the surgical procedure, and they have allowed low anastomoses where it would be technically difficult to achieve a hand-sewn anastomosis. Even in the patient in whom a descending end colostomy with a Hartmann pouch is initially created, the same techniques for low anastomosis may be carried out at a later point (e.g., at the second-look operation) to achieve colostomy take down and reanastomosis of the descending colon to the rectal stump.

Debulking of ovarian cancer may also require resection of segments of the colon, most commonly the transverse colon, which may be significantly involved with tumor metastatic to the omentum. In these situations the transverse colon may be resected and primary anastomosis of the right and left colon accomplished either using hand-sewn or stapling techniques. Finally, in the staging of early ovarian cancer, we recommend removal of the appendix as it is often involved with occult metastases from the ovarian cancer.

In performing an omentectomy in the course of staging or debulking ovarian cancer, the surgeon must be careful to avoid injury to the transverse colon. This is usually best accomplished by careful dissection along the undersurface of the omentum, where it is attached to the transverse colon. This portion of the omentum is relatively avascular and, unless invaded by cancer, can be easily separated from the transverse colon, mobilizing the omentum from the transverse colon. Thereafter, the primary blood supply to the omentum, which arises from the greater curvature of the stomach (the gastroepiploic vessels), may be clamped, divided, and ligated near the colon (infracolic omentectomy) or along the greater curvature of the stomach (total omentectomy). Again, it should be emphasized that when performing an omentectomy as the surgeon nears the splenic flexure of the colon, care should be taken to avoid pulling downward on the omentum or transverse colon to avoid injury to the splenic capsule.

Laparoscopic Injuries

The increase in use of the laparoscope for both diagnosis and surgical management of gynecologic disease has led to an increase in incidence of colonic injuries, the most common of which are in the transverse or rectosigmoid colon. Insertion of the Veress needle or laparoscopic trocar has the hazard of injury to the transverse colon. Immediate recognition of these injuries is paramount to the best outcome for the patient. Common signs of injury include obvious asymmetric filling of the abdomen with gas, the immediate passage of flatus while the gas is being insufflated, or stool on the laparoscopic trocar or sheath. As with injuries to the colon during open surgical procedures, if the patient has had an adequate mechanical bowel preparation, primary closure can be accomplished in nearly all instances without a diverting colostomy. Furthermore, given the evidence that penetrating wounds in an unprepared colon may be primarily closed without a diverting colostomy, most should be managed in this fashion. We would advocate exploratory laparotomy in most cases to fully assess the injury. Special attention and consideration must be given to the fact that this penetrating injury may have not only an entry site but also an exit site in the colon. Both the entry and exit sites need to be repaired. Because these

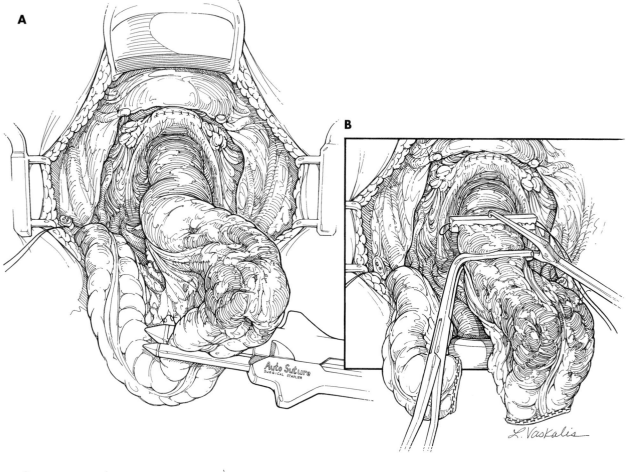

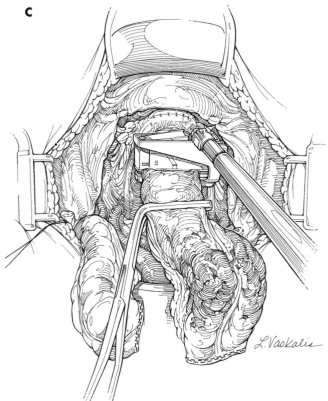

Fig. 51-5 Rectosigmoid colon resection. **A,** The diseased section of the rectosigmoid colon is isolated by dividing the mesocolon, with care being taken to avoid injury to the ureter or retroperitoneal vessels. The presacral space has been opened, again with care being taken to avoid the middle sacral artery and vein. With the sigmoid mobilized, its mesentery, including the sigmoid artery and vein, is divided, clamped, and suture ligated. The proximal sigmoid is divided between a GIA stapler. **B,** The rectum distal to the diseased portion to be resected is cross-clamped with the right-angle bowel clamp. A distal clamp may be either a purse-string device or **(C)** a TA55 Roticulator stapler. The colon is then divided between the two clamps. The descending colon may then be reanastomosed to the rectum (see Fig. 51-7) or the descending colon may be brought up as an end colostomy (see Fig. 51-6).

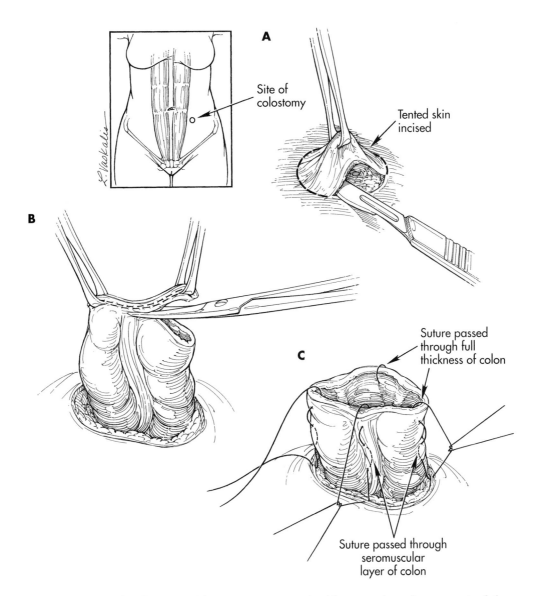

Fig. 51-6 End colostomy with a Hartmann pouch. After resection of a segment of the rectosigmoid colon, the fecal stream may be diverted by creating an end colostomy. The distal portion of the remaining rectum is either oversewn or closed by staples and left as a Hartmann's pouch. **A,** The colostomy stoma site is usually selected in the left lower quadrant on a flat portion of the abdominal wall to allow excellent adhesion of the stoma appliance. A circular piece of skin and subcutaneous fat and fascia are removed. **B,** The descending colon is brought through the stoma, and the staple line is excised. **C,** The stoma is "matured," creating a slight "rosebud" using absorbable suture.

are penetrating injuries, injury to other loops of small or large bowel or injury to the mesenteric blood supply should be considered and evaluated carefully. If the mesenteric blood supply is compromised, a segment of colon may need to be resected and reanastomosed. The basic principles of closure of these injuries in both open and laparoscopic procedures are the same. Good blood supply, healthy tissue, and tension-free approximation of the closure must be assured. We recommend a two-layer closure in this situation as well, although we are aware that some surgeons will perform a single-layer closure. Certainly, with good laparoscopic suturing and knot-

tying skills, the surgeon may find that an injury described previously could be closed through the laparoscope. Adequate peritoneal lavage should be achieved in either instance and treatment with broad-spectrum antibiotics for anaerobic and gram-negative bacteria coverage should be instituted.

The second area most likely to be injured in the course of laparoscopic surgery is the rectosigmoid colon. The most common reason for the injury is distorted anatomy from adhesions. Closure of the rectal injury in these settings may be achieved laparoscopically or with laparotomy, depending on the particular injury and the skill of the surgeon.

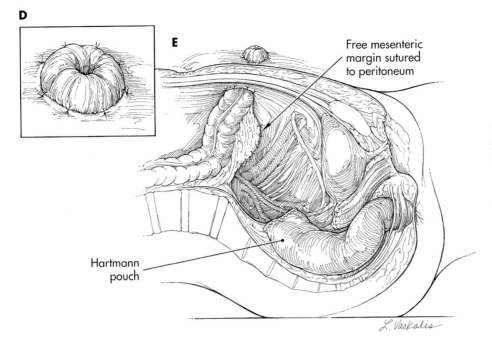

Free mesenteric margin sutured to peritoneum

Hartmann pouch

Fig. 51-6, cont'd   D, The "matured" stoma. **E,** The descending colon mesentery is sutured to the lateral peritoneum to prevent herniation lateral to the descending colon colostomy.

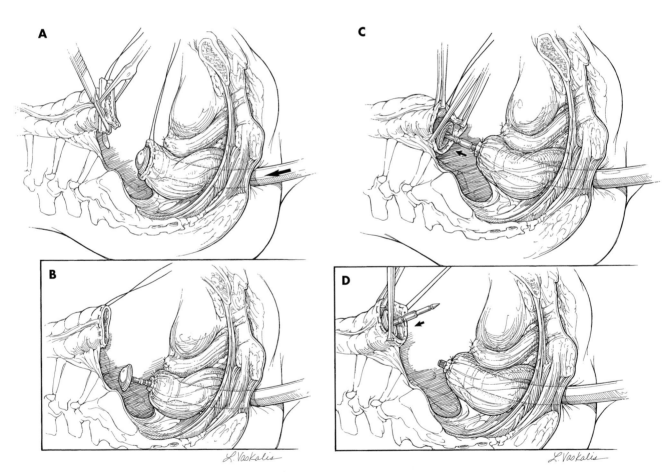

Fig. 51-7   Low rectal anastomosis. A, A purse-string suture has been placed around the distal rectum and the EEA circular stapling device has been passed transanally and exits through the rectum. **B,** The device is opened, and the purse-string suture is tied around the distal portion of the stapler. The descending colon has a purse-string suture placed around it and is brought into the pelvis. **C,** The anvil of the stapling device is introduced into the lumen of the descending colon and the purse-string suture is tied around the anvil. It is important that the purse-string suture incorporate all layers of the colonic wall yet not extend more than 5 mm from the cut edge to avoid incorporating excessive amounts of tissue in the stapling device, which might lead to a failed anastomosis. **D,** Alternatively, the anvil may be detached from the distal portion of the stapling device and the purse-string suture on the proximal colon tied more easily.

E

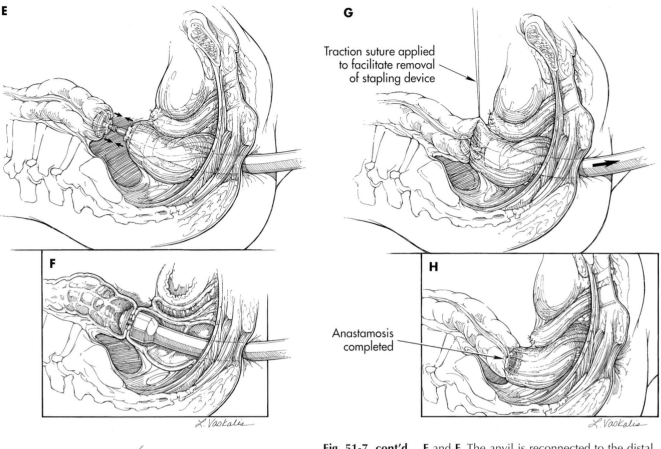

G

Traction suture applied to facilitate removal of stapling device

F

H

Anastamosis completed

L. Vaokalis

I

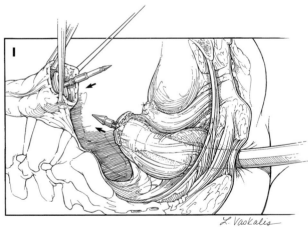

L. Vaokalis

Fig. 51-7, cont'd **E** and **F,** The anvil is reconnected to the distal stapling device. The stapler is closed until it has approximated the two segments of colon into the distance appropriate to the firing of the stapler. **G,** After the stapler has been fired, it is opened approximately 1 cm and then withdrawn from the anus. **H,** The circular anastomosis should be inspected with a proctoscope to make sure that there is no bleeding along the staple line, a bubble test should be performed to ensure that there is no leak along the staple line, and both "donuts" of the resected portion within the stapler should be inspected to be certain they are in total continuity. **I,** If the distal rectum had been divided between a stapling device, a purse-string suture is not necessary. Using the premium EEA stapler, a sharp trocar can be passed from the stapler through the distal rectum. With the trocars removed, the anvil portion that has been placed in the descending colon is attached to the stapler. The remainder of the anastomosis is created identically through the steps illustrated between **D** and **G** on the previous page.

Electrosurgical injury to the colon in the course of laparoscopic surgery should be managed in most cases by resection and reanastomosis. Because the electrosurgical thermal injury extends up to 4 cm beyond the site of initial injury, the surgeon should resect at least 4 cm on either side of the electrosurgical injury and then perform a reanastomosis.

The laparoscope has been used successfully to perform nearly all colon resections and anastomoses that can be performed with open laparotomy. It is beyond the scope of this chapter to outline each of those procedures, and the interested reader is referred to appropriate general surgical and laparoscopic surgical texts for further details.

Colonic Lesions Detected Intraoperatively

Despite careful history and physical examination and preoperative evaluation, the gynecologic surgeon may encounter unsuspected diseases of the colon. The two most common diseases encountered are diverticular disease and colon cancers.

Diverticulosis. Uncomplicated diverticulosis of the colon may progress to acute and chronic inflammatory disease (diverticulitis). The natural history of this process is thought to be secondary to an inspissated fecal plug, which obstructs the neck of the diverticulum. This obstruction then results in an inflammatory process called diverticulitis, which spreads into the paracolic fat. This inflammatory process in the colon, if not associated with an abscess and recognized intraoperatively, should be left alone, and no surgical treatment should be performed at that time. Patients should be treated with antibiotics postoperatively, and in most cases inflammation and infection will subside with this conservative management.

Diverticulitis may progress to the development of an abscess in the mesocolon or in adjacent tissues, which are often walled off by the mesocolon and omentum or other pelvic organs. Rupture of the abscess can lead to generalized peritonitis. An unruptured abscess recognized preoperatively may be managed with antibiotics and percutaneous drainage. Once the acute process has resolved, elected segmental resection of the involved bowel with primary anastomosis may be scheduled. Diverticular abscesses that are first recognized intraoperatively should be resected. A segmental resection of the involved colon is usually required. Primary anastomosis may be considered, but because of infection and inflammation in the adjacent tissues, diverting (protecting) colostomy is usually performed. Alternatively, the distal colon may be closed (Hartmann's pouch) and the proximal colon made into an end colostomy. Reanastomoses (colostomy take down) may be considered after the infection has resolved.

Colon Cancer. In the course of a pelvic operation, the gynecologist may encounter colon cancer in any segment of the colon, although the rectosigmoid colon is most often involved. Cancer of the colon is predominantly a disease of older women. It is the third leading cause of cancer death in American women, and the mortality rate has remained essentially stable through the last three decades. The cornerstone for therapy of colon cancer is surgical resection. Some excellent results with radiation therapy given in conjunction with chemotherapy for rectal carcinomas have been seen in recent years, and for many patients rectal resection and colostomy have been avoided. However, chemotherapy has limited effectiveness in patients with lesions outside of the rectum.

If colon cancer is unexpectedly found in the course of a gynecologic operation and the patient has had mechanical bowel preparation, appropriate resection should be carried out by a colorectal surgeon. On the other hand, if the patient has not had suitable bowel preparation or if an experienced colorectal surgeon is not available, the abdomen should be closed and definitive surgery performed at a later date after appropriate preoperative preparation.

Colonic Obstruction

Except for some advanced gynecologic malignancies, it is rare for a gynecologist to encounter an acute colonic obstruction secondary to gynecologic disease. Obviously, in patients with acute colonic obstruction, immediate surgical intervention is required despite the fact that mechanical bowel preparation cannot be accomplished. In these cases, broad-spectrum parenteral antibiotics should be given to the patient and exploratory laparotomy performed to identify the cause of the obstruction and at the same time to divert the fecal stream, creating either a loop colostomy (Fig. 51-8) or a descending end colostomy (see Fig. 51-6).

The decision about which type of colostomy should be performed should be made by an experienced colorectal surgeon. In general, for obstruction in the left colon, sigmoid colon, or rectum, a transverse loop colostomy is the simplest procedure to perform. The loop colostomy can remain as a permanent colostomy, although if a permanent colostomy is intended, an "end" colostomy is preferable because there is less chance of prolapse of the colostomy.

Postoperative Colonic Obstruction

Postoperative colonic obstruction must be distinguished from colonic ileus. Abdominal x-ray films may demonstrate significant distention of the colon. Although a colonic ileus is the most common diagnosis postoperatively, Ogilvie's syndrome should be considered and distinguished from mechanical obstruction. Both of these conditions are rare after gynecologic surgery, but it is certainly possible that the surgeon did not recognize a near-obstructing lesion in the descending, transverse, or right colon. Abdominal x-ray films should be followed carefully, and if the cecum (the segment most likely to perforate with colonic obstruction) approaches 9 cm in diameter, we would advise either colonoscopy or barium enema to exclude the possibility of a colonic obstruction. If a colonic obstruction is identified, the location and probable cause of the obstruction may be understood and appropriate surgical intervention selected to relieve the obstruction before perforation occurs. In situations such as when a patient has Ogilvie's syndrome, colonoscopy may be used to deflate the distended colon. If this cannot be accomplished, cecostomy may be necessary to avoid vascular compromise and perforation of the cecum.

Postoperative colonic perforation and intraperitoneal spill are often manifested by a septic course. Telltale signs of free air under the diaphragm on abdominal and chest x-ray films may be less accurate given the patient's recent surgery and the normal presence of air in the peritoneal cavity for a number of days postoperatively. Therefore the gynecologic surgeon must be aware of the possibility of colonic perforation, which might result from an unrecognized colonic injury or perforation of a diverticulum. The most common noninvasive diagnostic methods used are water-soluble contrast enema and a computed tomographic (CT) scan with contrast. Reexploratory surgery in the patient with pelvic abscesses of unknown cause should be accompanied by performance of a bubble test to ascertain the integrity of the rectosigmoid colon. Decisions regarding fecal diversion (colostomy) and repair versus resection should be made in conjunction with a colorectal surgeon.

Finally, a colovaginal fistula may be recognized in the immediate or delayed postoperative period. These fistulas are found most commonly between the rectosigmoid injury or a diverticular abscess and the vaginal cuff. Management of rectovaginal fistulas is discussed in Chapter 28.

THE APPENDIX

The appendix, being an organ located at the pelvic brim, often may be involved with gynecologic diseases (e.g.,

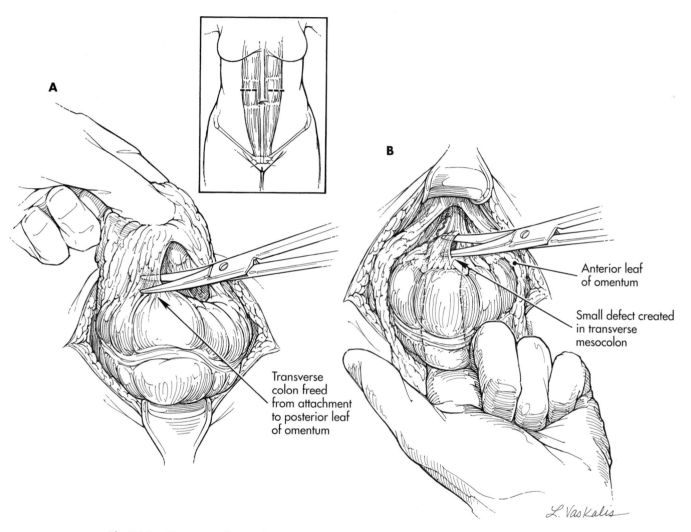

Fig. 51-8   Transverse loop colostomy. A segment of transverse colon used to create the co-lostomy is isolated. **A,** The omentum is dissected free from the distal surface of the colon. **B,** The transverse mesocolon mesentery is opened just beneath the serosa of the transverse colon.

Continued

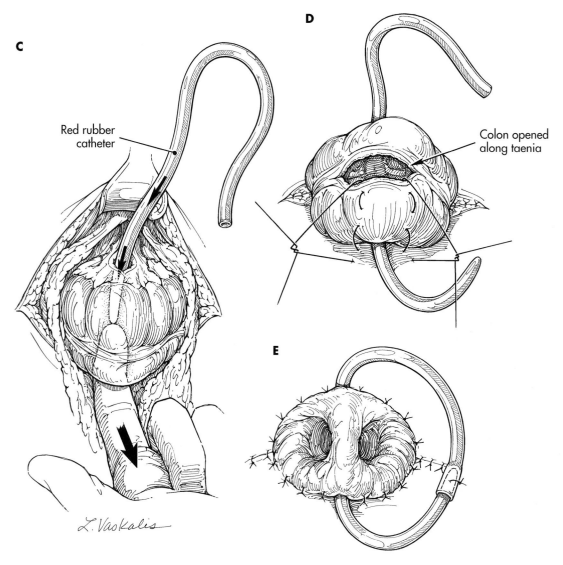

C

Red rubber
catheter

D

Colon opened
along taenia

E

L. Vaskalis

Fig. 51-8, cont'd **C,** A red rubber 16-Fr catheter is passed beneath the colon. **D,** The omentum and distal proximal colon are placed back into the abdominal cavity with the red rubber
catheter beneath the loop colostomy just at the skin level. The colon is opened along its
taeniae on the antimesentery border. **E,** Sutures are placed in the skin and colon, thus creating
a "double-barrel" colostomy.

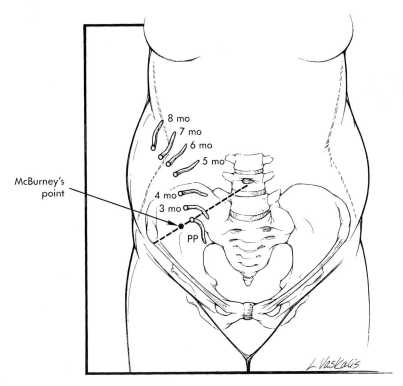

Fig. 51-9 The location of the appendix in relation to McBurney's point as pregnancy advances (*mo,* months; *pp,* postpartum). (Modified from Baer JL, Reis RA, Arens RA: *JAMA* 98:1359, 1932.)

endometriosis, pelvic inflammatory disease, ovarian carcinoma). Furthermore, diseases of the appendix may be mistaken for gynecologic disorders. It is therefore relevant for the gynecologic surgeon to have the surgical skills necessary to manage appendiceal disease.

Anatomy

The vermiform appendix arises from the cecum at variable distances from the ileocecal junction, usually approximately 2.5 cm from the ileocecal valve. On average, the appendix is 10 cm long, although it may attain twice this length. The base of the appendix is easily identified at the point of confluence of the three longitudinally oriented muscular bands of the colon (taeniae coli). The taeniae form the outer longitudinal muscle of the appendix. The appendiceal wall is composed of two perpendicular layers of smooth muscle. The narrow lumen is lined with mucinous epithelium; beneath the colonic epithelium are a number of lymphoid follicles, which diminish in number as we age.

The appendix may assume many locations in the right abdomen and pelvis and may change location, especially throughout pregnancy (Fig. 51-9). It is located in a retrocecal location in approximately 65% of individuals. When not easily identified, following the taeniae will invariably lead to the base of the appendix.

The primary arterial blood supply to the appendix is the appendiceal artery, which is a branch of the ileocolic artery (Fig. 51-10). The appendiceal artery courses to the appendix through the mesentery (mesoappendix).

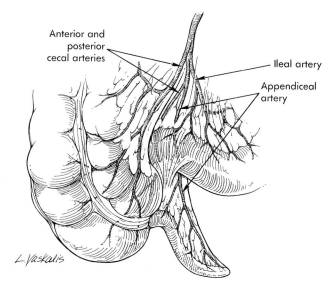

Fig. 51-10 The arterial blood supply to the appendix. Major branches from the superior mesenteric artery supply the ilium (ilial artery) and cecum. One branch from the center portion is the appendiceal artery, which courses behind the ileum or beneath the ileum and through the mesoappendix.

Elective (Incidental) Appendectomy

Although generally not a formidable procedure, appendectomy must be viewed strategically within the context of what is best for the patient (i.e., a very thoughtful consideration of the risk/benefit ratio for each particular person, which is indirectly the risk of future development of appendicitis). The hazards of elective appendectomy, although uncommon, must be considered and include postoperative infection, which may involve abscess formation either intraperitoneal or extraperitoneal, wound infection, or even peritonitis. Infection of the abdominal incision is certainly more common in patients who have had an appendectomy. Wound infection not only may disturb wound healing but also may weaken the abdominal scar, leading to evisceration and/or delayed hernia.

The "incidental" appendectomy has been advised as a means of preventing subsequent surgery and possible complications from appendicitis. However, when a cost-benefit analysis was performed by Addiss et al.,[1] they concluded that with the exception of the very youngest age groups, the preventative value of incidental appendectomy is relatively low. Furthermore, Sugimoto and Edwards[14] evaluated costs and concluded that the morbidity and mortality associated with appendicitis was not significant compared with the cost and complications of incidental appendectomies.

The patient's views concerning retention or removal of her appendix should be solicited preoperatively. If elective appendectomy is a consideration, the surgeon should outline his or her position and recommendation to the patient and her consent must be obtained.

Although the patient may express gratitude to the surgeon postoperatively for her unexpected appendectomy, in the absence of her informed consent for appendectomy, the surgeon is fully liable for any unexpected misfortune that may develop postoperatively as a consequence of appendectomy (e.g., bowel obstruction, abscess formation, peritonitis). Assault and battery is an almost indefensible charge against the surgeon in such a situation for having undertaken an elective procedure without the patient's knowledge and consent. The extent of liability will be proportionate to the pain, suffering, and damage produced. That a "routine appendectomy" may be the surgeon's "custom" would be of scant comfort to the surgeon and his or her legal defense during litigation. One simple preoperative statement by the surgeon may save a great deal of trouble: if the patient has given a positive response to the surgeon's question, "In the event that during the course of your operation it appears, in my judgment, that removal of your appendix is in your best interest, may I have your permission to do so?"

The location of the appendix should always be visualized as part of a laparotomy, the peritoneal surface should be inspected for inflammation, and the lumen should be palpated to detect any fecalith(s) present, which are thought by most to be precursors of appendicitis and by their very presence may constitute an indication for appendectomy. There are certain circumstances in which it is believed that elective appendectomy should be strongly considered:

1. With discovery of a retrocecal location of the appendix. In this situation, appendectomy may be warranted for two reasons: (1) the retrocecal location of the appendix may confuse and delay the diagnosis of future appendicitis, promoting increased risk of appendiceal abscess and peritonitis, and (2) future appendectomy

for an inflamed retrocecal appendix is invariably more difficult than when appendectomy is performed electively on the noninflamed appendix.

2. With palpation of one or more fecaliths within the lumen of the appendix (thought to be a precursor of appendicitis).
3. With carcinoid or mucocele of the appendix, as the lesion is usually of a low grade of malignancy.
4. With gross involvement of the appendix by endometriosis. This may predispose the patient to future symptomatology or mechanical obstruction.
5. In a patient with chronic or repeated episodes of right lower quadrant pain. However, the benefit from appendectomy is less certain when during exploratory laparotomy there is no explanation for the pain.
6. With laparotomy performed to remove a mucinous tumor of the ovary.
7. During staging operations for early ovarian malignancy, because metastases are not uncommon.[13]
8. Upon the patient's request for appendectomy.

Contraindications to elective appendectomy of a grossly normal, freely movable appendix are especially noteworthy in the patient who wishes to preserve her future fertility.[9] These include the following:

1. Surgical treatment of a coincident ectopic pregnancy.
2. Coincident pelvic operations to restore or enhance fertility (e.g., myomectomy, tubal reanastomoses, adhesiolysis, and fimbrioplasty, especially where there may be postoperative oozing of the surgical site).
3. Cesarean section, in a patient with uterine infection.
4. The patient having expressly forbidden the procedure.
5. A strong suspicion of Crohn's disease in a patient (e.g. weight loss, frequent bowel movements, and chronic crampy lower abdominal pains). Appendectomy in the face of active Crohn's disease is an invitation for postoperative enterocutaneous fistula.
6. A history of pelvic or abdominal radiation therapy.
7. Presence of vascular grafts or other "foreign" material in the abdomen or pelvis.

Relative contraindications to elective appendectomy include the following:

1. The patient's informed consent could not be obtained preoperatively.
2. The patient is already at greater than average medical risk for surgery.
3. The total operative time may be prolonged.
4. The surgeon lacks experience with the technical steps of the procedure and management of its possible complications.

It appears that the incidence of subsequent colon cancer, lymphomas, and leukemias is slightly increased in later years among women who had appendectomy in their youth. This is, of course, difficult to explain, but it has been suggested that the removal of lymphoid tissue at a younger age might deprive the patient of some protective influences.

Occasionally, after transvaginal colpotomy or vaginal hysterectomy, the appendix may appear in the operative field. Although it can be easily removed at this time using the same techniques that one might use abdominally, the surgeon must be assured that to do so is in the patient's best interest and that the procedure meets with her approval. The surgeon must inform the patient in such a circumstance that her appendix has been removed, lest future development of right lower quadrant pain be interpreted by another examiner as an indication for appendectomy, unaware because of the presence of an unscarred abdomen, that the appendix had been previously removed.

A history of previous appendectomy is not a guarantee against the future development of appendicitis because it may be seen in an appendiceal stump remaining after subtotal appendectomy.

Appendicitis

Symptoms and Pathogenesis. Appendicitis develops as a result of obstruction to the appendiceal lumen. In most instances, this is the consequence of submucosal lymphoid follicle hyperplasia secondary to infection anywhere in the body. The second most common cause of obstruction may be from a fecalith, and far more rarely obstruction is caused by a tumor or foreign bodies.

This obstruction may cause abscess formation within the lumen of the appendix. Progression of the abscess may diminish local circulation and produce edema, and as the vessels become obstructed, gangrene may develop. Perforation and peritonitis may then develop. Periappendicitis is less ominous because it may involve infection from without rather than within the appendix, secondary to an episode of pelvic inflammatory disease. As the inflammatory disease resolves, the periappendicitis may tend to resolve as well, without necessarily passing through a stage of luminal obstruction.

The symptoms of appendicitis generally begin with epigastric pain, which is followed by anorexia and possibly later by nausea and vomiting. As the area of inflammation comes in contact with the parietal peritoneum, the pain may seem to migrate to the right lower quadrant, where tenderness on deep palpation and rebound tenderness may be found. Fever may or may not be present before perforation. It is important to differentiate appendicitis from acute pyelonephritis, and a urinalysis should always be obtained. With pyelonephritis, the temperature tends to be higher than with appendicitis. Chills are more common with pyelonephritis, but leukocytosis is more common when the appendix overlies the patient's ureter because appendiceal inflammation here may generate ureteral inflammation and pyuria as well.

Differential diagnosis of appendicitis must include pyelonephritis, mesenteric adenitis, Crohn's disease, pelvic inflammatory disease (although the latter is usually bilateral), and adnexal torsion or hemorrhage.

Diagnosis. Anorexia, right lower quadrant pain, leukocytosis, and fever are characteristic of acute appendicitis, although periappendicitis will occasionally be seen unexpectedly during laparotomy for some other reason. The significance of the latter is unclear, but its presence should be recorded. In the patient who has episodes of right lower quadrant pain that subsides and recurs and borderline leukocytosis, further diagnostic study is indicated. Barium enema may be useful because an inflamed appendix will not fill, and the presence of visualized appendiceal filling tends to exclude appendicitis. There appears to be no hazard associated with barium enema, even in the patient with appendicitis, providing that perforation has not occurred before the procedure.

Other imaging techniques that may assist in the identification of periappendiceal inflammation or a mass (abscess) include ultrasound and CT scan.[8]

Diagnostic laparoscopy has also been used successfully in the evaluation of patients when diagnosis is uncertain. In a series reported by Deutsch et al.,[5] about one third of selected patients suspected of having appendicitis did not require appendectomy after laparoscopy was performed. Conditions other than appendicitis (e.g., tuboovarian abscesses, adnexal torsion) were occasionally recognized during laparoscopy.

Appendicitis in Pregnancy. Although appendicitis during pregnancy is uncommon, it can occur. The surgeon evaluating symptoms of possible appendicitis in a prenatal patient must be cognitive of the changes of the location in the site of the appendix coincident with the advancing state of pregnancy because it is displaced further toward the right upper quadrant. It is possible for appendicitis during pregnancy to have been undiagnosed and therefore untreated, and an appendiceal abscess may have formed. Labor with the presence of an appendiceal abscess can be deadly because the excursions of uterine contraction and later involution may rupture the wall of an appendiceal abscess, promoting a disseminated peritonitis.

Acute appendicitis is more common in women younger than 25 than in those older than 25. Because this is the age group of most reproduction, the incidence during pregnancy, 1 in 5000, will be that of the population as a whole. Appendicitis may occur at any time during pregnancy, although it is perhaps a slight bit more common in the first and second trimesters. The location of the appendix is altered considerably by displacement from the enlarged uterus, because the appendix is pushed laterally and cranially (see Fig. 51-8).[2] At times, the diagnosis may be difficult to establish, but Alders' sign may be helpful. Hereafter the right-sided tenderness has been localized in the supine position, the patient is turned on her left side, and if the tenderness or pain shifts to the left along with the pelvic organs, it is thought to be of gynecologic origin unassociated with appendicitis. Because the white blood cell count is generally elevated during the course of pregnancy, a mild leukocytosis is not pathognomonic, but a distinct left shift in the differential leukocyte count should be expected in the presence of appendicitis, particularly if the count is greater than 18,000 cells/mm.[3]

Removal of the unruptured appendix during pregnancy carries little risk for the fetus. However, rupture with abscess formation has grave consequences because, should labor start, the walls of the abscessed cavity are likely to be disturbed considerably by the movement of the uterus, risking purulent dissemination of the abscess contents and producing a generalized peritonitis. The toxins from the latter may be fatal for the baby, as well as for the mother.

When an appendiceal abscess is encountered, the cavity should be entered and cultures taken, but loculations should be broken up without disturbing the walls of the abscessed cavity or surrounding adhesions, lest the infection be disseminated. The appendix should be removed only if it is easy to do. The abscessed cavity should be emptied and irrigated, and closed drainage through a separate stab wound should be instituted. Appropriate antibiotics should be used. For the fetus younger than 33 weeks' gestation, concurrent cesarean section usually should not be performed because the risks of prematurity outweigh the risks of possible infection to the fetus; beyond the 33 weeks, concurrent cesarean section should be seriously considered if there is evidence of fetal compromise.[10]

Incidental appendectomy at the time of cesarean section is generally safe, although not widely practiced, because there is a very small risk of infection of the peritoneal cavity. If the surgeon contemplates incidental appendectomy, it would be wise to obtain the patient's permission preoperatively.[12]

Carcinoid of the Appendix

The appendix should always be examined at laparotomy or laparoscopy, and the presence or absence of adhesions should be noted as well as any signs of inflammation or tumors. Carcinoma of the appendix is quite rare; most tumors found will be carcinoid, although a few may be adenocarcinoma. The diagnosis is established by frozen section, and if positive for carcinoid tumor, the rest of the bowel must be inspected for other areas of tumor, and palpation of lymph nodes of the right colon and mesoappendix should be performed. If any nodes are positive, or if adenocarcinoma is found, right hemicolectomy is indicated. The characteristic appearance of a carcinoid tumor is a firm nodule at the tip of the appendix, which in cross-section appears as a yellow submucous ring encircling the appendix. Microscopically, there are masses of polyhedral cells with granulated or vacuolated cytoplasm. The tumors are chromaffinomas, or tumors of the endocrine system arising from Kulchitsky's cells of the intestinal mucosa, which are found between the columnar cells of the crypts of Lieberkühn and belong to the chromaffin system. Intestinal carcinoid, in contrast, is primarily a tumor of the ileum, where it may form a yellow mass partly encircling the bowel and projecting into the lumen. It is best treated by resection, although there may be secondary carcinoid growths in the liver, which may produce serotonin in the carcinoid syndrome.

Technique of Appendectomy

It is easy to remove an appendix if the cecum can be brought out of the abdomen and there are no complications. If the appendix is badly infected, bound down by adhesions, or retrocecal, its removal can be a very difficult operation.

"The inexpert will use numerous packs, retract forcefully, use sponge sticks on the intestine, injure the peritoneum and even tear the mesentery with the results of the postoperative course being marked by distention, often dangerous peritonitis and many later adhesions and even death. The worse the appendix and the more difficulty exposing, the greater the demands for gentleness and the more dangerous the gauze pack."[6]

There should be adequate preliminary operative exposure, making the organ accessible. If there is any peritoneal exudate, it should be cultured. As the appendix and cecum are visualized, moist packs should isolate this area from the rest of the abdominal cavity, often permitting the site for surgery to be delivered into the wound.

The mesoappendix at the tip of the appendix is grasped with the hemostat or Babcock clamp and gently elevated while traction is applied caudally and medially to the cecum. The mesoappendix is clamped perpendicular to the appendiceal axis, and the clamp is replaced by transfixion ligature. The appendiceal artery may be several millimeters from the base of the appendix (Fig. 51-11). In the event of infection and inflammation, the peritoneum overlying the mesoappendix should be incised on each side, the edematous fat should be removed, and the appendiceal artery should be clamped, cut, and ligated (see Fig. 51-11, C). The base of the appendix is ligated with an absorbable suture, the ends are held with the hemostat just beyond the knot and cut, and the second tie is placed a few millimeters distal to the first. A hemostat is placed across the body of the appendix and closed but not locked, stripping the appendiceal contents toward the distal tip, and when about 1 cm away from the tie, the hemostat is locked and the appendix (doubly tied at its base) is gently severed with the scalpel. Both appendix and scalpel are handed off the table.

An alternative method of handling the stump is to invert it and close the seromuscular layer by a series of interrupted mattress sutures. There seems to be no advantage to separate ligation followed by inversion of the stump because this would lead to postoperative formation of an intramural abscess, which would probably rupture into the intestinal lumen. If it was the surgeon's desire to use this combined treatment of the stump, it would be desirable to tie the stump off first with an absorbable suture in the area crushed by the hemostat and then invert this with a purse-string suture placed in the seromuscular layer of the bowel (see Fig. 51-11, D through G).

If the appendix is gangrenous, extending to its base, there may be considerable induration and edema of the cecum, making it desirable to reinforce the site of amputation of the stump with a series of interrupted mattress stitches. If the appendix has a retrocecal location, the cecum will have to be mobilized. Often, there is a small avascular band running from the tip of the appendix and ending close to the lower pole of the right kidney. This will have to be divided, with care being taken to divide the band and not the tip of the appendix.

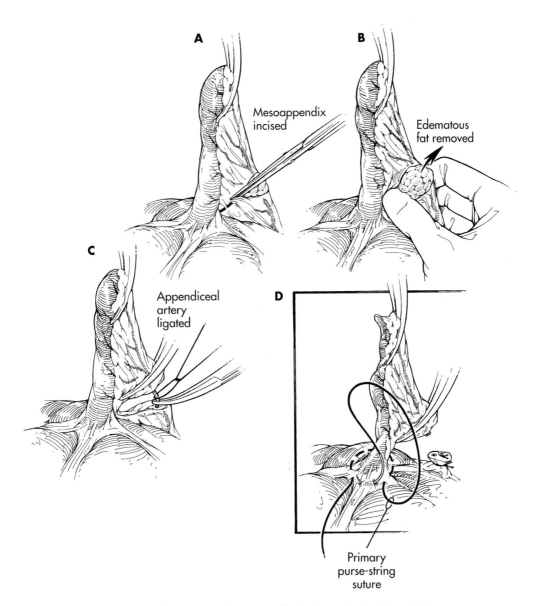

Fig. 51-11 Appendectomy. **A,** The appendix is elevated at its tip and the peritoneum overlying the mesoappendix is incised. **B,** In a patient with appendicitis, the fat is oftentimes edematous and may be squeezed and removed, thereby isolating the appendiceal vessels. **C,** The appendiceal vessels have been isolated, clamped, and ligated. **D,** A purse-string suture is placed in the cecum around the base of the appendix. *Continued*

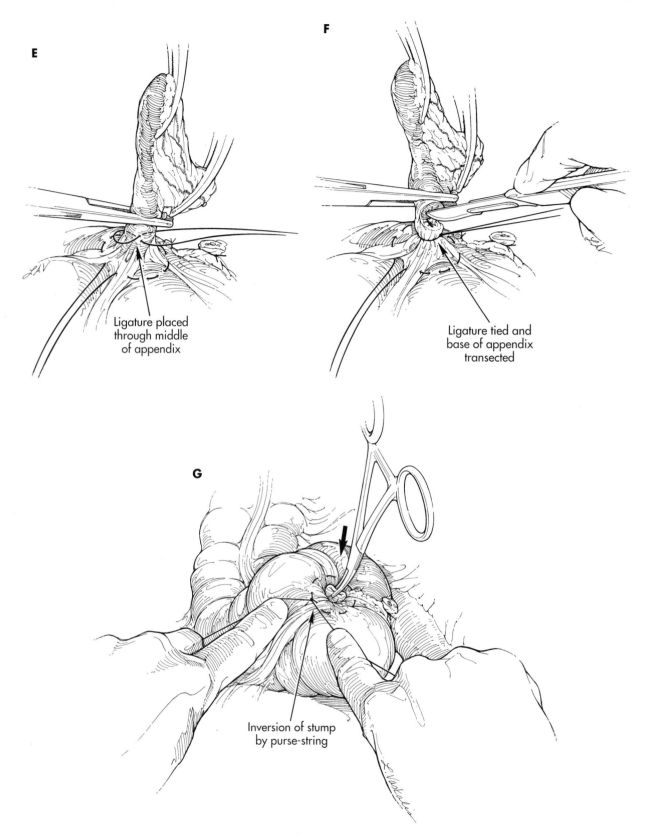

Fig. 51-11, cont'd **E,** The base of the appendix is crushed between the jaws of a hemostat and the hemostat is advanced distally a few millimeters. In the crush injury, a suture ligature is placed and tied. **F,** The appendix is then divided between the suture and the distal clamp. **G,** The appendiceal stump is inverted into the cercum, and the purse-string suture is tied.

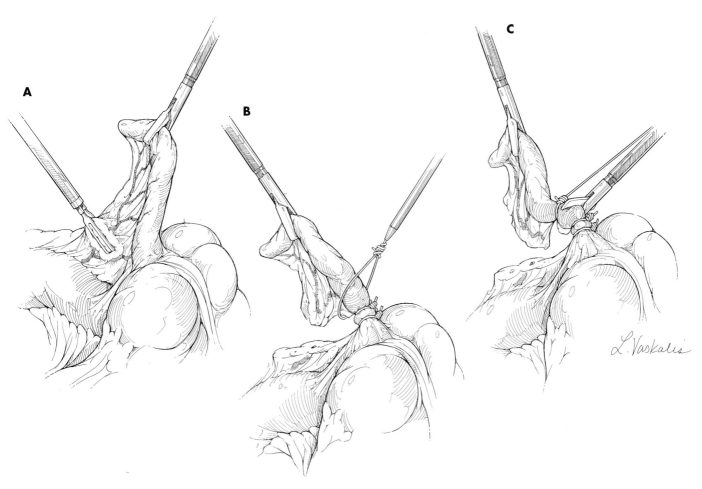

Fig. 51-12   Laparoscopic appendectomy. **A,** The mesoappendix and appendiceal vessels are cauterized using bipolar paddles. The cauterized mesentery is then incised. **B,** Three loop ligatures are placed along the base of the appendix. **C,** The appendix is divided between the second and third ligature and removed through the laparoscope port. (**A** through **C** and **G** through **I** from Gomel V, Taylor PJ: *Diagnostic and operative gynecologic laparoscopy,* St Louis, 1995, Mosby.)   *Continued*

Occasionally, a retrocecal appendix must be removed in a retrograde fashion, starting with the base of the appendix. With the stump now ligated, it may be possible to demonstrate the ill-defined mesoappendix; by blunt dissection the mesoappendix is clipped and cut until it has been removed.

Laparoscopic Appendectomy

Appendectomy may be safely performed using laparoscopic techniques (Fig. 51-12). Essentially, the same steps in performing an "open" appendectomy are followed. The appendix is identified, and traction is applied to the distal end either by grasping it with a grasping device or by ensnaring it with an endoloop suture. With the appendix elevated, the mesentery (mesoappendix) and the appendiceal artery may be controlled using several different methods:

- The mesoappendix and appendiceal artery may be cauterized using bipolar paddles. The portion of mesoappendix that has been cauterized will be divided with shears (see Fig. 51-12, *A*).

- Using sharp and blunt dissection, the mesoappendix is skeletonized and blood vessels are secured using the endoscopic clip device (see Fig. 51-12, *D*).
- A defect may be made in the distal mesoappendix using blunt and sharp dissection of a dissecting instrument. Through the defect, a suture is introduced, which encircles the appendix. Two sutures are placed proximally and one distally, and the appendix is divided. The mesoappendix and appendiceal artery are then ligated using an endoloop (see Fig. 51-12, *D* through *G*). (We find this technique to be the most technically challenging and prefer either of the first two methods.)

If one of the first two techniques just described was used to manage the mesoappendix, the appendix is now triply ligated using Endoloops (Ethicon, Inc., Somerville, NJ) and divided between the second and third ligature (see Fig. 51-12, *E*). The appendix is removed through the 10-mm port. Although many surgeons do not bury the appendiceal

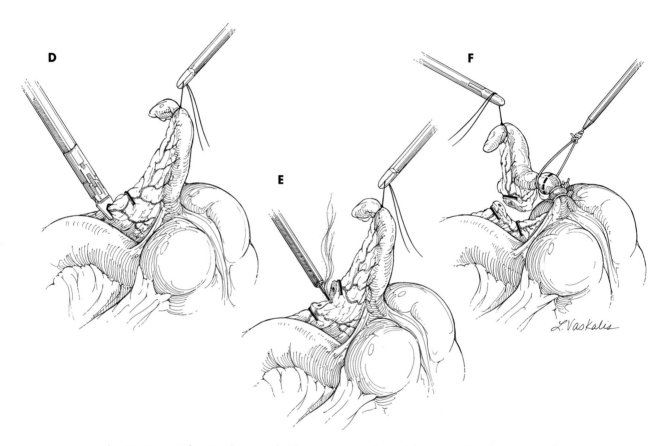

Fig. 51-12, cont'd   **D,** Alternatively, the mesoappendix and the appendiceal artery may be ligated using Ligaclips. **E,** Between the Ligaclips, the mesoappendix is divided using shears or, in this case, electrocautery. **F,** The base of the appendix is triply ligated and divided and removed. (**A** through **C** and **G** through **I** from Gomel V, Taylor PJ: *Diagnostic and operative gynecologic laparoscopy,* St Louis, 1995, Mosby.)

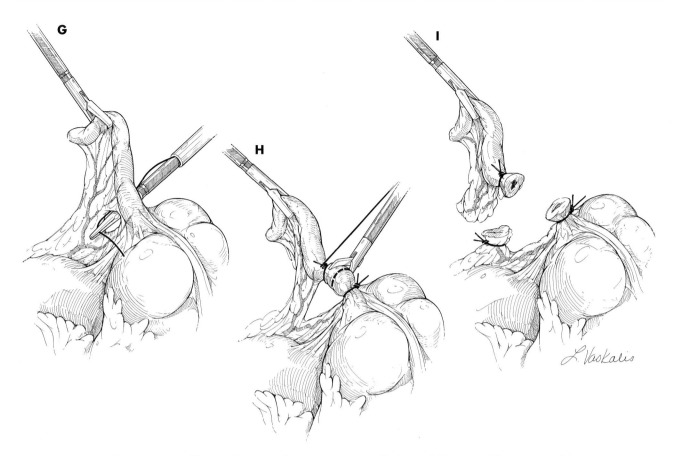

Fig. 51-12, cont'd   G, Alternatively, the mesoappendix is carefully opened in an avascular window isolating the appendiceal artery. Sutures are then passed through the window of the mesentery and around the appendix, thereby ligating the appendix. **H,** The appendix is then divided between these sutured ligatures. **I,** Finally, the appendiceal artery is controlled by another ligature tied around it.

stump, it may be buried by placing a figure-of-eight or a purse-string suture into the wall of the cecum using a laparoscopic needle holder. At the conclusion of the procedure, the pelvis and cecum are irrigated.

Appendiceal Abscess

A small percentage of patients have a right lower quadrant mass, and it is important to determine whether this represents a localized inflammation with edema or formation of an abscess. The latter invariably requires drainage because it has no effective circulation and it is difficult to deliver systemic antibiotics to the center of the abscessed cavity. Although some would favor bed rest with intravenous hydration and antibiotics (a cephalosporin and metronidazole or a gentamicin and clindamycin combination), it is important that the presence of abscess formation be identified because the abscess must be surgically drained. When surgery demonstrates an appendiceal abscess, it should always be drained through a separate stab wound and manipulation should be kept to a minimum. When clinical improvement is seen after 7 to 10 days of drainage and antibiotic administration, consideration should be given to interval appendectomy in 3 to 4 months because

appendicitis will recur in about 10% of such patients, usually within the year.

REFERENCES

1. Addiss DG, Shaffer N, Fowler BS, et al: The epidemiology of appendicitis and appendectomy in the United States, *Am J Epidemiol* 132:910, 1990.
2. Baer JL, Reis RA, Arens RA: Appendicitis in pregnancy with changes in position and axis of a normal appendix in pregnancy, *JAMA* 98:1359, 1932.
3. Cohen SM, et al: Prospective, randomized, endoscopic-blinded trial comparing precolonoscopy bowel cleansing methods, *Dis Colon Rectum* 37:689, 1994.
4. Condon RE, et al: Efficacy of oral and systemic antibiotic prophylaxis in colorectal operations, *Arch Surg* 118:496, 1983.
5. Deutch AA, Zelikovsky A, Reis R: Laparoscopy in the prevention of unnecessary appendectomies: a prospective study, *Br J Surg* 69:336, 1982.
6. Dudley G: The surgical assistant, *Surg Gynecol Obstet* 115:245, 1962.
7. Gonzalez RP, Merlotti GJ, Holevar MR: Colostomy in penetrating colon injury: is it necessary? *J Trauma Injury Infect Crit Care* 41:271, 1996.
8. Knishern JR, Eskin EM, Fletcher HS: Increasing accuracy in the diagnosis of acute appendicitis with modern diagnostic techniques, *Ann Surg* 52:222, 1986.

9. Mueller BA, et al: Appendectomy and the risk of tubal infertility, *N Engl J Med* 315:1506, 1986.

10. Newton M, Newton E: Surgical problems in pregnancy. In Dilts PV, Sciarra JJ, editors: *Gynecology and obstetrics,* vol 2, Philadelphia, 1991, JB Lippincott.

11. Nichols RL, Holmes JW: Prophylaxis in bowel surgery, *Curr Clin Top Infect Dis* 15:76, 1995.

12. Parsons AK, et al: Appendectomy at cesarean section: a prospective study, *Obstet Gynecol* 68:479, 1986.

13. Rose PG, et al. Appendectomy in primary and secondary staging operations for ovarian malignancy, *Obstet Gynecol* 77:116, 1991.

14. Sugimoto T, Edwards D: Incidence and costs of incidental appendectomy as a preventative measure, *Am J Public Health* 77:471, 1987.

52 Breast Biopsy

DOUGLAS J. MARCHANT

As I had noted in the introduction to this chapter for the first edition published in 1993, there had been at least the promise of a dramatic change in the role of the obstetrician/gynecologist in the diagnosis and treatment of breast diseases.[14] Although it is true that the American Board of Obstetrics and Gynecology indicated that "a knowledge of breast disease would be required for certification" and questions related to breast disease occur with regularity on the American Board examinations, regrettably the implementation of these objectives has never been completely realized.

Even as late at 1990, there were initiatives by the American College of Obstetricians and Gynecologists to provide training in the diagnosis of breast disease, including instruction in the techniques of breast surgery. One of my concerns at that time was the definition of "adequate training for breast surgery." My comments presented to the Committee on Gynecologic Practice are as follows[3]:

> I am concerned about who should be eligible for this training and under what conditions the obstetrician/gynecologist be permitted to practice surgery related to the breast.
>
> There is no question that the breast is an organ of reproduction and that the diagnosis and treatment of breast disease is within the responsibility of gynecologic practice as noted both by the American Board and the American College of Obstetricians and Gynecologists. The American Board has deliberately stopped short of recommending or suggesting training for major surgical procedures involving the breast because it was felt by a number of observers that the obstetrician/gynecologist should become involved in the diagnosis and treatment of breast disease in a step-wise fashion. As this concept is developed, consideration should be given to structuring residency programs to include such training and eventually outlining the surgical training required both for breast biopsy and the contemporary treatment of breast cancer.
>
> To immediately announce to our colleagues in general surgery, and radiation and medical oncology that the obstetrician/gynecologist should manage breast cancer including the surgical treatment seemed inappropriate. It was realized, however, that at some point, steps should be taken to outline surgical training and the conditions for which such surgical training and practice would be appropriate. There are several issues involved, not the least of which is the multifaceted nature of the current practice of obstetrics and gynecology. In my opinion,

while the proper examination of the breast is essential to the practice of good obstetrics and gynecology, and a knowledge of breast disease including breast cancer is necessary to advise patients and request appropriate referral, I do not believe that *every* obstetrician/gynecologist should proceed beyond simple diagnostic studies including breast examination, aspiration of cysts or fine-needle aspiration (FNA) when appropriate cytologic evaluation is available.

In 1965, I first began discussing these issues with the American College of Obstetricians and Gynecologists. At this time the management of breast cancer was a simple matter. Mammography had not yet been introduced, at least not on a widescale basis and there was only one treatment for breast cancer and that was radical mastectomy. Now, the situation is quite different. Mammography as a screening procedure is performed on a regular basis, frequently with the discovery of the occult lesion, and alternative treatments for breast cancer are available. Breast cancer is no longer a simple surgical problem. Appropriate treatment requires a multidisciplinary approach including the expertise not only of the surgical specialist but the medical oncologist, the radiation oncologist and, in many cases, the services of a well trained plastic surgeon. It must be understood that open biopsy often becomes part of the definitive treatment for breast cancer. In the past, a biopsy performed in any area of the breast and even one associated with local complications did not compromise the total treatment of breast cancer since the entire breast would be removed.

There is no lesion that is obviously benign, and every biopsy must be considered to be a cancer and appropriately handled by the pathologist. This means requesting immediate frozen section to determine whether cancer is present and, if so, the determination of estrogen and progesterone receptor values and the appropriate marking of the margins to facilitate discussion concerning conservative versus radical treatment.

Breast biopsy must be considered a plastic procedure, and the surgeon must be appropriately trained in tissue handling and the requirements of cosmetic surgery. The procedure is not difficult, but in must be practiced repetitively to produce satisfactory results. In terms of the definitive surgical procedures for breast cancer, the same philosophy applies. The radical mastectomy is no longer appropriate, and, in my opinion, the modified radical mastectomy is a more difficult procedure since there is less exposure when performing the lymph node dissection. Conservative management is even more difficult. The incisions must be carefully chosen and the surgery meticulously performed in accordance with the recommendations of the radiation therapist.

The position of the Board could be interpreted to indicate that *every* obstetrician/gynecologist should proceed with an open biopsy and surgical treatment, the only requirement being "approved surgical training." This is not the position of the Board nor the College, furthermore, in the average practice, breast cancer would occur so infrequently that the value of special training and skill so acquired soon would be lost. In dealing with this disease on a daily basis, it is my firm belief that the patient is best served by obtaining treatment from a multidisciplinary center with a sufficient volume to maintain a high level of surgical skill and appropriate interaction among the various disciplines associated with the treatment. This means that those obstetricians and gynecologists who wish to devote a significant amount of their practice to the diagnosis and treatment of breast disease should avail themselves of an approved training program and join their surgical colleagues as part of the multidisciplinary team in the diagnosis and treatment of this disease.

At about the same time that these discussions were taking place, dramatic changes occurred in the practice of medicine. Health maintenance organizations (HMOs) and the concept of managed care emerged as the operative language of medical practice. Hospitals began to merge to increase their market share and not surprisingly the primary care physician took center stage in this unfolding drama of new health care. In a society that had long been accustomed to a ratio of 70% specialists to 30% primary care physicians, it was now apparent that in due time the tables would be turned, and the primary care physician would become the gatekeeper in the new health care system.

Not willing to lose out on its market share the American College of Obstetricians and Gynecologists successfully lobbied to have the obstetrician/gynecologist designated as the primary care physician for women. Residency programs have been restructured to include training in primary care, including cardiovascular disease, gastrointestinal problems, and acute care, and predictably less time has been devoted to specialty areas, including developing subspecialties such as urogynecology and breast disease.

Beginning in 1993, the American College of Obstetricians and Gynecologists began publishing guidelines for primary care including routine assessment for women's health care.[1] The previous initiatives concerning the diagnosis and treatment of breast disease were not completely abandoned and the College did publish Committee Opinion 140 "The Role of the Obstetrician Gynecologist in the Diagnosis and Treatment of Breast Disease"[2] in 1994. The role of obstetricians/gynecologists as envisioned by this committee was more in keeping with their new capacity as primary care physicians. It was noted that breast examination, inspection, and palpation were integral parts of complete obstetric and gynecologic examinations, and it was also noted that the College encouraged both basic and clinical research into the cause, early diagnosis, and treatment of all breast disease. Postgraduate education, including residency training programs in obstetrics and gynecology, and continuing medical education should include education in the early diagnosis and management options of all forms of breast dis-

ease. Certainly this represents a watered down version of the original intent of both the College and the Board, although it is in keeping with the new mission of obstetricians and gynecologists as primary care physicians. The Council on Residency Education in Obstetrics and Gynecology (CREOG) made an attempt to establish minifellowships in four centers scattered throughout the country. One of these was based at the Breast Health Center at Women & Infants Hospital in Providence, Rhode Island. It was hoped that board-certified physicians would take advantage of this opportunity and participate in 2-week training courses intended to update the physician in the contemporary management of breast diseases. At this time it is unclear if these programs will be implemented because of competing pressures for the new demands on the obstetrician/gynecologist, especially in the area of primary care.

SCREENING

For several years the American College of Obstetricians and Gynecologists has reviewed the evidence supporting screening for breast cancer by mammography. In 1990, I was asked by the Jacobs Institute of Women's Health and the National Cancer Institute to assist in conducting a survey of mammography attitudes and usage (MAUS) of women 40 years of age and older to determine current attitudes and practices concerning mammography. This study revealed that 31% of the women were following the guidelines for screening.[15] Of the women, 41% were determined to be following the guidelines in 1992, and in 1997 the figure was 47%,[10,11] that is, almost 50% of the women studied were having mammography according to the currently recommended guidelines. There has recently been increasing debate about two issues: when to begin annual screenings—should women between the ages of 40 and 50 have an annual mammogram—and when to discontinue annual screenings. The available data suggest that screenings be continued until at least age 75 years.[12] Screenings beginning at age 40 remains controversial. Complete discussion of this debate is beyond the scope of this chapter, but the present situation can be summarized as follows. Advocates of screening beginning at the age of 40 refer to data from a number of meta-analyses that indicate a 15% decrease in mortality of breast cancer in this age group.[13,22] It was estimated that in 1997 breast cancer would be diagnosed in 30,000 women in their 40s, and by using annual screening, 1600 lives will be saved.[13,22] On the other hand, what is the cost? At an average cost of $125 for the 20 million women eligible and with 100% compliance the cost would be $2.5 billion. The entire budget of the National Cancer Institute is $2.15 billion. This figure does not take into account the additional diagnostic tests in the 10% of patients with false-negative results. Furthermore, what is the potential lost/ benefit to women older than age 50? If we could increase regular screening for women older than 50 by 15% to 20%, one third of deaths from breast cancer in the older than age 50 population would be prevented by early detection with mammography.[4] The real issue is one of public health policy. Is population screening by mammography of women between ages 40 to 49 an appropriate public health measure?

The American Cancer Society now recommends that annual screenings beginning at age 40. The American College of Obstetricians and Gynecologists has adopted the same recommendation. The National Cancer Institute now advises beginning screening every 1 or 2 years at age 40 for women at average risk. It is interesting to note that the American College of Physicians and the American Association of Family Practice continue to recommend annual screening beginning at age 50. Finally, it is important to remember that at the present time in the United States 50% of breast cancers are diagnosed by screening. Of these, 50% are ductal cancer in situ (DCIS). This represents 12% of all newly diagnosed breast cancers, approximately 23,000 to 36,000 cases annually.[21,23,24]

With the introduction of screening mammography, the discovery of an occult lesion (i.e., microcalcifications or an asymmetric density) is an increasing possibility. The decision to perform a biopsy is the responsibility of the radiologist.[1,6-9,17] These patients have no symptoms, and the physical examination is entirely negative. In my opinion the handling of the occult lesion is one of the most difficult aspects of the diagnosis and treatment of breast disease. A number of patients have been referred to our Breast Health Center with an "abnormal mammogram," and this has resulted in considerable anxiety for the patient and her family. When we have reviewed the films, in many cases the lesion is of no consequence and follow-up films to assess stability are all that are required.

When a patient has abnormal mammogram, three possibilities exist:

1. Additional studies are required to clarify the situation. These studies may include an additional mammogram with special reviews and/or ultrasound evaluation.
2. Follow-up films are needed in 4 to 6 months to assess stability.
3. A biopsy needs to be performed.

MAKING THE DIAGNOSIS

Once the decision has been made to perform a biopsy, the radiologist usually recommends either an open biopsy or a stereotactic or ultrasound procedure. This decision is based on a number of factors, including the experience of the radiology team, the location of the lesion, and the wishes of the patient.

An alternative to a needle-guided biopsy is the stereotactic core biopsy.[19] This uses sophisticated radiographic equipment with an automated biopsy "gun" containing a large-bore (12 to 14 gauge) needle.[20] Several cores may be taken from the area without the need for a surgical incision. Usually 5 and as many as 10 may be obtained. The specimens are then submitted for a radiographic examination to determine whether the lesion is present, in particular the presence of microcalcifications. The specimen is then carefully examined by the pathology department. Stereotactic biopsy is less costly, and the only incision is a small stab wound in the appropriate location in the breast. There is also less scarring in the breast that might interfere with subsequent interpretation of the mammogram.

Several studies are under way to determine the accuracy of the stereotactic core biopsy compared with the traditional needle-guided surgical biopsy.[16] A significant number of patients are required to obtain the skill necessary to perform the procedure and to interpret the core biopsy. There is a very definite learning curve. The efficacy of the core biopsy in patients with a localized area of microcalcifications continues to be debated. In this situation, multiple core biopsies must be taken, both from the area containing the microcalcifications and the adjacent tissue since occasional carcinomas are found adjacent to the microcalcifications associated with benign fibrocystic changes.

Improvements in ultrasound equipment have permitted the identification of smaller and smaller masses and the option to use ultrasonography for localization and biopsy of nonpalpable lesions. Ultrasound-guided core biopsy or FNA is well tolerated and usually takes less time to complete than the traditional stereotactic procedure; it is also less costly.[18]

Predictably, the increasing use of image-guided core needle biopsy by both stereotactic and ultrasound techniques, in addition to representing a major change in the diagnosis of mammographically detected abnormalities, has resulted in a credentialing controversy between the surgeons and the radiologists. As noted previously, approximately half of all breast cancers are now detected mammographically, and if the biopsy is now confirmed by image-guided core needle biopsy, the conventional needle-directed excisional biopsy performed by the surgeon will no longer be necessary. Should the surgeon with appropriate training and credentialing perform the image-guided biopsy or should this technique be performed by well-trained radiologists with a sufficient case load to maintain the expertise required for this procedure? At the Breast Health Center at Women & Infants Hospital, the image-guided biopsies are performed by the Department of Radiology. It is, after all, the radiologist who must make the decision whether the lesion should be biopsied. In my opinion the radiologist is in the best position to review the films and decide the technical issues involved in obtaining an adequate specimen. It is of some interest that the June 1997 bulletin of the American College of Surgeons proposes a centralized registry to prospectively document the consecutive experience of surgeons with image-guided biopsy.[5] However, it should be noted that the Food and Drug Administration (FDA) expects to develop national quality standards and regulations regarding image-guided biopsies as part of the authority granted under the Mammography Quality Standards Act of 1992.[5]

THE DOMINANT MASS

The diagnosis begins with a careful history and physical examination. The physician should note the chief complaint, including the date of onset. A thorough physical examination should be performed with the patient in both the sitting and the supine positions. Regrettably, a number of texts still discuss breast findings in terms of a mass, ulceration, erythema, edema, retraction, and other signs that indicate advanced disease. A cancer 1 cm in size with the average doubling time has been present for at least 7 to 8 years, ample time for the establishment of metastases. Therefore we must search for subtle changes that suggest smaller (or earlier) cancers for which conservative treatment may be appropriate. The most important feature of the physical examination of the breast is the time spent doing the examination, not the technique of examination.

If a dominant mass is discovered, it should be resolved within a reasonable time frame. No lesion is obviously benign. Resolution may include reexamination at another time during the menstrual cycle and additional appropriate diagnostic studies, including ultrasound evaluation or an attempt to aspirate. It is a mistake to assume that because a mass is firm, mobile, and nontender, it represents a fibroadenoma or a solid lesion, benign or malignant. I have seen a number of macrocysts from 5 mm to 2 cm in diameter, all of which had

the hallmarks of a solid lesion. They were firm, nontender, and mobile, but all were cysts.

In my opinion an attempt should be made to aspirate every dominant mass, the single exception being the obvious cancer for which FNA, as discussed in the following pages, is the appropriate procedure.

Aspiration is a simple procedure that does not require special equipment—only a plastic 10-ml syringe and a 23-gauge needle. The mass is stabilized as shown in Fig. 52-1, *A* through *C*, and the area over the mass is wiped with an alcohol sponge. Without the use of local anesthesia, the needle is quickly plunged into the mass. The surgeon should attempt to gauge the size of the mass so that the needle actually penetrates the cyst but does not pass through the opposite wall. This is particularly true with very small masses. The fluid is withdrawn until the mass has completely disappeared (see Fig. 52-1, *D* and *E*). An adhesive bandage is placed over the site.

It is important to note the exact location and size of the cyst and the date the aspiration was performed. With rare exceptions, the patient should be requested to return in 1 month to reevaluate this area. *If the mass returns, the phy-*

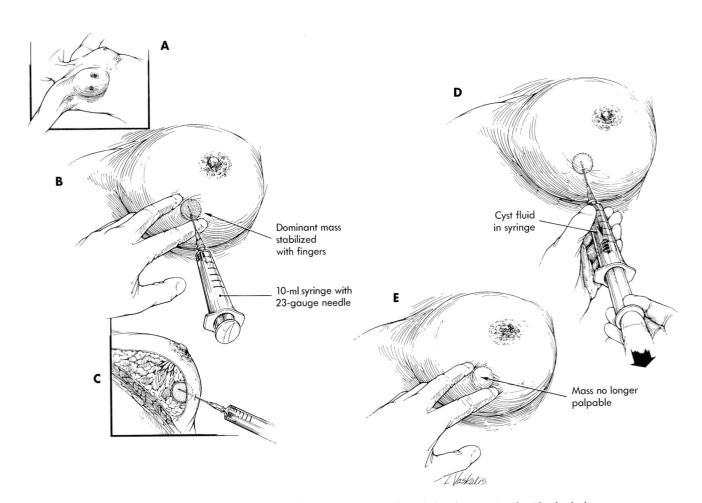

Fig. 52-1 Aspiration of cyst. **A,** The mass is palpated, and the skin is wiped with alcohol sponge. **B** and **C,** The needle penetrates the cyst without passing through opposite wall. (No local anesthesia is necessary.) **D** and **E,** Fluid is withdrawn until the mass disappears.

sician must suspect a carcinoma, and open biopsy is recommended. There are exceptions to this rule. It is almost impossible to aspirate completely a large (3 to 4 cm) cyst. The wall becomes quite flaccid, and inevitably, a few milliliters of fluid remain. Reexamination in 1 month often reveals a mass that can be completely emptied, and follow-up can again be recommended in 1 month.

Not every macrocyst requires aspiration. Often, a mammogram reveals asymmetric densities that on ultrasound prove to be multiple macrocysts. Many of these are nonpalpable. All that is required is a repeat mammogram or ultrasound to assess the stability of these lesions.

Should the aspirated fluid be sent for cytological evaluation? From a practical standpoint, no. The incidence of intracystic cancer is approximately 1 in 100,000. However, if the fluid is bloody or if the patient is in her late reproductive years without a longitudinal history, it is probably wise to submit the fluid for cytologic evaluation.

FINE-NEEDLE ASPIRATION AND CORE BIOPSY

Until recently, FNA has been considered a simple procedure, essentially a diagnostic study that can be performed by any physician. Special equipment is not required; however, the needle used should be of small caliber (23 to 25 gauge). It is a mistake to use a larger needle because the negative pressure available becomes much less and the specimen often is inadequate.

The recommendations for FNA or core biopsy are particularly relevant to obstetrician gynecologists. In many instances they are the first physicians to see patients with breast symptoms. In September 1996, a National Cancer Institute sponsored conference produced "The Uniform Approach to Breast Fine Needle Aspiration Biopsy." The final version of this conference may be found in *The Breast Journal,* volume 3, issue 4, pages 149-168, 1997.[7,25] I would recommend that every physician contemplating the use of FNA or core biopsy read the report in its entirety. The indications for performance of FNA or core biopsy in palpable breast lesions should be restricted to sufficiently defined palpable lesions. In my opinion, the routine aspiration of "breast thickenings" leads to confusion and often to unnecessary and inaccurate surgical biopsies. At the Breast Health Center, we often see patients referred after a FNA. Physical examination does not reveal a dominant mass. The report of the FNA indicates "atypical cells." Because there is no mass, it is impossible to determine from which area of the breast the cells have been recovered. Because most physicians perform these techniques only occasionally, it is best to refer the patient to a physician experienced in the diagnosis of breast lesions.

The accuracy rate for FNA varies considerably. The fine-needle sampling procedure is highly operator dependent. The National Cancer Institute report notes that fine-needle aspiration operators fall into roughly one of three categories:

1. The most common category consists of physicians who have no training in the FNA procedure beyond having read a description of it or having had a couple of occasions to watch a colleague perform it. Under these circumstances the noncontributory specimen rate is usually about 40% to 50%.

2. The second category is of physicians who have had the privilege of one on one training with an experienced operator and who have a good understanding of the pitfalls of the technique. However, their training is usually limited to less than 40 specimens and their volume of cases usually does not exceed 50 per year. The noncontributory specimen rate under these circumstances is usually 10% to 30%.

3. The third category is of operators with extensive, well-supervised training that included up to 150 to 200 cases. The volume of cases seen is at least 100 per year. Most of these operators are cytopathologists with special interest in FNA cytology, but some are radiologists and clinicians with the luxury of a high volume of cases. The noncontributory specimen rate in this category is less than 5%.

A noncontributory specimen in this sense is one that does not provide a specific diagnosis and does not contribute positively to the management of the patient. Some of these noncontributory specimens not only will fail to contribute useful information but will be misleading as when benign breast tissue adjacent to a cancer is sampled or when, for example, a sample contains scant atypical, perhaps distorted cells from what is actually a fibroadenoma. In such cases as this, the suboptimal sample may contribute to overinterpretation of the material. When abundant, well-preserved material is present, benignity or malignancy is much more easily determined.

Based on the previous section, it is recommended that FNA biopsy be performed by the most qualified personnel available.

At our Breast Health Center, because multiple "passes" must be made with the needle, we use local anesthesia (1% lidocaine without adrenaline). A small wheel is made, and the mass is immobilized with the fingers as shown in Fig. 52-2, A through C. A 10-ml syringe with a 25-gauge needle is used. It is important to test the needle before it is inserted into the breast. The needle is inserted into the breast, and suction is applied as the needle is withdrawn and replaced in a repetitive manner to cover a defined area of the lesion (see Fig. 52-2, D and E). It is important that the "tissue juice" not enter the syringe; it should remain in the needle. As the needle is withdrawn, the suction is released and the material is spread on a slide and processed according to the recommendations of the cytopathologist (Fig. 52-3). In our Breast Health Center the cytopathologist has requested that the aspirated material be immediately injected into a special solution, rather than placed on a slide. In some cases more than one sample is taken, and these are so labeled.

Consultation between the physician and the pathologist is essential. A FNA may provide cytologic evidence that the cells are malignant or benign and in some cases suggest whether the cells represent a ductal carcinoma or a lobular carcinoma. However, the "invasiveness" of the lesion can-

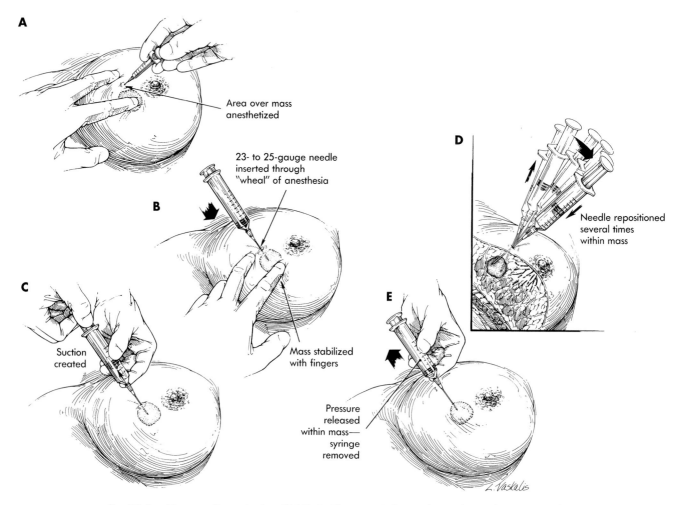

A, Area over mass anesthetized

23- to 25-gauge needle inserted through "wheal" of anesthesia

D, Needle repositioned several times within mass

Suction created

Mass stabilized with fingers

Pressure released within mass— syringe removed

Fig. 52-2 Fine-needle aspiration (FNA). **A,** The mass is located. Local anesthesia (1% lidocaine without adrenalin) is applied. **B,** The mass is stabilized and the needle inserted. **C,** Suction is created as the needle is withdrawn. **D,** The needle is repositioned several times. **E,** Suction is released as needle is withdrawn.

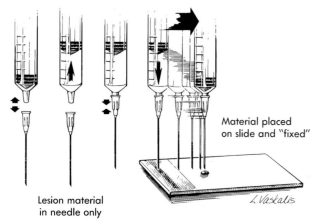

Material placed on slide and "fixed"

Lesion material in needle only

Fig. 52-3 Fine-needle aspiration being readied for processing. Note that "tissue juice" remains in the needle and does not enter the syringe.

not always be determined. If there is any question, an open biopsy should be performed as part of the local surgical management.

The core biopsy, as the name implies, removes a core of tissue. Appropriate needles (12 or 14 gauge) commonly are used. A local anesthetic is infiltrated over the lesion, and a small incision is made to admit the passage of the needle without undue pressure. One or more cores are removed and examined *histologically* by the pathologist. Obviously, the exact histologic type, grade, and invasiveness, together with the presence or absence of microcalcifications and other characteristics of the tumor can be determined. In addition, DNA analysis and receptor analysis can also be obtained. However, the core biopsy is not without complications. This is a large needle and occasionally moderate-sized hematomas are produced, which may interfere with the expeditious local treatment of the lesion.

The interested reader is urged to read the complete report developed and approved by the National Cancer Institute.

OPEN BIOPSY

Open biopsy often becomes part of the definitive treatment for breast cancer. In the past the choice of the incision was unimportant because if cancer was diagnosed, a radical mastectomy would be performed. With the advent of conservative management, the placement of the incision is crucial and the appearance of the wound may influence the timing and even the feasibility of conservative treatment.

Once the decision has been made to perform an open biopsy, the surgeon should discuss with the patient the type of anesthesia to be used and the immediate outcome of the biopsy procedure. With rare exception, almost all breast biopsies can be performed under local anesthesia. I have three exceptions. First, a teenager often is terrified of the operating room setting and the use of any type of needle. In this situation, I proceed with an open biopsy on a day-surgery basis under general anesthesia. In some cases, local anesthesia is no problem, but this should be discussed with both the patient and her parents. Second, patients with a language barrier are not ideally suited for local anesthesia. It is a frightening experience to be unable to understand the conversation in the operating room, and for these patients, unless an interpreter is available, I proceed on a day-surgery basis with general anesthesia. The final group of patients who are best operated on under general anesthesia are those with very large breasts and lesions deep within the breast for which extensive exposure is required to reach the lesion.

It is essential that breast biopsy be performed in a operating room setting with nurses familiar with the technique. Conversation must be kept to a minimum and be appropriate to the procedure being performed. In our day-surgery center, the draping is such that the patient is unable to watch the procedure (although if the patient looks directly at the reflection in the operating room light, a portion of the procedure can be seen).

It is important to examine the patient immediately before she is brought into the operating room. Occasionally, a mass

---

EQUIPMENT REQUIRED FOR OPEN BIOPSY PROCEDURE

EQUIPMENT	SUTURES
Mayo stand	3-0, 4-0 plain ties
Prep table	3-0, 4-0 chromic ties
2 arm boards	4-0 plain sutures
Bovie	4-0, 5-0 nylon sutures
Drapes	
Chux	**INSTRUMENTS**
Sponges	Small snaps—curved and
"Fluffs"	straight
Telfa	2 Allis clamps
6-in Ace bandage	2 small rake retractors
2-in silk tape	2 skin hooks
Specimen cup	1 curved Mayo scissors
1% lidocaine without	1 small Metzenbaum scis-
adrenaline	sors
0.25% bupivacaine	Knife handle and no. 15
without adrenaline	blades
Marking pencil and ruler	Small right-angle retractors
Suction (poole or plastic)	

---

that had been noted is no longer present, and of course, in this situation, the procedure is canceled.

I mark my incisions with the patient in the sitting position. The patient is brought into the operating room and placed in the supine position with the arm extended. The breast is carefully prepared. I use a Betadine preparation, but almost any standard operating room preparation can be used. It is important to include the nipple in the draped area for orientation. When the draping is complete, the Mayo tray with the appropriate instruments is brought over to the patient. The instruments most commonly used are listed in the box above.

It is important to explain to the patient that she will be told what is going to happen during the procedure, not in technical terms, but, for example, before the breast is touched or the needle for local anesthesia is inserted into the skin. For local anesthesia, I use 1% lidocaine without adrenaline. I believe it is important to identify any bleeding immediately, and because I do not use a drain, the wound must be absolutely dry before closure. The previously marked incision is infiltrated, noting the amount of anesthesia used (Fig. 52-4, *A* and *B*). While the local anesthesia is diffusing into the tissue, this is a good time to prepare the sutures and be certain that the Mayo tray contains all of the instruments required for the procedure. This delay has another practical application. For small lesions, the introduction of the local anesthesia often obscures the anatomy and the lesion no longer can be palpated.

The incision is made (see Fig. 52-4, *C*). I use a no. 15 blade. Bleeding is controlled with fine 4-0 plain catgut ligatures. I do not use the actual cautery near the surface nor during the excision of the specimen. Cauterization at the tissue results in coagulation artifacts that preclude the

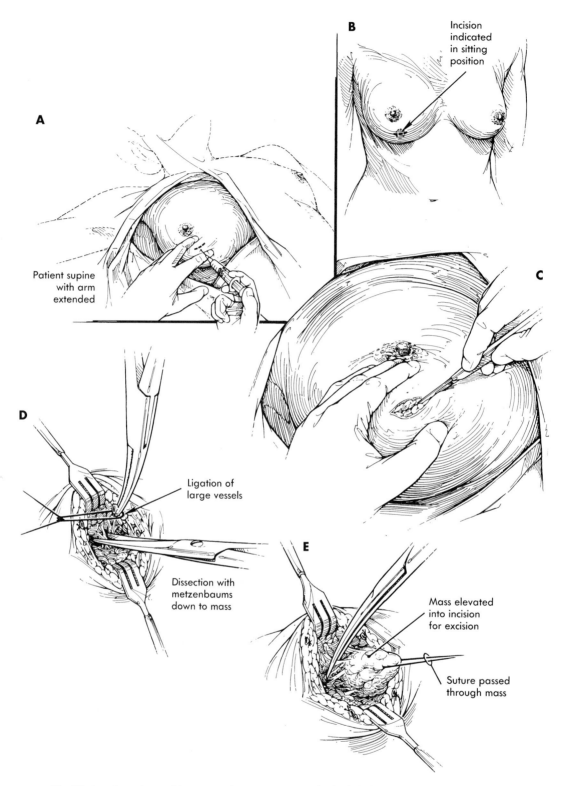

Fig. 52-4   Open breast biopsy. **A,** The incision is marked while the patient is in the sitting position. **B,** The patient is now in the supine position. The breast has been prepared and local anesthesia (1% lidocaine without adrenalin) administered. **C,** Incision is made. **D,** Large vessels are ligated and dissection proceeds. **E,** Suture is placed into the lesion, and the mass is elevated into the incision for excision.

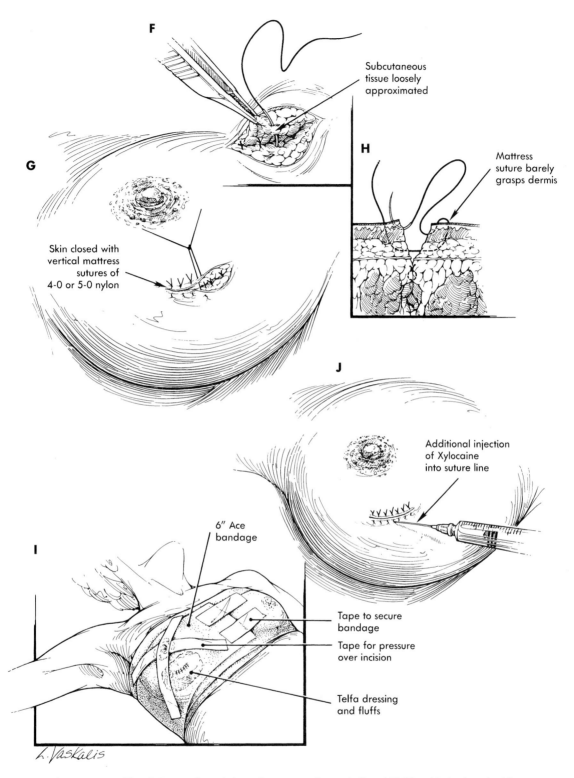

Fig. 52-4, cont'd   F, Breast tissue is loosely reapproximated. **G** and **H,** The skin is closed with vertical mattress sutures. **I** and **J,** Additional local anesthesia is injected and the pressure dressing is applied.

determination of accurate margins. Bleeding is controlled during the dissection with appropriate hemostats and fine catgut ligatures (see Fig. 52-4, *D*). Retraction is provided using either skin hooks or very small rake retractors. Every effort should be made not to damage the skin edges. To provide appropriate exposure, an assistant is essential. This may be a nurse or another physician.

The patient is instructed to indicate whether she has any discomfort during the procedure. It is essential that a minimal amount of normal tissue be removed. Most of the lesions are benign, and if cancer is present, this will be obvious in most cases. It is inappropriate to insert large Allis clamps to elevate tissue into the incision and blindly excise the breast tissue. Instead, the lesion should be directly identified. At this point, a suture of plain or chromic catgut can be placed into the lesion, and the lesion can be elevated into the incision (see Fig. 52-4, *E*). The lesion is easily excised by sharp dissection, and the bleeding points are clamped and ligated. The lesion is passed to the nurse and submitted to the pathology department for frozen section analysis. This is important because even the most benign-appearing lesion may contain cancer for which estrogen and progesterone receptors and the marking of margins are essential in the treatment planning process.

Once the lesion has been removed, the wound is inspected for hemostasis. It is at this point, particularly in the young patient with very dense breast tissue, that use of the actual cautery is appropriate. Small bleeding points can be cauterized. However, the major vessels are ligated with fine plain catgut. When the wound is dry, the breast tissue is *loosely* reapproximated with 4-0 plain catgut (see Fig. 52-4, *F*). No attempt is made to obliterate the cavity completely, The skin is closed with vertical mattress sutures of fine nylon (see Fig. 52-4, *G*). No drain is used. A close-up view of the skin closure is shown in Fig. 52-4, *H*. The sutures must be placed evenly along the incision line, and the most superficial suture should barely grasps the dermis. In this way, a cosmetic closure is achieved. The sutures should be removed in 5 to 7 days.

The most important part of this procedure is the placement of the pressure dressing. Once the skin has been closed, additional lidocaine without adrenaline is injected into the incision, and Telfa and a pressure dressing are applied directly over the incision and secured with a 6-inch Ace bandage for 48 hours (see Fig. 52-4, *I* and *J*). The use of the pressure dressing immobilizes the breast, reduces discomfort, and prevents ecchymosis and induration. The latter is essential if reexcision is required at a later date as part of the definitive surgical procedure for breast cancer.

Using this technique, I have not found it necessary to administer narcotics. The patient is simply told to take Tylenol (acetaminophen) and to begin normal activities once the dressing has been removed. I do not use prophylactic antibiotics.

It is helpful to show the patient the films and point out the lesion. I have found that patients are reassured by this procedure, and it also helps explain the localization process.

The patient is shown where and how the needle will be inserted.

On the day of localization, the patient reports to the radiology suite. No premedication is used because the films must be taken in the sitting position. The radiologist, noting the position of the lesion on the original films, places a small amount of lidocaine in the dermis (Fig. 52-5, *A*). We use a Homer mammalock needle as shown in Figs. 52-5, *B* through *D*, and 52-6. The illustrations show the technique of insertion of the needle and the final position of the needle relative to the occult lesion. The needle is inserted, and additional films are taken (see Fig. 52-6). If the needle is not within 5 mm of the lesion, it is withdrawn and reinserted to obtain the final position.

The films are reviewed by the radiologist and the surgeon, and the patient is taken to the day-surgery center for open biopsy. The films are brought to the operating room for review during the procedure. I use local anesthesia for this procedure as in the routine open biopsy and have found this to be quite satisfactory. My figures indicate that I obtain the lesion 96% of the time on the first operation and the other 4% in a second operation if this is required. I have had no significant complications using this technique, and because there is an appreciable amount of "down time" waiting for specimen radiography, I believe that the patient should be awake rather than subjected to the risk of general anesthesia.

The patient is placed in the supine position on the operating room table with the arm extended. In this case, a decision must be made where to make the incision. Should the incision be made at the entrance of the needle or should the needle be intercepted (Fig. 52-7, *A* and *B*)? This decision is based largely on the probability of the lesion being cancer and the need for additional surgery. An improperly placed incision may make a modified mastectomy difficult. A circumareolar incision is seldom used unless the lesion is directly beneath the incision.

The x-ray films are reviewed, and measurements are taken to locate the needle relative to the skin surface. This is helpful in deciding where to make the incision. The location of the occult lesion relative to the needle also is noted. Is it superior or inferior? Is it toward the midline or the axilla? The incision is chosen and marked. The 1% lidocaine without adrenaline is injected, and the incision is made as in the open biopsy. However, if the incision is made adjacent to the needle, it is essential to leave a small portion of dermis attached to the needle to provide stability during the dissection.

Using the films as a guide, sharp dissection is continued toward the lesion using appropriate retraction as in the open biopsy (see Fig. 52-7, *C* and *D*). Care must be taken not to disturb the needle. When the proper distance has been reached, the needle is freed from the dermis and the tissue is stabilized with a single Allis clamp. Using the films as a guide, the surgeon removes the area in question by sharp dissection (see Fig. 58-7, *E*). A fresh no. 15 blade is useful for this procedure, but appropriate scissors can be used as

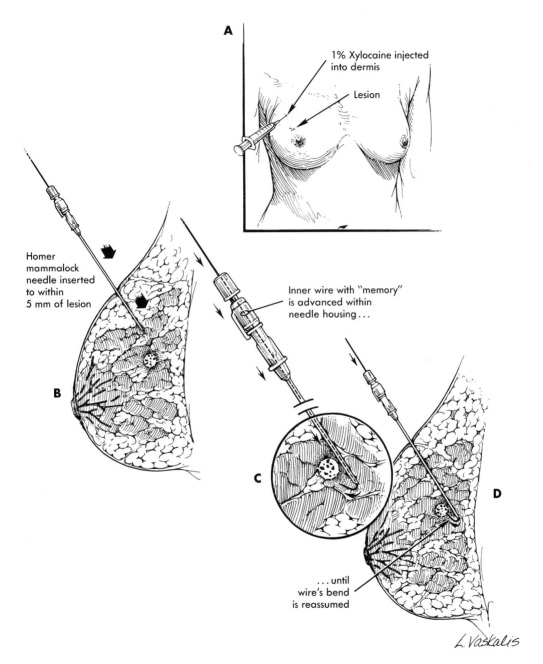

A

1% Xylocaine injected into dermis

Lesion

Homer mammalock needle inserted to within 5 mm of lesion

B

Inner wire with "memory" is advanced within needle housing...

C

D

...until wire's bend is reassumed

L. Vaskalis

Fig. 52-5   Localization and biopsy. **A,** Local anesthesia is injected. **B** through **D,** The Homer mammalock needle is inserted and positioned.

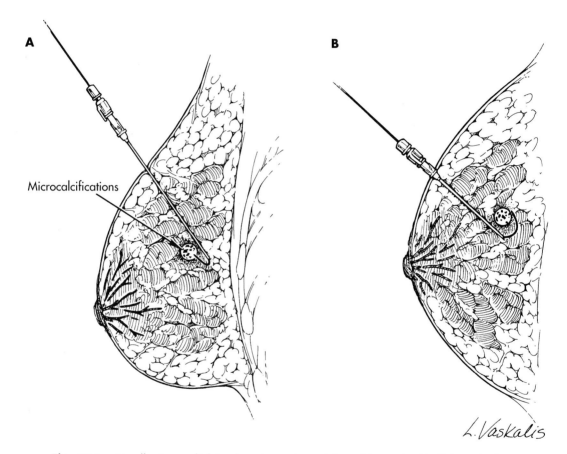

Fig. 52-6 Needle in mediolateral and craniocaudal positions. **A,** Mediolateral view. **B,** Craniocaudal view.

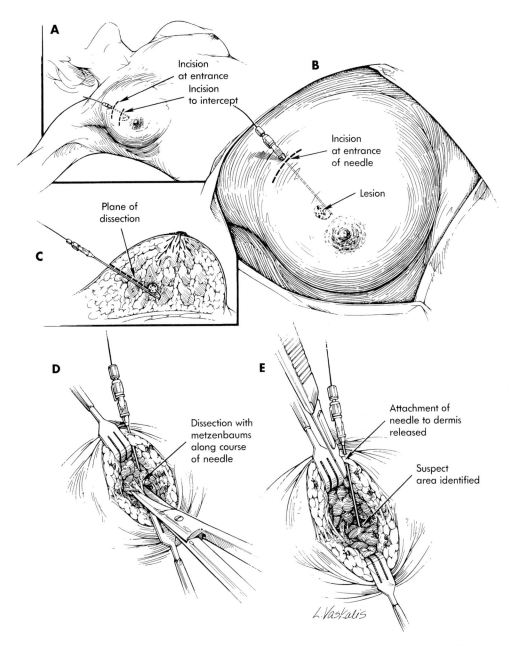

Fig. 52-7 Localization and biopsy, operative procedure. **A** and **B,** The incision site is chosen, and the incision is made. **C** and **D,** Sharp dissection continues along the needle toward the lesion. **E,** The needle is freed from dermis.

well. This is not an easy procedure, and it requires experience to know exactly when to stabilize the lesion and begin excision of the specimen. It must be remembered that the needle is placed with the patient in the *sitting* position and the operation is performed with the patient in the *supine* position; therefore there is displacement of the lesion, which must be considered during the dissection. In the very firm breast, little movement occurs. However, in a pendulous or fatty breast, the breast tissue may roll away from the midline and make identification of the lesion difficult.

If the incision is made midway between the needle and the nipple, once the dissection has reached the area in question, the needle is stabilized and withdrawn into the incision (Fig. 52-8, *A* through *E*). To perform this maneuver, the outer or larger needle is removed, leaving the wire, which is withdrawn through the incision and stabilized with the Allis clamp.

Once the lesion has been removed, preferably with the needle, it is placed on an appropriate tray with wet sponges and delivered with the films to the radiologist for specimen radiography (see Fig. 52-8, *F* through *H*). In most cases the wound is not closed until it has been confirmed that the lesion has been removed. No attempt should be made to use the actual cautery because if additional tissue is removed, the cautery may obscure the histology and make the definitive diagnosis difficult if not impossible.

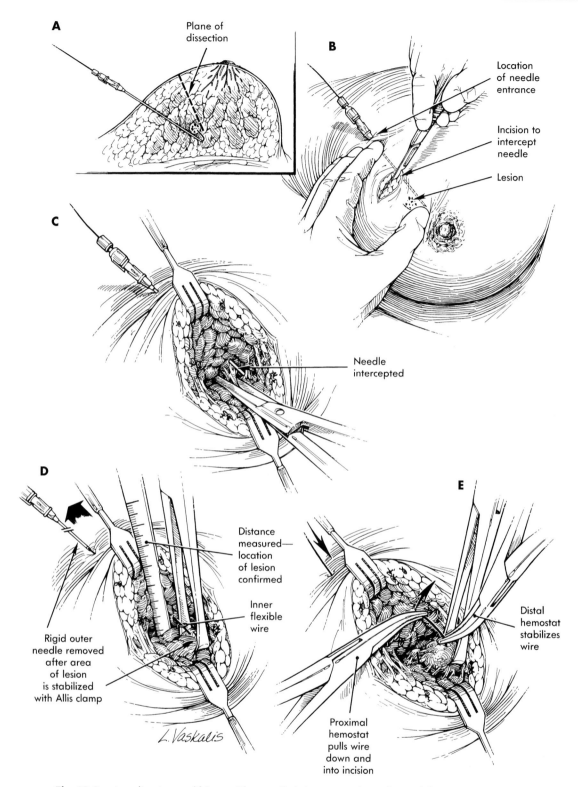

A Plane of dissection

B Location of needle entrance

Incision to intercept needle

Lesion

C Needle intercepted

D Distance measured—location of lesion confirmed

Inner flexible wire

Rigid outer needle removed after area of lesion is stabilized with Allis clamp

L. Vaskalis

E Distal hemostat stabilizes wire

Proximal hemostat pulls wire down and into incision

Fig. 52-8 Localization and biopsy. The needle is intercepted. **A,** Plane of dissection midway between needle and nipple. **B** and **C,** Incision and dissection made to intercept the needle. **D** and **E,** The needle is stabilized and withdrawn into the incision.

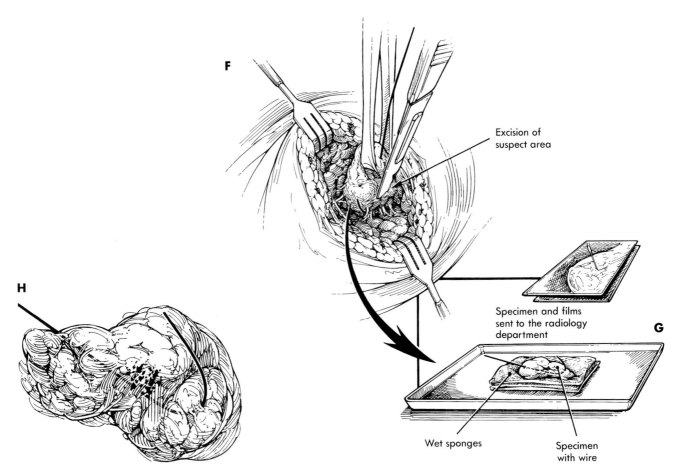

Fig. 52-8, cont'd **F** and **G**, The lesion is removed and sent with film to radiology. **H**, Specimen radiography showing microcalcifications.

If the lesion is not present in the specimen, additional tissue can be removed. I do not proceed beyond a second attempt because the landmarks are no longer available and successful removal is unlikely.

Once it has been determined that the lesion is present in the specimen, bleeding is controlled with the actual cautery or ligatures of fine plain catgut. Again, no drain is used. The breast tissue is loosely reconstructed, and the skin is closed with vertical mattress sutures of 5-0 nylon as in the open biopsy. Additional lidocaine without adrenaline is injected into the incision, and the pressure dressing is applied and left in place for 48 hours.

Successful removal of an occult lesion is not an easy procedure, particularly when local anesthesia is used. It should be performed only in a setting in which there is communication between an experienced radiologist and a skillful surgeon. In my institution, after radiography of the specimen has confirmed the presence of the lesion, the pathologist is called to the radiology suite and takes over responsibility for processing the specimen. In most cases a rapid section is not performed because of the small size of the lesion. The margins are marked to assist in treatment planning. In most cases, receptor analysis is impossible because of the small size of the specimen; however, this can be determined by immunocytochemical techniques. In some cases, a wide lo-

cal excision may be required for effective localization and biopsy, and this may constitute definitive treatment of the cancer. Obviously, this depends on the site and size of the lesion and the experience of the surgeon. In most cases, re-excision is required, and this is often performed at the time of the axillary dissection.

REFERENCES

1. American College of Obstetricians and Gynecologists: *Guidelines for women's health care,* 1996.
2. American College of Obstetricians and Gynecologists: *The role of the obstetrician/gynecologist in the diagnosis and treatment of breast disease,* Committee Opinion 140, Washington, DC, 1994.
3. Committee on Gynecologic Practice, American College of Obstetricians and Gynecologists, October 18, 1990.
4. Brawley O: Comments concerning national cancer advisory board guidelines for mammographic screening, *Am Med News* 3, May 5, 1997.
5. Edwards MJ, Israel PZ: Beyond the credentialling and privileging controversy surrounding image-guided breast biopsy, *Bull Am Coll Surg* 82:20, 1997.
6. Feig SA: Decreased breast cancer mortality through mammographic screening—results of clinical trials, *Radiology* 167:659, 1988.
7. Final version: The uniform approach to breast fine-needle aspiration biopsy, *Breast J* 3:149, 1997.
8. Homer MJ: Non palpable breast lesion localization using a curved-end retractable wire, *Radiology* 157:259, 1985.

9. Homer MJ, Marchant DJ, Smith TJ: The geographic cluster of breast microcalcifications—is it really intramammary? *Surg Gynecol Obstet* 161:532, 1985.

10. Horton JA, Romans MC, Cruess DF: Mammography attitudes and usage study, 1992, *Womens Health Issues WHI* 2:180, 1992.

11. Jacobs Institute: *Mammography attitudes and usage study, 1997,* personal communication, September 2, 1997.

12. Jos AA, et al: Efficacy of mammographic screening in the elderly: a case-referent study in the Nijmegen Program in the Netherlands, *J Natl Cancer Inst* 1986:934, 1994.

13. Leitch AM, et al: American Cancer Society guidelines for the early detection of breast cancer: update, 1997, *CA* 47:150, 1997.

14. Marchant DJ: Breast biopsy. In Nichols DH, editor: *Gynecologic and Obstetric Surgery,* St Louis, 1993, Mosby, p 947.

15. Marchant DJ, Sutton SM: Use of mammography: United States, 1990, *MMWR* 39:621, 1990.

16. Mikhail RA, et al: Stereotactic core needle biopsy of mammographic breast lesions as a viable alternative to surgical biopsy, *Ann Surg Oncol* 1:363, 1994.

17. Moscowitz M: Predictive value, sensitivity and specificity in breast cancer screening, *Radiology* 167:576, 1988.

18. Parker SH, et al: Ultrasound guided automated large core breast biopsy, *Radiology* 187:507, 1993.

19. Parker SH, et al: Stereotactic breast biopsy with a biopsy gun, *Radiology* 176:741, 1990.

20. Parker SH, et al: Non-palpable breast lesions, stereotactic automated large core biopsies, *Radiology* 180:403, 1991.

21. Parker SL, et al: Cancer statistics, 1997. *Cancer J Clin* 47:5-27, 1997.

22. Schwartz RM: Washington update, *J Oncol Manage* March-April:7, 1997.

23. Silverstein MJ, editor: Preface, *Ductal carcinomas in situ of the breast,* Baltimore, 1997, Williams & Wilkins.

24. Silverstein MJ, Lagios MD: Use of predictors of recurrence to plan therapy for DCIS of the breast, *Oncology* 11:393, 1997.

25. The uniform approach to breast fine-needle aspiration biopsy, *Diagn Cytopathol* 16:295, 1997.

53 Treatment Options for Breast Cancer

DOUGLAS J. MARCHANT

The American Cancer Society has predicted that, for 1998, breast cancer will represent 30% of the cancer incidence and 16% of the deaths. Lung cancer now surpasses breast cancer as the leading cause of cancer in women. It is also predicted that, for 1998, there will be 178,700 new cases and 43,500 deaths.[1]

HISTORY

Surgical removal of the breast was described in the first and second centuries AD. The lesions observed were far advanced, and the treatment was unsuccessful. Later refinements in surgical technique resulted in a lower operative mortality, but again, cures were uncommon. In 1867, Z.H. Moore[46] suggested that the entire breast be removed with a wide margin of skin. Halsted's mastectomy was first mentioned in 1891, and by 1894, he had performed 50 "complete mastectomies."[33] This radical mastectomy, as the operation came to be known, was enthusiastically adopted in the United States and abroad. Because the lesions for which the Halsted procedure was designed were far advanced, the operation was not associated with an increase in cure, although there was a dramatic decrease in chest wall recurrences. During the next several decades, the results of the radical mastectomy improved principally because of earlier diagnosis and more selective use of the operation. Because the radical mastectomy did not include resection of the internal mammary lymph nodes, it was suggested that the classic operation be extended to include resection of the internal mammary nodes and the chest wall. In 1951, Urban[73] described the extended radical mastectomy that included an en bloc dissection of the chest wall.

EVALUATION OF THE PATIENT

Treatment planning for breast cancer includes a multidisciplinary approach. Alternatives in treatment require the expertise not only of the surgeon but of the radiotherapist and the medical oncologist.

Once the diagnosis of breast cancer has been established, a number of preoperative studies should be obtained. Mammography is essential even in the most obvious case. Synchronous cancer is present in 5% of patients, and multicentric disease may be discovered in the involved breast. This may preclude wide local excision and radiation therapy. Patients should have a pretreatment chest radiograph, routine blood studies, and liver function tests. For invasive lesions, many surgeons recommend a bone scan; however, the yield is very low for T1 lesions. Because many patients are placed on protocol studies, bone scan may be required as part of the staging procedure for these studies. Clinical staging using the tumor, node, metastasis (TNM) system is recommended, although most students of breast disease recognize that this system does not adequately segregate patients nor does it help to select appropriate patients for surgical treatment (Table 53-1). The TNM system was designed so that patients could be categorized, thereby enabling centers to group patients similarly for intercenter comparison. It is well known that the clinical nodal status of the patient may be incorrect. In addition, it is difficult to obtain accurate tumor size either from the pathologist or from the surgeon. However, the TNM system is the best available and it does have some value in that it makes the physician record the patient and tumor information. Clearly, the future rests with some form of biologic staging.

Appropriate treatment planning requires formal consultation with a radiotherapist and a medical oncologist. This should not be presented to the patient as a competition among the specialities. This concept of pretreatment evaluation inevitably results in some delay in the treatment, but there is no evidence that a delay of 2 to 3 weeks or more between diagnosis and definitive treatment affects prognosis.

In addition, in the current era of managed care, patients must be prepared for surgery on an outpatient basis, and in many cases the total local treatment can be performed without admission to the hospital. In most states the maximum hospital time allowance for breast-conservation treatment—wide local excision and axillary dissection—is 24 hours and for mastectomy without reconstruction is 48 hours. This requires considerable pretreatment preparation and for some patients arrangements for in-home postoperative care.

The decision regarding outpatient surgery is a difficult one and will not be solved to everyone's satisfaction. It is clear that as the number of women screened according to current guidelines increases, smaller, and in many cases "earlier" cancers will be discovered. Most of these cancers probably could be treated on an outpatient basis. In selected patients sentinel lymph node biopsy may be indicated, again as an outpatient procedure performed under local anesthesia.

For patients who require more extensive surgery, either because of the extent of the lesion compared with the size of the breast or because they request mastectomy, outpatient surgery must be carefully planned with extensive psychological and emotional preparation, including arranging a

Table 53-1 The Staging of Cancer: Staging for Breast Carcinoma

Definitions

Primary tumor (T)

TX Primary tumor cannot be assessed

T0 No evidence of primary tumor

Tis Carcinoma in situ: intraductal carcinoma, lobular carcinoma in situ, or Paget's disease of the nipple with no tumor

T1 Tumor ≤2 cm in greatest dimension

  T1a ≤0.5 cm in greatest dimension

  T1b >0.5 cm, but not >1 cm in greatest dimension

  T1c >1 cm, but not >2 cm in greatest dimension

T2 Tumor >2 cm, but not >5 cm in greatest dimension

T3 Tumor >5 cm in greatest dimension

T4 Tumor of any size with direct extension to chest wall or skin

  T4a Extension to chest wall

  T4b Edema (including peau d'orange) or ulceration of the skin of breast or satellite skin nodules confined to same breast

    T4c Both T4a and T4b

    T4d Inflammatory carcinoma

Regional lymph nodes (N)

NX Regional lymph nodes cannot be assessed (e.g., previously removed or not removed for pathologic study)

N0 No regional lymph node metastasis

N1 Metastasis to movable ipsilateral axillary lymph node(s)

  N1a Only micrometastasis (none >0.2 cm)

  N1b Metastasis to lymph node(s), any >0.2 cm

    N1bi Metastasis in 1 to 3 lymph nodes, any >0.2 cm and all <2 cm in greatest dimension

    N1bii Metastasis to ≥4 lymph nodes, any >0.2 cm and all <2 cm in greatest dimension

    N1biii Extension of tumor beyond the capsule of a lymph node metastasis <2 cm in greatest dimension

    N1biv Metastasis to a lymph node ≥2 cm in greatest dimension

N2 Metastasis to ipsilateral axillary lymph nodes that are fixed to one another or to other structures

N3 Metastasis to ipsilateral internal mammary lymph node(s)

Distant metastasis (M)

MX Presence of distant metastasis cannot be assessed

M0 No distant metastasis

M1 Distant metastasis (includes metastasis to ipsilateral supraclavicular lymph node(s)

AJCC/UICC Stage Grouping

Stage 0	Tis	N0	M0
Stage 1	T1	N0	M0
Stage IIA	T0	N1	M0
	T1	N1	M0
	T2	N0	M0
Stage IIB	T2	N1	M0
	T3	N0	M0
Stage IIIA	T0	N2	M0
	T1	N2	M0
	T2	N2	M0
	T3	N1	M0
	T3	N2	M0
Stage IIIB	T4	Any N	M0
	Any T	N3	M0
Stage IV	Any T	Any N	M1

home environment that will permit recuperation. Several institutions have developed outpatient breast surgery programs. All emphasize careful preoperative preparation, an operating theater with the requirements for this type of breast surgery, and trained staff, including skilled anesthesiologists and an experienced operating team to reduce the amount of time required for surgery. Specially trained recovery room staff to provide the skilled support required during the immediate postoperative period and to determine in fact whether the patient is capable of being discharged are absolutely essential.

Predictably, health maintenance organizations (HMOs) have been willing to encourage outpatient "drive-through" mastectomies. The Department of Health and Human Services has taken a stand on this issue, essentially stating that "it will prohibit Plans from requiring that breast cancer surgeries be performed on an outpatient basis." The policy also forbids limiting hospital stays for beneficiaries undergoing breast cancer surgery.[52]

The American College of Surgeons in its April *Bulletin* stated the following: "It is the College's view that due to individual needs of patients and their response to treatment modalities, no one can accurately predict the appropriate length of stay for a given patient. Moreover, the College is opposed to the concept of identifying one specific number to represent a length of stay for a given procedure, believing that it is more accurate to define length of stay using a range of days. The College has always encouraged its Fellows to keep patient's length of stay as short as possible while recognizing the individual needs of patients and their families."[56] HMOs, however, continue to request surgeons to document a "medical necessity" that justifies even a one-night hospital admission.[47] The alternative is to send the patient home with adequate pain medication and instructions on caring for her wound. CIGNA Healthcare of Connecticut states that it finds outpatient mastectomies preferable because hospital stay may carry a "high risk of infection."[47] It is interesting to note that Connecticare's Chief Medical Officer has stated that "the plan never overrules doctors' recommendations on hospital stays—but merely tries to have educational discussions when physicians seek unneeded or overly long hospital stays."[47]

Fortunately, most patients are now being seen with smaller lesions, which in fact can be adequately treated by outpatient surgery as discussed in the following sections. However, the *standard* treatment basically follows the treatment guidelines of a number of contemporary organizations including the National Comprehensive Cancer Network

(NCCN),[71] The National Cancer Institute, the Department of Health and Human Services PDQ Statement on Breast Cancer,[54] the comprehensive breast cancer guideline programs of a number of breast cancer centers,[22] and the Breast Cancer Surgical Practice Guidelines of the Society of Surgical Oncology.[49]

The management plan adopted by the Breast Health Center is as follows.

We offer patients with all forms of breast cancer a contemporary treatment program that reflects the latest information and knowledge. Advances in therapy offer the best opportunity for survival, while achieving the least morbidity, hospitalization, pain, discomfort, and disfigurement. We particularly try to maintain normal function and appearance. We work with a multidisciplinary team that includes nurses, social workers, nutritionists, and support groups as well as physicians and surgeons skilled in operation procedures, use of radiotherapy, and administration of chemotherapeutic and hormonal agents.

Principles of Service to Our Patients

Each patient is an individual with a need for an individualized approach to her tumor. All patients will have a full explanation of management options. Emphasis is placed on a close and full interaction between doctor and patient, with use of all members of the treatment team.

All patients will have their situation presented to a prospective multidisciplinary tumor board for the most thorough and wide opinions regarding treatment. Patients will have the opportunity to discuss their situation with surgeons, radiotherapists, medical oncologists, nurses, and support groups, all of whom participate in our weekly tumor board and will be familiar with the patient's management options.

We will constantly emphasize the human as well as the technical aspects of care. Ample time for discussion and elaboration of treatment decisions is encouraged. Supportive and complementary care forms a regular part of our attention to patients.

We will maintain as close a relationship as possible to the patient's referring and primary doctors, as well as family members. We will always be available by telephone or personal office visit for discussion and explanation.

We will always be available for routine follow-up and care. Should the cancer recur, we will provide analysis, advice, and adequate treatment and support, and we will offer the very latest in technology, medication, and support in an atmosphere of caring and hope.

Table 53-2 is an overall guide to therapeutic recommendations for patients and doctors. Some aspects of these therapeutic recommendations may be considered "nonstandard" considering the current American treatment guidelines. These situations represent, in our opinion and based on substantial data from reports on breast cancer, less radical treatment that provides equivalent cure rates with considerably reduced discomfort, morbidity, complications, and time and are reasonable alternatives that we encourage, but leave open to patient selection. In all situations, patients will be given all options that we believe are safe and effective. Patients will be able to discuss options with all members of the team.

SURGICAL OPTIONS FOR LOCAL TREATMENT

A number of factors influence the definitive surgical treatment for breast cancer. Important considerations include the size and histology of the lesion, the skill and experience of the multidisciplinary team, and the wishes of the patient. Treatments discussed include:

1. Modified radical mastectomy
2. Simple mastectomy
3. Subcutaneous mastectomy
4. Conservative treatment including quadrantectomy or wide local excision with or without axillary dissection

There is no doubt that the conservative approach appeals to many patients; however, statistics clearly indicate that many patients are treated with the modified radical mastectomy.

The anatomy of the breast and axilla is shown in Figs. 53-1 and 53-2. For purposes of comparison, the extent of a radical mastectomy is demonstrated in Figs. 53-3 and 53-4 (pp. 974-978).

Modified Radical Mastectomy (Simple Mastectomy with Axillary Dissection)

Modified radical mastectomy, as the name implies, is, in essence, a total mastectomy (simple) and axillary node dissection with preservation of the pectoral muscles. There have been a number of modifications of this operation, including removal of the pectoralis minor muscle. Most contemporary surgeons agree, however, that the operation today is best performed with preservation of both the pectoralis major and minor muscles.

The modified mastectomy is the procedure of choice for patients with large operable lesions, for patients with smaller lesions in relatively small breasts, and for patients who refuse conservative treatment. It is also the procedure of choice for large lesions demonstrated by mammography and proven by biopsy.

For most patients, this operation is performed on an "admit after surgery basis." Therefore the workup, as previously described, is obtained on an outpatient basis. It is important that the operating surgeon supervise this evaluation to avoid cancellation of the procedure on the day of surgery because of an incomplete workup.

The procedure is performed using appropriate endotrachial anesthesia. I usually request a muscle relaxant, although some surgeons prefer no paralysis so that the nerves in the axilla can be stimulated if necessary during dissection. A transverse incision is ideal because it makes later reconstruction more cosmetic. However, the actual line of incision depends on the site of the primary tumor. A number of maneuvers can be used that result in a transverse incision. These include an S-shaped incision that includes not only the lesion but the nipple areolar complex as well. In some cases the lesion is in the midline, high in the breast

Table 53-2   Treatment Guidelines

Management of Duct Carcinoma In Situ (DCIS)*

Features specified: Size, grade, necrosis, margins, method of detection, and microinvasion
Strategy based on the Van Nuys Prognostic Index (VNPI)

The VNPI scoring system awards 1 to 3 points for each of three different predictors of local breast recurrence (size, margins, and pathologic classification). Scores for each of the predictors are totaled to yield a VNPI score ranging from a low of 3 to a high of 9.

Score	1	2	3
Size (mm)	≤15	16-40	≥41
Margins (mm)	≥10	1-9	>1
Pathologic classification	Non-high-grade without necrosis	Non-high-grade with necrosis	High-grade with or without necrosis

VNPI 3 or 4	*Primary cancer:*	Excision to 1-cm margins
	Axillary dissection:	None
	Adjuvant radiation therapy (RT):	None
VNPI 5, 6, or 7	*Primary cancer:*	Excision or reexcision to 1-cm margins, if possible
	Axillary dissection:	None
	Adjuvant RT:	Selection between observation or RT depending on excision margin
VNPI 8 or 9	*Primary cancer:*	Mastectomy with or without reconstruction
(implies 1-cm margin	*Axillary dissection:*	None
cannot be achieved)	*Adjuvant RT:*	None after mastectomy

Management of Invasive Ductal Carcinoma (IDC)

Features specified: Method of detection, size, grade, margin, histologic type, axillary lymph node status, other prognostic indices, age (estrogen receptor [ER], progesterone receptor [PR], lymph vessel invasion [LVI], DNA, and S-phase)
Strategy based on method of detection, size, lymph node metastases, and features of the primary cancer

T1a ≤5 mm diam-	*Primary cancer:*	Excision to 1-cm margin
eter (Not DCIS	*Axillary dissection:*	None
with micro-	*Adjuvant RT:*	Avoid if possible, but selective application
invasion)	*Adjuvant chemotherapy:*	None unless LVI and/or poor nuclear grade
T1b >5 ≤10 mm		
Mammographic	*Primary cancer:*	Excision to 1-cm margin
detection	*Axillary dissection:*	None unless poor nuclear grade: sentinel node (SN) biopsy
	Adjuvant RT:	Avoid if possible: selective application based on tumor features and margins.
	Adjuvant chemotherapy:	None unless LVI and/or poor nuclear grade
Palpable	*Primary cancer:*	Excision to 1-cm margin.
	Axillary dissection:	SN biopsy: axillary dissection if SN BX+
	Adjuvant RT	Selective: Yes—any margin, grade III. No—1-cm margin.
	Adjuvant chemotherapy:	Selection Based on SN Bx and primary tumor prognostic features

*Includes DCIS with microinvasion (≤1 mm invasive focus)

---

tissue or in the inframammary fold. In these cases, the tissue can be mobilized so that a vertical incision is avoided. In all cases the nipple areolar complex must be included in the incision. An alternative to mobilizing large flaps is to proceed directly with a transverse incision including the nipple areolar complex and leave the biopsy incision in situ. Because relatively thin flaps are obtained, there is little danger of local recurrence in this area.

To relax the pectoral muscles, I prefer to elevate the arm on a crossbar (see Fig. 53-4, *A*). It is secured with an Ace bandage and, after axillary dissection, is placed at the patient's side to complete the skin closure.

After the marking of the incision and the positioning of the arm, the chest, the upper arm, and the upper portion of the abdomen are carefully prepared, and the area is draped.

The incision is made, and the skin flaps are developed. This is accomplished by placing small Allis clamps in the subcutaneous tissue, not in the skin, and elevating these under slight tension as the flaps are developed by sharp dissection (see Fig. 53-4, *B*). Bleeding is controlled on the skin side with fine absorbable ligatures and on the breast side with the actual cautery (see Fig. 53-4, *C*). The dissection is carried to the chest wall superiorly, inferiorly, and medially (see Fig. 53-4, *D* and *E*). The breast is removed by sharp dissection from the sternum toward the latissimus dorsi muscle. As this is being accomplished, the perforating vessels appear. These are clamped and suture ligated with 3-0 chromic catgut or similar suture material (see Fig. 53-4, *F*). These vessels should be very carefully ligated because, if they retract, it is almost impossible to secure adequate hemostasis.

Table 53-2 Treatment Guidelines—cont'd

Management of Invasive Ductal Carcinoma (IDC)—cont'd

NB: For any patient with poor nuclear grade *and* LVI, or other poor prognostic features: consider systemic therapy.

T1c >10-≤20 mm	*Primary cancer:*	Excision or reexcision to negative (if extensive intraductal component positive) or only focally positive margin *or* mastectomy with axillary dissection
	Axillary dissection:	SN biopsy = axillary dissection if SN BX+
	Adjuvant RT:	Yes, if breast conservation: possible exception if low-grade, small size, mgm detection, and 1-cm margin
	Adjuvant chemotherapy:	Yes, generally; exception if primary tumor small, low-grade, SN BX− and prognostic features favorable
T2 >20-≤50 mm	*Primary cancer:*	Excision to negative or focally positive margin *or* mastectomy
	Axillary dissection:	If mastectomy, axillary dissection
		If breast conservation: SN biopsy; axillary dissection if SN BX+
	Adjuvant RT:	Yes, if breast conservation
	Adjuvant chemotherapy:	Yes
	Emphasize induction chemotherapy for all cancers ≥3 cm	
	If complete response (CR) or partial response (PR):	Excision and RT
	If no response (NR):	Consider mastectomy and axillary dissection; may elect breast conservation with radiation

NB: Axillary dissection if SN Bx positive for macrometastases.

T3 >50 mm	*Primary cancer:*	Induction chemotherapy
		Then if CR or PR: either mastectomy or excision plus radiation
		If NR: mastectomy
	Axillary dissection:	Induction chemotherapy
		Then CR or PR: either radiation or dissection
		NR: axillary dissection
	Adjuvant RT:	Yes, including chest wall and nodes after mastectomy
	Adjuvant chemotherapy:	Induction chemotherapy
N1, 2, or 3 (any T, N1, 2, 3, Mo) (clinically palpable and proved by positive fine needle aspiration)	*Primary cancer:*	Induction chemotherapy
		Then if CR or PR: either mastectomy or excision plus radiation
		If NR: mastectomy
	Axillary dissection:	Induction chemotherapy
		Then if CR or PR: radiotherapy or dissection
		If NR: axillary dissection
	Adjuvant RT:	Yes, including chest wall if mastectomy and lymph nodes
	Adjuvant chemotherapy:	Induction chemotherapy

Diffuse Invasive Lobular Carcinoma and Special Favorable Subtypes (i.e., Colloid, Medullary, Papillary, Tubular)

Features specified: Method of detection, size, grade, type of lobular carcinoma (i.e., diffuse or not) node status, prognostic indicators

Strategy based on method of detection, size, and features of primary cancer

Management scheme as for invasive ductal cancer generally, but with individual consideration

---

The dissection is carried to the latissimus dorsi muscle laterally, being careful not to proceed beneath the muscle. Bleeding points are clamped and ligated with fine chromic catgut. As this dissection proceeds, the lateral edge of the pectoralis major muscle is identified. The fascia of the muscle has been removed with the specimen, and, with dissection toward the axilla, the pectoralis minor muscle also comes into view (see Fig. 53-4, *F* and *G*).

At this point, the breast is wrapped in a moist towel and attention is turned to the axilla. The costocoracoid fascia is now visible and is incised with Metzenbaum scissors. The axillary fat is distinct from the adipose tissue noted during the breast dissection. It has a much lighter color and is obvious when one has entered the axilla. A small right-angle retractor is placed beneath the pectoralis major muscle. The axillary vein is identified, and the tissue immediately beneath and inferior to the vein is removed by sharp dissection (see Fig. 53-4, *H*). The intercostal brachial nerves may be sacrificed; however, if possible, at least some of the branches are spared to avoid lack of sensation on the medial surface of the upper arm. As the dissection proceeds, the thoracodorsal vessels and nerve become apparent at the floor of the axilla, and often the long thoracic nerve is visible along the chest wall, although, with the modified radical mastectomy, this is not always apparent (see Fig. 53-4, *I* and *J*). Bleeding in the axilla is controlled by using right-angle clamps and fine silk ligatures. As the dissection proceeds, an attempt should be made to remove at least some of the interpectoral (Rotter's) nodes. With the modified radical mastectomy, level 1 and 2 nodes can be removed, but, by definition, level 3 nodes are not routinely removed.

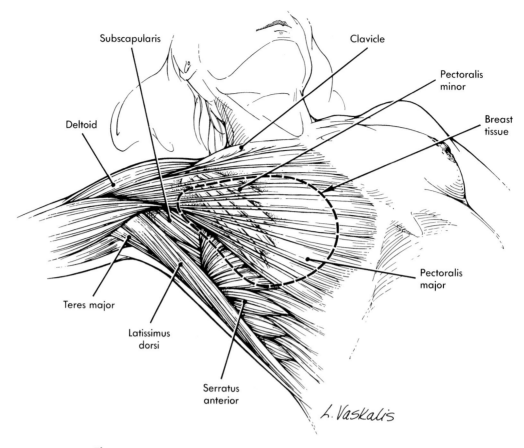

Subscapularis

Clavicle

Deltoid

Pectoralis minor

Breast tissue

Pectoralis major

Teres major

Latissimus dorsi

Serratus anterior

L. Vaskalis

Fig. 53-1 Anatomy and musculature of the chest wall and axilla.

With proper exposure and sharp dissection, a minimum of 12 to 15 axillary nodes will be recovered. The number of nodes actually removed depends on the thoroughness of the surgeon and the diligence of the pathologist at the surgical desk. Repeated recovery of but one to two nodes suggests either that the surgeon is not performing a true modified radical mastectomy or that the pathologist is careless in locating the lymph nodes in the specimen.

Because of the extensive elevation of the flaps, suction drainage is required (see Fig. 53-4, K); although, for some very thin patients, I have simply closed the incision and wrapped the patient in a pressure dressing using a 6-inch Ace bandage. If suction drainage is used, care must be taken in the placement of the drains. Some patients require external radiation therapy, and, if the exit incision is beyond the projected field of radiation, these patients may require extension of the radiation field to avoid local recurrence. The suction catheters are secured with a pursestring suture of silk (see Fig. 53-4, L).

The wound is inspected for bleeding. The axilla is irrigated with normal saline, and additional bleeding points are ligated. The bleeding points on the muscle may be cauterized with the actual cautery, and those in the subcutaneous tissue are ligated with fine absorbable suture material. When the wound is dry, the arm is brought to the patient's side and any redundant skin is excised.

The closure, in my opinion, is best achieved with a few sutures of absorbable catgut in the subcutaneous tissues to "line up" the skin edges. The skin is closed with vertical mattress sutures of fine nylon, although some surgeons prefer to use staples. I think a more cosmetic closure can be achieved with interrupted sutures, but this is a matter of personal preference (see Fig. 53-4, L).

A simple dressing is applied (see Fig. 53-4, M). No pressure dressing is required, and the hemovacs are secured with additional tape across the abdomen to prevent their inadvertent removal. The usual operating time is 2 to 3 hours. The blood loss depends, to some extent, on the size of the breast and the age of the patient. In older patients with very fatty breasts, there often is very little bleeding; however, in younger patients, the breast is definitely a functional organ and well supplied with vessels that require time-consuming hemostasis.

Most patients can be mobilized soon after the surgical procedure, and usually there is little discomfort, which can be controlled with analgesics. The suction drainage should be recorded, and the drains, in my opinion, should not be removed until the drainage is less than 10 to 15 ml/24 hours through each catheter. Premature removal invites seroma formation and the necessity for repeated aspiration. Orders should be written to have the patient seen by a physiotherapist so that arm and chest wall exercises can be established early in the postoperative period. *Text continued on p. 979*

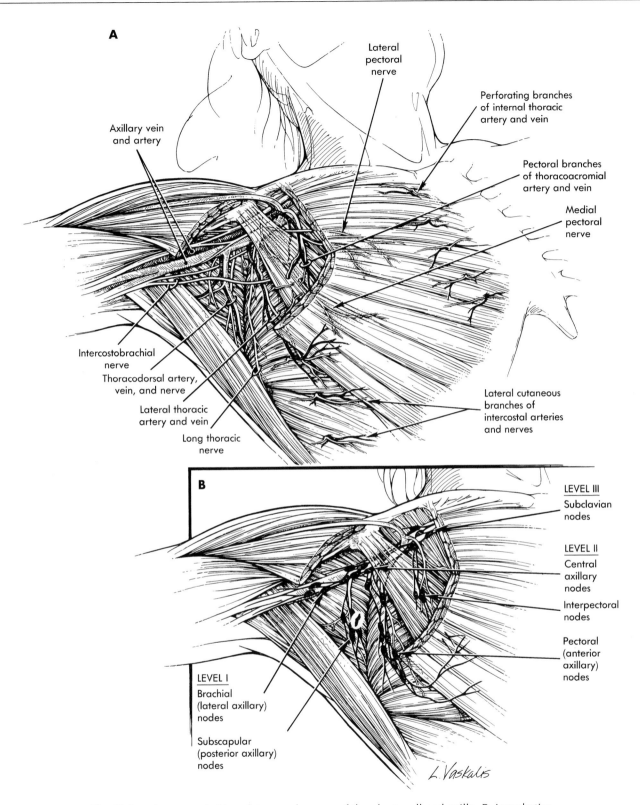

A

Lateral
pectoral
nerve

Perforating branches
of internal thoracic
artery and vein

Axillary vein
and artery

Pectoral branches
of thoracoacromial
artery and vein

Medial
pectoral
nerve

Intercostobrachial
nerve

Thoracodorsal artery,
vein, and nerve

Lateral thoracic
artery and vein

Long thoracic
nerve

Lateral cutaneous
branches of
intercostal arteries
and nerves

B

LEVEL III
Subclavian
nodes

LEVEL II
Central
axillary
nodes

Interpectoral
nodes

Pectoral
(anterior
axillary)
nodes

LEVEL I
Brachial
(lateral axillary)
nodes

Subscapular
(posterior axillary)
nodes

L. Vaskalis

Fig. 53-2   Anatomy. **A,** Vasculature and nerves of the chest wall and axilla. **B,** Lymphatics.
Level I, II, and III lymph nodes.

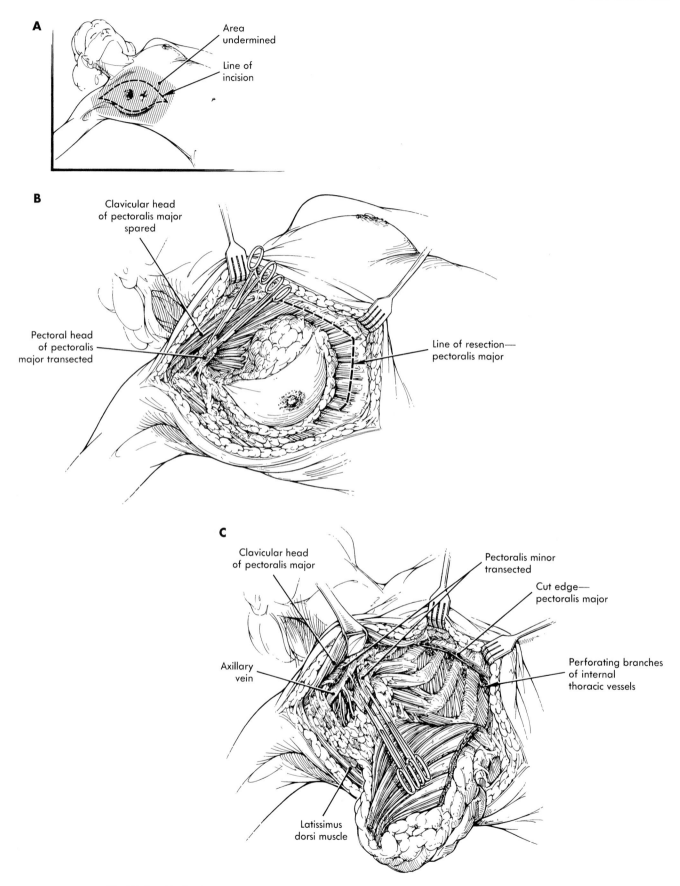

Fig. 53-3 Radical mastectomy. **A,** Line of the incision and area to be included in the dissection. **B,** Extent of muscular resection, pectoralis major and minor. **C,** Pectoralis major and minor resected. Exposure of axillary contents and anterior chest wall.

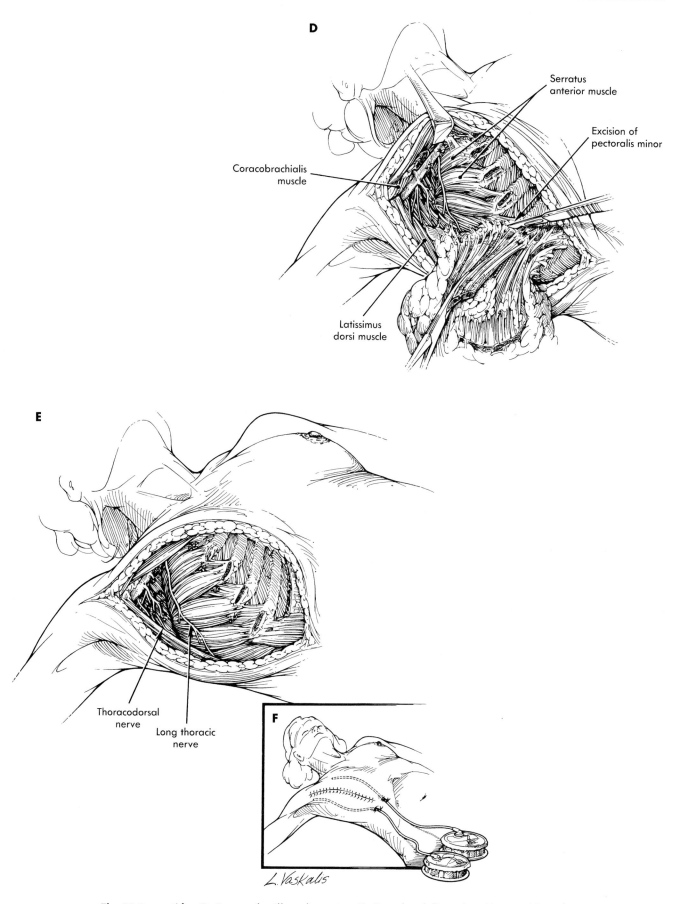

D

Serratus
anterior muscle

Excision of
pectoralis minor

Coracobrachialis
muscle

Latissimus
dorsi muscle

E

Thoracodorsal
nerve

Long thoracic
nerve

F

L. Vaskalis

Fig. 53-3, cont'd   **D,** Extent of axillary dissection. **E,** Completed dissection. Note position of the thoracodorsal and long thoracic nerves. **F,** Closure with suction drainage.

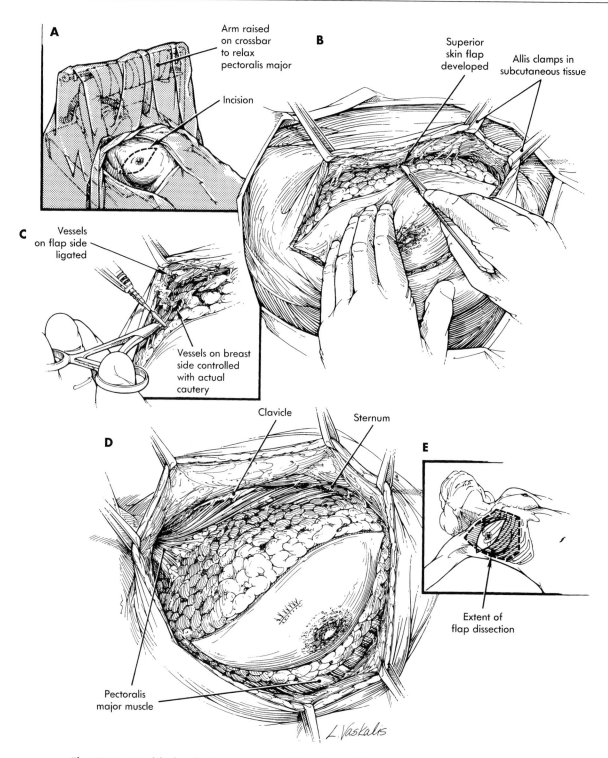

Fig. 53-4 Modified radical mastectomy. **A,** Position of the patient and extent of incision. Note the position of the arm to relax pectoralis major muscle. **B,** Development of the skin flap. The Allis clamps are on subcutaneous tissue, not skin. **C,** Control of bleeding. Vessels on the flap are ligated; vessels on the specimen are cauterized. **D,** Beginning removal of the breast. **E,** Extend of dissection.

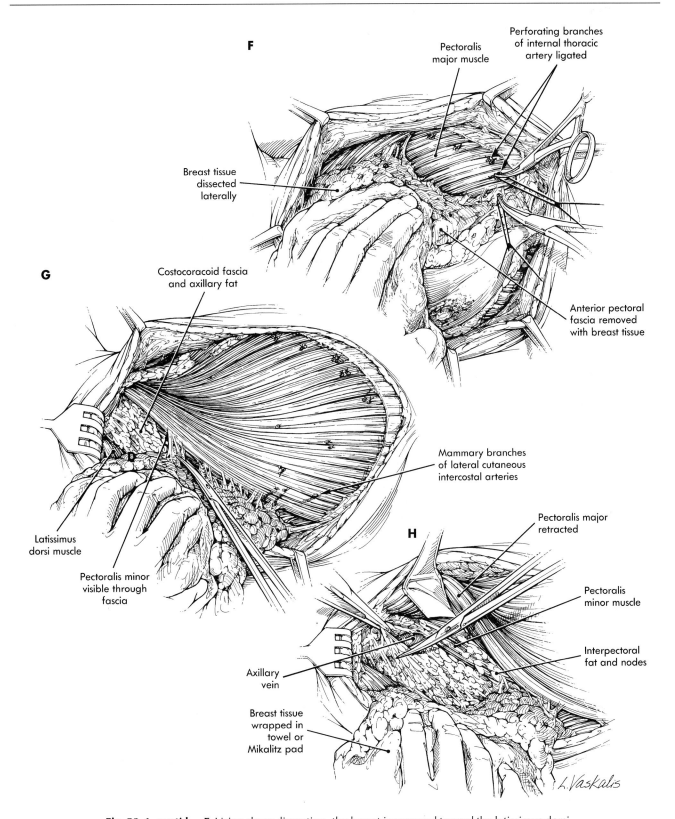

F

Pectoralis major muscle

Perforating branches of internal thoracic artery ligated

Breast tissue dissected laterally

Anterior pectoral fascia removed with breast tissue

G

Costocoracoid fascia and axillary fat

Mammary branches of lateral cutaneous intercostal arteries

Latissimus dorsi muscle

Pectoralis minor visible through fascia

H

Pectoralis major retracted

Pectoralis minor muscle

Interpectoral fat and nodes

Axillary vein

Breast tissue wrapped in towel or Mikalitz pad

L. Vaskalis

Fig. 53-4, cont'd   F, Using sharp dissection, the breast is removed toward the latissimus dorsi muscle. The perforating vessels are ligated. **G,** The costocoracoid fascia is exposed. **H,** The pectoralis major is muscle retracted medially, and axillary dissection begins.

Continued

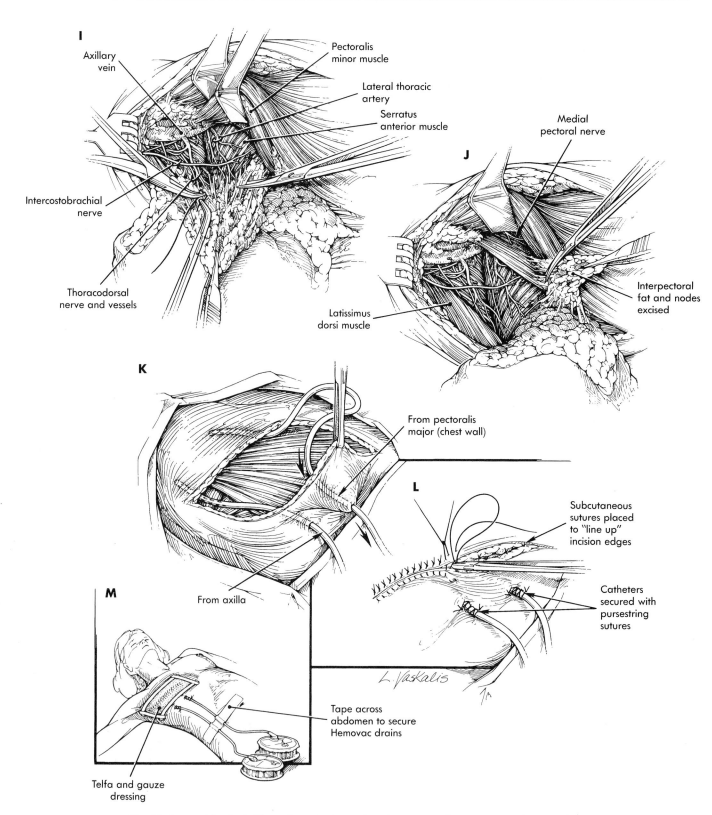

Fig. 53-4, cont'd   **I,** Axillary dissection completed. Note similarity to radical mastectomy. **J,** The pectoralis minor is exposed and interpectorial nodes are excised. **K,** Suction drainage is placed on the axilla and over the pectoral muscles. **L,** Skin closure with vertical mattress sutures of 4-0 nylon (staple closure optional). Note that drains are secured by pursestring sutures. **M,** Completed closure and small dressing applied to cover incision. Note that suction drainage is secured with tape.

The length of hospital stay varies with the surgeon and the requirements of the patient; it is usually no more than 4 or 5 days. Some surgeons send patients home with their drains. This may or may not be appropriate depending on the home situation.

Total (Simple) Mastectomy

Total mastectomy is performed the same as described for the modified radical mastectomy. It differs in that the axillary dissection is omitted, although level 1 nodes often are removed. The entire breast, including the nipple areolar complex and the fascia of the pectoralis major muscle, is removed (Fig. 53-5, *A* and *B*).

There are a number of indications for this procedure.

1. Patients with extensive ductal carcinoma in situ (DCIS) or lobular carcinoma in situ (LCIS)
2. Patients with recurrence after partial mastectomy or wide local excision with axillary dissection followed by radiation (i.e., conservative treatment)
3. Patients with bulky or ulcerated lesions or those with distant metastases when local control will improve quality of life
4. Elderly patients or those who are a poor operative risk and in whom there is no palpable axillary adenopathy and no evidence of distant disease
5. Selected patients in whom prophylactic removal of the opposite breast is recommended

Local recurrence after modified or simple mastectomy is unusual, occurring in fewer than 10% of cases. Lymphedema, which may occur in 30% of patients with the radical mastectomy, is unusual with the modified procedure.

Variations in surgical technique and length of hospital stay are the rule rather than the exception depending on the type of third-party reimbursement and the home situation of the patient. Some surgeons recommend prophylactic antibiotics and anticoagulation, but I have not used this in my own practice. One surgeon of my acquaintance has suggested that the modified mastectomy can be performed on a "day surgery" basis and has actually discharged patients immediately after the operation. My conversations with some of these patients indicate less than total satisfaction with this arrangement.

Subcutaneous (Prophylactic) Mastectomy

Total mastectomy is the operation of choice. It is the only operation that completely removes all of the breast tissue. Subcutaneous mastectomy is inadequate. Even with the most carefully performed subcutaneous procedure, breast tissue remains under the areola and is found in other locations in 80% of cases. Thus it is not a prophylactic procedure; however, there are no studies indicating whether removal of 80% of the breast tissue would yield an equivalent reduction in risk. In addition, the subcutaneous mastectomy may result in a less than satisfactory cosmetic result. A number of complications are associated with this operation including hematoma and subsequent scarring and fibrosis.

Breast Preservation (Conservative) Procedures

A number of consensus development conferences have dealt with the treatment of primary breast cancer in an effort to determine treatment recommendations that provide the best chance for disease-free survival. These conferences have dealt with the question whether conservative treatment including dissection of the axillary lymph nodes followed by irradiation to the breast is as effective as the modified mastectomy.

Although the concept of conservative treatment has gained favor, there has been continued controversy concerning the technical details of the surgery and the radiation therapy.

The use of breast conservation procedures involves four important criteria:

1. Patient selection
2. Surgery of the primary tumor
3. Surgery of the axilla
4. Radiotherapy to the retained breast

The principal advantage of conservative treatment is cosmetic. There are no data to indicate that the conservative approach provides improved survival compared to the radical procedure. Thus, the surgeon must select patients for whom an adequate resection results in an acceptable cosmesis. Patients who are poor candidates include those with widely separated tumors in the same breast, patients whose mammograms reveal diffuse disease in many quadrants, and patients with large tumors in relatively small breasts. Patients with central lesions involving the nipple areolar complex can be treated by resection of the nipple with careful attention to the final cosmetic result. Reconstruction of the nipple has been accomplished after radiation therapy. Advanced age is not a contraindication. Patients in their middle seventies often request conservative treatment for cosmetic reasons, and younger patients may request not only total mastectomy but prophylactic mastectomy "to avoid concern about recurrence of cancer in the treated breast and the development of new cancer in the opposite breast."

Adequate surgical resection implies grossly clear margins. The surgeon marks the specimen for orientation by the pathologist. The pathologist then "inks" the margins to assist in the examination of the permanent sections. The tissue is submitted for estrogen and progesterone receptor analysis without disturbing the resected margins.

I consider the margins positive if there is microscopic involvement within 2 mm of the margin. A 5-mm margin is adequate and does not require additional boost radiation therapy or reexcision.

A cosmetic incision is important. These incisions are marked with the patient in the sitting or the standing position. Often, a fold can be noted in the axilla and used for the axillary incision. Cosmetic skin lines in the breast are best observed in the sitting or the standing positions, and these should be marked immediately before the operative procedure (Fig. 53-6, *A*).

If no axillary dissection is contemplated, wide local excision can be performed under local anesthesia. However, in

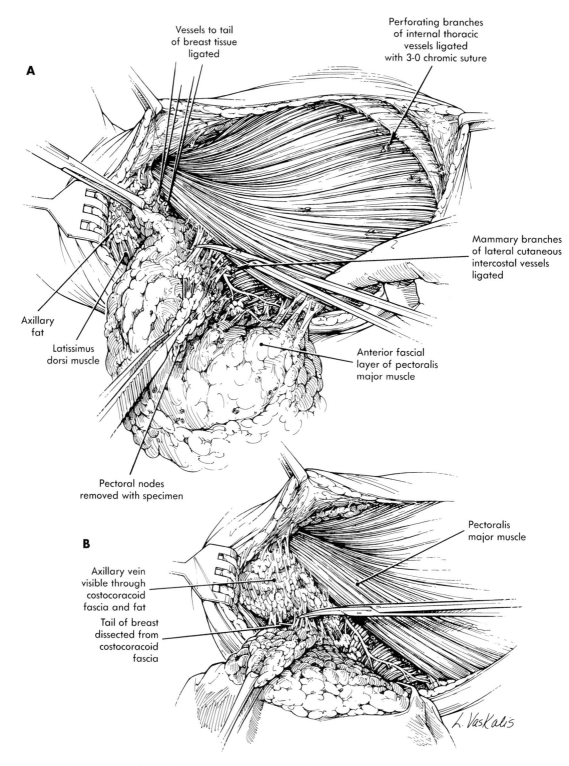

Vessels to tail
of breast tissue
ligated

Perforating branches
of internal thoracic
vessels ligated
with 3-0 chromic suture

Mammary branches
of lateral cutaneous
intercostal vessels
ligated

Anterior fascial
layer of pectoralis
major muscle

Axillary
fat

Latissimus
dorsi muscle

Pectoral nodes
removed with specimen

Pectoralis
major muscle

Axillary vein
visible through
costocoracoid
fascia and fat

Tail of breast
dissected from
costocoracoid
fascia

L. Vaskalis

Fig. 53-5   Total (simple) mastectomy. **A,** Extent of dissection. The costocoracoid fascia is not excised. **B,** The breast is removed, including the fascia and pectoralis major muscle. Exposure of axillary contents and lateral chest wall.

most cases, this is combined with an axillary dissection, and general anesthesia is required. Again, these patients fall under the category of "admit after" and must be carefully evaluated on outpatient basis before the surgical procedure.

Once the incisions have been marked, the patient is taken to the operating room suite and endotracheal anesthesia is

administered. Again, the arm is placed on a crossbar to relax the pectoralis muscles and facilitate exposure (see Fig. 53-6, *B*). The breast, upper arm, and upper abdomen are carefully prepared and draped as for the modified mastectomy. I usually perform the axillary dissection first, and the breast is covered with a drape. The previously marked incision is

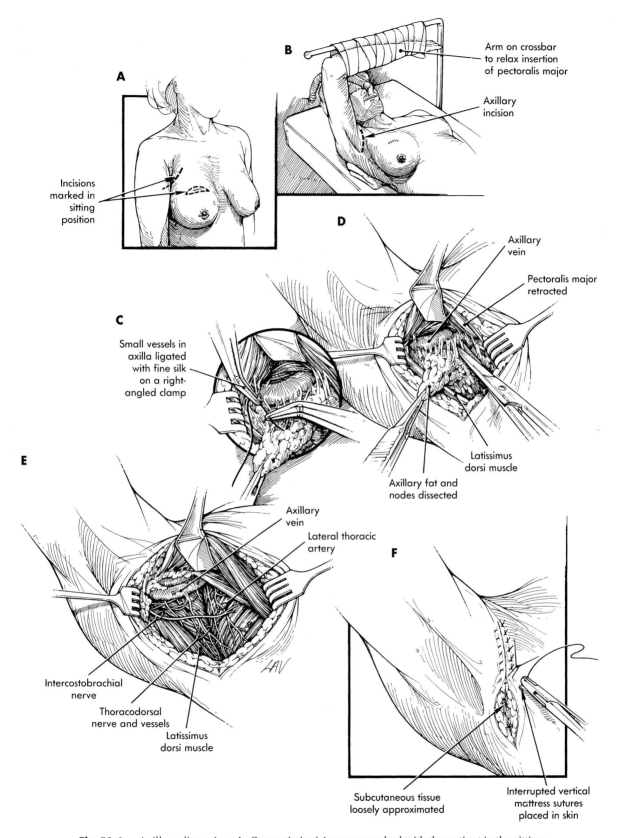

Fig. 53-6   Axillary dissection. **A,** Cosmetic incisions are marked with the patient in the sitting position. Note that the axillary incision can be placed in the "skin fold." **B,** Position of the patient before draping. Note that the arm is elevated on a crossbar to relax the pectoralis major muscle. **C,** The costocoracoid fascia is entered, and dissection is begun. **D,** the axillary vein and tributaries are exposed. Vessels are ligated with 3-0 silk (hemoclips optional). **E,** Axillary dissection is completed. Note similarity to modified radical mastectomy dissection. **F,** Skin closure with 4-0 or 5-0 nylon. No drain is used.

used, and bleeding is controlled with ligatures of fine absorbable catgut. The dissection is carried to the pectoralis major muscle, which is easily identified in the superior portion of the incision (see Fig. 53-6, *C* and *D*). It is not necessary to carry the incision beyond the muscle toward the midline. The costocoracoid fascia is identified as in the modified radical procedure and incised with Metzenbaum scissors. The axillary dissection is exactly the same as that performed with the modified radical mastectomy. The pectoral muscles are retracted by the assistant, and the tissue below the axillary vein, lateral to the pectoralis muscle and medial to the latissimus dorsi muscle, is removed (see Fig. 53-6, *E*). Bleeding is controlled with ligatures of fine silk. The same number of nodes should be recovered in this procedure as in the modified radical mastectomy. The elevation of the arm on a crossbar facilitates relaxation of the muscle and provides improved exposure for the axillary dissection. Once the dissection has been completed, the axilla is irrigated and inspected for hemostasis. If the wound is dry, I do not use any type of drainage. The subcutaneous tissue is simply closed with fine absorbable catgut, and the skin is closed with vertical mattress sutures of 4-0 or 5-0 nylon (see Fig. 53-6, *F*). A temporary pressure dressing is placed over the incision, and the arm is brought to the patient's side.

New instruments, drapes, and gloves are used, and the wide local excision is performed. It is helpful to have the original mammogram in the operating room because many of these cases represent an occult lesion. The wide local excision may be a "reexcision." It is important to know exactly where the original lesion was located so that grossly clear margins can be obtained. The previous incision is removed, and flaps are developed very similar to the modified radical mastectomy (Fig. 53-7, *A* and *B*). The subcutaneous tissues are grasped with the Allis clamp, and, using sharp dissection, superior and inferior flaps are developed on either side of the previous incision (see Fig. 53-7, *C*). With the mammogram as a guide, the dissection is carried to the chest wall, and all indurated tissue is removed (see Fig. 53-7, *D* and *E*). Bleeding is controlled with ligatures of fine absorbable catgut or the actual cautery. It is best to proceed quickly with the removal of the specimen so the anatomy is not distorted by repeated attempts to ligate vessels and reposition the retractors. Once the specimen has been removed, hemostasis can be achieved either with the actual cautery or ligatures of absorbable catgut.

The specimen is carefully marked usually before removal at least for the medial and inferior margins. I prefer to do this with a variety of sutures, for example, silk sutures for the medial margin, chromic catgut sutures for the inferior margin, and plain catgut for the deep margin (see Fig. 53-7, *F*). It is absolutely essential that some type of marking system be used and recorded on the pathology requisition. In most cases the specimens are sent in a fresh condition to the pathologist. This provides additional material for estrogen and progesterone receptor analysis.

Once hemostasis has been achieved, no attempt should be made to obliterate completely the dead space in the central portion of the excision. The subcutaneous tissues are closed with fine absorbable catgut, and the skin is closed with vertical mattress sutures of 4-0 or 5-0 nylon. A few milliliters of 0.5% Marcaine without adrenaline are injected into the incision (see Fig. 53-7, *G*). Before tying the last suture, I usually insert the suction to remove any fresh blooding, and then a pressure dressing is immediately applied (see Fig. 53-7, *H*). I do not use suction drainage, which inevitably results in retraction of the skin and a less than perfect cosmetic result. With the use of a pressure dressing, the breast is "molded" into its normal configuration. When the dressing is applied, compression of the axillary incision should be avoided (see Fig. 53-7, *I*).

Most of these patients can be discharged within 24 to 48 hours. I leave the pressure dressing on for a full 48 hours. When it is removed, there is seldom any ecchymosis and a relatively normal contour of the breast is achieved. Occasionally, there is some minor ecchymosis in the region of the axillary dissection as a result of the pressure dressing. Before discharge, the patient should be instructed in arm and chest exercises. This is important because of the fibrosis that may be associated with the subsequent radiation therapy.

These patients are treated over a 4- or 5-week period by the department of radiotherapy, receiving 180 to 200 cGy/day for a total of 45 to 50 Gy. Doses in excess of 50 Gy result in fibrosis and retraction and an unacceptable cosmetic result. This is particularly true for patients who require "boost" therapy. If possible, I prefer to reexcise the area to avoid this cosmetic complication. There is controversy concerning the technique for supplemental radiation. It can be delivered by insertion of radioactive nucleotides or by an electron beam. Whichever technique is used, it should not diminish the cosmetic result.

There are advantages and disadvantages associated with the conservative and radical approaches. In terms of the surgical procedure performed, wide local excision and axillary dissection require as much time as the modified mastectomy and, in my opinion, is a more difficult operation if a satisfactory cosmetic result is achieved. Obviously, the main advantage of the conservative approach is the preservation of the breast. However, the price to be paid is the extended radiation treatments and the real concern of some patients that future symptomatology in the retained breast may be associated with recurrent tumor. In the more radical approach, the treatment is accomplished in a few days and, obviously, the cancer cannot recur in the removed breast.

CONTEMPORARY ISSUES
The Timing of Surgery

The timing of surgery is an intriguing concept but upon reflection is a logistical nightmare. Most surgeons find it difficult to satisfy the request of the patient regarding the date for surgery. This combined with the surgeon's available operating time and the inevitable conflicts with a prospective tumor board often provides for the office staff an impossible challenge.

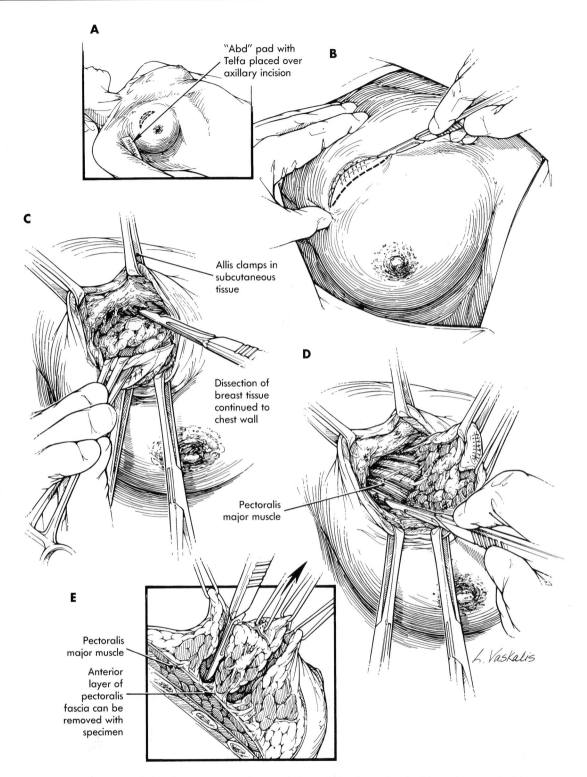

Fig. 53-7 Wide local excision. **A,** The arm is brought to the patient's side and covered with a temporary pressure dressing. **B,** Incision is made, removing a small amount of skin, including the previous incision. **C,** Skin flaps are developed by sharp dissection. **D,** Dissection continues to anterior chest wall. **E,** Sagittal view showing extent of dissection. *Continued*

It was noted in 1987 that the timing of breast resection within the fertility cycle affected the metastatic potential of mouse breast cancer,[57] and in 1989 Hrushesky et al.[37] reported a fourfold increase in the risk of recurrence and death from breast cancer for women who underwent resec-

tion during the perimenstrual period (days 0 to 6 and 21 to 36 of the menstrual cycle), compared with those who had surgery during the preovulatory period (days 7 to 20). Other studies have failed to confirm this finding; however, there is some biological plausibility to the "timing" hypoth-

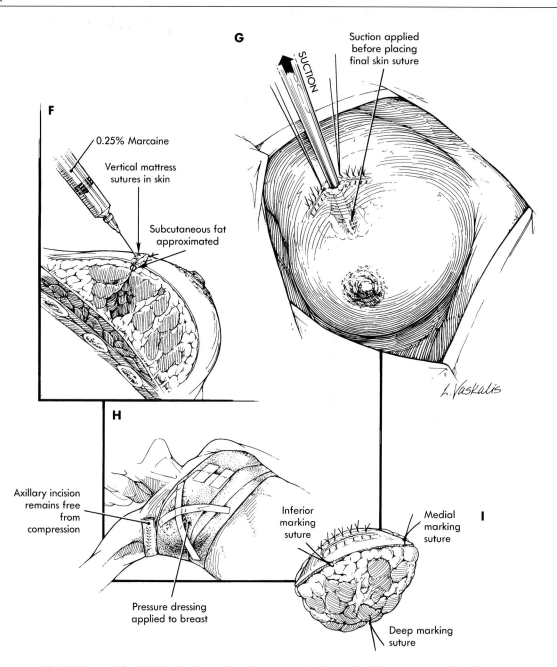

Fig. 53-7, cont'd **F,** The final specimen is appropriately marked for orientation by the pathologist. **G,** 0.25% Marcaine is injected. No attempt is made to obliterate the cavity. Only subcutaneous fat is approximated. **H,** The wound is partially closed with vertical mattress sutures of fine nylon. One suture is left "long" to permit suction before closure is completed. **I,** A pressure dressing with "fluffs" and a 6-inch Ace bandage are applied. Depending on the location of the axillary incision, this may or may not be included in the dressing.

esis. It has been noted that the mitotic activity of breast tissue peaks during the luteal phase with the presence of progesterone.[9] It has been speculated, however, that the heightened proliferation may be more than offset by a higher rate of programmed cell death (apoptosis), which may inhibit metastases.[62] A number of other plausible mechanisms, including decreased cell-to-cell adhesion as a result of unopposed estrogen during the follicular phase,[62] with high levels of follicle-stimulating hormone (FSH), which peak just before ovulation, and estradiol, producing insulin-like

growth factors that may promote metastases, have been suggested.[5]

Two large prospective trials to test these hypotheses are planned, one in Europe and one in the United States.[5] Many investigators have suggested defining the menstrual cycle through some agreed-on level of serum progesterone. This in turn might define the optimal hormonal environment that could be created pharmacologically, thus avoiding the logistical difficulties of attempting to plan surgery to coincide with a "favorable" point in a woman's cycle.[5]

Technical Issues

For patients who have chosen breast-conservation treatment, evaluation of the excised tissue may reveal close margins or minimally involved margins, necessitating either reexcision or boost therapy. Not all radiotherapists agree that the latter is appropriate, preferring instead to recommend reexcision or in some cases mastectomy. The skin incision and surgical induration are not reliable landmarks for boost field localization. Several studies have recommended the use of surgical clips to determine the placement and volume of interstitial boosts or tangential fields.[10]

The clips should be placed in the deepest portion of the excision cavity and each of the four cavity walls. At the Breast Health Center we routinely use clips to mark the excision cavity. There are few, if any, contraindications to this technique. The clips have not been demonstrated to migrate.[18] They do not interfere with subsequent mammography and may actually aid in the interpretation of the post-treatment films.[10]

Some surgeons prefer to use the cautery for dissection and to control blood loss. There is no question that the procedure can be performed more quickly using the cautery. However, when a cosmetic excision must be achieved and the resected margins evaluated for tumor involvement, the tissue artifacts associated with the cautery may preclude accurate margin assessment and uncertainty concerning the extent of local treatment. Recently, the CO_2 laser has been used in some surgical procedures, including mastectomy. Reports have indicated less bleeding, less pain, and earlier discharge in these patients.[4] However, there is little available information concerning tissue changes that may interfere with margin assessment and subsequent recommendations for local treatment.

Current Status of Axillary Node Dissection in Primary Breast Cancer: A Continuing Debate

The fiscal imperatives of managed care are nowhere more apparent than in the evolution of local treatment of primary breast cancer—less is better. "If the results of the test don't change what you do, don't do the test."[14] I have moved from the extended radical mastectomy of Urban to local removal of the tumor (wide local excision) with or without radiation therapy and with or without axillary dissection. The principal reasons for lymph node dissection in primary breast cancer are to prove the presence of nodal metastases, to fulfill nodal criteria in TNM staging, and to provide prognostic information to enable decisions regarding the use of adjuvant systemic therapy.

Chemotherapy and adjuvant hormonal therapy (tamoxifen) have been shown to proportionally reduce the risk of recurrence when they are administered after surgery and before (or after) radiation therapy.[70] The reduction is approximately 33% with standard chemotherapy (CMF [cyclophosphamide, methotrexate, and fluorouracil]) and 20% to 25% with tamoxifen. However, reduction in recurrence is proportional to risk and therefore is far less in patients with a good prognosis (stage T1a and T1b and low risk of recur-

rence) than in those at high risk. For example, a 33% reduction in a patient receiving adjuvant chemotherapy with a 9% risk of recurrence, lowers her risk of breast cancer recurrence to 6%. The 3% absolute gain from 9% to 6% indicates that 97% of such patients gained no benefit while subjected to the same risk of toxicity. Similarly, the use of tamoxifen with a 20% proportional risk means that a patient with a 10% risk of recurrence gains only 2% absolute benefit—with 98% of such patients receiving no benefit. It is apparent that the most logical use of adjuvant systemic therapy is in patients with a poor prognosis.

There is considerable debate about the risk of axillary node involvement in patients with "early" invasive breast cancer. Some argue that the risk is substantial even for patients with small tumors, and level I or II axillary dissection is recommended. Others note that in T1a (5 mm or smaller) invasive breast cancer, the rate of positive lymph nodes on routine histologic processing is 4% or less.[64] Even in patients with T1a and T1b invasive cancers detected by mammography without high nuclear grade or lymph vessel invasion, 35% will have an axillary node metastasis rate of only 3%. Therefore, defining this larger group of patients who have such a low rate of axillary metastasis as candidates for axillary dissection may not be justified.[8]

A number of studies have attempted to predict axillary node status by using prognostic indicators—tumor size, quantitative estrogen and progesterone receptor levels, flow cytometry, ploidy, and S-phase fraction. Other studies have included lymph vascular invasion (LVI). This information can refine estimates of whether a patient is likely to have nodes positive; however, no subsets can be identified as having a greater than 95% chance of being node negative or positive.[58] In other words, predictive models cannot alleviate the necessity of axillary dissection for staging of breast cancer in patients for whom *nodal status would affect therapeutic decisions.*[58]

To summarize the possibilities from the data currently available: there is no evidence that detecting the exact number of axillary lymph node metastasis is useful as a method of selecting distinctive adjuvant chemotherapy combinations, except in the context of clinical trials. Even if axillary lymph nodes remain the most important prognostic indicator, it may be that all that is required is to know whether the regional nodes are positive or negative to recommend appropriate adjuvant therapy. An exception might be the as yet undetermined prognostic implications of micrometastases.

Thus, approximately 30% of patients have an incidence of lymph node metastasis—so low that doing an axillary dissection cannot be justified (i.e., T1a stage, 3% to 4%). Forty percent of patients have primary tumors with features that suggest the use of adjuvant therapy such as high-grade tumors, LVI, etc., regardless of the lymph node status and, therefore, do not need an axillary dissection. In only 25% to 30% of patients do the results of the lymph node dissection alter the adjuvant treatment decision.

Concurrent with this debate, a new technique, the sentinel lymph node concept, promoted for melanoma has been suggested for breast cancer. This technique samples the physiologically defined "sentinel" node, which is the portal of entry to the remaining axillary lymph nodes and reliably differentiates between patients with lymph node positive and negative for disease.[31,39] This technique of sentinel node biopsy carries a false-negative rate of only 2% in reports summarizing recent experience.[31,39] One of the prerequisites for the successful completion of this procedure is the accurate identification of the sentinel lymph node. The node has traditionally been identified by injecting blue die into the dermis adjacent to the recently biopsied breast cancer.[50] To improve intraoperative identification of the sentinel node, a second method has recently been introduced. This method requires the injection of a radiocolloid that is absorbed into neighboring lymphatics and transplanted to the sentinel node where it can be intraoperatively detected by a sterile gamma probe.[12,45,76] This technique requires some experience and care in its application; however, the advantage is that it can be performed under local anesthesia, thus obviating the expense of general anesthesia and the morbidity of a formal axillary dissection. At the Breast Health Center we have performed sentinel node biopsy according to a strict protocol and a tutorial is offered to surgeons who wish to learn the technique. Credentialing and quality control are essential. This is a multidisciplinary procedure that requires quality control in nuclear medicine, surgery, and pathology.

As screening mammography increases in American women between the ages of 40 and 75, the median diameter of the primary tumor will decrease perhaps to less than 1 cm. This will set the stage for outpatient management of the majority of breast cancer patients. Three groups of patients will be defined:

1. Those with such a low risk of lymph node metastases based on primary tumor characteristics that no axillary nodes need to be sampled—DCIS, T1a, and T1b with special features.
2. Patients at such high risk of lymph node metastases and poor prognosis by analysis of primary tumor features that axillary sampling is not required because adjuvant systemic therapy will be given even in the presence of negative axillary nodes.
3. Those for whom axillary node information will be needed to complete the prognostic analysis. For these patients a sentinel node biopsy should be the initial procedure.

If the exact lymph node status is required, patients with micrometastatic disease in sentinel nodes might then require formal axillary dissection if the exact number of positive lymph nodes is important.

Finally, are there any other methods to assess axillary lymph node involvement? The use of positron emission tomography (PET) has allowed highly accurate detection of axillary metastasis in patients with locally advanced disease.[6] However, PET imaging does not provide the spacial resolution necessary to accurately assess the axillary node status in patients with small metastases. If only one lymph node is affected, the sensitivity of PET appears to be about 25%.[6]

Is Radiotherapy Necessary after Breast-Conserving Surgery?

Four randomized trials have convincingly demonstrated the value of radiotherapy in reducing the rate of local recurrence after breast-conserving surgery.[15,24,43,72,74] A number of studies have indicated risk factors associated with local recurrences for conservative surgery and radiotherapy. These include margin involvement, LVI, extensive intraductal component nodal involvement, and tumor size.[16,40,60]

A recently published prospective trial in selected patients with T1 node-negative breast cancer and without known risk factors for local recurrence has concluded that even in highly selected subgroups of patients with invasive breast cancer, the risk of local recurrence after wide local excision alone is substantial.[61] It still remains to be seen whether there is a small subgroup for whom radiation therapy can be safely omitted and in which patients themselves accept the possibility of recurrence and the necessity for salvage mastectomy. Some patients may be willing to take the risk.

There are several additional considerations that require discussion for patients selecting breast-conserving surgery: (1) The effect of reexcision; and (2) local recurrences and distant metastases after conservative breast surgery.

The success of breast-conserving surgery depends upon the removal of all gross disease. The significance of microscopically positive margins is less clear. Multiple studies have shown that the amount of tissue excised is a major determinant of cosmetic outcome. A single-stage lumpectomy with a removal of a conservative amount of breast tissue results in negative margins in the majority of patients. However, the use of excisional biopsy without margin evaluation should be abandoned.[38] A positive margin after single-stage wide local excision does not preclude reexcision and breast conservation.[38]

Local recurrences are a concern in breast-conservation surgery. It is important to distinguish local recurrences associated with increased risk of distant spread from those due to inadequate treatment. Studies have shown that local recurrences and distant metastases are partially independent events.[75] The relationship between local recurrence and distant metastases is complex. The timing of recurrence is different. The prognosis of patients with a local recurrence is approximately 70% survival in 5 years.[75] It is important to identify patients in whom local recurrence indicates a high-grade tumor and for whom aggressive systemic therapy is indicated. If the recurrence occurs during the first *2* years after surgery in young patients (younger than 35 years of age), who had LVI, systemic therapy is indicated in addition to consideration of salvage mastectomy to complete the local treatment.[75] If the local recurrence occurs *more than* 2 years after surgery and in patients with extensive intraductal components or questionable inadequate surgery, the indication for additional chemotherapy is less compelling.[75]

Decision Making for Early-Stage Breast Cancer

What are the factors associated with the decision between mastectomy and breast-conserving surgery? What resources do women use in making this decision? One study has shown that the surgeon's recommendation and the patient's perception of chance for cure were the most influential factors affecting her treatment decision.[66] A survey of these patients suggested that potential areas of intervention to improve the rate of breast-conservation therapy were a prospective tumor board, education of the primary care physician, and greater concern of family members.[66]

Another study showed that variation in the rate of breast-conserving surgery was related to factors other than the age and stage of disease and probably related more to local community factors than physician attitudes.[26] In the United States, there is a marked regional variation in the number of breast cancer patients who have breast-conservation treatment from a low of 5.9% to a high of 20%.[79] It has been shown that when informed of the diagnosis and treatment options in an unhurried, supportive setting and when encouraged to seek further consultations as desired, breast cancer patients tend to make appropriate therapeutic choices.[78]

Follow-Up

Traditional follow-up of breast cancer patients, including our own protocol at the Breast Health Center has included a clinical examination every 3 months for 2 years, every 4 months for 2 years, and every 6 months thereafter. Annual evaluation includes screening mammogram, chest x-ray, complete blood count, and liver function tests, plus carcinoembryonic antigen (CEA) and CA15-3.

Recent studies have recommended a sweeping change in posttreatment evaluation. They are summarized as follows. Follow-up should be individualized to reflect the patient's risk of recurrence. Women with one occurrence of breast cancer are at increased risk for the development of a new contralateral primary tumor. This risk is approximately 1% per year. The role of routine laboratory imaging studies to detect metastatic cancer when it is asymptomatic is controversial. A prospective, randomized trial has demonstrated no survival benefit for routine testing compared to a careful history and physical examination with further studies directed by symptoms. The clinical role of tumor markers such as CEA and CA15-3 is unproven. Patients receiving tamoxifen should have periodic, at least yearly, gynecologic examinations because of the increased risk of endometrial cancer.[48]

Recently under the auspices of American Society of Clinical Oncology (ASCO) and its health services research committee, recommendations have been developed regarding surveillance of breast cancer patients.[3] The goals of follow-up as defined by this panel were early detection of metastases, detection of secondary primary tumors, and informing and supporting the patient. As a result of these discussions, the current ASCO guidelines for breast cancer follow-up are: history and physical examination every 3 to 6 months for the first 3 years, every 6 to 12 months for 2 years, and then annually; monthly breast self-examination; and annual mammogram. Not recommended are routine complete blood count, automated chemistry testing, chest x-ray, bone scan, liver ultrasound, or computed tomography scan of the chest and abdomen or tumor markers. The panel, however, emphasized that new approaches to treatment and increased early detection of breast cancer may dramatically alter these recommendations over the next few years.[3]

These recommendations reflect the futility of extensive testing of asymptomatic breast cancer patients. At least one prospective randomized trial has demonstrated no survival benefit for routine testing compared with history and physical examination and annual mammogram.[25] The PDQ of the National Cancer Institute also has presented similar guidelines for follow-up, although admitting that such a step is controversial.[54]

My own experience is perhaps instructive. One of my patients, a registered nurse, who was treated for invasive breast cancer with breast-conservation surgery, radiation therapy, and adjuvant chemotherapy, had been followed every 3 to 4 months with semiannual laboratory studies and annual chest x-ray and mammogram. Based upon the "new guidelines," I suggested that in the absence of symptoms an annual examination and mammogram would be sufficient. She was "shocked" and clearly unhappy with my recommendation. The solution is to discuss the follow-up with the patient immediately after diagnosis as part of the overall treatment plan. If patients understand from the beginning that extensive follow-up is not required, they will accept it. Obviously one cannot tell a patient at a later date that follow-up will be discontinued because "it does not make any difference!"

DILEMMAS IN BREAST DISEASE
Ductal Cancer in Situ (DCIS)

From a historical perspective, it is of interest that the earliest investigations of malignant tumors focused on breast cancer and noted that carcinoma arises from normal epithelial cells. It was also observed that there was a histologic progression of breast epithelium into invasive carcinoma.[27] In 1932, this intraepithelial stage was labeled in situ breast cancer.[68] It was rarely diagnosed and considered a clinical oddity as late as the 1980s. Physical examination was the only means of detecting carcinoma of the breast, and DCIS was diagnosed rarely. In 1980, a survey of 28,000 breast biopsies by the American College of Surgeons documented only 202 cases (0.8%).[59] There were no screening programs and obviously no occult lesions. With the advent of widespread mammographic screening, DCIS has become a common diagnosis, representing 12% to 15% of all newly diagnosed breast cancers and in some institutions as many as 50%.[11] The age-adjusted incidence increased 17.5% annually from 1983 to 1992.[23] In the United States, 50% of breast cancers are diagnosed through screening and as many as 50% of these are DCIS,[11] representing 23,000 to 36,000 cases annually.[23]

The dilemma with DCIS is that as a noninvasive cancer it poses enough of a threat to be cautious about treatment recommendations, particularly because in many cases it will do no harm if left alone (undiscovered). Is it really a disease? By definition a disease is something that causes morbidity or mortality. Thus DCIS is more of a "condition" than a disease.[34] What then are the treatment options? Nearly all patients with the "condition" of DCIS can be cured by a radical prophylactic treatment—mastectomy. Many of these patients, perhaps 90% to 95% of them, do not need this procedure. Breast-conservation therapy, on the other hand, will cure most patients, but not quite as many as mastectomy. Breast-conservation treatment with radiation will cure more than breast conservation without radiation therapy. Tamoxifen may further decrease the risk of recurrence and might cure even more patients. Each of these slight gains in cure rate is accomplished at some expense—unsatisfactory cosmesis, side effects of radiation therapy and tamoxifen, increased cost, and possibly long-term toxic effects.[34] By using these treatments, however, we will prevent ultimately incurable disease (i.e., distant metastases). In other words, either we must overtreat all patients to benefit a few or we must undertreat a few patients to their detriment.

The key to successful treatment strategies involves acceptance of the fact that DCIS is a "condition" of incredible heterogeneity. Initial studies supported the multicentric nature of this disease. However, recurrence in the same breast and at the same site as the original biopsy has provided strong evidence of the *unicentric* nature of most cases of DCIS.[53] This view is also supported by careful three-dimensional reconstructions.[36] This concept suggests that small and low-grade tumors may be adequately treated by surgical excision alone, and indeed between 1983 and 1992 there was a dramatic decline in the proportion of DCIS treated by mastectomy (from 71% to 43.8%) and an increase in treatment by wide local excision to 30.2%.[23] There is compelling evidence, however, that both comedo or high-grade histology and large size are associated with greater likelihood of local recurrence and require more extensive treatment—wide local excision and radiation therapy or mastectomy.

Two major factors are responsible for the changes in the management of DCIS: (1) increased use of mammography and (2) breast-conservation therapy as the "standard" treatment.

The increasing acceptance of mammography has changed not only the way we detect DCIS but also the nature and extent of the neoplastic process. With the acceptance of breast-conservation treatment (i.e., wide local excision, axillary dissection, and radiation therapy) for invasive breast cancer, it is difficult to continue treating noninvasive disease with mastectomy. A number of treatment options have been suggested based on tumor size, histologic classification (including tumor architecture), nuclear grade, and margin status. One set of criteria, the Van Nuys Prognostic

Index (VNPI) scoring system, is used[65] by the Breast Health Center at Women and Infants Hospital and is summarized in Table 53-2.

In summary:

1. DCIS is relatively common and its frequency is increasing.

2. It is now known that not all microscopic DCIS will progress to clinical cancer. However, if DCIS is not treated, the patient is more likely to develop an ipsilateral invasive cancer than a patient without DCIS.

3. The separation of noninvasive cancer into architectural groups such as comedo versus noncomedo carcinoma may be an oversimplification and does not reflect the currently accepted histologic heterogeneity of the disease.

4. High-grade DCIS is more aggressive in its histologic appearance. It is more likely to be associated with a subsequent invasive cancer than non–high-grade tumors. It is more likely to have a high S-phase and when treated conservatively more likely to recur locally than non–high-grade disease.

5. As previously noted, most cases of noninvasive cancer detected today are not palpable and are detected by mammography, with microcalcifications being the most common finding.

6. Therefore preoperative evaluation should include film screen mammography with appropriate spot compression views. It is essential that the surgeon and the radiologist plan the treatment procedure together.

7. A critical member of the therapeutic team is the pathologist, who must reconcile the pathologic features of the disease and the clinical and diagnostic features.

8. The patient should be apprised of all of the features of her condition, and there should be a thorough discussion regarding the risks and advantages of the recommended therapeutic procedures. Using the VNPI scoring system, breast-conservation treatment is appropriate with a VNPI score of 3 or 4. If a patient has a VNPI score of 5, 6, or 7, reexcision may be considered. If this is not possible, radiation therapy should be considered. Actually, some patients with a high score (VNPI score of 7) are better treated by mastectomy. For patient with VNPI scores of 8 or 9, a mastectomy with or without reconstruction is recommended (see Table 53-2). The validity of these conclusions will require the test of time and confirmation of the VNPI score by additional independent evaluation. For now, the VNPI is the best available and illustrates the value of a well-designed protocol with data carefully collected and analyzed. This approach is ideally suited to the philosophy and mission of dedicated breast health centers.

Estrogen Replacement Therapy

The benefits and risk of estrogen replacement therapy have been debated for years. It is essential that the physician understand the rationale, especially in terms of the prevention of cardiovascular disease and osteoporosis, and at the same time be aware of the lack of solid data to support the unequivocal recommendation for estrogen replacement therapy, particularly in patients treated for breast cancer.

We live in an aging society. Two hundred years ago fewer than 30% of women lived long enough to reach menopause. Now 90% of women reach the climacteric. Approximately 56 million women in the United States are older than 35 years of age, and more than 30 million women have an average postmenopausal life expectancy of 28 years.[44] Furthermore, advances in the treatment of breast cancer have resulted in long-term survival, and premenopausal patients treated for breast cancer often receive adjuvant therapy that in many cases can result in premature menopause.

There are two aspects to estrogen replacement therapy: (1) *prevention*—osteoporosis and coronary heart disease, and (2) *treatment*—atrophic changes and vasomotor phenomenon.

There is no question that in the United States more women die of myocardial infarction than of breast disease. It is clear that the incidence of cardiovascular disease in women increases after menopause. A number of studies have suggested that estrogen replacement therapy reduces cardiovascular mortality by about 50%. Estrogen lowers low-density lipoprotein cholesterol and raises high-density lipoprotein cholesterol. However, this explains only 35% to 50% of the cardioprotective effect, and there is evidence that preservation of normal endothelial function also plays an important role.[69,80] However, many investigators are concerned about the validity of these data. The highly touted meta-analyses may have sample sizes too small to show an effect (i.e., a priori power calculations should always be done in quantitative research). The physician must weigh these data against the yet unknown information that may be available from the PEPI trial and the large Women's Health Initiative Study.[35,51]

In the meantime, there is increasing pressure to prescribe estrogen replacement therapy, but what are the risks? A number of interesting observations suggest a relationship between estrogen and breast cancer. It has been known for many years that oophorectomy in women younger than 35 years of age reduces the risk of breast cancer by 70%. Patients with metastatic cancer who are treated with aminoglutethimide (an aromatase inhibitor) have a significant reduction in estradiol: from 15 to 20 pg/ml to about 5 pg/ml because of the failure of conversion of hormones into estrogen. The level of estradiol is increased to 30 to 35 pg/ml with estrogen replacement therapy.[67] One article reported that patients receiving estrogen replacement therapy who developed metastatic breast disease had regression on withdrawal of estrogen therapy.[21] These data and a number of other studies clearly indicate that there is as yet an unknown relationship between estrogens and breast cancer.

The literature about the primary prevention of coronary heart disease, the risk factors for osteoporosis, and the use of estrogens and progestins and the risk of breast cancer is voluminous and often contradictory. Breast cancer is related to reproductive events. Increasing attention to the contemporary preventive approach to breast cancer focuses on the physiologic effects of the sex steroid hormones and their possible interaction with family history. One researcher has suggested vigorous exercise to delay puberty followed by hormone treatment to induce artificial menopause.[55] Adding to the potential risk of estrogen replacement therapy is the fact that current use of estrogen replacement therapy may be associated with lower specificity and lower sensitivity of screening mammography.[42] Clearly a risk-benefit analysis must be discussed with the patient, both in terms of prevention (including the uncertainty of the observational data and the lack of information from controlled, randomized trials on the risk of breast cancer) and in terms of the potential decreased accuracy of screening. Given the large number of women receiving estrogen replacement therapy, even a small risk could result in a public health problem.

A recent study discusses the effect of alcohol ingestion on estrogens in postmenopausal women.[30] It is interesting that some studies indicate that moderate ingestion of alcohol increases the risk of breast cancer. Apparently, acute alcohol ingestion may lead to significant and sustained elevations in circulating estradiol levels to 300% higher that those targeted in the clinical use of estrogen replacement therapy. Thus, although moderate alcohol consumption also appears to decrease the incidence of coronary artery disease, it may increase the incidence of breast cancer and the combination of estrogen replacement therapy and alcohol ingestion may be additive, increasing the risk of breast cancer more than either alone.[30]

Despite the reassuring data about the role of estrogens as an important determinant in breast carcinogenesis, there continues to be concern. A number of reports have reevaluated the role of a wide variety of pollutants in the ecosystem that have the ability to mimic the action of steroid hormones in the body. The principal concern centers around chemicals that can mimic the action of estrogens, termed environmental estrogens or "xenoestrogens."[63] DDT, for example, is the most effective organochlorine in regulating estrogen receptor-mediated response. One report has suggested that a detailed follow-up of breast cancer patients with estrogen receptor–positive breast tumors who have failed to respond to endocrine intervention therapy is crucial to establish whether xenoestrogens contribute to breast cancer risk and incidence.[63]

Other investigators question the role of environmental contaminants such as DDT in the development of breast cancer. Epidemiologic studies assessing regional variations in breast cancer incidence and mortality in the United States seem to suggest that known risk factors, age at menarche and menopause, and alcohol consumption rather than environmental exposures account in large part for the variations in geographic patterns of breast cancer in this country.[17] Nonetheless, there is growing enthusiasm for exploring the treatment of estrogen deficiency symptoms in menopausal patients and breast cancer survivors with tailored treatment strategies—the so-called designer estrogens. There is no question that the risk of breast cancer is related to reproductive events as has been mentioned: age at menarche and menopause, age at birth of first child, and other hormonally related conditions such as obesity. Therefore it is dangerous, in my opinion, to state that estrogen treatment is perfectly safe. This view is supported by the search for estrogen alternatives to treat the agreed-on problems related to menopause: vasomotor symptoms, urogenital symptoms (including frequent urinary tract infections and vaginal dryness), osteoporosis, increased risk of heart disease, and problems with memory, depression, and sleep. The recent development of a selective estrogen receptor modulator raloxifene, a therapy that potentially prevents postmenopausal bone loss and lowers serum cholesterol without stimulating reproductive tissue (uterus and breast), appears to offer considerable therapeutic benefits.[20] On the other hand, raloxifene does not appear to be useful therapy for hot flashes and possibly for atrophic changes as well.[20] Despite the beneficial effects of raloxifene on bone mineral density and serum lipoproteins, its effect in preventing fractures and cardiovascular events is yet to be determined.[28] On the practical side, it must be admitted that however desirable these designer estrogens are in preventing increased risk for breast and uterine cancer, it will be difficult to persuade women to take a drug that does not alleviate menopausal symptoms to prevent the development of osteoporosis and coronary heart disease 20 years later.

The issue of estrogen replacement therapy in patients treated for breast cancer presents a challenge because of lack of data. Whereas successful treatment of breast cancer depends on local control, there is always the potential for distant metastasis. If the patient is cured, the question is moot. Unfortunately, not all patients with breast cancer are cured even with the most effective treatment. The 10-year survival rate for the patients with the best prognosis—those with small tumors and negative nodes—is approximately 70%, indicating that 30% of these patients had metastatic disease that was unknown either at the time of the initial treatment or during the follow-up period. It is the effect of estrogen replacement therapy on occult metastatic disease that is the basis for caution regarding the use of this therapy in patients treated for breast cancer. Receptor data and other prognostic factors appear to be of little value at present, at least in deciding for or against estrogen replacement therapy in these patients. Finally, if overt metastatic disease is discovered, treatment, however aggressive, is ineffective. That is, none of these patients will survive.

In summary, when considering estrogen replacement therapy, the physician must discuss the benefits and risks, including the uncertainty of the available data. Patients must accept an unknown medical risk, and clinicians must accept an unknown medicolegal risk. It is essential that before estrogen replacement therapy is administered the oncology team be consulted for an opinion, which in some cases may be surprisingly liberal, particularly if quality of life issues are involved (vaginal atrophy and associated dyspareunia). It

should be noted that the vaginal administration of estrogen is not without risk. Estrogen is absorbed readily from the atrophic vaginal mucosa; however, there is decreased absorption with increasing vaginal cornification, but perhaps sufficient absorption to stimulate occult micrometastases.

Elderly Patients

One of the problems associated with recommendations regarding diagnostic studies and treatment for "elderly" patients is the definition of elderly. The life expectancy for a woman 75 years of age is 11.1 years and for a woman 85 years is 6.2 years, and even women reaching 90 can expect to live another 4.5 years.[19]

In Chapter 52 it was noted that there are no guidelines for continued screening beyond age 65 because there are no data. In the United States, more than 30 million people, or approximately 12% of the population, are older than age 65. It has been estimated that by the year 2000 this proportion will increase to 13% and by 2050 to 22% or 65 million Americans.[19] The biggest risk factor for breast cancer is age, and the need for better treatment and attention to quality of life issues will become an increasing consideration.

Older patients receive lesser treatments not only because of physician bias but also as a result of societal concerns. Chronologic age alone as a criterion for estimating operative risk does not appear to be a factor in postsurgical mortality. The American Society of Anesthesiologists classifies risk for perioperative mortality regardless of age—normal, healthy patients (ASA Class 1) older than age 80 have a 0% surgical mortality rate.[29]

Approximately half of all breast cancers occur in women older than 65 years of age.[41] Despite the high prevalence of disease, the elderly have largely been excluded from participating in trials that have defined state-of-the-art treatment for breast cancer. There are several important differences in breast cancer treatment in the elderly. The classification of diagnosis (stage) appears to be more advanced than in younger women. Surgical procedures also differ. Histologic documentation of cancer at presentation or before definitive treatment has not always been performed. In two series, more than 10% of elderly women had no histologic confirmation or biopsy before definitive treatment.[13] There is less frequent performance of axillary dissection and rare use of reconstructive procedures. Radiation is used less often; however, the local recurrence rates are similar to those in the younger group.

A number of recent publications in the *Journal of the National Cancer Institute* have addressed these issues,[7,32] and recent trials have demonstrated low recurrence rates with breast-conservation treatment among older women, suggesting that less aggressive treatment may represent good clinical judgment when viewed in terms of functional status and increasing importance of social support in older patients.[7] At the Breast Health Center at New England Medical Center, we initiated a prospective study to explore an approach of limited therapy in elderly patients with early clinical stage breast cancer.[77] Patients 65 years or older with American Joint Commission (AJC) stage I and II cancers and clinically negative nodes were enrolled in a treatment program consisting of tumor excision, breast and regional lymph node irradiation, and tamoxifen. Our results in terms of mortality and survival are encouraging but will require confirmation from other institutions.

At Women and Infants Hospital we have participated in multiinstitutional trials sponsored by the National Cancer Institute, the goals of which have been to optimize the proportion of women aged 60 and older who receive postsurgical treatment for breast cancer, including radiation treatment and tamoxifen. Our present recommendations for local treatment are based on stage of disease, the patient's functional status, and the availability of social support. Given the aging population, definitive guidelines for the treatment of breast cancer in this group of patients are urgently needed.

SUMMARY

To take advantage of the most recent advances in the local treatment of breast cancer, it is clear that the "Breast Health Center" concept—a group of surgeons with special training and high volume practice—is the best way to take advantage of cost-effective strategies and at the same time provide cutting-edge treatment. The institution with the occasional breast cancer patient can no longer provide the expertise required to take advantage of the latest technology. We are entering a new era in breast cancer treatment in which state-of-the-art treatment strategies contribute to the goal of cost-effective health care.

REFERENCES

1. American Cancer Society: Cancer facts and figures, *CA Cancer J Clin* 48:6, 1998.
2. American Joint Committee on Cancer: *Manual for staging of cancer,* ed 4, Philadelphia, 1992, JB Lippincott.
3. American Society of Clinical Oncologists (ASCO): Guidelines for breast cancer surveillance, *J Clin Oncol* 15:2149, 1997.
4. Ansanelli VW, Lesser ML: A prospective randomized trial of the use of the CO_2 laser vs. scalpel in breast cancer surgery, *Breast Dis* 9:125, 1996.
5. Astrow AB: The Scenie/Tenser article reviewed, *Oncology* 11:1518, 1997.
6. Avril N, et al: Assessment of axillary lymph node involvement in breast cancer patients with positron admission tomography using radiolabeled 2-(fluorine-18)-fluoro-2-deoxy-d-glucose, *J Natl Cancer Inst* 88:1204, 1996.
7. Ballard-Barbasch R, et al: Factors associated with surgical and radiation therapy for early stage breast cancer in older women, *J Natl Cancer Inst* 88:716, 1996.
8. Bath A, Craig PH, Silverstein MJ: Predictors of axillary lymph node metastases in patients with T_1 breast carcinoma, *Cancer* 79:1918, 1997.
9. Battersby S, et al: Influence of oral contraceptives on normal human breast epithelial proliferation. In Bresciani F, et al, editors: *Progress in cancer research and therapy,* vol 35 *Hormones and cancer 3,* New York, 1988, Raven.
10. Bedwinek J: Breast conserving surgery and irradiation: the importance of demarcating the excision cavity with surgical clips, *Int J Radiat Oncol Biol Phys* 26:675, 1993.
11. Blum E: Doctors strive to minimize DCIS treatment, *J Natl Cancer Inst* 89:1092, 1997.
12. Boak JL, Agwunnobi TC: A study of technetium-labelled sulfide colloid uptake by regional lymph nodes draining a tumor bearing area, *Br J Surg* 65:374, 1978.
13. Busch E, et al: Patterns of breast cancer care in the elderly, *Cancer* 78:101, 1996.
14. Cady B: Expert perspectives: current status of axillary node dissection in primary breast cancer, *Breast Dis* 8:87, 1997.
15. Clark RM, et al: Randomized clinical trial to assess the effectiveness of breast irradiation following lumpectomy and axillary dissection for node-negative breast cancer, *J Natl Cancer Inst* 84:683, 1992.
16. Clarke DH, Martinez AA: Identification of patients who are at high risk for locoregional breast cancer recurrence after conservative surgery and radiotherapy: a review article for surgeons, pathologists, and radiation and medical oncologists, *J Clin Oncol* 10:474, 1992.
17. Davidson NE, Yager JD: Pesticides and breast cancer: fact or fad, *J Natl Cancer Inst* 89:1743, 1997 (editorial).
18. Denham J, Carter M: Location of the excision site following segmental mastectomy for accurate post-operative irradiation, *Aust NZ J Surg* 56:685, 1986.
19. DiSilvestro PA, et al: You may think I'm too old, but can't you treat my cancer? *RI Med* 78:143, 1995.
20. Delmas PD, et al: Effects of raloxifene on bone mineral density, serum cholesterol concentrations, and uterine endometrium in postmenopausal women, *N Engl J Med* 337:1641, 1997.
21. Dhodapker MV, Ingle JN, Ahmann DL: Estrogen replacement therapy withdrawal and regression of metastatic breast cancer, *Cancer* 75:43, 1995.
22. Edge SB: Breast cancer practice guidelines: evaluation and quality improvement. *NCCN Proc* 11:151, 1997.
23. Ernster V, et al: Incidence of and treatment for ductal carcinoma in-situ of the breast, *JAMA* 275:913, 1996.
24. Fisher B, Redmond C: Lumpectomy for breast cancer: an update of the NSABP experience, *Monogr J Natl Cancer Inst* 11:7, 1992.
25. Fossati R, et al: The effectiveness of follow-up diagnostic testing in patients with curable breast cancer: results from a multi-center randomized trial, *Proc Am Soc Clin Oncol* 13:77, 1994.
26. Foster RS Jr, Farwell ME, Costanza MC: Breast-conserving surgery for breast cancer: patterns of care in a geographic region and estimation of potential applicability, *Ann Surg Oncol* 2:275, 1995.
27. Frykberg ER: An overview of the history and epidemiology of ductal carcinoma in-situ of the breast, *Breast J* 3:227, 1997.
28. Fuleihan G: Tissue-specific estrogens—the promise for the future, *N Engl J Med* 337:1686, 1997 (editorial).
29. Gilbert GH, Minaker KL: Principles of surgical risk assessment of the elderly patient, *J Oral Maxilofac Surg* 48:972, 1990.
30. Ginsburg ES, et al: Effects of alcohol ingestion on estrogens and postmenopausal women, *JAMA* 276:1747, 1996.
31. Giuliano AE, et al: Improved axillary staging of breast cancer with sentinel lymphadenectomy, *Ann Surg* 222:394, 1995.
32. Goodwin JS, Samet JM, Hunt WC: Determinants of survival in older cancer patients, *J Natl Cancer Inst* 88:1031, 1996.
33. Halsted WS: The results of operations for the cure of cancer of the breast performed at the Johns Hopkins Hospital, 1894.
34. Hayes DF: Ductal carcinoma in-situ of the breast: a new model, *J Natl Cancer Inst* 89:991, 1997.
35. Healey B, PEPI; In perspective good answers spawn pressing questions, *JAMA* 273:240, 1995.
36. Holland R, et al: Extent distribution and mammographic/histological correlations of breast ductal carcinoma in-situ, *Lancet* 335:519, 1990.
37. Hrushesky WJM, et al: Menstrual influence on surgical cure of breast cancer, *Lancet* 2:949, 1989.
38. Kearney TJ, Morrow M: Effective re-excision on the success of breast-conserving surgery, *Ann Surg Oncol* 2:303, 1995.
39. Krag DN, et al: Surgical resection and radiolocalization of the sentinel lymph node in breast cancer using a gamma probe, *Surg Oncol* 2:335, 1993.

40. Kurtz JM: Factors influencing the risk of local recurrence in the breast, *Eur J Cancer* 28:660, 1992.

41. Law TM, et al: Breast cancer in elderly women: presentation, survival and treatment options, *Surg Clin North Am* 76:289, 1996.

42. Laya MB, et al: Effect of estrogen replacement therapy on the specificity and sensitivity of screening mammography, *J Natl Cancer Inst* 88:643, 1996.

43. Liljetren G, et al: Sector resection with or without post-operative radiotherapy for stage I breast cancer: five year results of a randomized trial, *J Natl Cancer Inst* 86:717, 1994.

44. Marchant DJ: Dilemmas in breast disease. The impact of exogenous hormones on breast cancer risk, myth vs. reality: an overview, *Breast J*1:58, 1995.

45. Meyer CM, et al: Technetium-99m sulfa colloid cutaneous lymphoscintigraphy in the management of truncal melanoma, *Radiology* 131:205, 1979.

46. Moore ZH: On the influence of inadequate operations on the theory of cancer, *R Med Chir Soc (Lond)* 1:245, 1867.

47. More HMO's order outpatient mastectomies, *Wall Street J* Nov 6, 1996.

48. Morrow M: Breast cancer. In Fischer DS, editor: *Follow-up of cancer, a handbook for physicians,* Philadelphia, 1996, Lippincott-Raven.

49. Morrow M, Bland KI, Foster R: Breast cancer surgical practice guidelines, *Oncology* 11:877, 1997.

50. Morton DL, et al: Technical details of intraoperative lymphatic mapping for early stage melanoma, *Arch Surg* 127:392, 1992.

51. National Institutes of Health: Women's Health Initiative, 1994.

52. Opposition to outpatient mastectomy mounts, *Am Med News* 40:9, Mar 3, 1997.

53. Page DL, Jensen RA: Ductal carcinoma in-situ of the breast: understanding the misunderstood step-child, *JAMA* 275:948, 1996 (editorial).

54. PDQ Statement on Breast Cancer, Department of Health and Human Services, Public Health Service, National Institutes of Health, Oct 22, 1996.

55. Pike M: Cancer and genetic symposium, May 16, 1996.

56. Post-operative lengths of stay: can they be defined by a specific number of days? *Bull Am Coll Surg* 82:27, 1997.

57. Ratajczak HV, Sothern RB, Hrushesky WJM: Estrous influence on surgical cure of a mouse breast cancer, *J Exp Med* 168:73, 1988.

58. Ravdin PM, et al: Prediction of axillary lymph node status in breast cancer patients by use of prognostic indicators, *J Natl Cancer Inst* 86:1771, 1994.

59. Rosner D, et al: Non-invasive breast carcinoma: results of a national survey by the American College of Surgeons, *Ann Surg* 192:139, 1980.

60. Schnitt SJ: Pathologic factors predictive of local recurrence in patients with invasive breast cancer, treated by conservative surgery and radiation therapy. In Fletcher GH, Levitt SH, editors: *Non-disseminated breast cancer—controversial issues in management,* Berlin, 1993, Springer-Verlag.

61. Schnitt SJ, et al: A prospective study of conservative surgery alone in the treatment of selected patients with stage I breast cancer, *Cancer* 77:1094, 1996.

62. Senie RT, Tenser SM: The timing of breast cancer surgery during the menstrual cycle, *Oncology* 11:1509, 1997.

63. Shekhar PBM, Werdell J, Basrur VS: Environmental estrogen stimulation of growth and estrogen receptor function in preneoplastic and cancerous human breast cell lines, *J Natl Cancer Inst* 89:1774, 1997.

64. Silverstein MJ, et al: Axillary lymph node dissection for T_{1A} breast carcinoma, *Cancer* 73:664, 1994.

65. Silverstein MJ, et al: A prognostic index for ductal carcinoma in-situ of the breast, *Cancer* 77:2267, 1996.

66. Smitt MC, Heltzel M: Women's use of resources in decision-making for early stage breast cancer: results of a community based survey, *Ann Surg Oncol* 4:564, 1997.

67. Spicer D: National cancer survivor's day symposium, *NY Health Sci Center Prim Care* 15:10, 1995.

68. Stout AP: *Human cancer: etiological factors, precancerous lesions, growth, spread, diagnosis, prognosis, principles of treatment,* Philadelphia, 1932, Lea & Febiger.

69. Sullivan JM, Fowlkes LP: The clinical aspects of estrogen and the cardiovascular system, *Obstet Gynecol* 87:36, 1996.

70. Systemic treatment for early breast cancer by hormonal, cytotoxic, or immune therapy: 133 randomized trials involving 31,000 recurrences and 24,000 deaths among 75,000 women: Early Breast Cancer Trialists' Collaborative Group *Lancet* 339:1, 1992.

71. Update of the NCCN Guidelines for Treatment of Breast Cancer, NCCN Proceedings, *Oncology* 11:199, 1997.

72. The Uppsala-Örebro Breast Cancer Study Group: Sector resection with or without post-operative radiotherapy for stage I breast cancer: a randomized trial, *J Natl Cancer Inst* 82:277, 1990.

73. Urban JA, Marjani MA: Significance of internal mammary lymph node metastases in breast cancer, *AJR Am J Roentgenol* 111:130, 1971.

74. Veronesi U, et al: Radiotherapy after breast-preserving surgery in women with localized cancer of the breast, *N Engl J Med* 328:1587, 1993.

75. Veronesi U, et al: Local recurrences and distant metastases after conservative breast cancer treatments: partly independent events, *J Natl Cancer Inst* 87:19, 1995.

76. Wanebo HJ, Harpole D, Teates CD: Radionucleotide lymphoscintigraphy with technetium-99m antimony sulfide colloid to identify lymphatic drainage of cutaneous melanoma at ambiguous sites in the head and neck and trunk, *Cancer* 55:1403, 1985.

77. Wazer DE, et al: Breast conservation in elderly women for clinically negative axillary lymph nodes without axillary dissection, *Cancer* 74:878, 1994.

78. Weiss SM, et al: Patient satisfaction with decision-making for breast cancer therapy, *Ann Surg Oncol* 3:285, 1996.

79. Who gets breast-conserving surgery? *McCalls* 56, Aug 1993.

80. Wild RA: Estrogen: effects on the cardiovascular tree, *Obstet Gynecol* 87:227, 1996.

54 Breast Plastic Surgery and Reconstruction

SUMNER A. SLAVIN

A large segment of the average plastic surgeon's practice in the United States concerns the female breast. Increasingly, breast plastic surgery is emerging as a subspecialty of its own, mostly because of recent advances in breast augmentation, reduction, mastopexy, and reconstruction. This chapter describes the most common conditions for which women seek plastic and reconstructive surgery.

BREAST AUGMENTATION

Augmentation mammaplasty seems to satisfy the psychological and anatomic needs of women who are concerned about the small size of their breasts.[13] In North America it is a popular procedure despite its technical limitations and consumer alerts against the supposed dangers of silicone implants. At the outset, it should be stated that no study has demonstrated an increased incidence of cancer in women who have had breast augmentation with silicone prostheses. However, women who have had breast enlargement with implants do present a slightly greater difficulty in examination to some of their physicians as well as to mammographers who nevertheless have developed newer techniques for a more accurate depiction. When leakage or disruption of the silicone envelope of the prosthesis is suspected by clinical findings of encapsulation or a change in the appearance of the breast, a magnetic resonance study is the best diagnostic tool.

Patients for augmentation mammaplasty (Fig. 54-1) usually have one thing in common: a preoccupation with what they consider to be their inadequately developed breast. They commonly have poor self-esteem despite the fact that they may be very attractive and extremely accomplished. They may complain of the difficulty in purchasing the clothes they wish. Psychologically, they are usually not abnormal, but they may have a greater-than-normal concern with their bust size. During the initial consultation, the plastic surgeon must be certain that the patient is undertaking the operation for herself and is not doing it to please a partner or possibly to save a marriage. In those instances the patient would be better served by a psychotherapist than by a plastic surgeon.

In determining a woman's suitability for this procedure, it is important to inquire about the family history, especially whether a close relative—mother or sister—has had premenopausal breast cancer. It is also important to know whether the patient has had biopsies in the past or a history of breast masses that require frequent aspiration. Under these conditions the presence of a foreign body, such as a silicone implant, would be unwise. One cannot emphasize enough the need for a careful, thorough breast examination to rule out the presence of a malignancy. In patients 30 years or older, mammography is mandatory. In some instances it may be indicated with younger patients.

The plastic surgeon must inform the patient that regardless of which technique is used, the presence of a foreign body may induce an abnormal appearance and firmness to the breast, which results from the capsular and spherical contracture that occurs in a certain percentage of women having this procedure. If the patient expects that her breasts will be absolutely normal to inspection and examination, she is liable to be seriously disappointed. The fact that there are literally scores of different implants of various textures and sizes attests more to the inadequacy of the procedure than to the imagination of the manufacturer. Implants that may have an original tear-drop shape and a soft texture may become round and hard after operation. Also, because many saline devices are placed in a subpectoral position, the compressive forces of the overlying musculature tend to modify the implant's contour into a rounded form, despite its original shape.

Most plastic surgeons favor inserting a silicone gel implant under the muscle rather than immediately under the breast to lessen the incidence of a capsular contracture. Another previously popular alternative was to use a polyurethane- or silicone-textured implant (the so-called rough implant) rather than the smooth silicone gel implant with or without a saline component to obtain a more natural appearing breast and one that has less tendency to form a distorting, firm capsule. Implants may be inserted through the axilla, through or around the areola, or by way of an inframammary incision. The decision about what type of implant to use and how and where to insert it depends on the needs of the patient, the preferences of the patient and the surgeon, and the ruling of the Federal Drug Agency, which has determined that silicone-covered, saline-filled implants can now be used only for patients desiring augmentation. Since the Federal Drug Administration imposed a moratorium on the the use of silicone implants in 1992, saline inflatable prostheses have become the norm for both cosmetic and reconstructive breast surgery in the United States. However, in most other countries and in almost all of Europe, silicone gel implants remain popular. Whether these devices will be reintroduced in the United States for unrestricted use in breast plastic surgery is a subject of current debate.

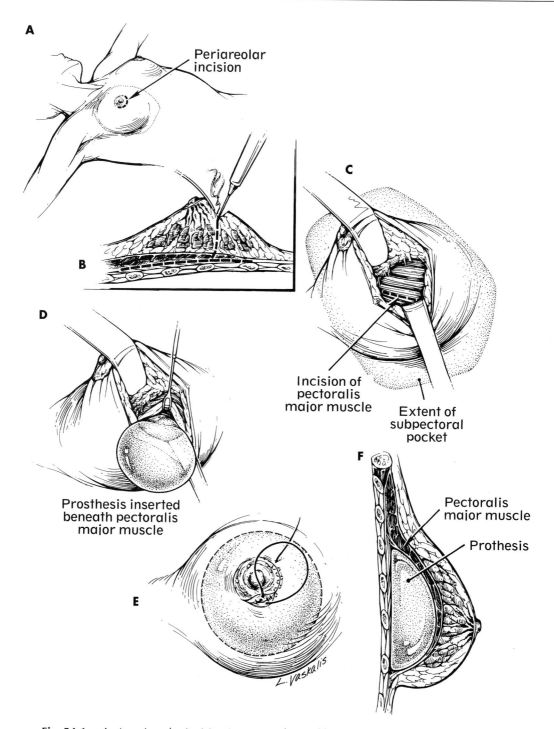

Fig. 54-1 **A,** A periareolar incision is commonly used because the scar may be concealed at the border of the pigmented areolar skin. **B,** The incision is carried through breast parenchyma to the level of the prepectoral fascia. **C,** The pectoralis muscle is divided along the oblique line of its muscle fibers. **D,** A subpectoral pocket is created for reception of saline prosthesis. **E,** Closure of the periareolar incision with a running subcuticular nonabsorbable monofillament suture can minimize scarring. **F,** The prosthesis is seated beneath the pectoralis muscle and its fascia continuation.

Saline implants combine a solid silicone shell with a hollow interior that can be filled to a predetermined volume by means of a specially designed fill tube and valve mechanism. Although patients must be advised of the possibility of deflation if there is a malfunction of the valve or a deterioration of the exterior shell, deflation rates of only 1% to 2% over 10 years have been observed. Saline implants can partially deflate, creating a wavy, irregular surface that may be manifested clinically by wrinkling of the breast skin and subcutaneous fatty layer. Therefore, along with the previously mentioned improved visualization on mammography, many plastic surgeons prefer a subpectoral positioning of the implant. The added soft tissue conceals surface irregularities and is particularly useful for the large number of patients seeking improved size and contour for postpartum breast changes. Because of atrophy of breast parenchymal volume, patients in this latter group are excellent candidates for augmentation mammaplasty.

Borrowing from gynecologists, plastic surgeons have been incorporating the endoscope into a wide variety of procedures, including endoscopic augmentation mammoplasty, abdominoplasty, reduction mammoplasty, mastectomy, and microsurgical donor tissue harvest. Of these, transaxillary subpectoral endoscopic augmentation mammoplasty has become extremely popular, based on the aesthetic appeal of a scarless breast with small incisions concealed in an axillary crease. Endoscopic placement facilitates the subpectoral dissection and reduces the likelihood of a sensory nerve injury. Visualization of the subpectoral space is excellent, and bleeding complications are uncommon. The ability to roll and fold the saline implant into a collapsed state has made it ideal for endoscopic breast augmentation and reconstruction using minimal incisions.

Before the operation, the plastic surgeon and patient must decide on the eventual size of the breast. Most patients do not want their breasts to be excessively large; if so desired, the plastic surgeon should warn the patient that the chance of getting abnormal firmness is greater if the pocket created for the implant can barely contain it. The operation is generally performed on an ambulatory basis, either under local anesthesia with intravenous sedation or under general anesthesia.

The patient should be aware not only of the possibility of abnormal firmness on one or both sides but also of the possibility of postoperative bleeding (less than 1%) and infection (less than 1%). Altered or decreased sensation in the nipple and areola may occur but is uncommon (less than 10%).

In the immediate postoperative phase, patients are instructed not to lift more than 10 pounds for 2 weeks, are usually asked not to drive for 5 days, but may return to work in 1 week or 10 days after operation. By 4 weeks, they are able to resume almost all activities, including the use of a Nautilus.

It is important that patients having had augmentation mammaplasty continue their periodic follow-up with their physician, who should continue to do careful breast examination and order mammograms on a regular basis, depending on the patient's age and other conditions intrinsic to the breast. In surveys of women who have had augmentation mammaplasty, satisfaction with the result is extremely high, about 96%, even in the presence of abnormal firmness and shape secondary to capsular contracture. This incidence varies from 3% to 10% with silicone implants placed below the pectoral muscle to 30% if silicone implants (not rough textured) are placed immediately below the mammary gland. The incidence of abnormal firmness in patients having the silicone-textured implant is less than 8%; long-term

follow-up with saline implants suggests encapsulation rates of less than 10%, but collection of the data did not begin until 1998 and a reliable figure is not yet known. It must be kept in mind that essentially all patients develop some internal encapsulation and that these rates are meant to infer a severe degree rather than an overall incidence.

The following case is typical of the kind of patient, the type of operation, and the outcome that one can usually expect.

CASE REPORT

A 32-year-old married woman complained of bilateral mammary hypoplasia (Fig. 54-2, *A*). She described herself as having a breast size of approximately an A cup bra and requested enlargement to a size B cup bra. She had no family history of breast cancer. The patient described her marital relationship as stable. Her primary reason for requesting the procedure was a self-motivated desire to improve her body image, which was supported by her husband.

A preoperative mammogram (the patient's first) disclosed no abnormalities. Bilateral subpectoral augmentation mammaplasties were performed under general anesthesia on an oupatient basis using 200-ml gel implants. Postoperatively (see Fig. 54-2, *B*), she noted some diminution of sensation medially on each breast, but nipple-areolar sensory function was unchanged. She has been followed for 3 years and has maintained a satisfactory breast form and natural softness. ▲

BREAST PTOSIS

Ptosis is literally sagging of the breast. Although ptosis can occur in women who have very large breasts, pure ptosis is a condition in which the elastic envelope of the breast has been stretched. Ptosis may be incipient, mild, moderate, or severe. Treatment may include correcting the ptosis and also augmenting the breast. This therapy would be for a woman whose breasts not only are sagging but, when elevated, are too small for her liking. Although the operation of correction of breast ptosis seems technically not difficult, it is not an easy procedure in terms of long-term results because the condition can recur as a result of the passage of time and the effect of gravity.[13] Patients whose ptosis has been corrected by excision of the skin and elevation of the breast on the chest wall (Fig. 54-3) present a less complicated problem than do those who have had augmentation as well. Often, these women's breasts tend to sag again, their breasts going downward over the implant, which by now has become fixed to the chest wall. This possibility must be completely and clearly explained to the patient. The correction of breast ptosis requires incisions; in some procedures the incision goes only around the areola; in others, additional incisions are made from the areola to the inframammary fold and then along the inframammary crease. Patients who have ptosis usually heal without thick scars. Perhaps that is evidence of the cause (still unexplained) of why their breast skin has

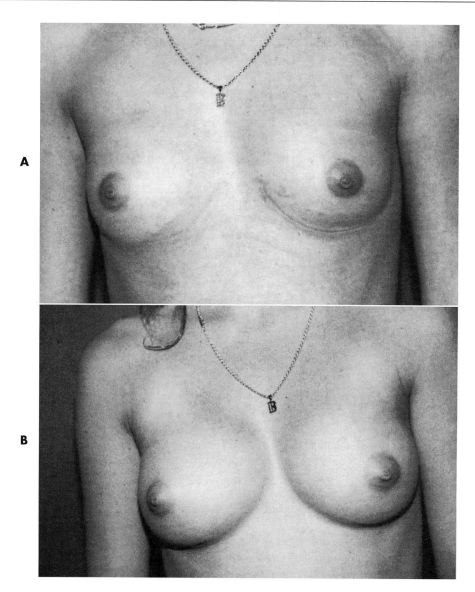

Fig. 54-2 **A,** A 32-year-old woman with mammary hypoplasia. **B,** Result after bilateral sub-pectoral augmentation mammoplasties.

stretched. Patients often complain that their breast ptosis and perhaps atrophy have occurred after childbirth, particularly after nursing. In some women it happens without pregnancy and often is a family trait.

The correction of breast ptosis, with or without augmentation, is usually done on an outpatient basis under local or general anesthesia. Patients are given approximately the same instructions for their postoperative activities as they are after augmentation mammaplasty even when no implant has been used. These patients with ptosis should be advised to wear a bra as much as possible after the operation and for years to come. Whether the bra decreases the chance of ptosis recurring is only conjecture. In this procedure, as in breast augmentation, infection and bleeding are possible, and if an implant has been used, unfavorable results or complications associated with the implant, particularly abnormal firmness, can also occur. In other countries, particularly Brazil, recurrent ptosis has been treated with the insertion of a hybrid mesh of polyglactine and polyester that encases the

mammary tissues. This fixes the breast parenchyma to the overlying skin brassiere and provides a longer-lasting correction. Unfortunately, its use in the breast raises legitimate concerns about the hazard of an inaccurate breast examination, and for that reason, it has not been accepted in the United States. The need for such a product underscores the difficulty of providing a lasting correction of breast ptosis. Many plastic surgeons are using a periareolar approach for this operation because of the favorable scar that it leaves on the breast, but continuing the incision into the inframammary crease remains popular and often necessary for removal of excess skin.

CASE REPORT

A 39-year-old woman complained of bilateral mammary ptosis (Fig. 54-4), which became more noticeable after the birth of her second child. Formerly, her breasts had a youthful form with a full shape of approximately size C cup bra.

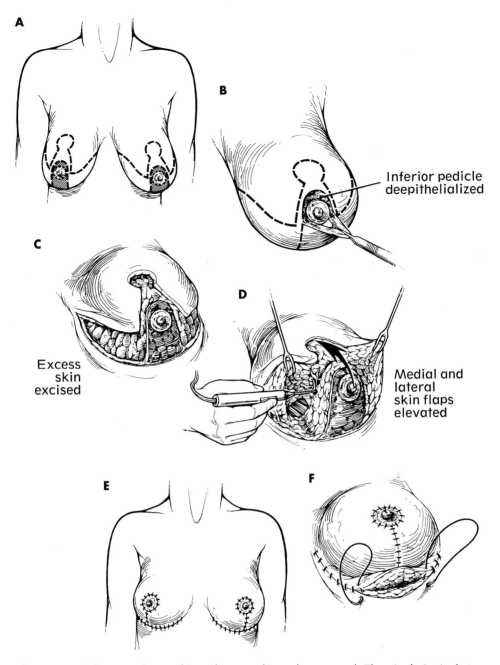

Fig. 54-3   **A,** Preoperative marking of excess skin to be removed. The nipple is sited at a more superior location. **B,** Deepithelialization of the inferior pedicle is commenced. Deeper blood vessels supplying the nipple are preserved. **C,** Excess skin has been resected. **D,** Medial and lateral flaps are elevated to facilitate wound closure. **E** and **F,** Wounds are closed to create an inverted T appearance. Most plastic surgeons prefer a subcuticular type of suture closure.

She had nursed both children for approximately 6 months each, noting loss of skin tone and atrophy of breast mass. Her breasts became increasingly ptotic, and she felt restricted in her choice of clothing. She had no family history of breast cancer. She had undergone a prior removal of a fibroadenoma at age 26.

Mastopexy was reviewed with the patient, emphasizing the location of incisions and the anticipated scarring. She requested concomitant breast augmentation to restore her former breast size. Under general anesthesia, bilateral mastopexies were performed along with subpectoral augmenta-

tion mammaplasties using 160-ml gel implants. She was discharged that same day. Results at 6 months after operation are shown in Fig. 54-5.   ▲

BREAST ASYMMETRY OR AGENESIS

Unilateral or bilateral agenesis of the breast or significant asymmetry can understandably distress a women. Many are so ashamed of the condition that they have kept it a secret even from their parents, as well as from their siblings and friends. Some adolescent girls have described

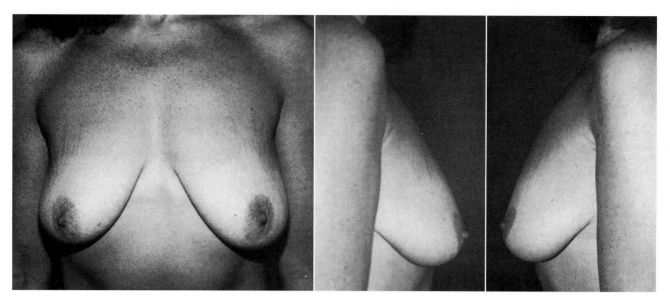

Fig. 54-4   A 39-year-old woman with bilateral mammary ptosis developing after the births of her two children.

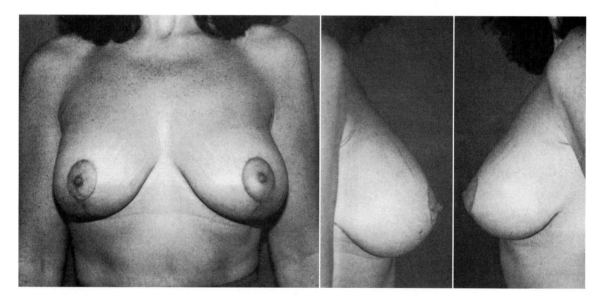

Fig. 54-5   Appearance of the patient 6 months after bilateral mastopexies with concomitant subpectoral augmentation mammoplasties.

the problem to their mothers but have never allowed a parent to see it.

Because those who seek plastic surgery have obviously not adjusted to their abnormality, they may not be representative of all those who have this problem.[13] Some teenage girls engage in promiscuous sexual activity almost to prove to themselves that they can still be women despite their abnormality. One of our patients stated that she wanted to get pregnant to see whether she could nurse.

Like the partners of patients for augmentation, reduction, or correction of ptosis, the partners of many women with mammary genesis or asymmetry do not believe that the woman has to undergo the operation.

In taking a history, it is important to elicit from the patient whether she prefers that the breast that is large be reduced or whether she wants the smaller one to be enlarged. It is easier technically to reduce the large breast to match the opposite but only if that breast is of normal development. The situation often involves a breast that is excessively large and one that is abnormally small. One may have to operate on both to get some kind of symmetry.

On physical examination, one must look carefully for abnormalities of the chest wall, pectoral muscles, and spinal column, such as scoliosis.

Informing the patient depends on what has to be done: reduce or augment, one breast or both; whether to use inflatable or gel prostheses or an expander or whether to make a moulage of the chest and breast and insert something that will not only augment the breast but restore the chest wall to relative normalcy. It is almost impossible in a significant case of asymmetry to obtain perfection. Perfection in plastic surgery is more often the ideal than the reality. One should stress to the patient, and to the parents if the patient is a teenager, that the operation hopefully will give improvement but only seldom, if ever, perfection. As with augmentation mammaplasty, the patient and family must understand the possibility of infection, hematoma, abnormal contour, and firmness if indeed the small breast is to be enlarged. These patients require general anesthesia, possibly an overnight stay in the hospital, and a postoperative recovery period similar to that of the patient undergoing augmentation mammaplasty or reduction mammaplasty, if one breast has been reduced. The patient should wear a bra for the initial few weeks after the operation.

If an expander is to be used, the patient is informed of the necessity for serial injections of fluid after the insertion of the implant and eventual replacement of the inflatable expander with a permanent implant. Some expanders are permanent, but these have not yet been developed without problems.

REDUCTION MAMMAPLASTY

Reduction mammaplasty, which is being performed increasingly, combines features of both aesthetic and nonaesthetic surgery (Fig. 54-6).[13,14] Although there may be controversy about how to classify reduction mammaplasty, there is little argument that most patients are pleased with the results. Indeed, the more severe the problem, the happier the patient is postoperatively, unless a complication has occurred. The age of patients wanting this operation ranges from adolescent to postmenopausal. Most women with very large breasts consider their condition a deformity.[6] They feel conspicuous and resent being singled out for this aspect alone. They complain that men fixate on their breasts to the exclusion of their personality or intellect. Buying clothes is frustrating and expensive. Bras also are costly. Commonly, these women avoid athletics or going to the beach. Many dread the summer. Some adolescent patients give a history of avoiding male contact, of overeating, or of encouraging in themselves obesity almost so that their large breasts are in proportion to their overweight body. (This is one of the few situations in which the plastic surgeon would be advised not to have the patient lose weight before he or she operates; weight loss usually follows reduction because the patient is more pleased with herself and has already reached a goal that can be further maximized.)

Not uncommonly, the father or partner opposes the operation. Many men like women with large breasts, despite the fact that the women suffer from this encumbrance. Patients often complain of pain in their neck and upper back and pain in pulling over the shoulders in the bra strap line.

The surgeon who treats the female breast not only for this condition but for others must be aware that the patient could have cancer, and every means—careful physical examination, history, and mammography if the patient is 30 years or older (or even younger if the patient has a strong family history of breast cancer)—must be taken to rule out its presence.

The patient, and the family if the patient is a teenager, must be informed that the operation inevitably produces scars and can sometimes alter or decrease nipple-areolar sensation. In addition, bleeding and infection are possible, for which antibiotics are usually given perioperatively. Surgery can interfere with the blood supply to the nipple and areola. This is obviously true if the nipple-areola are taken as a graft, a procedure less commonly done today unless the breasts are extra large. Even with transposing the nipple and areola on the pedicle, it is possible that the blood supply will be compromised. This is more likely to happen in a patient who is a smoker. Smokers should be encouraged to stop smoking at least 3 weeks before the operation (and hopefully forever). Breast reduction decreases the likelihood of nursing from about 98% to approximately 70%. It is impossible to predict which patients will nurse and whether it will be from one or both breasts.

The surgeon should show patients examples of what is considered excellent, good, and poor scarring. It must be emphasized that scars do not disappear, although they usually become less prominent. The patient should also be told that this operation, with its scars, should be discussed between her and her partner. Occasionally, the partner adamantly opposes the operation, putting the plastic surgeon "in the middle." Although the patient obviously has the right to have the operation, it might be wise not to perform surgery until the dissension can be worked out between the woman and partner, perhaps through the intervention of a psychotherapist. If this is not done, the patient and her partner may unite in unjustly condemning the plastic surgeon for having performed an operation that has caused them marital problems.

In an effort to reduce the scarring of breast reduction, which can produce hypertrophic or keloidlike scars in the inframammary location or in any portion of the incision, a new technique known as vertical mammaplasty was developed. This method leaves no inframammary scar and has produced a favorable breast contour that is adaptable to most kinds of mammary hypertrophy. However, the final result is not apparent for weeks or months after the operation, and during this waiting period, the breast shape can be displeasing. The operation has been available throughout the nineties, especially in Europe, where it originated, but it has not become as popular in the United States as might be expected. It relies on a superiorly based pedicle rather than on the inferior one with which most American plastic surgeons are familiar. The technique also requires considerable experience with its multitude of intraoperative variations and modifications. Finally, having to reassure the patient that the initial breast appearance will improve considerably over time strains the surgeon-patient relationship.

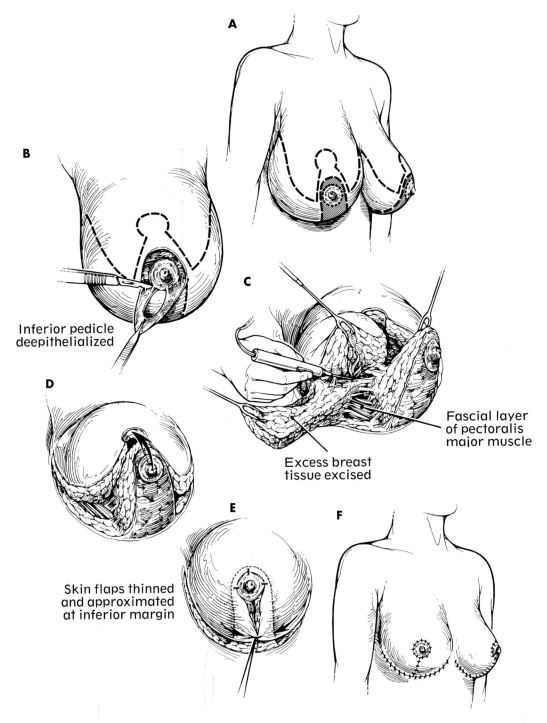

Fig. 54-6 **A,** Preoperative markings are similar to the technique for mastopexy. **B,** Deepithelialization of the inferior pedicle is performed. **C,** Excision of breast parenchyma from medial, lateral, and superior poles of the breast. Perforating vessels penetrating the inferior pedicle toward the nipple areolar complex are carefully preserved to maintain nipple vascularity. **D,** Reapproximation of the breast begins with elevation of the nipple to a more cephalad location. **E,** Excess skin is trimmed and contoured. **F,** Result demonstrates smaller size and improved contour after breast reduction.

In our practice, we almost never need to give a transfusion, but if it is a possibility, the patient should donate the blood herself (autotransfusion) so that it can be used at the time of surgery.

Insurance coverage must be discussed with patients. In-

surance plans have differing criteria, usually based on weight of tissue removed per breast. In Massachusetts, for example, Blue Cross/Blue Shield honors both the hospitalization and the surgeon's fee (without balance billing) if a weight of 300 g is removed per side. The patient and her family must determine their coverage, and the surgeon also should know whether the procedure and hospitalization will be covered. This can be a source of major disruption in the patient-doctor relationship. Increasingly, HMOs are requiring larger glandular removals to meet their own self-determined criteria for coverage. In extreme situations, some insurers will refuse to pay the hospital bill if the gram removal criteria—up to 700 g—are not proven on the patient's pathology report, in addition to rejecting the surgeon's fee.

The operation is almost always done under general anesthesia, and the patient will spend a day or two in the hospital. There is pressure on the surgeon as well as the patient to have the procedure done on an ambulatory basis. This is difficult for the patient, who needs careful watching postoperatively as well as medication to relieve pain. The operation generally lasts 3 to 4 hours.

Although most patients who have reduction mammaplasty are ultimately satisfied with the results, not every women is joyful immediately after operation. Despite their complaints about the large size of their breasts, some women experience transitory depression as a result of having their "badge" (although unwelcomed) of femininity removed. Many patients say they do not want to look at their incisions when their dressing is changed for the first time, but most eventually do. The reluctance to view their operative site is not only because of the presence of blood and stitches but also because of their need to accommodate to a new body image. In most patients, this takes just a few weeks.

Before the operation, the surgeon must know approximately what size the patient wants her breasts to be. No guaranteed size should be given, but one should hopefully achieve a size that pleases the patient. When in doubt, the surgeon should take less rather than more because it is always easier to take out more later than it is to enlarge the breast if one has been too zealous in performing the reduction.

Postoperatively, patients usually return to work in 2 weeks, although they are usually asked not to drive for 1 week and not to lift heavy bundles for 2 weeks. They are also usually told not to resume physical activity for 3 to 5 weeks, depending on what they wish to do and the surgeon's preferences.

If a women develops a mass after the operation, the surgeon or any physician who sees the patient must evaluate it carefully. It may be scar tissue, fat necrosis, or a reaction to a suture that has absorbed or is absorbing. A persistent lump, however, even in the presence of histologically normal tissue, may move during operation and requires a biopsy, particularly if the mass makes its appearance a few months later. Although mammograms are helpful, only the pathologist can provide the precise diagnosis.

CASE REPORT

A 26-year-old unmarried women with bilateral mammary hyperplasia was evaluated for reduction mammoplasty. She complained of neck, shoulder, and back pain in association with her extremely hyperplastic breasts. The patient confided that she was embarrassed by her appearance, lacked self-esteem, and generally avoided social interaction with men.

Her preoperative mammograms demonstrated dense glandular tissue but not abnormalities. On physical examination (Fig. 54-7), she was noted to have significant mammary hyperplasia, ptosis, and asymmetry. Her breast size was severely disproportionate for her slender frame of 5 feet 3 inches tall and 103 pounds. Bilateral reduction mammaplasties were performed with correction of the ptosis and asymmetry deformities. A final breast size of approximately a size B cup bra, as had been discussed with the patient preoperatively, was achieved (Fig. 54-8). Her satisfaction with the surgical result has been accompanied by psychological benefits of improved body image and social adaptation. ▲

SELECTING A MASTECTOMY INCISION— SKIN-SPARING MASTECTOMY TECHNIQUES

Optimal selection of an incision for mastectomy, whether it be simple or modified radical, requires close cooperation and careful planning by the surgeon performing the mastectomy and the plastic surgeon. Until the advent of skin-sparing mastectomy, most plastic surgeons preferred a low transverse or oblique incision because it preserved the integrity of the infraclavicular, medial, and superior native breast skin flaps. Moreover, it was less socially conspicuous and much more acceptable to patients. As breast conservation became the accepted method of treatment for early-stage breast cancer, patients began to compare both the oncologic and aesthetic results of two rival techniques: conservation with radiotherapy administered postoperatively versus mastectomy. Recognizing the supreme importance of the role of the skin brassiere in providing a satisfactory breast shape, plastic surgeons collaborated with their general surgical colleagues performing breast operations to modify mastectomy incisions. Beginning with smaller elliptical excisions around the nipple-areolar complex, these skin-preserving techniques have evolved into the popular periareolar (circular) mastectomy incision. This evolution developed out of the recognition that local recurrence is not related to the extent of the skin excision but rather to individual tumor biology. Studies have demonstrated that local recurrence is not increased by skin-sparing mastectomy using only a 5-mm border of normal skin around the nipple-areolar complex.

It is clear that mammary ducts can enter the areolar in an eccentric instead of a central direction. To completely excise ductal orifices and their epithelium, the areola must be sacrificed despite earlier attempts to save a thin core. Skin-sparing mastectomy's minimal incisions represent a natural outgrowth of confluent events influencing all aspects of surgical and surgical specialty practice. As endoscopic approaches have been refined for procedures as diverse as cholecystectomy and splenectomy to oophorectomy, more surgeons are reducing intraoperative scarring as they embrace these technological advances. The dovetailing of endoscopic surgery, minimal incisions, and breast conserva-

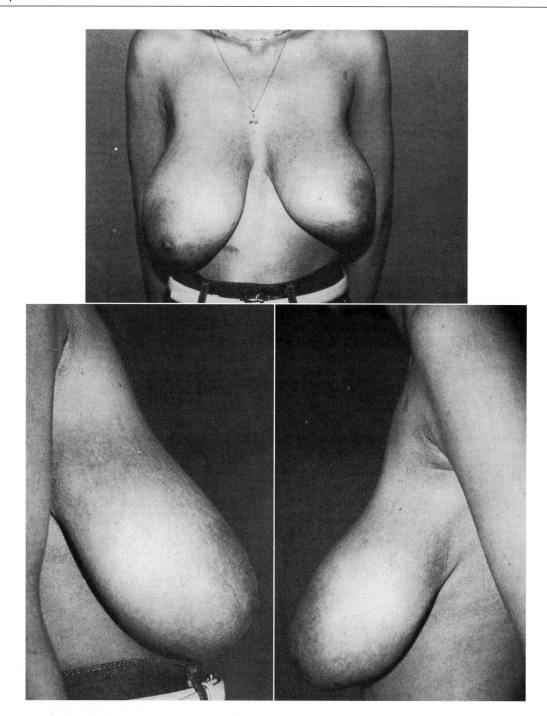

Fig. 54-7 Preoperative appearance of a 26-year-old woman with severe mammary hyperplasia, ptosis, and asymmetry.

tion has created a new generation of patients who eschew the disfigurement of large scars. If for no other reason than patient-driven consumerism, skin-sparing mastectomy has become established as the standard operative technique for the performance of mastectomy. It is particularly applicable to the increasing number of patients with ductal carcinoma in situ and early-stage breast cancer.

Despite these significant advances, wound complications have not been eliminated. Skin-sparing mastectomy techniques are prone to partial- or full-thickness necrosis of the native skin flaps, a complication that can result in the exposure or extrusion of an underlying implant. Even when a myocutaneous flap is providing soft tissue for breast glandular replacement, loss of skin adversely impacts the cosmetic result. Most breast cancer surgeons will be challenged initially by such a limited approach to the breast parenchyma, especially in patients with large breasts. Endoscopic or fiber optic instruments have facilitated the dissection in such instances, even allowing access to the axilla from the periareolar incision.

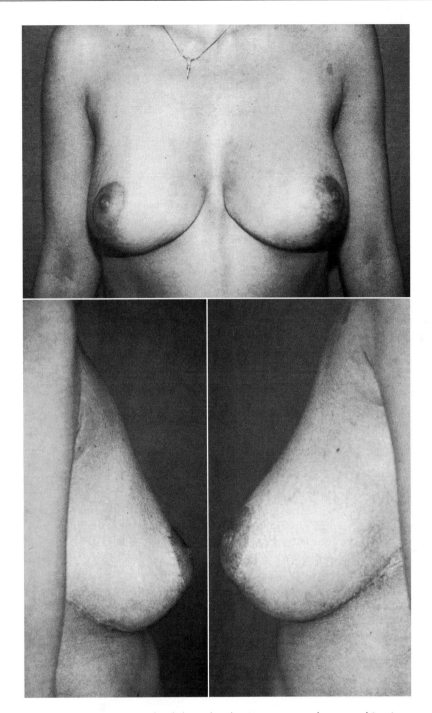

Fig. 54-8 Appearance 1 year after bilateral reduction mammoplasty, resulting in more appropriate breast size for patient's torso and alleviation of ptosis and asymmetry.

Re-creation of the breast's natural ptosis is also enhanced by these lower incisions. Any suture closure technique that leaves obtrusive suture marks on both borders of the incision should be avoided. In our experience the best technique has been a subcuticular, running nonabsorbable suture, usually of Prolene because of its tissue sliding properties. This can be removed in its entirety approximately 10 to 14 days later. Layered closures, which approximate the dermis with fine absorbable suture material (e.g., 5-0 Vicryl) may enhance the final scar appearance.

A number of factors can adversely affect incision placement. Breast lesions present along the medial, superior, or superolateral borders of the breast are the least favorable situations. When the tumor persists along the edges of wide excisional biopsies, encompassment of these incisions within the mastectomy incisional lines may result in a significant alteration of the anticipated scar. Extension of the incision medially onto parasternal or even sternal skin surface invites the formation of hypertrophic and keloidlike scar appearances. If possible, these types of incisional designs should be avoided. Similarly, incisions that extend superiorly to the axilla or infraclavicular hollow pose major aesthetic problems during breast reconstruction. Often, the prosthesis or flap appears displaced and unnatural. Because the efficacy of mastectomy in controlling or curing breast cancer supercedes all aesthetic considerations, unfavorably located incisions may accompany the removal of any lesion located outside of the lower pole or periareolar locations. The patient should be informed of these possibilities preoperatively so that she can anticipate a less-than-optimal scar placement or configuration.

Patients should also be informed of other local factors that can negatively influence the aesthetic result. The actual performance of the mastectomy may be associated with significant contour irregularities such as dimpling, retraction, thinning, atrophy, or inadvertent perforation of the cutaneous surface of the chest wall. In such instances the reconstruction can appear flawed. Postoperatively, skin necrosis and local wound infections contribute to widened scars healed by secondary intention or skin surfaces discolored by partial-thickness loss.

BREAST RECONSTRUCTION

Although the goal of breast reconstruction is to restore the patient to a more normal physical appearance, no procedure ever re-creates the unique aesthetic qualities and characteristics of a natural breast. However, the benefits of breast reconstruction far exceed considerations of anatomic form. Psychological benefits,[12,38] including improved self-image, have been documented by many authors. Most women describe a sense of well-being and self-confidence after undergoing such procedures. A diminished fear of the mutilation of mastectomy has been shown to encourage patients to seek earlier diagnosis and treatment for breast lesions. As breast reconstructive procedures have improved and the number of available techniques has increased accordingly, it seems likely that more women will choose from these reconstructive options.

Immediate versus Delayed Reconstruction

Until the last decade, most breast cancer patients were advised to forego breast reconstruction until some mandatory period of cancer surveillance had been completed. This philosophy of delaying the reconstructive procedure for some period, usually in the order of 5 years, was based not only out of concern that a combined mastectomy and reconstructive procedure was too formidable and stressful a surgical undertaking, but also out of fear that cancer recurrence might be concealed by the presence of the reconstructed breast. Fortunately, these fears have receded as evidence has emerged that recurrences can be expeditiously detected in the presence of the reconstructed breast. Although not all physicians are completely convinced, most oncologists support breast reconstruction undertaken immediately after completion of the mastectomy or delayed some period of months thereafter. The actual period of delay may be influenced by issues of wound healing or the necessity for adjuvant chemotherapy or radiation therapy. The leukopenia and thrombocytopenia of most chemotherapy regimens require waiting until normal cell levels have been achieved. Radiation therapy, now being given less commonly on a postoperative basis, significantly influences the selection of a reconstructive procedure and is reviewed elsewhere in this chapter.

The two-stage procedure—mastectomy followed by delayed reconstruction—remains popular with many plastic surgeons who cite the greater control over local wound conditions and the enhanced results that they can obtain. Immediate reconstruction may be associated with increased wound complications, such as skin necsosis, infection, hematoma, and exposure or extrusion of a prosthetic device. Nevertheless, immediate reconstruction has evolved to a point of proven safety.[10,26] It does require strenuous efforts by both the cancer surgeon and the plastic surgeon to plan and coordinate the two procedures. As the option of immediate breast reconstruction becomes more available to patients confronted by mastectomy, the trend toward choosing immediate reconstruction, observed in our practice for the past 10 years, will probably continue.

Neither term—*immediate* or *delayed reconstruction*—denotes a specific reconstructive technique. All procedures, including implants, inflatable expanders, and myocutaneous and microvascular flaps, can be performed on either basis. Although plastic surgeons initially preferred the simplest technique, insertion of a silicone implant beneath the pectoralis muscle for immediate breast reconstruction, improved inflatable expanders, and complex flap procedures have been reported as successful choices for immediate reconstruction.[7] More than any other factor, availability of skin and soft tissues on the chest wall determines the technique. The anatomy of the contralateral breast, if such exists, may also be a prime factor. In most patients, more than one breast reconstruction technique is appropriate for the patient's needs. The plastic surgeon who is most familiar with all of the available surgical options can customize the technique to the patient's unique reconstructive requirements.

Breast Reconstruction Techniques

Silicone Implants. The modern era of breast reconstruction began with the introduction of silicone implants made of medical grade dimethyl polysiloxane approximately 30 years ago. Although the silicone implant has undergone considerable modification since then and now includes an array of products that may or may not contain separate additional chambers for insertion of saline, the basis product has a silicone outer shell and liquid silicone fill. Recently, concern has focused on the issue of carcinogenicity, but no proven relationship exists between these products and breast cancer.

Originally placed subcutaneously, implants are now routinely placed in a subpectoral location.[3,39] Added coverage from the adjacent serratus anterior muscle and rectus fascia permits total enclosure in a myofascial envelope. When these elements of the chest wall are absent or the remaining chest wall skin at the mastectomy site is excessively tight and scarred, placement of the implant may be contraindicated. Ideal candidates for a silicone implant are women with a smaller breast size and healthy skin and soft tissues and no previous history of radiation therapy to the operative site.

Unlike augmentation mammaplasty, which can be performed under local or general anesthesia, dissection of the chest wall musculature almost always requires a general anesthetic. Given the relative paucity of soft tissues that characterizes most postmastectomy deformities, the procedure may be subject to complications of wound healing caused by skin necrosis, wound infection, exposure of the prosthesis, and ultimately extrusion. When compelled by local wound factors to remove the device, most plastic surgeons choose a different technique for subsequent reconstructive attempts. From an aesthetic view, silicone implants yield breasts that are small, rounded, and sometimes lacking definition in the area of the inframammary crease. The natural ptotic qualities of a normal breast may be absent. The simplicity of the technique is appealing to both the patient and plastic surgeon, and the quality of the match for a women with smaller breasts is usually satisfactory to excellent.

The major problem encountered with silicone implants is encapsulation, a process marked by deposition of fibrous tissue in a circumferential manner about the implant. A number of factors, including migration of molecules of silicone across the outer membrane of the posthesis, have been iden-tified in the causation of this process, but surface characteristics of the prosthesis and its interaction with surrounding local tissues appear to predominate.[2,5,17] Research directed at the surface kinetics and histology of the fibrous capsule suggests that alteration of the implant's outer envelope may reduce the incidence of encapsulation. Newer products (Fig. 54-9) designed to counteract the process of fibrous deposition contain roughened surfaces of textured silicone or are coated with a polyurethane foam to permit ingrowth of fibroblasts. Proof of the efficacy of such products remains elusive.

Inflatable Expanders. Recognition of the elastic and expandible qualities of skin and application of these concepts to the field of breast reconstruction were pioneered by a number of investigators during the past decade.[1,11,27] Specifically, the development of a hollow silicone device that could be injected percutaneously with saline in a step-wise manner (usually by weekly injections) represented a watershed breakthrough for the postmastectomy patient with tight skin and inadequate chest wall soft tissues. The device is inserted in a retropectoral position, just as is done for placement of a single implant (Fig. 54-10). As with all breast reconstruction techniques, inflatable expanders can be used on an immediate or delayed basis. The technique, called skin-expansion breast reconstruction, stretches the available cutaneous and muscular layers through weekly injections of saline in volumes averaging 50 to 75 ml. A process of skin expansion encompasing 12 weeks of injection, followed by

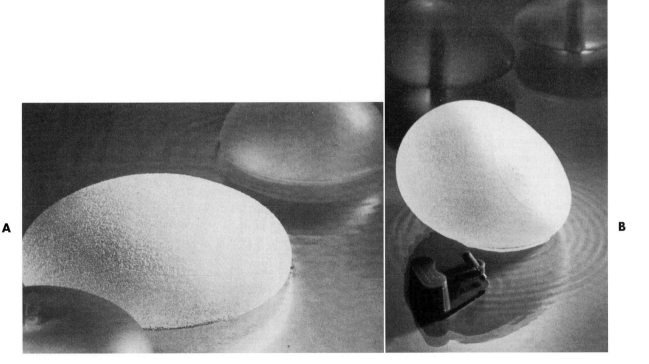

Fig. 54-9   A, Newer style of silicone implant has a roughened or textured surface designed to promote ingrowth of fibroblasts and decrease encapsulation. **B,** Inflatable expander with textured surface.

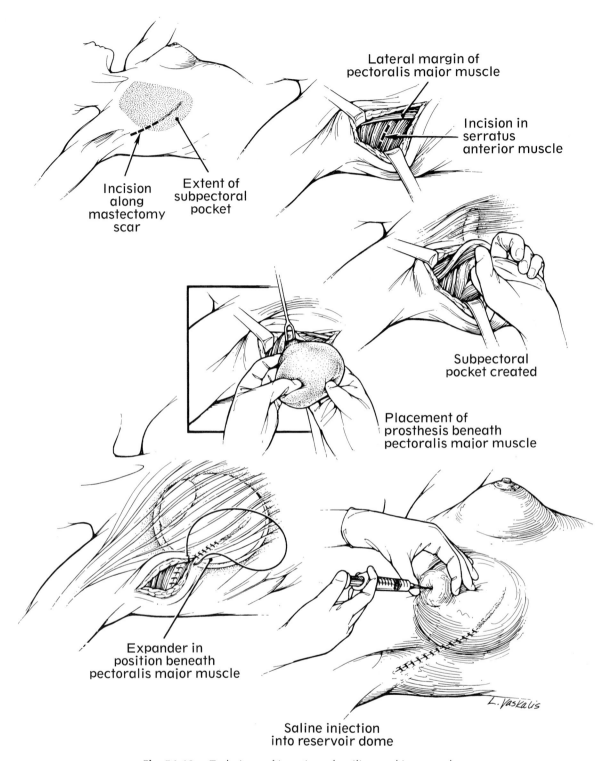

Lateral margin of
pectoralis major muscle

Incision in
serratus
anterior muscle

Incision
along
mastectomy
scar

Extent of
subpectoral
pocket

Subpectoral
pocket created

Placement of
prosthesis beneath
pectoralis major muscle

Expander in
position beneath
pectoralis major muscle

Saline injection
into reservoir dome

L. Vaskalis

Fig. 54-10 Technique of insertion of a silicone skin expander.

a sustained period of full inflation for 1 to 3 months, is the most common regimen. During the time of serial weekly injections or saline into a defined port valve located within or adjacent to the actual expander reservoir, the patient observes a full panorama of breast sizes evolving. The technique not only allows the patient to visualize these different sizes on the chest wall and select an optimal configuration based on this preview, but also deliberately overexpands the

skin and its underlying layers. After full saline expansion has been performed, a second operation involving removal of the expander and placement of the permanent implant completes the breast reconstruction. Because the final silicone implant is smaller than the maximal volume of saline used for expansion, an excess of skin and underlying muscle results. Unlike the original tissues at the start of the process, the final tissues have an augmented microcirculation. The expansion process is believed to inhibit capsule formation and provide durable and supple soft tissue coverage for the prosthesis. This technique appears to be appropriate for women requiring a breast of virtually any size; it has been particularly well suited for women in the mid to full breast size (bra size B or C) range. Some physicians have achieved the creation of extremely large breasts through filling the inflatable expander reservoirs up to volumes of 1000 ml or greater. Numerous modifications to the original inflatable expander design have occurred, including the addition of a textured surface, a self-enclosed valvular mechanism, preferential lower pole directional expansion, and a device that can be permanently left in place without silicone implant substitution.[3]

Despite its purported advantages, the inflatable expander has had its limitations. In general, it has not been proven suitable for placement in an irradiated field. These tissues not only lack the requisite vascularity for adequate wound healing over the device but also develop a fibrotic rigidity, which resists stretching. Nonradiated wounds have not been immune to complications. In some series, an overall complication rate of approximately 40% has been reported, with skin necrosis, infection, hematoma, seroma, and extrusion predominating.[22,25] Some patients require removal of the inflatable expander from an infected field and replacement after secondary wound healing is completed. Under these circumstances the aggregate number of procedures needed for the breast reconstruction may approach three (instead of two) in some instances.[32] Most plastic surgeons choose to reconstruct the nipple-areolar complex as a separate operation rather than add it to the final stage of the skin expansion breast reconstruction. General anesthesia is routinely used at each stage of the process, but hospitalization can usually be brief, involving a 1- or 2-day stay.

CASE REPORT

A 46-year-old woman was evaluated for bilateral breast reconstruction (Fig. 54-11, *A*). Three years earlier, she had undergone a left mastectomy for lobular carcinoma. A mirror biopsy on the right side was initially negative, but a subsequent excision also revealed lobular carcinoma, necessitating a right mastectomy. Her nodes tested negative on both sides, and no additional therapy was recommended. At the time of her consultation, she had bilateral postmastectomy defects characterized by tight skin. Her former breast size had been a bra size C, and she requested breast reconstructions of similar size. The first stage of the reconstruction was accomplished by placement of a 700-ml inflatable expander under bilateral pectoralis major serratus anterior muscle flaps. A 3-month course of weekly saline percutaneous injections of 60 ml into each expander reservoir was followed by the second-stage procedure. The expanders were removed, and 360-ml gel implants were inserted. One month after placement of gel implants, bilateral nipple-areolar complex reconstructions were performed as the third and final procedure (see Fig. 54-11, *B*).   ▲

From an aesthetic view, the result achieved with an inflatable expander is deemed superior to simple insertion (one stage) of a breast implant. Nevertheless, defects in breast contour, including a deficient inframammary crease, inadequate lower pole contour, and excess upper pole fullness, may be notable. Breast ptosis, although surpassing that of an implant, may be modest. To improve breast asymmetry, many plastic surgeons have found it necessary to alter the contralateral breast by means of an improving procedure, either an augmentation, reduction, or mastopexy, in more than half of their patients. Inflatable expanders, unlike flaps, preserve other areas of the body from use as potential donor sites, thereby reducing the total amount of scarring incurred. Encapsulation and its attendant deformity of breast shape appear lessened. The procedure has achieved its most satisfying results when bilateral breast reconstructions are necessary and the complex problems of symmetry with the contralateral breast do not exist.

Myocutaneous Flap. Myocutaneous flaps are composites of skin, subcutaneous fat, and muscle supplied by one or more dominant vascular pedicles. Although every muscle is potentially a flap donor site, not all are suitable for transfer. Depending on the specific donor site selected, myocutaneous flaps can consist of varying amounts of skin, fat, fascia, muscle, and bone. Some of the more common units were recognized for centuries, but the ability to transfer them with an intact blood supply was developed in the 1970s. Mobilization of these flaps requires careful preservation and dissection of the vascular pedicle to prevent any interruption of flow. Despite the abundance of myocutaneous flaps described for reconstruction or areas injured by neoplasm, infection, trauma, and radiation, two units—the latissimus and the rectus myocutaneous flaps—deserve special recognition.

Latissimus Dorsi Myocutaneous Flap. Considered the workhorse favorite of myocutaneous flaps, the latissimus dorsi flap (Fig. 54-12) is preferred for its proven safety, ample size, and superb vascularity.[4,23] Although recognized as the body's largest motor unit, the latissimus dorsi muscle is actually an expandable mass of soft tissue. Despite its location on the back, the muscle functions as a shoulder rotator. The extensive cutaneous surface overlying the muscle is vascularized by a multitude of direct perforating vessels that traverse the subcutaneous fat superficial to the muscle to enter the skin above. A dominant vascular pedicle, the thoracodorsal artery and vein, enter the hilum of the muscle in association with its motor innervation, the thoracodorsal nerve.

During the transfer of the flap, or "transposition" as it is customarily designated, the latissimus dorsi muscle is elevated off the posterior chest wall by dividing most, but not necessarily all, of its attachments to structures of origin and insertion. Its vascular pedicle is identified and carefully preserved throughout the procedure. Depending on the extent of dissection of the pedicle and its actual length, the muscle can be mobilized with portions of the overlying fat and skin. The cutaneous attachment is usually designed as an ellipse of varying dimensions; patients with redundant skin of the back will permit transfers of cutaneous islands large enough

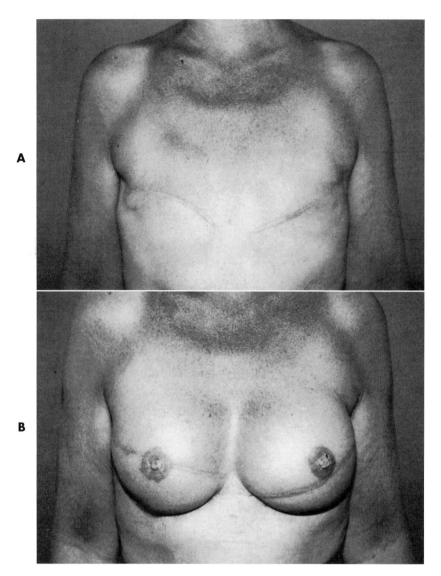

Fig. 54-11 **A,** A 46-year-old woman who underwent bilateral mastectomies for lobular carcinoma. **B,** Appearance of the patient after completion of a two-stage procedure using inflatable expanders.

to resurface extensive wounds. Closure of the elliptical skin defect creates a linear scar that tends to be located transversely in the area of the bra strap (see Fig. 54-12, *E*). Virtually any part of the ipsilateral hemithorax is accessible with this flap, as are defects involving sternum and proximal portions of the contralateral chest.

The latissimus dorsi myocutaneous flap has proven to be particularly useful for most postmastectomy defects. Its large expanse of muscle re-creates the natural fullness and contour of the pectoralis major muscle and anterior axillary fold when these structures are absent, while simultaneously providing a soft tissue complement to areas of deficiency in the infraclavicular hollow and the anterior axilla. Even the most formidale defect, such as the washboard chest deformity of a radical mastectomy, can be satisfactorily reconstructed with this technique. Placement of a silicone implant beneath the muscle enhances the breastlike contour of the flap unit while simultaneously facilitating the creation of a

breast of any desired size. Patients with radiated wounds and with extreme soft tissue loss are excellent candidates for reconstruction with this technique.[19] Loss of the latissimus muscle as a functioning motor unit is easily compensated by the remaining shoulder rotators. Most important, this myocutaneous flap has been distinguished by the reliability of its blood supply and a low incidence of either complete or partial necrosis. It is appropriate for use in any wound with diminished vascularity.

The addition of new skin, imported from the back and transferred by means of the cutaneous island of the flap, permits reconstruction of chest wall areas severely constricted by scarring after mastectomy. Latissimus flaps create a reconstructed breast with distinctly visible qualities of ptosis. For women who require a larger breast form, the latissimus reconstruction provides an excellence of symmetry and ptosis that matches the pendulousness of a generously proportioned remaining breast.

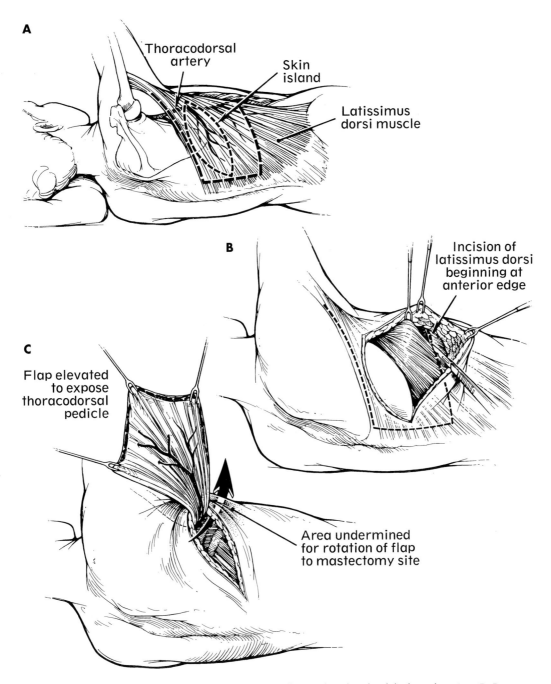

Fig. 54-12   **A,** Latissimus dorsi myocutaneous flap outlined on back before elevation. **B,** Borders of the latissimus dorsi muscle are elevated off the posterior chest wall by sharp dissection. **C,** The entire myocutaneous flap has been elevated. It will be transposed to the anterior chest wall by passing it subcutaneously beneath intact lateral chest wall skin.

Continued

This versatile myocutaneous flap has proven to be equally applicable for breast reconstruction undertaken on an immediate or delayed basis. The patient scheduled for immediate reconstruction must be alternately shifted from the supine position of mastectomy to a lateral decubitus position for the latissimus flap. The donor site is closed, and the patient is returned to a supine position. Some plastic surgeons prefer delayed reconstruction because it allows them to situate the flap in a precise and optimal manner on the chest wall. When a large amount of skin or large portions of the pectoralis muscle have been resected, the latissimus flap amply supplies the requisite tissues.

A major disadvantage of this technique is the encapsulation around the submuscular silicone prosthesis that normally accompanies the flap procedure. Although the exact incidence of this problem has not been determined, it occurs with enough frequency to compromise the result achieved.[24] Encapsulation may develop within months or years after the

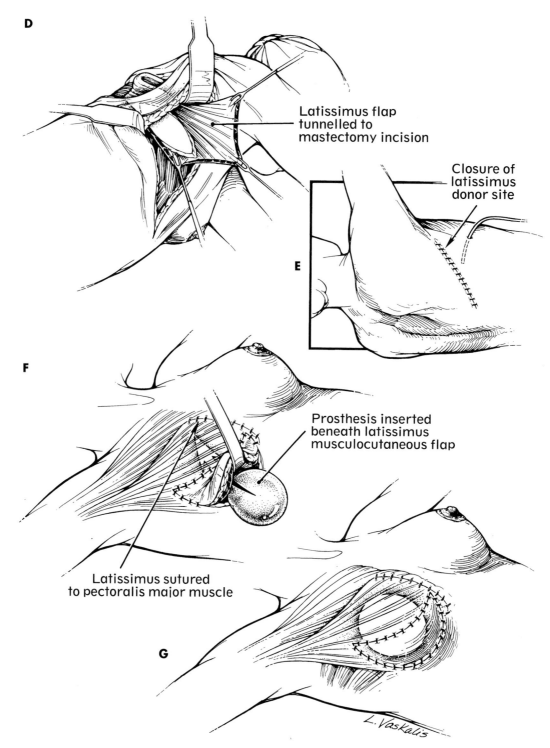

D

Latissimus flap
tunnelled to
mastectomy incision

Closure of
latissimus
donor site

E

Prosthesis inserted
beneath latissimus
musculocutaneous flap

Latissimus sutured
to pectoralis major muscle

F

G

L. Vaskalis

Fig. 54-12, cont'd **D,** Latissimus dorsi transposed anteriorly and sutured to anterior chest wall. **E,** Back donor site is closed after placement of suction catheters. **F,** An appropriately sized saline prosthesis is inserted beneath the flap but anterior to the pectoralis muscle. **G,** The flap is shaped to approximate the contralateral breast.

procedure, causing the reconstructed breast to be unnaturally firm in its consistency and distorted in contour. This process has been observed around different types of breast prosthesis, including a new model group with a roughened or textured surface. The hardened breast is characterized by pain,

superior pole prominence, and retraction of the entire reconstruction to a more cephalad position on the chest wall. Removal of the prosthesis, surgical incision of the fibrous capsule (or excision), and replacement with a different type of prosthesis sometimes can alleviate this unfavorable result.

Other objections to the latissimus flap point to differences in color tone and consistency between back and chest wall skin. Back skin tends to be slightly darker in tone and thicker than its anterior counterpart.

Complications. Seroma is by far the most common complication observed after latissimus dorsi breast reconstruction, developing in 20% or more patients.[30] The serous fluid accumulates in dependent portions of the back donor site wound and can cause pain or contribute to wound dehiscence. There is no agreement as to the optimal management of this problem, but many plastic surgeons aspirate large collections as an office procedure; smaller volumes of fluid gradually and spontaneously resorb. Infections appear to be uncommon problems, attesting to the superb vascularity of the flap and its elimination of scar and skin tension at the recipient site. Likewise, hematomas are unusual after this procedure. However, care must be taken to ensure that vessels along the border and undersurface of the latissimus muscle have been properly controlled. Dehiscence of the back donor site wound is unusual, but lesser degrees of wound separation are more common and tend to heal uneventfully. As mentioned, complete necrosis or even partial necrosis of the flap is rarely encountered.

CASE REPORT

A 41-year-old woman underwent a left mastectomy for infiltrating ductal carcinoma. Two nodes were positive, and a course of chemotherapy was commenced after the mastectomy. Two years after mastectomy, she was evaluated for reconstruction of the left breast. During the consultation, the patient requested that the opposite breast be lifted but that its size (bra size C) be maintained. On physical examination, she was noted to have a significant left-sided chest depression deformity characterized by an absence of skin and subcutaneous tissues (Fig. 54-13, *A*). Flexion of the pectoralis muscles revealed that the entire lower half of the left pectoralis either had been removed or was scarred and atrophic (see Fig. 54-13, *B*). Based on this finding, she was considered an unsatisfactory candidate for placement of a subpectoral implant or expander. Despite a slim body habitus and scarcity of abdominal soft tissues, she had adequate laxity of the skin overlying the left latissimus dorsi muscle. A latissimus dorsi myocutaneous flap breast reconstruction was performed with insertion of a 260-ml gel implant beneath the myocutaneous flap complex. Three months later, a right mastopexy was done in conjunction with a left nipple areolar reconstruction (see Fig. 54-13, *C*). ▲

Transverse Rectus Abdominis Myocutaneous Flap (TRAM Flap). The transverse rectus abdominis myocutaneous flap (Fig. 54-14) consists of a cutaneous island of abdominal skin attached to an underlying rectus abdominis muscle.[8,16] Usually, the cutaneous island is oriented transversely as an ellipse of varying sizes. It can incorporate upper, mid, or lower abdominal skin and extends as far laterally as the anterior superior iliac spine. Mobilization of this complex flap requires elevation of a rectus muscle with careful inclusion of the deep epigastric arterial pedicle located on its undersurface. A large subcutaneous tunnel is dissected between the abdominal donor site and the chest wall wound, which allows transposition of the flap to its new site. The flap's blood supply is derived from the internal mammary artery and its continuation beyond costal margin as the superior deep epigastric artery. Any encroachment of the internal mammary artery, by either surgical interruption or radiation injury, compromises the vascularity of the flap. In the absence of such factors, the TRAM flap is noteworthy for providing a large, well-vascularized mass of soft tissue. Abdominal fat included with the cutaneous island is strongly similar in consistency to breast tissue.

Because this particular myocutaneous flap provides such an abundance of tissue borrowed from the abdomen, it concomitantly creates a formidable defect at the donor site. After transposition of the flap, it is necessary to approximate residual fascial layers of anterior and posterior rectus sheath to avoid subsequent hernia formation. Additional buttressing of the abdominal closure has been achieved by placement of a sheet of synthetic mesh or by mobilization of adjacent flaps of external oblilque muscle. The entire operation may be lengthy and difficult.

Despite such obstacles of execution, the rectus abdominis myocutaneous flap is appropriate for reconstruction of most postmastectomy deformities. For extensive wounds of the chest wall characterized by osteomyelitis and radiation injuries, the rectus flap supplies a vast surface area of skin. The underpinning of this flap—the rectus muscle—is well suited to healing complex wounds injured by tumor, infection, or radiation. The entire procedure is performed with the patient in a supine position, an advantage for both immediate and delayed breast reconstruction. Like the latissimus flap, the rectus flap is also well suited for reconstruction of a radical mastectomy defect. Some plastic surgeons consider it a superior choice, based primarily on its abundant soft tissues and ease of filling areas of axillary and infraclavicular hollowing. The rectus flap is rouitinely used for total and modified radical mastectomy defects that require a moderate or large breast reconstruction for matching the contralateral side.[33] Elimination of the need for a breast implant, with its associated problems of encapsulation, is considered a major advantage of the technique.

Although a single-pedicled rectus flap is sufficient for most problems in breast reconstruction, augmentation of the flap and its blood supply has been accomplished by inclusion of the other rectus muscle. These double-pedicled rectus flaps are designed with a single overlying elliptical skin island.[18] They are most appropriate for salvage mastectomy in patients who have osteoradionecrosis of ribs and sternum with large associated skin deficiencies.

Complications. Given the complexity of this procedure, it is not surprising that an array of complications have been reported. Flap loss constitutes the most serious complication, followed by varying degrees of partial loss. The exact incidence of this complication is unknown, but it occurs

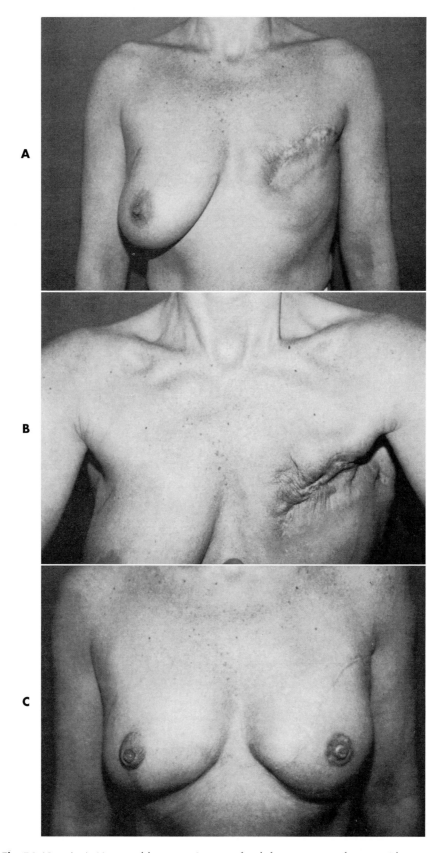

Fig. 54-13 **A,** A 41-year-old woman 2 years after left mastectomy for stage I breast cancer. **B,** During active contraction of the left pectoralis muscle, the lower pole of the muscle is noted to be absent. When significant portions of the pectoralis have been removed with the breast, the remaining muscle may provide inadequate soft tissue coverage for an implant or expander. **C,** Appearance of the patient after left-breast reconstruction using a latissimus flap and placement of an implant beneath the flap. A right mastopexy was also performed, as was left-nipple-areolar reconstruction.

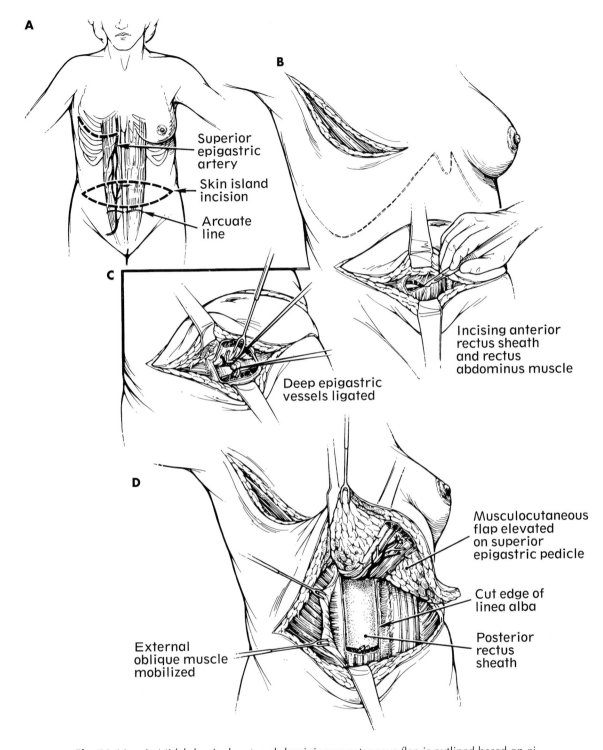

Fig. 54-14   **A,** Midabdominal rectus abdominis myocutaneous flap is outlined based on either the right or left deep superior epigastric arterial system. **B,** In this example the right rectus abdominis muscle is divided at the lower border of the flap. **C,** The deep epigastric vessels located on the undersurface of the rectus abdominis muscle are individually ligated. **D,** The entire transverse island rectus abdominis myocutaneous flap (TRAM flap) is elevated and transposed through a subcutaneous tunnel to the mastectomy site.   *Continued*

with enough frequency to warrant significant concern. Some plastic surgeons have attempted to select patients who are deemed to be high risk, but it is unclear precisely which patients are poor candidates. Obese patients, diabetic patients, and smokers have all been implicated. Pretreatment of these

patients using exercise regimens or corticosteroids has not been proven effective. Why some flaps develop complete or partial necrosis is not well understood, but vasospasm, venous obstruction, and microcirculatory failure have all been attributed. Strengthening of the pedicle by inclusion of the

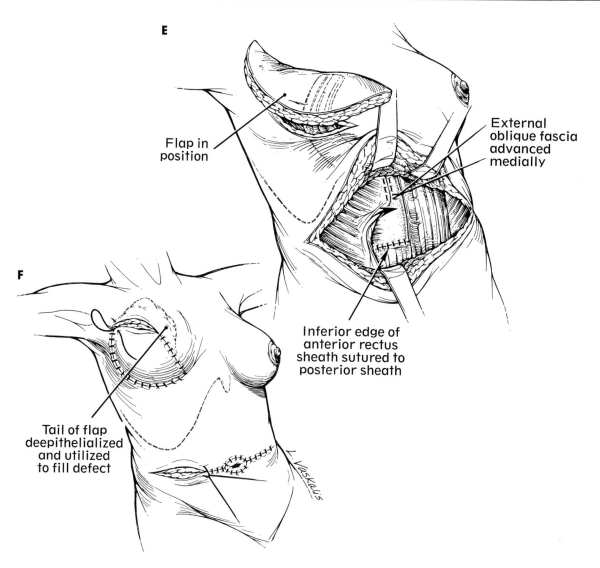

E

Flap in position

External oblique fascia advanced medially

Inferior edge of anterior rectus sheath sutured to posterior sheath

F

Tail of flap deepithelialized and utilized to fill defect

Fig. 54-14, cont'd **E,** Complete fascial closure of the donor defect is achieved by suturing the remaining anterior rectus sheath to the posterior sheath. The external oblique muscle is advanced medially to create a layered, stronger closure. Synthetic mesh is sometimes required to strengthen the closure. **F,** The flap is shaped and sutured to the chest wall. The abdominal donor site is closed and usually sutured with running subcuticular nonabsorbable monofilament.

opposite rectus muscle appears to create a flap of improved vascularity. In addition to double-pedicled vascular augmentation, microsurgical techniques have been tried that connect the inferior deep epigastric artery to a separate source of blood supply on the lateral chest wall. This particular method, called turbocharging the flap, results in a rectus flap with dual blood supply through the superior and inferior deep epigastric arteries.[15] Although successful for selected cases, it exposes the patient to a significantly lengthened operating room time and to the perils of a failed microvascular anastomosis.

Major problems of abdominal wall competence have occurred after rectus flap breast reconstruction. Mobilization of the rectus muscle with its anterior fascial sheath exposes the underlying posterior rectus to the forces of intraabdomi-

nal pressure. Although intact, this posterior fascial layer may become so severely attenuated in some middle-aged and older patients that a transitional zone of progressive fascial thinning extending from the level of the umbilicus to the arcuate line is observed. Extremely atrophied fascia is often located just cephalad to the arcuate line. This area of the abdomen, previously occupied by the muscle and its vigorous anterior sheath, constitutes a definite zone of vulnerability for subsequent hernia formation. Postoperative hernia incidence has ranged from 1% to 20%; concomitant loss of abdominal wall strength is another expected sequela of the procedure.[35] Patients need to be advised that the important spinal flexion function served by the paired rectus muscles is impaired by removal of either or both motor units. Postoperatively, patients may experience a decreased ability to elevate the head while lying supine or may have difficulty getting up from a sitting or lying position. Many patients spontaneously develop a number of compensatory mechanisms, such as grasping of a knee with both hands or rolling onto a side, to expedite rising from a reclining position. All patients should be examined carefully after the operation for signs of abdominal wall laxity or incompetence, which can predispose them to worsened abdominal wall function or outright herniation. In particular, patients with an established history of lower back pain who have required medical or surgical intervention for treatment may be unsuitable candidates for a rectus flap procedure. Finally, women of childbearing age should be informed of the paucity of information available regarding any increased risk during pregnancy or labor resulting from loss of portions of the rectus musculature. A case report[15] documented successful labor and delivery in one patient who had undergone previous rectus flap breast reconstruction, but more detailed information is lacking. Despite that apparently favorable outcome, some plastic surgeons are reluctant to recommend this procedure for women of childbearing age.

Other complications occurring after rectus flap procedures are fat necrosis, infection, hematoma, seroma, wound healing complications, and umbilical necrosis. When the flap is elevated on a single muscular pedicle, the contralateral portion of the transverse skin ellipse must derive its blood supply through a series of crossover myocutaneous perforators. Therefore the ipsilateral hemiellipse of skin has a superiority of blood flow compared with the marginal vascularity of the more distal (contralateral) skin segments. The contralateral skin can be discarded when ipsilateral sections are sufficient; when it is retained for the breast reconstruction, it may undergo necrosis and ultimately calcification. These calcifications may cause confusion and an inaccurate diagnosis if an inadvertent mammogram of the reconstructed breast is performed.

Given the diminished intrinsic blood supply of the lower abdominal skin and subcutaneous fat, delayed wound healing and skin dehiscence are not rare events. Most of these wounds heal secondarily but leave obtrusive scars that are permanently thickened. Whether located on mid or lower parts of the abdomen, donor site scars tend to be coarse and discolored. Hematomas are uncommonly reported in most series but may require operative intervention when the bleeding originates from the deep epigastric arterial pedicle. Seromas, however, commonly occur despite suction drainage. Most seromas resolve spontaneously, but some necessitate aspiration to relieve patient discomfort. Uncommonly, some seromas coalesce in the epigastrium, developing a fibrinous wall, which gradually forms a pseudocyst.[34] These established masses continue to grow unless they are drained and their anterior walls are excised.

Umbilical necrosis occurs when its blood supply is compromised during flap elevation. Because the embryologically derived umbilical blood vessels are obliterated in most adults, a cuff or periumbilical fat must be maintained for purposes of umbilical vascularity. Overzealous skeletoniza-tion of the umbilicus will risk its devascularization, and although functionally insignificant, the umbilicus exerts enough symbolic importance to many people to warrant its preservation.

CASE REPORT

A 54-year-old woman had undergone a left modified radical mastectomy for stage II breast cancer 6 years earlier. Her opposite breast was hyperplastic and pendulous—physical features that had not disturbed her before the mastectomy. Over the past 2 years, she had noticed progressive neck and shoulder pain, which both she and an orthopedic surgeon attributed to the unilateral pendulousness of the right breast. She requested reduction of the right breast and reconstruction of the left (Fig. 54-15, *A*). On physical examination, she had a large abdominal panniculus, which was considered optimal for a rectus abdominis myocutaneous flap breast reconstruction. After preoperative consultation with the patient, a left-breast reconstruction of approximately a bra size C/D was determined to be aesthetically appropriate for her body habitus and consistent with her desire for the full-breasted appearance to which she was accustomed. The left-breast reconstruction with a left rectus flap was performed as the first part of an anticipated two-stage procedure. Three months later, right-nipple reduction was accomplished in conjunction with left-nipple-areolar reconstruction (see Fig. 54-15, *B* and *C*).   ▲

Microvascular Free Flap Breast Reconstruction. For most mastectomy defects, adequate breast reconstruction can be achieved with the use of synthetic devices such as silicone implants and expanders or with autogenous tissue borrowed from the back or abdomen. The simplicity of using synthetic material is sometimes belied by complications of firmness, encapsulation, and extrusion. Autogenous techniques, exemplified by the latissimus dorsi and rectus abdominis myocutaneous, supply soft tissues of suitable bulk and warmth, which can be sculpted into a breast of virtually any size or contour. In certain situations, previous abdominal surgery may render that site unavailable for a rectus flap procedure, or the thoracodorsal arterial pedicle may have been previously ligated (during the course of a radical mastectomy) or heavily radiated, obviating use of a latissimus flap. Microvascular free flaps composed of abdominal or buttock skin, fat, and muscle were developed to remedy such situations. These exceedingly complete and challenging operations differ fundamentally from pedicled myocutaneous flaps. In free flap procedures, the donor tissues and their attendant nourishing vessels are dissected and divided. A recipient vessel on the chest wall is selected and prepared for the microvascular reanastomosis, which reestablishes flow into the donor flap. The donor site is closed primarily, just as is done for myocutaneous flaps. After successful reanastomosis, the microvascular flap is shaped and contoured to create the desired breast reconstruction.

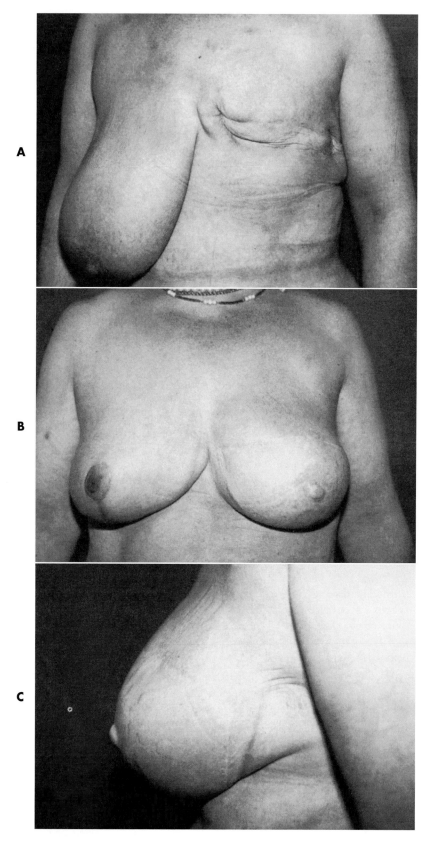

Fig. 54-15 **A,** A 54-year-old woman who had undergone previous left modified radical mastectomy. She complained of neck pain, which she and her orthopedist related to the right-breast hyperplasia. **B,** Appearance of the patient after a left rectus flap breast reconstruction was performed as the initial procedure, followed by right-breast reduction and left-nipple-areolar reconstruction 3 months later, (anterior view). **C,** Lateral view of the same patient.

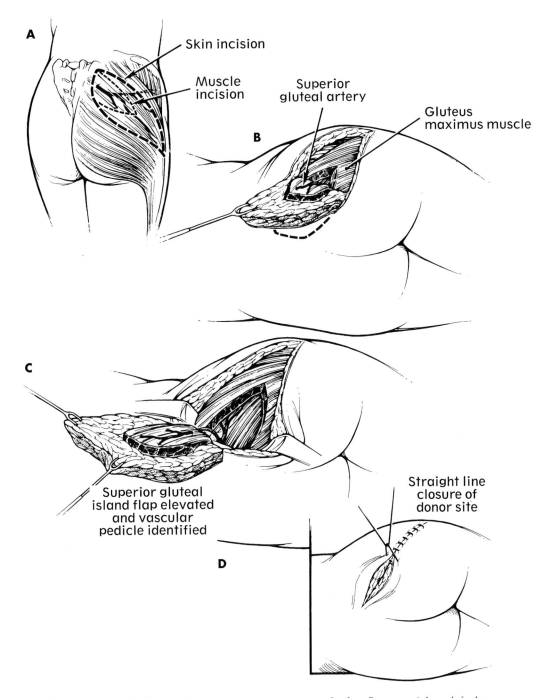

Fig. 54-16   **A,** Outline of gluteous maximus microvascular free flap over right or left gluteous maximus muscle. **B,** Careful dissection and preservation of the superior gluteal artery and vein as vessels enter the flap. **C,** The flap is ready for division of vascular pedicle and anastomosis of vessels at the breast recipient site. Primary closure of the flap donor site can be accomplished **(D).**   *Continued*

The Superior Gluteal Flap (Fig. 54-16). The superior gluteal flap of the upper portion of the gluteus maximus muscle, subcutaneous fat, and skin derives its blood supply from the superior gluteal artery.[28] Most patients have adequate or even generous amounts of tissue available for transfer from this site. The flap leaves an inconspicuous donor site scar on the upper portion of the buttock and little, if any, functional deficit. Inferior gluteal contributions to gait

controlled by the inferior gluteal neurovascular bundle remain largely intact.

Like all microvascular free flaps, the tissue must be attached to a suitable vessel in the vicinity of the breast reconstruction. Internal mammary, thoracodorsal, lateral thoracic, and external jugular vessels have been preferred for that purpose. Constraints created by the limited length of the donor vessels, or unsuitability of the recipient ones, have re-

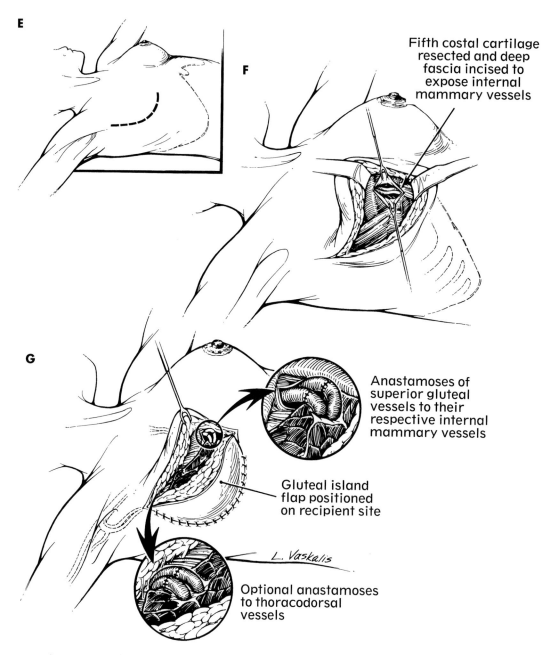

E

F

Fifth costal cartilage
resected and deep
fascia incised to
expose internal
mammary vessels

G

Anastamoses of
superior gluteal
vessels to their
respective internal
mammary vessels

Gluteal island
flap positioned
on recipient site

L. Vaskalis

Optional anastamoses
to thoracodorsal
vessels

Fig. 54-16, cont'd   E, The masectomy site is incised, and the native skin flaps of the chest wall are elevated. **F,** The superior gluteal vessels can be anastomosed to either the internal mammary or thoracodorsal vessels. **G,** After completion of the microvascular anastomoses, the flap is positioned and shaped.

stricted the placement or contouring of the flap into a breast mound. The relatively short vascular pedicle of the superior gluteal flap abetted the search for other free flap donor sites, as did the difficulty of the donor site dissection.

Transverse Rectus Abdominis Myocutaneous Free Flap. As a result of the extensive experience gained from pedicled TRAM flaps, this site became the next logical source of free flap donor tissue.[15] Unlike the superior gluteal flap, the TRAM flap contains donor vessels of superior caliber and length—the inferior deep epigastric artery and vein. The longer vascular leash obtained has eliminated

problems of tethering of the breast reconstruction and has greatly reduced episodes of microvascular thrombosis and flap loss. Another advantage of the rectus free flap—the use of the supine position for the entirety of the procedure—contrasts with the need for alternate positioning of the patient from lateral decubitus to supine when the superior gluteal procedure is performed. Also, in a free TRAM flap procedure, less muscle and fascia need to be taken, thereby facilitating closure of the abdominal wall and lessening the chance of subsequent hernia. Finally, the free TRAM flap supplies generous portions of abdominal skin and subcutaneous fat, which may exceed the availability of soft tissue in the upper buttock.

From an aesthetic view, microvascular free flaps harvested from the abdomen may provide a greater versatility of reconstruction than is usually possible with its gluteal counterpart. Like all microsurgical transfers, the free TRAM flap is vulnerable to major complications of thrombosis of the microvascular anastomosis and ultimate necrosis of the donor tissues. The possibility of complete loss of the breast reconstruction can be emotionally devastating to this group of patients who have already lost a breast to cancer. Although some microsurgeons have reported a 95% to 99% success rate of free tissue transfer, others indicate an overall complication rate, including reexploration for vascular problems, of 25% to 30%. Many plastic surgeons and their patients are daunted by these formidable statistics. Microvascular free tissue transfer is best accomplished at centers where the shear frequency of these procedures and the number of surgeons available to perform them and reoperate if necessary is adequate to ensure a high rate of success.

Free Perforator Flap. Because the major drawback of both pedicled myocutaneous flaps and their free flap counterparts is the need to incorporate muscle tissue, it was expected that new techniques would be developed that would preserve muscular function. Perforator flaps yield the ideal combination of skin and subcutaneous fat without muscle sacrifice. This is achieved by meticulous dissection of perforating blood vessels that arise from the muscle surface and enter the more superficially located fatty tissues to nourish both them and the overlying skin. Once dissected, microvascular anastomoses can be performed as is ordinarily done for free tissue transfer. A number of donor sites, including the abdomen, buttocks, back, and thighs, have been used for this approach. Concomitantly, there has been a significant lessening of postoperative hernia formation because weakening of the abdominal wall is much less likely when the musculature is preserved. Naturally, this type of procedure is more difficult to perform; only a small number of surgeons are expert at it, attesting to its difficulty 7 years after the original descriptions. Yet, it transfers the fatty tissues fo the abdomen, thighs, and buttock, where they may be in excess, to the deficient breast and chest wall areas. Surgeons comfortable with the perforator flap method report a success rate of 99%.

NIPPLE-AREOLAR RECONSTRUCTION

Reconstruction of the nipple-areolar complex is usually performed weeks or months after completion of the breast reconstruction.[21] This period of delay allows time for healing and descent of the reconstructed breast. However, the increasing popularity of immediate breast reconstruction has influenced the timing of the nipple-areolar reconstruction, with some plastic surgeons preferring to complete the entire process in a single stage. In addition to issues of size and symmetry, a reconstructed nipple should match the color, texture, and configuration of the existing contralateral structure, assuming such exists. When needed, bilateral nipple-areolar reconstructions optimize the opportunity for matching.

A variety of donor sites have been identified, including the opposite breast, medial thigh and labial skin, inguinal and buttock creases, ear, and toe. Most plastic surgeons prefer to harvest a full-thickness skin graft from the medial thigh because the increased pigmentation of this area creates a natural contrast of tone with the surrounding skin of the breast reconstruction. The tendency of a full-thickness skin graft to darken its color varies from patient to patient, but in most cases, the match is satisfactory. When the breast reconstruction is derived from a flap of abdominal soft tissues (TRAM flap), there may be excesses of skin along the lateral aspects of the abdominal donor site that can contribute for the creation of an areola and simultaneously allow correction of the dog-ear deformity. When significant tonal contrasts are necessary, intradermal tattooing with medical grade pigment is an excellent remedy.[37] The technique of tattooing has advanced to such a degree that it has become a routine part of breast reconstruction.

Creation of a projecting central nipple of approximately the same diameter and height as the other side can pose a significant challenge. Most techniques involve elevation of local flaps of skin and subcutaneous fat from the surface of a myocutaneous flap or from the residual native skin present after mastectomy and reconstruction with implants or expanders.[20] Depending on the particular design on the surface of the breast reconstruction site, these flaps have been dubbed *star, fishtail, quadrapod* (Fig. 54-17), *skate, pinwheel,* and other descriptive terms. Each design involves sculpting skin flaps based on the vascularity of the subdermal plexus. The star flap is unique because primary closure of its component flaps elevated from the surface of the reconstructed breast is achieved without a skin graft.

Application of a wide variety of techniques has resulted in the creation of aesthetically pleasing nipples that reasonably match the contralateral form. All of the techniques can be performed under local anesthesia and on an outpatient surgery basis, adding minimal morbidity for the patient. Major complications occurring after nipple reconstruction have consisted of partial or complete necrosis of the central nipple, combined with varying degrees of loss of the areolar graft. Fortunately, complete necrosis of the nipple has been uncommon. Donor site complications have involved wound separation, delayed healing, and infection. Long-term maintenance of nipple projection has been a problem that has been only partially solved by techniques incorporating larger volumes of soft tissue. It is also unclear what percentage of patients return for this final stage of breast reconstruction. However, those who do return express a high degree of satisfaction with the results achieved.

SENSATION AFTER BREAST RECONSTRUCTION

Most patients fail to ask about sensation after breast reconstruction, either because it may not have been discussed

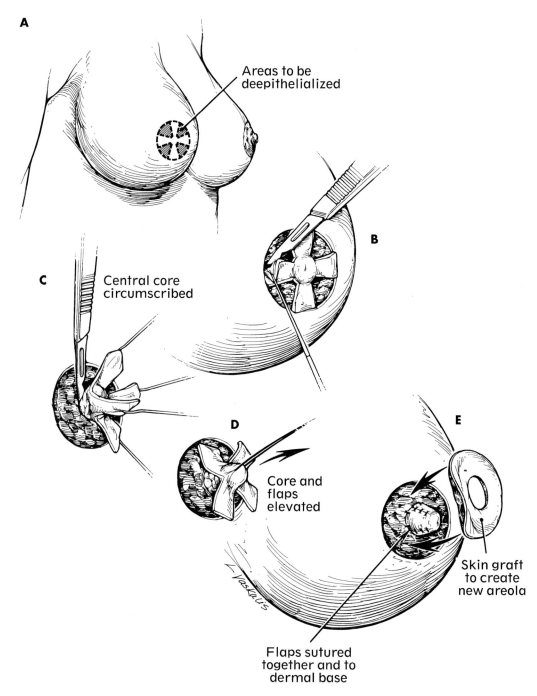

Fig. 54-17 **A,** Deepithelialization of the site chosen as the new areola. A quadrapod (four-limbed) flap is designed. **B** and **C,** The four limbs are elevated as epidermal-dermal flaps. A central core is preserved to maintain the vascularity of the flaps. **D,** Following gentle retraction on the central core, the four flaps are sutured together to create a projecting nipple reconstruction. **E,** A full-thickness skin graft can be harvested from a number of possible sites and sutured to the deepithelialization areolar site. As an alternative method, the areolar site can be tattooed.

with the plastic surgeon or because they mistakenly assume that there will be a complete absence of feeling. The normal surface sensuality of the breast is always diminished after mastectomy, a result of the removal of breast parenchyma and its associated sensory innervation. Among the intercostal nerves that penetrate the breast substance from the lateral pectoral border, the fourth intercostal directly innervates the nipple-areolar complex and underlying tissues. Unfortu-

nately, this important sensory nerve, along with other cutaneous contributors, is routinely removed during mastectomy. However, skin sensation is preserved in the superior and inferior native flaps, which are approximated at the conclusion of the procedure. Breast reconstruction procedures that re-create the breast mound by stretching the available chest wall skin tend to retain some qualities of light touch and pressure, but normal sensation is never present. When myocutaneous flaps are used from the back (latissimus dorsi) or abdomen (rectus abdominis), the transferred tissues lack sensory innervation. These flaps contain their respective motor nerves—thoracodorsal for the latissimus flap and intercostal for the rectus flap—but the cutaneous component of each flap has no sensory trunk. Although patients will gradually note some ingrowth of sensory branches around the periphery of the cutaneous island, usually appearing about 1 year later, they should be advised that the flap reconstruction is generally devoid of sensation. Chest wall recipient sites that have been previously irradiated or that require postoperative radiation therapy may not develop even a rudimentary level of sensory innervation. Similarly, the nipple-areolar complex reconstruction, usually sited centrally on the myocutaneous flap or the native skin flaps, will lack any appreciable surface sensory function.

BREAST RECONSTRUCTION AND RADIATION

The increasing popularity of conservative surgery and radiotherapy poses unique reconstructive challenges for the plastic surgeon. As the technique of lumpectomy and radiation has gained international recognition, more patients with radiation changes of the skin and soft tissues of the chest wall and residual breast parenchyma are requiring additional procedures. Two important groups are involved: (1) patients who have undergone lumpectomy or quadrantectomy and radiation therapy and (2) those who have failed conservative therapy because of cancer recurrence in the irradiated breast. In both situations, the reconstructive surgeon must understand the effects of radiation therapy on breast tissue.[31]

Physical findings after radiation consist of breast edema, retraction, fibrosis, induration, skin discoloration, and telangiectasia formation. Vascularity of the breast is significantly reduced by radiation, resulting in ischemic tissues prone to wound healing complications. Previously radiated chest wall skin is characterized by a leathery induration that is rigid and unyielding when subjected to stretching by an inflatable expander. Cutaneous sensory function is significantly reduced. Even the minimally increased skin tension occurring when a subpectoral implant is placed may abet skin necrosis and ultimate extrusion of prosthetic device. Such patients are generally poor candidates for techniques that use foreign body placement and must instead rely on the independent vascularity provided by a myocutaneous flap. In more extreme situations characterized by cancer recurrence in the irradiated breast or in the presence of ulceration and osteoradionecrosis, a myocutaneous flap is always necessary. Patients with these life-threatening problems become candidates for salvage mastectomy with immediate reconstruction using a myocutaneous flap.

Radiation therapy may create a zone of injury that encompasses skin and soft tissues extending from clavicle to costal margin and lateral chest wall to sternum. Microvascular free flap transfers can be especially hazardous in this group of patients because of radiation-induced injury of the intended recipient vessel and the increased probability of thrombosis. Therefore most plastic surgeons select a latissimus or rectus myocutaneous flap, based on availability of the particular unit and the requirements of the wound defect. If neither flap is available, a microvascular free flap procedure may have to be undertaken.

RECURRENCE AFTER BREAST RECONSTRUCTION

Breast cancer surveillance after mastectomy and reconstruction is an issue of critical importance for the patient and the physicians involved in her care. Earlier concerns that implants would impede the detection of breast cancer recurrence have not materialized. Gradually, the imposition of a mandatory waiting period for commencement of the reconstruction was replaced by the concept of immediate breast reconstruction. A number of studies have demonstrated that immediate breast reconstruction with implants or expanders does not affect cancer recurrence rates or survival rates in clinical stage I and II patients. Locoregional recurrences, usually manifested by visible and palpable cutaneous or subcutaneous tumor aggregates, are readily diagnosed by simple physical examination and can be treated by excision, radiation, or chemotherapy. Optimal cancer detection and management are not compromised.

When myocutaneous flaps were introduced for both delayed and immediate breast reconstruction, there was renewed concern that transfer of large masses of autogenous soft tissue could obscure a recurrence and lead to a delay in diagnosis. It was theorized that tumor cells would proliferate beneath the flap, escaping detection. Fortunately, a large review of this potential problem showed that breast cancer recurrences invariably developed on the native skin surface bordering the myocutaneous flap.[36] Again, all of the locoregional recurrences were detectable by physical examination, and no instances of occult recurrent cancer cells beneath the flap have been documented. These findings suggest that the use of myocutaneous flaps for immediate breast reconstruction does not interfere with the detection or treatment of a local recurrence. Furthermore, 90% of patients with local recurrence, whose incidence is about 9%, have systemic disease.

MANAGEMENT OF THE OPPOSITE BREAST

The basic premise of breast reconstruction is the achievement of symmetry with the remaining breast. When the opposite breast is aesthetically acceptable, all efforts are directed at creating a new breast of approximately the same size, shape, and configuration. The opposite breast can sometimes be altered by one or more of the techniques described earlier in this chapter—augmentation, mastopexy, or reduction. Some patients perceive in the plan to reconstruct the postmastectomy defect an opportunity to improve their opposite breast, which they might have spurned under other circumstances. The belief that they might look better than they did before mastectomy provides considerable psychological comfort.

Women who were not satisfied with a small breast size may choose to augment the opposite breast. After consultation with the patient's oncologist, it is usually permissible to place the breast implant in a subpectoral location that impedes to a lesser degree the mammographic or physical evaluation of the patient.

Similarly, patients with hyperplastic and pendulous breasts often choose either a reduction mammaplasty and mastopexy technique of breast correction, or they may prefer a breast reconstruction that attempts to match the opposite breast. Loss of a breast can lead to a protective stance in regard to any proposed surgical intervention for the other side. Scarring after breast reconstruction does not appear to interfere with the performance of an accurate physical examination.

In the most extreme situations, prophylactic mastectomy may be recommended for optimal management of high-risk patients. For these patients, whose breast pathology indicates a likelihood of bilaterality, total mastectomy is preferred to subcutaneous mastectomy. Total mastectomy achieves a more complete removal of breast parenchyma, leaving only residual microscopic foci of breast tissues at the limits of the dissection. The resulting bilateral mastectomy defects lend themselves to placement of implants or expanders because of the ease in attaining symmetry. Women whose genetic analysis suggests a predisposition to develop breast cancer may be advised to consider bilateral prophylactic mastectomies. As harsh as this approach may be, it can bring relief and cure to those at extraordinarily high risk.

REFERENCES AND SUGGESTED READING

1. Argenta LC: Reconstruction of the breast by tissue expansion, *Clin Plast Surg* 11:247, 1984.
2. Asplund O: Capsule contracture in silicone gel and saline filled breast implants after reconstruction, *Plast Reconstr Surg* 73:270, 1984.
3. Becker H: The expandable mammary implant, *Plast Reconstr Surg* 79:631, 1987.
4. Bostwick J III, Scheflan M: The latissimus dorsi myocutaneous flap: one stage breast reconstruction, *Clin Plast Surg* 7:71, 1980.
5. Caffee HH: The influence of silicone bleed on capsule contracture, *Ann Plast Surg* 17:284, 1986.
6. Cline CJ: Psychological aspects of breast reduction surgery. In Goldwyn RM (ed): *Reduction mammoplasty,* Boston, 1990, Little, Brown.
7. Cohen IK, Turner D: Immediate breast reconstruction with tissue expanders, *Clin Plast Surg* 14:491, 1987.
8. Dinner MI, Labandter HP, Dowden, RV: The role of the rectus abdominis myocutaneous flap in breast reconstruction, *Plast Reconstr Surg* 69:209, 1982.
9. Dowden RV, Dinner MI: Breast reconstruction without skin flaps, *Clin Plast Surg* 11:265, 1984.
10. Georgiade GS, et al: Long-term clinical outcome of immediate reconstruction after mastectomy, *Plast Reconstr Surg* 76:415, 1985.
11. Gibney J: The long-term results of tissue expansion for breast reconstruction, *Clin Plast Surg* 14:509, 1987.
12. Goin MK, Goin JM: Psychological reactions to prophylactic mastectomy synchronous with contralateral breast reconstruction, *Plast Reconstr Surg* 69:632, 1982.
13. Goldwyn RM: *The patient and the plastic surgeon,* Boston, Little, Brown.
14. Goldwyn RM, Courtiss EH: Inferior pedicle technique. In Goldwyn RM (ed): *Reduction mammoplasty,* Boston, 1990, Little, Brown.
15. Grotting JC, et al: Conventional TRAM flap versus free microsurgical TRAM flap for immediate breast reconstruction, *Plast Reconstr Surg* 83:828, 1989.
15a. Hartmann LC, et al: Efficacy of bilateral prophylactic mastectomy in women with a family history of breast cancer, *N Engl J Med* 340:77, 1999.
16. Hartrampf CR, Scheflan, M, Black PW: Breast reconstruction with a transverse abdominal island flap, *Plast Reconstr Surg* 69:216, 1982.
17. Hester TR Jr: Augmentation mammoplasty: polyurethane covered mammary implant. In Marsh JL (ed): *Current therapy in plastic and reconstructive surgery,* Toronto, 1989, BC Decker.
18. Ishii CH, et al: Double-pedicle transverse rectus abdominis myocutaneous flap for unilateral breast and chest wall reconstruction, *Plast Reconstr Surg* 76:901, 1985.
19. Larson DL, McMurtrey MJ: Musculotaneous flap reconstruction of chest wall defects: an experience with 50 patients, *Plast Reconstr Surg* 73:734, 1984.
20. Little JW: Nipple reconstruction by quadropod flap (letter), *Plast Reconstr Surg* 72:422, 1983.
21. Little JW: Nipple-areolar reconstruction, *Clin Plast Surg* 11:351, 1984.
22. Manders EK, et al: Soft-tissue expansion: concepts and complications, *Plast Reconstr Surg* 74:493, 1984.
23. Maxwell GP: Latissimus dorsi breast reconstruction: an aesthetic assessment, *Clin Plast Surg* 8:373, 1981.
24. Maxwell GP: Selection of secondary breast reconstruction procedures, *Clin Plast Surg* 11:253, 1984.
25. McCraw JB, et al: An early appraisal of the methods of tissue expansion and the transverse rectus abdominis musculocutaneous flap in reconstruction of the breast following mastectomy, *Ann Plast Surg* 18:93, 1987.
26. Noone RB, et al: A 6-year experience with immediate reconstruction after mastectomy for breast cancer, *Plast Reconstr Surg* 76:258, 1985.
27. Radovan C: Tissue expansion in soft tissue reconstruction, *Plast Reconstr Surg* 74:482, 1984.
28. Shaw WW: Breast reconstruction by superior gluteal microvascular free flaps without silicone implants, *Plast Reconstr Surg* 73:490, 1983.
29. Shaw WW: Microvascular free flap breast reconstruction, *Clin Plast Surg* 11:333, 1984.
30. Slavin SA: Drainage of seromas after latissimus dorsi breast reconstruction (letter to the editor), *Plast Reconstr Surg* 83:925, 1989.
31. Slavin SA: Salvage mastectomy and reconstruction. In Noone RB (ed): *Plastic and reconstructive breast surgery,* Toronto, 1991, BC Decker.
32. Slavin SA, Colen SR: Sixty consecutive breast reconstructions with the inflatable expander: a critical appraisal, *Plast Reconstr Surg* 74:493, 1990.
33. Slavin SA, Goldwyn RM: The midabdominal rectus abdominis myocutaneous flap: review of 236 flaps, *Plast Reconstr Surg* 81:89, 1988.
34. Slavin SA, Howrigan P, Goldwyn RM: Pseudocyst formation following rectus flap breast reconstruction: diagnosis and treatment, *Plast Reconstr Surg* 83:670, 1989.
35. Slavin SA, et al: Abdominal wall function after rectus flap breast reconstruction. Presented at the 55th Annual Scientific Meeting of the American Society of Plastic and Reconstructive Surgeons, Plastic Surgery Educational Foundation, American Society of Maxillofacial Surgeons, Los Angeles, Calif, Oct 27, 1986.
36. Slavin SA, Love SL, Goldwyn RM: Breast cancer recurrence and detection following immediate breast reconstruction with myocutaneous flaps. Presented at the 59th Annual Scientific Meeting of the American Society of Plastic Reconstructive Surgeons, Boston, Oct 23, 1990.
37. Spear SL: Intradermal tattooing. In Marsh J (ed): *Current therapy in plastic and reconstructive surgery,* Toronto, 1989, BC Decker.
38. Stevens LA, et al: The psychological impact of immediate breast reconstruction for women with early breast cancer, *Plast Reconstr Surg* 73:619, 1984.
39. Woods JE, Irons GB, Arnold PG: The case for submuscular implantation of prostheses in reconstructive surgery, *Ann Plast Surg* 5:115, 1980.

55 Invasive Fetal Diagnostic Procedures

DEVEREUX N. SALLER, Jr., and MARSHALL W. CARPENTER

The availability and choices of invasive prenatal diagnostic techniques have changed dramatically in recent years. These advances are particularly striking when one recalls that chromosome analysis has become widely available only within the last 30 years. Additional laboratory advances (including biochemical and microenzyme assay) have further widened the range of potential indications. The rapidly developing field of molecular biology has focused increasing attention on the development of safe clinical techniques of obtaining appropriate specimens for laboratory analysis. This chapter describes the development of these clinical techniques, their indications, and their risks.

AMNIOCENTESIS
Historical Perspectives

The use of amniocentesis was first described in the treatment of polyhydramnios as early as the 1880s.[50] These early interventions were unaided by any visualization of the internal anatomy. In the early 1900s, with the availability of ionizing radiation, Menees, Miller, and Holly[59] used amniocentesis to evaluate fetal anatomy and to localize the placenta by injecting contrast media into the amniotic cavity. It was not until the 1950s that broad clinical application of this technique became possible. At that time amniocentesis was reported in the evaluation of erythroblastosis fetalis. It was then noted that spectrophotometric analysis of amniotic fluid for bilirubin correlated with the severity of fetal anemia and the prognosis for the fetus in at-risk pregnancies.[8,52,90]

Amniocentesis was first used for prenatal diagnosis of congenital malformations in the late 1950s. Before the availability of chromosome analysis, the ability to identify the inactivated X chromosome (or Barr body) in amniotic fluid cells (and thereby to identify fetal sex) was reported.[33,45,57,77] With the advent of cytogenetic laboratory techniques that allow the counting of chromosomes in cultured cells from various tissues in the late 1950s and early 1960s, chromosome analysis from cultured amniotic fluid cells became possible. This allowed the use of amniocytes to provide prenatal diagnosis for fetal aneuploidy (including Down syndrome), which has become the most common indication for genetic amniocentesis. Successful karyotyping

of amniocytes was first reported by Steele and Breg[83] and quickly became commonly available. The development of chromosome banding techniques, high-resolution (or prometaphase) karyotyping, and most recently, fluorescent in situ hybridization (FISH) has further expanded the range of prenatal diagnosis.

Utility

Amniocentesis provides access to the amniotic fluid, which is essentially fetal urine (after 14 to 16 weeks' gestation). The amniotic fluid provides the substrate for three types of laboratory studies. First, after centrifugation the supranatant fluid may be studied directly by biochemical assay. The relative amounts of amniotic fluid α-fetoprotein (AFP) and acetylcholinesterase, for example, may be diagnostic in the prenatal evaluation for open neural tube defects.[74,80] Second, the cells in the pellet may be analyzed directly in biochemical studies (e.g., microenzyme assays for the diagnosis of certain inborn errors of metabolism) or molecular deoxyribonucleic acid (DNA) studies. Third, the cells may be cultured to provide material for similar biochemical or DNA studies, or they may be cultured for chromosomal analysis. At later gestations, amniotic fluid may be cultured for bacterial infection or may be used for biochemical studies such as fetal lung maturity studies or for spectrophotometric analysis (for bilirubin, in the evaluation of erythroblastosis fetalis).

Amniocentesis may be used for a variety of clinical indications (see the box on p. 1024). Currently the most common indication for genetic amniocentesis is an appreciation of an increased risk of a chromosomally abnormal fetus. Women of relatively advanced age (traditionally age 35 at EDC)[73] and couples with a known balanced chromosomal rearrangement (in either parent of the fetus) or with a history of a previous child with a chromosomal abnormality are at increased risk for a fetus with a chromosomal abnormality. Genetic amniocentesis may also be indicated in the evaluation of fetuses at risk for open neural tube defects[80] or for metabolic or other biochemical defects in which either the gene or gene product has been identified and can be quantitated.[60] Genetic amniocentesis is also indicated when a gross anatomic malformation that is associated with karyotypically abnormal pregnancies is prenatally diagnosed.

INDICATIONS FOR INVASIVE PRENATAL DIAGNOSIS

1. Increased risk of aneuploidy
   a. Advanced maternal age (traditionally ≥35 years old at EDC)
   b. Previous pregnancy complicated by a numerical chromosome abnormality
   c. Morphologic fetal anomaly noted (on ultrasound)
2. Increased risk of structural chromosomal abnormality
   a. Structural chromosomal abnormality in one of the parents
   b. Family history of structural chromosomal abnormality
3. Increased risk of genetic syndrome
   a. Previously affected child or positive family history
   b. Parent is a known (or suspected) carrier of a genetic disease for which prenatal diagnosis is possible
4. Increased risk of a neural tube defect
5. Maternal medical conditions associated with birth defects (e.g., diabetes mellitus)
6. Abnormal genetic or prenatal screening test

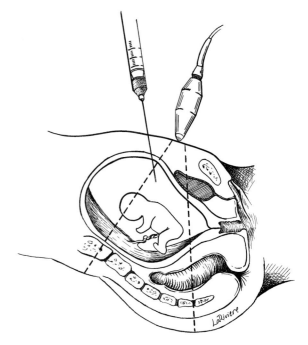

Fig. 55-1 Schematic representation of amniocentesis under ultrasonic guidance.

Recently, the application of the rapidly developing field of molecular biology to prenatal diagnosis has expanded the utility of amniocentesis. For example, several years ago the diagnosis of fetal blood type (in pregnancies at risk for isoimmunization) was possible only through fetal blood sampling. Presently, the fetal blood type may be determined by DNA analysis of amniocytes obtained through amniocentesis.[5] Thus current developments allow diagnoses to be made with less invasive, less expensive, and safer procedures.

Technique

The technique of amniocentesis (Fig. 55-1) involves the percutaneous insertion of a needle into the amniotic cavity and the aspiration of amniotic fluid. As with any other percutaneous biopsy procedure, care must be taken to assure asepsis. In addition, evidence suggests that sonographically monitored procedures result in a 74% reduction in the incidence of "dry" or unsuccessful needle insertions (7.7% in the guided group compared with 2% in the monitored group) and a 77% reduction in incidence of "bloody" specimens (5.2% in the guided group compared with 1.2% in the monitored group).[72] With the current availability of ultrasound, all amniocenteses should be performed with continuous ultrasound guidance by experienced personnel.

Several methods of insertion have been described. Jeanty et al.[46] have described needle insertion immediately adjacent to the side of a linear array transducer at a slight angle. The tip of the needle is kept within the ultrasound beam and is thereby visualized throughout the insertion, but the entire length of the needle cannot be visualized. The transducer may then be placed in a sterile glove (or sheath) and held by the single surgeon (at least initially).

Benacerraf[4] suggested inserting the amniocentesis needle at one end of a sector probe (or a curvilinear array transducer). With this method, the entire needle is within the ultrasound beam and can be visualized throughout the procedure, thereby enhancing the surgeon's spatial orientation. However, this technique may require an assistant to hold the ultrasound transducer adjacent to the sterile field. Although this technique does not require that the transducer be placed within a sterile sheath, it does depend on successful coordination of the sonographer and the surgeon.

Amniocentesis may be performed in the second or third trimesters (after 14 to 16 weeks' gestation). The technical aspects of the procedure and laboratory evaluations are the same in either trimester. Because the laboratory studies may take several weeks, however, amniocentesis in the first 20 weeks provides the option for termination of pregnancy.

"Early Amniocentesis"

The safety and feasibility of amniocentesis as early as 10 weeks have been more recently investigated.[29,38,47] In these procedures, the surgeon removes a larger volume of amniotic fluid relative to the total amniotic fluid volume and the total intrauterine volume; thus the size of the amniotic cavity may change to a greater extent than is seen in more traditional second trimester amniocentesis. These changes in intrauterine volume may theoretically impact uterine contractility, placental perfusion, or embryologic development.

A number of studies have now been published describing the technique, efficacy, and success rate of early amniocentesis.[40,79,84] Most of the literature comes from small case series with one or a few surgeons. Large series with complete follow-up are more difficult to find. Recently, Nicolaides[61] has published preliminary data from a prospective partially randomized study. In this study, patients could choose early amniocentesis (N = 493), chorionic villus sampling (CVS) (N = 320), or randomization (N = 488). This report suggested a 3% increase in spontaneous losses after early amniocentesis overall, and a 4.7% increase in spontaneous losses in the randomized patients after early amniocentesis. Although this study has been criticized,[26] it provides the best data currently available. Although in certain hands early amniocentesis may be safe, the safety of widespread general use has yet to be proven.

Risks

The recognized maternal risks of amniocentesis include chorioamnionitis, hemorrhage, injury to abdominal viscera, and blood group isoimmunization. Fetal risks include premature rupture of membranes, abortion or preterm labor, abruptio placentae, injury from needle trauma, orthopedic deformities, and possibly respiratory difficulties.

Several investigators[54,85,86] have addressed the precise risks of second trimester amniocentesis. A prospective nonrandomized study of more than 2000 pregnancies in the United States was coordinated by the National Institutes of Child Health and Human Development.[54] Ultrasound "was used in only about one-third of the taps." Of the 1040 pregnant women undergoing amniocentesis, 950 (91.3%) were having the procedure performed for cytogenetic analysis, whereas 90 (8.7%) were having the procedure to evaluate the possibility of an inherited metabolic disorder (e.g., Tay-Sachs disease). Patients referred for abnormal AFP were excluded. This study reported that immediate complications (including bleeding and amniotic fluid leakage) were noted in 2.4% of patients, and 3.5% of the pregnancies were lost after amniocentesis, compared with 3.2% lost in the control group. This 0.3% difference has now become a commonly quoted "procedure-related loss rate." No other physical problems were noted more commonly after amniocentesis. A report of a Canadian collaborative group[58] suggested similar complication rates in a study of 1020 pregnancies, but the study did not have a control group.

A collaborative British study[86] of more than 4800 pregnancies was reported in 1978. The use of ultrasound in conjunction with the amniocentesis was considered optional. Of 3131 patients undergoing amniocentesis, 1632 (52.1%) were having it for chromosomal analysis and 1282 (40.9%) for an increased risk of neural tube defects. This study suggested that the risks of spontaneous midtrimester abortion after amniocentesis were about 2.6%, compared with 1.1% in the control group. In addition, approximately 1.2% of newborns in the amniocentesis group were reported to have nonfatal respiratory difficulties compared with 0.4% in matched control subjects. Orthopedic postural deformities (including talipes equinovarus and congenital hip dislocations) were noted in 1.4% of newborns in the amniocentesis group and in none of the matched control subjects. The rate of orthopedic defects in the control group was unexpectedly low, however. It is also noteworthy that significant differences were seen between the amniocentesis group and the control group in maternal age. In addition, this study included a large number of patients (30%) for whom the indication for amniocentesis was elevated maternal serum α-fetoprotein, which in the absence of open fetal defects has been associated with poor pregnancy outcome.[36] Whether these factors account for the differences between this study and the U.S. and Canadian studies is unclear.

A more recent randomized, controlled Danish study of 4606 pregnant women[85] reported a pregnancy loss rate of 1.7% in the patients undergoing amniocentesis, whereas the control group had a loss rate of 0.7%. Respiratory distress and pneumonia were also more common in neonates from the amniocentesis group. No differences were noted in orthopedic problems, however. Although all of the amniocentesis procedures in this study were done with ultrasound guidance, an 18-gauge needle was used to aspirate the fluid. In the other reports, a 20- or 22-gauge needle was usually used for the amniocentesis.

The long-term follow-up of children whose mothers had second trimester amniocentesis has also been studied. Several case-control studies[2,27,35] now suggest that children who were exposed to amniocentesis did not have increases in hearing deficits, learning disabilities, limb anomalies, fine motor coordination, speech, visual-perceptual-motor ability, or behavioral problems. One study[2] did suggest an increased rate of ABO isoimmunization after amniocentesis.

Although the precise risks of amniocentesis remain unclear, it may be considered a generally safe procedure with attributable risks of less than 1% and probably less than 0.5%. However, its use must be weighed in each case against the need and value of the information to be gained and risk of an unexpected or abnormal result (e.g., a chromosomal abnormality).

CHORIONIC VILLUS SAMPLING
Historical Perspectives

Although investigations into placental biopsy for prenatal diagnosis date back to the late 1960s,[37] prenatal diagnosis for chromosomal abnormalities was almost exclusively carried out through amniocentesis until the 1980s. This preference was primarily based on assumptions about the safety and technical ease of amniocentesis compared with that of CVS at a time when high-resolution ultrasound was unavailable. By the early 1980s, high-resolution ultrasound was able to adequately image the developing placental tissue and provide guidance for a biopsy catheter or needle.[49] This, as well as technical cytogenetic laboratory advances, made CVS an attractive alternative to amniocentesis for genetic prenatal diagnosis.

Utility

CVS provides tissue for prenatal diagnosis of a wide variety of indications. After careful cleaning, the tissue may be assayed directly (similar to amniocytes) for biochemical studies (e.g., microenzyme assays for the diagnosis of inborn errors of metabolism) or molecular DNA studies. In addition, because the cells in the developing placenta (chorion) are rapidly dividing, the cells may be directly analyzed for karyotype,[78] with the results available within 72 hours. The tissue may also be placed into culture to provide material for similar biochemical or DNA studies or for chromosomal analysis. Early studies suggested that the directly analyzed cells offer the advantage of less maternal cell contamination, whereas the cultured cells show fewer incorrect predictions of fetal cytogenetic status.[51] The combination of both methods is considered optimal and has resulted in no incorrect predictions of fetal status in a large collaborative trial.[51] Many laboratories now rely exclusively on the culture technique. Typically, karyotype results from such cultures are generally available within 10 to 12 days.

A major advantage of CVS over amniocentesis is the earlier gestational age at which this procedure can be performed. CVS appears to have a lower attributable risk when performed between 9 and 11 weeks' gestation.[42] This earlier gestational age may be an important advantage to patients at increased risk for specific types of genetic abnormalities because the results of this diagnostic test allow termination of pregnancy before 14 weeks' gestation. Termination of pregnancy at this early stage offers a lower risk of hemorrhage and uterine or cervical trauma than later terminations. There may also be social and emotional advantages to earlier prenatal diagnosis for certain patients, relating to the fact that a first trimester pregnancy is not obvious to social contacts and therefore may remain private. In addition, awareness of fetal movement has not occurred in the first trimester, and such awareness, after second trimester amniocentesis, may make decisions about pregnancy termination more difficult.

CVS may be used for any prenatal diagnostic indication for which amniocentesis (see the box on p. 1024) is used except for the diagnosis of neural tube defects (in which the biochemical evaluation of amniotic fluid is advantageous).[80] Because CVS is typically performed between 10 and 12 weeks' gestation, it is of less use in evaluation of second or third trimester pregnancies. Currently, CVS is most commonly used for karyotypic evaluation of pregnancies at risk for chromosomal abnormalities (usually related to the increasing risk of nondisjunction with advancing maternal age or previous aneuploidy).

Technique

CVS involves a biopsy of chorionic villi, which is the fetal tissue of the developing placenta. CVS is usually performed either by a transabdominal route (Fig. 55-2) using percutaneous needle biopsy of the placenta[12,63] or by transcervical passage of a catheter (Fig. 55-3) into the chorion or developing placenta.[42]

The performance of second or third trimester chorionic villus biopsy by the percutaneous transabdominal approach has been described by several authors.[43,65,87] Although late CVS has been shown to be feasible, its safety compared with amniocentesis has not been critically evaluated. Nevertheless, in selected cases when chromosomal abnormalities

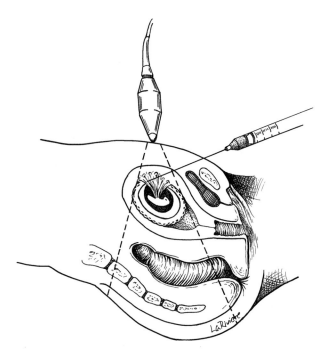

Fig. 55-2 Schematic representation of transabdominal chorionic villus sampling.

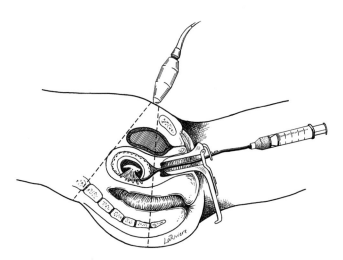

Fig. 55-3 Schematic representation of transcervical chorionic villus sampling.

are highly suspected and when amniocentesis is deemed difficult or impossible (as in cases of oligohydramnios), late CVS is currently a viable alternative.

Risks

Risks related to CVS can be categorized into maternal risks and fetal risks. The maternal risks of CVS are rare but mainly involve intrauterine infection presenting as acute chorioamnionitis.[42] Fetal risks mainly involve oligohydramnios, with or without a clear history of amniotic fluid leakage,[42] and fetal loss.

The results of two large collaborative trials are now available. The Canadian Collaborative Trial[94] was a multicenter trial of 2787 women aged 35 or older, randomized to CVS or amniocentesis. Of these women, 396 were excluded after randomization because of a nonviable fetus, multiple gestation, infection, or incorrect gestational age. The report suggested that the excess risk of pregnancy loss in patients undergoing CVS (compared with patients undergoing amniocentesis) was 0.6% (7.6% in the CVS group compared with 7% in the amniocentesis group). However, this difference was not statistically significant (the 95% confidence interval for the total pregnancy loss rate for CVS was 6.2% to 9.3%, whereas the 95% confidence interval for the amniocentesis group was 5.6% to 8.6%).

A similar collaborative multicenter trial from the United States[69] reported on 2278 pregnant women undergoing CVS. This report suggested that the total loss rate for women undergoing CVS was 0.8% greater than that for women undergoing amniocentesis, after adjustment for slight differences in maternal and gestational age at enrollment. Again, a higher loss rate was seen after CVS, but this was not statistically significant (the 80% confidence interval for the excess total loss in the CVS group was −0.6% to 2.2%).

Ämmälä et al.[1] reported on a randomized trial of first trimester CVS and second trimester amniocentesis. They noted no difference in diagnostic accuracy or fetal loss rate between CVS and amniocentesis. More recently, Blakemore et al.[9] reported on 4105 patients undergoing CVS with the Cook catheter and found no increase in major birth defects (or specific categories of birth defects) after CVS.

Jackson et al.[44] reported on a randomized comparison of transcervical and transabdominal CVS and suggested that both appeared equally safe in the first trimester. Other retrospective studies have suggested that there may be a lower risk for transabdominal CVS than for transcervical CVS.[16] The addition of transabdominal CVS availability (along with experience) also reduced loss rates after both approaches.[16] These reports emphasize the importance of the availability of both methods, as well as surgeon experience. Both the transabdominal and transcervical techniques have achieved clinical acceptance and are believed to be equally safe.[11,56]

Limb Reduction Abnormalities

In 1991, Firth et al.[28,29] reported on a cluster of five babies with transverse limb reduction abnormalities in pregnancies exposed to CVS at 56 to 66 days' gestation. This was followed by the report by Burton et al.[13] of four babies with transverse limb reduction deformities after CVS. These two reports resulted in a reevaluation of data from centers around the world. However, other authorities found no association in their data. Many other authorities were unimpressed with the data and noted other data sets without the association. The use of CVS has decreased since the recognition of this possible association.[20]

Attempts to review large data sets and reach consensus on the possible association of CVS and transverse limb reduction abnormalities have met with mixed success. The National Institutes of Child Health and Human Development

convened a Workshop on the issue in 1992.[17] The participants were unable to reach consensus and suggested further studies. The National Center for Environmental Health of the Centers for Disease Control and Prevention reported a population-based, multistate case-control study.[66] This study suggested a sixfold increased risk of transverse limb reduction abnormalities after CVS. In 1996, Froster and Jackson[31] reported on the World Health Organization international CVS registry. This dataset showed no association between CVS and transverse limb reduction abnormalities.

CVS performed before 10 weeks' gestation has now largely been abandoned. Whether a cause-and-effect relationship exists between CVS at 10 weeks or later and transverse limb reduction abnormalities remains controversial. If such a relationship exists, the risk of transverse limb reduction abnormalities after CVS appears small (1 in 2900 births).[66] Thus CVS remains an appropriate option for patients seeking invasive prenatal diagnosis. Until consensus exists, however, it appears prudent for patients to be counseled about the potential risks.[17]

FETAL BLOOD SAMPLING
Historical Perspectives

Fetal blood provides material for analysis of cellular characteristics, DNA, metabolic status, biochemical markers, and physical characteristics. Fetal blood sampling has been described since the early 1970s.[88] Early use of sampling via a 1.7-mm fetoscope was performed in only a few centers and was associated with a high risk of preterm birth and fetal mortality.[6,82] Its greatest use was for the diagnosis of fetal hemoglobinopathies, which now can be performed on amniocyte DNA.[5]

Today, sonographic image quality now provides precise localization of fetal vasculature, which has resulted in a relatively low risk of complications from cordocentesis. Percutaneous umbilical blood sampling (PUBS) was first reported by Daffos et al. in 1983,[22] in which 66 samples were taken from 63 pregnant women.

Utility

PUBS has been used in the evaluation and treatment of fetal hematologic abnormalities, growth restriction with or without abnormal fetal velocimetry, nonimmune hydrops, and fetal anatomic abnormalities. PUBS has also been used for fetal metabolic evaluation of fetuses who are at risk for hypoxia, endocrinopathies, or inborn errors of metabolism.

Hematologic Abnormalities. Evaluation of fetal anemia can serve several clinical purposes (see the box on p. 1028). A high a priori risk of anemia and the need for transfusion may be apparent (including fetal hydrops, high amniotic fluid optical density with maternal isoimmunization, Kell isoimmunization, and elevated maternal blood concentration of fetal red cells). Under these circumstances, fetal venous access allows transfusion to be done as soon as significant anemia is identified. Documentation of fetal anemia is also helpful if such findings help confirm a diagnosis

---

FETAL HEMATOLOGIC ABNORMALITIES SUBJECT TO FETAL BLOOD SAMPLING

Anemia
  Hydrops
  Maternal isoimmunization with high amniotic fluid
    optical density
  Kell isoimmunization
  Congenital hypoplastic anemia
  Fetal-maternal transfusion
  Parvovirus infection
Thrombocytopenia
  Maternal alloimmunity to platelet antigens (e.g.,
    Pl^A1)
  Maternal autoimmune thrombocytopenia (idiopathic
    thrombocytopenic purpura)
  Thrombocytopenia, absent radius (TAR) syndrome
Coagulopathy
  Hemophilia A and B
  von Willebrand disease
  Kasabach-Merritt syndrome
  Disseminated intravascular coagulation
Immunodeficiency diseases
  Severe combined immunodeficiency disease
  Chédiak-Higashi syndrome
  Wiskott-Aldrich syndrome
  Chronic granulomatous disease

---

when the patient has a family history of syndromes associated with fetal anemia or if the fetus has a fetal infection that is likely to cause anemia such as parvovirus or cytomegalovirus.

Fetal thrombocytopenia, if severe, may pose significant risk (10%) of fetal exsanguination and death during and after umbilical blood sampling.[67] Umbilical blood sampling for fetal alloimmune thrombocytopenia may be valuable, however. Clinical trials[14] suggest that maternal treatment with immunoglobulin G (IgG) reduces fetal hemorrhagic morbidity; thus knowledge of the fetal platelet count and phenotype is helpful to case management. The utility of fetal blood sampling in the context of maternal immune thrombocytopenia is less clear. The probability of fetal platelet count less than $50,000/mm^3$ in the context of maternal idiopathic thrombocytopenic purpura has been estimated to be $10.1 \pm 3.5\%$ and the probability of fetal platelet count less than $20,000/mm^3$ to be $4.2 \pm 2.3\%$.[10] The fetal platelet count at which internal bleeding is a significant risk is unknown in this condition, but it is probably fewer than $20,000/mm^3$. No effective fetal treatment exists for this condition, which generally has a low risk of fetal hemorrhage. Finally, the utility of one route of delivery over another with respect to fetal risk for internal bleeding has not been established. Secondary morbidity rates of approximately 40% are noted among infants born with platelet counts of less than $50,000/mm^3$, regardless of route of delivery.[10] Of 557 liveborn infants in one review, 5 had intracranial hemorrhage, 2

of whom died. If fetal blood studies are performed for infections known to cause thrombocytopenia, a fetal platelet count should also be performed.

Reports[25] have described timely diagnosis of other fetal coagulopathies such as hemophilia A and B, von Willebrand disease, Kasabach-Merritt syndrome, or disseminated intravascular coagulation with twin-to-twin perfusion abnormalities by use of umbilical vein sampling. Occasionally, thrombocytopenia can serve as a marker to differentiate among fetal structural abnormalities such as absent radius syndrome. Also, fetal blood sampling has been reportedly used in the antenatal diagnosis of congenital (usually X-linked) immunodeficiency diseases.

Fetal Karyotype and DNA Studies. Fetal lymphocytes provide a source of tissue for karyotyping and DNA molecular genetic diagnoses.[62] Fetal blood may be used when karyotype from fetal amniocytes or chorionic villus samples suggests fetal mosaicism. In one report of 23 fetuses with true mosaicism, fetal blood sampling demonstrated mosaicism in only 3 fetuses. The remainder, all of whom had normal anatomic sonographic surveys, were normal at term birth.[76]

Fetal karyotype from blood lymphocytes can generally be available within 72 hours. This may be advantageous when fetal anatomic malformations are identified sonographically (suggesting a high probability of chromosomal abnormality), late in the previable period so that pregnancy termination can be obtained, or in the third trimester when delivery is immanent.

Evaluation of Fetal Growth Restriction. Gestational age less than 32 weeks at birth is associated with significant neonatal and long-term morbidity. Several methods have been used to identify which fetuses with growth restriction at an early gestational age would benefit from delivery. These methods include the nonstress test, contraction stress test, biophysical profile scoring, Doppler velocimetry, and fetal blood sampling. All of these tests have moderate to poor sensitivity for fetal hypoxia. Abnormal velocimetry has a high positive predictive value for fetal hypoxia among growth-restricted fetuses. Given the overall 1% to 2% risks of cordocentesis that may be higher in these fetuses, the role of fetal blood sampling is uncertain. It seems to add little to the management of fetuses with absent end-diastolic umbilical artery flow and would be used to excess in fetuses who had equivocal biophysical testing. Its main utility may be for karyotype assessment in severe or early growth restriction or in fetuses who have structural abnormalities that are associated with growth restriction.

Evaluation of Fetal Hypoxia and Other Metabolic Abnormalities. The norms for fetal pH and gas values have been established; the values in fetuses with a high risk of hypoxia can be compared with these norms.[81] The uncertain prognostic value of mild hypoxia or acidosis in fetuses without attributes that otherwise suggest significant placental dysfunction limits the utility of fetal blood sampling for this indication.

Fetal blood sampling has allowed correlation of varying fetal observations with fetal acid-base status and blood gas measures. The fetal middle cerebral artery pulsatility index appears to be associated with fetal hypoxia, for example.[70] Erythropoietin has been found to correlate with fetal pH and Po_2 in both the term and preterm fetus but does not appear to identify fetal growth deficiency or fetal hematocrit.[71]

DNA analysis is available for prenatal diagnosis of an ever-increasing number of metabolic diseases. However, some families have DNA that is uninformative for a particular mutation. In these patients, examination of fetal hepatic or blood enzymes or metabolic products may be diagnostic. For example, abnormal fucose metabolism (Rambam-Hasharon syndrome) has been identified in utero by documenting fucosylated proteoglycan deficiency manifested as Bombay blood type in the fetus.[32]

Diagnosis of Fetal Infection. PUBS has also been used for the evaluation of viral, bacterial, and parasitic fetal infections, usually in the context of serologic evidence of maternal infection or sonographic findings suggestive of fetal infection. Fetal antibody titers, direct culture of fetal blood, or DNA studies for microorganisms have been reported. Fetal blood sampling has been used extensively in Europe for the evaluation of patients at risk for toxoplasmosis.[24] In the latter instance, 746 such pregnant women were evaluated with PUBS. If the fetus was demonstrated to be infected, the mother was treated with antimicrobial agents.

Other Uses. Fetal blood sampling may improve the evaluation of fetal renal failure. Compared with unaffected control subjects and fetuses with milder urinary tract abnormalities, fetuses with bilateral severe renal dysplasia or agenesis have been observed to have elevated blood α_1-microglobulin concentration.[18] Such observations, in concert with information about fetal urine osmolality, and electrolyte excretion patterns may be useful in assigning in utero therapy for fetal urinary tract dysfunction.

Technique

The technique of umbilical blood sampling (Fig. 55-4) involves the insertion of a needle into the umbilical vein with sonographic guidance using both two-dimensional and color Doppler imaging.[21,23,41,91] We find it preferable to perform all PUBS in the same suite to ensure the same team of nurses, technicians, and physicians. Because many procedures are performed in late gestation, all PUBS are performed in the operating room so that emergency delivery of the fetus can be accomplished when appropriate. Local anesthesia alone is usually sufficient for patient comfort. In cases of maternal obesity, difficult access to the cord insertion site, or a posterior placenta, or when PUBS transfusion is being performed, maternal sedation and transient fetal paralysis may be helpful. Fetal paralysis may be accomplished by fetal intramuscular or intravenous injections of pancuronium bromide.[75] PUBS is usually performed in the umbilical vein, preferably near the placental insertion site, where mechanical stability is optimal.

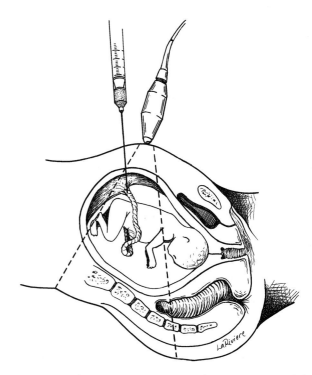

Fig. 55-4 Schematic representation of percutaneous umbilical blood sampling.

Possible contamination of the fetal blood specimen by amniotic fluid or maternal blood can be identified by demonstrating a lower "shoulder" or bimodal red cell volume distribution on an automated cell counter.[30] Such contamination will confound most diagnostic tests but can usually be avoided by stable needle placement before aspiration.

Differential staining of fetal cells in the maternal circulation by the Kleihauer-Betke test and post-PUBS rise in maternal serum α-fetoprotein have both been documented to identify sufficient fetal blood in the maternal circulation to elicit a maternal immune response (0.25 ml or more in 46% of cases).[89]

Successful PUBS has been reported in five of eight attempts in first trimester pregnancies scheduled for elective termination using a transcervical endoscope.[68] PUBS has been performed as early as at 18 weeks' gestation in ongoing pregnancies and becomes technically easier as gestation advances.

Risks

The maternal complications of percutaneous umbilical blood sampling include chorioamnionitis, hemorrhage, injury to abdominal viscera, and blood group isoimmunization. Fetal complications include fetal bleeding, infection, and bradycardia.[3,21,55] Persistent bradycardia is reported to occur 3% to 12% of fetuses and is associated with umbilical artery puncture, antecedent fetal anemia, and growth retardation.[34] Procedure-related fetal death is usually preceded by fetal bradycardia, but most cases of fetal bradycardias are self-limited and brief.

The risks of PUBS appear to be low in the hands of experienced surgeons. Daffos[23] reported an in utero fetal death rate of 1.1%, an abortion rate of 0.8%, and a premature delivery rate of 5% among 606 consecutive PUBS. More recent data on more than 2000 PUBS (including the 606 previously reported cases) suggest that the combined risk of abortion and fetal death in experienced hands is between 0.5% and 1%.[21] Weiner et al.[92] reported on a series of 1260 PUBS procedures performed at two active centers at a mean of 29 weeks. Of 12 procedure-related loses (0.9%), 11 were associated with fetal bradycardia. Losses were also associated with umbilical artery puncture. When fetal chromosomal abnormalities and growth restriction were excluded, the procedure-related loss rate was 0.2%. This reflects the relatively increased PUBS-related risk sustained by chromosomally abnormal fetuses compared with normal control subjects noted by Wilson et al.,[93] who calculated a procedure risk of fetal death of 3.25% and 1.25%, respectively, in 214 procedures.

PUBS-associated fetal bradycardia has stimulated investigation about fetal hemodynamics during umbilical blood sampling. In one report,[15] amniocentesis with or without transplacental needle insertion was not associated with a decrease in Doppler pulsatility index (PI). However, cordocentesis was associated with a significant decrease of PI values in fetal vessels. Furthermore, with respect to the uterine artery, the amplitude of this decrease was greater in cases in which the umbilical vein was accessed through the placenta. This was not found in other fetal arteries. Because fetal heart rate in this study was not affected by cordocentesis, changes in fetal vascular impedance, increased cardiac contractility, or increased fetal pressure may account for the observed changes. Further insight will depend on animal experiments.

Although more active sites and later reports note lower fetal loss rates and other complications from PUBS, examination of the loss rate within surgeons as they gain experience in these larger centers does not show increased safety with advancing surgeon experience.[7,92] This suggests that a well-organized team, appropriate supervision, and prudent selection of cases for intervention may impact fetal safety more than individual surgeon experience.

CONCLUSIONS
Risk-Benefit Analysis

Diagnostic procedures in pregnancy, whether invasive or not, require consideration of the value of the information to be obtained versus the possible risks of the procedure. The physician not only must consider the risks and benefits, but he or she also must clearly explain the risks and benefits to the patient and document the discussion. The availability of a variety of techniques (amniocentesis, CVS, and fetal blood sampling) now allows a choice of which fetal tissue might be most appropriate to make a given diagnosis. Other considerations in the choice of procedure include the gestational age at the time of procedure and the risk of a given procedure in relation to the risk of a suspected diagnosis (Table 55-1).

Because these procedures are used at differing gestational ages, it is important to consider (and to discuss with the patient) the background risks of spontaneous pregnancy loss, to which the procedure-related risks are added. It is also true that the prevalence of fetal chromosomal abnormalities decreases with advancing gestational age. Therefore the risk of finding aneuploidy increases when prenatal diagnostic tests are applied at earlier gestational ages.

The Future

These invasive diagnostic procedures have dramatically changed the practice of obstetrics. Future developments, which are certain to continue this process, are likely to include less invasive and less risky diagnostic procedures for prenatal diagnosis. For example, there is renewed interest in isolating fetal cells directly from the maternal circulation.[95] If this becomes possible, only a maternal venipuncture would be required to obtain fetal DNA for diagnostic purposes. However, the technical feasibility of fetal lymphocyte isolation remains to be demonstrated. In addition, the use of

Table 55-1 A Brief Comparison of Prenatal Diagnostic Techniques

	Amniocentesis	Chorionic Villus Sampling	Purcutaneous Umbilical Blood Sampling
What can be diagnosed	Chromosome problems Some inherited diseases Open spina bifida	Chromosome problems Some inherited diseases	Chromosome problems Some inherited diseases Fetal blood studies (hematocrit, platelets)
	ΔOD450 Lung maturity studies Studies for chorioamnionitis		Fetal drug levels
When test is performed	>14 wk	10-12 wk	After 18-20 wk
Availability of results	7-14 days	7-14 days	Similar to adult blood studies (some in 48 hr)
Procedure-related risk	<1% (probably 0.2%-0.5%)	~1.1% (0.8% greater than amniocentesis)	>1%

newer laboratory techniques such as fluorescent in situ hybridization[48] may allow the diagnosis of certain cytogenetic abnormalities, within hours, from any fetal tissue (including amniotic fluid cells).

Options for in utero therapy, other than transfusion, may also become available. However, recent attempts at open fetal surgery during ongoing pregnancy have met with limited success and must be considered investigational.[39,53] The role of fetal surgery in humans will be further constrained by the requirement for timely diagnosis and referral of suitable cases for effective intervention. These issues continue to generate a lively debate about the clinical utility of fetal treatment.

REFERENCES

1. Ämmälä P, et al: Randomized trial comparing first-trimester transcervical chorionic villus sampling and second-trimester amniocentesis, *Prenat Diagn* 13:919, 1993.
2. Baird PA, Yee AML, Sadovnick AD: Population-based study of long-term outcomes after amniocentesis, *Lancet* 344:1134, 1994.
3. Benacerraf BR, et al: Acute fetal distress associated with percutaneous umbilical blood sampling, *Am J Obstet Gynecol* 156:1218, 1987.
4. Benacerraf BR, Frigoletto FD: Amniocentesis under continuous ultrasound guidance: a series of 232 cases, *Obstet Gynecol* 62:760, 1983.
5. Bennett PR, et al: Prenatal determination of fetal RhD type of DNA amplification, *N Engl J Med* 329:607, 1993.
6. Benzie R, et al: Fetoscopy and fetal tissue sampling, *Prenat Diagn* 1(suppl):29(special issue), 1980.
7. Bernaschek G, et al: Complications of cordocentesis in high-risk pregnancies: effects on fetal loss or preterm delivery, *Prenat Diagn* 15:995, 1995.
8. Bevis DCA: The antenatal prediction of haemolytic disease of the newborn, *Lancet* 1:395, 1952.
9. Blakemore K, et al: Cook obstetrics and gynecology catheter multicenter chorionic villus sampling trial: comparison of birth defects with expected rates, *Am J Obstet Gynecol* 169:1022, 1993.
10. Borrows RF, Kelton JF: Pregnancy in patients with idiopathic thrombocytopenic purpura: assessing the risks for the infant at delivery, *Obstet Gynecol Surv* 48:781, 1993.
11. Bovicelli L, et al: Transabdominal versus transcervical routes for chorionic villus sampling, *Lancet* 1:290, 1986.
12. Brambati B, Oldrini A, Lanzani A: A transabdominal chorionic villus sampling: a freehand ultrasound-guided technique, *Am J Obstet Gynecol* 157:134, 1987.
13. Burton B, Schultz CJ, Burd LI: Limb anomalies associated with chorionic villus sampling, *Obstet Gynecol* 79:726, 1992.
14. Bussel JB, et al: Fetal alloimmune thrombocytopenia, *N Engl J Med* 337:22, 1997.
15. Capponi, A, et al: The effects of fetal blood sampling and placental puncture on umbilical artery and fetal arterial vessels blood flow velocity waveforms, *Am J Perinat* 13:185, 1996.
16. Cheuh JT, et al: Comparison of transcervical and transabdominal chorionic villus sampling loss rates in nine thousand cases from a single center, *Am J Obstet Gynecol* 173:1277, 1995.
17. Clinical Opinion: Report of National Institute of Child Health and Human Development Workshop on Chorionic Villus Sampling and Limb and Other Defects, October 20, 1992, *Am J Obstet Gynecol* 169:1, 1993.
18. Cobet G, et al: Assessment of serum levels of α-1-microglobulin, α-2-microglobulin, and retinol binding protein in the metal blood: a method for prenatal evaluation of renal function, *Prenat Diagn* 16:299, 1996.
19. Reference deleted in proofs.
20. Cutillo DM, et al: Chorionic villus sampling utilization following reports of a possible association with fetal limb defects, *Prenat Diagn* 14:327, 1994.
21. Daffos F: Fetal blood sampling, *Annu Rev Med* 40:319, 1989.
22. Daffos F, Capella-Pavlovsky M, Forestier F: Fetal blood sampling via the umbilical cord using a needle guided by ultrasound: report of 66 cases, *Prenat Diagn* 3:271, 1983.
23. Daffos F, Capella-Pavlovsky M, Forestier F: Fetal blood sampling during pregnancy with the use of a needle guided by ultrasound: a study of 606 consecutive cases, *Am J Obstet Gynecol* 153:655, 1985.
24. Daffos F, et al: Prenatal management of 746 pregnancies at risk for congenital toxoplasmosis, *N Engl J Med* 318:271, 1988.
25. Daffos F, et al: Prenatal diagnosis and management of bleeding disorders with fetal blood sampling, *Am J Obstet Gynecol* 158:939, 1988.
26. Eiben B, et al: Safety of early amniocentesis versus CVS, *Lancet* 344:1303, 1994 (letter to the editor).
27. Finegan JK, et al: Children whose mothers had second trimester amniocentesis: follow-up at school age, *Br J Obstet Gynecol* 103:214, 1996.
28. Firth HV, et al: Analysis of limb reduction defects in babies exposed to chorionic villus sampling, *Lancet* 343:1069, 1994.
29. Firth HV, et al: Severe limb abnormalities after chorion villus sampling at 56-66 days' gestation, *Lancet* 337:762, 1991.
30. Forestier F, et al: The assessment of fetal blood samples, *Am J Obstet Gynecol* 158:1184, 1988.
31. Froster UG, Jackson L: Limb defects and chorionic villus sampling: results from an international registry, 1992-94, *Lancet* 347:489, 1996.
32. Frydman M, et al: Prenatal diagnosis of Rambam-Hasharon syndrome, *Prenat Diagn* 16:266, 1996.
33. Fuchs F, Riis P: Antenatal sex determination, *Nature* 117:330, 1956.
34. Ghidini, A, et al: Complications of fetal blood sampling, *Am J Obstet Gynecol* 168:1339, 1993.
35. Gilberg C, Rasmussen P, Wahlstrom J: Long-term follow-up of children born after amniocentesis, *Clin Genet* 21:69, 1982.
36. Haddow JE, et al: Data from an alpha-fetoprotein screening program in Maine, *Obstet Gynecol* 62:556, 1983.
37. Hahnemann N, Mohr J: Genetic diagnosis in the embryo by means of biopsy from extraembryonic membranes, *Bull Eur Soc Hum Genet* 2:23, 1968.
38. Hanson FW, et al: Amniocentesis before 15 weeks gestation: outcome risks and technical problems, *Am J Obstet Gynecol* 156:1524, 1987.
39. Harrison MR, et al: Successful repair in utero of a fetal diaphragmatic hernia after removal of herniated viscera from the left thorax, *N Engl J Med* 332:1582, 1990.
40. Henry GP, Miller WA: Early amniocentesis, *J Reprod Med* 37:396, 1992.
41. Hobbins JC, et al: Percutaneous umbilical blood sampling, *Am J Obstet Gynecol* 152:1, 1985.
42. Hogge WA, Schonberg SA, Golbus MS: Chorionic villus sampling: experience of the first 1000 cases, *Am J Obstet Gynecol* 154:1249, 1986.
43. Holzgreve W, et al: Safety of placental biopsy in the second and third trimester, *N Engl J Med* 317:1159, 1987.
44. Jackson LG, et al: A randomized comparison of transcervical and transabdominal chorionic-villus sampling, *N Engl J Med* 327:594, 1992.
45. James F: Sexing foetuses by examination of amniotic fluid, *Lancet* 1:202, 1956.
46. Jeanty P, et al: How to improve your amniocentesis technique, *Am J Obstet Gynecol* 146:593, 1983.
47. Johnson A, Godmilow L: Genetic amniocentesis at 14 weeks or less, *Clin Obstet Gynecol* 31:345, 1988.
48. Julien C, et al: Rapid prenatal diagnosis of Down's syndrome with in-situ hybridisation of fluorescent DNA probes, *Lancet* 2:863, 1986.
49. Kazy S, Stigar AM, Bakharev VA: Chorionic biopsy under immediate real-time (ultrasound) control, *Orv Hetil* 121:2765, 1980.
50. Lambl D: Ein seltener Fall von Hydramnios, *Zentralbl Gynakol* 5:329, 1881.

51. Ledbetter DH, et al: Cytogenetic results of chorionic villus sampling: high success rate and diagnosis accuracy in the United State collaborative study, *Am J Obstet Gynecol* 162:495, 1990.

52. Liley AW: Liquor amnii analysis in the management of the pregnancy complicated by rhesus sensitization, *Am J Obstet Gynecol* 82:1359, 1961.

53. Longaker MT, et al: Maternal outcome after open fetal surgery: a review of the first 17 human cases, *JAMA* 265:737, 1991.

54. Lowe CU, et al: The NICHD amniocentesis registry: the safety and accuracy of mid- trimester amniocentesis, DHEW Pub. no (NIH) 78-190. Washington, DC, 1978, US Department of Health, Education, and Welfare.

55. Ludomirsky A, et al: Percutaneous fetal umbilical blood sampling: procedure safety and normal fetal hematologic indices, *Am J Perinatol* 5:264, 1988.

56. MacKenzie W, Holmes D, Newton J: A study comparing transcervical with transabdominal chorionic villus sampling (CVS), *Br J Obstet Gynaecol* 95:75, 1988.

57. Makowski EL, Prem K, Kaiser IH: Detection of sex of fetuses by the incidence of sex chromatin body in nuclei of cells in amniotic fluid, *Science* 123:542, 1956.

58. Medical Research Council: *Diagnosis of genetic disease by amniocentesis during the second trimester of pregnancy,* Rep no 5, Ottawa, Canada, 1977.

59. Menees TO, Miller JD, Holly LE: Amniography: preliminary report, *Am J Roentgenol Radium Ther* 24:363, 1930.

60. Nadler HL, Gerbie AB: Role of amniocentesis in the intrauterine detection of genetic disorders, *N Engl J Med* 282:596, 1970.

61. Nicolaides KH, et al: Comparison of chorionic villus sampling and amniocentesis for fetal karyotyping at 10-13 weeks' gestation, *Lancet* 344:435, 1994.

62. Nicolaides KH, Rodeck CH, Gosden GM: Rapid karyotyping in nonlethal fetal malformations, *Lancet* 5:283, 1986.

63. Nicolaides KH, Soothill PW, Rosevear S: Transabdominal placental biopsy, *Lancet* 2:855, 1987.

64. Nicolaides KH, et al: Have Liley charts outlived their usefulness? *Am J Obstet Gynecol* 155:90, 1986.

65. Nicolaides KH, et al: Why confine chorionic villus (placental) biopsy to the first trimester? *Lancet* 1:543, 1986.

66. Olney RS, et al: Increased risk for transverse digital deficiency after chorionic villus sampling: results of the United States multistate case-control study, 1988-1992, *Teratology* 51:20, 1995.

67. Paidas MJ, et al: Alloimmune thrombocytopenia: fetal and neonatal losses related to cordocentesis. *Am J Obstet Gynecol* 172:475, 1995.

68. Reece EA, et al: Gaining access to the embryonic-fetal circulation via first-trimester endoscopy: a step into the future, *Obstet Gynecol* 82:876, 1993.

69. Rhoads GG, et al: The safety and efficacy of chorionic villus sampling for early prenatal diagnosis of cytogenetic abnormalities, *N Engl J Med* 320:609, 1989.

70. Rizzo G, et al: The value of fetal arterial, cardiac and venous flows in predicting pH and blood gases measured in umbilical blood at cordocentesis in growth retarded fetuses, *Br J Obstet Gynaecol* 102:963, 1995.

71. Rollins MD, et al: Cord blood erythropoietin, pH, PaO_2 and haematocrit following caesarean section before labour, *Biol Neonate* 63:147, 1993.

72. Romero R, et al: Sonographically monitored amniocentesis to decrease intraoperative complications, *Obstet Gynecol* 65:426, 1985.

73. Schreinemachers DM, Cross PK, Hook EB: Rates of trisomy 21, 18, 13 and other chromosome abnormalities in about 20,000 prenatal studies compared with estimated rates in live births, *Hum Genet* 61:318, 1982.

74. Second report of the UK collaborative study on alpha-fetoprotein in relation to neural tube defects: Amniotic fluid alpha-fetoprotein measurement in antenatal diagnosis of anencephaly and open spina bifida in early pregnancies, *Lancet* 2:652, 1979.

75. Seeds JW, Corke BC, Speilman FL: Prevention of fetal movement during invasive procedures with pancuronium bromide, *Am J Obstet Gynecol* 155:818, 1986.

76. Shalev E, et al: The role of cordocentesis in assessment of mosaicism found in amniotic fluid cell culture, *Acta Obstet Gynecol Scand* 73:119, 1994.

77. Shettles LB: Nuclear morphology of cells in human amniotic fluid in relation to sex of infant, *Am J Obstet Gynecol* 71:834, 1956.

78. Simoni G, et al: Efficient direct chromosome analyses and enzyme determinations from chorionic villi samples in the first trimester of pregnancy, *Hum Genet* 63:349, 1983.

79. Smidt-Jensen S, Sundberg K: Early amniocentesis, *Curr Opin Obstet Gynecol* 7:117, 1995.

80. Smith AD, et al: Amniotic fluid acetylcholinesterase as a possible diagnostic test for neural tube defects in early pregnancy, *Lancet* 1:685, 1979.

81. Soothill PW, et al: Effect of gestational age on fetal and intervillous blood gas and acid-base values in human pregnancy, *Fetal Ther* 1:168, 1986.

82. Special Report: The status of fetoscopy and fetal tissue sampling, *Prenat Diagn* 4:79, 1984.

83. Steele MW, Breg WR Jr: Chromosome analysis of human amniotic fluid cells, *Lancet* 1:383, 1966.

84. Sundberg K, et al: Experience with early amniocentesis, *J Perinatal Med* 23:149, 1995.

85. Tabor A, et al: Randomized controlled trial of genetic amniocentesis in 4606 low risk women, *Lancet* 1:1287, 1986.

86. Turnbull AC, et al: Report to the Medical Research Council: an assessment of the hazards of amniocentesis, *Br J Obstet Gynaecol* 85:1, 1978.

87. Vachon F, et al: Second trimester placental biopsy versus amniocentesis for prenatal diagnosis of ß-thalassemia, *N Engl J Med* 322:60, 1990.

88. Valenti C: Antenatal detection of hemoglobinopathies, *Am J Obstet Gynecol* 115:851, 1973.

89. Van Selm, M, Kanhai, HH, Van Loon AJ: Detection of fetomaternal haemorrhage associated with cordocentesis using serum alpha-fetoprotein and the Kleihauer technique, *Prenat Diagn* 15:313, 1995.

90. Walker A: Liquor amnii studies in the prediction of haemolytic disease of the newborn, *Br Med J* 2:376, 1957.

91. Weiner CP: Cordocentesis for diagnostic indications: two years' experience, *Obstet Gynecol* 70:664, 1987.

92. Weiner CP, Okamura K: Diagnostic fetal blood sampling-technique related losses, *Fetal Diagn Ther* 11:169, 1996.

93. Wilson RD, et al: Cordocentesis: overall pregnancy loss rate as important as procedure loss rate, *Fetal Diagn Ther* 9:142, 1994.

94. Wilson E, et al: Multicentre randomised clinical trial of chorionic villus sampling and amniocentesis, *Lancet* 1:1, 1989.

95. Yeoh SC, et al: Detection of fetal cells in maternal blood, *Prenat Diagn* 11:117, 1991.

56 First and Second Trimester Abortion

PHILLIP G. STUBBLEFIELD

Abortion is a common procedure, yet most abortions are performed in free-standing clinics, out of the mainstream. Physicians in training may not understand the central role safe, legal abortion plays in the health of women. Before the technology for abortion is considered, it is important to describe something of the social and medical background of pregnancy termination.

Pregnancy carries a risk of illness and death. The U.S. maternal mortality rate was 9.2 per 100,000 live births in 1987 through 1990.[41] Annual fatality rates for all legal abortions in the United States from 1980 through 1991 were less than or equal to 1.2 per 100,000 abortions, and in the first trimester were far less than 1 per 100,000.[41,42] Young women are especially in need of abortion because fertility is greater and intercourse without contraception more common than for older people.[23] For women 15 to 19 the abortion ratio was 400 per 1000 live births in 1994, and the ratio was 650 per 1000 for girls younger than age 15.[41] Without legal abortion, births to teenaged mothers would almost double. For all age groups, contraception fails more often than medical personnel usually realize. For this reason and because of fear of side effects, sterilization is the most common method of contraception among U.S. couples.[48] Deaths from complications of illegal abortion were a major cause of maternal mortality until the 1960s. With the increasing availability of legal abortion, the number of these deaths fell dramatically. In 1991, 6 deaths occurred in the United States from spontaneous abortion, 11 from legal abortion, and 1 from illegal abortion (abortion induced by a nonphysician).[41]

The problems of fertility control and health are far worse in the Third World. Maternal mortality rates are significantly higher, typically 300 to 500 per 100,000 births; access to contraception is limited; and illegal abortion is widely practiced. In many countries half or more of pregnancy-related deaths are from complications of illegal abortions. However, safe abortion services can be provided at low cost and reduce maternal mortality.[2]

The risk of death from abortion increases with gestational age, and after 16 weeks abortion is probably no safer than continuing pregnancy (Table 56-1).[43] For individual women with high-risk conditions, even late abortion is undoubtedly safer than continuing pregnancy. More than 90% of U.S. abortions are performed in the first trimester when they are safest.[49]

FIRST TRIMESTER ABORTION
Surgical Techniques

Virtually all first trimester abortions in the United States are performed by vacuum curettage. The technique was first reported in China in 1954.[73] It spread to Eastern Europe and was then introduced into England in the 1960s. It was introduced into the United States through the efforts of Laylor Burdick. Standard vacuum curettage uses a rigid plastic cannula, 8 to 12 mm in diameter, with an electric pump. A more recent innovation is the menstrual regulation, or minisuction, technique with smaller, flexible cannula, often used with only a modified 50-ml syringe as vacuum source.[39]

Standard Vacuum Curettage. A medical history is taken, and a physical examination is performed to rule out complicating factors. There are no absolute contraindications to first trimester vacuum curettage performed under local anesthesia, but some conditions will dictate additional consultation and preparation or referral. The patient deserves the opportunity to discuss her decision with a nonjudgmental person and to have full information about her options and time to make an informed choice.[59] However, because complications increase with gestational age, providing abortion services should be regarded as urgent, once the patient has reached a decision.

Pelvic Examination. A bimanual examination is performed, noting uterine size, position, tenderness, and the presence of adnexal masses. Suspicion of abnormality or size-date discrepancy calls for an ultrasound examination. A speculum is inserted, and specimens are taken for cervical cytological analysis, gonorrhea culture, and *Chlamydia* antigen test. For local anesthesia procedures, the familiar weighted speculum is uncomfortable, and the short, Moore modification of the Graves speculum is preferred. It requires some experience to easily expose the cervix with this speculum, but once in place and the cervix is grasped with a tenaculum, it is easy to draw the cervix down to the introitus, facilitating safe introduction of instruments through the cervical canal (Fig. 56-1).

Next, the cervix is cleansed with a germicide such as povidone iodine. Full sterile technique is not necessary. Most U.S. abortions are carried out following the "no-touch technique." The surgeon wears sterile gloves and works from a small sterile instrument kit, but sterile drapes and gowns are not used.[9] The surgeon takes care never to touch that portion of an instrument that will enter the uterus.

Paracervical Block. I use a 1% lidocaine solution containing 0.5 mg of atropine in 20 ml. Atropine is added to

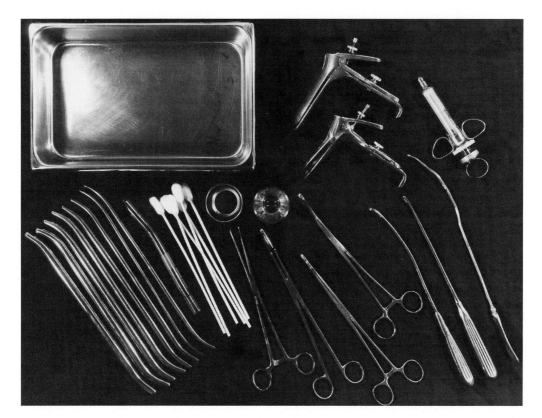

Fig. 56-1   Instrument kit for vacuum curettage abortion. *Left to right:* sterile tray, Graves speculum, Moore speculum, control syringe, uterine sound, no. 1 curette, no. 3 curette, curved Foerster forceps, straight Foerster forceps, Moore ovum forceps, single tooth tenaculum, medicine glasses, cotton swabs, plastic Vacurette, Pratt cervical dilators. (From Stubblefield PG: Surgical techniques for first trimester abortion. In Sciarra JJ, Zatuchni GI, Daly MJ, editors: *Gynecology and obstetrics,* vol 6, Hagerstown, Md, 1993, Harper & Row.)

Table 56-1   Legal Abortions, Deaths, Case-Fatality Rates, and Relative Risks by Gestational Age at Time of Procedure, United States 1972-1987

Weeks of Gestation	Deaths	Abortions	Rate*	Relative Risk Referent
≤8	33	8,673,739	0.4	
9-10	39	4,847,321	0.8	2.1
11-12	33	2,360,768	1.4	3.7
13-15	28	962,185	2.9	7.7
16-20	74	794,093	9.3	24.5
≥21	21	175,395	12.0	31.5

From Lawson HW, et al: *Am J Obstet Gynecol* 171:1365, 1994.
*Number of legal abortion deaths per 100,000 abortions. Deaths with unknown gestation excluded.

prevent "cervical shock," a form of vasovagal syncope that can be seen with cervical dilation. Some have advocated the use of epinephrine-containing solutions, but these can cause cardiac arrhythmias even at concentrations as low as 1:200,000, and in asthmatic patients the metabisulfite preservative in all epinephrine solutions can cause fatal anaphylaxis.[65] There are several variations in technique for the block. In the past I used the superficial technique, in which the local anesthetic is injected submucosally. I am convinced that the combination of superficial and deep technique introduced by Glick[25] is superior. Weibe[70] has con-

firmed this in a comparative study. I use a modification of Glick's technique, injecting at three sites rather than the multiple locations he described. The cervix is infiltrated superficially with 2 to 3 ml at the 12-o'clock position, and the needle is then advanced through the anesthetized area for approximately 3 cm to reach the junction of the cervix and lower uterine segment, where an additional 2 ml is injected. This allows for painless placement of the tenaculum. The procedure is repeated at the 4- and 8-o'clock positions, injecting 2 to 3 ml superficially and then advancing the needle 3 cm to infiltrate the lower uterine segment on each side

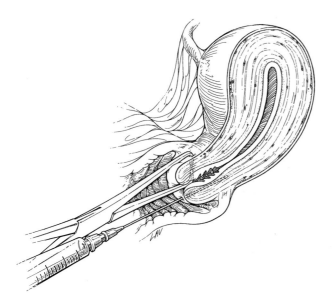

Fig. 56-2   Deep technique for paracervical block. Infiltrating the lower uterine segment at the 4-o'clock position.

with 4 to 5 ml. Care is taken to aspirate before each injection to avoid intravascular injection. This is important. Deaths have been reported with paracervical block. A 22-gauge 3½-inch spinal needle or a needle extender with a 1½-inch needle is used (Fig. 56-2). I use a total of 20 ml of 1% lidocaine (200 mg) in patients who weigh 100 lb or more. One should not exceed 2 ml/lb as an initial dose, so the amount is reduced in smaller patients.[27] Occasionally, the block is less effective on one side. If this occurs, an additional 5 to 6 ml of 1% lidocaine is injected deeply into the junction of cervix and lower uterine segment on that side.

Tenaculum Placement. I use a single-tooth, square-jaw tenaculum, placed vertically with one branch inside the cervical canal. Placement of the tenaculum in this fashion, grasping the cervix about 2 cm proximal to the external os, provides traction near the internal os, the region of greatest resistance. Outward traction with the tenaculum then serves to reduce the angle between the cervical canal and the uterine cavity, making it easier to insert dilators in the proper direction to avoid perforation (Fig. 56-3).

Sounding and Dilation. When forcible dilation will be performed, I favor sounding the uterus in the conventional fashion. Some view the sound as a "perforator" and do not use it. In my opinion, the use of the sound is optional. If the first dilator is easily inserted without resistance, sounding adds little. On the other hand, if any difficulty is encountered with the first dilator, using the sound can provide additional information regarding uterine size and position. With the uterine sound, dilator, or any instrument inserted through the cervical canal, it is important to avoid excessive force. The rule to follow is "If it isn't easy, something isn't right." The surgeon should not push harder. The cervical opening should be checked to ensure that it has been correctly identified, that the tenaculum is properly placed, and that the cervix is pulled well down toward the introitus. The

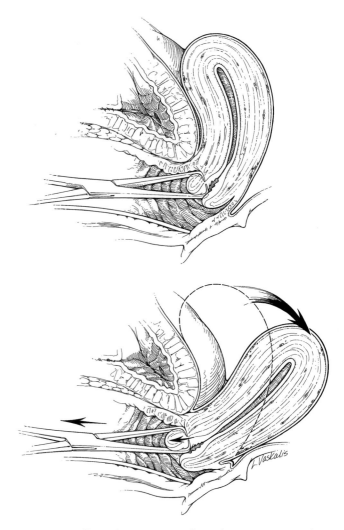

Fig. 56-3   Effect of proper tenaculum placement in straightening the angle between the cervix and the uterus by traction.

surgeon should bend the sound to a gentle curve, then slowly rotate it around its axis while pressing it gently through the canal. This allows the sound to find the true passage. Especially in the young nulligravida and in early pregnancy, the cervix can be tortuous and firm. Caution is required. Dilation is accomplished with gently tapered dilators; Pratt's or Denniston's plastic modification of the Pratt dilator is recommended (Fig. 56-4). Full-sized Hegar dilators should not be used because their blunt design requires excessive force. Half-sized Hegar dilators, with increases of only 0.5 mm between them, are an excellent choice, although rarely seen in U.S. operating rooms. Each dilator is inserted slowly and carefully, keeping in mind that the dilator tip must negotiate a curve where the cervix and uterus join. With an anteflexed uterus, the surgeon's hand must follow a downward curve to properly direct the dilator (Fig. 56-5). The direction is reversed when the uterus is retroverted. Failure to incorporate these simple concepts can lead to perforation. Sometimes placement of the tenaculum on the posterior lip of the cervix is helpful if the uterus is significantly retroverted.

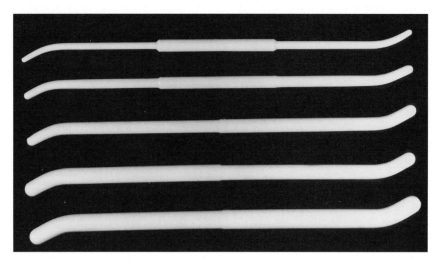

Fig. 56-4 Denniston dilators. (Photo courtesy of International Projects Assistance, Chapel Hill, NC.)

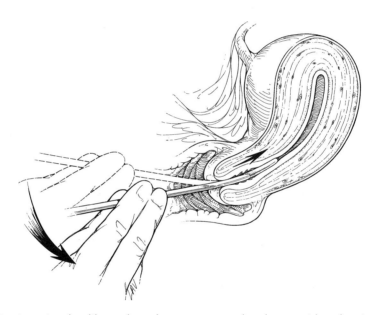

Fig. 56-5 Inserting the dilator along the proper curved path to avoid perforation. The tenaculum is omitted.

If much resistance is encountered during dilation, one should stop, reassess the position of tenaculum and cervix, and redirect the dilator along the proper curve. If there is still excessive resistance, the dilator should be removed and the next smallest dilator to that previously used should be inserted to confirm the correct angle. This smaller dilator should be inserted so that its widest portion traverses the internal os; it should be left in place for a minute or two before proceeding to the next larger dilator. There may come a point where continued dilation will require considerable force. At this point the surgeon should consider whether the abortion can be successfully completed with a smaller vacuum cannula than originally intended. Ordinarily, I use a cannula that is 1 mm smaller than the gestational age in menstrual weeks (e.g., 9 mm for 10 weeks). However, the 6-mm flexible Karman cannula used for minisuction (see the following section) works for pregnancies of 8 and 9 weeks, although the aspiration takes longer and more cannula action is required. At times use of the flexible cannula allows safe evacuation of the pregnancy from a significantly anteverted or retroverted uterus where the rigid cannula cannot negotiate the curve from cervical canal into uterine cavity. An 8-mm cannula can evacuate 10-week pregnancies, and a 9-mm rigid cannula will suffice through 12 weeks, although the procedure takes longer and requires more of the surgeon to avoid an incomplete procedure than would a larger cannula. Angulated cannulas are used in first trimester procedures. After 12 weeks I prefer straight cannulas because the uterine size is large relative to the cannula and the curve of the angulated cannula just gets in the way.

Uterine Evacuation. After insertion of the selected cannula, a vacuum is established. An electric vacuum pump is used at its maximum setting. Initially, the cannula is rotated vigorously around its long axis. This usually ruptures the membranes and begins the aspiration of amniotic fluid and tissue. After 30 seconds or so, tissue may block the cannula. At this point an in-and-out motion is combined with rotation. As the cannula is pulled back almost to the internal os, the lower uterine segment serves as a funnel, linearizing the tissue into the cannula orifice and helping to shear off pieces of placenta and membranes so that they can be evacuated. Depending on cannula size relative to gestational size, uterine evacuation is essentially complete in 1 to 2 minutes. When all tissue has been aspirated, the surgeon sees only a pink foam entering the cannula and notices the gritty feel of the cannula passing over the endometrial surface. The vacuum cannula is removed and a light curettage is performed, using the curette as one would use a finger, to palpate and confirm that the cavity is empty. Forceful curettage should be avoided because it is unnecessary. Pregnancy tissue is only lightly adherent to the uterine wall. If tissue has been retained, it is best to continue evacuation with the vacuum cannula. After the check with the sharp curette, the vacuum cannula should be reinserted for a final few seconds. The tenaculum is then removed, and the tenaculum site is observed for bleeding. Such bleeding will stop with pressure. Sometimes, it is necessary to compress the full thickness of the cervix with the ring forceps for 2 to 3 minutes to stop tenaculum site bleeding. Rarely, the tenaculum will have slipped off during the procedure and lacerated the cervical mucosa. If so, the laceration should be inspected to make sure it does not extend into the lower uterine segment and should be immediately repaired with a figure-of-eight suture of an absorbable material.

Tissue Examination. Next, the surgeon must carefully examine the aspirated tissue to be sure complete abortion has been performed and rule out ectopic or molar pregnancy.[10] The tissue is placed in a strainer, rinsed with normal saline, and then poured into a clear glass or plastic dish with a small amount of saline. Inspection over a light source facilitates identification of chorionic villi. From 8 weeks onward, fetal parts are also identified, and for later first trimester procedures (11 to 12 weeks), care must be taken to identify the calvarium, the axial skeleton, and extremities. Routine pathologic examination is unnecessary if the surgeon rigorously performs and documents the fresh inspection. Pathologic consultation is mandatory when the gestational sac is not identified, when tissue is scant for gestational age, or when abnormality is suspected.

Rhesus-negative patients not already sensitized are given Rh immunoglobulin immediately after the procedure.

Prophylactic Antibiotics. Perioperative antibiotics are commonly used in U.S. clinics. Two large nonrandomized studies showed benefit.[33,56] Others found the benefit limited to patients with a history of previous pelvic inflammatory disease.[58] A subsequent large randomized study found that although most of the benefit accrued to patients colonized

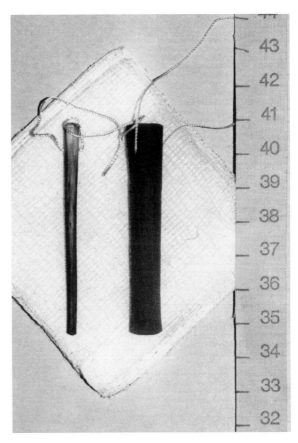

Fig. 56-6 Tents of *Laminaria japonicum*. Dry tent *(left)* as it would be just before insertion. Wet tent *(right)* as it would be after several hours of exposure to water. (Courtesy Mildred Hanson, M.D.)

with *Chlamydia*, *Chlamydia*-negative patients also benefitted.[45] On the other hand, antibiotics were not routinely used in Hakim-Elahi et al.'s[29] large series, yet serious infection was rare. Tetracycline, doxycycline, and minocycline have been most used. When cultures for gonorrhea and *Chlamydia* can be conveniently taken in advance, this should be done and therapy should be started for patients with positive screening results. I use single-dose oral azithromycin for *Chlamydia*-positive patients, or intramuscular (IM) ceftriaxone for gonorrhea-positive patients, and then perform the abortion procedure 1 to 2 hours later. My patients routinely receive doxycycline, 100 mg twice a day for 3 days, starting on the evening before the procedure when feasible.

Alternative Means for Cervical Dilation. Osmotic dilators can be used instead of forcible dilation. Presently, three types are available: laminaria tents, magnesium sulfate sponges (Lamicel), and synthetic tents of polyacrylonitrile (Dilapan). *Laminaria* is a genus of seaweed. When inserted into the cervical canal, *Laminaria* take up water from the cervix, causing it to swell and exert gentle pressure that produces dilation (Fig. 56-6). Only tents of *L. japonicum* should be used. The other medical laminaria, *L. digitata*, become too soft when wet and easily fragment with removal. Two or more small tents should be used rather than a single larger tent. A single tent may swell above a resistant internal cervical os and be difficult to remove.

Early studies found that use of laminaria reduced cervical laceration[55] and perforation[26] without increasing the risk of postabortal infection. In current U.S. practice, rates of cervical laceration and perforation are very low for experienced surgeons using conventional forcible dilation with Pratt dilators.[29] In my own practice, the main use of osmotic dilators is for the midtrimester. The main drawback of laminaria is that several hours are needed for dilation to be accomplished. Lamicel acts more quickly to pull water from the cervix and produce softening but exerts little force. Dilapan swells rapidly and exerts more force than natural laminaria. Analogs of prostaglandin produce useful dilation within 2 to 3 hours, but gastrointestinal side effects and pain are common. In a three-way trial, Dilapan produced more dilation than laminaria, whereas a prostaglandin analog produced less dilation and more side effects of vomiting and pain.[17]

Minisuction. In U.S. practice the minisuction technique is not used beyond 7 weeks. The procedure begins with a careful bimanual examination, and as with standard vacuum curettage, the cervix is exposed with a speculum, grasped with a tenaculum placed vertically, and then infiltrated with 20 ml of 1% lidocaine containing 0. 5 mg of atropine. Flexible Karman cannulas of 4 and 5 mm are passed through the cervical canal as dilators and used to sound the uterus. Then, a 6-mm cannula is inserted and attached to the evacuated 50-ml syringe to establish suction. The 4- and 5-mm cannulas are too small to dependably evacuate the uterus in pregnancy but are useful in treatment of anovulatory bleeding. The 6-mm cannula is rotated and pushed in and out with gentle strokes. The cannula must not be rotated when it is pushed against the fundus because the flexible tip can be twisted off. When no more tissue comes through, the cannula is withdrawn, its tip is cleared in a sterile fashion, and vacuum is reestablished to prove that the uterus is empty. Optionally, a small sharp curette can also be used to check, as with standard vacuum curettage. Fresh examination of the aspirated tissue is even more important with these early procedures because ectopic pregnancy is seen more often before 8 weeks than after and failed abortion is more likely as well. To prevent failed abortion, it is not enough to identify a few chorionic villi. The gestational sac must be seen.[22] Fig. 56-7 shows the appearance of an early pregnancy.

Edwards and Carson[18] have modified the minisuction technique and applied it to pregnancies as early as 3 weeks from last menstrual period. The cervix is dilated to 7 mm with Pratt dilators and then a 7-mm rigid curved Vacurette is used with a handheld 60 ml syringe as vacuum source (Mylex, Chicago). An intracervical block of 20 ml of 0.5% lidocaine with 2 U of vasopressin and conscious sedation with intravenous (IV) midazolam and nalbuphine are used for analgesia. A series of 1530 patients were treated before 6 weeks from the last menstrual period after preoperative ultrasound and with careful examination of the aborted tissue and follow-up with serial β-human chorionic gonado-

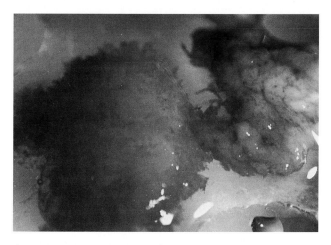

Fig. 56-7 Tissue specimen from 6-week pregnancy, as seen without magnification. The conceptus is on the *left*. To the *right* is the decidual lining of the uterus. (From Stubblefield PG: Surgical techniques for first trimester abortion. In Sciarra JJ, Zatuchni GI, Daly MJ, editors: *Gynecology and obstetrics,* vol 6, Hagerstown, Md, 1982, Harper & Row.)

tropic hormone titers to ensure diagnosis of ectopic pregnancy. No serious complications occurred, and nine unsuspected ectopic pregnancies were diagnosed and treated.

Minisuction at 8 Weeks and Beyond. In the Third World, minisuction instrumentation may be the only modern technology available. In some countries physicians have modified the procedure to successfully terminate pregnancy throughout the first trimester. Rigid dilators are used, usually half-sized Hegar, to dilate the cervix to 8 to 9 mm. The 6-mm Karman cannula is advanced to the fundus and back to just above the internal os several times to begin shearing the gestational sac off the uterine wall. The syringe plunger is then withdrawn to create a vacuum, rupture the sac, and aspirate the amniotic fluid. When the cannula tip plugs with tissue, cannula and tissue are withdrawn together without breaking the vacuum. Some of the pregnancy tissue will pass through the lumen of the cannula, but larger portions are removed in this fashion, held in the cannula tip by the vacuum. A small, sharp curette is used as well, alternating with the vacuum. When the syringe is partially full, the vacuum becomes reduced. The syringe is emptied and reevacuated to again establish a vacuum. This is repeated until the cavity feels empty. A 12-week procedure done in this fashion may take 10 to 15 minutes, much longer than is needed with an 11-mm rigid cannula and electric pump as is standard in U.S. practice. Nevertheless, an experienced surgeon can provide abortion services successfully and safely under field conditions with only the simple instruments described: 6-mm flexible cannula and syringe, dilators, and a small steel curette. With the addition of a slender ovum forceps, early midtrimester dilation and evacuation (D&E) procedures can be performed as well.[65]

Medical Abortion. Prostaglandins are effective abortifacients at any gestational age, and three forms are available in the United States that could be used in the first trimester: vaginal suppositories of prostaglandin E_2 (PGE_2), and carboprost tromethamine, the 15-methyl analog of prostaglandin $F_{2\alpha}$ ($PGF_{2\alpha}$) (Hemabate) given by IM injection, are approved by the Food and Drug Administration (FDA) for induction of abortion. Misoprostol, a 15-methyl analog of prostaglandin E_1, is FDA-approved for other indications and is being investigated for use as an abortifacient. These agents often cause side effects, and because of the widespread availability of surgical abortion, they are not often used in the first trimester. The first practical medical abortifacient was mifepristone (RU486), an analog of the progestin norethindrone. Mifepristone is an antagonist to progesterone, acting at the level of progesterone receptors in the nucleus of steroid-sensitive tissues. A single oral dose given to women in early pregnancy produces complete abortion in about 85% of cases. The addition of a single small dose of prostaglandin greatly improves efficacy. In a large French experience, 2115 women at or before 49 days of amenorrhea were given 600 mg of mifepristone as a single dose on day 1.[57] On day 3 they were treated with a prostaglandin, either 1 mg of gemeprost given vaginally or IM sulprostone (0.25 to 0.5 mg). Altogether, 96% aborted completely; 1% required urgent vacuum curettage for heavy bleeding, but only 1 of the 2115 patients had to be given a transfusion; 2% aborted incompletely and required a later curettage; 1% failed to abort and needed vacuum curettage. Later in pregnancy, the drug becomes less effective and there is a greater chance of incomplete abortion that will require curettage. Mifepristone can also be used to trigger cervical softening and dilation before surgical abortion.[44] The drug is widely used in France and England and, although approved by the FDA, is not yet available in this country.

Methotrexate, a folic acid antagonist, is being studied for medical abortion. In initial studies the same dose that is used to treat ectopic pregnancy, 50 mg/m^2 of body weight was given IM, and then followed 3 days later with 800 μg of misoprostol given vaginally.[14] In a multicenter study, 300 women received methotrexate at or before 56 days' gestation, followed 7 days later with 800 μg of misoprostol vaginally.[15] The misoprostol was repeated after 24 hours if the patient had not aborted. After the first dose of misoprostol, 53% aborted, an additional 15% aborted after a second dose; and a total of 92% aborted by 35 days. The methotrexate-misoprostol combination requires a longer interval to achieve the high efficacy of mifepristone-methotrexate; however, the regimen is very inexpensive, and both drugs are available in the United States.

Reduction of Multifetal Pregnancies

Extreme prematurity and perinatal loss are likely with multifetal pregnancy. In recent years there has been considerable interest in reduction of multifetal pregnancies and in selective termination of twin gestations where one fetus has major anomalies. The most often used technique is ultrasound-guided intracardiac injection of potassium chloride. Using high-resolution ultrasound, a 22-gauge spinal

needle is advanced through the abdominal and uterine walls toward the cardiac echo. A 2-mmol solution of KCl is used. In the first trimester, 0.2 to 0.4 ml are injected at a time until cardiac asystole is observed. In the series reported by Wapner et al.,[68] 0.2 to 1.8 ml total volume was required. Visualization is continued until 2 minutes of asystole have been observed. The needle is then withdrawn and redirected into another gestational sac as needed. Usually two gestations are left intact because the morbidity of diamniotic twins is not unacceptably greater than that of singletons. For second trimester procedures, 0.5 ml is injected at a time and total doses of 0.5 to 3 ml are required. In Wapner et al.'s series, 2 of 42 first trimester cases and 1 of 4 second trimester cases showed resumed cardiac activity 30 minutes later despite 2 minutes observation of asystole. These were successfully reinjected the same day. In Berkowitz et al.'s initial series[6] of 12 patients treated, 4 went on to abort the entire pregnancy, 7 delivered twins, and 1 delivered a singleton at term. All were healthy. Wapner et al.[68] treated 46 pregnant women. Of 80 fetuses remaining after reduction, 75 (94%) survived. They caution that monoamniotic twins should not be treated because this usually results in death of the remaining normal fetus. Similarly, treatment of twin-twin transfusion syndrome by selective termination of one fetus has been troublesome, with the occurrence of infarctions resulting from embolism of tissue from the dead fetus through the shared circulation. The maternal serum α-fetoprotein level is elevated after selective termination. Maternal coagulation defects were not seen, but most of the patients were treated in the first trimester, when risk for this phenomenon is very low. Maternal coagulation surveillance is warranted after second trimester procedures. In a large multicenter trial, Evans et al.[20] reported on 463 patients treated for multifetal gestations. Of the women, 83% delivered at 33 weeks or later, and 16% of the fetuses were lost before 24 weeks. The same group reported a series of 183 cases of selective termination for anomalies. Termination of the anomalous fetus was successful in all cases. In 12% of the pregnancies miscarriage occurred after the termination procedure and before 24 weeks.[21]

Complications of First Trimester Abortion

Postabortal Triad. The syndrome of pain, bleeding, and low-grade fever is the most common complication of first trimester abortion. The symptoms may respond to treatment with ergot preparations and oral antibiotics; however, in most cases the symptoms indicate some amount of retained tissue or blood clot in the uterine cavity. Repeat evacuation is readily accomplished under local anesthesia without need for the operating room and usually resolves the problems quickly. Because some amount of endometritis is usually present, I use a 7- to 10-day course of oral antibiotics after reevacuation.

Hematometra. In hematometra, a type of uterine atony, the patient experiences increasing lower abdominal pain soon after the abortion.[54] The symptoms can be dramatic, with severe lower midline pain, diaphoresis, and tachycardia. On examination the uterus is enlarged, tense, and tender. This could be mistaken for perforation with a broad ligament hematoma except that the mass is midline. Immediate reevacuation is the treatment of choice. In Hakim-Elahi et al.'s large series,[29] 1 in 500 experienced this complication and were managed with reaspiration of the uterus in the clinic on the same day. It has been suggested that perioperative use of an IM ergot preparation will reduce the incidence.[54] The same syndrome can develop more slowly with symptoms of pain and bleeding a few days after the abortion.

Hemorrhage. Excessive bleeding with vacuum curettage may be caused by uterine atony, perforation, or a pregnancy of more advanced gestational age than anticipated. Rare causes are low-lying implantation or cervical pregnancy and disseminated intravascular coagulopathy. General anesthesia leads to additional concerns because all of the potent anesthetic gases will relax the uterus in proportion to the inhaled concentration. Management of excess bleeding requires a rapid reassessment of gestational age by examination of the fetal parts already extracted and gentle exploration of the uterine cavity with curette or forceps to confirm that there is no perforation. IV oxytocin is administered, and the abortion is completed. The uterus is massaged between two hands to ensure contraction. Intracervical administration of 10 U of vasopressin diluted to 10 ml and intracervical or IM administration of 250 μg of carboprost tromethamine are helpful. Misoprostol, 800 μg, can be given rectally if carboprost is unavailable. As a temporizing measure, a Foley catheter with a 30-ml balloon can be inserted through the cervix and the balloon inflated to tamponade the lower uterine segment. If these measures fail, the patient should be transferred immediately to the hospital with IV fluids running. Continued brisk bleeding from atony persisting after complete evacuation is uncommon, as is coagulopathy with first trimester procedures. If bleeding persists, coagulopathy is ruled out and the patient is prepared for laparoscopy and repeat curettage. Cervical pregnancy and cervical perforation (described in the following section) are special cases, best managed by arteriography and selective embolization of the bleeding vessels.[66] Selection of this form of treatment requires prompt and accurate assessment to rule out other causes and volume support for the patient while arrangements are made for the radiologic procedure.

Perforation. The rate of perforation was 0.9 per 1000 in a multicenter study of 67,175 abortions.[28] The risk of perforation was greater for patients at more advanced stages of pregnancy and for parous women than for women with no previous delivery. Use of laminaria reduced risk, as did physician skill. Resident physicians were more likely than attending physicians to cause a perforation. A much lower rate, only 1 per 10,000, was reported in the series of 170,000 procedures through 14 weeks from the Planned Parenthood Clinic of New York City, where all procedures were performed by a small number of experienced physicians.[29] In that series dilation was achieved with Pratt dilators. Laminaria were not used.

In my own experience with patients hospitalized for perforation, the perforations were lateral and usually occurred either at the junction of the cervix and lower uterine segment or were perforations of the cervix itself (Fig. 56-8).[4] These lateral perforations produced different clinical syndromes depending on the anatomic location of the injury. Lateral perforations at the junction of the cervix and lower uterine segment can lacerate the ascending branch of the uterine artery within the broad ligament, causing severe pain, a broad ligament hematoma, and intraabdominal bleeding. This type of injury is usually recognized immediately. Laparoscopy is required to confirm the injury, with laparotomy to ligate the severed uterine artery and repair the uterine injury. Hysterectomy should not be required and may not stop the bleeding should the surgeon fail to perceive that the vascular injury is lateral to the site where the vessels are ligated in standard hysterectomy technique. Low cervical perforations, on the other hand, may injure the descending branch of the uterine artery within the dense collagenous substance of the cardinal ligaments. In this case there is only external bleeding through the cervical canal, and no broad ligament hematoma will form. Bleeding from this injury will cease as the arteries temporarily go into spasm, but it recurs. Deaths have occurred when a low cervical perforation was not recognized and began bleeding again several hours later when the patient was at home.

Hysterectomy has usually been required for management, but other options are available if the injury is suspected. Freiman[24] described a patient managed by laparotomy and placement of sutures through the cardinal ligaments after downward mobilization of the bladder and identification of the ureter. Arteriography and selected embolization of the injured vessel can be attempted.[66] Both types of injuries undoubtedly occur during dilation. Midline and fundal perforations generally do not cause heavy bleeding, but if they are not recognized and curettage is continued, extensive damage to the bowel or bladder may result. Management requires laparoscopy to assess the extent of injury, and then laparoscopic-guided completion of evacuation and coagulation of the bleeding site on the uterus. Antibiotics are administered, and the patient is observed overnight in the hospital.

Bowel Injury. When bowel injury is suspected, as when the bowel has been drawn into the perforation, it is essential to completely visualize the affected area. Often, this can be accomplished during laparoscopy by an experienced physician, but if there is difficulty in visualizing the site of injury, laparotomy is indicated. Failure to recognize and adequately treat a bowel injury can be fatal. If the patient has a full-thickness injury or the mesentery has been stripped, segmental resection and anastomosis are required. Small areas of injury can be managed successfully by oversewing the lesion, irrigating the peritoneal cavity, and leaving a large intraabdominal drain. High-dose antibiotics are given prophylactically. Larger injuries to the colon require a diverting colostomy after resection and anastomosis.

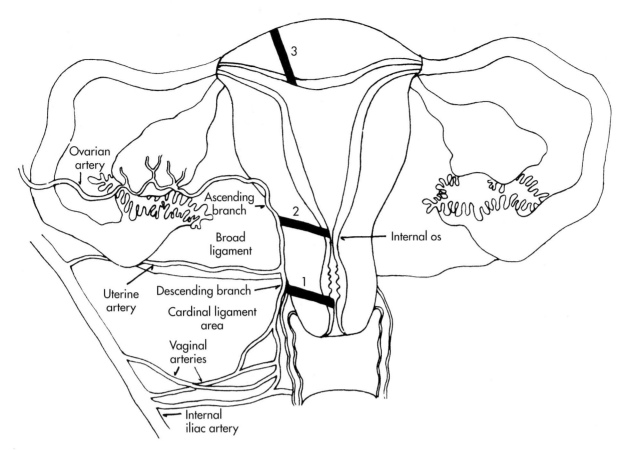

Fig. 56-8   Possible sites of uterine perforation at abortion. *1,* Low cervical perforation with laceration of descending branches of uterine artery. *2,* Perforation at junction of cervix and lower uterine segment with laceration of ascending branch of uterine artery. *3,* Fundal perforation. (From Berek IS, Stubblefield PG: *Am J Obstet Gynecol* 135:181, 1979.)

Bladder Injury. Anterior perforations can lacerate the bladder trigone. Part of the evaluation of a major perforation is bladder catheterization to look for gross hematuria. The injury is confirmed at laparoscopy, but laparotomy is needed for management. Direct repair should not be attempted for injury to the trigone. An ample cystotomy incision is made on the dome, the ureters are catheterized, and the rent is then repaired in two layers with absorbable suture. It is important to obtain the best possible operative consultation with a general surgeon or urologist for management of these more extensive injuries. Inadequate initial management of major injury adds greatly to the patient's problems and may jeopardize survival.

Failed Abortion, Continued Pregnancy, and Ectopic Pregnancy. Failure to interrupt the pregnancy is more often a problem with very early abortions. Therefore many U.S. clinics refuse to accept patients before 8 weeks from the last menstrual period. In contrast, abortion services in the Third World, having equipment only for minisuction procedures, prefer operating at 6 or 7 weeks. With early procedures the gestational sac must be identified with a fresh examination of the tissue.[18,22] When no chorionic villi are found in the fresh examination, the patient is at risk for ectopic preg-

nancy. Patients are considered either high-risk or low-risk for ectopic pregnancy based on symptoms and physical findings. High-risk patients should have immediate laparoscopy. Low-risk patients are followed with serial quantitative assays for β-chorionic gonadotropin with frequent contact until the problem is resolved.[10] Vaginal probe ultrasound is often helpful.

Incomplete and Septic Abortion. Preexisting colonization with pathogenic bacteria, retained pregnancy tissue, and uterine perforation are the principal causes of postabortal sepsis. Because septic abortion has become rare as a cause of death since the legalization of abortion, physicians may no longer appreciate how rapidly this problem can progress to death if not adequately treated without delay.[60] Treatment of the postabortal syndrome with immediate repeat vacuum curettage and antibiotics as described previously will prevent more serious infection from developing.

Patients seen with signs of more established infection, such as fever higher than 38° C (100.4° F) and pelvic peritonitis, need to be hospitalized. Therapy involves eradication of the infection with high-dose multiple-agent antibiotic therapy, uterine evacuation, and skilled supportive care. Maternal tissue for culture and Gram stain can be obtained from the endometrial cavity with a small endometrial vacuum cannula (e.g., Pipelle), and then antibiotic treatment is started. There should be no delay in emptying the uterus beyond the time needed to begin fluid resuscitation and initiate antibiotic therapy.

Evacuation of the first trimester uterus can be accomplished with vacuum curettage using conscious sedation in most patients. A retained midtrimester fetus poses a challenge. An experienced practitioner who regularly performs D&E procedures can usually evacuate the uterus by curettage with ultrasound guidance. If a practitioner with the required skills is not immediately available, the uterus can be emptied by medical means: high-dose oxytocin infusion[71] or IM carboprost, 250 μg every 2 to 3 hours. Obvious improvement in the patient's status should be expected within 12 to 24 hours after uterine examination. If severe sepsis is still present as manifested by the continued need for pressor drugs or continuing metabolic acidosis despite maximal ventilation, laparotomy is needed and almost certainly hysterectomy with bilateral salpingo-oophorectomy if the patient is to survive. Other indications for laparotomy are uterine perforation with a suspected bowel injury, a pelvic abscess, or clostridial myometritis. Clostridial sepsis is rare after legal abortion but should be suspected from the presence of large gram-positive rods on Gram stain of the cervical secretions or curetted tissue, when tachycardia seems out of proportion to the fever, or when hemolysis develops. Hematuria, shock, and severe adult respiratory distress syndrome can develop rapidly. The initial treatment is high-dose IV penicillin, curettage, and fluid management. A superficial clostridial infection will respond to these measures. If hemolysis is present, indicating systemic release of clostridial toxins, prompt hysterectomy.[34]

Supportive Care. Severe sepsis should be managed in an intensive care setting with the help of critical care specialists. An arterial line, a balloon-flotation right-sided heart catheter, and an indwelling urinary catheter are inserted. Fluid resuscitation is given in large volumes to maximize perfusion. Vasopressors, dopamine, and dobutamine are added if the pulmonary capillary wedge pressure becomes elevated before the target mean arterial blood pressure is reached. Of patients with septic shock, 25% to 50% will develop respiratory distress syndrome. Tissue oxygenation is monitored, and mechanical ventilation is started if oxygen saturation falls to less than 90%.[60]

SECOND TRIMESTER OR MIDTRIMESTER ABORTION
Dilation and Evacuation

Surgical evacuation is the most common method for midtrimester abortion in the United States.[11] Hence, this procedure is described in detail.

Technique. After adequate counseling, complete medical history, and physical examination, laminaria tents are placed in the cervical canal and held in place with two 4 × 4 gauze sponges tucked into the fornices. At 13 to 15 weeks,

2 small tents will suffice, but at 16 to 20 weeks 4 or more small tents are inserted, and after 20 weeks, 8 to 10 small tents are needed. Paracervical anesthesia is produced with 10 ml of 1% lidocaine for the insertion. To avoid syncope, the patient is kept lying on her side for a few minutes after insertion and then goes home. If the membranes are ruptured during insertion, the abortion is performed as scheduled the next day. I leave the tents in place for 12 to 24 hours. Dilapan tents provide about the same dilation as two medium *L. japonicum* tents and can be used instead of or in combination with laminaria. An analgesic is prescribed because some patients will have moderate abdominal discomfort through the night. I routinely give doxycycline, 100 mg after insertion, 100 mg at bedtime, and then 100 mg twice a day for 2 days after the procedure.

Ultrasound examination is advisable if there is a discrepancy between menstrual dates and uterine size or if there is an abnormality on bimanual examination and for all patients at gestation of 20 weeks and beyond. Operative ultrasound guidance is helpful for the more advanced pregnancies.[16]

Uterine evacuation is performed as follows.[1] An IV line is established. Infusion of the anesthetic of choice is begun. The patient is placed in the lithotomy position, and the previously placed vaginal sponges and laminaria are removed. The vagina and cervix are cleansed with a germicide. Paracervical block is administered with 20 ml of 1% lidocaine containing 10 U of vasopressin.[13] When a general anesthetic is used, the lidocaine is omitted but the same dose of vasopressin is given in 10 ml of saline at the 4- and 8-o'clock positions deep into the cervical stroma to reach the junction of cervix and lower uterine segment. Great caution is exercised to avoid intravascular injection. Two single-tooth tenaculums are placed vertically side by side, each with one branch inside the cervical canal. A large dilator is gently inserted to confirm dilation. IV oxytocin is started, 40 U/1000 ml solution, at 150 to 200 ml/hr.

The vacuum cannula is then inserted, and the vacuum is established briefly to rupture the membranes and drain amniotic fluid. The 12- or 14-mm cannulas are used for 13- to 15-week procedures; the 16-mm system is used for more advanced pregnancies (16-mm vacuum systems are available from Rocket of London, Inc., Branford, Conn.). The cannula is then removed, and evacuation is begun with the ovum forceps. A Foerster forceps is adequate for 13 to 15 weeks. Beyond this, the small Sopher forceps and the Kelly placental forceps are used for most procedures (Fig. 56-9). If there is difficulty in locating fetal parts, the uterine cavity is explored with the Kelly placental forceps, preferred for its rounded contour and light feel to the heavier Sopher instrument. When the fetal parts are located, they may be extracted with the Kelly forceps, but more often the Sopher or Bierer forceps will be needed. Fetal parts are extracted slowly and carefully, rotating the instrument as they are brought through the cervical canal to avoid lacerating the cervix. The Bierer forceps are used for larger gestations. The vacuum cannula is reinserted as needed to pull tissue downward, where it can be grasped with the forceps. When

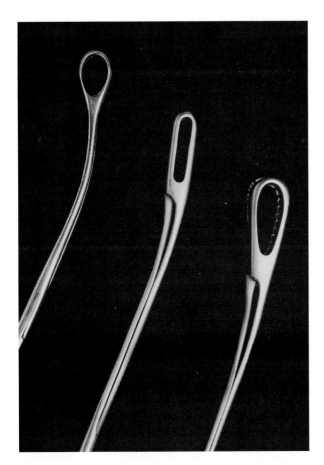

Fig. 56-9   Instruments for dilation and evacuation: Kelly placental forceps, Sopher forceps, and Bierer forceps.

the procedure feels complete, the Vacurette is gently inserted all the way to the fundus and slowly rotated for 1 to 2 minutes; then a large sharp curette is used to explore the cavity. If any additional tissue is encountered, the forceps or cannula is reinserted to remove it. After the procedure the surgeon carefully examines the fetal parts to be sure all have been evacuated. On occasion the fetal calvarium is retained in the uterus. If exploration with the Kelly placental forceps does not locate it, the vacuum cannula is inserted and slowly rotated as described previously, producing a strong uterine contraction that may push the retained parts downward, where they can be grasped with the forceps. If these attempts are unsuccessful, it is best to stop, administer an oxytocin infusion for 2 hours, and then try again. By then, the remaining fetal parts will be pushed down to the internal os, where they can be easily extracted. Hern's monograph[31] provides a more detailed description of the procedure.

Attempting evacuation of a pregnancy beyond the surgeon's skill and experience poses serious risk and mandates liberal use of preoperative ultrasound. If the cervix has been widely dilated by multiple laminaria tents, the experienced surgeon can satisfactorily extract a pregnancy up to 20 or 21 weeks. Beyond this, I believe that the procedure should be abandoned unless the surgeon regularly performs more advanced procedures. IV oxytocin or systemic prostaglandins can be used instead.

Modifications of technique are often used to facilitate D&E in the late midtrimester. Hern[32] has described a combination method. After multistage laminaria treatment over 2 days, urea is injected into the amniotic sac to produce fetal demise and initiate labor. When expulsion begins, an assisted delivery is performed under local anesthesia. Wright[72] practices another approach. Multiple laminaria or four Dilapan tents are inserted into the cervix, and under ultrasound guidance, a fetal intracardiac injection of 1.5 mg of digoxin is given. The D&E is carried out under brief general anesthesia on the following day. Oxytocin is administered as 50 to 100 U/1000 ml during the procedure. As noted in the next section, digoxin has been used to produce fetal death before prostaglandin abortion. Wright described 2400 procedures performed at 19 to 23 weeks with no perforations.

Intact D&E. This variation of D&E described in 1992 is typically used at 20 to 24 weeks. Paracervical block is placed, the cervix is dilated to 9 to 11 mm with Pratt dilators and then several laminaria or Dilapan dilators are inserted, and the patient is discharged. On the next day, the original osmotic dilators are removed, 15 to 25 Dilapan dilators are inserted into the cervical canal, and the patient is again discharged. On the third day, uterine evacuation is performed. Ultrasound is used to determine fetal position and presentation. In the variation described by Haskell,[30] the membranes are ruptured and a large grasping forceps such as Hern or Bierer forceps is inserted through the dilated cervix. A fetal foot is grasped and pulled downward, converting the presentation to breech. The surgeon manually delivers the second lower extremity into the vagina, then the torso, and then the upper extremities, rotating the fetus so the dorsum remains up. The calvarium remains at the internal cervical os. Next, traction is applied to the shoulders of the fetus with the surgeon's fingers while elevating the cervical lip with one finger, and a scissors is advanced into the base of the fetal skull. A suction catheter is introduced and the central nervous system is aspirated. With the calvarium thus decompressed, the fetus is delivered intact.

McMahon[47] described a similar procedure, with dilation followed by laminaria placement twice a day for 2 days or more, followed by rupture of the membranes, administration of 250 mg of carboprost, and then 20 minutes later, fetal evacuation, as already described if the fetus is breech or transverse. If the fetus is in vertex presentation, the calvarium is allowed to descend into the cervical canal by uterine contractions and then decompressed by insertion of a trocar and aspiration of the cerebrospinal fluid and central nervous system followed by forceps extraction of the collapsed calvarium and intact fetus.[48] The breech extraction variation of intact D&E, described in the lay press as "partial birth abortion" has been made illegal in several states.

Anesthesia. With good psychological support from trained counselors, midtrimester D&E can be performed under paracervical block with low-dose IV sedation. This may be difficult to provide in the operating rooms of a busy general hospital, oriented toward use of major anesthetics. In a multicenter study, general anesthesia increased the risk for cervical laceration and hemorrhage with D&E.[46] On the other hand, large series have been reported in which very low rates of uterine injury occurred with general anesthesia.[38,72] When general anesthesia is used, it is even more critical to have adequate preparation of the cervix with laminaria or Dilapan tents. Suitable regimens for IV sedation are diazepam (5 mg) followed by fentanyl (0.05 mg), repeated after several minutes if needed. Alternatively, midazolam (2 to 4 mg) is given, 1 mg at a time, followed with 200-μg doses of alfentanil given at 3- to 4-minute intervals during the procedure. Use of a pulse oximeter is advisable with these regimens because all of these agents depress respiration and when combined have the potential to cause greater respiratory depression.[3] Fentanyl can cause chest wall rigidity and respiratory arrest, especially at higher dosages. Treatment is immediate administration of the narcotic antagonist naloxone and respiratory support.[67] If general anesthesia is used, full compliance with current standards for monitoring tissue oxygen levels, end-expiratory CO_2, and vital signs are mandatory.[19] When these procedures take place out of the hospital, more stringent patient selection is required. Combinations of short-acting barbiturates, nitrous oxide, and oxygen are preferred. Potent inhalant agents are avoided altogether or used in very low concentrations. Close observation during recovery is essential. Use of IV sedation or general anesthesia requires personnel trained in cardiorespiratory support.

Labor-Induction Methods

Many techniques are used for labor-induction abortion. The more common primary methods are described in the following section. In practice, primary methods are often combined with adjunctive methods to improve efficacy, shorten the interval from treatment to delivery, and prevent delivery of a living fetus. These adjunctive methods include laminaria tents or other osmotic dilators placed into the cervical canal, combinations of prostaglandins with reduced dosages of hypertonic saline or urea, intrafetal injection of digoxin or potassium chloride, and IV oxytocin.

Hypertonic Saline. Intraamniotic instillation of saline, the most common method for midtrimester abortion in the 1970s, has largely been replaced as a primary method, but saline is sometimes used at lower dosages to augment other labor-induction methods. Hypertonic saline has unique hazards: Cardiovascular collapse, pulmonary and cerebral edema, and renal failure occur if there is intravascular injection, and disseminated intravascular coagulopathy is a risk for all patients. Intravascular injection is avoided by careful amniocentesis and instillation of the saline through a catheter placed in the amniotic sac. Given alone, hypertonic saline produces mean times to abortion of 33 to 35 hours.[5,40] The addition of oxytocin at 17 to 67 mU/min reduces the mean time to 25 to 26 hours; thus there are fewer failed abortions, fewer retained placentas, less blood loss, and less risk of infection.[5] However, the addition of oxytocin increases the rate of occurrence of disseminated intravascu-

lar coagulation (DIC) and requires caution to avoid water intoxication.

Intraamniotic Urea. Urea is safer than saline because inadvertent intravascular injection of small amounts is harmless. Urea requires augmentation to avoid prolonged intervals from injection to abortion. The combination of 80 g of urea plus 5 mg of $PGF_{2\alpha}$ instilled into the amniotic sac produces abortion in a mean time of 17.5 hours, with 80% of patients aborting within 24 hours. The urea-prostaglandin combination offers a shorter injection-to-abortion interval than hypertonic saline and has fewer serious complications.[7]

Intrauterine Prostaglandins. $PGF_{2\alpha}$ was the first prostaglandin approved by the FDA. Initial problems were the need for a second injection in many cases, transient fetal survival in some cases, failure of the primary technique, incomplete abortion, and in the primigravida, risk for cervical rupture. Overnight treatment with laminaria tents reduces the mean times to abortion from 29 to 14 hours, reduces the risk for cervical injury, and reduces the need for a second dose.[61] Routine exploration of the uterine cavity with forceps and vacuum curette reduces postabortal hemorrhage and injection from retained products.

$PGF_{2\alpha}$ is no longer available in the United States. An alternative is the 15-methyl analog of $PGF_{2\alpha}$, carboprost tromethamine (Hemabate). For intraamniotic injection, 2 mg of this drug replace 40 mg of $PGF_{2\alpha}$, and 0.250 mg replaces the 5-mg dose of $PGF_{2\alpha}$, used to augment intraamniotic urea. Osathanondh[50] described extensive experience with intraamniotic carboprost in a combination method. Patients are treated overnight with multiple laminaria tents packed around one Lamicel tent. The next morning, the tents are removed and an intraamniotic injection of 2 mg of carboprost is given in combination with 64 ml of 23.4% sodium chloride. After 4 hours the membranes are artificially ruptured, and unless the cervix is already well dilated, a 20-mg PGE_2 (Prostin E_2) suppository is placed into the cervical canal on the end of a Dilapan tent. Subsequently, PGE_2 vaginal suppositories are given at 3-hour intervals until abortion. All patients have a brief exploration of the uterine cavity and curettage under low-dose sedation after expulsion of the placenta. If the patient has not aborted by 14 hours, a D&E procedure is performed. A mean time from instillation to abortion of 8 hours was reported, and neither cervical laceration nor uterine rupture occurred in more than 4000 consecutive cases after this protocol.

Systemic Prostaglandins. PGE_2 vaginal suppositories and IM carboprost are available in the United States. Both are highly effective. With vaginal PGE_2 (20 mg every 3 hours), the mean time to abort is 13.4 hours, and 90% of patients abort within 24 hours.[63] Mean times to abort are 15 to 17 hours with carboprost given as 0.25 mg IM injections at 2-hour intervals and 80% abort within 24 hours.[52] Vomiting and diarrhea commonly occur with both, usually more often with carboprost. PGE_2 produces a temperature elevation of 1° C or more in about one third of patients. Overnight treatment with laminaria shortens the length of prostaglandin treatment, reduces the dose of drug required, and hence reduces prostaglandin-related side effects.[62] Transient fetal survival is a problem with all prostaglandin methods. One group has reported ultrasound-guided intracardiac injection of digoxin to ensure fetal death.[69]

Misoprostol. Misoprostol, the PGE_1 analog, has been compared with PGE_2 suppositories in a randomized trial. Misoprostol, 200 μg administered vaginally every 12 hours, was as effective as 20 mg of PGE_2 every 3 hours, but with many fewer side effects.[35] Misoprostol is inexpensive and stable at room temperature.

Oxytocin. Oxytocin is used to augment other methods but is generally considered to be poorly effective by itself. In fact, oxytocin can be a primary method for abortion in the midtrimester, but very high infusion rates are required. Winkler et al.[71] compared a high-dose oxytocin protocol with vaginal PGE_2 suppositories at 17 to 24 weeks and found the oxytocin just as effective and with fewer side effects. Their protocol was as follows. Oxytocin, 50 U in 500 ml of 5% dextrose and normal saline, is given over 3 hours (approximately 278 mU/min), followed by a 1-hour rest period off oxytocin. Then, 100 U in 500 ml is given over 3 hours, followed by a 1-hour rest, and repeated, adding 50 U of oxytocin to each infusion until the patient aborts or a final solution of 300 U in 500 ml (1667 mU/min) is reached. Of 59 patients in the PGE_2 group, 2 experienced severe bronchospasm. No signs of water intoxication were seen with the oxytocin. This report is instructive and offers more options for managing late abortion, fetal death, and premature rupture of the membranes. However, the lessons we have learned from high-dose oxytocin used to augment saline or prostaglandin must be remembered. Uterine rupture, cervicovaginal fistula, and annular detachment of the cervix can be seen when the uterus is overstimulated without adequate cervical preparation.

Midtrimester Complications

Failed Abortion. Labor-induction methods share the common problem that not all patients abort from the primary method within a reasonable time and so have an increasing risk for bleeding and infection. For these methods, a graph showing cumulative percentage of patients aborted versus time shows a plateau (Fig. 56-10). At this point a second method is indicated. High-dose IV oxytocin can be used, but caution is required to avoid uterine rupture in multigravida[51] and cervical rupture in primigravida. A better alternative is to change to a different prostaglandin or a different route of administration (e.g., if the primary method was intraamniotic carboprost, change to vaginal suppositories of PGE_2). If the second prostaglandin is unsuccessful after a defined period, D&E is performed.[8] Because failure of a second prostaglandin is uncommon and may indicate a uterine anomaly, it is wise to consider an ultrasound examination before surgical intervention if this was not already done.

Disseminated Intravascular Coagulopathy. DIC is rare after first trimester vacuum curettage, occurring in approximately 8 per 100,000 procedures, but the incidence is higher after midtrimester D&E (191 per 100,000 proce-

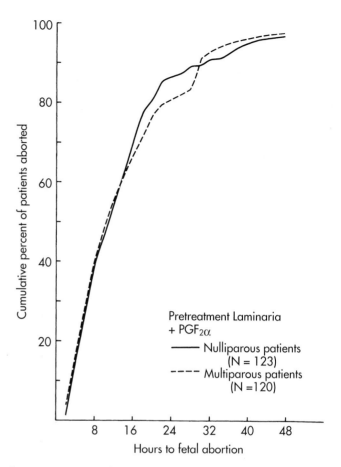

Fig. 56-10 Curve showing the cumulative percentage of patients undergoing abortions as a function of time since the start of prostaglandin therapy. (From Stubblefield PG, et al: *Contraception* 13:723, 1976.)

dures) and highest for saline instillation (658 per 100,000 procedures).[36] DIC is much more common when abortion is performed after fetal death in utero than with the same procedure done with an intact pregnancy. DIC must be considered when postabortal hemorrhage is seen and, if present, requires aggressive management. Carboprost given in IM doses of 0.25 mg is often effective in controlling uterine bleeding and is the first step in treatment. It is likely that 0.800-mg doses of misoprostol given rectally would be equally effective, but this has not been studied. If bleeding persists after prostaglandin administration, therapy is begun with cryoprecipitate, fresh frozen plasma, and packed red cells. Heparin therapy is not helpful in these patients.

Others. Perforation with midtrimester D&E is more likely to result in major visceral injury than in the first trimester and usually requires laparotomy for management. Inexperienced surgeons may confuse the maternal small intestine for late midtrimester fetal bowel, although the diameters are different, and fail to recognize a perforation until considerable harm has resulted. The labor-induction methods can lead to fetal expulsion through a rent in the cervix above the external os, a cervicovaginal fistula. This is repaired by debridement of the avascular edges and primary closure of the defect. Uterine rupture can occur when saline, urea, or prostaglandin is augmented with high-dose oxytocin. Uterine rupture is suspected because of severe pain followed by falling blood pressure and rising pulse from intra-abdominal bleeding. Management requires blood replacement and laparotomy with repair of the uterine laceration.

Choice of Midtrimester Procedure

The mortality risk for different methods is shown in Table 56-2. Early midtrimester D&E is the safest method. Labor-induction methods and D&E are comparable in the later midtrimester, and both are much safer than hysterotomy or hysterectomy for abortion. The labor-induction methods all involve overnight hospitalization, which in the United States greatly increases expense and limits accessibility. The D&E technique can be safely provided on an outpatient basis and in well-equipped free-standing clinics at much reduced cost. Also, the psychological impact on the patient is much less than with labor-induction techniques.[38] In the early midtrimester, D&E has fewer complications than labor induction.[37] Several skilled surgeons offer D&E to 24 weeks. Indeed, the lowest reported rate of complications for any late abortion technique is that of Hern[32] for his combination method of laminaria, intraamniotic urea, and D&E. For the surgeon faced with the occasional need to provide midtrimester abortion, I would suggest ultrasound-guided fetal intracardiac injection of 1.5 mg of digoxin and intra-cervical laminaria, followed the next day by vaginal suppositories of PGE$_2$. If abortion is prolonged beyond 24 hours, carboprost injections of 0.25 mg at 2-hour intervals would be substituted. If the initial good experience with vaginal misoprostol, 0.200 mg every 12 hours, is confirmed, this method may become the method of choice for labor-induction abortion.

Fetal Death in Utero. Fetal death in utero can be managed as abortion of an intact pregnancy, with either D&E techniques, vaginal PGE$_2$, or IM carboprost. The intraamniotic route is not advised because increased permeability of the membranes and the greater difficulty of amniocentesis may result in systemic reaction to saline or prostaglandin. The response of the uterus to prostaglandin is quicker after fetal death. With PGE$_2$ suppositories, the mean time to abortion is about 10 hours. Special caution is required for use of prostaglandins after 28 weeks. The full dose of 20 mg of PGE$_2$ is too much and has produced fatal uterine rupture on occasion. My facility's protocol, used successfully for many years, is to cut the suppository into quarters and administer one quarter of the full dose (approximately 5 mg of PGE$_2$) at 1- to 2-hour intervals, titrating uterine activity to avoid hyperstimulation. This also greatly reduces gastrointestinal side effects and fever. We have used this same low-dose protocol successfully in patients with active asthma. In patients with ruptured membranes or much vaginal bleeding, vaginal PGE$_2$ may be poorly effective because dilution by blood or amniotic fluid may limit absorption. IM carboprost (0.25 mg every 2 to 3 hours) is a better choice in these patients. Patients who will receive prostaglandins are given antiemetics and antidiarrheal agents on a routine basis to reduce vomiting and diarrhea. Acetaminophen suppositories are given at 4-hour intervals to block the febrile response to PGE$_2$.

When laminaria are used to prepare the cervix after fetal death, labor can sometimes be triggered by the laminaria alone. This is not a problem if the patient knows it may happen and has been instructed to return to the hospital. Because DIC is more common with abortion for fetal death than with the same procedure and an intact pregnancy, preoperative evaluation of the clotting system is advised before intervention for fetal death.

ABORTION IN THE THIRD TRIMESTER

Viability is the limit for abortion based on the decision of the woman in most U.S. jurisdictions, following the Supreme Court's ruling in *Roe v. Wade*.[53] Viability is a legal concept, usually meaning the ability to survive indefinitely, with or without medical support. Fetuses with major mal-

Table 56-2 Case-Fatality Rates[a] for Legal Induced Abortion, by Type of Procedure and Weeks of Gestation, United States, 1972-1987[b]

	Weeks of Gestation						
	≤8	9-10	11-12	13-15	16-20	≥21	Total
Dilation and curettage[c]	0.3	0.7	1.1	—[d]	—	—	—
Dilation and evacuation	—	—	—	2.0	6.5	11.9	3.7
Instillation[e]	—	—	—	3.8	7.9	10.3	7.1
Hysterectomy/hysterotomy	18.3	30.0	41.2	28.1	103.4	274.3	51.6
Total[f]	0.4	0.7	1.1	2.2	6.9	10.4	1.0

From Lawson HW, et al: *Am J Obstet Gynecol* 171:1365, 1994.
[a]Legal induced abortion deaths per 100,000 legal induced abortions.
[b]Excludes data for 1972-1973 because gestational age by method data were not collected.
[c]Includes all suction and sharp curettage procedures.
[d]Not applicable.
[e]Includes all instillation methods (saline, prostaglandin, other).
[f]Excludes five deaths by "other" methods.

formations incompatible with life thus could be considered as previable at any gestational age, and intervention to induce labor could be considered to spare the woman the prolongation of a pregnancy that will have no fetal benefit. Chervenak et al.[12] have explored the ethical dimensions of the issue and concluded that third trimester abortion is ethical, provided two conditions are met: (1) the fetus has a condition with no prospect for prolonged survival after birth, and (2) there exists a completely accurate way to diagnose this condition. Anencephaly is one such condition.

REFERENCES

1. Altman A, et al: Midtrimester abortion by laminaria and evacuation (L & E) on a teaching service: a review of 789 cases, *Adv Plan Parent* 16:1, 1981.
2. Begum SF, Jalif K: Problems of septic abortion in Bangladesh and the need for menstrual regulation. In Landy U, Ratnam SS, editors: *Prevention and treatment of contraceptive failure,* New York, 1986, Plenum.
3. Bell GP, et al: A comparison of diazepam and midazolam as endoscopy premedication: assessing changes in ventilation and oxygen saturation, *Br J Clin Pharmacol* 26:595, 1988.
4. Berek JS, Stubblefield PG: Anatomical and clinical correlations of uterine perforations, *Am J Obstet Gynecol* 135:181, 1979.
5. Berger GS, Edelman DA: Oxytocin administration, instillation to abortion time, and morbidity associated with saline instillation, *Am J Obstet Gynecol* 121:941, 1975.
6. Berkowitz RL, et al: Selective reduction of multifetal pregnancies in the first trimester, *N Engl J Med* 318:1043, 1988.
7. Binkin NJ, et al: Urea-prostaglandin versus hypertonic saline for instillation abortion, *Am J Obstet Gynecol* 146:947, 1983.
8. Burkeman RT, et al: The management of midtrimester abortion failures by vaginal evacuation, *Obstet Gynecol* 49:233, 1977.
9. Burnhill M: *Physician's manual: standard medical procedures,* ed 3, Newton, Mass, 1975, Preterm Institute.
10. Burnhill MS, Armstead JW: Reducing the morbidity of vacuum aspiration abortion, *Int J Gynaecol Obstet* 16:204, 1978.
11. Centers for Disease Control and Prevention: *Abortion surveillance 1979-80,* Atlanta, Jan 1983, CDC.
12. Chervenak FA, et al: When is termination of pregnancy during the third trimester morally justifiable? *N Engl J Med* 310:501, 1984.
13. Christensen D: Use of vasopressin to reduce D & E blood loss. Paper presented at the 8th Annual Meeting of the National Abortion Federation, Los Angeles, May 14, 1984.
14. Creinin MD, Darney PD: Methotrexate and misoprostol for early abortion, *Contraception* 48:339, 1993.
15. Creinin MD, et al: Methotrexate and misoprostol for early abortion: a multicenter trial. I. Safety and efficacy, *Contraception* 53:321, 1996.
16. Darney PD: Midtrimester abortion under ultrasound guidance. Postgraduate course presented by the National Abortion Federation, Tampa, Fla, Jan 31, 1983.
17. Darney PD, Dorward K: Cervical dilatation before first trimester elective abortion: a controlled comparison of meteneprost, laminaria, and hypan, *Obstet Gynecol* 70:397, 1987.
18. Edwards J, Carson SA: New technologies permit safe abortion at less than six weeks gestation and provide timely detection of ectopic gestation, *Am J Obstet Gynecol* 1076:1101, 1987.
19. Eichhorn JH, et al: Standards for patient monitoring during anesthesia at Harvard Medical School, *JAMA* 256:1017, 1986.
20. Evans MI, et al: Efficacy of transabdominal multifetal pregnancy reduction: collaborative experience among the world's largest centers, *Obstet Gynecol* 82:616, 1993.
21. Evans MI, et al: Efficacy of second trimester selective termination for fetal anomalies: international collaborative experience among the world's largest centers, *Am J Obstet Gynecol* 171:90, 1994.
22. Fielding WL, et al: Continued pregnancy after failed first trimester abortion, *Obstet Gynecol* 63:421, 1984.
23. Forrest JD, Henshaw SK: What U.S. women think and do about contraception, *Fam Plann Perspect* 15:157, 1983.
24. Freiman M: Personal communication, April 2, 1982.
25. Glick E: Paracervical and lower uterine field block anesthesia for therapeutic abortion and office D & C. Paper presented at the 11th Annual Convention of the National Abortion Federation, Salt Lake City, Utah, May 18, 1987.
26. Gold J, et al: The safety of laminaria and rigid dilators for cervical dilatation prior to suction curettage first trimester abortion: a comparative analysis. In Naftolin F, Stubblefield PG, editors: *Dilation of the uterine cervix: connective tissue biology and clinical management,* New York, 1980, Raven.
27. Grimes DA, Cates W: Deaths from paracervical anesthesia used for first trimester abortion, 1972-1975, *N Engl J Med* 295:1397, 1976.
28. Grimes DA, Schulz KF, Cates WJ: Prevention of uterine perforation during curettage abortion, *JAMA* 251:2108, 1984.
29. Hakim-Elahi E, Tovell HMM, Burnhill MS: Complications of first trimester abortion: a report of 170,000 cases, *Obstet Gynecol* 76:129, 1990.
30. Haskell M: Dilatation and extraction for late second trimester abortion. Presented at the National Abortion Federation Risk Management Seminar, Dallas, Texas, Sept 13, 1992.
31. Hern WM: *Abortion practice,* Philadelphia, 1984, JB Lippincott.
32. Hern WM: Serial multiple laminaria and adjunctive urea in late outpatient dilatation and evacuation abortion, *Obstet Gynecol* 63:543, 1984.
33. Hodgson JE, et al: Prophylactic use of tetracycline for first trimester abortions, *Obstet Gynecol* 45:574, 1975.
34. Hoyme UB, Eschenbach DA: *Postoperative infection.* In Iffy L, Charles D, editors: *Operative perinatology,* New York, 1984, Macmillan.
35. Jain JK, Mishell DR: A comparison of intravaginal misoprostol with prostaglandin E_2 for termination of second trimester pregnancy, *N Engl J Med* 331:290, 1994.
36. Kafrissen ME, et al: Coagulopathy and induced abortion method, rates and relative risks, *Am J Obstet Gynecol* 147:344, 1983.
37. Kafrissen ME, et al: A comparison of intraamniotic instillation of hyperosmolar urea and prostaglandin $F_{2\alpha}$ vs dilatation and evacuation for midtrimester abortion, *JAMA* 253:916, 1984.
38. Kaltreider NH, Goldsmith S, Margolis AJ: The impact of midtrimester abortion techniques on patients and staff, *Am J Obstet Gynecol* 135:235, 1979.
39. Karman H, Potts M: Very early abortion using syringe as vacuum source, *Lancet* 1:7759, 1972.
40. Kerenyi TD, Mandelaman N, Sherman DH: Five thousand consecutive saline abortions, *Am J Obstet Gynecol* 116:593, 1973.
41. Koonin LM, et al: Pregnancy related mortality surveillance-United States, 1987-90, *MMWR* 46:17, 1997.
42. Koonin LM, et al: Abortion surveillance—United States, 1992, *MMWR* 45:1, 1996.
43. Lawson HW, et al: Abortion mortality, United States, 1972-1987, *Am J Obstet Gynecol* 171:1365, 1994.
44. LeFebre Y, et al: The effects of RU38486 on cervical ripening, *Am J Obstet Gynecol* 162:61, 1990.
45. Levallois P, Rioux JE: Prophylactic antibiotics for suction curettage abortion: results of a clinical controlled trial, *Am J Obstet Gynecol* 158:100, 1988.
46. MacKay HT, Schulz KR, Grimes DA: The safety of local versus general anesthesia for second trimester dilatation and evacuation abortion, *Obstet Gynecol* 66:661, 1985.
47. McMahon JT: Intact D & E, the first decade. Presented at National Abortion Federation Annual Meeting, New Orleans. La, Apr 2, 1995.
48. Mosher WD: Fertility and family planning in the United States: insights from the national survey of family growth, *Fam Plann Perspect* 20:207, 1988.
49. National Center for Health Statistics: *Monthly Vital Statist Rep* 39(suppl 11):7, 1990.

50. Osathanondh R: Conception control. In Ryan KJ, Barbieri R, Berkowitz RS, editors: *Kistner's gynecology,* ed 5, St Louis, 1990, Mosby.

51. Propping D, Stubblefield PG, Golub J: Uterine rupture following midtrimester abortion by laminaria, prostaglandin $F_{2\alpha}$ and oxytocin: report of two cases, *Am J Obstet Gynecol* 128:689, 1977.

52. Robins J, Mann LI: Second generation prostaglandins: midtrimester pregnancy termination by intramuscular injection of a 15 methyl analog of prostaglandin $F_{2a\alpha}$, *Fertil Steril* 27:104, 1976.

53. *Roe v. Wade,* 410 U.S. 113, 1973.

54. Sands RX, Burnhill MS, Hakim-Elahi E: Post-abortal uterine atony, *Obstet Gynecol* 43:595, 1974.

55. Schulz KF, Grimes DA, Cates W Jr: Measures to prevent cervical injury during suction curettage abortion, *Lancet* 1:1182, 1983.

56. Schutz KF, et al: Prophylactic antibiotics to prevent febrile complications of curettage abortion. Paper presented at the 8th Annual Meeting of the National Abortion Federation, Los Angeles, May 15, 1984.

57. Silvestre L, et al: Voluntary interruption of pregnancy with mifepristone (RU486) and a prostaglandin analogue: a large scale French experience, *N Engl J Med* 322:645, 1990.

58. Sonne Holme S, et al: Prophylactic antibiotics in first trimester abortion: a clinical controlled trial, *Am J Obstet Gynecol* 139:693, 1981.

59. Stubblefield PG: Induced abortion indications, counseling, and services. In Sciarra JJ, Zatuchni GI, Daly MJ editors: *Gynecology and obstetrics,* Philadelphia, 1982, Harper & Row.

60. Stubblefield PG, Altman AM, Goldstein SP: Randomized trial of one versus two days of laminaria treatment prior to late midtrimester abortion by uterine evacuation: a pilot study, *Am J Obstet Gynecol* 143:481, 1982.

61. Stubblefield PG, et al: Laminaria augmentation of intraamniotic $PGF_{2\alpha}$ for midtrimester pregnancy termination, *Prostaglandins* 10:413, 1975.

62. Stubblefield PG, et al: Combination therapy for midtrimester abortion: laminaria and analogues of prostaglandin, *Contraception* 13:723, 1976.

63. Surrago EJ, Robins J: Midtrimester pregnancy termination by intravaginal administration of prostaglandin E_2, *Contraception* 26:285, 1982.

64. U.S. Food and Drug Administration: Warning for prescription drugs containing sulfite, *Drug Bull* 17:2, 1987.

65. VanLith DAF, et al: Aspirotomy. In Berger GS, Brenner WE, Keith LG, editors: *Second trimester abortion: perspectives after a decade of experience,* Boston, 1981, John Wright PSG.

66. Vedantham, S, Goodwin SC, McLucas B, et al: Uterine artery embolization: an underused method of controlling pelvic hemorrhage, *Am J Obstet Gynecol* 176:938, 1997.

67. Viscomi CM, Bailey PL: Opioid induced rigidity after intravenous fentanyl, *Obstet Gynecol* 89:822, 1997.

68. Wapner RJ, et al: Selective reduction of multifetal pregnancies, *Lancet* 335:90, 1990.

69. Waters JL, Pitts-Hames M: Digoxin induction abortion. Paper presented at the 8th annual meeting of the National Abortion Federation, Los Angeles, May 14, 1984.

70. Weibe ER: Comparison of the efficacy of different local anesthetic techniques in therapeutic abortions. Paper presented at the Annual Meeting of the Canadian College of Family Physicians, Vancouver, BC, Nov 24, 1990.

71. Winkler CL, et al: Mid second trimester labor induction: concentrated oxytocin compared with prostaglandin E_2 vaginal suppositories, *Obstet Gynecol* 77:297, 1991.

72. Wright PC: Late midtrimester abortion by dilatation and evacuation using Dilapan and digoxin. Paper presented at the 13th Annual Meeting of the National Abortion Federation, San Francisco, Apr 4, 1989.

73. Wu YT: Suction in artificial abortion: 300 cases, *Chin J Obstet Gynecol* 6:447, 1958.

57 Cervical Cerclage

DONALD R. COUSTAN

Cervical incompetence was described by Palmer and La-Comme[70] in 1948. The placement of a suture around the cervix, known as cerclage, was first popularized by Shirodkar[81] in 1955, when he described the use of fascia for this procedure. Numerous other procedures have been proposed and popularized during the past four decades, and virtually every obstetrician has a favorite approach. What is most striking is the relative dearth of data addressing the supposed condition for which this procedure is used, the *incompetent cervix*. This diagnosis is often applied but rarely proven. Although it has been estimated to complicate as many as 1% of all pregnancies,[64] its true prevalence is more likely to be in the range of 0.05% to 0.2%.[6,31,89] Textbooks of obstetrics define incompetent cervix as the functional inability to retain a pregnancy in utero until term. The "classic history" of painless dilation of the cervix resulting in delivery between 16 and 28 weeks' gestation (or later) is obviously a retrospective diagnosis. Attempts to make the diagnosis prospectively, whether in the nonpregnant state by passage of a no. 8 Hegar dilator or a no.16 Foley catheter or in the pregnant woman by serial digital examination of the cervix, remain unproven. Floyd[25] performed serial vaginal examinations of 100 women whose pregnancies went to at least 36 weeks. By the sixth month of pregnancy, 15% of nulliparas were 1 cm dilated, as were 72% of parous women. In fact, 36% of parous women manifested cervical dilation of 2 cm or more. Similarly, Parikh and Mehta[71] found that 16% of nulliparas and 17% of parous women had an "open" cervix (dilation of at least one fingertip) at 21 to 28 weeks. Such women manifested a prematurity rate of 14%, not much different from the 11% among those with closed cervixes. Schaffner and Schanzer[77] examined 299 women at 28 to 32 weeks' gestation. At 28 weeks, the cervixes of 7% were dilated 2 to 3 cm at the internal os, and by 32 weeks, 32% were dilated to this extent. Premature births occurred in 6.1% of the dilated group and 6.9% of those with closed cervixes, despite the fact that no treatment was provided those with dilated cervixes. Bouyer et al.[8] reported a townwide, population-based study in which women were examined at each prenatal visit. Among nulliparous women, 3% had an "open" cervix (at least one fingertip at the internal os) at 25 to 28 weeks, as did 6.5% at 29 to 31 weeks and 9.6% at 32 to 34 weeks. For parous women, the corresponding figures were 5.6%, 13.3%, and 14%. This variable (open cervix) carried with it a relative risk for preterm birth of 4.6 at 25 to 28 weeks in nulliparas and 3 in parous women. However, no mention is made of incompetent cervix or cer-

clage in the paper, and the open cervix was generally treated with increased rest. Thus, in this study, one cannot distinguish between cervical dilation and incompetent cervix as a risk factor for preterm labor.

The ideal way to test the hypothesis that incompetent cervix is an entity that is appropriately treated by cerclage would be a randomized trial of the procedure in patients deemed to have the condition by virtue of the classical history. Most published studies compare pregnancy outcome among women undergoing cerclage with past pregnancy performance. Such studies are bound to demonstrate an apparent benefit for the procedure because studies of subsequent pregnancies among women with one[72] or two[4] consecutive midtrimester losses demonstrate term birth rates of approximately 70%, even without intervention. Thus any procedure applied to a group of women with previous midtrimester losses would be expected to have a 70% success rate even if the procedure were no better than a placebo. This lesson should have been learned from studies on the use of progestational agents to prevent spontaneous abortion[32,80] and from the diethylstilbestrol (DES) tragedy. If incompetent cervix is a distinct entity, correctable by cerclage, one would expect that patients with this condition undergoing the procedure would demonstrate better reproductive performance than patients without the condition, whose previous losses were caused by preterm labor. In fact, Barford and Rosen[5] found just the opposite. Two randomized trials of cerclage have been published.[44,75] Because of ethical concerns about the use of an untreated control group, neither study focused on patients with a classical history or signs of incompetent cervix. Instead, both studies were of patients at high or moderate risk for preterm delivery. In neither study did cerclage provide any benefit, and in both studies there was increased morbidity among patients receiving cerclage. Because patients with classical histories were not the subjects of these investigations, the only conclusion that could be drawn is that pregnancies of women at high risk for preterm labor who do not have such classic incompetent cervix histories do not benefit from cerclage. This finding is particularly important in light of published recommendations for "aggressive" prophylactic use of this procedure to prevent pregnancy wastage.[17]

In 1993, a final report was published by the MRC/RCOG Working Party on Cervical Cerclage.[63] In this multicenter prospective trial, 1292 pregnant women without classical histories but whose obstetricians were uncertain whether to recommend cerclage were randomly assigned to treatment;

approximately half (647) received cervical cerclage and half (645) did not. Although preterm delivery rates (before 37 weeks) were not significantly different (26% versus 31%, $p = 0.07$), those treated with cerclage manifested a slightly but significantly lower likelihood of delivery after 13 but before 33 weeks than did the untreated women (11% versus 16%, $p = 0.015$) and a similar decrease in the likelihood of delivering a baby weighing less than 1500 g (10% versus 13%). Puerperal fever occurred significantly more often among patients receiving cerclage than among control women (6% versus 3%, $p = 0.03$). Perinatal mortality rates did not differ between the two groups (2% versus 3%). When data were stratified by indication for cerclage, only those with three previous second trimester miscarriages or preterm deliveries showed a statistically significant benefit from cerclage (delivery before 33 weeks in 15% versus 32% of control women, $p < 0.05$). The authors caution that stratification led to fairly small group sample sizes, making interpretation problematic. For example, no association could be found between the number of previous losses or preterm deliveries and the likelihood of a protective effect of cerclage. The authors conclude the following:

> The results of this trial do therefore suggest that the operation of cervical cerclage can have an important beneficial effect in a minority of pregnant women. Although the operation is associated with increased intervention during pregnancy (and doubles the risk of puerperal pyrexia . . .), its use should be considered when there is a high likelihood of benefit (e.g. for women who have had three or more second trimester miscarriages or preterm deliveries). Nevertheless, the challenge to identify other women at high risk remains.

An understanding of the pathophysiology of incompetent cervix should form the basis for approaches to diagnosis and intervention strategies. The cervix is primarily composed of fibrous and connective tissue, with a small amount of smooth muscle. The smooth muscle is more abundant at the upper portion of the cervix, as the isthmus is approached. As the second trimester begins, the isthmus starts to unfold and the functional internal os moves downward. Before this time the uterus and cervix grow ahead of the enlarging conceptus, and the cervix is apparently not responsible for retaining the pregnancy.[18] Thus incompetent cervix is not believed to be responsible for pregnancy loss before 14 to 16 weeks' gestation. An understanding of the genesis of the incompetent cervix may well have to wait for elucidation of the biochemical changes that occur in the cervix during pregnancy, particularly as term approaches, a process usually referred to as "ripening." This poorly understood process, which transforms the cervix from a firm, unyielding structure to a buttery soft, easily negotiated portal for fetal egress, is almost certainly mediated by the hormonal changes of pregnancy. Possible candidates for this role include estrogens, prostaglandins, and relaxin. Another promising area of investigation is the chemical composition of the cervix. Leppert et al.[47] have demonstrated decreased elastin content in cervical biopsies of women with classical

incompetent cervix compared with normal pregnant and nonpregnant control women. Rechberger et al.[73] found evidence of increased collagen turnover in cervical biopsies from presumed incompetent cervixes compared with normal controls. Kiwi et al.,[42] using a cervical balloon, found the "elastance" of the cervixes of nonpregnant women with clinical histories of incompetent cervix to be significantly lower than that of normal controls. The clinical applicability of this elastance test is not yet clear.

Studies of incompetent cervix are made difficult by the likelihood that both congenital and acquired forms exist. Trauma to the cervix, as may occur from forceful dilation, cone biopsy, or obstetric laceration, may be associated with this condition. There is also evidence that DES exposure in utero may lead to congenital predisposition toward this problem. Whether multiple causes may lead to a common problem, such as loss of elastin content in the cervix, remains to be established.

INDICATIONS FOR CERCLAGE

Despite the relatively nihilistic view of incompetent cervix that emerges from a review of the scientific literature, it remains true that cerclage is commonly performed in patients suspected of having this abnormality. The clinician must decide, on an individual basis, when to place a cerclage. Some guidelines may be useful in making such a decision. What follows is based on my approach to this clinical problem, with reference to the pertinent literature where data are available.

The patient whose most recent previous pregnancy ended in painless dilation of the cervix, culminating in relatively painless and rapid labor in the midtrimester, presents little problem in decision making. Most clinicians would place a cerclage in the cervix of such a patient. It was previously the practice to wait until the first trimester had passed to lessen the chance of an operative procedure being followed by a spontaneous first trimester abortion unrelated to incompetent cervix. However, the identification of fetal heart motion by ultrasound allows earlier intervention, if desired, because the odds of miscarriage decrease greatly once fetal viability is documented.

The patient with a previous midtrimester or early third trimester delivery but without a classic history presents more of a problem. In patients at an advanced state of cervical dilation but with painful contractions during the midtrimester, there always remains the possibility that silent cervical dilation went undetected and that cervical stretching ultimately caused uterine contractions. Thus the typical clues to incompetent cervix may have been missed. Similarly, patients with preterm premature rupture of membranes and a dilated cervix may have experienced this problem because of cervical dilation, with exposure of the membranes to mechanical and bacteriologic stimuli leading to disruption of membrane integrity. Finally, it seems possible that preterm labor and delivery leading to forceful dilation of a cervix that may be "unripe" could cause cervical trauma.

Thus, at least theoretically, such patients may be at risk for subsequent pregnancy loss related to incompetent cervix. The data cited in the first section of this chapter lend little support to the concept of "prophylactic" cervical cerclage in such patients, except perhaps when there have been three or more previous second trimester losses or preterm births. A reasonable approach, then, is to consider such pregnancies at risk for incompetent cervix. McDonald's early description of incompetent cervix[59] cited symptoms of vaginal discharge, lower abdominal discomfort, or the sensation of a lump in the vagina. Such complaints should always prompt a vaginal examination in a patient believed to be at risk. Cervical examinations performed at weekly intervals may allow the placement of a cerclage in a timely fashion once cervical softening and dilation, or effacement combined with palpable thinning of the lower uterine segment, occur. This approach leaves open the possibility that cervical change may occur and precipitate labor and delivery during the interval between examinations. On the other hand, the placement of a cerclage without clear-cut indications entails definite risk without definite benefit. Risks include those inherent with anesthesia, whether general or conduction. In addition, maternal sepsis[36] and even death[23] have been reported. Other risks include preterm labor, rupture of membranes, cervical injury, and cervical stenosis.[1]

As ultrasound equipment has advanced, yielding better and better resolution, there has been increasing interest in the use of this modality to visualize the lower uterine segment and internal cervical os, structures that are relatively inaccessible to the examining finger. Sarti et al.[76] described a patient with already diagnosed incompetent cervix, in whom cerclage had been performed and ultrasound demonstrated a distended upper cervix that appeared closed when the urinary bladder was filled. Brook et al.[10] reported that the internal os was significantly wider among patients scheduled for cerclage (2.57 ± 0.36 cm) than in normal controls (1.67 ± 0.23 cm). A number of subsequent investigators have reported ultrasonic evidence of incompetent cervix, including prolapse of the membranes into the upper portion of the cervix,[86] shortening of the cervix, and a dilated endocervical canal.[40] Mahran[57] suggested that an internal os diameter of 15 mm or more during the first trimester or 20 mm or more during the second trimester was diagnostic for incompetent cervix. Varma et al.[87] found that a "short cervix" (less than 2.5 cm) was not a particularly bad sign so long as the cervical canal was closed (less than 5 mm in width) and the width of the entire cervix at the level of the internal os was less than 3 cm. A canal width greater than 7 mm with herniation of the amniotic membrane containing fetal parts was considered an ominous sign. Measurement of cervical canal width was felt to be the most useful predictor of incompetent cervix. It seems eminently reasonable that ultrasound would be useful in making the diagnosis of incompetent cervix in individuals without a classic history, and this approach is gaining popularity. However, it must be borne in mind that no series has reported the function of this diagnostic tool in directing the

use of cerclage in a blinded fashion. Ultrasonographic diagnosis of incompetent cervix leading to cerclage becomes a self-fulfilling prophecy, and data are not available on the fate of such patients if left untreated. Furthermore, at least one case has been reported of an ultrasonographic examination showing a somewhat short but closed cervix followed by a vaginal examination 20 minutes later revealing 4 to 5 cm dilation.[91] Thus not all cases of incompetent cervix can be detected with ultrasonography. Brown et al.[11] published preliminary data suggesting that vaginal sonography may have advantages compared with more traditional transabdominal sonography with respect to cervical evaluation.

In a cross-sectional study of cervical length measured by transvaginal ultrasound Iams et al.[38] found a continuous relationship between cervical length at 20 to 30 weeks and the gestational age at previous preterm delivery. They hypothesized that cervical competence is a continuous rather than a categoric variable. Subsequently Iams et al.[39] reported a large longitudinal study from the National Institutes of Child Health and Human Development Maternal-Fetal Medicine Unit Network in which cervical length at various gestational ages was a strong predictor of subsequent preterm delivery. It should be noted, however, that the preterm deliveries were not specifically related to classical signs and symptoms of incompetent cervix, and no evidence has emerged as yet that basing interventions such as cerclage on cervical length is effective in preventing preterm births.

The indications for cerclage thus far described have been based on previous pregnancy performance; the recommendation has been placement of a suture when the history is classic, and close observation in other cases. Digital and sonographic examinations may be helpful in determining which of the latter group of patients require intervention. However, another group of patients considered for cerclage by many clinicians includes women who have not experienced a reproductive loss as yet but whose histories contain certain risk factors believed to be associated with cervical incompetence. Whether cerclage should be performed prophylactically to minimize the likelihood that cervical dilation will advance between examinations and thus preclude treatment is controversial. Risk factors that have been cited in the literature include DES exposure in utero, previous cone biopsy of the cervix, previous voluntary interruption(s) of pregnancy, structural uterine abnormalities, placenta previa, and multiple gestation.

Exposure to DES in utero has been associated with reproductive wastage, particularly prematurity and midtrimester loss,[16] but not specifically with incompetent cervix except in the form of case reports or series.[30,83] In one case-control study,[85] DES-exposed gravidas were significantly more likely to have a cerclage than normal control subjects, but the diagnosis of incompetent cervix was not always clear. In a prospective but nonrandomized study, Ludmir et al.[53] followed 63 DES-exposed patients using a standard protocol. Cerclage was placed prophylactically in 26 who had a previous midtrimester loss or hypoplastic cervix on examination. The other 37 patients were managed expectantly. Of the latter, 16 (44%) underwent emergency cerclage because of cervical change. All of the 5 perinatal deaths occurred in the 21 patients who received neither an elective nor an emergency cerclage. These patients also delivered significantly earlier than those who received cerclage did. The authors concluded that strong consideration should be given to early cerclage placement in DES-exposed gravidas. Because of the nonrandomized nature of the study, confirming data would be helpful; none have been reported as yet. Levine and Berkowitz[49] subsequently published a series of 120 pregnancies in daughters of DES-treated women managed conservatively over 10 years. Only three pregnancies were treated with cerclage. Although there were a large proportion of first trimester losses (35%), 92% of pregnancies reaching the second trimester culminated in a liveborn baby who survived to discharge. All 5 of the losses at 16 to 25 weeks (among 94 pregnancies reaching the second trimester) were among the individuals with gross upper or lower tract lesions, as were all 14 preterm births. These authors concluded that prophylactic cerclage for all DES-exposed patients was not to be recommended. Fortunately, most daughters of DES-treated women have completed their reproductive years, so these issues are becoming moot.

A history of cervical cone biopsy is often considered a risk factor for cervical incompetence. It stands to reason that removal of a large portion of the cervix may weaken the structure, particularly if the internal cervical os is included in the biopsy. However, determination of the amount of risk associated with a particular individual's biopsy remains problematic. Lee[45] noted that 14% of 106 pregnancies after cone biopsy ended in midtrimester abortions or premature births. In a 1979 literature review, Weber and Obel[88] noted that when all series including 25 or more patients were combined, 7% of 577 pregnancies resulted in premature delivery, with only 2 patients receiving cerclage. Because the various studies considered included patients with differing depths and widths of cone biopsy, it is still impossible to conclude that cone biopsy carries no risk for incompetent cervix. Leiman et al.[46] reviewed 88 pregnancies occurring after cone biopsy, dividing the cone biopsy procedures into large (maximum cone height more than 2 cm and/or cone volume more than 4 ml) and small cones. Large cone biopsies (by height) were performed in 23 patients and small ones in 65. Patients having large cone biopsies experienced a 52% rate of second trimester abortion or preterm delivery, whereas those with small cone biopsies experienced a 21% rate of these complications. Tests of statistical significance were not applied in this article. Buller and Jones[12] found no effect of cone biopsy on second trimester abortion or prematurity rates, using the patients' pregnancy performance before conization as their own controls. Moinian and Andersch,[62] on the other hand, reported a sevenfold increase in second trimester abortion after conization, with 19% of patients ultimately receiving cerclage. The latter two studies did not report on the extent of the cone biopsy procedures, and this may be the critical issue. In the final report of the MRC/RCOG randomized trial of cerclage,[63] the data were

subjected to a secondary analysis by various subgroups. Among the 138 subjects with previous cone biopsy or cervical amputation, 70 were assigned to undergo cerclage and 68 were controls. The likelihood of delivery before 33 completed weeks of gestation was 19% versus 22% in the two groups, a difference that was not statistically significant. In fact, when the likelihood of delivery before 37 weeks was the outcome variable, the nonsignificant differences went in the opposite direction, with 36% of those undergoing cerclage and 32% of control women delivering prematurely. Kristensen et al.[43] used the population based Danish birth registry to establish a cohort of 170 women who had undergone cervical conization and subsequently conceived. Preterm birth (less than 37 completed weeks) occurred in the first childbirth after conization in 18% of patients, compared with 5% of first births of control women who did not undergo conization ($p < 0.01$). For second births, the figures were 8% versus 4%, but the difference was not statistically significant. Surprisingly, prematurity rates for deliveries occurring *before* cervical conization were significantly higher than in control women (8% versus 4%, $p < 0.05$). These data suggest that not all preterm births after conization are caused by the conization.

Cold knife conization has been largely supplanted by loop electrosurgical excision. Many clinicians, myself included, have anecdotes of patients with little or no cervix remaining after such a procedure who experienced pregnancy loss and did well after cerclage. Ferenczy et al.[24] followed 574 women who had undergone that procedure (to a maximum depth of 1.5 cm and a mean frontal diameter of 1.8 cm), who subsequently experienced 54 pregnancies. No preterm births occurred in this series, although there were three first trimester spontaneous abortions and two stillbirths. Spitzer et al.[84] compared pregnancy outcomes in a group of 433 women who had undergone laser procedures to their cervices with 433 matched control women. There was no difference in pregnancy losses or prematurity between groups. However, only approximately one fourth of pregnancies were in patients undergoing laser excisions, and it is unclear how many of these were the equivalent of cone biopsies. It appears reasonable that patients with a previous cone biopsy and no intervening term pregnancies be managed expectantly with weekly or biweekly cervical examinations after the 16th week of pregnancy.

Goldberg et al.[29] reported a procedure for combining cone biopsy during pregnancy with cervical cerclage.

It seems logical that cervical trauma caused by induced abortion might predispose to incompetent cervix in subsequent pregnancies. Bracken[9] reviewed the world's literature pertaining to perinatal complications in pregnancies subsequent to induced abortion. Although some studies showed increased rates of second trimester spontaneous abortion compared with control pregnancies, others did not. No conclusion could be reached, although the authors suggested that abortion by dilation and curettage (D&C) may carry a higher risk for subsequent pregnancy loss than abortion by suction aspiration. Harlap et al.[35] found a relative risk of

3.27 for midtrimester losses among nulliparous women who had induced abortion by D&C, a risk that disappeared after cervical dilation with laminaria was introduced. Levin et al.[48] found a significantly increased likelihood (relative risk 4.7) of two or more previous induced abortions among women with pregnancy loss between 20 and 27 weeks compared with women with term pregnancies but no increased likelihood of having had only one previous induced abortion. In the latter series the method of abortion and degree of cervical dilation could not explain the subsequent losses. In another group of women, Schoenbaum et al.[78] confirmed no apparent increase in risk with one previous induced abortion. Unfortunately, none of the available studies addressed the issue of incompetent cervix. We are thus left with the possibility that multiple induced abortions may increase the risk of subsequent midtrimester pregnancy loss, and we can speculate that some of these losses might possibly be related to incompetent cervix. Clearly there is inadequate evidence to support prophylactic cerclage in such patients. Whether women with two or more previous induced abortions require frequent cervical examinations remains to be elucidated.

Abramovici et al.[2] reported on 15 women with congenital uterine anomalies and previous reproductive losses who were treated with cerclage despite the absence of clinical or radiologic evidence of incompetent cervix. All of the patients delivered surviving infants, 13 of them at term. The authors concluded that the reproductive outcomes were so much better than in previous pregnancies that cerclage should be performed in such patients before surgical correction of the anomalies is attempted. Unfortunately, no control group was available for comparison, so we do not know how these 15 women would have done without the surgery. Golan et al.[27] reported a case series of 98 women with various uterine anomalies; in 30%, most often in those with bicornuate uterus, cervical incompetence was diagnosed clinically and radiologically. Cerclage appeared to improve the prognosis markedly in patients with cervical incompetence. However, the series contained a limited sample size after stratification, and there is also a concern about selection bias because patients were more likely to be seen for diagnosis if they had experienced a problem pregnancy. Routine cerclage cannot be recommended for such patients at the present time.

Arias[3] performed a randomized trial of McDonald cerclage in 25 patients with bleeding at 24 to 30 weeks and sonographic evidence of placenta previa. The 13 patients treated with cerclage had later deliveries (35 versus 32 weeks), larger birth weight (2709 versus 1812 g), and fewer neonatal complications than did the 12 patients not receiving cerclage. Patients receiving cerclage also spent less time in the hospital. Although Arias concluded that his results support the use of cervical cerclage in patients with placenta previa, no confirmatory data have yet become available.

Multiple gestation represents a clinical situation in which preterm birth is an ever-present risk. Although incompetent cervix has not been shown to occur with increased frequency in such pregnancies, it is not surprising that cerclage has been applied as a possible means of preventing prematurity. Zakut et al.[94] performed cerclage at 12 to 15 weeks' gestation on 20 women with multiple pregnancies induced by gonadotropin therapy. The pregnancy outcomes were compared with those of 20 other women with similar gonadotropin-induced multiple gestations, not treated with cerclage. Women treated with cerclage had significantly more surviving offspring and significantly longer duration of gestation.

Admirably, because therapy was not randomly allocated in the latter study, some of the same authors[20] later carried out a randomized trial of cerclage in 50 women with ovulation-induced twin pregnancies. The perinatal outcomes were remarkably similar: 45% of pregnancies in women treated with cerclage and 48% in nontreated women ending in premature delivery and 18% and 15%, respectively, ending in neonatal death. These studies point out the tremendous importance of using appropriate control groups when studying clinical interventions. A subsequent study[19] found no difference in outcomes between women with twin pregnancies who were treated with cerclage and those treated with bed rest. Cerclage was associated with a significantly increased incidence of premature rupture of membranes, but perinatal outcomes were otherwise similar. The authors concluded that cerclage offered an improved quality of life over bed rest, but another conclusion would be that since the efficacy of bed rest in twin gestation remains unproven, neither therapy is superior. Currently available evidence does not support the routine use of cerclage to prevent prematurity in multiple gestations.

One situation that may cause consternation is the patient with a previous pregnancy loss or preterm delivery whose caregiver made the diagnosis of incompetent cervix at the time, but whose history does not otherwise seem typical. On the one hand, it would be inappropriate to ignore the opinion of an apparently trained observer who was present at the scene. Conversely, many clinicians are loathe to carry out an operation when the indications do not seem clear. Under such circumstances it is best to gather as much data as possible, ideally by talking directly with the previous caregiver. Failing that, a diligent attempt should be made to review the birth records from the pregnancy in question. The decision whether to proceed with cerclage versus careful observation can then be undertaken with as much information as possible. As with all clinical decision making, the patient should be included in the process and should be fully informed about the uncertainties involved.

Contraindications to cerclage include active labor, active uterine bleeding, rupture of membranes, intraamniotic infection, and the known presence of major congenital anomalies incompatible with life. The use of bed rest and/or vaginal pessaries has been advocated as an alternative to cerclage but has not gained widespread popularity.

In summary, cerclage appears to be an appropriate intervention when the history for incompetent cervix is classic (i.e., a previous pregnancy culminating in delivery during the second or early third trimester, in which painless cervical dilation was followed by relatively painless labor). Other situations, such as DES exposure, previous second or early third trimester birth without a classic history, multiple previous pregnancy terminations, or multiple gestations, merit frequent cervical examinations and perhaps ultrasound examinations, with cerclage reserved for those patients demonstrating cervical change.

PROCEDURES

The choice of one cerclage procedure over another has no clear scientific foundation. At present, no randomized "head-to-head" comparison studies have been carried out. Outcomes of the two most common procedures, the Shirodkar and McDonald, appeared to be similar in one retrospective review of 251 cerclage operations.[34] Therefore this section describes the commonly performed procedures and recounts the apparent advantages and disadvantages of each.

Shirodkar Procedure

As originally described by Shirodkar,[81] this operation was performed as follows:

1. A strip of fascia lata ¼ inch wide and 4½ inches long is removed from the outer side of the thigh, and each end of this strip is transfixed with a linen suture.
2. The cervix is pulled down, a transverse incision is made above the cervix as in anterior colporrhaphy, and the bladder is pushed well up above the internal os.
3. The cervix is then pulled forward, toward the symphysis pubis, and a vertical incision is made in the posterior vaginal wall, again at and above the internal os, going only through the vaginal wall.
4. Through the right and left corner of the anterior incision an aneurysm needle is passed between the cervix and the vaginal wall until its eye comes out of the posterior incision.
5. The linen attached to each end of the fascia is passed through the eye of the aneurysm needle, and the right end of the fascia is pulled retrovaginally forward into the anterior incision. The same thing is done from the left side.
6. The two ends of the strip cross each other in front of the cervix and are tightened to close the internal os. The surgeon's left index finger in the internal os will indicate how much to pull on the strips. The assistant should be holding one end of the strip with an artery forceps.
7. The two ends are stitched together by a number of stitches that take a bite of the muscle fibers of the lowest part of the lower uterine segment, using a small curved needle and fine linen.
8. Extra portions of the fascia are cut out, and the anterior and posterior incisions are closed with 0 chromic catgut.

Later refinements by Shirodkar[82] included switching from fascia lata to a no. 2 Dacron suture and tying the suture posteriorly.

A number of other modifications to Shirodkar's original operation have been suggested. Fascia has been replaced by newer synthetic materials, most often a Mersilene band 5 mm in width or no. 2 Mersilene thread.[82] Druzin and Berkeley[21] suggested the use of a White tonsil forceps with medium curve to grasp the tissue between the anterior and posterior incisions and retract it laterally, allowing the use of an atraumatic Mayo needle swedged onto the Mersilene band (rather than the aneurysm needle previously recommended) to place the suture through the paracervical tissue on each side. Caspi et al.[14] described a modification wherein a single transverse incision in the anterior fornix is used. A monofilament nylon suture 0.6 mm in diameter is passed on each side, under the mucosa at the level of the internal os, from the anterior incision to exit through the mucosa of the posterior cervix, and is then tied. The procedure was compared with the modified technique of Shirodkar[82] in a randomized fashion, the subjects being 90 patients who previously had a McDonald procedure that failed or with cervical anatomy felt to be unfavorable for McDonald cerclage. Similar pregnancy outcomes were noted with the two procedures. The investigators believe that the newer modification has the advantages of simplicity, ease of removal, and lower incidence of severe vaginal discharge.

Advantages often cited for the Shirodkar procedure center around the fact that the anterior mucosal incision and reflection of the bladder upward allow the stitch to be placed high on the cervix, near the location of the internal os. In addition, most of the suture is buried under the mucosa. Disadvantages include occasional difficulty in removal of the suture at term, particularly if a Mersilene band is used. Although at one time many surgeons left the suture in place and performed cesarean section delivery, I favor removal of the stitch at term with vaginal delivery planned.

Following is a description of the Shirodkar procedure as I perform it:

1. I prefer to use regional anesthesia because patients awakening from general anesthesia sometimes cough and retch, which may put particular strain on the cerclage and membranes. Nevertheless, either method of anesthesia is acceptable, and the choice should be made in a collaborative manner, with the patient, anesthesiologist, and obstetrician involved in the process.
2. The patient is placed in the lithotomy position in stirrups. Assuming that the procedure is being done before cervical dilation, the vagina is prepared with Betadine in the usual fashion. The bladder is not emptied unless it is overdistended; a semifilled bladder allows easier visualization of the cervicovesical reflection.
3. A long, weighted speculum is placed in the posterior vagina. The anterior and posterior lips of the cervix are grasped with ring forceps or with tenacula if the former is impossible. Care should be exercised not to lacerate the cervix if tenacula are used.
4. Because bleeding from the anterior mucosal incision may obscure the surgeon's view of the posterior cer-

vix, the posterior mucosal incision is made first (Fig. 57-1). A 2-cm vertical incision is begun approximately 2.5 cm proximal to the external os and carried upward. The plane between the cervical mucosa and the cervical substance is entered using blunt dissection.

5. The cervicovesical reflection is identified by moving the cervix cephalad and caudad, allowing visualization of the slight ballooning of the bladder. The anterior mucosal incision, approximately 2 cm long, is made transversely at the reflection (Fig. 57-2). The appropriate tissue plane is identified by blunt dissection. The bladder is reflected superiorly bluntly, exposing the cervix as close to the level of the internal os as possible.

6. A large tonsil forceps with medium curve or a long curved Allis clamp is used to bring the mucosa and paracervical tissue laterally (Fig. 57-3, *A* and *B*). One blade of the clamp is inserted in the anterior incision and the other in the posterior incision on the left side of the cervix. As the clamp is closed, the tissues are drawn away from the substance of the cervix.

7. Although many obstetricians prefer a Mersilene strip, I have noted difficulty in the removal of such sutures once they have become scarred into the substance of the cervix. Therefore I prefer to use a 0.6-mm monofilament nylon suture, swedged onto a medium-sized atraumatic curved needle. Because the suture will be tied posteriorly to prevent erosion of an anterior knot into the bladder, the first bite of tissue is taken from posterior to anterior (Fig. 57-4). The needle is grasped at about its midpoint in a long, preferably curved, needle holder. The needle tip is placed just beyond the tip of the clamp holding the paracervical tissue, with the needle's curvature going in a direction opposite to the curvature of the cervix. This orientation helps avoid the needle tip's "wandering" into the endocervical canal. The needle is driven directly upward through the paracervical tissue, emerging in the anterior mucosal incision.

8. The process just described is repeated on the right side of the cervix, except that the needle is driven from anterior to posterior, emerging in the posterior mucosal incision (Fig. 57-5).

9. The nylon suture is then anchored to the anterior cervical substance at the level of the internal os. Although a permanent silk suture is preferred by many for this step, I believe it is better to use an absorbable suture to avoid leaving a foreign body in the area after the pregnancy has been completed. Therefore, 0 chromic or 2-0 polyglycolic acid (or some similar substance) suture is used for this purpose (Fig. 57-6). It is assumed that by the time the absorbable suture has deteriorated, the nylon suture will have scarred in so that slippage will be unlikely.

10. The cerclage should now be tied. The assistant should insert a fingertip into the endocervical canal to the level of the internal os. A surgeon's knot is then tied, and the knot is snugged down as the assistant slowly withdraws the fingertip. The internal os should be very slightly open once the procedure is completed. Four or five more throws are taken in the knot. The long ends of the suture are then held in a small mosquito forceps.

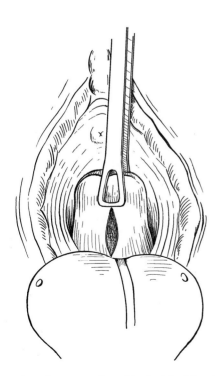

Fig. 57-1 Shirodkar procedure. Vertical incision in the posterior mucosa of the cervix.

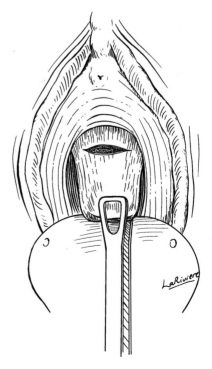

Fig. 57-2 Shirodkar procedure. Transverse incision in the anterior mucosa of the cervix.

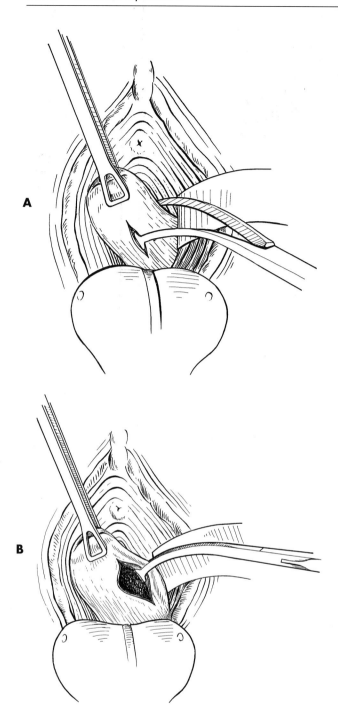

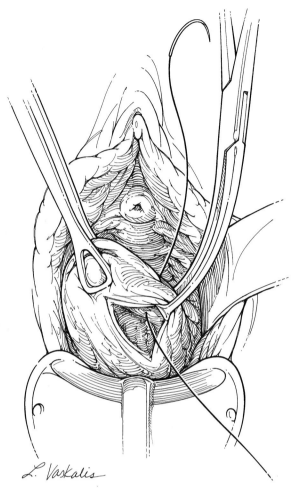

Fig. 57-4 Shirodkar procedure. A suture is placed through cervical tissue on the patient's left side, with the needle inserted from posterior to anterior.

Fig. 57-3 Shirodkar procedure. Long, curved Allis clamp encompassing tissue between anterior and posterior mucosal incisions on the patient's left side. **A,** Jaws of the clamp are opened. **B,** Jaws of the clamp have been closed, drawing paracervical tissues laterally.

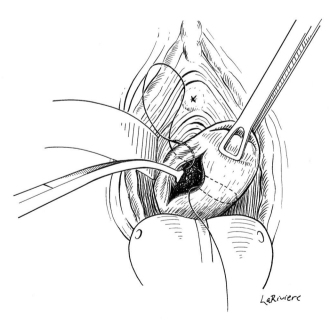

Fig. 57-5 Shirodkar procedure. A suture is placed through cervical tissue on the patient's right side, with the needle inserted from anterior to posterior.

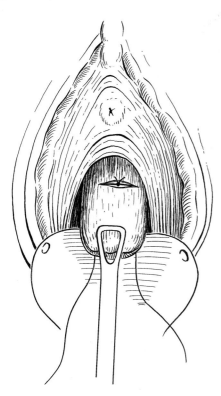

Fig. 57-6 Shirodkar procedure. Absorbable suture is used to anchor the cerclage stitch to cervical substance under the anterior mucosal incision.

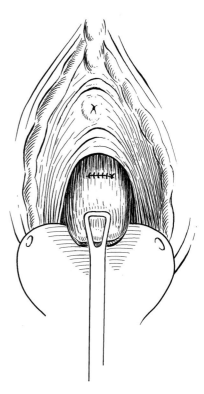

Fig. 57-7 Shirodkar procedure. The anterior mucosal incision is closed with running absorbable suture, burying the cerclage stitch.

11. The edges of the anterior mucosal incision are then approximated using a running, locking 2-0 chromic suture for hemostasis (Fig. 57-7).

12. The edges of the posterior incision can be approximated using interrupted 2-0 chromic sutures on each side of the emerging cerclage stitch.

13. The cerclage suture ends are then trimmed but left approximately 3 cm long (Fig. 57-8) to allow easy identification and manipulation when it is time to remove the suture.

14. The patient should be warned of the likelihood that pieces of absorbable suture material may be discharged from the vagina in 1 to 2 weeks after the procedure and that these do not represent the cerclage coming out.

15. Once the patient has fully recovered from the anesthesia, she may be kept in the hospital for overnight observation of possible uterine activity and discharged the next morning.

Perioperative antibiotics and/or tocolysis are not used routinely in my center when Shirodkar cerclage is performed before cervical effacement and/or dilation. Although Novy et al.[68] identified increases in circulating prostaglandin metabolite levels immediately after vaginal and abdominal cerclage procedures, these were generally transient and returned to baseline levels within 6 to 8 hours of the procedure. They were not associated with adverse outcomes unless the cervix was in an advanced state of dilation and

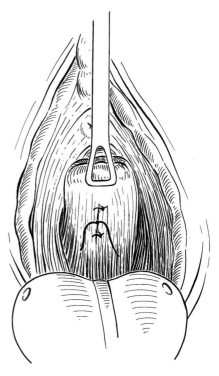

Fig. 57-8 Shirodkar procedure. Posterior view of the completed cerclage.

effacement, the uterus was already irritable, or the membranes were prolapsed or ruptured. The authors concluded that routine tocolysis was not indicated after nonemergency cerclage.

McDonald Procedure

As originally described by McDonald,[59] who reported on 70 patients in whom cerclage was performed at an advanced state of dilation with a 43% success rate (surviving babies), this procedure was accomplished in the following manner:

> The bladder having been emptied, the cervix is exposed and grasped at each quadrant by Allis' or Babcock forceps. If necessary the bulging bag of membranes is reduced by one or two dampened swabs held on sponge forceps . . . . A purse-string suture of no. 4 Mersilk on a Mayo needle is inserted around the exo-cervix as high as possible to approximate the level of the internal os. This is at the junction of the rugose vagina and smooth cervix. Five or six bites with the needle are made, with special attention to the stitches behind the cervix. These are difficult to insert and must be deep. If the ligature pulls out later, it is always from this portion, the silk remaining attached to the anterior lip. The stitch is pulled tight enough to close the internal os, the knot being made in front of the cervix and the ends left long enough to facilitate subsequent division.

McDonald[60] later reported an 80% success rate with his subsequent 25 procedures, an improvement that he attributed to prophylactic suturing at 14 weeks' gestation. He also switched from silk suture to no. 4 braided Mersilene suture material.

Advantages of the McDonald procedure may include its relative simplicity and bloodlessness, compared with the Shirodkar cerclage. Mucosal incisions are not required.

Although some authorities recommend the Shirodkar procedure when the cervix is markedly effaced, I have found the McDonald procedure more practical under these difficult circumstances. Occasionally, it is helpful to place a second McDonald suture above or below the first after the initial cerclage has initiated the reconstitution of the cervix. Disadvantages of the McDonald procedure include the fact that generally it is not placed as high on the cervix, and it is not anchored as well into the cervical substance as is the Shirodkar. Therefore it may be more likely to pull through or slip (although controlled studies addressing this issue have not been reported).

Following is a description of the McDonald operation as I perform it:

1. I prefer to use regional anesthesia because patients awakening from general anesthesia sometimes cough and retch, which may put particular strain on the cerclage and membranes. Nevertheless, either method of anesthesia is acceptable, and the choice should be made in a collaborative manner, with the patient, anesthesiologist, and obstetrician involved in the process. McCulloch et al.[58] compared 20 patients undergoing McDonald cerclage under pudendal anesthesia with 49 receiving regional anesthesia. There were no differences in pain perception or complications be-

tween the two groups. Pudendal anesthesia may be a viable alternative.

2. The patient is placed in the lithotomy position in stirrups. Assuming that the procedure is being done before cervical dilation, the vagina is prepared with Betadine in the usual fashion. If the cervix is already dilated the preparation is applied to the vulva but not into the vaginal cavity itself.

3. A long, weighted speculum is placed in the posterior vagina. The anterior and posterior lips of the cervix are grasped with ring forceps or with tenacula if the former is impossible. Care should be exercised not to lacerate the cervix if tenacula are used.

4. A 0.6-mm monofilament nylon suture, swedged to a medium-sized curved atraumatic needle, is grasped at its midportion with a long, curved needle holder. The curvature of the needle is oriented opposite the curvature of the cervix. The first bite of tissue is taken as high on the cervix as possible by entering the needle into the submucosa of the posterior cervix at approximately the 6-o'clock position and bringing it out at approximately the 4-o'clock position (Fig. 57-9). The needle is reinserted into the cervical mucosa at the 2-o'clock position and emerges at the 12:30 position. It is reinserted at the 11:30 position and reemerges at the 10-o'clock position. It is finally reinserted at the 8-o'clock position and reemerges at the 6-o'clock position. Care must be taken to obtain adequate purchase of the cervical connective tissue but not to bury

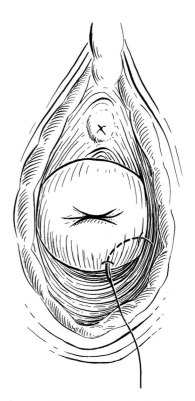

Fig. 57-9 McDonald procedure. The first bite of cervical substance is taken from the 6- to the 4-o'clock position.

the needle too deeply in the cervix lest the endocervical canal be traversed. Such a "transcervical" suture might lead to sawing through of the membranes and is also bound to be less effective than the usual cerclage.

5. Once the needle has been removed from the end of the suture, the purse-string can be drawn closed. First, a finger should be inserted into the endocervical canal to ascertain that the suture has not violated this space. Then the surgeon places a surgeon's knot into the stitch and cinches it down on the posterior aspect of the cervix (Fig. 57-10) as the assistant's finger is slowly withdrawn from the canal. A slight opening should remain at the internal os. Four or five more throws are placed into the knot, and the ends are trimmed to about 2 to 3 cm in length to allow easy identification and manipulation at the time removal is planned.

6. Once the patient has fully recovered from the anesthesia, she may be kept in the hospital for overnight observation to detect signs of labor and discharged home the next morning. Alternatively, Golan et al.[28] reported no difference in complication rates between 125 patients undergoing elective outpatient cerclage and 101 patients undergoing elective inpatient cerclage in a retrospective, nonrandomized study.

Abdominal Cerclage

Some patients manifest severe cervical injuries, and others have apparent congenital absence of the portio vaginalis of

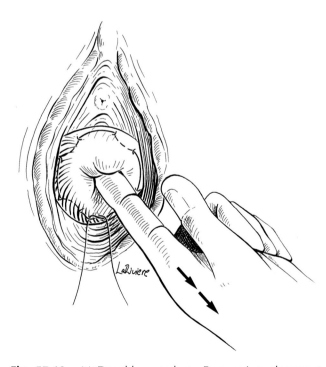

Fig. 57-10 McDonald procedure. Purse-string placement has been completed. The knot is tied posteriorly and snugged down as the assistant withdraws the finger from the cervical canal.

the cervix, rendering Shirodkar or McDonald cerclage technically difficult or impossible. Benson and Durfee[7] described an abdominal approach to cerclage, a procedure that was applied to congenitally short or surgically amputated cervixes and those with marked scarring, deep notching, multiple defects, or penetrating lacerations of the fornices. Novy[65] has popularized this procedure and added the indications of "wide or extensive cervical conization, cervicovaginal fistulas following abortion, or a previously failed vaginal approach to cervical cerclage." In addition, Novy suggested using this procedure in pregnant patients with cervical effacement that precluded high placement of a vaginal cerclage. Although his first report described only 4 patients, Novy[66] later reported on 16 patients treated with transabdominal cerclage during a 14-year interval, including 22 pregnancies, 21 of which resulted in living children. Indications for the procedure in these patients included marked scarring after failed vaginal cerclage ($N = 6$), abnormally short or amputated cervix ($N = 5$), deep forniceal lacerations ($N = 3$), and significant cervical effacement with dilation less than 4 cm and intact membranes ($N = 3$). The last 3 patients are of great interest because the procedures were performed at 22 to 26 weeks and all 3 went to term. Mahran[56] reported 10 instances of abdominal cerclage placed for very short or absent cervix with poor reproductive history, 7 of which resulted in perinatal survival. Herron and Parer[37] reported on 9 abdominal cerclage procedures on 8 patients in whom vaginal cerclage had failed. They had deep traumatic defects ($N = 6$) or extremely short cervix ($N = 2$) and a previous fetal salvage rate of only 5 of 25 pregnancies going beyond the first trimester. After cerclage, 13 pregnancies resulted in 11 births at 36 weeks or more and 2 fetal losses. In 1991, Novy[67] reported the results of an additional 20 abdominal cerclage procedures performed since 1982. The perinatal survival rate was 90%. Cammarano et al.[13] reported on a series of 24 abdominal cerclage procedures with a live birth rate of 93%. Indications for such a procedure are exceedingly rare; Novy[67] noted that in his center there was 1 abdominal cerclage for every 6 vaginal cerclage procedures, and it should be noted that his center presumably receives referrals specifically for this procedure. My own guidelines for patient selection include the following: (1) previous failed vaginal cerclage with scarring or lacerations rendering vaginal cerclage technically very difficult or (2) absent or very hypoplastic cervix with history of pregnancy loss fitting the classical description of incompetent cervix.

Specifically, I have only once placed an abdominal cerclage in a patient with a scarred or apparently absent cervix who has not had a previous typical pregnancy loss. A high proportion of such patients go through pregnancy successfully because, although the portio vaginalis of the cervix is apparently lacking, the internal os is presumably intact. In a single case I placed an abdominal cerclage without a previous pregnancy loss because the patient had undergone two previous cone biopsies and had been advised to have a postpartum hysterectomy because of persistent severe dysplasia.

She requested an abdominal cerclage because the current pregnancy would be her last no matter what the outcome.

Whether a diagnosis can be made in such patients by ultrasound before their first pregnancy loss cannot be answered without controlled studies.

Ludmir et al.[52] described the use of transabdominal ultrasound-guided dissection of the cervix and placement of sutures transvaginally, at the level of the internal cervical os, in four patients with extremely hypoplastic cervices who would otherwise have qualified for abdominal cerclage. All were successful. I have not had any personal experience with this approach, but it certainly sounds promising.

Advantages to abdominal cerclage include the obvious fact that it is performed in patients who cannot be treated successfully with vaginal cerclage. Clearly, the cerclage can be placed higher on the cervix, at the level of the internal os, with the abdominal approach. Theoretically, the risk of infection should be lower because the procedure is done through the peritoneal cavity, a clean operative field. The main disadvantage of abdominal cerclage—an important problem—is that the patient must undergo two laparotomies because most authors advocate delivery by cesarean section. An even greater problem is the pregnancy that results in fetal death or preterm labor before viability after abdominal cerclage; here a laparotomy is usually necessary even though no living child will result. Novy[67] has reported 2 patients in whom spontaneous abortions at 13 and 14 weeks were treated with dilation and evacuation, with abdominal cerclage sutures left in place. I have had two similar experiences. Infection, hemorrhage, injury to intraabdominal structures, and disfigurement from the abdominal incision are all potential complications. Thus the procedure must be reserved for highly selected cases.

Following is my approach to abdominal cerclage, which is based upon Novy's descriptions[65-67] and my own preferences:

1. The procedure is planned for the end of the first trimester or the early second trimester, after fetal viability has been documented. It is important to wait until the highest risk of spontaneous first trimester abortion has passed so that the necessary laparotomy is unlikely to be followed immediately by a second laparotomy.

2. An indwelling catheter is placed in the bladder. Although conduction anesthesia is my preference because of the decreased likelihood of postoperative retching, general anesthesia is also commonly used. Both Pfannenstiel and vertical abdominal incisions have been advocated. Because of my experience with what seemed to be the excessive manipulation necessary to bring the gravid uterus up and into a Pfannenstiel incision in two cases, I strongly favor the vertical abdominal incision.

3. Once the peritoneal cavity is opened, the bladder flap is incised transversely for approximately 5 cm at its reflection on the uterus, just above the level of the internal cervical os (Fig. 57-11). The bladder flap is advanced downward bluntly for only about 5 cm.

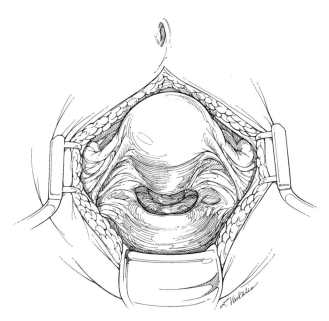

Fig. 57-11 Transabdominal cerclage. The bladder flap is created.

4. The uterine fundus is wrapped in a laparotomy pad moistened with warm saline, and the uterus is brought up into the abdominal incision, putting the cervix on some degree of traction. The uterine artery on one side of the cervix is palpated and then visualized, splitting into ascending and descending branches (Fig. 57-12). The relatively avascular space lateral to the cervix but medial to the branches of the uterine artery is identified. This space is then enlarged by the assistant, using gentle lateral traction on the uterine vessels.

5. A 5-mm Mersilene tape swedged onto a needle is then placed through the avascular space from anterior to posterior. Occasionally, this "avascular" space contains so many vessels that I have found it necessary to place the needle medial to the space, hugging and just digging into the substance of the cervix.

6. If bleeding is encountered at this point, it is usually controlled by gentle pressure. On one occasion I found it necessary to use hemostatic clips for this purpose.

7. The same process is repeated on the other side of the uterus except that the needle carrying the Mersilene tape is now passed from posterior to anterior so that the knot can be placed anteriorly (Fig. 57-13). Although a posterior knot might enable the removal of the cerclage through a posterior colpotomy, the manipulations necessary to tie and secure the knot are much more difficult when attempted posterior to the gravid uterus.

8. Care must be taken to ensure that the Mersilene tape is flat all the way around and not twisted. A square knot is placed anterior to the internal os, compressing the cervical tissue but not too tightly. The free ends of the tape are secured to the band by 3-0 silk sutures

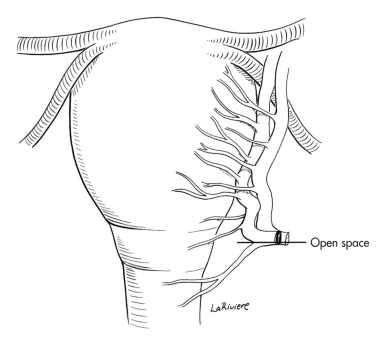

Fig. 57-12 Transabdominal cerclage. Relatively avascular space at the level of the internal cervical os. The paracervical tissue is drawn laterally to enlarge the space, and the suture is placed through avascular space.

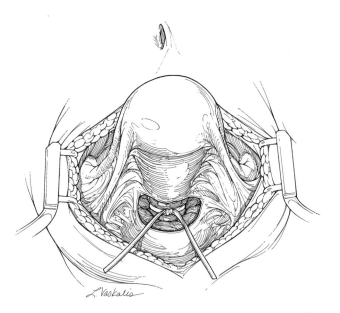

Fig. 57-13 Transabdominal cerclage, anterior view. The Mersilene strip has been placed and tied. The free ends have not yet been sutured down and trimmed.

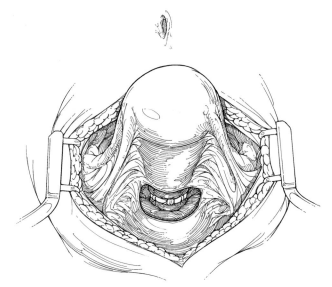

Fig. 57-14 Transabdominal cerclage, anterior view, just before closure of the bladder flap and completion of the procedure.

placed approximately 1 to 2 cm distal to the knot. The remaining free ends are then cut away (Fig. 57-14). The posterior portion of the band passes around the isthmus of the uterus at about the level of insertion of the uterosacral ligaments and is easily palpable and visible from behind as the uterus is drawn into the incision. Later it will become encased in scar tissue.

9. The bladder flap, peritoneal cavity, and abdominal incision are closed routinely.

Emergency Cerclage

All three of the aforementioned procedures for cervical incompetence are best performed before cervical dilation and effacement. However, as noted previously under "Indications for Cerclage," many patients do not have the classic history that indicates prophylactic cerclage in the late first or early second trimester. Such patients are managed expectantly, with cerclage reserved for those who manifest cervical change demonstrated clinically or by ultrasound. Therefore many cerclage procedures are performed as emergencies rather than prophylactically. At least two comparative studies have reported a lower success rate (50% and 59%) with emergency cerclage than with prophylactic cerclage (86% and 81%), although in neither was the number of cases sufficient to reach statistical significance.[31,34] Various case series report perinatal survival rates ranging from 56%[92] to 63%[55] to 77%[51] when the cervix was dilated 3 cm or more at the time of the procedure. In one series of 40 consecutive emergency cerclage procedures with the cervix dilated at least 1 cm, the perinatal survival rate was 83%.[61] In fact, 15 of 19 women with bulging membranes at the time of cerclage carried for an additional 4 weeks or more, and 12 reached 28 or more weeks' gestation. If emergency cerclage procedures truly have a lower success rate, the supposition is that the cervical incompetence advanced too far before intervention. However, an alternative explanation would be that some prophylactic procedures are done in patients who do not need them and are thus bound to have favorable outcomes.

The most important step in performing emergency cerclage is making the diagnosis. Other causes of premature cervical dilation must be ruled out, specifically preterm labor. Thus external monitoring of uterine contractions should be performed. If regular uterine contractions are present, tocolysis should be considered. Abruptio placentae should be part of the differential diagnosis and is considered a relative contraindication to tocolysis and probably an absolute contraindication to cerclage. In the absence of evidence of abruption, tocolysis can be initiated. Only if uterine contractions can be successfully inhibited, and the clinician is convinced that preterm labor was the result of cervical dilation rather than the cause of it, should emergency cerclage be considered. Steps should be taken to rule out chorioamnionitis if contractions are present. Even in the absence of contractions, cervical cultures should be obtained to rule out specific organisms such as group B streptococci, although the cerclage procedure need not be delayed pending results. In one study, microbial invasion of the amniotic cavity was detected on amniocentesis in 52% of 33 patients admitted with cervical dilation of 2 cm or more with intact membranes, not in active labor.[74] Organisms included *Ureaplasma, Gardnerella, Candida,* and *Fusobacteria.* Bacterial isolates portended a worse prognosis for cerclage.

The choice of procedure for emergency cerclage is not universally agreed on. Although the Shirodkar procedure unquestionably gains access to "higher territory," closer to the internal os, it may be particularly difficult to carry out successfully in a markedly effaced and dilated cervix. Novy[66] advocates the abdominal procedure in such cases. In my experience, the McDonald procedure has worked well, although I have not attempted an abdominal cerclage under conditions of cervical dilation and effacement. Schulman and Farmakides[79] recommend a modification of the McDonald procedure for patients with failed cerclage needing reoperation. Prolene suture, no. 0, is used, and multiple small bites are taken. Two circumferential sutures are placed and tied anteriorly. No comparative results are available.

Cerclage is clearly contraindicated in the presence of ruptured membranes. However, a number of investigators have published descriptions of approaches to the dilated cervix with bulging, unruptured membranes. In his original description of the procedure, McDonald[59] suggested using a moistened swab on a sponge forceps to reduce the bulging membranes. Goodlin[33] suggested transabdominal amniocentesis to reduce the tension in the amniotic cavity and allow retraction of "hour glassing" membranes. I have used this approach on occasion, with limited success. Olátunbosun and Dyck[69] recommended the placement of such patients in steep Trendelenburg position under general anesthesia and the use of 6 to 10 cervical stay sutures of 2-0 silk, then using traction on these sutures to cause the membranes to fall back into the uterine cavity before placing the cerclage. Katz and Chez[41] suggested that filling the bladder by instilling 400 to 500 ml of normal saline may lead to a retraction of the amniotic sac into the uterine cavity, thus allowing cerclage.

Charles and Edwards[15] recommended the use of prophylactic antibiotics when emergency cerclage is performed. They found a 2.6-fold increase in chorioamnionitis when cerclage was performed after, compared with before, 18 weeks' gestation and a tripling in the likelihood of preterm premature rupture of membranes (PROM). It is our practice to prescribe a 3-day course of broad-spectrum antibiotics beginning just before emergency cerclage, although data are not available to allow a specific rational choice of type or duration of therapy.

Similarly, it has been our practice to use tocolysis with terbutaline subcutaneously (0.25 mg every 4 to 6 hours) for the first 24 hours in patients undergoing emergency cerclage with a dilated cervix, particularly if uterine irritability is present. No controlled trials are available to evaluate this practice.

Although maternal sepsis[22,36,50] and death[23] have been reported, particularly with ruptured membranes and a cerclage left in place, Yeast and Garite[93] reported on 32 patients managed expectantly with cerclage in place at the time of preterm PROM. The cerclage was removed immediately in each case. The patients were compared with 32 matched control subjects with PROM but without cerclage in place. Latency periods and infectious complications were similar in both groups, suggesting that the presence of a preexisting cerclage in the face of preterm PROM is not a contraindication to expectant management as long as the cerclage is removed. Ludmir et al.[54] compared the outcomes in 20 patients whose cerclage was removed immediately after PROM with 10 whose cerclages were left in place despite PROM, with PROM occurring at an average of 28 weeks in both groups. Although delivery was more likely to be delayed for at least 48 hours (90% versus 50%) when the cerclage was left in place, perinatal mortality was significantly higher also (70% versus 10%), with most of the poor outcomes being caused by sepsis. The management of preterm PROM with an abdominal cerclage in place remains speculative. Although I have not personally encountered this situation, my inclination would be to manage with nonintervention because removal of the abdominal cerclage would involve a laparotomy and the intraabdominal location of the suture should not predispose to infection with ruptured membranes.

FOLLOW-UP CARE

Patients who have undergone vaginal cerclage prophylactically are usually discharged from the hospital on the day of[28] or the day after the procedure, provided that their condition is stable. Patients who have undergone elective abdominal cerclage are kept in the hospital as for any laparotomy, 2 to 4 days if there are no complications. When emergency cerclage has been performed for a dilated and/or effaced cervix, the patient may require a longer period of rest and observation to detect preterm labor if it supervenes. Once discharged, patients with cerclage in place are usually asked to observe "pelvic precautions," avoiding coitus or the placement of any object in the vagina. Those who have had an elective procedure are allowed to resume other normal activities and are examined weekly to ascertain the integrity of the cerclage. Women whose cervixes were dilated and effaced, particularly if they were at an advanced state of dilation, are often asked to restrict their activities and may require bed rest at home. This advice is individualized. All patients with cerclage are instructed to report any signs of cervical change, including vaginal or back pressure, increased discharge, pelvic ache, or cramps.

The timing of cerclage removal has not been studied in a controlled manner. However, it seems reasonable that the cerclage be removed at such a time as the clinician would be willing to deliver the baby electively (i.e., at 38 weeks or beyond). Although some patients may ask that the cerclage be removed at an earlier point, for convenience, this approach could lead to early delivery with its attendant risks. On the other hand, it has been my practice to remove the cerclage in any patient with significant contractions at a gestational age when we would not ordinarily be willing to institute tocolysis (i.e., 36 weeks or beyond). The logic behind such a policy is that uterine contractions in the face of a sutured cervix could lead to rupture of the uterus or avulsion of the cervix. Patients should be prepared for the possibility that their pregnancies may extend postterm despite the removal of the cerclage. Whether this phenomenon represents scarring of the cervix from the cerclage or mistaken diagnosis of incompetent cervix or neither remains unknown. Weissman et al.[90] reported normal labor patterns in 114 women with cerclage, with no cases of cervical dystocia. When an abdominal cerclage has been placed, I generally plan elective cesarean section at term. If labor supervenes the cesarean section can be performed on an emergency basis, or tocolysis can be used if the onset of labor is before term.

Finally, it is worth mentioning that the very name of the condition for which cerclage is prescribed is an unfortunate choice of words. In his essay "The Incompetent Cervix: Words That Can Hurt," Fox[26] notes that the definition of *incompetent* includes "lacking in qualities (as maturity, capacity, initiative, intelligence) necessary to effective independent action . . . one incapable of doing properly what is required." He concludes, "In light of these last meanings, it is easy to see how a mother grieving over the death of her premature infant might be additionally upset by being told by her physician that the premature birth resulted from her 'incompetent cervix.'" Fox cites several examples of patients reporting a tremendous sense of guilt and worthlessness because of this diagnosis and experiencing real relief when the nature of the condition was better explained to them. My own experience has been similar, and I support Fox's suggestion that the name be changed to some less judgmental term such as *premature cervical dilatation,* although the latter is not specific enough to convey the absence of labor or other causes.

REFERENCES

1. Aarnoudse JG, Huisjes HJ: Complications of cerclage, *Acta Obstet Gynecol Scand* 58:255, 1979.
2. Abramovici H, Faktor JH, Pascal B: Congenital uterine malformations as indication for cervical suture (cerclage) in habitual, abortion and premature delivery, *Int J Fertil* 28:161, 1983.
3. Arias F: Cervical cerclage for the temporary treatment of patients with placenta previa, *Obstet Gynecol* 71:545, 1988.
4. Bakketeig L, Hoffman HJ, Harley EE: The tendency to repeat gestational age and birth weight in successive births, *Am J Obstet Gynecol* 135:1086, 1979.
5. Barford DA, Rosen MG: Cervical incompetence: diagnosis and outcome, *Obstet Gynecol* 64:159, 1984.
6. Bengtsson LP: Cervical insufficiency, *Acta Obstet Gynecol Scand Suppl* 47:9, 1968.
7. Benson RC, Durfee R: Transabdominal cervicoisthmic cerclage during pregnancy for the treatment of cervical incompetence, *Obstet Gynecol* 25:145, 1965.
8. Bouyer J, et al: Maturation signs of the cervix and prediction of preterm birth, *Obstet Gynecol* 68:209, 1986.
9. Bracken MB: Induced abortion as a risk factor for perinatal complications: a review, *Yale J Biol Med* 51:539, 1978.
10. Brook I, et al: Ultrasonography in the diagnosis of cervical incompetence in pregnancy—a new diagnostic approach, *Br J Obstet Gynaecol* 88:640, 1981.
11. Brown JE, et al: Transabdominal and transvaginal endosonography: evaluation of the cervix and lower uterine segment in pregnancy, *Am J Obstet Gynecol* 155:721, 1986.
12. Buller RE, Jones HW III: Pregnancy following cervical conization, *Am J Obstet Gynecol* 142:506, 1982.
13. Cammarano CL, Herron MA, Parer JT: Validity of indications for transabdominal cervicoisthmic cerclage for cervical incompetence, *Am J Obstet Gynecol* 172:1871, 1995.
14. Caspi E, et al: Cervical internal os cerclage: description of a new technique and comparison with Shirodkar operation, *Am J Perinatol* 7:347, 1990.
15. Charles D, Edwards WR: Infectious complications of cervical cerclage, *Am J Obstet Gynecol* 141:1065, 1981.
16. Cousins L, et al: Reproductive outcome of women exposed to diethylstilbestrol in utero, *Obstet Gynecol* 56:70, 1980.
17. Cromblebolme WR, et al: Cervical cerclage: an aggressive approach to threatened or recurrent pregnancy wastage, *Am J Obstet Gynecol* 146:168, 1983.
18. Danforth DN: The fibrous nature of the human cervix and its relation to the isthmic segment in the gravid and nongravid uteri, *Am J Obstet Gynecol* 53:541, 1947.

19. Del Valle G, et al: Comparison between the use of prophylactic cerclage and bedrest in twin gestation, *Am J Obstet Gynecol* 164:408, 1991.
20. Dor J, et al: Elective cervical suture of twin pregnancies diagnosed ultrasonically in the first trimester following induced ovulation, *Gynecol Obstet Invest* 13:55, 1982.
21. Druzin ML, Berkeley AS: A simplified approach to Shirodkar cerclage procedure, *Surg Gynecol Obstet* 162:375, 1986.
22. Dubouloz P, Maye D, Béguin F: Cerclage et infections: etude clinique et thérapeutique, *J Gynecol Obstet Biol Reprod* 9:671, 1980.
23. Dunn U, Robinson JC, Steer CM: Maternal death following suture of the incompetent cervix during pregnancy, *Am J Obstet Gynecol* 78:335, 1959.
24. Ferenczy A, et al: The effect of cervical loop electrosurgical excision on subsequent pregnancy outcome: North American experience, *Am J Obstet Gynecol* 172:1246, 1995.
25. Floyd WS: Cervical dilatation in the mid-trimester of pregnancy, *Obstet Gynecol* 18:380, 1961.
26. Fox HA: The incompetent cervix: words that can hurt, *Am J Obstet Gynecol* 147:462, 1983.
27. Golan A, et al: Cervical cerclage—its role in the pregnant anomalous uterus, *Int J Fertil* 35:164, 1990.
28. Golan A, et al: Outpatient versus inpatient cervical cerclage, *J Reprod Med* 39:788, 1994.
29. Goldberg GE, Altaras MM, Bloch B: Cone cerclage in pregnancy, *Obstet Gynecol* 77:315, 1991.
30. Goldstein DP: Incompetent cervix in offspring exposed to diethylstilbestrol in utero, *Obstet Gynecol* 52(suppl):73s, 1978.
31. Goldstein PJ, Wolff RJ: The incompetent cervix: a survey of survivors, *Obstet Gynecol* 23:752, 1964.
32. Goldzieher JW: Double-blind trial of a progestin in habitual abortion, *JAMA* 188:651, 1964.
33. Goodlin RC: Cervical incompetence, hourglass membranes, and amniocentesis, *Obstet Gynecol* 54:748, 1979.
34. Harger JH: Comparison of success and morbidity in cervical cerclage procedures, *Obstet Gynecol* 56:543, 1980.
35. Harlap S, et al: Prospective study of spontaneous flat after induced abortion, *N Engl J Med* 301:677, 1979.
36. Heinemann M, Tang C, Kramer EE: Placental bacteremia and maternal sepsis complicating Shirodkar procedure, *Am J Obstet Gynecol* 128:226, 1977.
37. Herron MA, Parer, JT: Transabdominal cerclage for fetal wastage due to cervical incompetence, *Obstet Gynecol* 71:865, 1988.38.
38. Iams JD, et al: Cervical competence as a continuum: a study of ultrasonographic cervical length and obstetric performance, *Am J Obstet Gynecol* 172:1097, 1995.
39. Iams JD, et al: The length of the cervix and the risk of spontaneous premature delivery, *N Engl J Med* 334:567, 1996.
40. Jackson G, et al: Diagnostic ultrasound in the assessment of patients with incompetent cervix, *Br J Obstet Gynaecol* 91:232, 1984.
41. Katz M, Chez RA: Reducing prolapsed membranes, *Contemp Ob/Gyn* 35:48, 1990.
42. Kiwi R, et al: Determination of the elastic properties of the cervix, *Obstet Gynecol* 71:568, 1988.
43. Kristensen J, Langhof-Roos J, Kristensen FB: Increased risk of preterm birth in women with cervical conization, *Obstet Gynecol* 81:1005, 1993.
44. Lazar P, et al: Multicentred controlled trial of cervical cerclage in women at moderate risk of preterm delivery, *Br J Obstet Gynaecol* 91:731, 1984.
45. Lee NH: The effect of cone biopsy on subsequent pregnancy outcome, *Gynecol Oncol* 6:1, 1978.
46. Leiman G, Harrison NA, Rubin A: Pregnancy following conization of the cervix: complications related to cone size, *Am J Obstet Gynecol* 136:14, 1980.
47. Leppert PC, et al: Decreased elastic fibers and desmosine content in incompetent cervix, *Am J Obstet Gynecol* 157:1134, 1987.
48. Levin AA, et al: Association of induced abortion with subsequent pregnancy loss, *JAMA* 243:2495, 1980.
49. Levine RU, Berkowitz KM: Conservative management and pregnancy outcome in diethylstilbestrol-exposed women with and without gross genital tract abnormalities, *Am J Obstet Gynecol* 169:1125, 1993.
50. Lindberg BS: Maternal sepsis, uterine rupture and coagulopathy complicating cervical cerclage, *Acta Obstet Gynecol Scand* 58:317, 1979.
51. Lombardi SJ, et al: Advanced cervical dilatation: the role of cervical cerclage, *J Matern Fetal Med* 2:48, 1993.
52. Ludmir J, et al: Management of the diethylstilbestrol-exposed pregnant patient: a prospective study, *Am J Obstet Gynecol* 157:665, 1987.
53. Ludmir J, Jackson GM, Samuels P: Transvaginal cerclage under ultrasound guidance in cases of severe cervical hypoplasia, *Obstet Gynecol* 78:1067, 1991.
54. Ludmir J, et al: Poor perinatal outcome associated with retained cerclage in patients with premature rupture of membranes, *Obstet Gynecol* 84:823, 1994.
55. MacDoudall J, Siddle N: Emergency cervical cerclage, *Br J Obstet Gynaecol* 98:1234, 1991.
56. Mahran M: Transabdominal cervical cerclage during pregnancy: a modified technique, *Obstet Gynecol* 52:502, 1978.
57. Mahran M: The role of ultrasound in the diagnosis and management of the incompetent cervix. In Kurjak A, editor: *Recent advances in ultrasound diagnosis,* vol 2, New York, 1980, Excerpta-Medica.
58. McCulloch B, et al: McDonald cerclage under pudendal nerve block, *Am J Obstet Gynecol* 168:499, 1993.
59. McDonald IA: Suture of the cervix for inevitable miscarriage, *J Obstet Gynaecol Br Emp* 64:346, 1957.
60. McDonald IA: Incompetent cervix as a cause of recurrent abortion, *J Obstet Gynaecol Br Commonw* 70:105, 1963.
61. Mitra AG, et al: Emergency cerclages: a review of 40 consecutive procedures, *Am J Perinatol* 9:142, 1992.
62. Moinian M, Andersch B: Does cervical conization increase the risk of complications in subsequent pregnancies? *Acta Obstet Gynecol Scand* 61:101, 1982.
63. MRC/RCOG Working Party on Cervical Cerclage: Final report of the Medical Research Council/Royal College of Obstetricians and Gynaecologists multicentre randomized trial of cervical cerclage, *Br J Obstet Gynaecol* 100:516, 1993.
64. Niebyl J: Detecting signs and symptoms of incompetent cervix, *Contemp Ob/Gyn* 28:37, 1990.
65. Novy MJ: Managing reproductive failure by transabdominal isthmic cerclage, *Contemp Ob/Gyn* 10:17, 1977.
66. Novy MJ: Transabdominal cervicoisthmic cerclage for the management of repetitive abortion and premature delivery, *Am J Obstet Gynecol* 143:44, 1982.
67. Novy MJ: Transabdominal cervicoisthmic cerclage: a reappraisal 25 years after its introduction, *Am J Obstet Gynecol* 164:1635, 1991.
68. Novy MJ, Ducsay CA, Stmczyk FZ: Plasma concentrations of prostaglandin $F_{2\alpha}$ and prostaglandin E_2 metabolites after transabdominal and transvaginal cervical cerclage, *Am J Obstet Gynecol* 156:1543, 1987.
69. Olátunbosun OA, Dyck F: Cervical cerclage operation for a dilated cervix, *Obstet Gynecol* 57:166, 1981.
70. Palmer R, LaComme M: Le beance de l'orifice interne, cause d'avortement s repitition? Une observation de dechirure cervicoisthmique reparee chiurgicalement, avec gestation a term consecutive, *Gynecol Obstet (Paris)* 47:905, 1948.
71. Parikh MN, Mehta AC: Internal cervical os during the second half of pregnancy, *J Obstet Gynaecol Br Commw* 68:818, 1961.
72. Ratten GJ: Etiology of delivery during the second trimester and performance in subsequent pregnancies, *Med J Aust* 2:654, 1981.
73. Rechberger T, Uldbjerg N, Oxlund H: Connective tissue changes in the cervix during normal pregnancy and pregnancy complicated by cervical incompetence, *Obstet Gynecl* 71:563, 1988.
74. Romero R, et al: Infection and labor. VIII. Microbial invasion of the amniotic cavity in patients with suspected cervical incompetence: prevalence and clinical significance, *Am J Obstet Gynecol* 167:1086, 1992.

75. Rush RW, et al: A randomized controlled trial of cervical cerclage in women at high risk of spontaneous preterm delivery, *Br J Obstet Gynaecol* 91:724, 1984.

76. Sarti DA, et al: Ultrasonic visualization of a dilated cervix during pregnancy, *Radiology* 130:417, 1979.

77. Schaffner F, Schanzer SN: Cervical dilatation in the early third trimester, *Obstet Gynecol* 27:130, 1966.

78. Schoenbaum SC, et al: Outcome of the delivery following an induced or spontaneous abortion, *Am J Obstet Gynecol* 136:19, 1980.

79. Schulman H, Farmakides G: Surgical approach to failed cervical cerclage, *J Reprod Med* 30:626, 1985.

80. Shearman RP, Garrett WJ: Double-blind study of effect of 17-hydroxyprogesterone caproate on abortion rate, *Br Med J* 1:292, 1963.

81. Shirodkar VN: A new method of operative treatment for habitual abortions in the second trimester of pregnancy, *Antiseptic* 52:299, 1955.

82. Shirodkar VN: Discussion following Barter RH et al: Further experience with the Shirodkar operation, *Am J Obstet Gynecol* 85:795, 1963.

83. Singer MS, Hochman M: Incompetent cervix in a hormone-exposed offspring, *Obstet Gynecol* 51:625, 1978.

84. Spitzer M, et al: The fertility of women after cervical laser surgery, *Obstet Gynecol* 86:504, 1995.

85. Thorp JM Jr, et al: Antepartum and intrapartum events in women exposed in utero to diethylstilbestrol, *Obstet Gynecol* 76:828, 1990.

86. Vaalamo P, Kivikoski A: The incompetent cervix during pregnancy diagnosed by ultrasound, *Acta Obstet Gynecol Scand* 62:19, 1983.

87. Varma TR, Patel RH, Pillai U: Ultrasonic assessment of cervix in "at risk" patients, *Acta Obstet Gynecol Scand* 65:147, 1986.

88. Weber T, Obel E: Pregnancy complications following conization of the uterine cervix, *Acta Obstet Gynecol Scand* 58:259, 1979.

89. Weingold AB, Palmer JI, Stone ML: Cervical incompetency: a therapeutic enigma, *Fertil Steril* 19:244, 1968.

90. Weissman A, et al: The effect of cervical cerclage on the course of labor, *Obstet Gynecol* 76:168, 1990.

91. Witter FR: Negative sonographic findings followed by rapid cervical dilatation due to cervical incompetence, *Obstet Gynecol* 64:136, 1984.

92. Wong JP, Farquharson DF, Dansereau J: Emergency cervical cerclage: a retrospective review of 51 cases, *Am J Perinatol* 10:341, 1993.

93. Yeast JD, Garite TR: The role of cervical cerclage in the management of preterm premature rupture of the membranes, *Am J Obstet Gynecol* 158:106, 1988.

94. Zakut H, Insler V, Serr DM: Elective cervical suture in preventing premature delivery in multiple pregnancies, *Isr J Med Sci* 13:488, 1977.

58 Episiotomy, Repair of Fresh Obstetric Lacerations, and Symphysiotomy

DAVID H. NICHOLS

EPISIOTOMY

Episiotomy with or without forceps or vacuum extraction was the most common operative procedure for patients discharged from short-stay units in the United States for 1995 (1.41 million).[3,37]

A significant drop in the number of episiotomies performed has paralleled a coincident drop in the number of babies delivered by forceps and a simultaneous increase in the number of deliveries by cesarean section in the 1980s and 1990s both in the United States and, to an even greater extent, in the United Kingdom. This trend is also parallel to an increase in the numbers of deliveries attended by midwives during this period.

There is much concern about the risk/benefit ratio of episiotomy. The risks include the possibility of third- or fourth-degree perineal laceration and a resultant incidence in postpartum anal incontinence; the benefit is a lesser degree of obstetric damage to the perineum and a shorter and safer second stage of labor.[42] It is suggested that a prolonged second stage of labor will, by distending the perineum, actually stretch the pudendal nerves to a pathologic degree, inviting a future predictable and clinically significant neuropathy.[35] Much of the data of the 1990s draws on the performance of midline episiotomies, citing their ease of repair in reuniting symmetrically incised perineal connective tissues rather than muscle and lessened patient discomfort.[27,38]

Mediolateral episiotomies are more complex to repair correctly, requiring retrieval and reunification of the bulbocavernous and the transverse perineal muscles if severed, and causing a greater level of postpartum patient discomfort. But at the same time, there is minimal risk of sphincter damage and anal incontinence.[26] From my previous experience as an obstetrician and in following the aging process of my patients over many years, my prejudice in general is for the mediolateral episiotomy *anatomically repaired* over the perineotomy or midline episiotomy—a view shared with Poen et al.[32] Their studies have shown no relation between anal sphincter tears and mediolateral episiotomy, but a "strong association between midline episiotomy and anal sphincter tears," and note that ". . . in most European countries this type of episiotomy has been replaced by the mediolateral type," and conclude ". . . mediolateral episiotomy may be sphincter saving, especially in nulliparous women, and therefore prevent them from chronic faecal incontinence." Haadem et al.[20] studied by anal pressure profilometry women who had sustained anal sphincter rupture and repair 2 to 7 years earlier and noted significant trouble (gas incontinence, dyspareunia, and pain) in more than half of them.

Although episiotomy was intended to prevent perineal tearing, providing the alternative of repair of a fresh surgical "incision" to that of the jagged edges of the perineal tear, there were large areas of interest in using episiotomy as a safe aid in shortening the second stage of labor. At the height of its popularity, this operation, often combined with "prophylactic" low forceps application, was practiced on women of all ages in the Western world—in America in particular[8]—at a time when the relative inelasticity of tissues of the parturient now in her 30s was not as commonly encountered as it has become during the 1980s and 1990s.[6]

The first truly significant, objectively documented study that correlated the management of labor and delivery with subsequent evidence of maternal soft tissue injuries was reported by Gainey[14] in 1943. No equally significant study appeared in the U.S. literature until 1955, when Gainey[15] reported the results of his comparison of specific, documented injuries in two series of 1000 patients each. Gainey had personally delivered and assessed the postpartum evidence of injury in each patient in both series. However, there was an essential difference in the management of labor in patients in the two series. He had performed an episiotomy in the first group only when there was a maternal or fetal indication for it—either to avoid "impending" perineal laceration or to hasten delivery because of "fetal distress." In every instance in the second series, he had performed an episiotomy at the outlet station of the presenting part, after which he had accomplished all deliveries by low or outlet forceps (except in 27 instances that required forceps rotation and 40 breech presentations in which the fetuses were delivered by "breech assists" with forceps to the aftercoming head). Gainey found that performing episiotomy and controlling the delivery of the fetal head by "outlet" or "prophylactic" use of forceps provided significant protection for the vagina, urogenital diaphragm, and perineum.

Almost any obstetric procedure that had become "routine" has lost much of its popularity, and episiotomy, as such, is no exception.

An Argentine study by Lede et al.[28] strongly recommended against *routine* episiotomy despite the reduced number of labial tears and cystocele among women who received episiotomy. Although Ecker et al.[10] recorded a decrease in episiotomies at operative delivery from 93.4% to 35.7% over 10 years (1984 to 1994), the incidence of vaginal lacerations increased from 16.1% to 40% during this same period. However, during this period the management of patients in labor changed considerably with an increase in cesarean section rates and a decrease in the rate of forceps delivery.

Handa et al.[21] have emphasized their view that serious pelvic floor injuries may be minimized by allowing passive descent of the presenting part during the second stage of labor, using only specific indications for forceps and episiotomies, and selectively recommending elective cesarean section.

Although there is no clear-cut objective evidence that episiotomy significantly reduces the incidence of soft tissue damage requiring future reconstructive surgery, one is mindful of the large number of current parturients who have chosen to have their babies later in life, often starting their families after they have reached the age of 30. Because the "aging" tissues have apparently lost some of their elasticity, it appears that the obstetric incidence of significant vaginal and perineal tears and soft tissue damages is increased in this group, suggesting the long-range desirability of a more liberal application of timely episiotomy. Once performed and anatomically repaired, the applicability of episiotomy with future deliveries for the same patient remains the same. This thinking presumes that the timeliness of the episiotomy was such that it was performed before the soft tissue damage had occurred, and occasionally this requires that it be done during the end of the second stage of labor but before crowning of the fetal head.

The duration of the second stage of labor to some extent determines the capability of the vaginal and perineal musculature to respond safely to stretching. If labor has been short or precipitate, such ability to stretch is usually compromised, suggesting further the desirability of timely episiotomy, and similarly the episiotomy may be "protective" in the case of a prolonged second stage of labor. Some indication of good elastic distensibility of the pelvic soft tissue may be inferred by observation of the extent and width of striae appearing on the patient's abdomen and breast. This was observed and reported by Magdi,[29] who coined the phrase *elastic index*, as he suggested clinical relevance between many wide striae and decreased elasticity with increased likelihood of parturient tearing.

Gentle manual dilation of the perineum near the end of the second stage of labor, by downward and side-to-side pressure of the examiner's well-lubricated hand, has been described as an "ironing out" maneuver. It takes several minutes to accomplish, and one may start with the introduction of two fingerwidths, palm down, and gentle side-to-side pressure. A third (and then a fourth) finger is inserted when it can be accommodated, and the process is gently continued with emphasis on making posteriorly directed pressure.

Types of Episiotomy

If one has decided to perform episiotomy, usually coincident with some lack of elasticity of the perineal tissues, the choice between a midline and mediolateral site for the episiotomy incision depends largely on the experience of the

obstetrician or gynecologist. The obvious site of a previous episiotomy, the position of the baby's presenting part, the thickness or rigidity of the patient's perineum, and the obstetric perception of an impending severe laceration that risks fourth-degree extension, are all factors.[19] Intentional midline episioproctotomy was recommended by Cunningham and Pilkington[7] in the late 1960s. Although the long-term results were most satisfactory and associated with a reduced incidence of subsequent rectocele and soft tissue damage, the increased amount of immediate postpartum pain and discomfort, especially in the current presence of almost mandatory reduction in length of hospital stay, has caused the procedure to be abandoned. Given a parturient patient who has had successful repair of a previous rectovaginal fistula, many obstetricians would opt for a subsequent *mediolateral* episiotomy, performed before crowning of the presenting fetal part. When a midline episiotomy or perineal tear threatens to interrupt the external sphincter or extend to become a fourth-degree perineal laceration, a deliberate and timely incision can be made at the base of the opened perineum off to one or both sides (the "hockey stick" extension), directing the extension away from the rectal lumen.

There appears to be no indication for a bilateral mediolateral episiotomy.

Infibulation

Ritualistic mutilation of female genitalia has been practiced in certain African and Middle-Eastern cultures for thousands of years. Even today this forms the basis for serious health issues among those who have undergone the procedure. Although the severe scarring present has little effect on the first stage of labor, it exerts a profound influence on the second stage by creation of a soft tissue dystocia and obstruction. Anterior as well as separate posterior episiotomy, if necessary, is usually required to prevent severe tearing, fistula production, and hemorrhage. The technique of deinfibulation is shown in Fig. 58-1, and the result after reinfibulation and episiotomy repair is shown in Fig. 58-2. As emphasized by Elchalal et al.,[11] repair or reinfibulation of this scar tissue after delivery should be discussed with the patient, who might for cultural reasons demand reinfibulation.

Technique of Repair

The technique of repair is as important as the choice of site for episiotomy. The goal is to put back together the soft tissues that had been incised, having arrested by ligation the free bleeding that was created. The anatomy of the undamaged perineum is shown in Fig. 58-3. Administration of a pudendal block is shown in Fig. 58-4. This approximation is far easier to do with a midline episiotomy repair (Figs. 58-5 through 58-11) than a mediolateral one because the incised tissues with the former are bilaterally symmetrical. With repair of a mediolateral episiotomy (Figs. 58-12 and 58-15), in contrast, the bulbocavernosus muscle often has been incised and the anterior extremity has retracted into the labia

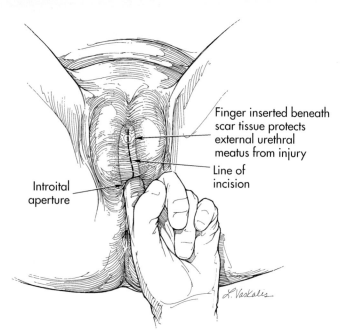

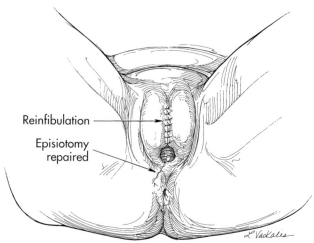

Fig. 58-1 Anterior episiotomy or deinfibulation. During the second stage of labor, the dense band of scar tissue enclosing the upper part of the vestibule is incised along the path indicated by the dashed line over a protective finger, which has been inserted through the introital aperture as shown. The incision is carried upward until the urethral meatus has been exposed. A posterior episiotomy is then performed.

Fig. 58-2 Reinfibulation. After any posterior episiotomy has been repaired, and if the patient requests reinfibulation, it is repaired by interrupted absorbable sutures, as shown.

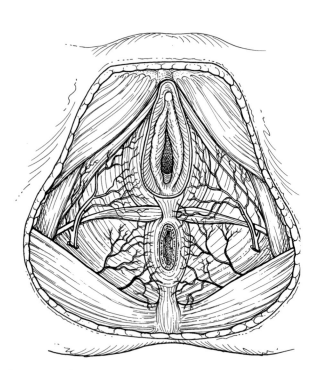

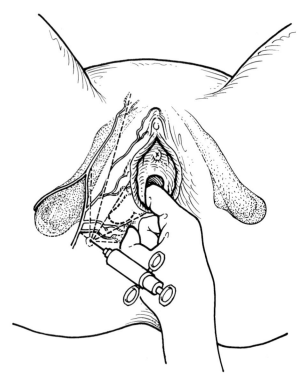

Fig. 58-3 The anatomy of the perineum after removal of the skin and subcutaneous tissue. The perineal body is the center of the hub of a wheel that includes the transverse perineal muscles, the capsule of the external anal sphincter, and the bulbocavernosus muscles. The blood vessels enter from the side, and their branches may be cut by episiotomy at the 5-, 6-, and 7-o'clock positions. Mediolateral episiotomy transects the superficial muscles of the perineum, but the midline episiotomy does not.

Fig. 58-4 The pudendal block. The pudendal nerves can be effectively blocked by a local anesthetic, thereby anesthetizing the perineum. The tip of the obstetrician's right index finger is placed overlying the right ischial spine. The pudendal nerve and artery are directly behind the spine. A pudendal block, to be effective, must be done on each side. The tip of a long needle attached to a syringe of local anesthetic is injected through the skin medial to the ischial tuberosity and headed toward the ischial spine, which is identified by palpation. The anesthetic is injected into the tissues around the pudendal nerve, and additional anesthetic agent may be injected along the site of the *dashed lines,* as shown.

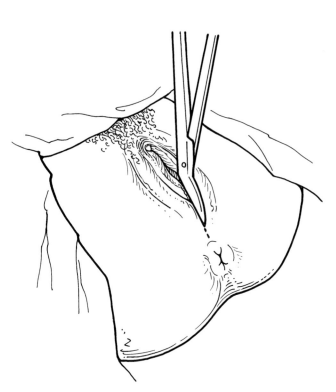

Fig. 58-5   A midline episiotomy (perineotomy) is made through the anterior portion of the perineal body in the 6-o'clock position as shown.

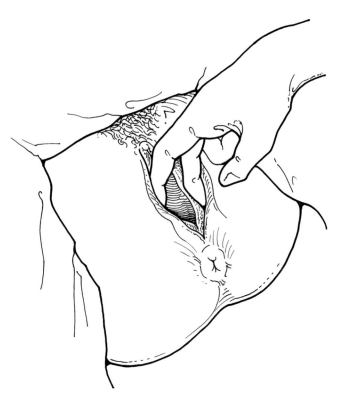

Fig. 58-6   The temporarily gaping introitus after midline episiotomy.

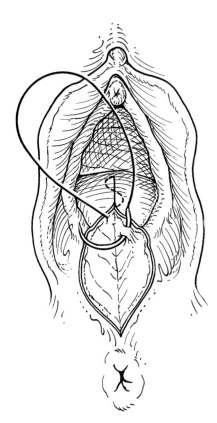

Fig. 58-7   Midline episiotomy is repaired by a running sub-cuticular suture beneath the vaginal incision and starting at its very top. This is carried down to the hymenal margin.

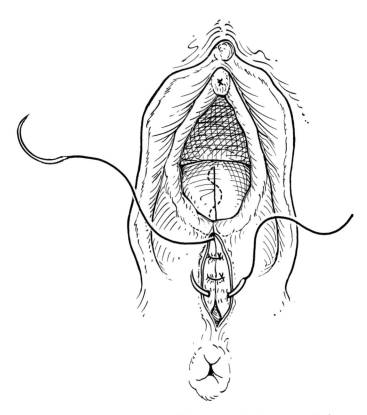

Fig. 58-8   Bisected portions of the perineal body are reunited by a series of interrupted sutures.

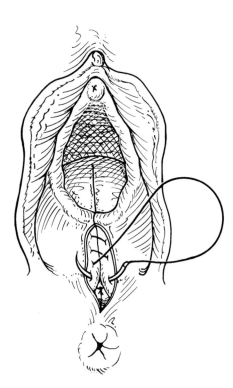

Fig. 58-9 If desired, the vaginal suture may be continued as a running layer to reunite the sides of the perineal body.

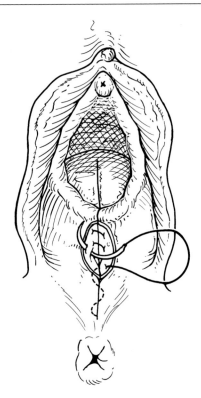

Fig. 58-10 When the suture has reached the bottom of the episiotomy, it is returned to the hymenal margin as a running subcuticular suture.

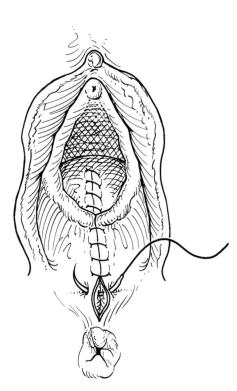

Fig. 58-11 Alternatively, the skin of the vagina and other perineal body may be reunited by a series of interrupted sutures.

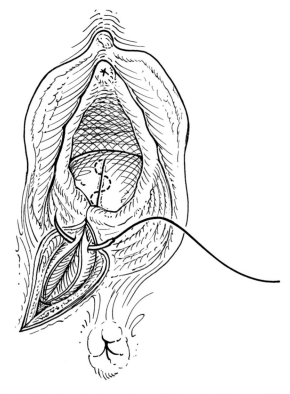

Fig. 58-12 Repair of a right mediolateral episiotomy. The vaginal portion of the incision is reunited by a running subcuticular suture placed according to the path indicated by the *dashed line.* The series of deep interrupted stitches reunite the deeper tissues of the perineal incision as shown. It is important to search for and unite the severed ends of bulbocavernosus and the transverse perineal muscles.

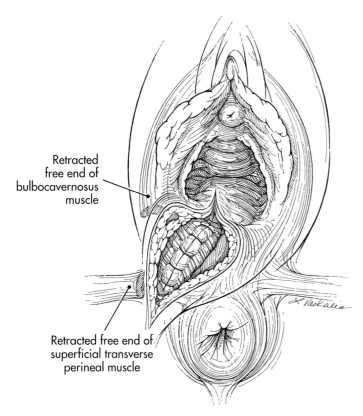

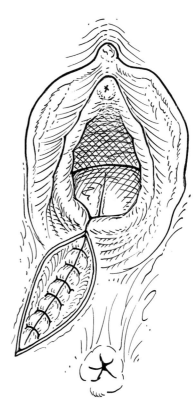

Retracted free end of bulbocavernosus muscle

Retracted free end of superficial transverse perineal muscle

Fig. 58-13 A special effort is made to find the retracted free end of the bulbocavernosus muscle and reattach it to the perineal body. The retracted ends of the cut muscle are shown. These must be reunited to the perineal body if an anatomic restoration is to be accomplished. The same is true for the transverse perineal muscles.

Fig. 58-14 When the deeper tissues have been reunited, as shown, the subcutaneous layer is closed by a running subcuticular suture.

(Fig. 58-13). To a less obvious extent the cut transverse perineal muscle has retracted into the surrounding tissues and should be sought and surgically reunited or sought and anchored to the perineum by a separate suture. The vaginal wall can be approximated by either running subcuticular stitching, using a small-gauge (2-0 or 3-0) chromic or polyglycolic acid suture, or either running or interrupted through-and-through sutures (Fig. 58-14). The subepithelial tissues are best approximated by buried interrupted stitches, and the perineal skin is closed by a running subcuticular suture or through-and-through suture, according to the surgeon's preference (Fig. 58-15). The pelvic muscles are displaced laterally after delivery (Fig. 58-16).

After repair of an episiotomy, a rectal examination should be done, and if a stitch in the rectum is discovered, it should be cut, usually on the rectal side, after which the ends fully withdraw and disappear into the deeper tissues. Cutting such a suture not only lessens the amount of postpartum pain and discomfort but also reduces the tendency for local necrosis at the suture site, lessening the chance of a postpartum rectovaginal fistula.

Aftercare

In many patients the postpartum perineal pain may induce some degree of spasm of the levator ani muscle, inhibiting

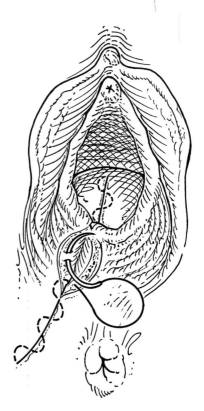

Fig. 58-15 When the deeper tissues have been reappproximated, the skin of the perineum is reapproximated by a running subcuticular suture placed as shown.

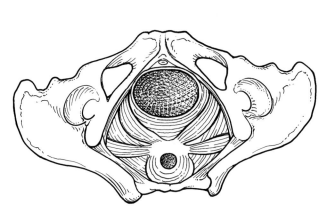

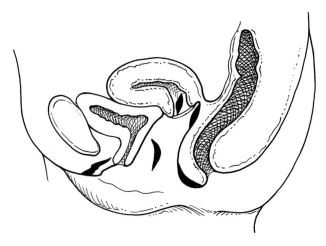

Fig. 58-16 The introitus and subcutaneous muscles at the time of vaginal delivery. Compare this with Fig. 58-1, and notice the lateral displacement of the muscles during obstetric delivery.

Fig. 58-17 The various sites of laceration that may occur with vaginal delivery are identified by the blackened areas. Note that laceration may occur in the cervix and lower uterine segment, the vault of the vagina, the perineum, the lateral wall of the vagina, and anterior to the urethra.

the spontaneous voiding process and making catheterization necessary. Should this become evident, the administration of an α-adrenergic blocking agent usually relaxes the "reflex" urethral spasm sufficiently to permit voiding, provided that the bladder has not become temporarily paralyzed by having become overdistended. An example of such a blocking agent (also useful for the same purpose after any procedure that by pain inhibits muscular relaxation, i.e., hemorrhoidectomy, appendectomy, or herniorrhaphy) is phenoxybenzamine (Dibenzyline), 10 mg/dose, by mouth. Adequate postpartum analgesia inhibits perineal pain, often precluding the necessity for catheterization. Early ambulation also has a salutary effect in reestablishing voiding because many women are unable to void when lying down. Application of ice packs to the perineum is comforting during the first 18 hours postpartum while the patient is hospitalized. Local applications of cotton balls saturated with witch hazel are soothing to the perineum.

The perineum should be inspected daily during hospitalization, usually with the patient in the lateral recumbent or Sims' position, and if the perineum is unusually tender or inflamed, local heat is helpful after the first postpartum day. Heat may be in the form of a heat lamp or the heat from a blow-type hair dryer initially because the skin incision does not become watertight until after the second postpartum or postoperative day. After the second day, warm water sitz baths, two or three times a day, may be comforting.

Attention to bowel habit is important because perineal pain may inhibit defecation and it is important to avoid the development of a fecal impaction. Stool softeners and gentle laxatives and the use of a rectal laxative suppository (glycerin or Dulcolax) may be necessary.

Perineal infection, although rare, should be taken seriously because the severe consequence, development of synergistic bacterial gangrene or even necrotizing fasciitis, is

possible. The latter may develop unexpectedly after discharge from the hospital so attention must be given to postpartum communication from the patient concerning her perineum.

Postpartum hematoma of the vulva and episiotomy site produces local disfigurement and pain. The site should be watched carefully because the veins of the vulva have no valves and continued bleeding can occur, distending all of the soft tissues and compartments of the pelvis. Progressive enlargement is evident, often with accompanying discoloration. Such sutures are taken out as necessary to provide exposure and evacuation of clots, and the raw surfaces are inspected. Any bleeding vessels that can be identified are clamped and tied, and the hematoma cavity is packed, for which iodoform gauze is useful.

LACERATIONS OF THE PELVIS

The cervix and vagina should be inspected for the presence of lacerations (Fig. 58-17), which may be repaired promptly, with adequate visualization provided by appropriate retractors, usually using interrupted sutures of absorbable material. Blood vessels that are found bleeding should, of course, be clamped and tied. Most lacerations should be repaired as soon after delivery as possible.

Degrees of Tearing

A first-degree laceration of the perineum is one that extends through the vaginal and perineal skin and superficial tissues of the perineal body. Debridement is rarely necessary, and a single layer of interrupted sutures placed about 1 cm apart suffices in most patients.

A second-degree perineal laceration, on the other hand, extends deeply into the soft tissues of the perineum, sometimes down to but not including the external anal sphincter,

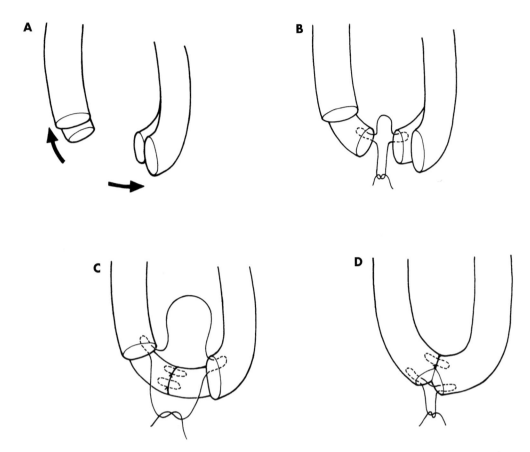

Fig. 58-18 The details of suture placement reuniting the severed ends of the perineal muscles are shown. **A,** The ends of the muscles tend to retract from the site of their incision, as indicated by the black arrows. **B,** The ends of the muscle are identified and reapproximated by a series of interrupted sutures, the deeper ones being placed first. **C,** When these have been tied, additional interrupted sutures are placed in the ends of the transected muscle in its more superficial portion. **D,** The appearance when these are tied.

and generally involves disruption of some fibers of the transverse perineal muscles. A layer of buried interrupted sutures is placed, and a superficial layer of through-and-through absorbable interrupted stitches finishes the repair. Damage to the smooth and striated muscles and soft unexposed tissues from unexposed stretching of the perineum has already been done and will not likely be repaired or restored by repair at this time.

A third-degree laceration extends through the skin and tissues of the perineum and portions or all of the external anal sphincter. This should also be repaired by a series of interrupted sutures reuniting the sides of the perineal body. Each severed end of each component of the external anal sphincter is identified and grasped by an Allis clamp and brought together by two interrupted mattress sutures of long-lasting absorbable suture material such as Maxon or polydioxanone (PDS), placed at right angles to one another (Fig. 58-18). Each stitch should include the connective tissue of the muscle capsule, if possible.

Although the patient may consume a regular house diet, special attention should be given to keeping the stool on the soft side, using stool softeners as necessary duringthe first month postpartum, and restoration of bowel habits with regular movement is the immediate goal. Appropriate laxative stimulation, if necessary, helps avoid fecal impaction. Perineal resistive exercises of the Kegel type (15 squeezes of 3 seconds' duration six times a day) are useful for 3 months postpartum. A mental or a written note is appended to the patient's chart to consider strongly a mediolateral episiotomy with the next birth.

A fourth-degree laceration, although occasionally unavoidable, is an obstetric tragedy, and its repair and the aftercare require the undivided attention of the patient's obstetrician. Laceration is more common in the presence of a relatively inelastic perineum, especially during a violent labor, that has compromised the ability of the perineal tissues to stretch slowly to accommodate the passage of the fetal presenting part.

A fourth-degree laceration may occur within a few seconds, usually followed by the explosive delivery of the fetus. The laceration should be repaired immediately after delivery of the placenta and inspection of the birth canal.

Repair of Fourth-Degree Laceration

Any necessary debridement should he accomplished, the injury site should be irrigated with sterile saline, and the necessary components for anatomic reconstruction should be identified and tagged if necessary. The full extent of the laceration in the anterior rectal wall is exposed (Figs. 58-19 and 58-20) and approximated from side to side by submucosal running suture all the way down to the margin of the anal skin. A second layer of running suture will invert the first, taking some of the tension from the first layer closure, which may be helpful during the healing process. If not previously accomplished, the retracted ends of the external anal sphincter and its connective tissue capsule, if it can be identified, are grasped with Allis clamps, and mattress sutures of long-lasting absorbable polyglycolic acid type are placed, but not yet tied (Fig. 58-21). The vaginal wall is approximated from side to side by suture, and careful side-to-side placement of interrupted absorbable sutures begins the reconstruction of the perineal body and perineum. These stitches are carefully tied as they are placed, with the tension sufficient to approximate the tissues, but not so tightly that the tissues in which they have been placed are strangulated. When all stitches have been placed and tied, the sutures previously placed uniting the ends of the severed anal sphincter are tied, and the perineum and skin are closed, usually using interrupted absorbable sutures. The occurrence of rectovaginal fistula after a fourth-degree laceration is highly litigious! Fistula formation should be prevented by careful control of

diet and resumption of good bowel habits postpartum and until the tissues have fully healed. A low-residue diet is initiated, and daily doses of stool softeners and bulk producers are started. Careful attention must be given to initiation of the first bowel movement, and if this has not occurred after 48 hours postpartum, a mild laxative is given, such as milk of magnesia with cascara. After the first bowel movement, a regular diet may be initiated, although daily stool softeners and laxatives should be continued for 1 month until a history of regular daily bowel movements has been reported.

Immediately after the repair of even a routine episiotomy, rectal examination should be done to check for an unexpected hole between the rectum and vagina above the site of the episiotomy repair, and if one is found, it should be repaired at this time. If a stitch is found transgressing the rectum, it should be cut transrectally to lessen the chance of rectovaginal fistula.

Failure to heed the tremendous intrarectal pressures that can be generated during forceful evacuation of the first large bolus of hard stool some 7 to 10 days after delivery and repair may compromise the integrity of the anterior rectal wall portion of the repair—with disruption of its cranial portion, through both rectal and vaginal wall, and the production of a rectovaginal fistula. The patient will date her incontinence of gas and feces to that first postpartum bowel movement. In general, I believe this unwelcome eventuality results from mismanagement of postpartum bowel habits more than from any technical imprecision in the repair of the fourth-degree laceration.

When breakdown of a fourth-degree laceration has been noted while the postpartum patient is still in the hospital, there is usually much coexistent edema, local infection, pain, and some necrosis. Most obstetricians and gynecologists have elected in the past to recommend repair after some 3 months postpartum, when pain, infection, and edema have subsided and provision has been made for the care of the newborn baby. Early repair of an episiotomy dehiscence associated with infection was successful in 94% of patients in a civilian hospital after debridement and removal of all infected or necrotic tissue and suture fragments, after the patient had been afebrile for more than 24 hours.[24,36]

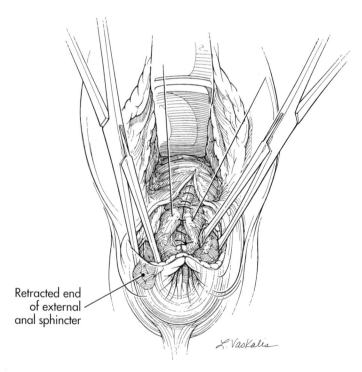

Fig. 58-19 Repair of a fourth-degree laceration. The torn edges of the rectal submucosa and muscularis are reunited by the series of interrupted sutures as shown, and the cut edges of the external anal sphincter and its capsule are grasped with Allis clamps.

Retracted end of external anal sphincter

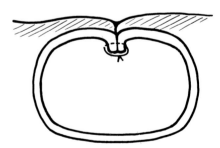

Fig. 58-20 When there is considerable bleeding from the rectal edges of the tear in the rectal mucosa, it may be controlled by a series of stitches that invert the mucosa into the rectal lumen. These stitches are tied so that the suture knot is on the internal surface of the rectum.

This was corroborated by Arona et al.[1] who studied patients with third- and fourth-degree lacerations and episiotomy breakdown, debrided as outpatients, and then admitted for short-stay reconstruction, dramatically reducing patient suffering and disability and avoiding prolonged hospitalization.

Postpartum Rectovaginal Fistula

Postpartum rectovaginal fistula is more common in patients older than age 40, in whom tissue elasticity and distensibility are reduced, after breakdown of the repair of a fourth-degree laceration, or it may come from unrecognized buttonholing of the anterior rectal and posterior vaginal wall coincident with episiotomy. In this instance, incontinence of gas should be noted within the first 2 postpartum days. A postpartum rectovaginal fistula that is not recognized for 7 to 14 days after delivery may be more likely caused by necrosis at the site of an episiotomy suture placed through the posterior vaginal wall and inadvertently through the anterior wall of the rectum. A digital examination of the rectum should always be done after episiotomy repair so that any such transgressing suture can be identified and promptly cut. Usually, if it is cut on the rectal side, it retracts promptly from the rectum toward the vagina and out of harm's way.

These fistulas are repaired without the coincident performance of a complementary colostomy, using an appropriate repair as described in Chapter 28. Generally speaking, if the perineal repair and anal sphincter reunification have healed effectively, it is *not* essential to redivide the healed areas by recreation of a fourth-degree laceration for the repair because on occasion the rerepair may break down with disruption of previously healed strategic tissue. Should the

patient request and be prepared for an "immediate rerepair," this can be offered as a consideration, although she must understand that a small percentage do not heal properly and require another rerepair some months in the future. Should the patient be prepared to take her chances with "immediate rerepair," she should be immediately given a clear liquid diet, frequent sitz baths, and heat to the perineum, rinsing the area twice daily with 5% hydrogen peroxide solution, and experiencing gentle daily debridement of any necrotic tissue, until purulence, pain, and edema have subsided. Preoperative mechanical and appropriate antibiotic bowel preparation (Nu-LYTELY and erythromycin-neomycin or Mefoxin) is also given. Because healing of the uninfected tissues is incomplete, a fresh wound is recreated at surgery and repaired. Antibiotics and a clear liquid diet are continued postoperatively, along with abundant analgesia, local heat, and daily stool softeners such as Colace. Beginning the third postoperative day, a low-residue diet may be started, but the patient is not discharged until after the first bowel movement. The low-residue diet is continued for 3 weeks after discharge, with periodic phone calls from the office staff to the patient to solicit and answer any relevant questions and to inquire and advise concerning bowel evacuations.

Paravaginal Hematoma

A paravaginal hematoma may be found, usually unexpectedly, immediately after delivery and will be present as a discreet and spongy localized fullness in the region of the ischial spine. Paravaginal hematomas are usually unilateral and may represent unexpected trauma to the pudendal blood vessels. Because of their arterial component and the lack of counterpressure on the cranial side of the hematoma, expansion within the vaginal and subvaginal tissues and more particularly into the retroperitoneal tissues of the pelvis is to be expected, which can give rise to a most disproportionate degree of pelvic pain if undetected. These hematomas can contain up to 1200 ml of blood clot. There is no place for expectant treatment of these hematomas. If they are detected immediately after delivery, the full thickness of the vaginal wall should be incised longitudinally and the clot should be evacuated. If individual bleeding vessels are encountered, they should be clamped and the clamp should be replaced by a transfixion ligature. If they have retracted within the sidewall of the pelvis and are not visible, the hematoma cavity should be tightly packed with gauze, preferably iodoform, which is shortened in 12 hours and generally removed in 24 hours. This compression effectively controls residual bleeding by counterpressure, and the wound and vaginal incision generally heal promptly and with no sequelae.

If the hematoma occurs on the side or at the site of an episiotomy, the stitches are removed, the clot is evacuated, and the episiotomy is rerepaired using interrupted sutures. Postpartum purplish discoloration of the vulvar skin is to be expected, but the associated edema rapidly subsides. Supravaginal hematomas, although uncommon, may be sus-

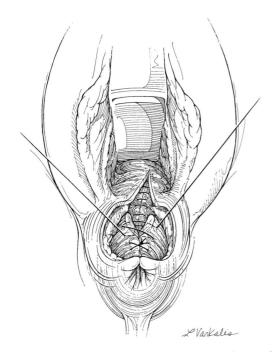

Fig. 58-21 The Allis clamps are replaced with transfixion ligatures, reuniting the ends of the external anal sphincter.

pected by an unexplained rise in the pulse rate and coincident drop in blood pressure. Such a hematoma can be confirmed by a falling hematocrit, and an ill-defined pelvic fullness, usually unilateral, may be perceived with bimanual examination. These should be watched carefully, and if palpable suprapubically, the height should be marked on the patient's abdominal skin so that one can observe objectively whether an increase in size evolves. If it does not, expectant treatment may suffice, but if the mass enlarges, laparotomy should be performed, the clot should be evacuated, and the area should be drained.

SYMPHYSIOTOMY

In usual North American practice situations, emergency symphysiotomy is not a substitute for cesarean section, but it is a welcome solution to obstructed labor in many parts of the world (underdeveloped regions including South America, Central Africa, Asia, and various parts of Australia and New Zealand) where facilities for emergency cesarean section are unavailable. Timely symphysiotomy not only may be lifesaving for the fetus but also may spare the mother the incalculable pain and suffering of massive disability or death.[16,23,41]

Although this operation was documented more than 200 years ago, it was reintroduced into obstetric technology by the South American Zarate,[45] who published detailed experience and description of the operation in 1955. Important but somewhat sporadic contributions have been published in the international literature since then.

Indications for Symphysiotomy

Indications for symphysiotomy are as follows:

- A modest degree of fetal pelvic disproportion, with the membranes ruptured and the cervix fully dilated; progress of fetal descent has become arrested, either inlet midpelvic or, more rarely, outlet (in the latter circumstance, separation of the pubis does not ensure appreciable separation of lines at the outlet).
- Unexpected arrest of a nonhydrocephalic aftercoming head during breech delivery through a fully dilated cervix. Delivery of a living, undamaged fetus is otherwise improbable in a clinical setting in which emergency cesarean section is neither safe nor technically feasible.
- Most of the patients will be primigravidas. An occasional indication is the unmolded aftercoming head of a baby presenting by breech that may become trapped within the bony pelvis and may be salvaged. If it is to be effective, symphysiotomy must be implemented without delay.

Technique for Symphysiotomy

The operation is simple, although it requires technical precision. For a proper indication, it can be performed under local anesthesia in about 5 minutes. The technique is a modification from Zarate's[45] description and is as follows. The patient is in the lithotomy position, and her legs should

be firmly held by two assistants (Fig. 58-22, *A* through *C*). A local anesthetic solution is infiltrated into the skin above the symphysis and then around the joint, and a transurethral catheter is passed and left in place.

The skin and tissues of the mons pubis are infiltrated, and the needle is directed into the joint of the symphysis pubis where more local anesthetic is injected. This step, as pointed out by Menticoglou,[30] identifies the joint space and the needle can be left in situ as a guide wire if desired as mentioned by Chrichton and Seedat[4] (see Fig. 58-22, *D* and *E*). The index and middle fingers of the left hand are introduced palm side up into the vagina. The index finger pushes the catheter and urethra to one side, and the middle finger remains on the posterior aspect of the pubic joint to make sure the scalpel blade, when it is almost through the joint, does not penetrate too deeply. The scalpel (an old-type, one-piece scalpel without detachable blade is desirable, or a modern scalpel with a no. 20 blade) is used to make a short incision 0.5 cm above the upper edge of the pubis and directly toward the center of the joint.

According to Zarate,[45] the scalpel is held in the right hand, and the hypothenar eminence may rest on the pubic region to keep strict control over the movements of the knife. The scalpel is grasped like a pencil, except that the ring and the little fingers are maximally flexed with their tips pressed against the palm of the hand. The scalpel is kept in a strict sagittal plane, resisting the natural tendency to give the hand the lateral inclination used for writing.

This method is a subcutaneous partial symphysiotomy, which is simple, rapid, and associated with a minimum of complications. The two vaginal fingers monitor the position of the scalpel blade to make sure it does not penetrate too deeply.[22]

The knife is held perpendicular to the skin overlying the symphysis. The cutting edge of the blade faces the surgeon, and the knife enters 1 cm below the upper edge of the pubis. If the knife is placed perpendicularly and in the midline, it meets little resistance and only minimal force is needed to direct it posteriorly until the tip of the blade is felt by the vaginal fingers. If resistance is encountered, the blade has deviated laterally and is hitting the articular surface of one of the pubic bones; the blade is withdrawn a few millimeters, recentered, and readvanced.

The knife is carried down to the center of the upper part of the joint in an almost vertical position (see Fig. 58-22, *F*). With gentle rocking movements, the superior and anterior ligaments are divided with the joint down to and including the upper part of the arcuate ligament. When the scalpel tip is felt through the anterior vaginal wall (which must not be pierced), the knife handle is lowered toward the maternal abdomen and, using the upper part of the symphysis pubis as a fulcrum, the blade cuts through the lower half of the symphysis. The knife is removed, turned 180 degrees so that the cutting edge faces away from the surgeon, and reintroduced through the same stab incision in the skin. By lowering the handle toward the surgeon, the upper half of the symphysis will be divided (see Fig. 58-22, *G*). The vaginal

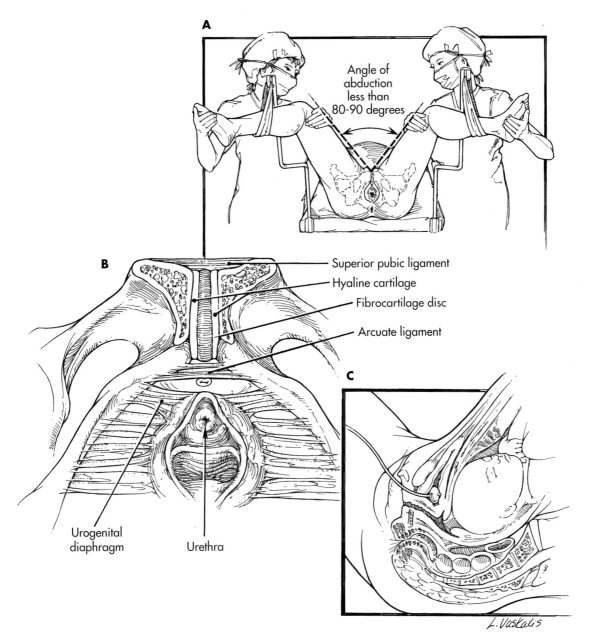

Fig. 58-22   Symphysiotomy. **A,** The patient's legs are supported. The angle of abduction must be between 80 and 90 degrees. **B,** Basic anatomy of the pubis symphysis. **C,** Sagittal section of the pelvis during labor. A catheter has been inserted into the bladder.

finger can identify any ligaments left to be divided. When the middle finger in the vagina can fit into the space created by the separation of the pubic bones, the symphysiotomy is complete. Alternatively, the joint may be only partially divided, the posterior ligament and lower fibers of the arcuate ligament being left intact. These subsequently rupture either by gentle abduction of the legs by the assistants or as the presenting part descends with continuing labor. The separation of the pubis should not exceed 3.5 cm and is controlled by counterpressure by the leg holders. The skin is closed by one or two interrupted sutures, and any bleeding is controlled by external tamponade.

After the operation, delivery of the fetus is often sponta-

neous and rapid. Forceps should be avoided if possible, although use of the vacuum extractor during a uterine contraction can be recommended should further interference with the progress of labor be required. A generous episiotomy should be made in the primigravida and, when necessary, in the multipara. Postpartum, a tight binder is applied around the pelvis at the level of the trochanters and a catheter is left in place for 4 or 5 days.

Postoperative Care

Ambulation should be encouraged as soon as the patient wishes to get up, although she should be aided in walking as she should use short, shuffling steps. The patient should

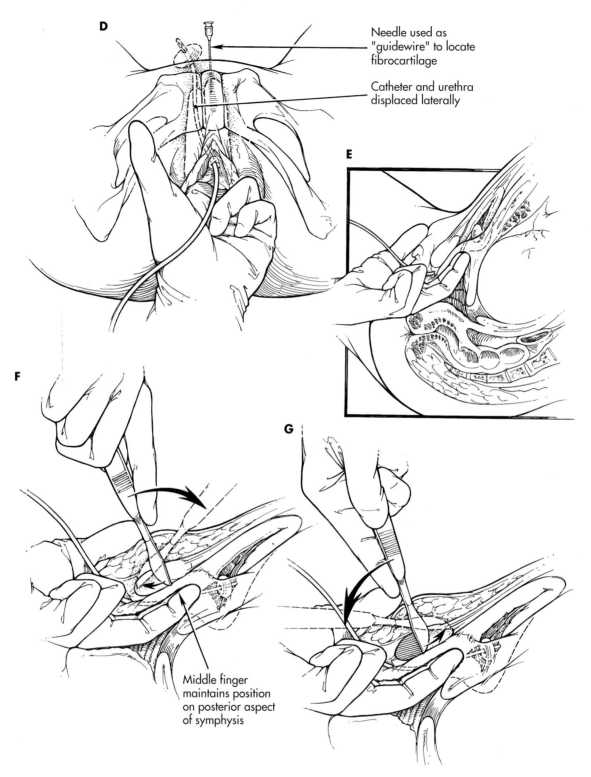

D

Needle used as "guidewire" to locate fibrocartilage

Catheter and urethra displaced laterally

E

F

G

Middle finger maintains position on posterior aspect of symphysis

Fig. 58-22, cont'd   D, An anesthetic has been injected, and the needle of the syringe is used as a guide wire to locate the pubic fibrocartilage. The fingers of the surgeon's left hand displace the catheter and urethra to one side. This is shown in sagittal drawing in **E. F,** A scalpel is held perpendicular to the skin, with the cutting edge toward the surgeon, and is directed posteriorly until it can be felt by the vaginal fingers. With a gentle rocking motion, as indicated by the arrows, the superior and anterior ligaments are divided down to the upper part of the arcuate ligament. The knife handle is lowered toward the maternal abdomen, and, using the upper part of the symphysis as a fulcrum, the knife cuts through the lower half of the symphysis. **G,** The knife is removed, turned 180 degrees, and reintroduced through the same stab incision, and the handle is lowered, cutting the upper half of the symphysis. The maximal separation of the pubis should not exceed 3.5 cm and is controlled using counterpressure by the leg holders.

be warned against undue exercise for at least 3 months postpartum.

Immediate complications from symphysiotomy are uncommon. Hemorrhage from the vascular bed over the pubis is sometimes profuse and is said to always stop as soon as the baby is born and may be controlled before delivery by firm pressure. Infection at the operative site may occur but may usually be prevented by appropriate antibiotics. Soft tissue injury is rare. The patient may sustain damage to the urethra, usually consequent to a technical error during the procedure, and rarely, the patient may develop urinary stress incontinence.

The operation should not be undertaken before labor in the patient with obvious disproportion, nor early in labor, because it may be unnecessary if there is adequate molding of the head. Occasionally, the patient has spontaneous separation of the symphysis during labor.[5]

The one exception to this rule is that, in patients with modest disproportion, the operation may be undertaken earlier in the second stage of labor in a patient with breech presentation, provided that the baby's buttocks have descended at least to the midcavity. If the baby is dead, it is better delivered by a destructive operation on the fetus. In the patient with a scar from a previous cesarean section, repeat cesarean section is by far the safest choice. Similarly, the head of a hydrocephalic infant is better delivered by decompression of the skull (often by needling through the occipital foramen) than by symphysiotomy, unless the obstetrician wishes to perform cesarean section.

Long-term orthopedic disability is reported to be uncommon. Occasional cases of spontaneous pubic separation are seen during antepartum care or in early labor in any large obstetric practice.

Complications of Symphysiotomy

Recorded complications of symphysiotomy include the following:

1. Cystotomy or urethrotomy with or without formation of a subsequent vesicovaginal or urethrovaginal fistula
2. Urinary stress incontinence
3. Fever with abscess formation
4. Severe hemorrhage.
5. Orthopedic disability when intrapartum pubic separation improperly exceeded 2.5 cm, thus subjecting the sacroiliac articulation to permanent and symptomatic damage from avulsion or overstretching

Once performed, however, symphysiotomy is a logistic situation in which the patient will be likely to continue to be able reproduce in the future. The accommodation of reseparation of the pubis during subsequent labor may occur "automatically," negating the requirements for cesarean section at a site where this operation is not available, or for repeat cesarean section if the patient's problem resulting from the initial disproportion had been solved previously by primary cesarean section.

REFERENCES

1. Arona AJ, et al: Early secondary repair of third- and fourth-degree perineal lacerations after outpatient wound preparation, *Obstet Gynecol* 86:294, 1995.
2. Reference deleted in proofs.
3. Buxton BH, Muram D: *Episiotomy.* In Sciarra J, editor: *Gynecology and obstetrics,* vol 2, Philadelphia, 1991, JB Lippincott, p 1.
4. Chrichton D, Seedat EK: The technique of symphysiotomy, *S Afr Med J* 37:227, 1963.
5. Cibils LA: Rupture of the symphysis pubis, *Obstet Gynecol* 38:407, 1971.
6. Combs CA, Robertson PA, Laros RJ: Risk factors for third-degree and fourth-degree perineal lacerations in forceps and vacuum deliveries, *Am J Obstet Gynecol* 63:100, 1990.
7. Cunningham CB, Pilkington JW: Complete perineotomy, *Am J Obstet Gynecol* 70:1225, 1955.
8. DeLee JB: The prophylactic forceps operation, *Am J Obstet Gynecol* 1:34, 1920.
9. Reference deleted in proofs.
10. Ecker JL, et al: Is there a benefit to episiotomy at operative vaginal delivery? Observations over ten years in a stable population, *Am J Obstet Gynecol* 176:411, 1997.
11. Elchalal U, et al: Ritualistic female genital mutilation: current status and future outlook, *Obstet Gynecol Surv* 52:643, 1997.
12. Reference deleted in proofs.
13. Reference deleted in proofs.
14. Gainey HL: Postpartum observation of pelvic tissue damage, *Am J Obstet Gynecol* 45:457, 1943.
15. Gainey HL: Postpartum observation of pelvic tissue damage: further studies, *Am J Obstet Gynecol* 70:800, 1955.
16. Gebbie D: Symphysiotomy, *Clin Obstet Gynaecol* 9:663, 1982.
17. Reference deleted in proofs.
18. Reference deleted in proofs.
19. Graham ID: *Episiotomy,* London, 1997, Blackwell Scientific.
20. Haadem K, et al: Anal sphincter function after delivery rupture, *Obstet Gynecol* 70:53, 1987.
21. Handa VL, Harris TA, Ostergard DR: Protecting the pelvic floor: obstetric management to prevent incontinence and pelvic organ prolapse, *Obstet Gynecol* 88:470, 1996.
22. Hartfield VJ: Subcutaneous symphysiotomy—time for a reappraisal? *Aust NZ J Obstet Gynaecol* 13:147, 1973.
23. Hartfield VJ: Symphysiotomy for shoulder dystocia, *Am J Obstet Gynecol* 155:228, 1986 (letter to the editor).
24. Hauth JC, et al: Early repair of an external sphincter ani muscle and rectal mucosal dehiscence, *Obstet Gynecol* 67:806, 1986.
25. Reference deleted in proofs.
26. Inmon WB: Mediolateral episiotomy, *South Med J* 53:257, 1960.
27. Klein MC, et al: Relationship of episiotomy to perineal trauma and morbidity, sexual dysfunction, and pelvic floor relaxation, *Am J Obstet Gynecol* 171:591, 1994.
28. Lede RL, Belizan JM, Carroli G: Is routine use of episiotomy justified? *Am J Obstet Gynecol* 174:1399, 1996.
29. Magdi I: Obstetric injuries of the perineum, *J Obstet Gynecol Br Emp* 49:687, 1942.
30. Menticoglou SM: Symphysiotomy for the trapped aftercoming parts of the breech: a review of the literature and a plea for its use, *Aust NZ J Obstet Gynaecol* 30:1, 1990.
31. Reference deleted in proofs.
32. Poen AC, et al: Third degree obstetric perineal tears: risk factors and the preventive role of mediolateral episiotomy, *Br J Obstet Gynaecol* 104:563, 1997.
33. Reference deleted in proofs.
34. Reference deleted in proofs.
35. Rageth JC, Buerklen A, Hirsch HA: Long-term sequelae of episiotomies, *Z Geburtshilf Perinatol* 193:233, 1989.

36. Ramin SM, et al: Early repair of episiotomy dehiscence associated with infection, *Am J Obstet Gynecol* 167:1104, 1992.

37. Seward WF: The hospital industry, *Bull Am Coll Surg* 83:15, 1998.

38. Shiono P, et al: Midline episiotomies: more harm than good? *Obstet Gynecol* 75:765, 1990.

39. Reference deleted in proofs.

40. Reference deleted in proofs.

41. van Roosmalen J: Safe motherhood: cesarean section or symphysiotomy? *Am J Obstet Gynecol* 163:1, 1990.

42. Willson JR: Prophylactic episiotomy to minimize soft tissue damage, *Infect in Surg* July:399, 1987.

43. Reference deleted in proofs.

44. Reference deleted in proofs.

45. Zarate E: *Subcutaneous partial symphysiotomy* (English edition), Buenos Aires, 1955, TICA.

59 Instrumental Delivery:
A Critique of Current Practice

JOHN PATRICK O'GRADY

The chirurgeon must have a good eye and a stedfast hande . . . Chirurgeons ought to be wyse and gentil, sober and circumspect.

. . . Nor must they promise more than they can perform with God's helpe.

Breviary of Health
Andrew Boorde
(1490-1549)

INTRODUCTION
Role of Instrumental Delivery

Since its inception in the seventeenth century, instrumental delivery has remained controversial. Establishing the appropriate role for this traditional technology in modern obstetrics is the challenge. Although most practitioners use one or more methods of assisted delivery for at least some obstetric indications, there are great international and local variations.[8,11,71,110,176] Even within the same country birth attendants are surprisingly inconsistent in how they use delivery instruments. Techniques for instrumental delivery have also changed rapidly in the last decade. The title of this chapter reflects the complexity of current practice. Both forceps and the vacuum extractor are now in common use and controversy exists concerning when to conduct operative deliveries and which instrument is best.[27,49,92,114,163-167]

In prior years the principal use of instrumental delivery was to save the baby and the mother from potentially serious complications of prolonged second-stage labor. Other common uses included rapid extractions in situations of presumed fetal jeopardy. "Prophylactic" forceps use was also common for maternal and fetal "protection." In experienced hands the forceps and the vacuum extractor are still well suited for at least the first two of the tasks. But, what is best now? Obstetrics is not the same now as practiced by DeLee, when he introduced "protective," elective forceps use in 1920 and profoundly different from that experienced by the original developers of forceps in the eighteenth century.[40] Current management of labor and delivery is even substantially different from that practiced just two decades ago. The introduction of fetal monitoring, increasing medicolegal concerns about maternal or fetal injuries, new data suggesting long-term maternal morbidity from childbearing, improvements in anesthesia, the availability of potent uterotonics, and the discovery of new, broad-spectrum antibiotics have permanently changed our approach to labor and delivery.* These innovations have challenged traditional thinking about practice while providing new management alternatives. Various types of monitoring now permit safe lengthening of the second stage if prognosis and fetal condition are good,[34] cesarean delivery is now easily and safely performed, and the concepts of active management of labor prompt surgeons to an earlier and more liberal use of uterine stimulation in desultory labors.[2,112]

The safe alternatives for labor management and new concerns about potential long-term complications of vaginal birth have led to a progressively more selective and critical view of instrumentation.† Thus, in instances where in prior years an instrumental delivery would have been the immediate choice, alternatives in labor/delivery management are now routinely considered by clinicians. Some practitioners have gone even further to either restrict their practice to use only vacuum extraction or outlet forceps or to abandon assisted delivery entirely.

In this chapter the principal controversies concerning risks and benefits of delivery instrumentation are reviewed, the available data are critiqued, and recommendations for current practice using both forceps and the vacuum extractor are made. Furthermore, the specific dissimilarities between instrument types and the relative importance of these differences are discussed in some detail. This review of instrument design and the discussion of the choice between delivery instruments are not to obscure the larger issue of the general *desirability* and *safety* of instrumental delivery, which remains our principal focus.

The review of this subject is difficult. In so far as it is possible, the basis of clinical decision-making should be objective data rather than simple opinion. Finding the best, unbiased data on which to base decisions concerning instrumental delivery is the problem. Unfortunately, many basic forceps and vacuum extraction techniques have not been subjected to systematic study.[113,175] Much of the voluminous literature on this subject is anecdotal, uncontrolled, or retrospective. Despite these limitations our problems as obstetric practitioners remain the same. Neither dystocia nor fetal distress has disappeared and management choices must be made. By necessity, our guides in judging appropriate clinical behavior will be several: information derived from properly conducted prospective trials, the outcome data from various prospective and retrospective clinical studies,

---

*References 8, 19, 25, 39, 49, 57, 86, 114, 146-149, 151.
†References 27, 49, 92, 115, 174, 175.

and the collective experience of prior practitioners as reflected in the obstetric literature.

Two questions are pertinent. Is instrumental delivery merely a dramatic remnant of past practice that is increasingly of historic interest only? Or is instrumental delivery a valuable adjunct to modern obstetric management in need of reassessment? If the first observation is true, these techniques should be relegated to obscurity and progressively abandoned. But, if the latter is correct, techniques of instrumental delivery must be refined and improved so that they can be carefully retained in the armamentarium available to practitioners.

History of Forceps Operations

The history of instrumental delivery is filled with unusual characters, colored by political intrigue and medical politics and influenced by the prevailing social mores and the obstetric philosophy of the time.[113,128,142] The different approaches surgeons have taken toward instrument-assisted delivery mirrors the permanent tension in obstetric practice between contending philosophies concerning parturition: the willingness to intervene versus the concept of leaving to nature. Before the invention of forceps, birth attendants lacked much that is now routinely available to obstetric surgeons, including intravenous fluids and transfusion, potent antibiotics, and safe and effective uterotonics and tocolytics. When progress in labor slows or stops, choices were starkly limited. The mother could be permitted to continue to labor at high risk for her own injury and for the loss of her child. Alternatively, version and extraction or a fetal destructive procedure could be performed.[89] Such procedures might save the mother but often did so at the cost of severe if not fatal fetal injuries. Before the midnineteenth century and before the discovery of anesthesia and other advances in medical science, surgery was brutal and far from safe and often was delayed until the situation was nearly hopeless. Cesarean delivery, the principal modern answer to unremitting dystocia, was not a feasible option until the late nineteenth century because of the initially insurmountable risks of hemorrhage and infection and the absence of safe and effective anesthesia.[128] It was in this formidable setting that nondestructive delivery instruments were first invented.

The Chamberlens, a family of displaced French Huguenots working in England, developed delivery forceps about 1630, possibly from urologic instruments originally designed for the removal of bladder stones. The process of their invention is not known.[113,128,142] The Chamberlen forceps was maintained as a family trade secret for three generations. This monopoly ended in the mideighteenth century, when the secret device—a scissorlike, two-bladed instrument—was finally publically released. Between 1720 and 1750, a number of practitioners who recognized the utility of this new delivery instrument, including Edmund Chapman (1680?-1750), Paulus De Wind (1714-1771), William Giffard (1660?-1731), William Smellie (1697-1763), and John Palfyn (1650-1730), experimented with or proposed various instrument designs and publicized their ideas

and experiences. After technical improvements to the instrument and with the development of techniques of application by William Smellie, André Levret (1703-1770), Benjamin Pugh (1710?-1775), and others, forceps became remarkably popular. Here at last was an alternative to the dreary triad of heroically prolonged labors, attempted version and extraction, and destructive operations that had characterized earlier practice.[37] Unfortunately, indiscriminate use led rapidly to various abuses. Knowledge of techniques for safe application and training to disseminate advances lagged well behind the enthusiastic application of these new instruments. Inevitably, many partially trained or untrained practitioners applied forceps inappropriately with damage to mother and child. This led to a backlash. In the early decades of the nineteenth century a conservative school of obstetric management developed in England. Practitioners in this school, especially Thomas Denman (1733-1815), William Osborn (1736-1808), and Richard Croft (1762-1818), favored even extreme prolongations of labor rather than any resort to instrumental assistance. In their view the risks attendant to instrumentation outweighed any potential benefits. Inevitably these practitioners experienced obstetric disasters from failure to intervene in extreme cases. These events eventually discredited this conservative school and led to a more balanced view of the role of assisted delivery.[128]

After major improvements in the science of medicine introduced by Ignaz P. Semmelweis (1818-1865), James Young Simpson (1811-1870), Walter Channing (1786-1876), Joseph Lister (1827-1912), F. W. Scanzoni (1821-1891), Charles Pajot (1816-1896), and many others, the heyday for instrumental delivery was the late nineteenth and early twentieth centuries. By this time the problems of aseptic surgery, anesthesia, and basic techniques for forceps application and fetal cranial rotation were well established, vacuum extraction was only rarely performed, and abdominal delivery still remained risky. In the early decades of the twentieth century, Bolivar DeLee (1920) proposed the "prophylactic forceps operation."[40] Forceps delivery was recommended once the fetal head had reached the pelvic floor. This concept of routine operative delivery for both maternal and fetal reasons—even though unsupported by data—strongly influenced North American practice for more than four decades. Since DeLee, there have been two major trends. Specialized delivery instruments have been developed with the aim of better ensuring maternal and fetal safety by design. Such devices have been invented by Shute, Laufe, Salinas, Piper, Barton, Kjelland, Hays, Nagolkar, and many others. A recent event has been the publication of various prospective and retrospective studies in the attempt to judge the safety and effectiveness of forceps or vacuum extraction operations and determine the role they should play in practice. These data are discussed in detail later.

History of Vacuum Extraction

The technique of vacuum extraction has deeper historical roots than forceps operations. Its origin was in "cupping," an ancient therapeutic technique in which a heated metal or glass cup is applied to a lesion or skin puncture.[114,138,154] As the cup cools, a vacuum develops, extracting blood or other fluids. As a medical procedure, cupping predated Hippocrates. However, surgical applications of cupping including assistance at deliveries were not reported until the seventeenth century, when James Younge (1646-1721) and other surgeons recorded vacuum deliveries in their case notes. However, these practitioners failed to publicize their successes. Nothing is known concerning the details of these instruments, which apparently did not influence later designs.

Cupping faced certain technical limitations. Originally, cups were constructed of metal or glass and were heated over an open flame. As obstetric use required a vaginal application of the cup, a different technology was obviously required! Successful cup design needed to incorporate two important features: easy insertion into the birth canal, and the capacity to form a seal to the fetal head while retaining the ability to sustain traction. There was also a requirement for continuous regeneration of the suction because leaks inevitably occurred as a result of imperfections in the seal. The first practical vacuum extractor was invented by the noted obstetrician, James Young Simpson in 1849.[26] Simpson's enthusiastic reports concerning the use of his device evoked considerable attention and some opposition. However, Simpson promptly became interested in other projects, including his design for obstetric forceps and lost interest in his "suction tractor." A number of vacuum delivery devices were invented and tested in subsequent decades, but vacuum extraction essentially disappeared until the mid 1950s, when Malmström introduced his stainless steel extractor cup.[87] Malmström's device incorporated several important features now found on all vacuum devices. A protective disc was fitted in the cup to avoid injury to the fetal scalp. There was a separate vacuum source capable of continuous vacuum production protected by a collecting bottle or trap. Finally, a pressure gauge was fitted to determine the degree of force generated.

The Malmström extractor rapidly became popular, especially in Europe, because of its ability to function as a substitute for forceps. Other rigid cup extractors were subsequently invented by Bird, Lovset, Party, O'Neil, Halkin, and others.[115,164] These various modifications were introduced to reduce the likelihood of cup detachment, facilitate application, or better protect the fetal scalp.[115,154,164]

Metal cup extractors had a variable reception in the United States. After widespread interest in the early 1960s, vacuum extraction fell into disfavor for two decades, partially because of reports of serious scalp injuries and other complications. Interest in vacuum extraction was revived after introduction of low-cost, flexible plastic, and improved design metal suction cups, coupled with changes in physician attitudes concerning assisted delivery. This renewed interest and the development of new instruments have contributed to a better understanding of vacuum technique, improving both success and safety. Interested readers are referred to standard texts for a full discussion of currently available vacuum instruments and extraction techniques.[85,115,164]

CLINICAL ISSUES

The central issues in the modern practice of instrumental delivery are which operative procedures are appropriate and how should these procedures be conducted? These subjects are the focus of the remainder of this chapter.

Assessment of which assisted delivery procedures are appropriate requires close review of published data combined with a clinical perspective.* In the following sections, elements common to all instrumental delivery procedures (see the first box below), a review of prerequisites (see the second box below),† guidelines for conducting operations (see the box on p. 1084), data on outcomes, various methods for the evaluation of dystocia, examinations of maternal and fetal anatomy favoring or contraindicating a trial of instrumentation, and the various alternatives in management are considered (Fig. 59-1).

Common Elements

An instrumental delivery is best considered as a major intervention akin to any other surgical operation. An ap-

---

*References 19, 27, 49, 79, 114, 116, 165, 175.
†References 44, 45, 48, 84, 113, 115, 116.

> **BASIC ELEMENTS IN THE CONDUCT OF AN INSTRUMENTAL DELIVERY**
>
> - Case analysis
>   Review of progress
>   Determination of fetal/maternal condition
>   Clinical examination
>   Consideration of alternatives
> - Review of prerequisites (see the box below)
> - Patient counseling
> - Meticulous performance of the operation (see the box on p. 1084)
> - Documentation

> **PREREQUISITES FOR INSTRUMENTAL DELIVERY**[44,45,48,84,85,113,115,116]
>
> - Patient consent
> - Appropriate indication(s)
> - Prepared physician
>   Knowledge of instrument
>   Willingness to abandon, if operation is difficult
> - Prepared patient
>   Ruptured membranes
>   Empty bladder (voiding, Credé maneuver, catheterization)
>   Full cervical dilation
>   Engaged fetal head
> - Acceptable analgesia/anesthesia
>   Pudendal
>   Spinal/epidural
>   Other

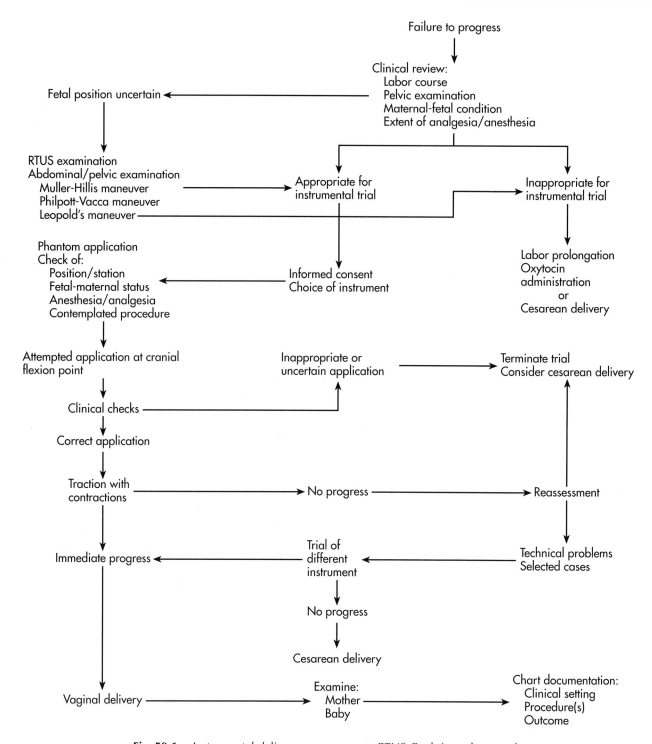

Fig. 59-1   Instrumental delivery: management. *RTUS,* Real-time ultrasound.

propriate indication and the consent of the mother are mandatory. Careful choice of cases, close review of the intended technique, adequate anesthesia and analgesia, meticulous technique, and the willingness to abandon the attempt if it does not proceed easily are additional, basic requirements for proceeding. The most important part of the process is the consideration of *alternatives.* In the following sections each of these elements is reviewed in detail.

Course in Labor

The principal clinical problem leading to assisted delivery is poor labor progress. The course in labor is unpredictable, and there are extreme differences in the speed and ease of parturition. Important variables include the size of the baby, the bony architecture of the maternal pelvis, the resistance provided by maternal soft tissue, the strength and frequency of uterine contractions, and a multitude of poorly understood features of fetal cranial positioning (e.g., deflection, delayed rotation).[2]

CONDUCTING THE OPERATION (SEE TEXT FOR DETAILS)

- Phantom application (ghosting)
  Instrument checked/tested before the application attempted
  Correct orientation established
  Appropriate setting reviewed
- Assurance of correct cranial application
  Instrument positioned over the flexion (pivot) point
  Specific checks performed
- Traction in correct vector, timed to spontaneous/induced uterine contractions
- Limited effort
  Initial progress mandatory
  Number of cup pop-offs/traction efforts limited by protocol
- Full medical record documentation
  Clinical setting
  Alternatives considered
  Procedures/results
  Complications

When the fetal bulk is simply too large to traverse the birth canal, *fetopelvic* or *cephalopelvic disproportion* exists, precluding vaginal delivery. True disproportion is uncommon. Dystocia or poor progress usually occurs when a relatively normal-sized baby is malpositioned in an otherwise normal-sized pelvis or when uterine activity is inefficient for any reason. A slow or difficult labor also occurs when a large baby traverses through an otherwise normal-sized pelvis. An important and insufficiently emphasized role for instrumentation is to assist progress by correcting fetal malpositioning such as cranial deflection by applying a traction force to the fetal head, directed in a specific direction. Such small corrections in the attitude or positioning of the fetal head are often associated with a resumption of descent and a successful delivery. This observation emphasizes that the principal for any delivery instrument is to *safely assist but not necessarily replace* the natural forces of labor. Furthermore, *instrumental delivery is appropriate only when fetopelvic disproportion is not present.* The question immediately arises, how is disproportion excluded?

Evaluation of Pelvic Adequacy

Traditionally, the course of labor is followed by serial pelvic examinations with cervical dilation, effacement and descent of the presenting part recorded graphically as a *partogram.*[12,52,125,145] Once progress is slow or stops, additional means of evaluation are needed because simple review of the course in labor progress cannot alone accurately diagnose the cause for dystocia or determine the correct treatment. In cephalic presentations, if disproportion is excluded, a trial of oxytocin stimulation with progress followed by serial examination is the best measure of pelvic adequacy. Despite prior beliefs, current evidence suggests that with close attention to fetal condition labor prolongation, despite problems such as prolonged active phase, protractions, or arrests and failure to descend, are not associated with long-term neurologic abnormalities.[17,54,132] The risk is not so much in labor prolongation as it is in attempting an instrumental delivery in the face of a disproportion between the passenger and the birth passages[112] (see the box on p. 1086). Clinical evidence for disproportion can include (1) a protracted or arrested labor, (2) significant cranial deflection, (3) progressive cranial molding unaccompanied by descent of the presenting part, (4) non-engagement of the presenting part despite adequate uterine activity, (5) a fetal head that overlies the pubic symphysis, or (6) other malpresentations.

In labor management, we must obey the rule of reason. When advancement of the fetal head ceases after adequate uterine stimulation combined with pain relief, maternal encouragement, and/or repositioning, spontaneous vaginal delivery is no longer an option and intervention is required. The surgeon must then decide between a method of operative delivery—either a cesarean delivery or a vaginal trial of an instrumental delivery. If the problem is disproportion, an inappropriately positioned head or a high presenting part, a cesarean is best. Else, the options of an instrumental delivery by forceps or vacuum extraction may be considered.

Clinical evaluation for poor progress is a fairly complex matter. It includes a review of the partogram notation of the maternal and fetal status; a pelvic examination, including clinical pelvimetry; judgment of fetal station and position and the extent of cranial molding; a Hillis-Müller (Mueller) maneuver (estimating descent of the presenting part with fundal pressure, once full dilatation and effacement have occurred)[88]; abdominal palpation for fetal size, positioning, and cranial engagement (Leopold's and Crichton's maneuvers) (Table 59-1)[36]; and increasingly, real-time ultrasound scanning.

As commonly practiced, clinical pelvimetry is of little assistance in making clinical decisions, except in the rare case of absolute disproportion or when fetal malpresentation such as a transverse lie is present. More specialized evaluations such as outlined in the following paragraphs are required.

During the pelvic examination the degree of cranial molding is estimated by judging the overlap of the bones of the fetal skull at the occipitoparietal and parietal-parietal junctions.[125,164] If the bones are overriding and cannot be easily separated by the surgeon's finger, molding is advanced and relative disproportion is suspect (Fig. 59-2). If so, an instrumental delivery is best avoided. Similarly, on Leopold's maneuvers a high or irregularly shaped presenting part may be palpated, suggesting a deflexed (brow or face) presentation or an oblique or transverse lie. Uncommonly, it may be noted that the fetal head overrides the pubic symphysis. Crichton[36] describes another useful technique. He judges the desirability/feasibility of an instrumental delivery by estimating the degree to which the fetal head has descended into the pelvis, calculated in fifths based on abdominal palpation. He argues that this method avoids the distractions of cranial molding and is a more reliable indication of station than pelvic examination—at least

---

INSTRUMENTAL DELIVERY: POSSIBLE MATERNAL BIRTH INJURIES[114]

DIRECT INJURIES	INDIRECT INJURIES
Birth canal lacerations	Perineal scarring, dyspareunia
Episiotomy extensions	Venous thrombosis, embolism
Bladder, paraurethral, or urethral injuries	Rectal sphincter dysfunction
Vaginal, vulvar, or perirectal hematomas	Pelvic instability
Uterine rupture	Fistula formation
Rupture of the symphysis pubis	Rectovaginal
Fracture or subluxation of the coccyx	Vesicovaginal
Nerve injuries	Infection
Sural	Cellulitis or local abscess
Iliac	Necrotizing fasciitis/myonecrosis
Other	Endometritis
Vessel injuries	Bladder atony, inability to void
	Uterine atony
	Anemia, hemorrhagic shock, vascular collapse

Table 59-1 Leopold's Maneuvers

Maneuver	Procedure
First maneuver	The surgeon stands at the patient's side (traditionally the right) and palpates the contents of the uterine fundus. The fetal size is estimated, and the contents of the fundus are evaluated.
Second maneuver	Using both hands, the surgeon judges the contents of the midportion of the uterus. The fetal back versus small parts can normally be distinguished by kneading the uterus back and forth gently, noting the contour of the fetus and the resistance to digital pressure.
Third maneuver	The surgeon grasps the lower uterine segment with the right hand and attempts to move it back and forth. This helps judge engagement and identify the presenting part, establishing the presentation.
Fourth maneuver	The surgeon turns toward the patient's feet and passes his or her hands longitudinally along the presenting part, noting whether the fingers diverge immediately suprapubically (suggesting engagement) or dip into the pelvis, displacing the presenting part (indicating lack of engagement). Unusual lateral masses (e.g., occiput) are also palpable during this examination.

Modified from O'Grady J: Instrumental delivery. In O'Grady J, Gimovsky M, McIlhargie C, editors: *Operative obstetrics,* Baltimore, 1995, Williams & Wilkins.

as pelvic examinations for station are commonly conducted.

When heavy molding or caput succedaneum is present, other clinical findings become important. Failure of the fetal head to fill the hollow of the sacrum or the inability of the surgeon to easily palpate the fetal ear are strong suggestions that the head lies higher than expected and has not negotiated the midpelvis.

Some knowledge of normal pelvic anatomy is also useful. A platypelloid pelvis precludes a rotation, except on the perineum, whereas an anthropoid configuration usually mandates delivery as an occiput posterior. This subject is beyond the scope of the current discussion and interested readers are referred to standard texts.[144] There are other approaches to judging the fetopelvic relationship, including imaging techniques. In cephalic presentations, radiographic pelvimetry as currently practiced is not helpful in evaluating labor progress or the possibility of disproportion, except in breech presentation. However, some experienced surgeons believe otherwise.[96,97,159-161] Also, ultrasound estimation of fetal weight or between specific fetal measurements have also especially not proven useful in clinical management. This is because of both the inaccuracy of the technique and the fact that only the fetus and *not the fetus and pelvis* is evaluated. Ultrasound data concerning fetal weight estimates should not be ignored but must be interpreted with caution and combined with other information. Real-time ultrasound is still of considerable assistance in doubtful or uncertain cases for other reasons. In obese or uncooperative patients, when palpation is difficult, the presentation is immediately determined by scanning. By using combined abdominal and perineal scanning, the surgeon can easily visualize the orbits of the fetal head, the extent of cranial bone overlap, the presence or absence of caput succedaneum, and the position of cranial falx. This helps the surgeon identify the cranial position, judge the extent of disproportion, and to a lesser degree, station.

Conduct of the Operation

The essential prerequisites for an operative delivery include a clear idea of the procedure to be undertaken, knowledge of the dynamics of how the delivery is to be accomplished (e.g., mechanism of labor, vector of force, required rotation), and a favorable clinical setting (appropriate baby size, position, adequate maternal pelvic anatomy, patient consent).* The procedure begins with a ghosting or phantom application (Fig. 59-3). The surgeon holds the delivery instrument in front of the maternal pelvis and rotates it to the position that it will occupy when a correct cephalic application is made. The proposed procedure and the direction of the vector of traction are mentally reviewed. The instrument is then introduced into the birth canal. Once the correct application is ensured, traction is applied. After delivery, the appropriate paperwork is prepared. Additional details are discussed in the following section.

---

*References 43, 44, 84, 85, 113, 115, 116.

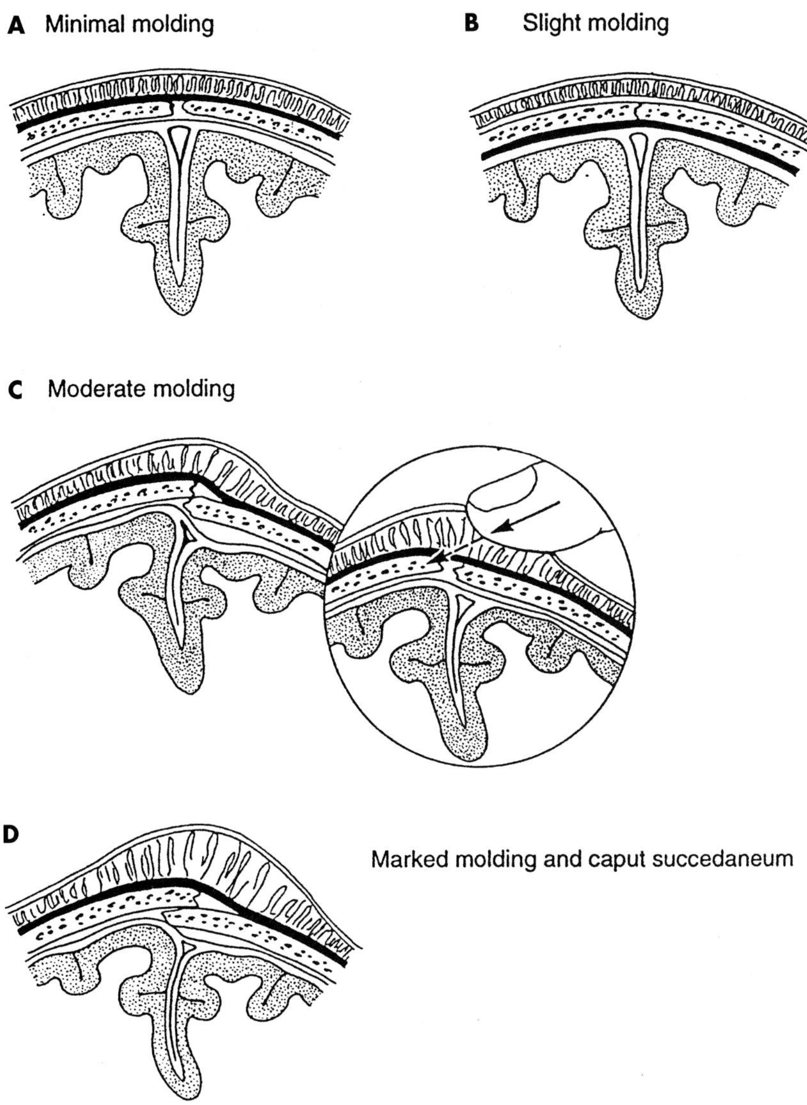

A Minimal molding

B Slight molding

C Moderate molding

D

Marked molding and caput succedaneum

Fig. 59-2   Cranial bone overlap. Clinical evaluation of cranial molding by digital examination is depicted (Philpott-Vacca maneuver). As molding progresses from minimal **(A)** through slight **(B)** to moderate **(C)** and finally to marked **(D),** the cranial bones progressively overlap, and additional caput succedaneum is formed. Palpation judges the extent of cranial bone overlap and the ease of its reduction. See text for details. (Redrawn from Vacca.[164])

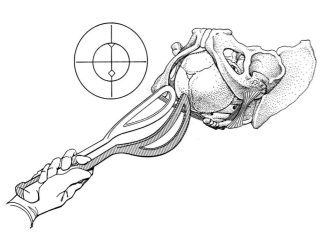

Fig. 59-3   Ghosting (phantom application) for an outlet forceps operation. A Simpson forceps is depicted. In the phantom or ghosting application the surgeon holds the articulated forceps in front of the perineum in the altitude and position the instrument will occupy when correctly applied to the fetal head. The application and the proposed operation are then mentally reviewed *before the forceps is introduced into the birth canal.* This maneuver is *never* omitted. The circular image to the left indicates the relative position of the fontanelles in the maternal pelvis when the mother is in dorsal lithotomy position. (Redrawn from O'Grady JP.[113])

Equipment

The principal methods for instrumental delivery are vacuum extraction and forceps operations.[49,92,113,115,164] The vacuum extractor is simply a plastic and/or metal cup fitted with a traction handle and a vacuum port for attachment to a vacuum pump (Fig. 59-4). In use, the extractor is positioned against the fetal scalp and held in place by the vacuum continuously regenerated by the pump. Traction applied to the handle of the instrument pulls the fetal scalp at its attachments to the cranium and, secondarily, the fetal head. Forceps are especially modeled metal or plastic instruments that are applied to the fetal cranium (Fig. 59-5). Pulling on the handles directly applies traction to the fetal skull. Other various instruments for assisted delivery are also occasionally used in clinical practice. These instruments include vectis blades (e.g., the Murless extractor) and other unique obstetric instruments used for traction or other specialized functions.[113-115]

For purposes of discussion, the delivery devices available for general use are conveniently classified into eight types: five of forceps, two of vacuum extractors, and one for miscellaneous instruments.[114] For full details the reader is referred to standard texts.*

1. *Classic outlet forceps:* These instruments include Elliot's and Simpson's cross-bladed, English lock designs, incorporating a pelvic and cephalic curve (see Fig. 59-5). These blades are most often used for outlet and low pelvic rotational operations.

2. *Modified classic forceps:* These instruments are designed with overlapping, extended, or shortened shanks; varying cephalic and pelvic curves; and solid, fenestrated, or pseudofenestrated blades; they use a

---

*References 43, 44, 48, 84, 85, 113, 115.

variety of locks. Common examples include the Tucker-McLean and Luikart-Simpson instruments. These forceps are usually applied in low to midpelvic procedures primarily for rotation and are also often used for simple outlet operations.

3. *Parallel or divergent blade forceps:* These instruments are designed to limit fetal cranial compression. Intended for low or outlet applications, they include designs developed by Salinas, Shute, Leff, Laufe, and many others. Shute also suggests that his parallel blade instrument is also useful in shoulder dystocia.

4. *Axis-traction forceps:* These instruments include offset or axis traction and, commonly, French or German locks in their design. Axis traction is incorporated in the DeWees, Hawks-Dennen, and Hays forceps, among others. If axis traction is desired, it is usually easiest to attach a traction handle (Bill's) to a standard forceps than to apply one of these rarely used instruments.

5. *Specialized forceps:* These designs include instruments modified for specific clinical situations. Examples include the Kjelland forceps for midpelvic rotation and correction of asynclitism, Barton forceps for transverse arrest in a flat pelvis, and Piper forceps for the aftercoming head in breech presentations.

6. *Vacuum extractors—soft cup:* The vacuum instruments now most popular are the disposable extractors manufactured by CMI (Midvale, Utah) and Mityvac (Phoenix, Ariz.). The CMI/Mityvac devices are successful in most outlet or low extraction procedures. They are also cheap and disposable, do not require assembly, and apparently have a lower incidence of fetal scalp injury than rigid cup extractors. The other available soft cup extractors, including the Ameda/Egnell Silc cup extractor and the Kobayashi cone, are less commonly used. Specially modified plastic cups, designed for use with deflexed or poste-

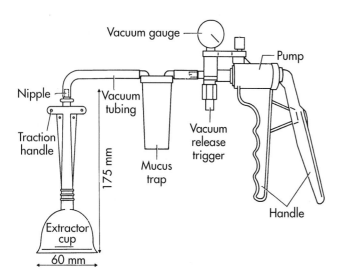

Fig. 59-4 A soft cup vacuum extractor. A hand vacuum pump, connecting tubing, and vacuum trap with an attached standard extractor cup are depicted. The combination of cup, tubing, trap, and vacuum source is common to all extractors. See text for details. (Redrawn from O'Grady JP.[113])

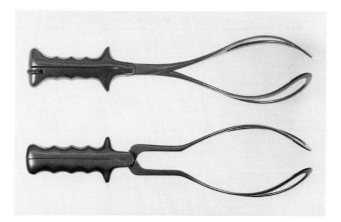

Fig. 59-5 Classic outlet type forceps. Elliot forceps (ca. 1858) are depicted *above* and Simpson forceps (ca. 1849) *below*. (Redrawn from O'Grady JP.[113])

rior positioned fetal heads, are now also available. New soft cup design is guided by the dictates of commerce, not of science. For most of the "new or improved" soft cup designs, there are no data to favor the use of any one type over another.

7. *Vacuum extractors—rigid cup:* Rigid cup extractions include the original Malmström stainless steel vacuum cup as well as various modifications of this design (Bird, O'Neil). Several different instruments exist, varying in details of the cup and in the arrangement of the traction attachment or the vacuum port. Although currently less popular than the soft cup extractors, rigid metal and plastic cups remain the instruments of choice for posterior and lateral presentations involving marked deflection or asynclitism.

8. *Other delivery instruments:* This category includes a variety of uncommonly used obstetric instruments such as vectis blades, the obstetric bonnet of Elliot, and a heterogenous collection of other devices, none of which has yet gained wide popularity, except perhaps the Murless vectis blade, which is commonly used to assist cranial extraction during cesarean delivery.[50,98,113]

Definitions for Procedure Coding

The standard definitions suggested by the American College of Obstetricians and Gynecologists (ACOG) for instrumental delivery operations include *outlet, low,* and *mid* operations, depending on clinical examination, assessing the position and station of the fetal head at the commencement of the procedure (see the box below).[1,3,5] These ACOG guidelines were originally written for forceps operations, but the same descriptions with minor modifications may be applied to vacuum extraction operations (Table 59-2).

ACOG DEFINITIONS: FORCEPS OPERATIONS[1,3,5]

Outlet forceps—the application of forceps when:
- The scalp is visible at the introitus without spreading the labia
- The fetal skull has reached the pelvic floor
- The sagittal suture is in the anterior/posterior diameter or in the right or left occiput anterior or posterior position
- The fetal head is at or on the perineum

Low forceps—the application of forceps when the leading point of the skull is at station $\geq +2/\pm 5$ cm.* There are two subdivisions:
- Rotation is 45 degrees or less.
- Rotation is more than 45 degrees.

Midforceps—the application of forceps when the fetal head is engaged but the leading point of the skull is above station $< +2/\pm 5$ cm.

---

*Note that *station* is defined as the distance from the bony presenting part to the plane of the ischial spines, recorded in centimeters (± 5 cm). See text for details.

The retrospective analyses of Bashore et al.[7] and Robertson et al.[131] and the prospective study of Hagadorn-Freathy et al.[63] indicate the utility of current 1988-1989 ACOG coding criterion. This coding better identifies procedures that carry an increased risk for fetal/maternal morbidity than the prior system, in which all operations that were not outlets were coded as midforceps. The problem for the surgeon is to determine whether either differences in the instrument applied (i.e., blade type or vacuum extractor versus forceps) or an alternative procedure (cesarean delivery) is the best choice in a given clinical situation.

The subclassifications suggested for the basic vacuum operations are of limited utility as in vacuum extraction rotation occurs spontaneously with descent and is not imposed by the surgeon as in forceps procedures. A simple distinction between occiput posterior and anterior positions is pro-

Table 59-2 Proposed Classification for Vacuum Extraction Procedures

Type of Operation*	Description of Classification
Outlet vacuum operation	• The fetal head is at or on the perineum.
	• The scalp is visible at the introitus without separating the labia.
	• The fetal skull has reached the pelvic floor.
Low vacuum operation	• The position/station of the fetal head does not fulfill the criteria for an outlet operation.
	• The leading edge of the fetal skull is at station $\geq +2/\pm 5$ cm.
	• The fetal skull has not reached the pelvic floor.
Subdivisions	(1) Occiput anterior (OA, LOA, ROA)
	(2) Occiput posterior (OP, LOP, ROP) or transverse (LOT, ROT)
Midvacuum operation	• Station is $< +2/\pm 5$ cm.
	• The fetal head is engaged, but the criterion for outlet or low operations are not fulfilled.
Subdivisions	(1) Occiput anterior (OA, LOA, ROA)
	(2) Occiput posterior (OP, LOP, ROP) or transverse (LOT, ROT)
Vacuum-assisted cesarean delivery	This includes all vacuum-assisted cesarean deliveries; technique is not specified.
Special vacuum operations	This includes vacuum extraction operations; technique is not specified.
	Full details are described in a dictated operative note.
High vacuum operation	Such procedures are not included in the classification.

From O'Grady J: Instrumental delivery. In O'Grady J, Gimovsky M, McIlhargie C, editors: *Operative obstetrics,* Baltimore, 1995, Williams & Wilkins.

OA, Occiput anterior; *LOA,* left occiput anterior; *ROA,* right occiput anterior; *OP,* occiput posterior; *LOP,* left occiput posterior; *ROP,* right occiput posterior; *LOT,* left occiput transverse; *ROT,* right occiput transverse.

*The type of operation coded is determined by pelvic examination, noting the position and station of the fetal head at the time the extraction is performed.

posed. Because of frequent cranial deflection, occiput transverse positions are included in the OP category.

Note that the estimation of *station* in these protocols is reported in centimeters (±5). This is the clinical estimate of the distance between the leading bony part of the fetal skull and the plane of the maternal ischial spines. When station is discussed, two numbers should be recorded (e.g., +2/±5 cm). The first number indicates the station as estimated by pelvic examination—+2 in the example given. The second number in this example indicates that the 5 cm scale for reporting station is the one used by the examiner. Stations in this ±5 point scale do not correspond with station as classically reported on the ±3 point scale originally taught and still commonly used by many obstetricians (Table 59-3).

Table 59-3 Estimation of Station of the Presenting Part: Comparison between Methods*

Classic Three Station Scale	ACOG Centimeter Scale	Cranial Position
−3	−5	Pelvic inlet
−2	−4	
−1	−3	
	−2	
0	0	Ischial spines (engagement)
+1	+1	
	+2	
+2	+3	
+3	+5	On the perineum

Modified from Rosen MG: *Management of labor,* New York, 1990, Elsevier.

Application Safety

The initial technical issues to consider in application safety are the condition of the instrument and the accuracy of the cranial positioning of the device. Before attempting to apply any delivery instrument, the surgeon should carefully examine it to exclude a mismatch in blades (forceps) or a technical malfunction (vacuum extractor).[70,113,115] An accurate cephalic application of both the forceps and the vacuum extractor is critical to safety and success.* Correct application for either the forceps or the vacuum extractor requires close attention to fetal cranial anatomy. The fit between the fetal head and the fenestration of the blades, the location of the posterior fontanel, and the position of the sagittal suture are the components of the classic "checks" for forceps.[43,113] There are similar checks for the vacuum extractor.[115,164]

A correct forceps application (biparietal or bimalar) evenly distributes the compressive force generated by the blades over the fetal head. This *cephalic* application is distinguished from a *pelvic* application, in which the forceps are applied independently of knowledge of the exact position of the fetal head. The only currently acceptable pelvic application is the placement of Piper or Kjelland forceps to the aftercoming head in a breech presentation.

When the forceps blades are correctly applied, the tips of the forceps blades lie over the fetal cheeks with the upper or concave border of the blade directed either toward the fetal occiput in anterior positions or toward the face in posterior positions (Fig. 59-6). The largest diameter of the fetal head—the biparietal—fits in the center of the cephalic curve of the instrument. The plane of the blades is positioned to pass through the occipitomental diameter of the fetal head—

*References 43, 44, 84, 85, 113, 114, 152, 164.

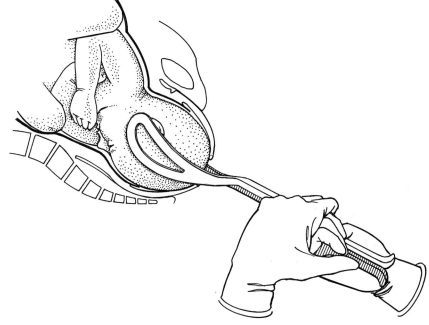
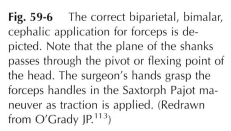

Fig. 59-6 The correct biparietal, bimalar, cephalic application for forceps is depicted. Note that the plane of the shanks passes through the pivot or flexing point of the head. The surgeon's hands grasp the forceps handles in the Saxtorph Pajot maneuver as traction is applied. (Redrawn from O'Grady JP.[113])

the cranial flexing point. The importance of this application site is discussed next.

For both the vacuum extractor and forceps, proper application ensures that the vector of traction force passes through the flexing or pivot point of the fetal skull (Fig. 59-7). This is an imaginary site 6 cm behind the edge of the anterior fontanel or approximately 1.5 to 2.5 cm in advance of the posterior fontanel, centered over the sagittal suture. When the forceps are applied correctly, the pivot point lies in the middle of a plane that connects the center or widest diameter of the cephalic curve of the blades and the plane of the shanks. If the pivot point of the head is not in the center of the blades, the fetal head is either overextended or alternatively excessively flexed when traction is applied.

A correct forceps application also requires attention to the fit of the blades to the fetal head. Normally, only one fingertip can be inserted between the fenestration of the blade and the fetal head. If too much of the fenestration is palpable, the blade is not correctly applied or the fetal head is very small. Correctly applied, the forceps will fit easily and not slip with normal traction, and the risk of fetal injury is believed to be reduced.

In a vacuum extraction operation, cranial traction is also vectored through the pivot point, *with the center of the cup applied over this site.*[12,164] The pull is directed over the center of the sagittal suture, to avoid an oblique rotation of the fetal head, which increases the work of extraction and risks cup displacement[165] (Fig. 59-8). When correctly placed, the edge of a standard 60-mm vacuum cup lies approximately 3 cm from the *anterior fontanel.* Thus, in vacuum extraction

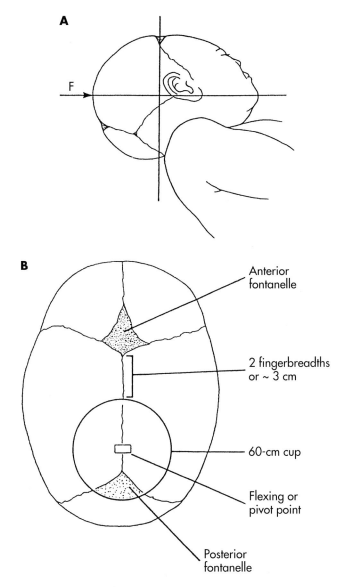

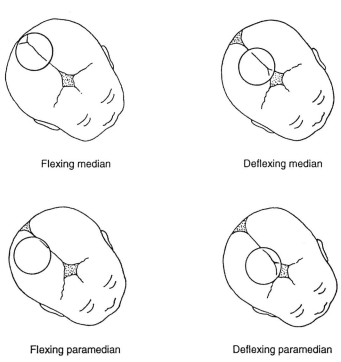

Fig. 59-8   Suction cup placement is important to extraction success. The circle inscribed on the fetal head indicates the diameter of a 60-mm vacuum cup. Ideally, the cup center should be positioned over the cranial flexing point approximately 6 cm from the edge of the anterior fontanel or 2 cm (two fingerbreadths) anterior to the posterior fontanel. Traction over the flexing point in a median application promotes cranial flexion and synclitism; other applications do not. Extraction failure rates are: flexing median 4%, deflexing median 29%, flexing paramedian 17%, and deflexing paramedian 35%. Note that because of the cup position in vacuum extraction, the *anterior* fontanel is the principal landmark for correct cup placement. See Fig. 59-7. (Redrawn from O'Grady JP.[115])

Fig. 59-7   The pivot point of the fetal head is depicted. **A,** The flexing or pivot point *(F)* of the fetal head is located midsagittally, approximately 6 cm from the center of the anterior fontanel or 2 cm in advance of the posterior fontanel. When a standard vacuum cup is applied, the cup edge will lie approximately 3 cm or two fingerbreadths behind the anterior fontanel. The posterior fontanel is often covered by a correctly applied cup and is thus not useful as a landmark. **B,** The same site is viewed from above. Traction centered over this site promotes cranial flexion, other applications do not. (Redrawn from O'Grady JP.[115])

operations, the anterior and not the familiar posterior fontanel becomes the reference point for checking instrument application. Access to the posterior fontanel is usually partially blocked by the extractor cup, making this familiar landmark unusable.[114]

RISKS AND BENEFITS

Instrumental deliveries must be performed at minimal maternal and fetal risk. The potential risks of any obstetric intervention including an instrumental delivery involve (1) *risks specific to the procedure or technique* and (2) *risks inherent in the pregnancy complication compelling intervention.* As is discussed later, these latter risks are little influenced by the eventual mode of delivery. Knowledge of both the specific and the situational risks is important. Education and refinement of technique may reduce the risk of an instrument specific risk but is powerless in changing an inherent risk. The question for the practitioner concerns the danger of injury associated with specific procedures and how such risk(s) are minimized.

Risk translates into maternal and fetal injuries. The avoidance of trauma requires an understanding of potential mechanisms for birth injury. *Infant birth injuries are abnormalities of the baby found to be present at or soon after delivery and thought to be related to the process of labor/delivery* (see the box below).[114]

Most injuries occurring to mothers and babies during labor and delivery are inconsequential.[79,115,116] There are rare central nervous system injuries (cord accidents/ hemorrhages) or uncommon complications such as subgaleal hemorrhages, which are potentially serious and can even prove fatal.[94,113,126] However, our principal concern is the much more common injuries that might result in permanent damage and/or serious morbidity. Despite our prior beliefs, permanent neurologic impairment (e.g., cerebral palsy, intellectual deficits) are uncommon and even rare after mechanical birth trauma unless the original injury is combined with major birth asphyxia or complicated by prematurity. Many, if not most, serious or permanent fetal/neonatal neurologic abnormalities result from complex in utero problems that either precede parturition or are not under the control of the surgeon.* Furthermore, difficulties in labor, such as episodes of fetal distress, can be the *effect* of occult injury rather than the *cause* of an abnormality. Not surprisingly, the uncertainties in establishing clear causes for many injuries still leaves ample grounds for honest dispute.

Still, based on current data, surgeons in all specialties should hesitate before confidently ascribing an observed neonatal injury to an event at parturition unless the cause is obvious, such as a laceration. In an individual case close review of all clinical data, including the clinical and family history, genetic data, careful examination of the neonate, and placental pathologic examination, is prudent before a final determination is made.[99,123,124,134]

Viewed in the largest sense, maternal or fetal injuries during parturition may occur from either *direct* or *indirect* causes. Both must be considered when the morbidity of intervention is considered.[114]

Direct injuries are the immediate consequences of the process of spontaneous or assisted parturition (see the box below). These injuries are reasonably associated with the intervention performed and may be avoided or lessened by case choice and surgical skill. An example is a subgaleal hematoma after a vacuum extraction operation. However, even this apparently straightforward association may not be as simple as it seems. Subgaleal hemorrhages are uncommon and usually restricted to pregnancies complicated by obstructed labor, those with prior unsuccessful efforts at vaginal instrumental delivery, or infants with a preexisting coagulation abnormalities. This injury can also occur in infants delivered abdominally. Also, a similar injury could result from assisted delivery with forceps or even spontaneously after a precipitate labor. Finally, although some type of cranial trauma is a common association, subgaleal bleeding can also occur in spontaneous, uninstrumented, apparently normal deliveries.

Indirect injuries have a more complex cause. These are neonatal and maternal conditions or injuries resulting from the interactions between birth events. These injuries might be considered the indirect morbidity resulting from direct injuries. An example of an indirect injury is neonatal jaundice accompanying the resorption of a subgaleal hematoma. Necrotizing fasciitis after a perinatal birth laceration might also be viewed as a serious indirect maternal birth injury.

In judging the risks, serious considerations must be given to both the maternal *and* the infant birth injuries accompanying instrumental delivery. By far, the most common of the

---

INSTRUMENTAL DELIVERY: POSSIBLE FETAL/NEONATAL BIRTH INJURIES[114]

DIRECT INJURIES

Bruises/superficial abrasions
Lacerations
Pericranial injuries
    Caput succedaneum
    Chignon
    Subaponeurotic hemorrhage
    Subperiosteal hemorrhage
    Extradural hemorrhage
    Subdural hemorrhage
    Tears of falx tentorium/ intracerebral hemorrhage

Skull fracture
    Linear or depressed
    Occipital osteodiastasis
Spinal cord injury
Nerve injury (e.g., brachial plexus)
Long bone fracture
Hepatic or other visceral injury
Unusual injuries (e.g., eye, cerebral embolization)

INDIRECT INJURIES

Anemia
Hemorrhagic shock, vascular collapse
Infection/septicemia
Jaundice

---

*References 4, 22, 56, 61, 62, 69, 74, 75, 81, 90, 100-105.

maternal injuries are episiotomy extensions and lacerations of the birth canal. Although both cervical and vaginal vault lacerations can result after spontaneous deliveries, these complications are more common and usually more extensive after instrumental delivery and may result in long-term symptoms.[57,86] In general, the more complex the extraction and the higher the station of the fetal head at the beginning of the procedure, the greater the risk. In the following sections, several major risk factors are reviewed and their possible contribution to maternal or fetal injury is considered.

Risk Factors

Fetal macrosomia (weight more than 4500 g or more than 2 standard deviations [SD] from the mean) is an important and recently much discussed risk factor for obstetric injuries. Despite the fact that most large infants are delivered without complication, they remain a problem because of their increased risk of shoulder dystocia and other traumatic injuries.[93,114,118] Big babies are now common. Approximately 10% of infants weigh 4000 g or more at birth, and 2% will reach 4500 g or more.[133] Problems with big infants and instrumental delivery occur when descent of the fetal head proceeds far enough to entrap the unwary into attempting a delivery that proves difficult and/or traumatic.

Large infants are surprisingly difficult to diagnose, except in extreme cases (or in retrospect!).* Physical examination, ultrasonic measurements at or near term, and various clinical parameters (e.g., fundal height, weight gain) are notoriously imprecise in the accurate prediction of macrosomia, however defined. Ultrasonically derived weight estimates have been suggested as indications for cesarean delivery. The use of ultrasound weight estimates for the elective induction of pregnancies to "avoid" problems of excessive fetal size are even more questionable. As an example, in the randomized, prospective trial of Goven et al.,[60] term labor indication for diagnosis of "suspected macrosomia" neither decreased the cesarean rate nor reduced neonatal morbidity. The most important of the several problems with this and similar schemes include the inaccuracy of ultrasound weight estimates ($\pm6\%$ to 15% at term)† and the limits of clinical evaluation of fetopelvic proportion. The latter issue is reviewed in detail later.

A common obstetric procedure that is a risk factor for permanent birth-related injury is *episiotomy.* Reliable and unbiased data concerning the outcome of episiotomy are difficult to obtain, but recent information is bothersome. Despite prior beliefs concerning the benefit of episiotomy, there is little, if any, convincing evidence to support the traditional claims that this procedure, as routinely practiced, protects the mother.‡ In fact, it is now generally conceded that an episiotomy increases the risk of third-degree (rectal sphincter) and fourth-degree (rectal mucosal) injuries while providing some protection against periurethral lacerations.

Beyond discomfort with healing, the newly identified risk from these obstetric lacerations is chronic rectal/pelvic floor dysfunction.

Recent studies of women with pelvic floor dysfunction and fecal incontinence have implicated childbearing as an important cause.[86,146-149,151] Two problems have been identified: denervation of pelvic musculature and direct damage to the rectal sphincter. In a series of papers, Sultan et al.[146,148] identify the culprits as large babies, long second-stage labors, and instrumental delivery. In these reports, there appears to be a relationship between the length of the second stage of labor and the degree of pudendal nerve injury. The most interesting discovery is that some women delivering vaginally *without* overt sphincteric injury still have occult disruption of the internal or external anal sphincter. What mechanisms are at work here?

Some clinical observations are pertinent. New-onset postpartum fecal incontinence has not been observed after elective cesarean deliveries in which labor has not occurred. This implicates either the labor or the physical passage of the infant through the birth canal as the principal cause of trouble. This effect is probably not caused by instrumentation alone. A controlled series evaluating women with equally prolonged second stages who either had cesarean or instrumental deliveries is needed to better understand the cause of these injuries.

What should be recommended for obstetric practice? Episiotomy should not be performed *routinely,* even when an instrumental delivery is anticipated.[114] However, if maternal soft tissue interferes with instrument application or impedes the descent of the presenting part when traction is applied in the correct vector of force, an episiotomy then becomes necessary. Extractions from the midpelvis or those involving cranial malpositioning (e.g., OP, deflexed position) require an angle of traction that applies heavy pressure to the perineum and are most likely to result in the need for episiotomy and/or a laceration.

The effects of episiotomy in potentially reducing the force required for instrumental delivery or in shielding the premature fetal head from injury require further study as the data to support this approach are neither extensive nor entirely convincing.[19]

OUTCOME SERIES

Information on outcomes in instrumentally delivered pregnancies comes from several sources. There are a few randomized trials, most comparing a specific delivery technique (vacuum extractor) against another (forceps) or evaluating one extraction cup against a competitive design. There are retrospective studies in which instrumentally delivered infants are paired with others of similar clinical characteristics but who were subjected to an alternative form of delivery. Finally, there are several longitudinal studies in which a large cohort of neonates was followed for a defined period and then reexamined or surveyed to determine the prevalence of certain morbidities. Examples of

---

*References 29, 30, 65, 109, 133, 169.

†References 60, 42, 45, 115, 127, 133.

‡References 6, 15, 59, 66, 80, 137, 139, 140, 153, 158, 171.

each of these types of study are briefly reviewed in the following section.

Long-Term Follow-Up Studies

Studies including long-term follow-up of instrumentally delivered infants have limitations such as nonrandom selection and the loss of infants experiencing the most serious complications (Table 59-4). However, these studies also have large numbers and have been conducted in quite different populations, providing some reassurance concerning the reliability of the findings. In general, such investigations confirm the safety of instrumental deliveries. However, because the type of delivery procedures involved in these series are heavily weighted toward the more common outlet/low operations, good results should be anticipated.

A recent example of this type of study is the report of Wesley et al.[170] In this investigation, a cohort of 3413 children from a prepaid health plan service were studied at age 5 years by a battery of cognitive tests. No significant differences were detected between the 1192 children delivered by forceps (including 114 delivered by midforceps) versus 1499 who were delivered spontaneously.

McBride et al.[90] studied a cohort of Australian children at ages 4 to 5 years who were born between 1970 and 1974. In this group, there were no statistically significant intelligence quotient (IQ) differences between spontaneously delivered infants and those who were delivered by forceps.

Seidman et al.[136] retrospectively studied outcomes in 52,282 children born in Jerusalem between 1964 and 1972. The method of delivery and other birth events were correlated with intelligence testing administered at age 17 years. The author reported no demonstrable adverse effects from instrumental delivery.

Drawing from Collaborative Perinatal Project Data, Broman et al.[21] administered Stanford-Binet Intelligence tests to 26,760 children at age 4 years and correlated the results with perinatal events. On analysis, the major variables found to affect IQ scores were not obstetric, indicating that events of delivery were not the critical variables in cognitive function.

Table 59-4   Selected Studies of Long-Term Follow-Up after Instrumental Delivery

Author	Patients	Comparison Group	Follow-Up (yr)	Outcome/Comment
McBride et al., 1979[90]	188 low forceps* 51 midforceps 57 forceps rotation	101 elective cesarean deliveries	5	Insignificant differences between groups
DeCosta, 1982[38]	127 vacuum extraction	127 "next spontaneous" delivery matched for parity/gestational age	≥2	Insignificant differences between groups
Friedman et al., 1984[55]	70 midforceps* 82 low forceps*	70 spontaneous deliveries 82 spontaneous deliveries	7	In the midforceps group, IQ lower by 5.76 ± 2.17 Low forceps—no difference in IQ
Nilsen, 1984[107]	62 low, mid, and high forceps (Kjelland and Simpson forceps)*	38 low, mid, and high Malmström vacuum extractor deliveries	18	Forceps deliveries associated with signficantly elevated mean intelligence score than Norwegian mean
Dierker et al., 1986[47]	110 midforceps	110 cesarean deliveries	≥2	Insignificant difference between groups; subjects matched for sex, age, weight, race, dystocia, and fetal distress
Seidman et al., 1991[136]	567 forceps 1207 vacuum	1335 cesarean deliveries 29,136 spontaneous deliveries	17	Insignificant differences between groups in intelligence scores at age 17†
Wesley et al., 1993[170]	114 midforceps 1078 low/outlet forceps	1499 spontaneous deliveries	5	Insignificant differences between groups; forceps operations coded as low, low-mid, or mid, but criteria were not specified.
Ngan et al., 1990[106]	295 vacuum extractions	302 spontaneous deliveries	10	Insignificant differences between groups

IQ, Intelligence quotient.
*By pre–1988-89 ACOG definitions.
†6.6% of original cohort lost. Possible selection bias.

Specific Procedure Studies

Low/Outlet Operations. In a series of reports, regardless of the instrument chosen, fetal and maternal outcomes in outlet operations are similar to those of spontaneous deliveries. Specifically, there are no differences in perinatal outcome for either forceps or the vacuum extraction and the incidence of injury is very low.* From these data, we may confidently conclude that outlet procedures are safe.

Midpelvic Procedures. The incidence of fetal injury with midforceps is approximately 5% to 10%, with maternal risk related to the difficulty of the operation. This observed incidence of injury must be compared against that occurring among infants with similar obstetric problems (e.g., dystocia, jeopardy) delivered by a cesarean. In general, when this is done, most authors report that outcomes are roughly the same (Table 59-5).

However, midpelvic operations are much more controversial than outlet procedures.* The most influential studies concerning forceps outcome were those of Friedman et al.[53,55] (see Table 59-4). These data were derived from the Collaborative Perinatal Project. Both studies involved the evaluation of IQ in midforceps-delivered infants compared with spontaneously vaginally delivered infants. On review, the mean difference between the groups was approximately 6 IQ points with the forceps group doing less well. The 1984 study was controlled for race, parity, sex, type of delivery, labor pattern, and birth weight but not for family socioeconomic status. These data have always presented problems in interpretation. First, because Broman et al.'s 1975 study[21] of essentially the same population did not find events of labor/delivery to be major factors in influencing IQ. Furthermore, it seems difficult to argue that IQ differences of ±6 points are of significance, especially if the critical variable of socioeconomic class is not controlled. Finally, and perhaps most important, was the comparison fair? Specifi-

*References 19, 24, 56, 63, 108, 111, 120, 131, 135, 136, 173.

*References 18-20, 35, 46, 47, 67, 73.

Table 59-5   Midforceps Procedures versus Cesarean Delivery: Selected Comparison Studies

	N		Outcome	
Authors	**Midforceps Delivery**	**Cesarean Delivery**	**Neonatal**	**Maternal**
Bowes and Bowes, 1980[18]	40	37	4× neonatal morbidity, including lacerations, asphyxia, meconium aspiration	No difference
Cardozo et al., 1983[23]	65	127	Higher 5 min Apgar score Fewer NICU admissions	NA
Traub et al., 1984[162]	132	101	No difference	NA
Gilstrap et al., 1984[56]	234	111	No significant differences in fetal acidosis, low 5-min Apgar scores, trauma or neurologic defect at discharge when matched for indication	In forceps group: lower incidence of endometritis and blood transfusion; higher incidence of perineal trauma
Dierker et al., 1985[46]*	176	165	Increased incidence of cephalhematoma, low 1-min Apgar scores; with diagnosis of fetal distress or dystocia: equal neonatal morbidity present	In forceps groups: higher incidence perineal trauma
Bashore et al., 1990[7]	358	486	Minor and transient neonatal injuries with forceps; cord gasses equal when cases matched by indication	Decreased postpartum febrile morbidity in forceps group
Robertson et al., 1990[131]	505 Forceps 455 Vacuum	828	Decreased Increased incidence of pH <7.10, high base defect, birth trauma and admission to NICU	Decreased postpartum hospital stay and blood transfusion in instrumented group
Cibils and Ringler, 1990[33]	274	106	Increased admission to NICU for cesarean babies	Increased incidence perineal lacerations (third- and fourth-degree); increased length of stay and febrile morbidity in cesarean group

NICU, Neonatal intensive care unit.

*Infants matched for weight, gestational age, dystocia, and heart rate abnormalities. Total population = 21,414 deliveries.

cally, the comparison group for midforceps operations should be infants delivered by a cesarean, matched for fetal condition and gestational age and with similar obstetric indications for delivery. In fact, when just this comparison was made by Dierker et al.,[46,47] there were no differences observed in neonatal outcome observed. It is also true that Dierker et al.'s patients were derived from a population in which difficult midplane procedures were avoided, and fetal condition was followed by electronic monitoring.

Other data are available for review. Bashore et al.[7] retrospectively compared the immediate results of 358 midforceps operative deliveries and 486 cesarean deliveries occurring in their institution (UCLA) over a 7-year period.[7] They reported no increase in significant *short-term* neonatal morbidity in this comparison, but they did report increased morbidity among mothers in the cesarean delivery group. It should be noted that the definition of type of operative vaginal delivery in both this study and that of Dierker et al. was that in use before the 1988-1989 ACOG revision. Thus, in these series, any nonoutlet procedure was a "midforceps" delivery. It is important to point out that although the Bashore article included rotational forceps deliveries, it excluded instances of vacuum extraction at station +1 to +3/±5 cm. Also, in the Bashore study, there was considerable maternal morbidity, with approximately 25% of mothers sustaining a third- or fourth-degree episiotomy extension and 18% having cervical or vaginal lacerations.

SPECIAL ISSUES
Contraindications

In certain clinical settings an instrumental delivery is contraindicated. Skill must have a role in avoiding risk; however, this is difficult to evaluate.[68] Obviously, uncertainty or inexperience of the surgeon or the inability to achieve a proper application of the instrument are cogent reasons not to attempt an instrumental delivery. An inadequate trial of labor, uncertainty concerning fetal position and/or station, an incompletely dilated cervix, or a high presenting part are additional, basic contraindications.

There are circumstances in which a specific instrument is best, as is discussed in detail later. For example, forceps may be used for the aftercoming head in a breech presentation—an application inappropriate for the vacuum extractor.[95] The vacuum extractor should be used with caution in preterm pregnancies because the data on safety are limited.[16,115,155] My recommendation, which is admittedly conservative, is not to perform vacuum extraction operations on infants of less than 32 weeks' gestation and to use a soft cup extractor if a procedure is performed.

Neither scalp sampling nor electrode use are absolute contraindications to a vacuum operation.[76,92,115,130] Many safe extractions have occurred despite prior scalp sampling or electrode placement. As long as the scalp electrode does not interfere with correct cap placement, it is simply left in place on the fetal scalp during the vacuum operation. As an

extra caution, clear vacuum tubing is used and should be occasionally checked during the operation to be certain that the discharge is not bloody.

Unless there has been a technical failure or misapplication, failure in prompt descent is an *absolute indication* for abandoning an operative procedure. Also, *if either a vacuum extraction or forceps operation fails despite correct application and appropriate technique, a subsequent trial with the alternate instrument is generally not recommended.*[113,115] If the forceps is substituted for the vacuum extractor or vice versa and additional efforts are made, such procedures are limited to only the most experienced of surgeons because the risk of fetal or maternal injury is probably increased.

Special Applications

At cesarean delivery the vacuum extractor or forceps can be used to assist cranial extraction.[10,115,121,141] In most circumstances, either vaginal displacement of the fetal head by an assistant or uterine relaxation (e.g., with nitroglycerin) is best for cranial extraction. However, when instrumental assistance is needed, a vectis blade such as a Murless or a classic forceps is usually the most convenient instrument.[91,168] A number of types of delivery forceps may also be used on occasion. Many operative delivery kits contain short or "baby" Simpson forceps or a short Hale forceps or a similar instrument. Specific techniques utilizing the Kjelland[168] and Barton forceps[91] are described in the literature.

When the fetal head is difficult to extract, the immediate question is why. If the problem is an inadequate skin or fascial incision, it is simply extended. When the difficulty is a deeply impacted fetal head, elevation from below by a gloved assistant is best. An instrumental extraction makes the most sense when the presenting part is high in the uterus and difficult to grasp. The application of a forceps or the vacuum extractor to such floating heads is usually easy and the subsequent delivery rapid and atraumatic. If the uterus has firmly contracted around the baby, particularly if the lie is oblique or transverse, uterine relaxation by the intravenous administration of a β mimetic or (preferably) nitroglycerin commonly permits an easy and safe extraction.

Anesthesia/Analgesia

With proper coaching and a cooperative patient, a pudendal block and verbal encouragement is often adequate for outlet forceps procedures and sufficient for low vacuum extraction. Higher or rotational forceps operations require spinal or epidural anesthesia. In selected patients, outlet vacuum extraction operations can be performed with only local or no anesthesia. If the contemplated procedure involves a forceps rotation, if the presenting part is midpelvic, or if there is any uncertainty concerning the likelihood of success, epidural analgesia/anesthesia is best. General anesthesia should not be used except in unique circumstances. General anesthesia may unnecessarily depress the infant in a delayed extraction, and it increases the traction required for delivery by denying the surgeon the voluntary assistance of the mother.

The use of anesthesia and its potential effects on second-stage labor progress is controversial. There is a consensus among clinicians that epidural anesthesia predisposes patients to second-stage labor arrest or prolongation, a contention denied by anesthesiologists.[32,156,157] An important and often overlooked detail is the decision concerning how dense a block should be administered. During normal labor, it is *analgesia* that is required, not surgical *anesthesia.* In general, the denser the anesthetic blockade, the more the interference with normal progress. Multiagent, low-dose continuous infusion anesthetic techniques have been developed to address this issue. Dense epidural blockade paralyzes the pelvic musculature and interferes with endogenous oxytocin release, predisposing to poor prognosis and delayed rotation. Thus, in the absence of fetal jeopardy or disproportion, oxytocin may be indicated in the second stage once an epidural blockade is given.[9,58,117]

Traction

There is little solid research concerning how to apply traction in an instrumental delivery. The following comments derive principally from clinical experience and obstetric tradition. Although no data exist to substantiate this general approach, it seems reasonable. Traction in instrumental deliveries is timed to uterine contractions. Tension on the blades or to the vacuum extractor handle is patterned as an incremental pull building slowly to full pressure to parallel the uterine contractions. There is a parallel relaxation in force as the contraction abates. Traction applied without accompanying contractions or the verbal recruitment of maternal bearing down efforts or by jerking of the blades or vacuum cup is imprudent and believed to increase the risk of injury.

For forceps, the surgeon's elbow is bent at a right angle with the arm close against the body. As traction is applied, the surgeon's other hand rests on the shank of the blades and presses downward (Saxtorph-Pajot or Osiander maneuver). This helps create the vector of force guiding the fetal head through the pelvic curve (Carus' curve). The angle of pull is slowly varied either toward the symphysis or, alternatively, in the direction of the perineum as resistance is felt and the presenting part descends.

Although a firm pull is at times required, the average surgeon is easily capable of a forceps delivery without ever taxing one's strength. Any difficult pull is one that requires immediate reassessment.

Several other points are worth emphasis. The forceps handles should not be moved up and down as traction is applied because the posterior toe of the blade can injure the posterior vaginal vault as descent of the fetal head occurs. A mild side-to-side rocking motion is used by some surgeons to assist descent if the fit is tight. The fetal heart should be either auscultated or checked by real-time ultrasound, a handheld Doppler device, scalp electrode recording, or di-

rect auscultation *before* the operation begins *as well as between contractions/pulls.* A folded towel can be placed between handles to reduce cranial compression. The blades may disarticulated between contractions at the surgeon's discretion.

For all vacuum extractions a two-handed technique is suggested with the vector of traction force following the pelvic curve in the same fashion as for forceps.[115] During extraction, using the nondominant hand, the surgeon palpates the fetal scalp with one or more fingers while placing a thumb and the remaining fingers on the extractor cup. So positioned, the surgeon can better judge the appropriate angle for traction while detecting early cup separation. The bimanual technique reduces the risks from sudden cup displacement and is recommended for all vacuum extraction operations.[113,115]

If a rigid metal or plastic cup is chosen, it should not be left applied for more than 20 to 25 minutes. Prolonged extraction times risk scalp injury.[152] The time limits for plastic or soft cup applications are not established. Nonetheless, it is prudent not to exceed 20 to 25 minutes, although the level of risk for a scalp injury is arguably lower with soft cups than with the rigid cup devices.[72,82] Twenty-five minutes is usually ample time for four or more traction efforts. Full vacuum can be either maintained or reduced between contractions. Vacuum reduction may lessen the risk of scalp injury and is recommended.

Failure to make progress as force is applied requires immediate reassessment. If no advance is made, the surgeon carefully rechecks the application, reviews the vector of traction, and considers the force applied. If the fetal head has failed to move, either there is a technical problem or disproportion is present. If true disproportion is suspected, the vaginal procedure is abandoned and cesarean delivery performed.

The Use of Force

In theory, as long as station is continually reevaluated and the fetal heart rate and pattern are acceptable, there is no absolute limit to the period of a forceps application nor to the number of traction efforts. However, the incidence of trauma and failure increases rapidly if the number of tractions exceeds four (Table 59-6). Delivery usually occurs within four pulls.[76,138] If delivery has not occurred or is not imminent after the fourth complete traction effort, careful reconsideration is mandatory. As previously emphasized, *if no descent occurs on the initial attempt after adequate traction with a correctly applied instrument, the procedure is immediately reassessed.*

The limitations of vacuum extractors in applying force have long been argued as an inherent safety factor. This limitation in available traction force is a mixed blessing. An extraction failure can be dangerous. The unjudicious may be tempted to follow failed extraction by multiple, unsuccessful, and possibly traumatic efforts or to substitute with forceps. Meddlesome midwifery in situations of undiagnosed

Table 59-6 Number of Tractions Required to Achieve Delivery in 1497 Assisted Vacuum Extraction and Forceps Delivery Procedures*

No. Traction Efforts	Malmström Vacuum Extractor (N = 433)	Forceps (Type Unspecified) (N = 555)
1-2	296 (68.4%)	213 (38.4%)
3-4	108 (24.9%)	270 (48.6%)
≥5	29 (6.7%)	72 (12.9%)

*Neonates <600 g were excluded; other exclusions include breech presentations, cesarean deliveries, transverse lies, and multiple gestations. Twins were included if each weighed ≥600 g and if one was delivered spontaneously/cephalically.
Modified from Sjöstedt JE: *Acta Obstet Gynecol Scand* 46(suppl 10):3, 1967.

disproportion or malpresentation risks serious fetal/maternal injury.

Trial and Failed Operations

Among the most difficult of obstetric procedures is a *trial of instrumental delivery.*[20,113] Although all instrumental deliveries are to some extent trials, it is also true that in most instances, the surgeon believes at the onset that the operation will prove successful. However, there are circumstances in which success is less certain. In these instances, there remains a role for a *trial of instrumental delivery.* It is important to distinguish such *trials* from *failed procedures* and to conduct the operation to minimize the risks of maternal or fetal injury.

A *failed procedure* occurs when an instrument is applied under circumstances in which the surgeon does not anticipate failure and no alternative preparations have been made. Uncommonly, there are accompanying maternal and/or fetal injuries. As clinical medicine is an imperfect combination of art and science, all surgeons will encounter such cases at some time in their career. Yet, judicious use of accepted protocols and clinical judgment will avoid many, if not most, of these events.

The setting for a *trial* procedure is unique. Here, it is unclear to the surgeon whether it is possible or prudent to deliver the infant vaginally. Nonetheless, there remains a reasonable likelihood of success. For this operation, the patient is moved to an area where it is possible to perform a prompt cesarean delivery. The consent process and medical record documentation for these procedures must be meticulous. Appropriate assistants, including an anesthesiologist, are recruited. In the operating room the surgeon conducts a careful reexamination. The decision is then made whether to apply an instrument and to attempt traction. If the judgment is that an application is inappropriate, if an instrument cannot be applied, or if one is applied and with traction there is no descent of the presenting part, the instruments are removed, any perineal injuries are sutured, and the surgeon simply proceeds with a cesarean operation. If traction has been applied, it is prudent to manually displace the head upward before proceeding with the cesarean.

After an unsuccessful trial of vaginal delivery *with any instrument and regardless of the extent of the effort,* an internal fetal monitoring clip is attached and continuous heart rate monitoring commenced while awaiting cesarean delivery. If this is not technically possible, the fetal heart should be auscultated after every contraction or every 5 minutes until the surgical skin preparation is begun. Bradycardias after traction are common. Failure of the fetal heart to promptly resume a normal rate alerts the surgeon that an emergency delivery rather than a simple urgent delivery is needed.

Forceps versus Vacuum Operations

For many applications, the forceps and the vacuum extractor are interchangeable. There are at present strongly divergent opinions concerning which device is best. Thus the choice of instrument remains controversial.[49] Differences in training and experience are often much more important than the technical features of the available instruments in determining the device(s) actually used. Nonetheless, certain circumstances favor the use of one device over the other. Important considerations include the surgeon's expertise, the extent of analgesia/anesthesia, the position and station of the presenting part, and the equipment available. In specific circumstances as, for example, the assisted delivery of the second twin or applications when anesthesia is limited, the vacuum extractor has clear advantages over the forceps. In other settings, such as a breech delivery, there is no role for the extractor but occasionally an important one for forceps.

If presumed fetal jeopardy (fetal distress) is diagnosed at low station, many surgeons prefer to apply forceps rather than the vacuum extractor, believing that a forceps operation is faster. However, when tested in a prospective trial, neither the extractor nor the forceps is superior in either safety or speed.[166] Theoretical concerns aside, in difficult circumstances the best chance for success occurs when the surgeon uses a familiar instrument.

Vacuum extractors are also arguably better than forceps in midpelvic procedures in which cranial deflection is inconsequential, in low operations when no anesthesia has been given, and in trials of instrumental delivery when fetal jeopardy is not an issue.

There are a number of studies comparing forceps and vacuum extraction performance for similar indications (Table 59-7). Johanson et al.[76,77] recently published an analysis of randomized controlled trials of vacuum extraction versus forceps. In summary, the pooled data showed

Table 59-7 Forceps versus Vacuum Extractor: Selected Comparison Studies

Author	Study Type (Vacuum Extractor/Forceps)	N Vacuum Extractor	Forceps	Results/Comments
Lasbrey et al., 1964[83]	Prospective, randomized (Malmström/Kjelland and unspecified)	121	131	More maternal perineal trauma with forceps; more fetal lacerations and scalp trauma with vacuum extraction (VE)
Vacca et al., 1983[166]	Prospective, randomized (Bird/Haig Ferguson, Kjelland)	152	152	More maternal perineal trauma and blood loss with forceps; more neonatal jaundice and scalp lesions with VE, including cephalohematoma and subgaleal hematoma
Dell et al., 1985[41]	Prospective, randomized (Mityvac, Silastic/Tucker-McLane)	73*	45	More maternal perineal injuries with forceps; more minor infant scalp injuries with VE; increased failure with VE
Johanson et al., 1989[76]	Prospective, randomized (Silc-cup, Bird cup/Neville-Barnes, Kjelland)	132	132	More failures with VE; more perineal and rectal injuries with forceps
Williams et al., 1991[172]	Prospective, randomized (CMI Soft Touch/Simpson, Tucker-McLane)	48	51	Equal maternal trauma; slight increase in fetal trauma with VE
Johanson et al., 1993[77]	Prospective, randomized (Silicone elastomer cup for occiput anterior; Malmström cup for occiput posterior [Neville-Barnes, Kjelland])	296	311	Maternal trauma increased with forceps; more cephalohematomas with VE, other lacerations reduced

*Silastic, 36; Mityvac, 37.

that the vacuum extractor (VE) compared with forceps had the following characteristics:

- VE was significantly more likely to fail at vaginal delivery (odds ratio [OR] 2.0; 95% confidence interval [CI] 1.54 to 2.71).
- VE was significantly less likely to be associated with cesarean delivery (OR 0.5; 95% CI 0.27 to 0.95).
- VE was significantly less likely to be associated with maternal regional/general anesthesia (OR 0.30; 95% CI 0.24 to 0.37).
- VE was significantly less likely to be associated with significant maternal perineal and/or vaginal trauma (OR 0.44, 95% CI 0.33 to 0.58).
- VE was significantly more likely to be associated with cephalhematomas (OR 2.7; 95% CI 1.71 to 4.25).
- VE was significantly more likely to be associated with retinal hemorrhages (OR 1.88; 95% CI 1.74 to 2).
- VE was more likely to be associated with low 5-minute Apgar scores (OR 1.67; 95% CI 0.99 to 2.8).
- VE was no more likely than forceps to be associated with need for phototherapy (OR 0.98; 95% CI 0.47 to 2.05).

A similar pattern emerges from these and other studies of vacuum extraction. Maternal perineal injuries are more likely to occur with forceps deliveries, whereas fetal scalp injuries are more common after vacuum extraction operations.[126] Transitory neonatal jaundice and retinal hemorrhages are more common in vacuum-extracted neonates than in those delivered by forceps, but these complications

are usually inconsequential. It is suspected that the likelihood of neonatal vacuum extractor complications is lessened depending on the type of instrument chosen.[31]

Some of these vacuum extraction data need close consideration. The increased incidence of cephalhematomas, retinal hemorrhages, and subgaleal hemorrhages found in many studies and the trend toward lower Apgar scores deserve further study, specifically with long-term follow-up.

Aside from the issue of maternal trauma, the vacuum extractor has several potential advantages. The cup can be inserted and adjusted on the fetal head and traction initiated with minimal or no maternal analgesia. This makes the instrument particularly useful when the patient refuses a major anesthetic, when a regional anesthetic has failed or has proven only partially successful, or when only a pudendal block is in place. The fact that the extractor does not occupy space lateral to the fetal head is a potential advantage in comparison with forceps. Forceps blades must occupy some space and cannot be safely introduced if the fit of the fetal cranium to the birth canal is "too tight." Of interest, there is a suggestion from the literature that vacuum extraction operations are associated with an increased incidence of shoulder dystocia.[115] This is probably because of the preferential use of vacuum extraction in patients with suspected disproportion, in whom it is easier to apply a vacuum cup as opposed to the forceps. A feature of vacuum extraction that is sometimes stated as an advantage is the limited ability of the instrument to generate traction. However, this presumed safety factor may actually constitute a risk. Although not proven, it is suspected that recurrent episodes of cup displacement with traction (pop-offs) predispose to scalp injury. Also, the apparent ease of application of current extractors and the surgeon's belief in the safety of the device may lull the unwary into repeated efforts or borderline applications in which persistence overpowers prudence, thus increasing and not diminishing risk.

Not all vacuum extractors are the same. As with forceps operations, the type of vacuum instrument chosen is best tailored to the specific clinical requirements. In outlet procedures, any cup type can be used. However, the use of rigid metal cups risks a chignon that is usually avoided with soft cups. The unusual cranial distortion of the chignon often distresses families and even pediatricians. Although these deformities are only transient, they are best avoided if other, equally effective, delivery alternatives exist.

If the fetal head is in transverse arrest in the midpelvis, deflection is common and a metal OP cup (Bird-Malmström or O'Neil) or the Mityvac M cup is usually the best choice. In cases of minimal cranial deflection, any soft cup is equally successful. If extraction from an occiput posterior or near posterior position (ROP, LOP) is attempted, an OP metal cup is clearly superior.[77] A modified plastic cup such as the Mityvac M model may also prove effective in the OP position. There is an important technical issue here. When the fetal head is more than minimally deflexed or directed posteriorly, many extractors cannot be correctly applied. Their rigid handles preclude correct positioning of the cup over the cranial pivot point and make it impossible to apply traction evenly, requiring oblique traction, predisposing to cup pop-offs.[164]

Education

There are important questions concerning the adequacy of training in techniques of operative delivery.* Survey studies of North American resident education programs and international studies of obstetric practice report both important and concerning trends.[14,92,110,129,176] Virtually all programs (95%) in the most recent North American survey (95%) offered instruction in instrumental delivery.[14] Education in vacuum extraction has become increasingly popular, with approximately 70% of North American residencies now providing this training. Plastic or silicone soft cups from various manufacturers were the choice of 86% of programs using vacuum extraction. Approximately 65% of training programs continue to teach midpelvic operative vaginal delivery with two thirds of respondents favoring forceps use and one third the vacuum extractor for these procedures. For training programs that no longer teach midpelvic procedures, safety concerns (70%) and litigation risks (38%) were listed as the reasons.

As these data are more deeply analyzed, several bothersome trends emerge. Bofill et al.'s data[14] confirm a continued decline in the teaching of midpelvic operative procedures. In

their 1990 survey, Ramin et al.[129] reported that 14% of programs had abandoned instruction in midpelvic procedures. In a 1995 survey this number had risen to 36%. In the 1995 data only half of responding programs would attempt a forceps rotational operation, with the remainder favoring either vacuum extraction (22%) or cesarean delivery (28%).[14]

What are the implications of these findings for the profession? The time-honored methods of teaching instrumentation in the operating room will almost certainly need to be changed. There are too few cases for all residents to gain good instruction in the less frequent vaginal operations and too few qualified instructors. Also, modern practice is increasingly (and appropriately) resistant to "teaching" forceps (or vacuum extraction) procedures, conducted without a clear clinical indication. If the specialty wishes to retain instrumental delivery, new methods of teaching—whether by better use of existing cases, computer simulation, or other educational means—must be developed.[165] Otherwise, within a generation, a potentially valuable obstetric technique will be lost simply because of the progressive retirement from practice of experienced obstetric surgeons. The dismal cycle involves progressively decreased opportunities for application, leading to inexperienced instructors and poorly supervised procedures. Skilled practitioners are progressively lost, decreasing the opportunities for education, progressively lessening the chances that vaginal instrumental procedures will either be considered or attempted.

These data raise additional issues for educators. Given the declining number of procedures and the recognized risk, what techniques should residents be taught? Unless midpelvic forceps procedures are conducted with reasonable frequency within an institution, most young practitioners will never experience a sufficient number of cases either to feel comfortable with these operations or to be safe in their performance. For most education programs, perhaps it is better to intensively teach the more frequent low and outlet forceps operations, restricting true midpelvic procedures to trials of vacuum extraction. This should be accompanied by special emphasis on basic fetopelvic evaluation and correct instrument application. These choices will limit forceps operations but better ensure fetal and maternal safety while retaining basic skills. Midpelvic forceps procedures do not need to be abandoned by the profession but must be limited to experienced obstetric surgeons.

Documentation

All operative or assisted deliveries, whether by forceps or vacuum extraction, require full documentation in the medical record. It is best for the responsible physician to dictate these cases into the medical record in the same fashion as any surgery. This approach is most likely to result in a detailed and complete report.

If the outcome is less than perfect or an occult injury is suspected, a discussion with the pediatrician is best. Obviously, when problems occur, careful patient and family

---

*References 14, 19, 28, 79, 113, 129, 165.

counseling is always required. When presumed fetal jeopardy (fetal distress) was the principal indication for the operation or when there is an unanticipated poor neonatal outcome, it is prudent to obtain umbilical arterial and venous pH values and to submit the placenta for histologic examination.

CONCLUSIONS

Human labor and birth are imperfect and incompletely understood processes. Nonetheless, in recent decades, great strides have been made in our understanding of the physiology of labor and delivery, leading to major changes in practice. Potent uterotonic and tocolytic drugs are now available, as are highly sophisticated techniques for in utero visualization and for the evaluation of fetal condition. Also, new knowledge of maternal physiology permits safe anesthesia and surgical delivery for even severely compromised women. Yet, to a degree, we are overconfident and have become the victims of our own success. We have belatedly discovered that despite our best intentions, electronic assessments do not invariably ensure a good outcome, complications still occur and many birth injuries, including cerebral palsy, are poorly understood and are not preventable. As difficulties with the birth process are inevitable and prevention of *all* complications not possible, it is a comfortable assertion that some form of delivery assistance will always be required. Cesarean delivery will never be the only answer to obstetric difficulties. In many situations such a major intervention is both unnecessary and unduly risky. Alternatives, including instrumental delivery, must also be considered.

We must use the medical literature with caution in our efforts to improve practice. Most of the well-fought-over data concerning instrumental delivery no longer reflect what is actually done in perinatal medicine.[25] Management has changed profoundly in the last 20 years and substantially in the last 10. We have witnessed rapid improvements in neonatal intensive care, pushing the period of potential viability back to 23 to 24 weeks with concomitant pressures on obstetric management. New biophysical and ultrasonic techniques are available for fetal assessment. High cesarean delivery rates are common, albeit under intense scrutiny and reassessment. In this setting and despite controversy, there has been a growing realization over the last 10 years that a reassessment of what might be termed traditional obstetric interventions—including instrumental delivery—is appropriate.

What general conclusions can we reach after our review? There are several important points to consider concerning maternal and neonatal condition, instrumental delivery, and appropriate clinical conduct.

1. *The method of delivery is not the most important factor in determining neonatal outcome.* The evidence is strong that antepartum events have the greater influence. Although infants are injured intrapartum, most of these injuries are inconsequential and most permanent neurologic injuries are not caused by trauma at parturition.*

2. *Determining the best mode of delivery requires careful examination, evaluation of maternal and fetal status, knowledge of possible techniques, and most important, a consideration of alternatives.* Instrumental delivery may be the best answer to an obstetric difficulty, but it is rarely the *only* answer.[19,112,116]

3. *Forceps operations and vacuum extraction procedures are often but not always interchangeable.* In general, maternal injuries are more common with forceps and infant injuries with the vacuum extractor.[115,164] Recent comparative series favor vacuum extraction as opposed to forceps, but this issue is far from settled.[27,41,76,77] In my opinion, modern practitioners should become skilled in both techniques.

4. *Outlet and low forceps operations are safe for the infant but do have an increased incidence of maternal perineal trauma.*[173] Maternal perineal injury from delivery may have long-term consequences.[78,146-149,151] Perineal lacerations involving the rectal sphincter are of special concern. The relationship of these and other pelvic floor injuries to labor events and delivery technique needs close scrutiny.

5. *Complications with midpelvic operative delivery procedures are more common than with low or outlet procedures, but regardless of the method of delivery, the outcome for these infants is essentially equal.* I, along with other reviewers, believe the available data may be fairly read to support the continued use of selected instrumental delivery techniques.[19,25,113-115,164] In considering which operations are prudent, the general rule is to avoid difficult procedures (especially midpelvic rotational procedures), with reconsideration of labor management in terms of the length of the second stage, type of analgesia/anesthesia, administration of oxytocin, and maternal positioning (see Fig. 59-8). For most practitioners, reliance on vacuum extraction is indicated for the more difficult deliveries, especially for trials of midpelvic delivery. These settings result in a higher incidence of injured mothers and babies if forceps are applied by all but the most experienced surgeons.

6. *For all assisted deliveries, a detailed description in the medical record is mandatory.* The intentions of the surgeon, indications for the operation, and the actual procedures performed should be included.

7. *Education of patients, birth attendants, and birth educators concerning the appropriate use of instrumental delivery is an important responsibility for all obstetric surgeons.* If valuable procedures are to be retained, serious educational efforts are needed by training programs and by surgeons along with active support for

---

*References 3, 13, 51, 62, 64, 74, 75, 81, 100, 103-105, 108, 119, 122-124, 143, 150.

clinical research, especially studies involving long-term maternal and infant follow-up.

Obstetrics remains an art of the possible, aided by science and limited by various restrictions. These constraints are imposed by the limits of nature, ethical concerns, the constraints of facilities, finance and medicolegal risks, the standards of practice/practice guidelines that we embrace, and patient consent. As the population and society change and medical science advances, continuous reevaluation and reassessment of all current obstetric practices including instrumental delivery will occur. In the future, this process will undoubtedly alter management in directions impossible to predict.

REFERENCES

1. American College of Obstetricians and Gynecologists Committee on Obstetrics, Maternal and Fetal Medicine: *Obstetric forceps,* Committee Opinion no. 71, Washington DC, 1989, American College of Obstetricians and Gynecologists.
2. American College of Obstetricians and Gynecologists: *Dystocia,* Technical Bulletin no. 137, Washington DC, 1989, American College of Obstetricians and Gynecologists.
3. American College of Obstetricians and Gynecologists: *Operative vaginal delivery,* Technical Bulletin no. 152, Washington DC, 1991, American College of Obstetricians and Gynecologists.
4. American College of Obstetricians and Gynecologists: *Fetal and neonatal neurologic injury,* Technical Bulletin no. 163, Washington DC, 1992, American College of Obstetricians and Gynecologists.
5. American College of Obstetricians and Gynecologists: *Operative vaginal delivery,* Technical Bulletin no.196, Washington DC, 1994, American College of Obstetricians and Gynecologists.
6. Banta D, Thacker S: The risks and benefits of episiotomy: a review, *Birth* 9:25, 1982.
7. Bashore RA, Philips WH, Brinkman CR: A comparison of the morbidity of midforceps and cesarean delivery, *Am J Obstet Gynecol* 162:1428, 1990.
8. Baskett TF: Operative vaginal delivery in the 21st century, *J Surg Obstet Gynaecol Can* 19:355, 1997 (editorial).
9. Bates RG, et al: Uterine activity in the second stage of labour and the effect of epidural analgesia, *Br J Obstet Gynaecol* 92:1246, 1985.
10. Bercovici B: Use of the vacuum extractor for head delivery at cesarean section, *Isr J Med Sci* 16:201, 1980.
11. Bergsjo P: Differences in the reported frequencies of some obstetrical interventions in Europe, *Br J Obstet Gynaecol* 90:628, 1983.
12. Bird GC: The use of the vacuum extractor, *Clin Obstet Gynaecol* 9:641, 1982.
13. Blair E, Stanley FJ: Intrapartum asphyxia, a rare cause of cerebral palsy, *J Pediatr* 112:515, 1988.
14. Bofill JA, et al: Forceps and vacuum delivery: a survey of North American residency programs, *Obstet Gynecol* 88:622, 1996.
15. Borgatta L, Piening S, Cohen W: Association of episiotomy and delivery position with deep perineal laceration during spontaneous delivery in nulliparous women, *Am J Obstet Gynecol* 160:294, 1989.
16. Bottoms SF: Delivery of the premature infant, *Clin Obstet Gynecol* 38:780, 1995.
17. Bottoms SF, Hirsch VJ, Sokol RJ: Medical management of arrest disorders of labor: a current overview, *Am J Obstet Gynecol* 156:935, 1987.
18. Bowes WA, Bowes C: Current role of the midforceps operation, *Clin Obstet Gynecol* 23:549, 1980.
19. Bowes WJ, Katz V: Operative vaginal delivery forceps and vacuum extractor, *Curr Prob Gynecol Fertil* 17:82, 1994.
20. Boyd ME, et al: Failed forceps, *Obstet Gynecol* 68:779, 1986.
21. Broman SH, Nichols PL, Kennedy WA: *Preschool IQ prenatal and early developmental correlates,* Hillsdale, NJ, 1975, Lawrence Erlbaum Associates (John Wiley & Sons).
22. Bryce R, Stanley F, Blair E: The effects of intrapartum care on the risks of impairments in childhood. In Chalmers I, Eukin M, Keirse M, editors: *Effective care in pregnancy and childbirth,* Oxford, 1989, Oxford University Press, p 1313.
23. Cardozo LD, et al: Should we abandon Keilland's forceps? *Br Med J* 287:315, 1983.
24. Carmona F, et al: Immediate maternal and neonatal effects of low-forceps delivery according to the new criteria of the American College of Obstetricians and Gynecologists compared with spontaneous vaginal delivery in term pregnancies, *Am J Obstet Gynecol* 173:55, 1995.
25. Carpenter M: Safety of forceps vaginal delivery and principles of application. In Nichols D, editor: *Gynecologic and obstetric surgery,* St Louis, 1993, Mosby, p 1061.
26. Chalmers J: James Young Simpson and the "suction-tractor," *J Obstet Gynaecol Br Commonw* 70:94, 1963.
27. Chalmers JA, Chalmers I: The obstetric vacuum extractor is the instrument of first choice for operative vaginal delivery, *Br J Obstet Gynaecol* 96:505, 1989 (commentary).
28. Charles A: Forceps delivery and vacuum extraction. In Sciarra J, editor: *Gynecology and obstetrics,* vol 2, Philadelphia, 1997, Lippincott-Raven, p 1.
29. Chauhan SP, et al: Intrapartum clinical, sonographic, and parous patients' estimates of newborn birth weight, *Obstet Gynecol* 79:956, 1992.
30. Chauhan SP, et al: Intrapartum prediction of birth weight: clinical versus sonographic estimation based on femur length alone, *Obstet Gynecol* 81:695, 1993.
31. Cheney R, Johanson RB: A randomised prospective study comparing delivery with metal and silicone rubber vacuum extractor cups, *Br J Obstet Gynaecol* 90:360, 1992.
32. Chestnut DH, et al: Does early administration of epidural analgesia affect obstetric outcome in nulliparous women who are receiving intravenous oxytocin? *Anesthesiology* 80:1193, 1994.
33. Cibils LA, Ringler GE: Evaluation of midforceps delivery as an alternative, *J Perinat Med* 18:5, 1990.
34. Cohen WR: Influence of the duration of second stage labor on perinatal outcome and puerperal morbidity, *Obstet Gynecol* 49:266, 1977.
35. Cosgrove RA, Weaver OS: An analysis of 1,000 consecutive midforceps operations, *Am J Obstet Gynecol* 73:556, 1957.
36. Crichton D: A reliable method of establishing the level of the fetal head in obstetrics, *S Afr Med J* 48:784, 1974.
37. Cutter I, Viets H: *A short history of midwifery,* Philadelphia, 1964, WB Saunders.
38. DeCosta C: The vacuum extractor. a re-appraisal, *Ir J Med Sci* 151:105, 1982.
39. DeLancey J: Childbirth, continence, and the pelvic floor, *N Engl J Med* 329:1956, 1993 (editorial).
40. DeLee J: The prophylactic forceps operation, *Am J Obstet Gynecol* 1:34, 1920.
41. Dell DL, Sightler SE, Planche WC: Soft cup vacuum extraction: a comparison of outlet delivery, *Obstet Gynecol* 66:624, 1985.
42. Delpapa E, Mueller-Heubach, E: Pregnancy outcome following ultrasound diagnosis of macrosomia, *Obstet Gynecol* 78:340, 1991.
43. Dennen E: *Forceps deliveries,* ed 2, Philadelphia, 1964, FA Davis.
44. Dennen P: *Dennen's forceps deliveries,* ed 3, Philadelphia, 1989, FA Davis.
45. Deter RI, Hadlock F: Use of ultrasound in the detection of macrosomia: a review, *J Clin Ultrasound* 13:519, 1985.
46. Dierker LJ, et al: The midforceps: maternal and neonatal outcomes, *Am J Obstet Gynecol* 152:176, 1985.
47. Dierker LJ, et al: Midforceps deliveries: long term outcome of infants, *Am J Obstet Gynecol* 154:764, 1986.

48. Dill L: *The obstetrical forceps,* Springfield, Ill, 1953, Charles C Thomas.

49. Drife J: Choice and instrumental delivery, *Br Obstet Gynaecol* 103:808, 1996 (editorial).

50. Elliot B, et al: The development and testing of new instruments for operative vaginal delivery, *Am J Obstet Gynecol* 167:1121, 1992.

51. Freeman JM, Nelson KB: Intrapartum asphyxia and cerebral palsy, *Pediatrics* 82:240, 1988.

52. Friedman EA: *Labor, clinical evaluation and management,* New York, 1967, Appleton-Century-Crofts.

53. Friedman EA: Midforceps delivery: no? *Clin Obstet Gynecol* 30:93, 1987.

54. Friedman EA, Sachtebon MR, Bresky PA: Dysfunctional labor. XII. Long-term effects on infant, *Am J Obstet Gynecol* 127:779, 1977.

55. Friedman EA, et al: Long-term effects of labor and delivery on offspring: a matched pair analysis, *Am J Obstet Gynecol* 150:941, 1984.

56. Gilstrap LC, et al: Neonatal acidosis and method of delivery, *Obstet Gynecol* 63:681, 1984.

57. Glazener C, et al: Postnatal maternal morbidity: extent, causes, prevention and treatment, *Br J Obstet Gynaecol* 102:282, 1995.

58. Goodfellow CR, et al: Oxytocin deficiency at delivery with epidural analgesia, *Br J Obstet Gynaecol* 90:214, 1983.

59. Goodlin R: On protection of the maternal perineum during childbirth, *Obstet Gynecol* 62:393, 1983.

60. Goven O, et al: Induction of labor versus expectant management in macrosomia: a randomized study, *Obstet Gynecol* 89:913, 1997.

61. Gresham E: Birth trauma, *Pediatr Clin North Am* 22:317, 1975.

62. Grether JK, Nelson KB: Maternal infection and cerebral palsy in infants of normal birth weight, *JAMA* 278:207, 1997.

63. Hagadorn-Freathy A, Yeomans E, Hankins G: Validation of the 1988 ACOG forceps classification system, *Obstet Gynecol* 77:356, 1991.

64. Hagberg B, Kyllerman M: Epidemiology and mental retardation—a Swedish survey, *Brain Dev* 5:441, 1983.

65. Hanretty K, Neilson J, Fleming J: Re-evaluation of clinical estimation of fetal weight: a comparison with ultrasound, *J Obstet Gynecol* 10:199, 1990.

66. Harrison R, et al: Is routine episiotomy necessary? *Br Med J* 288: 1971, 1984.

67. Hayashi RH: Midforceps delivery: yes? *Clin Obstet Gynecol* 30:90, 1987.

68. Healy DL, Quinn MA, Pepperell RJ: Rotational delivery of the fetus: Kielland's forceps and two other methods compared, *Br J Obstet Gynaecol* 89:501, 1982.

69. Hensleigh P, Fainstat T, Spencer R: Perinatal events and cerebral palsy, *Am J Obstet Gynecol* 154:978, 1986.

70. Hibbard BM, McKenna DM: The obstetric forceps—are we using the appropriate tools? *Br J Obstet Gynecol* 97:374, 1990.

71. Hillier C, Johanson R: Worldwide survey of assisted vaginal delivery, *Int J Gynecol Obstet* 47:109, 1994.

72. Hofmeyr GJ, et al: New design rigid and soft vacuum extractor cups: a preliminary comparison of traction forceps, *Br J Obstet Gynaecol* 97:681, 1990.

73. Hughey MJ, McElin TH, Lussy R: Forceps operations in perspective. I. Midforceps rotation operations, *J Reprod Med* 20:253, 1978.

74. Illingworth R: Why blame the obstetrician? A review, *Br Med J* 1:797, 1979.

75. Illingworth R: A paeditrician asks—why is it called birth injury? *Br J Obstet Gynaecol* 92:122, 1985.

76. Johanson R, et al: North Staffordshire/Wigan assisted delivery trial, *Br J Obstet Gynaecol* 96:537, 1989.

77. Johanson RB, et al: A randomised prospective study comparing the new vacuum extractor policy with forceps delivery, *Br J Obstet Gynaecol* 100:524, 1993.

78. Kamm M: Obstetric damage and faecal incontinence, *Lancet* 344:730, 1994.

79. Katz V, Bowes WJ: Operative vaginal delivery: do forceps and vacuum extraction have a place in modern obstetrics? *Female Patient* 22:39, 1997.

80. Klein M, et al: Relationship of episiotomy to perineal trauma and morbidity, sexual dysfunction, and pelvic floor relaxation, *Am J Obstet Gynecol* 171:591, 1994.

81. Kuban KCK, Leviton A: Cerebral palsy, *N Engl J Med* 330:188, 1994.

82. Kuit JA, et al: A randomized comparison of vacuum extraction delivery with a rigid and a pliable cup, *Obstet Gynecol* 82:280, 1993.

83. Lasbrey AH, Orchard CD, Crichton D: A study of the relative merits and scope for vacuum extraction as opposed to forceps delivery, *S Afr J Obstet Gynaecol* 2:1, 1964.

84. Laufe L: *Obstetric forceps,* New York, 1968, Harper & Row.

85. Laufe L, Berkus M: *Assisted vaginal delivery,* New York, 1992, McGraw-Hill.

86. MacArthur C, Bick D, Keighley M: Faecal incontinence after childbirth, *Br J Obstet Gynecol* 104:46, 1997.

87. Malmström T: The vacuum extractor: an obstetrical instrument and the parturiometer, a tocographic device, *Acta Obstet Gynecol Scand* 36:7, 1957.

88. March MR, et al: The modified Mueller-Hillis maneuver in predicting abnormalities in second stage labor, *Int J Gyneol Obstet* 55:105, 1996.

89. Mauriçeau F: *Traité des maladies de femmes grosses,* Paris, 1694, Quatièrne Edition.

90. McBride W, et al: Method of delivery and developmental outcome at five years of age, *Med J Aust* 1:301, 1979.

91. Megison J: Save the Barton forceps, *Obstet Gynecol* 82: 313, 1993.

92. Meniru G: An analysis of recent trends in vacuum extraction and forceps delivery in the United Kingdom, *Br J Obstet Gynaecol* 103:168, 1996.

93. Menticoglou SM, et al: Must macrosomic fetuses be delivered by a cesarean section? A review of outcome for 786 babies >4500 g, *Aust NZ J Obstet Gynaecol* 32:100, 1992.

94. Menticoglou SM, Perlman M, Manning FA: High cervical spinal cord injury in neonates delivered with forceps: report of 15 cases, *Obstet Gynecol* 86:589, 1995.

95. Milner ROG: Neonatal mortality of breech deliveries with and without forceps to the aftercoming head, *Br J Obstet Gynaecol* 82:783, 1975.

96. Morgan M, Thurnau G: Efficacy of the fetal-pelvic index in nulliparous women at high risk for fetal-pelvic disproportion, *Am J Obstet Gynecol* 166:810, 1992.

97. Reference deleted in proofs.

98. Murless RC: Lower segment cesarean section: a new head extraction, *Br Med J* 1:1234, 1948.

99. Naeye R: *Disorders of the placenta, fetus, and neonate: diagnosis and clinical significance,* St Louis, 1992, Mosby.

100. Nelson K: What proportion of cerebral palsy is related to birth asphyxia? *J Pediatr* 112:572, 1988.

101. Nelson K: Relationship of intrapartum and delivery room events to long-term neurological outcome, *Clin Perinatol* 16:995, 1989.

102. Nelson K, Ellenberg J: Apgar scores as predictors of chronic neurologic disability, *Pediatrics* 68:36, 1981.

103. Nelson K, Ellenberg J: Obstetric complications as risk factors for cerebral palsy or seizure disorders, *JAMA* 251:1843, 1984.

104. Nelson K, Ellenberg J: Antecedents of cerebral palsy, *N Engl J Med* 315:81, 1986.

105. Nelson K, Ellenberg J: The asymptomatic newborn and risk of cerebral palsy, *Am J Dis Child* 141:1333, 1987.

106. Ngan HYS, et al: Long-term neurological sequelae following vacuum extractor delivery, *Aust NZ J Obstet Gynaecol* 30:111, 1990.

107. Nilsen ST: Boys born by forceps and vacuum extraction at 18 years of age, *Acta Obstet Gynecol Scand* 63:549, 1984.

108. Niswander K, Gordon M: Safety of the low forceps operation, *Am J Obstet Gynecol* 117: 619, 1973.

109. Nocon JJ, Weisbrod L: Shoulder dystocia. In O'Grady JP, Gimovsky ML, McIlhargie CJ, editors: *Operative obstetrics,* Baltimore, 1995, Williams & Wilkins.

110. Notzon FC: International differences in the use of obstetric interventions, *JAMA* 263:3286, 1990.

111. Nyirjesy I, Pierce W: Perinatal mortality and maternal morbidity in spontaneous and forceps vaginal deliveries, *Am J Obstet Gynecol* 89:568, 1964.

112. O'Driscoll K, Meagher D, Boylan P: *Active management of labor,* ed 3, Aylesbury, England, 1993, Mosby, Europe Limited.

113. O'Grady J: *Modern instrumental delivery,* Baltimore, 1988, Williams & Wilkins.

114. O'Grady JP: Instrumental delivery. In O'Grady JP, Gimovsky M, McIlhargie C, editors: *Operative obstetrics,* Baltimore, 1995, Williams & Wilkins.

115. O'Grady JP: *Vacuum extraction in modern obstetric practice,* New York, 1995, Parthenon.

116. O'Grady JP, Gimovsky M: Instrumental delivery: a lost art? In Studd, J, editor: *Progress in obstetrics and gynaecology,* vol 10, Edinburgh, 1993, Churchill-Livingstone, p 183.

117. O'Grady JP, Youngstrom P: Must epidurals always imply instrumental delivery? *Contemp Ob/Gyn* 35:19, 1990.

118. O'Leary J: *Shoulder dystocia and birth injury: prevention and treatment,* New York, 1992, McGraw-Hill.

119. Paneth N, Stark RI: Cerebral palsy and mental retardation in relation to indicators of perinatal asphyxia: an epidemiologic overview, *Am J Obstet Gynecol* 147:960, 1983.

120. Pearse WH: Forceps versus spontaneous vaginal delivery, *Clin Obstet Gynecol* 8:813, 1965.

121. Pelosi M, Apuzzio J: Use of soft, silicone obstetric vacuum cups for the delivery of the fetal head at cesarean section, *J Reprod Med* 29:289, 1984.

122. Perkins RP: Selected perinatal events and follow-up studies. In Tejani N, editor: *Obstetrical events and developmental sequelae,* ed 2, Boca Raton, Fla, 1994, CRC Press, p 1.

123. Phelan JP: Nucleated red blood cells: a marker for fetal asphyxia? *Am J Obstet Gynecol* 173:1380, 1995.

124. Phelan JP, Ahn MO: Perinatal observation in forty eight neurologically impaired term infants, *Am J Obstet Gynecol* 171:424, 1994.

125. Philpott RH, Castle WM: Cervicographs in the management of labour in primigravidae. I. The action line and treatment of abnormal labour, *J Obstet Gynaecol Br Commonw* 79:592, 1972.

126. Plauché WC: Fetal cranial injuries related to delivery with the Malmström vacuum extractor, *Obstet Gynecol* 53:750, 1979.

127. Pollack R, Pollack G, Divon M: Macrosomia in postdates pregnancies: the accuracy of routine ultrasonographic screening, *Am J Obstet Gynecol* 167:7, 1992.

128. Radcliffe W: *Milestones in midwifery and the secret instrument,* San Francisco, 1989, Norman.

129. Ramin SM, Little B, Gilstrap LC: Survey of operative vaginal delivery in North America in 1990, *Obstet Gynecol* 81:307, 1993.

130. Roberts IF, Stone M: Fetal hemorrhage: complication of vacuum extractor after fetal blood sampling, *Am J Obstet Gynecol* 132:109, 1978.

131. Robertson PA, Laros RK, Zhao RL: Neonatal and maternal outcome in low-pelvic and mid-pelvic operative deliveries, *Am J Obstet Gynecol* 162:1436, 1990.

132. Rosen MG, et al: Abnormal labor and infant brain damage, *Obstet Gynecol* 80:961, 1992.

133. Sandmire H: Whither ultrasonic prediction of fetal macrosomia, *Obstet Gynecol* 82:860, 1993.

134. Schindler N: Importance of the placenta and cord in the defense of neurologically impaired infant claims, *Arch Pathol Lab Med* 115:685, 1991.

135. Schwartz OB, Miodovnik SM, Thompson K, et al: Abnormal labor and infant brain damage, *Obstet Gynecol* 80:961, 1992.

136. Seidman D, et al: Long-term effects of vacuum and forceps deliveries, *Lancet* 337:1583, 1991.

137. Shiono P, Klebanoff M, Carey J: Midline episiotomies: more harm than good? *Obstet Gynecol* 76:765, 1990.

138. Sjösted J: The vacuum extractor and forceps in obstetrics; a clinical study, *Acta Obstet Gynecol Scand* 46:203, 1967.

139. Sleep J, et al: West Berkshire perineal management trial: three year follow up, *Br Med J Clin Res Ed* 295:749, 1984.

140. Sleep J, Roberts J, Chalmers I: Care during the second stage of labour. In Chalmers I, Eukin M, Keirse M, editors: *Effective care in pregnancy and childbirth,* Oxford, 1989, Oxford University Press, p 1129.

141. Solomons E: Delivery of the head with the Malmström vacuum extractor during cesarean section, *Obstet Gynecol* 19:201, 1962.

142. Speert H: The obstetric forceps, *Clin Obstet Gynecol* 3:761, 1960.

143. Stanley FJ, Watson L: The cerebral palsies in Western Australia: trends, 1968-1981, *Am J Obstet Gynecol* 158:89, 1988.

144. Steer CM: *Moloy's evaluation of the pelvis in obstetrics,* ed 3, New York, 1975, Plenum.

145. Studd J: Partograms and normograms of cervical dilatation in management of primigravid labour, *Br Med J* 24:451, 1973.

146. Sultan A, et al: Anal sphincter trauma during instrumental delivery, *Int J Gynecol Obstet* 43:263, 1993.

147. Sultan A, et al: Third degree obstetric anal sphincter tears: risk factors and outcome of primary repair, *Br Med J* 308:887, 1994.

148. Sultan A, Kamm M, Hudson C: Pudendal nerve damage during labour: prospective study before and after childbirth, *Br J Obstet Gynaecol* 101:22, 1994.

149. Sultan A, et al: Anal sphincter disruption during vaginal delivery, *N Engl J Med* 329:1905, 1993.

150. Sunshine P: Epidemiology of perinatal asphyxia. In Stevenson D, editor: *Fetal and neonatal brain injury: mechanisms, management, and the risks of practice,* Philadelphia, 1989, BC Decker, p 2.

151. Swash M: Faecal incontinence: childbirth is responsible for most cases, *Br Med J* 307:636, 1993.

152. Teng FY, Sayne JW: Vacuum extraction: does duration predict scalp injury? *Obstet Gynecol* 89:281, 1997.

153. Thacker S, Banta H: Benefits and risks of episiotomy: an interpretive review of the English literature, 1860-1980, *Obstet Gynecol Surv* 38:322, 1983.

154. Thiery M: Obstetric vacuum extraction, *Obstet Gynecol Annu* 14:73, 1985.

155. Thomas SJ, et al: The risk of periventricular intraventricular hemorrhage with vacuum extraction of neonates weighing 2000 grams or less, *J Perinatol* 17:37, 1997.

156. Thorp JA, et al: Epidural analgesia and cesarean section for dystocia: risk factors in nulliparas, *Am J Perinatol* 8:402, 1991.

157. Thorp JA, et al: The effect of intrapartum epidural analgesia on nulliparous labor: a randomized, controlled, prospective trial, *Am J Obstet Gynecol* 169:851, 1993.

158. Thorp JJ, Bowes WJ: Episiotomy: can its routine use be defended? *Am J Obstet Gynecol* 160:1027, 1989.

159. Thurnau G, Haless K, Morgan M: Evaluation of the fetal pelvic relationship, *Clin Obstet Gynecol* 35:570, 1992.

160. Thurnau G, Morgan M: Efficacy of the fetal-pelvic index as a predictor of fetal-pelvic disproportion in patients with abnormal labor patterns requiring labor augmentation, *Am J Obstet Gynecol* 159:1168, 1988.

161. Thurnau G, Scates D, Morgan M: The fetal-pelvic index: a method of identifying fetal-pelvic disproportion in women attempting vaginal birth after previous cesarean delivery, *Am J Obstet Gynecol* 165:353, 1991.

162. Traub AI, et al: A continuing use for Keilland's forceps? *Br J Obstet Gynaecol* 91:894, 1984.

163. Vacca A: The place of the vacuum extractor in modern obstetric practice, *Fetal Med Rev* 2:103, 1990.

164. Vacca A: *Handbook of vacuum extraction in obstetric practice,* London, 1992, Edward Arnold.

165. Vacca A: Choice and instrumental delivery, *Br J Obstet Gynaecol* 103:1269, 1996 (letter to the editor).

166. Vacca A, et al: Portsmouth operative delivery trial: a comparison of vacuum extraction and forceps delivery, *Br J Obstet Gynaecol* 90:1107, 1983.

167. Vacca A, Keirse M: Instrumental vaginal delivery. In Chalmers I, Eukin M, Keirse M, editors: *Effective care in pregnancy and childbirth,* Oxford, 1989, Oxford University Press, p 1216.

168. Warenski J: A technique to facilitate delivery of the high-floating head at cesarean section, *Am J Obstet Gynecol* 139:625, 1981.

169. Watson W, Soisson A, Harlass F: Estimated weight of the term fetus: accuracy of ultrasound vs. clinical examination, *J Reprod Med* 33:369, 1988.

170. Wesley BD, van der Berg B, Reece EA: The effect of forceps delivery on cognitive development, *Am J Obstet Gynecol* 169:1091, 1993.

171. Wilcox L, et al: Episiotomy and its role in the incidence of perineal laceration in a maternity center and tertiary hospital obstetric service, *Am J Obstet Gynecol* 160:1047, 1989.

172. Williams M, et al: A randomized comparison of assisted vaginal delivery by obstetric forceps and polyethylene vacuum cup, *Obstet Gynecol* 78:789, 1991.

173. Yancey MK, et al: Maternal and neonatal effects of outlet forceps delivery compared with spontaneous vaginal delivery in term pregnancies, *Obstet Gynecol* 78:646, 1991.

174. Yeomans E, Gilstrap L: The role of forceps, *Clin Obstet Gynecol* 37:785, 1994.

175. Yeomans E, Hankins G: Operative vaginal delivery in the 1990's, *Clin Obstet Gynecol* 35:487, 1992.

176. Zahniser SC, et al: Trends in obstetric operative procedures, 1980 to 1987, *Am J Public Health* 82:1340, 1992.

60 Advanced Ectopic Pregnancy

JOHN R. OLIVER and RICHARD H. PAUL

Often, the terms *ectopic pregnancy* and *abdominal pregnancy* are used interchangeably. In this chapter, however, *ectopic pregnancy* is a general term used to encompass any pregnancy that develops after implantation of the blastocyst anywhere other than the endometrium lining the uterine cavity. On the other hand, abdominal pregnancy is a form of ectopic pregnancy, specifically, pregnancy that develops in any portion of the peritoneal cavity. *Extrauterine* is synonymous with *ectopic*.

In 1903, J. Whitridge Williams, in the first edition of Williams' *Obstetrics*,[42] wrote regarding ectopic pregnancy that, "the operation is still one of the most dangerous which the gynaecologist is called upon to perform." This statement is still true today. Many of the controversies about the management of advanced ectopic pregnancies that existed in 1903 still exist today. Fortunately, this condition is rare. The key to optimizing maternal morbidity and mortality is the early detection and treatment of all extrauterine gestations. With the advent of ultrasound and other methods of early pregnancy detection, the incidence of advanced ectopic pregnancies should decline. When an advanced ectopic pregnancy is encountered, the surgeon is faced with decisions about the timing of delivery and the management of the placenta, which may have a significant impact on both maternal and fetal outcomes.

The reported maternal mortality rate for ectopic pregnancies in 1886 was about 89%. By 1933, the mortality rate had dropped to 32%. As blood transfusions became available, the mortality rate continued to decrease and by 1948 was 15%. As antibiotics became available to treat the severe infections that occurred in these patients, mortality declined even further. By 1957, the mortality rate for patients with abdominal pregnancies was 2%.[20]

There are six types of extrauterine pregnancy:

1. *Primary ovarian pregnancy:* The incidence of ovarian pregnancies has been reported to be about 1 per 6970 deliveries or 0.7 to 1.0 per 100 ectopic gestations.[31] In 1878, Spiegelberg defined ovarian pregnancies using four strict pathologic criteria that are still in use today: (1) the tube on the affected side must be intact, (2) the gestational site must occupy the normal position of the ovary, (3) the gestational site must be connected to the uterus by the ovarian ligament, and (4) histologically identified ovarian tissue must be identified in the sac wall.[3,16,31] Usually, ovarian pregnancies are identified in the first trimesters.[23,43] King[23] described one study of ovarian pregnancy in which 60 cases were diagnosed in the first trimester, 11 cases in the second trimester, and 11 in the third trimester. Seven third-trimester fetuses were stillborn, and four were living (two with gross deformities).

2. *Primary abdominal pregnancy:* This type of ectopic pregnancy is rare, with only 24 cases of primary abdominal pregnancy reported in 1968.[14] In 1942, Studdiford gave a strict definition for primary abdominal pregnancy that is still used today: (1) normal tubes and ovaries, (2) no evidence of uteroplacental fistula, and (3) pregnancy implanted only on the peritoneal surface and early enough in the gestation to eliminate the possibility of secondary implantation of a ruptured tubal gestation.[3,6,14,31] This third definition makes it impossible to distinguish advanced primary abdominal pregnancies from advanced secondary ectopic pregnancies because the placental implantation usually involves the uterus tubes and ovaries to some extent in both types of abdominal pregnancies. Most primary abdominal pregnancies are implanted in and around the cul-de-sac.[14,17] However, in a recent case at Los Angeles County University of Southern California (USC) Medical Center, a primary abdominal pregnancy was implanted on the infundibulopelvic ligament about 6 cm above the ovary. This points out the need for careful, detailed abdominal exploration when performing laparoscopy or celiotomy on a patient suspected of having an ectopic gestation, especially if the tubes appear to be normal. Perhaps the most unusual locations for implantation of a primary abdominal pregnancy are the liver and spleen. Six cases of splenic and four of hepatic pregnancies have been reported.[7,19,22,27,31,33]

3. *Secondary abdominal pregnancy:* This is the most common type of advanced ectopic pregnancy.[3,23,31] The gestation ruptures through the tube, aborts out of the end of the tube, or ruptures through a previous uterine scar retaining enough placental function to continue supporting the pregnancy. The reported incidence ranges from 1 per 782 deliveries[45] to 1 per 50,820 deliveries.[39] Recent reports have ranged from 1 per 7095[11] deliveries to 1 per 10,200.[32] Approximately 1 in 70 ectopic pregnancies are abdominal, although this incidence may be higher in regions where early prenatal care is not obtained.[1,11] In advanced extrauterine pregnancies that result from tubal rupture or abortion, the placenta usually involves portions of the

uterus, tubes, ovaries, cul-de-sac, broad ligament, and other pelvic structures. Bilateral ureteral obstruction has even been reported in cases of advanced abdominal pregnancy.[12] In advanced extrauterine pregnancies that result from a rupture of a uterine scar, the placenta might remain completely inside the uterine cavity.[9]

4. *Primary tubal pregnancy:* Most tubal pregnancies rupture in the first trimester. However, King[23] reported on five cases that had advanced to term. All of these were located in the interstitial portion of the tube. Interstitial pregnancies are often incorrectly called cornual pregnancies.

5. *Intraligamentous pregnancy:* This occurs when a tubal pregnancy ruptures into the broad ligament with the pregnancy growing between the anterior and posterior leaves of the broad ligament. The incidence is reported to range from 1 per 49,765 to 1 per 183,900 pregnancies.[3] As the pregnancy progresses, the placenta may erode and invade the sigmoid colon, rectum, vagina, bladder, and anterior abdominal wall. The placenta may form fistulous tracts with these structures. King[23] describes an example with the patient having passed per rectum what she thought was chicken bone. Careful examination revealed that this was a fetal femur. At surgery, the patient was found to have an intraligamentous pregnancy demise that had formed an amniocolic fistula.

6. *Rudimentary horn (cornual) pregnancy:* This type of pregnancy is rare. The reported incidence is 1 per 100,000 pregnancies.[3] It occurs when the pregnancy develops in the noncommunicating horn of a bicornuate uterus. For this to occur, the spermatozoa or the fertilized ovum must migrate transperitoneally. O'Leary[29] reported that only 11% of cornual pregnancies went to term, whereas 89% ruptured before term. Only seven surviving infants have been reported.[3] A recently managed pregnancy of this type at Los Angeles County USC Medical Center occurred in the noncommunicating right horn with its tube and ovary located adjacent to the cecum. This case emphasizes the need for careful exploration when performing laparoscopy or exploratory celiotomy for a suspected ectopic gestation.

The risk for advanced extrauterine gestations depends on the type and site of implantation. Primary abdominal pregnancy is so rare that cases probably represent spontaneous incidents and no significant identifiable risk factors are present. Primary tubal pregnancies, secondary abdominal pregnancies, and intraligamentous pregnancies present similar historic risk factors. A history of salpingitis or prior tubal surgery is an identifiable risk factor.[6,9,11] Low gravidity and long-standing secondary infertility are additional risk factors. These women tend to be older, with an average age of about 30 years.* Primary ovarian pregnancy has risk factors similar to tubal pregnancies in general, except that women with ovarian pregnancies are less likely to have a history of infertility.[16] Obviously, for a rudimentary horn pregnancy to occur, a woman must have a bicornate uterus with a noncommunicating horn.

It should be emphasized that hysterectomy does not preclude the occurrence of an extrauterine pregnancy. Ectopic pregnancies that have occurred years after hysterectomy have been reported.[26,28]

DIAGNOSIS

Much progress has been made in the diagnosis of extrauterine and abdominal pregnancies. The first report of an ectopic pregnancy was made by Albucasis (936-1013), a famous Arabic physician who lived in Cordova, Spain. One of his patients developed an abscess near the umbilicus and started to pass bones from the wound. Realizing that the abdomen does not contain bones, he explored the wound, removed many more bones, and made the diagnosis of ectopic pregnancy. The patient survived. Most ectopic pregnancies were diagnosed in this manner or at autopsy until the late nineteenth century, when reports describing successful delivery of live fetuses with survival of the mother began to appear.[23] The most important contribution to decreasing maternal morbidity and mortality from ectopic pregnancies was early diagnosis and treatment.[3,17] Patients with an ectopic pregnancy that can be treated in the first trimester or early second trimester should have morbidity and mortality rates similar to those of the more common tubal gestation.

Patient history

The history can be helpful in establishing the diagnosis of ectopic pregnancy. King[23] described five stages through which abdominal pregnancies pass:

1. *The symptoms of early pregnancy:* These are similar to the symptoms of a normal pregnancy (e.g., missed menses, morning sickness, breast tenderness).

2. *A phase of threatened or actual rupture*[3,6,13,23,45]*:* King was able to obtain a history of onset of severe low abdominal pain in 6 of 12 patients he reported on. The onset of pain occurred between 6 and 16 weeks' gestation. The patient may have some vaginal bleeding at this time.[23] An excellent example of this stage was recently encountered at the Los Angeles County USC Medical Center. The patient presented 9 weeks after her last normal menstrual period with symptoms of low abdominal pain and vaginal bleeding. She had developed sudden onset of lower abdominal pain 2 weeks earlier and was seen by a physician who told her she had an infection and prescribed antibiotics. She sought further treatment at our facility because her symptoms had not resolved. Her urine pregnancy test was positive, and ultrasonography revealed a fetus with cardiac motion in the left adnexa. At exploratory celiotomy, the patient was found to have a ruptured left fallopian tube with implantation of the

*References 3, 4, 6, 13, 18, 31.

gestational sac on the posterior leaf of the left broad ligament. A left salpingo-oophorectomy was performed, and the patient's postoperative course was uncomplicated. As exemplified by this case, morbidity and mortality can be minimized if operative intervention occurs during these first two phases.

3. *Symptoms of continuation of the pregnancy:* King[23] points out that most patients have sought treatment before this stage occurs. Delke et al.[11] reported that 8 of the 10 patients in their study had care before 16 weeks' gestation. Patients in this phase may complain of abdominal pain and painful fetal movements. They also commonly have nausea and vomiting that persist throughout pregnancy. The patient notes increasing abdominal size as expected with a normal intrauterine pregnancy. Patients with abdominal pregnancies do not experience Braxton Hicks contractions. They may complain that the fetus is unusually high in the abdomen.[3,4,8,9,13,23,31,32,45]

4. *A history of false labor:* King obtained this history in 6 of his 12 patients, with passage of a decidual cast in 5 of the 6. This false labor usually occurs near term, and fetal movements may decrease or cease.[4,8,13,23,45]

5. *Later clinical manifestations:* Should the fetus die, the patient has a decrease in abdominal size, but she may continue to have abdominal pain and gastrointestinal complaints (frequent bowel movements, tenesmus). Eventually, menses returns, and the patient might conceive again.[8,23,45]

Physical Examination

The physical examination can be helpful in making the diagnosis of ectopic pregnancy. It would seem that the fetal parts should be easily palpable in an abdominal pregnancy. However, this is rarely the case. The presence of easily palpable fetal parts should raise one's suspicion about the possibility of an ectopic pregnancy, but the absence of this finding in no way excludes the diagnosis. If a mass is palpable separate from the uterus, ectopic pregnancy should be suspected. The fetus is often in an abnormal presentation. If fetal heart tones are auscultated, they may be unusually loud. If the patient has a fetal demise, the diagnosis of ectopic pregnancy should be considered. The cervix may be unusually high and displaced either laterally or anteriorly. It is usually closed and uneffaced. Historically, patients with intraligamentous pregnancies often form fistulous tracts with the rectum, vagina, bladder, or abdominal wall, through which they pass the fetal bones and tissue.[3,4,6,8,9,11,13,18,23,31,32,45]

Diagnostic Tests

Several tests can aid in the diagnosis of ectopic pregnancy. The patient usually has a positive urine or serum β-human chorionic gonadotropin (β-hCG) unless the fetus has been dead for a long time. About 70% of the patients are anemic.[31] There has been a report of an ectopic pregnancy with maternal serum α-fetoprotein values in a range usually only

seen with hepatomas and endodermal sinus tumors (greater than 20 multiples of the median).[40] The elevated maternal serum α-fetoprotein values seem to correlate with the extent of placental involvement with the abdominal viscera. If the pregnancy is otherwise normal, the amniotic fluid α-fetoprotein is normal.[37] Culdocentesis and paracentesis have been used to diagnose ectopic pregnancies. However, a negative test does not rule out the diagnosis.[18] Measuring the uterine depth with a sound should be avoided. If the diagnosis is incorrect, the membranes may be ruptured with potential harm of the fetus. A case has been reported in which the uterus was perforated into the sac of an abdominal pregnancy with the subsequent development of amnionitis in the pregnancy.[8] Failure of the cervix to dilate in response to oxytocin or prostaglandins is also suggestive of ectopic pregnancy.[3,4,6,11,13,31,32,45]

Historically, several radiographic tests have aided in the diagnosis of ectopic pregnancy. The simplest is the abdominal x-ray study, which Hibbard[18] did not find to be very useful. However, Clark and Guy[9] recommended an anteroposterior view and an upright lateral view. The anteroposterior view might show the maternal bowel intimately associated with the fetus. The pathognomonic x-ray finding for ectopic pregnancy is presence of the fetal skull behind the anterior border of the maternal spine. Hysterosalpingography has been used to confirm the diagnosis of ectopic pregnancy. However, it should be used with great caution and is largely supplanted by ultrasonography.[4,6,8,9,11,13,23,31,32,45]

Ultrasound is extremely valuable in diagnosing extrauterine pregnancy, particularly early in the gestation. The diagnosis becomes more difficult as the pregnancy progresses. Delke et al.[11] reported that of five patients with ectopic pregnancies undergoing ultrasound evaluation, two were misdiagnosed as having intrauterine pregnancies (at 28 weeks and 39 weeks). Important ultrasound findings include (1) a small uterus with minimal internal uterine echoes, (2) the fetal head and body located outside of the uterus, (3) an ectopic placenta, (4) the fetal body and maternal bladder not separated by uterine wall, and (5) the identification of fetal parts close to the maternal abdominal wall (Fig. 60-1).[3,31] Magnetic resonance imaging (MRI) may also prove to be of benefit in diagnosing ectopic pregnancy.[15,38]

Management

There has been much controversy about the optimal management of ectopic pregnancies. First, there has been controversy about the timing of delivery. Should the patient have surgery as soon as the ectopic pregnancy is diagnosed, or should the delivery be delayed if the fetus is close to viability so that its chances for survival are improved? This question may be complicated by the fact that there is a simultaneous intrauterine pregnancy in a patient who has been treated for infertility. This may be her only chance for a successful pregnancy outcome.[2] Additional controversy has focused on the management of the placenta. Should the placenta be removed or left in the abdomen at the time of surgery? If the placenta is left in the abdomen, should the

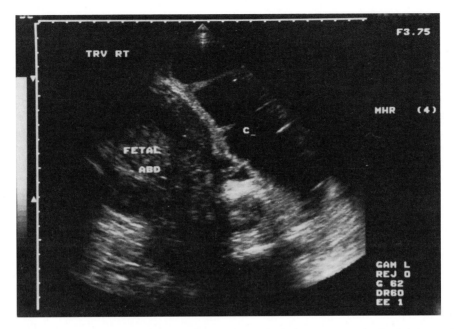

Fig. 60-1 Ultrasound of an abdominal pregnancy, which demonstrates the fetal abdomen in close proximity to the maternal colon *(C)* with no intervening uterus. (Courtesy Richard E. Frates, M.D.)

patient in contemporary practice receive methotrexate to accelerate the resorption of the fetal placenta? These issues may be addressed by reviewing the history of advanced extrauterine pregnancies.

The first successful delivery of an ectopic pregnancy occurred in Sigerhausen, Switzerland, in 1500. Elizabeth Nufer, whose husband Jacob was the local swine-gelder, had been in labor for several days. She was attended by 13 midwives and several lithotomists without success. In an act of desperation, her husband decided to deliver the baby abdominally. After receiving permission from the local magistrate, he placed his wife on a table and after one stroke with his knife delivered a healthy, crying infant. He closed the incision, and Elizabeth recovered. She subsequently had five intrauterine pregnancies, including twins. The first reported successful delivery of an ectopic pregnancy in the United States was in 1759 by a surgeon in New York, Dr. John Bard.[23] In London in 1791, Tumbul was the first to recommend leaving the placenta in situ at the time of surgery for an abdominal pregnancy.[20]

In 1888, Dr. Lawson Tait published his *Lectures on Ectopic Pregnancy and Pelvic Hematocele,* which firmly established surgery as the preferred treatment for ectopic gestations. He was one of the first to recognize the management dilemma of the placenta in advanced ectopic pregnancy and described this as the "crux of the discussion." He left the placenta in situ in three and removed the placenta in two; all patients survived.[23]

The surgical management of an advanced extrauterine gestation is determined somewhat by the type of gestation. Patients with a pregnancy in a rudimentary horn require resection of the horn along with the tube on that side. Obviously, if the fetus is potentially viable, it should be delivered

before resection of the rudimentary horn. Otherwise, it may be left intact to prevent unnecessary blood loss. If the patient does not desire fertility and is hemodynamically stable, a total hysterectomy may be considered. These patients should have an intravenous pyelogram performed postoperatively because of the association of renal anomalies with this condition.[3,31]

Similar recommendations can be made for advanced interstitial pregnancies. If the fetus is viable, it should be removed through a large linear salpingostomy incision before the salpingectomy is performed. Otherwise, the fetus and tube may be removed intact. In the patient who does not desire future fertility, a total abdominal hysterectomy with salpingo-oophorectomy of the involved side is probably the safest procedure. This might be best performed by first performing a salpingo-oophorectomy followed by hysterectomy with the interstitial pregnancy out of the way.

Ovarian pregnancies often are associated with hemoperitoneum at the time of diagnosis because of the vascularity of the ovary. Hallatt[16] reported that 81% of the ovarian pregnancies in his series had more than 500 ml of hemoperitoneum at the time of surgery. Most cases, if diagnosed early, can be treated by performing ovarian wedge resection or ovarian cystectomy.[16] Williams et al.[43] reported on the delivery of a live infant from a term ovarian pregnancy.

Intraligamentous pregnancies are much more likely than ovarian or interstitial pregnancies to progress to term. Paterson and Grant[30] reviewed 48 cases and found that there were 23 live births (with 6 subsequent neonatal deaths). It is unusual to have significant hemoperitoneum with an intraligamentous pregnancy because the pregnancy is confined between the leaves of the broad ligament. Adhesions are often present between the omentum and bowel and the superior aspect of the gestational sac. The placenta is usually not a problem in intraligamentous pregnancies and should be removed at the time of surgery.[3,31] Paterson and Grant[30] reported a single maternal death in their series of 48 cases. This occurred as a result of hemorrhage in a patient whose placenta was not removed. It should be remembered that intraligamentous pregnancies are the most likely to form fistulous tracts between the gestational sac and the rectum, vagina, bladder, or abdominal wall, especially when the demise has been present for some time.[23] In such patients, Gastrografin enemas and cystograms before surgery may identify fistulous tracts to the bladder, rectum, or abdominal wall. These patients also benefit from bowel preparation with laxatives and antibiotics should rectal or sigmoid resection be necessary. Obviously, these recommendations apply only to the patient who is stable before surgery.

Of all advanced extrauterine pregnancies, the abdominal pregnancy is by far the most complex and challenging to manage. It is also the most controversial. The patient is at significant risk for developing massive hemorrhage at the time of surgery and is also at risk for developing hemoperitoneum before delivery. This raises an important management question: Should an abdominal pregnancy be delivered as soon as it is diagnosed, or should delivery be delayed to enhance fetal viability?

If the pregnancy is diagnosed in the first trimester or the early second trimester, surgery should be performed without delay. In more advanced abdominal gestations, with patient consent and willingness to spend the remainder of her pregnancy in the hospital, it is not unreasonable to delay delivery for several reasons: (1) The fetus may achieve relative maturity. (2) The patient can be delivered immediately should bleeding or deterioration occur. (3) There is no evidence that expectant management increases the risk of massive hemorrhage at the time of delivery. In patients who elect expectant management, the physician should obtain serial hemoglobin or hematocrit determinations. There must always be at least 4 units of blood typed and crossmatched. Symptoms of false labor should lead to delivery because false labor historically has often preceded fetal death. Fetal surveillance should be done twice weekly. Amniocentesis has unwittingly been performed in abdominal pregnancies, but the risk of rupture of the gestational sac contraindicates the use of this procedure. Ultrasound dating criteria for fetal maturity are likely to be of questionable value because the fetus' growth is probably retarded. Therefore relative maturity has to be assessed, and the fetus is delivered as deemed maturationally appropriate.

In abdominal pregnancy with a fetal demise, there is also controversy about the timing of delivery. Waiting has been advocated because the placenta is easier to remove at the time of surgery and would less likely be associated with massive hemorrhage. However, massive hemorrhage has been reported as long as 7 years after the demise occurred.[8,20] Therefore delay is probably of little value in such patients. If delay is necessary for any reason, the patient must

be observed in the hospital. Serial hematocrits must be performed, and blood must be immediately available.

In patients presenting initially in shock with evidence of massive hemoperitoneum, surgery must be performed as soon as possible. In elective, planned procedures, the patient should have a bowel preparation with laxatives and antibiotics. Although bowel injury rarely occurs in patients with abdominal pregnancy, when it does, the results can be devastating.[18] All patients should have antibiotic prophylaxis and postoperative therapy because of the significant risk of infection, particularly when the placenta is not removed.

At the time of surgery, adhesions between the gestational sac omentum and abdominal wall are likely to be encountered.[23] Once the infant has been delivered, the surgeon is faced with the next management decision: Should the placenta be removed or left inside the abdomen at the time of delivery? Often, the placenta separates on its own after delivery of the fetus, thus answering the question for the surgeon.[44] A surgeon who decides to remove the placenta should be prepared for massive hemorrhage. If possible, the blood supply to the placenta should be identified and ligated before the placenta is removed. The surgeon should not hesitate to perform salpingo-oophorectomy or even hysterectomy if either is necessary to control the bleeding, particularly if the patient does not desire future fertility. If the blood supply to the placenta involves a loop of bowel, the surgeon should be prepared to resect a portion of the bowel to control the bleeding. Control of bleeding from arteries and veins is vital; however, the surgeon should expect some continued arteriolar and capillary oozing from the placental bed. Many surgeons are uncomfortable enclosing the abdomen without achieving total hemostasis. However, strict hemostasis is often impossible in these patients. Application of coagulation-enhancing agents such as Gelfoam, Avitene, or Surgicel alone or in combination with gauze packing to tamponade the placental bed has been used to control the bleeding.[4,9,18,45] An umbrella packing brought out through the posterior cul-de-sac has not been reported but might be useful for controlling blood loss.

Sandberg and Pelligra[35] reported on the use of the medical antigravity suit or Medical Anti-Shock Trousers (MAST; David Clark Co., Inc., Worcester, Massachusetts) to control hemorrhage in three patients with abdominal pregnancies. Two of the patients underwent surgery at 30 weeks' gestation, and the third patient underwent surgery at about 20 weeks' gestation. In two of the patients, complete spontaneous separation of the placenta occurred at the time of surgery. One of the patients had partial separation of the placenta at the time of surgery. In all three patients, complete hemostasis was not possible at the time of surgery. These patients were placed in a MAST suit at a pressure of 20 to 30 mm Hg. All of the patients showed a dramatic improvement in their hemodynamic status while the MAST suits were in place. Two of the patients remained intubated while the suits were inflated. One of the patients required reexploration to ligate a bleeding artery 2 days later. This emphasizes the importance of initial control of arterial bleeding at the time of surgery because the medical antigravity suit cannot effectively control arterial bleeding once the suit is deflated. Another patient required reexploration 14 days later to remove the placental tissue that had been left behind at the initial surgery. Other complications encountered included adult respiratory distress in one patient, the formation blisters on the thighs of one patient, and the inadvertent ligation of a ureter at the initial surgery that resulted in a subsequent nephrectomy for a nonfunctioning kidney.

If the patient continues to demonstrate evidence of intraperitoneal bleeding after surgery, angiographic arterial embolization can be considered to control hemorrhage. Kivikoski et al.[24] reported on a case in which this was done with satisfactory results. If successful, this procedure may prevent a second celiotomy.

Our opinion supports initial placental removal at the time of surgery. Review of the literature clearly demonstrates that both maternal morbidity and mortality rates are reduced when the placenta is initially removed. Hibbard[18] reported on 23 cases of abdominal pregnancy that occurred at Los Angeles County USC Medical Center. The placenta was left in situ in four of these patients, all of whom developed subsequent significant infections. Only 2 of the remaining 19 patients in whom the placenta was removed developed infections. Furthermore, there was no evidence that leaving the placenta in situ reduced the need for blood replacement. The four patients in whom the placenta was left in situ received an average of 2835 ml (range of 2000 to 5000 ml) of blood. The remaining 19 patients in whom the placenta was removed received an average of 2132 ml (range of 500 to 5000 ml) of blood. The one death occurred in a patient in whom the placenta had implanted into the wall of the rectosigmoid colon. The placenta spontaneously separated at the time of surgery, and a 2-cm perforation of the rectosigmoid colon was identified and repaired. This patient died 4 days later from sepsis caused by overwhelming fecal peritonitis despite antibiotic therapy.

Hreshchyshyn et al.[20] reviewed the world literature and found 101 cases of abdominal pregnancy between 1950 and 1957. The placenta was completely removed in 65 patients and partially removed in another 7 patients. Only 17.5% of these patients required more than 20 days of hospitalization. In the remaining 29 patients, the placenta was left in situ, and 47.5% of these patients required hospitalization for more than 20 days. Most of the patients in whom the placenta was left in situ had symptoms of abdominal pain, intermittent fever, and general malaise for months to years. These patients often required repeat celiotomies to remove the placenta because of hemorrhage, persistent pain, and intermittent partial intestinal obstruction, and to drain abscesses. Two maternal deaths occurred in patients whose placentas were left in situ. A higher mortality rate when the placenta was left in situ had previously been reported. Beacham et al.,[4] in their review of the literature and their personal experience at Charity Hospital in New Orleans, found a higher maternal mortality rate when the placenta was left in situ. The usual causes of death in all patients with

abdominal pregnancies include hemorrhage, sepsis, renal failure, and chronic blood loss.[6]

Although the literature and our opinion suggest initial removal, we cannot say that the placenta should never be left in situ. One can imagine a case of an unstable patient in whom the blood loss expected from attempted removal of the placenta would result in an exsanguination death on the operating table. Obviously, clinical judgment is required on the part of the surgeon to determine whether the patient falls into this category. However, when the placenta is left in situ, it can spontaneously separate postoperatively, resulting in massive hemorrhage. We recommend that when the placenta is left in situ, the placenta should be drained of as much blood as possible and the umbilical cord should be cut at its insertion site into the placenta. Plans should be made to reoperate under stable conditions to remove the placenta to minimize the morbidity anticipated in these patients. Ultrasound and gallium scanning have been used to follow resorption of the placenta when it was left in the abdomen after celiotomy.[5,34,38]

In 1965, Hreshchyshyn et al.[21] reported the first case in which methotrexate was given to a patient in whom the placenta was left in situ after removal of an abdominal pregnancy. The goal was to promote destruction of the trophoblast, resulting in a decrease in life span and vascularity for the placenta. The patient was followed with serial hCG titers until a return to a nonpregnant value was seen. Four months later, the patient was reexplored and the placenta was removed with minimal blood loss. Three more case reports that involved four patients in whom the placenta was left in situ and methotrexate was given followed.[25,36,41] Methotrexate was given to one of these patients even though the hCG titers had returned to a nonpregnant value. It should be stressed that two of these patients were reexplored to remove the placenta; the two not reexplored had palpable masses at the time of examination 1 year after therapy. The value of methotrexate was questioned in one of the reports.[41]

Not all of the reports of methotrexate use have satisfactory outcomes. Rahman et al.[32] in Saudi Arabia reported on 10 cases of abdominal pregnancy. In three of the patients, the placenta was removed. The placenta was partially removed in one patient, and in six the placenta was left in situ. Five of the six were treated with methotrexate. Two of these patients died from sepsis. These authors rightfully questioned the efficacy of methotrexate. Methotrexate does cause myelosuppression and may pose unacceptable risks in patients prone to sepsis.

The literature contains little information about fetal outcome. Perinatal mortality rates as high as 95% have been reported.[4] However, these rates can be deceiving because intervention often occurred as soon as the diagnosis of abdominal pregnancy was made. This resulted in the delivery of many infants who subsequently died from the effects of preterm delivery. Survival rates as high as 50% to 70% are reported when only viable infants are considered. The most thorough discussion of fetal outcome is by Tan and Wee in

Singapore. They evaluated eight cases of abdominal pregnancy that occurred between 1958 and 1968. Three of the fetuses were stillborn. Of the five living infants, one had microcephaly and died at 8 months of age. Three of the infants had deformities, which were believed to be pressure deformities resulting from oligohydramnios. These deformities included talipes equinovarus; webbing of the neck, elbows, and knees; torticollis; and facial asymmetry (Fig. 60-2). The incidence of such deformities has been reported to be about 20% to 40%.[29,31,39] All four of the surviving infants showed normal development.[39]

In cases of demise, the fetus is initially macerated like any other demise. It will gradually become mummified or develop into adipocere (degeneration into a greasy yellow substance). Fetuses retained in the abdomen for years become lithopedions (calcified). King[23] describes three types of lithopedions:

1. Lithotecnon (43%) is calcification of the fetus only.
2. Lithokelyphopedion (31%) is calcification of the fetus, membranes, and placenta.
3. Lithokelyphos (26%) is calcification of the membranes only. The fetus becomes mummified or skeletonized.

In conclusion, the operation for abdominal pregnancies is "still one of the most dangerous which the gynaecologist is called upon to perform."[42] The key to preventing significant maternal morbidity and mortality is early diagnosis and treatment. Patients with advanced abdominal pregnancies may be closely monitored in the hospital until 36 to 38 weeks in an effort to optimize fetal outcome. At the time of surgery, every effort should be made to remove the placenta and control the arterial bleeding. Continued bleeding may respond to treatment with the MAST suit or angiographic embolization. If the placenta is initially left in situ, it should be removed after the patient becomes stable. There is minimal evidence to support actively the use of methotrexate in abdominal pregnancies. Living infants delivered near term can usually be expected to have normal development. There are no easy cookbook recipes for management of advanced extrauterine pregnancies. Sound clinical judgment must be applied to each case.

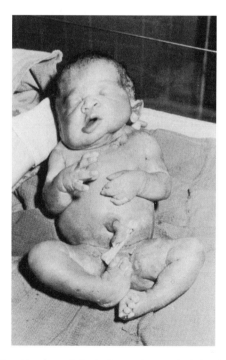

Fig. 60-2 Newborn infant of an advanced abdominal pregnancy. Notice the facial asymmetry and the limb deformities.

REFERENCES

1. Alto W: Is there a greater incidence of abdominal pregnancy in developing countries? Report of four cases, *Med J Aust* 151:412,1989.
2. Bassil S, et al: Advanced heterotopic pregnancy after in-vitro fertilization and embryo transfer, with survival of both babies and the mother, *Hum Reprod* 6:1008, 1991.
3. Bayless RB: Nontubal ectopic pregnancy, *Clin Obstet Gynecol* 30:8l, 1968.
4. Beacham WD, et al: Abdominal pregnancy at Charity Hospital in New Orleans, *Am J Obstet Gynecol* 84:1257, 1962.
5. Belfar HL, Kurtz AB, Wapner RI: Long-term follow-up after removal of an abdominal pregnancy: ultrasound evaluation of the involuting placenta, *J Ultrasound Med* 5:521, 1986.
6. Bendvold E, Raabe N: Abdominal pregnancy: a case report and brief review of the literature, *Acta Obstet Gynecol Scand* 62:377, 1983.
7. Caruso V, Hall WHJ: Primary abdominal pregnancy in the spleen: a case report, *Pathology* 16:93, 1984.
8. Charlewood GP, Culiner A: Advanced extrauterine pregnancy: fifty two cases, *J Obstet Gynaecol Br Emp* 62:555, 1955.
9. Clark JFJ, Guy RS: Abdominal pregnancy, *Am J Obstet Gynecol* 96:511, 1966.
10. Reference deleted in proofs.
11. Delke I, Veridiano NP, Tancer ML: Abdominal pregnancy: review of current management an addition of 10 cases, *Obstet Gynecol* 60:200, 1982.
12. el Kareh A, Beddoe AM, Brown BL: Advanced abdominal pregnancy complicated by bilateral ureteral obstruction: a case report, *J Reprod Med* 38:900, 1993.
13. Foster HW, Moore DT: Abdominal pregnancy: report of 12 cases, *Obstet Gynecol* 30:249, 1967.
14. Friedrich EG Jr, Rin CA Jr: Primary pelvic peritoneal pregnancy, *Obstet Gynecol* 31:649, 1968.
15. Hall JM, et al: Antenatal diagnosis of a late abdominal pregnancy using ultrasound and magnetic resonance imaging: a case report of successful outcome, *Ultrasound Obstet Gynecol* 7:289, 1996.
16. Hallatt JG: Primary ovarian pregnancy: a report of 25 cases, *Am J Obstet Gynecol* 143:55, 1982.
17. Hallatt JG, Grove JA: Abdominal pregnancy: a study of twenty-one consecutive cases, *Am J Obstet Gynecol* 152:444, 1985.
18. Hibbard LT: The management of secondary abdominal pregnancy, *Am J Obstet Gynecol* 74:543, 1957.
19. Hietala SO, Andersson M, Emdin SO: Ectopic pregnancy in the liver: report of a case and angiographic findings, *Acta Chir Scand* 149:633, 1983.
20. Hreshchyshyn MM, Bogen B, Loughran CH: What is the actual present-day management of the placenta in late abdominal pregnancy? Analysis of 101 cases, *Am J Obstet Gynecol* 81:302, 1961.
21. Hreshchyshyn MM, Naples JD, Randall CL: Amethopterin in abdominal pregnancy, *Am J Obstet Gynecol* 93:286, 1965.
22. Huber DE, Martin SD, Orlay G: A case report of splenic pregnancy, *Aust NZ J Surg* 54:81, 1984.

23. King G: Advanced extrauterine pregnancy, *Am J Obstet Gynecol* 67:712, 1954.

24. Kivikoski AL, et al: Angiographic arterial embolization to control hemorrhage in abdominal pregnancy: a case report, *Obstet Gynecol* 71:456, 1988.

25. Lathrop JC, Bowles GE: Methotrexate in abdominal pregnancy: report of a case, *Obstet Gynecol* 32:81, 1968.

26. Metzner I, et al: Abdominal pregnancy following hysterectomy, *Isr J Med Sci* 19:283, 1983.

27. Mitchell RW, Teare AJ: Primary hepatic pregnancy: a case report and review, *S Afr Med J* 65:220, 1984.

28. Niebyl JR: Pregnancy following total hysterectomy, *Am J Obstet Gynecol* 119:512, 1974.

29. O'Leary IL, O'Leary JA: Rudimentary horn pregnancy, *Obstet Gynecol* 22:371, 1963.

30. Paterson WG, Grant KA: Advanced intraligamentous pregnancy: report of a case, review of the literature and a discussion of the biological implications. *Obstet Gynecol Surv* 30:715, 1975.

31. Peterson HB: Extratubal pregnancies: diagnosis and treatment, *J Reprod Med* 31:108, 1986.

32. Rahman MS, et al: Advanced abdominal pregnancy—observations in 10 cases, *Obstet Gynecol* 59:366, 1982.

33. Reddy KSP, Modgill VK: Intraperitoneal bleeding due to primary splenic pregnancy, *Br J Surg* 70:564, 1983.

34. Rettenmaier MA, et al: The use of gallium scanning and determination of human chorionic gonadotropin to evaluate resorption of an abdominal placenta, *Am J Obstet Gynecol* 146:471, 1983.

35. Sandberg EC, Pelligra R: The medical antigravity suit for management of surgically uncontrollable bleeding associated with abdominal pregnancy, *Am J Obstet Gynecol* 146:519, 1983.

36. St. Clair JT, Wheeler DA, Fish SA: Methotrexate in abdominal pregnancy, *JAMA* 208:529, 1969.

37. Shumway JB, et al: Amniotic fluid alpha fetoprotein (AFAFP) and maternal serum alpha fetoprotein (MSAFP) in abdominal pregnancies: correlation with extent and site of placental implantation and clini, *J Matern Fetal Med* 5:120, 1996.

38. Spanta R, et al: Abdominal pregnancy: magnetic resonance identification with ultrasonographic follow-up of placental involution, *Am J Obstet Gynecol* 157:887, 1987.

39. Tan KL, Wee JH: The paediatric aspects of advanced abdominal pregnancy, *J Obstet Gynecol Br Commonw* 76:1021, 1969.

40. Tromans PM, et al: Abdominal pregnancy associated with an extremely elevated serum alphafetoprotein: case report, *Br J Obstet Gynaecol* 91:296, 1984.

41. Weinberg PC, Pauerstein CJ: Methotrexate and the abdominal placenta, *Obstet Gynecol* 33:837, 1969.

42. Williams JW: *Obstetrics,* Norwalk, Conn, 1903, Appleton.

43. Williams PC, Malvar PC, Kraft JR: Term ovarian pregnancy with delivery of a live female infant, *Am J Obstet Gynecol* 142:589, 1982.

44. Yu S, et al: Placental abruption in association with advanced abdominal pregnancy. A case report, *J Reprod Med* 40:731, 1995.

45. Zuspan FP, Quilligan EJ, Rosenblum JM: Abdominal pregnancy, *Am J Obstet Gynecol* 74:259, 1957.

61 Cesarean Section

RAPHAEL DURFEE

Cesarean Section—"That smash and grab raid"!

Lawson Tait

Removal of a child from the body of its mother by an abdominal incision was the first incision of the abdominal wall in history; the only other so-called major surgery from prehistoric and ancient times was trepanation. Early abdominal deliveries were done for religious or mythologic reasons and almost invariably on dead or agonal women. It is possible that the concept of abdominal delivery was introduced by one or both of two means: one, the discovery of a live unborn fetus at the time of animal sacrifice; or, two, the deliberate or accidental evacuation of a human pregnant uterus by a sword of a conqueror. There are some factual records of cesarean section in legal documents, mythologic poems and prose, and written legends of several peoples.

The earliest record of performance of cesarean section in ancient times is from Sumer, where it was reported that the operation was performed on slaves in the second millennium BC. In a cuneiform written tablet, which was a legal document also from Sumer, there was reference to precedence of inheritance. This was to remain with the first child born by normal vaginal delivery rather than by abdominal means. A statement was made that "the child was pulled out," an inference that this was from the abdomen and not the pelvis. There is another illustration from Sumer of a seal on which there are depicted surgical instruments and a figure stated to be a person who delivered children. These artifacts establish the fact that the operation was done earlier than 2000 BC.

The use of cesarean was involved in innumerable problems not all medical. Laws were created to control its use, and medical discussions and confrontations have continued to the present day. The procedure developed very slowly and painfully, and it was not until the later part of the 1700s but especially in the 1800s that its use became accelerated because of the advances in anesthesia, hemostasis, antisepsis, and the application of uterine suture.

In the early to middle 1900s, the operation became acceptable and has been so ever since. The cesarean operation is so widely used today that it may well be a matter of abuse. Modern challenges to 24% to 26% cesarean section rates may bring about an effort to reduce this operative furor!

ORIGIN OF THE TERM: CESAREAN SECTION

"That operation is called Cesarean by which any way is opened for the child than that destined for it by nature" (L. Baudelocque, 1790). *Vaginal cesarean* was not a term preferred by Williams, who stated in 1903 that "vaginal hysterotomy" is correct. The term *cesarean section* should not be applied to a laparotomy for abdominal pregnancy. Confusion about this matter led to false reports of early successful cesarean operations. Many texts that deal with the cesarean section present misinformation about the origin of the term. Etymologists are fascinated with this term because it is a unique word formation. There is a persistent repetition of error by historians who have simply followed their predecessors' statements for information without the authenticity of such material. *Cesarean section* is a phrase that uses two words with similar meanings. This is defined as a pleonasm (or tautology). The derivation of each of these words is complex because of the ancient historic references to the matter.

Pliny, who some refer to as a "lying historian," was in error when he stated that some of the Caesars, Julius in particular, were delivered by an abdominal incision. *"Caesar"* is derived from the Latin verb *caedo*—to cut. Eventually the word *Caesar* was assumed by several Roman emperors and became a synonym for *imperator*—emporer. *Caesus*—cut, from the same Latin root, *caedo*—to cut, may have been the origin of the term *Caesar*. Festus stated that those persons delivered by abdominal incision were called *"caesones."* Isidorus of Seville firmly and erroneously established the relationship between the operation and the person Julius Caesar and referred to such persons as *"Caesares."* According to Pundel, Rousset, author of the first text on the subject, became confused with Pliny's Latin text. de Chauliac and Roesslin both perpetuated the story, and it has been repeated in print as late as March 1985. The myth was preserved in the Middle Ages in many manuscripts in the 1300s in *The Faits des Romains*. The first printed version of *The Twelve Caesars* written in the second century, printed in 1506, and includes a woodblock print that purports to be the first picture of a cesarean section. This is an error (Fig. 61-1) because Aurelia was present at his triumps. This picture also was not repeated in later printings.

More probable origins for this elusive pleonasm are derived from some form of Latin words meaning to cut or to kill. The Latin verb *caedo, caedere, cecidi, caesum* means to cut or to kill. An adverb form *caesium*, from *caedo*, means

1114

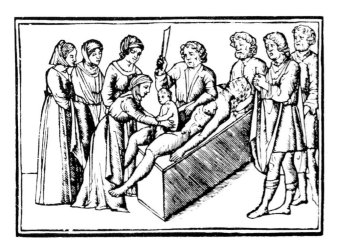

Fig. 61-1   Birth of Caesar. (From Suetonius C: *The Twelve Caesars,* 1506, first printing.)

with cutting. There is no identifiable word *caesones* or *caesares* in Cassell's Latin Dictionary.

Another possibility is that the term arose from the *Lex Regia* or *Lex Caesara* (The King's Law), ascribed to Numa Pompilius in 716 BC.

There is also some confusion about the second part of the phrase, which probably arose from the verb *seco, secare, secui, sectum,* meaning to cut. The noun for this is *sectio* (f).

It is stated that Rousset used "section" in his first book but in the author's copy are the words "enfantement cesarien." Bauhin, about a year later, published Rousset's book, and in the index of that text are listed the following: *Caesarea sectio,* page 163; *Casaream sectione,* page 188; *Caesarei partus,* page 3; and *Partus Caesarei definito,* page 1. Guillemeau in 1598 used the phrase "cesarienne section" thus discrediting the point that this combination was first used by Raynaud in 1737 and as is indicated it was Bauhin who first used the combination.

Modern terminology is an Anglicized version of the French spelling *cesarienne;* thus we are provided with the words cesarean section, which eliminates the confusion over Caesar and this operation for all time.

CESAREAN SECTION FROM 2000 BC TO THE EIGHTEENTH CENTURY

There are few records of the cesarean operation from 120 AD to 1115. Gestein von Gerstadt was delivered by postmortem cesarean in 1115. The earliest confirmed delivery of a living child by the abdominal route was Gorgias of Leontine, Sicily, in 508 BC. Gebhardt, the Bishop of Constance, was delivered in 919 AD; Count Linsgow, known as Ingentius the Abbey of Saint Gall, was delivered in 949. Both were postmortem deliveries of premature infants, and the children were placed in the abdomen of a newly killed pig because the pig fat stayed warm and moist for a longer time than any other animal. These served as excellent rural incubators.

de Castro reported the birth of Sancho Garcia or Mayer of Navarre who was delivered by a brave strong Spanish nobleman when Sancho's mother was killed by the Saracens; he saw the child's arm had protruded through the wound in the mother's abdomen, pulled it free, and it lived and breathed at once. The nobleman educated his little miracle who later became the King of Navarre in the twelfth century.

One of the more controversial royal deliveries concerned Edward VII, son of Henry VIII and Jane Seymour. Because of a failed labor, the king was questioned about whether such an operation should be done because it was usually fatal. He presumably replied, "Proceed, for it is easier to find another wife than a son and heir." There were several songs and ballads about this sung in the pubs and ale houses in London in 1537, which mirrored popular opinion, but apparently was not true.

Cesarean for the Live Woman

The first unquestioned successful cesarean section for a live woman performed by a physician was by Trautmann and Seest in 1610 AD in Wittenberg. From this time the operation was used rarely, but as time passed, its use increased despite high maternal mortality. Cesarean section for the live woman is truly an operation of the late 1800s and the twentieth century. When the first cesarean section was done for a live woman is unknown, unless the statement in the Sushruta Samhita is acceptable. The reference to cesarean section for women slaves in Sumer probably involved live women to ensure live children, otherwise why sacrifice the slave? Reference was made to Hua T'o, a great surgeon in the Han Dynasty in China, who purportedly performed cesarean section in 120 AD. This operation was mentioned again in the Tang Dynasty and was a postmortem procedure.

deLee wrote that in the Talmud, *Kareth Habetan* was the term used for midline delivery postmortem and *Jotze Dophan* was the term used for delivery through a flank incision for live women. In the Misnah of the Talmud, there are several references to cesarean section; the Talmud is not a medical manuscript but rather an interpretation of the rules and customs of human conduct. For many years, the records have been debated by scholarly rabbis, and it is apparent that the operation was performed on both live and dead women. For example, it is stated that a woman who delivered by cesarean section did not have to undergo the postpartum purification rites usually associated with vaginal delivery. These rites were very specific and strictly enforced. If the operation had not been done, there would have been no reason to include it in the Talmud. There are no other reports of the operation for a live woman that can be verified with certainty until about 1500 AD.

The cesarean birth of Julius Caesar caught the fancy of the miniature printers of the 1300s particularly in a text entitled *The Faits des Romains* where there is a print in an edition in the late 1200s of the birth of Caesar that because of the valid date establishes this as the first illustration of cesarean section in the literature. There were several other prints in later editions of *The Faits des Romains* in the 1300s.

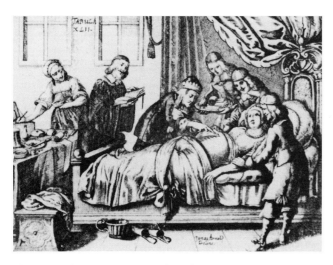

Fig. 61-2 Cesarean section for a live woman. (From *Armamentarium chirururgicum*, Frankfurt, 1666, J Scultetus. In Ricci V: *The development of gynecological surgery and instruments*, Philadelphia, 1949, The Blakiston Co.)

In 1500, there was the famous case of the pig gelder, Nufer, who recorded that he performed a cesarean section for his wife who had an apparent unsolvable labor condition; she and the child survived. This documented operation is the first proven case known to have been successfully done for a live woman not by a physician.

van Roonhuyze, 1663, one of the more famous of the early surgeons who performed operations on women, produced a text that illustrated the technique of cesarean for live women. He illustrated a postmortem laparotomy for a ruptured uterus. Scultetus in 1666 published the first text on this matter in detail (Fig. 61-2), in which he described a cesarean for a live woman.

CLASSICAL, FUNDAL, AND CORPOREAL CESAREAN SECTION

In the eighteenth century the cesarean operation had undergone many influences affecting its use. These varied from absolute forbiddance to use for religious purposes (e.g., baptism of the child as fostered by the strong Christian church). Most physicians involved in obstetric care were strongly opposed to the use of cesarean except in the obviously moribund or recently expired woman. The few who advocated the use of cesarean when the mother was alive and in good condition were severely castigated by their peers but, nevertheless, persisted in their attitude. Of these pioneers, Levret and Baudelocque in France were the leading protagonists for cesarean and each realized that a contracted pelvis beyond a certain reasonable point indicated one of two possibilities for evacuation of the fetus: embryotomy with decapitation or cesarean section. Opinions concerning destruction of a living child in utero were as divided and as vehement as attitudes in contemporary times are about abortion. Severe desperation brought about unusual solutions; one of the most unique was the operation of symphysiotomy

proposed by Sigault in 1768. This procedure, which is still used in modern times in Third World countries, permitted an increase in size of the inner bony pelvis but was accompanied by several risks, one of the worst of which was the compromise in the ability of the patient to walk normally after delivery. There were decades of public and private discussions about these matters, especially in England. However, Hull was a strong advocate of cesarean in uterine rupture and even in cases of abdominal pregnancy if the child was alive. He received some support from Smellie, but in general, the operation was not popular in England. One occurrence in the eighteenth century could have decreased the high mortality of the cesarean operation and that was the introduction of suture placement in the uterine wound by Lebas in 1769. Strangely, this concept was not used for nearly 70 years!

Most of the first cesarean sections in England and America were done by midwives, charlatans, or women themselves. Bennett presumably was the first to do cesarean section in the United States in 1794 in Virginia. King in 1975 disproved the Bennett priority very conclusively and stated unequivocally that the first cesarean section in the United States was done by Richmond in 1827 in Newton, Ohio. In the nineteenth century, obstetrics, gynecology, and general surgery all began to proliferate and prosper because of the solution to the three absolute requirements for successful surgery. These were and still remain: control of bleeding—hemostasis; control of pain—anesthesia; and control of infection—asepsis.

Despite the amazing difference produced by the three solutions to surgical problems, the mortality rate for the cesarean operation was inordinately high. This was not the result as much of the inherent possible fatality of the procedure as of the timing of the operation. The search continued for an improved operation, and one of the first and most dramatic was the postdelivery hysterectomy created by Porro in 1876. The idea for such a procedure was originated by Porro's predecessors and actually a cesarean delivery was followed by a hysterectomy for hemorrhage from myomas by Storer in Boston in 1869. Unfortunately, Storer's patient died; otherwise, he would have had the famous name that accompanies cesarean hysterectomy. There were many additions to the Porro operation, but the fact that it was considered to be a mutilation made it unacceptable to many operators. The last hysterectomy with abdominal exteriorization of the cervical stump after cesarean section was done by Davis in the 1920s in the United States. Modifications of abdominal and uterine incisions were abundant in these years; packs and drains both cervical and through the wounds were also numerous and not very successful. In 1817, Barlow was the second to suture the uterine wound in England. Very few followed this addition except in the United States, where it was often used successfully. The next important contribution to the cesarean operation occurred in 1882.

Uterine suture was a very controversial matter in 1882 when two German surgeons, Kehrer and Sanger, introduced

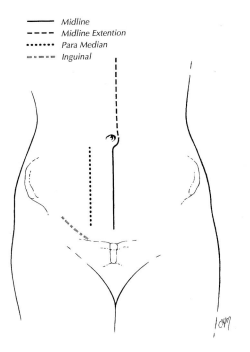

Fig. 61-3 Vertical and oblique abdominal incisions. (Adapted from several illustrations.)

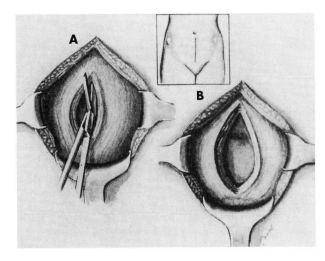

Fig. 61-4 Vertical uterine incision. (From Bonica J: *Principles and practice of obstetric analgesia and anesthesia,* vol 2, Philadelphia, 1967, FA Davis.)

adequate and entirely useful methods for closure of the uterine wound. The Sanger operation closed the uterine fundus, and the Kehrer operation closed a transverse lower uterine segment. If Kehrer had been more aggressive in reporting his procedure, the lower uterine segment operation probably would have been used 40 years before it was recognized. Various modifications of the Sanger closure have been introduced to contemporary times. Management of the abdominal wound is another area in which many modifications have been introduced.

Fundal cesarean has an important but limited use in modern obstetrics. Another procedure closely associated with an incision in the uterine fundus is one used in certain cases of indicated late abortion or early prematurity and is referred to as abdominal hysterotomy.

Another answer to the problem of the high mortality and morbidity of fundal cesarean was to pursue a method of entering the uterine cavity extraperitoneally. These are discussed in the section entitled "Extraperitoneal Cesarean Section." Still another solution was the use of an intraperitoneal lower uterine segment incision.

Fundal or Classical Technique

Fundal cesarean is performed usually with a vertical abdominal incision (Fig. 61-3). The peritoneum is opened vertically, and a vertical incision is made, usually in the upper middle of the anterior uterine fundus. This is done with a scalpel and completed with a blunt-nosed scissors (Fig. 61-4). The delivery is accomplished with the placenta and membranes (Fig. 61-5), the uterine cavity is explored, and the wound is closed with either 2-0 chromic catgut or poly-

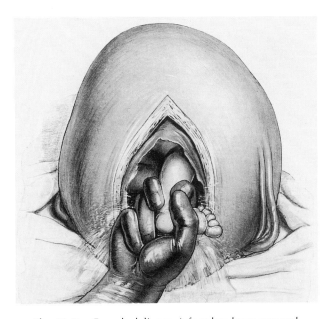

Fig. 61-5 Breech delivery. A foot has been grasped.

glycolic acid suture by the surgeon's choice. A running stitch or interrupted figure-of-eight sutures may be placed in the deep portion of the wound (Fig. 61-6). The endometrial layer should not be included in the suture, and if possible, a two-suture closure of the uterine wall is desirable if the tissues can be well approximated and hemostasis is complete. The serosa may be inverted or closed with a fine 5-0 or 6-0 suture to reduce the number of postoperative adhesions (Fig. 61-7).

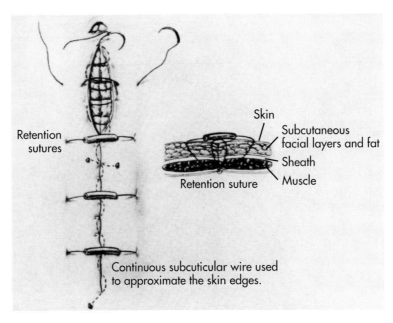

Fig. 61-6 Classical cesarean section: uterine incision closure with retention sutures. (From Riva H: *Clin Obstet Gynecol* 2:954, 1959.)

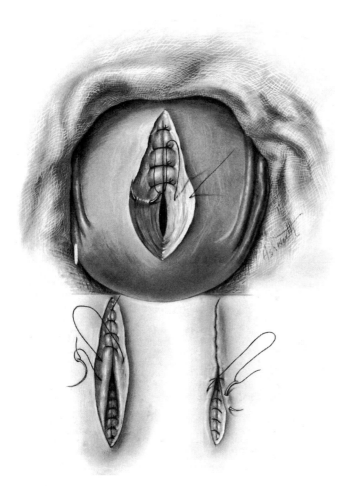

Fig. 61-7 Classical cesarean section: uterine incision closure. Three layers: interrupted; continuous; subserosal or through-and-through.

Fundal cesarean is indicated in most premature births in which the fetus is at risk, all premature abnormal presentations especially breech, in cases of high anterior implantation of the placenta, term gestation transverse presentation with the back anterior or down, in many anomalies such as fused twins, in cases in which an anterior myoma blocks the low uterine segment, and in cases of extreme emergency when time is all important and the delivery must be accomplished as soon as possible. Fundal cesarean should probably be repeated if a second or more pregnancies ensue, but a low-segment operation has been suggested. Vaginal delivery in a subsequent pregnancy is a controversial point; if certain prerequisites are present, normal onset of labor may be carefully followed and, if the previous indication is absent, the presentation is vertex, and labor progress rapidly, then normal vaginal delivery can be accomplished. The risk of uterine rupture, however, is higher than with the low-segment operation, and many are of the opinion that labor should not be induced in these patients.

More blood may be lost with a fundal cesarean, hemostasis may be difficult, and the wound may be difficult to close (Fig. 61-8). Regional anesthesia probably cannot be used, and the uterus should be eventrated postdelivery to facilitate wound closure.

Abdominal hysterotomy has a limited use, but it should be used for indicated late abortion when vaginal delivery is impossible. The procedure is a miniclassical operation and is best conducted under general anesthesia. A vertical incision is usually made, but a high transverse incision can be made in the interest of aesthetics. The uterine incision is vertical but can be lower than for fundal cesarean. Management is much the same, but usually the patient can be dismissed early (Figs. 61-9 and 61-10).

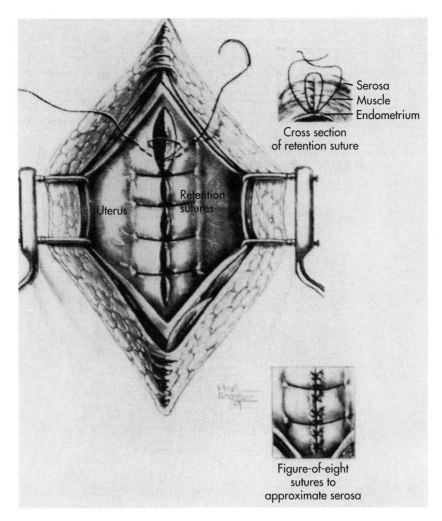

Cross section
of retention suture

Figure-of-eight
sutures to
approximate serosa

Fig. 61-8 Classical cesarean section: abdominal incision closure with retention sutures. (From Riva H: *Clin Obstet Gynecol* 2:954, 1959.)

LOW-SEGMENT CESAREAN SECTION

Not until 1805 was there any reference to a low uterine approach for delivery; deLee gives Osiander credit for being the originator of the low-segment cesarean. Osiander decided that there were many advantages to making an incision in the dependent portion of the uterus and performed such an operation, according to deLee, in 1915.

Kehrer outlined and illustrated the technique for low-segment cesarean section with a plan for closure of the uterine wound in 1882. Pfannenstiel failed in 1908 to perform an extraperitoneal dissection; he then cut the uterine serosa as in hysterectomy, advanced the bladder downward, entered the low portion of the uterus, and successfully delivered a child. He resurrected the transperitoneal, easy low uterine segment cesarean section in this manner. By 1912, he reported 33 cases with only 1 maternal death. In 1911, Opitz used a vertical abdominal incision, dissected the uterine serosa, used a vertical low-segment incision, and closed the serosa carefully over the sutured uterine incision. A year later, Kronig introduced another precursor to the modern operation: he raised the bladder serosa high over the tip of

the closed vertical uterine incision, which theoretically sealed the uterine cavity completely. However, a failed procedure done in this manner that resulted in mortality from peritonitis induced Beck and deLee in 1919 to perform what came to be known as a "two-flap" closure for low-segment operations.

de Lee and Cornell reported on 145 cases in 1922 with remarkable results. The procedure became popular in England where St. G. Wilson in 1931 proposed the use of a *transverse incision* in the low uterine wall and declared that this brought about a return to a single-flap closure of the uterine wound and furthermore the entire incision was in the lowest part of the uterus or even in the dilated cervix. This was the first known transverse uterine incision since Kehrer. Wilson was supported in his contention by Kerr who curved the incision downward for some time but eventually curved it upward as did all his colleagues.

There are several small detailed modifications of this operation, but only one is of true importance. It is now recognized that peritoneal cuts or separations heal from inside the area, which eliminates the serosal closure after low-

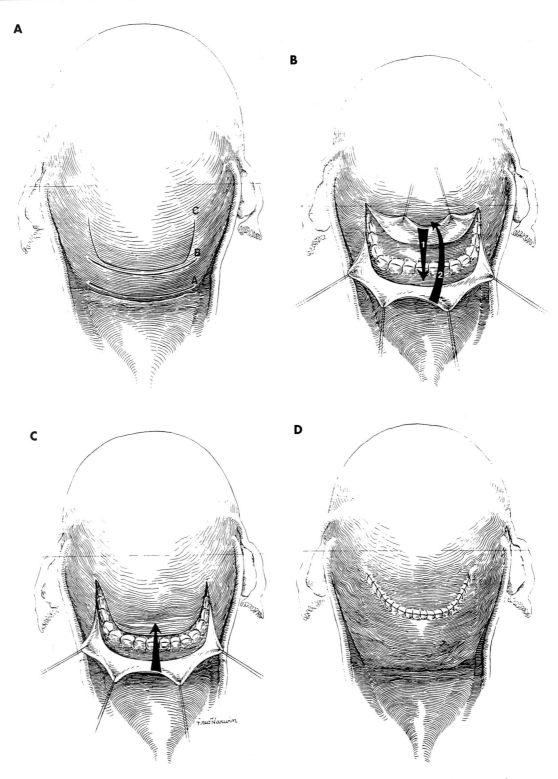

Fig. 61-9 "Low classical" cesarean. **A,** *A* and *B,* Two possible incisions are too low. *C,* In the lower third of uterine fundus, a modified Bailey incision. **B,** Fundal incision, serosal closure: *1,* upper serosal flap; *2,* lower serosal flap. **C,** Serosal flaps for suture. **D,** Serosal suture closure. (From Durfee R: *Obstet Gynecol Surv* 21:210, 1970.)

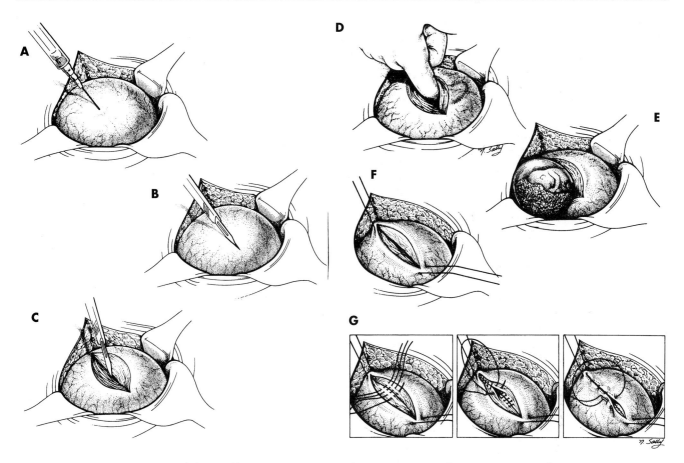

Fig. 61-10   Abdominal hysterotomy. **A,** Serosal injection. **B,** Initial incision. **C,** Second incision. **D,** Finger dissection of placenta. **E,** Evacuation of pregnancy. **F,** Traction sutures for closure. **G,** Three-step uterine incision closure. (From Quilligan and Zuspan: *Douglas-Stromme operative obstetrics,* Norwalk, Conn, 1982, Appleton-Century-Crofts.)

segment cesarean. This means that the bladder will not be used to cover the surgical area but will remain in its normal anatomic area. This should prevent dense adhesion formation between the bladder and the anterior uterine wall and help eliminate that problem at the time of hysterectomy at a later date.

Modern technique for this operation appears below. Preoperative management of an elective low-segment operation is fairly simple.

Cesarean Section and Human Immunodeficiency Virus

One very important and difficult matter is the problem of how to manage the prenatal care and ultimate delivery of the fetus exposed to human immunodeficiency virus (HIV) through its mother. Some, but not all fetuses are infected in utero and several are protected by the placenta enhanced by modern drug combinations. There is considerable limitation as to what drugs may be used in this situation because of undesirable effects of the chemicals on the developing embryo. The method of delivery may well expose the infant to the HIV-positive maternal blood, and this may be especially so at the time of cesarean section.

In reports from various sources in 1994 and later, the use of zidovudine during pregnancy and delivery apparently reduced the number of transmissions of HIV type I from mother to fetus. Exposure to maternal fluids, especially blood, however, always puts the fetus at risk. To reduce this contact at cesarean, a technique for reduction of blood loss at the time of the operation has been devised by Towers et al. This is referred to as a "bloodless cesarean." Here is a summary of the technique for this interesting procedure. An abdominal incision is made, and all blood vessels are carefully occluded; the area is rinsed with sterile saline so that the wound is dry and free of any blood. The area is redraped with fresh uncontaminated materials, and the surgeon's gloves are cleaned with a soap solution or better yet are changed. The uterine incision is made without rupture of the membranes, which are then stripped back from the wound edges at which time Allis clamps are placed on the wound edges for traction and an Auto Suture Poly CS-57 stapling device is used to close both wound edges tightly. This results in a hemostatic incision line. The child is then delivered with membranes intact as far as possible; the newborn and the field are continuously washed with sterile warm saline solution so that no blood of any kind comes in contact with the baby. Once the child is delivered, he or she is immediately bathed with warm Hibiclens soap solution and passed to the attending pediatrician who completes the cleansing process.

Further use of this unusual procedure should decide its value in the prevention of newborn HIV infection.

Surgical Technique for Cesarean Section

Low uterine segment (LUS) cesarean section is the most frequently used operation for abdominal delivery in contemporary obstetrics. The usual preoperative preparations are made with attention to any unusual details. The patient's position must not be supine and is best shifted approximately 15 degrees to the left; this is easily accomplished by the use of one or more towels under the buttocks on the opposite side. A catheter should be placed in the bladder, and the fluid should be emptied; the catheter is left in situ. Bath towels are frequently placed bilaterally along the lower body to absorb any overflow of amniotic fluid or blood. An adherent plastic drape is often used to help keep the operative field dry. When the peritoneum has been opened, large laparotomy sponges may be placed along the uterine adnexal gutters to prevent spill of uterine contents into the peritoneal cavity.

Transverse abdominal incisions began to be used in the early 1900s. Anatomic studies of the muscle orientation in the uterine body, the low uterine segment, and the cervix by Goerttler (Fig. 61-11) provided information for the evolution of transverse incisions in the low uterine segment or the completely dilated cervix.

A high straight transverse abdominal incision was inherited from the past but was not adaptable to the LUS operation (Fig. 61-12). In 1881, Bardenhaer described a wide curved lower abdominal incision in which the rectus muscles were transected after ligation of the inferior hypo-

gastric vessels to provide maximal exposure of the lower abdomen and pelvis. Maylard modified this extensive transverse incision by reduction of its length and also transected the rectus muscles. Pfannenstiel changed the location of the incision, slightly altered the curve, dissected the abdominal fascia from the anterior recti in both directions, retracted the muscles with Fritsch abdominal retractors, and did not transect the muscle. Cherney further modified these incisions by excision of the rectus muscles at the insertion of the conjoined tendon on the superior aspect of the pubic symphysis. Various incisions for the lower uterine area have been proposed (Fig. 61-13). Each of these was used for specific purposes and to adapt to different situations such as available space for delivery of the child, the presence of large aberrant vessels, and a large or several undiagnosed myomas. A scar from previous surgery, either abdominal or uterine, is almost always excised. Most transverse incisions

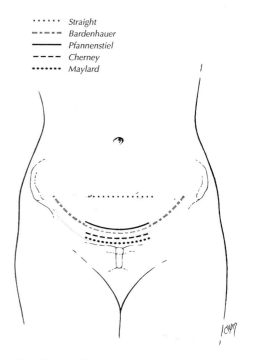

Fig. 61-12   Transverse abdominal incisions.

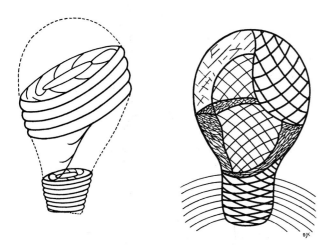

Fig. 61-11   Diagrammatic representation of muscle arrangement in the uterus and cervix. (From Goettler. In Marshall CM: *Cesarean section: lower segment operation,* London, 1939, John Wright & Sons, Bristol & Simpkin Marshall.)

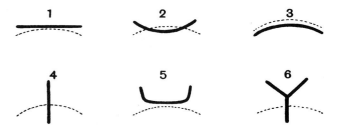

Fig. 61-13   Some incisions shown in relation to the uterovesical reflection of peritoneum. *1,* Doerfler; *2,* type used by many, including the author; *3,* Munro Kerr's incision; *4,* vertical incision; *5,* Bailey's "trapdoor" incision; *6,* Drüner's incision. (From Marshall CM: *Cesarean section: lower segment operation,* London, 1939, John Wright & Sons, Bristol & Simpkin Marshall.)

are made when the fetal pole is vertical; vertical incisions are made for premature breech, for patients with an unformed lower uterine segment or a contraction ring, and for hysterotomy (Fig. 61-14).

Care must be taken with use of a transverse incision not to extend the cut into the lateral uterine vessels. The incision can be made with a scalpel (Fig. 61-15) followed by bilateral extension with finger traction (Fig. 61-16). The incision can also be made with a blunt-nosed scissors, but one must

be sure not to cut too far laterally. Figure-of-eight sutures can be placed at both ends of the incision, but it is easy to perforate a vessel with a needle. A clamp can be used bilaterally to limit the extent of the incision as well. If more space is needed, the incision can be converted into a partial vertical extension. It is better to convert the incision into a form of "trap door" with vertical extensions bilaterally (Fig. 61-17, *A*) or with a single laterally placed vertical J-shaped incision on one side or the other. A single central incision

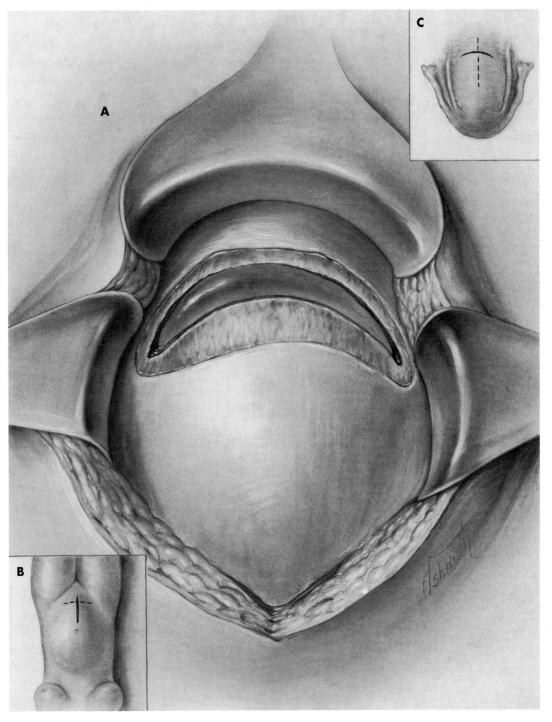

Fig. 61-14   **A,** Transverse incision for low uterine segment cesarean section. **B,** Indicates vertical incision. **C,** Two abdominal incisions.

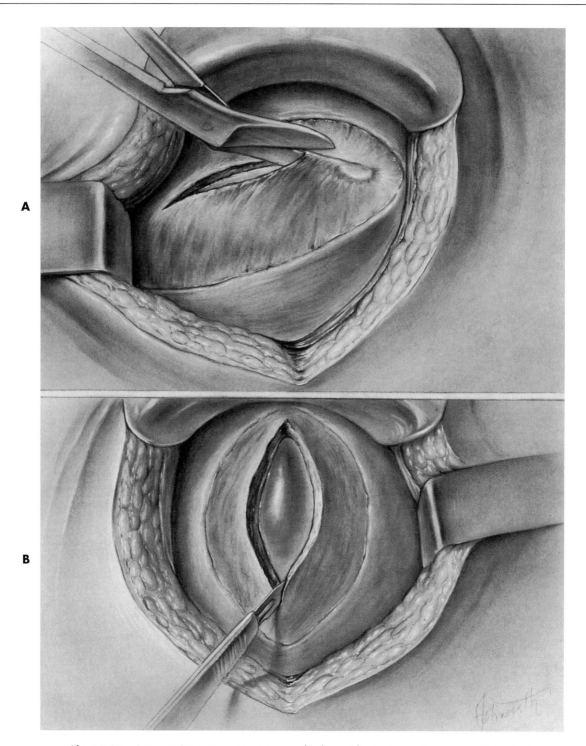

Fig. 61-15   Low uterine segment incision methods. **A,** Blunt scissors, transverse. **B,** Scalpel, vertical.

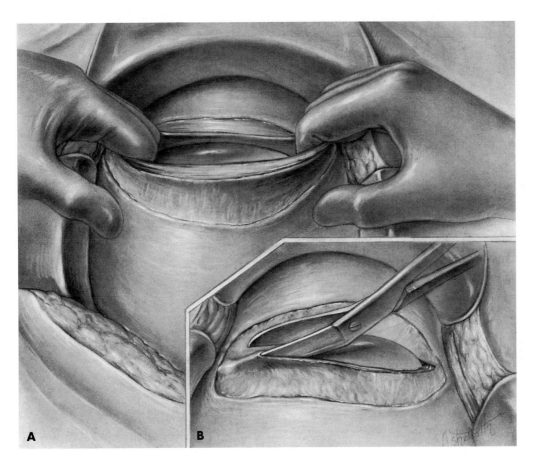

Fig. 61-16 Low uterine segment transverse incision extension. **A,** With finger traction. **B,** With blunt scissors.

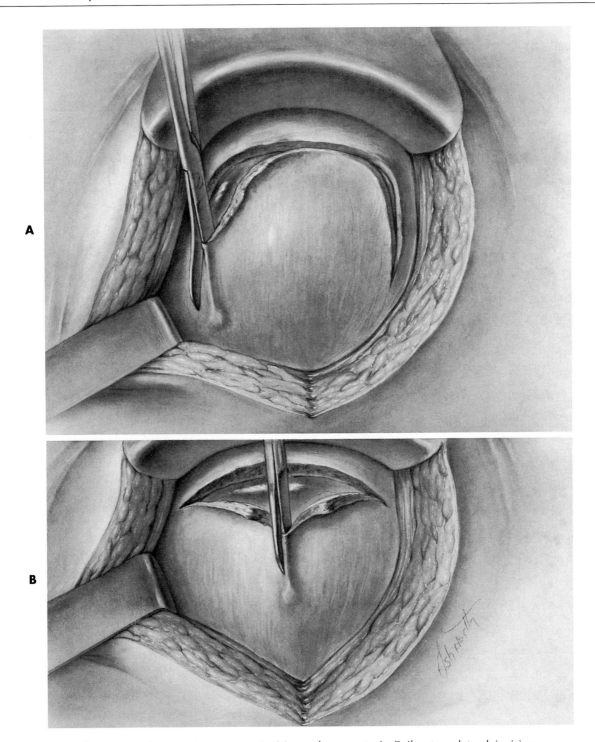

Fig. 61-17 Low uterine segment incision enlargement. **A,** Bailey type lateral incisions. **B,** Vertical or "T" extension.

cephalad toward the fundus may be made (see Fig. 61-17, *B*). This T-shaped incision does not heal as readily as the trap door or J type of extension because of the nature of the wound edges. A vertical incision or extension should not enter either the fundus or the vagina if at all possible. A fundal extension may compromise the possibility for vaginal delivery at a later date. An extremely rapid delivery can be accomplished with a good transverse incision and may readily avoid a fundal delivery. All areas of blood loss are

clamped but not ligated until after the delivery just as in the case of a fundal incision made for the same reason, speed.

Regardless of the type of transverse low-segment incision that has been selected, it is ordinarily retrovesical. The vesical plica is dissected with the uterine and bladder serosa, and the bladder is directed downward. This is a simple but very important move and may only be complicated by dense adhesions between the posterior bladder wall and the anterior low uterine segment wall. These are usually from a pre-

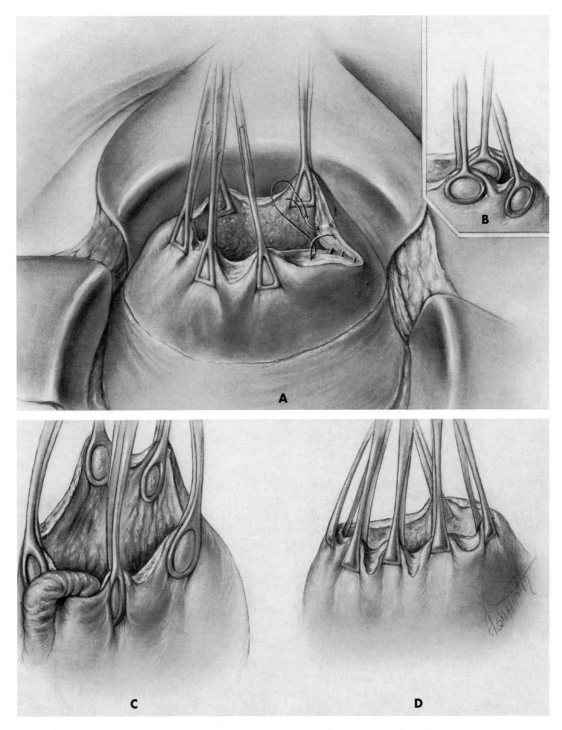

Fig. 61-18 Various instruments for traction on uterine wound edges for suture closure. **A,** Pennington clamps. **B,** Oval clamps. **C,** Long ring forceps. **D,** Long Allis forceps.

vious cesarean. If this is exceptionally difficult, a layer of so-called uterine fascia may be available and the dissection can be performed under this layer, which permits mobilization of the tissues. Care must be taken not to split or thin the bladder muscle and, of course, not to perforate the vesical mucosa. If this should occur, it should be repaired immediately if there is no reason for immediate delivery. Sharp dissection may be effective, but the curved portion of the scissors must face the uterine tissues.

When the uterine tissue is thin, incision of the fetus is possible and should be guarded against. If there is a considerable wide, thin scar, this can be excised at the time of uterine closure. The edges of the uterine wound can be held with any one of four or five kinds of clamps (Fig. 61-18), many of which have been made for this purpose. Ring clamps in the corners of the uterine wound may prevent blood loss. The membranes are ruptured if intact, and delivery is accomplished. The uterus may be eventrated at this point to make it easier to close the wound or massage the uterine body if it is not contracted from previous medication. The wound edges can be trimmed at this point, if, as noted previously, there is excessive scar tissue or if there has been a silent rupture or division of the previous scar.

Delivery of a Child from a Uterine Incision

Neurophysiologists are convinced that each human brain comes with a given number of nerve cells that are never replaced nor do they heal if injured. If these irreplaceable cells are damaged in a vulnerable portion of the brain, they are gone forever. Everyone who takes a child out of the uterus through an incision must remember that fact. If the performance of a cesarean operation is done to preserve the baby's brain as opposed to a traumatic vaginal delivery or because of an obstetric accident, the care with which the child's body and especially its brain are removed from the uterus must be absolute. There is no excuse for trauma to a child in cesarean section delivery—*none!* Methods for such delivery need to be reviewed and analyzed constantly to improve the results of cesarean delivery. If a child's brain, spine, clavicles, abdominal contents, or limbs are damaged by inept delivery through uterine and abdominal incisions, the operator is absolutely liable for the consequences.

There are several methods for cesarean delivery. It is common to place a finger in the child's mouth, turn the face into the wound (Fig. 61-19), and deliver the head by gentle flexion over the bottom of the wound. It is frequently helpful to pass two fingers of each hand bilaterally along the sides of the head (Fig. 61-20). A simple and safe method is to apply carefully a forceps that has been specially made for this purpose to the proper area of the fetal head (Fig. 61-21), then use gentle traction. If the fit of the instrument is too tight or the traction too difficult, the incisions should be enlarged as needed. Vacuum traction is a viable alternative to forceps. The head may be guided into the incision by a scalp forceps as suggested by Kustner. A vectis may be applied carefully using one blade of a small fenestrated forceps or a Murless type or Torpin blade. Occasionally, bilateral gentle pressure from above on the mother's flanks may facilitate removal of the head, but it should *never* be done with the aftercoming head of a breech.

Delivery of a breech at cesarean requires equal or more skill than a vaginal delivery; this is even more important when dealing with a premature breech presentation. Both incisions may be made a little larger in the beginning when one knows that a breech is presenting; a vertical incision may be especially advantageous with a premature frank breech or a transverse presentation. Conversion of frank breech to a single footling requires intrauterine manipulation, which can frequently be easier than when attempted vaginally. All traction must be very gentle. There should be absolutely *no twisting of the spine at any time.* Each arm must be delivered without force, traction, or direct pressure. The aftercoming head must be managed under complete control; it is especially important not to allow a sudden expulsion of the head through the wound because such sudden

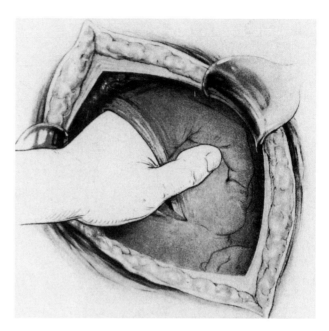

Fig. 61-19 Finger to mouth maneuver to change position of the fetal head. (From Doderlein A: *Doderlein-Kronig operative gynakologie,* Leipzig, 1924, Georg Thieme.)

decompression produces trauma to the base of the brain. Very careful use of small forceps with the aftercoming head may be most helpful but requires experience and skill. Pressure must *never* be put on the aftercoming head from above because of the danger of herniation of brain tissue through the foramen!

Delivery of an impacted presenting part may prove to be difficult and can damage the fetus. A molded, tightly impacted head deep in the pelvis, as seen after a long, difficult labor, sometimes requires vaginal assistance (Fig. 61-22). Two suggestions to solve the problem are: relief of the impaction before the cesarean, or simultaneous relief of the impaction from above and below at the time of the cesarean. Such manipulations must be unusually gentle because of the increased vulnerability of the fetal head and risk of trauma to the maternal soft tissues. Larger than usual incisions are mandatory in complicated cases. If transverse abdominal incisions are used, those designed by Bardenhauer, Maylard, or Cherney should be considered.

In cases of impacted shoulder and arm especially with the back down, a long vertical incision is the best to allow for unusual intrauterine manipulation. If the vertical abdominal incision is made long enough, total uterine eventration may be used to complete difficult intrauterine manipulation for delivery. Fortunately, these situations are extremely rare.

Another situation that may require vaginal assistance is the upward pressure against a fetal part to hold it out of the pelvis in a case of prolapsed umbilical cord. If the membranes have not been ruptured, this may not be as important.

After a child has been delivered, mucus and fluids are aspirated by a bulb syringe or a deLee trap, the cord is doubly clamped and divided on the mother's abdomen, and blood specimens are taken. If contamination is suspected, the cord

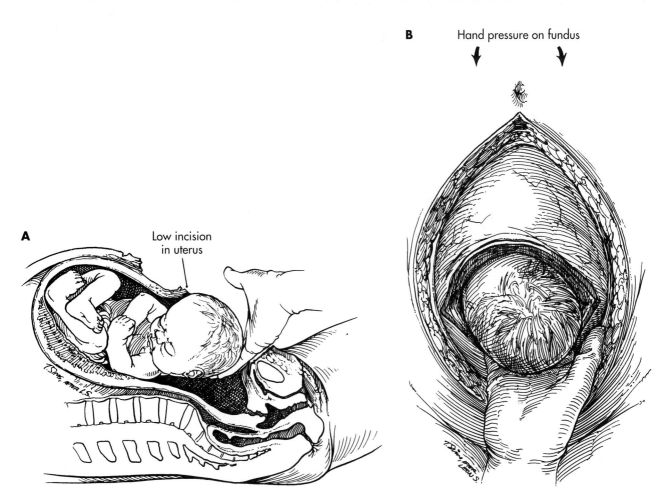

Fig. 61-20 Manual delivery of fetal head at LUS cesarean section. **A,** Lateral view. **B,** Anterior view. (From Pritchard J, MacDonald P, Gent N: *Williams' obstetrics,* ed 17, Norwalk, Conn, 1985, Appleton-Century-Crofts.)

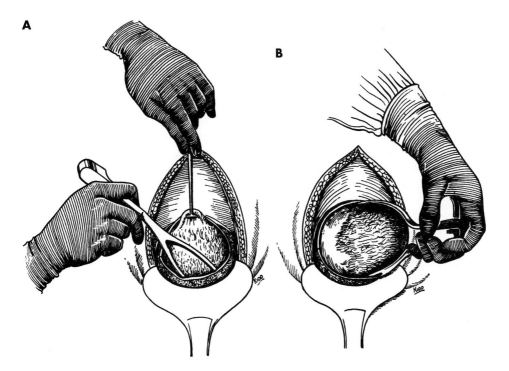

Fig. 61-21 Forceps delivery at LUS cesarean section. **A,** Scalp forceps and application of Obs forceps. Single blade can be used as a vectis. **B,** Forceps application to transverse fetal head position. (From Marshall CM: *Cesarean section: lower segment operation,* London, 1939, John Wright & Sons, Bristol & Simpkin Marshall.)

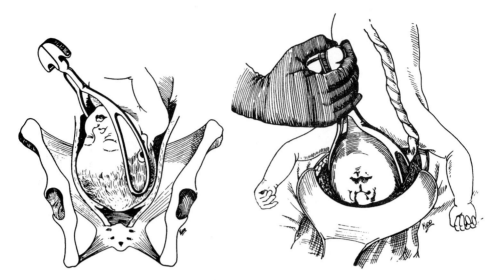

Fig. 61-22 Forceps application to impacted fetal head at LUS cesarean section. (From Marshall CM: *Cesarean section: lower segment operation,* London, 1939, John Wright & Sons, Bristol & Simpkin Marshall.)

can be divided 6 inches from the fetal abdomen before the child is passed to the receiving team; the placental side of the cord is left inside the uterus. This is a moot point in modern obstetrics because of the efficiency of antibiotics in cases of potential or actual infection. The infant's introduction to the mother is done when expedient, and when she is awake. Oxytocin has been given in the intravenous (IV) system by this time, and the placenta is delivered, not by traction on the cord but usually manually with gentleness. The uterine cavity is inspected to be sure all the placental tissues have been removed. At this time, any areas of blood loss are clamped. In cases in which the cervix is tightly closed, a long, curved forceps can be passed through the cervical canal to allow for drainage later; suggestions have been made that a small drain or wick be placed in this area to be removed vaginally 12 hours later. There is no longer any mention of the use of a de Lee shuttle for this purpose.

If cesarean section hysterectomy is contemplated in a grave emergency, the uterine vessels are bilaterally clamped, cut, and tied. The adnexal structures and ligaments are all clamped but not ligated, and the body of the uterus may be easily removed by extension of the transverse incision around posteriorly, which quickly removes the uterine tissue mass; this allows the surgeon to proceed with the removal of the cervix and ligation of the various pedicles with much more space and better visualization of the pelvis. This procedure is especially helpful if there has been massive hemorrhage or abruptio placenta, where speed in removal of the uterine body facilitates hemostasis. Identification of the ureters and bladder is much more accurate as is location of the cervix and vagina, which can be difficult if the cervix has been completely dilated for some time. Ligation of all the pedicles is also much more accurate and without pressure to hurry unnecessarily.

Suture of the Uterine Incision

Suture closure of the uterine incision is a matter of some controversy. Alternatives are as follows:

1. Close the angles of the wound bilaterally with a single figure-of-eight suture of 2-0 polyglycolic or 0 chromic catgut. Follow with interrupted sutures of either material to close the myometrial layer; avoid the endometrial cavity and use a minimal amount of suture material to accomplish the closure. Or follow with a continuous suture of either material, and avoid the endometrial cavity but not with a locked stitch unless there is unusual blood loss, as may be the case if there has been some form of placenta previa. In this instance, interrupted figure-of-eight sutures may produce the best hemostasis without as much potential for tissue necrosis as with locked stitch.

2. Close the entire incision with a continuous or locked stitch of either 2-0 polyglycolic material or 0 chromic catgut. Avoid the endometrial cavity and keep the suture placements even, with traction that is neither too tight nor too loose. Make only one needle placement each time.

3. A second closure of superficial uterine tissues, not the serosa, may be performed at this time. This may be more indicated in elective cesarean section in which there has been no dilation of the cervix than in cases in which the reverse is true, because in the latter the tissues may be very thin and a single closure will suffice. Hemostasis is one of the important points, and this may be accomplished with a single figure-of-eight suture as indicated.

4. No second closure is indicated if the first is properly done, with the exception of the rare figure-of-eight suture for bleeding.

5. The serosa may not be closed at all (Fig. 61-23).

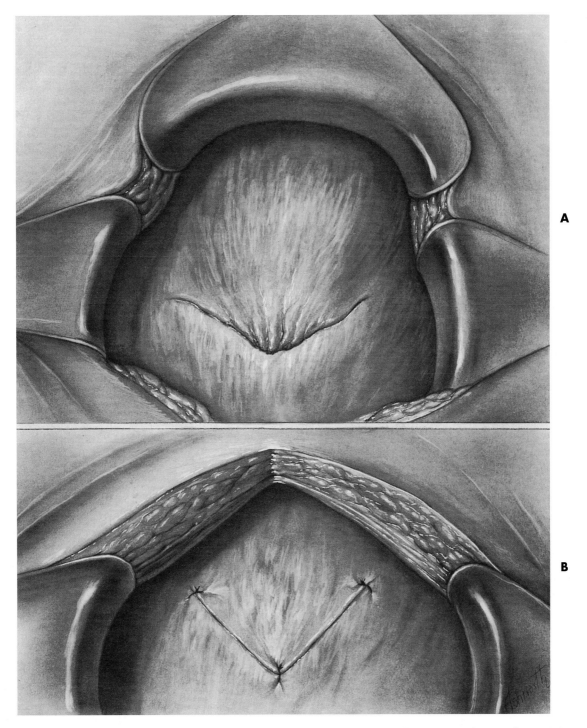

Fig. 61-23   **A,** Nonsutured serosal flap over sutured incision. **B,** Three-suture closure of serosa.

6. The serosa may be sutured above the closed incision line with three interrupted sutures of 4-0 polyglycolic material or 3-0 chromic catgut. The intent of these alternative methods is to prevent the formation of an undue amount of scar between the bladder and the lower uterine segment, which might seriously compromise either vaginal or abdominal hysterectomy at a later date.

7. Close the serosa, avoid the bladder, and use a fine continuous suture carefully applied to seal the uterine suture line to prevent drainage from the uterus into the peritoneal cavity; this is particularly true in patients with gross or potential severe intrauterine infection.

If eventrated, the uterus is returned to the pelvic cavity; the uterus should be kept moist at all times while it is external to the abdominal cavity.

In the past 4 or 5 years, there has been increased interest in a single-suture closure of the LUS wound after cesarean section. This use is limited by the anatomic site and the presence of increased vasculature, extension into lateral blood vessels, and hemorrhage. Suture material has varied from 1 chromic catgut to 0 or 2-0 Dexon or other suture materials. The use of large catgut or perhaps any catgut is archaic. Locked stitches or numerous single or figure-of-eight sutures except in rare instances for hemostasis or when placed laterally to ligate large vessels are not good technique.

Certain provisions for single suture apply. The LUS incision should be transverse and within the lateral uterine blood vessels. With vertical incisions the thickness of the uterine muscle is often irregular, and these generally are not adaptable to single-suture closure. There should not be an anterior placental lie.

There is also continued promotion of nonsuture closure of either the visceral uterine or the parietal peritoneum in uncomplicated cases where no infection is present. Because closure of both these tissues has been the method of choice for so many years, acceptance of new procedures may be in doubt for some time. Closure of the uterine peritoneum in the presence of actual or predicted uterine infection with enough fine suture to seal the area superficially is a method of choice. Such suture must be placed with a minimum of involvement of the underlying uterine muscle. Great care with this suture placement prevents the formation of a kind of fistulous tract with the infected endometrium so there is no direct access to the peritoneal cavity.

Laparoscopic examination or direct observation with a second entrance to the abdominal cavity often indicates excellently healed peritoneal wounds with no or minimum adhesions. It is clear that the presence of suture material in the peritoneal tissues for approximation actually may inhibit proper healing.

Comparison of Two Techniques for Cesarean Section

One difference in methods of performing cesarean section is the manner of entrance into the abdominal cavity and the uterus. The advantage of the Joel-Cohen technique is a more rapid incision for entry followed by no peritonization of the uterus or closure of the parietal peritoneum. The standard transverse lower abdominal and uterine incisions with the usual uterine closure and peritonization of uterine serosa and parietal tissues with polyglactin 2-0 suture result in longer operation times. This difference results in a shorter postoperative stay with the first technique and fewer wound infections. Otherwise, there is no difference in other possible complications of the two techniques. Even patients undergoing the standard operation without peritonization have a shortened postoperative stay. It would appear from several reviews of the literature about not closing either the visceral or parietal peritoneum that this produces some advantages. However, there are some situations that require peritoneal closure to prevent possible severe problems.

Closure of the Abdominal Wound

The abdominal wound is closed by the surgeon's choice. Some do not close the parietal peritoneum. The fascia is closed with a continuous suture of 2-0 polyglycolic material. The subcutaneous tissue may be closed with one or two interrupted sutures if the area is unusually thick; otherwise, the skin is closed with surgical clips or a fine subcuticular polyglycolic suture. Drains may be placed in the presence of obvious infection, and the wound is closed with interrupted sutures in the skin; in some rare cases, the abdominal wound may be left open down to the closed parietal peritoneum.

Results

This operation has been modified many times in small details, and these are merely a matter of choice. The basic procedure is as outlined. Low-segment cesarean is a very efficient successful procedure with minimal postoperative problems and can be repeated several times. Rupture of the scar is not common, and when it occurs, there is usually no hemorrhage and often there is no pain. The size of the rupture may vary from 1 to 2 cm to the entire length, but rarely is the fetus found in the abdominal cavity. These weakened tissues have been dissected free at the ends of the operation, and freshened edges have been approximated with no repetition of the rupture at a later pregnancy. It is hoped that by avoiding the use of suture to cover the area of the uterine incision with serosa, scar formation between the bladder and anterior uterine wall may not occur.

Postoperative Management

Postoperative care after a simple, uncomplicated cesarean section is usually not difficult. The patient is taken to a post-surgical care unit where she is carefully monitored for at least 4 to 6 hours. Observation is made of fundal height, respiratory activity, blood pressure, and any possible evidence of hemorrhage. In modern obstetrics, pain control is frequently accomplished by repeated doses of the regional anesthetic that was used for the operation. Another method is the use of epidural or intrathecal Fentyl or another drug of choice. When this is no longer used, pain control is usually accomplished with parenteral opiates, which often are not needed, or by oral medications such as aspirin or acetaminophen and codeine or the synthetic codeines such as Percocet. When possible, the doses should be minimal and frequent rather than large, loaded doses. It should be kept in mind that lactation may prevent the use of these drugs for very long.

Modern operative technique saves blood and prevents contamination of the peritoneal cavity by blood and amniotic fluid or meconium so that problems with nausea or bowel stasis are minimal. The bladder catheter is removed as soon as possible, and the patient is ambulated usually in 6 hours after she has left the postoperative unit. IV hydrations and supplemental glucose are administered until the patient takes solid food. She should be fed a diet as near to her usual normal intake as soon as possible. Such management with encouragement generally rehabilitates most normal women quickly. Bowel functions return rapidly, and convalescence can be carried out at home. Minor difficulties can be controlled with specific medication and treatment that varies to some extent by a physician's choice. A competent staff of nurses is invaluable in such cases, and the proper combination has the patient in a normal condition in a few days at the most. Management of the breast and lactation is especially dependent on knowledgeable nurses, and such help and encouragement are essential for an ideal nursing experience. Combined team effort returns the patient in good health and spirits to her home with minimal hospital stay, which is the goal of obstetrics today. This provides emotional and financial benefits.

EXTRAPERITONEAL CESAREAN SECTION

As the earliest of the concepts of low uterine segment operations were developed simultaneously, other ideas had evolved. These were more concerned with protection of the abdominal cavity from infection than the approach to the low segment of the cervix for delivery of the child. The information gained from these various dissections made the evolution and performance of true low-segment transperitoneal cesarean seem simple (Fig. 61-24). Throughout this time, extraperitoneal, peritoneal exclusion, uteroabdominal fistula, vaginal cesarean, and pseudoextraperitoneal operations were being introduced along with uterine eventrations that included a posterior fundal incision.

The true extraperitoneal operation involved dissections near the bladder in the adjacent tissues that admitted entrance to the dilated cervix or low uterine segment external to the peritoneal cavity (Fig. 61-25). There are two basic varieties: one is to dissect the vesical peritoneum from the anterior bladder wall and expose the low segment or dilated cervix to incisional entrance of sufficient size to permit delivery of a child; the other is to accomplish the same result by a lateral dissection of the vesical peritoneum and lateral exposure of the same anatomical area for the same purpose. At this point, it should be noted that the anatomy of the area inferior to the bladder and superior to the low uterine segment, dilated cervix, and vagina is distorted by the changes brought about by pregnancy and labor. Because most of these operations were performed at the end of a long and often complicated labor, some after attempted vaginal delivery, it was impossible to discern where the fully dilated and edematous cervix, vagina, and thin low uterine segment actually were, in relation to each other. This accounts for the discussions in regard to the terminology of these operations, extraperitoneal or not: were these truly low-segment or cervical cesarean sections? The question is moot. As noted, the supravesical procedure was first conceived by Physick in 1824 in the United States (Fig. 61-26). A technique somewhat similar was proposed by Bell in 1837 in England, but was not quite as clearly defined. The extraperitoneal approach thus suggested was not accepted, and it was not until Skene and Thomas in 1874 and 1878 reviewed the operation of gastroelytrotomy, which was so named by Baude-

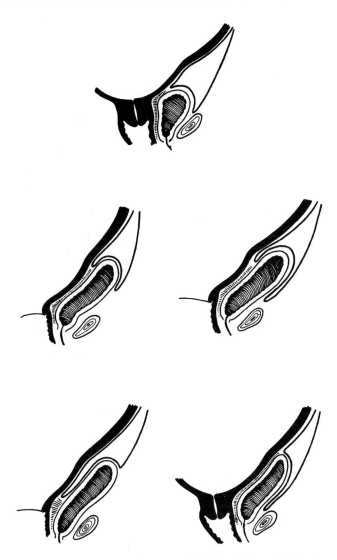

Fig. 61-24 Variations in peritoneal relationships to the bladder. (From Marshall CM: *Cesarean section: lower segment operation,* London, 1939, John Wright & Sons, Bristol & Simpkin Marshall.)

locque in 1823. In 1870, Thomas described an operation much like that of Ritgen in which, after the proper dissection and manual dilation of the cervix, the cervix was brought through the vaginal incision and the child was delivered. This revived operation had a brief acceptance and then yielded to the other less exotic attempts at extraperitoneal cesarean. German and American surgeons were the most active in the development of both supravesical and lateral approaches for delivery without peritoneal invasion.

In summary, the following are examples of these various methods:

1. *Gastroelytrotomy* was begun by Ritgen, prompted by Baudelocque and Thomas.
2. *Extraperitoneal* methods include retrovesical and paravesical techniques. Paravesical dissection approaches the low uterine segment by lateral tissue manipulation, which extends behind the bladder and below the peritoneum, followed by lateral retraction of

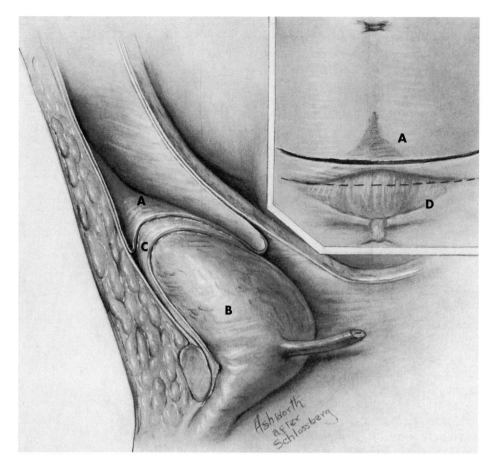

Fig. 61-25   Lateral anatomical view of anterior pelvic area. **A,** Peritoneum. **B,** Bladder. **C,** Perivesical "fascia." **D,** Anterior abdominal wall and incision relationship.

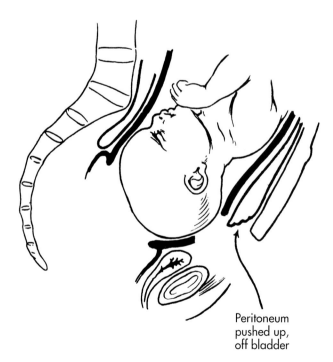

Fig. 61-26   Physicks' suprasymphysial supravesical approach to the low uterine segment. (From DeLee J: *Am J Ob/Gyn* 10:610, 1925.)

the bladder, which exposes the area of the anterior uterine wall for the incision for delivery. This was created by Latzko, who used one of Sellheim's several methods (Fig. 61-27). Since that time, 1908, Burns (1930), Norton (1935), and the author (1965) have simplified the dissection and allowed for increased space for delivery (Fig. 61-28). Doderlein in Europe used an inguinal incision.

3. *Retrovesical or supravesical dissection:* originated with Physick in the United States and was securely established by Sellheim (Fig. 61-29). The operation was promoted by Waters, Leavitt, Cartwright, and Ricci. In this operation, the peritoneum is dissected from the anterior wall of the bladder through a T-shaped superficial incision, which permits it to be retracted inferiorly to expose the lower uterine segment for incision after the uterine peritoneal fold has been retracted anteriorly (Fig. 61-30). It has an advantage of increased space for delivery but has a high failure rate because of injury to the peritoneum. The anatomical relationships of these low operations are seen in Fig. 61-30, *A (3), B (2),* and *C (2).*

4. *Peritoneal exclusion* was created by Frank in 1906. In this operation the parietal peritoneum was sutured to the upper visceral peritoneum, which closed off the

Text continued on p. 1139

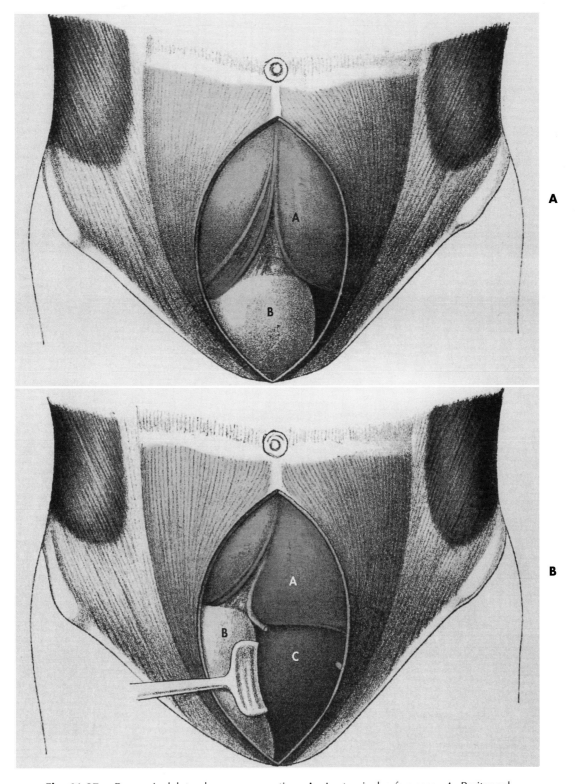

Fig. 61-27   Paravesical lateral cesarean section. **A,** Anatomical references. *A,* Peritoneal folds; *B,* bladder. **B,** Uterine wall exposure. *A,* Peritoneum; *B,* bladder; *C,* uterine wall. (Adapted from Latzko W: *Wein Klin Wochenschr,* 22:477, 1909, and in Ricci J, Marr J: *Principles of extraperitoneal cesarean section,* Philadelphia, 1939, The Blakiston Co.).

Continued

C

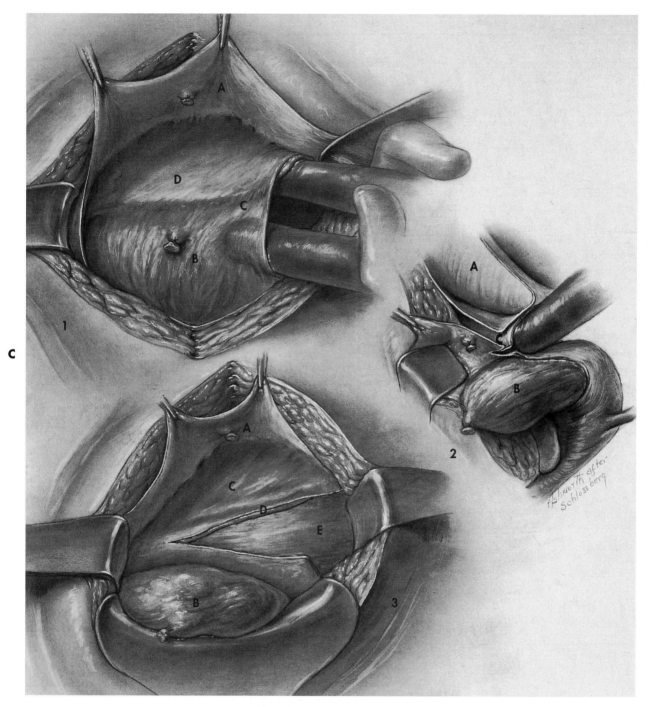

Fig. 61-27, cont'd **C,** Dissecting the vesical peritoneum from the lower uterine segment. (Adapted from Latzko W: *Wein Klin Wochenschr,* 22:477, 1909, and in Ricci J, Marr J: *Principles of extraperitoneal cesarean section,* Philadelphia, 1939, The Blakiston Co.).

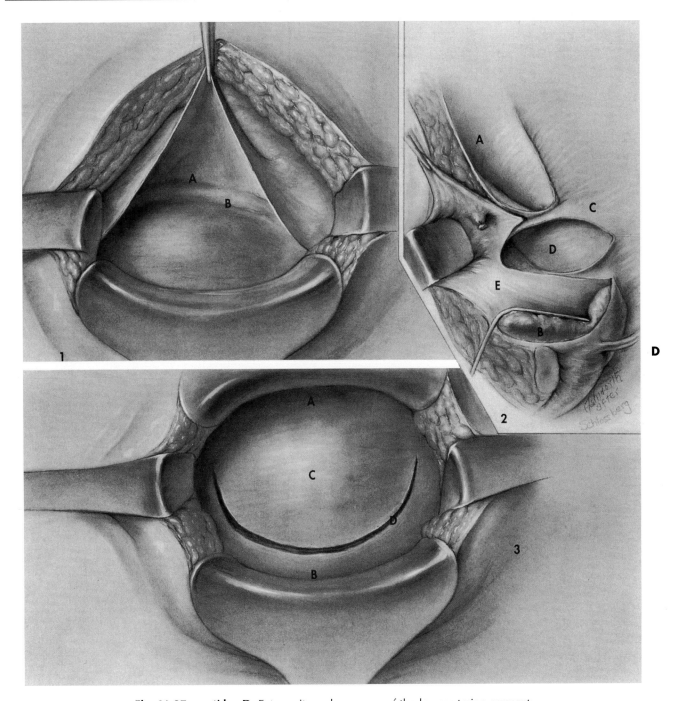

Fig. 61-27, cont'd   D, Extraperitoneal exposure of the lower uterine segment.

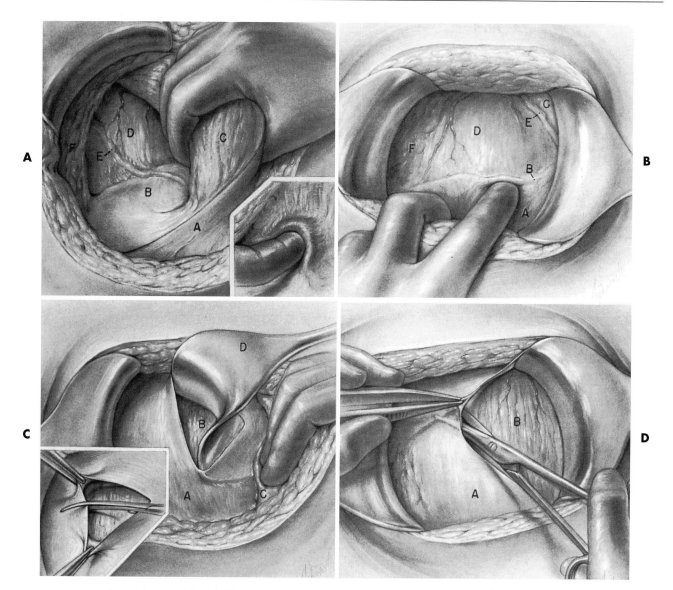

Fig. 61-28 **A,** The bladder is gently retracted medially with the fingers. *A,* Parietal peritoneum. *B,* Posterior peritoneal fold. *C,* Bladder. *D,* Lower uterine segment. *E,* Obliterated hypogastric artery. *F,* Fatty tissue and large vessels in the lateral pelvic space. *Inset,* Method of
dissecting with fingertip. **B,** Further progression in the blunt dissection of the area. *A,* Parietal
peritoneum. *B,* Posterior peritoneal fold. *C,* Bladder retracted laterally. *D,* Lower uterine segment. *E,* Obliterated hypogastric artery. *F,* Fatty tissue and large vessels in the lateral pelvic
space. **C,** *Inset,* Method of extending the fascial incision. *Main illustration,* Extension of the
fascial dissection using the Fritsch retractor. Shows the next step in extension of the dissection
enlarging the operative field. *A,* Superficial uterine fascia. *B,* Lower uterine segment. *C,* Edge
of posterior peritoneal fold. *D,* Fritsch retractor. **D,** *A,* Superficial uterine fascia. *B,* Lower uterine segment. (From Durfee R: *Surg Gynecol Obstet* 110:173, 1960.)

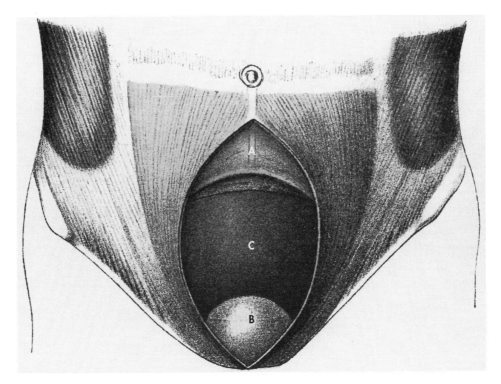

Fig. 61-29 Supravesical extraperitoneal cesarean section by Sellheim. *A,* Peritoneum. *B,* Bladder. *C,* LUS uterine wall. (Adapted from Latzko W: *Wein Klin Wochenschr,* 22:477, 1909, and in Ricci J: *Principles of extraperitoneal cesarean section,* Philadelphia, 1939, The Blakiston Co.)

peritoneal cavity (Fig. 61-31). There were several variations of this type of peritoneal suture placement, but, in reality, no sutured tissue was free from bacterial invasion and permeation. Peritoneal exclusion continued with many variations, which included ingenious methods using clamps, packing with various materials, and the use of a rubber dam.

5. *Uteroabdominal fistula formation* was first created by Pillore in France in 1845. He sutured the uterine incision edges to the abdominal incision, which allowed the uterine cavity to drain its contents exterior to the peritoneal cavity. This was followed by others, but it remained for Sellheim, who was disappointed by his previous three procedures, to establish this method.

6. *Pseudoextraperitoneal operations* have not been well accepted because they violate the principle of extraperitoneal surgery. It was first introduced by Aldridge in 1937 and performed in several different ways by others, which included the injection of methylene blue dye intraperitoneally to identify it for dissection.

7. Duhrssen and Solms in 1909 *combined vaginal cesarean with a supra-Poupart's ligament approach.* The abdominal operation was first done with exposure of the area, the vaginal incision was then performed, and the delivery was accomplished through the abdominal wound extraperitoneally.

All of the exotic procedures have yielded to either a paravesical or supravesical operation. When these operations are

properly performed with care, skill, and knowledge of the anatomy of the area and the possible variations in the peritoneal folds, the procedure is successful.

INDICATIONS FOR CESAREAN SECTION

The primary indication for a cesarean section was to remove a child from a dead woman perhaps to save it, but more so for satisfaction of rituals and religious reasons. With the appearance of Christianity, a child was removed for the purpose of baptism. Almost all of these were postmortem, but the use of cesarean section for the dying woman produced more living children and led directly to the use of the operation in the living.

In 1581, Rousset outlined the following indications for abdominal delivery: very large child, large twins, complications from myomas, fetal monstrosities, abnormal irreducible presentations, a contracted pelvis, a strictured uterus, a large vesicle stone, and an aged woman or one too young. These are familiar and clearly were situations designed for cesarean sections for live women.

Despite such a wide variety of indications, the high mortality associated with the operation reduced the indications for cesarean for the live woman to a totally contracted pelvis and nothing else. A very few intrepid physicians used the operation for more than this single indication, but by 1747 Levret summed it all up into "an extreme contraction of the pelvis which caused the absolute impossibility for delivery

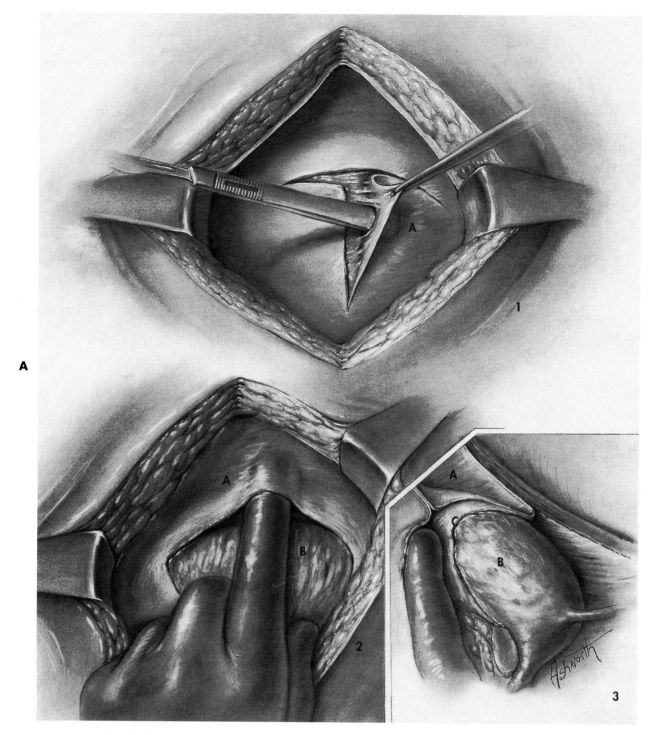

Fig. 61-30   Supravesical extraperitoneal cesarean section. **A,** *1A,* "T" incision over bladder; *2A,* paravesical "fascia"; *B,* bladder; *3A,* peritoneal cavity; *B,* bladder; *C,* paravesical "fascia."

through the natural passages." There were other conditions that had to be met. The child had to be alive and the pelvis so contracted that the obstetrician could not pass a hand through it to perform a version or embryotomy. Levret did not acknowledge blockage by fleshy tumors or the restraint caused by stenosis or constriction of the cervix or vagina because there were methods to circumvent these problems by less hazardous procedures than cesarean section. What these were is not clear. This opinion included placenta

previa. By 1756, Crantz added the occasion of imminent uterine rupture as an indication. But neither this nor the presence of placenta previa was generally reason for performance of cesarean section.

The situation remained static until 1890 when Tait advocated the cesarean operation without question for hemorrhage from placenta previa followed by hysterectomy; he did one of these in 1898 and succeeded in safe delivery of the mother, but the child died after 1 month of pneumonia. In the

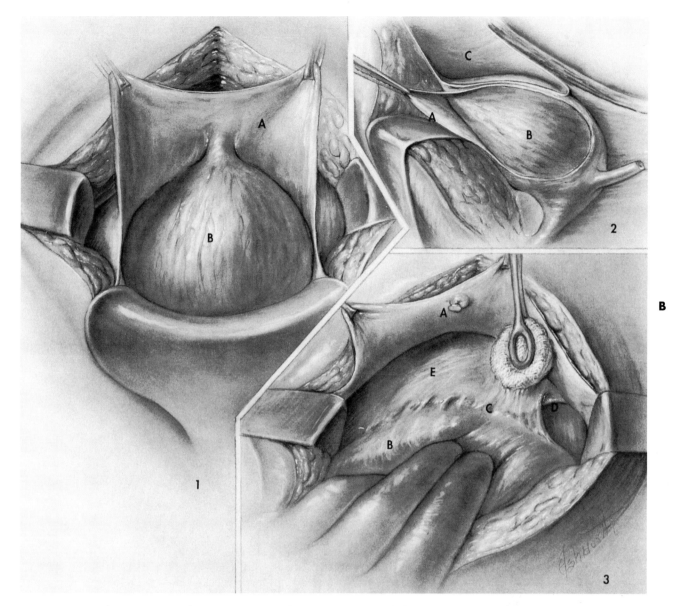

Fig. 61-30, cont'd **B,** *1A,* Dissected superior paravesical "fascia"; *B,* bladder; *2A,* paravesical "fascia"; *B,* bladder; *C,* peritoneal cavity; *3A,* paravesical "fascia"; *B,* bladder; *C,* deep paravesical "fascia"; *D,* uterine wall; *E,* peritoneum.

United States in 1892, cesarean section for placenta previa was suggested by Ford; it was done by Hypes and Hulbert with no details. A child was delivered from a badly over-manipulated patient by Sligh in 1892, but she was in such poor condition that she had no chance for survival. Bernays in the United States did the first successful operation in 1894, without hysterectomy; three other operations had been done in the United States before Tait's successful case. By 1901, Zinke advocated cesarean for central placenta previa, for women with a closed cervix, in a primigravida not in labor, and for women with hemorrhage not controlled by conservative methods. Kerr was opposed to this indication, but from 1902 to 1921 he changed his mind completely. In the next 50 years, the indication was more or less as it is today.

Another often fatal situation in obstetrics has been eclampsia. In 1788, Lauverjat suggested the use of cesarean for a convulsive woman; he did the operation four times in 1780. Each of these was postmortem, and a dead child was delivered each time. He stated that clearly the operation should be done while the mother was alive because apparently the child would die before she did. In 1827, Richmond performed cesarean section for an eclamptic woman in the backwoods of the United States with success; Bennett's wife also had toxemia. In 1904, Pollack reported that Van de Akker in 1875 was the first to perform the operation for eclampsia, but this is clearly not true. Foster reported a case in 1870, but it was Halbertsma in 1881 who established the real basis for cesarean in eclampsia. He repeated his opinion in 1889. There was much divided attitude about this practice, and, by 1937, it was agreed that a high percentage of the maternal deaths after cesarean section for this indication was because of absence of treatment, or the failure thereof, before surgery. Once again, the cesarean was an operation of last resort.

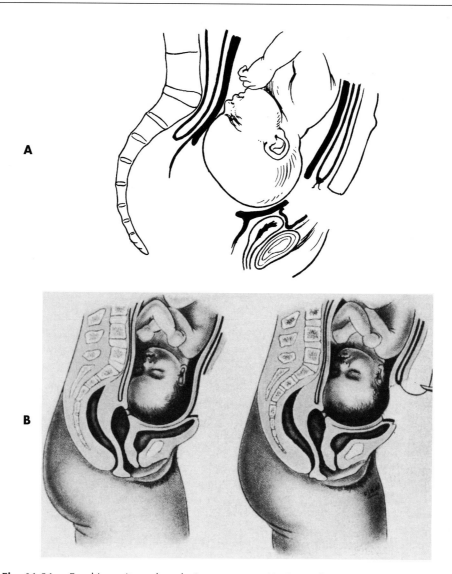

Fig. 61-31   Frank's peritoneal exclusion cesarean. (**A,** From de Lee: *Am J Ob/Gyn* 10:51, 1925. **B,** From Marshall JM: *Cesarean section: lower segment operation,* London, 1939, John Wright & Sons, Bristol & Simpkin Marshall.)

In the years that followed, cesarean section became safer with the recognition of the importance of "timing" in application of the procedure for all indicated situations.

From 1940 to the present day, indications have been categorized by such definitions as "absolute" and "relative" for want of better terms. In some reports there are special divisions for fetal or maternal indications only. The following are some examples of the trends for the use of the operation.

"Absolute" Indications in the Era from 1940

1. A completely contracted pelvis
2. Central placenta previa with blood loss
3. Transverse presentation not amenable to version
4. Breech presentation in a primipara with borderline pelvis
5. Severe increasing toxemia with progression to eclampsia
6. Imminent uterine rupture

7. Premature separation of the placenta with severe abruption
8. Complete obstruction of the pelvis by nonremovable tumors or cysts
9. Prolapsed fetal cord without cervical dilation above 3 cm
10. Severe threat to life or progressive maternal disease (e.g., severe uncontrollable diabetes, some cardiac diseases)
11. Previous pregnancy loss in labor or nonviable premature more than three times
12. Failed labor of 18 to 24 hours in women older than 40 or younger than 14 years of age
13. Moribund woman after pulmonary aspiration, with asphyxia; symptoms of amniotic fluid embolus; massive cardiovascular accident with coma
14. Invasive cervical carcinoma diagnosed at term
15. Paralytic poliomyelitis with paralysis to C-6 no longer an indication

16. Coma or brain death within range of fetal viability
17. Diagnosed uterine rupture, symptomatic with hemorrhage
18. Total soft tissue obstruction of the lower birth canal (e.g., nearly complete vaginal atresia, massive vulvar edema, or scar formation from trauma or severe genital burns)
19. Multiple pregnancy with unengaged fetal parts (e.g., triplets)
20. Massive fetal monstrosities not amenable to embryotomy

"Relative" Indications from 1940

1. Cervical dystocia (i.e., failed dilation)
2. Failed onset of labor after attempted induction with ruptured membranes over 12 hours
3. Uterine atony in second stage of labor with high station of the presenting part, unengaged
4. Uterine contraction ring unresponsive to treatment
5. Failed forceps or vacuum extraction delivery
6. Premature separation of the placenta with severe abruption with failed response to conservative therapy
7. Unmanageable psychiatric disease (e.g., wild mania or sustained hysteria, not amenable to treatment); this may be questionable in contemporary obstetrics
8. Evidence of severe intrauterine infection and fetal distress with poor labor
9. Emergency development of extensive maternal disease (many examples)
10. Prolonged painful red degeneration of a large myoma
11. Abnormal fetal presentations in overdue elderly primipara with firm undilated cervix
12. Extensive pelvic plastic repair of extremely severe previous vaginal, cervical, or perineal trauma that included the rectum and/or bladder with fistula formation, successfully repaired
13. Extensive intraabdominal pelvic surgery, such as exenteration of extragenital organs
14. Moribund woman with severe chronic disease (e.g., carcinoma anywhere, advanced tuberculosis)
15. Highly valuable child with any complication
16. Failed test of labor
17. Prolapse of fetal arm or arm and leg
18. Obvious evidence of increased fetal distress diagnosed by electronic devices
19. Repeat cesarean section if original indication is still present
20. Any number of rare and exotic situations

Questionable Indications from 1940

1. Patient and relatives request for cesarean section
2. Elective cesarean section to preserve tissues of the genital canal (e.g., Harris in Hollywood to preserve the sexual attractiveness of actresses)
3. Malingering hysteria and purported fear of labor and vaginal delivery
4. Herpes virus disease not active in the genital tract
5. Acquired immunodeficiency syndrome (AIDS)

6. "Once a cesarean always a cesarean"
7. Delivery of a child on a special date (e.g., a relative's birthday, anniversary, or sibling's birthday, or by decision of an astrologist)
8. Guarantee a live child for royal succession or in some cases of involved inheritance
9. Nonpermanent cervical cerclage, with dilation
10. Healed vesicovaginal fistula in multipara with history of easy labor

Contraindications from 1940

1. For a patient with a dead child and no other indication
2. For severe intrauterine infection, before antibiotic era, and now with severe maternal disseminated intravascular coagulation (DIC)
3. In a woman dead more than 1 hour
4. For the purpose of baptism only
5. Where any risk of cesarean section would be fatal for the mother
6. Where there is no available anesthesia of any kind
7. For the purpose of sterilization only
8. In the presence of intraabdominal infection, nonobstetric

Contemporary Fetal Indications

1. Abnormal fetal heart rate pattern that persists and a fetal scalp pH of less than 7.2
2. Abnormal fetal heart rate with cardiac abnormalities
3. Low birthweight child with abnormal fetal heart rate or any other added problem, such as a position other than a normal vertex, multiple gestation, long duration membrane rupture not responsive to amnioinfusion, any suspected evidence of even mild asphyxia
4. Abruptio placentae with live child and no maternal DIC
5. Placenta previa, central, or with worrisome blood loss if near viability; failure of conservative treatment and presence of hemorrhage
6. Active genital tract maternal herpes simplex virus
7. Idiopathic thrombocytopenic purpura (ITP) with low platelet count in fetus
8. Hydrocephaly in certain cases
9. Highly valuable child
10. Prolapsed cord without labor, or prolapsed arm or arm and leg together

Contemporary Maternal Indications

1. Mechanical obstructions to the birth canal
2. Genital tract malignancy; cervical or vaginal carcinoma
3. Permanent cervical cerclage
4. Massive abruption of the placenta with imminent shock and potential interference with the blood clotting mechanism
5. Obstetric situations that require delivery not necessarily only for the fetus

For almost all the indications from the era of 1940 to 1975 with few exceptions, the term *absolute,* is not ruled out.

The extraperitoneal operation can be used for debilitated patients with infection after long labor in whom prevention of gross contamination of the abdominal cavity may be the difference between life and death. It is acknowledged that it may not totally prevent peritonitis, but at least it prevents an overload of contaminated material. It can be done electively for purposes of instruction in a medical school environment.

The low-segment operation is the method of choice for most cesarean sections. Variations in techniques are essentially a matter of choice by the obstetrician.

The fundal operation is chosen for selected patients for whom delivery through a low-segment incision would be compromised and especially with premature fetal malpresentations.

Abdominal hysterotomy is done for indicated late abortion when labor induction is not feasible or possible.

Although vaginal hysterotomy is rarely used, it can be valuable in certain situations in which removal of a fetus is essential to save its life when it is not feasible to subject the patient to an abdominal operation.

COMPLICATIONS OF CESAREAN SECTION
Intraoperative Complications

Uterine Hemorrhage. Heavy sudden blood loss in the course of or at the start of the operation disturbs the surgeon-obstetrician and arises from several causes:

1. Uterine atony
2. Extension of incision into uterine vessels
3. Anterior implantation of the placenta or placenta previa
4. Premature placental separation with or without abruption
5. Myometrial damage from severe placental abruption
6. Incomplete removal of the placenta includes placental anomalies
7. Presence of myomata uteri
8. Suspected or unsuspected uterine rupture
9. Cervical or vaginal lacerations from attempts to deliver vaginally
10. Partial or complete placenta accreta
11. Failure of the blood clotting mechanism
12. Uterine trauma at the time of delivery of the fetus

The intraoperative collection of the patient's own blood at cesarean section with the use of modern techniques is safe and in many cases may be life saving. Such a process eliminates the problems associated with transfusion of stored, banked blood from an outside source. A cell saver and filtration system allow the collection of blood from the operative field with the elimination of potential difficulties with contents of the amniotic fluids. Autologous blood collection should be available in every center in which obstetric hemorrhage at cesarean is a strong possibility or a reality. An automatic cell saver is prepared before surgery, and the blood collected is properly processed. At the time of autotransfusion additional filtration is provided in the transfusion line to remove any other debris from the red cell mass, and anticoagulation is provided with a citrate solution rather than heparin. It is obvious that this process will save lives and reduce postoperative anemia caused by hemorrhage. This has become a safe transfusion and can also be used for Jehovah's Witness patients who may be at serious risk, since the patient's own blood is the transfusion source. Probably all collected red cells obtained in this manner should be returned within a few hours. Contraindications include known bacterial contamination, such as with bowel perforation. Known documented malignancy or the presence of much amniotic fluid also precludes its use.

Acute Hemodilation in Patients at Cesarean Section. It is generally accepted that maternal mortality today is primarily caused by hemorrhage, and much of this occurs with cesarean section. In the United Kingdom hemorrhage is the third cause of maternal mortality, some of which is due to the associated risks with homologous transfusion. The actual figure is 6.4 per 1 million pregnancies. Grange et al. reported in 1998 that postpartum hemorrhage accounts for approximately half of these deaths and is not necessarily due to a cesarean operation itself but is usually attributed to the pathologic conditions associated with the indication for the cesarean.

Autologous transfusion is most desirable, and there are several techniques to accomplish this. According to Grange et al. these are predonation over several weeks, immediate preoperative blood collection, and normovolemic hemodilution. Hemodilution is attained by the removal of blood immediately before the operation, which is replaced with an equal amount of 10% pentastarch (Pentaspan, DuPont Pharma). This reduces the blood cell mass lost at the time of surgery and maintains normal volemia. All of this is monitored by an experienced anesthesiologist. Collected blood is carefully prepared and properly stored. After the preoperative blood removal, the patient is preloaded with intravenous fluid and anesthetized for the cesarean delivery. It has been estimated that the average blood loss at cesarean is 1000 ml according to Williams in 1989 and may be considerably higher.

It is obvious that patients for this procedure must be picked with zealous care, which includes immediate detailed studies of the blood chemistry values. It also includes careful and accurate analysis of pathologic conditions that indicate high risk for excessive blood loss such as placenta previa, placenta accreta, anterior position, presence of myomata, and uterine atony not responsive to stimulation. The risks of homologous transfusion are immunologic problems and potential infection. These are avoided by exceedingly careful management of blood that is obtained for future use. Hemoglobin levels must be monitored during surgery and corrected as indicated. Two veins must be catheterized to facilitate the administration of these fluids.

Acute normovolemic hemodilution as an adjunct to a previous autologous blood program is suggested and can be used in the absence of such a program. Previous donation of the patient's blood makes retransfusion possible and is safe but can also stimulate erythropoiesis. Acute hemodilution is used only in those patients who show an immediate need.

Apparently the procedure has no deleterious effect on the fetus.

This procedure is well tolerated, is safe, and is feasible for patients at risk for or in the process of hemorrhage.

Each of these complications above is managed in a specific and individual manner. Uterine atony is managed by injection of oxytocic drugs, systemic and local, uterine massage and the use of hot packs, and eventration and temporary or permanent occlusion of the uterine vessels; hysterectomy is a last resort. Uterine trauma, incision extension, and rupture are all managed by local hemostasis, the use of clamps and suture repair; vessel obstruction or hysterectomy may be necessary. Blood clotting problems are usually managed by the hematologist and anesthesiologist.

Placental Abnormalities and Hemorrhage. The position of the placenta in the uterus can cause any number of difficulties before, in the course of, and after delivery (Fig.

61-32). The posterior low level is an incursion into the pelvic space. The importance of recognizing this was emphasized by Stallworthy, who also strongly recommended detailed care in such cases because the low level posterior placental position was potentially very dangerous. Not only can the placenta prematurely separate in this position, but the presence of the tissue mass prevents engagement of the fetal pole into the pelvic inlet. The latter may compromise management of placental separation blood loss. An anterior low-level placenta may cause similar problems but has the added disadvantage of impeding a surgical approach through the anterior uterine wall at low-segment cesarean (Fig. 61-33). Management usually depends on the degree and frequency of blood loss, the position of the fetal pole at the onset of labor, and whether the presentation is vertex or breech. Encroachment of the placenta into the cervix with subsequent interference with normal labor and delivery to-

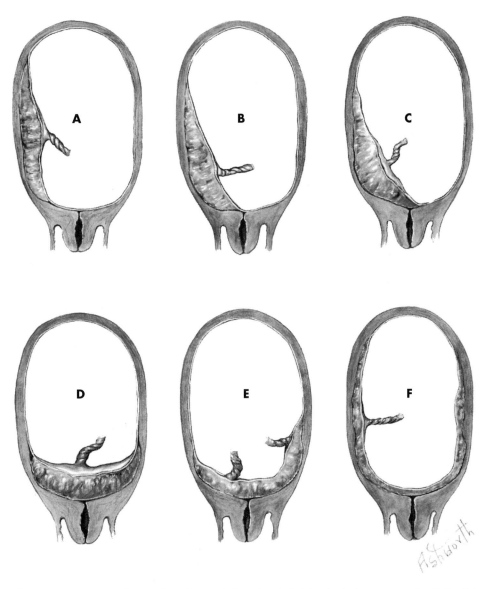

Fig. 61-32   Various placental positions. **A,** Low level. **B,** Marginal placenta previa. **C,** Partial placenta previa. **D,** Central placenta previa. **E,** Twin placenta previa. **F,** Placenta membranacea.

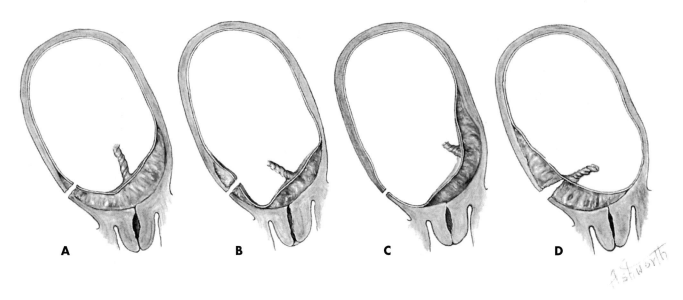

Fig. 61-33 Placental injury by an incision in the low uterine segment wall. **A,** Placental edge entered. **B,** Placental lobe entered. **C,** Placenta missed. **D,** Center placenta entered.

gether with the increased incidence of hemorrhage is a frequent indication for cesarean. This is known as placenta previa. A central placenta previa almost always is an indication for operative delivery (see Fig. 61-32). A delivery through a LUS incision may require premature placental removal, incision of placental tissue, and penetration of the tissue mass to reach the fetal pole. Extensive hemorrhage can occur at this time. Rapid dissection, delivery, and immediate placental removal are mandatory (Fig. 61-34). In contemporary obstetrics, the diagnosis often can be made by ultrasound (US) examination.

When there is premature separation of the placenta, regardless of its position (which is known as abruption in certain circumstances), the surgeon must be prepared for unusual blood loss. Abruption is usually associated with a normally implanted placenta, and there may be several stages of severity (Fig. 61-35). In such cases, blood replacement is often necessary, hysterectomy may be required, the fetus may be compromised especially when premature, and the mother can be seriously involved. When possible, all eventualities must be communicated to the patient and her relatives in detail before the operation. Massive intrusion of blood into the uterine wall may cause such trauma that the uterus cannot contract and a condition known as uteroplacental apoplexy (Couvelaire uterus) is observed. This often leads to the intense onset of shock, complicated by interference of the formation of normal blood clots and DIC, which may be a threat to the mother's life. Treatment involves the entire surgical team, which includes hematologists and laboratory personnel. If further surgery is necessary after the condition is brought under control, uterine or hypogastric artery ligation may be sufficient to stop the hemorrhage. If the uterus has been badly damaged, hysterectomy is indicated.

If the situation is not so severe, sustained external pressure may control blood loss from the open placental bed after cesarean; if this does not suffice, sutures placed in the

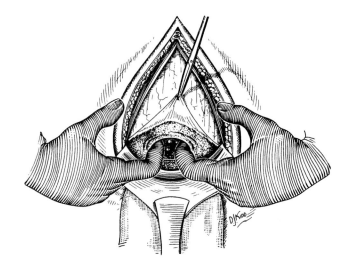

Fig. 61-34 Finger dissection of low uterine segment cesarean section placenta previa. (From Marshall JM: *Cesarean section: lower segment operation,* London, 1939, John Wright & Sons, Bristol & Simpkin Marshall [from Geppert and Hauser].)

area may control blood loss. Intrauterine or intravenous medications may bring about sustained uterine contraction; hot packs may also be used.

Magnetic resonance imaging (MRI) has been suggested as a method of choice for diagnostic analysis of the pelvis, the fetal size and presentation, the fetal position in the pelvis, and any unsuspected pathologic conditions. MRI has the advantage of elimination of the potential undesirable effects of ionizing irradiation from x-ray pelvimetry or computed tomography scan. Reports have been recorded of the value of MRI in the predelivery evaluation of abnormal fetal presentation such as breech and the subsequent method of delivery whether after a labor trial or an elective cesarean. This may influence the incidence of cesarean and if the

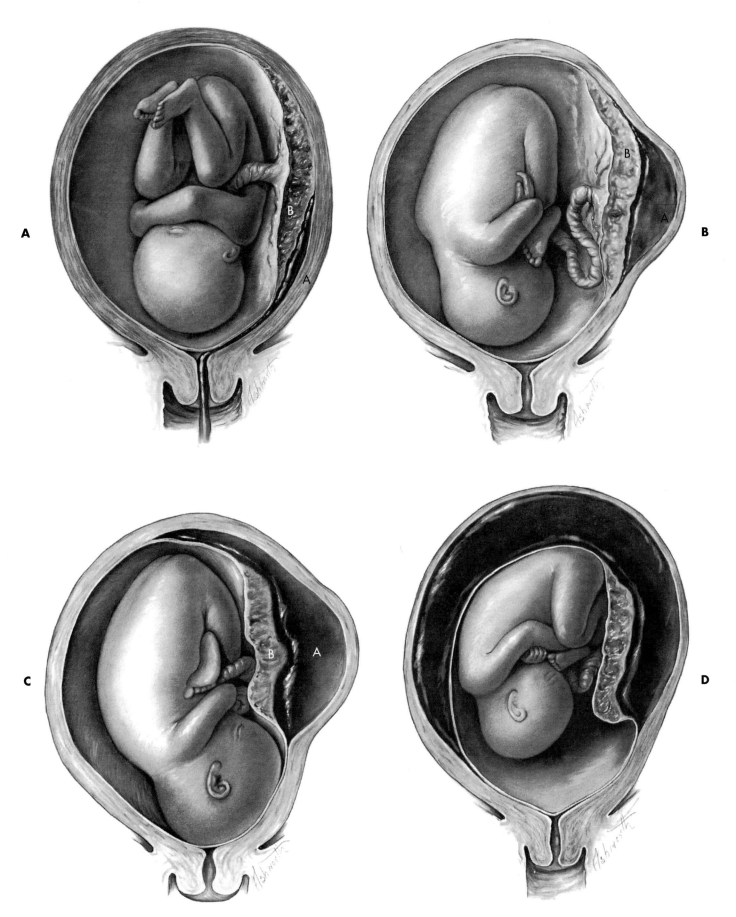

Fig. 61-35 Placental abruption. **A,** Early placental separation with blood loss. *A,* Area of minor separation; *B,* placenta. **B,** Early occult placenta separation. *A,* Blood clot; *B,* placenta. **C,** Moderately severe separation. *A,* Large blood clot; *B,* separated placenta. **D,** Total placental separation with uteroplacental apoplexy.

indications are proper increase vaginal delivery in selected patients. One aspect of the MRI that is a deterrent for its use is cost and another is the sense of claustrophobia that some patients feel when undergoing MRI.

Another instance of the value of MRI has been recorded in a patient with placenta percreta that involved the bladder. The original diagnosis was made in the first trimester. The same author used MRI for diagnosis of abnormal placental position in 1992 for placenta previa. This diagnosis alerts the attending physician to the problem and may avert a disaster.

Other uses for MRI in obstetrics are feasible, and this modality is one more added contribution to accuracy of pre-delivery diagnoses.

If there should be a placenta accreta in association with placenta previa and blood loss persists after removal of all but the adherent portion, hysterectomy may be indicated (Fig. 61-36). Occasionally, if blood loss stops, the accreta may be left intact to be treated with methotrexate. This should begin immediately postoperatively. The patient should not nurse. She should be observed carefully with almost constant follow-up, and if there are no complications, the methotrexate can be stopped as indicated. If one is fortunate, the placental tissue can be seen with a high-resolution US or MRI scan, and, if it disappears rapidly, the treatment may be successful.

Another use for US is the application of color Doppler US as a guide for transabdominal autoinfusion in patients with second-trimester oligohydramnios. This method has many possibilities for increasing successful treatment in

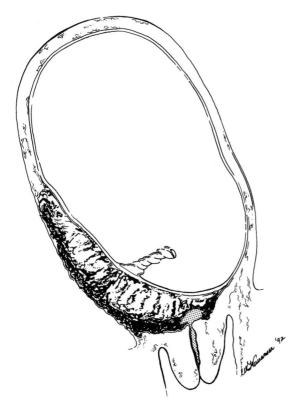

Fig. 61-36 Placenta accreta with mild blood loss.

some patients related to the proof and finding of reduced amniotic fluid. Unrecognized premature rupture of the membranes may be present, or there may be fetal anomalies associated with reduced amniotic fluid. The procedure permits accurate needle placement for injection as indicated.

Progress can be followed with hormonal tests and charts of hormone concentration curve, as in the management of hydatid mole or choriocarcinoma. If hemorrhage or other complications such as infection, severe constant pain, or reaction to the chemotherapeutic agent increase in severity, hysterectomy may have to be done. Actinomycin can be used, but its action is not reversible; sequential measureable titers are mandatory.

If a myoma that has undergone red degeneration is pedunculated, it may be removed without much difficulty. However, attempts to perform intramural myomectomy are not usually recommended because of excessive blood loss and additional creation of thinness of the uterine wall; there almost always is prolonged postoperative recovery. Use of the laser has future possibilities, and it remains to be seen if dissolution of myomatous tissue with the laser followed by polyglycolic suture closure of the wound will permit myomectomy especially for control of blood loss at cesarean.

Urinary Tract Injury. Vesical laceration is easily repaired if recognized early in the operation; this can be done with a mucosal inversion suture in the bladder wall followed by a second layer for reinforcement. The bladder should be tested for integrity after closure and before suture closure of the abdominal cavity. It is more secure to use a serosal cover procedure over the uterine suture line and close the parietal peritoneum in such cases; drainage is arbitrary.

Ureteral avulsion, or partial or complete severance, usually can be successfully repaired if diagnosed at the time of the accident. Although all operators should know more than one method for ureteral anastomosis or repair, consultation with the urologist is recommended, especially in the litigious atmosphere of modern practice. Drainage is always provided, and wound closure is meticulous, *never by use of permanent sutures.*

Uterine Infection. Infection of the uterus at the time of the cesarean is usually due to long and difficult labor, with extended time of membrane rupture and some trauma from attempted vaginal delivery. There is obvious endometritis and chorioamnionitis, which is treated during and after the operation with rigorous antibiotic therapy. Minimal amounts of nonreactive absorbable suture material are used for closures, and, in such cases, the peritoneum is closed and the proper areas are drained; if the infection is extremely severe, the abdominal wound may be left open down to the peritoneal or fascial layer. Severe acute thrombophlebitis associated with extensive uterine infection is rarely seen in the United States but is seen in Third World countries. This requires intensive, detailed, complicated care and generally is not an intraoperative problem.

Gastrointestinal Problems. Intraoperative problems with the bowel usually have to do with adhesions and possible bowel injuries associated with lysis of these tissues.

This may occur with trauma associated with adhesion separation from previous surgery. Instant repair is indicated; if bowel resection is needed, this should be done by a general surgeon. As a rule, bowel surgery is contraindicated with cesarean section.

Lethal or Near-Lethal Accidents. Amniotic fluid embolism, with a sudden pulmonary crisis, is usually a problem for anesthesia; minimal manipulatory termination of the cesarean is indicated (Fig. 61-37). Other severe accidents such as vascular or fatty pulmonary embolism, cardiac arrest, severe convulsions, or coma require the immediate attention of a team, which presumably is available in every modern operating suite. Attention to the child, if undelivered, is essential; hemostasis should be complete. Placental removal is best allowed to be spontaneous, and wound closures are delayed until the patient's condition permits such activity. The wounds should be closed routinely if the patient expires.

Postoperative Complications

Most postoperative problems are postanesthesia complications, which are often pulmonary difficulties. Situations such as postspinal headache or paresthesias related to conduction anesthesia are not ordinarily cared for exclusively by the obstetrician. The development of endometritis with or without peritonitis requires extensive supportive treatment and specific high-dose combinations of antibiotics. Ileus is not common in modern times, but when it occurs, treatment should be IV hydration, no oral intake, careful and complete laboratory studies, and close observation. US or x-ray studies may reveal the severity of the problem and lead to more active treatment such as nasogastric suction or, in severe cases, the passage of a Miller-Abbott tube. Urinary tract infection is common postoperatively and is usually managed with specific antibiotics after culture and hydration; failure to respond to usual treatment leads to suspicion of urinary tract injury. Wound infection that appears 2 or 3 days after cesarean may be from an unsuspected infected uterus before the operation or, more commonly, from a contaminant at the time of surgery. With the meticulous care with which surgery is done today, none of these should occur. Usually a break in technique is the responsible factor, and every effort should be made to prevent wound infection in otherwise clean cases. Details of the methods of performance of the operation must be reviewed and examined constantly. Wound infections are now related to a classification of the conditions of the genital tract at the time of surgery.

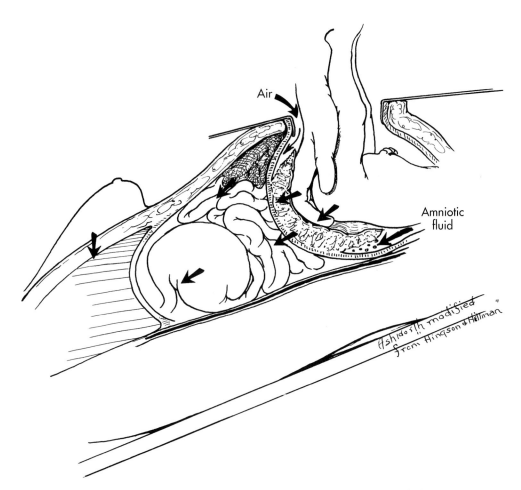

Fig. 61-37 Theoretical cause of an amniotic fluid embolus or an air embolus at cesarean section.

There is and always has been considerable postoperative wound infection in obese women after cesarean section. Attempts to control this with antibiotics and other methods have never been entirely satisfactory. These complications include postoperative fever, seroma, hematoma, and separation of the wound. Women with 2 cm or more of fatty tissue are more prone to these complications. Some have been treated with subcutaneous suture, some have been left open with no sutures, and some have a subcutaneous drain with suction. Closed drainage in this manner greatly reduces the incidence of these complications and should be considered for any obese patient.

Wounds vary from primary clean to totally infected. Some wounds may be predicted to break down with infection on this basis, and prophylactic antibiotics may be effective in the reduction of the severity and numbers of these. Drainage should be properly used in wounds in which infection is probable. An infected wound should be treated by exposure to the fascia and the use of local, established methods for management. Wounds may be closed by first or second intention. In cases of dehiscence, the wound should be debrided if necessary, closed loosely with Smead-Jones or retention sutures, and managed with local methods. In cases in which there is bowel protrusion, closures should be accomplished in the operating room. Supportive measures of all kinds are available for use in these cases. Necrotizing fasciitis is the most formidable of wound problems and requires early diagnosis, extensive debridement (several times), a combination of at least three antibiotics, and hyperbaric oxygen. Final treatment may require skin grafts.

Postsurgical convulsions in patients with eclampsia are managed as aggressively as before surgery. Postsurgical hemorrhage may be due to uterine atony, incomplete placental removal or accreta, or blood loss from the wound. US often makes the diagnosis for a probable specific cause of the blood loss. Treatment includes exploration, as indicated, to produce hemostasis in the uterine wound.

ANESTHESIA FOR CESAREAN SECTION

General inhalation anesthetics discovered in the early 1800s by Morton et al. were introduced early by Simpson into use in conduct of labor and delivery. Ether, chloroform, and nitrous oxide were used until the early 1900s, when cyclopropane and thiopentothal were added. Potential risks for both mother and child were recognized, so when the regional anesthetic agents were developed, they were promptly adopted for use for cesarean section. All anesthetic agents virtually removed the agony of abdominal surgery and solved most of the problems of pain control with operative procedures. Most important was the recognition of the effect of these agents on the fetus as well as the mother. The adoption of anesthesia for cesarean section with this knowledge facilitated the rise of the anesthesia specialist, especially in obstetrics, such as Apgar.

Conduction anesthesia was used in cases in which the fetus or the mother was in a grave situation and in which a rapid delivery was mandatory. Induction with intravenous pentothal in small doses, the addition of nitrous oxide and oxygen followed by intravenous curare, and perhaps the addition of one of the halogenated agents as indicated is a method of choice for certain emergency cesarean sections. Regional anesthesia is more popular for most operations and often can be used both for a test of labor and the subsequent cesarean sections when necessary.

Regional anesthesia began with carefully administered and monitored intrathecal or spinal anesthesia for cesarean section. This was followed by caudal anesthesia, known as a "low-lying" epidural. Continuous caudal epidural was then developed with use of a catheter in the caudal space to replenish the anesthetic agent as needed; this could be successfully used for labor and also for a cesarean section when necessary without the addition of another medication. In contemporary obstetrics, this has been replaced with epidural anesthesia, which accomplishes a similar result and may be easier to administer with reduced risks.

Anesthesia for Labor

The increased use of epidural anesthesia has been analyzed critically in several recent studies. The results are summarized here. When epidural anesthesia is properly used at 4 cm or more dilation with good labor and the maintenance of a T10 level, there was no increase in cesarean rate. Most fetuses delivered by either abdominal or vaginal method had good Apgar scores, and the mother had very acceptable pain relief. One study done with patient-controlled analgesia (PCA) revealed that the PCA group had a reduced number with very good pain relief, and several infants required naloxone for respiratory depression, which was probably because of the meperidine-Fentyl combination. There are controversial reports concerning the prolongation of labor with epidural anesthesia, but none of these indicate any complications nor an increased cesarean rate. One difficulty with such an analysis is that some patients with incomplete analgesia in a PCA group crossed over to epidural use, but the number was small.

Patients given inhalation anesthesia must be monitored for the inherent risks of inhalation of gastric contents, anoxia, hypotension, and concentration of anesthetic agents in the fetus. Patients given regional anesthesia must be monitored for inherent risks of hypotension, a possibly fatal elevation level, and postanesthesia complications such as headache, meningeal irritation, and other rare problems. Position of the patient for cesarean section is paramount to prevent compression of the great vessels and is prevented by turning the patient's body to the left approximately 15 to 20 degrees (Fig. 61-38). IV lines are mandatory, and, in the case of conduction (inhalation) anesthesia, *so is tracheal intubation, the only sure method to prevent aspiration.*

The use of local infiltration anesthesia for cesarean section has specific indications. Certain points with its use must be considered. The patient should have a minimal nonthreatening amount of sedation—just enough to alleviate anxiety and fear. She should be verbally encouraged throughout the

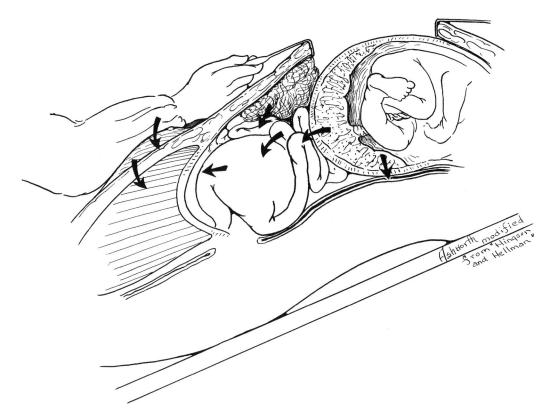

Fig. 61-38 Effect of pressure from several sources to produce hypotension with flat supine position at cesarean section.

procedure with explanation as to what is going on and what to expect in the way of sensation from time to time. At best, the operation should be considered less painful than vaginal delivery without anesthesia. The choice of local anesthetic is arbitrary, but what must be always carefully considered, as with continuous epidural or spinal techniques, is the *quality and quantity* as well as low concentration of the agents used. The primary indications for local anesthesia are (1) circumstances in which there is no anesthesiologist available or perhaps not even another physician obtainable; (2) patients in whom endotracheal intubation is impossible and it is important to provide exceedingly light anesthesia with a high oxygen content combined with the use of local injection; (3) patients with neuromuscular diseases such as myasthenia gravis in which muscular relaxation medications should be avoided; and (4) patients who wish to be awake in whom attempts to provide regional spinal or epidural anesthesia have failed (Fig. 61-39).

Special application of anesthesia is needed for patients who are high risk (e.g., patients with toxemia, eclampsia, chronic hypertension, any heart disease, hepatitis, diabetes, pulmonary disease, placental abruption, or severe chronic or acute anemia).

Regional anesthesia for cesarean section for breech delivery appears to be the method of choice. Because epidural or spinal anesthetics have been observed to affect the fetal brain, these side actions are prevented as much as possible. Any deleterious effect from regional anesthesia is probably due to an unexplained overdose of the metabolites of the anesthetic agent, hypotension, or sedative drugs. Because the morbidity of breech delivery by cesarean section is not yet acceptable, this could be corrected by improved management of the delivery at the time of the operation. There is no question that the brain can be easily traumatized by a careless or unnecessarily difficult delivery of a breech infant through the cesarean wounds. The same skill and art of obstetric management of these presentations must be used in these cases as much or more than in vaginal delivery. All of these factors are highly increased and magnified for a premature breech birth. The outcome of vaginal delivery of a premature breech baby is also not acceptable, and, for many reasons, the usual performance of cesarean section in these cases can be very different. Difference in placement and size of both incisions is essential, and the care with which anesthesia and manipulation at delivery are done need to be greatly intensified. Occasionally, a uterine muscle-relaxing agent will facilitate removal of the child, especially when there is an unformed low uterine segment.

Evaluation of the Child at Delivery

At delivery, the child has been very carefully monitored throughout labor or evaluated before an elective operation. Abdominal and scalp records have been taken, and blood studies have been done. Characteristic tracings are seen by monitor. At delivery, some idea of the child's condition ex-

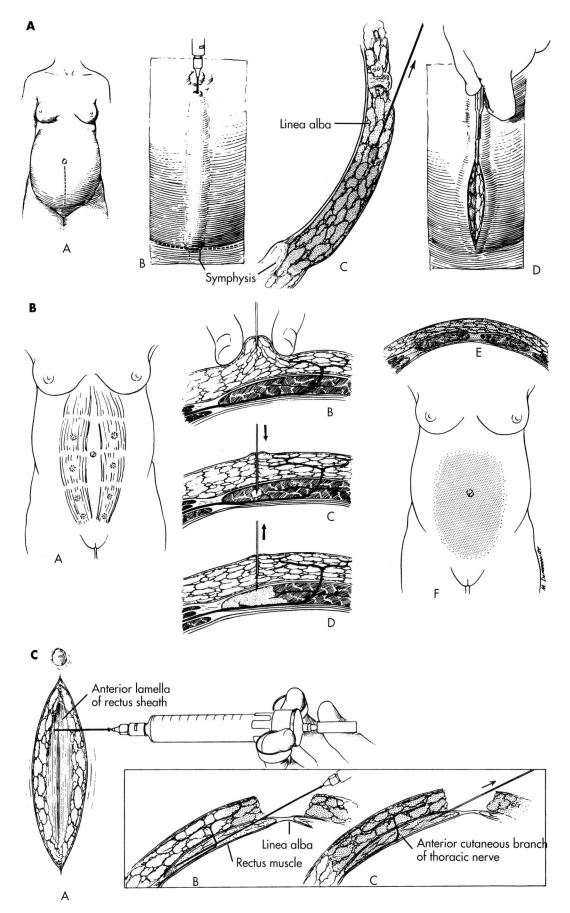

Fig. 61-39 Local anesthesia for cesarean section midline incision. **A,** *A,* Incision line; *B,* superficial injection; *C,* detailed illustration; *D,* superficial incision. **B,** *A,* Areas for injection; *B-E,* details of injection; *F,* area of anesthesia. **C,** Details of injection. (From Bonica J: *Principles and practice of obstetric analgesia and anesthesia,* vol 1, Philadelphia, 1967, FA Davis.)

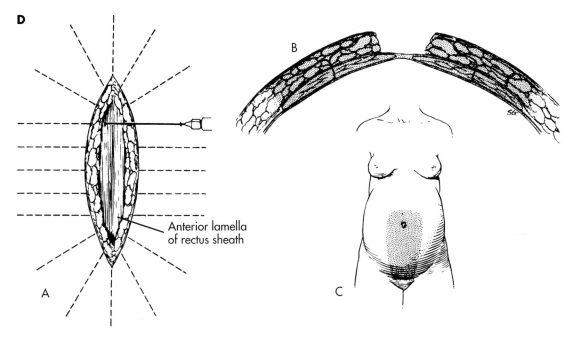

Fig. 61-39, cont'd **D,** *A,* Extended injection; *B,* detail; *C,* area of anesthesia.

ists. The Apgar score is taken immediately either before or after the cord is cut. An Apgar score reads:

Sign	0	1	2
Heart rate		Slow (<100)	>100
Respiratory effort	Absent	Slow, irregular	Good, crying
Muscle tone	Absent	Some extremity flexion	Active motion
Reflex irritability	Flaccid	Grimace	Vigorous cry
Color	Blue or pale	Extremities blue Body pink	Completely pink

The original Apgar score used 0-3 for 0, 4-7 for 1, 8-10.

There must be an integrated, close relationship between all members of the team that is prepared to care for the vulnerable child in many obstetric matters. This team includes the perinatologist, who is the keystone of modern obstetric practice. Unquestionably, the presence of a highly trained specialized anesthesiologist for all cesarean sections will reduce morbidity even more.

ADJUNCTIVE SURGERY WITH CESAREAN SECTION

Questions about surgery other than the cesarean section arise with regard to appendectomy, herniorrhaphy, ovariectomy, myomectomy, gastrointestinal surgery, panniculectomy, correction of uterine anomalies, and tubal ligation. In general, each of these has a very specific indication. Routine appendectomy at every operation is not recommended. Excision of ovarian cysts or paraovarian cysts is indicated if there are no complicating factors related to the primary operation. If the cesarean section has been elective without any complications, excision of pedunculated myomata may be performed without risk. Subserous myomata, unless they interfere with closure of the uterine wound, should not be removed. Uterine anomalies should not be repaired, with the exception of a small uterine horn or sacculation. Excision of a previous defective myometrial scar may be performed.

Tubal ligation must be done with attention to the increased vascularity of the mesosalpinx; the more simple procedures such as Pomeroy or Parkland are the most popular. The tube should be ligated with at least *1-0 and preferably 1 plain catgut;* this produces the greatest immediate local tissue reaction, which is desirable. The Uchida procedure is the most dependable with an almost nonexistent failure rate (when properly performed). On the other hand, if poorly performed, it requires more time and skill and can result in local bleeding or hematoma formation. Ampullary fimbriectomy, such as the Kroner procedure, with use of 1-0 plain catgut as a ligature, double tied, is simple and effective; except in rare circumstances, an Irving procedure is not indicated at cesarean section. Because of the added time of operation and the increased blood loss, total hysterectomy at the time of cesarean section is not usually indicated for sterilization. Good postoperative recovery is directly related to operating time, low tissue trauma, minimal blood loss, and reduced size and amount of suture material.

Any severe gastrointestinal disease that includes the gallbladder should be dealt with by a consultant. Panniculectomy should not be done; repair of a symptomatic hernia, if small and simple, can be done at cesarean section. Umbilical hernia, which is common in pregnancy, can be repaired very easily. Superficial plastic surgery can be done currently with the cesarean under local anesthesia, but extensive tissue dissection and any surgery on the breasts should be avoided.

ELECTIVE CESAREAN SECTION AND POSTCESAREAN VAGINAL DELIVERY

Elective Cesarean Section

A repeated cesarean section is performed for conditions in which a trial of labor is not indicated. Some examples of this are previous classical operation, poorly healed postcesarean section scar, the presence of the same indication for which the previous operation was done, evidence of imminent uterine rupture, fetal indications that preclude vaginal delivery at any time, and central placenta previa.

The single most important consideration in elective or repeated cesarean section is "timing." The maturity of the fetus must be established without any doubt. This is one of the most serious failures in the use of the elective operation and should be one that never occurs in modern obstetric practice. Fetal pulmonary maturity can be determined by several factors. When possible, the determination of accurate gestational dates is essential. Reliable dates can be supported by records of ovulation when available. Early pregnancy tests done by the patient have become common and are reliable when positive on a given date in relation to the last menstrual period. Pelvic examination, accurate estimation of fundal height, determination of a fetal heart, and "quickening" all indicate accuracy of conception time. US determinations are more reliable to determine fetal age and size at various times in the pregnancy and are used with increased accuracy to judge overall fetal maturity. Invasive studies such as amniocentesis with determination of lecithin/sphingomyelin (L : S) ratio, while moderately risky, are nevertheless very valuable markers of lung maturity. It is obvious that careful prenatal care and exact records together with the information from fetal maturity determinations are absolutely necessary to establish both fetal whole body and lung maturity. It may be necessary to allow the patient to go into labor and then perform the operation with further estimation of fetal maturity whenever possible. Failure to be particularly precise about this matter may be disastrous, for respiratory distress syndrome and hyaline membrane disease may produce a damaged child, which could have been avoided and will lead, if nothing else, to indefensible litigation.

Postcesarean Vaginal Delivery

Now that the "once a cesarean section always a cesarean section" theory has been put to rest, the practice to permit vaginal delivery after a previous cesarean section has reached a proportion of approximately 65%. This is true even after the patient has had more than one previous cesarean section in the past 10 years. If the original indication is absent, the previous postoperative course was uneventful, and there are no other contraindications, vaginal delivery after cesarean section has become very successful. Rupture of the uterine scar is relatively rare. The use of very dilute oxytoxic agents to enhance labor has been without event; vaginal delivery has progressed readily. If the patient has had a vaginal delivery either before or after a previous cesarean section, her chances of success are high. Prostaglandin gels have been used to ripen the cervix in several patients without noticeable deleterious effect. If there are suspicions that the scar may have ruptured, an immediate cesarean section can be performed. This means that vaginal delivery after cesarean section should be done in an adequate environment with a full backup team available for major surgery.

Cesarean Section: Contemporary Aspects

In the past 7 years, more and more emphasis has been placed on two important but controversial points: (1) the role of vaginal delivery after previous cesarean, which is an unsolved dilemma, and (2) combined methods to reduce the ever increasing use of cesarean section, which involves such matters as an alternative method and what is an acceptable operation rate.

At a symposium under the auspices of the San Diego Gyn Society in March of 1998, Jeffrey Phelan, holder of both M.D. and J.D. degrees made the statement that if the rate of use of cesarean section for delivery continues, the national average may well reach 50%! It was also stated that more than 90% of women with a previous operation had another cesarean for subsequent deliveries. In view of this, the present application of vaginal birth after cesarean (VBAC) has not significantly lowered the overall cesarean rate. Consideration of VBAC warrants reevaluation.

VBAC has been used since 1934. There was an increase through 1984 but even then more than 50% of women with a history of a previous cesarean had an elective repeat operation. However, by 1994 the increase in VBAC trials of labor with successful fetal and maternal outcome had increased to 70% in some large institutions. The overall incidence of uterine rupture in these patients ranged from 0.5% to 0.8%. Not all such ruptures resulted in catastrophic outcome for either mother or child. There were no maternal deaths and whether the fetus survived depended on prematurity, previous fetal compromise from many causes, and failure to promptly diagnose the uterine rupture. A high success rate for VBAC depends on several factors:

1. Knowledge of details of the prior cesarean, such as indication, pathologic condition of mother or child, the presence of infection, and postoperative recovery as well as the kind of operation done
2. Detailed information on the present pregnancy
3. Position and status of the fetus
4. Condition of the cervix (Is it favorable for induction of labor?)
5. Progress of the trial of labor and the condition of the fetus throughout (This implies normal progress and normal presentation.)
6. Absence of any signs of abnormal uterine function or symptoms suggestive of actual or impending uterine rupture, placental accident, or sudden excessive vaginal bleeding
7. Favorable outlook of the mother for trial of labor and vaginal delivery

The favorable aspects of trial of labor and VBAC may encourage the increased use of this method to reduce the incidence of routine repeat cesarean sections. However, an important point is that VBAC with labor induction must be done in a setting where immediate cesarean section or exploratory laparotomy can be provided with expert anesthesia, available blood, and preferably a pediatric consult as needed.

Combined methods to reduce the incidence of cesarean delivery aside from VBAC have been studied and discussed recently at a symposium in Chicago, most of which is found in an article by Flamm published in June 1998. He points out that doctors and nurses should provide the clinical leadership to reduce the cesarean rate to 15% by the year 2000. This goal is timely, ethical, and in the best interests of childbearing women in America. The outcome of these collaborative projects may be summarized as follows.

Reduction of the overall cesarean rates safely involves several concepts as well as specific practices for primary operations and subsequent repeat cesareans. These are an expectant trial of labor, prevention of cesarean section for failed trial of labor, more effective management of labor pain, no hospital admissions for false labor, and cultivation of nurses to improve their impact on the labor process. These points can be divided into two categories: prevention of unnecessary primary operations and prevention of repeat procedures. For prevention of primary cesarean sections do the following: break the chain of unnecessary intervention, do not admit a patient in false labor, improve pain management in labor, use the physiologic model for labor support, and control specific conditions to reduce the use of cesarean for delivery. For avoidance of a repeat cesarean section make the following changes: educate clinicians to expect and conduct a trial of labor under controlled conditions; educate pregnant women to expect a trial of labor and vaginal birth; and use counseling to eliminate medically unnecessary operations.

Some, if not all, of this reduction depends upon changes in staff organization. This may be accomplished by identifying the processes that establish the safety of a reduced cesarean rate for the staff, improving communication and teamwork among clinicians, and creating policies more conducive to vaginal birth.

Elements that basically work against reduction of the rate of cesarean section are: (1) failure of intention by obstetricians to reduce the operation rate; (2) fear of malpractice litigation; (3) failed coordination between obstetricians and nurses; (4) the practice of a schedule for repeat operations and on-call services that promote cesareans; and (5) persistent myths about management of labor.

To reach the appropriate cesarean rate and overcome some of the resistance to change, it is necessary for the physician staff, including the chief and the hospital administrator, to set a goal to improve. Some actions to take include increasing cooperation between the leaders of obstetrics and labor and delivery nurses, monitoring rates for all individuals and publishing results in a visible report, promoting change in all concepts as described above, and particularly addressing the problems of malpractice litigation.

Cesarean Section versus Vaginal Delivery

Recent comparisons of maternal mortality rates for both vaginal and abdominal delivery have resulted in not surprising statistics: the maternal mortality rate for vaginal delivery is 3.6 per 100,000; for all cesareans is 21 per 100,000; for emergency cesareans is 30 per 100,000; and for elective cesareans is 2.8 per 100,000. Elective cesarean sections and vaginal deliveries theoretically should have a lower maternal mortality rate in modern hospitals. Cesarean section maternal mortality rates depend on the circumstances that surround the indication for the abdominal operation. In emergency cesareans, the condition of the mother may be marginal or becomes so during the operation. Other conditions appear with indicated cesareans such as failed labor or debilitation from disease or an impacted fetus. As always, these indications for cesarean influence the outcome of the operation.

CESAREAN SECTION ETHICAL AND LEGAL CONSIDERATIONS
Definitions

ethics: right or wrong, good or bad, moral obligation (Webster Law); a rule of conduct imposed by authority (Oxford Dictionary)

life: animate existence (Oxford Dictionary)

murder: to kill a human being intentionally, unlawfully, with malice aforethought; to kill wickedly or inhumanely (Oxford Dictionary); to kill a person secretly as opposed to openly (old English law); to kill a person under circumstances defined by statute (Webster's Dictionary)

In the sense of ethics, a decision between two of its elements and the concept of moral obligation, a third element, is involved in questions of the correct use of the cesarean operation. In the earliest of times, moral obligation was the primary consideration in these decisions. In India, a child was removed postmortem by abdominal incision to provide it with a separate burial in the ground rather than by cremation with its mother. In Sumer, 2000 BC, female slaves were delivered by cesarean section, details unknown; legal preference for inheritance was given to the child born by "normal" means. According to the Talmud, a child was removed from an agonal woman in childbirth even on the occasion of the Sabbath. In 1751, when cesarean mortality was extremely high, Burton stated that to abandon an undeliverable live woman with a live child to certain death was unpardonable; because to neglect to save a person when one has the power to save her makes him an accessory to her death, and to decline the operation under the circumstances described above made him an accessory to the death of two persons.

Questions are raised by these historic references.

Questions

What was the justification of the separation of two persons at the time of death during childbirth?

Was there religious custom that required the establishment of independence for the child?

What was the importance that the identification of the unborn child be verified by release from the prison of its dead mother's body?

Whatever the reasons were for the separation of child and mother postmortem, the infant was removed by abdominal incision in most cases for many centuries without emphasis or reference to the principle of right or wrong. The first legal reference to this practice is in the *Lex Regia* of Numa Pompilius 715 BC (see Chapter 1). The child should always be removed from a dead woman's body.

The strongest impact of thought on this matter was by the Christian church and the importance of the right of baptism. Before and all through the Middle Ages, there was movement of the nuns into midwifery; males were excluded even from the examination of a female except in rare instances of embryotomy by instrumentation. Questions arose in the minds of these midwives that concerned certain situations.

If there is no clear evidence of fetal movement, how can one be certain that a child is still alive after the death of its mother?

How can one be sure the mother is truly dead and the child is not alive?

How long after a mother's death can a child survive in utero?

Does baptism of a newly dead child entitle it to the proper quality of life after death?

If no knowledgeable person is present at a woman's death with a viable child in utero, can a "lay" person perform postmortem cesarean section?

Does any public or religious authority or relative have to give permission for postmortem operation in such cases?

What is the punishment for failure to rescue a live child postmortem?

Most of these questions, until very recently, have never been adequately answered, and there are those who are still not sure of all the answers. One of the motivations to write about obstetric matters was ostensibly for the education of midwives; almost all of the earliest obstetric texts were for this purpose. There was intense pressure to remove a child for baptism, if not to save its life, and this led to many strange practices including the pretense of life in a postmortem child so that it could be baptized and properly buried. It has been suggested that maternal death was even hurried to allow for abdominal delivery. In the 1500s, Estienne was the first to suggest cesarean section in the moribund woman. He depicted a certain area and kind of abdominal incision for this purpose. In the past, ethics, the law, and religious matters came into conflict, and Estienne's suggestion of the agonal cesarean, as it was referred to, helped solve some of this dilemma.

Even in contemporary times, "when does the soul enter the fetus?" is the most vexatious question. Is an unborn fetus a person? When does a fetus really become *viable* without life support in a highly technical neonatal intensive care nursery? Aside from this point in the decision for cesarean, consider the incredible impact of this matter in questions of abortion.

The matter of the soul was debated by literally thousands of religious people in the Western world and millions in the Eastern world and still is. For an historic landmark in the West, there is the philosophic attitude of Tertullian in 200 AD who was the greatest protagonist of the soul for many years. His opinion was that the fetus was a living organism from conception and did not acquire life at birth. He was convinced that the soul was in the fetus from the beginning and considered various obstetric procedures such as embryotomy on a living child. He referred to an instrument that caused a violent secret intrauterine death without the obvious dismemberment of embryotomy. This was a long, bronze, sharp, stylet, called a "foeticide," which was inserted into the fetal head in utero, which caused a fetal death. Later in this same reference, Tertullian referred to the use of an abdominal incision to deliver a child for preservation of its "soul." This adherence to the concept of the soul caused an ethical problem when embryotomy was considered because, if it was carried out with a live child, it can be judged as being murder.

Should a woman be sacrificed to preserve a child, if not for life, at least for baptism? An English translation of Trotula leaves little doubt how the midwives were advised: "When the woman is feeble and the chylde may naught comyn out, then it is better that the chylde be slayne than the moder of the chylde also dye." According to St. Paul (Rom. 3:8) no woman should be sacrificed for the purpose of saving the child: "Evil should not be done that good may come." In the 1500s, on the other hand, is the famous quote of Henry VIII regarding the fate of Jane Seymour: "Save the child by all means, for it is easier to get wives than male heirs." In 1513, Roesslin in his text on advice to midwives implied the presence of males at the time of cesarean section, even though one midwife in the 1300s had apparently performed seven successful operations.

At a meeting of the faculty of Doctors of Theology in France in 1733, four questions were asked for solution:

1. Can one use the cesarean operation to save a mother and child when there is a good prognosis to save one or the other by the procedure? The answer: One can use the operation when the best prognosis is good for both mother and child.

2. Can one prejudice a mother, to obtain a secure salvation for the child when her certain death will be caused by the operation? The answer: If the operation will cause certain death, one cannot use it as a remedy. There is more in the answer, but, in summary, it was said that God who gives us life, alone can dispose of it; one cannot do evil to do good; the mother's consent does not make the operation legal; she is not in a state to give away that which is not hers to give; one cannot compare the temporal life of the mother with the spiritual life of the child, because one compares the mother's homicide with the child's misfortune and this assures the homicide is a crime without excuse, whereas the child's misfortune, deplorable as it is, does not charge anyone.

3. When the loss of both mother and child is anticipated because of the circumstances that surround them, can one be expected to use the cesarean section for the one who has the better chance of survival? The answer: In such a case, even if there is no certainty of success with the operation for either, it is permissible to use it. One can certainly use a doubtful cure in a hopeless disease. One would not use the operation, however, to accelerate a death to obtain a life.

4. Finally, if one can save only the mother or the child by the use of the operation, with good prognosis for the other, which of the two is preferable? The answer: In response to this, the Council regarded the respect for the question to a court of law, but there is always the requirement of mercy. If one does not abide by the law, one can sacrifice the child's life for that of the mother; but mercy demands that a mother may prefer the preservation of the child's rightful life. We have the right to preserve the life God has given us, and we are empowered to take away the refuge when to do so rejects that which needs it. (This is a rough translation from Pundel.)

In 1752, Fra Cangiamila in his text, "Embryologie Sacree," very strongly indicated the opinion of the Christian church about the absolute importance of salvation of the soul through baptism. There were implications of the tendency to favor the child in this writing, and he reported on more than 112 cases of postmortem cesarean section with successful infant baptism. This historic background provides consideration of some aspects of these heavy decisions in contemporary obstetrics. For example, from a legal point of view, a physician who dismembers a live child in utero because it cannot be delivered vaginally or another who performs a cesarean section for a live child with full knowledge that such an operation will kill the mother could be liable for a charge of murder. Murder charges have never been brought probably because of the involuntary nature of inescapable circumstances. However, if either child or mother or both die because of neglect, ignorance or failure to perform the duties of an obstetrician in accord with established minimum standards, or if the physician is under the influence of drugs or alcohol and is totally incompetent to accomplish *anything* properly, such a person may be liable for more than just malpractice.

In the 1700s, every possible solution was explored and Sigault, in 1768, proposed a method to increase the size of the internal bony pelvis by splitting the cartilage of the pubic symphysis. This procedure has many sequelae but is still used in some countries. For more than 150 years, the discussions raged as to the ultimate anterior-posterior internal measurement that would not permit even an embryotomy. Several women were left to die with a partially dismembered dead fetus still in utero in the mistaken belief that such treatment did not constitute murder as much as the use of the cesarean operation. As of 1843, the cesarean was considered the most brutal operation in medicine, condemned by every principle of humanity, philosophy, and religion. No one understood that long difficult labors with ruptured membranes and multiple internal and external manipulations before performance of a cesarean *compromised the operation completely.* By 1865, Radford stated that no physician had cause to commit murder of the unborn and that the lack of reasonable estimate of the child's value had led to destruction of infants for which there was no compensation. Barnes, who greatly favored embryotomy, was of the opinion that physicians should not employ vengeance against the woman who could not deliver vaginally, by use of cesarean section as punishment. In 1880, Kinkead in Ireland remarked that a live unborn child has as much a right to life as the mother has to hers. At that time, the earlier philosophy was repeated that, in the end, the mother has the inalienable right of survival even if it means destruction of the child, because both she and the physician were answerable to God and the child was not. The impact of anesthesia, antisepsis, hemostasis, and suture of the uterine wound was immeasurable and between 1880 and 1940 cesarean section mortality was 5% or less. The operation became more improved as to "timing," and indications were observed early in labor or often even before.

Injudicious use of the operation arose with improvement, and this may be a problem in modern times. Two major problems still existed in the early twentieth century: the continued risk and presence of intraabdominal infection and uterine rupture with a subsequent pregnancy. This led to the dictum, "once a cesarean always a cesarean" and stimulated invention of the low uterine segment and extraperitoneal operations and caused investigation of certain indications. As the safety of the operation increased, these questions became more important from the standpoint of the ethical use of cesarean:

1. Should cesarean be performed when the child is dead?
2. Can the parents or relatives demand that the operation be done?
3. Should cesarean section be done without a medical indication, such as high social value of the child?
4. Is preservation of the soft tissue of the pelvis a reason for performance of the operation?
5. Are most abnormal fetal presentations always delivered by cesarean?
6. Should the operation ever be performed for gross fetal abnormalities?
7. What are the ethics of performance of a cesarean for a moribund woman?
8. Is a failed induction of labor with ruptured membranes after 48 hours an indication for the operation?
9. Are severe psychoses or unstable personalities contraindications for vaginal delivery?
10. Is an abnormal fear of labor or the loss of three premature infants compensated by elective cesarean?

All of these reasons have been used for performance of cesarean many times. The ethical considerations of these various problems are rarely discussed with the parents; some overly conservative obstetricians would not consider most of these at any time for cesarean section. The moral integrity of the obstetrician in attendance has been questioned on occasion, and absence of it may have been correct. The importance of truth as one sees it, with all the available information and perhaps the opinion of another, equally ethical physician, may solve some of these unacceptable practices. Instruction of the importance of absolute personal integrity in medicine has been considered since before the second millennium BC. In cases involving two or more lives, this integrity must be complete.

As this century moves on, lawsuits and open criticism in the media; ethical considerations by the public in other areas of reproductive medicine such as abortion, in vitro fertilization, surrogate parents, preservation of fertilized ova, use of fetal organs for transplantation, artificial insemination especially in parents of the same sex; and improvements in intrauterine surgery have all influenced the use of cesarean section in the United States.

Terms such as right to life, right for perfection, wrongful life, and maternal denial of the operation are now in the public eye almost on a daily basis. Consideration of court-ordered cesarean section regardless of the parent's wishes is a potential devastation in obstetric practice. Incursion of the law into medicine in obstetrics began, as has been seen, with the *Lex Regia* in 715 BC. This was preserved in the Justinian Code, and the principle was reviewed in 1139. Rules of conduct in relation to cesarean section were established in Europe in various countries. One of the most extensive was the decree in 1749 by Charles III of Spain made in Sicily, which empowered priests and other laypersons in the Catholic Church to perform postmortem cesarean in the absence of a physician. This decree was the basis for postmortem cesarean performed by Catholic priests in the early days of California and Mexico.

In France, postmortem cesarean was decided by the physician and the family; if the Catholic Church insisted on the operation, *it was never supported by the law.* In the early 1800s, there was punishment for burial of a woman with a viable child without an examination by an expert to decide to save the child.

In another country, cesarean operations could only be done by a specialist unless there was sudden death, in which case any physician could do it. Viability was set at 6 months' gestation. Postmortem cesarean had to be performed with the same care and diligence as if the woman was alive. Some of the laws in Europe were enacted as late as 1835. The multiplicity and sometimes discrepancy in these legal decrees indicated the confusion over the ethics of performance of cesarean section. The only law still known in the United States is a state law that requires the permission of a husband or near relative to allow a postmortem operation when possible.

In contemporary practice there are several items for consideration; for example, negligence, which is composed of duty, breach, causation, injury. It is the obligation of the obstetrician to use all knowledge, skill, care, and diligence in management of all decisions with regard to the kind of birth required for the best outcome. When is referral indicated? Should there always be a second opinion? Informed consent should always contain at least the reason for the operation, the risks, the potential complications, alternatives, consequences if not performed, and recuperation. Other matters are concerned with the timely cesarean, the failure to perform it at all or at the wrong time, failure to perform the operation properly, the problems of the broken instruments, presence of a foreign body in the uterus or peritoneal cavity, and the principle that the surgeon is still responsible for everything and everyone in the operating room.

Some situations must be considered in the use of the cesarean operation that might not be usually recognized: What is the legal status of a child who is killed in utero by a bullet, dies during intrauterine fetal surgery, dies because its mother is killed or injured either accidentally or maliciously, dies from prematurity because of elective cesarean, or dies from maternal drug overdosage or extreme alcoholism? These are mostly matters for attorneys, and, yet, this begins another dilemma: What are the mother's rights to permit or request a cesarean, and what are the child's rights for delivery by cesarean rather than by vaginal delivery no matter how difficult?

Cases have been filed in the courts in which the person who caused the violent death of the child either directly or indirectly is indicted for second-degree murder. Recent cases reported in the media with potential if not actual legal consequences are as follows:

1. A young woman was admitted in labor in an emergency room, with no prenatal care, in deep coma, and with knowledge that she had taken a recent heavy dose of crack cocaine. There was fetal tachycardia. She delivered a newly dead infant in 3 hours. The mother may be indicted for manslaughter or murder on the basis of violation of the fetal right to life.

2. A young woman, who was an intense chronic drug user throughout her pregnancy, delivered a newly stillborn child. She was not indicted because of very low mentality and an inability to recognize the gravity of her situation. She was recommended for custodial care.

3. A young male was arrested, indicted, and convicted of second-degree murder of an unborn child. He struck the automobile in which the mother was being driven while he was under the influence of drugs and alcohol. She had severe injuries and deep hemorrhagic shock, which led to the death of her 7-months' premature child delivered by emergency cesarean section. The defendant showed no remorse and was sentenced to a long prison term without parole. At issue were the rights of the unborn child and whether a 7-months' premature child could survive outside the mother's body.

4. A case is under consideration for indictment of a severely chronic alcoholic young woman, drunk throughout her pregnancy, who delivered a child so severely compromised by fetal alcohol syndrome that it could not survive. There are no extenuating circumstances.

5. There are two recent cases of trauma to an unborn infant by gunfire. One was a "drive-by shooting," which resulted in trauma to the abdomen and uterus and an injury to the fetal zygomatic arch and the external ear on the same side. The mother survived. The second was a gunshot trauma of the abdomen at the time of the Los Angeles riots. This random bullet lodged in the fetal arm, which prevented it from entrance to vital areas. Both of these involve questions of assault with a deadly weapon upon the unborn child.

The precedence for these cases is not strong, and it remains to be seen what the law will ultimately do with such conditions. It is the role of any physician who is involved in obstetrics to enter into discussion of all of these things, and it is also the role of obstetric organizations to impact as strongly as possible the creation of solutions that are reasonable, moral, ethical, and correct for all concerned.

CONTEMPORARY CESAREAN SECTION

The primary concern with the use of cesarean delivery, aside from life itself, is the preservation of the fetal brain. Everyone who conceives is entitled to a perfect child regardless of any of the factors that work against this. This single element is probably the most important reason for the high cesarean rate in modern American obstetrics. Litigation involves the liability of the obstetrician in cases of the imperfect child and almost never its parents, especially the mother (see Chapter 12).

The human brain develops as the largest single organ in the embryo and at 38 to 40 weeks weighs an average of 350 g. It doubles in size by the sixth month of neonatal life, averaging about 700 g. It doubles again by 3 years of age. Preservation of this remarkable organ must begin early in prenatal life. During this time, critical influences that affect the brain occur. These may be beneficial under normal conditions but may produce devastation when adverse environmental factors are present. Toxic poisons can enter the fragile vulnerable brain cells as a result of almost all drugs ingested by the mother. The more toxic the drug, the greater is the damage. The effects of so-called benign medication or foods that may impair these cells are not reversible. Nerve cell damage is observed in cases of starvation or inadequate diet, irradiation, and trauma. Neurophysiologists state that millions of nerve cells never reproduce. They cannot repair themselves. They cannot be replaced. Once injured or killed, these cells are lost (see Chapter 5).

The effects of prenatal care, no matter how exact and careful, may be negated by the rigors of labor, trauma of delivery, obstetric accident, uteroplacental insufficiency, or inherent genetic defects, among other things. Modern obstetric practice uses an incredible array of scientific devices and chemical materials to facilitate the care of the fetal brain before, during, and after labor and delivery. This includes the judicious use of cesarean section to respond to indicators of fetal trouble, failing labor, or maternal physiologic problems.

Knowledge of predictable difficulty in the obstetric situation is essential in the never-ending battle for preservation of the fetal brain. Information derived from US and numerous other testing methods may lead to cesarean section as the method of choice for delivery even without a test of labor or trial of induction of labor. This obviously is in the interest of preservation of the fetal brain. Obstetric accidents such as premature separation of the placenta, prolapse of the fetal cord, sudden or increased development of fetal distress, or uterine hemorrhage with central placental previa, for example, all indicate immediate surgical intervention, again, especially for preservation of the fetal brain. Some maternal illnesses may have a profound influence on developing brain cells, and the progression or intensification of such disease leads to the performance of elective cesarean, even premature, rather than induced premature labor. Otherwise, obstetric situations are obvious, such as failed labor, disproportion between the fetus and maternal pelvis, and several others, as indicators for avoidance of traumatic vaginal delivery by performance of cesarean.

Some of the effects of instrumental delivery on the fetal brain are incompletely known, and there are undoubtedly subtle effects on the fetal brain by these maneuvers that are as yet unknown, regardless of the skill and competence of the specialized obstetrician.

In 1942, Ricci and Marr stated: "Of what value is the adroit forceps (or vacuum extractor) delivery of a woman in prolonged labor if every muscle and every fiber is stretched and attenuated beyond resiliency, if the perineal body becomes relaxed, scarred and functionless, initiating a trial of distressing pelvic symptoms? Of what value is a type of delivery which (thus) destroys the natural tone of the vagina and starts the gradual descent of the cervix and fundus necessitating an eventual drastic repair." The author would add, perhaps of even greater importance, of what value are such deliveries and ill-timed interventions if there is permanent damage to the fragile cells of the infant brain, with the recollection that a high percentage of "nerve cells" never replace themselves; once damaged, forever damaged, they are not restored. The disastrous effects of asphyxia, internal cerebral blood loss either gross or microscopic, and laceration or distortion of brain tissues by trauma and edema set the stage for the tragedy of the kind of damage in which all variations of cerebral palsy are only partial results.

Cesarean section is, of course, no panacea against damage to the fetus by any means, but, if its use is judicious as to "timing," true indication, and other factors, it is potentially a positive influence in the production of a healthy child. External elements such as prematurity, poor surgical ability, careless delivery of the child through abdominal or uterine incisions of improper size or placement, improper anesthesia producing anoxia or toxic effects, maternal hypotension, excessive blood loss before delivery all influence the success of cesarean delivery.

The inability to guarantee a perfect child by abdominal delivery is cause for careful deliberation with regard to frivolous or convenient use of the operation. One must be prepared to defend both sides of the case; the operation should have been done earlier, or electively, or later, or not at all!

The passage of time and the potential increase in knowledge and sophistication in the management of the reproductive process from start to finish, which includes cesarean section, should assist all physicians to reach a much higher success with the product being "the perfect child."

SUGGESTED READING

Allaire A, Fisch J, McMahon M: A prospective randomized trial of subcutaneous drain versus subcutaneous suture in obese women undergoing cesarean section, *Am J Obstet Gynecol* 178(1, part 2):578, 1998 (abstract 250).

Apgar V: Proposal for a new method of evaluation of the newborn, *Anesth Analg* 32:260, 1953.

Baas J: *Outlines of the history of medicine,* Huntington, NY, 1971, Robert E Kreiger (Translated by H Handerson; originally published in 1889).

Baudelocque J: *L'art des accouchements,* ed 3, Paris, 1796, Chez Mequignon.

Bauhin C: *Hysteromotokia by Francisco Rousset,* Basle, Conrad Valdkirch, 1581 (Translated by C Bauhin).

Beck A: Low segment cesarean section, *Am J Obstet* 79:179, 1919.

Benirshke K: *Pathology of the placenta,* New York, 1991, Springer-Verlag.

Bhishagratna K: *The Sushruta Samhita Varanasi,* ed 2, India, 1963, Chowkhamba Sanskrit Series Office.

Blumenfeld-Kosinski R: *Not of woman born,* Ithaca, NY, 1990, Cornell University Press.

Boley J: Caesarean section, *Can Med Assoc J* 32:557, 1935.

Bonica J: *Principles and practice of obstetrical analgesia and anesthesia,* Philadelphia, 1967, FA Davis.

Bumm E: *Geburtshulfe,* ed 17.

Burns H: The Latzko extraperitonial caesarean section, *Am J Obstet Gynecol* 19:759, 1930.

Cangiamila F: *Embryologica sacra,* Milan, 1751 (abridged into French, 1762, Chez Nyon).

Cartwright E: Retrovesical extraperitoneas cesarean section, *Am J Obstet Gynecol* 39:423, 1940.

de Lee J: Newer methods of cesarean section, *JAMA* 73:91, 1919.

de Lee J: An illustrated history of the low or cervical cesarean sections, *Am J Obstet Gynecol* 10:503, 582, 1925.

Dionis M: *Cours d'operation de chirurgie,* Paris, 1740, Chez d'Henry.

Doderlein A: *Operative Gynakologie Doderlein-Kronig,* ed 5, Leipzig, 1924, Georg Thieme.

Duhrssen A: Vaginaler Kaiserschnitt bei Eklampsie, *Arch Gynakol* 39:235.

Durfee R: Extraperitoneal cesarean section, *Surg Gynecol Obstet* 1962.

Durfee R: "Low classical" cesarean section, *Obstet Gynecol Surv* 27:624, 1972.

Estienne C: *La dissection de partis du corps,* Paris, 1546, Chez Simon de Colines.

Finan M, et al: The "Allis" text for easy cesarean delivery, *Surg Gynecol Obstet (Int Abstr Surg Suppl)* 174:22, May 1992.

Flamm BL: Once a cesarean, always a cesarean controversy, *Obstet Gynecol* 90:312, 1997.

Flamm BL, Geiger AM: Vaginal birth after cesarean delivery: an admission scoring system, *Obstet Gynecol* 90:907, 1997.

Flamm BL, et al: Elective repeat cesarean delivery versus trial of labor: a prospective multicenter study, *Obstet Gynecol* 83:927, 1994.

Franchi M, et al: A randomized clinical trial of two surgical techniques for cesarean section, *Am J Obstet Gynecol* 178(1, part 2):S31, 1998 (abstract 71).

Grange CS, et al: The use of hemodilution in parturients undergoing cesarean section, *Am J Obstet Gynecol* 178(1, part 1):156, 1998.

Hudon L, Belfort MA, Broome DR: Diagnosis and management of placenta percreta: a review, *Obstet Gynecol Surv* 53:509, 1998.

Kehrer F: Ueber ein modifiziertes Verfahren beim Kaiserschnitte, *Arch Gynakol* 19:177, 1882.

King A: The legacy of Jesse Bennet's cesarean section, *Bull Hist Med* 2:242, 1976.

Kinght A: Life and times of J Bennett, MD, *S Hist Mag* 2:1, 1892.

Lagrew DC, Adashek JA: Lowering the cesarean section rate in a private hospital: comparison of individual physicians' rates risk factors and outcomes, *Am J Obstet Gynecol* 178:1207, 1998.

Latzko W: Extraperitonealer Kaiserschnitt, *Wien Klin Wochenschr* 22:477, 1909.

Marshall C: *Caesarean section lower segment operation,* Bristol, 1939, John Wright & Sons.

Maygrier J: *Midwifery illustrated 1833* (Translated by A. Doane).

Mercurio S: *La comare o raccoglitrice,* ed 2, Venice, Italy, 1713, Domenico, Lovisa.

Norton J: Latzko extraperitoneal caesarean section, *Am J Ob/Gyn* 30:209, 1935.

Opitz E: Die Kaiserschnitt, *Zentralb Gynäkol* 35:270, 1911.

Osiander F: *Handbuch der Entbindungkunst,* Tubingen, Germany, 1820.

Phelan J: Prevention of fetal/neonatal brain injury: three simple techniques, presented at the San Diego Gyn Society Symposium, 1998, p 1.

Phelan JF: Vaginal birth after cesarean—when is it informed consent? Presented at the San Diego Gyn Society Symposium, 1998, p 30.

Phelan J, Clark S: *Cesarean delivery,* New York, 1988, D Appleton.

Poidevin L: *Caesarean section scars,* Springfield, Ill, 1956, Charles C Thomas.

Porro E: Dell'amputazione utero-ovarica come complemento di taglio caesareo, *Ann Univers Med Chirurg* 5:237, 1876.

Preuss J: *Biblical and talmudic medicine,* New York, 1978 Sanhedrin Press (Translated by F Rosner).

Pundel G: *Histoire de l'operation cesarienne,* Brussels, 1969.

Rasmussen S, Irgens LM, Dalaker K: The effect on the likelihood of further pregnancy of placental abruption and the rate of its recurrence, *Br J Obstet Gynaecol* 104:1292, 1997.

Rebarber A, et al: The safety of intraoperative autologous blood collection and autotransfusion during cesarean section, *Am J Obstet Gynecol* 179(3, part 1):715, 1998.

Ricci J: *The development of gynecological surgery and instruments,* Philadelphia, 1949, The Blakiston Co.

Ricci J: *The geneology of gynecology,* Philadelphia, 1950, The Blakiston Co.

Ricci J, Marr J: *Principles of extraperitoneal caesarean section,* Philadelphia, 1942, The Blakiston Co.

Roonhuyze H: *Heel-konstige aanmerkkingen betreffende de gebrekken der vrouwen,* Amsterdam, 1663 (translated into English, London, 1676).

Rosslin E: *Rosengarten,* Munich, 1910, reprint G Klein & Carl Kuhn (originally published 1513).

Rueff J: *De conceptu et generatione hominis.*

Sanger M: Die kaiserschnitt, *Arch Gynak* 19:370, 1882.

Scultetus J: *Armamentarium chirurgicum,* Frankfort, 1666.

Sharma SK, et al: Cesarean delivery: a randomized trial of epidural versus patient controlled meperidine analgesia during labor, *Anesthesiology* 87:487, 1997.

Siebold EV: *Geschichte der geburtshulfe,* ed 2, Tubingen, 1901, Franz Pietzcker.

Suetonius C: *The historie of twelve caesars,* London, 1931, Frederick Etchells & Hugh Macdonald (reprint by Oxford University Press; originally published in English 1606).

Sushruta. In *The Sushruta Samhita Varanasi,* ed 2, India, 1963, Chowkhamba Sanskrit Series Office.

Tertullian: In Ricci: *The geneology of gynecology,* Philadelphia, 1950, The Blakiston Co.

Thorp JM, et al: First trimester diagnosis of placenta previa percreta by magnetic resonance imaging, *Am J Obstet Gynecol* 178:616, 1998.

Towers CV, et al: A "bloodless cesarean section" and perinatal transmission of the human immunodeficiency virus, *Am J Obstet Gynecol* 179(3, part 1):708, 1998.

van Loon AJ, et al: Randomized controlled trial of magnetic resonance pelvimetry in breech presentation at term, *Lancet* 350:1799, 1997.

Waters E: Retrovesical extraperitoneal cesarean section, *Am J Ob/Gyn* 39:423, 1940.

Wax JR, Gallagher MW, Eggleston MK: Adjunctive color Doppler ultrasonography in second-trimester transabdominal amnioinfusion, *Am J Obstet Gynecol* 178:622, 1998.

Williams J: *Obstetrics,* ed 17, Baltimore, 1989, Williams & Wilkins.

Yoles L, Maschiach S: Increased maternal mortality in cesarean section as compared to vaginal delivery? Time for re-evaluation. *Am J Obstet Gynecol* 178(1, part 2):S78, 1998 (abstract 249).

Young J: *Caesarean section,* London, 1944, HK Lewis & Co.

DICTIONARIES

1. *Cassell's New Latin Dictionary,* New York, 1960, Funk & Wagnalls (originally published in 1854).
2. *Cassell's New German Dictionary,* New York, 1959 Funk & Wagnalls.
3. *Cassell's New French Dictionary,* New York, Funk & Wagnalls.
4. *Klein's Etymological Dictionary.*
5. *Oxford Dictionary.*
6. *Webster's Dictionary.*
7. *The Holy Bible,* King James version.

62 Cesarean Hysterectomy

DAVID L. BARCLAY and PAUL J. WENDEL

EVOLUTION OF THE OPERATION

Cesarean hysterectomy evolved as a lifesaving procedure to prevent death after cesarean section. When the uterus, with a gaping wound, was returned to the peritoneal cavity after cesarean section, maternal mortality approached 100% as a result of intraperitoneal hemorrhage and spillage of infected uterine contents. Animal experiments suggested that the uterus was not an essential organ, and it was thought that removal might reduce the prohibitive postoperative mortality. In 1876, Porro reported on the first successful hysterectomy at the time of cesarean section. However, within 6 years, Sanger introduced closure of the uterine incision with multiple sutures, which obviated the need for a hysterectomy. The Sanger operation became known as the conservative cesarean section. The Porro operation was reserved for the treatment of uncontrollable hemorrhage and uterine infection after cesarean section.

Interest in the operation as an elective procedure was rekindled with the advent of improved antimicrobial agents and relatively safe blood banking procedures in the 1940s. These developments expanded the indications for all elective operations, including cesarean hysterectomy. During the next two decades, reports from major clinics showed elective cesarean hysterectomy to be considered a suitable procedure for sterilization at the time of an obstetrically indicated cesarean section. In addition, total cesarean hysterectomy was recommended in place of the Porro procedure, which consisted of a subtotal hysterectomy and bilateral salpingo-oophorectomy. This enthusiasm began to wane in the latter part of the 1970s. By the 1980s, publications reflected an adverse attitude to the elective operation, and in many major centers the operation was reserved for emergency indications only.

ERA OF SPECULATION: 1768-1868

In 1768, Joseph Cavallini published his experience with experiments on dogs and sheep in which he removed the uterus at the time of delivery. His conclusions were as follows: "All which things having been duly weighed, I do not doubt that the uterus is not at all necessary to life; but whether it may be plucked out with impunity from the human body, we cannot be certain without a further series of experiments of this kind which perhaps a more fortunate generation will attain."[54]

In 1809, Dr. G.P. Michaelis of Marburg suggested that amputation of the uterus after removal of the fetus might make cesarean section a less dangerous operation. Although Dr. James Blundell confined himself to experiments on animals, in 1828, he suggested in his lectures on obstetrics at Guy's Hospital that he was inclined to believe that the dangers of the cesarean operation might be considerably diminished by removal of the uterus. He encouraged adoption of this change in the method of operating in successive lectures and editions of his book on obstetrics. Despite the great mortality accompanying cesarean sections in Great Britain, no surgeon in that country ever tested the value of his suggestion. He died at the age of 87, in the year 1878, by which time other surgeons had proved his views to be correct. The history of cesarean section has been reviewed in great detail by Young.[54]

The First Operations: 1868-1876

Horatio Robinson Storer performed the first cesarean hysterectomy on a woman.[48] Storer was a strong individualist who received his degree from the Harvard Medical School in 1853 and continued his training in Paris and London. In 1855, he entered general practice in Boston but soon broke with tradition and announced himself a specialist in the diseases of women. He became the first American physician to teach gynecology as a separate subject and was the first surgeon to wear rubber gloves while operating. His staunch independence resulted in his removal from the Harvard faculty in 1866, which was the year in which he performed the fourth successful abdominal hysterectomy in the United States.

Storer and his associate Bixby performed the first cesarean hysterectomy on July 21, 1868. Storer had seen the patient on July 16, 1868, and determined that vaginal delivery would be impossible, even with craniotomy, because of a large abdominal tumor obstructing the birth canal. The onset of labor occurred on July 18, and despite active labor and rupture of the membranes, the presenting part could not enter the pelvis. Surgery was delayed until the morning of July 21, when the operation was performed using chloroform anesthesia. A large uterine fibroid tumor complicated the operation and caused extensive hemorrhage. The male child and placenta were badly decomposed, and hemorrhage was profuse. After cesarean section, a metallic cord was firmly tied around the lower uterine segment. The corpus and adnexa were excised and the cervical stump exteriorized. The patient succumbed to the infection on the third postoperative day.

In contrast to Storer's unplanned emergency operation, Eduardo Porro of Pavia, Italy, carefully planned and executed the 26-minute operation that he performed on May 21, 1876.[48] Before that operation, no woman had ever survived a cesarean section in Pavia. The patient was a 25-year-old primigravid dwarf who had a skeletal deformity complicated by rickets, resulting in absolute disproportion. Porro thought that a cesarean section was mandatory, discussed the matter with his colleagues, and planned the operation very carefully. The patient, Julia Cavallini, sought religious support and finally consented to the operation after 6 hours of labor. Essentially, a classical cesarean section was performed, after which there was profuse hemorrhage from the uterine incision. The corpus and adnexa were delivered through the incision, and a wire snare of Cintrat was placed around them and drawn tightly at the level of the internal os. The structures could then be excised and the cervical stump exteriorized through the lower pole of the incision. Peritoneal toilet was accomplished, and a large curved clamp was placed through the vagina and cul-de-sac into the peritoneal cavity for insertion of a large drainage tube. The uterine stump was incorporated into the lower angle of the wound and painted with an antiseptic. The snare was removed with the gangrenous portion of the uterine stump on the fourth postoperative day, and the vaginal drain was removed the following week. By definition, a Porro operation is a subtotal hysterectomy and bilateral salpingo-oophorectomy.

Porro assumed the Chair of Obstetrics at the university at Pavia in 1875 and remained until 1882, when he became head of the School of Obstetrics of Milan. In 1902, he wounded his hand during an operation on an infected patient and died from sepsis. His statue stands in the courtyard of the Women's Hospital at the University of Milan (Fig. 62-1).

There was serious question about the morality of the operation; he discussed the issue at great length with the bishop of Pavia, who sanctioned the hysterectomy as a procedure for saving the patient's life. Only with this backing could Porro present his operation to the Medical Congress of Turin. The keys to his success were planning of the operation before prolonged labor and rupture of the membranes, use of chloroform anesthesia, and adherence to Lister's principles of asepsis. The operation was accepted in European countries but was not favorably considered in Great Britain or the United States. At the Vienna Lying In Hospital during the previous 100 years, not a single woman had recovered after cesarean section. From 1787 until the first successful Porro operation in Paris 1879, all cesarean section patients had died at the Maternity Hospital at Paris. Nevertheless, in 1879, Harris of the United States was not ready to accept the operation and called it an "unsexing and mutilating procedure."[54]

Evolution of Operative Technique

Modifications of the operative procedure began shortly after the report of Porro's operation. In 1878, Muller delivered the uterus through the abdominal incision and constricted the lower uterine segment with an elastic tube, after which the uterus was incised, delivery effected, and the corpus am-

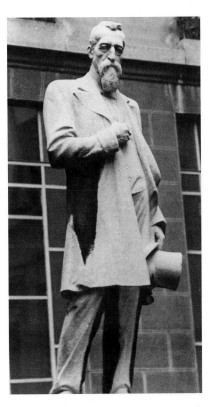

Fig. 62-1 Statue of Professor Eduardo Porro in the courtyard of the Instituto Obstetrico Ginecologico L. Mangiagalli Dell 'Universita' Di Milano. (Courtesy Professor G.B. Candiani.)

putated. The concept was that the peritoneal cavity would be protected from contamination.[19] However, the constrictor caused asphyxia of the child. Isaac Taylor of New York performed the first Porro-type cesarean hysterectomy in the United States in 1880. The cervical stump was returned to the abdominal cavity after hemostasis had been secured, and no drains were used. Unfortunately, the patient died of a pulmonary embolus on the twenty-sixth postoperative day. The first 50 cases of "cesarean ovariohysterectomy" from the world literature were reported by Harris[27] of Philadelphia in 1880: there were 29 maternal deaths and 7 fetal deaths; 23 of the operations had been performed in Italy and 11 in Australia. The first successful cesarean hysterectomy in the United States was performed using the Porro-Muller technique by Richardson in 1881. In that same year, Spencer Wells performed the first total cesarean hysterectomy for cancer of the cervix. Goodson performed the first in the United Kingdom in 1884, using a transverse incision that was extended laterally by traction; this was the first reference to the low segment operation. In addition, he summarized 134 Porro operations, indicating that return of the cervical stump to the peritoneal cavity was associated with a 77% mortality rate compared with a 53% mortality rate for exteriorization.[19] In 1892, Von Waerz introduced specific vessel ligation and returned the cervix to the peritoneal cavity in patients without infection; otherwise it was exteriorized. By 1901, the overall maternal mortality rate was 24.8% in the 1097 operations that had been reported.[19]

Only 6 years after the first successful Porro operation, Max Sanger, a German surgeon, introduced the use of a large number of sutures, deep and superficial, to secure perfect closure of the uterine wound and prevent spillage of blood and lochia into the peritoneal cavity. As noted previously, this came to be called the conservative cesarean section, or Sanger operation, whereas the Porro operation was called the radical cesarean operation. Although Sanger was not the first to close the uterine incision, he described the procedure in detail. The conservative cesarean section became the procedure of choice, and cesarean hysterectomy in the United States was limited to emergency situations such as infection after prolonged labor and hemorrhage. Cesarean hysterectomy was replaced by the low cervical or extraperitoneal procedure for the treatment of intrauterine infection.[54] The Johns Hopkins experience was reported by J.W. Harris[26] in 1922: 64 of 223 cesarean sections were followed by a subtotal hysterectomy, with a maternal mortality of 4.68%. Interestingly, eight operations were performed for sterilization. Sterilization was also listed as an indication for cesarean hysterectomy by Lash and Cummings[31] in 1935.

Evolution of Indications

Until the early 1940s, little emphasis was placed on elective sterilization by hysterectomy at the time of cesarean section. At the University of Rochester in 1945, Wilson[53] reported that 8.7% of all cesarean sections included a hysterectomy; indications were hemorrhage, uterine pathologic conditions, intrapartum infection, and also sterilization. A review in 1947 indicated that in the United States about 2.54% of cesareans were terminated by hysterectomy, with a maternal mortality of 5.2% in contrast to 3.42% for cesarean birth.[46] The results of 153 cesarean hysterectomies performed since 1931 were reported by Dieckman in 1948.[17] Again, some operations had been performed strictly for sterilization.

In the early 1940s, expansion of indications for all elective operations, including elective cesarean hysterectomy, was fostered by the increased availability of antimicrobial drugs and the introduction of blood banking procedures. Davis,[17] of Chicago, advocated total cesarean hysterectomy for elective sterilization, removal of a diseased uterus, or removal of the uterus no longer functionally useful for a woman near the climacteric. At the Chicago Lying In Hospital, form July 1, 1947, to April 1, 1951, 140 of 700 cesarean sections were terminated by hysterectomy. In 1953, Dyer et al.[21] emphasized the fact that cesarean hysterectomy was the preferred method for surgical removal of a diseased uterus and reported 84 cases of total hysterectomy. They strongly advocated total cesarean hysterectomy, and they described the technique of passing a finger into the vagina through the cervical canal to identify the lower limits of the cervix. In 1951, it became the policy of the Tulane service, Charity Hospital, New Orleans, to perform a total operation. This decision was made after review of three patients who had died after a subtotal operation for a ruptured uterus that had extended into the cervix and vaginal fornix, resulting in postoperative hemorrhage.[3] Refinements of the operative

technique of total hysterectomy were described by Bradbury[10] in 1955. A radical hysterectomy and pelvic lymphadenectomy for treatment of cancer of the cervix were reported by Brunschweig and Barber[12] in 1958. Cesarean hysterectomy was openly advocated as a sterilization procedure during the remainder of the 1950s.[4]

Cesarean hysterectomy, primarily for elective reasons, was further advocated in the 1960s, although most authors thought that a cesarean section should not be performed simply for the purpose of removing the uterus. In 1963, Pletsch and Sandberg[42] raised the question of whether or not cesarean hysterectomy should replace cesarean delivery and tubal ligation for sterilization. The "posttubal ligation syndrome" was a concern to some, and Weed[52] questioned the fate of the postcesarean uterus. Half of the September 1969 issue of *Clinical Obstetrics and Gynecology* was devoted to articles on the subject.[50] From January 1, 1938, to September 1, 1959, 1000 cesarean hysterectomies were performed at the Charity Hospital in New Orleans.[3] All operations were performed after 28 weeks' gestation and after abdominal delivery. The operations were further classified as either elective or emergency procedures; the latter designation included only operations performed to prevent exsanguination from profuse hemorrhage. If uterine rupture had occurred, the case was included as abdominal delivery and emergency hysterectomy. There were 800 elective and 200 emergency hysterectomies, which constituted 15.3% of all cesarean sections performed during that period.

During the 1970s, the incidence of cesarean hysterectomy decreased throughout the country, and although some private institutions retained enthusiasm for it, teaching services were losing interest. The first article appeared that compared the characteristics of elective cesarean hysterectomy with cesarean birth, with or without tubal ligation.[9] Two articles[1,8] reported on the use of primary cesarean hysterectomy to accomplish delivery and removal of the uterus for carcinoma in situ of the cervix. Three review articles were published during that decade.[4,29,37] Altogether, 866 cesarean hysterectomies performed between 1938 and 1967 were reported from the Tulane service, Charity Hospital in New Orleans.[4] The changing indications and modifications of the operative procedure over that 30-year period were reviewed with particular reference to discontinuance of the subtotal operation in 1951. Despite the continued popularity of the operation during that decade, notes of caution were voiced, particularly in a article by Haynes and Martin.[29]

During the decade of the 1980s, publications emphasized the role of cesarean hysterectomy for management of uncontrolled hemorrhage and perhaps for the treatment of concurrent uterine pathologic conditions identified at the time of an obstetrically indicated cesarean section.[4] The latter was only a relative indication, depending on the surgeon's experience. A review[25] from Charity Hospital in New Orleans indicated that between 1984 and 1988, a total of 129 cesarean hysterectomies were performed after 4891 cesarean sections; 107 were classified as elective and 22 as emergency operations. In a recent updated tape,[7] Barclay et al., from the University of Southern California, indicated that at their institution a cesarean hysterectomy was performed in roughly 1 of 200 cesarean sections, primarily for control of hemorrhage. During this decade, concern was voiced about the adequacy of residency training for the young physician who might be confronted with the need to perform an emergency postpartum hysterectomy. In summary, outside of a few institutions, cesarean hysterectomy has again become a rather uncommon procedure.

CURRENT INDICATIONS FOR CESAREAN HYSTERECTOMY

Emergency Hysterectomy

An emergency cesarean hysterectomy is by definition a life-saving procedure performed to control hemorrhage. The causes of postpartum hemorrhage fall into roughly four categories: uterine atony, placental disorders, ruptured uterus, and extension of the cesarean incision into the uterine vessels. In 1984, Clark et al.[16] reported that 43% of emergency hysterectomies in their series were performed for uterine atony. This is somewhat less than the 67% incidence reported by O'Leary and Steer.[37,38] In the Tulane series,[4] extending from 1938 to 1967, 31.6% of operations were performed for that indication. In the early years of that study, the Couvelaire uterus associated with abruptio placenta and a consumption coagulopathy was a common indication. Hysterectomy is, of course, an option of last resort, and this is currently an uncommon indication. Clark et al.[16] found that hysterectomy for atony had a statistically significant association with amnionitis, oxytocin augmentation of labor, cesarean section for labor arrest, preoperative magnesium sulfate infusion, and increased fetal weight. In 23% of their patients there was no identifiable risk factor causing the atony. A hysterectomy for uterine fibroids in a patient who has undergone an obstetrically indicated cesarean section would be classified as elective. However, uterine fibroids may interfere with closure of the uterine incision and contractility of the corpus, causing hemorrhage.

Bleeding from the placental site usually involves the noncontractile lower uterine segment in a patient who has undergone a cesarean section for placenta previa. The lower segment is less resistant to penetration by the placenta, causing placenta accreta, increta, or percreta; the last may result in laceration of the uterine vessels when the placenta is removed. The placenta may penetrate through a previous low segment incision and into the base of the bladder. Placenta accreta in excess of that noted in the older literature is emerging as a major indication for hysterectomy, particularly in patients who have undergone a previous cesarean section.[33,45,55] The sharp rise in the cesarean section rate in this country during the past decade may account for this increase. The incidence of placenta accreta is increased when there is the coexistence of a placenta previa and at least one previous cesarean section. Miller et al.[33] from L.A. County Hospital recently reviewed the topic of placenta accreta in more than 155 thousand deliveries over the past 10 years. In the 186

women with both a placenta previa and at least one prior cesarean section, the incidence of placenta accreta was 22%.

Uterine rupture is currently the third most common indication for emergency cesarean hysterectomy. The prevalence of uterine rupture has changed considerably over the last 20 years as the rate of cesarean section has increased. The presence of a scar through the muscle of the uterus represents the greatest risk factor for subsequent uterine rupture. *Uterine rupture* is defined as disruption of the uterine wall along with chorioamniotic membranes and resultant extrusion of fetal parts into the peritoneal cavity. *Uterine dehiscence* is a more common event and is defined as separation of a prior scar without rupture of the chorioamniotic membranes. In a large 10-year retrospective review from Sweden involving women with a prior cesarean section, the incidence of uterine dehiscence was 4% and that of true rupture was 0.6% in women undergoing the trial of labor.[36] In a more recent review from Los Angeles, a similar 10-year retrospective analysis showed the risk of uterine rupture to be 0.6% in laboring women with one prior cesarean section. However, when two or more prior cesarean scars were present, the risk of rupture tripled (1.7%).[34] It has been suggested that puerperal infection after the initial cesarean section contributes to poor healing of the uterine scar and subsequent rupture of the uterus in labor. However, there appears to be little evidence to support this concept.[36]

Spontaneous rupture of an unscarred uterus in labor is a rare event and thought to occur in roughly 1 in every 16,849 deliveries.[35,49] Other causes of obstetric uterine rupture include trauma,[20] use of oxytocic agents,[28] and multiparity. Trauma to the uterus can be either direct or indirect. Examples of direct trauma to the uterus include forceps applications and rotations (i.e., internal and external versions), postpartum curettage, or intrauterine manipulations. Indirect trauma to the uterus would involve blows to the abdomen incurred in falls, domestic violence, or motor vehicle accidents.[20] Uterine rupture associated with oxytocic agents is clearly associated with oxytocin stimulation of labor. However, the use of prostaglandin agents (E_1, E_2, $F_{2\alpha}$) are commonly used in midtrimester abortions. These agents are potent stimulants of uterine contractibility. Their methods of administration produce erratic absorption and potentially tetanic contractions, which cannot be remedied by withdrawing the medication.[28]

Extension of a low transverse incision into the uterine vessels or the cervix and vagina is an uncommon occurrence. In patients of low parity, an extended incision can usually be repaired. Care must be taken to prevent damage to the ureter or bladder. Bleeding is not completely controlled by ligation of the anterior division of one or both hypogastric arteries, although pulse pressure in the uterine artery is decreased.[13,16,39] Ligation of the uterine artery at its origin is usually necessary and can be accomplished by developing the pararectal and paravesical spaces. The ureter is identified and the vessels are secured with clips, but venous bleeding remains a problem because of the increased vascularity of the pelvis in pregnancy. Throughout the repair procedure, the ureters must be identified by palpation or visualized before placing ligatures or clips.[23]

Elective Cesarean Hysterectomy

Indications for elective cesarean hysterectomy fall into two categories: pathologic conditions in the pelvis and elective or medically indicated sterilization. These indications are relative, and the frequency with which the operation is performed depends on the philosophy of the particular obstetric unit. In some obstetric units, an elective cesarean hysterectomy has never been performed. Primary cesarean section to allow an associated hysterectomy may occasionally be performed for uterine pathologic conditions such as leiomyomata or carcinoma in situ of the cervix. Early invasive cancer of the cervix can be treated by a primary cesarean delivery and radical hysterectomy with pelvic lymphadenectomy.[12,47,51]

Since 1980, few publications have suggested elective cesarean hysterectomy as a means of sterilization. In 1980, Britton[11] reported 112 elective cesarean hysterectomies, of which 74 were planned and performed for sterilization; the remaining patients underwent hysterectomy for uterine or other gynecologic pathologic conditions or for medically indicated sterilization. In 1981, Plauche et al.[40] reported on 108 cesarean hysterectomies performed in a private practice setting; 46.3% were for the purpose of sterilization. There is little current support for this method of sterilization without the presence of associated uterine or pelvic pathologic conditions. Although the failure rate of tubal ligation performed at the time of cesarean section is somewhat higher than that of an interval operation, it is considered to be the method of choice in conjunction with abdominal delivery. Although the fate of the postcesarean uterus has been questioned, it has been suggested that 25% of these patients will undergo a subsequent hysterectomy.[52] In general, interval hysterectomy is though to present fewer complications.

Uterine pathologic indications for cesarean hysterectomy are usually listed as carcinoma in situ of the cervix, uterine fibroids, or severe intrauterine infection. The advent of improved antibiotic therapy has obviated the need for hysterectomy in patients with infection, although with advanced pelvic sepsis it is an important adjunctive form of therapy, particularly in diabetic and otherwise medically compromised patients.

Carcinoma in situ of the cervix can usually be accurately diagnosed during pregnancy by colposcopy. If invasive disease has been excluded, vaginal delivery is allowed and the cervix is treated by an appropriate means after the postpartum period. However, some patients who would be candidates for hysterectomy may wish to proceed with completion of treatment at the time of delivery. In 1977, a satisfactory fetal and maternal outcome was reported for 32 patients treated by cesarean hysterectomy for carcinoma in situ of the cervix.[8] The operations were planned and performed before the onset of labor; therefore adequate removal of the cervix was accomplished without difficulty.

Uterine leiomyomata are seldom an indication for cesarean delivery unless there is interference with the labor and delivery process. If an interval hysterectomy were planned for treatment of large uterine fibroids, hysterectomy after an obstetrically indicated cesarean section would be appropriate in the hands of an experienced surgeon. This approach appeals to patients and is cost-effective.

A controversial indication for elective cesarean hysterectomy is the "thin uterine scar."[4] Cesarean section scars may vary from thin, white avascular scars to asymptomatic complete dehiscences. Most low-segment scars can be repaired, but a defective vertical scar extending into the corpus or a T incision may not heal well. Most surgeons would choose to perform a tubal ligation to prevent future pregnancies; however, in the past, hysterectomy was performed in hospitals where tubal ligation was prohibited.

Interval vaginal hysterectomy and repairs would be the treatment of choice for uterine prolapse and vaginal relaxation. If a cesarean hysterectomy is performed for this indication, the uterosacral ligaments should be plicated and a suprapubic urethrovesical suspension performed.[5,9]

If bilateral adnexal pathology is identified at the time of cesarean section, a hysterectomy is ordinarily performed also. Care must be taken not to misinterpret bilateral adnexal enlargement that is due to benign hyperactio luteinalis or luteoma of pregnancy.

Other reported indications for elective cesarean hysterectomy are dysfunctional uterine bleeding, adenomyosis, endometriosis, and other forms of pelvic pathologic conditions that would be infrequently identified at the time of cesarean section.

THE SURGICAL PROCEDURE

A cesarean hysterectomy is distinctly different from a hysterectomy in the nonpregnant patient. The tissues are soft and pliable, and the uterine and paravesical veins are greatly distended. Constant tension on the uterine corpus attenuates the very engorged uterine vessels and allows sharp dissection throughout.

Preparation for the operation is that usually undertaken for a patient undergoing an elective cesarean section. Vaginal cleansing has not been routinely carried out. The patient's blood is typed and screened so that blood will be available if needed. For a planned operation, autologous blood can be stored.[14] A short course of prophylactic antibiotics is prescribed and is the same as that used by the surgeon for cesarean delivery. Consent-to-sterilization forms are completed, and the patient is counseled about the irreversibility of the infertility that is a secondary consequence of this operation.

Basic surgical principles that facilitate the operation are as follows:

1. The skin incision may be vertical or transverse.
2. Dissection of the vesicouterine space is carried out before incision of the uterus.

3. A vertical or transverse uterine incision in the lower segment can be used, although the vertical incision facilitates constant tension on the corpus.

4. The uterine corpus is placed on constant tension by the first assistant.

5. Sharp dissection allows the uterine vessels, particularly the veins, to be skeletonized.

6. Vascular pedicles are secured with clamps and cut but not ligated until the uterine vessels on both sides have been secured.

7. Low ligation of the uterine vascular pedicles requires that the ureters be identified by palpation.

8. Compression of the lower uterine segment between the thumb and forefinger allows one to "milk" the soft dilated cervix above the fingers and secure the vagina with angle clamps.

Either general or conduction anesthesia is used, whichever is ordinarily used for cesarean section.[15,30] A vertical or low transverse abdominal incision can be used. It is usually easier to develop the bladder flap over the presenting part before the uterine cavity is opened; adhesions from a prior cesarean section require sharp dissection. Although the dilated veins over the bladder may appear formidable, sharp dissection and gentle blunt dissection can usually avoid entry into the venous channels.

After delivery of the newborn, the uterus is delivered from the abdominal cavity. The placenta is removed only if it separates easily; otherwise it is left in place. If the uterine incision tends to bleed, it can be secured with large sutures or simply clamped with small ring forceps. It is important to move quickly and secure vascular pedicles without delay. The corpus is placed on constant tension by the first assistant, which maintains anatomic relationships and decreases blood loss (Fig. 62-2). If the need for cesarean hysterectomy has been determined preoperatively, a vertical incision facilitates delivery of the newborn, and the first assistant's finger can be placed into the upper pole of the incision to maintain constant traction on the uterus throughout the procedure. A self-retaining retractor is placed.

If oophorectomy is not indicated, the operation is begun on one side by placing a clamp on the round ligament, which is cut, and the anterior leaf of the broad ligament is incised to join the bladder flap incision. The avascular space in the broad ligament is penetrated, and the uteroovarian ligament and fallopian tube are doubly clamped and cut, with a third clamp securing the proximal pedicle to prevent back bleeding. With constant tension on the corpus, the broad ligament is incised sharply with the scissors and the uterine vessels skeletonized (Fig. 62-3). This dissection progresses so quickly and easily that the uterine vessels may be skeletonized to the cardinal tunnel, jeopardizing the ureter. The clamp is placed on the uterine vessels quite low on the cervix. As a consequence, the vesicouterine space should be reinspected to be certain that the angle of the bladder has been adequately mobilized and perhaps elevated with a retractor. Because the tissues of the cardinal ligament are quite soft and pliable, the ureters can be readily rolled between the thumb and forefinger for precise identification

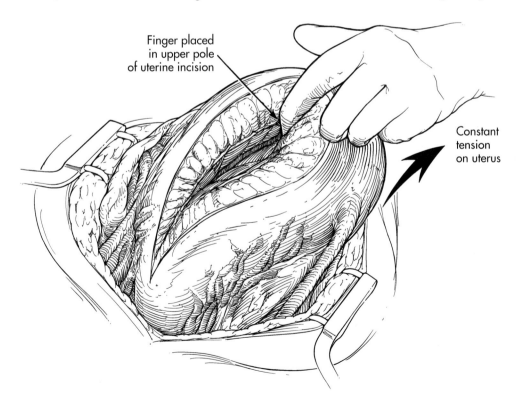

Finger placed
in upper pole
of uterine incision

Constant
tension
on uterus

Fig. 62-2 Constant tension on the uterus maintains anatomic relationships and attenuates the uterine vessels, which facilitates sharp dissection.

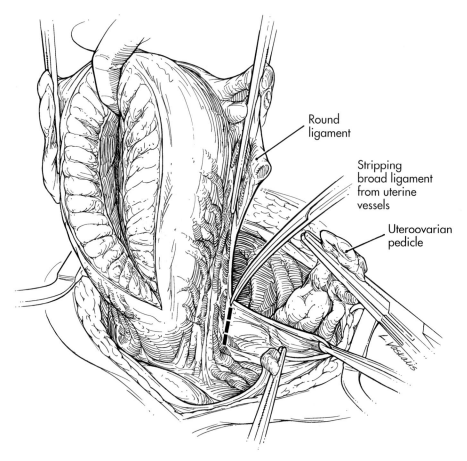

Round
ligament

Stripping
broad ligament
from uterine
vessels

Uteroovarian
pedicle

Fig. 62-3 Vascular pedicles are clamped but not ligated until the uterine vessels are secured. Uterine vessels are skeletonized by sharp dissection.

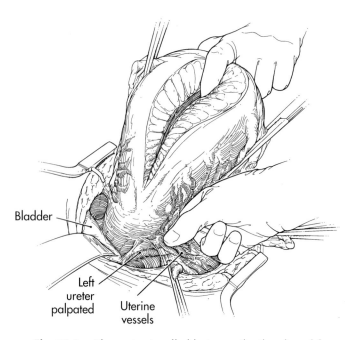

Bladder

Left
ureter
palpated

Uterine
vessels

Fig. 62-4 The ureter is rolled between the thumb and forefinger, and the bladder is retracted before the uterine vessels are clamped.

before the clamp is placed on the uterine vessels (Figs. 62-4 and 62-5).

After a similar dissection is performed on the opposite side and the uterine vessels are clamped, the major vascular pedicles have been secured. A proximal clamp is placed on the uterine vessels on either side to prevent back bleeding, after which the uterine vascular pedicles are cut and secured with a stick tie. The round ligament pedicle is secured in a similar manner. However, the uteroovarian pedicle is large and requires a free tie followed by a stick tie. If the ties are placed too close to the ovary, there is a tendency for the suture to cut through the ovarian parenchyma, resulting in intraoperative or postoperative bleeding. As a consequence, about 6% to 10% of patients receive a unilateral salpingo-oophorectomy.[4,9] If the pedicle is entirely too large, the ovarian portion may be secured separately.

The need for additional pedicles can be determined by compressing the lower uterine segment between the thumb and forefinger. This assists in identification of the very soft cervix, which is difficult to define, particularly in the patient who has undergone much cervical dilation and effacement. Compression of the lower segment tends to "milk" the uterine cervix upward for identification (Fig. 62-6). The adequacy of dissection of the bladder from the upper vagina is again assessed. An additional pedicle is usually required

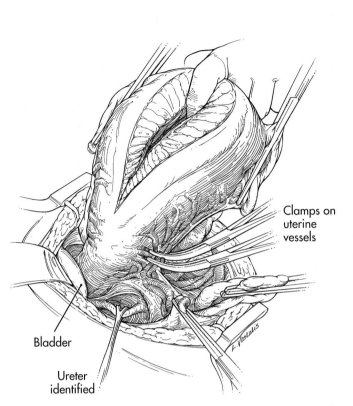

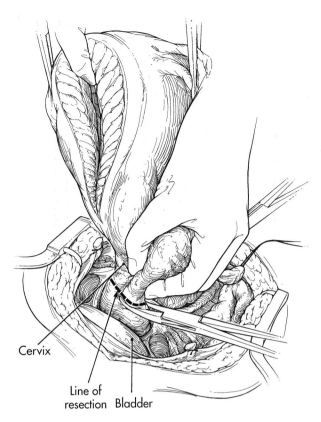

Fig. 63-5 A Babcock clamp is placed on the distal ureter for demonstration purposes. The ureter and bladder are at risk when the uterine vessels are clamped.

Fig. 63-6 With constant traction on the uterus, the upper vagina is compressed to "milk" the soft cervix above the fingers. A clamp can then be placed on each angle of the vagina.

at the base of the cardinal ligament and may include the attenuated uterosacral ligament. The pedicle is grasped with a straight Kocher or Heaney clamp that is allowed to slide off the lateral portion of the cervix and grasp the base of the cardinal ligament. A knife is used to cut a wedge-shaped pedicle that is tied with a suture ligature, which may include and retie the adjacent uterine vascular pedicle. A retractor is placed beneath the bladder reflection to assure that space has been adequately developed, and the cervix is again identified by palpation. A curved Heaney clamp can then be placed on each angle of the vagina, the vagina incised, and the specimen removed. If there is uncertainty about the cervix, the anterior vaginal wall can be opened and the Heaney clamps can then placed on each angle of the vagina before the remainder of the vagina is circumscribed.

The mucosa of the cut edge of the vagina tends to retract; therefore Kocher clamps are placed on the anterior and posterior vaginal walls. A figure-of-eight suture is placed at each angle of the vagina, making certain that the angle of the vaginal mucosa is included and secured to the base of the cardinal ligament. The remainder of the vaginal cuff is closed with figure-of-eight sutures. If the surgeon prefers to leave the vaginal cuff open, the entire edge can simply be run with a locking suture. (Within 24 to 48 hours postoperatively, the vaginal cuff that is left open is probably functionally closed, although it is easier to open if there is a pelvic hematoma.) The pelvis is thoroughly inspected and irri-

gated, and hemostasis is secured. The ovarian pedicle is secured to the adjacent round ligament and not attached to the vaginal cuff. A transvaginal T-tube or extraperitoneal drain is used at the surgeon's discretion. Ordinarily drainage is not necessary if prophylactic antibiotics are used. We do not reperitonealize the pelvis after any hysterectomy, although this is a debatable issue and the surgeon's choice.

The described surgical technique represents our own bias.[5] A low transverse uterine incision may decrease blood loss from the cesarean section, but constant tension on the corpus is easier with a vertical incision. There may be hesitancy in developing the vesicouterine space before incising the uterus for delivery, but the space is more easily and thoroughly developed over the presenting part, particularly if there have been prior cesarean sections and there is scar tissue in the space. If there is uncertainty about identification of the ureters by palpation, the uterine vessels can be taken at a higher lever; however, this requires several pedicles along each side of the uterus, close to the cervix. The lower limits of the cervix can be identified by incising the cervix anteriorly or by entering the vagina posteriorly. This causes additional contamination of the operative field, however, and delineation of the cervix, if well effaced, may still be difficult. Extrusion of mucus from the cervical glands has been suggested by Plauche et al.[40,41] as a helpful indicator of the lower edge of the cervix. Particularly with emergency cesarean hysterectomies, a variable number of patients reportedly have retained a remnant of cervix. Absorbable polyglycolic and/or chromic catgut suture is used throughout the operation.

In an emergency situation, in the hands of a surgeon who has had little experience with the operation, subtotal hysterectomy is an acceptable alternative. However, one must be certain that a uterine tear has not extended into the cervix or fornix of the vagina, a problem not resolved by subtotal hysterectomy. After ligation of the uterine vessels, the corpus is amputated and the cervix simply closed.

OPERATIVE COMPLICATIONS

The surgical complications of cesarean hysterectomy are not unique to the operation, but their frequency of occurrence is greater. Operating time may be prolonged, and the frequency of blood transfusion and urinary tract injury is increased. In experienced hands the average elective operation takes less than 90 minutes, which is approximately 30 minutes longer than a cesarean section, with or without tubal ligation.[6,9] Plauche et al.[40,41] reported an average operating time of about 65 minutes for a series of elective operations that Plauche performed. The duration of emergency operations depends primarily on the amount of time spent attempting to stop bleeding before a decision is made to remove the uterus. Clark et al.,[16] reporting on a series of emergency operations, noted an approximately 3-hour operating time.

The incidence and quantity of blood transfusion depend on the indications for the operation, whether emergency or elective, the surgeon's experience, and the extent of pelvic pathologic conditions. A hysterectomy performed after a cesarean for a bleeding complication, such as placenta previa, obviously increases the need for blood replacement. In our series,[9] approximately 20% of the patients undergoing elective cesarean hysterectomy received a transfusion, but 4% of those undergoing cesarean delivery, with or without tubal ligation, were given transfusions. The mean preoperative hematocrit in patients undergoing cesarean hysterectomy was 35.6% ± 3.5%; 13 of the 47 patients given transfusions were admitted to the hospital with a hematocrit of 30% or less, and 1 had undergone a cesarean delivery for bleeding. Plauche et al.[40] reported that 11.8% of private patients undergoing an elective operation received a transfusion. Fluid administration during the operation can often maintain vital sign stability until equilibration in the recovery room necessitates transfusion. Pritchard et al.[44] demonstrated that a gravida at term can lose 1 L of blood with little or no hemodilution in the postpartum period. It may be reasonable for the patient scheduled to undergo a planned elective cesarean hysterectomy to store a unit of her own blood several weeks preoperatively.[14] Some authors[24,39] have recommended ligation of the anterior division of the hypogastric artery prior to hysterectomy, but this has had little influence on the amount of blood loss or incidence of transfusion. Clark et al.[16] have also found this to be true during emergency hysterectomy for hemorrhage. On the other hand, if a uterine vessel retracts into the cardinal ligament adjacent to

the ureter or there is excessive bleeding for other reasons, the surgeon should open the pararectal and paravesical spaces and place a clip on the anterior division of the hypogastric artery and on the uterine artery at its origin. Pulse pressure in the uterine artery is decreased after ligation of the anterior division and may assist in defining the site of bleeding.[13] The importance of operative technique cannot be overemphasized: constant tissue tension, sharp dissection, and development of the vesicouterine space before delivery of the presenting part are imperative if one is to maintain control of the operation and minimize blood loss.

Bladder entry and ureteral injury are recognized complications of cesarean hysterectomy but also occur with cesarean section. In our series,[9] 4 of 390 patients undergoing repeat cesarean section without hysterectomy sustained bladder entry and repair with satisfactory healing; 4 of 242 patients undergoing an elective cesarean hysterectomy sustained bladder entry, all among the 114 patients undergoing a repeat cesarean birth. Eisenhop et al.[23] reported 23 bladder entries and 29 diagnostic cystotomies in a series of 5376 primary and 2151 repeat cesarean sections. The diagnostic cystotomies were performed to evaluate for ureteral injury. Bladder entry is ordinarily recognized, repaired, and heals uneventfully; most fistulas probably result from inclusion of bladder wall during closure of the vaginal cuff or separation of bladder muscle such that the adjacent mucosa undergoes subsequent necrosis. Leakage of urine usually occurs within the first 10 days postoperatively. Some authors[31] have recommended that the bladder be partially distended with methylene blue or sterile milk before or after the hysterectomy to detect an unrecognized entry. A lacerated bladder wall is closed in two layers, using absorbable suture, and the catheter is left in place for approximately 7 to 10 days.

Ureteral injury is a greater risk during cesarean hysterectomy than during abdominal or vaginal hysterectomy in the nonpregnant patient. The ureter is most often injured with ligation of the uterine vessels. However, when salpingo-oophorectomy is performed, the ureter should be identified at the pelvic brim before the infundibulopelvic ligament is secured. Our technique of cesarean hysterectomy can be used only if the surgeon is confident that the course of the ureter can be identified by palpation. If there is a question of ureteral injury, the surgeon can open the bladder extraperitoneally, identify the ureteral orifice, and pass a retrograde ureteral catheter. Another alternative is to perform a linear ureterotomy at the pelvic brim and thread a ureteral catheter into the bladder. Partial severance of the ureter may be detected by injection of methylene blue into the ureteral lumen at the pelvic brim. In our series of 242 elective cesarean hysterectomies,[9] there was injury to 1 ureter, which was recognized and repaired and which healed satisfactorily, and the hospital stay was not prolonged. In the Tulane series of 866 cesarean hysterectomies performed over a 30-year period,[4] there were 4 ureteral injuries, of which 3 were recognized and repaired and healed satisfactorily and 1 was repaired during the postoperative period. Plauche et al.[40] reported no ureteral injuries in a series of 108 elective and emergency operations performed in a private hospital. Mickal and Plauche[32] reported 808 consecutive operations at the Charity Hospital in New Orleans; there were 30 bladder entries, 7 vesicovaginal fistulas, and 2 ureteral fistulas. It should be emphasized again that because dissection and skeletonization of the uterine vessels progress easily in pregnancy, there is a tendency to clamp the uterine vessels quite low. If the surgeon cannot be certain of the location of the ureter by palpation, the uterine vessels should be taken high, but this means multiple pedicles on each side of the uterus.

It should be noted that Eisenhop et al.[23] reported on 7 patients who sustained ureteral injury among 7527 who underwent cesarean section: 5 of the ureteral ligations occurred during control of bleeding from extension of a uterine incision into the broad ligament; in 1 patient the uterine incision extended into the trigone of the bladder; in another patient the ureter was compromised during evacuation of a retroperitoneal hematoma. Because the ureters are always at risk during a pelvic operation, the importance of learning to visualize the ureter or define its course by palpation is obvious.

POSTOPERATIVE COMPLICATIONS

Febrile morbidity secondary to infection of the operative site and bleeding are the primary postoperative complications. In most studies the incidence of febrile morbidity is less after cesarean hysterectomy than after cesarean delivery. This is particularly true if there has been prolonged labor or evidence of intrauterine infection. In our series,[9] febrile morbidity after elective cesarean hysterectomy was 31% compared with 55% after cesarean and 34% after cesarean delivery and tubal ligation. The cesarean tubal ligation and cesarean hysterectomy patients, by and large, underwent a planned operation before the onset of labor. In addition, the study was made during an era when prophylactic antibiotics were not used. In a recent study, Gonsoulin et al.[25] reported an 18.3% incidence of febrile morbidity after elective cesarean hysterectomy when prophylactic antibiotics were used. Although vaginal cuff infection is the most common source of febrile morbidity, urinary tract infection, pulmonary atelectasis, wound infection, thrombophlebitis, and breast inflammation must all be considered.

Postoperative ovarian abscess is a special cause of postoperative febrile morbidity after cesarean hysterectomy: 6 of 12 cases reviewed by one of the authors (DB) had occurred after cesarean hysterectomy. The latent period between the operation and acute symptoms was as long as 300 days. The ovary in pregnancy is particularly susceptible to infection. Sutures on the uteroovarian ligament may cut through and fracture the ovarian cortex sufficiently to allow entry of organisms.

The incidence of postoperative bleeding after abdominal hysterectomy is approximately 0.7% and after a vaginal hysterectomy is approximately 2% in the nonpregnant patient.[2,18,22,43] Postoperative bleeding, consisting of intraabdominal or vaginal hemorrhage, expanding vaginal cuff or retroperitoneal hematoma or incisional bleeding that requires suturing, occurs after approximately 3% to 4% of elective cesarean hysterectomies.[4,7,9,32] Intraperitoneal hemorrhage necessitates secondary surgery in approximately 1% to 2% of patients. The site of bleeding is most often the uteroovarian ligament, which may require unilateral salpingo-oophorectomy. Bleeding from the area of the vaginal cuff or uterine vessels is difficult to identify immediately. A pack can be placed in the pelvis and the retroperitoneal space entered for identification of the anterior division of the hypogastric and uterine arteries at the pelvic sidewall on either side, and the vessels can be secured with clips. The hypogastric venous system is markedly dilated during pregnancy, and care must be taken to avoid injury to those vessels. This approach ordinarily slows bleeding sufficiently to allow specific identification and ligation of bleeding points. Again, the ureter must be identified and protected. After a number of transfusions, a consumption coagulopathy is a consideration. Treatment of large vaginal or retroperitoneal hematomas must be individualized as one would after any type of hysterectomy. After an emergency operation for uterine rupture, care should be taken not to overlook an extension of the uterine tear into the vaginal fornix; this is particularly true if a subtotal operation has been performed.

Addition of hysterectomy to cesarean delivery should increase the average hospital stay by 1 day or less. Currently, that would mean approximately a 4-day postoperative hospital stay.[7,9]

One would expect a no greater postoperative death rate after cesarean hysterectomy than after an elective cesarean section alone, or for that matter, abdominal or vaginal hysterectomy in the nonpregnant patient. The indication for the operation, such as uterine rupture or severe intrauterine infection, is usually the determining factor in postoperative outcome.

SUMMARY

The evolution of the cesarean hysterectomy operation has been reviewed. The operation was devised to prevent death from hemorrhage and sepsis after cesarean section. Need for the operation was obviated by closure of the uterine incision, aseptic surgical techniques, and extraperitoneal cesarean section.

Performance of an emergency cesarean hysterectomy, defined as an operation to prevent death from hemorrhage, has not been questioned. Introduction of transfusion therapy and antibiotics in the 1940s expanded indications for all elective surgery, including elective cesarean hysterectomy. Until perhaps the mid-1970s, the elective operation, even for sterilization only, was advocated by many authors. That enthusiasm has now waned, and the question is whether or not enough operations are being performed to maintain surgical skills.

The surgical technique of cesarean hysterectomy is different from that of hysterectomy in the nonpregnant patient.

Those differences must be recognized and taught, preferably during an elective operation. An emergency operation in untrained hands can be hazardous.

The complications of cesarean hysterectomy, primarily hemorrhage and urinary tract injury, are well recognized. Approximately 10% to 20% of patients undergoing an elective operation, particularly those in an indigent population, require transfusion—often 1 U of packed red blood cells. The incidence of postoperative bleeding is approximately 4%, and 1% of patients require reoperation. Bladder entry occurs even during cesarean section, but if recognized, repair is usually successful. An occasional vesicovaginal fistula or ureteral injury occurs in association with cesarean hysterectomy. The incidence of these complications should be interpreted in the context of similar occurrences during or after abdominal or vaginal hysterectomy in nonpregnant patients.

Each surgeon, on the basis of surgical experience, must decide in conjunction with each patient whether elective hysterectomy at the time of cesarean section is in the patient's best interest.

REFERENCES

1. Abitbol MM, Benjamin F, Gastillo N: Cesarean hysterectomy in the treatment of carcinoma in situ of the cervix diagnosed during pregnancy, *Am J Obstet Gynecol* 117:909, 1973.
2. Amirikio H, Evans TN: Ten year review of hysterectomies: trends, indications and risks, *Am J Obstet Gynecol* 134:431, 1979.
3. Barclay DL: Cesarean hysterectomy at the Charity Hospital in New Orleans—1000 consecutive operations, *Clin Obstet Gynecol* 12:635, 1969.
4. Barclay DL: Cesarean hysterectomy—thirty years experience, *Obstet Gynecol* 35:120, 1970.
5. Barclay DL: Current ob/gyn techniques. *Surgical communications,* vol 1, no 3, Ortho Pharmaceutical Corp., 1976.
6. Barclay DL: Cesarean hysterectomy. In Phelan JP, Clark SL, editors: *Cesarean delivery,* New York, 1988, Elsevier.
7. Barclay DL, Clark SL, Plauche WC: Cesarean hysterectomy, update tape, *Am College Obstet Gynecol* 11, 1986.
8. Barclay DL, Frueh DM, Hawks BL: Carcinoma in situ of the cervix in pregnancy: treatment with primary cesarean hysterectomy, *Gynecol Oncol* 5:357, 1977.
9. Barclay DL, et al: Elective cesarean hysterectomy: a 5 year comparison with cesarean section, *Am J Obstet Gynecol* 124:900, 1976.
10. Bradbury WV: Cesarean hysterectomy, *West J Surg* 63:232, 1955.
11. Britton JJ: Sterilization by cesarean hysterectomy, *Am J Obstet Gynecol* 173:887, 1980.
12. Brunschwig A, Barber HR: Cesarean section immediately followed by radical hysterectomy and pelvic node excision, *Am J Obstet Gynecol* 76:199, 1958.
13. Burchell CR: Physiology of internal iliac artery ligation, *J Obstet Gynecol Br Commonw* 75:642, 1968.
14. Chestnut DH: Autologous blood for elective cesarean hysterectomy, *Am J Obstet Gynecol* 150:796, 1984 (letter).
15. Chestnut DH, Redick LF: Continuous epidural anesthesia for elective cesarean hysterectomy, *South Med J* 78:1168, 1985.
16. Clark SL, et al: Emergency hysterectomy for obstetric hemorrhage, *Obstet Gynecol* 64:376, 1984.
17. Davis ME: Complete cesarean hysterectomy: logical advance in modern obstetric surgery, *Am J Obstet Gynecol* 63:838, 1951.
18. Dicker RC, et al: Complications of abdominal and vaginal hysterectomy among women of reproductive age in the United States, *Am J Obstet Gynecol* 144:841, 1982.
19. Durfee RB: Evolution of cesarean hysterectomy, *Clin Obstet Gynecol* 12:575, 1969.
20. Dyer I, Barclay DL: Accidental trauma complication pregnancy and delivery, *Am J Obstet Gynecol* 83:907, 1962.
21. Dyer I, Nix FG, Weed JC: Total cesarean hysterectomy at cesarean section and in the immediate puerperal period, *Obstet Gynecol* 65:517, 1953.
22. Easterday CL, Grimes DA, Riggs JA: Hysterectomy in the United States, *Obstet Gynecol* 62:203, 1983.
23. Eisenhop SM, et al: Urinary tract injury during cesarean section, *Obstet Gynecol* 60:591, 1982.
24. Evans S, McShane P: The efficacy of internal iliac artery ligation in obstetric hemorrhage, *Surg Gynecol Obstet* 160:250, 1985.
25. Gonsoulin W, Kennedy RT, Guidry KH: Elective versus emergency cesarean hysterectomy cases in a residency program setting: a review of 129 cases 1984-1988, *Am J Obstet Gynecol* 165:91, 1991.
26. Harris JW: A study of the results obtained in sixty-four cesarean sections terminated by supravaginal hysterectomy, *Bull Johns Hopkins Hosp* 33:318, 1922.
27. Harris RP: Results of the first fifty cases of "caesarean ovaro-hysterectomy," 1869-1880, *Am J Med Sci* 80:129, 1880.
28. Hawe JA, Olah KS: Posterior uterine rupture in a patient with a lower uterine segment caesarean section scar complicating prostaglandin induction of labour, *Br J Obstet Gynaecol* 104:857, 1997.
29. Haynes DM, Martin BJ Jr: Cesarean hysterectomy: a twenty-five year review, *Am J Obstet Gynecol* 134:393, 1970.
30. LaPlatney DR, O'Leary JA: Anesthetic considerations in cesarean hysterectomy, *Anesth-Analg* 49:328, 1970.
31. Lash AF, Cummings WG: Porro cesarean section, *Am J Obstet Gynecol* 30:199, 1935.
32. Mickal A, Plauche WC: Cesarean hysterectomy, *Mediguide to ob/gyn,* vol 4, no 1, Lawrence DellCorte Publications, Inc., Miles Pharmaceuticals, 1985.
33. Miller DA, Chollet JA, Goodwin TM: Clinical risk factors for placenta previa-placenta accreta, *Am J Obstet Gynecol* 177:210, 1997.
34. Miller DA, Diaz FG, Paul RH: Vaginal birth after cesarean: a 10-year experience, *Obstet Gynecol* 84:255, 1994.
35. Miller DA, et al: Intrapartum rupture of the unscarred uterus, *Obstet Gynecol* 89:671, 1997.
36. Nielson TF, Ljungblad U, Hagberg H: Rupture and dehiscence of cesarean section scar during pregnancy and delivery, *Am J Obstet Gynecol* 160:569, 1989.
37. O'Leary JA: Cesarean hysterectomy: a 15 year review, *J Reprod Med* 4:231, 1970.
38. O'Leary JA, Steer CE: A 10 year review of cesarean hysterectomy, *Am J Obstet Gynecol* 90:227, 1964.
39. Pelosi M, Langer A, Hung C: Prophylactic internal iliac artery ligation at cesarean hysterectomy, *Am J Obstet Gynecol* 121:394, 1975.
40. Plauche WC, Gruich FG, Bourgeois MO: Hysterectomy at the time of cesarean section: analysis of 108 cases, *Obstet Gynecol* 48:459, 1981.
41. Plauche WV, et al: Cesarean hysterectomy at Louisiana State University, 1975 through 1981, *South Med J* 76:1261, 1983.
42. Pletsch TD, Sandberg EC: Cesarean hysterectomy for sterilization, *Am J Obstet Gynecol* 85:254, 1963.
43. Pratt JH: Common complications of vaginal hysterectomy, *Clin Obstet Gynecol* 19:645, 1976.
44. Pritchard JA, et al: Blood volume changes in pregnancy and the puerperium. II. Red blood cell loss and changes in apparent blood volume during the following vaginal delivery, cesarean section and cesarean section plus total hysterectomy, *Am J Obstet Gynecol* 84:1271, 1962.
45. Read JA, et al: Placenta accreta: changing clinical aspects and outcome, *Obstet Gynecol* 56:31, 1980.
46. Reis RA, DeCosta EF: Cesarean hysterectomy, *JAMA* 134:775, 1947.
47. Sall S, Rini S, Pineda A: Surgical management of invasive carcinoma of the cervix in pregnancy, *Obstet Gynecol* 118:1, 1974.
48. Speert H: Eduardo Porro and cesarean hysterectomy, *Surg Gynecol Obstet* 106:245, 1958.

49. Sweeten KM, Graves WK, Athanassiou A: Spontaneous rupture of the unscarred uterus, *Am J Obstet Gynecol* 172:1851, 1995.

50. Symposium: Cesarean hysterectomy, *Clin Obstet Gynecol* 12:652, 1969.

51. Thompson JD, et al: The surgical management of invasive cancer of the cervix in pregnancy, *Am J Obstet Gynecol* 121:853, 1975.

52. Weed JC: The fate of the post cesarean uterus, *Obstet Gynecol* 14:780, 1960.

53. Wilson KM: The role of Porro cesarean section in modern obstetrics, *Am J Obstet Gynecol* 50:761, 1945.

54. Young JH: *Cesarean section: the history and development of the operation from earliest times,* London, 1944, Lewis & Co.

55. Zelop CM, et al: Emergency peripartum hysterectomy, *Am J Obstet Gynecol* 168:1443, 1993.

63 Inversion of the Uterus

DAVID H. NICHOLS

DEFINITION AND TYPES

A turning inside-out, or inversion, of the uterus may be incomplete, in which only the uterine fundus is inverted to varying degrees, or complete, in which the entire endometrial cavity is everted. Das' historic review[8] of uterine inversion notes that it was recorded as long ago as 2500 BC.

Degrees[33]

First-degree inversion of the uterus is incomplete, and the inverted cavity is said to extend to the cervix, but not beyond the cervical ring. Because at times it may be self-correcting, its frequency may be greater than reported.

Second-degree uterine inversion is the most common type reported. The inverted endometrial cavity extends through the cervical ring, but it does not descend as far as the perineum.

Third-degree, or complete, inversion extends to the perineum. The fundus has descended through the cervix and the os presents upwards.

NONOBSTETRIC INVERSION OF THE UTERUS
Cause and Diagnosis

Downward traction to the uterine fundus from an attached pedunculated submucosal leiomyoma or other neoplasm, combined with long-standing myometrial contraction as an attempt by the uterus to rid itself of such a perceived "foreign body" may invert the uterine fundus along with the tumor. The lesion may be found on routine examination often in the presence of a chronic bloody discharge.[17]

Treatment

This condition should be treated initially by transvaginal amputation of the tumor, being careful that the surgery be extraperitoneal at this time, because the prolapsed lesion is usually infected. If subsequent hysterectomy is contemplated, the uterus should be given several weeks for the infection to subside to lessen the risk of peritonitis.

Fundal inversion coincident with a prolapsed leiomyoma can be identified by careful bimanual pelvic or rectal examination whereby the gynecologist, while palpating the top of the uterine fundus, feels for the characteristic dimple in the fundus. Finding such a dimple forewarns of the possibility of unexpectedly transecting the inverted fundus along with removal of the prolapsed tumor and, by opening into the peritoneal cavity, risking peritonitis (Fig. 63-1).

When such a dimple has been identified, the stalk of the pedicle should be transected *near its attachment to the prolapsed tumor.* The base of the stalk may be ligated or cauterized for hemostasis, and the remaining stalk is permitted to retract within the uterine cavity. Freed of the tumor, the partially inverted uterine fundus usually reverts to normal over a few weeks.

PUERPERAL UTERINE INVERSION
Cause and Diagnosis

Most of the uterine inversions that are encountered are accidents of labor and delivery. The frequency with which obstetric uterine inversion is encountered varies from 1 per 1000 to 1 per 6500 deliveries,[27,35,38] the different rates possibly reflecting the rate of detection and diagnosis.

Obstetric uterine inversion occurs unexpectedly during the third stage of labor, possibly when a portion of the uterine fundus becomes indented (as from cord traction to an unseparated placenta or the presence of a short umbilical cord), and the remaining muscle of the uterus contracts around the invaginated portion as it would around a foreign body[25,26] and, in attempting to expel it, turns itself inside-out.[21] It has even been reported to occur at cesarean section.[12]

Puerperal inversion is most common among the primiparous[2,3,31] and is seen more often among patients who were receiving intravenous $MgSO_4$ for treatment of preeclampsia.[27,35,37] In most instances, the condition occurs spontaneously without demonstrable obvious cause, although it is more common among nullipara, especially those with a previous pregnancy loss in the first trimester.

Subsequent recurrence of inversion in the same patient has been reported.[41] Deep anesthesia causing uterine relaxation after delivery has been noted.[2,19,30] Plaut[36] cautions against membrane traction during delivery of the placenta as possibly etiologic, and Catanzarite and Grossman[5] and Harris[18] recommend routine exploration of the uterine cavity after every delivery to detect early inversion and treat it immediately. An association with prolonged labor has been suggested.[43]

Careful management of the third stage of labor is the most important factor in preventing this serious complication.

Treatment

Acute Obstetric Uterine Inversion. Acute obstetric uterine inversion is noted at the time of delivery or within

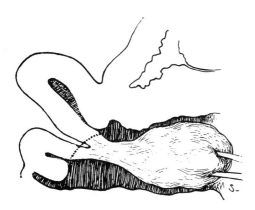

Fig. 63-1 One of the dangers of myomectomy in the presence of a partial uterine inversion is shown. If the pedicle stalk is divided at the site of the *dotted line,* the peritoneal cavity would be opened, risking peritonitis. (From Crossen HS, Crossen RJ: *Operative gynecology,* ed 6, St Louis, 1948, Mosby.)

the first 24 hours postpartum. Immediate recognition of the inversion with prompt reposition of the uterus may prevent the alarming hemorrhage and consequent shock associated with the condition.[29,31] Often, deep general anesthesia may be required, such as with the fluorinated hydrocarbon halothane (Fluothane) given in high concentration to provide rapid, maximal relaxation.[1,5]

Of the reported deaths from postpartum uterine inversion, 90% occur within the first 2 hours after delivery[11] and are caused by hemorrhage or shock.[21] Administration of an oxytocic agent to the patient with uterine inversion before it is reduced makes replacement of the fundus more difficult.[4]

When acute uterine inversion is first recognized, two large-bore intravenous lines carrying Ringer's lactate are immediately started,[5,6] and immediate professional assistance including an anesthetist is requested. A transfusion of whole blood should be started, instilled under mechanical pressure if necessary, as soon as the need has become evident. To lessen the size of the raw endouterine surface from which hemorrhage can arise, the surgeon may leave the unseparated placenta attached to the fundus until the latter has been replaced within the abdomen.[2,5,14,27]

Transvaginal Treatment of Acute Inversion. The Johnson technique[24] of applying steady pressure to the periphery of the inverted fundus, usually posteriorly, is useful, especially if it can be performed before the myometrium becomes contracted. The entire hand of the surgeon is placed in the vagina, with the fingertips at the uterocervical junction and the fundus in the palm. Pressure is applied so the entire uterus is lifted out of the pelvis to the level of the umbilicus where countertraction of the uterine ligaments exerts pressure to widen the cervical ring pulling the fundus back through it.[21] If myometrial spasm and contraction rings impede the reinversion, tocolytic agents as well as deep general anesthesia may be helpful. MgSO$_4$ may be given intravenously, 1 g/min for 4 minutes, to relax the uterus.[6,14] If this is not effective, 0.125 to 0.25 mg of terbutaline may be given intravenously.[28,42]

Before the hand is removed from the repositioned uterus, the uterine fundus may be elevated against the anterior abdominal wall and an oxytocic agent or prostaglandin is injected through the abdominal wall directly into the uterus. The hand is withdrawn only when the uterus has contracted firmly.[5,6,38] If bleeding persists and examination has ruled out rupture or perforation of the uterus, an intrauterine packing may be inserted for 24 hours.[34]

If the aforementioned technique is not successful in repositioning the uterus, the Jones' method[25,26] may be attempted. The gloved fingers are placed in the center of the inverted fundus while pressing slowly upward. Countertraction with ring forceps applied to the cervix may be helpful.[21]

O'Sullivan[34] suggested another method whereby the obstetrician's hand replaces the inverted uterus within the vagina, and with the hand and wrist occluding the introitus, an intravenous infusion tube is passed into the posterior vaginal fornix. Saline is run rapidly into the upper vagina, and the hydraulic pressure created reverts the uterus.[16] In 1997, Ogueh and Ayida[33] described success with hydrostatic uterine replacement using a 6-cm Silastic ventouse cup. The cup was inserted into the vagina and the palm of one of the surgeon's hands was used at the introitus to maintain the seal between cup and vagina. The cup was connected through an intravenous set to the first of two bags of saline placed about 1 m above the patient. This technique seems more gentle than that described by Sher[39] in which the surgeon "forcefully applied his forearm to the vagina introitus, while an assistant pressed the labia to the surgeon's forearm to occlude the vaginal orifice." Unless the repositioned uterus contracts firmly, it may reinvert,[22] requiring that the patient be watched carefully postpartum.

Whichever method seems to be most effective in the individual case should be used.

Unlike the reports of Kitchen et al.[27] and of Donald,[9] Platt and Druzin's review[35] of their own cases did not support the view that prophylactic antibiotic use is indicated in patients with uterine inversion.

Transabdominal Surgical Approach. If the transvaginal methods of repositioning the acutely inverted uterus fail, laparotomy should be considered.

The Huntington procedure[21,25] should be tried first, in which the abdominal peritoneal side of the uterus is grasped on both sides by thick bites with Allis clamps about 2 cm below the ring and upward traction is applied. Additional forceps are placed below the original pair, successively picking up portions of the uterus until the inversion is completely repositioned. Simultaneous transvaginal pressure by an assistant's hand in the patient's vagina may be helpful.

If success cannot be achieved by the Huntington maneuver, as might be noted when the inversion is of longer duration, the Haultain[20] procedure may be used.[10,20,21] In this transabdominal operation, a longitudinal incision of a size sufficient to reduce the prolapse is made in the posterior uterine wall over and through the contraction ring. A finger may be introduced through the uterine incision to a point below the inverted fundus, and reduction is effected by ap-

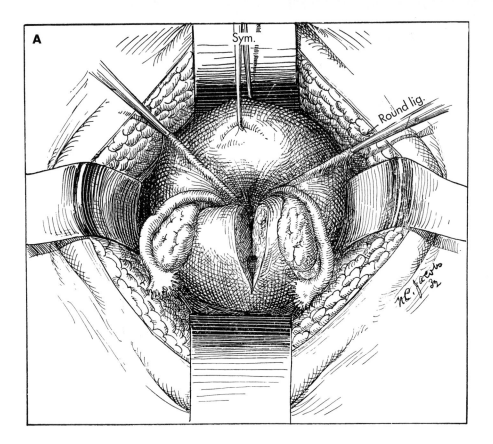

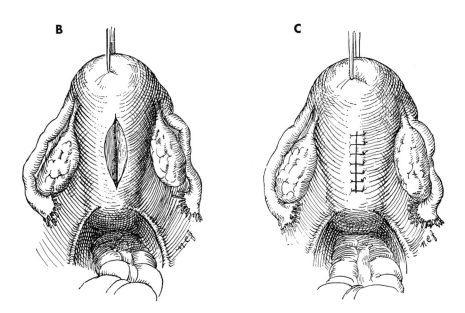

Fig. 63-2   A, The site and the extent of the incision made in the middle of the posterior portion of the constricting ring are shown. The inverted fundus can be replaced by pressure from below, through the vagina, or by traction from above, according to the method of Huntington and Irving. An incision of approximately 1 inch in length usually suffices, but if necessary, this can be enlarged somewhat. The constricting ring should be incised as it lies; the incision will then be in the region of the lower uterine segment rather than in the upper portion, thus rendering the uterus safer for future childbearing. **B,** Diagrammatic illustration of the uterus after it has been replaced. The incision in the posterior wall will be closed by two layers of sutures: an intramuscular layer of interrupted sutures and a continuous seromuscular layer. (In the diagram, the incision is represented at a rather higher level than usual.) **C,** The uterine incision is closed. If there is any tendency toward backward displacement, some form of uterine suspension may be used. (From Wilson K: *Am J Obstet Gynecol* 28:738, 1934.)

plying pressure with this finger against the fundus[7] or by simultaneous pressure from the fingers of an assistant, which are placed in the patient's vagina. When the reposition is completed, the uterine incision is repaired transabdominally by a series of interrupted stitches (Fig. 63-2).

Chronic Obstetric Uterine Inversion. Chronic obstetric uterine inversion is discovered more than 1 month postpartum. When a patient with an undetected uterine inversion has survived for months, a large degree of uterine involution will have taken place in the postpartum uterus, and the condition may be described as "chronic" inversion. When the condition is associated with a nonobstetric cause, it may be present for years. The patient may describe a bloody vaginal discharge of long duration, and upon pelvic examination the presence of a dusky dark red mass protruding from the uterine cervix will be noted, as well as the palpable dimple at the top of the shortened uterine fundus, perhaps best identified by bimanual palpation of the uterus during rectal examination.

Transvaginal Surgery. A vaginal approach to reposition of the inverted fundus may be preferable for the patient with chronic inversion because of better access to the operative site and the more limited intraperitoneal manipulation than would be necessary with the transabdominal operation.

In the older Küstner operation,[15,32] a transvaginal transverse colpotomy and incision of (Küstner O: *Zentalbl Gynäkol* 41:17, 1893) the full thickness of the cervix at the

6-o'clock position carried up through the posterior uterine wall are made (Fig. 63-3) and the inversion is repositioned. The incision in the posterior uterine wall and cervix is repaired, as is the original transverse incision and colpotomy in the vagina. Disadvantages of the Küstner operation are the greater risk of pelvic adhesion formation to the recently sutured posterior uterine wall than for a similar incision in the anterior wall, and the posterior uterine incision not being available for palpation during subsequent pregnancy, possibly masking a silent or impending uterine rupture.

These objections are overcome when the somewhat newer transvaginal Spinelli operation[7,13,32,40] is performed (Fig. 63-4). The anterior vaginal wall is made tense against the countertraction of a retractor and is incised transversely just above the anterior, cervical lip. The bladder is separated by dissection from the cervix and lower uterine segment. A midline incision is made through the cervix at the 12-o'clock position, completely dividing the constriction ring. The incision is carried in the midline to the uterine fundus. The uterus is reverted by hooking the forefingers on the peritoneal side into the incision and making counterpressure with the thumbs on the exposed endometrial surface, forcing the fundus upward much in the manner that one would use to turn a cut tennis ball inside-out (see Fig. 63-4, *A* through *C*). As much myometrium and endometrium as bulge into the uterine incision are trimmed by longitudinal wedging to permit coaptation of all layers of myometrium

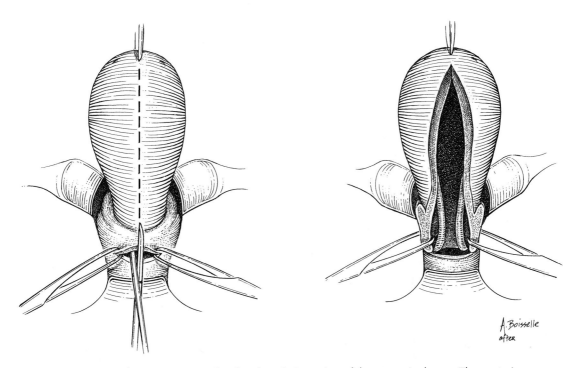

Fig. 63-3 The Küstner operation for chronic inversion of the uterus is shown. The posterior cul-de-sac has been opened, and the cervix and posterior wall of the uterus should be incised along the path of the broken line as shown in the drawing on the left. When this has been completed, as shown in the drawing to the right, thumb pressure along the sides of the uterus produce reversion, the wounds are closed with interrupted sutures, and the uterus is replaced in the pelvic cavity. The colpotomy is then closed. (From Nichols DH, Randall CL: *Vaginal surgery,* ed 4, Baltimore, 1996, Williams & Wilkins.)

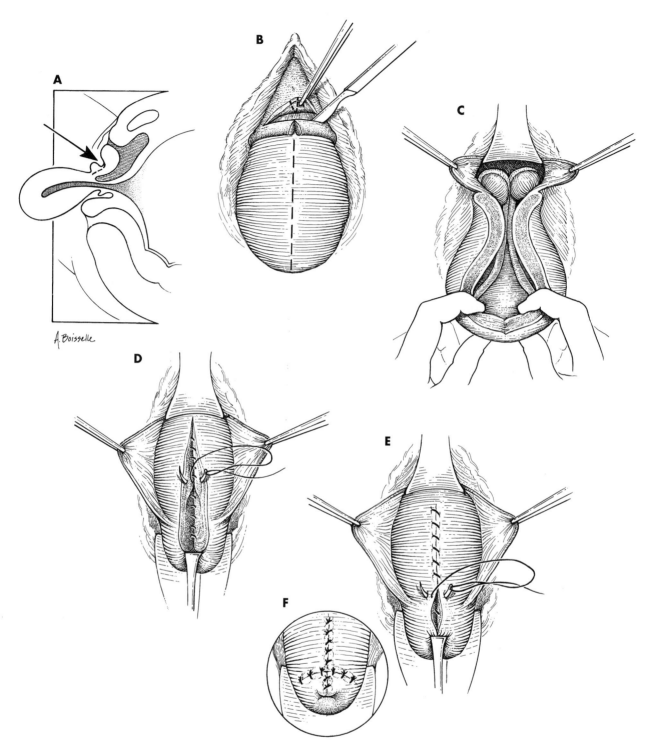

Fig. 63-4 The Spinelli operation for chronic inversion of the uterus is illustrated. The cervix is split in the midline and carefully separated from the bladder as shown by the dotted line in **A.** The anterior wall of the everted uterus is split along the path of the dotted line in **B. C,** By pressure with the surgeon's index fingers and thumbs, the uterus is turned outside-in. **D,** The myometrium is reapproximated by two layers of running PGA suture. **E,** The serosal surface is reapproximated by a single layer. **F,** The vaginal mucosa is reapproximated with interrupted sutures, as is the full thickness of the cervix. (From Nichols DH, Randall CL: *Vaginal surgery,* ed 4, Baltimore, Williams & Wilkins, 1996.)

and peritoneum without tension. The vertical incision in the cervix is closed by side-to-side interrupted sutures, and the transverse vaginal skin is approximated as shown (see Fig. 63-4, *D* through *F*). The technique permits some transabdominal palpable evaluation and assessment of the anterior uterine scar during a subsequent pregnancy.

Future obstetric delivery should be by elective cesarean section 2 weeks before term in most patients who have experienced such a hysterotomy.

Hysterectomy. Vaginal or abdominal hysterectomy may be advised for the patient in whom reinversion continues or in whom extensive tissue necrosis and infection are observed.

REFERENCES

1. Albright GA, et al: *Anesthesia in obstetrics—maternal, fetal, and neonatal aspects,* ed 2, Boston, 1986, Butterworths.
2. Bell JE Jr, Wilson GF, Wilson LA: Puerperal inversion of the uterus, *Am J Obstet Gynecol* 66:767, 1953.
3. Bunke JW, Hofmeister FJ: Uterine inversion—obstetrical entity or oddity, *Am J Obstet Gynecol* 91:934, 1965.
4. Burrus JH, Lampley CG Jr: Acute puerperal inversion of the uterus, *NC Med J* 26:502, 1965.
5. Catanzarite VA, Grossman R: How to manage uterine inversion, *Contemp Ob/Gyn* 28:81, 1986.
6. Catanzarite VA, et al: New approaches to the management of acute puerperal uterine inversion, *Obstet Gynecol* 68:75, 1986.
7. Crossen HS, Crossen RJ: *Operative gynecology,* ed 6, St Louis, 1948, Mosby, p 424.
8. Das P: Inversion of the uterus, *Br J Obstet Gynecol* 47:525, 1940.
9. Donald I: *Practical obstetric problems,* ed 4, Philadelphia, 1969, JB Lippincott, p 609.
10. Easterday CL, Reid D: Inversion of puerperal uterus managed by Haultain technique, *Am J Obstet Gynecol* 78:1224, 1959.
11. Eastman NJ, Hellman LM: *Williams' obstetrics,* ed 13, New York, 1966, Appleton-Century-Crofts.
12. Emmott RS, Bennett A: Acute inversion of the uterus at cesarean section, *Anesthesia* 43:118, 1988.
13. Greenhill JP: *Surgical gynecology,* ed 2, Chicago, 1957, Mosby, p 198.
14. Grossman RA: Magnesium sulfate for uterine invention, *J Reprod Med* 26:261, 1981.
15. Halban J: *Gynäkologische Operationslehre,* Wien, 1932, Urban & Schwarzenberg, p 196.
16. Halles RW: The use of intravaginal hydrolic pressure douches, *Am J Obstet Gynecol* 56:133, 1948.
17. Hanton EM, Kempers RD: Puerperal inversion of the uterus, *Postgrad Med* 36:541, 1964.
18. Harris BA: Acute puerperal inversion of the uterus, *Clin Obstet Gynecol* 27:134, 1984.
19. Harris RE, Dunnihoo DR: Inversion of the uterus in a patient under halothane anesthesia, *Obstet Gynecol* 27:655, 1966.
20. Haultain FWN: The treatment of chronic uterine inversion by abdominal hysterotomy, with a successful case, *Br Med J* 2:974, 1901.
21. Hess H: Uterine inversion, *Female Patient* 7:1, 1982.
22. Heyl PS, Stubblefield PG, Phillippee M: Recurrent inversion of the puerperal uterus managed with 15(S)-15-methyl prostaglandin F2-alpha and uterine packing, *Obstet Gynecol* 63:263, 1984.
23. Huntington JL: Acute inversion of uterus, *Boston Med Surg J* 184:376, 1921.
24. Johnson AB: A new concept in the replacement of the inverted uterus and a report of nine cases, *Am J Obstet Gynecol* 57:557, 1949.
25. Jones WC: Inversion of the uterus with report of a case occurring during the puerperium and caused by a fibroid, *Surg Gynecol Obstet* 16:632, 1913.
26. Jones WC: Reports of two cases of postpartum inversion of the uterus with discussion of the pathogenesis of obstetrical inversion, *Am J Obstet* 69:982, 1914.
27. Kitchen D, et al: Puerperal inversion of the uterus, *Am J Obstet Gynecol,* 123:51, 1975.
28. Kovacs VW, DeVore GR: Management of acute and subacute puerperal uterine inversion with terbutaline sulfate, *Am J Obstet Gynecol* 150:784, 1984.
29. Lee W, et al: Acute inversion of the uterus, *Obstet Gynecol* 51:144, 1978.
30. Marcus MB, Brandt ML: Acute puerperal inversion of the uterus complicated by lower nephron nephrosis, *Obstet Gynecol* 9:725, 1957.
31. Mehra U, Ostapowicz F: Acute puerperal inversion of the uterus in a primipara, *Obstet Gynecol* 47:30, 1976.
32. Nichols DH, Randall CL: *Vaginal surgery,* ed 4, Baltimore, 1996, Williams & Wilkins, p 547.
33. Ogueh O, Ayida G: Acute uterine inversion: a new technique of hydrostatic replacement, *Br J Obstet Gynaecol* 104:951, 1997.
34. O'Sullivan JV: Acute inversion of the uterus, *Br Med J* 2:282, 1945.
35. Platt LD, Druzin ML: Acute puerperal inversion of the uterus, *Am J Obstet Gynecol* 141:187, 1981.
36. Plaut GS: Chronic puerperal inversion of the uterus, *Postgrad Med J* 37:164, 1961.
37. Pritchard JA, MacDonald PC, Gant NF: *Williams obstetrics,* ed 17, Norwalk, Conn, 1985, Appleton-Century-Crofts, p 715.
38. Shah-Hosseini, Evrard JR: Puerperal uterine inversion, *Obstet Gynecol* 73:567, 1989.
39. Sher G: Correction of postpartum uterine inversion by the application of intravaginal hydrostatic pressure, *Am J Obstet Gynecol* 143:601, 1979.
40. Spinelli PC: Cura chirurgica conservative dell' inversione cronica dell' utero col processo kehrer, *Arch Ital Ginecol* 2:7, 1899.
41. Steffen E: Puerperal inversion of the uterus occurring in consecutive pregnancies in the same patient, *Am J Obstet Gynecol* 74:655, 1957.
42. Thiery M, Delbeke L: Acute puerperal uterine inversion: two step management with a mimetic and a prostaglandin, *Am J Obstet Gynecol* 153:891, 1985.
43. Watson T, Besch N, Bowes WA Jr: Management of acute and subacute puerperal inversion of the uterus, *Obstet Gynecol* 55:12, 1980.

Surgical Therapy of Gestational Trophoblastic Disease

JOHN T. SOPER and CHARLES B. HAMMOND

INTRODUCTION

The term *gestational trophoblastic disease* (GTD) includes a wide range of clinically and histologically defined neoplasms derived from the human trophoblast, ranging from benign molar pregnancies with spontaneous resolution after evacuation to highly malignant gestational choriocarcinoma. Several factors have contributed to GTD becoming among the most curable forms of human solid tumors, including the widespread availability of sensitive and specific assays for human chorionic gonadotrophin (hCG), development of effective chemotherapy, integration of appropriate surgical intervention with chemotherapy, and individualization of chemotherapeutic regimens for patients with malignant GTD based on recognized risk factors. Although GTD afflicts young women during their prime reproductive years and can be a potentially devastating illness, most women with malignant GTD can be cured using contemporary approaches to management. The primary management of women with partial and complete hydatidiform mole is through surgical evacuation coupled with close monitoring of hCG. In patients who develop postmolar GTD or gestational choriocarcinoma, chemotherapy has largely replaced surgery as the primary therapeutic modality. However, surgical procedures are often useful in managing women with malignant GTD. Specific surgical techniques are not reviewed in detail in this chapter, but the integration of surgery into the management of women with GTD is presented.

HYDATIDIFORM MOLE

Two distinct entities of molar gestations, partial and complete moles, have been defined on the basis of cytogenetic, histopathologic, and clinical characteristics (Table 64-1). Most partial moles have a 69, XXX or 69, XXY karyotype derived from both maternal and paternal genome.[2,17,40-44] Often, partial moles have clinical or histologic evidence of a fetus (e.g., amniotic membranes, fetal vessels with fetal red blood cells) and have hydropic changes of chorionic villi with focal trophoblastic proliferation.[2,17,40-44] Because of the only modest increases in placental size and trophoblastic mass, the uterus is usually enlarged less than would be anticipated from the duration of gestation. Clinically and ultrasonographically, partial moles most often present as threatened or missed spontaneous abortions. Malignant sequelae, usually consisting of persistent (nonmetastatic) GTD, develop in less than 5% of patients after evacuation of partial hydatidiform moles.[5]

In contrast, complete hydatidiform moles have a 46, XX or 46, XY karyotype derived from the paternal genome.* Histologically, these are characterized by absence of fetal development and diffuse, often massive hydropic degeneration of chorionic villi, coupled with diffuse trophoblastic proliferation.[40,41] The uterus is often enlarged more than would be expected based on gestational age. The clinical and ultrasonographic diagnosis is most often that of hydatidiform mole. In contrast to partial moles, patients with complete moles have approximately a 20% incidence of malignant sequelae after evacuation, with 10% to 20% of these having metastatic disease.[8,24,31]

Despite these differences, the management and surveillance of partial and complete molar gestations are similar. Once the diagnosis is made, the workup of a patient with a molar gestation involves screening for metastatic disease and stabilizing the patient for evacuation. The evaluation consists of a complete physical examination, baseline hCG level, chest x-ray film, hematologic profile, renal and liver function tests, and thyroid function tests. If the uterus is larger than 14 to 16 weeks' size or the patient has pregnancy-induced hypertension, arterial blood gas measurements should be obtained preoperatively because many of these patients develop respiratory insufficiency after evacuation. A baseline ultrasound should be obtained to screen for the presence of the calutein cysts.

EVACUATION OF HYDATIDIFORM MOLE

Several techniques for evacuation of hydatidiform moles have been used, including induction of labor with oxytocin or prostaglandins, hysterotomy, cervical dilation with suction curettage (D&C), and hysterectomy. Of these, we recommend suction D&C or, if the patient desires sterilization, abdominal hysterectomy.

Suction Curettage

The patient should be hemodynamically stable, with correction of preoperative anemia and stabilization of pregnancy-induced hypertension or systemic manifestations of hyperthyroidism. If the uterus is more than 14 to 16 weeks' gestational size, a central line should be placed for intraoperative central venous pressure monitoring and rapid administration of fluids or blood products during the procedure. At least 2 U of blood and a laparotomy set should be available

---

*References 1, 4, 16, 18, 40, 41.

Table 64-1   Partial versus Complete Hydatidiform Mole

	Partial Mole	Complete Mole
Cytogenetic Analysis	69,XXX	46,XXX
	Occasional 69,XXY	Occasional 46,XY
	Paternal + maternal origin	Paternal origin
Pathologic features		
Fetus, amnion, fetal vessels	Frequent	Rare
Hydropic villi	Variable, irregular	Diffuse, often pronounced
Trophoblastic proliferation	Focal, slight to moderate	Variable, often pronounced
Clinical Features		
Clinical/ultrasound diagnosis	Missed abortion	Molar pregnancy
Uterus large for dates	Rare	25%-50%
Malignant sequelae	<5%	10%-30%

in the operating room. We follow these steps for suction D&C of a hydatidiform mole:

1. The cervix is dilated gently with Pratt dilators.
2. The largest available suction cannula (14 to 16 mm) is introduced through the cervix into the midendometrial cavity. Because the myometrium is often softened, predisposing to uterine perforation, no attempt is made to sound the uterus to the fundus. During curettage, one hand is placed on the fundus (to sense involution of the uterus during evacuation of the uterine contents and to assist in achieving uterine contraction through fundal massage).
3. Suction is applied, and the cannula is initially rotated to evacuate the uterine contents. Most of the mole will be removed using this maneuver without requiring vigorous curettage. Pitocin (oxytocin) in a concentration of 20 U/L is begun only after cervical dilation has been completed and the suction curettage is started to prevent contractions against an undilated cervix.
4. As the uterine fundus involutes with evacuation and myometrial contraction, completion of evacuation is performed by using gentle curettage with the suction cannula.
5. After evacuation of uterine contents with the suction cannula, the endometrium is gently curetted using a large sharp curette to ensure complete evacuation. Also, this may yield the diagnosis of invasive mole (chorioadenoma destruens) if villi are seen invading the myometrium directly without intervening endometrium. The diagnosis of invasive mole is an indication for chemotherapy, but it is extremely difficult to make from the uterine curettage samples.

Pitocin infusion is continued for 12 to 24 hours after evacuation, until vaginal bleeding is minimal.

Hysterectomy

In women who desire sterilization, hysterectomy offers the advantages of simultaneous evacuation of hydatidiform mole and sterilization. In addition, performance of hysterectomy decreases the risk of malignant sequelae to approximately 3.5% from the 20% anticipated for those treated with D&C.[8] However, because hysterectomy does not eliminate the potential for malignant sequelae, all women must be monitored for hCG levels after hysterectomy. We recommend a simple total abdominal hysterectomy as the procedure of choice in women with hydatidiform mole because of uterine enlargement and, rarely, adnexal or intraabdominal metastases. Most women with hydatidiform mole are younger than 40 years; therefore the adnexa should not be removed unless the patient is perimenopausal or there are obvious adnexal metastases. Theca-lutein cysts usually regress spontaneously after evacuation or hysterectomy and do not need to be drained or removed unless torsion or intraoperative rupture has occurred.

Other Techniques of Molar Evacuation

Induction of labor with oxytocin or prostaglandins produces theoretical increased risk of disseminating trophoblast through the systemic circulation caused by uterine contractions against an undilated cervix. Blood loss may be great, and evacuation is often incomplete, requiring suction D&C. Hysterotomy is also associated with increased blood loss compared with suction D&C.[32] The vertical uterine incision often results in a need for cesarean section to deliver subsequent pregnancies. This is an important consideration in the majority of these patients, who are in the prime reproductive age group. In addition, Tow[47] found that evacuation of hydatidiform mole with hysterotomy resulted in a greater incidence of postmolar malignant sequelae than did suction D&C.

COMPLICATIONS ASSOCIATED WITH EVACUATION
Theca-Lutein Cysts

Clinically evident (larger than 5 cm) theca-lutein cysts are detectable in approximately one fourth of women with hydatidiform mole, with additional smaller cysts often detected by ultrasound alone.[8,36] Histologically and physiologically, these are similar to iatrogenic ovarian hyperstimulation caused by exogenous gonadotrophin/hCG administration for ovulation induction. These cysts will usually spontaneously regress with evacuation of the hydatidiform mole and diminishing hCG levels. It is rare for a patient to develop overt ovarian hyperstimulation with fluid retention and/or ascites. However, patient will occasionally develop ovarian torsion or rupture and bleeding from the cysts, requiring oophorectomy.[26]

Montz et al.[26] studied the natural history of theca-lutein cysts. They reported that they were associated with both acute complications of molar evacuation and subsequent development of postmolar malignant GTD. Although cyst size did not affect the incidence of postmolar GTD, bilaterality or theca-lutein cysts associated with a complication of molar evacuation increased the risk of postmolar GTD to approximately 75%, with a risk of 52% for patients who had theca-lutein cysts but lacked bilaterality. In addition, 16% of the theca-lutein cysts developed 2 to 13 weeks after evacuation, and these were also associated with a 75% risk of postmolar GTD. Others have documented an increased risk of postmolar GTD when theca-lutein cysts are associated with uterine enlargement greater than dates.[8,31]

Theca-lutein cysts usually regress spontaneously with diminishing hCG levels, but approximately 30% enlarge in response to the rising hCG levels associated with postmolar GTD.[26] Occasionally, theca-lutein cysts persist for several months beyond normalization of hCG levels.[26]

Respiratory Distress Syndrome

Causes for respiratory distress during evacuation of molar gestation include trophoblastic deportation, high-output congestive heart failure caused by anemia or hyperthyroidism, preeclampsia, and iatrogenic fluid overload. Pulmonary complications appear in approximately one fourth of all patients with uterine size more than 16 weeks' gestation.[48] In a small series of patients studied with invasive central monitoring during suction D&C, a transient impairment of left ventricular function was observed during general anesthesia.[7] This might contribute to the development of pulmonary edema in unmonitored patients given large volumes of crystalloid during the procedure. In general, pulmonary complications should be managed with ventilator support and pulmonary wedge pressure monitoring. A Swan-Ganz catheter can accurately determine fluid status and the need for blood products or diuresis. All patients should have a chest x-ray study after evacuation of hydatidiform mole to rule out significant trophoblastic deportation or pulmonary edema.

Uterine Perforation

Fortunately, uterine perforation rarely occurs as an acute complication during suction D&C for hydatidiform mole.[32] If perforation is recognized, the suction should be immediately discontinued and the rate of Pitocin infusion increased. Laparoscopy or laparotomy should be performed to assess the site of perforation. If hemostasis is adequate and the gastrointestinal organs are not damaged, curettage can be completed under direct visualization.

Rarely, uterine perforation occurs during or after suction D&C in a focus of deep myometrial penetration by invasive mole.[4] Perforation occurs most commonly in the midline of the uterine fundus. Although some patients require hysterectomy, anecdotal case reports have suggested that individual patients with invasive moles can be treated with segmental resection and repair of the affected myometrium. The full-thickness myometrial incision usually requires cesarean section for delivery in subsequent pregnancies. Surgical management should be individualized based on the site and extent of perforation.

MANAGEMENT AFTER MOLAR EVACUATION

Monitoring of serial quantitative serum hCG levels is the only reliable means for detecting malignant sequelae of hydatidiform mole.[8,24,31] One of any number of sensitive assays using polyclonal or monoclonal antibodies on either whole-molecule or total β-hCG fragments can be used for monitoring. A baseline level should be obtained within 48 hours of evacuation and serial levels followed at 1- to 2-week intervals until normal hCG levels are attained. Levels should then be followed at 1- to 2- month intervals to ensure that spontaneous remission is sustained beyond 6 to 12 months. It is rare to observe reelevation of hCG caused by malignant GTD after more than 6 months of normal hCG levels without an intercurrent pregnancy. Physical examination and a chest x-ray study should be repeated every 2 to 4 weeks as long as the hCG level is more than 1000 mIU/ml. Patients who have not undergone hysterectomy should use active contraception until sustained hCG regression has been documented. Oral contraceptives are usually recommended because these do not increase the risk of malignant sequelae.[4]

Malignant sequelae after hydatidiform mole are diagnosed if the hCG levels rise acutely or if they plateau (+10%) over more than 2 to 3 weeks. In addition, the histologic diagnosis of choriocarcinoma or invasive mole or the appearance of metastatic disease is an indication for chemotherapy.

Patients with malignant sequelae after hydatidiform moles often develop vaginal bleeding and uterine enlargement. The efficacy of a secondary D&C to remove additional trophoblastic tissue and allow spontaneous regression has never been prospectively evaluated. Schlaerth et al.[30] retrospectively reviewed their experience with secondary D&C among women with GTD. Most exhibited either a transient decrease in hCG levels followed by a subsequent rise or no effect upon hCG levels. Only 20% entered spontaneous remission after secondary D&C. Others[11,19] have observed that secondary D&C affects management in only 10% of patients. We have been reluctant to recommend secondary therapeutic D&C unless there is significant hemorrhage because of the documented lack of success, increased chance of uterine perforation or infection, and possible risk of delaying therapy, which might result in uterine perforation or metastases from clinically occult intrauterine or extrauterine foci of malignant GTD.

SURGICAL MANAGEMENT OF MALIGNANT GTD

The development of effective chemotherapy has diminished the role of surgery for therapy of women with malignant GTD. However, many procedures are useful adjuncts when integrated into the management of patients with malignant GTD. Primary or delayed hysterectomy may remove central disease, and removal of distant metastases may result in the cure of highly selected women with isolated foci of drug-resistant disease. We perform extirpative procedures (e.g., hysterectomy) under coverage of chemotherapy to minimize the possibility of metastasis induced by surgical manipulation of tissues. There does not appear to be an increase in morbidity using this combined modality approach.[12,20,21] In approximately 30% of patients with high-risk metastatic disease, one or more surgical procedures will be performed during therapy, either as a planned therapeutic maneuver or to treat complications of the disease, such as hemorrhage or abscess, and allow continuation of chemotherapy.[12] Finally, we have used indwelling double- or triple-lumen central catheters for prolonged venous access in most women with high-risk disease, who often require prolonged chemotherapy, blood product support, or total parenteral nutrition during therapy.

GENERAL MANAGEMENT

Approximately one half to two thirds of cases of malignant GTD follow molar pregnancies. Gestational choriocarcinomas derived from term pregnancies, spontaneous abortions, and tubal pregnancies account for the reminder. Although the diagnosis of malignant GTD after hydatidiform mole is usually made promptly, malignant GTD resulting from other pregnancies is often diagnosed later in the course of the disease, and patients are commonly seen first with nongynecologic signs and symptoms.[13,25] It should be emphasized that in any woman in the reproductive age group with abnormal uterine bleeding or metastases to distant sites from an unknown primary site of malignancy the diagnosis of GTD must be excluded with a screening test for hCG.

Malignant GTD initially invades the myometrium and penetrates small uterine vessels. Venous metastasis then occurs, resulting in pulmonary and/or vaginal metastases. Usually, systemic hematogenous metastases occur only after pulmonary metastases have become established.[38] Occasionally, pulmonary metastases are not detected by conventional chest x-ray study.[27] Therefore all women with malignant GTD should have a complete metastatic survey before initial therapy, consisting of chest x-ray film or computed tomography (CT) scan and CT scans of the brain, abdomen, and pelvis. A pretherapy hCG level should be obtained in addition to complete blood count and renal and liver function tests.

The anatomic stage of malignant GTD is assigned by International Federation of Gynecology and Obstetrics (FIGO) criteria.[28,37] The recently revised FIGO staging system (see the box above, top) includes some clinical prog-

---

FIGO STAGING OF GTD

Stage I: Disease confined to the uterine corpus
Stage II: Vaginal or pelvic metastases
Stage III: Pulmonary metastases
Stage IV: Other systemic metastases
Substages—assigned within each stage:
  A: No risk factors
  B: One risk factors
  C: Two risk factors
Risk factors used to assign substage:
  1. Pretherapy human chorionic gonadotropin level >100,000 mIU/ml
  2. Interval from antecedent pregnancy >6 mo

From Soper JT, et al: *Obstet Gynecol* 84:969, 1994.

CLINICAL CLASSIFICATION OF GESTATIONAL TROPHOBLASTIC DISEASE (GTD)

  I. Nonmetastatic GTD: no evidence of disease outside of uterus—not assigned to prognostic category
 II. Metastatic GTD: any metastases
    A. Good-prognosis metastatic GTD
      1. Short duration (<4 mo)
      2. Low human chorionic gonadotropin (hCG) level (<40,000 mIU/ml serum β-hCG)
      3. No metastases to brain or liver
      4. No antecedent term pregnancy
      5. No prior chemotherapy
    B. Poor-prognosis metastatic GTD: any high-risk factor
      1. Long duration (>4 mo)
      2. High pretreatment hCG level (>40,000 mIU/ml serum β-hCG)
      3. Brain or liver metastases
      4. Antecedent term pregnancy
      5. Prior chemotherapy

From Hammond CB, Weed JC, Currie JL: *Am J Obstet Gynecol* 136:844, 1980.

---

nostic information to assign substage, but the many substages do not correlate well with treatment outcome.[37] However, initial therapy is assigned on the basis of the risk for failure of primary single-agent chemotherapy. Either the Clinical Classification System[12] (see the box above, bottom) or the World Health Organization (WHO) prognostic index score[51] (Table 64-2) are used to determine whether the patient has low- or high-risk disease. In general, single-agent regimens of methotrexate or dactinomycin are used to treat patients with nonmetastatic or low-risk metastatic GTD, whereas those with high-risk metastatic GTD should be treated initially with multiagent chemotherapy.* Triple therapy with methotrexate-dactinomycin-chlorambucil or

---

*References 9, 12, 14, 23, 35, 37.

Table 64-2 World Health Organization Prognostic Index Score for Gestational Trophoblastic Disease

Prognostic Factors	Score*			
	0	1	2	4
Age (yr)		>39		
Antecedent pregnancy	Hydatidiform mole	Abortion	Term	
Interval+ (mo)	<4	4-6	7-12	>12
hCG level (IU/L)	<10	10-10	10-10	>10
ABO groups (female × male)		O × A	B	
		O × A	AB	
Largest tumor, including uterine tumor		3-5 cm	>5 cm	Brain
Site of metastases		Spleen, kidney	Gastrointestinal tract, liver	
Number of metastases identified		1-4	4-8	>8
Prior chemotherapy			Single drug	≥2 agents

From World Health Organization Scientific Group: *Gestational trophoblastic disease,* Technical Report Series 692, Geneva, 1983, World Health Organization.
*The total score for a patient is obtained by adding the individual scores for each prognostic factor. A total score of 0-4 = low risk, 5-7 = intermediate risk, >8 = high risk. Months from antecedent pregnancy.

Table 64-3 Management Summary for Gestational Trophoblastic Disease

Category*	Therapy	Survival (%)
Nonmetastatic	Primary: methotrexate regimens	>99
Metastatic GTD, good prognosis (WHO PI <4)	Primary: methotrexate or dactinomycin	>99
Metastatic GTD, poor prognosis (WHO PI >4)	Primary MAC or EMA-CO	60-85
	Salvage: combination regimens; individualized surgical resection(s)	

GTD, Gestational trophoblastic disease; *WHO PI,* World Health Organization prognostic index score; *MAC,* methotrexate-dactinomycin-chlorambucil/cytoxan; *EMA-CO,* alternating cycles of etoposide-methotrexate-dactinomycin/cyclophosphamide-vincristine.
*Clinical criteria. Selected patients may receive brain or liver radiation therapy.

cyclophosphamide (MAC) is often used, but patients with high WHO prognostic index scores are probably best treated with etoposide-containing regimens, because their prognosis is very poor when MAC chemotherapy is used.[9] Table 64-3 displays clinical groupings, therapy, and expected outcome. In general, most women with malignant GTD can be cured with available chemotherapeutic regimens.

PRETHERAPY D&C

The theoretical benefits of a pretherapy D&C before the first cycle of chemotherapy for malignant GTD include "debulking" of the intrauterine tumor and detection of histologic changes that might correlate with response to chemotherapy. Potential disadvantages include perforation and the introduction of infection during uterine manipulation. The efficacy of routine pretherapy D&C for the purpose of debulking intrauterine disease has never been tested prospectively. Berkowitz et al.[3] evaluated their experience with pretherapy D&C in 37 patients with nonmetastatic postmolar GTD: 20 (54%) had no tissue detected by pretherapy D&C, and 19 of these achieved sustained remission with limited chemotherapy. Patients having intrauterine disease with a worsened histologic diagnosis were at risk for failure of initial chemotherapy. None of their patients had uterine perforation or other complications. However, Schlaerth et al.[30] documented an 8.1% incidence of uterine perforation during

D&C performed in this setting, and two of the three patients with perforation required hysterectomy. We prefer to reserve secondary D&C for patients who experience significant uterine bleeding and anemia during chemotherapy.

HYSTERECTOMY

Before effective chemotherapy was widely available, Brewer et al.[5] reported a 2-year survival rate of 40% for women with nonmetastatic choriocarcinoma and only 15% for those with metastatic choriocarcinoma who were treated with hysterectomy alone. Although chemotherapy has markedly improved the outlook for women with malignant GTD, both primary and delayed hysterectomy continues to play a role in the management of patients with malignant GTD. However, primary hysterectomy is not indicated for younger patients who wish to preserve childbearing capacity.

Among 194 women with nonmetastatic or good-prognosis metastatic malignant GTD reported from out institution,[12] there was a 100% sustained remission rate whether patients were initially treated with chemotherapy alone or chemotherapy combined with hysterectomy. Of those who wished to retain fertility, 89% were able to, and many had subsequent viable pregnancies. Patients who underwent primary hysterectomy had decreases in the total hospitalization, total number of courses of chemotherapy, and total chemotherapy dosages compared with those treated with chemotherapy alone. Therefore primary hysterectomy is indicated for patients with nonmetastatic or good-prognosis metastatic GTD who do not wish to preserve childbearing capacity.

Delayed hysterectomy may be considered for patients who fail to respond to initial chemotherapy. In our experience,[12] almost all patients with nonmetastatic and good-prognosis metastatic GTD who were treated with delayed hysterectomy after the failure of primary single-agent chemotherapy achieved a sustained remission without requiring multiagent chemotherapy.

Primary or delayed hysterectomy may be considered in selected patients with poor-prognosis metastatic GTD who have a small extrauterine tumor burden, but in general, the procedure is not as beneficial as in those with more limited disease.[12] This reflects the relatively large amount of extrauterine disease present in many of these patients. Nevertheless, primary or delayed hysterectomy may be beneficial for selected patients in this disease category.

Most women undergoing hysterectomy for malignant GTD have been treated with total abdominal hysterectomy, with or without preservation of the adnexa. This allows visualization of intraabdominal organs to assess for extrauterine metastases, which are rarely encountered in patients with limited disease. We occasionally perform vaginal hysterectomy in women with low-risk nonmetastatic GTD who have a small uterus and desire primary hysterectomy as sterilization during their initial course of chemotherapy. We have not encountered any significant complications using standard vaginal hysterectomy techniques.

PULMONARY RESECTION

Thoracotomy with pulmonary wedge resection or partial lobectomy is the most commonly performed surgical procedure for extirpation of distant drug-resistant metastases of GTD. Pulmonary resection can be performed safely under the coverage of chemotherapy, but it is not necessary to resect pulmonary disease in most patients. Although those with persistent pulmonary nodules on chest x-ray film after chemotherapy may be at increased risk for recurrent GTD, radiographic evidence of tumor regression may lag far behind the hCG level response.[22,50] Some patients have persistent pulmonary nodules that gradually resolve over several months of follow-up after completion of therapy. Therefore there is no justification for the indiscriminate resection of pulmonary metastases that persist on chest x-ray during chemotherapy in a patient with a satisfactory hCG level response or after induction of hCG level remission. Resection of pulmonary nodules in highly selected women with drug-resistant disease may be successful in inducing remission.[10,33,34,46] Before thoracotomy is performed, however, it is important to exclude the possibility of active disease elsewhere. We recommend rescreening these patients with CT evaluation of the brain, thorax, and abdomen to search for occult extrapulmonary metastases. If the patient has not undergone hysterectomy, active pelvic disease should also be excluded radiographically with angiography

or magnetic resonance imaging (MRI). Tomoda et al.[46] reviewed indications for planned resection of pulmonary metastases of GTD. They proposed the following criteria for successful resection: (1) good surgical candidate, (2) primary malignancy controlled (uterus excised or no evidence of pelvic disease on angiographic studies), (3) no evidence of other metastases, (4) solitary pulmonary lesion, and (5) persistent hCG level of less than 1000 mIU/ml. In their series, 14 (93%) of 15 patients who satisfied these criteria survived after pulmonary resection compared with none of the 4 patients who had one or more unfavorable clinical feature. Other investigators have also reported that prompt hCG level remission after resection of an isolated pulmonary nodule predicts a favorable outcome.[10,33,34,46]

CRANIOTOMY

Central nervous system metastases are clinically or radiographically detected in 8% to 15% of women with metastatic GTD and are associated with a worse prognosis than lung or vaginal metastases.* These metastases are highly vascular and have a tendency for hemorrhage, often early in the course of therapy, when patients may develop acute neurologic deterioration. The major goals of therapy are early detection of brain metastases through complete radiographic evaluation of the patient before chemotherapy is initiated, stabilization of neurologic status, and institution of appropriate therapy. Craniotomy to obtain tissue for the diagnosis of GTD is not indicated. Any women of reproductive age with brain metastases or cerebral hemorrhage of unexplained cause should be screened for GTD with an hCG level.[12,31] If the hCG level is elevated and pregnancy is excluded, therapy can be instituted without a tissue diagnosis. In the United States, whole brain irradiation has been used in an attempt to prevent hemorrhage from brain metastases.[12,14,35,39,49] In contrast, Rustin et al.[29] recommend early craniotomy and intrathecal methotrexate in an attempt to eradicate brain lesions. Both approaches appear to be fairly successful, and in stark contrast to patients with brain metastases from other solid tumors, the majority of women who are seen with primary brain metastases of malignant GTD will survive.

Craniotomy for resection of drug-resistant lesions is justified only rarely and then only for carefully selected patients who do not have evidence of metastatic disease elsewhere. In general, we reserve craniotomy for patients who require acute decompression of hemorrhagic lesions to allow stabilization and institution of therapy.

OTHER EXTIRPATIVE PROCEDURES

Occasionally, surgical extirpation of disease involving other sites is beneficial in treating women during primary or salvage therapy of malignant GTD.[12] Vaginal metastases are highly vascular, originating via metastasis through the submucosal venous plexus,[38] and should not be undergo resec-

---

*References 1, 9, 12, 14, 29, 35, 37, 39, 49.

tion or biopsy unless they represent the only site of drug-resistant disease. Rare patients seen with intraabdominal metastasis or gastrointestinal involvement will require resection of involved structures for stabilization during therapy.[12] In addition, a few patients with unilateral renal metastasis and limited systemic disease burden have been successfully managed by integrating primary or salvage nephrectomy with chemotherapy.[36]

CENTRAL VENOUS CATHETERS

We generally use a tunneled Hickman-Broviac catheter for central venous access in women with high-risk metastatic GTD.[6,15,45] This provides reliable venous access in patients who require long-term chemotherapy, nutritional support, and support with antibiotics or blood components. The catheter is inserted under fluoroscopic guidance and tunneled subcutaneously to reduce infectious complications. Each patient is instructed in the care of the catheter site, and the catheters are maintained by a special nursing team while the patient is in the hospital to reduce infectious complications. Despite the use of strict aseptic techniques, some catheter-related sepsis, skin infections, or thrombosis will occur, requiring removal of the catheter.[6,15,45] Nevertheless, these catheters aid in the care of patients with high-risk disease.

SUMMARY

Although the development of effective chemotherapy has resulted in improved survival of patients with GTD, surgery remains an important part of the integrated management of these women. The coordination of chemotherapy, surgery, and radiation therapy requires the availability of sensitive hCG assays and physicians with experience in the treatment of these diseases. Patients undergoing intensive therapy for poor-prognosis GTD are best managed by physicians with experience in coordinating a multidisciplinary approach to the treatment of GTD.

REFERENCES

1. Bagshawe KD: Risk and prognostic factors in trophoblastic neoplasia, *Cancer* 38:1373, 1976.
2. Berkowitz RS, Goldstein DP, Bernstein MR: Natural history of partial molar pregnancy, *Obstet Gynecol* 66:677, 1983.
3. Berkowitz RS, et al: Pretreatment curettage a predictor of chemotherapy response in gestational trophoblastic neoplasia, *Gynecol Oncol* 10:39, 1980.
4. Berkowitz RS, et al: Oral contraceptives and post-molar trophoblastic disease, *Obstet Gynecol* 58:474, 1981.
5. Brewer JI, Smith RT, Pratt GB: Choriocarcinoma: absolute survival rates of 122 patients treated by hysterectomy, *Am J Obstet Gynecol* 85:84, 1963.
6. Broviac JW, Cole JS, Scribner BH: A silicone rubber atrial catheter for prolonged parenteral alimentation, *Surg Gynecol Obstet* 136:602, 1972.
7. Cotton DB, et al: Hemodynamic observations in evacuation of molar pregnancy, *Am J Obstet Gynecol* 138:6, 1980.
8. Curry SL, et al: Hydatidiform mole: diagnosis, management and long-term follow up in 347 patients, *Obstet Gynecol* 45:1, 1975.
9. DuBeshter B, et al: Metastatic gestational trophoblastic disease: experience at the New England Trophoblastic Disease Center, 1965-1985, *Obstet Gynecol* 69:390, 1987.
10. Edwards JL, Makey AR, Bagshawe KD: The role of thoracotomy in the management of pulmonary metastases of gestational choriocarcinoma, *Clin Oncol* 1:329, 1975.
11. Flam F, Lundstrom V: The value of endometrial curettage in the follow up of hydatidiform mole, *Acta Obstet Gynecol Scand* 67:649, 1988.
12. Hammond CB, Weed JC, Currie JL: The role of operation in the current therapy of gestational trophoblastic disease, *Am J Obstet Gynecol* 136:844, 1980.
13. Hammond CB, et al: Diagnostic problems of choriocarcinoma and related trophoblastic neoplasms, *Obstet Gynecol* 29:224, 1967.
14. Hammond CB, et al: Treatment of metastatic trophoblastic disease: good and poor prognosis, *Am J Obstet Gynecol* 115:451, 1973.
15. Hickman RO, et al: A modified right atrial catheter for access to the venous system in marrow transplant recipients, *Surg Gynecol Ostet* 148:871, 1979.
16. Jacobs PA, et al: Mechanism of origin of complete hydatidiform moles, *Nature* 286:714, 1980.
17. Jacobs PA, et al: Human triploidy: relationship between paternal origin of the additional haploid complement and development of partial hydatidiform mole, *Ann Hum Genet* 46:223, 1982.
18. Kajii T, et al: XX and XY complete moles: clinical and morphologic correlations, *Am J Obstet Gynecol* 150:57, 1984.
19. Lao TT, Lee FH, Yeung SS: Repeat curettage after evacuation of hydatidiform mole: an appraisal, *Acta Obstet Gynecol Scand* 66:305, 1987.
20. Lewis J Jr., Ketcham AS, Hertz R: Surgical intervention during chemotherapy of gestational trophoblastic neoplasms, *Cancer* 19:1517, 1966.
21. Lewis J Jr, et al: The treatment of trophoblastic disease with the use of adjunctive chemotherapy at the time of the indicated operation, *Am J Obstet Gynecol* 96:710, 1966.
22. Libshitz HI, Barber CE, Hammond CB: The pulmonary metastases of choriocarcinoma, *Obstet Gynecol* 49:412, 1977.
23. Lurain JR, et al: Gestational trophoblastic disease: treatment results at the Brewer Trophoblastic Disease Center, *Obstet Gynecol* 60:354, 1982.
24. Lurain JR, et al: Natural history of hydatidiform mole after primary evacuation, *Am J Obstet Gynecol* 145:591, 1983.
25. Magrath IT, Golding PR, Bagshawe KD: Medical presentation of choriocarcinoma, *Br Med J* 2:633, 1971.
26. Montz FJ, Schlaerth JB, Morrow CB: The natural history of the calutein cysts, *Obstet Gynecol* 72:247, 1988.
27. Mutch DG, et al: Role of computed axial tomography of the chest in staging patients with non-metastatic gestational trophoblastic disease, *Obstet Gynecol* 68:348, 196.
28. Petterson F, et al, editors: *Annual report on the results of treatment in gynecologic cancer*, vol 19, Stockholm, 1985, International Federation of Gynecology and Obstetrics.
29. Rustin GJS, et al: Weekly alternating etoposide, methotrexate and actinomycin/vincristine and cyclophosphamide chemotherapy for the treatment of CNS metastases of choriocarcinoma, *J Clin Oncol* 7:900, 1989.
30. Schlaerth JB, Morrow CP, Rodriguez M: Diagnostic and therapeutic curettage in gestational trophoblastic disease, *Am J Obstet Gynecol* 162:1465, 1990.
31. Schlaerth JB, et al: Prognostic characteristics of serum human chorionic gonadotropin titer regression following molar pregnancy, *Obstet Gynecol* 58:478, 1981.
32. Schlaerth JB, et al: Initial management of hydatidiform mole, *Am J Obstet Gynecol* 158:1299, 1988.
33. Shirley RL, Goldstein DP, Collins JJ Jr: The role of thoracotomy in management of patients with chest metastases from gestational trophoblastic disease, *J Thorac Cardiovasc Surg* 63:545, 1972.

34. Sink JD, Hammond CB, Young WG: Pulmonary resection in the management of metastases from choriocarcinoma, *J Thorac Cardiovasc Surg* 81:830, 1981.
35. Soper JT, Clarke-Pearson DL, Hammond CB: Metastatic gestational trophoblastic disease: prognostic factors in previously untreated patients, *Obstet Gynecol* 71:338, 1988.
36. Soper JT, et al: Renal metastases of gestational trophoblastic disease: a report of eight cases, *Obstet Gynecol* 72:796, 1988.
37. Soper JT, et al: Evaluation of prognostic factors and staging in gestational trophoblastic tumor, *Obstet Gynecology* 84:969, 1994.
38. Sung H, et al: A staging system of gestational trophoblastic neoplasms based on the development of the disease, *Chin Med J* 97:557, 1984.
39. Surwit EA, Hammond CB: Treatment of metastatic trophoblastic disease with poor prognosis, *Obstet Gynecol* 55:565, 1980.
40. Szulman AE: Syndromes of hydatidiform moles: partial versus complete, *J Reprod Med* 29:788, 1984.
41. Szulman AE, Surti U: The syndromes of hydatidiform moles. I. Cytogenetics and morphologic correlations, *Am J Obstet Gynecol* 131:665, 1978.
42. Szulman AE, Surti U: The syndromes of hydatidiform moles. II. Morphologic evolution of the complete and partial mole, *Am J Obstet Gynecol* 132:20, 1978.
43. Szulman AE, Surti U: The clinicopathologic profile of the partial hydatidiform mole, *Obstet Gynecol* 59:597, 1982.
44. Szulman AE, et al: Triploidy: association with partial moles and nonmolar conceptuses, *Hum Pathol* 12:1016, 1981.
45. Thomas HJ, et al: Hickman-Broviac catheters, *Am J Surg* 140:791, 1980.
46. Tomoda Y, et al: Surgical indications for resection in pulmonary metastases of choriocarcinoma, *Cancer* 46:2723, 1980.
47. Tow WSH: The place of hysterotomy in the treatment of hydatidiform mole, *Aust NZ J Obstet Gynaecol* 7:97, 1967.
48. Twiggs CB, Morrow CP, Schlaerth JB: Acute pulmonary complications of molar pregnancy, *Am J Obstet Gynecol* 135:189, 1979.
49. Weed JC, Hammond CB: Cerebral metastatic choriocarcinoma: intensive therapy and prognosis, *Obstet Gynecol* 55:89, 1980.
50. Wong LC, Ma HK: Persistent chest opacity in trophoblastic disease: is thoracotomy justified? *Aust NZ J Obstet Gynaecol* 23:237, 1983.
51. World Health Organization Scientific Group: *Gestational trophoblastic disease,* Tech Rep Series 692, Geneva, 1983, World Health Organization.

DAVID H. NICHOLS

GENERAL CONSIDERATIONS

The presence of the pregnant uterus modifies the type of injury that is sustained from objects penetrating the abdominal wall and perineum. The pregnant uterus affords protection to the other viscera and displaces the abdominal and pelvic contents to somewhat different locations, depending on the duration of the pregnancy. Many pregnant women have been injured by bullets, shrapnel, and other objects capable of inflicting a penetrating wound during recent military conflicts, in which attacks on military targets in the vicinity of large cities were commonplace. It is expected that many more such accidents will happen in any future conflict because it would not be possible, at least in the early stages of an attack, to single out pregnant women for evacuation. Other factors that increase the likelihood that these injuries will occur include the trend for women to remain actively employed during pregnancy, an increase in women undertaking jobs that are considered more hazardous, and the increase in violence in society in general.

CAUSE AND PATHOLOGIC ANATOMY

In civilian accidents the most common penetrating object is an accidentally discharged bullet. The accidents occurring during the bombing of large cities place secondary objects in motion by the explosion. The change in the position of the peritoneal reflections of the bladder, uterus, and bowel in the various months of pregnancy is the most important factor in determining the type of injury. The protection given to other abdominal organs by the pregnant uterus and fetus varies with the duration of pregnancy, and organs that are ordinarily vulnerable to penetrating wounds of the abdomen are less so in the presence of a term pregnancy.

The site of entry of a high-velocity missile to a large extent determines the presence of visceral injury. Visceral injuries are expected when the entry site was in either the upper abdomen or back and are rarely seen when the site of entry was anterior and below the uterine fundus. In the latter the missile usually does not cross the posterior uterine wall. Therefore fortified by appropriate radiographic views, which should show the location of the bullet, and by careful observation of the patient, the surgeon should weigh carefully whether a conservative approach is warranted versus an emergency exploratory laparotomy. Awwad et al. have

noted that preterm delivery of a live fetus with no evidence of acute distress or injuries may expose it unduly to the risks and complications of prematurity. In 1960, Shaftan described his experience with selective surgical intervention, believing that unnecessary emergency surgery was potentially harmful to the injured patient (pulmonary complications, wound infection, ileus, bowel obstruction). Selective laparotomy for these patients was proposed in 1980 by Iliya et al., who pointed out that the gravid uterus acts as a shield, protecting more vital maternal structures from injury. If the entrance wound is below the uterine fundus, the infant is dead, the bullet can be shown radiographically to be in the uterus, the patient's vital signs remain stable, the abdomen is soft, and there is no blood in the urinary or gastrointestinal tract, a conservative treatment without laparotomy is warranted. Most patients with a bullet hole in the uterus can deliver their baby vaginally, and as noted by Buchsbaum and Stapes, "The only indication for performing cesarean section with a dead infant is a pregnant uterus that compromises the surgeon's ability to repair maternal visceral injuries." Awwad et al. have provided a comprehensive review of this subject and for those patients being observed have recommended having continuous fetal monitoring with immediate cesarean delivery and exploration should fetal distress supervene. "Early recognition and treatment of abdominal injury are crucial," and they recommend that "When in doubt, exploratory laparotomy remains the safest approach."

Fig. 65-1 shows some of the common wounds that may occur with the fetus at term. The bowel is crowded into the upper abdomen at this time, and a penetrating wound entering above the fundus might be expected to penetrate several loops of bowel. Perforations of the bowel, whether in the presence of a pregnancy or not, tend to occur in multiples of two. This fact should be remembered in exploring the abdomen after accidents, because fragments passing through a segment of bowel have a wound of entrance and a wound of exit. The fragment may pass through the bowel and the uterine wall to lodge in the placenta. This may cause a premature separation of the placenta, with concealed bleeding. The fragment may enter the uterus and cause a laceration of the cord, with death of the fetus. The deflection of fragments from bony structures within the pelvis, with the creation of secondary fragments of bone, causes many bizarre wounds. Wounds from missiles in which the entrance is in the perineum are less serious if they are below the levator muscle (see Fig. 65-1). The possible course of these missiles is de-

---

*Modified from Ball TL: *Gynecologic surgery and urology,* ed 2, St Louis, 1963, Mosby.

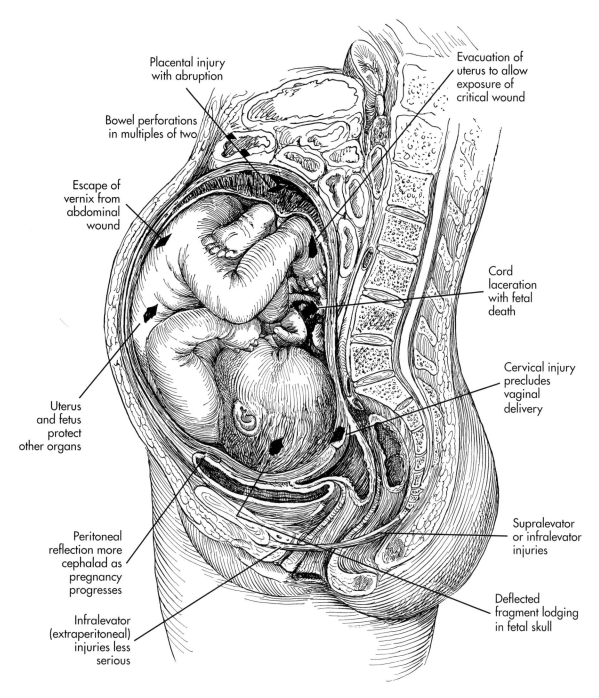

Placental injury
with abruption

Evacuation of
uterus to allow
exposure of
critical wound

Bowel perforations
in multiples of two

Escape of
vernix from
abdominal
wound

Cord
laceration
with fetal
death

Cervical injury
precludes
vaginal
delivery

Uterus
and fetus
protect
other organs

Supralevator
or infralevator
injuries

Peritoneal
reflection more
cephalad as
pregnancy
progresses

Deflected
fragment lodging
in fetal skull

Infralevator
(extraperitoneal)
injuries less
serious

Fig. 65-1   Common wounds to the uterus and fetus.

termined to decide whether supralevator or infralevator injuries or a combination of both has occurred. Lacerations of
the cervix and vagina occur and may preclude vaginal delivery. There is almost an unlimited combination of wounds
that may occur in addition to those injuries sustained by the
fetus. In assessing the probable damage, the surgeon constantly keeps in mind the change in the peritoneal reflection
and the position of the fetus, placenta, and abdominal and
pelvic viscera at the various weeks of pregnancy. Despite
the apparent vulnerability of the fetus and pregnant mother
to such penetrating wounds, the number of case reports is
relatively small and the survival rate is reasonably good. No

statistical studies are available to suggest the number of casualties that may be anticipated among pregnant women
during a mass attack. They have undoubtedly occurred in
considerable numbers, but seldom, under wartime conditions, does the physician stop to analyze the individual factors resulting from the pregnancy that may have influenced
the type of wounds observed.

SYMPTOMS AND DIAGNOSIS

The wounds of entrance and exit are noted on all parts of the
chest, abdomen, and perineum. The wound of entrance is

usually smaller than the wound of exit and may be further identified by threads of cloth or grease from the object along the edges of the entrance hole. Amniotic fluid, as well as vernix, may escape from the abdominal wound, confirming a perforation of the uterine wall. The passage of meconium in the abdominal wound suggests severe injury, with death of the fetus or severe injuries to the fetus. If x-ray facilities are available, the fetus and placental site are studied to locate objects or bullets that may have lodged in either the fetus or placenta. Fragments of shrapnel and other objects have been passed in the lochia after penetrating wounds of the pregnant uterus and subsequent delivery. Injuries to other organs in conjunction with the pregnant uterus may not show the characteristic signs and symptoms seen in the nonpregnant state because of their displacement and the added confusing factors resulting from injury to the pregnant uterus or fetus. Many injuries are not diagnosed until the uterus is emptied and an exploratory laparotomy is performed.

SURGICAL PRINCIPLES

The surgical principles in dealing with penetrating wounds during pregnancy are discussed under four headings: (1) abdominal injuries involving the pregnant uterus with the fetus alive and viable, (2) abdominal injuries not affecting the pregnant uterus with the fetus alive and viable, (3) abdominal injuries that have a favorable prognosis but with a fetus that is premature or not viable, and (4) abdominal or perineal injuries with no involvement of the uterus itself in which labor is either in progress or imminent. Many other possible situations exist, each of which must be evaluated individually. If the fetus is alive and viable, the abdominal injuries are repaired, usually after evacuation of the uterus by cesarean section. The obstetrician decides at this time whether a Porro section or a section hysterectomy should be done, depending on the extent of the damage to the uterus. The judgment of the obstetrician in this decision is the result of many years of experience and skill in determining the future capabilities of the uterus and the possible complications that would result from its retention. Injuries that do not affect the uterus, in which the fetus is alive and viable, are managed by evacuating the uterus to facilitate the repair of other organs. In exceptional cases the pregnant uterus is removed to manage wounds in the pelvis in which the presence of the recently evacuated uterus causes technical difficulties. The presence of a premature fetus and an abdominal injury with a favorable prognosis again requires the skill and judgment of the obstetrician to decide whether the pregnancy can be allowed to continue or whether the uterus must be evacuated and the fetus lost. Many factors enter into the final decision, but if it appears that the patient is going into premature labor, the most conservative course is to evacuate the uterus at the time of abdominal surgery. If study of the abdominal wounds and uterus indicates that the prognosis is just as favorable with the uterus remaining, the uterus is left and measures are taken to prevent premature labor. Subsequently, the patient can be expected to deliver vaginally provided there are no injuries to the perineum or vagina that would contraindicate this method of delivery. The problem of managing abdominal injuries while labor is in progress requires judgment as to the mode of delivery. The presence of abdominal hemorrhage or perforation of the bowel or other vital organs cannot await the termination of labor and a vaginal delivery. A cesarean section is done and uterine contractions are stopped by a general anesthetic, regardless of the cervical dilation. If delivery is imminent, one might be faced with the problem of delivering the infant vaginally and immediately proceeding with a laparotomy for multiple abdominal injuries that may not have seriously affected the uterus.

PROCEDURE FOR EMERGENCY LAPAROTOMY

In the event that the bullet has entered the abdomen above the uterine fundus and visceral injury is likely, the abdomen should be entered through a long midline incision. Gross blood is evacuated, and exploration conducted in an orderly manner, as Thal et al. have emphasized, to minimize hemorrhage and contamination and facilitate the identification of injuries. The uterus should be exteriorized, if possible, and if necessary for visualization of visceral repair, emptied by cesarean section or removed by Porro hysterectomy.

Most gastric wounds can be repaired primarily as can small bowel injuries that occupy less than 50% of the circumference of the bowel after debridement. A single-layer closure is less likely to compromise luminal size. Solitary colonic injuries not associated with shock or significant contamination may be repaired primarily, but large or multiple injuries to the right colon may require hemicolectomy with ileocolic anastomosis. Injuries to the left colon usually require resection and proximal temporary diversion. The liver and spleen are visualized; then the retroperitoneum and its contained organs and vessels, with repair and drainage as necessary.

When hemorrhage and visceral contamination have been controlled (remembering the therapeutic advantage of tight but temporary packing as necessary), and if a coagulopathy or deep shock supervenes, it may be necessary to temporarily close the abdomen as swiftly as possible. Fascia can be bridged with nonabsorbable plastic mesh or even sterile intravenous bags. A series of surgical towel clips can bring and hold the skin edges together. Reoperation is planned when it is safe, and stability has been restored.

PROGNOSIS

Some of the factors influencing the outcome of the patient with a perforating wound of the abdomen in the presence of a pregnant uterus are as follows: the greater the number of perforations and the greater the length of time between injury and treatment, the higher the mortality; the further advanced the pregnancy and therefore occupying more space, the greater the chance of uterine injury. However, the contractility of the uterine musculature permits severe lacerations without exsanguinating the patient. Experience in labor with a previously myomectomized uterus has taught us that the organ need seldom be sacrificed for any lacerations caused by perforating objects. The patient's age is a consideration. Older gravidas do not tolerate abdominal wounds as well as younger patients because of arteriosclerotic changes in the vessel walls that prevent vasoconstriction. The location of wounds in the abdominal viscera is an important factor. A tear in the left colon, with the escape of formed fecal material, does not produce the dramatic symptoms of a lacerated stomach, with the escape of a large quantity of gastric contents. It likewise does not produce symptoms as soon as lesions of the small bowel, with pouring of liquid contents into the peritoneal cavity. Lack of symptoms due to the escape of formed fecal material may delay surgery, and time is a factor in the ultimate prognosis. In reviewing many of these injuries one cannot help but be impressed with the remarkably safe locale the fetus occupies in utero, compared with the rest of us on the outside.

RUPTURE OF THE PREGNANT UTERUS BY EXTERNAL VIOLENCE

Rupture of the pregnant uterus by external violence, such as automobile accidents, falls, and crushing injuries from other accidents, is uncommon despite the large number of pregnant women exposed to these possibilities. Patients usually show a laceration or contusion of the abdominal wall. The signs of primary shock, loss of fetal heartbeat, and a tetanic contraction of the uterus indicate an intraabdominal and uterine catastrophe. Examination of the abdomen reveals the tender uterus and signs suggesting intraabdominal hemorrhage. The pulse rate continues to rise, whereas the blood pressure falls, and immediate preparations must be made to combat shock and prepare the patient for operation. Treatment consists of a laparotomy, with the decision about the preservation of the uterus being made by the obstetrician for each individual case. The fetus is often lost, and the placenta and fetus may be found free in the abdominal cavity. After expulsion of the fetus into the peritoneal cavity, the uterus contracts down around the point of rupture and serious hemorrhage is less likely to occur. The obstetrician must decide whether the uterus can be preserved as a functional organ. If

so, the rent in the uterus is repaired in layers, and systematic examination of all of the pelvic and abdominal viscera is done to exclude injury to any other organs. If not, immediate hysterectomy is performed.

SUGGESTED READING

Armstrong CL, Andreson PS: Metallic intrauterine foreign body in term pregnancy, *Am J Obstet Gynecol* 78:442, 1959.

Awwad JT, et al: High-velocity penetrating wounds of the gravid uterus: review of 16 years of civil war, *Obstet Gynecol* 83:259, 1994.

Beattie J, Daly R: Gunshot wound of the pregnant uterus, *Am J Obstet Gynecol* 80:772, 1960.

Belkap R: Gunshot wound of the pregnant uterus, *J Maine MA* 30:13, 1939.

Black B: Surgical treatment with recovery in a case of perineo-abdominal shotgun wounds fare close range with multiple injuries to viscera, *Surg Clin North Am* 24:952, 1944.

Buchsbaum HJ, Staples PP Jr: Self-inflicted gunshot wound to the pregnant uterus: report of two cases, *Obstet Gynecol* 65(suppl):32S, 1985.

Echerling B: Obstetrical approach to abdominal war wounds late in pregnancy, *J Obstet Gynecol Br Emp* 57:747, 1950.

Elias M: Rupture of the pregnant uterus by external violence, *Lancet* 2:253, 1950.

Flamrich E: Gunshot wounds of the pregnant uterus, *Zentralbl Tynak* 65:25, 1941.

Fowler R: Gunshot wounds of the pregnant uterus, *NY J Med* 11:525, 1911.

Gourlay N: Accidental rupture of the female urethra, *J Obstet Gynecol Br Emp* 67:991, 1960.

Helsper J: Nonperforating wounds of the abdomen, *Am J Surg* 90:580, 1955.

Holters O, Daversa B: Bullet wound of a gravid uterus with intestinal perforation, *Am J Obstet Gynecol* 56:985, 1948.

Iliya FA, Hajj SN, Buchsbaum HJ: Gunshot wounds of the pregnant uterus: report of two cases, *J Trauma* 20:90, 1980.

Jacobus W: Gunshot wound of the gravid uterus, *Am J Obstet Gynecol* 63:687, 1952.

Koback AJ, Hurwitz CH: Gunshot wounds of the pregnant uterus, *Obstet Gynecol* 4:383, 1954.

Motta M, Vianna C: Bullet wound in a pregnant uterus, *Rev Gynecol Obstet* 23:319, 1929.

Placintianu G, Turcanu G: Bullet wound in a pregnant uterus at term, *Spitalul* 48:224, 1928.

Shaftan GW: Indications for operation in abdominal trauma, *Am J Surg* 99:657, 1960.

Souter RJ de N: Penetrating gunshot wound of a pregnant uterus, *Med J Aust* 2:111, 1947.

Thal ER, Eastridge BJ, Milhoan R: Operative exposure of abdominal injuries and closure of the abdomen. In Wilmore, et al, editors: *Scientific American surgery*, vol 1, New York, 1997, Scientific American.

Zondek B: Shrapnel shot through the placenta, *Lancet* 1:674, 1947.

66 Laparoscopically Assisted Radical Vaginal Hysterectomy or Trachelectomy

DANIEL F. G. DARGENT

The vaginal radical hysterectomy (VRH) can be regarded at the top of the specific repertoire of the qualified gynecologist. Unfortunately, as was written by Luigi Carenza in the chapter devoted to the topic in the first edition of this book,[7] "the number of surgeons capable of performing this operation properly is declining as a result of the smaller number of patients requiring this form of surgery." Since that time the landscape has changed considerably. In fact, if one postulates that VRH has to be reserved for "contained" cervical cancers, one can say that such cancers today are more numerous because they can be identified very accurately thanks to the improvements in two techniques: magnetic resonance imaging (MRI) and laparoscopy. MRI enables us to determine the volume of a tumor with great precision, and laparoscopy makes a low-cost lymph node assessment possible at the same time with great accuracy. A tumor of less than 4 cm in diameter (MRI) with no lymph nodes involvement (laparoscopy) can be considered a "contained" tumor. This is an appropriate application for VRH, and one can guess that this field of opportunity will broaden when forthcoming imaging and/or biologic technologies will make definition easier and more precise. Now is an appropriate time for the decline in use of VRH to be reversed and for gynecologic oncologists again to be trained in the vaginal surgical approach.

My aim in this chapter is to describe VRH in the form I consider appropriate in the contemporary context of technology and concept: the laparoscopically assisted radical vaginal hysterectomy or trachelectomy. However, before describing it, I will review the different techniques used in the preceding decades and present these operations in the historic order in which they appeared. Those choices are not proof of a nostalgic attachment to the past, but reviewing their history makes it easier for us to understand our practice of today.

THE EARLY SCHAUTA'S OPERATION

After centuries of empiric use of procedures aiming to debulk tumors with cold knives, thermocautery, or various corrosive mixtures or to remove the intravaginal part of the uterus, the vaginal hysterectomy was the first sensitive intervention proposed for curing a patient with cervical cancer. On July 26, 1829, Recamier was the first to do it. The place was at the Hotel Dieu Hospital in Paris, and the patient was 50 years of age. The picture of the operative specimen[48] shows that the tumor was a bulky endocervical cancer with no involvement of the vagina and no involvement of the paracervical ligament: stage IB2 by today's International Federation of Gynecologists and Obstetricians (FIGO) classification. Recamier operated without anesthesia! After ligating the uterine arteries he cut the paracervical ligaments. The operation lasted 20 minutes. The patient survived, was discharged after 21 days, and was still alive 1 year later.

Unfortunately, the results obtained in the following years by Recamier himself and those who followed him were much less spectacular. The operation was condemned by the professional authorities and abandoned. The surgical movement started again only after anesthesia and antisepsis became available. The vaginal approach was the preference of most surgeons, but some took the risk of operating through laparotomy. Freund[19] in 1878 is considered the first who did this. Not surprisingly, the outcomes were even worse. In the survey published by Hegar and Kaltenbach in 1886[24] the number of postoperative casualties was 80 for 119 abdominal operations and only 1 patient was surviving after 1 year. In the survey on vaginal hysterectomy published in 1887 by Hache[21] postoperative casualties were only (!) 24% and the rate of 2-year survival was 26%.

Despite the high postoperative mortality, surgeons did not give up the prospect of curing patients using surgery (it is fair to say that no alternate existed). In this perspective the concept of radical surgery was devised and "extended hysterectomy" was proposed in place of the extrafascial hysterectomy that was carried out by the "vaginalists" and by the "laparotomists" as well. Pawlik,[41] who was in Prague and head of the Czech-speaking Surgery Institute in 1890 published a report on the first three hysterectomies performed with simultaneous removal of part of the vagina and pelvic cellular tissue. The operation was carried out transvaginally after stents had been placed in the ureters. Pawlik was able to put the stents in without endoscopy (which did not exist) and without intravesical palpation of the ureteral papillae, the methods surgeons used at this time after first dilating the urethra. Clark,[10] at the time a 24-year-old resident at the Johns Hopkins Hospital in Baltimore, in 1895 published the first report of a similar operation performed transabdominally.

Once launched by the pioneers, the radical hysterectomy rapidly became popular. Amazingly, the abdominal route, which continued to be the more hazardous, developed more quickly than the vaginal one. At the time Wertheim[64] presented his communication to the Medical Society in Vienna (October 14, 1904) he had performed 250 abdominal radical hysterectomies, while Schauta had performed only 113 vaginal radical hysterectomies (it is fair to mention that Wertheim started performing radical hysterectomies in November 1898 as did Schauta in June 1901).

The debate between the two leaders of this new surgery is worth the renown it enjoys. Knowing that Wertheim was the pupil of Schauta is meaningful from the psychological point of view. Knowing that their collaboration dated from the time that Schauta was the head of the German speaking Institute of Gynecology and Obstetrics in Prague is important for one who seeks the historical truth (it is clear that the technique of VRH was born in the Czech province and not in the capital of the Hapsburg's empire). However, the content of the debate itself is most important for the contemporary gynecologic oncologist. This content is considerable (the debate was not closed after the October 14th session; the October 21st session was also devoted to it), and is of great interest as well.

The comparatively lesser danger of the vaginal approach was the first point of discussion. The first patient operated on by Wertheim died within 8 hours of surgery. Of the 32 patients he subsequently operated on, only 22 survived. In the series presented in October 1904, the postoperative casualties remained as high as 26% (30 for the 100 first patients operated on and 22 for the next 100 patients). At this time the surgical mortality in Schauta's series was only 12%. Despite its greater danger, the abdominal approach appeared to have a higher curative value. The global survival rate was 22.5% in Wertheim's series and 5.9% in Schauta's series. However, Schauta's data at this time were for the simple vaginal hysterectomy, which could not be compared fairly to Wertheim's data. Nevertheless, it became obvious in the following years that the abdominal approach was therapeutically superior to the vaginal one.

Comparison of the data reported in the monographs published by Schauta in 1908[51] and by Wertheim in 1911[65] confirmed the first feelings. In Schauta's 1901 to 1902 series, of 116 referred patients, 47 were operated on, 9 died postoperatively, 4 died later with intercurrent disease, and 21 had a recurrence within the 5 years of follow-up. In Wertheim's 1898 to 1904 series, of 607 referred patients, 250 were operated on, 63 died postoperatively, 3 died later with intercurrent disease, and 78 had a recurrence within the 5 years of follow-up. The postoperative mortality rate of Wertheim's operation was twice that of Schauta's operation, but the rate of recurrence was less: 78 of 184 patients who

survived the operation and did not die with intercurrent disease versus 21 of 34 (ratio: −1.5).

A century later the first observation remains true: the vaginal approach is less dangerous than the abdominal one.[66] The difference for the second point no longer exists. The rate of recurrence is no longer higher after vaginal surgery, but this result has been obtained only after advanced technical and strategic modifications.

PEHAM-AMREICH'S OPERATION

The poorer oncologic value of Schauta's original operation obviously was linked to reduced radicality. During the October 1904 discussion, Wertheim stressed that he was able to remove the enlarged pelvic lymph nodes, and in this ability he saw the source of his improved outcome. But Schauta remarked that in the Wertheim series not a single patient with a positive lymph node survived without recurrence. The issue of lymphadenectomy would be discussed again some decades later, but at the turn of the century the question was elsewhere: the original Schauta operation clearly was not radical enough as far as the resection of vagina and pelvic cellular tissue were concerned. A more radical operation was necessary. Schauta himself and then Peham and Amreich (his successors as leaders of the second University Clinic in Vienna) developed and performed it. Their operation is described in full detail and magnificently illustrated in their book published in 1934.[42] This description has been paraphrased many times, and I will give here only a short summary, stressing the points that identify the specificity of this fully radical operation.

Amreich's operation starts with a so-called Schuchardt's incision. Schuchardt was an Austrian gynecologist whose name should have been mentioned in the pioneer's gallery because in 1893,[54] he started performing extended vaginal hysterectomies. The approach he proposed included a "paravaginal incision." This incision is made on the left side. It is a sort of large mediolateral episiotomy completed by an incision in the levator muscle. The division of the muscle leads to a large opening into the ipsilateral pararectal space and gives access to the vaginal cuff and to the surrounding dense pelvic cellular tissue, the removal of which is an aim of the extended hysterectomy.

The second step of the operation is preparation, separation, and grasping of the so-called vaginal cuff. The preparation is made at a level depending on the extent of the tumor and is performed using a cold knife. The cuff is grasped using Chrobak's forceps, and the vesicovaginal space and then the paravesical spaces are opened.

The opening of the paravesical space and the subsequent exposure of the bladder pillar identify the specificity of Amreich's procedure. Taking advantage of the large opening of the left pararectal space, the surgeon enters the ipsilateral paravesical space while moving around the inferior border of the paracervical ligament, first using curved scissors with closed tips and then the finger. Once opened, the space is enlarged so that two or, better, three fingers can move easily from the pelvic wall to the lateral aspect of the bladder, acting as one would for maneuvering outside the bladder itself. This preparation largely frees the lateral aspect of the bladder pillar, whose dissection is the second specific point of Amreich's technique.

Strictly speaking the bladder pillar is not an anatomic structure. It is just a condensation of the pelvic cellular tissue but which by surgical preparation gives the appearance of an autonomous structure. In fact, the pelvic cellular tissue surrounding the bladder, which is very smooth in the so-called dry spaces (the vesicovaginal space and the paravesical spaces), becomes more dense on each side of the midline in front of the sites where the ureters course into the bladder floor. This densification gives rise to the so-called vesico-uterine ligaments (or anterior parametrium) whose insertion onto the vagina are marked by two dimples that Pawlik was able to identify to catheterize the ureters without cystoscopy. Traction to the vaginal cuff makes the pseudoligaments stronger and draws the ureters into the operative field, giving them a convex curvature: identifying and mobilizing the "knee of the ureter" is the first concern in the dissection of the bladder pillar.

Identification and mobilization of the knee of the ureter is decisively made in Amreich's operation. The ureter is first identified while the pillar is palpated between one finger in the paravesical space and one other finger in the vesicovaginal space. Once the "snap" has been perceived, the tissues lying lateral to the ureteral knee are cut with a cold knife. These are fibers surrounding the collateral vessels that the uterine and vaginal vessels send to the lateral aspect of the bladder. They constitute the "lateral bladder pillar" as opposed to the "medial bladder pillar" (i.e., the vesicouterine ligament itself). The division of the lateral pillar must be done cautiously. Although preventive hemostasis is impossible, secondary hemostasis is easy, if needed (surprisingly, it is not needed in all cases). Once the lateral bladder pillar has been divided and the knee of the ureter identified, the medial bladder pillar is divided after appropriate exposure. At this time the knee of the ureter and the next part of the bladder can be pushed into the depth, freeing the ventral aspect of the paracervical ligament for its full length: from the pelvic wall to the vaginal cuff. The uterine artery, which comes into the operative field inside the knee of the ureter, can be prepared, ligated, and cut.

The ventral aspect of the specimen being free, the same dissection is carried out on the dorsal aspect: opening into Douglas' pouch, section of the rectal pillars, and clamping and section of the paracervical ligaments as close as possible to their pelvic extremities.

The radicality of the Peham-Amreich procedure is evidenced by the data published by the few surgeons using the procedure who followed them. In 1956, Van Bouwdijk Bastiaanse[63] reported on 76 patients operated on during the years 1947 and 1948 with a rate of disease-free survival of 75% for patients with stage I disease and 65.2% for those with stage II disease. In 1963, Navratil[38] reported on 808 patients operated on during the years 1947 to 1956: 83.3% 5-year disease free-survival for stage I, 79.9% for stage IB,

and 51.7% for stage II. In the same year, McCall[35] reported about 50 patients with stage IA, IB, and IIA disease operated on 5 years or more before of whom 45 survived. In 1961, Scheele[52] gave results for Fauvet's Clinic in Hanover: 71.7% relative cure rate for patients with stage I and II disease operated on during the years 1944 to 1955 (759 patients). In 1966, Inguilla[28] released the results for 327 patients: the rate of 5-year disease-free survival was 81% for patients with stage I disease and 56% for stage II. In the chapter he wrote for the first edition of this book, Carenza[7] reported results obtained for 217 patients operated on during the years 1968 to 1984: the 5-year survival was 51 of 53 patients with stage IA disease, 90 of 103 for stage IB, and 43 of 61 for stage IIA. In 1993, Massi published[34] results of the Florence experience for 458 patients operated on during the years 1968 to 1983: for patients with stage IB disease, the rate of 5-year disease-free survival was 79.5% for the Schauta Amreich vaginal procedure (356 patients) and 76.7% for the for the Wertheim-Meigs abdominal operation (288 patients).

The data reflected in the preceding paragraph are often biased. Most of the surgeons using the Schauta-Amreich procedure did it while trying to exclude poor-risk patients (e.g., Carenza, starting from 1972, operated only on patients with normal lymphography). Nevertheless, one knows that none of the tools of patient selection (including lymphangiography) is perfect. The series of patients operated on by the Schauta-Amreich procedure certainly includes patients with positive lymph nodes, and it is striking to see that the results obtained (without complementary lymphadenectomy) approximate the results obtained from use of the Wertheim-Meigs procedure (the Florence experience in which no selection was used is, from this viewpoint, especially enlightening). That means that the Schauta-Amreich procedure is at least equivalent to the abdominal procedure as far as the local regional radicality is concerned.

STOECKEL'S OPERATION

As a consequence of its radicality, the Amreich procedure carries a risk of urinary complications and especially urinary bladder retention or voiding difficulties. In fact, most of the surveys devoted to this issue underline the significant increase of such complications in patients operated on through the vaginal approach rather than the abdominal one.[2,40,46] The difference generally is attributed to the vaginal approach itself. It is possible that the Schuchardt incision plays some negative role. However, in certain series the difference between the two approaches is reversed, as is the case in Burghardt's series[47]: dysuria in 81.4% of the patients undergoing abdominal operations versus 17% of the patients undergoing transvaginal operation and average urethral pressure 58.2 cm H_2O versus 53.6 cm H_2O. In this series Amreich's technique is used for the vaginal procedure and the abdominal procedure is performed using an original technique after which the vessels making the skeleton of the paracervical ligament are divided one after another between staples put at the contact with the pelvic wall. In other words, the technique used for the abdominal approach is a Piver 4 technique, which accounts for the difference. If one compares the Schauta-Amreich procedure with a Piver 3 abdominal procedure (Wertheim-Meigs), the difference is in favor of the abdominal approach. If one compares it with a Piver 4 abdominal procedure, the difference is reversed, and this observation enables us to end the debate concerning radicality: the Amreich procedure is more radical than a Piver 3 procedure but less so than the Piver 4 procedure.

Bladder floor denervation is the cause of the bladder problems one sees after the radical hysterectomy. The innervation of the bladder floor is carried by a branch of the hypogastric autonomous nervous plexus called nervus pelvicus accessorius. It originates alongside the pelvic wall at various levels: either dorsal to the paracervical ligament or ventral to it. It then crosses the upper vagina laterally and touches the bladder floor and the posterior urethra. It is endangered at two levels during the radical hysterectomy: at the crossing of the paracervical ligament and at the crossing of the vagina. The closer to the pelvic wall the paracervical ligament is divided, the greater the danger (it depends on the anatomy as well). The more extensive the vaginal removal, the greater the danger.

Tailoring the vaginal removal can be impossible in patients with stage IIA disease or higher, but this tailorization is perfectly possible in those with stage IB disease. Concerning the paracervical ligament, one can ask if a dissection such as the Piver 4 is mandatory in every patient. The giant sections done in Piver 4 radical hysterectomy specimens[20] show that lymph nodes do exist everywhere in the paracervical ligaments: in the distal (lateral) part as well as in a proximal (medial) one. These lymph nodes can be involved by the cancer in its very early phase of development. However, a direct relationship also exists between the risk of involvement and the morphologic features. The most significant feature (after Burghardt) is the cervical coefficient (i.e., the ratio volume of the tumor to the volume of the cervix). If the coefficient is less than 20%, the risk is 3%, but it becomes 15% for a coefficient of 40 to 60% and 35% for a coefficient of 80 to 90%. This coefficient can now be assessed quite accurately using MRI.

Stoeckel was unaware of the data collected thanks to today's technologies. He described his variant of the genuine Schauta procedure, but he was conscious of the dangers of the maximalist operation and at the same time of its uselessness in early patients. This idea is the core of the rationale of the operation he described in 1928.[60] This operation is worth bearing the name Stoeckel's operation. Here I stress only the points that make it different from the Peham-Amreich operation. The details of the technique are described later because they are part of the operation I use and recommend today.

The first difference in Stoeckel's operation is to not include a Schuchardt incision. One or two episiotomies can be performed. Stoeckel did it, but there is no need to extend them to the pararectal spaces. By not making a Schuchardt incision, the surgeon avoids a major source of postoperative pain and, perhaps, bladder retention and subsequent dys-

urias. The vaginal cuff is tailored economically (1.5 cm on the ventral aspect and 3.0 cm on the dorsal one for stage IB1 disease); this also prevents postoperative voiding difficulties. The vesicovaginal space is developed as in the Amreich procedure, but the opening of the paravesical spaces is carried out differently, resulting in a more economical development (for the technical details see the following section). The bladder pillars as well are managed in another way: only the most caudal fibers of the lateral part of each are divided, and finally the clamps placed on the paracervical ligaments are located closer to the vaginal cuff (i.e., medial to the origin of the so-called lateral bladder pillar). For these reasons, the bladder floor remains connected to the pelvic wall, lessening the risk of persistent bladder dysfunction.

Although less traumatizing, the modified VRH (or Stoeckel's operation) is obviously less radical. Its radicality is like that of the Piver 2 operation, which seems to be enough for patients with stage IB1 disease. Two prospective and randomized studies[32,59] have demonstrated that the cure rates are the same after the Piver 2 and 3 operations in patients with stage IB1 disease. However, specific data concerning this vaginal approach are missing, and it seems wise to restrict the operation to patients with a tumor diameter of less than 2 cm.

MITRA'S OPERATION

The lymph node issue was on the agenda of the 1904 discussion between Wertheim and Schauta. At the time the lymphadenectomy carried out by Wertheim was only a "selective lymphadenectomy" as we name it today. Only the enlarged lymph nodes were removed. As previously stated, the therapeutic value of such a lymphadenectomy is doubtful. Because of the uncertainties concerning the value of the lymphadenectomy, the gynecologists who continued, during the following decades, to use surgery in the management of cervical cancer used either the abdominal or the vaginal route, depending on the training they had received or on the patient's general condition. Thanks to improvement in technique the vaginal operation gave the same results as the abdominal one.

In fact, after World War I, only a minority of gynecologists went on using surgery for treatment of cervical cancer. As soon as the first results were obtained from the application of Marie Curie's radium, the new treatment spread like a flash all over the world. The misfortune of Wertheim during the German meeting of gynecology held in Halle an der Saale in 1913 is symptomatic of the size of the revolution that happened at this time. Doderlein, who reported the results obtained in Germany with the new tool, declared that Wertheim's operation, starting from this date, was only a historical souvenir. Wertheim withdrew the communication he was scheduled to give. However, despite this public scandal, use of the new tool did not expand very fast in Germany and Austria because of the difficulties the gynecologists had in obtaining radium, difficulties that increased after World War I.

It was in France (Curie's country), the United Kingdom,

and the United States where the maximal development of radiotherapy occurred. This development led paradoxically to the revival of surgery at the beginning of the 1940s. The results obtained from radiotherapy were not as good as expected, especially in patients with stage II disease, in whom pelvic recurrences were numerous, even if the tumor response to radiation was apparently complete. Leveuf in France[31] and Taussig in the United States[61] stressed the high frequency of occult lymph nodal metastases and suspected their role in the failures of radiotherapy. They proposed integration of a lymphadenectomy in the therapeutic policy. It was no longer the Wertheim selective lymphadenectomy, but they performed a "systematic pelvic lymphadenectomy." Now that surgery was again accepted as having a role to play, many gynecologists went back to it as the first-choice therapy. Among this new phalanx of surgeons, the name of Joe Vincent Meigs deserves to be celebrated as the father of the "new" Wertheim operation.[36]

At the same time as the Meigs operation gained more and more popularity, the "vaginalist" surgeons devised new policies, combining the Leveuf and Taussig extraperitoneal systematic pelvic lymphadenectomy and Schauta's operation. Navratil was the first to do this, but he never reported his data. He operated on his patients in two stages, performing the VRH first and the extraperitoneal lymphadenectomy about 3 weeks later. Mitra[37] slightly modified the Navratil policy. He operated in one stage instead of two and took advantage of the extraperitoneal abdominal incision for adding to the lymphadenectomy the preparation of the VRH (i.e., division of the infundibulopelvic ligaments, uterine arteries, and paracervical ligaments). This operation, described in a 1960 monograph, is called Mitra's operation. It was imitated by other surgeons, including Inguilla[27] and Von Bouwdijck Bastiaanse.[61] The data afforded by Mitra and followers demonstrate that the effectiveness of the combined "extraperitoneal systematic pelvic lymphadenectomy-Schauta operation" equaled that of the Meigs operation, even in patients with stage II disease.

Arriving at this point of the history, one can say that the debate between Wertheim and Schauta was over at last. The Schauta operation modified by Amreich and Stoeckel and combined with a systematic pelvic lymphadenectomy is not different from the modern Meigs variant of the Wertheim operation as far as the chances of cure are concerned. The choice between the two operations seems a question of training and circumstances. This is a pity because Mitra's operation surely better fits certain patients, especially those who are poor surgical risks. The operating room time is longer, and there are more scars (three instead of one). However, Mitra's operation is less traumatic and the postoperative complications are fewer. The technical changes introduced to the genuine Schauta operation have improved its radicality without impairing its advantage of lessened danger.

Mitra's operation did not lose all of its supporters in the contemporary era. The Indian gynecologists (Chowdury[9]) remain faithful to an operation that fits their population op-

portunely. Some gynecologists working in developed countries use it as well either routinely or for selected patients and either in its original manner or with some modifications. The Amsterdam school[30] systematically uses the variant described by Sindram[57] in 1959 as AVRUEL (abdominal and vaginal radical uterus extirpation and lymphadenectomy). The abdominal part is performed through a midline laparotomy, and the vaginal part starts with a bilateral Schuchardt incision. Although the aim is to lessen the radicality, there is no lessening of the danger. Imparato et al.[26] perform the abdominal part using the extraperitoneal approach and open the peritoneum at the very last moment, just before moving to the vaginal part. Delgado et al.[17] use a similar strategy, which lessens the danger. Massi[33] uses a technique that is very close to Mitra's but modulates the length of the abdominal extraperitoneal incision and the radicality of the vaginal operation, depending on the characteristics of the tumor. Massi, as do the other gynecologists mentioned, reserves the indications for Mitra's operation to patients who are poor surgical risks.

THE LAPAROSCOPICALLY ASSISTED VAGINAL RADICAL HYSTERECTOMY

At the time the new era of laparoscopic surgery began, Mitra's operation in my experience was carried out in one of three patients.[12] It was reserved for old, obese, and disabled patients and those who were poor surgical risks. In my series collected between 1972 and 1989, I operated on 807 patients with uterine cancer using the Wertheim operation in 531 patients and the Schauta operation in 276 patients. In the Schauta series there were twice as many patients who were older than 70, who weighed more than 80 kg, and who had hypertension. The patients who had experienced thromboembolic disease after delivery or previous operations constituted 7.6% versus 3.0% in the Wertheim series. Despite these differences, the rate of postoperative complications was not different in the two series except that the rate of thromboembolic complications was more than twice as high in the lower-risk Wertheim series: 4.3% versus 1.4%. As a consequence the number of casualties was lower in the high-risk series, the Schauta one: 0.3% versus 0.9%. On the other hand, the cure rates in the patients with stage I and stage II cervical cancer were the same in the two series.

Although it appeared to be an appropriate solution in the management of selected patients, Mitra's operation was not the solution of choice in my opinion. The infectious risk seems to be higher in my series (the standard infectious morbidity was not increased, but the only death was from sepsis as a consequence of pelvic cellulitis caused by a contamination of the extraperitoneal space by *Bacteroides fragilis*). Operating in two stages lessens the risk, but it makes the treatment more complex. In addition, leaving three scars instead of one is not really satisfying from the psychological viewpoint. For all of these reasons, I was in search of a more "patient friendly" solution to avoid the bilateral abdominal incisions. Assessing the pelvic lymph nodes without laparotomy or simple or double extraperitoneal abdominal incisions was possible using the Carlens mediastinoscope or instruments derived from it. Bartel in 1969 was the first to do it.[3] He called the new tool retroperitoneoscopy. Some surgeons followed him,[22,67] and in 1986, I decided to try using this technique in management of cervical cancer. Having neither the instrument nor training in its use, I used the laparoscope instead of the mediastinoscope and bilateral inguinal microincisions, following a technique that was a mixture of the retroperitoneoscopy (digital preparation of the retroperitoneal space) and open laparoscopy (CO_2 insufflation through the sheath of the laparoscope). The lymph nodes could be "palpated," inspected, and punctured. The first experience, on December 15, 1986, was demonstrative enough for treating a patient using VRH (she was afflicted by a IB1 adenocarcinoma of the cervix, and the lymph nodes appeared normal; she is still alive and well more than 10 years after the surgery). This experience suggested to me that it was possible to perform a true lymphadenectomy using a laparoscope instead of a simple endoscopic lymph nodal sampling or assessment.

After my first laparoscopic assessment of the pelvic lymph nodes I developed with Jacques Salvat a technique of laparoscopic preperitoneal assessment of the pelvis that we named retroperitoneal panoramic pelviscopy (PRPP). We described this technique in a monograph published in 1989.[15] The operation was performed through a suprapubic midline minilaparotomy (Fig. 66-1). The preperitoneal space was prepared with the forefinger moving along the iliopubic bone. Then the laparoscopic trocar was introduced, and the opened dry space was insufflated with CO_2. The CO_2 insufflation was made through the sheath of the trocar whose external surface was covered with a rubber drain, making a more efficient pneumostasis, which was further enhanced by a continuous suture made on the edge of the cutaneous incision. From this moment the surgery proceeded under direct endoscopic guidance. The two lateral pelvic walls were assessed consecutively, the surgeons staying on the opposite side and working with two instruments introduced through

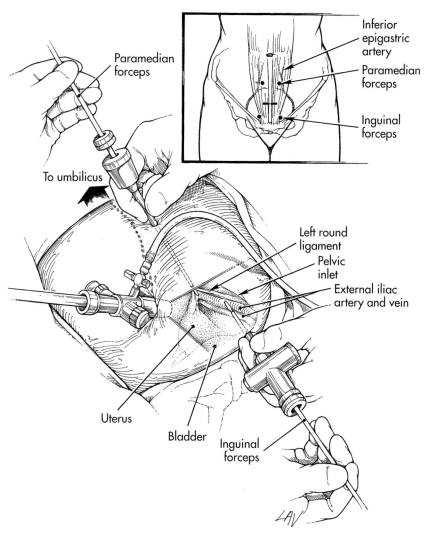

Fig. 66-1 The panoramic retroperitoneal pelviscopy for assessment of the pelvic lymph nodes.

two ports opened lateral to the midline (ipsilateral to the pelvic wall to assess). The two instruments were used first to free up the pelvic wall and then to clean the iliac vessels from the lymph node–bearing tissues by which they are surrounded. A complete description of this technique can be found in our chapter in the first edition of this book. Fig. 66-2 demonstrates the quality of the job that can be done: at the end of the procedure we completely remove the adventitia from the iliac vessels.

The aim of PRPP and videoendoscopic pelvic lymphadenectomy was to avoid Mitra's bilateral abdominal incisions before making the VRH. Long before the data arrived (which later confirmed the value of the laparoscopic dissection[16]), it was clear after the simple inspection of the operative field at the end of the procedure that the result of such a dissection could be trusted. Starting with this observation we saw the indications for the combined procedure differently. Mitra's operation, because of its above-mentioned drawbacks, was reserved for selected patients. On the opposite, the "new Mitra's operation" (which means the combination of laparoscopic lymphadenectomy and Schauta operation) could be applied as the first-choice solution in the management of cervical cancer. In this way the answer to the question we asked as the title of the first communication we proffered about the topic "A new future for Schauta's operation through presurgical retroperitoneal pelviscopy?[11]" was yes!

In the years after our first communication, the concept of laparoscopic lymphadenectomy grew in many ways. First, Querleu[43] devised and described a transumbilical transperitoneal technique. This technique rapidly became a large success because it was much more simple for the gynecologist using this way with which he or she was familiar than with the preperitoneal technique which seemed to be quite odd. Shortly afterwards the field of laparoscopic lymphadenectomy was extended to the aortic area. Querleu,[45] Childers,[8] and Nezhat[39] described the technique at almost the same time. A wavering was observed concerning the use of the new tool during the first years. Querleu used the laparoscopic

lymphadenectomy for selecting patients with positive lymph nodes, who were referred to the radiotherapist, whereas the others were operated on through laparotomy. Because the latter patients were much more numerous (85% in stage IB1), the costs were higher than the benefits. In that context attempts to perform radical hysterectomy using the laparoscopic tool appeared logical. Canis[6] in 1990 was the first to do it. This pioneer was quickly followed by other gynecologists[55,58] who progressively developed the laparoscopic radical hysterectomy (LRH). Today this technique appears to be more time-consuming, more hazardous, and less radical than the Schauta operation combined with laparoscopic lymphadenectomy. As a consequence, a growing number of gynecologists* currently have moved to the laparoscopically assisted radical vaginal hysterectomy (LAVRH).

My own experience with the techniques and strategies has increased significantly during the past decade. I still use the preperitoneal approach for performing the lymphadenectomy (a transumbilical transperitoneal approach is used only in patients bearing a scar from previous laparotomy), but I do it starting from an infraumbilical incision. This modification became possible with the availability of new laparoscopic trocars whose tip is both cutting and transparent (Optiview7 Ethicon, Visiport7 USSC), a characteristic that makes direct entry into the preperitoneal space possible through a 10-mm cutaneous incision without digital preparation. Another instrumental advancement led us to modify the strategy. When Endostaplers became available I started using them for performing an operation, which was both simpler and more radical at the same time. This operation, named the coelio-Schauta,[13] is described elsewhere.[14] It is very similar to the operation devised by Kadar at about the same time[29]: division of the uterine arteries and paracervical ligaments at their contact with the pelvic wall, using Endostaplers introduced through the ipsilateral iliac ports after the lymphadenectomy had been carried out, and the paravesical and pararectal spaces were opened. This operation is not described here because it is no longer used because of the high rate of bladder dysfunction we had observed: even higher than after the classical Amreich procedure. It now appears that the Amreich procedure is clearly too radical for tumors less than 2 cm in diameter (Stoeckel's procedure is enough), and it can be replaced, for the tumor more than 2 cm in diameter, by an operation I have devised jointly with Querleu that we named laparoscopic vaginal radical hysterectomy (LVRH) for the role of the laparoscopy is as important as the role of the vaginal approach in the tailorization of radicality. This is the operation described in the following section.

LAPAROSCOPIC VAGINAL RADICAL HYSTERECTOMY

The LVRH is a variant of the LAVRH. It differs from the other variants of the operation in two ways. The preference given to the extraperitoneal approach in the performance of

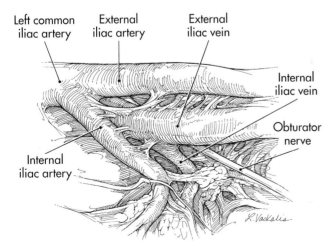

Fig. 66-2 View of the left sidewall of the pelvis after pelvic lymphadenectomy performed using PRPP.

Left common iliac artery
External iliac artery
External iliac vein
Internal iliac vein
Obturator nerve
Internal iliac artery

*References 5, 23, 44, 46, 49, 50, 53.

the laparoscopic part of the operation is only a detail. I mention it only as testimony about the relationship between the new Mitra's operation and the original one, but recognizing that the laparoscopic step of the LVRH can be performed using the transumbilical intraperitoneal approach as well. Anyway, it is the solution I adopted for patients with an abdominal scar. Both approaches enable one to perform the pelvic lymphadenectomy with the same accuracy. They also enable management of the paracervical ligaments and the uterine arteries in the same way. In fact, the main differentiation of our method is in the way we manage these structures more than in the way we approach them.

The most important goal of the extended hysterectomy is removing the lymphatic structures located around the uterus as completely as possible. Those structures, lymphatic channels, lymphatic clusters, and lymph nodes of various size are borne by the celluloadipose tissue surrounding the vessels and nerves that constitute the skeleton of the paracervical ligaments (and to a lesser degree the sacrouterine ligaments as well). Using giant sections, Girardi[20] demonstrated that lymph nodes located in the paracervical ligaments are present in 78% of patients. Their localization is ubiquitous, and all of them can be involved by the cancer. Over the decades the challenge was to divide the ligaments closer to the pelvic wall, the most radical way being to cut the vessels one after the other at the level of their origin. Using this technique one definitely obtains a larger operative specimen, but a higher rate of bladder dysfunction as well![47]

The surgical anatomy of the paracervical ligaments is quite different in its median and lateral parts. In the median part the venous network is rich and complex: plexoid. In the lateral part it becomes more and more simple as one arrives closer to the pelvic wall. Separating the lymph node–bearing tissues from the vessels is absolutely impossible in the median part, but it is perfectly possible in the lateral part. Such a job could probably be done through laparotomy but is much easier to do it through laparoscopy thanks to the magnification provided by the endoscopic tool. That is a rationale for our LVRH, which combines microsurgical dissection of the lateral part of the paracervix (cardinal ligament) performed during the laparoscopic step and a division of it made halfway during the vaginal step of the operation. Such management of the paracervical ligament provides the same radicality as the most radical Wertheim or Schauta operation without leading to the same vesical consequences, for the bladder's nerve supply is respected as well as its vascular supply.

TECHNIQUE OF THE LVRH

The LVRH starts with a laparoscopic operation, which can be accomplished through either the transumbilical transperitoneal approach or the infraumbilical preperitoneal one. Because the transumbilical transperitoneal pelvic and aortic lymphadenectomies are described elsewhere in this book (see Chapter 38), I describe here the preperitoneal procedure, which is my technique of first choice. All details of the

Schauta-Stoeckel technique concerning the vaginal part of the operation, which was only mentioned in the preceding pages, are described here.

The Laparoscopic Part

The laparoscopic part of the LVRH is performed after having put the patient in the frog-leg or ski position. The surgeon stays on the left side of the patient. The first assistant stays in front of the surgeon and the second assistant stays between the legs of the patient. The nurse stays at the left of the surgeon. The video monitor is placed at the right of the first assistant (if possible a second video monitor is placed in the background, between the surgeon and the nurse: it enables the first assistant to easily follow the operation). The instrumentation (Figs. 66-3 and 66-4) is now precisely settled. I mentioned my preference for the two forceps designed by Manhes (Micro-France Fab): the crocodile forceps and the cobra forceps are used as the primary working instruments (scissors, bipolar coagulation instrumentation, washing and aspiration tool, and staplers are used as well but much less often). The Lyonnese coelioextractor (Lépine Fab) is very useful as well: it works as "a sugar forceps" operated through an unpalpable handle and is used for the delivery of the prepared lymph node–bearing tissues.

The Infraumbilical Preperitoneal Approach

The cutaneous incision is performed along the inferior brim of the umbilicus and is just large enough to admit the tip of the Visiport (USSC Fab) (Fig. 66-5). This trocar has been

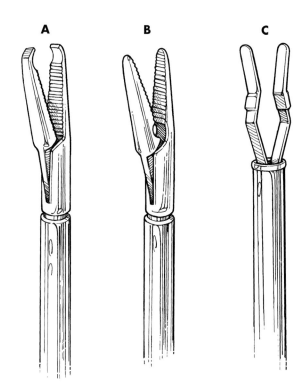

Fig. 66-3 The Mahnes forceps. **A,** Cobra forceps (grasping forceps). **B,** Atraumatic hemostatic forceps (dissecting forceps). **C,** Bipolar coagulation forceps.

devised to watch the progress through the successive layers of the abdominal wall as it is penetrated. The laparoscope is introduced in the trocar itself and the video camera is focused on the blade. One identifies the subcutaneous fat, then aponeurosis, then the muscular bundles on each side of the aponeurotic incision, and finally, the fascia parietalis at which level one stops handling the trigger, which operates the cutting part (the blade) of the trocar. At this time the whole instrument can be pushed vertically since the tip of it makes contact with the pubic bone.

The trocar is moved away once this pubic contact is obtained. The CO_2 insufflation tube is linked to the sheath of the laparoscopic trocar, and one starts insufflating the blindly created tunnel. The video camera is focused on infinity. The laparoscope is reintroduced in the tunnel, which is enlarged slightly by little lateral movements. Finally, a fine-needle puncture is performed in the midline 3 to 4 cm above the pubis. Being sure one is in the appropriate space, a 10- to 12-mm trocar is introduced, taking care not to injure the fascia parietalis, which constitutes the posterior aspect of the tunnel. This trocar enables one to introduce a scissors

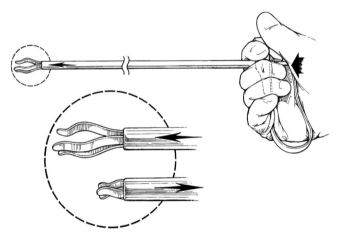

Fig. 66-4   Lyonese "coelioextractor."

with which the preparation of the preperitoneal space will be carried out under direct visual surveillance.

The development of the preperitoneal space is first made on the right side. Cooper's ligament is the first landmark to identify. Once this ligament is seen, one proceeds directly to the external iliac vessels, then proceeds to the inferior epigastric ones, which are their upward collaterals. One has to proceed laterally backward to the origin of the inferior epigastric vessels. The detachment of the fascia parietalis has to be started at the lowest level (starting too high could lead to working in front of the vessels, into the space located between them and the abdominal wall, with a risk of tearing the collaterals). As soon as the epigastric vessels are crossed one meets the round ligament at the level it enters the inguinal canal. The ligament is crossed frontally. One proceeds laterally at the contact of the posterior surface of the abdominal wall. A new port can be opened in the McBurney area at the time one reaches the junction between the aponeurotic and muscular parts of the transverse muscle.

The port (10- to 12-mm trocar) opened in the McBurney area enables one to introduce a second instrument into the operative field. Using this instrument and the scissors, one more easily develops the preperitoneal space to the left of the midline (an operation that is more difficult for the right-handed surgeon to perform). The third port is opened symmetric to the McBurney port. Before opening the door, the surgeon must not hesitate to watch on both sides of the abdominal wall, putting the tip of the endoscopic instrument at the selected point and watching and palpating it on the cutaneous aspect and not forgetting to make a fine-needle assay before using the endoscopic trocar. An injury made by the fine needle does not need to be repaired, which is *not* the case with an injury made by a 10- to 12-mm trocar! The three ancillary ports being opened, the surgeon widens the operative field while cutting the two round ligaments in their preperitoneal part. Making them free for roughly 2 cm is necessary (and detaching them from the external iliac arteries), but they should be cut using only the monopolar electrocautery.

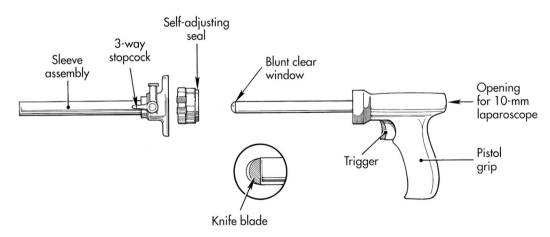

Fig. 66-5   The Visiport system (USSC Fab) used for the laparoscopic transumbilical preperitoneal pelvic lymphadenectomy.

To gain space and have an unobstructed view onto the most dorsal part of the pelvic wall, it is mandatory to detach the natural adhesions that bind the fascia parietalis to the abdominal wall at the level of the line joining the two iliac spines (arcade of Douglas). To make this possible I recommend use of the laparoscope through one of the lateral ancillary ports and use the two other ones for the instruments, the surgeon moving from the laparoscopic position for pelvic surgery to the laparoscopic position for upper abdominal surgery (he or she stays between the legs of the patient). The adhesiveness of the tissues that one has to divide is very strong. The risk is injuring the fascia parietalis and opening the peritoneum. To avoid this embarrassing complication, one has to cut at the direct contact of the muscular bundles. Once this job is completed on both sides, the surgeon returns to the pelvic surgery position with the laparoscope introduced through the infraumbilical port to get a panoramic view into the pelvic cavity. The preliminary preparations take longer using the transumbilical preperitoneal approach but one gains time afterwards by encountering no difficulties with the gut and enjoying a better "pneumatic" hemostasis.

The Lymphadenectomy

As far as the lymphadenectomy itself is concerned I refer the reader to Chapters 37 and 38 devoted to this topic. I will stress only two points. The first relates to the extent of the dissection. In my conception this dissection has to be limited to the so-called interiliac lymph nodes, which means to the obturator and hypogastric lymph nodes of the classical nomenclature. In fact, the lymphatic spread of uterine cervical cancer follows a regular pathway in most patients. If the interiliac lymph nodes are not involved, the risk of metastatic involvement elsewhere is less than 2%.[4] Therefore I recommend removing only the interiliac nodes. This removal has to be limited but at the same time be very thorough: at the end of the dissection the adventitia covering the bifurcation of the common iliac artery and the convergence of the external iliac vein and internal iliac vein(s) has to be removed completely. This job can be done easily using the simplest technique: a so-called crocodile forceps attracts the lymph node–bearing tissues and the so-called cobra forceps tears the fine filaments that join them to the surrounding structures. No laser, Cavitron, nor electrocautery is needed. A good knowledge of the surgical anatomy is essential because if one works in the good spaces no preventive hemostasis is needed. That is the second point I wanted to make about the lymphadenectomy.

Preparation of the VRH

The preparation of the VRH is the second aim of the laparoscopic part of the operation. This preparation is made while opening the two lateropelvic so-called dry spaces (paravesical and pararectal) and then managing the paracervical ligaments that lie between.

Opening the paravesical space is the natural continuation of the pelvic lymphadenectomy. In fact, at the time one pushes the obliterated umbilical artery (continuation of the superior vesical artery) medially to free the medial surface of the external iliac vessels one pushes the lateral aspect of the bladder, on which the artery is dependent, at the same time, and opens the paravesical space. Once the so-called superficial obturator lymph nodes have been removed and the obturator vessels and nerves demonstrated, the surgeon has to push the preparation deeper to join the bottom of the space (i.e., the levator ani muscle insertion onto the arcus tendineus pelvici [linea alba pelvici]). Doing this is not difficult. The surgeon just has to be careful not to injure the vessels going transversally from the pelvic wall to the vagina and the urethra and vice versa. These vessels are arranged in a plane whose obliquity is more than that of the instruments with which one works. As far as the pararectal space is concerned, the surgeon opens it while pushing the lateral aspect of the rectum medially. This step must be started beneath the point where the uterine artery crosses the ureter. The ureter generally has already been found at the very beginning of the operation at the time one detaches the peritoneum from the dorsolateral part of the pelvis: it is adherent to the peritoneum. One can follow it (while letting it remain attached to the peritoneum) from back to front to find its crossing by the uterine artery. Conversely, one can follow the superior vesical artery from front to back to arrive at the same point. In any event it is just lateral and dorsal to the crossing that one has to push the peritoneum medially to enter the pararectal space. This space is more restricted than the paravesical space because of the projection on the fifth lumbar vertebra, but the axis one works along is less dangerous and one arrives quickly at its bottom (i.e., the ventral aspect of the last sacral vertebra).

The paracervical ligament is managed by the same technique used for the pelvic lymphadenectomy. The lymph node–bearing tissues are grasped and detached using two forceps. The only difference is that the structures to which the lymph nodes are attached are the vessels forming the skeleton of the paracervical ligament. The surgeon has to be very careful while freeing these vessels, mostly veins, whose walls are thin and fragile. At the end of the procedure the collaterals of the internal iliac artery and veins must be completely cleared (Fig. 66-6): uterine, vaginal, and vesicourethral vessels in the same time as obturator vessels, which are often dependent from the same common trunks. The other "parietal vessels" (psoaic and gluteal vessels) have to be cleared as well at the same time as the dorsal part of the obturator nerve and sacrolumbar nerve (Fig. 66-7). Finally, the hypogastric nervous plexus must be demonstrated crossing the lateral aspect of the rectum at the bottom of the pararectal space (Fig. 66-8). The demonstration of all these anatomic structures provides proof that the dissection is complete, but the vessels and nerves are preserved and their functions as well.

Cutting the uterine artery (Fig. 66-9) at its origin is the last step of the laparoscopic preparation for VRH. I favor the use of staples and "cold" scissors. Two details must be stressed. First, finding the origin of the artery deserves special attention if a preperitoneal approach is used: the origin

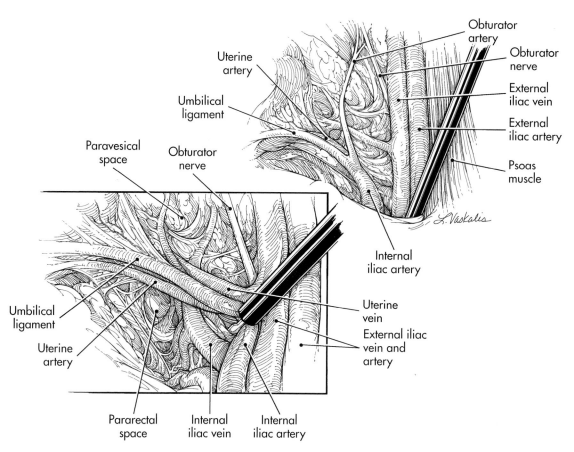

Fig. 66-6 Views of the right sidewall of the pelvis after complete pelvic and paracervical lymphadenectomies performed using the preperitoneal approach (the umbilical ligament goes dorsalward due to the development of the preperitoneal space). The paravesical and pararectal spaces are widely opened. The visceral and parietal collaterals of the internal iliac artery and vein are seen.

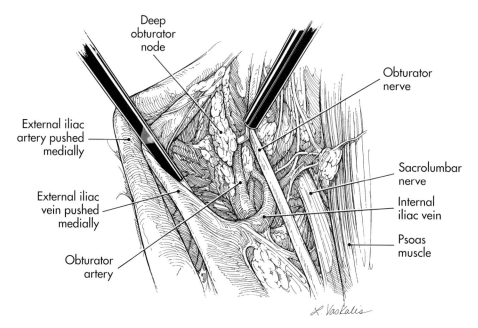

Fig. 66-7 The external iliac artery and vein are pushed medially *(left)*. The obturator and lumbosacral nerves are visible. The psoas muscle forms the lateral *(right)* border of the picture.

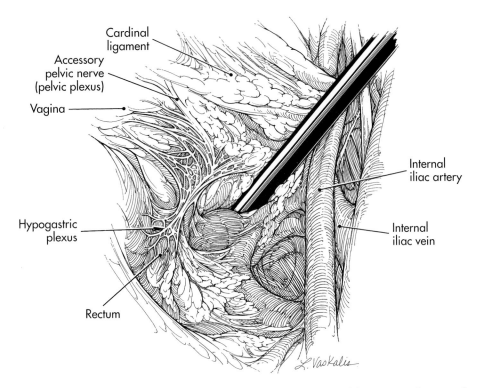

Fig. 66-8   Demonstration of the hypogastric plexus at the bottom of the pararectal space. The collaterals the plexus sends to the lateral aspect of the rectum then to the lateral aspect of the vagina are visible. The nervus accessorius going further ventrally (up) is visible as well.

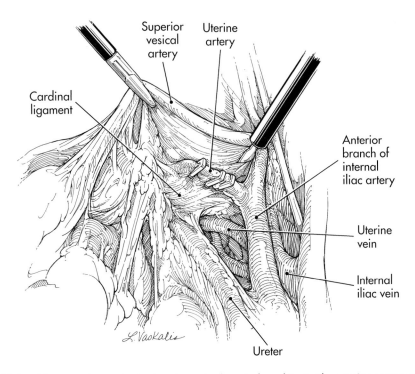

Fig. 66-9   The superior vesical artery is pushed ventralward (up). The uterine artery crosses the ureter transversely. Three clips have been put on the artery. This artery will be cut between the two lateral clips and the medial one. A uterine vein is visible, which crosses the ureter caudally.

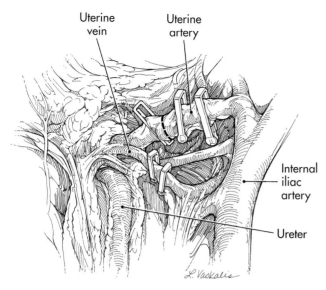

Fig. 66-10 If a uterine vein crosses the ureter cranially, it has to be secured and cut in the same time as the uterine artery during the laparoscopic part of the laparoscopic vaginal radical hysterectomy.

of the uterine artery is hidden by the superior vesical artery whose pathway is inverted because the bladder has been detached from the abdominal wall. Second, the uterine artery can be accompanied by a second artery or a so-called superficial uterine vein (Fig. 66-10), which crosses the ureter as the main artery does. Those vessels have to be cut as the main vessel (the uterine artery) and the so-called deroofing of the ureter has to be initiated, which will be achieved later (during the vaginal step of the procedure).

The Vaginal Part

The vaginal part of the operation is performed with the patient in the classical lithotomy position. The surgeon is sitting in front of the operative field, and the two assistants are standing at either side. All three operators are placed between the legs of the patient. The nurse is standing back and to the surgeon's right. The instrumentation includes a complete set of Breisky retractors. The Chrobak (Krobach) forceps are mandatory. The other instruments are the ones used in simple vaginal surgery to which we add the O'Schaugnessy right-angle dissector and the Roger's clamps. No Schuchardt incision is needed for the vaginal part of this operation. The operation includes three main steps, of which making the vaginal cuff is the first.

Making the Vaginal Cuff

The separation of the vaginal cuff is made at roughly the level of the junction of the upper and middle thirds of the vagina. A series of Kocher forceps is put onto the vaginal wall at the chosen level. The first four forceps are put onto the anterior wall, the most lateral of them being inserted lateral to the two extremities of the base of the Pawlik triangle. The last four forceps are put onto the posterior wall symmetric to the first ones. Traction is exerted onto the forceps, creating a sort of internal vaginal prolapse or intussuscep-

tion. The incision is made on the superficial surface of this iatrogenic prolapse.

Dividing the vagina is done after the leading point of the prolapse has been infiltrated using saline to which synthetic vasopressin has been added (if no contraindications). The aim of this infiltration is to provide preventive hemostasis. It also helps separate the two sheaths of the folds that one creates while pulling on the forceps. Therefore the infiltration has to be performed just in the center of each of the folds. The vagina is then incised just above the tip of the pulling forceps. The anterior aspect is managed first. The three layers of the vaginal wall have to be divided, opening into the vesicovaginal space, while taking care to not injure the inferior pole of the bladder which lies beneath and which is displaced in the vaginal fold on which one is pulling. The posterior aspect is then managed the same way, opening into the rectovaginal space (with a lesser risk; the rectum is relatively far). Only the skin is cut at the level of the lateral aspects to maintain the relationship between the vaginal cuff and the paracervical ligaments whose extensions are attached to the deep layers of the vaginal fornices.

Managing the Ventral Aspect of the Specimen

Managing the ventral aspect of the specimen to be developed is the most delicate part of the operation. As explained before, the bladder floor and the terminal part of the two ureters follow the vaginal cuff at the time it is separated and pulled downward. To free the ventral aspect of the vagina and the cervix at the same time as the two paracervical (cardinal) ligaments that continue lateral to them, it is necessary to divide the connections that bind the bladder floor and ureters to them: the supravaginal septum and bladder pillars. This is harder to do in Stoeckel's operation than in Amreich's because one does not have the large opening of the paravaginal incision. In the LVRH, the laparoscopic preparation (opening of the paravesical and pararectal spaces and division of the uterine arteries) makes the surgery easier.

Opening the supravaginal septum is done while pulling the vaginal cuff downward as it is grasped by the Chrobak forceps. At the same time the upper vaginal flap is pulled upward with a forceps put onto the midline. The opening is made on the midline close to the base of the triangular pseudoaponeurotic structure, which artificially appears, thanks to the divergent traction. It is made with the scissors whose handle is held vertically. As soon as the pseudoaponeurotic fascia (the "supravaginal fascia") is opened and the underlying soft reticular tissue seen, the scissors handle can be lowered to a more horizontal position. Then a tunnel can be established by dissection beneath the inferior pole of the bladder and by passing the level of the vesicouterine peritoneal fold, which I recommend not be opened yet.

The next portion of the ventral part of the Stoeckel's-like operation is opening the paravesical spaces. One starts on the left side while placing two forceps, one at 1 o'clock and the other at 3 o'clock, on the margin of the upper vaginal flap. One of the assistants applies countertraction to these forceps. A little depression appears close to the forceps at 3 o'clock. Here is the entry to the left paravesical space, which one opens with the tip of the Metzenbaum scissors by pushing laterally and ventrally. The scissor blades are introduced in the closed position and removed in the outspread position. The smallest of the Breisky retractors is introduced. The structure lying between it and the previously opened vesicovaginal space is the left bladder pillar. The ureter can be identified by palpating the pillar against the Breisky speculum by putting a finger in the vesicovaginal space. The bladder pillar is managed while the two parts are separated. To succeed, the anatomic structure has to be presented in the correct way. The specimen is pulled downward by one of the assistants. The second assistant pulls onto the forceps at the 1-o'clock position and pushes the small Breisky retractor laterally. This way the bladder pillar appears to be vertical. An incision with the scissors is made in the middle of the inferior margin of the pillar. This first aperture cannot be made too close to the bladder (risk of bleeding and/or bladder injury), nor too close to the vagina (risk of opening a wrong, intrafascial, path). Although the aperture cannot be too ventral and too dorsal, it must not be made too medial nor too lateral, but precisely in the middle of the inferior margin of the pillar. Once this aperture is made, the closed scissors are pushed ventrolateral into the depths of the pillar in such a way that the lateral part of the pillar is separated from the pillar itself. After having palpated the pillar against the instrument to be sure the ureter stays medial to it, one removes the instrument and divides the fibers halfway. The laterovesical space becomes wider. A larger retractor can be placed and the knee of the ureter becomes visible or foreseeable. At this time the medial fibers of the pillar can be divided after appropriate traction has been exerted on it (a Breisky retractor placed in the vesicovaginal space substitutes for the forceps at the 1-o'clock position).

Finding and managing the uterine artery is the next step in this part of the operation. Having pushed the terminal part of the ureter and the adjoining part of the bladder backward, the surgeon identifies the arch of the uterine artery whose descending branch arrives in the operative field just inside the knee of the ureter. If the arch is not visually identifiable, the place where it lies can be identified by palpation. This place is the "paraithmic window" (i.e., the depression that can be felt lateral to the isthmus of the uterus above the superior brim of the paracervical ligament). The "paraisthmic window" being located, the surgeon half blindly takes the structures lying in the lateral part of it, using a forceps and a right-angle dissector (O'Schaugnessy). When the descending branch of the arch is isolated, gentle traction is exerted on it and the vessel suddenly appears in the operative field. Its extremity shows the clip put on during the laparoscopic preparation before the artery was divided. The same is done on the other side. Then one can move to the dorsal and lateral preparation of the specimen.

Managing the Dorsal and Lateral Aspects of the Specimen

Managing the dorsal and lateral aspects of the specimen starts with reversal of direction of the traction exerted onto the vaginal cuff. As the vaginal cuff is drawn upward, the lower vaginal flap is pulled downward and the pouch of Douglas is dissected free and then opened. Once the peritoneal cavity has been opened and an adequate retractor placed, the retrouterine ligaments or rectal pillars are cut halfway (not too close to the rectum). This division can be made without prior clamping (no bleeding), if the surgeon does not cut too close to the rectum. This leads directly to the medial part of the pararectal space (on the dorsal aspect of the paracervical ligament whose upper brim can be located by palpation through the paraisthmic window). When the paraisthmic window is located, the O'Schaugnessy forceps is applied to it and the traction exerted onto the Chrobak forceps is inverted: the tip of the right-angle dissector, guided by a finger put on the ventral aspect of the ligament, goes through the window. Then the dissector is opened, and the superior brim of the paracervical ligament becomes free.

The last step of the operation is freeing the inferior brim of the paracervical ligament and then dividing the ligament at the appropriate level. For freeing the inferior margin of the ligament one deepens the shallow incision made on the lateral part of the vagina at the beginning of the operation. After this deepening has been carried out, the lateral flap is pushed backward about 2 cm. At this time the ligament is freed on its two aspects, ventral and dorsal, and on its two margins, superior and inferior. Two clamps can be placed after having pushed the knee of the ureter backward and displaced the rectum using appropriate retractors. The lateral clamp is placed after traction has been exerted onto the medial clamp. In this way, a larger paracervical removal can be achieved. However, the second clamp must not be placed too far laterally, lest its tip endanger the knee of the ureter, requiring one to be vigilant while tightening the instrument. After division of the ligament and control of its lateral stump, the same is done on the other side, and the specimen can be extracted while the last ties are cut (i.e., the dorsal sheets of the broad ligaments). One must be mindful of the ureters, which are adherent to them, and must never divide the ligaments without having formally identified the ureters. Afterward the remainder of the operation is routine. I need not describe the routine division of the infundibulopelvic ligaments, the peritonization, the hemostasis, and finally, the circular pursestring suture one places on the vagina to close it but not close it totally. Neither drain nor gauze is put in the vagina. A Foley catheter is inserted for 6 days.

INDICATIONS FOR LVRH

As stated in the beginning of this chapter, VRH is performed for tumors contained within the cervix, which means tumors that are known to be cured by so-called wide local excision. One can hope that with forthcoming technological improvements, this prediction will soon be 100% accurate. At the moment we rely on two markers: tumor volume and the state of the lymph nodes. Selection based on these two criteria is not 100% accurate, but one arrives close to this goal: if the tumor diameter is less than 4 cm and the lymph nodes are negative the rate of failure is no more than 10% after surgery only. Now MRI enables us to assess the tumor volume with great accuracy[18] and even more the so-called cervix coefficient. On the other hand, laparoscopic assessment is accepted today as an accurate tool for evaluating the lymph nodes. Thus the indication for VRH is defined by using MRI as the first selection tool and then performing laparoscopy, which is used both for selecting patients and at the same time for preparing the VRH.

One Stage or Two?

Earlier in my experience with the laparoscopic-assisted vaginal radical hysterectomy I operated on patients in two stages. It was impossible at that time in my institution to obtain frozen sections of the numerous lymph nodes one removed during the pelvic lymphadenectomy. After frozen sections became available, I changed to a one-stage procedure, which obviously shortens the hospital stay with all the advantages linked to this shortening. However, I soon renounced this course because of the high rate of false-negative results! The literature shows that this rate is on average 7% to 27.5%,[25] which is not acceptable. Therefore I returned to the two-stage procedure.

In addition to its greater safety, the two-stage procedure appears to be definitely better from the psychological viewpoint. In fact, it is a source of great psychological stress to a patient to have the rest of the operation canceled because of findings during the surgery. It is much better to first make the assessment on which the indication for hysterectomy depends, to then discuss the indication with the patient, and finally to operate. Before the laparoscopic era such a protocol was not conceivable, but today it is. If we want to take full advantage of the laparoscopic tool, we must operate in two stages even if it is economically less advantageous.

The only real problems with the two-stage procedure are the management of uterine arteries and the interval between the two stages. Dividing the uterine arteries at the end of the laparoscopic operation in the LVRH technique induces a uterine hypoxia, which can reduce the tumoral sensitivity to radiation if this therapy has to be finally chosen. This problem seems to me to be more theoretical than practical. Nevertheless, I recommend canceling the division of the uterine arteries if the lymph nodes appear positive or suspicious on endoscopic examination. In cases where Schauta operation is finally chosen, experience has taught us that 7 to 14 days is the most appropriate interval between the two stages: the paravesical and pararectal spaces are not yet obliterated and the pelvic cellular tissue is still edematous and soft.

Conservation of Uterine Body, Tubes, and Ovaries in Young Women: Radical Trachelectomy

The basic concept of LVRH is that "wide local excision is enough for contained tumors." The correctness of this concept is largely confirmed by the data collected about early cervical cancer treated only by surgery (either abdominal or vaginal). If the division of the surrounding tissues is made on the vaginal and paracervical verges at an interval of roughly 2 cm, the cure rate is the same as that obtained with more extended operations and/or radiotherapy. This concept being accepted, the question can be asked, "Why remove the uterine body, tubes, and ovaries if the cranial pole of the tumor is more than 2 cm beneath the isthmus?" The Romanian gynecologist Aburel[1] was the first to answer this question while proposing an operation that can be named "radical trachelectomy" for young women desiring to preserve their capacity for childbearing. This operation was performed through laparotomy.

The operation I recommend to achieve this goal is performed using the laparoscopic vaginal approach. The laparoscopic part of the operation is performed using the LVRH technique except that the uterine arteries are not cut. The uterine arteries are preserved as well during the vaginal part of the operation. Only the collaterals going to the cervix and the vagina are cut after the paracervical ligaments have been divided. The uterus is then divided just underneath the isthmus. A prophylactic cerclage is put onto the isthmus and an isthmovaginal anastomosis is performed. Thanks to great precision in the performance of the anastomosis and to the absence of peritoneal adhesion, the laparoscopic vaginal approach allows the patient to become pregnant and deliver, which never occurred after the genuine Aburel operation.

As far as radicality is concerned, the radical trachelectomy seems to be an adequate operation. The rate of pelvic recurrences does not seem to be increased. However, the rules of safety have to be strictly respected. The preoperative workup includes MRI and colposcopy: this therapy should only be used for tumors growing exophytically onto the superficial aspect of the cervix. Frozen sections have to be requested during the operation, and the patient must be aware that a classical operation will be performed if doubt exists about the tumor-free margins of the specimen. The postoperative anatomic and laboratory assessment of the specimen could lead to a second opportunity for "totalization."

Postoperative Management

The postoperative management after LVRH is theoretically easy to define. Because the operation is restricted to "contained" tumors, no adjuvant therapy is needed. However, false-negative results can occur at each step of the procedure, and assessment of the embedded specimen can afford surprises. It is imperative that this assessment be done using the technique of semiserial giant sections. The best way to do it is the technique used at Munich's First University Clinic of OBGYN.

It is not rare that an unsuspected extrauterine involvement is detected in the paracervical ligaments and/or in the vagina. The direct infiltration is unusual in the paracervical ligament, but tumor deposit can be found at some distance from the tumor in the lymphatic channels and/or lymph nodes. The same is true for the vaginal cuff. In patients who show evidence of such involvement, adjuvant radiotherapy is recommended (radiotherapy combined with brachytherapy). It is unclear whether such adjuvant therapy improves the chances of survival, but it does lessen the risk of pelvic and vaginal recurrences. Being aware of these facts, some patients choose only the follow-up policy, especially if a radical trachelectomy has been performed.

Whatever the choice of postoperative management it seems appropriate to assess the aortic lymph nodes in the patients with unexpected extrauterine spread of the tumor. This assessment can be done by laparoscopy. During this laparoscopy the ovaries and tubes can be transposed to a higher iliac position, especially if radiotherapy is scheduled for young patients whom one had chosen to treat while preserving their ovarian function.

REFERENCES

1. Aburel E: Colpohisterectomia largita subfundica (1956). Cited in Sirbu P, editor: *Chirurgia Ginecologica—Tehnica si tactica operatorie*, vol II, Bucharest, 1981, Editura Medicala.
2. Barclay DL, Roman-Lopez JJ: Bladder dysfunction after Schauta hysterectomy, *Am J Obstet Gynecol* 123:519, 1975.
3. Bartel M: Die Retroperitoneoskopie, *Zentralbl Chir* 12:377, 1969.
4. Berman ML, et al: Survival and pattern of recurrence in cervical cancer metastatic to the periaortic lymph nodes (a Gynecologic Oncology Group Study), *Gynecol Oncol* 19:8, 1984.
5. Bojahr B, et al: Erste Erfahrungen und Ergebnisse mit der gaslosen laparoskopischen pelvinen, Lymphnodektomie in Kombination mit der vaginalen radikalen hysterektomie nach, Schauta beim Zervix Karzinom Stadium IB, *Zentralbl Gynäkol* 119:493, 1997.
6. Canis M, et al: La chirurgie endoscopique a-t-elle une place dans la chirurgie radicale du cancer du col utérin? *J Gynecol Obstet Biol Repr* 19:221, 1990.
7. Carenza L, Nobili F, Lukic A: The Schauta Amreich radical vaginal hysterectomy. In Nichols D, editor: *Gynecologic and obstetric surgery*, St Louis, 1993, Mosby.
8. Childers JM, et al: Laparoscopic para-aortic lymphadenectomy in gynecologic malignancy, *Obstet Gynecol* 82:741, 1993.
9. Chowdury: Personal communication, 1996.
10. Clark JG: A more radical method for performing hysterectomy for cancer of the uterus, *Bull Johns Hopkins Hosp* 6:120, 1985.
11. Dargent D: A new future for Schauta's operation through the pre-surgical retroperitoneal pelviscopy, *Eur J Gynecol Oncol* 8:292, 1987.
12. Dargent D, Kouakou F, Aadeleine P: L'opération de Schauta 90 ans après, *Lyon Chir* 8:45, 1987.
13. Dargent D, Mathevet P: Hystérectomie élargie laparoscopico-vaginale, *J Gynecol Obstet Biol Repr* 21:709, 1992,
14. Dargent D, Mathevet P: Radical vaginal hysterectomy in the primary treatment of invasive cervical cancer. In Rubin S, Hoskins W, editors: *Cervical cancer and preinvasive neoplasia*, Philadelphia, 1996, Lippincott-Raven.
15. Dargent D, Salvat J: *Envahissement ganglionnaire pelvien: place de la pelviscopie retropéritonéale*, Paris, 1989, Medsi McGraw-Hill.
16. Dargent D, et al: L'association "lymphadénectomie coelioscopique-opération de Schauta" dans le traitement des cancers invasifs du col utérin, *J OB/GYN* 5:353, 1993.
17. Delgado G, Potkul RK, Dolan JR: Retroperitoneal radical hysterectomy, *Gynecol Oncol* 56:197, 1995.
18. Ebner F: Magnetic resonance imaging. In Burghardt E, editor, *Cervical cancer in surgical gynecologic oncology*, New York, 1993, G Thieme.
19. Freund WA: Zu meiner Methode der Total Uterus Exstirpation, *Zentralbl Gynäkol* 2:265, 1878.
20. Girardi F, et al: The importance of parametrial lymph nodes in the treatment of cervical cancer, *Gynecol Oncol* 34:206, 1989.
21. Hache M: De l'hystérectomie vaginale pour cancer, *Rev Sci Méd* 29:724, 1887.
22. Hald T, Rasmussen F: Extraperitoneal pelviscopy, a new aid in staging of lower urinary tract tumors: a preliminary report, *J Urol* 124:245, 1980.
23. Hatch KD, Nour M, Hallum AV: New surgical approaches to treatment of cervical cancer, *J Natl Cancer Inst Monogr* 21:71, 1996.
24. Hegar A, Kaltenback: *Die operative Gynaekologie*, ed 3, 1886.
25. Hermansen DK: Frozen section lymph node analysis in pelvic lymphadenectomy for prostate cancer, *J Urol* 139:1073, 1988.
26. Imparato E, et al: La linfoadenectomia extraperitoneale secondo Mitra come intervento complementare nella operazione di Schauta Amreich et nella vulvectomia radicale: In *Atti del convegno di chirurgia vaginale del guigno, 1983 a Porto Cervo*, Sassari, 1983, Gallizzi.
27. Ingiulla W: Il metodo vaginale di Amreich nel trattamento chirurgico del cancro del collo uterino, *Riv Ostet Ginecol* 7:49, 1952.
28. Ingiulla W: Five year results of 327 Schauta Amreich operations for cervical cancer, *Am J Obstet Gynecol* 96:188, 1966.
29. Kadar N, Reich H: Laparoscopically assisted radical Schauta hysterectomy and bilateral laparoscopic pelvic lymphadenectomy for the treatment of bulky stage IB carcinoma of the cervix, *Gynecol Endosc* 2:135, 1993.
30. Ketting BW, Bleker OP: Surgical treatment of cervical cancer by the AVRUEL procedure. In Heintz APM, Griffiths CTh, Trimbos JB, editors: *Surgery in gynecological oncology*, Boston. 1984, Martinus Nijhoff.
31. Leveuf J: L'envahissement des ganglions lymphatiques dans le cancer du col de l'utérus, *Bull Mem Soc Natl Chir* 57:662, 1931.
32. Maneo A, et al: Radical hysterectomy in cervical cancer stage IB-IIA: a randomized study. In Benedetti Panici P, editor: *Wertheim's radical hysterectomy*, Rome, 1996, Societa Editrice Universo.
33. Massi GB: La linfoadenectomia extraperitoneale nell'approcio chirurgico vaginale alle neoplasie uterine, *Riv Ostet Ginecol* 8:51, 1995.
34. Massi G, Savino L, Susini T: Schauta Amreich vaginal hysterectomy and Wertheim Meigs abdominal hysterectomy in the treatment of cervical cancer: a retrospective analysis, *Am J Obstet Gynecol* 3:928, 1993.
35. McCall ML: A modern evaluation of the radical vaginal operation for carcinoma of the cervix, *Am J Obstet Gynecol*, 85:295, 1963.
36. Meigs JV: Wertheim operation for carcinoma of the cervix, *Am J Obstet Gynecol* 49:542, 1945.
37. Mitra S: The treatment of cervix cancer by radical vaginal operation, *Arch Gynaekol* 179:166, 1951.
38. Navratil E: Indications and results of the Schauta Amreich operation with and without postoperative roentgen treatment in epidermoid carcinoma of the cervix of the uterus, *Am J Obstet Gynecol* 146:141, 1963.
39. Nezhat CR, et al: Laparoscopic radical hysterectomy with para-aortic and pelvic node dissection, *Am J Obstet Gynecol* 166:864, 1992.
40. Omr H: Fortschritte bei der Verhutung und Bekampfung urologischer, Komplikationen des Zervix Karzinoms, *Zentralbl Gyneakol* 100:1320, 1978.
41. Pawlik A: Uber exstirpation der ganzen Gebärmutter sammt Theilen des Beckenbidegewebes, *Zentralbl Gynäkol* 1:22, 1889.
42. Peham H, Amreich J: *Operative gynecology*, Philadelphia, 1834, JB Lippincott (translated by LK Ferguson).
43. Querleu D: Laparoscopic pelvic lymphadenectomy in the staging of early carcinoma in the cervix, *Am J Obstet Gynecol* 164:579, 1991.
44. Querleu D: Laparoscopically-assisted vaginal hysterectomy, *Gynecol Oncol* 51:248, 1993.
45. Querleu D: Laparoscopic para-aortic lymphadenectomy: a preliminary experience, *Gynecol Oncol* 68:90, 1993.
46. Raatz D: Laparoscopic assisted vaginal radical operation: 4th Congress of the European Society for Gynecological Endoscopy. In Donnez J, Brossens I, editors: *The uterus throughout the woman's life*, Bologna, 1997, Monduzzi.
47. Ralph G, et al: Funktionelle Störungen des unteren Harntraktes nach der abdominalen und vaginalen Radikaloperation des Zervixkrebses, *Geburtshilfe Frauenheilkd* 47:551, 1987.

48. Recamier JCA: *Recherche sur le traitement du cancer,* Paris, 1829, Gabon.

49. Roy M, et al: Vaginal radical hysterectomy versus abdominal radical hysterectomy in the treatment of early stage cervical cancer, *Gynecol Oncol* 62:336, 1996.

50. Sardi J, DiPaola G: Personal communication, 1997.

51. Schauta F: *Die erweite vaginale Totalextirpation des Uterus bei Kollumkarzinome,* Vienna-Leipzig, 1908, J Safar.

52. Scheele R: Die Behandhungsergebnisse bösartiger Geschwülste der Jahre, 1944 bis 1955, *Geburtshilfe Frauenheilkd* 21:854, 1961.

53. Schneider A, et al: Laparoscopy-assisted radical vaginal hysterectomy modified according to Schauta-Stoeckel, *Obstet Gynecol* 6:1057, 1996.

54. Schuchardt K: Eine neue Methode der Gerbärmutter extirpation, *Zentralbl Chir* 20:1211, 1893.

55. Sedlacek TV, et al: Laparoscopic radical hysterectomy: a feasibility study, *Gynecol Oncol* 56:126, 1995 (abstract).

56. Seski JC, Dioknu AC: Bladder dysfunction after radical abdominal hysterectomy, *Am J Obstet Gynecol* 128:43, 1977.

57. Sindram IS: A new combined approach in the treatment of cancer of the uterine cervix, *Acta Union Int Contre Cancer* 15:403, 1959.

58. Spirtos NM, et al: Laparoscopic radical hysterectomy (type III) with aortic and pelvic lymphadenectomy, *Am J Obstet Gynecol* 6:1763, 1996.

59. Stark G: Zum operativen Therapie des collum carcinoms stadium IB, *Geburtshilfe Frauenheilkd* 47:45, 1987.

60. Stoeckel W: Die vaginale Radikaloperation des Collumkarzinomes, *Zentralbl Gynäkol* 52:39, 1928.

61. Taussig FJ: Iliac lymphadenectomy for group II cancer of the cervix, *Am J Obstet Gynecol* 15:733, 1943.

62. Van Bouwdijck Bastiaanse MA: Voorlopige medelingen over de behandeling va, jet cervixcarcinome met radium, operatie en röntgenbestraling, *Ned Tijdschr Geneeskd* 31:22, 1952.

63. Van Bouwdijk Bastiaanse MA: Treatment of cancer of the cervix uteri, *Am J Obstet Gynecol* 72:100, 1956.

64. Wertheim E: Bericht über die mit der erweiterten Uteruskrebsoperation zu erwartenden Dauerheilungen, *Weiner Klin Wochensclovift* 42:1128, 1904.

65. Wertheim E: *Die erweite abdominale Operation bei Carnino ma Colli uteri,* Berlin, 1911, Urban und Schwarzenberg.

66. Wingo PA, et al: The mortality risk associated with hysterectomy, *Am J Obstet Gynecol* 164:579, 1992.

67. Wurtz A, et al: Bilan anatomique des adénopathies retropéritonéales par endoscopie chirurgicale, *Ann Chir* 41:258, 1987.

67 Therapeutic and Endoscopic Perspectives

LEILA V. ADAMYAN

The elaboration of principally new methods of surgical intervention and the improvement of traditional techniques characterize the modem period of operative gynecology. A number of advances in the fields of polymeric chemistry and physics during the twentieth century have contributed to these developments in operative gynecology. Together, these developments have widened significantly the possibilities for surgical intervention in cases of varying cause and severity, even making surgical treatment effective in some patients in whom it had previously been considered inappropriate.

Among the most promising developments are (1) the use of biologic glues, such as fibrin glue; (2) the embolization of internal iliac arteries; (3) the use of preserved dura mater; (4) the use of laparoscopy in the treatment of, for example, congenital disorders, endometriosis, and postoperative rehabilitation; and (5) colpopoiesis (formation of a new vagina) in patients with both vaginal and uterine aplasia.

BIOLOGIC GLUES

Despite the use of modem suturing instruments (e.g., electrical and laser devices) in reconstructive surgery, patients often develop adhesions and other complications postoperatively, partly because traditional methods of suturing wound edges may deform tissues, disturb the microcirculation, and cause local ischemia as a result of tension along the suture lines. Infections along puncture routes and local tissue reactions to suture materials may result in excessive adhesion formation and may lead to subsequent malfunction of the involved organ. Surgeons in many different countries have been seeking some means of nonsuture anastomosis and wound sealing that does not have such disadvantages.

Biologic glues may be used not only in reconstructive operations on the genital organs (e.g., reconstruction of the uterine tubes) but also for hemostasis (i.e., in the place of hermetic sutures) in patients with a high risk of hemorrhage or with abnormalities of coagulation. The medical glues used in gynecologic surgery are cyanoacrylate, sulfacrylate, and fibrin sealants. For the last 30 years, the use of cyanoacrylate sealants has been widespread in different fields of surgery all over the world. These sealants have a number of disadvantages, however. For example, they resolve slowly, and toxic decomposition products may have an adverse effect on tissue regeneration. Studies conducted to find ways to resolve these problems led to the development of biocompatible biologic glue.

The sealing and hemostatic properties of fibrinogen have attracted physicians' attention for several centuries; the use of blood preparations with such properties dates back to the end of the eighteenth century. In 1909, Bergel[5] reported the use of fibrin as a protective and curative preparation, and in 1915 to 1916, Grey[10] and Harvey[11] reported using it to control hemorrhage from parenchymatous organs. Since highly purified blood plasma factors became commercially available, the problems of the use of blood products have been extensively studied in Western Europe, the United States, and the former Soviet Union.

Fibrin glue is a two-component sealant. The primary component is human fibrinogen produced by cryoprecipitation or lyophilization; this component contains factor XIII dissolved in aprotinin. The second component is an application solution that contains lyophilized thrombin and calcium salts.

Mechanism of Fibrin Glue Action

In the end phase of the biologic process of blood coagulation, fibrinogen becomes unstable fibrin, which is then stabilized by the action of factor XII in the presence of calcium ions. Aprotinin prevents the lysis of the fibrin, resulting in the formation of a fibrin clot. The mechanism of fibrin glue action is similar. After the application of fibrin glue, numerous fibrin fibers attach themselves to the wound edges, sealing the edges and controlling diffuse bleeding from small vessels. The network of fibers provides sufficient tension strength and acts as a framework for the ingrowing fibroblasts from which connective tissue is formed, thus ensuring firm adherence of the wound edges.

In their experimental work, Hedelin et al.[12] implanted both Teflon cylinders that were empty and Teflon cylinders that were filled with 0.5% to 1% fibrin clots in the backs of rats. Microscopic and histologic examinations 1, 2, and 4 weeks after the implantation showed that all the cylinders were completely filled with granulation tissue. As early as 2 weeks after the implantation, however, granulation tissue with growing capillary buds had begun to replace the fibrin clots.

Applications of Fibrin Glue

Used as separate components, fibrin glues are sometimes applied with the help of the Duploject double syringe, which consists of a holder for two disposable syringes of equal volume operated simultaneously by pistons; in this case, volumes of the two components are mixed in the joining piece of the syringe clip. The fibrin glue components can also be applied in succession. When bleeding is diffuse, fibrin glue may be applied using a spray.

Surgeons in European countries such as Austria, Germany, Italy, and Great Britain generally use different modifications of commercial fibrin glue (e.g., Tissucol, Tissel, Beriplast, Sony-I, Sony-2), but those in the United States usually prefer fibrin glue made of fresh-frozen plasma obtained from a single donor or from the patient. Russian surgeons sometimes use fibrin glues that are commercially produced by the Tissucol and Beriplast companies, but may use a homemade fibrin glue.

Fibrin glue is appropriate for use in reconstructive operations on uterine tubes for infertility[2,3] in wedge-shaped resection of ovaries, myomectomy, and metroplasty; in procedures to achieve hemostasis in the parametrium; in excisions for retrocervical endometriosis; and in a one-stage operation of colpopoiesis in which pelvic peritoneum is used.

Fibrin glue has been used successfully to treat premature rupture of the amniotic sac in the second trimester of pregnancy.[4,7-9,13,14] Fibrin glue injected into the cervical canal 3 to 4 cm above the internal cervical os and introduced from several syringes, in combination with tocolytic and antibiotic therapy, was effective for sealing the amniotic sac. Electron microscopy had shown that after the sac has been sealed, amniotic membrane regeneration was promoted at the site of the defect. Baumgarten believed that fibrin sealing of the amniotic membranes, although safely attempted at an earlier stage of gestation, was most successful after week 32. Fibrin glue has been shown to be advantageous for control of diffuse capillary bleeding when no specific bleeding source can be identified.[15] It has been used to close a small vesicovaginal fistula after the epithelial lining had been removed by a sharp curette.[16] Some authors believed that fibrin formed a scaffolding for migratory fibrinoblasts and promoted the ingrowth of capillaries.[6,12] The article by Adamyan et al.[1] reviewing the literature concerning the use of fibrin glue in obstetrics and gynecology is followed by an extensive and comprehensive bibliography.

Reconstructive Surgery on Uterine Tubes. Fibrin glue may be used for implantation of uterine tubes into the uterus, isthmus-isthmus anastomosis, ampulla-ampulla anastomosis, and fimbrioplasty. In all these procedures, surgeons may use fibrin glue either to unite tissues without sutures or to stabilize suture lines.

In the implantation of tubes into the uterus after the primary procedures of the operation, fibrin glue can join the serous coat of the uterine tube and the serous coat of the uterus. In a tubal anastomosis that involves a silicon stent, the surgeon may use fibrin glue for a sutureless anastomosis of the tubes or in a combined technique of suture strengthening and tubal anastomosis. In fimbrioplasty, fibrin glue completely replaces suture materials.

Fibrin gluing for a tubal anastomosis requires the following:

- Thrombin, two ampules, 800 units each
- Calcium chloride solution, 5.0 ml (40 mmol/L)

- Fibrinogen, 1 ampule (0.7 g of coagulating protein)
- Water for injection, 10 ml
- Two disposable syringes
- Four disposable needles

Each of the two ampules of thrombin is dissolved in 1.5 ml of calcium chloride. To ensure the complete dissolution of the thrombin, it is necessary to shake the ampules well. Then 0.7 g of lyophilized fibrinogen is dissolved in 10 ml of water for injection. Before the solution is made, the ampule must be shaken well to separate the powder from the wall; when the water has been added, the mixture should be shaken again. The components are applied to the tissue surface in the following sequence: thrombin, fibrinogen, thrombin, fibrinogen.

When the patient is under general anesthesia, the surgeon brings both uterine tubes out through the anterior abdominal wall incision and dissects them in the area of the occlusions. Then, to approximate the cut edges of the uterine horns, the surgeon inserts polyvinyl chloride plastic (PM-1/92) stents that are 1.33 to 2 mm in diameter and 22 cm in length. For a sutureless anastomosis, the surgeon places fibrin glue in the gap between the uterine tubes and presses the cut margins closely together for 2 to 3 minutes. Another application of fibrin glue over the serous coat increases the strength of the anastomosis. If a combined method is appropriate, two sutures, one in the area of attachment of the mesosalpinx and the other on the opposite side, may be placed, but not tied, before the first application of fibrin glue; the sutures are tied before the second application of fibrin glue.

Clinical data on more than 700 operations completed with the use of fibrin glue and more than 450 microsurgical procedures performed on the uterine tubes of infertile women indicate that this new biologic adhesive is a promising tool for gynecologic surgeons. Fibrin glue has been found to have several advantages, perhaps because it is made of natural blood components. It is absorbed within 10 to 15 days after the operation, never causes foreign body tissue reaction, and stimulates wound healing. In addition, fibrin glue reduces the number of postoperative adhesions, decreases the operating time required, and as shown by the pregnancy rate among women who have undergone procedures in which fibrin glue was used, effectively maintains the anatomic patency and functional activity of the uterine tubes. Fibrin glue also contributes to hemostasis, controlling capillary oozing and making it possible to use fewer sutures. The clinical applications of fibrin glue for sutureless tissue connection are not widespread, however, because of the high cost of the commercial preparations.

Ovarian Surgical Procedures. In resection or biopsy of the ovaries, the surgeon may use fibrin glue to achieve hemostasis or to seal the layer of the resected ovaries. The operative technique is rather simple in laparotomy. It is more difficult in laparoscopy because the glue components undergo polymerization very rapidly and the application of fibrin glue through a laparoscope requires a long syringe and a large amount of glue. In the future, hemostasis by means of fibrin glue may become more important in laparoscopy because surgeon-endoscopists are likely to be performing more and more procedures that require hemostasis in areas where the placement of sutures risks coagulation difficulties.

Myomectomy and Metroplasty. During myomectomy and metroplasty, fibrin glue is useful for uniting the uterine serous coat without sutures, strengthening the suture lines, maintaining hemostasis, and creating a single suture-glue complex on the surface of the uterus. In most patients, postoperative adhesions that lead to disorders of the female reproductive system complicate surgery for uterine myomata. These adhesions may be associated with ischemia of the uterine tissue caused by multiple sutures. A well-performed anastomosis with fibrin glue may prevent or reduce the number of serous sutures and thus eliminate ischemia. Furthermore, the application of additional fibrin glue on the uterine suture reduces the possibility of adhesion formation, provided polymerization has occurred.

The use of fibrin glue after the excision of the retrocervical endometrium or the rectouterine hollow enables a surgeon to stop bleeding without the use of dangerous sutures in the parametrium and the rectovaginal septum.

EMBOLIZATION OF INTERNAL ILIAC ARTERIES

The commonly used hemostatic techniques (e.g., ligation, electrocoagulation, excision of bleeding tissues, or even removal of the whole organ) involve an external approach to vessels. In the practice of medicine, however, situations sometimes arise in which the usual methods of hemostasis either are impossible or require difficult procedures that risk the life of the patient. A new approach to hemostasis in surgery—intravascular blockade of a bleeding vessel by means of artificial emboli made of hydrogel—is reducing the risks of surgery for patients in these situations.

In obstetrics and gynecology, embolization is indicated in patients with pelvic angiodysplasia and angioma in combination with any genital pathologic condition that requires operative intervention, such as the following:

- Uterine and adnexal tumors
- Congenital abnormalities
- Genital fistulas
- Large extraperitoneal tumors
- Pregnancy and labor associated with pronounced disorders of the pelvic vascular system
- Varicosity of pelvic veins
- Profuse coagulopathic postpartum uterine hemorrhage in association with disseminated intravascular coagulation syndrome caused by blood diseases (e.g., Werlhof's disease, von Willebrand's disease)

Although extraperitoneal tumors make up only 0.03% to 0.3% of all growths, extraperitoneal tumors and pelvic hemangiomas are of particular concern, especially in women of reproductive age. The presence of these pathologic processes near the internal genitals, bladder and urinary canals, rectosigmoid part of the intestine, and iliac arteries (at the level or after their bifurcation) presents a high risk for hemorrhage both intraoperatively and postoperatively and was once considered a contraindication for pregnancy and labor. Embolization of the internal iliac arteries decreases this risk.

The search for optimal occlusive materials has accompanied the resolution of the clinical problems that have arisen in the development of this technique. The main requirement is "medical cleanliness," the absence of low molecular weight additives that can have a negative effect on the patient. In addition, the material should be biocompatible; it should cause minimal inflammatory reaction and must cause no general toxic, carcinogenic, or allergic disturbances. Finally, it should be highly resistant to the influence of body substances.

Emboli made of hydrogel (poly-2-hydroxyethylmetankrilat), created in collaboration with coworkers of the Vishnevsky Institute of Surgery, the Institute of Macromolecular Chemistry, and the Institute of the Chemical Physics attached to the Russian Academy of Medical Science, appear to be the most promising. As a rule, the emboli are in the form of small balls that are 0.05 to 1.5 mm in diameter or cylinders that are 0.5 to 4 mm in diameter and vary in length. They have a spongelike structure; the pores make up approximately 50% to 60% of the volume and may be altered in form and diameter.

Mechanism of Embolic Action

When introduced into a vessel, an embolus swells and blocks the vessel. Despite the pressure that it exerts on the vessel walls, the swollen embolus does not irritate or damage them. It induces hypercoagulation as early as the first day after its implantation into the vessel bed. The trigger factor for the hypercoagulation in the first hours after embolization appears to be the aggregation of thrombocytes, followed by the activation of other factors. Thrombus-forming factors are activated even in patients who have severe hypercoagulation disorders and whose hemorrhage may be life-threatening. With a reduction in anticoagulation parameters, hypercoagulation may last as long as 3 days; coagulation then decreases and becomes normal 10 to 15 days after embolization.

Simultaneously with hypercoagulation, blood proteins are absorbed along the surface of the embolus, strengthening the process of local thrombus formation. Later, connective tissue penetrates the pores of the embolus, making repatency of the vessel impossible and preventing hemorrhage.

Therapeutic Embolization Procedures

Patients with angiodysplasias and extraperitoneal tumors need angiography to determine the peculiarities of vascularization of the tumor, as well as the diameter and topography of the vessels. The location of the tumor and its proximity to other organs and tissues determine the appropriate route of surgical access: laparotomy line, vaginal access, or combined abdominovaginogenital access. The new generation of roentgenocontrast emboli has facilitated the medical procedure because their movement is easier to monitor and control than was that of emboli used in the past. In addition, roentgenocontrast emboli with silver iodide are bactericidal, thus eliminating the risk of local tissue infection around them.

There are two methods of embolization: closed selective and open intraoperative. The two methods do not compete with each other and are sometimes used in the treatment of a single patient. The indication determines the method used.

Closed selective embolization is performed in a special operating room equipped with an electronic optical transformer that has a television device. In the first step of the procedure after the administration of local anesthesia, the surgeon inserts a catheter into the femoral artery. The surgeon then uses angiography to determine the character of the disorder, identify the site of bleeding, and control the position of the catheter in the vessel space. After introducing the emboli into the catheter lumen, the surgeon pushes them into the vessel until occlusion is complete. In general, 3 to 5 ml of saline and 30 to 40 emboli are required for one embolization. Control angiography follows the procedure so that the surgeon can determine precisely the locations and effect of the emboli.

In open intraoperative embolization, which is useful for patients with angiodysplasias of the pelvis and extraperitoneal tumors, the surgeon introduces the emboli through a special syringe inserted into the great vessel exposed during the operative procedure.

Effectiveness of Embolization

Nine patients with pelvic hemangiomas who underwent embolization of the internal iliac arteries up to their third or fourth branches for prophylaxis of hemorrhage in the period from 1 to 5 years before pregnancy were able to deliver infants successfully, although cesarean delivery was indicated. There was a significant decrease in the amount of hemangiomic tissue in the uterus, permitting preservation of the uterus in six patients; extravaginal extirpation of the uterus was necessary in only three patients. None of the patients experienced hemorrhage in the postoperative period.

Similarly, preliminary embolization, arteriography, and endovascular occlusion of the branches of the internal iliac artery with the help of hydrogelic emboli in four patients with extraperitoneal tumors permitted operative treatment for the tumors with minimum hemorrhage. Observations indicate that patients with extraperitoneal pelvic tumors can undergo surgery either in inpatient gynecologic facilities with the assistance of a general or vascular surgeon or in general surgical facilities with the assistance of a gynecologist. When the extraperitoneal tumor is in the small pelvis (and has the form of sand glass) and has encroached on the perineal tissues, two surgical teams should be ready for two operative approaches: abdominovaginal or abdominoperineal.

These studies have proved the effectiveness of preoperative angiography with subsequent endovascular occlusion of major vessels in preventing intraoperative complications. Preoperative embolization of the internal iliac artery on the side affected by an extraperitoneal tumor or angiodysplasia not only ensures minimum hemorrhage but also improves visualization and reduces trauma, which is especially important for surgery of the small pelvis. Embolization of the

internal iliac arteries has also been shown to be extremely effective in arresting massive postnatal hemorrhage (2.5 L) in women with von Willebrand's disease when other methods of coagulation were unsuccessful.

USE OF PRESERVED DURA MATER

In a number of patients, surgical interventions fail to produce the desired results, especially reoperations associated with defects and scars in the tissue. Because the introduction of polymeric materials (e.g., Lavsan and Capron) has not always been successful in reconstructive and plastic operations in patients with uterine myoma and cervicovaginal, urogenital, and intestinovaginal fistulas, preserved tissues from the dura mater are being used to repair defects of the muscular tissue and to strengthen sutures placed during gynecologic operations.

Since World War II, when surgeons first noted that dura mater is an effective barrier capable of preventing infections, neurosurgeons; abdominal, thoracic, cardiac, and vascular surgeons; traumatologists; otolaryngologists; ophthalmologists; and urologists have found transplants of these tissues to be useful in various types of operations. For example, such tissue can be used to repair extensive defects of breast and abdomen, to close hermetically the stumps of bronchi, to recreate the cardiac valve apparatus, to block terminal defects of blood vessels, and to eliminate fistulas and defects of the digestive system.

The dura mater is preserved by freezing, by lyophilization, or by chemical treatment with a mixture of 0.5% to 4% solution of formalin, 96% of glycerol, and 0.5% to 2% of ethylene oxide solution or β-propiolactone to retain its structural and functional features up to the moment of the operation. The many collagenic and elastic fibers that interlace in various directions give the dura mater its mechanical properties of strength, elasticity, and solidness. Because its cellular elements are limited in number, dura mater transplants have rather low immunologic activity and produce no clinical and morphologic signs of transplant rejection or sensitization of a recipient.

My personal experience with 63 patients indicates that dura mater transplants are appropriate for gynecologic reconstructive and plastic operations in patients with pronounced defects and scarring changes (e.g., defects of uterine development, uterine myomata, vaginal operations, uterine prolapse, or prolapse of the vaginal stump).

EARLY POSTOPERATIVE LAPAROSCOPY

The role of laparoscopy in gynecology in the past has been limited primarily to the diagnosis of disease in the internal reproductive organs. During recent years, surgeons have found laparoscopy to be a useful route for surgery and useful in planning a postoperative rehabilitation program, in evaluating reparative regeneration processes after different surgical procedures, and in determining the prognosis for restoration of reproductive function after surgery. All of these aspects are of the utmost importance in modern gynecologic surgery because of the increasing number of reconstructive procedures performed in an effort to establish or restore fertility in sterile women. However, in some myomectomies, repairs of incorrect uterine development, and partial resections of the uterine tubes, the results are still unsatisfactory.

Despite the recent large-scale introductions of microsurgery, areactive sutures, lasers, and different dextrans in various surgical procedures, the incidence of adhesion development after gynecologic surgical procedures remains high. Laparoscopic reinspection by means of traditional techniques long after surgery is less effective and because of dense adhesions can be dangerous. Only an early postoperative laparoscopy can provide the information required to correct any "fresh," reversible deviations that have followed surgery. Even if the surgery has been unsuccessful and the early laparoscopic inspection reveals the reocclusion of the uterine tubes or bowel adhesions, the surgeon can at least inform the patient of the prognosis at an early date.

After completing the initial laparotomy, the surgeon inserts two-channel silicon drainage tubes, 8 and 11 mm in diameter, through the counterapertures in the left and right hypogastric areas and fixes them to the skin of the front abdominal wall with Capron sutures. The inner part of the drainage tubes is 5 cm long; the outer part is 10 to 15 cm long. The outer openings of the tubes are connected to hermetic and sterile devices for draining the wound secretions under negative pressure.

Laparoscopic inspection takes place on the fourth or fifth day after the reconstructive procedure. The surgeon first closes one of the tubes. The other tube, after being shortened and washed both inside and out, serves for the carbon dioxide pneumoperitoneum. As for the usual diagnostic laparoscopy, 1.5 to 2 L of gas is generally enough.

To begin the procedure, the surgeon inserts an optical system through the wide (11 mm) drain and a manipulator through the narrow drain. The surgeon examines the condition of the peritoneum of the small pelvis, the quantity and character of the exudate in the abdomen, and the condition of the tissues on which surgery was performed (e.g., the presence of hyperemia or edema, the status of sutures and adhesions). The patency of the tubes is tested by means of indigo carmine hydrotubation. Fresh adhesions are separated, and hemostasis is achieved with bipolar coagulation of the blood vessels in the area. The abdomen is irrigated with isotonic saline solution, 0.01% chlorhexidine solution, or dextran.

After completing the laparoscopy, the surgeon removes the drains from the peritoneal cavity. There have been no reported complications associated with early postoperative laparoscopy.

COLPOPOIESIS IN VAGINAL AND UTERINE APLASIAS

Over the last century, gynecologic surgeons have tried a variety of methods to create an artificial vagina for patients with vaginal and uterine aplasias, but none has been completely satisfactory. In an effort to develop a simpler, more effective technique, surgeons have devised a one-stage colpopoiesis in which the pelvic peritoneum is used as a reconstructive material.

As in all methods of operative treatment for vaginal aplasia, the most important stage is the creation of the bed for the future vagina, because there is always a danger of wounding the bladder or rectum. The patient is placed on the table in the supine position with the legs wide apart. The patient's pelvis is placed so that the surgeon can manipulate the tissues with a vaginal retractor.

One-Stage Colpopoiesis of Pelvic Peritoneum

After the labia minora are spread wide apart, the surgeon makes a 3- to 4-cm incision in the vaginal orifice along the lower edge of the labia minor between the urethra and the rectum (Fig. 67-1, *A* and *B*). The surgeon dissects not only the epithelial coat, but also 1 to 1.5 cm of the deeper fascia (see Fig. 67-1, *C*). When the fascial plate is open (see Fig. 67-1, *D*), the surgeon inserts two fingers and moves them straight ahead as far as the peritoneum of the small pelvis, dividing the tissues between the bladder and the rectum (see Fig. 67-1, *E*). (In another technique, the surgeon may insert a speculum deeper and deeper to separate these tissues.) The movement of the fingers (or the speculum) from side to side creates a rather wide canal in which the operator will subsequently place the transplant.

In some cases, the surgeon can separate the tissues between the bladder and the rectum rather easily; if the tissue must be dissected near the bladder or the rectum, however, there is a risk that the adjacent organ may be injured. Although this injury is the most commonly occurring complication of the procedure, its incidence is actually very low (approximately 1% in 500 patients). In the event of such an injury, the surgeon sutures the wound and continues the procedure. When pulled down later, the peritoneum will cover a wound in the rectum and facilitate healing. If the bladder is injured, a catheter should remain in the bladder for 5 to 7 days. After an injury to the rectum, the patient should be given antibiotic therapy, placed on a liquid diet, and followed as if she had undergone a rectovaginal fistula repair. The dissection is continued until the pelvic peritoneum has been exposed and incised transversely (see Fig. 67-1, *F*).

The pelvic peritoneum appears as a sagging, thin, pale yellow plate. The most difficult stage of the operation is the identification of the peritoneum. To make it easier, the surgeon may use one of the following procedures:

1. Injection of indigo carmine solution into the bladder so that the bladder mucosa can be identified before it is inadvertently opened.
2. Puncture of the abdominal cavity through the vagina and aspiration of its contents. If the needle is placed into the abdominal cavity, light, amber peritoneal fluid is always seen.
3. Traction on the peritoneum applied with the manipulator of a laparoscope to avoid trauma to the adjacent organs.

The surgeon takes the peritoneum with long forceps, opens it, pulls it down (see Fig. 67-1, *G*), and sutures it to

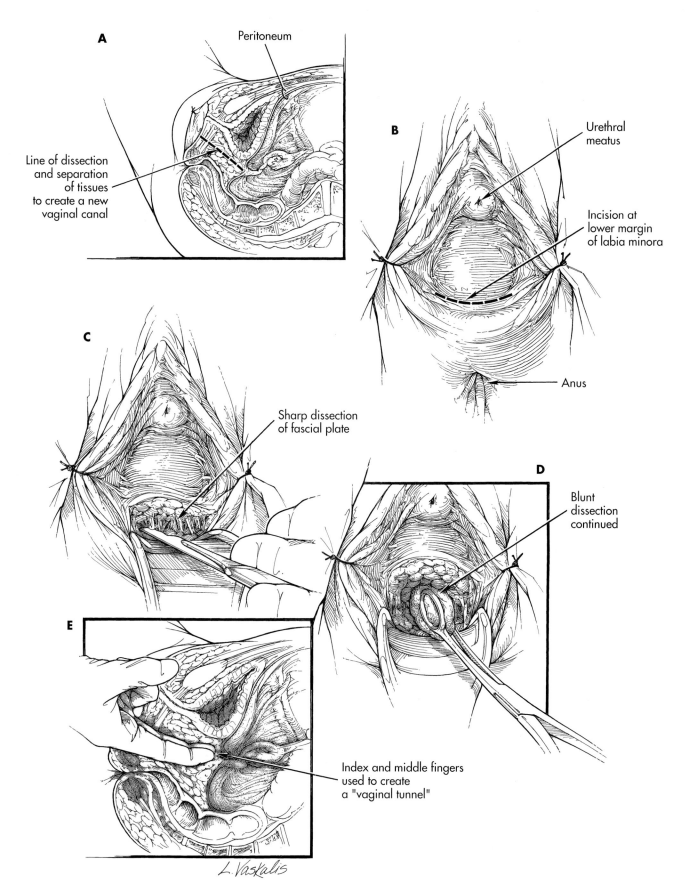

Fig. 67-1 One-stage colpopoiesis using peritoneum to line the new vagina. **A,** Sagittal view of a patient with vaginal agenesis. The pathway of dissection to create a new vagina is shown by the *broken line*. **B,** A transverse incision between the lower edges of the labia minora is made at the site indicated by the *broken line*. **C,** Sharp dissection of the subepithelial fascial plate begins as shown. **D,** It is continued bluntly in a cranial direction. **E,** The tissues between bladder and rectum are divided by dissection using two fingers, palm side up.

Within the figure:

A

Peritoneum

Line of dissection and separation of tissues to create a new vaginal canal

B

Urethral meatus

Incision at lower margin of labia minora

Anus

C

Sharp dissection of fascial plate

D

Blunt dissection continued

E

Index and middle fingers used to create a "vaginal tunnel"

L. Vaskalis

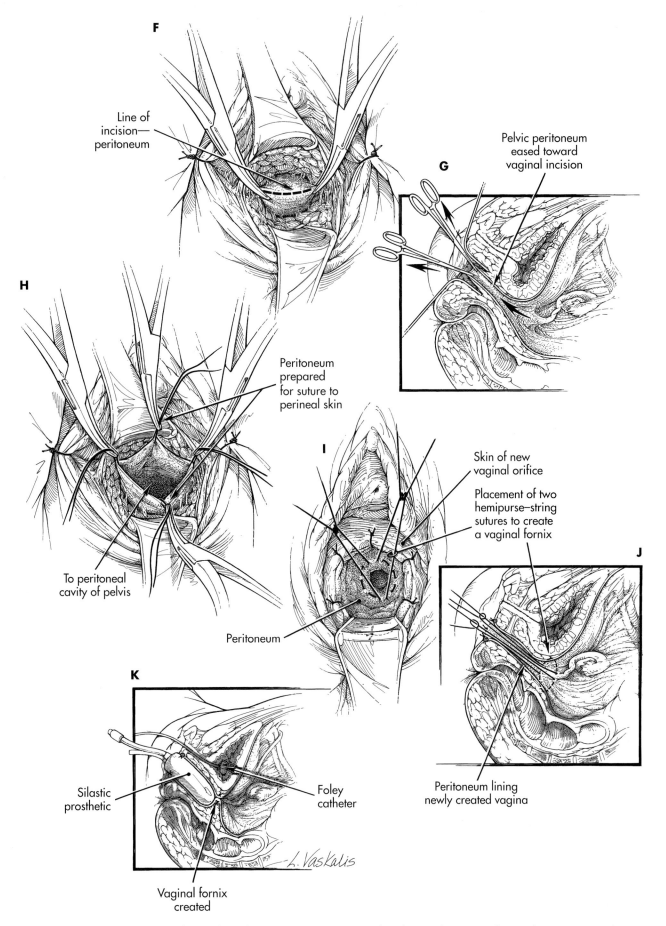

F

Line of incision—peritoneum

G

Pelvic peritoneum eased toward vaginal incision

H

Peritoneum prepared for suture to perineal skin

To peritoneal cavity of pelvis

I

Skin of new vaginal orifice

Placement of two hemipurse–string sutures to create a vaginal fornix

Peritoneum

J

Peritoneum lining newly created vagina

K

Silastic prosthetic

Foley catheter

Vaginal fornix created

—L. Vaskalis

Fig. 67-1, cont'd   **F,** The pelvic peritoneum is exposed and incised transversely. **G,** The circumference of peritoneum is gently drawn into the canal of the neovagina. **H,** The edges of the peritoneum are sewn to the skin of the vaginal orifice. **I,** The peritoneal cavity is closed by two hemipurse-string sutures placed high in the neovagina **J,** Closing of the peritoneal cavity is shown in sagittal drawing. **K,** A Foley catheter is inserted into the bladder, and a silicone prosthesis is inserted into the vagina.

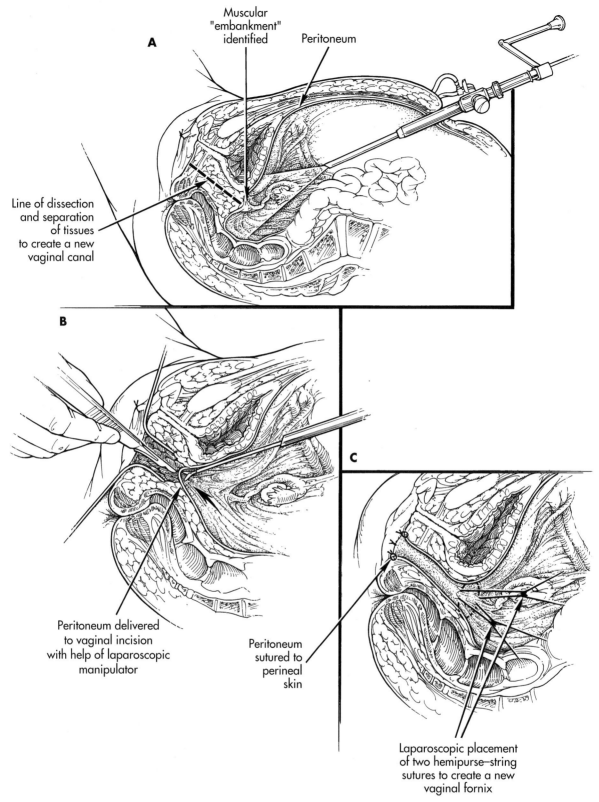

A, Muscular "embankment" identified

Peritoneum

Line of dissection and separation of tissues to create a new vaginal canal

B

C

Peritoneum delivered to vaginal incision with help of laparoscopic manipulator

Peritoneum sutured to perineal skin

Laparoscopic placement of two hemipurse–string sutures to create a new vaginal fornix

Fig. 67-2 Laparoscopy-assisted colpopoiesis. **A,** Laparoscopic examination of the pelvis is performed. The site of transvaginal dissection for creation of a neovagina is shown by the *dashed line.* **B,** Using a laparoscopic probe or manipulator may help deliver the peritoneum to the new tunnel. The peritoneum is opened transversely. **C,** The cut edges of peritoneum are sewn to the skin of the vaginal orifice, and the peritoneal cavity is closed by two hemipurse-string sutures placed through the laparoscope.

the skin in the vaginal orifice (see Fig. 67-1, *H*). Then, using the rudiment of the uterus, the surgeon forms a vaginal fornix from the side of the vagina by placing three or four catgut sutures with a small round needle. If there is no uterine rudiment, the surgeon sutures the peritoneum separately to the bladder walls, rectum, and back wall of the pelvis with separate catgut sutures (see Fig. 67-1, *I* through *K*). If there are any difficulties in forming the vaginal tunnel, the surgeon should also use a laparoscope.

Laparoscopic Colpopoiesis

A laparoscopic examination is helpful to determine the precise abnormality of genital development. In patients with vaginal and uterine aplasia, laparoscopy may reveal a muscular "embankment" positioned in the center of the small pelvis transversely between the bladder and the rectum (Fig. 67-2, *A*). The peritoneum of the small pelvis in this area has ample mobility. Generally, the most mobile part of the peritoneum is approximately 5 to 7 cm behind the muscular embankment.

The surgeon incises the perineum midway between the urethra and anus transversely. In general, the best place for this incision is the lower edge of the labia minora, where they meet the skin of the perineum. Using both blunt and sharp dissection to make a tunnel between the bladder wall and the rectum, the surgeon reaches the small pelvis peritoneum. The surgeon then uses a laparoscopic manipulator to move the peritoneum so that he or she can open it from the vaginal side, dissect it, and pull it to the dissected skin of the vagina (see Fig. 67-2, *B*).

The peritoneum is fixed with separate catgut sutures to the perineal skin around the full circumference, and the vaginal fornix is created from the small pelvis peritoneum that covers the bladder and front wall of the rectum (see Fig. 67-2, *C*). The surgeon can perform the latter reconstructive procedure either from the peritoneal cavity, by using the laparoscope, or from the vaginal side. Separate purse-string sutures of absorbable material (e.g., Dexon, Vicryl) are placed longitudinally 10 to 12 cm from the vaginal orifice. In some cases the surgeon creates the fornix center by connecting the muscular embankment to the bladder peritoneum.

Results of Surgery

A one-stage colpopoiesis with the use of the pelvic peritoneum seldom takes more than 25 to 45 minutes, but it results in a new vagina, which, when lined up with growth of squamous epithelium from the orifice, is physiologically similar to a natural one. It has an acid pH, for example. Furthermore, after epithelialization, the new vagina has the same cyclic changes. Coitus is permissible 10 to 15 days after the surgery.

REFERENCES

1. Adamyan LV, Myinbayev OA, Kulakov VI: Use of fibrin glue in obstetrics and gynecology: a review of the literature, *Int J Fertil* 36:76, 1991.
2. Akuns KB: Nonsuture method of salpingo-salpingoanastomosis using fibrin tube, *Sov Med* 1:82, 1965.
3. Akuns KB: Salpingostomy using fibrin tube, *Akusherstvo Gynecol* 7:71, 1968.
4. Baumgarten K, Moser S: The technique of fibrin adhesion for premature rupture of the membranes during pregnancy, *J Perinat Med* 14:43, 1986.
5. Bergel S: Uber Wirkungen des Fibrins, *Deutsch Med Wochenschr* 35:663, 1909.
6. Bruhn H, et al: Regulation der Fibroblastenproliferation durch Fibrinogen/Fibrin, Fironectin und Faktor XIII. In Schimpf K, editor: *Fibrinogen, fibrin and fibrin glue,* Stuttgart, 1980, FK Schattauer, p 217.
7. Genz HJ: Die Behandlung des vorzeitigen Blasensprungs durch Fi brinklebung, *Med Welt* 30:1557, 1979.
8. Genz HJ, Gerlach H, Metzger H: Behandlung des vorzeitige Blasensprungs durch Fibrinklebung. In Deutscher E, Zechner, editors: *Fibrinolyse, thrombose, hamostase,* Stuttgart, FK Schattauer, p 698.
9. Genz HJ, et al: Antibiotikahaltiger Fibrinkleber zur Behandlung des vorzeitigen Blasensprungs in Perinatale Medizin. In Dudenhausen JW, Saling E, editors: *Perinatale medizine,* band IX, Stuttgart, 1982, Tieme.
10. Grey EC: Fibrin as a hemostatic in cerebral surgery, *Surg Gynecol Obstet* 21:452, 1915.
11. Harvey SC: The use of fibrin paper and forms in surgery, *Boston Med Surg J* 174:6, 1916.
12. Hedelin H, et al: Influence of fibrin clots on development of granulation tissue in preformed cavities, *Surg Gynecol Obstet* 154:521, 1982.
13. Kulakov VI, et al: The use of fibrin glue in gynecological reconstructive plastic operations, *Akusherstvo Gynecol,* 1990.
14. Kurz CS, Huch A: Fibrin sealing: an advanced therapy in dealing with premature rupture of membranes, *J Perinat Med* 10:66, 1982.
15. Moront MG, et al: The use of topical fibrin glue at cannulation sites in neonates, *Surg Gynecol Obstet* 166:358, 1988.
16. Petersson S, et al: Fibrin occlusion of a vesicovaginal fistula, *Lancet* i:933, 1979.

68 Horizons

DANIEL L. CLARKE-PEARSON

In this edition of *Gynecologic, Obstetric, and Related Surgery,* the authors have endeavored to bring to our students, residents, fellows, and surgical colleagues the most up-to-date information in our field of surgery. Looking back to the horizon behind us, we recognize that since the first edition of this text, the field of laparoscopic surgery has expanded tremendously and therefore new chapters have been added to address the current status of laparoscopic surgery in gynecology. New techniques for the management of cervical intraepithelial neoplasia and modified methods for restoring pelvic floor support are also notable additions to the current text.

The horizon ahead of us, I am sure, will bring new techniques and methods of management of gynecologic and obstetric disorders. Although it is difficult to prognosticate the specific changes that we will see in the next decade, there are current issues that I believe will impact the gynecologic and obstetric surgeon in the very near future.

SURGICAL EDUCATION AND TRAINING

The basis for the continued improvement in the surgical care offered to women with gynecologic and obstetric conditions rests on the training of future generations of pelvic surgeons. This education is a lifelong process and clearly begins only at the completion of residency or subspecialty fellowship training. No matter what the future holds for changes in surgical procedures, methods, or equipment, the basics of gynecologic surgery must always be firmly implanted in the surgeon's mind. That education should follow the advice of David Nichols: "Knowing how to perform surgery is important, but knowing when, what, and why to perform it is even more important."[6] Our challenges in the next decade rest on continued excellence in the education of medical students and residents. I am concerned with the current emphasis on primary care in the field of obstetrics and gynecology and with the increasing requirements for nonsurgical educational experiences for our residents. The time a resident spends in the operating room, in the evaluation of preoperative and postoperative care of women with gynecologic conditions, should not be trivialized or diminished. Furthermore, with the decreasing number of major surgical procedures being performed and with an increasing emphasis to avoid expensive surgical procedures, the resident's training experience diminishes further. Given the disparity between the clinical acumen required of a physician delivering the primary care in obstetrics and gynecology versus

the subspecialists performing gynecologic surgery, I believe that we should strongly consider modifications in our residency and certification programs to allow tracking to different types of obstetricians and gynecologists. This will allow excellence in both primary care providers and in the surgical subspecialists. Many others have spoken to this concern over the past decade. For example, Charles Hammond, M.D., has proposed a tracking system wherein after a core residency curriculum, some residents are trained in a primary care of women's health and others receive additional subspecialty training. As he has stated, "Although we would like for all graduates of our programs to be both generalists and specialists, it does not seem likely that this can still occur."[4]

Further pressures are likely to diminish our ability to fully train surgical specialists in the residency program, not the least of which are medicolegal- and federal government–mandated requirements. As resident and fellowship training progresses, the opportunities to make independent decisions both in the preoperative and postoperative management of patients as well as in the operating room is critical to the learning process. This has been a traditional step in the development of senior residents but is now being severely impacted by "teaching physician guidelines" imposed by the Health Care Financing Administration as well as medicolegal pressures wherein the "attending faculty physician" must legally remain closely involved with the entire surgical procedure. Although I would not suggest that a surgical procedure be performed fraudulently and although the attending physician must always bear final responsibility for the patient, we must work to find ways of allowing those in training to develop independent decision-making skills and establish an autonomous status as a gynecologic surgeon. "Senior residents finish their years of formative experience with a lifetime of learning ahead, confident because of their learning experience, but clearly aware of their limitations."[8]

Because the surgical learning process is a lifelong matter, we need to seek methods to improve postgraduate medical education (continuing medical education). This is particularly important as new surgical techniques and new technology are brought to the surgeon who has completed his or her formal residency training program. The traditional continuing medical education lecture format courses seem to be inadequate to teach surgical skills. The experience gained from brief "weekend" courses that offer "animal wet labs" are also inadequate to fully train a surgeon in new or advanced surgical techniques. We need to further define the extent of training, experience, and competence necessary to credential a surgeon in a particular technique. After having basic training in a new technique, should the surgeon be mentored by a colleague for a given number of cases or until certain competency criteria have been established? If the mentor certifies that his or her colleague is now competent to perform a procedure, does the mentor likewise assume medicolegal risks for poor outcomes of the colleague? What criteria will be established to define competency? Clearly, evaluation of surgical outcomes would be optimal. However, given the current state of affairs in which a surgeon may perform major procedures infrequently, it may take several years to be able to amass a large enough "caselist" to evaluate the outcomes of an individual surgeon. I would hope that the horizon for postgraduate education would reveal new methods for surgical training and credentialing. Certainly, the potential for computer-aided training and evaluation and virtual reality experiences could provide excellent training and evaluation of surgeons in a safe environment where a patient's health is not jeopardized.

With regard to general hospital credentialing of gynecologic surgeons, the use of outcome research and individual assessment of certain outcomes will play an ever-increasing role in the credentialing process. For example, if a surgeon has a complication rate that is 2 standard deviations from the mean (by either a regional or national standard), will his or her credentials be limited in specific surgical procedures? Furthermore, given the increasing specialization that now includes recognition of urogynecologists, reproductive endocrinologists and gynecologic oncologists, better definition of the roles of the general obstetrician and gynecologist as compared with the subspecialist needs to be achieved. Although there is clearly overlap in procedures performed by the generalist and the subspecialist, it must be acknowledged that there are procedures that should be limited to be performed by subspecialty trained and certified surgeons.

NEW TECHNOLOGY AND SURGICAL TECHNIQUES

The inevitable emergence of new technologies will offer a wealth of new opportunities for gynecologic surgeons in the next decade. Despite pressures to contain costs and to evaluate outcomes discussed subsequently, I have no doubt that opportunities abound to afford women improved health care and surgical care by technologies to be brought to medicine and surgery in the near future. The improvement of imaging techniques steadily expands, and I expect will allow much better definition of pelvic anatomy. The field of urogynecology will continue to refine its understanding of the structure and interconnected support in the pelvis as tissue planes and facial planes can be better imaged preoperatively. Using this information, the pelvic surgeon of the future will be able to better plan a specific reconstructive surgical procedure based on specific anatomic criteria and would follow the advice of Dr. Nichols in that they will "choose an operation

that best fits the needs of a particular patient."[9] New imaging technologies will also add to the understanding of anatomic relationships between malignant and normal tissues, thus allowing the gynecologic oncologist to select patients who will have the best surgical outcome from resection of a malignancy. Conversely, patients who might have better outcome by being provided other cancer therapy such as radiation therapy or chemotherapy might be saved a surgical procedure.

Increasing understanding of cellular biology and molecular biology will allow us to manipulate angiogenesis to promote or control wound healing. Tissue glues and growth factors will likely also be brought into the operating room, allowing the combination of "medical" as well as traditional surgical reconstruction of tissues. Transplantation technology will likely improve, allowing new sources of tissues which may replace synthetic materials currently used in some pelvic surgical procedures.

Our increasing understanding of molecular biology and genetics will likely impact a number of conditions and may even eliminate the need for surgery in some cases. Given that some of the most common reasons for hysterectomy include management of uterine fibroids and endometriosis, these surgical procedures may be diminished considerably in the future as we come to a better understanding of the growth and control of these benign conditions that might be manipulated medically. In gynecologic oncology, gene therapy and immunotherapy as well as understanding of tumor associated angiogenesis will likely reduce the need for radical pelvic surgery in some malignancies.

The surgical aspects of reproductive endocrinology and infertility seemed to have diminished even in this past decade. The improved fertility rates associated with the new reproductive technologies have considerably reduced the need for surgical intervention to attempt to establish tubal patency. We would expect this trend to continue.

The emerging subspecialty field of urogynecology seems dedicated to more objectively evaluating the various surgical procedures that have been developed and advocated for the management of pelvic floor defects and urinary incontinence. The ability to communicate staging of pelvic organ prolapse[1] will allow future surgeons to more clearly describe anatomic defects to be repaired as well as to quantitate the reestablishment of normal anatomy and function. As noted previously, new imaging techniques will also allow more objective quantification of anatomic defects. Therefore we believe that selection of specific surgical procedures may be more objectively based on anatomic and radiographic criteria, and at the same time, the outcomes of specific surgical procedures may be more objectively evaluated so that specific surgical procedures can be more confidently recommended to correct specific problems.

The careful study of the pelvic floor and a variety of surgical procedures has also taken on a more objective evaluation in that many of these procedures are being evaluated carefully and in some cases in randomized clinical trials. Organized research programs, as part of urogynecology training, will also substantially add to our basic understanding of not only the pathophysiology of the pelvic floor but also the molecular biology of defective tissue. Preventive strategies and nonsurgical medical management may subsequently follow for the care of some women.

The evolution of gynecologic oncology surgery over the past three decades since it became a recognized subspecialty in the United States has substantially changed the surgical management of a number of gynecologic malignancies. Although the pendulum swung toward more aggressive surgical debulking, including intestinal, splenic, diaphragm, and hepatic resection for advanced ovarian cancer, the advent of more effective systemic chemotherapy will likely result in less aggressive surgery to manage advanced ovarian cancer. The current investigation of "neoadjuvant chemotherapy" administered before surgical debulking appears to result in the need for less radical surgery and possibly diminished surgical morbidity. Earlier detection of cervical, endometrial, and vulvar carcinoma appears to be the trend and in this respect it is appropriate to perform less radical surgery. Further delineation in the next decade as to the criteria that will allow less radical surgery for early invasive cervical cancer and a better definition of the role of pelvic and paraaortic lymphadenectomy in the management of endometrial cancer will define a specific surgical procedure needed to result in the most cost-effective management of early gynecologic malignancies. We would also expect that the number of pelvic exenterations would diminish as the use of chemotherapy concurrently with radiation therapy (as radiation sensitizers) appears to reduce central pelvic failures. In centers of excellence where pelvic exenterations will continue to be performed, surgeons will continue to collaborate with their urologic, plastic reconstructive surgery, and general surgery colleagues, exchanging ideas and techniques to allow improved quality of life after pelvic exenteration. This has advanced rapidly over the past decade with the addition of continent urinary conduits, vaginal reconstruction, and low rectal anastomosis to our surgical armamentarium.

HEALTH CARE FINANCING

Demographics of the American population forecast an ever-increasing elderly population in whom we would expect to encounter increasing numbers of gynecologic malignancies and difficulties with urogynecologic defects. Emphasis will be placed on the perioperative management of this elderly population and a search for nonsurgical management of elderly women who are at poor medical risk to undergo surgical therapy.

This ever-increasing elderly population will likely continue to have the health care funded through managed care mechanisms such as Medicare and Medicare-HMOs. Furthermore, American demographics speaking to the lack of access to health care include the fact that some 40 million Americans have no health insurance at present, and 35 million are estimated to have too little insurance. This problem

with lack of funding for health care for a significant portion of our population in addition to the impact of managed care programs that have diminished reimbursement to physicians and hospitals will continue to impact and change the practice of medicine over the next decade. The ability of the health care system, physicians, and hospitals to adapt to this change in reimbursement and to react appropriately to the trends in health care management are critical issues that may influence our view of pelvic surgery in the near future.[2] The impact of managed care will influence the training programs, and at this time, it is uncertain who will accept the ever-increasing cost of medical education. Presently, American medical school graduates enter their residency training programs with substantial debt incurred in financing their medical education. With the diminishing physician reimbursement caused by managed care, it is suspected that there will be fewer physicians taking the additional time to receive subspecialty training and fewer entering academic practice of medicine where reimbursement has been traditionally lower than that in the private practice sector. Diminishing physician satisfaction is linked not only to diminished reimbursement but also to other issues of control and autonomy, which have traditionally been hallmarks of the medical profession. This diminished satisfaction may have a substantial impact on the desire of some gynecologists to undertake more difficult and risky surgical procedures.[5] The future of pelvic surgery in a managed care environment is uncertain, and I worry that "incentives" presented by managed care companies to physicians may limit women's access to the best gynecologic care. Will surgeons with inadequate skills or who are inexperienced be expected to manage the "lives" in their care plan without access to more extensive subspecialty care? Will the menopausal woman with a complex adnexal mass that is suspicious for ovarian cancer be required to undergo surgery by her general obstetrician and gynecologist rather than being allowed to be referred to a gynecologic oncologist who is most familiar with the proper staging and management of ovarian cancer? There is clear evidence that depending on the surgeon's level of experience and skill, patients will have different outcomes. Recent practice pattern analysis have clearly demonstrated that women with ovarian cancer are more often properly staged if a gynecologic oncologist is performing the surgical procedure rather than a general obstetrician and gynecologist or general surgeon.[10]

EVIDENCE-BASED MEDICINE AND ECONOMIC ANALYSIS

"When the benefits and risks of current therapy are counter balanced, the benefits should decisively outweigh the risks. If they do not, then the surgeon's philosophy of practice should be modified to fit the facts."[7]

Most surgical procedures have been developed based on good surgical principles and a desire to improve the patient's quality of life. In evaluating these surgical procedures, most have been compared with prior procedures (historical controls) and judgments made as to the outcome when compared with other techniques. However, because of significant biases that have included patient selection as well as biases by a particular surgeon, it is difficult to truly evaluate one surgical technique compared with another. Ideally, one would base these decisions on randomized clinical trials that eliminated potential biases. Unfortunately, this has not been the case. Therefore we are challenged to use critical thinking and evaluation before considering acceptance of new medical innovation.[3] As new techniques and instruments are developed, we must insist that a surgical procedure be evaluated in the context of risks and benefits. The role of economic analysis plays into this issue, where we must be interested and concerned not only with regard to the surgical outcome, and operative morbidity, but also with the costs of a new procedure. Before performing a cost-benefit analysis, however, there must be good evidence that a procedure is effective. We are hopeful that randomized clinical trials, such as have been performed by Stovall in evaluating the role of laparoscopically assisted hysterectomy[11] and the Gynecologic Oncology Group in evaluating laparoscopy for the surgical staging of endometrial cancer, will more objectively answer questions as to the best surgical technique. The future decade will no doubt see substantial increase in these types of analyses. Clearly, there will be an emphasis by managed care companies to identify techniques that are least costly. However, other analyses are important and must also be considered with regard to both short- and long-term consequences. This critical evaluation of what we do, what works, and what works best will be guiding principles in the future as we evaluate new and old surgical techniques.

Finally, we must continue to recall our basic goals as gynecologic surgeons, which have been clearly stated by Dr. Nichols[9]:

1. Relief of symptoms
2. Restoration of normal anatomic relationships
3. Restoration of function

These have been our goals and objectives in caring for women with gynecologic conditions and must remain our ultimate objective in the years ahead.

REFERENCES

1. Bump RC, et al: The standardization of terminology of female pelvic organ prolapse and pelvic floor dysfunction, *Am J Obstet Gynecol* 175:10, 1996.
2. Drukker BH: Envelopes, *Am J Obstet Gynecol* 179:1400, 1999.
3. Grimes DA: Technology follies: the uncritical acceptance of medical innovation, *JAMA* 269:3030, 1993.
4. Hammond CB: Future directions for academic obstetrics and gynecology, *Am J Obstet Gynecol* 172:1, 1995.
5. Kassirer JP: Doctor discontent, *N Engl J Med* 339:1543, 1998.
6. Nichols DH: Preface. In Nichols DH, editor: *Gynecologic and obstetric surgery,* St Louis, 1993, Mosby.
7. Nichols DH: Preoperative and postoperative care. In Nichols DH, editor: *Gynecologic and obstetric surgery,* St Louis, 1993, Mosby.
8. Nichols DH: The role of the surgical assistant. In Nichols DH, editor: *Gynecologic and obstetric surgery,* St Louis, 1993, Mosby.
9. Nichols DH: Vaginal hysterectomy. In Nichols DH, editor: *Gynecologic and obstetric surgery,* St Louis, 1993, Mosby.
10. Nguyen HN, et al: National survey of ovarian cancer, part V. The impact of physician's specialty on patient's survival, *Cancer* 72:3663, 1993.
11. Summitt RL, et al: A multicenter randomized comparison of laparoscopically assisted vaginal hysterectomy and abdominal hysterectomy in abdominal hysterectomy candidates, *Obstet Gynecol* 92:321, 1998.

Index

Page numbers in italics indicate illustrations;
t indicates tables.